ANDERSON'S
PATHOLOGY

VOLUME ONE

ANDERSON'S PATHOLOGY

Edited by

JOHN M. KISSANE, M.D.

Professor of Pathology and of Pathology in Pediatrics,
Washington University School of Medicine;
Pathologist, Barnes and Affiliated Hospitals,
St. Louis Children's Hospital, St. Louis, Missouri

Former editions edited by

W.A.D. ANDERSON,
M.A., M.D., F.A.C.P., F.C.A.P., F.R.C.P.A. (Hon.)

Emeritus Professor of Pathology and Formerly Chairman
of the Department of Pathology,
University of Miami School of Medicine,
Miami, Florida

EIGHTH EDITION

with **2949** *illustrations and 8 color plates*

THE C. V. MOSBY COMPANY

ST. LOUIS • TORONTO • PRINCETON   1985

MOSBY

A TRADITION OF PUBLISHING EXCELLENCE

Editors: Rosa L. Kasper, Don E. Ladig
Assistant editor: Anne Gunter
Manuscript editor: Patricia Tannian
Design: Staff
Production: Carol O'Leary, Teresa Breckwoldt, Mary Stueck

Two volumes

EIGHTH EDITION

Copyright © 1985 by The C.V. Mosby Company

Previous editions copyrighted 1948, 1953, 1957, 1961, 1966, 1971, 1977

Printed in the United States of America

The C.V. Mosby Company
11830 Westline Industrial Drive, St. Louis, Missouri 63146

Library of Congress Cataloging in Publication Data

Pathology (Saint Louis, Mo.)
  Anderson's Pathology.

  Rev. ed. of: Pathology / edited by W.A.D. Anderson,
John M. Kissane.   7th ed. 1977.
  Includes bibliographies and index.
  1. Pathology.   I. Anderson, W.A.D. (William Arnold
Douglas), 1910-   .   II. Kissane, John M., 1928-
III. Title.   IV. Title: Pathology.   [DNLM: 1. Pathology.
QZ 4 A5521]
RB111.P3   1984   616.07   84.9868
  ISBN 0-8016-0191-6

TS/VH/VH 9 8 7 6 5 4 3 2 1   01/B/001

Contributors

ARTHUR C. ALLEN, M.D.

Professor of Pathology, State University of New York, Downstate Medical Center; Director of Laboratories, Jewish Hospital and Medical Center (currently Interfaith Medical Center), Brooklyn, New York

ROBERT E. ANDERSON, M.D.

Professor and Chairman, Department of Pathology, The University of New Mexico, Albuquerque, New Mexico

FREDERIC B. ASKIN, M.D.

Professor of Pathology, University of North Carolina School of Medicine; Director of Surgical Pathology, North Carolina Memorial Hospital, Chapel Hill, North Carolina

SAROJA BHARATI, M.D.

Chairperson, Department of Pathology, Deborah Heart and Lung Center, Browns Mills, New Jersey; Clinical Professor of Pathology, Temple University Medical School, Philadelphia, Pennsylvania; Clinical Professor of Pathology, The Pennsylvania State University, The Milton S. Hershey Medical Center, Hershey, Pennsylvania; Research Professor of Medicine, University of Illinois, Abraham Lincoln School of Medicine, Chicago, Illinois

CHAPMAN H. BINFORD, M.D.

Consultant to the Leprosy Registry, American Registry of Pathology; Formerly Chief, Special Mycobacterial Diseases Branch, Geographic Pathology Division, Armed Forces Institute of Pathology, Washington, D.C.

FRANCIS W. CHANDLER, D.V.M., Ph.D.

Chief, Experimental Pathology Branch, Center for Infectious Diseases, Centers for Disease Control, Atlanta, Georgia

JACOB L. CHASON, M.D.

Neuropathologist, Department of Pathology, Henry Ford Hospital; Clinical Professor of Pathology (Neuropathology), Wayne State University School of Medicine, Detroit, Michigan

MASAHIRO CHIGA, M.D.

Professor of Pathology, Departments of Pathology and Oncology, University of Kansas College of Health Sciences and Hospital, School of Medicine, Kansas City, Kansas

A.R.W. CLIMIE, M.D.

Chief of Pathology, Harper-Grace Hospitals; Associate Professor of Pathology, Wayne State University School of Medicine, Detroit, Michigan

JOSE COSTA, M.D.

Professor of Pathology, University of Lausanne, Lausanne, Switzerland; Formerly Chief, Pathologic Anatomy Branch, National Cancer Institute, National Institutes of Health, Bethesda, Maryland

CHARLES J. DAVIS, Jr., M.D.

Associate Chairman, Department of Genitourinary Pathology, Armed Forces Institute of Pathology; Professor of Pathology, Uniformed Services, University of Health Sciences, Washington, D.C.

KATHERINE DeSCHRYVER-KECSKEMETI, M.D.

Associate Professor, Division of Surgical Pathology, Washington University School of Medicine, St. Louis, Missouri

GEORGE Th. DIAMANDOPOULOS, M.D.

Professor of Pathology, Department of Pathology, Harvard Medical School, Boston, Massachusetts

HUGH A. EDMONDSON, M.D.

Professor of Pathology, University of Southern California, School of Medicine, Los Angeles, California

ROBERT E. FECHNER, M.D.

Royster Professor of Pathology and Director, Division of Surgical Pathology, University of Virginia Medical Center, Charlottesville, Virginia

GERALD FINE, M.D.

Chief, Division of Anatomic Pathology, Department of Pathology, Henry Ford Hospital, Detroit, Michigan

KAARLE O. FRANSSILA, M.D., Ph.D.

Chief of Pathology Laboratory, Department of Radiotherapy and Oncology, Helsinki University Central Hospital, Helsinki, Finland

ROBERT J. GORLIN, D.D.S., M.S.

Regents' Professor and Chairman, Department of Oral Pathology and Genetics, and Professor, Departments of Pathology, Dermatology, Pediatrics, Obstetrics-Gynecology, and Otolaryngology, Schools of Dentistry and Medicine, University of Minnesota, Minneapolis, Minnesota

ROGERS C. GRIFFITH, M.D.

Assistant Professor of Pathology and Surgical Pathology, Washington University School of Medicine; Assistant Pathologist, Barnes and Affiliated Hospitals, St. Louis Children's Hospital, and The Jewish Hospital of St. Louis, St. Louis, Missouri

JOE W. GRISHAM, M.D.

Professor and Chairman, Department of Pathology, University of North Carolina, School of Medicine, Chapel Hill, North Carolina

PAUL GROSS, M.D.

Adjunct Professor, Department of Pathology, Medical University of South Carolina, Charleston, South Carolina

DONALD B. HACKEL, M.D.

Professor of Pathology, Department of Pathology, Duke University Medical School, Durham, North Carolina

GORDON R. HENNIGAR, M.D.

Professor and Chairman, Department of Pathology, Medical University of South Carolina, Charleston, South Carolina

CHARLES S. HIRSCH, M.D.

Director of Forensic Pathology, Hamilton County Coroner's Office; Professor of Pathology, University of Cincinnati College of Medicine, Cincinnati, Ohio

DAVID B. JONES, M.D.

Professor of Pathology, Department of Pathology, State University of New York, Upstate Medical Center, Syracuse, New York

HAN-SEOB KIM, M.D.

Associate Professor of Pathology, Baylor College of Medicine; Attending Pathologist, The Methodist Hospital; Attending Pathologist, Harris County Hospital District, Houston, Texas

JOHN M. KISSANE, M.D.

Professor of Pathology and of Pathology in Pediatrics, Washington University School of Medicine; Pathologist, Barnes and Affiliated Hospitals, St. Louis Children's Hospital, St. Louis, Missouri

FREDERICK T. KRAUS, M.D.

Director of Laboratory Medicine, St. John's Mercy Medical Center; Professor of Pathology (Visiting Staff), Washington University School of Medicine, St. Louis, Missouri

CHARLES KUHN III, M.D.

Professor of Pathology, Washington University School of Medicine, St. Louis, Missouri

MICHAEL L. KYRIAKOS, M.D.

Professor of Pathology, Washington University School of Medicine; Surgical Pathologist, Barnes Hospital; Consultant to St. Louis Children's Hospital and Shriner's Hospital for Crippled Children, St. Louis, Missouri

PAUL E. LACY, M.D.

Mallinkrodt Professor and Chairman, Department of Pathology, Washington University School of Medicine, St. Louis, Missouri

MAURICE LEV, M.D.

Director, Department of Pathology, Deborah Heart and Lung Center, Browns Mills, New Jersey; Clinical Professor of Pathology, Temple University Medical School, Philadelphia, Pennsylvania; Clinical Professor of Pathology, The Pennsylvania State University, The Milton S. Hershey Medical Center, Hershey, Pennsylvania

CHAN K. MA, M.D.

Staff Pathologist, Department of Pathology, Henry Ford Hospital, Detroit, Michigan

VINCENT T. MARCHESI, M.D.

Professor and Chairman, Department of Pathology, Yale University, School of Medicine, New Haven, Connecticut

MANUEL A. MARCIAL, M.D.

Research Fellow in Pathology, Department of Pathology, Brigham and Women's Hospital and Harvard Medical School, Boston, Massachusetts

RAÚL A. MARCIAL-ROJAS, M.D., J.D., M.P.H., M.P.A.

Professor of Pathology and Dean, School of Medicine, Universidad Central del Caribe, Cayey, Puerto Rico; Formerly Chairman, Department of Pathology, University of Puerto Rico, School of Medicine, San Juan, Puerto Rico

ROBERT W. McDIVITT, M.D.

Professor of Pathology, Washington University School of Medicine; Director of Anatomic Pathology, Jewish Hospital of St. Louis; Associate Pathologist, Barnes Hospital; Consultant, Children's Hospital of St. Louis, St. Louis, Missouri

WILLIAM A. MEISSNER, M.D.

Emeritus Professor of Pathology, New England Deaconess Hospital, Harvard Medical School, Boston, Massachusetts

F. KASH MOSTOFI, M.D.

Chairman, Department of Genitourinary Pathology, Armed Forces Institute of Pathology, Washington, D.C.; Professor of Pathology, Uniformed Services University of Health Sciences, Washington, D.C.; Associate Professor of Pathology, Johns Hopkins University, School of Medicine; Clinical Professor of Pathology, University of Maryland Medical School, Baltimore, Maryland; Clinical Professor of Pathology, Georgetown University School of Medicine, Washington, D.C.

WAYKIN NOPANITAYA, Ph.D.

Professor, Department of Pathology, Prince of Songkla University, Songkla, Head-Yai, Thailand

JAMES E. OERTEL, M.D.

Chairman, Department of Endocrine Pathology, Armed Forces Institute of Pathology, Washington, D.C.

ROBERT L. PETERS, M.D.

Professor of Pathology, University of Southern California, School of Medicine, Los Angeles, California; Chief Pathologist, Rancho Los Amigos Hospital, Downey, California

R.C.B. PUGH, M.D., F.R.C.S., F.R.C. Path.

Consulting Pathologist, St. Peter's Hospitals and Institute of Urology, London, England

ALAN S. RABSON, M.D.

Director, Division of Cancer Biology and Diagnosis, National Cancer Institute, Bethesda, Maryland

JUAN ROSAI, M.D.

Professor of Laboratory Medicine and Pathology and Director of Anatomic Pathology, University of Minnesota Medical School, Minneapolis, Minnesota

ARKADI M. RYWLIN, M.D.

Director, Department of Pathology and Laboratory Medicine, Mount Sinai Medical Center; Professor of Pathology, University of Miami School of Medicine, Miami, Florida

DANTE G. SCARPELLI, M.D., Ph.D.

Ernest J. and Hattie H. Magerstadt Professor and Chairman, Department of Pathology, Northwestern University Medical School; Chief of Service, Northwestern Memorial Hospital, Chicago, Illinois

THOMAS M. SCOTTI, M.D.

Formerly Professor of Pathology, University of Miami School of Medicine, Miami, Florida

STEWART SELL, M.D.

Professor and Chairman, Department of Pathology and Laboratory Medicine, University of Texas Health Science Center at Houston, Houston, Texas

HERSCHEL SIDRANSKY, M.D.

Professor and Chairman, Department of Pathology, The George Washington University Medical Center, Washington, D.C.

RUTH SILBERBERG, M.D.

Visiting Scientist, Department of Pathology, Hadassah Hebrew University School of Medicine, Jerusalem, Israel

MORTON E. SMITH, M.D.

Professor of Ophthalmology and Pathology, Washington University School of Medicine, St. Louis, Missouri

SHELDON C. SOMMERS, M.D.

Clinical Professor of Pathology, Columbia University College of Physicians and Surgeons, New York, New York; Clinical Professor of Pathology, University of Southern California, School of Medicine, Los Angeles, California

STEVEN L. TEITELBAUM, M.D.

Professor of Pathology, Washington University School of Medicine and The Jewish Hospital of St. Louis, St. Louis, Missouri

JACK L. TITUS, M.D., Ph.D.

Professor and The Moody Chairman, Department of Pathology, Baylor College of Medicine; Chief, Pathology Service, The Methodist Hospital; Pathologist-in-Chief, Harris County Hospital District, Houston, Texas

DAVID H. WALKER, M.D.

Associate Professor, Department of Pathology, University of North Carolina, School of Medicine; Associate Attending Pathologist, North Carolina Memorial Hospital, Chapel Hill, North Carolina

NANCY E. WARNER, M.D.

Hastings Professor of Pathology, University of Southern California, School of Medicine, Los Angeles, California

JOHN C. WATTS, M.D.

Attending Pathologist, Department of Anatomic Pathology, William Beaumont Hospital, Royal Oak, Michigan; Clinical Assistant Professor of Pathology, Wayne State University School of Medicine, Detroit, Michigan

ROSS E. ZUMWALT, M.D.

Associate Professor of Pathology, University of Cincinnati College of Medicine; Associate Pathologist, Hamilton County Coroner's Office, Cincinnati, Ohio

Preface to eighth edition

Readers and followers of this book will have noticed that this is the first edition in which Dr. W.A.D. Anderson ("Wad" to his innumerable friends) has not actively participated. He remains vigorous and active, however, and has offered welcome encouragement and advice. We all wish him well.

Since the preparation of the seventh edition, spectacular advances have occurred in the basic sciences and in clinical medicine, on which pathology depends and to which it contributes. Advances in immunopathology and hematopathology, to mention only two general areas, and in diseases of the breast and of somatic soft tissues, to mention only two organ systems, have compelled revision of the text.

My first responsibility as editor was to examine the organization of the book to see if major structural revision was in order. I have retained the initial presentation of mechanisms both as a didactically effective transition between the basic sciences and pathology and as a review for readers whose exposure to the basic sciences has not been recent. This section of the book is followed by considerations of diseases of the various organ systems. The emphasis throughout is on the mechanisms whereby normal phenomena and processes become disturbed, giving rise to diseases and lesions.

The seventh edition introduced a chapter on geographic pathology. Even by that time, however, the Jet Age had made geographic pathology an authentic sub-specialty with a language and information base of its own. It deserves separate consideration without the duplication of language and concepts that its introduction in a primary pathology text would impose. Thus, with some regret, I decided to remove the chapter on geographic pathology and rely on contributors of organ-system chapters to include geographic factors in their discussions of the epidemiology of various disorders. This effort I believe has been effectively addressed in this edition.

I chose also not to include a separate chapter on venereal diseases. Such a chapter has, over several decades, come to include sociologic and public health considerations that transcend the mechanisms and morphologic expressions of the venereal diseases. These aspects are more appropriately dealt with in works directed to public health or preventive medicine than in a work on pathology. In this edition venereally transmitted diseases are considered along with other agent-mediated diseases.

In the preparation of this edition I have been fortunate in being able to recruit several new contributors. I welcome their contributions and at the same time express my appreciation to previous contributors.

Finally, I would like to express my gratitude to the generation of supporters of *Anderson's Pathology*. I hope the eighth edition continues to merit their support.

John M. Kissane

Preface to first edition

Pathology should form the basis of every physician's thinking about his patients. The study of the nature of disease, which constitutes pathology in the broad sense, has many facets. Any science or technique which contributes to our knowledge of the nature and constitution of disease belongs in the broad realm of pathology. Different aspects of a disease may be stressed by the geneticist, the cytologist, the biochemist, the clinical diagnostician, etc., and it is the difficult function of the pathologist to attempt to bring about a synthesis, and to present disease in as whole or as true an aspect as can be done with present knowledge. Pathologists often have been accused, and sometimes justly, of stressing the morphologic changes in disease to the neglect of functional effects. Nevertheless, pathologic anatomy and histology remain as an essential foundation of knowledge about disease, without which basis the concepts of many diseases are easily distorted.

In this volume is brought together the specialized knowledge of a number of pathologists in particular aspects or fields of pathology. A time-tested order of presentation is maintained, both because it has been found logical and effective in teaching medical students and because it facilitates study and reference by graduates. Although presented in an order and form to serve as a textbook, it is intended also to have sufficient comprehensiveness and completeness to be useful to the practicing or graduate physician. It is hoped that this book will be both a foundation and a useful tool for those who deal with the problems of disease.

For obvious reasons, the nature and effects of radiation have been given unusual relative prominence. The changing order of things, with increase of rapid, worldwide travel and communication, necessitates increased attention to certain viral, protozoal, parasitic, and other conditions often dismissed as "tropical," to bring them nearer their true relative importance. Also, given more than usual attention are diseases of the skin, of the organs of special senses, of the nervous system, and of the skeletal system. These are fields which often have not been given sufficient consideration in accordance with their true relative importance among diseases.

The Editor is highly appreciative of the spirit of the various contributors to this book. They are busy people, who, at the sacrifice of other duties and of leisure, freely cooperated in its production, uncomplainingly tolerated delays and difficulties, and were understanding in their willingness to work together for the good of the book as a whole. Particular thanks are due the directors of the Army Institute of Pathology and the American Registry of Pathology, for making available many illustrations. Dr. G.L. Duff, Strathcona Professor of Pathology, McGill University, Dr. H.A. Edmondson, Department of Pathology of the University of Southern California School of Medicine, Dr. J.S. Hirschboeck, Dean, and Dr. Harry Beckman, Professor of Pharmacology, Marquette University School of Medicine, all generously gave advice and assistance with certain parts.

To the members of the Department of Pathology and Bacteriology at Marquette University, the Editor wishes to express gratitude, both for tolerance and for assistance. Especially valuable has been the help of Dr. R.S. Haukohl, Dr. J.F. Kuzma, Dr. S.B. Pessin, and Dr. H. Everett. A large burden was assumed by the Editor's secretaries, Miss Charlotte Skacel and Miss Ann Cassady. Miss Patricia Blakeslee also assisted at various stages and with the index. To all of these the Editor's thanks, and also to the many others who at some time assisted by helpful and kindly acts, or by words of encouragement or interest.

W.A.D. Anderson

Contents

Color Plates

CHAPTER 1 Cellular Basis of Disease

JOE W. GRISHAM
WAYKIN NOPANITAYA

During the past several centuries prevailing medical opinion variously emphasized different levels of organization of the human body as the primary locus at which disease was initiated.[25] Generally this emphasis reflected the store of anatomic and physiologic knowledge then current and the methods available to study the diseased organism. Early physicians saw disease only at the level of the body as a whole. Morgagni and other incipient pathologists attempted to locate the origin or seat of disease in the different organs of the body. Subsequently, Bichat and his followers emphasized the importance of the fabrics, or tissues, in development and expression of disease. Virchow called attention to the importance of individual cells as the primary locus at which abnormal function and structure arise. In our own time, Peters has established the role of disturbances in specific biochemical processes,[31] and many contemporary investigators have found that the various subcellular organelles, and the biochemical reactions that go on within and around them, are sites for initiating disease.

The various functional and structural properties of cells and tissues provide the critical points for induction of disease. Disease is not caused by the acquisition of a new and different set of properties by the affected cell, but rather by quantitative alterations in existing functions and structures. The goal of this chapter, which is necessarily brief and incomplete, is to direct the reader's thoughts to the multiple overlapping levels of cell structure and function that are the ultimate loci of the many pathologic lesions discussed in the subsequent chapters. Although this presentation emphasizes the cell and its parts, disease as it afflicts a person is much more than simply an abnormality of organelle structure and function within some particular cell. The mechanisms by which a critical subcellular lesion leads to a cascade of abnormal reactions in different cells and tissues, ultimately expressed at the organismic level as disease, are the essence of modern pathology.

GENERAL ASPECTS OF CELL STRUCTURE

Although cells are described as having fixed, unchanging structure, this is a static distortion of the living state, wherein cellular structures are dynamic and constantly changing. The fixed, sectioned cell represents a mere shadow of reality—a thin slice of a cell that has been killed in action and embalmed. Because cells are killed at moments when they are occupied with different functions, static structural views vary. Only by sampling and fixing cells according to a precise schedule and by correlating structure and function in the same sample can an appreciation of the true dynamics of cell structure and function be gained.

The cell may be viewed simplistically as a membrane-enclosed compartment, subdivided into several smaller compartments and surfaces by further internal ramifications of membrane; these membranes and compartments provide distinctive domains that allow a wide variety of mutually incompatible biochemical processes to occur simultaneously. The major subcellular compartments are nucleus, mitochondria, endoplasmic reticulum, Golgi apparatus, lysosomes, and cytosol (Fig. 1-1).

Cell membranes

All cellular membranes are complex mixtures of lipids, proteins, and carbohydrates and have a generally similar morphologic appearance in fixed, sectioned specimens.[40] The morphologic pattern usually seen, termed the *unit membrane*, consists of two electron-dense lines, each 2 to 3 nanometers (nm) thick, separated by an electron-lucent line 3 to 4 nm thick. The total thickness of this trilayer structure is 7.5 to 10 nm. Despite the general morphologic similarity of all fixed and sectioned membranes, there is a considerable diversity in both the chemical composition and the width of the layers of trilaminar membranes taken from various cells and from different membranes of the same cell. In fact, some studies suggest that true layers do not exist, but rather that

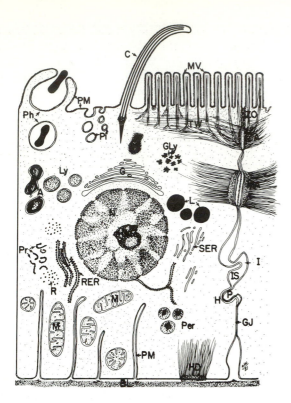

Fig. 1-1. Schematic representation of substructures of generalized mammalian cell. Plasma membrane, *PM*, and its modifications: *BL*, basal lamina; *C*, cilia; *GJ*, gap junction; *H*, hole; *HD*, hemidesmosome; *I*, interdigitation; *IS*, intercellular space; *MA*, macula adherens (desmosome); *Mv*, microvilli and their "glycocalyx" coats; *P*, protrusion or peg; *Ph*, phagocytic vesicles; *Pi*, pinocytic vesicles; *ZA*, zonula adherens (intermediate junctions); *ZO*, zonula occludens (tight junction). Cell organelles: *A*, autophagosome; *G*, Golgi apparatus; *Gly*, glycogen particles; *L*, lipid droplets; *Ly*, lysosome; *M*, mitochondria; *N*, nucleus; *Nu*, nucleolus; *Per*, peroxisome; *Pr*, polyribosomes; *R*, ribosome; *RER*, rough endoplasmic reticulum; *SER*, smooth endoplasmic reticulum; *TW*, terminal web and its microfilaments.

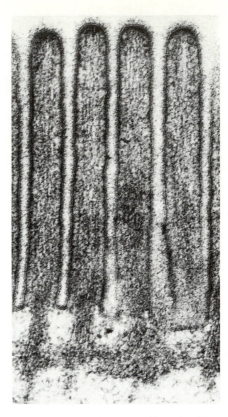

Fig. 1-2. Microvilli on cell surface. Outer membrane of all microvilli, seen in longitudinal section, is covered with fine filamentous material (glycocalyx). Core of individual microvilli consists of microfilaments that interweave with those of the terminal web at their base. (88,000×.)

certain membranes may be composed of globular units. Ultramicroscopic examination of surface replicas prepared from membranes split through their core also shows tiny, membrane-associated particles whose distribution varies in different cells. These intermembranous particles are laterally mobile within the plane of the membrane and can be caused to aggregate by environmental manipulation. Some particles in the core of the plasma membrane appear to be continuous with a variety of receptors on the outer surface of the membrane and, perhaps, with a protein "tail" that projects from the cytoplasmic side. Membrane-associated particles have been related to receptors for phytohemagglutinin and influenza virus, to ABO blood group antigens, to sites of oxidative phosphorylation, and to sites of active transport. The outer surface of the cell membrane contains a partial coating of mucopolysaccharides, such as sialic acid.[17] Properly fixed, this surface coat appears on some types of cells as a fuzzy layer, termed the *glycocalyx* (Figs. 1-2

and 1-3). Membrane proteins and glycoproteins are responsible for antigenic characteristics of intact cells, including blood group determinants.

The precise molecular structure of cellular membranes is still unknown, and theorists have been challenged to provide a hypothesis for the biophysical configuration of membranes that explains morphologic observations, biochemical composition, and functional characteristics such as permeability, antigenicity, and electrical conductivity. A variety of theories now exists, but the oldest still retains considerable credibility in its recently modified form. This lipid-bilayer theory postulates that lipid molecules are oriented in two layers in cell membranes, with their hydrophilic ends turned outward and their hydrophobic ends turned inward. An early version of this theory postulated that lipid-lined pores penetrate the bilayer (to explain permeability) and that the hydrophilic surfaces are covered by protein molecules in the extended form. More recent variations postulate the presence within the membrane of globular proteins that are exposed on one or both surfaces and that mediate transport and other membrane functions. Other theories hold that the cell membrane is composed

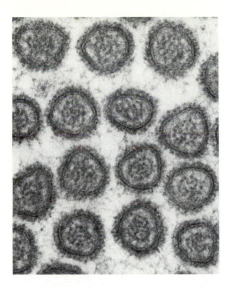

Fig. 1-3. Cross section of microvilli showing glycocalyx on outer surface of their surface membranes and central filamentous cores. (145,000×.)

of lipid either in the liquid-crystalline state or in the form of micelles in which globular proteins are partly or completely embedded. The fluid lipid-protein mosaic model is consistent with most current data. Such a model accounts for major properties of cell membranes, including fluidity, structural and functional asymmetry, and the inclusion of specialized molecular components that function as receptors.

A major structural feature of the plasma membrane, which accounts for many of its functional properties, is the presence of receptors and of markers that are not yet known to have a receptor function. Receptors, which may be composed of proteins, carbohydrates, or lipids, may be broadly defined as a class of molecules that are able to form high-affinity complexes with complementary molecules (ligands). The macromolecular combination of a ligand and a receptor causes a chemical or physical response in the cell, resulting in a functional change. Receptors exist in great variety and may participate in enzyme reactions, active transport of metabolites, and recognition and communication phenomena. Membrane receptors that have been well defined include those for peptide hormones, bacterial products, viruses, lectins, and immunoglobulins. Receptors for polypeptides are of two major types: those that lead to a change in metabolism when occupied by a ligand without requiring internalization of the ligand-receptor complex and those in which internalization of the receptor-ligand complex is required for a physiologic response. A large number of enzymes are also located within membranes, where they are important in determining that biochemical reactions occur in spatially appropriate parts of the cell.

On many cells the surface area of the plasma membrane is increased by folds or projections. *Microvilli* are cylindrical protrusions of membrane 1 μm long by 0.1 μm wide, surrounding a cytoplasmic core containing a bundle of microfilaments (Figs. 1-2 and 1-3). The microfilaments in the cores of microvilli merge with the submembrane microfilamentous web (terminal web). Microvilli are especially numerous on absorptive and secretory surfaces of cells, where they vastly increase the cell's surface area. Membranes of cells involved in the movement of large amounts of water may exhibit complex foldings distinct from microvilli; these also augment the cell's surface.

Cytosol

Cytosol is the cytoplasmic ground substance, the watery, gel-like mixture in which the cell's organelles and inclusions are suspended. The cytosol provides the matrix in which all the subcellular organelles are embedded. Many enzymatic reactions occur outside formed organelles, mediated by enzymes suspended or dissolved in the cytosol. Some processes occurring in the cytosol may be linked to enzymatic steps taking place in organelles. The cytosol has a highly organized structure, which we are unable to observe in detail with currently available techniques. The cytoskeleton (discussed later in the chapter) appears to be the major determinant of the spatial organization of the cytosol and the organelles it contains.

Mitochondria

Although the general morphologic features of mitochondria are similar in all mammalian cells, their precise structural details (especially the arrangement of their internal cristae) vary considerably.[37] Typical mitochondria (Fig. 1-4) are 0.5 to 1 μm in diameter and 3 to 5 μm in length. A cell may contain from a few score to more than 1000 mitochondria. They are enveloped by a smooth outer membrane and contain a variably folded inner membrane.[24] The inner membrane may be composed of shelflike ridges, tubules, or concentric layers. The elaborate foldings of the inner membrane are termed *cristae*. Outer and inner membranes delimit several actual or potential spaces: the matrix space within the inner membrane, the intercristal space between the two unit membranes of cristae, and the peripheral space between outer and inner membranes. In the so-called orthodox or typical configuration, outer and inner mitochondrial membranes are closely apposed and peripheral and intercristal spaces are minimal.

Mitochondria are composed mainly of lipid and protein. Nearly half of the protein appears to be enzymes that are components of integrated pathways. All of the lipid is in the membrane. The outer membrane closely resembles other cytomembranes, both chemically and structurally. The inner membrane is unusual in that it contains no cholesterol and a large amount of acidic phos-

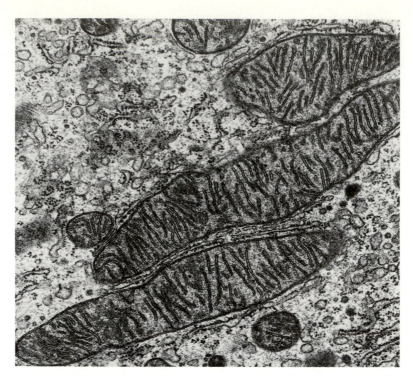

Fig. 1-4. Mitochondria sectioned both longitudinally and across. (25,000×.)

pholipid, a condition reminiscent of bacterial membranes. Both membranes are ultrastructurally trilaminar in sections, but the inner membrane shows a prominent globular substructure when negatively stained. Within the inner membranes are cylindric globular subunits about 6 by 10 nm. Apparently attached to the membrane are other globular subunits, which are shaped like "lollipops" and project into the matrix. These structures consist of a stalk, which measures about 4 nm long by about 2 to 3 nm wide, and a "headpiece" at the end of the stalk, which measures 7 to 10 nm in diameter. These globular structures and the adjacent particles in the inner membrane are the locus of the components of the electron-transfer chain. The "lollipops" are thought to contain adenosine triphosphatase, and other components of the respiratory assemblies (succinic dehydrogenase and the cytochromes of the respiratory chain) are embedded in the inner membrane. Other enzymes found in mitochondria include those belonging to the Krebs cycle and enzymes of fatty acid oxidation. The matrix often contains a variety of fibrillar or particulate inclusions, including fibrils of deoxyribonucleic acid (DNA), ribosomes, calcium-containing crystals, and glycogen.

Although this morphologic description delineates a static structural configuration, in vitro studies of isolated organelles suggest that in metabolically active mitochondria the configurations of internal membranes and spaces shift dramatically. The orthodox configuration, typically seen in fixed cells, is characteristic of the nonenergized state in vitro, when the rate of dissipation of high-energy intermediates exceeds their production. In the energized state, when production of high-energy intermediates exceeds their dissipation, the matrix space swells. Configurational changes in energized and nonenergized mitochondria predominantly involve relative shifts in the volumes of matrix and peripheral spaces, with little net change in total mitochondrial volume. The outer membrane is relatively inelastic, and when it breaks, the matrix space may balloon greatly; this event, termed *high-amplitude swelling*, heralds the complete deterioration of integrated mitochondrial function.

Mitochondria are self-replicating organelles that contain their own structurally distinct genetic apparatus. Mitochondrial DNA forms closed circles and lacks histones; mitochondrial ribosomes are smaller than are cytoplasmic ribosomes. The mitochondrial genome appears to direct the synthesis of membrane-bound proteins of this organelle, whereas soluble proteins and lipids are synthesized in the surrounding cytoplasm.

Nucleus

The nuclear contents are enclosed in an envelope composed of two layers of unit membrane (Fig. 1-5) separated by a 20 to 70 nm wide space continuous with the interstices of the endoplasmic reticulum.[21] The outer leaf of the nuclear membrane is studded with ribosomes. At many points the outer and inner unit membranes of the nuclear envelope are fused into a thin diaphragm

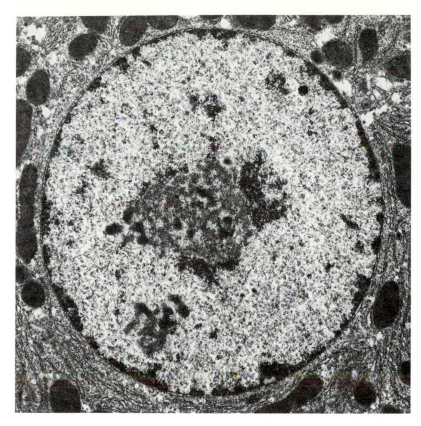

Fig. 1-5. Nucleus. Nuclear chromatin contains a few aggregates of heterochromatin around inner nuclear membrane; most of nucleolus is composed of euchromatin. Nucleolus is visible in center of nucleus. (11,000×.)

over an area about 50 to 80 nm in diameter. These foci, called *nuclear pores*, are distributed more or less uniformly over the nuclear surface (Figs. 1-6 and 1-7). When sectioned tangentially, they appear to contain a central dense granule and tiny filaments (Fig. 1-8). Surface views of freeze-cleaved specimens suggest that an octagonal thickening about 100 nm across, called the *annulus*, surrounds each pore. Pores always occur over areas of euchromatin (see the following paragraph) and are believed to represent the pathway by which ribosomes are transported from the nucleus.

Except for mitochondria, nuclei contain all of the DNA in mammalian cells. Diploid human nuclei each contain about 6 picograms (pg) of DNA, 1 to 3 pg of RNA, and 30 to 35 pg of protein. Nuclear proteins include several varieties of basic proteins (histones), which have an important role in chromatin structure, and a large group of neutral and acidic proteins.[19] At distances of about 200 base pairs, DNA in both euchromatin and heterochromatin is associated with histone proteins to form 10 nm nucleosomes.[9] Most of the associated DNA is wound over the surface of the nucleosome, with a smaller piece separating adjacent nucleosomes. Nucleosomes are arrayed along DNA strands like beads on a string. Included among the neutral and acidic proteins are the

several forms of RNA and DNA polymerases and other enzymes involved in the synthesis and processing of RNA and DNA. In addition, histones and acidic nuclear proteins may have a mutually important role in the regulation of gene expression. The diploid mammalian nucleus of 6 to 8 μm contains coiled fibers of DNA complexed to protein (*chromatin*), which if fully extended would measure more than 1 m in length. Interphase chromosomes are composed of tangled webs of extended, relatively uncoiled fibers (*euchromatin*), interspersed with areas in which fibers are highly coiled (*heterochromatin*). Extended strands of DNA in euchromatin are available for transcription of messenger RNA, whereas heterochromatin is believed to be transcriptionally inactive.[9] One of the X chromosomes in female cells is visible in most somatic cells as a highly condensed mass of heterochromatic DNA lying next to the nuclear membrane (*Barr body*). The ultramicroscopic appearance of the chromatin in sectioned nuclei is disappointingly uninformative. Except that heterochromatin is more electron dense than is euchromatin, little detail can be discerned other than profiles of fibers varying in diameter from 2 to 10 nm.

Coordinated with the onset of mitosis, the chromatin strands of individual chromosomes undergo supercoiling

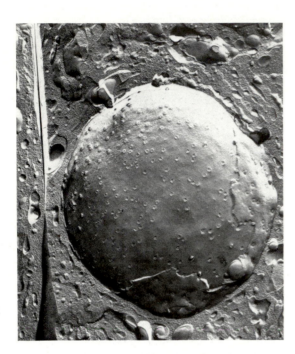

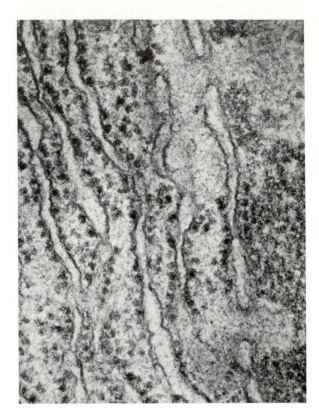

Fig. 1-6. Replica of nucleus showing its surface and nuclear pores. (8700×.)

Fig. 1-7. Two nuclear pores are seen in envelope of portion of nucleus occupying lower part of this figure. Nuclear chromatin at pores is euchromatic. Rough endoplasmic reticulum and outer nuclear membrane are continuous. (144,000×.)

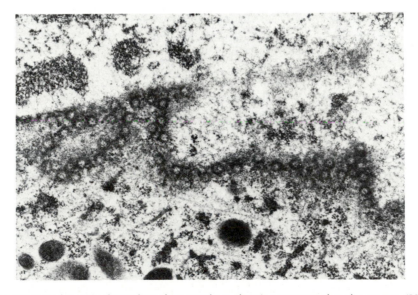

Fig. 1-8. Tangential section through nuclear envelope showing transected nuclear pores. (30,000×; courtesy W. Hanton and D.W. Misch, Chapel Hill, N.C.)

to give rise to the 46 mitotic chromosomes in human diploid cells.[9] Based on the total length of the chromosomes and on the location of their centromeres, human metaphase chromosome doublets can be categorized morphologically. In this arrangement there are seven groups (conventionally designated A to G) containing the 44 paired autosomes, plus two sex chromosomes, either XX (female) or XY (male). These morphologic criteria allow certain identification of only six individual chromosomes within these groups. Recently developed techniques to evaluate the patterns of crossbanding of chromosomes permit identification of each individual chromosome and even allow the origin of chromosome fragments to be ascertained.[5] Hundreds of bands can be discerned in highly condensed metaphase chromosomes, and thousands can be distinguished on more extended prophase chromosomes. Chromosomes are separated by the action of microtubules of the mitotic spindle.

The *nucleolus* (Fig. 1-9) is the most prominent internal feature of most interphase mammalian nuclei; its size varies in relation to the intensity of protein synthesis in the cell in which it is located. This relationship exists because the nucleolus is the site of synthesis of ribosomal RNA and, perhaps, of the complete assembly of ribosomal subunits. Nucleoli are composed of intermixed fibrillar and granular components, both of which are largely RNA. Fibrils measure about 5 to 8 nm in cross section and granules are about 15 nm in diameter. It is believed that fibrils and granules represent newly synthesized ribosomal RNA at different stages in its processing.

Ribosomes

Individual mammalian ribosomes are flattened, spheroid particles that measure about 15 by 25 nm.[29] Monomeric ribosomes are composed of one small subunit about 9 nm in diameter (40S) and one large subunit about 15 nm in diameter (160S). (S is the Svedberg unit, a sedimentation constant of 10^{-13} second.) The small subunit sits on the large subunit as a flattened cap, with a cleft or groove marking their point of attachment. Ribosomes are composed of approximately equal parts of RNA and a variety of proteins. About 80% to 85% of the cell's total RNA is included in ribosomes. Small subunits contain a single 18S piece of RNA; large subunits contain one 28S piece and one 5S to 7S piece of RNA.

Polyribosomes (Fig. 1-10) are the protein-synthesizing units. They consist of several monomeric ribosomes attached to a single linear molecule of messenger RNA, which may vary from 300 to 600 nm in length, depending on the size of the protein molecule for which it codes.[29] Ribosomes are attached to messenger RNA by binding sites in the cleft between subunits. Polyribosomes may be randomly located in the cytosol where they appear as characteristic spirals, or they may be attached by the large ribosome subunits to specific binding sites on membranes of the rough endoplasmic reticulum. Membrane-attached ribosomes and unattached ribosomes are usually designated as "bound" and "free," respectively. A canal has been postulated to penetrate the large subunit through which the nascent protein molecule is extruded.

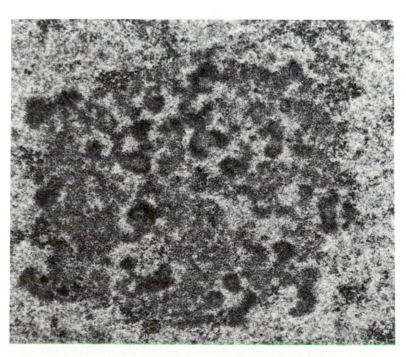

Fig. 1-9. Nucleolus showing filamentous and granular components. (45,000×.)

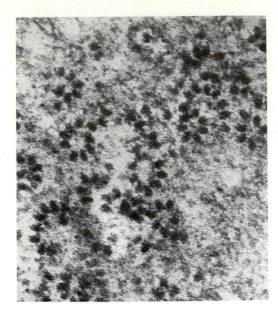

Fig. 1-10. Characteristic spiral form of polyribosomes in cytoplasm of cell. (136,000×.)

Endoplasmic reticulum

The endoplasmic reticulum is a variable structure of anastomosing tubules, flattened parallel sacs, and vesicles, which pervades the cytoplasm of most metabolically active cells. It is composed of typical unit membranes, which enclose cisterns that vary in cross section from 30 to 70 nm and in most cells comprise the major fraction of cytomembranes. It is widely continuous with both the nuclear envelope and the Golgi apparatus. According to some investigators its membranes are also continuous with the plasma membrane of the cell. There are two general morphologic forms of endoplasmic reticulum, rough (or granular) and smooth (or agranular); these structural variations mirror differences in function. *Rough endoplasmic reticulum* is so named because its outer membrane is studded with ribosomes (Fig. 1-11), which bind to specific sites on the membrane. Rough endoplasmic reticulum is the site of synthesis of many proteins and is especially abundant in cells that synthesize large quantities of protein for export (such as plasma cells). Protein newly synthesized by polyribosomes attached to endoplasmic reticulum is extruded into the cisterns of the reticulum.[4] *Smooth endoplasmic reticulum* lacks ribosome-binding sites and therefore ribosomes (Fig. 1-12). It often appears to be more highly twisted or vesicular than is rough endoplasmic reticulum with which it is widely continuous. Smooth endoplasmic reticulum is the locus of enzymes that metabolize steroids, chemicals and drugs,[13] lipids, and glycogen.[8] The sarcoplasmic reticulum in striated and cardiac muscle cells is a modification of smooth endoplasmic reticulum, which serves as a channel for transporting and distributing energy-rich materials required for sustained muscle contraction.

Golgi apparatus

The Golgi apparatus (or complex, as it is sometimes known) is the second major part of the cell's cytomembranes, and it freely opens into the endoplasmic reticulum.[33] Morphologically the Golgi apparatus consists of several lamellar stacks or large flattened sacs of unit membrane, typically in a cup-shaped configuration (Fig. 1-13). Golgi complexes are often located at the so-called cell center near the nucleus, but in some secretory cells they are near the secretory pole. The structure of the lamellae of the Golgi apparatus is asymmetric, giving rise to two distinct faces; the cis (or forming) face is continuous with the rough endoplasmic reticulum and the trans (or maturing) face is on the opposite side. Enzymes are differentially located within the cisterns between the two faces. Cisterns are thin at the centers of stacks and are progressively dilated toward the lateral ends, which are bulbous (Fig. 1-13). Often adjacent to these bulbous ends are a number of vesicles of varying sizes. Some of the vesicles may contain slightly electron-dense fibrillar material, lysosomal enzymes, or immature specific granules (the latter in cells that synthesize packaged specific granules, such as polymorphonuclear leukocytes or beta cells of the pancreatic islets).

The Golgi apparatus is involved in the synthesis of complex proteins (particularly the addition of carbohydrates), the sorting of different types of proteins, and the packaging of some synthesized materials into vesicles of unit membrane.[33] Studies on the morphologic tracing of protein synthesis in a variety of cells in which the protein is packaged in a membrane have demonstrated the essential involvement of the Golgi apparatus.[4] Radioactivity from amino acids appears first in protein located in the cisterns of the rough endoplasmic reticulum. From this site it moves to the cisterns of the laminar part of the Golgi apparatus, then into the bulbous ends, and finally into membrane-surrounded vesicles in the vicinity of the Golgi apparatus.

Lysosomes

Lysosomes are oval or round bodies, which measure 5 to 10 nm in diameter, delimited by a single unit membrane (Fig. 1-14). The contents of lysosomes are structurally heterogeneous and may consist of amorphous material of varying electron density, multiple tiny vesicles, membranous materials, and degenerating cellular organelles. Common to all lysosomes are a number of hydrolytic enzymes, maximally active at acid pH.[10] Several types of lysosomes have been morphologically categorized: primary lysosomes or storage vacuoles; digestive and autophagic vacuoles, both secondary lysosomes; and residual bodies. *Primary lysosomes,* or *storage vacuoles,*

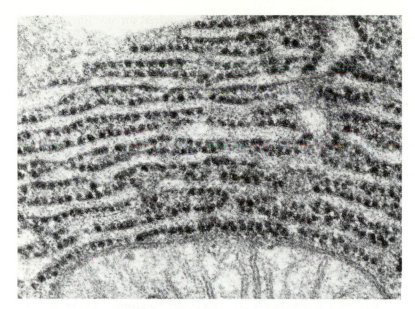

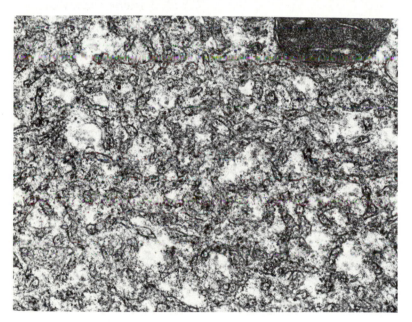

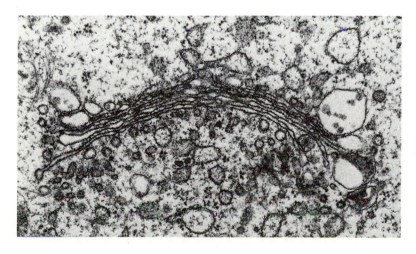

Fig. 1-11. Rough endoplasmic reticulum with ribosomes attached to outer layer of reticular unit membranes. (88,000×; courtesy W. Hanton and D.W. Misch, Chapel Hill, N.C.)

Fig. 1-12. Twisted tubules of smooth endoplasmic reticulum. (60,000×.)

Fig. 1-13. Golgi apparatus, illustrating complex structure of its lamellae and vesicles. (38,500×.)

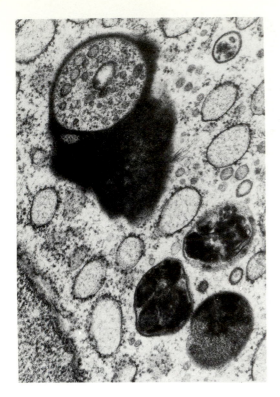

Fig. 1-14. Lysosomes and an autophagosome *(at top)*. (27,200×.)

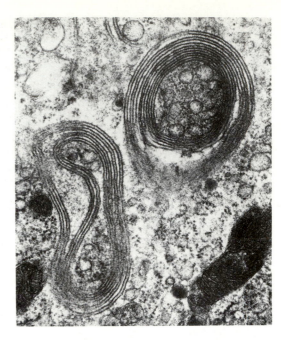

Fig. 1-15. Autophagic vacuoles are surrounded by several layers of membrane and contain partly degraded cytoplasmic material. (30,000×.)

are virgin organelles that have not yet been active in intracellular digestion. Primary lysosomes are packaged in the Golgi apparatus after the various hydrolytic enzymes are synthesized in the rough endoplasmic reticulum. Primary lysosomes may fuse with phagosomes containing extracellular particulate materials that have been ingested or with areas of focally sequestered cytoplasm to become *secondary lysosomes (digestive* and *autophagic vacuoles,* respectively) (Fig. 1-15). During the degradation process some materials may not be completely digested. The remaining undegradable material encased in a single membrane is known as a *residual body.* Residual bodies are the brown pigment lipofuscin, which may remain in cells for long periods or may be ejected from the cell by the process of emiocytosis. Lysosomal contents may leak from actively phagocytic cells and damage surrounding tissue structures. Some investigators have proposed that lysosomal membranes have special stability properties. Certain agents appear to specifically stabilize the lysosomal membrane, whereas others may render it more vulnerable to lysis.

Cytoskeleton

Microfilaments, intermediate filaments, and microtubules are involved in maintaining cellular form and movement.[1] These structures are frequently referred to collectively as the cytoskeleton because they form prominent scaffoldlike structures that permeate the cell and appear to determine its shape and the location of organelles.

Microfilaments are chemically and functionally heterogeneous,[20] having in common only their size, a diameter of 5 to 7 nm (Figs. 1-2 and 1-3). Their possible composition may include substances as diverse as dispersed subunits of microtubules and ribonucleoprotein fibers. Although the composition of many cellular microfilaments is uncertain, an important class of microfilaments is composed of the contractile protein actin.[32] These filaments are especially prominent in an ill-defined layer just beneath the plasma membrane, called the *terminal web*. Submembranous filaments, which extend into cores of microvilli, insert into the inner leaflet of the plasma membrane. *Intermediate filaments*, about 10 nm thick, are prominent cytoplasmic features of most types of cells, and they are especially prominent in epithelial cells. Intermediate filaments are composed of proteins, many of which are related chemically to prekeratin. Filamentous proteins from various cells have been given different names.

Microtubules are hollow, nonbranching tubules 20 to 24 nm in diameter and up to several micrometers long (Fig. 1-16). They are made of globular subunits of the protein tubulin, which are 4 nm in diameter and are closely packed into a helix containing 13 subunits per turn.[3] Microtubules are physically unstable, and when they break down, their subunits may reaggregate in the form of stacks of 5 nm filaments or of 35 nm tubules. *Cilia* and *flagella* are specialized structures involved in the locomotion of some single cells and in the movement of

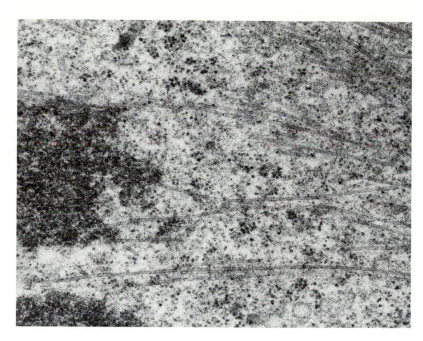

Fig. 1-16. Microtubules of mitotic spindle. *Left,* Portions of two condensed chromosomes. (55,000×.)

substances (such as secretions) along cells lining a surface. Both cilia and flagella, which project from the cell's surface, consist of a complex core composed of nine microtubule doublets oriented around two central microtubules, all enclosed by plasma membrane; the entire structure is 5 to 10 μm long by about 0.2 μm in diameter. Peripheral tubules terminate in the basal body located in the cytosol at the base of each cilium or flagellum. Closely associated with many microtubules are structures that appear to be involved in their local occurrence and function. These structures are variously known as centrioles or basal bodies, depending on their location. *Centrioles* (Fig. 1-17) are associated with the mitotic spindle, and *basal bodies* are involved in the function and duplication of cilia. Centrioles and basal bodies are morphologically similar, consisting of cylinders of nine microtubule triplets 0.2 to 1 μm long by about 0.2 μm in diameter. Often a smaller but nearly identical satellite body is oriented at a right angle to the major structure.

Peroxisomes

Peroxisomes or microbodies are present in a minority of mammalian cells, predominantly hepatocytes and renal epithelial cells.[16] The morphologic appearance of peroxisomes from different species varies considerably, the only common feature being a biochemical characteristic, the presence of the enzyme catalase and at least one oxidase. The variety of oxidases may include urate oxidase, amino acid oxidases, and glycolate oxidase.

Most peroxisomes are spherical, are enclosed by a single layer of unit membrane, and are about the same

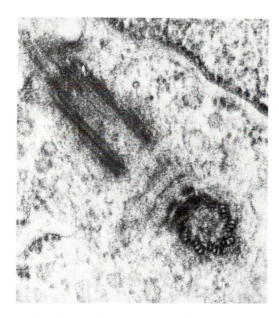

Fig. 1-17. Pair of centrioles oriented at right angles to each other. (68,000×.)

diameter as mitochondria (0.5 to 1 μm). The matrix is granular and moderately electron dense, and in some species the peripheral membrane shows a focal, plaque-like thickening. If the microbodies in a species contain urate oxidase, this enzyme is present in the form of a crystalloid structure, consisting of an array of closely packed tubules. Peroxisomes in humans do not contain urate oxidase. Peroxisomes may participate in the oxidation of lipids.

MAJOR CELLULAR FUNCTIONS

This section considers some of the most important cellular functions and relates them to specific cellular substructures. The minimum functions of a "typical" mammalian cell can be generalized into eight processes: (1) ingestion and egestion, (2) communication and excitation, (3) energy production, (4) synthesis, (5) storage, (6) digestion and detoxication, (7) movement, and (8) reproduction. To a lesser or greater extent, all mammalian cells carry out these basic functions, and malfunction of any of these processes may lead to cellular disability or death. In the adult animal certain cells are altered in such a way that one or more functions become their preeminent occupation; such cells are commonly said to be specialized or differentiated.

Ingestion and egestion

The plasma membrane, with its associated receptors, serves a major role in recognizing external stimuli and determining the cellular responses to these stimuli. An essential function of the cell membrane is the control of movement of substances from one side to the other (that is, from the exterior into the cell and the reverse).

Cells have several mechanisms available for moving substances across membranes. The nature of the mechanism employed depends to a great extent on the character of the substance to be transported. Small solutes readily diffuse through membranes, with the diffusion rate depending on their solubility in the membrane and on their concentrations on either side. Movement of water across a cell membrane is determined by the net flux of ions. Transport of many substances through membranes is effected by carrier molecules (receptors) in the membrane, which have a high affinity for the molecule or ion to be transported at one side of the membrane and a lowered affinity for the molecule or ion on the other side.[30] Often the movement of one substance in an inward direction is coupled with movement of another substance in an outward direction. Carrier-mediated ion transport mechanisms are often termed *membrane pumps*. Such a process is energy consuming, since it must usually function against a gradient of concentration of the substance to be transported. Lipid-soluble substances penetrate membranes freely by virtue of their ability to dissolve in the lipid of membranes.

Larger molecules and particulate materials are transported across membranes either by a complex process of membrane infolding, which produces internalized compartments that surround the substance,[18] or by the reverse process whereby an internal compartment fuses with the cell's outer membrane and breaks, releasing its contents outside the cell.[11] Transport to the interior of the cell is termed *endocytosis* and that in the opposite direction is *exocytosis*. Endocytosis is often subdivided into two processes, *pinocytosis* (cell drinking) and *phagocytosis* (cell eating). Exocytosis, at least operationally,

appears to be the reverse of endocytosis. It is the mechanism by which certain secretory cells transfer their synthetic product (enzyme, hormone, and so on) to the outside of the cell. Excretion of specific hormone granules is often termed *emiocytosis*.[23] Endocytosis and exocytosis involve, in addition to the cell membrane, the coordinate action of cytoplasmic microfilaments and microtubules.[1]

Pinocytosis and phagocytosis are morphologically similar processes, distinguishable by the character of the material ingested and the sizes of the vacuoles formed. Both processes involve the envelopment of substances to be ingested in infoldings of the cell's plasma membrane, and in both the infolded unit membranes fuse to form a spherical compartment that separates completely from the plasma membrane.

Pinocytosis appears to be directed mainly to the bulk transport of fluids and dissolved solids into and through cells.[18] Small vesicles (20 to 30 nm) with smooth unit membranes (Fig. 1-18) bud inward from the luminal plasma membrane, move to the surface membrane at the base or side of the cell with which they fuse, and discharge their contents into the extracellular space. Their directional movement has been deduced from carefully timed studies employing microparticles. Alternatively, the contents of pinocytic vesicles may be emptied into the cytosol. Fluid-phase pinocytosis is nonselective, the uptake rate of solutes being a linear function of their extracellular concentration.

A variant of pinocytosis, in which selected uptake of ligands is mediated by their binding to membrane receptors before internalization, is seen in a wide variety of epithelial cells. This type of pinocytic vesicle appears to form only at morphologically distinct sites on the plasma membrane, where the specific surface receptors are presumably located. Plasma membranes at these points have a prominent glycocalyx on their exterior, as well as tiny perpendicular bristlelike structures attached to their interior. The bristlelike structures are associated with actin-containing and clathrin-containing microfilaments. Materials to be ingested appear to bind to the membrane at these points, after which a vesicle is formed by membrane infolding. Such vesicles are morphologically distinct, since their outside (cytosol) surface contains the bristles (Fig. 1-19). This appearance has caused them to be called "coated" vesicles. Their size ranges from 50 to 250 nm.

Phagocytosis results in the ingestion by cells of much larger particulate materials than can be accommodated in pinocytic vesicles.[36] Such materials may be as large as bacterial or small eukaryotic cells (or their parts). Therefore phagosomes resulting from this process may be several micrometers in diameter. As with pinosomes, they are bounded by a single layer of unit membrane. The capacity for copious phagocytosis is limited to a relatively small number of mammalian cells, which are termed

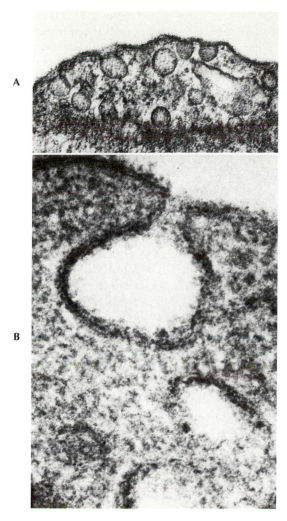

Fig. 1-18. A, Pinocytic vesicles opening onto cell surface *(top)* and within cytoplasm. **B,** Pinocytic vesicles at higher magnification showing that they are composed of infolded surface unit membrane. (**A,** 52,000×; **B,** 225,000×.)

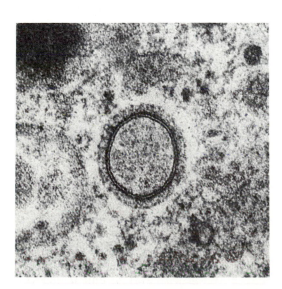

Fig. 1-19. "Coated" pinocytic vesicle showing the bristlelike material on its cytoplasm-facing side. (150,000×.)

phagocytes or *macrophages*. The process of phagocytosis is complex, involving not only the phagocyte and the particulate material to be ingested but also extracellular factors including plasma fibronectin (opsonin), antibodies, and surfaces of adjacent tissues. Within the cell, phagosomes fuse with primary lysosomes and the contents are partially or completely digested. *Autophagocytosis* is a variant process that does not involve the plasma membrane in the production of the vacuole. In this process a group of the cell's own organelles is enclosed by membranes of the endoplasmic reticulum, perhaps by infolding into a cistern analogous to phagocytosis at the cell's surface. Presumably the organelles so segregated are effete or acutely damaged. Such membrane-bound areas of cytoplasm then fuse with one or more primary lysosomes. Autophagocytosis appears to be an important mechanism for the "turnover" of cellular organelles, their component substrates being reutilized in the building of new organelles.

Communication and excitation

In the general sense all cells communicate through their microenvironments by the mutual interchange of metabolites across membranes. However, cells communicate with each other in a much more specific sense; such communication causes the cell receiving the message to act in a specified manner, for example, to depolarize, to contract, to alter its metabolic state, or to secrete its stored product.

Perhaps the most pervasive form of communication between cells is that mediated by the binding of certain compounds, especially hormones, to receptors. A given hormone may produce effects in only certain cells, and it may produce varying effects in different cells. The ability of a cell to respond to a particular hormone depends on the presence of specific receptors on its surface membrane,[22] and how it responds depends on the characteristics of its metabolic machinery and whether the surface receptor and the specific organelles are linked (often by the adenyl and guanyl cyclase systems). Because of these variations, hormones have characteristic and widely divergent effects on different types of cells.

A more direct form of communication between cells takes place through physical coupling.[26] Adjacent cells in all epithelia are joined by so-called *nexus junctions* (see the discussion of junctional complexes and basal laminae), which allow the ready passage of an electrical current between them (low-resistance coupling). Fluids and solutes up to about 10,000 molecular weight may also transit this junction. Neurons have elaborated a more highly varied means of communicating with cells (other nerve cells, muscle cells, or gland cells). Axons lead from the neuron cell body to the cell with which it communicates. Communication takes place through synapses, muscle spindles, and a variety of sensing structures. The forms of communication are electrical and chemical.

Electrical coupling takes place through structures similar to nexus junctions, which allow the low-resistance flow of electrical current between adjacent cells. Synaptic communication on a chemical basis is effected by neurotransmitter substances (acetylcholine or norepinephrine), which pass into the receptor cell and cause the propagation of an electrical current.

The external surface of the outer membranes of all cells is electrically polarized relative to the inner surface. In certain cells, notably nerve and muscle, the cell surface can be focally depolarized and the local depolarization propagated along the cell. By this means an action potential, which may lead to muscle contraction, glandular secretion, and so on, is produced.

Energy production

Energy is produced in the cell from the derivatives of food (amino acids, fatty acids, glucose, and so on). The major fraction of cellular energy is produced as a result of metabolic events taking place in the cytosol near and within mitochondria.[37] For example, glucose is glycolytically converted to pyruvic acid, which in turn is oxidized to form acetyl coenzyme A. Oxidation of fatty acids contributes more acetyl coenzyme A. Within mitochondria, acetyl coenzyme A is enzymatically converted through various steps of the Krebs tricarboxylic acid cycle to carbon dioxide and water. At several points along the Krebs cycle electrons are captured by the electron-transfer chain of mitochondria (NAD, FAD, and cytochromes b, c_1, a, and a_3), ultimately giving rise to high-energy intermediates. Energy is stored in the form of adenosine triphosphate (ATP), from which it can be enzymatically released as needed. ATP apparently is transported by a carrier protein from mitochondria into the adjacent portions of the cell where it is required.

Anaerobic metabolism accounts for only a small fraction of the energy produced in mammalian cells, and alone it is incapable of sustaining most cellular functions. When mitochondrial energy production is blocked or when ATP is sequestered, mammalian cellular functions rapidly deteriorate and the cells may die. Transformation of the latent energy of foods to ATP is only fractionally efficient, and the lost energy is converted to heat.

Synthesis

Mammalian cells synthesize all of their own cellular macromolecules from building blocks derived from food. Synthesis, as a general cellular process, is extremely diverse and complicated. Even so, it occurs almost entirely in three locations in the cell: mainly in the nucleus, in the endoplasmic reticulum–Golgi complex, and to a much lesser extent in mitochondria. Replacement synthesis for organelles and membranes that wear out takes place constantly. When new cells are formed, virtually the entire contents of the cell are duplicated before the daughter cells separate. Some cells are specialized to synthesize and secrete great quantities of a substance (usually a protein in the form of an enzyme, a hormone, or a metabolic substrate) to be used by other cells in distant sites.

With minor exceptions, all of the cell's nucleic acids are synthesized within the nucleus. DNA, which is completely duplicated only when new cells are formed, is enzymatically synthesized by use of the preexisting strands of this macromolecule as a template from which to form an exact copy.[12] Complex replication apparatuses containing several coordinated enzyme activities, including DNA replicative polymerase, are associated with chromatin. Replication occurs in multiple sites throughout the chromatin at forklike structures where the DNA helix is transiently unwound. Ribonucleic acid (RNA) is also synthesized by use of a portion of the nuclear DNA as a template.[39] In this instance the enzyme responsible for copying the template (an RNA polymerase) forms the new molecule from ribonucleoside triphosphates, rather than from the deoxyribonucleoside triphosphates found in DNA. This process whereby an analog of DNA is made in the form of RNA is called *transcription*. The types of RNA made in the nucleus are messenger RNAs (which contain the information content of a defined segment of DNA), transfer RNAs (each specific for a single amino acid), and ribosomal RNAs (28S, 18S, and 5S to 7S molecules, which are included in ribosomes). Ribosomal RNAs are synthesized in the nucleolus. All the types of RNA mentioned are transferred to the cytoplasm where they participate in the synthesis of proteins and complex macromolecules, which include protein moieties.

Protein synthesis occurs in the cytoplasm on polyribosomes.[15] Ribosomes attach to the "front" end of the strand of messenger RNA, which determines the amino acid sequence of the protein to be synthesized, and progress three bases (a *codon*, which specifies an amino acid) at a move down the messenger. Movement is coordinated with the attachment of the proper amino acid–charged transfer RNA to the next coded nucleotide trio on the messenger. As this progression occurs along the messenger strand, a peptide bond is formed between adjacent amino acids and the transfer RNA is released. The protein molecule grows as a strand elongating from each ribosome. As one ribosome moves along the messenger strand away from the origin, another one attaches until the messenger is fully covered. One ribosome detaches from the end of the strand with a completed protein molecule, as a new ribosome attaches at the beginning to start the synthesis of another molecule. This process by which the information contained in a molecule of messenger RNA is converted to a protein molecule is known as *translation*.

Protein synthesis occurs on both "free" and "bound" polyribosomes; in the first instance the newly synthesized protein molecule is discharged into the cell sap, and in the second situation it is discharged into the interstices of the endoplasmic reticulum. Although the significance of these two categories of protein synthesis is not entirely clear, evidence suggests that proteins synthesized on unattached polyribosomes can be used without further modification within the cell where they are produced. Proteins that require further modification (such as the addition of a second protein chain, the excision of a portion of the chain originally synthesized, or the addition of lipids or carbohydrates) or that must be purified and packaged in membrane-bound vesicles for use within the cell (such as lysosomes) or for export outside the cell (such as hormones or enzymes) are synthesized on polyribosomes attached to membranes of the endoplasmic reticulum. The protein strands extruded into the cisterns of the endoplasmic reticulum pass on through the tubules of the smooth endoplasmic reticulum into the sacs and vesicles of the Golgi apparatus, where they are chemically modified or packaged into vesicles. The complex lipoproteins that constitute cell membranes are themselves synthesized in this way.[28]

Lipids are synthesized within and around the smooth endoplasmic reticulum. Glycogen is also synthesized and stored in the general vicinity of the smooth endoplasmic reticulum.[12] Small amounts of DNA and RNA are synthesized in mitochondria.

Storage

A variety of metabolic products are stored in cells before their ultimate utilization. Secretory granules of endocrine and exocrine glandular cells, lysosomes, leukocytic granules, fat, and glycogen are examples of the diverse forms of stored products. Many of the specific granules have characteristic ultrastructural forms that facilitate their morphologic identification. Other major storage particles represent indigestible remnants of lysosomal degradation, retained in cells in a membrane-enclosed vesicle. Such residual bodies contain a morphologically heterogeneous variety of materials.

Certain cells are able to store carbohydrate and lipid for subsequent metabolic use as glucose and fatty acids. Glucose is stored as glycogen, a highly branched polymer, and fatty acids are stored as neutral lipids. Both metabolic substrates can be quickly released enzymatically when the need arises. Glycogen occurs in two morphologic patterns, termed alpha and beta particles (Fig. 1-20). Beta particles are roughly spherical irregular granules that measure 30 to 40 nm in diameter. Alpha particles are aggregates of beta particles and can reach 0.1 μm in diameter. Glycogen is stored in areas of cytoplasm that contain smooth endoplasmic reticulum, although individual particles appear to be free in the cytosol.

Neutral lipid is formed in the cisterns of endoplasmic reticulum and is seen initially as small electron-dense

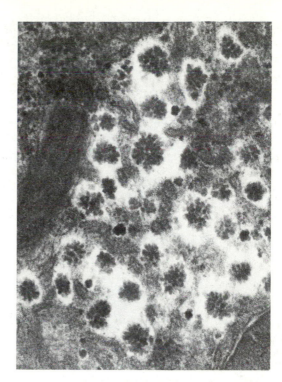

Fig. 1-20. Glycogen particles. Most of the particles are rosettes or alpha particles. (60,000×.)

spheres. These small liposomes can fuse to form lipid drops up to 2 μm in diameter (Fig. 1-21).

Digestion and detoxication

Digestion and detoxication are processes by which the mammalian cell attempts to rid itself of effete membranes and organelles, of particulate materials that it has ingested (including microbes), and of toxic chemicals that have been transported into its cytoplasm. Digestion of cellular membranes or phagocytized particles is analogous to the intracellular digestion of food by more primitive unicellular organisms. Indeed, the mammalian cell reutilizes the building blocks that it derives from digestion of intracellular membranes and extracellular debris. Furthermore, the metabolism of exogenous toxins is similar to that of certain compounds (especially steroids) that mammalian cells normally encounter.

Digestion takes place in membrane-enclosed vacuoles that fuse with lysosomes. The various lysosomal hydrolases catabolize a number of macromolecules. Phagosomes may arise from the ingestion of particulate material through the cell membrane (*heterophagy*)[10] or from focal cytoplasmic sequestration of effete organelles (*autophagy*).[11] In either situation these phagosomes fuse with primary lysosomes, which empty their hydrolytic enzymes into the phagosomes. Indigestible residual materials may remain in the cytosol in membrane-enclosed vacuoles, or they may be extruded from the cell.

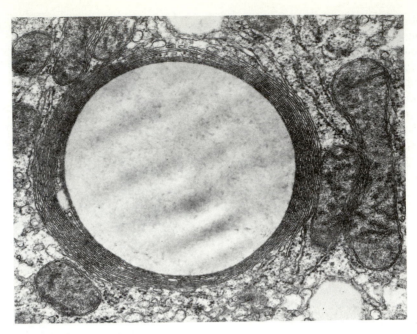

Fig. 1-21. Lipid droplet surrounded by closely packed profiles of smooth endoplasmic reticulum. (25,000×.)

Detoxication of a variety of foreign, lipophilic chemicals is mediated through the cytochrome P450–linked mixed-function oxidases,[14] located on some parts of the smooth endoplasmic reticulum.[13] The action of these enzyme sequences is to render nonpolar chemicals water soluble and therefore excretable. It is ironic that, during the enzymatic process that converts them to a water-soluble form, some chemicals are activated to a more toxic state. Cells that have an abundance of mixed-function oxidases (such as hepatocytes) may be extremely vulnerable to the cytotoxic effects of toxins that are metabolically activated.

Movement

Movement of cells includes the locomotion of cells along surfaces, the translocation of organelles within cells, and the contraction of cells.

It is well known that the contraction of muscle fibers, both smooth and striated, results from the action of two types of microfilaments composed of *actin* and *myosin*.[32] Both the spatial arrangement and the functional character of actin and myosin filaments in smooth and striated muscle differ. In essence, contraction (shortening of the muscle fiber) in both types of muscle appears to occur because of directed movement of each type of fibril past the other. This type of movement is associated with the energy-dependent making (and breaking) of chemical bonds between actin and myosin. It is perhaps less well appreciated that many types of general cell movement are also caused by microfilaments of actin, which are present in all mammalian cells.[1] Actin microfilaments are responsible for movement of the cell membrane, including cellular locomotion, movement of microvilli (and perhaps their projection), and ingestion in membrane-bound vesicles, such as pinocytosis and phagocytosis.

Microtubules are related to some of the directed movements of subcellular particles within cells and also may have other functions. For instance, they appear to be responsible for cellular rigidity, acting in essence as a cytoskeleton. Organelles and packaged secretory products (and perhaps dissolved solids) appear to move along microtubular tracks in the cytosol. This form of directed intracytoplasmic movement receives one of its highest expressions in mammalian neurons, where organelles and secretory vacuoles may be transported for long distances down axons along microtubules. Microtubule-oriented movement is also involved in the excretion of some membrane-enclosed secretory products by the process of emiocytosis. Perhaps the most notable function of microtubules is the separation of chromosomes by the mitotic spindle, which is composed of thousands of tubular substructures. Another type of motion that depends on microtubular action is the whipping or beating motion of cilia and flagella.

Reproduction

Reproduction is the most complex of cell functions, and yet it is virtually universal; only a few specialized mammalian cells have totally lost the ability to reproduce. In essence, cellular reproduction involves the manufacture of a nearly complete set of membranes and organelles and, most important, a complete and accurate reproduction of the nuclear DNA, combined with a mechanism to split the parent cell in half. Each daughter cell receives exact copies of the nuclear DNA and about half of the various organelles and membranes; a deficiency of organelles and membranes may be corrected by synthesis after division if an accurate distribution of the nuclear DNA is effected.

The life cycle of a mammalian cell (the *cell cycle* or *proliferative cycle*), which exists between the occurrence of two consecutive divisions, is divisible into four phases or stages based on the occurrence of two specific events.[2, 7] These events are the synthesis of the nuclear DNA (*S phase*) and the mitotic apportionment of the DNA and cytoplasm to daughter cells (*M phase*). Preceding the S phase is the so-called *G_1 phase*, and the *G_2 phase* separates S and M phases. During each of the G phases (or gaps), highly characteristic metabolic events occur. During the G_1 phase, messenger RNAs for a variety of enzyme proteins are synthesized, and then the proteins themselves are synthesized. These proteins are those required for the cell to commence and complete the S phase and include DNA polymerase and ligase, proteins that initiate DNA synthesis, "unwind" the DNA helix, and so on. Initiation of DNA replication, which starts the S phase, is poorly understood but may include the synthesis of a small primer segment of RNA. Replication occurs in multiple small segments of DNA, called replicons, and its continuation requires the coordinate synthesis of certain proteins. During the G_2 phase, messenger RNAs are synthesized and direct the synthesis of proteins required for mitosis. At the same time, during the premitotic phases, all of the cell's constituents (membranes, organelles, and so on) are essentially doubled.

Cell division consists of both chromosome separation and splitting of the cytoplasm. The onset of mitosis is heralded by division of the centriole and migration of the two daughter centrioles to opposite poles of the nucleus. Chromosomes condense from the dispersed nuclear chromatin, and the nuclear membrane disintegrates (*prophase*). The microtubules of the mitotic spindle polymerize and arrange themselves between the centrioles while the chromosomes align at the equatorial plate of the spindle (*metaphase*). Chromatids separate and move toward the opposite poles of the spindle; cytokinesis begins by a constriction of the cytoplasm in the region of the spindle equator (*anaphase*). Nuclear membrane reforms around each mass of chromosomes, which melt into a chromatin network, the nucleolus reaggregates, spindle microtubules depolymerize, and the cytoplasm of the two daughter cells completely separates (*telophase*). Continuity of the cell cycle is usually interrupted after a cell has divided. Thus, noncycling cells are considered to be blocked in early G_1 or to be located in a hypothetical out-of-cycle phase, termed G_0. However, even under physiologic conditions some cells may be temporarily or permanently arrested in some other stage of the cycle, most frequently G_2.

After completing a proliferative cycle, which can vary greatly in length, a cell must take one of two courses, either to continue or to temporarily or permanently stop cycling. The frequency with which cells cycle is highly variable, determined by a multiplicity of poorly understood factors.[6] Organization of cells in tissues constrains their uncontrolled proliferation (see the discussion of cellular population kinetics in tissues). When continued proliferation is incompatible with function, the cell stops cycling to develop specialized functional and structural properties.

CELLULAR ENVIRONMENT

Most mammalian cells are capable of an independent autonomous existence under optimum environmental conditions. However, they are totally dependent on the quality of their immediate environment (microenvironment), tolerating only a limited range of variation in concentrations of hydrogen ions, salts, oxygen, carbon dioxide, and temperature. In mammals, cells are bathed by interstitial fluid, a product of blood plasma processed by filtration and percolation through vascular endothelium, basement membrane, and interstitial connective tissue. Interstitial fluid is the pathway by which both nutrients and toxins are brought to the cell. In multicellular tissues other cells are part of the total microenvironment of a given cell, as are connective tissue fibers. Various cells in a tissue or organism constantly alter the quality of the interstitial fluid by adding or subtracting materials. Water is the major component of the environment surrounding cells (as it is of the cells themselves), and significant depletion or excess of intracellular or extracellular water is incompatible with cellular viability. In fact, much cellular work is spent in controlling the water distribution between cell and environment, which is effected by controlling cation distribution. In addition to providing the solvent phase for various chemical entities around and within cells, water stabilizes temperature through its capacity to absorb and conduct heat. Alterations in the composition of fluids surrounding cells rapidly affect cell structure and function.

CELLS IN TISSUES

Cells rarely function as individuals in the mammalian organism. More commonly groups of cells, each specialized to perform a limited number of functions, are aggregated into tissues. The framework for tissues is composed of connective tissue macromolecules, mainly collagen types, including basement membrane, and proteoglycans. Fibronectin, a molecular "gluelike" substance, helps bind cells to collagen fibers, to basal laminae, and to each other.[27]

Location of a cell in a tissue affects both its structure and its pattern of behavior. Furthermore, segregation of highly specialized cells in tissues, where their viability is dependent on blood supply, nervous function, drainage of secretions, and so on, creates opportunities for initiation of disease that are not found in single cells. In addition, narrow specialization of a cell makes it more vulnerable to injurious agents that affect that special function and also limits its range of reparative response. Specialization results in loss of self-sufficiency, making certain cells exquisitely dependent on the continued functioning of supporting cells, often equally highly specialized. Such dependent relationships suggest the manner in which the death of a single type of cell in an organism can produce a ripple or cascade effect extending to far distant cells.

Tissue-determined cellular aggregations

In addition to one or more groups of similarly specialized cells, essential components of tissues include the supporting framework of connective tissue, vessels, and nerves to supply nutrients and information from other sites in the body and to remove wastes and endocrine products, and in the case of exocrine glandular tissues, excretory ducts. Thus, tissues are structurally complex supracellular organizations. Parenchymal, or specifically functioning, cells have structural specializations associated with their organization in a tissue, including junctional complexes and basal laminae.

Junctional complexes and basal laminae

Plasma membrane of apposed epithelial and endothelial cells contains several modifications that have a role in cell adhesion and local intercellular communication.[35] These specializations of the cell's lateral surface membrane, collectively known as junctional complexes (Fig. 1-22), occur in four forms: (1) the occluding zone, (2) the adhering zone, (3) the adhering plate or desmosome, and (4) the gap junction.

Occluding zones and *adhering zones* are belt-shaped modifications of juxtaluminal cell membranes, which completely encircle the cell. Occluding zones, located immediately at the luminal margin, seal the space between adjacent cells, preventing the passage of tracer materials. Outer leaflets of the adjacent plasma membranes focally touch, often appearing in sections as a single line. Freeze-etched preparations of the surface of a disrupted occluding zone show an anastomosing pattern of tiny ridges; the apices of these ridges are points at which adjacent membranes touch. Adhering zones are located just distal to occluding zones. The space separating the outer leaflets of the plasma membranes at an adhering zone is uniformly narrowed to about 20 nm, but membranes do not touch at any point and the junction is permeable to tracer particles. On the cytoplasmic side of the inner leaflet of the plasma membrane overlying an adhering zone, there typically occurs an ill-defined, electron-dense plaque.

Desmosomes (adhering plates) occur as tiny plates ("spot welds") focally distributed along the abutting plasma membranes of a variety of epithelial cells. They are especially numerous in epidermis. Adjacent to desmosomes the intercellular space is narrowed to about 20 nm and typically contains a flocculent material bisected by a central dense line. On the cytoplasmic side of each membrane there is a plaque of electron-dense material from which a mass of intermediate filaments (termed *tonofilaments* in epidermis) radiates into the cytoplasm. Desmosomes do not block the passage of microparticulate materials through the narrowed intercellular space. A *hemidesmosome* is a desmosomal variant that occurs at the basal plasma membrane of epithelial cells next to bas-

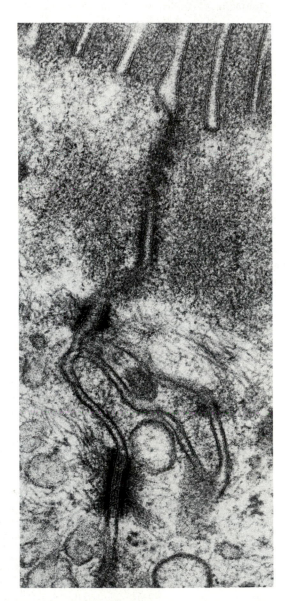

Fig. 1-22. Junctional complexes joining two cells. From top to bottom are shown an occluding zone or tight junction, an adhering zone or intermediate junction (two are shown), and an adhering plate or desmosome. (45,000×.)

al laminae. In structure it appears to be one half of a desmosome, as its name implies.

The *gap junction*, or *nexus*, is a platelike modification of plasma membrane that occurs on the deep lateral surface of all electronically coupled epithelia. The nexus consists of an array of hexagonal particles with a center-to-center spacing of about 9 nm, which forms a precisely registered polygonal lattice on the outer surfaces of adjacent plasma membranes. Each particle appears to have a tiny pit or hole in its center. Adjacent membranes are separated by a 2 nm gap, rendering the nexus permeable only to very small tracer particles. In addition to electri-

cal currents, the nexus allows the free passage between connected cells of water and solutes up to 10,000 molecular weight.

Adjacent epithelial cells occasionally exhibit mutually interlocking membrane pits and projections about 0.1 to 0.3 μm in diameter and up to 0.5 μm long (Figs. 1-23 and 1-24). These structures, sometimes called peg-and-hole processes, may hold adjacent cells in apposition.

Basal laminae are specific appendages of most epithelial and endothelial cells in tissues.[38] The basal lamina or basement membrane is a moderately electron-dense band 50 to 100 nm thick that separates epithelial and endothelial cells from other types of cells and from connective tissue fibers (Fig. 1-25). It follows the contour of the cell membrane but is separated from it by an electron-lucent zone about 40 nm wide. The basal lamina is composed of mucopolysaccharide and an amorphous form of collagen. Epithelium apparently synthesizes its own basal lamina, which appears to function as an anchoring support for cells, as well as a semipermeable filter for dissolved and particulate substances.

Cellular population kinetics in tissues

In young organisms, tissues continue to grow until the organism reaches adulthood, after which time tissue size normally remains constant. The size of a tissue is determined by the number and size of the cells and by the amount of intercellular substance the tissue contains. Populations of cells that do not change in number are referred to as steady-state populations, a term that encompasses a variety of mechanisms for maintaining a constant population.[7] In essence, two general situations

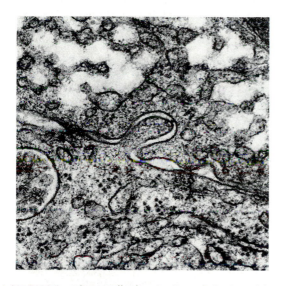

Fig. 1-23. Portions of two cells showing interdigitation of their lateral membranes in peg-and-hole configuration. (27,000×.)

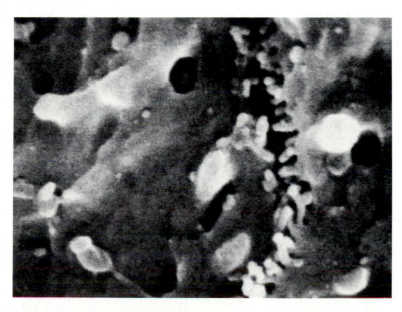

Fig. 1-24. Scanning electron micrograph of surface of cell showing pegs and holes in surface view. (21,000×.)

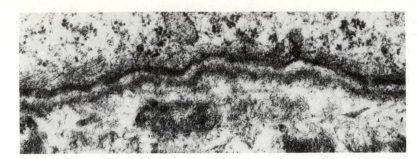

Fig. 1-25. Basal plasma membrane of epithelial cell and underlying basal lamina. (52,000×.)

reflect the mechanism by which most cell populations in vivo are maintained in a steady state: populations in which there is neither cell production nor cell loss and populations in which cell loss is precisely balanced by cell gain. The situation in the organism is more complicated than this, but three designations include the cell populations in most tissues. *Stable* or *static populations* produce virtually no new cells in adult animals. An example of such a population is the neurons of the central nervous system. The germ cell population in the ovary is usually included in this category, but in the adult female this group of cells steadily declines to total depletion at menopause. *Expanding populations* show little cell loss, coupled with a small but appreciable formation of new cells throughout adulthood. An example of such a population is the hepatocytes of the liver; the liver continues to grow slowly but perceptibly throughout life. *Renewing populations* include those tissues in which there is an appreciable physiologic death of cells apparently because of their functional obsolescence. In such a population, cell formation just balances cell loss and the size of the population remains nearly constant.

The mechanism by which the number of cells in a population is regulated is unknown, but it involves control of the cell life cycle.[6] The size of the functioning pool of mature cells in a population must be sensed in some way by the proliferating pool where new cells are produced, but the sensing mechanism is unexplained. It has been proposed that mature cells manufacture substances that suppress cell formation in the proliferating pool (such substances have been called *chalones*); another theory postulates the occurrence of factors that stimulate proliferation, such factors being normally catabolized by the functioning pool of cells. In either instance a sudden decrease in the number of functioning cells would allow a comparably rapid increase in cell formation by decreasing the production of an inhibitor or by allowing the buildup of a stimulator.

It is clear that most cellular populations can respond to the loss of functional capacity (caused by a decreased number of cells or by the inability of some cells to work) or to the demand for more work (that is, greater function) by producing more cells or by increasing the size of cells already present. Cells in different types of populations meet this demand in different ways. Stable or static populations, in which cell formation is impossible, can meet this emergency only by increasing the size of the already existing cells (*hypertrophy*). Both of the other major types of cell population (expanding and renewing) can meet the increased functional need by augmenting the rate of formation of new cells (*hyperplasia*) or by combined hypertrophy and hyperplasia. Renewing cell populations, in which new cells are already being rapidly formed, can increase the rate of formation to some extent by shortening the duration of the cell cycle (achieved mainly by speeding transit through G_1). This type of cell population can also increase its functioning population by decreasing the rate of physiologic or programmed cell death. For near steady-state expanding populations, in which physiologic cell death is practically nil, the number of cells in the population can be increased only by augmenting the proliferative pool (sometimes termed the *growth fraction*, that is, the fraction of cells that is progressing through the cell cycle).

Integration of cellular functions

Integration of cellular functions is effected by the coordination of chemical activities within cells. Control of cellular functions is accomplished mainly by regulatory proteins that have special properties (allosteric proteins). Regulatory proteins are able to associate selectively and reversibly with two or more molecular species that do not show any mutual chemical reactivity. Reactivity between these two hypothetical species takes place only through the mediation of a regulatory protein. Regulatory proteins function as allosteric molecules with at least two functional domains. One domain gives the protein the capacity to recognize and bind to a particular chemical species, causing the bound chemical to alter its action in the cell. The second domain binds an entirely different compound, and this binding modifies the reactivity of the first domain. Depending on whether the modifying compound is bound to the second domain, the protein oscillates between two states, activity and inactivity, and acts as a chemical "on-or-off" switch. By coupling different functions of cells, allosteric regulatory proteins form the basis of feedback loops that connect enzymatic processes with, for example, substrates or metabolic products. Through such feedback loops, the level of substrate or metabolic product can be made to control the rate of an enzyme reaction.

At the organismic level, similar regulatory circuits coordinate the interaction of different cells and tissues in various parts of the body. Coordinating networks involve direct contact between cells or indirect contact by "chemical messengers." In each instance, cells receive signals through specific receptors. When a signal is not transmitted or a receptor is blocked, one of the circuits ensuring the social behavior of the organism may be interrupted, leading to the deterioration of integrated function.

CELLULAR INJURY AND DISEASE

Cells may be injured by any of a variety of agents acting on cellular structures and metabolic processes. The nature of some of these agents and the types of lesions they produce will be explored in subsequent chapters. Detection of cellular injury is a problem that constantly confronts students of disease. Although lesions produced in subcellular metabolic machinery can be exquisitely precise, the interdependence of functional pathways causes the initial injury, if sufficiently severe, to rapidly broaden and amplify. Cells readily adapt to differing functional and environmental conditions, and injury is normally detectable only when steady-state function and structure are not maintained. The frequent difficulty of precisely identifying an injured cell stems from the fact that the injured cell is not characterized by new types of metabolic pathways, but only by the increase, decrease, or loss of those that are present in an uninjured cell. This situation often causes the detection of functional and structural abnormality in cells and tissues to be a subtly difficult, intellectually challenging task.

REFERENCES

1. Allison, A.C.: The role of microfilaments and microtubules in cell movement, endocytosis, and exocytosis, Ciba Found. Symp. **14:**110, 1973.
2. Baserga, R., and Wiebel, F.: The cell cycle of mammalian cells, Int. Rev. Exp. Pathol. **7:**1, 1969.
3. Bryan, J.: Biochemical properties of microtubules, Fed. Proc. **33:**152, 1974.
4. Caro, L.G., and Palade, G.E.: Protein synthesis, storage and discharge in the pancreatic exocrine cell: an autoradiographic study, J. Cell Biol. **20:**473, 1964.
5. Caspersson, T., et al.: The use of fluorescence techniques for recognition of mammalian chromosomes and chromosome regions, Int. Rev. Exp. Pathol. **11:**1, 1972.
6. Clarkson, B., and Baserga, R., editors: Control of proliferation in animal cells, Cold Spring Harbor, N.Y., 1974, Cold Spring Harbor Laboratory.
7. Cleaver, J.E.: Thymidine metabolism and cell kinetics, Amsterdam, 1967, North-Holland Publishing Co.
8. Coimbra, A., and LeBlond, C.P.: Sites of glycogen synthesis in rat liver cells as shown by electron microscope autoradiography after administration of glucose-H³, J. Cell Biol. **30:**151, 1966.
9. Comings, D.E.: The structure and function of chromatin, Adv. Hum. Genet. **3:**237, 1972.
10. de Duve, C., and Wattiaux, R.: Functions of lysosomes, Annu. Rev. Physiol. **28:**435, 1966.
11. Ericsson, J.L.E.: Mechanism of cellular autophagy. In Dingle, J.T., and Fell, H.B., editors: Lysosomes in biology and pathology, vol. 2, Amsterdam, 1969, North-Holland Publishing Co.
12. Fansler, B.S.: Eukaryotic DNA polymerases, their association with the nucleus and relationship to DNA replication, Int. Rev. Cytol. **4**(suppl.):363, 1974.
13. Fouts, J.R., Rogers, L.A., and Gram, T.E.: The metabolism of drugs by hepatic microsomal enzymes: studies on intramicrosomal distribution of enzymes and relationships between enzyme activity and structure of the hepatic endoplasmic reticulum, Exp. Mol. Pathol. **5:**475, 1965.
14. Gillette, J.R., Davis, D.C., and Sasame, H.A.: Cytochrome P_{450} and its role in drug metabolism, Annu. Rev. Pharmacol. **12:**57, 1972.
15. Haselkorn, R., and Rothman-Denes, L.B.: Protein synthesis, Annu. Rev. Biochem. **42:**397, 1973.
16. Hruban, Z., and Recheigl, M.: Microbodies and related particles: morphology, biochemistry, and physiology, Int. Rev. Cytol., suppl. 1, 1969.
17. Ito, S.: Form and function of the glycocalyx on free cell surfaces, Philos. Trans. R. Soc. Lond. (Biol.) **268:**55, 1974.
18. Jacques, P.J.: Endocytosis. In Dingle, J.T., and Fell, H.B., editors: Lysosomes in biology and pathology, vol. 2, Amsterdam, 1969, North-Holland Publishing Co.
19. Johnson, J.D., Douvas, A.S., and Bonner, J.: Chromosomal proteins, Int. Rev. Cytol. **4**(suppl.):273, 1974.
20. Kalnins, V.I.: The fiber systems of cells, Bull. Microscop. Soc. Canada **6:**4, 1978.
21. Kay, R.R., and Johnston, I.R.: The nuclear envelope: current problems of structure and function, Subcell. Biochem. **2:**127, 1973.
22. Kornfeld, S., and Kornfeld, R.: Cell surface receptors—structure and function, Prog. Hematol. **7:**161, 1971.
23. Lacy, P.E.: Endocrine secretory mechanisms: a review, Am. J. Pathol. **79:**170, 1975.
24. Lehninger, A.L.: The molecular organization of mitochondrial membranes, Adv. Cytopharmacol. **1:**199, 1971.
25. Long, E.R.: A history of pathology, New York, 1965, Dover Publications, Inc.
26. Lowenstein, W.R.: Intercellular communication, Sci. Am. **222**(5):78, 1970.
27. McDonagh, J.: Fibronectin, a molecular glue, Arch. Pathol. Lab. Med. **105:**393, 1981.
28. Morre, D.J., Keenan, T.W., and Huang, C.M.: Membrane flow and differentiation: origin of Golgi apparatus membranes from endoplasmic reticulum, Adv. Cytopharmacol. **2:**107, 1974.
29. Nanninga, N.: Structural aspects of ribosomes, Int. Rev. Cytol. **35:**135, 1973.
30. Oxender, D.L.: Membrane transport, Annu. Rev. Biochem. **41:**777, 1972.
31. Peters, R.: Biochemical lesions and lethal synthesis, London, 1963, Pergamon Press, Inc.
32. Pollard, T.D., and Weihing, R.R.: Actin and myosin and cell movement, CRC Crit. Rev. Biochem. **2:**1, 1974.
33. Rothman, J.E.: The Golgi apparatus: two organelles in tandem, Science **213:**1212, 1981.
34. Singer, S.J., and Nicolson, G.L.: The fluid mosaic model of the structure of membranes, Science **175:**720, 1972.
35. Staehlin, L.A.: Structure and function of intercellular junctions, Int. Rev. Cytol. **39:**191, 1974.
36. Stossel, T.P.: Phagocytosis: recognition and ingestion, Semin. Hematol. **12:**83, 1975.
37. Tandler, B., and Hoppel, C.L.: Mitochondria, New York, 1972, Academic Press, Inc.
38. Vracko, R.: Basal lamina scaffold—anatomy and significance for maintenance of orderly tissue structure, Am. J. Pathol. **77:**314, 1974.
39. Weinberg, R.A.: Nuclear RNA metabolism, Annu. Rev. Biochem. **42:**329, 1973.
40. Weissman, G., and Claiborne, R., editors: Cell membranes: biochemistry, cell biology, and pathology, New York, 1975, HP Publishing Co., Inc.

CHAPTER 2

Inflammation and Healing

VINCENT T. MARCHESI

INFLAMMATION

Inflammation is the characteristic response of mammalian tissue to injury. Whenever tissue is injured, there follows at the site of injury a series of events that tend to destroy or limit the spread of the injurious agent. The early events in this so-called *inflammatory response* are mainly vascular and are usually succeeded by repair and healing of the injured tissue. The inflammatory response might therefore be taken to include the subsequent healing and repair processes, but it is preferable to consider inflammation and healing as separate events while remembering that inflammation and subsequent repair do merge and overlap and that a clear-cut chronologic distinction is impossible.

The agents that injure tissues and therefore evoke the inflammatory response include bacteria and other types of microorganisms and nonliving agents such as trauma, heat, cold, radiant and electrical energy, and chemicals. Because of the diversity of the causative factors, inflammation is one of the most common and important conditions with which the physician has to deal.

Definition and signs of inflammation

A definition of inflammation is complicated because the local vascular and tissue reactions may be accompanied by systemic effects that include malaise, fever, leukocytosis, metabolic disturbances, and shock.

According to its duration, inflammation is described as acute or chronic. Sometimes the acute process subsides but the stimulus persists sufficiently to evoke a subsequent chronic inflammation. In other cases, with a stimulus that typically induces chronic inflammation, the tissue response may be acute for the first day or so. The tissue response differs considerably in acute and chronic inflammation. However, when inflammation or the inflammatory response is mentioned in this chapter without qualification, it is acute inflammation that is being discussed.

Main events in an acute inflammatory process— a vascular reaction

The following account of acute inflammation describes the main events comprising the inflammatory process, discusses the mechanism of these events, and indicates how the events are responsible for the clinical signs of inflammation.

The early features of the inflammatory response result from reactions of the small blood vessels in the injured tissue. Some of the features are demonstrated by the events induced by firm stroking of the skin on the inner aspect of the forearm. The line of the stroke is accurately marked by a red line that appears in 3 to 18 seconds and reaches a peak in 30 to 50 seconds. When the stroking is heavy or repeated several times in succession, the red line becomes bordered by a spreading flush that appears in the first minute and intensifies into a bright red flare. Finally, the red line becomes replaced by a pale wheal, which begins 1 to 3 minutes after the stroking and becomes maximal in 3 to 5 minutes. Next, the wheal and then the flare become pale, but it is 1 or several hours before the wheal subsides.

The red line results from local vasodilatation of capillaries and small venules, the flare is caused by dilatation of the neighboring arterioles, and the wheal represents local edema. The local *vasodilatation* and the *flare* and *wheal* constitute what Lewis[6] termed the "triple response."

Similar effects can be obtained by pricking or scratching, by freezing or burning, or by inducing electrical or chemical injury. With cold, electrical, or chemical injury, the triple response is often accompanied by itching or pain. These simple experiments therefore elicit the four classic signs of inflammation—redness, swelling, heat, and pain. They also demonstrate that the same events are evoked by various kinds of stimuli and that the events themselves are predominantly vascular in nature.

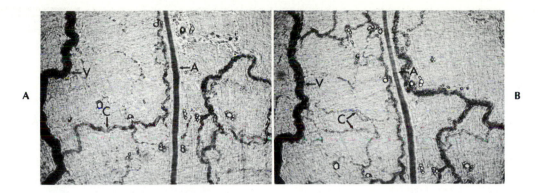

Fig. 2-1. A, Arteriole, *A,* capillary, *C,* and venule, *V,* in periphery of uninjured rabbit ear chamber. **B,** Same area shown in **A** 24 hours after injury. Note engorgement of additional capillaries, *C.* (65×; from Allison, F., Jr., Smith, M.R., and Wood, W.B., Jr.: J. Exp. Med. **102:**655, 1955.)

Microscopic observations

When the early vascular events in injured tissue are observed microscopically, it becomes apparent that the responses of the vessels[2,3] are far more complex than might be thought from macroscopic observation.

The events can be demonstrated in the vessels of the exposed frog tongue or mesenteric loops of rats. Both tissues are thin enough to be examined in the living state with the light microscope. The connective tissue beds of rabbit ears have also proved to be a valuable experimental model. Special chambers (called ear chambers) are inserted into rabbit ears to allow one to see the vascular bed with great clarity and watch what happens when it is injured. A typical view of the microvessels obtained in this way is shown in Fig. 2-1, *A.*

Immediately after injury, regardless of the stimulus, there is transient vasoconstriction of the arterioles. With mild injury, blood flow may be reestablished in a few seconds. With strong thermal injury, however, the vasoconstriction lasts about 5 minutes. Then follows a progressive dilatation of the blood vessels, which involves mainly the arterioles but also, to less extent, the venules and capillaries. Within 30 minutes, the arteriolar dilatation is evident, and blood flow through the injured tissues is greater than before injury. The arteriolar dilatation continues to increase, so that by 24 hours after injury the blood vessels of the area are engorged, and the capillaries and veins in which there was previously little or no blood flow now carry a rapid stream (Figs. 2-1 and 2-2). Arteriolar pulsation becomes so strong that it is transmitted to the capillaries and venules, and the whole area visibly pulsates.

Two further events are important in the development of the inflammatory response. The first is the exudation of plasma from blood vessels in the injured tissues. This exudation is accompanied by a decrease in blood flow. As the bloodstream slows, the formed elements become redistributed in the local circulation as a preliminary to

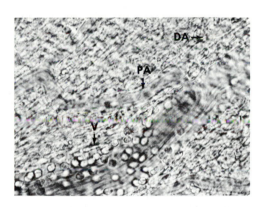

Fig. 2-2. Vascular shunt in which blood flow bypasses lesion located at upper right. Blood is flowing from proximal arteriole, *PA,* to venule, *V,* and bypassing distal arteriole, *DA.* Sticking of leukocytes is pronounced in venule. (250×; from Allison, F., Jr., Smith, M.R., and Wood, W.B., Jr.: J. Exp. Med. **102:**655, 1955.)

the second important event—the emigration of neutrophilic leukocytes into the injured tissues.

Exudation of plasma. From microscopic examination, the tissues in and adjacent to the injured areas appear increasingly dense from the accumulation of edema fluid, which indicates the escape of plasma through the wall of the peripheral vascular bed. Immediately adjacent to the site of injury, edema begins to develop in the first 10 to 15 minutes. Farther afield, where the intensity of the stimulus is less, edema appears more slowly. Edema causes swelling of inflamed tissue. Edema is also recognizable in blisters, such as occur in second-degree burns, and exudation also results in the accumulation of fluid in cavities lined by inflamed serosal membranes (for example, pleurisy with effusion).

Edema fluid in inflamed tissue is characterized by high protein content (1 to 6 g/dl) and ready coagulability (because of the content of fibrinogen and other clotting factors). In contrast to exudate, the term *transudate* refers to fluid that leaks out of vessels in noninflammatory conditions such as congestive cardiac failure. Transudates have a protein content less than 1 g/dl and less tendency to coagulate. The protein is mainly albumin.

The local exudation of plasma in inflammation can be demonstrated by intravenous administration of a marker dye to animals fitted with ear chambers. Such dyes become bound to plasma albumin, so that their accumulation provides an indicator of the exudation of plasma protein. By this technique,[12] dye is observed to begin escaping in ear chambers as early as 3 minutes after injury. Coloration of the lesions by dye reaches a peak 3 hours after injury. As vascular stasis spreads from the center to the periphery of the lesions and adjacent tissues, the vessels exhibiting stasis cease to exude dye. Finally, as stasis becomes more prominent, hemorrhage occurs adjacent to the obstructed vessels.

Changes in formed elements of blood. In the early stages of the inflammatory response, blood flow through the dilated vessels becomes accelerated, so that the movement of the individual blood cells is too rapid to be followed by the eye. But after some hours, the rate decreases and flow may even cease. The early acceleration is readily explained by the dilatation of the arteriolar bed, which results in an increase in hydrostatic pressure at the proximal end of the capillaries and hence an increased gradient of hydrostatic pressure in the capillary bed. The subsequent slowing of blood flow has been attributed to an increase in blood viscosity. It has been hypothesized that the escape of plasma into the tissues has the effect of increasing the concentration of red cells in the circulating blood that enters the venules. The consequent rise in the viscosity of the blood increases the resistance to flow in the venules with a corresponding rise in hydrostatic pressure in the capillary bed. The latter effect assists the expulsion of more plasma and therefore further increases viscosity, the slowing of venular blood flow, and the ensuing cycle of events that terminate in stasis.

While stasis is developing, the distribution of the red and white cells changes within the affected vessels (Fig. 2-3). As blood flow slows in the dilated vessels, the axial column of blood cells becomes relatively wider and the plasmatic zone much narrower—as might be expected from the loss of plasma by exudation. The redistribution of the blood cells is followed by striking behavior on the part of the neutrophilic leukocytes.

Emigration of neutrophilic leukocytes. The peripheral leukocytes begin to stick to the vascular endothelium. At first they stick momentarily and then move on with the flow of the blood. But the duration of sticking gradually increases, and finally some of the neutrophils remain adherent to the endothelium.

In rabbit ear chambers, neutrophils begin adhering to the endothelium within a few minutes, the response becoming quite distinct in 15 to 30 minutes (Fig. 2-2).

Ear chamber studies following thermal injury have revealed that vasodilatation is the rule, although not a

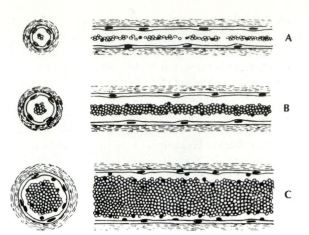

Fig. 2-3. Progressive changes in caliber of blood vessels and character of blood flow in an area of inflammation. **A,** Normal venule with its axial stream of cells. White cells *(closed circles)* tend to lie centrally among column of red cells *(open circles)*, surrounded by wide plasmatic zone. **B,** Early stage of inflammation showing vascular dilatation and broader axial stream of cells. Leukocytes are now more peripheral in column, but plasmatic zone is still conspicuous. **C,** Later stage of inflammation showing still further vascular dilatation. Central column of cells is now much broader and plasmatic zone correspondingly reduced. Peripherally placed white cells are now close or even adhering to endothelium. (From Wright, G.P.: An introduction to pathology, ed. 3, London, 1958, Longmans, Green & Co. Ltd.)

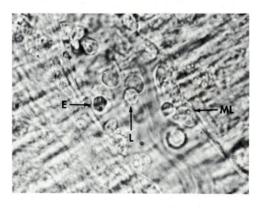

Fig. 2-4. Leukocytes migrating on endothelial surface before emigrating through wall of blood vessel. Motile cells, *ML,* have lost their usual globular shape, *L.* One erythrocyte, *E,* is adhering to endothelium. (250×; from Allison, F., Jr., Smith, M.R., and Wood, W.B., Jr.: J. Exp. Med. **102:**655, 1955.)

necessary precursor for the adherence of neutrophils. Another point is the frequent sticking of white cells to one another. Furthermore, when leukocytes sticking to endothelium become dislodged, the displaced cells do not attach themselves to uninjured endothelium farther along the same vessel.

Soon after the onset of sticking of neutrophils to endothelium, the cells begin to migrate through the vascular wall into the adjacent tissues. The adherent cells first move over the endothelium (Fig. 2-4). When a suitable site is found, the process of emigration commences, with each cell taking several minutes to migrate through the wall of a blood vessel. After a cell has passed through the vessel wall, a defect seems to exist in the vessel wall and additional cells often follow the same route.

Initially, emigration of neutrophils is more evident in vessels nearer the lesion than in those farther removed. But as stasis develops adjacent to the lesion, emigration becomes more noticeable in vessels farther afield.

Hemorrhage. Hemorrhage often occurs in severe inflammation. In the ear chamber, thermal burns cause noticeable hemorrhage 3 to 6 hours after injury, particularly adjacent to vessels that are dilated and exhibiting stasis. Red cells escape through the vessel wall by a seemingly passive process termed diapedesis. Often they become trapped in the endothelial defects left by emigrating leukocytes, and one or several erythrocytes "trickle" through the wall of the vessel.

• • •

In summary, acute inflammation is characterized by three main vascular events: (1) vasodilatation and changes in blood flow, (2) exudation of plasma, and (3) emigration of neutrophilic leukocytes. These events will now be considered in some detail.

Vasodilatation and changes in blood flow

In the triple response, vasodilatation involves first the capillaries and small venules at the site of injury and then the adjacent arterioles.

The mechanism responsible for the local dilatation of capillaries and venules was examined by Lewis[6] in a series of experiments whose simplicity is a lesson in experimental technique. The response can be compared on both forearms of the same subject, with one arm having its circulation occluded by an inflated sphygmomanometer cuff above the elbow. Firm stroking of the skin of both forearms results in vasodilatation of each. Vasodilatation on the unobstructed arm lasts about 10 minutes. On the arm with the cuff, the vasodilatation lasts as long as the arterial obstruction is continued, with the longest test period being 25 minutes. As soon as the sphygmomanometer cuff is released, the erythema behaves like that on the unobstructed arm and fades during the ensuing 10 minutes. With heating at 43° to 44° C, the duration of the initial erythema can be similarly prolonged by arterial obstruction.

Lewis interpreted these results to indicate that injury leads to the local release of a substance responsible for the dilatation of the capillaries and venules. When blood is circulating freely in the vessels of the injured tissues, the vasodilator substance is removed by the flowing blood in about 10 minutes. But when the arterial circulation is obstructed, the liberated substance is retained locally as long as the circulation is occluded. Lewis obtained strong support for these conclusions by obtaining similar results when low doses of histamine were pricked into the skin. Not only did histamine induce a typical triple response, but the fading of the initial erythema was also delayed by arterial obstruction as with injury by stroking.

There are other substances, apart from histamine, that play a role in mediating vasodilatation. Kinins,[19,23,25,26] in particular, have attracted attention because (1) kinin-forming enzymes appear to be associated with physiologic vasodilatation and (2) kinins accumulate in inflammatory exudates.[22] Since kinins are vasodilators under physiologic conditions, they may well play a similar role in pathologic conditions such as inflammation. These and other substances are discussed in the following.

Exudation of plasma

Under physiologic conditions the endothelium of the capillaries and proximal portion of the venules permits free movement of water and small molecules to and fro across the endothelium but normally restricts the passage of plasma protein. According to Starling's theory, fluid equilibrium across this endothelial barrier is maintained by the hydrostatic pressure of the capillary blood being balanced by the equal and opposite restraint of the osmotic pressure of the plasma proteins. In inflammation, there is a net movement of fluid into the tissues that has been estimated to be five to seven times greater than that from a normal vessel with similar levels of hydrostatic pressure and plasma protein. The fluid exudate of inflammation characteristically contains 1 to 6 g of plasma protein per 100 ml. The protein content of the exudate may even reach that of plasma itself.

Demonstration of permeability responses in inflammation. A simple method of identifying and quantifying increased vascular permeability depends on the use of vital dyes. When circulating in the blood, such dyes accumulate in skin sites that have been damaged by injury. Vital dyes all form complexes with plasma albumin and other plasma proteins, so that their local accumulation in tissues indicates a movement of plasma protein across vascular endothelium.

For experimental injury, one can assess a permeability response by measuring the amount of dye that exudes into the injured tissue (Fig. 2-5).[58] When factors thought to increase permeability are tested by injection into skin, the exuded dye forms a round blue lesion at the injection site, with the mean diameter of the lesion being proportional to the dose of factor injected.

The dye technique is performed by giving a standard dose of dye intravenously to experimental animals from which the fur on the back of the trunk has been removed. Experimental injury (such as by heating) can be obtained by applying a heated metal disk to the skin, as described in the legend for Fig. 2-5. Dye accumulates locally in a few minutes after injury, but the coloration then remains unchanged for some hours, so that subsequent fluctuations in the permeability of the local vascular bed cannot

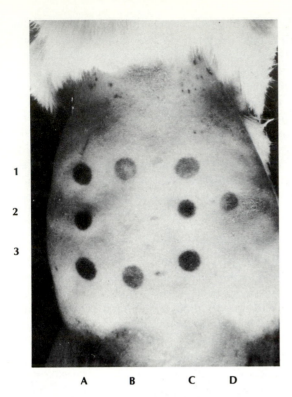

Fig. 2-5. Method of demonstrating increased vascular permeability. Metal disk (8.5 mm in diameter) heated to 54° C was applied for 5 seconds to depilated skin of back of trunk of guinea pig previously given Evans blue dye intravenously. Dye exudes into injured sites, and intensity of permeability response can be assessed by estimating amount of dye extracted from each lesion. (From Wilhelm, D.L., and Mason, B.: Br. J. Exp. Pathol. **45:**487, 1960.)

be discerned. This disadvantage is easily overcome by withholding the intravenous injection of dye until the animal bears a number of sites heated at intervals beforehand to give lesions of different ages. Intravenous dye will now exude only into sites where vascular permeability is still increased. The technique therefore allows us to map the life history or time course of the permeability response.

Permeability factors. Much effort has gone into identifying substances produced at sites of injury that might be responsible for the characteristic increase of vascular permeability. Since histamine and other factors did not provide all the answers to the problem, the continuing search has resulted in an ever-growing list of so-called permeability factors that were isolated from normal and inflamed tissues. These substances fall into four main groups:

1. Pharmacologically active amines, such as histamine and 5-hydroxytryptamine
2. Polypeptides such as bradykinin, together with various proteolytic enzymes whose activity probably results in the production of these polypeptides; such enzymes include kallikrein, plasmin, and possibly trypsin

3. Prostaglandins, particularly E_1 and E_2 and leukotrienes
4. Derivatives of the third and fifth components of complement such as the anaphylatoxins

Histamine. Histamine is still the first substance considered in any discussion of the natural mediators of inflammation. Histamine is widespread in the tissues and is associated particularly with the granules of mast cells.[21,24]

Tissue histamine is probably obtained from three main sources[17,18]: (1) decarboxylation of histidine in the tissues, (2) decarboxylation of histidine by bacteria in the bowel, and (3) the diet. Although the actual mechanism of the release of histamine is unclear, this agent is readily released as a result of various kinds of tissue injury, including anaphylaxis. Histamine causes dilatation of capillaries and increases the permeability of venules to plasma protein.

Claims that histamine is a natural permeability factor in injury are based on three main pieces of evidence:

1. Lewis's work[6] on the triple response
2. Its widespread distribution, ready release, and high activity as a permeability factor, particularly in guinea pigs, rabbits, and humans
3. Suppression of the permeability response in mild inflammation by histamine antagonists[9,29](Fig. 2-5)

5-Hydroxytryptamine. 5-Hydroxytryptamine (5-HT, serotonin) was found to be a potent permeability factor in rats.[9] Rats have long been popular for experimental work on inflammation, but the low activity of histamine as a permeability factor in this species provided at least one good reason for doubting the overall importance of histamine in inflammation. When 5-HT was demonstrated to have high activity in both rats and mice, it seemed possible that a family of amines might be involved rather than histamine itself.

As with histamine, 5-HT is widely distributed in the body tissues, with the highest concentrations occurring in the intestine, blood, spleen, and nervous system. In rats its activity as a permeability factor is exceeded only by bradykinin.

Recent studies with the electron microscope have revealed that the increased permeability of injured small blood vessels is associated with intercellular changes in vascular endothelium.

In addition to dyes, circulating colloidal carbon also identifies vessels having increased permeability by becoming deposited in the walls of the involved vessels. In animals given india ink intravenously, deposits of carbon quickly fill venules and capillaries in the injured tissues (Fig. 2-6). After treatment of cremaster muscle of the rats with histamine or 5-HT, the labeling is confined to venules 7 to 100 μm in diameter, with the heaviest labeling in venules 20 to 30 μm in diameter. The capil-

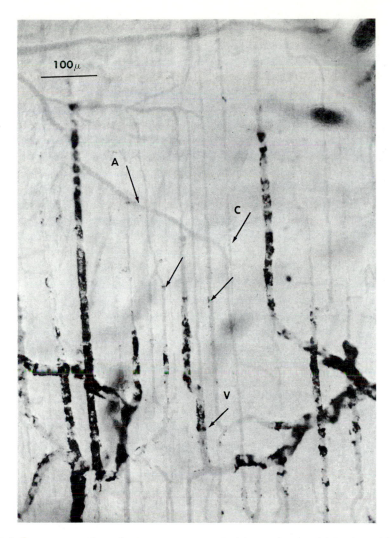

Fig. 2-6. From preparation of rat cremaster muscle 1 hour after local injection of histamine and intravenous injection of colloidal carbon. This field shows arteriole, *A*, branching into capillaries, *C*, with latter draining into venules, *V*. Histamine-induced leaks are marked by deposits of carbon. Note that there are no deposits at arterial end of capillaries, that occasional small deposits appear along venous end, and that heavy deposits occur only in venules *(arrows)*. (140×; from Majno, G.: Mechanism of abnormal vascular permeability in acute inflammation. In Thomas, L., Uhr, J.W., and Grant, L., editors: International symposium on injury, inflammation and immunity, Baltimore, 1964, The Williams & Wilkins Co.; copyrighted by Miles Laboratories, Inc.)

laries do not exhibit labeling. Electron microscopic examination of the labeled venules reveals that the endothelial cells become separated by gaps 0.1 to 1 µm in width (Fig. 2-7), which appear as early as 1 minute after histamine or 5-HT is applied. The affected endothelial cells appear to be partially disconnected along their intercellular junctions, whereas the basement membrane remains intact and serves as an additional barrier.

The gaps between the endothelial cells provide a ready passage for the escape of plasma through the vessel wall to the basement membrane. The plasma passes on, but if the circulating blood contains a "marker" substance such as colloidal carbon, particles of the marker are restrained by the basement membrane. The mechanism responsible for the separation of the endothelial cells remains to be identified.

Kinins and proteolytic enzymes. The generation of biologically active peptides from larger inactive precursor proteins by specific proteolytic enzymes is a biologic principle that is encountered frequently in living systems. This biochemical mechanism recurs repeatedly throughout all stages of the inflammatory reaction. An extremely active peptide generated by proteolytic cleavage of a plasma protein is the nonapeptide bradykinin. Bradykinin is generated by the action of a class of pro-

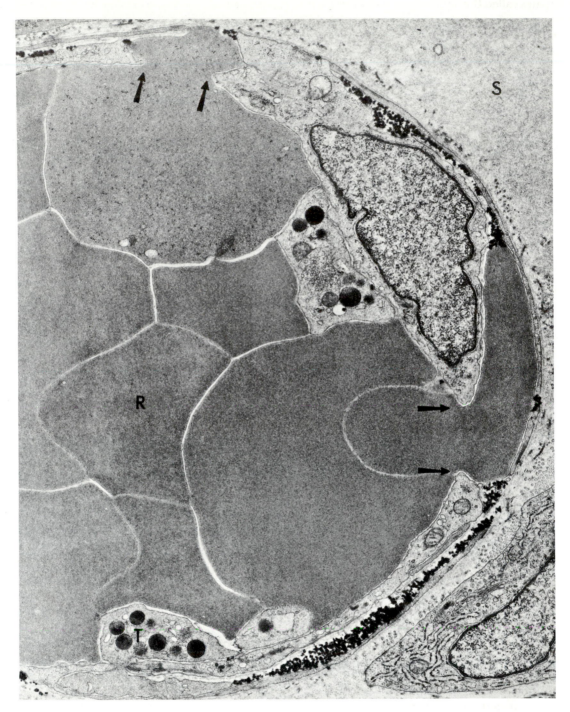

Fig. 2-7. Interendothelial gaps in venules induced by agents such as histamine, 5-hydroxytrypta-mine, or bradykinin. Electron micrograph of venule in rat striated muscle 6 minutes after treatment with bradykinin. Lumen is packed with red blood cells, *R*. Three gaps have formed in venular wall by separation of endothelial cells: one at top *(between arrows)* plugged by reticulocyte; one at right *(between arrows)* plugged by red blood cell; one at bottom plugged by thrombocyte, *T*. Dark granules in venular wall represent carbon particles, which had been administered intravenously just before local injection of bradykinin. Basement membrane, which is holding back components of blood that have passed through endothelial gaps, is visible as faint gray line just outside endo-thelium. *S*, Extracellular space. (19,400×; courtesy Prof. Guido Majno; from Wilhelm, D.L.: Rev. Can. Biol. **30:**153, 1971.)

teolytic enzymes called the kallikreins. These act on larger proteins, generating either the nonapeptide bradykinin or the decapeptide kallidin, which is simply bradykinin containing an extra lysine residue.

Kallidin

H.Lys.Arg.Pro.Pro.Gly.Phe.Ser.Pro.Phe.Arg.OH

Bradykinin

All kallikreins are proteolytic and esterolytic enzymes, and most share with trypsin the ability to hydrolyze certain peptide bonds. Kallikreins are widely distributed in the body and fall into two groups: (1) tissue kallikreins, which occur particularly in glandular organs (such as the salivary glands, the pancreas, and the sweat and lacrimal glands), as well as in the kidney and intestinal mucosa, and (2) plasma kallikrein. Although closely related, the tissue kallikreins appear to be distinct. They are produced in the various tissues as the active enzyme or the inert precursor.

Kinins[19,23,25,26] are formed from high–molecular weight glycoproteins termed kininogens. Kinins have an extremely short half-life in circulating blood, being hydrolyzed by kininases to inactive peptides. The interrelation of the kinin system can therefore be summarized as follows:

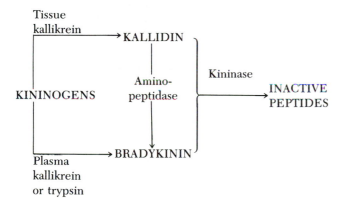

Bradykinin, kallidin, and other kinins have high activity as permeability factors,[27] their high potency being apparent whatever the species of test animal. The technique of vascular labeling with colloidal carbon given intravenously (Fig. 2-6) and subsequent examination by electron microscopy indicates that the effects of bradykinin (Fig. 2-7) parallel those of histamine and 5-HT in causing interendothelial gaps in venules.[15]

Leukotrienes. The leukotrienes are complex lipid molecules that are derived enzymatically from the breakdown of phospholipid molecules of cell membranes. Leukotrienes were originally described as being derived from leukocytes (hence the name), but it now appears that leukotrienes of different types can be generated from macrophages, tissue mast cells, and other connective tissue cells as well. Leukotrienes are generated first by the action of phospholipases on membrane phospholipids that release arachadonic acid, which is in turn converted by a series of enzymes to many complex forms, among them prostaglandins, thromboxanes, and the family of molecules called leukotrienes. Some of the leukotrienes are extremely potent bronchoconstricting and vasoconstricting agents, and some have actions similar to histamine but are far more powerful. When applied to appropriate vascular beds, some of the leukotrienes cause transient vasoconstruction that is followed by a marked increase in the leakiness of the venules of the treated vessels. The leukotrienes seem to act directly on the vessel wall, rather than acting through the liberation of histamine. Another class of leukotrienes, distinct from those that act on blood vessels, appears to act directly on leukocytes, causing effects that mimic those found in inflammatory reactions. This particular class of leukotrienes promotes adhesion of leukocytes to the walls of venules and their subsequent extravasation into the tissue spaces. These leukotrienes are also chemotactic for neutrophils, eosinophils, and monocytes. Finally, such leukotrienes stimulate leukocytes to release lysosomal enzymes, consistent with the idea that these leukotrienes play an important role in activating many of the cellular reactions found in acute inflammation. The leukotrienes of the bronchoconstricting and vasoconstricting type are now known to be the biologically active agents that were once referred to as the slow-reacting substances of anaphylaxis (SRS-A).

Pattern and mechanism of increased vascular permeability. The permeability responses in various examples of experimental injury fall into three main categories, according to their onset after injury: (1) immediate, (2) delayed, and (3) early. For each category the response may have a shorter or longer duration, so that there is a total of six main types of response (Fig. 2-8).

Immediate responses (Fig. 2-8, curves A and B) are exhibited in thermal injury and injury from ultraviolet light, as well as in anaphylaxis in both guinea pigs and rats. The provocative stimuli are usually mild or short lived, although for injury to occur from ultraviolet light the stimulus needs to be quite strong. The permeability response is transient, with peak effects being reached in 5 minutes and normal permeability usually restored in 10 to 15 minutes. The same type of response is also obtained with histamine, 5-HT, and bradykinin.

The immediate response is usually mediated in injury by histamine or 5-HT released from the injured cells. This response is readily suppressed by antihistamines or antagonists of 5-HT. As might be expected, the lesion (for example, in mild thermal injury of skin) is the interendothelial gap in venules (Figs. 2-6 and 2-7).

Some immediate responses are slightly prolonged as illustrated by curve B in Fig. 2-8.

Delayed responses have a comparatively late onset,

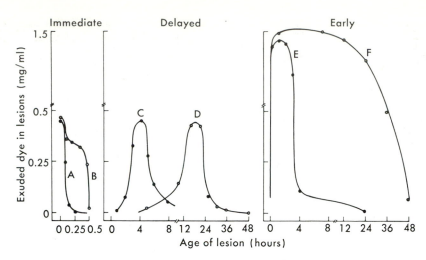

Fig. 2-8. Main types of vascular permeability responses induced in skin of guinea pig. Animals had previously received Evans blue dye, and exudation was induced by thermal injury of varying intensity, by ultraviolet injury, and by intracutaneous injection of the histamine liberator, compound 48/80. Immediate responses *(left side)*: curve A (heating at 54° C for 5 seconds); curve B (intracutaneous injection of compound 48/80). Delayed responses *(center)*: curve C (heating at 54° C for 20 seconds); curve D (ultraviolet radiation for 20 seconds). Early responses *(right side)*: curve E (heating at 58° C for 20 seconds); curve F (heating at 60° C for 60 seconds). (From Wilhelm, D.L.: Pattern and mechanism of increased vascular permeability in inflammation. In Zweifach, B.W., Grant, L., and McCluskey, R.T., editors: The inflammatory process, vol. 2, ed. 2, New York, 1973, Academic Press, Inc.)

being preceded by a latent interval of normal low permeability. Peak effects occur at about 4 hours (Fig. 2-8, curve C) or 24 hours (Fig. 2-8, curve D).

A typical delayed response of short duration is elicited by thermal injury (54° C for 20 seconds) in guinea pig skin. As illustrated in Fig. 2-9, this pattern is often combined with a preceding early response to give a diphasic effect. For thermal injury, the initial responses depend to some extent on the animal species. The same pattern of increased permeability is also induced by bacterial infection[13] and the alpha toxin of *Clostridium welchii*,[16] one of the organisms that causes gas gangrene (Fig. 2-9).

Delayed responses of prolonged duration (Fig. 2-8, curve D) are observed in mild ultraviolet light or chemical injury, in delayed hypersensitivity, and in skin sites injected with various bacterial toxins. Carbon labeling indicates that both venules and capillaries are affected. Electron microscopically, the venules show intercellular gaps in the endothelium of small and medium-sized vessels, whereas the smaller capillaries contain thrombi that plug their lumina and often show damage and disruption of the endothelium.[14] This type of response is also usually part of a diphasic effect.

The results suggest that such responses involve pharmacologic mediation affecting venules, as well as direct damage of vascular endothelium, particularly of capillaries.

Early responses seem to represent the effects of relatively strong stimuli[28] such as surgical incision, heating (for example, at 60° C), or the application of organic solvents such as xylol, benzene, or chloroform. A strong permeability response may begin within a few minutes of injury and reach a peak in 15 to 30 minutes, or in about 60 minutes with weaker stimuli (Fig. 2-8). Early responses may last 1 to several hours or may be greatly prolonged as in the case of severe burns. As might be expected, endothelial disruption is a prominent feature. Carbon labeling indicates that venules, capillaries, and even arterioles are involved. Electron microscopically, there is injury to endothelium and pericytes, as well as fragmentation and sloughing of endothelial cells. Leaking vessels, particularly capillaries, often are occluded by thrombi consisting of platelets and fibrin.

Summary. The permeability effects in acute inflammation may include six types of response. Under particular circumstances, each of the six types may occur alone as a monophasic permeability response, but an immediate response or a short-term early response may be succeeded after a latent interval by a delayed response to give a diphasic response.

As for the mechanisms involved, immediate responses are usually mediated by amines such as histamine and 5-HT. Electron microscopic evidence suggests that pharmacologic mediation is mainly responsible for lesions in the faster type of delayed response but is accompanied by endothelial damage in the slower type. Kinins have been proposed as the natural mediators of delayed

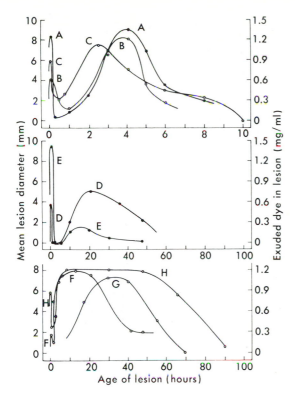

Fig. 2-9. Patterns of vascular permeability responses induced by various types of injury in skin of guinea pig. Patterns represent various combinations of the type responses illustrated in Fig. 2-8. *Open circles*, Mean lesion diameter (mm). *Closed circles*, Exuded dye (mg/ml). Curve *A*, thermal injury (54° C for 20 seconds); curve *B*, acute bacterial infection; curve *C*, *Clostridium welchii* toxin; curve *D*, delayed hypersensitivity (tuberculin reaction); curve *E*, xylol injury; curve *F*, *C. welchii*, type E, ι toxin; curve *G*, *C. oedematiens* toxin; curve *H*, *Vibrio cholerae* toxin. (From Wilhelm, D.L.: Pattern and mechanism of increased vascular permeability in inflammation. In Zweifach, B.L., Grant, L., and McCluskey, R.T., editors: The inflammatory process, vol. 2, ed. 2, New York, 1973, Academic Press, Inc.)

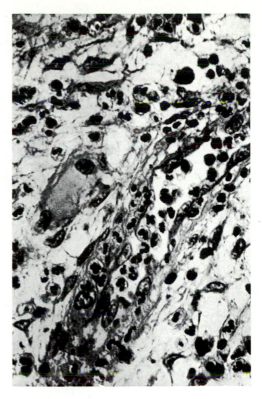

Fig. 2-10. Emigration of leukocytes in nasal polyp. Neutrophilic leukocytes are present in lumen of vessel in center, but number of neutrophils are emigrating through vessel wall or have reached tissues immediately around vessel. (640×.)

responses, but there is no convincing evidence for this proposal. Endothelial damage is prominent in lesions of early responses.

Emigration of neutrophilic leukocytes

The emigration of neutrophilic leukocytes through the wall of blood vessels into the adjacent tissues represents the main cellular phase of acute inflammation.[20]

Reference has already been made to the evidence from studies of transparent preparations and rabbit ear chambers that neutrophils bind to the endothelium of venules and, to a lesser extent, of capillaries before migrating through the vascular wall (Fig. 2-10). *Adherence* and *emigration* of neutrophils will now be discussed in the light of additional information obtained with the electron microscope.

Sticking of neutrophils. With the light microscope, neutrophils are seen to adhere to the walls of *venules*.

The cells behave as though attached to a sticky surface, along which they are slowly being pushed by the bloodstream.

As leukocytes come into contact with the endothelium of venules in injured tissue, the cells adhere to the endothelium, and the margin of the cell in contact with the endothelium becomes flattened. Some of these neutrophils appear to move on the inner surface of the endothelium by ameboid motion.

The phenomenon of leukocytic adhesion seems to be attributable to a change in the endothelial cells, but the biochemical mechanisms are unknown.

Escape of neutrophils. Once a neutrophil becomes closely apposed to the endothelium of venules, it extrudes a pseudopod preparatory to migrating (Fig. 2-11). If extrusion occurs at or near a cell junction, the neutrophil forces its way through the junction down to the basement membrane of the endothelium (Figs. 2-12 and 2-13). Serial sections of neutrophils in different stages of emigration indicate that the pseudopod separates the intercellular junctions between the endothelial cells. The advancing pseudopod is then followed by the main body of the cell. How the pseudopod separates the junction is not understood, but it may be the result of physical force or be associated with enzymatic activity.

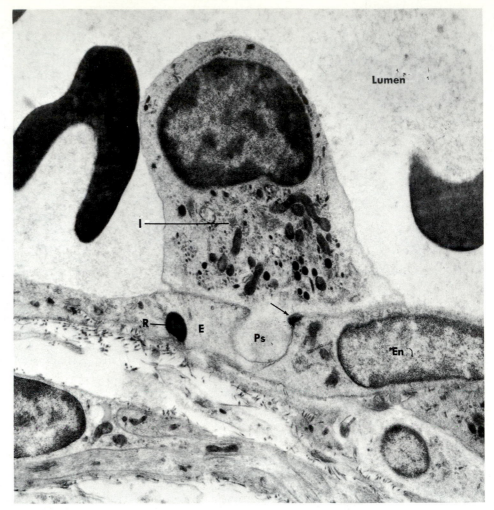

Fig. 2-11. Pseudopod *(Ps)* of neutrophil, *I*, in endothelium of inflamed venule. Electron-dense material *(arrow)* may be part of attachment belt. *R*, Part of red blood cell within cytoplasm of endothelial cell, *E. En*, Nucleus of endothelial cell. (11,700×; from Marchesi, V.T., and Florey, H.W.: Q. J. Exp. Physiol. **45:**343, 1960.)

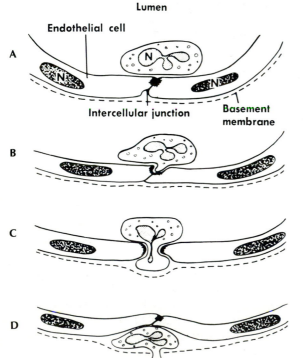

Fig. 2-12. Progressive stages in migration of neutrophil, *N*, through venule in acute inflammation. Cell penetrates intercellular junction and separates endothelial cells. (From Marchesi, V.T., and Gowans, J.L.: Proc. R. Soc. Lond. [Biol.] **159:**283, 1964.)

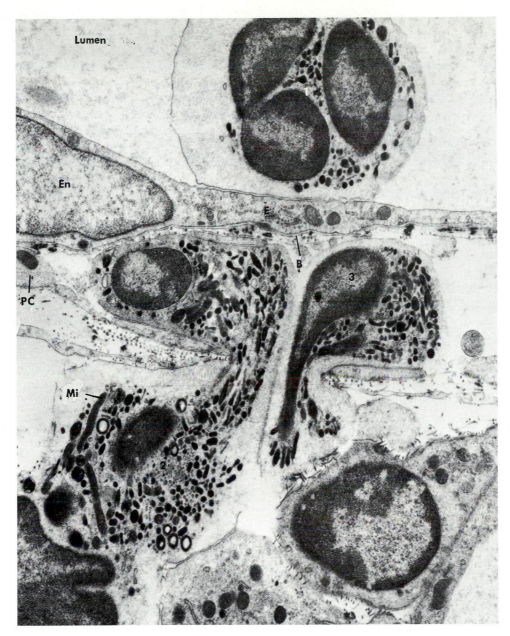

Fig. 2-13. *1*, Neutrophil adherent to endothelium, *E*. *2* and *3*, Neutrophils streaming through periendothelial sheath into adjacent connective tissue. *En*, Nucleus of endothelial cell. *B*, Basement membrane of endothelium. *Pc*, Periendothelial cell. *Mi*, Mitochondria. (14,000×; from Marchesi, V.T., and Florey, H.W.: Q. J. Exp. Physiol. 45:343, 1960.)

Neutrophils that manage to emigrate between the endothelial cells come against a second barrier—the basement membrane[39]—which, with the periendothelial cells and connective tissue, collectively forms the periendothelial sheath. This barrier hinders the continued migration of the neutrophil so that its pseudopod usually changes course to take up a position between an endothelial cell and its basement membrane. Eventually, the neutrophil penetrates the periendothelial sheath and emerges into the connective tissue around the venule (Fig. 2-13). Penetration of the wall takes about 3 to 9 minutes. Once clear of the wall, the neutrophils move in the perivascular tissues at rates of up to 20 μm per minute. Eosinophils and monocytes migrate through the venular wall in the same manner as neutrophils.

The migration of neutrophils does not appear to leave a breach in the endothelium. The edges of the adjacent endothelial cells that are separated keep in contact with the emigrating cell and apparently come together again after the leukocyte has escaped through the endothelium.[34,39] Nevertheless, the escape of a neutrophil is sometimes followed by a trickle of erythrocytes from the same site in the endothelium. This process, diapedesis of the red cells, appears to be passive.

Sequential accumulation of cells in inflamed tissues. Practically any type of tissue injury evokes an initial accumulation of neutrophilic leukocytes. If the lesion persists for some time, these polymorphonuclear cells often become replaced by mononuclear cells (monocytes, macrophages, and their derivatives), as well as by lymphocytes. Such a transition is typically illustrated by the cellular accumulation in lobar pneumonia: the initial dense accumulation of neutrophils exhibits an increasing proportion of mononuclear phagocytes. Although not invariable, such a transition is common, whatever the type of infection or cause of injury, but differs in time of onset, rate of development, and the proportion of mononuclear cells in the inflamed tissue. If some infections, either acute (such as typhoid fever) or chronic (tuberculosis), the cellular reaction is characteristically "mononuclear"—but even in these cases there is an initial transient infiltration by neutrophils, which quickly gives way to a substantial and persistent accumulation of mononuclear cells.

Since the initial cellular reaction is similar whatever the type of injury, how does the cell type change from predominantly neutrophils to mononuclear cells?

Chemotaxis and leukocytic emigration. When grains of starch are injected into the tail of a tadpole, leukocytes adhere to the vascular endothelium, emigrate through the vessel wall, and move toward the starch grains.[33] Such a directional response is referred to as *chemotaxis*[40]—the phenomenon being defined as a response in which the direction of locomotion of a cell or organism is determined by a substance in its environment. Chemotaxis ensures that, rather than wandering at random, the leukocytes move toward the site of injury and therefore concentrate in the infected or injured tissues.

Work on chemotaxis has been stimulated by a technique developed by Boyden.[32] A Perspex chamber is separated into two compartments by a millipore filter membrane through which leukocytes can pass only by active migration. Blood cells are allowed to settle on one side of the membrane, and a solution of a substance to be tested for chemotactic activity is placed in the chamber on the other side of the membrane. After incubation for suitable periods, the membrane is removed and the cells that have migrated through it are counted microscopically.

In a medium containing normal rabbit serum, Boyden observed that human albumin was strongly chemotactic in the presence of its own antiserum. The chemotactic substance appeared to be a heat-stable product released into the solution in the chamber, although not produced when the rabbit serum was "inactivated" by heating at 56° C for 30 minutes.

Boyden's results recalled an earlier finding that immune precipitates were capable of inducing the chemotaxis of neutrophils in vitro in the presence of fresh plasma. The incubation of serum with minced liver or a suspension of neutrophils also produces a chemotactic factor.[36] The clue to the problem appears to be the presence of *fresh* plasma because the results become inconsistent with aged plasma and negative when the plasma is replaced by serum, whether fresh or aged.

The nature of the chemotactic factors in fresh plasma is now beginning to emerge. The key factors appear to be various components of complement, since chemotactic activity is not obtained when complement fixation is prevented by the heating of serum, by removal of divalent cations, or by the use of antibodies that fix complement poorly. Three factors derived from complement and chemotactic for neutrophils have been identified—a trimolecular complex of components C5, C6, and C7 of complement, and two factors with low molecular weight (C3a and C5a), which correspond respectively to cleavage products of C3 and C5.[46] However, chemotaxis for neutrophils has also been demonstrated for kallikrein, products of virus-infected cells, and bacterial products of both high and low molecular weight.[48] The exhibition of chemotaxis by rabbit neutrophils involves the activation of an esterase with serine in its active site.[31] Such activation has been demonstrated for C$\overline{567}$, C5a, C3a, and a chemotactic factor from culture filtrates of *Escherichia coli*. In detail, the inert proesterase exists in or on the leukocyte, being activated to the esterase by any of the chemotactic factors just mentioned. In addition to activation of proesterase, chemotaxis requires metabolic energy provided mainly or wholly by anaerobic glycolysis and also requires the presence of Ca^{++} and Mg^{++} in the external medium. The process of chemotaxis possibly involves the contractile mechanism of the cell.[31]

Experiments with these chemotactic factors associated with complement suggest that neutrophils move toward regions of greatest concentration of the chemotactic factors. On the other hand, the addition of activated C$\overline{567}$ complex to the cells themselves prevents their migration through the filter membrane. It may be that chemotactic factors induce neutrophil migration toward the source of activated factor. Once the cells have accumulated, however, they may be unable to move away from the higher concentration of chemotactic factor.[53]

Eosinophilic granulocytes are particularly associated with immunologic lesions and parasitic infestations. Eosinophils seem particularly involved in immunologic responses when antigen is persistently present as in chronic infections or is subsequently reintroduced into the body.[44] They are chemotactically attracted to specific memory cells that contain components of both the priming antigen and the challenge antigen, being later engulfed by macrophages before the formation of plasma cells. A factor chemotactic for eosinophils has been isolated from human lung sensitized with IgE antibody.[37]

Factors inducing the accumulation of eosinophils in

tissues harboring parasites have received little attention. One such factor has been recovered, however, from *Ascaris suum*, as well as the wall and fluid of hydatid cysts. The factor is a lecithin plasmalogen.[30]

The numerical paucity of *basophilic granulocytes* in human blood is matched by our lack of knowledge of their function. Nothing is known of factors chemotactic for basophils, although these cells seem implicated in certain types of immediate and delayed hypersensitivity.[55]

Factors chemotactic for *monocytes* overlap with those for neutrophils and include cleavage products of C3 and C5, other serum factors that are distinct from C$\overline{567}$, and soluble bacterial products.[47] *Lymphocytes* do not respond chemotactically to substances that induce directional movement in other varieties of leukocytes. Nevertheless, a substance that can influence the movement of lymphocytes in vitro has been identified among the products released by lymphocytes stimulated with antigen.[59]

Leukocytes in inflammation

Neutrophils. Neutrophils have a diameter ranging from 10 to 15 μm.[35] Phase-contrast microscopy reveals the cells to be actively motile and constantly changing in shape, with the leading margin having the form of a ruffled border or pseudopod. The cytoplasm contains 50 to 200 granules, which vary in size and shape according to species, but lack other organized structures. The granules contain various proteases, carbohydrases, lipases, and miscellaneous enzymes such as nucleotidase, peroxidase, oxidases, esterases, arylsulfatase, and acid and alkaline phosphatases. Nonenzymatic components of the granules include sulfated and nonsulfated mucopolysaccharides, as well as cationic proteins.

In the adult mammal, neutrophils arise in the bone marrow from a population of stem cells. Mature neutrophils from the bone marrow are released into the bloodstream, in which about half the neutrophils comprise a circulating pool and the other half provide a reserve pool in blood vessels at sites of slow or stagnant circulation. The latter cells are concentrated on the endothelial surface of the corresponding vasculature. Neutrophils in the peripheral blood leave the circulation in a random one-way migration into the tissues, after a mean half-life in the circulation of 6 to 7 hours. In the tissues the cells die of senility or are excreted in the stool and respiratory tract secretions. Alternatively, they may be lyzed during combat with infecting microorganisms or in dealing with other forms of tissue injury.

The neutrophil utilizes glucose as a source of energy and has a reserve supply of glycogen in its cytoplasm.[35] But even under aerobic conditions, neutrophils derive 90% of their energy supply from glycolysis. They also exhibit an active turnover of various types of lipids, although practically no metabolism of deoxyribonucleic acid, in keeping with the inability of the mature cell for mitosis.

The function of neutrophils is associated mainly with the initial phagocytosis of microorganisms and other foreign material introduced into the tissues. To meet this function, the neutrophil adheres to vascular endothelium and exhibits locomotion on endothelium or in the tissues, emigration through the vascular wall, chemotaxis, phagocytosis, degranulation, and digestion or egestion of the foreign material. The importance of neutrophils in the defense of the host against microbial invaders is illustrated by the high incidence of infection in persons with agranulocytosis. In other examples of lowered host resistance (such as after massive x radiation or excessive levels of certain adrenal corticosteroids), there is a decrease in the availability or functional capacity of neutrophils.[35] In these latter circumstances, however, host resistance is also decreased by the concurrent impairment of antibody formation. Unusual forms of neutrophilic granulocytes in certain congenital disorders also leave the individual highly vulnerable to infection.

Neutrophils also engulf antigen-antibody complexes, as well as nonmicrobial material introduced into the tissues. Undigested materials are engulfed by neutrophils or by mononuclear phagocytes. Besides this role of scavenger, neutrophils also seem to play a key role in various types of immunologic injury. Many examples are known in which the leukocytes contribute to the breakdown of the host's own tissue.

Deleterious effects of neutrophils seem particularly directed at the internal elastic lamina of arteries and the basement membrane of smaller vessels and glomeruli.[53] The accumulation of neutrophils on or near these membranes is succeeded by damage and lysis of the membrane. To date, this field of study has been confined to the Arthus and Shwartzman reactions, acute experimental glomerulonephritis, and the arteries in serum sickness. But as the scope of investigation is widened, it seems that a similar picture will be revealed in various acute clinical conditions with an immunologic basis.

Eosinophils. Larger than the neutrophil although less numerous, the eosinophil has much in common with the neutrophil, both structurally and functionally.[4] Both types of cell are produced in the bone marrow, have a short life in the bloodstream, and pass into the tissues. Both exhibit locomotion and phagocytosis, and both carry cytoplasmic granules that are disrupted during the phagocytosis of particulate material. Even many of their enzymes are similar, although the granules of eosinophils have a higher content of peroxidase and contain an unidentified crystalline structure but no lysozyme.

The function of eosinophils remains unknown. In health they are present in large numbers in the skin, lungs, and bowel. It may be relevant that these parts of the body have contact either with the outside world or with substances from the exterior. The blood and tissue levels of eosinophils are elevated in allergies, parasitic infestations, skin diseases, and some types of malignant lymphoma. However, the long-recognized association of eosinophilia with parasitic infestation may be part of an immunologic phenomenon. This possibility is suggested by the finding that, in infestation of the rat by the nematode *Trichinella spiralis*, the eosinophil response is sharply decreased by procedures that deplete or inactivate the pool of circulating lymphocytes.[51]

The distribution of these cells is strikingly affected by hormonal secretion, particularly of the adrenal cortex. High levels of cortisone lead to decreased numbers or even disappearance of eosinophils from the blood.

Basophils. In humans, basophils comprise about 1% of circulating leukocytes. Their large basophilic granules contain heparin and histamine, which are released when the cells degranulate. Reference has already been made to the apparent involvement of basophils in both immediate and delayed types of hypersensitivity. Human homocytotropic antibody (IgE) is bound specifically to basophils and sensitizes them for antigen-induced release of histamine. Basophils therefore seem likely to participate in atopic allergic disease.[55] Furthermore, several varieties of delayed hypersensitivity are characterized in both humans and animals by intense infiltration of tissue by basophils (so-called cutaneous basophil hypersensitivity). Such reactions are particularly prominent in the guinea pig but also occur in humans. Lymphocytes play an essential role in such reactions.[55] The morphologic and pharmacologic similarities of basophils with tissue mast cells and the predominance of one or the other type of cell in various species suggests that basophils and mast cells may well have allied functions.

Lymphocytes. In histologic sections, lymphocytes are rather smaller than neutrophils and consist almost entirely of nucleus, with little or no cytoplasm (Fig. 2-14). The living cell, however, has a distinct and more abundant cytoplasm. Lymphocytes comprise the major variety of cells in normal lymph nodes, white pulp of the spleen, and the lymphoid tissue of the alimentary tract and lungs. They also comprise 15% to 30% of the leukocytes in peripheral blood, being more numerous in children than in adults, and are the predominant type of cell in lymph that has passed through lymph nodes. Their number in blood increases little or not at all in acute infections, although their number may increase relatively during convalescence or in chronic infections such as tuberculosis. In the tissues, lymphocytes are particularly numerous in chronic inflammation (for example, renal interstitial tissue in chronic pyelonephritis). They are prominent as a perivascular infiltration in the brain in syphilis and various types of viral encephalitis (Fig. 2-15) and at the periphery of tuberculous lesions. Periportal infiltration by lymphocytes is common in cirrhosis of the

liver, and the cells often occur at the periphery of neoplasms. They form a feature of the tissue reaction in delayed hypersensitivity and transplanted organs.

Monocytes. In most species, monocytes seldom comprise more than 8% to 10% of the circulating leukocytes. These cells in the blood belong to a system of mononuclear phagocytes, which are widely distributed in the body, being found in bone marrow, blood, liver, lym-

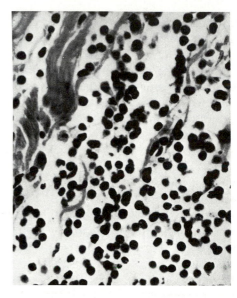

Fig. 2-14. Lymphocytes infiltrating connective tissue. In tissue preparations, cells exhibit little cytoplasm. (510×.)

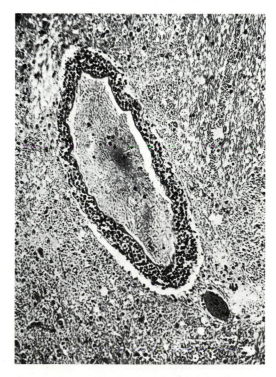

Fig. 2-15. Lymphocytes forming perivascular "cuff" of cells in brain in lethargic encephalitis. (130×.)

phoid tissue, lungs, connective tissue, and serous cavities. Important because of their phagocytic ability, the cells share a common morphology, origin, function, and other properties that have prompted their designation collectively as the "mononuclear phagocyte system," which includes the following elements[38]:

Promonocyte (bone marrow)
↓
Monocyte (blood)
↓
Macrophage (tissues)
   Histiocyte (connective tissue)
   Kupffer cell (liver)
   Alveolar macrophage (lung)
   Free and fixed macrophage and sinusoidal lining
     cell (spleen)
   Free and fixed macrophage (lymph node)
   Macrophage and sinusoidal lining cell (bone
     marrow)
   Peritoneal macrophage (serous cavity)
   Osteoclast (bone tissue)
   Microglia? (nervous system)

Accordingly, "the monocytes of the peripheral blood form a population of young cells on the way from their place of origin, the bone marrow, to their ultimate location, the tissues."[46]

Circulating monocytes[84] arise in the bone marrow by division of promonocytes, which in turn are derived from an unidentified precursor stem cell.[45] Under normal conditions the tissue macrophages have a relatively long life, with the normal turnover of Kupffer cells taking about 60 days; of alveolar macrophages, about 50 days; and of peritoneal macrophages, about 30 to 40 days.

Reference has already been made to the emigration of monocytes through postcapillary venules in inflammation and to the concurrence of their emigration with that of neutrophils.

Phagocytosis. Many cells possess the ability to ingest material by engulfment.[49] The ingested matter is usually particulate, such as bacteria, protozoal parasites or other microorganisms, tissue cells (usually necrotic), dust, pigment, and other foreign material. When engulfment involves such particulate matter, the process is termed *phagocytosis*.

Phagocytes comprise two main classes of cells: those that are capable of migrating to the site where their phagocytic ability is required (such as neutrophilic and eosinophilic leukocytes and circulating mononuclear phagocytes) and those that are fixed in tissues during all or most of their life and therefore depend on chance encounter with foreign materials (such as Kupffer cells in liver and lining sinusoid of lymph node).

In the act of phagocytosis, small particles such as a grain of charcoal may be ingested in an instant. In the rapid engulfment of a small particle viewed with a light microscope, the particle appears to pass directly through the cell membrane. But electron microscopy indicates that this is not the case; firm contact is first established between cell membrane and particle. The area of contact is then extended by invagination of the cell membrane until the apposing membrane surfaces meet and fuse (Fig. 2-16). Larger objects such as tissue cells, clumps of bacteria, or a single large bacterium (such as *Bacillus megaterium*) are ingested by a more active response. Fig. 2-16 illustrates the sequence of events in the phagocytosis of *B. megaterium* by a neutrophilic leukocyte; the leukocyte flows slowly about the bacillus until ingestion has been completed. This process is similar for neutrophils (microphages), monocytes, and tissue macrophages.

The process of phagocytosis involves two stages:
1. The attachment stage, in which the particle becomes bound to the surface of the phagocyte
2. The ingestion stage, involving invagination of the surface membrane and the surrounding of the particle

The fate of ingested particulate matter is closely related to the process of degranulation and the discharge of granule contents into the newly formed digestive pouch (Fig. 2-16) or phagosome. The nature of the surface of the object to be ingested (whether bacterium, cell, or foreign body) determines whether there can be firm fixation to the neutrophil surface as the necessary prelude to phagocytosis. Since both bacteria and neutrophils usually have a net surface charge that is negative and therefore repellent, some form of physical or chemical bond must be established between particle and cell membrane. Opsonins are factors that act on the surface of many bacteria, presumably by adsorption, and render them susceptible to phagocytosis. In the absence of opsonins (as in serum), ingestion of most microorganisms by neutrophils proceeds slowly or not at all. Besides the coating of bacteria with a film of opsonin, the beneficial effects of serum on phagocytosis also include colloid osmotic effects and the binding or inactivation of toxins.

The physical nature of the environment also influences phagocytosis by neutrophils. Even encapsulated unopsonized microorganisms are engulfed, provided the cells can trap the bacteria "in corners" or between cells. This phenomenon of "surface phagocytosis" may have considerable importance in the tissues.[50]

Phagocytosis is accompanied by degranulation of the neutrophils (Fig. 2-16), resulting in the liberation of digestive enzymes and antibacterial substances. The degranulation seems to result from contact of the membranes of the cytoplasmic granules with the membranes of the "phagocytic pouch" surrounding the ingested particle. The hydrolases released by the granules are discharged into the pouch, and so the cell's cytoplasm is protected from its own ferments. The antibacterial substances released include lysosome, hydrogen peroxide, basic peptides (leukins), and a basic protein (phagocytin)

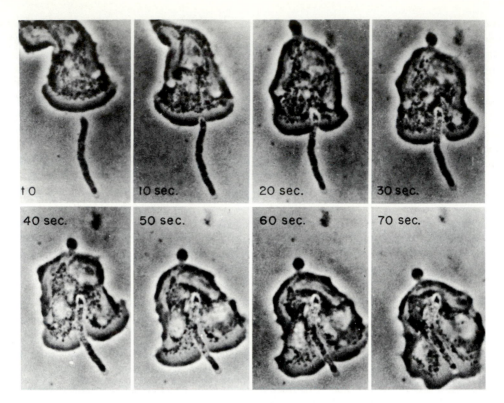

Fig. 2-16. Timed sequences from motion picture of human neutrophil engulfing *Bacillus megaterium*. Note invagination of cell membrane and formation of digestive pouch. There is overall reduction in cytoplasmic content of granules by the time ingestion has been completed. (Phase contrast; approximately 1400×; from Hirsch, J.G.: J. Exp. Med. **116:**827, 1962.)

that kills a wide range of organisms without lyzing them.[35]

Lymph flow in inflammation

The fluid exudate that accumulates in inflamed tissues is mainly drained away by the lymphatics.[1] The regional lymph nodes are admirably constructed as a filtering mechanism,[52] with the efficiency of filtration being improved when the rate of flow of incoming lymph is decreased. This factor assumes considerable importance in the management of inflamed tissues by rest and immobilization.[79]

Cardinal signs of inflammation

The cardinal signs of inflammation are redness, swelling, heat, and pain.

The *redness* is caused by vasodilatation. The *swelling* results mainly from the accumulation of fluid exudate consequent to increased vascular permeability, with smaller contributions from the cellular infiltration of the affected tissues and the engorgement of their blood vessels.

The sensation of *heat* is attributable to the rapid inflow of relatively warm blood through dilated vessels in the inflamed area, the incoming blood from the deep tissues being warmer than that in the superficial tissues and skin. It is hard to believe that the strong sensation of heat in a carbuncle or infected wound corresponds to a comparatively small temperature difference between the inflamed area and neighboring skin, but such is the case.

Various factors contribute to the *pain*. Distension of tissue, particularly when there is little room for expansion, results in the all too familiar throbbing pain of an infected nail bed of the finger or toe. But other factors such as kinins, histamine, and metabolites, which are liberated or activated by injured cells, probably also play a role in causing the pain felt in acutely inflamed lesions.

Varieties of acute inflammation
Factors in variation of inflammatory response

Inflammation is referred to as *acute* when it lasts days or 2 to 3 weeks and as *chronic* when more prolonged. The typical case of acute inflammation is characterized by vasodilatation, exudation of plasma, and emigration of neutrophilic leukocytes into the injured tissues. But not all examples of acute inflammation exhibit neutrophilic infiltration, and conversely, neutrophils may be associated with prolonged and therefore chronic inflammation. Typhoid fever represents an acute inflammatory process in which the cellular response in the submucous lymphoid tissue of the small bowel is typically mononuclear, and chronic osteomyelitis is an example of prolonged chronic inflammation in which the cellular response is mainly neutrophilic. Between acute and chronic inflammation is a wide range of overlapping processes.

The main events in acute inflammation are vascular in origin and remarkably consistent for a wide range of stimuli. Nevertheless, the response exhibits considerable differences that depend, first, on factors related to the injury or infection and, second, on the condition of the host and nature of the tissue involved.[8] For example, skin reacts to the virus of herpes simplex by forming a vesicle (or blister), to staphylococci with an abscess (such as a boil), and to streptococci with a diffuse brawny red swelling known as erysipelas. Furthermore, there is a remarkable difference in the way the lung reacts to pneumococci in lobar pneumonia and to mycobacteria in chronic tuberculosis.

The site of an inflammation also modifies the inflammatory response—the lung with its loose texture would be expected to exhibit a response differing from that in dense compact tissue such as bone. But, in general, the picture of inflammation in an organ depends largely on the predominance of one of three processes: exudation, proliferation of tissue cells, or necrosis caused by the injurious agent. Although these three processes are combined in varying proportions, all are usually present to a greater or lesser extent. They may be combined in various proportions to produce recognizable types of inflammation that are influenced by the character and site of the tissue involved in the inflammatory process.

Exudation. The term *exudation* is preferably limited to the escape of plasma rather than emigrating leukocytes, but both can be conveniently included in the present context. The exudate is described as *serous* when it resembles serum (that is, consists of water, solutes, and plasma protein but with scanty fibrin and neutrophils). Serous exudates are found in tuberculous pleurisy.

A *fibrinous* exudate has a high content of fibrin. It is common on the pleura when pneumonia extends to the pleural surface and on the pericardium in pneumococcal or rheumatic pericarditis. Fibrinous inflammation frequently involves serous membranes and the meninges (Fig. 2-17). The exudate has a gray, lusterless appearance and can be readily peeled off with forceps or by rubbing with the finger.

The terms *purulent* and *suppurative* refer to the presence of pus. It seems noteworthy that pus consists of both dead and still viable neutrophils, with a contribution of necrotic cells and tissue, as well as exuded plasma. Initially thick and creamy, pus becomes thinner in consistency after the proteolysis that results from the activity of proteolytic enzymes released from dying and dead neutrophils.

In severe inflammation there is often sufficient vascu-

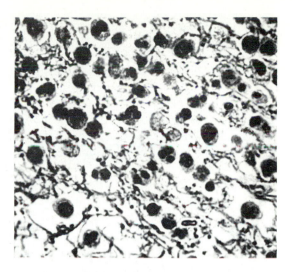

Fig. 2-17. Fibrinocellular exudate in pneumococcal meningitis. Neutrophils and macrophages lie in mesh of fibrin. (760×.)

lar damage to cause hemorrhage, the inflammation then being referred to as *hemorrhagic*. Some degree of hemorrhage is common in severe or advanced inflammation such as acute appendicitis.

Proliferation. Cell proliferation is usually inconspicuous in acute inflammation caused by bacteria, but a notable exception is typhoid fever, in which there is considerable multiplication of large mononuclear cells in the intestinal lymphoid tissue. Viral infections have a characteristic ability to stimulate cell division, so that the early stages of a number of viral diseases show cellular proliferation. This is particularly true for epidermis, with proliferation occurring in the early stages of herpes simplex, chickenpox, smallpox, and vaccinia. Another example of proliferation in inflammation is the formation of "crescents" resulting from proliferation of glomerular capsular epithelium in glomerulonephritis.

Proliferation is also a common feature of chronic inflammation, with cellular multiplication particularly involving macrophages and fibroblasts.

Necrosis. Although necrosis often involves individual cells in inflammation, it sometimes dominates the picture, as in gas gangrene. In this condition the tissues may be discolored and foul, with microscopic evidence of nuclear fragmentation. Leukocytes are scarce. Necrosis results from the action of toxins of the responsible organisms that belong to the genus *Clostridium*.

Some microorganisms are associated with necrotizing inflammation in the mouth and throat. In other instances, necrosis may result from vascular obstruction caused by bacterial infection. Such obstruction is a common cause of acute appendicitis progressing to gangrenous appendicitis and rupture of the appendix. Necrosis is often prominent in chronic inflammation, a common example being the caseous necrosis (caseation) that characteristically occurs in tuberculous lesions (Fig. 2-18).

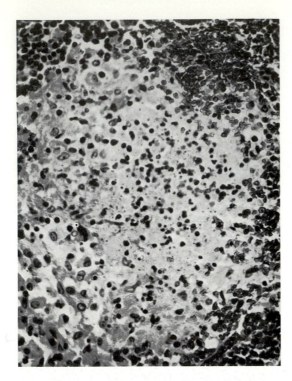

Fig. 2-18. Necrosis in inflammation. Necrotic area is in center of tubercle. Such necrosis is referred to as caseation and contains nuclear remnants and debris. Pale cells at periphery of necrosis are macrophages (so-called epithelioid cells), with lymphocytes still farther afield, particularly in upper and lower right-hand corners. (760×.)

Pseudomembranous inflammation

Pseudomembranous inflammation is a response of mucous surfaces (as in the pharynx, larynx, trachea, bronchi, and bowel) to necrotizing agents such as the toxin of diphtheria bacilli or irritant gases. The surface epithelium is destroyed, a condition that allows the irritant to penetrate the underlying tissues, where it increases the permeability of the blood vessels. Plasma therefore exudes onto the eroded surface, coagulates, and encloses the necrotic epithelium in its fibrinous meshes. This coagulum of necrotic tissue constitutes the false membrane that gives this type of inflammation its name.

Such inflammation in the trachea is typical of diphtheria. At this site, the formation of a false membrane carries a particular risk of respiratory obstruction and hence the need for relief by tracheotomy. With the present-day programs of immunization against diphtheria, the condition has become uncommon except where immunization is not the rule.

Ulceration

The term *ulceration* means a circumscribed loss of substance from the surface of an organ, usually accompanied by inflammation of the adjacent tissue (Fig. 2-19). Ulceration results from necrosis occurring as the sequel to cell destruction by toxins and poisons or from interference with blood supply. The necrotic tissue becomes

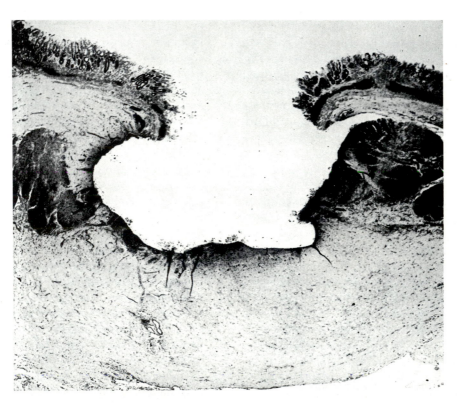

Fig. 2-19. Chronic ulcer of stomach extending through muscularis mucosae. Fibrosis of submucosa and base of ulcer provides evidence of long-continued process. (8×.)

loosened and finally separated from the adjacent viable tissue.

Frequent sites of ulceration are the stomach and first part of the duodenum. Intestinal ulcers are a common feature of typhoid fever, intestinal tuberculosis, and both bacillary and amebic dysentery. On the legs, ulcers are associated with varicose veins. Ulcers are among the most common and important inflammatory lesions.

Abscess formation

An abscess is a localized collection of pus in a tissue, organ, or confined space. Common sites of abscess formation include the dermis of skin, the lung, brain, kidney, and liver, or a cyst. Abscesses are often caused by strong irritants that remain localized rather than spreading diffusely. Examples are the ingress of staphylococci through hair follicles to cause a boil or the embolism of infected thrombi in pyemia.

The established focus of infection incites an outpouring of large numbers of neutrophilic leukocytes (Fig. 2-20). These become concentrated in the infected area and liberate proteases that digest damaged and dead tissues and so convert it into the semiliquid material known as pus.

An abscess therefore consists of a collection of pus surrounded by inflamed tissue heavily infiltrated with neutrophils. As long as the irritant (such as staphylococcus) persists, more leukocytes are attracted, more tissue is liquefied, and further pus is formed. Proteolysis results in the splitting of larger molecules into smaller ones, with a consequent increase in osmotic pressure, which attracts more water from the surrounding tissues. The increasing pressure in the abscess often causes the pus to "track" or burrow through adjacent tissues along lines of least resistance, such as intermuscular septa. Eventually, the pus reaches a surface, where it is discharged. Tracking and erosion cause considerable damage, which the surgeon tries to prevent by opening the abscess to establish drainage of the pus.

Suppuration (formation of visible pus) involves the destruction of tissue. It is therefore an irreversible process that cannot be restored to normal by resolution but rather results in healing with scarring. The healing process is described later in this chapter.

Sometimes the irritant is overcome by natural defenses before pus reaches a surface. Under these circumstances pus may be absorbed. If too abundant, however, it may persist as a collection of sterile fluid (a cyst) or become dehydrated and circumscribed by a fibrous tissue capsule.

Cellulitis (diffuse inflammation)

By contrast with the circumscription of an abscess, other inflammatory lesions may be diffuse (Fig. 2-21). The diffuseness results when the irritant, such as bacteria causing infection, is equipped with factors that aid the

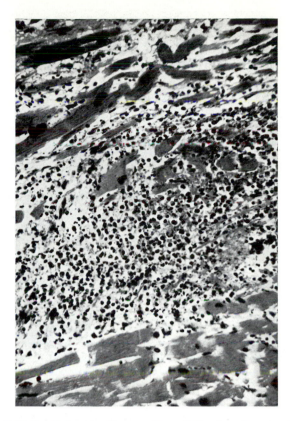

Fig. 2-20. Small abscess of myocardium. Collection of neutrophils has replaced muscle fibers. Fragments of dead muscle are present near periphery of abscess. (370×.)

spread of the infection. For example, the rapid spread of infection by hemolytic streptococci is largely attributable to their production of hyaluronidase, or "spreading factor," which breaks down hyaluronic acid in the ground substance of connective tissue.

Inflammation in hypersensitivity

An important part of our defense mechanism involves the production of antibodies against antigens such as bacterial toxins. But the union of antigen with antibody is not always advantageous to the host. Sometimes the outcome is unfavorable, with a result worse than the effects of the antigen itself. When such conditions are acquired and have a specific immunologic basis, they constitute examples of hypersensitivity. The current usage of the term *hypersensitivity* is synonymous with *allergy*. Allergic reactions are, then, defined according to common usage as those immunologic reactions that damage the tissues or disrupt the physiology of the vertebrate host. Although we carefully distinguish in words and in fact between allergy and immunity, the same mechanisms operate in both; the fundamental difference in any individual reaction is who or what is the primary target of the given immunologic mechanism—whether the invading organism and its products are affected in the case of immunity or the host itself in the case of allergy.

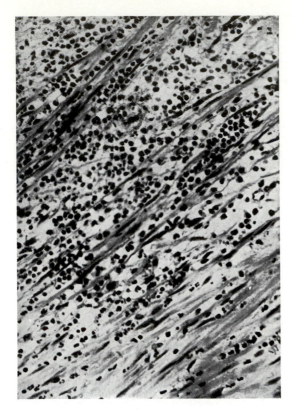

Fig. 2-21. Acute inflammation of appendix. Muscle fibers are separated by inflammatory exudate in which many neutrophils are recognizable. Lesion is example of diffuse type of inflammation. (270×.)

Disorders that come within the category of hypersensitivity include a wide range of conditions that may be conveniently divided into immediate type and delayed type of hypersensitivity, on the basis of rapidity of onset and duration. Immediate-type reactions begin seconds or minutes after contact of antigen with antibody, although the effects may take minutes or even hours to become apparent. Delayed-type reactions are slower in onset and take at least some hours, usually 24 to 48 hours, to become obvious. They run a prolonged course, which is often associated with chronic disease.

Although the division of hypersensitivity into immediate type and delayed type is based simply on the time course of the disorder, such a division corresponds to important differences in the underlying mechanisms. Of these, the most fundamental is the dependence of immediate-type hypersensitivity on the presence of circulating antibody. Delayed-type hypersensitivity undoubtedly involves the immune mechanism, but the presence of circulating antibody is not essential for the exhibition of the disorder, although often accompanying it. Delayed-type hypersensitivity is mediated by sensitized lymphoid cells and is transferable by means of such cells, although not by serum. Hypersensitivity reactions that may evoke damage of tissues have been classified into four types[54]:

1. *Type I* (anaphylactic) reactions result from the interaction of antigen with antibody "fixed" on tissue cells, particularly mast cells. In humans, atopic or reaginic antibodies (IgE) are mainly responsible. Challenge by antigen locally or systemically results in an acute release of short-lived factors such as histamine, 5-hydroxytryptamine, kinins, and "slow-reacting substance" (SRS), having both local and systemic effects.[57]

2. *Type II* (cytotoxic) reactions are initiated by heterologous or autologous antibodies that provoke complement-dependent lysis of target cells or a local inflammatory response (transient or persistent) in the target tissue.[57] The antibody is usually IgG or IgM.

3. *Type III* (damage by immune complexes) reactions involve aggregation of antigen-antibody under two sets of circumstances: first, in the bloodstream when relatively large amounts of antigen persist until corresponding antibody is formed and then combine with that antibody; second, when antibody is circulating in the blood and antigen is introduced locally in the tissues in high concentration.[54] The first situation results in "serum sickness," and the second in an *Arthus reaction.* The antibodies are IgG or gamma globulin.

4. *Type IV* (delayed hypersensitivity) reactions are cell mediated and include bacterial or tuberculin type of hypersensitivity and contact dermatitis.

Types I, II, and III therefore represent varieties of immediate types of hypersensitivity, whereas type IV corresponds to the delayed type.

Hypersensitivity constitutes another form of injury that evokes the nonspecific inflammatory response. The picture varies, however, according to whether the inflammation is provoked by antigen-antibody reactions without the presence of additional agents, as in the Arthus and Shwartzman reactions,[57] or results from an agent that is also the provocative antigen, as in many bacterial infections.

When hypersensitivity provides the only factor responsible for inflammation, the tissue reaction is a rapid development of edema resulting from increased vascular permeability and an accumulation of neutrophils, macrophages, and often eosinophils. Vascular lesions may be prominent and particularly include arteriolar necrosis and extensive thrombosis. In addition to its acute exudative onset, hypersensitivity differs qualitatively from other varieties of inflammation in provoking rapid proliferation of macrophages and plasma cells.

A good example of the tissue reaction in delayed-type hypersensitivity is the response to the intradermal injection of old tuberculin in a person previously infected with tubercle bacilli. In contrast to the edema and comparatively sparse cellular infiltration of the immediate type of reaction, the delayed type of reaction histologically shows a dense accumulation of cells, mainly lymphocytes and macrophages. The relation of delayed-type hypersensitivity to chronic granulomatous inflammation, necrosis, and immunity (as in tuberculosis) is a complex subject that warrants further reading.[57,60]

Systemic effects of acute inflammation

The present account of the acute inflammatory response has purposely been concentrated on the local responses at the site of injury. This approach, however, should not be taken to indicate that systemic responses have little magnitude or importance. On the contrary, as noted early in this chapter, the systemic effects are both complex and comprehensive. They include malaise, fever, leukocytosis, fibrinolysis, metabolic disturbances, shock, and endocrine and immunologic responses.

Functions of inflammatory response

The exudation of plasma and the accumulation of neutrophilic leukocytes in foci of inflammation provide important protective mechanisms in the defense of the host. The outpouring of plasma dilutes bacterial toxins or other noxious factors, while the protein content of the plasma includes specific and nonspecific antibodies that antagonize the toxins. The benefits of the fluid phase of the response overlap with those of the emigrated neutrophils. These leukocytes comprise the first wave of phagocytes that arrive to deal with invading bacteria, but their role as phagocytes is considerably facilitated by the presence of antibodies in the fluid exudate. In addition, the fibrin mesh that is formed from the exuded fibrinogen probably provides an important framework on which the neutrophils move about in the tissues.

The role of inflammation is not as obvious in nonbacterial inflammation. The increased vascularity ensures that both sites involved by infection and those of noninfective injury have a blood supply adequate for the local metabolic demands. In addition, the close relation of repair to inflammation suggests that the latter process may act as a stimulus for subsequent healing and regeneration.

Nevertheless, inflammation in certain circumstances may have disadvantages.[10] Phagocytosed bacteria may survive within phagocytes and even be protected against antibodies or antibiotics. Or again, the "successful" outcome of the inflammatory response may extract a high price in terms of functional loss in organs such as the eye.

In the final summing up, however, the definite advantages of inflammation seem amply illustrated by the harmful effects that follow experimental suppression of vasodilatation in bacterial infection. After the experimental inoculation of bacteria in skin, the number of bacteria capable of establishing infection is considerably greater in sites treated with a vasoconstrictor, such as epinephrine, than in control sites with a normally responsive vasculature.[7]

Chronic inflammation

Textbook accounts of acute and chronic inflammation often separate the two conditions by a description of healing and regeneration. An understanding of the histologic picture of chronic inflammation is certainly assisted by a knowledge of the processes involved in repair, but the separation from acute inflammation leaves the impression that these two varieties of inflammation are distinct from each other, although sharing the term "inflammation" in their names. This is not the case. In general, the term *acute*, as applied to inflammation, refers to a response with a rapid onset and relatively short duration characterized by particular vascular phenomena. The common sequel is resolution of the inflammatory exudate and restoration of normal structure and function. In some cases, however, the acute events lose their intensity, so that the process continues as a smoldering chronic condition. In other cases the initial infection may be attributable to an organism of low pathogenicity, which therefore evokes a less intense response from the outset. Such is the case with *Mycobacterium tuberculosis*. Even so, the experimental introduction of this organism into the tissues evokes an initial response of acute inflammation for the first 24 hours; then there is a rapid change to the picture of chronic inflammation.

Besides infection by bacteria and other microorganisms of low-grade pathogenicity, causes of chronic inflammation include physical agents of mild intensity or chemical agents of low concentration. Examples of such agents are particles of sand entering the tissues through an abrasion or laceration, and talc powder from a surgeon's glove contaminating an operative incision. The pneumoconioses are a group of diseases of the lung in which chronic inflammatory lesions result from the inhalation of dust containing silica or other irritants. Sometimes the agent is a chemical factor of plant or occupational origin to which a low-grade sensitivity has developed, usually after continued exposure, as in some types of contact or occupational dermatitis.

Other circumstances favoring the development of chronic inflammation include minor trauma or infection involving tissues that are handicapped by restricted blood supply attributable to arterial disease or by poor venous return as in varicose veins of the legs. In such cases an injury or infection that normally would evoke no more than transient acute inflammation is followed by a persistent chronic inflammation.

As long as irritation persists, the lesion should be considered inflammatory. Once the irritation abates or is removed, the process becomes reparative. The ensuing process of repair commonly takes the form of fibrosis with the formation of "scar tissue," adhesions, and fibrous bands. Such lesions are relatively common as the outcome of chronic inflammation of serous membranes but should not be labeled "chronic peritonitis" or "chronic pericarditis." The chronic inflammation has subsided and the condition is one of peritoneal or pericardial adhesion or fibrosis, respectively.

Features of chronic inflammation

Inflammation is said to be chronic when its duration is relatively prolonged—often for months or years. Its prolonged course is provoked by persistence of the causative factor in the tissues, whether the factor be an infection or an inanimate foreign body. The tissues are infiltrated by cells derived from three lines: mononuclear phagocyte, lymphoid cell, and fibroblast. In addition, there may be granulocytic leukocytes, particularly eosinophils.[43] Mononuclear phagocytes are represented by macrophages, epithelioid cells, or multinucleated giant cells. Lymphoid cells are present as lymphocytes, plasma cells, or immunoblasts. Fibroblasts produce collagen and ground substance and proliferate to form more fibroblasts. At varying stages during the course of the lesion, lymphocytes, fibroblasts, or granulocytes may predominate, but the most important unit of chronic inflammation is almost always the macrophage and its derivatives, the epithelioid cell and the giant cell.[43]

Necrosis is also common in chronic inflammatory lesions. Quite often, there are episodes of necrosis that stimulate the formation of granulation tissue and hence of fibrous tissue, even to such extent that fibrosis becomes a feature of older lesions. The overall participation of the "dividing" tissue cells and their efforts in producing new tissue have resulted in chronic inflammation being described as *proliferative,* in contrast to the *exudative* features of acute inflammation.

The accumulation of macrophages, lymphocytes, and plasma cells may be diffuse or focal. Although the histologic picture can be variable, a distinctive pattern often occurs in conditions such as tuberculosis, leprosy, syphilis, sarcoidosis, brucellosis, rheumatic fever, and certain mycoses. A proliferative type of reaction, which is focal in distribution, results in a lesion that is often described as a "granuloma." When the condition is caused by infection, the lesion is referred to as an "infective granuloma." The term *granuloma* is alleged to have two origins: (1) that it goes back to the time when the nodular foci were considered to be neoplastic—hence the name "granule-*oma*"—and (2) that the term refers to the tumorlike nodules of proliferating granulation tissue.

Granulomatous inflammation. The development of granulomatous inflammation is well illustrated by the tissue response to the primary lodgment of tubercle bacilli in the lungs of guinea pigs or rabbits. When the bacilli are injected intravenously, those that lodge in the pulmonary capillaries evoke a transient neutrophil response. After 12 hours, however, the immigrant neutrophils are overshadowed by incoming macrophages that predominate throughout the remaining life of the lesion. When the tubercle bacilli are inspired into the pulmo-

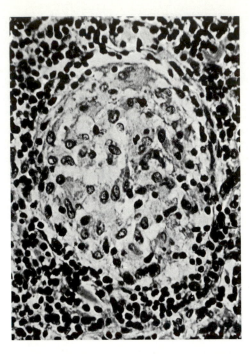

Fig. 2-22. Macrophages in tubercle, which is circumscribed ovoid focus in center. Peripheral cells are mostly lymphocytes. Fig. 2-18 illustrates caseous necrosis subsequently developing at center of tubercle. (510×.)

nary alveoli, macrophages predominate from the outset. In either case the macrophages proceed to engulf the tubercle bacilli and, by the second or third day, they form clusters of elongated cells that are closely packed at the center of the lesion (Fig. 2-22). In these macrophage clusters, adjacent cells often fuse to form multinucleated giant cells, containing up to 50 to 100 nuclei; these are the so-called Langhans' giant cells (Fig. 2-23) that are common in tuberculosis.

Beyond 10 to 12 days, the central macrophages begin to undergo a characteristic necrosis termed *caseation* (Fig. 2-18), a term that refers to the caseous or cheeselike appearance and consistency of the necrotic tissue. The development of such necrosis in tuberculosis appears to be related to the onset of tissue hypersensitivity resulting from an immunologic response to the microbial invader. By 2 or 3 weeks, each lesion usually exhibits a central area of necrosis surrounded by macrophages and often one or several multinucleated giant cells. Surrounding the macrophages is a zone of lymphocytes (Figs. 2-18 and 2-22). The periphery of the granulomatous focus is bounded by fibroblasts and fibrous tissue. In tuberculosis each such lesion is about 1 mm in diameter and is known as a "tubercle." The focal lesions gradually coalesce, while much of the remaining tissue becomes infiltrated by mononuclear cells (lymphocytes, plasma cells, and macrophages) and exhibits progressive fibrosis. But even at an advanced stage of the disease, the microscopic picture usually shows some evidence of the focal lesions.

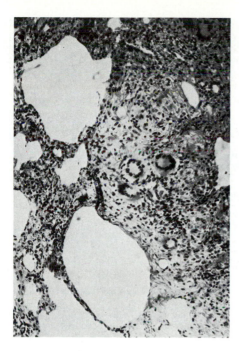

Fig. 2-23. Multinucleated giant cells of Langhans type in lipid pneumonia. (110×.)

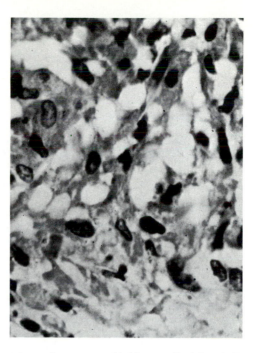

Fig. 2-24. Macrophages, more highly magnified than in Fig. 2-22, in sarcoidosis. (1130×.)

Granulomatous inflammation is provoked by various infections, particularly by tuberculosis, leprosy, syphilis, and actinomycosis, and less commonly by brucellosis and various mycoses. In other cases the condition is associated with diseases having an allergic (or hypersensitive) background, such as rheumatic fever and rheumatoid disease. Still other examples are provided by beryllium poisoning and by the presence of foreign bodies such as talc, grit, sutures, or splinters of wood. Finally, the condition named "sarcoidosis" includes a number of conditions that share the feature of granulomatous lesions resembling tubercles, but with minimal or no necrosis (Fig. 2-24).

It should be emphasized that the histologic picture of granulomatous inflammation is both variable and nonspecific. In some cases a causative organism is established, in others the lesion probably results from hypersensitivity associated with infection, and in still others there is no suggestion of an association with infection. Some of the diseases have widespread systemic manifestations, whereas for others the clinical features remain almost entirely local. The focal proliferative lesions may predominate or may be infrequent—for example, the tubercle is common in tuberculosis, whereas the gumma is much less common in syphilis. Under various conditions of dosage, virulence, and host resistance, some of the organisms responsible for granulomatous inflammation produce tissue responses that are nongranulomatous. The tubercle bacillus, for example, usually evokes the formation of a tubercle, but occasionally it incites a distinctively exudative inflammation.

The giant cells also exhibit considerable variation in incidence and morphology. In tuberculosis they are relatively large and contain many rounded nuclei, arranged either peripherally or at one or both poles. Their cytoplasm is acidophilic and finely granular and contains fine filaments. In sarcoidosis the giant cells sometimes contain cytoplasmic inclusions, whereas in "foreign body" reactions the giant cells tend to be variable in size and morphology (Fig. 2-25).

Two points warrant reiteration:

1. The histologic picture in granulomatous inflammation is seldom specific, although the Aschoff nodule in rheumatic heart disease may be one exception to this rule. In general, however, the microscopic appearances are inconclusive.

2. There is a strong tendency for granulomatous inflammation to be associated with hypersensitivity. This association is established for some conditions and seems probable in others. Such a relation may appear less likely for reactions to foreign bodies, but so many foreign bodies are chemical in nature, endogenous or plant in origin, that an associated delayed type of hypersensitivity cannot be entirely excluded.

Macrophages. The circulating monocyte is the main precursor of the mononuclear macrophage in inflamed tissues. However, the infiltration of inflamed tissues by macrophages may be transient or persistent, according to the cause of the lesion. In acute inflammation, macrophages disappear in a few days because of death of the cells, their removal by lymphatics, or migration elsewhere. In chronic inflammation the persistence of macrophages may result from their local proliferation, from

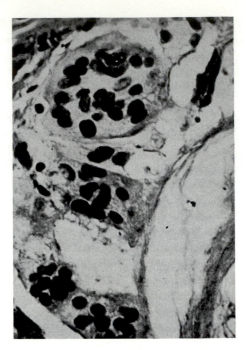

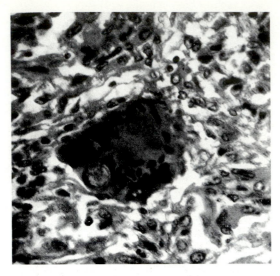

Fig. 2-26. Phagocytosis of pathogenic fungus, *Coccidioides immitis*, by multinucleated giant cell in human lung. Doubly contoured organism is seen at lower left-hand side of giant cell. (420×.)

Fig. 2-25. Three multinucleated giant cells of "foreign body" type in response to keratin that was retained in hair follicle. (450×.)

longevity of the cells in the tissues, or from their continuing mobilization from the bone marrow. There is, in fact, evidence for all three possibilities.[43]

Functionally, the macrophage has a high capacity for phagocytosis and a highly developed system for digesting engulfed material. These features are best illustrated in infections by large facultative bacteria such as *Mycobacterium tuberculosis* or by fungi, or in lesions provoked by the introduction of foreign bodies. Compared with the neutrophil as a phagocyte, the macrophage has a longer life, greater hardiness, and different functions.[42]

Epithelioid cells provide a major feature of various examples of granulomatous inflammation, such as tuberculosis (Fig. 2-22), leprosy, and sarcoidosis (Fig. 2-24). They are relatively large cells (Fig. 2-22), polygonal or somewhat elongate, with a pale nucleus and the cell membranes of adjacent cells in apposition. Epithelioid cells are derived from macrophages by natural maturation, provided that (1) the macrophage survives and remains in situ for long enough, (2) it is not required to undertake phagocytosis, or (3) if it does so, the particle is completely degraded or eliminated. Macrophages that ingest poorly degradable material (such as mycobacteria) do not mature into epithelioid cells.[42]

Epithelioid cells in the mouse normally live for 1 to 4 weeks and are nonphagocytic but retain high pinocytic activity. Epithelioid cells divide to produce small round cells that develop, in turn, into typical macrophages that are phagocytic but that mature into epithelioid cells when appropriate conditions prevail.[42]

Giant cells are large multinucleate cells formed by fusion of macrophages (Fig. 2-26). They are common in granulomatous inflammation, particularly when the lesions are caused by the following:

1. Infection such as tuberculosis, syphilis, and fungal infections
2. Insoluble exogenous substances such as talc, ligatures, and other foreign bodies
3. Insoluble endogenous substances such as fat, keratin, and sodium biurate crystals

The morphology of giant cells is variable. Nuclei arranged peripherally in the cell are characteristic of the so-called Langhans' giant cell (Fig. 2-23), which is common in tuberculosis, whereas nuclei positioned centrally in the cell are more common in giant cells in foreign-body reactions (Fig. 2-25). All the nuclei of these multinucleated cells exhibit synchronous synthesis of DNA.[41]

Lymphocytes and plasma cells. The occurrence of lymphocytes and plasma cells (Fig. 2-27) in chronic inflammation, particularly in granulomatous lesions, and their role in antibody formation raise the question of the part that immune mechanisms play in chronic inflammation, especially where the lesions are granulomatous.

The possible importance of such immunologic mechanisms is highlighted by the number of diseases exhibiting granulomatous inflammation for which an associated delayed type of hypersensitivity provides the basis for a diagnostic skin test. The list of conditions includes infection by the following:

1. Bacteria—tuberculosis, leprosy, syphilis, and brucellosis
2. Viruses—lymphogranuloma inguinale and cat-scratch fever
3. Fungi—dermatomycosis, coccidioidomycosis, and histoplasmosis
4. Metazoa—hydatid disease
5. Protozoa—leishmaniasis

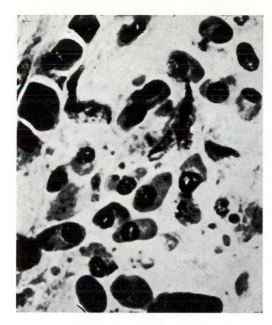

Fig. 2-27. Plasma cells have eccentric nucleus with chromatin arranged peripherally to give "cartwheel" or "clock face" appearance. Large cells are macrophages. (1070×.)

Eosinophils. Eosinophils are common in chronic inflammatory lesions, particularly when the disease is associated with hypersensitivity or attributable to parasitic infestation. Reference has already been made in this chapter to the decrease of the eosinophil response that occurs in trichinosis when there is depletion or inactivation of the pool of lymphocytes normally recirculating in the body.[51]

Fibroblasts are prominent in chronic inflammation when organization is in process (such as at the periphery of a tubercle) or when the reaction is fibrogenic (as in silicosis).[42] Fibroblasts arise by proliferation of other local fibroblasts and synthesize collagen. Their fate and life span have not been established.

Causes of chronicity of inflammation

Experimental work with various irritants labeled with radioactive isotopes indicates that persistence of a granulomatous reaction is accompanied by the intracellular presence of irritant. Disappearance of irritant results in disappearance of the reaction.[42] Persistence of irritant within cells may result from survival of viable microorganisms or from failure of macrophages to degrade dead organisms to diffusible breakdown products.

The development of hypersensitivity is frequently put forward as a cause of chronicity. An excess of antibody over antigen in the formation of immune complexes certainly provokes a granulomatous reaction rather than an acute inflammation, but the reaction is nevertheless exhibited by thymectomized animals. Recurrent reactions of immediate-type hypersensitivity (for example, to circulating antigen-antibody complexes as in allergic vas-

culitis) may provoke chronic inflammation, but the evidence also indicates that delayed-type hypersensitivity may accompany chronic inflammation and may also cause it.[42]

HEALING

The resolution of inflammation involves the removal of exudate and dead cells by enzymatic dissolution and phagocytosis. These events are followed by healing: the replacement of the killed or damaged tissue by cells derived from the parenchymal or connective tissue elements of the injured tissue. When healing is accomplished mainly by proliferation of the parenchymal elements, the process is termed *regeneration* and often results in complete restoration of the original tissue. When the main contribution is made by the nonspecialized elements of connective tissue, fibrosis or scarring results, and the process is called *repair*. The same principles are involved in the restoration of destroyed tissue whether the process involves mainly regeneration or repair.

Regeneration

The cells of the body can be divided into three groups according to their capacity to regenerate[64,72]:
1. *Labile cells* continue to multiply throughout life, even under normal physiologic conditions. They include the epithelial cells of the skin and mucous membranes and the cells of the bone marrow and lymph nodes.
2. *Stable cells* have a decrease or loss of ability for physiologic regeneration in adolescence but retain the ability to proliferate throughout adult life. They include parenchymatous cells of the liver, pancreas, kidney, adrenal, and thyroid.
3. *Permanent cells* lose their ability to proliferate around the time of birth. The most important example is the neuron of the central nervous system.

Regeneration of labile cells

The process of regeneration is basically similar whatever the tissue involved. The events are well illustrated after the curettage of a longitudinal strip 2 mm wide from the mucosal epithelium of the trachea. The rings of tracheal cartilage prevent distortion of the injured tissue and hence make it easy to follow the regeneration of the thin layer of specialized cells in the mucosa.

Regeneration proceeds in four stages[80]: (1) thrombosis and inflammation, (2) regeneration of epithelium over the denuded surface, (3) multiplication of the new cells, and (4) differentiation of the new epithelium.

In *thrombosis and inflammation* the denuded surface is quickly covered by fibrin clot (Figs. 2-28, *A*, and 2-29) with entangled blood cells, while the adjacent underlying tissues exhibit an acute inflammatory response that

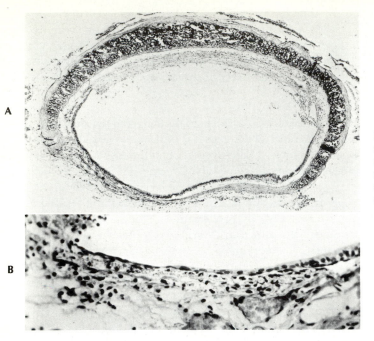

Fig. 2-28. A, Regeneration of tracheal mucosa in rat. Two fifths of mucosa has been removed by curettage. Six hours after curettage, migration of epithelial cells has commenced at margins of residual mucosa. B, Higher magnification of migrating epithelial cells illustrated in A. (A, 35×; B, 150×; from Wilhelm, D.L.: J. Pathol. Bacteriol. 65:543, 1953.)

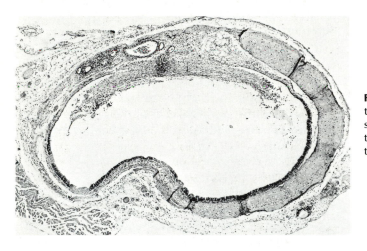

Fig. 2-29. Regeneration of tracheal mucosa 18 hours after curettage. Advancing epithelium is undermining fibrin clot on curetted surface. Peritracheal tissues exhibit inflammatory edema and infiltration by neutrophils. (35×; from Wilhelm, D.L.: J. Pathol. Bacteriol. 65:543, 1953.)

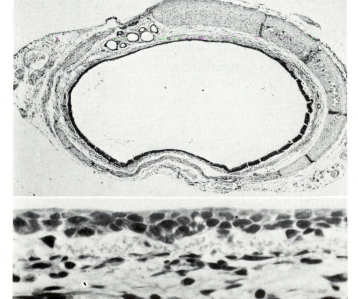

Fig. 2-30. A, Regeneration of tracheal mucosa 48 hours after curettage. Curetted surface is reepithelialized by shallow epithelium. B, Higher magnification of new epithelium illustrated in A. New epithelium is simple and stratified. (A, 35×; B, 625×; from Wilhelm, D.L.: J. Pathol. Bacteriol. 65:543, 1953.)

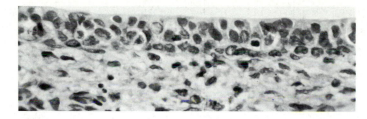

Fig. 2-31. Regeneration of tracheal mucosa 96 hours after curettage. New epithelium shows evidence of redifferentiation. (550×; from Wilhelm, D.L.: J. Pathol. Bacteriol. **65**:543, 1953.)

reaches a peak in 24 to 36 hours and then subsides over the next few days.

Regeneration of epithelium over the denuded surface occurs by the migration of cells from the margin of the wound. The tracheal mucosa consists of a pseudostratified ciliated epithelium with intervening goblet cells and a basal layer of germinal cells. Under physiologic conditions it is the basal cells that proliferate, migrating toward the surface as they mature.

In regeneration the resurfacing of the denuded area is performed by the mature cells at the wound margin (Fig. 2-28). These cells lose their cilia and then migrate laterally as a sheet of cells that are noticeably thinned as though each were covering as great an area as possible. Some cells still exhibit cilia as they begin to migrate, but not for long. Such migration (or thigmotaxis, as it is called) begins as early as 1 hour after injury and is usually well established in 6 hours. The migrating cells cover distances of about 200 μm in the first 8 hours and 400 μm to 1200 μm in 24 hours, with the migrating cells at both edges of a longitudinal curettage together covering the 2 mm defects within 48 hours (Fig. 2-30, *A*). Cells from the curetted necks of submucosal glands make smaller contributions to the sheet of spreading cells.

When the lesions are about 24 hours old, the original mucosal cells just lateral to the initial margin of the wound exhibit a sudden wave of mitotic activity. The proliferation begins six to eight cells behind the margin of curettage and involves both ciliated columnar cells and basal cells. This mitotic activity provides a population of cells to replace those lost by thigmotaxis and ensures a continuing supply of cells for migration. Mitosis involves most of the original mucosa. Another factor of importance in regeneration is the requirement of an appropriate surface on which the spreading cells can migrate. In the case of the tracheal mucosa, the elastic layer of the lamina propria serves very well. But if it is breached by the curettage, migration is correspondingly delayed. The advancing cells undermine the superficial blood clot, presumably by fibrinolytic activity, and continue migrating until the defect is covered. With migration complete, the retromarginal mitosis ceases abruptly. The migrating cells are therefore derived mainly from the original mucosal cells, although lesser numbers arise by mitosis of the spreading cells themselves.

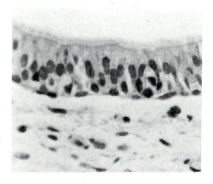

Fig. 2-32. Regenerated tracheal mucosa 6 weeks after curettage. Normal mucosal epithelium with mitosis in basal cell. (550×; from Wilhelm, D.L.: J. Pathol. Bacteriol. **65**:543, 1953.)

Multiplication of the new cells follows as soon as the defect has been covered by the new "emergency" epithelium. A fresh wave of mitotic activity appears in the regenerated mucosa. This second wave is strictly confined to the new mucosal epithelium, occupies the next 24 to 48 hours, and results in the new mucosa's becoming multilayered, the cells at this stage being simple and stratified in type.

Differentiation of the new epithelium begins by the time the whole process is 4 days old. The new cells are rearranged into a superficial layer of cuboid cells and a basal layer of flattened germinal cells (Fig. 2-31). In 5 to 7 days, differentiation is advanced, with the cuboid cells already becoming columnar and some containing droplets of mucin. Differentiation into goblet cells takes 12 to 14 days. Cilia begin to form during the second week, but more so in the third week. The final restoration of normal tissue may take up to 6 weeks (Fig. 2-32).

The same sequence of events is evident in regeneration of columnar cell epithelium of other organs and of *squamous cell epithelium* of the epidermis and cornea. In the skin there is no regeneration of specialized structures such as sweat glands, sebaceous glands, or hair follicles unless viable remnants of these structures persist in the dermis.

With *burns,* the severity of destruction is closely related to the depth of the tissue affected. Burns are described as *first degree* (epidermal) when the superficial epidermis is involved but its continuity is maintained; as *second degree* (dermal) when the epidermis is virtually destroyed so that the underlying dermis with its sweat glands, nerve endings, and bulbs of hair follicles is exposed; and as *third degree* (full thickness) when all epithelial structures in the dermis have been destroyed. In second-degree burns the epidermis is largely reformed from surviving cells of the dermal appendages. Without this possibility in third-degree burns, reepithelialization can occur only from the edges, while the depth of the burn results in substantial scarring.

Regeneration of stable cells

The liver has remarkable powers of regeneration that have been repeatedly described after surgical resection or exposure to chemical poisons causing hepatic necrosis. Regeneration after the resection of healthy liver was originally demonstrated in rabbits by Ponfick[74,75] in the 1890s. In a series of animals of comparable body weight, he estimated the proportional weight of the liver lobes to that of the whole liver and therefore could calculate the proportion that was surgically excised.

The liver has a striking regenerative capacity. Successful regeneration can occur even when nearly 90% of the organ is removed. A residuum of 10% of the liver might be expected to be too little for postoperative survival, but it proved adequate for Ponfick's rabbits, as well as for rats and dogs in later studies by other workers.

A wide range of chemical poisons and biochemical and metabolic disorders, as well as certain viral infections, all produce liver necrosis that may be focal, zonal, or diffuse in distribution. For example, the hepatic necrosis induced by exposure to carbon tetrachloride chiefly involves the parenchyma around the central veins.[65] The necrotic cells are removed by lysis and phagocytosis, but the supporting mesenchymal stroma survives. Proliferation soon occurs in the surviving liver cells throughout each lobule, and new cells migrate into the centrilobular zones, being guided by the persistent reticulin framework, which normally supports the columns of hepatocytes. Remarkably satisfactory regeneration is achieved within 2 weeks. But if necrosis is again induced before regeneration is complete, or the lesion results in damage of the supporting stroma, "regeneration nodules" of liver tissue are formed without restoration of normal hepatic architecture.

Regeneration of permanent cells

Permanent cells occur predominantly in the central nervous system. At birth the nervous system already has its full complement of neurons, which lack a capacity for regeneration. For peripheral nerves, however, limited regeneration can occur, although it is confined to the axons (the cytoplasmic extensions of the neurons).

Regeneration of peripheral nerves. The divided ends of a sectioned nerve[83] become united by proliferating Schwann cells and fibroblasts, which arise from the cut ends, although mainly from the distal stump. On about the third day, the myelin sheath and axon of the remaining intact nerve degenerate back as far as the next node of Ranvier of the proximal surviving axon. From the peripheral end of the viable axon appear numerous new sprouts; 25 to 50 such fibrils emerge from the central stump, but most become lost in the "union scar" joining the cut ends of the fiber.

Meanwhile, in the peripheral stump, there are breakdown and phagocytosis of the axon and myelin, as well as proliferation of the surviving Schwann cells. About 50 days after injury, the peripheral stump consists of tubes filled with elongated Schwann cells. Of the fibrils emerging from the proximal stump, one or more enter the old neural tube; one of the entering fibrils in turn grows in diameter, becomes medullated, and develops into the new functional axon. After crushing or division and suture of a nerve, function is restored after an initial lag of 20 to 40 days, the rate of advance being 2 to 3 mm per day.

The success of regeneration depends on the width of the union scar and the alignment of the cut ends; the nature of any intervening tissue; and suturing of the cut ends. Suturing is well worthwhile, even some time after a nerve is sectioned, although the results are unsatisfactory if suture is delayed more than 6 months.

Regeneration of muscle. Regeneration of striated muscle[68] resembles that of peripheral nerve in that each fiber must be regarded as a unit that can be regenerated only when there is survival of a reasonable part of the unit. When muscle fibers are divided, the subsequent retraction of the cut ends seriously handicaps regeneration. But after crushing, the ends of injured fibers are held together by the connective tissue stroma. The injured site is first filled with fibrinous exudate containing neutrophils and macrophages. The damaged portions of the fibers are soon removed, with short lengths of sarcolemmal tubes filled with histiocytes being left. At about 3 days, outgrowths of sarcoplasm extend from the fiber stumps along these tubes. These outgrowths contain numerous nuclei and have a characteristic pointed tip. The regenerating strands meet, overlap, and anastomose, although complete restoration of muscle architecture is slow and individual fibers may be disoriented for up to 3 months. When the sheath of the fibers is destroyed, the outgrowth of sarcoplasm may be obstructed by connective tissue and therefore forms a multinucleated mass.

With muscle damage from ischemia or bacterial toxins, new endomysial tubes are formed on the scaffolding of the dead fibers and provide the channels that guide the new fibers. Regeneration is independent of an intact nerve supply.

Smooth muscle (as of the ureter, bladder, and bowel)

has similar, although lesser, capacity for regeneration than does striated muscle.

• • •

This discussion of regeneration has been purposely restricted to only a few tissues and organs because the process basically consists of (1) cell migration, with proliferation of the original cells to maintain a population of cells available for migration, and (2) proliferation of the migrated cells constituting the regenerated tissue and their subsequent differentiation and maturation. These processes are modified for the various parenchymal cells, according to their morphologic features and functional requirements.

Repair

Repair refers to the replacement of tissue defects by fibrous tissue, whereas *regeneration* should be restricted to the replacement of a single type of parenchymatous cell by proliferating survivors of the same kind. Both terms come under the more general one of *healing*.

The most common example of healing is the healing of wounds. Before considering the healing process, however, it is helpful to discuss two aspects of the process: the formation of granulation tissue and the contraction of wounds.

Formation of granulation tissue

Much of our information on the formation of granulation tissue comes from the work of E.R. and E.L. Clark,[66,67] who microscopically observed the events provoked by injury of the tail of the tadpole, and from Sandison,[77] who studied repair in mammalian tissues in the rabbit ear chamber. After insertion of an ear chamber, the central table of the chamber is soon covered by blood clot containing strands of fibrin, erythrocytes, and a few leukocytes. During the next day or two, the fibrin becomes more evident, the red cells less so, and the central table covered by a light brown granular mass. Concurrent with these preliminary changes, *macrophages* appear on the table, invade the blood clot, and begin to ingest and digest cellular debris, fragments of fibrin, and red cells. Some of the macrophages fuse to form giant cells. The digestion of the fibrin clot is also facilitated by extracellular enzymes derived from the macrophages, as well as from disintegrated neutrophils.

The advancing macrophages are soon followed by *capillaries* that arise from blood vessels at the periphery of the table where preexisting tissue adjoins the blood clot. The young capillaries usually reach the edge of the table by the seventh day after insertion of the chamber and continue to advance at a rate of 0.1 to 0.6 mm daily. The new capillaries are formed by migration and mitosis of endothelial cells of adjacent preexisting blood vessels in a manner analogous to that for regeneration of mucosal epithelium. Endothelial cells at the line of severance of blood vessels migrate forward beyond the cut vessel to form a small sprout with a fine terminal prolongation. This new capillary is initially solid (Fig. 2-33), but within a few hours it develops a lumen and carries blood. The tips of proliferating vessels have blunt, plump, or even bulbous ends, into the lumen of which are forced red cells, platelets, and a few white cells. However, the fluid exhibits no movement other than oscillations imparted by the heartbeat and respiration. The new capillaries gradually proliferate into the areas of the blood clot cleared by the scavenging macrophages and sometimes join one another or anastomose to form capillary loops.[77] The outcome is an advancing margin of delicate vascular arches through which blood flows (Fig. 2-34). The newly formed capillaries are abnormally permeable at or near the advancing tip, the interendothelial junctions being tenuous and exhibiting distinct gaps. The newly formed vessels also bleed readily, their fragility possibly being attributable to the morphologic features underlying their abnormal permeability.[78]

The new blood vessels initially consist of endothelial cells alone. Within a few days they develop into arterioles, true capillaries, or venules, possibly according to intravascular pressure and the amount of blood flow.[4] During the next weeks the new vessels continue to differentiate until after some months the field on the table of an ear chamber exhibits a whole range of vascular elements—artery, arterioles, true capillaries, venules, and vein.[66,67] While the vascular bed is differentiating, there is a constant remodeling of the vasculature. This remodeling particularly involves obliteration of many of the initial capillaries, consequent to absence of blood flow through these vessels. The process begins by a decrease in diameter and then a loss of lumen. The solid cord so produced breaks in two, and the ends retract to the level of the next patent vessel.[77]

Vasomotor nerves appear on the arterioles as early as 2 to 3 days after the formation of endothelial tubes. The development of muscle cells in the vascular wall imparts tone, but contraction is not evident until the cells are reached by vasomotor twigs.[4]

Lymphatics proliferate in much the same manner as blood vessels, although the growth of lymphatic vessels is slower and less labile.[4]

Fibrous tissue. At the stage when the formed elements of the initial blood clot have been removed from an ear chamber, the cells and proliferating elements are supported by an amorphous gelatinous matrix ("ground substance"). This matrix has a relatively high content of mucopolysaccharide, the concentration of which begins to decrease when the first young fibrils of collagen are produced by fibroblasts. The fibroblasts probably arise from fibrocytes or some less differentiated precursor in the tissues around the table of the chamber, particularly

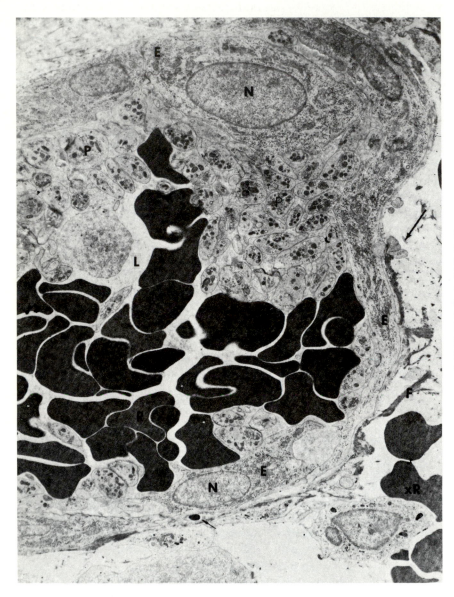

Fig. 2-33. Vascular sprout in 3-day-old wound of rat muscle. The sprout has a blunt extremity, and lumen, *L*, is filled with platelets, *P,* and red blood cells, *R. Lower right,* Extravasated red cells, *xR.* Note cytoplasmic extrusion *(right arrow)* of endothelial cell, *E.* Shreds of fibrin, *F,* coat adventitial aspect of vessel. *Bottom arrow,* Portion of red cell in cleft in vascular wall. *N,* Nucleus of endothelial cell. (Karnovsky stain; 3800×; from Schoefl, G.I.: Virchows Arch. [Pathol. Anat.] **337**:97, 1963.)

Fig. 2-34. Cornea of rat, 5 days after silver nitrate injury. Arcades of new blood vessels appear in healing wound. Abnormal permeability of new vessels is indicated by escape of circulating colloidal carbon into the perivascular tissue *(arrow).* (22×; from Schoefl, G.I.: Virchows Arch. [Pathol. Anat.] **337**:97, 1963.)

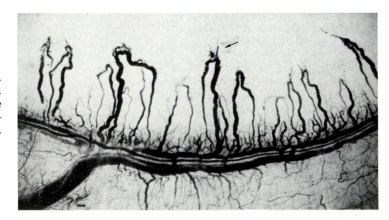

the loose connective tissue. Fibroblasts enter the clot just after the macrophages and at about the same time as the blood vessels, advancing at a rate of about 0.2 mm a day. Their number is constantly increased by further cells from the surrounding tissue, as well as by mitotic division of fibroblasts already on the scene. Collagen fibers become identifiable by about the sixth day. At first they are radially disposed and lie in a single plane, but other layers of fibers subsequently appear, roughly at right angles to the first. The direction of the fibers seems to be determined by lines of tension during the laying down of the fibers.

The outcome of these processes is the formation of vascular young connective tissue containing a variable number of inflammatory cells. This so-called *granulation tissue* (Fig. 2-35) derives its name from its appearance, as in the base of a large open wound. The new tissue has a slightly granular surface with each "granule" corresponding to a vascular arcade of new capillaries, elevating their thin covering of young collagen slightly above the adjacent unsupported matrix. The term *granulation tissue* refers to the consequent impression of granularity of the surface.

Chemical estimations of the constituents of healing wounds reveal two phases of activity: (1) an initial pro-

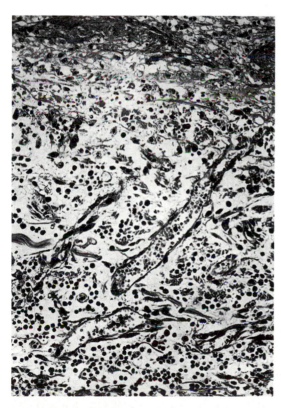

Fig. 2-35. Granulation tissue in pericarditis. Newly formed blood vessels are supported by loosely arranged connective tissue, in interstices of which lie inflammatory cells. Fibrinous exudate *(at top)* obscures outline of serosal pericardium. (170×.)

duction phase, during which there is accumulation of proteins and an increase in content of hexosamine, the latter possibly corresponding to the entry of glycoproteins with the inflammatory exudate, succeeded by (2) a collagen phase. The level of hexosamine in the healing tissue decreases with the progression of fibroplasia.[69,70] The amount of collagen formed, assessed by the wound's content of hydroxyproline, increases as the argyrophilic reticulin fibers disappear. For some weeks the amount of collagen parallels the increasing tensile strength of the healing tissue.

Repair with organization

The process whereby coagulated blood becomes replaced by granulation tissue is known as *organization*. The same process occurs in four main sets of circumstances:

1. *Repair*. This was just described.
2. *Inflammation*. Acute inflammation generally resolves, leaving little or no evidence of the episode. Occasionally, however, resolution is incomplete or delayed, whereupon fibrinous exudate in particular becomes invaded by proliferating fibroblasts and blood vessels, with the enhanced vascular supply being required to meet the heightened metabolic needs of the granulation tissue. This process of organization may complicate unresolved pneumonia, being associated with persistence of fibrin in lobar pneumonia and with mixed bacterial infections in bronchopneumonia. It also occurs in rheumatic pneumonia, bronchiectasis, and lung abscess. Organization also complicates inflammatory lesions of serous membranes, such as fibrinous pericarditis (Fig. 2-35), empyema of the pleural cavity, and inflammation of the peritoneal cavity. The process results in adhesions, bands, and scarring.
3. *Thrombosis*. Thrombi that persist at their site of formation are often invaded by granulation tissue and converted into fibrous tissue.
4. *Infarction*. A slow ingrowth of granulation tissue frequently occurs at the periphery of infarcts exhibiting coagulative necrosis, such as in the kidney, spleen, myocardium, and lung. The infarct is eventually converted into a fibrous scar.

Contraction of wounds

The rapidity of the healing of wounds depends to considerable extent on the contraction that begins a few days after injury and continues for several weeks. The magnitude of such contraction is not always appreciated. In rats the scar occupies about 20% to 30% of the area of the original wound, and in rabbits the process is even more successful. But until quite recently, the mechanism of wound contraction remained uncertain. Dehydration was claimed to contribute, although the main factor was alleged to be contraction of the mature reparative collagen.[11] Nevertheless, the theory of contraction of collagen was acknowledged to be inconsistent with the fact that contraction proceeds at a stage when the collagen content of granulation tissue is negligible. An even greater difficulty is the fact that formation of collagen is decreased in scorbutic animals, although wound contraction in such animals proceeds as in normal controls.

The observation that contraction occurs when granulation tissue is being formed prompted various workers to regard granulation tissue as an *organ of contraction*,[62,63] a proposal that gained support from the observation that comparable contraction occurs in scorbutic animals.[61] The puzzle concerning the element responsible for contraction seems resolved by work in Majno's laboratory.[71,76] In wounds of the rat's skin, fibroblasts increase in number from the third day onward. Between 7 and 21 days, according to the type of lesion, many of the fibroblasts in granulation tissue develop three morphologic modifications: (1) bundles of fibrils in the cytoplasm, resembling those of smooth muscle cells, as well as opaque areas among the bundles or beneath the plasmalemma, resembling "attachment sites" of smooth muscle; (2) nuclear indentations, comparable to those on nuclear membranes of contracted muscle cells; and (3) differentiation of the cell's surface to provide numerous intercellular connections resembling desmosomes. The morphologic similarity of these modified fibroblasts to smooth muscle cells is supported by other observations. The cytoplasm of the modified cells exhibits immunofluorescent labeling with human anti–smooth muscle serum, and strips of granulation tissue respond to various drugs in vitro similarly to smooth muscle. Furthermore, the extraction of granulation tissue yields quantities of actomyosin (with the same adenosine triphosphate activity) similar to those obtained from nonstriated muscle of the pregnant rat uterus. The overall results therefore indicate that modified fibroblasts ("myofibroblasts") are responsible for the process of contraction of granulation tissue in healing wounds.[71] Similar myofibroblasts have been identified in granulation tissue from human lesions.[76]

Healing by first intention

When the surgeon sutures a clean incision, healing takes place with minimum loss of tissue and without significant bacterial infection. This is referred to as *healing by first intention* or *primary union* (Fig. 2-36). The space between the opposing surfaces of the incised skin becomes filled with blood from *hemorrhage* of severed vessels; the blood then coagulates to form a clot that seals the incision against dehydration and infection.

Acute inflammation quickly ensues, and within 24 hours the margins of the incision are infiltrated by neutrophils and monocytes, and swollen by fluid exudate. Autolytic enzymes liberated by dead tissue cells, proteolytic enzymes from neutrophils, and phagocytic activity by monocytes and tissue macrophages combine to clear away the necrotic tissue, debris, and red blood cells. The ingested hemoglobin becomes converted into hemosiderin and hematoidin.

The early events in healing by first intention include an important contribution by the *epidermis*.[73] At both margins of the incision, the epidermis responds within hours by becoming thickened and migrating from the margins of the wound down into the upper part of the incisional gap and uniting in the upper dermis. The advancing epidermis cleaves the overlying necrotic epithelium and associated necrotic dermis from underlying viable dermis (Fig. 2-36), so that the scab over the migrated epidermis finally contains dry blood clot, fragments of dead epidermis, and fibers of collagen and elastin. Throughout the invasion by the epidermis, the migrating cells are nondividing. Mitotic activity is confined to basal cells adjacent to the margins of the wound.

With well-approximated wounds, a continuous layer of epidermis usually forms in 48 hours (Fig. 2-36). During the next day or so, the new epidermis may further invade the dermal breach to form a downward-pointing spur (Fig. 2-37). Thereafter, the new epidermis takes on the morphologic features of the adjacent uninjured epidermis, and the epidermal spurs are remodeled from early in the second week onward.

Organization proceeds meanwhile in the incisional deficit of the dermis, protected by the overlying new epidermis. By about the third day, the dermal lesion contains fibroblasts and capillary buds emigrating from the edges of the wound. Reticulin is demonstrable by the second or third day, and new collagen by the fifth day. During the fourth week (and even earlier in the tissue adjacent to the margins of the wound site), the cellular and vascular elements are decreasing in both number and concentration.

Response to sutures. Healing by first intention of a wound more than minimal in size requires that the wound be sutured. However, the suture material itself evokes a complex and often prolonged reaction.[73] During the initial 3 days, the epidermis and the epithelium of dermal appendages react to the presence of the foreign material by advancing along the suture track to form an incomplete tube of epithelium two to three cells thick around the whole length of the suture (Fig. 2-37). Between the epithelial tube and the suture lie fibrin, neutrophils, and erythrocytes. Externally, the epithelium initially lies on the collagen of the dermis, although in a day or two, mononuclear cells come to surround the epithelial tube. Deep to the advancing margin of downgrowing epithelium, the suture is encased by (1) leuko-

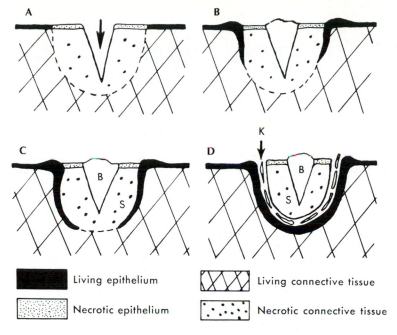

Fig. 2-36. Healing by first intention of a shallow incised wound of skin. **A** (8 hours): Incision *(arrow)* is flanked by a zone of necrotic tissue. **B** (16 hours): Epidermis is thickened near line of demarcation between viable and necrotic tissue. Tongue of epithelial cells is invading underlying dermis, separating necrotic from viable tissue. **C** (24 hours): Epithelial invasion is advanced, with two tongues moving toward each other. **D** (40 to 48 hours): Epithelial tongues have met and severed necrotic tissue (incorporated in scab) from underlying viable tissue. Keratinization of epithelium leads to dislodgment of scab. *B,* Blood clot and necrotic debris in track of incision; *K,* keratin; *S,* scab. (Modified from Croft, C.B., and Tarin, D.: J. Anat. **106:**63, 1970.)

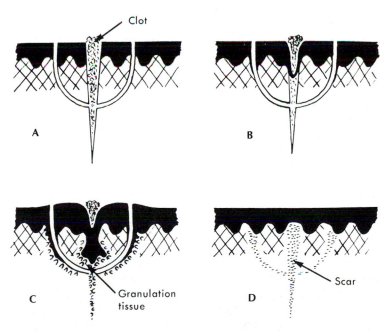

Fig. 2-37. Healing of incised wound that has been sutured. Track alone of suture is illustrated. **A,** Wound rapidly fills with blood clot. **B,** Soon afterwards, epidermis *(black)* migrates both into wound and around suture track. **C,** Epithelial tongues or spurs are formed, and granulation tissue begins to be formed. For convenience, zone of necrotic tissue flanking incision (see Fig. 2-36) is not illustrated but is nevertheless present and becomes separated from underlying viable dermis by invading epithelial cells from the epidermis. These epithelial cells are represented in **B** and **C** by the centrally placed spur. **D,** Suture has been removed and scar tissue marks sites of incision and of suture track. Epithelial tongues and spurs have degenerated. (From Walter, J.B., and Israel, M.S.: General pathology, ed. 3, Edinburgh, 1970, J. & A. Churchill.)

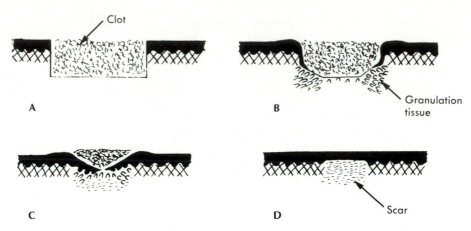

Fig. 2-38. Healing of excised wound by second intention. **A,** Blood clot rapidly fills the wound. **B,** Epidermal cells migrate into the wound as a tongue of cells, separating blood clot and zone of necrotic tissue from underlying viable dermis. **C,** In center of wound, clot becomes organized and rising body of granulation tissue elevates tongues of epithelium until they meet and reform the surface. **D,** Most or all of the clot is cast off without being organized. Contraction of wound results in relatively small scar. (From Walter, J.B., and Israel, M.S.: General pathology, ed. 3, Edinburgh, 1970, J. & A. Churchill.)

cytes and nuclear debris, (2) foreign-body granulation tissue containing macrophages and giant cells, and (3) young collagen.

Removal of sutures at about the tenth day usually results in part or much of the epithelial tube being left in the suture track. The epithelium so isolated in the dermis provokes a strong foreign-body reaction. However, the epithelium is resorbed during the next week and the breach in the epidermis is healed by regeneration (Fig. 2-37).

In summary, the insertion of sutures itself entails incisional damage. To this damage is added a brisk granulomatous reaction evoked by both the suture material and the downgrowing epithelium, which arises particularly from dermal appendages injured by suturing. The tissue reaction is equally severe for monofilament nylon as for polyfilament Mersilk of equivalent caliber. The earlier the sutures are removed, the less will be the granulomatous response. However, the use of adhesive tape avoids even the lesser granulomatous response obtained by early removal of sutures.[73]

Healing by second intention

Not all wounds can or should be sutured. In either case the edges gape and the open wound has a red base and margins that become swollen from inflammatory edema. The floor of the wound exudes a yellowish pink fluid that contains protein, including fibrinogen, and therefore coagulates over the wound.

The relatively wide separation of the wound edges means that healing has to progress from the base upward. Nevertheless, the basic events in healing by second intention resemble those for first intention. Acute inflammation and clearing of debris are accompanied chronologically by downgrowth of epidermis to form a layer of epithelium that separates viable preexisting collagen of the dermis from injured necrotic collagen at the wound's margin (Fig. 2-38).

Meanwhile, the base of the coagulum becomes replaced by granulation tissue, produced by fibroblasts and vascular sprouts from the adjacent viable dermis (Fig. 2-39, *A*). The surface of the young granulation tissue is deep red, granular, and fragile. Concurrent with the development of the granulation tissue, there is contraction of the wound induced by myofibroblasts. The advancing sheets of epidermis finally cover the granulation tissue so that the scab is separated and cast off. Progressive contraction decreases the size of the wound, and the new epidermis is elevated by the increasing amount of granulation tissue (Fig. 2-38). The scar is at first pink but becomes pale and whitish because of a decrease in vasculature over the succeeding months (Fig. 2-39).

The *presence of infection* is an important factor in handicapping the healing of wounds. The increased amount of exudate enlarges the wound, bacterial toxins provoke necrosis and suppuration, and the fibrinolytic enzymes in pus destroy the framework of fibrin, which is so important for the ingrowth of fibroblasts and capillaries. Finally, bacterial toxins may induce thrombosis of blood vessels and therefore interfere with the blood supply of healing tissue.

Metaplasia

Metaplasia ("transformation") is usually defined as the transformation of fully differentiated cells of one kind into differentiated cells of another kind in response to

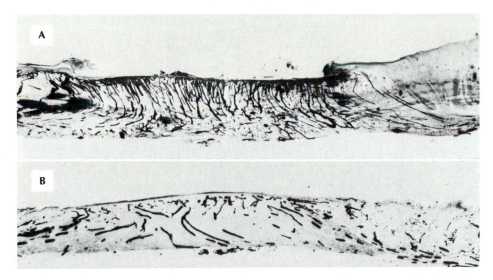

Fig. 2-39. Vasculature of wounds healing by second intention. Full thickness of disk of skin was excised from back of trunk of rats, and regenerated blood vessels were demonstrated by intra-arterial injection with opaque colloidal medium. **A,** Numerous new blood vessels supplying wound that has been filled by granulation tissue. **B,** Decreased vasculature in wound healed in rat 2 months after injury.

abnormal stimuli. This definition is misleading, however, because the change in form of the mature cells results from a *change in the usual line of differentiation*, not a transformation of the fully differentiated cell. For example, the progeny of the germinal cells of tracheal mucosa normally differentiate into ciliated columnar and goblet cells, but in rats deficient in vitamin A the proliferating cells abandon their usual line of differentiation for one that results in squamous cells.[80] The term *metaplasia* therefore refers to a change in the line of differentiation of proliferating cells, such that the type of fully differentiated cell usual for a tissue becomes replaced by a different variety of differentiated cell. Since metaplasia is confined to proliferating cells, the condition is associated mainly with regeneration or neoplasia. It particularly involves epithelium or connective tissue[82] (see also p. 517.)

Metaplasia in epithelium

Under various circumstances, columnar cell and transitional cell epithelia are transformed into squamous cell epithelium resembling epidermis, the process being referred to as *squamous* or *epidermoid metaplasia*. Squamous metaplasia of a transitional cell epithelium, such as the mucosa of the urinary tract, represents little substantial change in character of the epithelium. On the other hand, squamous metaplasia of the pseudostratified ciliated columnar cells lining the respiratory tract (Fig. 2-40) results in an epithelium that is entirely different morphologically and has lost important features of the normal mucosa that make it such an effective guardian against

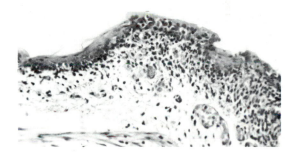

Fig. 2-40. Early squamous metaplasia of ciliated columnar epithelium of tracheal mucosa from 35-day-old rat fed diet deficient in vitamin A. Metaplasia begins in small foci that extend and coalesce until whole circumference of tracheal mucosa is involved. (185×; from Wilhelm, D.L.: J. Pathol. Bacteriol. **67:**361, 1954.)

the entry of inhaled bacteria and foreign material. Such metaplasia is common in the presence of chronic bronchitis and bronchiectasis and in smokers. Squamous metaplasia is reasonably common in the ducts of the salivary glands (Fig. 2-41) and pancreas, in the mucosa of prolapsed bowel, in endometrial polyps, in hyperplasia of the prostate, and in chronic inflammation of the epididymis and thyroid gland.

The same process of squamous metaplasia is common in neoplasms, particularly in adenocarcinoma of the lung, uterus, breast, and gallbladder, as well as in pleomorphic salivary adenoma. It occurs occasionally in carcinoma of the stomach, large bowel, pancreas, and prostate and in transitional cell cancers of the urinary tract.

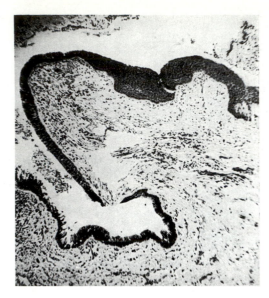

Fig. 2-41. Metaplasia of epithelial lining of salivary duct. Columnar epithelium *(bottom left)* has been replaced by squamous epithelium *(upper right).* (50×.)

Metaplasia in connective tissues

The extraosseous formation of bone or cartilage has been frequently observed in scars, chronic inflammatory and degenerative lesions, sclerotic arteries, and muscle. Ossification sometimes occurs in scars from operative incisions, particularly of the upper abdomen, in or near the linea alba. In degenerative necrotic lesions, ossification is preceded by the deposition of calcium. Myositis ossificans is frequently related to previous injury, with ensuing fibrosis and vascularization of the injured muscle.

The most surprising example of osseous metaplasia is that associated with the mucosa of the urinary tract. The process occurs in connective tissues closely related to the transitional cell epithelium of the mucosa of the bladder, ureter, or renal pelvis, being possibly related to the phosphatase activity of regenerating epithelium of the urinary tract.

Bony or cartilaginous metaplasia is not unusual in the connective tissue stroma of neoplasms and has been described in carcinoma of the stomach, bowel, gallbladder, salivary gland, and prostate. Less commonly, muscle may exhibit metaplasia, in which nonstriated muscle becomes striated.[82]

• • •

Metaplasia therefore represents a change in the direction of cellular differentiation, resulting in the development of mature cells having a character different from that usually occurring in a particular tissue. On the other hand, when tissue occurs in an unusual site as the result of alleged "primary displacement" or developmental abnormality, the foreign tissue is termed a *heterotopia* (for example, the presence of gastric mucosa in a congenital Meckel's diverticulum of the terminal ileum).

In conclusion, attention should be drawn to the disadvantages that may follow the development of metaplasia. The replacement of the usual cell by another type of cell often results in decreased function of the affected organ or in impairment of mechanisms that are important in defense against infection (as in the respiratory tract).

REFERENCES
General

1. Casley-Smith, J.R.: An electron microscopic study of injured and abnormally permeable lymphatics, Ann. N.Y. Acad. Sci. **116**:803, 1964.
2. Chambers, R., and Zweifach, B.W.: Capillary endothelial cement in relation to permeability, J.Cell. Physiol. **15**:255, 1940.
3. Chambers, R., and Zweifach, B.W.: Topography and junction of mesenteric capillary circulation, Am. J. Anat. **75**:173, 1944.
4. Florey, H.W., editor: General pathology, ed. 4, London, 1970, Lloyd-Luke (Medical Books) Ltd.
5. Hunter, J.: A treatise on the blood, inflammation and gunshot wounds, vol. 1, London, 1974, G. Nicoll.
6. Lewis, T.: The blood vessels of the human skin and their responses, London, 1927, Shaw & Sons Ltd.
7. Miles, A.A.: Ann. N.Y. Acad. Sci. **66**:356, 1956.
8. Robbins, D.L.: Pathologic basis of disease, Philadelphia, 1974, W.B. Saunders Co.
9. Spector, W.G., and Willoughby, D.A.: The inflammatory response, Bacteriol. Rev. **27**:117, 1963.
10. Thomas, L.: Inflammation as a disease mechanism. In Zweifach, B.W., Grant, L., and McCluskey, R.T., editors: The inflammatory process, ed. 2, vol. 3, New York, 1974, Academic Press, Inc.
11. Walter, J.B., and Israel, M.S.: General pathology, ed. 4, Edinburgh, 1974, Churchill Livingstone.

Inflammation
Exudation of pus

12. Allison, F., Jr., and Lancaster, M.G.: Studies on the pathogenesis of acute inflammation. II. The relationship of fibrinogen and fibrin to the leucocyte sticking reaction in ear chambers of rabbits injured by heat, Br. J. Exp. Pathol. **40**:324, 1959.
13. Burke, J.F. and Miles, A.A.: The sequence of vascular events in early infective inflammation, J. Pathol. Bacteriol. **76**:1, 1958.
14. Cotran, R.S., Suter, E.R., and Majno, G.: The use of colloidal carbon as a tracer for vascular injury: a review, Vasc. Dis. **4**:107, 1967.
15. Majno, G.: Mechanism of abnormal vascular permeability in acute inflammation. In Thomas, L., Uhr, J.W., and Grant, L., editors: International symposium on injury, inflammation and immunity, Baltimore, 1964, The Williams & Wilkins Co.
16. Miles, A.A.: Large molecular substances as mediators of the inflammatory reaction, Ann. N.Y. Acad. Sci. **116**:855, 1964.
17. Paton, W.D.M.: Histamine release by compounds of simple chemical structure, Pharmacol. Rev. **9**:269, 1957.
18. Paton, W.D.M.: The release of histamine, Progr. Allerg. **5**:79, 1958
19. Pierce, J.V.: Fed. Proc. **27**:52, 1968.
20. Pullinger, B.D., and Florey, H.W.: Some observations on structure and functions of lymphatics: their behavior in local edema, Br. J. Exp. Pathol. **16**:49, 1935.
21. Riley, J.F., and West, G.B.: Tissue mast cells: studies with histamine-liberator of low toxicity (compound 48/80), J. Pathol. Bacteriol. **69**:269, 1955.
22. Rocha e Silva, M.: The physiological significance of bradykinin, Ann. N.Y. Acad. Sci. **104**:190, 1963.
23. Schachter, M.: Kallikreins and kinins, Physiol. Rev. **49**:509, 1969.

24. Uvnäs, B.: Mechanism of histamine release in mast cells, Ann. N.Y. Acad. Sci. **103:**278, 1963.
25. Webster, M.E.: Fed. Proc. **27:**84, 1968.
26. Webster, M.E.: Kinin system. In Movat, H.Z., editor: Cellular and humoral mechanisms in anaphylaxis and allergy, New York, 1969, S. Karger.
27. Wilhelm, D.L.: Pattern and mechanism of increased vascular permeability in inflammation. In Zweifach, B.W., Grant, L., and McClusky, R.T., editors: The inflammatory process, ed. 2, vol. 2, New York, 1973, Academic Press, Inc.
28. Wilhelm, D.L., Bertelli, G., and Hoceck, J.C., editors: Symposium on inflammation, biochemistry, and drug interaction, Amsterdam, 1969, Excerpta Medica Foundation.
29. Wilhelm, D.L., and Mason, B.: Vascular permeability changes in inflammation: the role of endogenous permeability factors in mild thermal injury, Br. J. Exp. Pathol. **45:**487, 1960.

Blood cells and inflammation

30. Archer, G.T., Robson, J., and Thompson, A.R.: Proc. Aust. Biochem. Soc. **8:**96, 1975.
31. Becker, E.L.: Enzyme activation and the mechanism of neutrophil chemotaxis, Antibiot. Chemother. **19:**409, 1974.
32. Boyden, S.: The chemotactic effect of mixtures of antibody and antigen on polymorphonuclear leucocytes, J. Exp. Med. **115:**453, 1962.
33. Clark, E.R., and Clark, E.L.: Anat. Rec. **24:**127, 1922.
34. Florey, H.W., and Grant, L.H.: Leucocyte migration from small blood vessels stimulated with ultraviolet light: an electron-microscope study, J. Pathol. Bacteriol. **82:**13, 1961.
35. Hirsch, J.G.: Neutrophilic leukocytes. In Zweifach, B.W., Grant, G., and McCluskey, R.T., editors: The inflammatory process, ed. 2, vol. 1, New York, 1973, Academic Press, Inc.
36. Hurley, J.V.: Incubation of serum with tissue extracts as a cause of chemotaxis of granulocytes, Nature (Lond.) **198:**1212, 1963.
37. Kay, A.B., and Austen, K.F.: The IgE-mediated release of an eosinophil leukocyte chemotactic factor from human lung, J. Immunol. **107:**899, 1971.
38. Langevoort, H.Z., et al.: Classification of mononuclear phagocytic cells. In van Furth, R., editor: Mononuclear phagocytes, Oxford, 1970, Blackwell Scientific Publications, Ltd.
39. Marchesi, V.T., and Florey, H.W.: Electron micrographic observations on the emigration of leucocytes, Q. J. Exp. Physiol. **45:**343, 1960.
40. McCutcheon, M.: Chemotaxis in leukocytes, Physiol. Rev. **26:**319, 1946.
41. Ryan, G.B., and Spector, W.G.: Natural selection of long-lived macrophages in experimental granulomata, Proc. R. Soc. Lond. (Biol.) **175:**269, 1970.
42. Spector, W.G.: Chronic inflammation. In Zweifach, B.W., Grant, L., and McCluskey, R.T., editors: The inflammatory process, ed. 2, vol. 3, New York, 1974, Academic Press, Inc.
43. Spector, W.G., and Willoughby, D.A.: Recruitment of macrophages in granuloma. In van Arman, C.G., editor: White cells in inflammation, Springfield, Ill., 1974, Charles C Thomas, Publisher.
44. Speirs, R.S., and Speirs, E.S.: Eosinophils in granulomatous inflammation. In van Arman, C.G., editor: White cells in inflammation, Springfield, Ill., 1974, Charles C Thomas, Publisher.
45. Steinman, R.M., and Cohn, Z.A.: Metabolism and physiology of mononuclear phagocytes. In Zweifach, B.W., Grant, L., and McCluskey, R.T., editors: The inflammatory process, ed. 2, vol. 1, New York, 1974, Academic Press, Inc.
46. van Furth, R., editor: Mononuclear phagocytes, Oxford, 1970, Blackwell Scientific Publications, Ltd.
47. Ward, P.A.: Chemotaxis of mononuclear cells, J. Exp. Med. **128:**1201, 1968.
48. Ward, P.A.: Mechanisms of phagocytosis. In Lepow, I.H., and Ward, P.A., editors: Inflammation: mechanisms and control, New York, 1972, Academic Press, Inc.

Phagocytosis

49. Elsbach, P.: Phagocytosis. In Zweifach, B.W., Grant, L., and McCluskey, R.T., editors: The inflammatory process, ed. 2, vol. 1, New York, 1974, Academic Press, Inc.

50. Wood, W.B., Jr.: Phagocytoses with particular reference to encapsulated bacteria, Bacteriol. Rev. **24:**41, 1960.

Hypersensitivity and inflammation

51. Basten, A., and Beeson, P.B.: Mechanism of eosinophilia. II. Role of the lymphocyte, J. Exp. Med. **131:**1288, 1970.
52. Burnet, M.: Self and non-self, Cambridge, Eng., 1969, Cambridge University Press.
53. Cochrane, C.G.: Immunologic tissue injury mediated by neutrophilic leukocytes, Adv. Immunol. **9:**97, 1968.
54. Coombs, R.R.A., and Gell, P.G.H.: Classification of hypersensitivity. In Fell, P.G.H., and Coombs, R.R.A., editors: Clinical aspects of immunology, ed. 2, Oxford, 1968, Blackwell Scientific Publications, Ltd.
55. Dvorak, H.F., and Dvorak, A.M.: Basophils, mast cells, and cellular immunity in animals and man, Hum. Pathol. **3:**454, 1972.
56. Ford, W.L., and Gowans, J.L.: The traffic of lymphocytes, Semin. Hematol. **6:**67, 1969.
57. Humphrey, J.H., and White, R.G.: Immunology for students of medicine, ed. 3, Oxford, 1970, Blackwell Scientific Publications, Ltd.
58. Lykke, A.W.J., and Cummings, R.: Increased vascular permeability in the primary cutaneous allograft response in the rat, Experientia **24:**1287, 1969.
59. McGregor, D.D., and Mackaness, G.B.: Life history and function of lymphocytes. In Zweifach, B.W., Grant, L., and McCluskey, R.T., editors: The inflammatory process, ed. 2, vol. 3, New York, 1974, Academic Press, Inc.
60. Waksman, B.M.: In Wolstenholme, G.E.W., and O'Connor, M., editors: Cellular aspects of immunity, Ciba Foundation Symposium, Boston, 1960, Little, Brown & Co.

Healing

61. Abercrombie, M., Flint, M.H., and James, D.L.: J. Embryol. Exp. Morphol. **4:**167, 1956.
62. Abercrombie, M., James, D.L., and Newcombe, J.F.: Wound contraction in rabbit skin, studied by splinting the wound margins, J. Anat. **94:**170, 1960.
63. Billingham, R.E., and Russell, P.S.: Studies on wound healing, with special reference to the phenomenon of contracture in experimental wounds in rabbits' skin, Ann. Surg. **144:**961, 1951.
64. Bizzozero, G.: Accrecsimento e rigeneragione nell' organismo, Arch. Sci. Med. (Torino) **18:**245, 1894.
65. Cameron, G.R., and Karunaratne, W.A.E.: Massive necrosis ("toxic infarction") of liver following intra-portal administration of poisons, J. Pathol. Bacteriol. **44:**297, 1937.
66. Clark, E.R., and Clark, E.L.: Microscopic observations on growth of blood capillaries in living mammal, Am. J. Anat. **64:**251, 1939.
67. Clark, E.R., et al.: General observations on ingrowth of new blood vessels into standardized chambers in rabbit's ear, and subsequent changes in newly grown vessels over period of months, Anat. Rec. **50:**129, 1931.
68. Clark, W.E.L.: Experimental study of regeneration of mammalian striped muscle, J. Anat. **80:**24, 1946.
69. Dunphy, J.E.: On the nature and care of wounds, Ann. R. Coll. Surg. Eng. **26:**69, 1960.
70. Edwards, L.C., and Dunphy, J.E.: Wound healing (in two parts), N. Engl. J. Med. **259:**224, 275, 1958.
71. Gabbiani, G., et al.: Granulation tissue as a contractile organ: a study of structure and function, J. Exp. Med. **135:**719, 1972.
72. Leblond, C.P., and Walker, B.E.: Renewal of cell populations, Physiol. Rev. **36:**255, 1956.
73. Ordman, L.J., and Gillman, T.: Studies in the healing of cutaneous wounds (in three parts), Arch. Surg. **93:**857, 883, 911, 1966.
74. Ponfick, E.: Verh. Dtsch. Ges. Chir. **19:**28, 1890.
75. Ponfick, E.: Experimentelle Beiträge zur Pathologie der Leber, Virchows Arch. (Pathol. Anat.) **138**(suppl.):81, 1895.
76. Ryan, G.B., et al.: Myofibroblasts in human granulation tissue, Hum. Pathol. **5:**55, 1974.
77. Sandison, J.: Observations on growth of blood vessels as seen in transparent chamber introduced into rabbit's ear, Am. J. Anat. **41:**475, 1928.

78. Schoefl. G.I.: Studies on inflammation. III. Growing capillaries: their structure and permeability, Virchows Arch. (Pathol. Anat.) **337**:97, 1962.

79. Trueta, R.J.: The principles and practice of war surgery, ed. 3, London, 1946, Hamish Hamilton, Ltd.

80. Wilhelm, D.L.: Regeneration of tracheal epithelium, J. Pathol. Bacteriol. **65**:543, 1953.

81. Wilhelm, D.L.: Regeneration of tracheal epithelium in vitamin-A–deficient rats, J. Pathol. Bacteriol. **67**:361, 1954.

82. Willis, R.A.: In King, E.S.J., Lowe, T.E., and Cox, L.B., editors: Studies in pathology, Melbourne, 1950, Melbourne University Press.

83. Young, J.Z.: Functional repair of nervous tissue, Physiol. Rev. **22**:318, 1942.

CHAPTER 3 Cell Injury and Errors of Metabolism

DANTE G. SCARPELLI
MASAHIRO CHIGA

The study of morphologic and functional reactions of cells and tissues to various types of injurious agents forms the basis on which our fundamental knowledge of disease rests. In recent years such studies have increasingly emphasized molecular mechanisms and their correlation with morphologic changes, an approach that has been termed molecular pathology. Cells are complex units in which vital processes occur continuously and whose "normal" function depends on the fine integration of numerous intracellular metabolic reactions. Injury occurs when noxious chemical, physical, or biologic elements in the environment alter these processes to the extent that cells lose their capacity to generate energy, mediate transport of small molecules of biologic importance such as electrolytes, glucose, and amino acids, and finally synthesize vital macromolecules and cell membranes. A few of the more common elements in the environment that are known to cause cell injury in humans are classified and listed below. In recent years our environment has been fouled by an increasing number of chemical toxicants, many of which are man made. Elements in the environment capable of causing cell injury in humans include the following:

Chemical
  Chlorinated hydrocarbons and other industrial compounds
  Heavy metal compounds
  Ethyl alcohol
  Aflatoxins and other natural products
  Nitrites and other food additives
Physical
  Mechanical trauma
  Ultraviolet light
  Ionizing radiation
  Heat
  Cold
Biologic
  Bacteria
  Fungi
  Viruses

With the advent of cell biology and, in particular, molecular genetics, knowledge of metabolic disturbances that are genetically predetermined has blossomed. Diseases attributable to errors of gene function are included in this chapter because they are both a form of cell injury and, as they are expressed, ultimately a cause of cell injury. Whenever possible, one must approach the study of cell injury by correlating structural with functional alterations of the cell and by describing these in the terms of modern biology and biochemistry. Such an approach must in part be an intuitive reconstruction and synthesis of events because of considerable gaps in our current state of knowledge, but it should be pursued because such exercises will prepare the student for the practice of modern medicine, which increasingly depends on a firm understanding and correlation of cell biology, biochemistry, microbiology, and cell physiology with the clinical sciences.

CELL CONTROL MECHANISMS AND HOMEOSTASIS

Cells exist in an *external milieu* that requires virtually continuous work against chemical gradients with the expenditure of energy so that they can maintain close regulation of their internal environment. Thus, cell control systems are of vital importance for optimal function and survival of cells.

Points of control of cell metabolism exist throughout the various compartments of the cell and at different levels of structural organization. These range from the interaction of free molecules in the cell sap, which apparently do not require spatial or oriented relationships, to highly ordered arrays of macromolecules embedded in cell membranes, where function and structures are intimately interrelated. In the case of unbound catalytic molecules such as those involved in glycolysis, organization and coordination of multisequential reactions are afforded solely by their *chemical* specificity for a particular substrate. Thus the product of one reaction can continue along a particular metabolic pathway by virtue of its specificity for the next enzyme in the sequence. Contrast this with the citric acid cycle enzymes, many of which are physically embedded in the inner membrane of mitochondria. The distances between one enzyme and the next, as well as other components of the respiratory chain, are sufficiently close to facilitate movement of electrons produced by oxidation along the chain, and control can also be accomplished by regulating the *amounts* of enzymes and other macromolecules synthesized by cells.[105] The means by which control is effected by regulating the amount of an enzyme is so obvious that it need not be discussed further. Regulation of metabolism by synthesis of various molecular forms (isoenzymes) of the same enzyme is a more complex mechanism. An excellent example is the stimulation of glycolysis in mammalian liver by insulin, in which a special isoenzyme of pyruvate kinase, so-called liver pyruvate kinase, is synthesized. This enzyme possesses catalytic and regulatory properties that are better able to meet the increased demand for glycolysis imposed by a high-carbohydrate diet than is another form of pyruvate kinase

also present in liver, muscle, brain, heart, and other tissues that is less responsive to insulin.[98] Another example of hormone-mediated control of metabolism involves the stimulation of glycogenolysis by epinephrine in which the hormone simultaneously exerts different effects, namely inhibition of glycogen synthetase and activation of gluconeogenesis. Such regulation is modulated by a variety of environmental factors, notable among which is the concentration of specific substrates and certain hormones. This means of control is necessarily slow, because it involves protein synthesis, and coarse, because it precludes fine adjustments of metabolism. On the other hand, modulation of the activity of enzyme molecules offers both a rapid response and a fine degree of regulation, which allow cells to effect smooth metabolic control. Such modulation can be achieved by conformational changes in the enzyme protein molecule, termed allosteric regulation,[69] in which the enzyme-substrate affinity is altered. Slight changes in the enzyme-substrate affinity can result in significant alterations in the rate of catalysis.[3,87]

At the highest level of organization, metabolic control

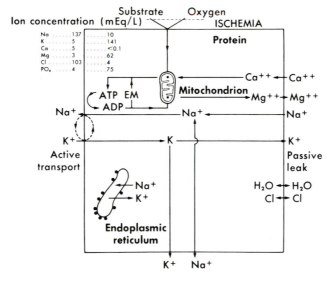

Fig. 3-1. Diagram of various factors responsible for control of cell volume. High intracellular concentration of protein requires continuous active pumping of ions (largely sodium and potassium ions) and passive outward diffusion of water to counteract the tendency for water to enter cells because intracellular osmolality is higher than that in the extracellular space. Control is mediated by vectorial transport enzymes associated with cell membranes, particularly the plasma membrane, that are driven by dephosphorylation of high-energy compounds such as adenosine triphosphate (ATP). *Upper left,* Extracellular and intracellular concentrations of various ions in "normal" cells are shown; maintenance of the intracellular concentration of various ions requires expenditure of considerable work against a chemical gradient. Energy in the form of ATP is supplied by aerobic glycolysis and mitochondrial phosphorylation (oxidative phosphorylation). The latter reaction or reactions are highly sensitive to alterations of substrate and oxygen concentration and are interrupted by ischemia. When the pump is effective, it pumps sodium ions at a rate to balance their entry into the cell by passive leak, which in turn regulates inward passive diffusion of water and thus the cell volume. Note that active transport of sodium and potassium ions also occurs in intracellular membrane systems such as endoplasmic reticulum. *EM,* Embden-Meyerhof pathway. (From Scarpelli, D., and Trump, B.F.: Cell injury, Bethesda, Md., 1974, Universities Associated for Research and Education in Pathology, Inc.)

depends on the functional integrity of the various membranes and compartments of the cell,[91] such as the plasma membrane, endoplasmic reticulum, Golgi complex, mitochondria, lysosomes, peroxisomes, nuclear membrane, chromatin, nucleoplasm, and nucleolus. These regulate the types and amounts of substances that enter the cells, their metabolic interactions (synthetic or catabolic), intracellular incorporation, transport, concentration and storage of synthesized products (secretory granules), and finally export. Membrane-bound and unbound cytoplasmic receptors capable of recognizing a variety of hormones and other molecules by specific binding of high affinity represent a major mechanism by which cell function, including cell-cell interaction, is regulated and integrated. The foregoing summary emphasizes the extent to which normal control of cell metabolism and function are closely dependent on molecular, supramolecular, and anatomic levels of cell structure.

A cell's capacity rapidly and effectively to regulate its internal environment and function in order to adapt to a variety of external environments is a property that has obvious selective advantages. The fine regulation of cell volume depends on the continuous function of active transport systems for a variety of ions. The ionic composition and protein concentration of the cell interior differ greatly from those of the extracellular fluid. These differences in ion and protein concentration would lead to a passive diffusion of water into the cell, which would be considerable if unopposed by active transport of sodium ions into the extracellular fluid and intracellular uptake of potassium ions by the adenosine triphosphatase (ATPase)–sodium pump in the plasma membrane (Fig. 3-1). Only by continuous chemical work and expenditure of energy is the cell prevented from reaching the Gibbs-Donnan equilibrium in which ingress of water into the cell would lead to massive cell swelling and eventual death.

CELL INJURY AND DEATH

The remarkable and brilliant intuitive insight of Rudolph Virchow, a German pathologist whose treatise *Cellular Pathology*, published in 1855, revolutionized the scientific basis of medicine, is revealed in the following excerpt from his writings: "All diseases are in the last analysis reducible to disturbances, either active or passive, of large groups of living units whose functional capacity is altered in accordance with the state of their molecular composition and is thus dependent on physical and chemical changes of their contents."[103] This statement presaged by some 50 years the wealth of scientific developments in the biology of medicine that began in the early 1900s and continues at an ever increasing pace. With our current state of knowledge concerning the biology of disease, terms such as "degeneration" to denote progressive deterioration of cells or "infiltration" to

describe intracellular or extracellular accumulations of normal or abnormal substances are of little more than historical interest and should not be used. The various responses of cells to injury are being increasingly described in the more precise and quantitative terms of modern biology.

Cellular reactions to injury vary depending on the type, duration, and severity of damage (Fig. 3-2). The response can range from a minimal and reversible disturbance of cell volume to massive irreversible swelling with a concomitant loss of cell function, followed by death.[101] When injury develops rapidly, it is conventionally referred to as "acute." The factor or factors that ultimately determine whether a cell will survive or succumb after injury remain to be unequivocally established. Irreversibility is probably attributable to the effect of the loss of a number of vital functions coupled with increased degradation of intracellular components. Recent studies indicate that in the early stages of cell injury there are significant losses of phospholipids from cell membranes. This leads to functional alterations of the cell, possibly resulting from activation of intracellular phospholipases.[11] Clearly the impaired capacity to generate adenosine triphosphate (ATP) and synthesize protein is insufficient to cause death of liver cells. Experimental studies have shown that hepatocytes faced with such dire events are capable of down-modulating their functional demands, thereby decreasing their requirement for ATP generation to the extent that they can survive short periods of stress. If stress is sufficiently prolonged, cells will certainly die; perhaps this occurs when the synthesis of a certain vital molecule or molecules is sufficiently compromised that the renewal of cell substance is critically impaired. The point beyond which survival is no longer possible, aptly referred to as the "point of no return," has not been determined because we still do not know pre-

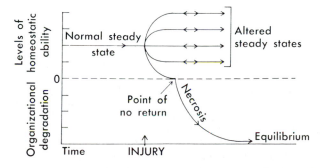

Fig. 3-2. In the "normal" steady state a cell is able to maintain a homeostasis (internal milieu) that allows optimum function. When injury occurs, the cell alters its steady state and function; if injury is sufficiently intense and protracted, it is unable to maintain its homeostasis at a level sufficient for function compatible with life, and cell death results. (From Scarpelli, D., and Trump, B.F.: Cell injury, Bethesda, Md., 1974, Universities Associated for Research and Education in Pathology, Inc.)

cisely what vital functions must be compromised before a cell dies. In less intense and prolonged forms of injury, termed "chronic," cells are able to adapt to environmental abnormalities to the extent that they are capable of augmented rather than diminished function. Cases in point are (1) the increase in cell mass (hypertrophy) of muscle cells after increased demands for work, as occurs in the heart after pathologic stress or in peripheral striated muscle of athletes as a consequence of increased physiologic stress, and (2) the enlargement of hepatocytes, accompanied by an increase in smooth-surfaced endoplasmic reticulum membranes and the associated drug-metabolizing enzyme systems, following exposure to compounds such as phenobarbital and other drugs.

The response of cells to an adverse environment is conditioned by numerous intracellular and extracellular factors. These can be classified into four broad categories: (1) extracellular and intracellular milieu, (2) pattern and degree of metabolic activity, (3) level of cell differentiation, and (4) type, amount, and expression of information contained in the genome. A brief discussion of each of these follows.

Several experimental models have demonstrated that manipulation of either the intracellular or extracellular milieu can to some degree protect cells from the deleterious effects of injury. Perfusion of isolated rat heart with a high concentration of glucose in the oxygenated perfusate sharply diminishes ischemic injury of myocardium induced subsequently by 30 minutes of perfusion with perfusate charged with nitrogen. Protection is characterized by a return of nearly normal cardiac function as well as ultrastructural integrity of myocardial cells after reperfusion with perfusate containing oxygen. Presumably protection is afforded by the glycolytic pathway's ability to generate sufficient ATP to maintain myocardial cells until they are again supplied with oxygen.[107] Intracellular acidosis appears to offer some protection to Ehrlich ascites tumor cells by stabilizing their cell membranes and delaying the membrane damage characteristic of ischemic injury.[72] However, as might be expected, this protection is limited because continued acidosis cannot be tolerated for long periods.

The pattern and degree of metabolic activity of a cell also determine to some extent its response to certain types of injury. For example, the high sensitivity of cardiac muscle cells to ischemia is largely due to their dependence on aerobic metabolism for a continuous supply of high levels of ATP required for their contractile and other functions. When ATP generation is interrupted for as short a period as 20 to 30 minutes, injury is irreversible and cardiac cell death ensues. Cells such as hepatocytes and fibroblasts appear to be somewhat more resistant to ischemic injury, since they apparently do not require such a steady and high level of ATP to survive. As mentioned previously, such cells can apparently mod-

ulate their energy requirements for extended periods and thus adapt to an adversely altered environment.

Increased resistance of the poorly differentiated neuronal cell layers of the developing infant brain to hypoxic injury, as contrasted to the increased susceptibility of differentiated neurons in the brain of growing and adult animals, including humans, is an example of the altered response to injury that differentiation confers on cells. The increased sensitivity of differentiated cells is probably related to their more complex metabolic machinery and greater dependence on oxidative metabolism than is true for less differentiated cells.

The role of the genome in determining how and to what extent a cell population will respond to an injurious agent is an area in which there is a small but growing fund of information. For example, the inability of individuals with xeroderma pigmentosum to repair injury to DNA of squamous epithelium of skin after exposure to ultraviolet light is apparently caused by a genetically determined lack of the necessary repair enzymes[12] and is probably closely related to the high incidence of skin cancer in such persons. In this case, the absence, abnormality, or inexpression of a specific bit of genetic information has made exposure to sunlight a serious hazard.

Studies of acute injury caused by a variety of noxious agents on both isolated cells and tissue have shown a striking similarity in the types and sequence of morphologic changes, regardless of the nature of the injurious agent. Some of the most impressive findings have resulted from time-lapse cinematographic phase-contrast microscopy of cells in culture[5] because these have emphasized the rapidity, variety, and extent of cytologic changes incident to injury. The initial event, occurring almost immediately after exposure of a cell to a noxious environment, is a loss of cell volume control, which is followed by a decrease in the optical density of the cytoplasm owing to intracellular swelling (hydropic change) and eventual accumulation of lipid droplets (fatty change). If the noxious agent is particularly toxic and the exposure is sufficiently prolonged to be lethal, additional alterations are seen: violent movements of the plasma membrane followed by the development of bizarre pseudopods and blebs of the plasma membrane, nuclear swelling, condensation of nuclear chromatin (pyknosis), dissolution of the nucleus (karyolysis), and finally lysis of the cell (cytolysis).

Cell death, autolysis, and necrosis

Cell death is that state in which cells are incapable of *any function*, including homeostatic control, motility, uptake of materials, synthesis, export, and reproduction. Within minutes after cell death, hydrolytic enzymes are released from lysosomes in the cytoplasm and activated by the increasingly acid pH arising from diminished or absent oxidative metabolism. Hydrolytic enzymes rapid-

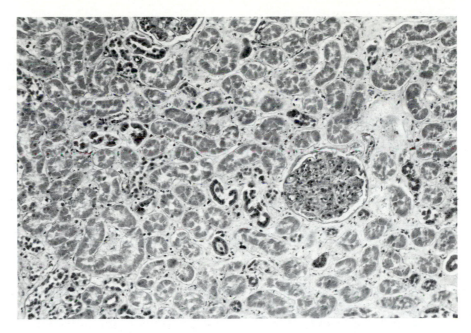

Fig. 3-3. Autolysis of kidney removed from body 72 hours after death. Epithelial cells lining the renal tubules are no longer attached to basement membrane (desquamated) and are devoid of nuclei. Absence of inflammatory cells indicates that cell death and necrosis did not occur during life of the patient.

ly degrade intracellular materials including organelles and other cell membrane systems; this process of self-digestion is referred to as *autolysis*. As autolysis proceeds, the cell cytoplasm becomes homogeneous in appearance and intensely eosinophilic. Eventually cellular details are lost and cell debris remains. The onset of autolysis is rapid in cells with a high content of hydrolytic enzymes such as those of the pancreas and gastric mucosa; intermediate in the heart, liver, and kidney; and slow in fibroblasts, which have relatively few lysosomes and a corresponding low level of hydrolytic enzymes. When focal death and autolysis of a tissue occur in a living body, the process is referred to as *necrosis;* since the focus rapidly incites activation of body cellular defenses, it is quickly surrounded by inflammatory cells. Autolysis of normal tissues in a dead body, termed postmortem change, can be distinguished from autolysis in the living body by the fact that the former is diffuse rather than focal and does not invoke an inflammatory reaction (Fig. 3-3). When sufficiently advanced, both autolysis and necrosis result in softening and eventual liquefaction of tissues.

Types of necrosis

Based on the gross appearance of tissues obtained from autopsy or surgery, three different major types of necrosis have been described. Each type also has characteristic microscopic features. In *coagulation necrosis* the tissue has an opaque appearance likened to that of boiled meat and is drier than surrounding normal tissue (Fig.

3-4). This type of necrosis in humans is most frequently caused by irreversible focal injury after sudden cessation of blood flow (ischemia) in organs such as the heart, kidney, or spleen. Less common causes are potent bacterial toxins and phenol, mercurials, and other corrosive chemicals. Foci of coagulation necrosis vary in their gross appearance depending on their age. Areas of fresh coagulation necrosis are pale, firm, and slightly swollen; as it progresses, the tissue becomes more yellowish as a result of increasing numbers of inflammatory cells and softer as a result of autolysis. Foci of early coagulation necrosis contain cells that are slightly more eosinophilic than normal with little or no alteration of cellular detail. As the necrosis progresses, eosinophilia becomes intense and cells swell and undergo the changes described previously. Eventually the focus becomes infiltrated with inflammatory cells, which help to digest the dead cells, leaving residual cellular debris.

Caseation necrosis (Fig. 3-5) is a variant of coagulation necrosis encountered when cell death is attributable to certain microorganisms such as *Mycobacterium tuberculosis*. Grossly, such foci are yellowish white and sharply circumscribed from the surrounding normal tissues. The necrotic tissue is soft, granular, and friable, reminiscent of dry cheese (hence the name). The necrosis is in part attributable to the severe histotoxic effects of high–molecular weight lipoid substances present in tubercle bacilli. Because of limited growth of capillary-size blood vessels from the surrounding normal tissues into the area of necrosis, intense scarring around such foci, and inhi-

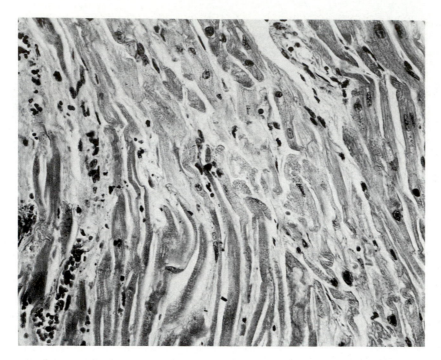

Fig. 3-4. Coagulation necrosis of cardiac muscle. Contrast deeply staining necrotic muscle fibers devoid of nuclei at lower left with more normal-appearing muscle fibers at upper right.

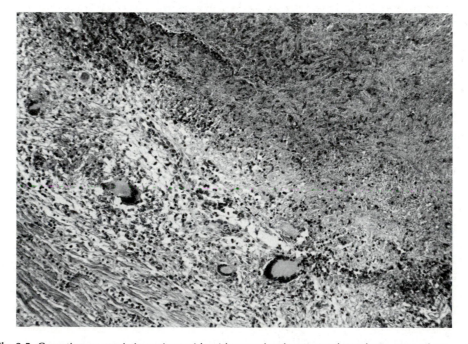

Fig. 3-5. Caseation necrosis in patient with widespread pulmonary tuberculosis; area of necrosis appears at the right with an adjacent zone of inflammation including multinucleated giant cells.

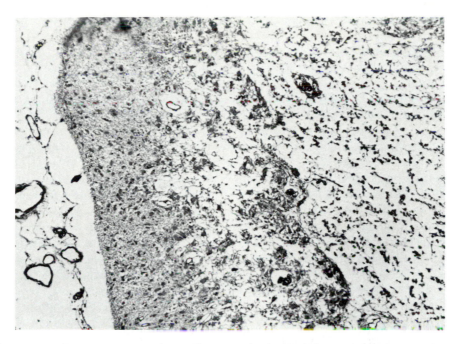

Fig. 3-6. Liquefaction necrosis in brain of patient who had had numerous cerebrovascular accidents. Liquefaction necrosis, present at right, consists of cellular debris and numerous glial cells; the cyst is limited by a thin rim of brain substance at left.

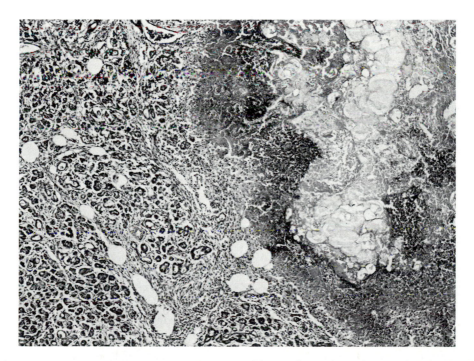

Fig. 3-7. Fat necrosis of pancreas. Necrotic area, visible at right, consists of accumulations of pale amorphous material (sodium, magnesium, and calcium salts of fatty acids).

bition of intracellular hydrolytic enzymes by certain chemical components of mycobacteria, the caseous material remains for long periods.

Liquefaction necrosis (Fig. 3-6) is the focal degradation of tissue that rapidly undergoes softening and liquefaction. It is most frequently encountered in the central nervous system after ischemic injury resulting from primary occlusion of an artery, or after massive cerebral trauma. Grossly, the necrotic area is soft and the center is liquefied. As time passes, a cystic space whose walls are defined by nonnecrotic tissue develops. Histologically, the cystic space contains necrotic cell debris, among which can be seen free glial cells containing phagocytized material, and the cyst wall is lined by a network of proliferating capillaries and numerous glial cells.

Fat necrosis (Fig. 3-7) is encountered in adipose tissue contiguous to the pancreas as a result of leakage of lipase following acute injury to pancreatic acinar tissue, most commonly from obstruction of pancreatic ducts. Grossly, fat necrosis appears as firm, minute, yellow-white deposits in peripancreatic and mesenteric adipose tissue. When the extent of pancreatic injury is severe, fat necrosis may be widespread, affecting extra-abdominal adipose tissue such as that in the anterior mediastinum and bone marrow. The necrotic foci consist of necrotic fat cells in which the triglycerides have been hydrolyzed by pancreatic lipase into fatty acids and glycerol. The fatty acids are subsequently converted into soaps (saponification) by reaction with calcium, magnesium, and sodium ions. As the concentration of calcium and magnesium soaps increases, the deposits become firmer and chalky white. Histologically, necrotic fat cells are distinguishable as pale outlines, and their cytoplasm is filled with an amorphous-appearing, faintly basophilic material (soap).

Some details of cell injury caused by chemical, physical, and biologic agents

Although the basic pattern of cellular response tends to be similar for injury caused by different types of noxious agents, there are significant variations, especially in the early stages of injury. These appear to be related to the nature of the injurious agent, including the mechanism by which it exerts its effects, its severity, and its duration. In this discussion we consider the sequential biochemical and other functional and structural changes that occur in injury caused by several chemical toxins, ischemia, ionizing radiation, and virus.

Toxic chemical injury

Toxic injury of the liver is a common outcome of ethanol abuse; exposure to certain industrial chemicals or, to a lesser extent, to therapeutic drugs or naturally occurring toxicants such as the aflatoxins may also be the cause. In this discussion we consider cell injury by carbon tetrachloride and ethanol, the former because it has been well studied and is a classic example of an industrial toxicant, and the latter because of its obvious clinical significance.

Toxic injury of liver induced by carbon tetrachloride (CCl_4) is a model system of toxic injury. Toxic injury of liver by CCl_4 and other foreign compounds is the result of their metabolic conversion by a complex of enzymes bound to membranes of the smooth-surfaced endoplasmic reticulum (SER). Action of these enzymes is the major mechanism by which toxic compounds are converted to less toxic or nontoxic ones. However, in some instances nontoxic substances are metabolized to toxic ones; such is the case for CCl_4. CCl_4 is converted by homolytic cleavage to a highly reactive haloalkane free radical and a chlorine free radical in the following reaction: $CCl_4 \rightarrow CCl_3^{\cdot} + Cl^{\cdot}$. These in turn react with a variety of intracellular molecules, notably the unsaturated fatty acids that constitute membranes and organelles. Polyenoic fatty acids, for example, are converted to organic free radicals, which in turn react with molecular oxygen to form organic peroxides. These compounds are highly unstable and decompose spontaneously to form aldehydes, ketones, and other products. Free radicals are also capable of reacting with methylene bridges to form unstable peroxides, which can also form free radicals. Finally, $CCl_3^{\cdot}$ reacts with sulfhydryl groups, which mediate the function of many cell proteins, including a number of important enzymes, and this reaction leads to their alkylation and subsequent loss of function. The free radicals formed react rapidly with other molecules to form additional free radicals; such reactions are autocatalytic and tend to spread from a small focus to involve larger areas of cytoplasm. The earliest change that has been detected in rat liver cells is a functional one that occurs 30 minutes after the intragastric administration of a single dose of 0.25 ml of CCl_4. It consists of a rapid decrease in synthesis of the export protein albumin, as well as the cytochrome c.[94,95] The liver grossly and histologically appears entirely normal; ultrastructural studies, however, indicate a slight dilatation of the cisternae of the endoplasmic reticulum (ER), suggestive of very early swelling, and dissociation of ribosomes from the ER membrane. Ultracentrifugal analysis of ribosomes from experimental animals supports the morphologic findings and demonstrates a progressive loss of 200S polysome aggregates and a concomitant increase in 54S subunits, indicating that disaggregation has occurred. The diminution of protein synthesis after CCl_4 intoxication appears to be linked to disaggregation of the polysomes and probably represents a physical disruption of their association with messenger RNA. Significantly, in this early phase of CCl_4-induced injury, mitochondria appear morphologically intact and are capable of normal oxidative phosphorylation and fatty acid oxidation among their many functions.

Within a few hours after administration of CCl_4, neu-

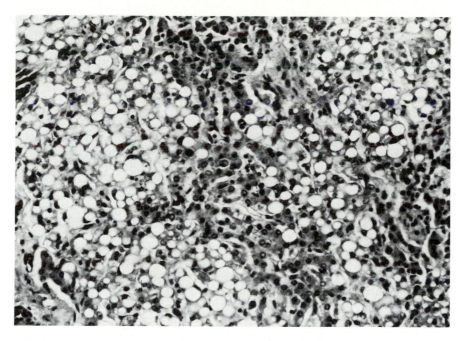

Fig. 3-8. Fatty liver in a patient after a protracted alcoholic debauch. Hepatocytes are vacuolated; these represent accumulations of neutral lipids that have been removed by lipid solvents during tissue processing.

tral lipids (triglycerides) begin to accumulate in the cytoplasm, making their first appearance as osmiophilic droplets in the ER cisternae. These coalesce to form larger droplets, which ultimately fill the entire cytoplasm. Approximately 10 to 12 hours after CCl_4 administration, the liver is grossly enlarged and pale because of accumulated fat (Fig. 3-8). This experimental model, which reproducibly leads to the development of fatty liver, has been of signal importance in elucidating one of the major pathogenetic mechanisms responsible for this condition.[59] Impairment of protein synthesis leads to a rapid diminution of lipoprotein secretion by the liver because the synthesis of the protein (lipid acceptor protein) necessary for the coupling of triglyceride to phospholipids to form lipoprotein has been interrupted (Fig. 3-9). This results in the accumulation of lipid in the form of triglycerides, since these can be secreted into the blood from the liver only as lipoproteins. Lipid can also accumulate in the liver by other mechanisms, such as by increased mobilization of free fatty acids from depot fat, as occurs in early starvation and following the excessive ingestion of ethanol such that the capacity for its metabolism and secretion by liver is exceeded, or by concomitant stimulation of synthesis and decreased oxidation of fatty acids as occurs in toxic injury by ethanol. Mitochondrial injury occurs somewhat later than that of ER and appears first as a loosening of the coupling between oxygen consumption and the esterification of adenosine diphosphate (ADP) to form ATP, which may progress to total uncoupling. The cells then undergo progressive swelling, which begins in the early phases of injury and

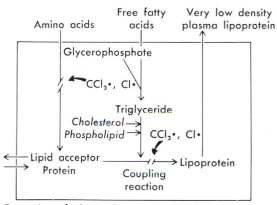

Formation of plasma lipoproteins by the hepatocyte showing sites of CCl_4 effect

Fig. 3-9. Diagram of lipid metabolism involved in development of fatty liver. (From Scarpelli, D., and Trump, B.F.: Cell injury, Bethesda, Md., 1974, Universities Associated for Research and Education in Pathology, Inc.)

becomes more severe as they lose their capacity to oppose the passive inward diffusion of sodium ions and water owing to decreased function of the plasma membrane. The swollen cells have a pale, almost clear-appearing cytoplasm and are referred to as balloon cells. At about this time, dense basophilic granules appear in the cytoplasm, becoming progressively larger as injury continues (Fig. 3-10). These have been shown to be the result of an increased influx of calcium ions from the extracellular compartment into the cells, which are in turn actively accumulated by mitochondria through an energy-dependent process.[79] Although injured mito-

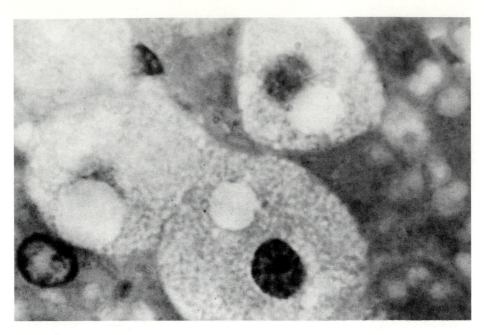

Fig. 3-10. Liver cells 8 hours after administration of CCl₄. Hepatocytes are large and swollen with a finely granular cytoplasm; clear vacuoles probably represent early accumulation of neutral lipids (triglycerides). Nuclei appear unaltered.

chondria can no longer generate ATP, they continue to actively accumulate calcium ions. A high intramitochondrial concentration of calcium ions delivers a coup de grace to mitochondria, since the ions uncouple oxidative metabolism. Ultimately calcium ions are precipitated as intramitochondrial deposits of hydroxyapatite salt. In addition to the functions just mentioned, mitochondria also lose others, among which is their capacity to oxidize fatty acids and other metabolites.

Nuclear and nucleolar injury also occurs; however, the sequence of injury is difficult to describe because structure-function relationships for these organelles are still poorly understood. Clumping and margination of nuclear chromatin may be related to sharp alterations of electrolytes and pH resulting from injury and are accompanied by impaired DNA and RNA synthesis. Thus, impaired transcription is superimposed on the previously described defects of translation. Hepatocytes may die at this time for reasons that are not entirely clear. Dead hepatocytes appear in increasing numbers, undergo necrosis (structural and chemical dissolution), and are characterized by a flocculent eosinophilic cytoplasm and a dense basophilic nucleus that becomes progressively shrunken (pyknosis), fragmented, and ultimately totally digested (karyolysis). Digestion of necrotic liver cells is due to activation of enzymes by the high hydrogen ion concentration in the cytoplasm resulting from the accumulation of lactic acid following the loss of oxidative metabolic activity. These and other metabolic alterations that characterize toxic cell injury by CCl₄ are summarized schematically in Fig. 3-11. Note how these various events are linked both chemically and temporally.

Ethanol is a less potent toxicant than CCl₄, although a single bout of excessive ingestion can induce significant functional disturbances of the liver, which subside rapidly with abstinence. Chronic ethanol abuse leads to severe hepatotoxicity and liver cell death. Although ethanol is a normal metabolite of the mammalian organism, formed both from the reduction of acetaldehyde in tissues and in the gut by bacteria, a high level of ethanol is toxic to cells. Recent evidence indicates that unmetabolized ethanol can inhibit amino acid uptake by liver cells.[81] Since ethanol is metabolized rapidly following its ingestion, attention has been focused on the cellular effects of its metabolism. Ethanol is metabolized largely in the liver via three pathways. The first and primary one involves alcohol dehydrogenase; the second, catalase; and the third, the drug-metabolizing enzyme system localized on membranes of smooth-surfaced endoplasmic reticulum (SER). All of these lead to the formation of acetaldehyde, which in turn is oxidized to acetate by acetaldehyde dehydrogenase. The overall result of sustained ethanol metabolism, which involves NAD⁺-linked oxidation in two major steps, its oxidation to acetaldehyde and subsequently to acetate and acetyl coenzyme A (CoA), is to produce an excess of intracellular NADH and a concomitant decrease in the ratio of NAD⁺ to NADH. The sustained increase in NADH leads to enhanced reduction of pyruvate to lactate, decreased gluconeogenesis, and a higher concentration of α-glycerophosphate, which in turn lead to increased esterification of fatty acids to triglycerides. It also causes inhibition of mitochondrial beta-oxidation of fatty acids and an increased synthesis of fatty acids by the coupling of eth-

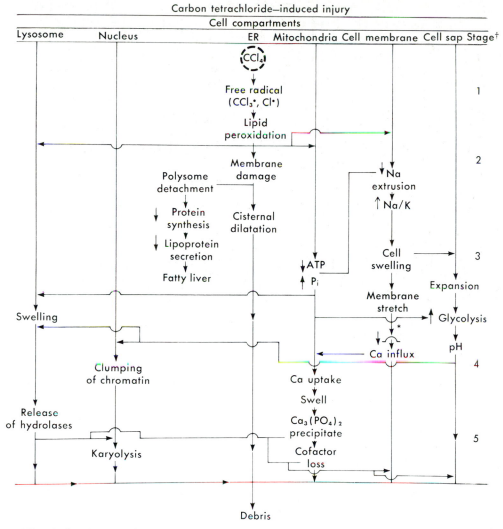

Carbon tetrachloride—induced injury

*Electrical resistance of membrane.

†Numbers at the right correspond to the temporal sequence of events.

Fig. 3-11. Flow sheet of sequential events during acute CCl_4 intoxication. (From Scarpelli, D., and Trump, B.F.: Cell injury, Bethesda, Md., 1974, Universities Associated for Research and Education in Pathology, Inc.)

anol oxidation with the oxaloacetate-malate cycle and the production of NADPH necessary for lipogenesis. These changes together are responsible for the accumulation of triglyceride in liver cells, a cardinal although not exclusive sign of alcohol-induced liver cell injury.

Chronic excessive ingestion of ethanol leads to enhanced synthesis of drug-metabolizing enzymes and membranes of SER. Such adapted hepatocytes have an increased capacity for the metabolism of ethanol and as a consequence produce excessive amounts of acetaldehyde. On the other hand, chronic ingestion of ethanol significantly impairs the capacity of liver mitochondria to oxidize acetaldehyde,[37] so that the net effect is an increased level of the metabolite in the liver and other tissues and in the blood. As a class, aldehydes are highly reactive compounds capable of a variety of chemical reac-

tions, including oxidation, reduction, addition, substitution, and polymerization. In tissue, acetaldehyde reacts with the active hydrogen atoms of the amines of protein to form cross-linking methylene bridges. It is also capable of reacting with other chemical groups of living matter such as amide, peptide, hydroxyl, carboxyl, imine, thiol, disulfide, and indole. It is not surprising, then, that acetaldehyde has been suggested as the toxic metabolite involved in ethanol toxicity. Recent studies have shown that chronic ingestion of ethanol adversely affects mitochondria by inducing decreased fluidity of their inner membranes, changes in the temperature dependence of respiration and ATPase activity,[82] and impaired mitochondrial protein synthesis.[9] In addition to the implication of acetaldehyde in ethanol toxicity, there is increasing evidence that free radicals causing lipid peroxidation of cell membranes may be involved. Some of these effects are no doubt responsible for the toxic injury and cell death in the liver and in some cases other organs, such as the heart and brain, in chronic alcoholic patients. Whatever the mechanisms responsible for ethanol toxicity, it should be clear that continued abuse of ethanol leads to serious disease and eventual death.

Ischemic injury

Injury resulting from ischemia differs considerably from that caused by chemical toxicants in both the initial focus of dysfunction and the general sequence of events, especially in the early phases of injury. Ischemic injury and subsequent death are all too frequently encountered in clinical medicine. They occur when the vascular supply of an organ is interrupted by spontaneous formation of an occluding blood clot or thrombus, a process discussed in Chapter 4. Ischemic injury has been studied most profitably in two experimental models, the heart and the kidney, in which the blood supply has been suddenly interrupted by ligation of the coronary arteries or the renal artery, respectively. The heart is the simpler of the two models because of its less complex blood supply, and it has been studied much more extensively. Experimental ischemia of the heart induced by arterial ligation is characterized initially by a number of functional changes that are followed by morphologic ones.[44,45] The earliest gross change occurs within a few beats after liga-

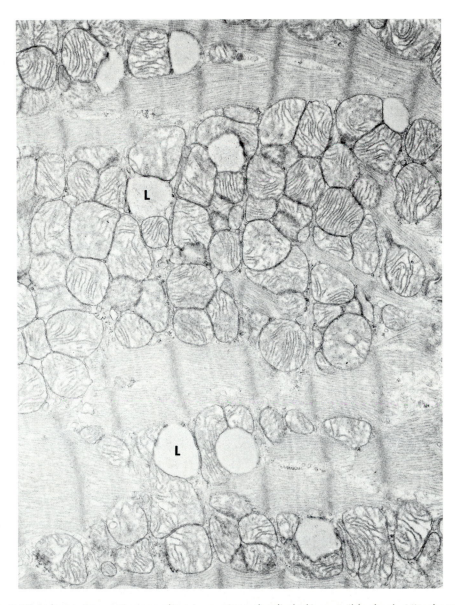

Fig. 3-12. Ischemic injury of myocardium in a patient who died of irreversible shock. Mitochondria are swollen, and numerous droplets of neutral lipid *(L)* are present. (From Scarpelli, D., and Trump, B.F.: Cell injury, Bethesda, Md., 1974, Universities Associated for Research and Education in Pathology, Inc.)

tion; the myocardium becomes cyanotic and ceases to contract, so that the ischemic focus bulges passively with each contraction. This is thought to be due to either depletion of the small pool of ATP that shuttles Ca^{++} from the sarcoplasmic reticulum to the myofibrils and supports contraction, or to an accumulation of H^+, which displaces calcium from binding sites on the myofibrils. As soon as the oxygen supply is interrupted, mitochondrial phosphorylation diminishes rapidly, leading to depletion of creatine phosphate and ATP. This in turn stimulates phosphorylase and phosphofructokinase activity and an increase in anaerobic glycolysis. However, since no new substrate is available, this regulatory mechanism for the generation of ATP in the face of a low oxygen tension ceases in a few minutes when myocardial

stores of glycogen are depleted and low ATP levels and acidosis inhibit anaerobic glycolysis. As ATP levels continue to fall, the sodium-potassium pump ceases to function, the electrical potential of the cells decreases as Na^+, Cl^-, K^+, and water freely cross the sarcolemmal membrane, and edema ensues. The sarcoplasmic reticulum and mitochondria also fail to control the transport of ions and water, and they swell (Fig. 3-12). ATP deprivation also leads to the development of severe focal contractures of heart muscle fibers characterized by the formation of "rigor" bonds of actin and myosin. As ATP levels are almost totally depleted, the permeability of the sarcolemma increases to the point that large protein molecules, including enzymes, and other cellular components leak into the extracellular space and the cells are

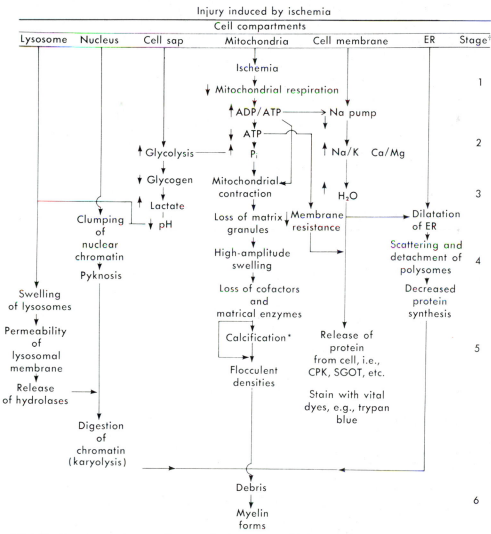

*Calcification does not generally occur in the centers of infarcts unless reflow of blood is permitted.

†Numbers at the right correspond to the temporal sequence of events.

Fig. 3-13. Flow sheet of sequential events in ischemic injury. (From Scarpelli, D., and Trump, B.F.: Cell injury, Bethesda, Md., 1974, Universities Associated for Research and Education in Pathology, Inc.)

lethally injured. Flocculent densities representing precipitated lipid and protein complexes appear in swollen mitochondria within 40 to 60 minutes after the onset of ischemia. These are morphologic evidence of irreversible injury. In contrast to toxic injury of liver, the initial salient effects of ischemic injury seem to involve energy production and ion transport by cell membranes (Fig. 3-13). As the duration of ischemic injury increases, the sequence of events tends to resemble that seen in toxic injury of liver—failure of protein synthesis, alterations of membrane structure, activation of lysosomes, and ultimately death and self-digestion.

An understanding of the events that follow the return of blood flow to ischemic myocardium is important because of the dire consequences. At the interface between ischemic and normally perfused heart muscle, return of blood to irreversibly injured myocardium induces a sudden contraction of muscle cells with a clumping of sarcomeres followed by an explosive swelling of the cells, sarcolemmal rupture, and a rapid intracellular influx of Ca^{++}, which accumulates in mitochondria as granular dense deposits of hydroxyapatite. As one would expect, these changes are accompanied by a massive loss of myoglobin and intracellular proteins including creatine kinase and other enzymes. Knowledge of these effects, coupled with the demonstration that the viability of heart muscle cells can be maintained for several hours in the absence of blood flow if high intracellular levels of ATP are preserved, has led to the methodology routinely employed in open-heart surgery. Hypothermia and stilling of the heart (cardioplegia) are used to drastically diminish energy requirements of the heart and thus conserve cellular ATP levels. The protective effects of hypothermia and cardioplegia are additive, and the early recovery of heart function appears directly related to the cellular ATP levels remaining at the end of the ischemic interval.

Disturbances in intracellular ion homeostasis

There are major differences in the early phases of cell injury depending on the nature of the insult and the target cell affected. In contrast, the later phases, in which the biochemical and structural events are similar regardless of the toxicant and cell involved, have been referred to as the final common pathway. One common thread in cell injury and death is the major disturbances in intracellular ion homeostasis that have been identified in cells lethally injured by a toxicant or by sustained ischemia. Recent evidence suggests that an abnormality in intracellular levels of Ca^{++} may be a central event in coagulation necrosis. This is based on the demonstration that cultured hepatocytes remain viable in the presence of a variety of potent chemical toxins as long as they are kept in calcium-free medium and that cell death rapidly follows exposure to Ca^{++}.[84] The lethal event has been postu-

lated to be the massive influx of Ca^{++} across the damaged plasma membrane, rather than the preexisting membrane damage. Other studies of freshly isolated hepatocytes, however, suggest that uncontrolled fluxes of other ions such as Na^+ and K^+ may be involved.[93] Although it has been known for many years that abnormally high accumulations of Ca^{++} and other ions are present in severely injured and dead cells, only recently have studies focused on the kinetics of their intracellular accumulation and the biochemical effects that follow.

Ionizing radiation

Exposure to ionizing radiation is a fact of life that has become increasingly important in the latter half of the twentieth century. In addition to natural sources of ionizing radiation in the environment over which we have little control, such as cosmic radiation, terrestrial radiation, and natural radioisotopes in our bodies, we are exposed to radiation from a variety of man-made sources, which we can control; these include diagnostic radiology, therapeutic, industrial, and fallout radiation. The physician may encounter injury from excessive exposure to ionizing radiation as a complication of intensive radiation therapy for the treatment of cancer or more rarely from industrial accidents in facilities that produce fissionable materials or generate electrical power by atomic energy.

Ionizing radiations are classified according to their physical properties into two general categories: radiations that are electromagnetic, nonparticulate, and devoid of mass and charge, and those that are particulate, have mass, and may be charged as shown in Table 3-1. The physician should be aware of the general characteristics and source of x rays, gamma rays, and beta rays and to a lesser extent of alpha rays, protons, and neutrons. This section deals with the physical and chemical events that occur in irradiated cells and ultimately lead to their injury.

The effects of ionizing radiation on cells begin with the absorption of energy by cell substance. This leads to the formation of ions when the energy is sufficient to expel external electrons from constituent atoms, causing them to become positively charged. The ejected electrons may interact with a nearby atom so that it becomes negatively charged, and thus an ion pair is formed. When x rays or gamma rays are the source of radiation, the expelled electrons are so highly energized that they give rise to multiple ion pairs before their energy is sufficiently reduced to make them incapable of displacing electrons. Alpha and beta rays may also dislodge electrons if their energy is sufficient; such electrons become secondary ionizing particles. Chemical bonds in molecules are broken when the absorbed energy is greater than that of the bond. Thus, in brief, the interaction of ionizing radiation with cell matter leads to excitation of atoms to form

Table 3-1. Various types of ionizing radiation of importance to medicine

Type	Mass	Charge	Description	Tissue penetration
X rays	None	None	Electromagnetic and nonparticulate	High (ft)
Gamma (γ) rays	None	None		High (ft)
Beta (β) rays (particles)	1/1836	Either + or −	Charged electrons	Low (mm-cm)
Alpha (α) rays	4	+2	Ionized helium atoms	Very low (< mm)
Protons	1	+1	Hydrogen nuclei	Intermediate between α and β
Neutrons	1	None	Neutrons	High (ft)

ions,[53] resulting in a series of localized physicochemical perturbations in the cell.

Studies of the radiochemistry of water have been of salient importance in elucidating the reactions that probably occur in irradiated cells. Cell substance is a dilute complex mixture of proteins, carbohydrates, and lipids, present either in aqueous solution or in suspension. Water, the major component of cell substance, absorbs energy from ionizing radiation to a greater extent than do solute molecules, which are more infrequent. The interaction of ionizing radiation with water leads to the formation of ionized water molecules, H_2O^+ and H_2^-, which dissociate to form the free radicals $H^{\cdot}$ and $OH^{\cdot}$; subsequently these react with each other, with water molecules, with their own reaction products, and finally with other substances in the cell, including organic molecules.[18] Interactions of free radicals with each other, their reaction products, and cell macromolecules are largely dependent on their volume concentration, that is, how closely together the free radicals are formed.[15] As the energy transfer from ionizing radiation to surrounding matter in a given volume increases, the number of free radicals formed and the ensuing interactions also increase. Various types of ionizing radiation differ in the amounts of energy they lose as they pass through matter; this property is referred to as linear energy transfer (LET). Highly penetrating gamma rays, for example, have a low LET; they lose their energy over a long distance and thus generate a very low ion concentration. Conversely, radiations with low penetration such as alpha rays have a high LET and generate a high ion concentration. X rays and beta rays or particles have intermediate LET values and generate moderate ion concentrations. H_2O^+ and H_2O^- are unstable ions that dissociate in about 10^{-16} second; the resultant free radicals react with nearby molecules in about 10^{-5} second.[4] These various reactions are summarized in Table 3-2.

Irradiation of deaerated solutions of simple organic molecules leads to their decomposition, a reaction that may also occur in irradiated cells. The decomposition of the amino acid glycine in irradiated water, for example, is as follows:

Table 3-2. Summary of various reactions that occur during the irradiation of water molecules

Initial reactions	$H_2O \longrightarrow$	$H_2O^+ + e^-$
	$H_2O^+ \longrightarrow$	$H^+ + OH^{\cdot}$
	$e^- + H_2O \longrightarrow$	H_2O^-
	$H_2O^- \longrightarrow$	$H^{\cdot} + OH^-$
Reactions of free radicals	$H^{\cdot} + OH^{\cdot} \longrightarrow$	H_2O
	$H^{\cdot} + H^{\cdot} \longrightarrow$	H_2
	$OH^{\cdot} + OH^{\cdot} \longrightarrow$	H_2O_2
Reactions with reaction products	$H_2O_2 + OH^{\cdot} \longrightarrow$	$HO_2^{\cdot} + H_2O$
	$HO_2^{\cdot} + HO_2^{\cdot} \longrightarrow$	$H_2O_2 + O_2$
	$HO_2^{\cdot} + OH^{\cdot} \longrightarrow$	$H_2O_2 + O_2$
Reactions with organic molecules	$HO_2^{\cdot} + RH \longrightarrow$	$R^{\cdot} + H_2O_2$
	$RH + HO_2^{\cdot} \longrightarrow$	$RO^{\cdot} + H_2O$

$$OH^{\cdot} + {}^+NH_3CH_2COO^- \rightarrow OHCH_2COO^- + NH_3^+$$
$$NH_3^+ + H_2O \rightarrow NH_4^+ + OH^{\cdot}$$

Irradiation of proteins, including enzymes, leads to their denaturation through attack on their peptide linkages and oxidation of sulfhydryl groups to disulfide bonds; the latter reaction appears to be enhanced by the presence of oxygen dissolved in the water. Ionizing radiation rapidly depolymerizes DNA and decreases its viscosity; in addition, chemical changes occur because of the rupture of glycoside and phosphate ester linkages and the ring opening of heterocyclic bases.[86]

High doses of ionizing radiation rapidly induce cell injury characterized by swelling and vacuolization of the cytoplasm, rupture of the nucleus and nucleolus, pyknosis, karyorrhexis (nuclear fragmentation), karyolysis, and cytolysis. These changes are of course identical to those seen in any acutely injured cell and must be considered nonspecific reactions to injury. Elegant experiments with amphibian eggs have shown that injection of minute amounts of cytoplasm from previously irradiated cells into nonirradiated ones promptly induces nuclear injury. These experiments also demonstrated that nuclei freed of cytoplasm by microdissection are very radioresistant, withstanding dose levels of x irradiation as high as 30,000 roentgens (R), whereas nuclei surrounded by cytoplasm in cells are injured by a dose of only 3000 R, suggesting that toxic substances that promote radiation injury arise in irradiated cytoplasm.[26] These experiments also point out that at least part of the injury induced by irradiation must be indirect in nature; that is, the injury must be mediated through chemical alterations of the cytoplasm that secondarily affect the nucleus. In view of the extremely short half-life of ions and free radicals and the short life of hydrogen peroxide at body temperature, it is doubtful that these can be implicated in injury induced by injection of cytoplasm from irradiated cells into normal cells. Radiobiologists have also postulated that cell injury can be caused by a "direct" effect of ionizing radiation in which the radiation effect is localized totally to the smallest structural unit in the cell. Considering the diffuse nature of the physical interaction of ionizing radiation with matter and the complexity of biologic organization of cells, it seems fruitless to attempt to explain the mechanism(s) of injury induced by ionizing radiation in this manner.

The most thoroughly studied effects of ionizing radiations on cells are those that are localized in the nucleus and more especially the chromosomes. This is so because it became apparent to the early workers in radiobiology that these organelles were altered by very small doses of radiation and that the changes were readily detectable by light microscopy. All phases of the cell cycle can be affected by ionizing radiation, depending on the intensity and duration of exposure. Sensitivity of the cell appears to be greatest in G_2, that phase of the cycle just preceding mitosis (M); irradiation during this phase leads to a temporary block and retards the onset of cell division. Irradiation during mitosis induces chromosome aberrations, which differ depending on when exposure occurred. Exposure during or after metaphase and before S phase when DNA is synthesized induces lesions of the whole chromosome that become apparent at the first mitotic division *after* exposure. These lesions consist of breaks in the continuity of chromosomes, which may remain broken (deletion) or may be rejoined (repair). The rejoining may be such that no visible lesion is apparent, or it may be grossly abnormal if different broken ends are rejoined, leading to a so-called exchange. If, on the other hand, exposure to irradiation occurs late in the S phase, or early in G_2, after the chromosomes have doubled, the lesions involve one of a pair of chromatids of the replicated chromosomes. Chromatid lesions range from simple breaks to complex rejoining of various fragments, which may be symmetric or asymmetric. Chromosome lesions may lead to mutations because of structural changes in the purine and pyrimidine bases. These may result from the formation of hydrogen bonds between two bases after ionization or from the deletion of bases as a result of their interaction with free radicals. Such "errors" are replicated, and the functional disturbance, which more often than not is a negative one such as the deletion of an enzyme, is perpetuated in the daughter cells. If the mutation involves the deletion of a critical function or functions, it may be lethal. One of the most dreaded complications of mutation is the transformation of a previously normal cell to a malignant one. Radiation-induced damage of chromosomes becomes especially apparent morphologically during the metaphase, anaphase, and telophase stages of mitosis when their movements in the cytoplasm are more pronounced. Lesions at these latter stages consist of so-called lagging chromosomes where whole or fragments of chromosomes bridge the gap between the two separated masses of chromosomes. These are believed to be attributable to an increased stickiness of the chromosomes, a view consonant with the fact mentioned earlier that DNA is depolymerized by ionizing radiation. Aberrant movement of chromosomes may also be attributable to radiation-induced injury to the microtubules of the mitotic spindle, especially at the centromeres where they are attached to the chromosomes. This injury probably involves denaturation of tubulin, the major protein component of microtubules. Exposure of cells to ionizing radiation in the G_1 phase immediately after mitosis or in the S phase leads to a temporary inhibition of DNA synthesis. Such cells eventually enter the S phase and synthesize DNA even when they are exposed to high doses of radiation. Thus, cell injury after irradiation is manifest at one or more of the following levels of biologic organization: structural damage to its DNA; breaks in the continuity of the chromosome, the organelle responsible for replication and transmission of genetic material; and finally denaturation of the proteins of the spindle, the organelle involved in distribution of genetic material to daughter cells.

As a result of inhibition of mitosis and DNA synthesis and premature cell death after irradiation of a cell population, there is a rapid decline in the number of cells that are in mitosis at any given time. The extent and duration of the overall effect are dependent on the dose of irradiation. A classic series of experiments,[77] studying the ability of single HeLa cells in culture to replicate and form clones after exposure to x irradiation as a biologic index of radiation effect, showed that mammalian cells respond in one of three ways. Irradiated single cells that cannot proliferate to give rise to colonies capable of continued growth die, survive as single cells, or undergo a limited number of mitotic divisions (abortive colonies) and develop into cells that eventually become giant cells (Fig. 3-14). These reactions appear to be dose related. The average number of cells in an abortive colony varies inversely with the dose; the number of giant cells appears to vary directly with the dose. In abortive colonies the mitotic rate is reduced in direct proportion to the dose. Such studies have important clinical relevance because they form a basis for rational approaches to radiotherapy.

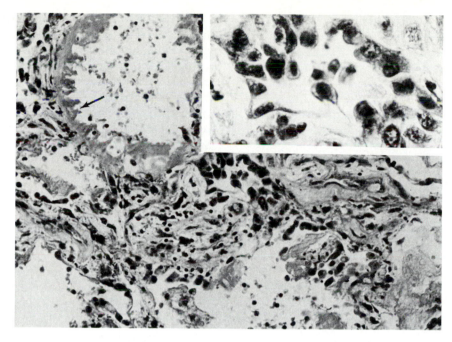

Fig. 3-14. Radiation-induced giant cells in the lung of patient who received radiation therapy for disseminated cancer. Note fibrin deposits resulting from increased vascular permeability *(arrow)* and the cluster of large deeply staining cells *(center)*, which are much larger than other cells in the lung. *Inset,* At higher magnification these appear to be giant cells with large basophilic nuclei probably derived from pneumocytes.

Virus

Viruses are a class of infectious particles that are obligate intracellular parasites. They consist of a core of either DNA or RNA surrounded by a protein coat that both protects the core and facilitates its entry into a host cell. In view of the large number of viruses and the numerous variations encountered in their interactions with susceptible cells, this section is limited to a general discussion of virus–host cell interactions and a presentation of a few examples in detail.

In contrast to many other noxious agents, the interaction of virus with host cells can be modulated by numerous factors such as immune competence, tolerance, genetic variation in host susceptibility, and age and body temperature of the host. Viruses can rapidly produce irreversible and lethal injury in highly susceptible cells in an immunosuppressed host. On the other hand, if a symbiotic equilibrium is reached between the virus and host cell, persistent inapparent infection may result. In the latter instance, cell injury does not develop and virus persists. This occurs when immune tolerance is present, as in the case of the common "fever blister" caused by the DNA virus herpes labialis. The virus remains latent or occult in apparently healthy ganglion cells until it is activated to replicate,[34] giving rise to lethal cell injury of epithelial cells of the lip characterized by the blisters.

The earliest stage of interaction between virus and a sensitive host cell begins with primary attachment of viral particles to the cell surface.[19,50] The initial binding involves ionic, van der Waals' forces and hydrogen bonds. Adsorption becomes stable when sufficient complementarity exists between specific-receptor molecules on the protein coat of the virus and the cell surface. Such virus-specific receptors have been identified and studied with appropriate host cells for the myxoviruses, rhabdoviruses, and poliovirus.

Once stable adsorption has occurred, the virus is internalized by phagocytosis. The cell membrane adjacent to the virus flows around it, the invaginated membrane separates from the plasma membrane, and the vesicle moves into the cytoplasm of the virus particle. A series of complex reactions follows that ultimately uncoats the virus or virion and releases viral nucleic acid into cytoplasm. The complexity of the uncoating phenomenon appears to depend on the number of coats possessed by the virus. In vaccinia, a poxvirus that contains several coats, uncoating has been studied in detail from both a biochemical and a morphologic point of view. Within 20 minutes after phagocytosis the large (250×300 nm), brick-shaped virions begin to break down. This begins with dissolution of phospholipid of the outer coat and vacuolar membrane; since it occurs almost immediately after ingestion, it probably involves already existing hydrolytic enzymes of the host cell. The nucleoprotein core is freed from the outer coat, and approximately 1 hour later its protein coat begins to undergo digestion. This lag period is apparently the time required for synthesis of a specific proteolytic enzyme. This enzyme seems to be coded for

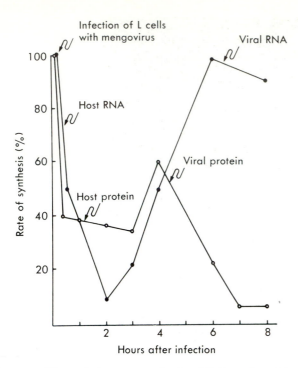

Fig. 3-15. Effect of virus on synthesis of RNA and protein by infected host cells. Synthesis of host cell RNA and protein is greatly inhibited almost immediately after infection. Return of synthesis of these macromolecules represents synthesis of viral RNA and protein by parasitized host cells. (Modified from Franklin, R.M., and Baltimore, D.: Cold Spring Harbor Symp. Quant. Biol. **27**:175, 1962.)

in the host cell genome, but its expression is continuously repressed and is derepressed only by the presence of specific viral protein made available by digestion of the core outer coat. The viral DNA that is liberated into the cytoplasm collects in pools, and information encoded in it is transcribed and translated. The truly parasitic nature of viruses becomes evident as the synthesis of vital macromolecules by the host cell is progressively inhibited while the synthetic machinery of the cell is utilized to form viral DNA and proteins (Fig. 3-15).[27] In vaccinia infection the rate and extent of inhibition of protein synthesis are more pronounced than those observed with actinomycin D, a potent antibiotic that interferes with transcription. Since inhibition of protein synthesis by virus reaches a level of about 10% of normal in 2 hours after infection, inhibition is mediated either by inactivation of host messenger RNA, which normally has a half-life of about 3 hours, or by prevention of its translation. The rate of host DNA synthesis decreases to approximately one third of normal within the first hour after infection because of virus-induced changes in host DNA, which impair its function as a template, after which viral DNA synthesis proceeds at a rate several times greater than that of the host cell. Such synthesis is mediated in the cytoplasm by a new virus-induced DNA polymerase synthesized by a specific messenger RNA copied from

viral DNA released from the virion. Vaccinia-specific thymidine kinase is also synthesized at this time. These synthetic events are closely regulated temporally by specific information encoded in the viral genome. In the case of thymidine kinase, its synthesis is terminated at the appropriate time by the synthesis of an inhibitory protein. Similar on-off controls are encoded in viral DNA for initiation and termination of synthesis of nucleic acid and protein components of the virion so that their synthesis is complete in time for final assembly of the mature virus particle. Assembly of vaccinia virus is characterized morphologically in the cytoplasm of infected cells by the appearance of membranelike structures adjacent to the pools of newly synthesized viral DNA. These subsequently form the protein coats of the immature viral particles, which in turn are surrounded by an additional coat of protein forming the brick-shaped mature virions. Pools of DNA accumulate, giving rise to large cytoplasmic structures, or "inclusion bodies," visible by light microscopy.

Multiplication of single- and double-stranded RNA viruses differs in a variety of ways. The genome of poliovirus, a small, single-stranded RNA virus, functions as messenger RNA once it has been uncoated. It is translated into a large, high–molecular weight protein, which subsequently splits into several small ones. These include the enzymes required to replicate viral RNA and capsid proteins. Replication of viral RNA begins shortly after synthesis of the appropriate polymerases. The entire cycle from formation of progeny RNA molecules to encapsidation is complete in about 30 minutes.

Double-stranded RNA viruses are modified in the phagosome after phagocytosis by partial degradation of their capsid. An RNA polymerase present in the modified viral particle transcribes information encoded in the genome into messenger RNA, which in turn is translated into viral proteins. Single-stranded messenger RNA serves as a template for synthesis of complementary RNA strands with which it associates into double-stranded RNA. At no time during these replicative and translational events does parental double-stranded RNA leave the modified particle. The partially digested capsid shell is sufficiently permeable to allow passage of the requisite amino acids for the synthesis of new viral particles.

Although the foregoing events ensure replication of virus at the expense of synthesis of host macromolecules, they do not injure the cell. This is precisely what one would expect from a nearly perfectly adapted parasite. The means by which cell injury, or a cytopathic effect,[73] is produced by virus is not altogether understood. Although viral infections significantly inhibit synthesis of vital host macromolecules, this is short lived, so that interference with the normal turnover of macromolecules necessary for cell survival is an unlikely explanation. Two facts tend to support this: first, the amount of

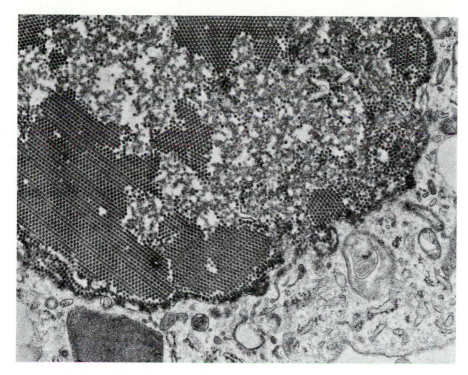

Fig. 3-16. Intranuclear inclusion of virus in a glial cell of patient with progressive multifocal leukoencephalopathy. Virions are in a tightly packed crystalline arrangement. (Courtesy Dr. Itaru Watanabe, Kansas City, Mo.)

viral components synthesized is approximately 15% of total host cell material so that a critical paucity of precursor molecules for synthesis of host molecules probably does not develop; second, in some virus infections, such as vaccinia and poliovirus, increased synthesis of host membrane phospholipids and lipids has been observed. During the course of virus replication, inclusion bodies (intracellular accumulations of virus particles) (Fig. 3-16) may reach such proportions that they make up a large percentage of the host cell volume and could conceivably interfere with normal function of cell organelles and intracellular transport to cause cell injury. A number of observations suggest that viral coat protein, especially that synthesized in the late stages of viral replication, may exert a toxic effect on host cells by increasing the permeability of lysosomal and plasma membranes through mechanisms that remain obscure. For example, it has been observed that high concentrations of vaccinia virus can rapidly injure host cells in culture. Furthermore, intravenous injections of concentrated vaccinia or mumps virus into mice cause death within 24 hours, without evidence of viral multiplication or at most with synthesis of incomplete viral particles, which in the case of vaccinia virus consist largely of the outer protein coat. Increased permeability of cell membranes develops, leading to cell injury and death by mechanisms presented in previous sections of this chapter.

Viruses can cause cell injury indirectly through medi-ation of the host immune response, rather than by a direct cytopathic effect. This mechanism has been most extensively studied in experimental infections of the central nervous system involving lymphocytic choriomeningitis[13] and more recently Theiler's, Chandipura, vesicular stomatitis,[17] and herpes simplex viruses. The latter viruses cause demyelination by mechanisms that are at present poorly understood. In recent years a number of so-called degenerative central nervous system diseases in humans have been shown to be the result of chronic infection by viruses that may also induce injury by indirect mechanisms. Indirect immune-mediated injury could be due to one or several of the following: (1) insertion of viral antigen into the plasma membrane of infected host cells; (2) presence of common antigenic determinants in viruses and host cells; (3) damage to host tissues as a result of an immune reaction occurring in their proximity. In each instance an immune response mounted by the host would lead to injury of the host's own cells, a perverse twist of a defense mechanism.

In addition to necrosis, viruses can induce fusion of an infected cell with its neighbors, ultimately leading to the formation of multinucleated giant cells, or polykaryocytes. This can be considered a nonlethal expression of cell injury. The giant cells induced in lymphoid tissue by measles virus and in other tissues by herpesvirus and Sendai virus, a parainfluenza virus that causes respiratory disease in humans, are cases in point. Augmented cell replication is another nonlethal effect of certain viruses; the pocks induced by variola (smallpox) and vaccinia (cowpox) viruses growing on the chorioallantoic membranes of chick embryos in the laboratory and on the skin of human hosts are the result of numerous focal nodular aggregations of proliferated cells. Cell proliferation is a salient feature of certain groups of DNA and RNA viruses that cause or are closely associated with neoplasms in animals and perhaps humans and that are appropriately classified as oncogenic or tumor viruses. Much experimental evidence suggests that polykaryocytosis and cell proliferation are phenomena mediated in large part by basic alterations in the structure and function of the plasma membrane, an organelle that appears to be significantly involved in both lethal and nonlethal effects of virus on host cells.

Cellular reactions to sustained sublethal injury

As pointed out previously, a fundamental property of cells is their capacity to adapt to an adverse environment, especially when the environmental alterations develop slowly and are not of sufficient intensity to be lethal, at least at their onset. Such adaptations are mediated through feedback control mechanisms that initiate and modulate structural and functional alterations to allow cell survival under adverse conditions. Cellular adaptations are a common and integral part of many disease states. In some instances it is difficult to ascertain what is a pathologic response and what represents an extreme adaptation to an excessive functional demand. It should be recalled that, in the early stages of a successful adaptive response, cells may be capable of enhanced function.

Cellular accumulations

When injury is sublethal and sustained, cells and tissues tend to accumulate substances in abnormal quantities, a phenomenon referred to as "infiltration" in the older literature. Most commonly such accumulations consist of molecules that are normally present, such as triglycerides, glycogen, calcium, uric acid, melanin, and bilirubin. In the preceding section on acute cell injury, a few examples of these were described. More uncommonly the accumulated substances are abnormal, as in amyloidosis or more rarely in diseases attributable to defective genes in which abnormal metabolites accumulate because of faulty synthetic or degradative pathways. In addition, exogenous materials such as mineral dusts, pigments, and certain heavy metals may accumulate in the cytoplasm of cells after their introduction into the body by inhalation, ingestion, or injection. In contrast to these accumulations in which the materials are distinct chemical entities, there are morphologic alterations in injured cells that are referred to collectively as *hyaline change* because of the cells' homogeneous glasslike appearance when viewed by light microscopy. Hyaline change is included in this section because it tends to involve tissues extensively and when severe appears to fill the cytoplasm; certain varieties apparently develop extracellularly.

The basic processes of ingestion, digestion, and storage of materials by cells are well known, since they are encountered at all levels of phylogeny and biologic organization.[22,23] They involve complex interactions of cell membranes with lysosomes, cytoplasmic particles that contain a spectrum of acid hydrolases capable of hydrolyzing a variety of macromolecules including nucleic acids, proteins, and carbohydrates (Fig. 3-17). Ingestion involves the inward flow of plasma membrane so that it eventually encloses either fluid (pinocytosis) or particulate material (heterophagocytosis) that is internalized in the cytoplasm although still enclosed in a membrane-limited vacuole. As the vacuole (phagosome) moves inward, its membrane fuses with that of a preexisting lysosome whereupon hydrolytic enzymes are released into the phagosome, interacting with and digesting the enclosed material. Because of the rapidity of pinocytosis, phagocytosis, phagosome movement, and fusion with lysosomes, certain types of cells may ingest and digest prodigious amounts of material. When the material is ingested in amounts so large that they exceed the capacity of lysosomes to digest them, or if the material is degraded slowly or not at all, it tends to accumulate in the cytoplasm, a condition referred to as "lysosomal overloading."

Lysosomal overloading may occur rapidly if not all the ingested material is subject to attack by digestive enzymes or more slowly, sometimes a matter of years, if only a small proportion of ingested material is undigested. Digestion of biologic material leads to the formation of soluble substances such as small peptides, amino acids, and sugars, which are reutilized by the cell. Accumulation of material may cause the organs involved to become enlarged and firm; in the case of pigments the tissues may be strikingly colored. When the storage of material is excessive, cells may be mechanically compromised and their functions may be impaired to the point that cell death occurs. Lysosomal overloading can also result from material originating within the cell (Fig. 3-18), for example, the indigestible material produced by focal cytoplasmic degradation, a process referred to as autophagy ("self-eating"). Autophagy is probably a normal cellular event responsible for the turnover of cell organelles and membranes, a sober reminder that "living" is dying.

Intracellular accumulation of glycogen, complex lipids, and carbohydrates

Pathologic accumulations of glycogen occur in the tissues of patients with diabetes mellitus in whom the normal cellular uptake of glucose is impaired. Excessive storage of glycogen is also found in genetic diseases in

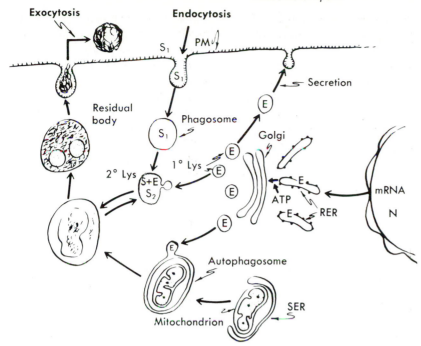

Fig. 3-17. Diagram of the lysosome system. Note the interrelationships of endocytosis, phagosomes, primary lysosomes, secretion granules, autophagosomes, and residual bodies. *E,* Acid hydrolase; *mRNA,* messenger RNA; *N,* nucleus; *PM,* plasma membrane; *RER,* rough endoplasmic reticulum; S_1, substrate; S_2, partially digested substrate; *SER,* smooth endoplasmic reticulum; *Lys,* lysosome. (From Scarpelli, D., and Trump, B.F.: Cell injury, Bethesda, Md., 1974, Universities Associated for Research and Education in Pathology, Inc.)

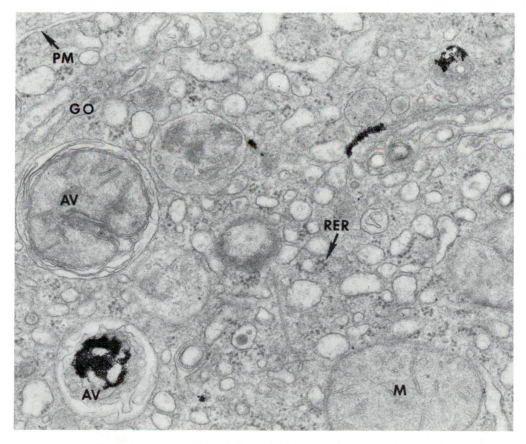

Fig. 3-18. Autophagy induced experimentally in rat liver by administration of catabolic hormone glucagon. Dense deposits represent sites of acid phosphatase activity in membranes of the Golgi apparatus at upper right. Mitochondrion is enclosed in a newly formed autophagic vacuole at middle left. Beneath it a second autophagic vacuole containing membrane arrays and exhibiting acid phosphatase activity may be seen. *AV,* Autophagic vacuoles; *GO,* Golgi apparatus; *M,* mitochondrion; *PM,* plasma membrane; *RER,* rough-surfaced endoplasmic reticulum. (From Scarpelli, D., and Trump, B.F.: Cell injury, Bethesda, Md., 1974, Universities Associated for Research and Education in Pathology, Inc.)

which there is absence of one or another of the enzymes that constitute the Embden-Meyerhof glycolytic pathway, or when an abnormally structured glycogen that cannot be degraded by glycolytic enzymes is synthesized. Intracellular accumulations of glycogen impart a vacuolated appearance to the cytoplasm. Since accumulations of glycogen resemble those of water (hydropic swelling) and fat (triglyceride), one of the following tests is necessary to establish that the deposit is glycogen: (1) application of the periodic acid–Schiff test in which glycogen is stained a reddish purple (tissues previously digested with diastase serve as negative controls) or (2) quantitative analysis of the glycogen content of affected tissues.

In diabetes mellitus, glycogen deposits are encountered in epithelium of the distal segment of the proximal convoluted renal tubules and the descending loop of Henle, hepatocytes, beta cells of pancreatic islets, and cardiac muscle. Accumulation in the kidney occurs when the degree of glycosuria leads to levels of glucose in the glomerular filtrate that exceed the rate at which glucose is reabsorbed by epithelial cells of the renal tubules (tubular mass). Massive intracellular deposits of glycogen occurring in glycogen storage disease cause affected organs such as the liver, kidney, or heart to be greatly enlarged and their function to be ultimately compromised.

Excessive intracellular deposits of lipids, glycolipids, mucolipids, and mucopolysaccharides develop in patients with genetic disorders, leading to faulty metabolism of these substances. Such patients show a variety of symptom complexes depending on the pattern and extent of organ involvement. Since the central nervous system is commonly involved, severe mental retardation and neurologic dysfunction occur in many of these diseases. In addition to accumulation of abnormal metabolites in neurons of the central nervous system, as well as parenchymal cells of the liver, kidney, and heart, cells of the reticuloendothelial system are also affected, and so massive enlargement of the spleen and to a lesser degree the lymph nodes and liver occurs. As in the other storage diseases attributable to gene defects, involvement ultimately becomes so severe that it is incompatible with life. These and similar diseases will be considered in greater detail in a subsequent section dealing with inborn errors of metabolism.

Pigments

Pigments are colored substances present in the majority of living forms, including humans, and are widely distributed in our environment both as pollutants and as artifacts of cultural practices such as smoking tobacco and tattooing the skin. Pigments are generally classified into two broad categories: (1) endogenous pigments, which are normal constituents of cells and tissues, for example, tyrosine- and tryptophan-derived pigments, such as mel-

anin, argentaffin substances, and adrenochromes; hemoproteins, which include porphyrins, hemoglobin, and hemosiderin (ferritin); and lipid-rich pigments such as lipofuscin and ceroid; and (2) exogenous pigments introduced into the body from without, such as anthracotic pigments, mineral dusts containing silica and oxides of iron, ingested iron, lead, and silver salts, and the various pigments that are used in tattoos of the skin.

Melanin. Melanin is a brown-black pigment synthesized by melanocytes from tyrosine. In humans, as in lower animals (the ink of cuttlefish and the cutaneous pigment cells of some animals), melanin serves a protective function. The skin of individuals adapted to long exposure to sunlight contains much more melanin than does the skin of those living in northern latitudes where such exposure is much less. This is believed to be an important factor in the widely differing incidences of skin cancer in these two population groups; skin cancer, which is virtually unknown among blacks, is a very common neoplasm in fair-skinned whites. Measurements of sheets of stratum corneum for their effectiveness in screening out ultraviolet light have shown that such material derived from blacks is much more effective than that from less-pigmented people.[100] Ultraviolet light, which stimulates the synthesis of melanin, is also highly absorbed by the pigment as part of the protective mechanism. In addition, since melanin's properties indicate that it is a stable free radical and that its free radical content increases after exposure to ultraviolet light, it may protect by capturing injurious free radicals formed by the action of ultraviolet light on skin.[20,63]

Melanin is formed by the oxidation of tyrosine to dihydroxyphenylalanine (dopa), a reaction catalyzed by tyrosinase, a copper-containing enzyme. Dopa is further oxidized to indole-5,6-quinone (dopachrome), which in turn is converted by oxidation-reduction to 5,6-dihydroxyindole, which is polymerized to a highly insoluble substance.

A generalized increase in skin melanin commonly occurs with continued exposure to sunlight; more rarely it is seen in individuals with Addison's disease, an adrenocortical insufficiency resulting from destruction of the adrenal cortex. The mechanism by which melanogenesis is stimulated in such cases is an interesting facet of comparative endocrinology. In the lower animals, melanin formation is under control of a polypeptide hormone called melanin-stimulating hormone (MSH), which is localized in the pars intermedia of the pituitary. Its existence has not been unequivocally established in humans, in whom melanogenesis appears to be stimulated by adrenocorticotropic hormone (ACTH). The loss of adrenocortical hormones in Addison's disease leads to a loss of feedback control of ACTH secretion so that it continues to be secreted at high levels. The melanin-stimulating properties of ACTH are no doubt related to the fact that a segment of the molecule bears a strong chemical homology to MSH through an identical amino acid sequence.

Increased melanogenesis is also seen in patients with proliferative lesions of melanocytes. The benign form includes the commonly occurring "pigmented moles" (nevi). The malignant equivalent, malignant melanoma, is a highly malignant neoplasm that invades normal tissues early and widely and that almost invariably terminates in death. Such tumors are highly pigmented because of the synthesis of excessive amounts of melanin, which may accumulate in serum and urine, making them gray to black. An interesting although less common variant is the so-called amelanotic melanoma, in which the neoplastic melanocytes have lost their capacity to produce melanin pigment because of the deletion of one or more of the enzymes necessary for its synthesis.

Albinism is an inherited disorder of melanin metabolism in which there is a decrease or absence of the pigment in the skin and choroid of the eye. It occurs in both lower animals and mammals, including humans. Careful histologic and ultrastructural studies of the skin of albinos have definitely established that, although melanocytes are present and show an essentially normal structure and complement of cell organelles, including premelanosomes, the latter are devoid of melanin. The condition may be diffuse, involving all the skin, the eyes, and the hair, or it may be localized to a certain site or sites (piebalding). Such curious distributions are attributable to the fact that the genetic defect is limited to only a specific group or groups of precursor melanocytes that migrate during embryonic development from the neural crest to peripheral sites where albinism is localized. Patients with oculocutaneous albinism have poor vision and severe photophobia. The hair is blond, often with a slight reddish cast, and the skin is exquisitely sensitive to sunlight, becoming rapidly erythematous on exposure. Chronic exposure invariably leads to the development of precancerous lesions of the skin that ultimately evolve into squamous and basal cell cancers.

A melanin-like pigment is produced in large amounts in alkaptonuria, a rare metabolic disorder involving abnormal metabolism of homogentisic acid, an intermediate product formed in the metabolism of phenylalanine and tyrosine. The metabolic block is caused by the lack of homogentisic acid oxidase, an enzyme that converts homogentisic acid to methylacetoacetic acid. The black pigment, a polymer derived from homogentisic acid, accumulates in the skin and connective tissues, especially cartilage of the nose, ears, ribs, joints, and the tendons of the hands; such pigmentation is referred to as ochronosis. The pigment also appears in perspiration and is excreted in the urine.

Pigments derived from hemoproteins. Hemoproteins constitute some of the most important normal endogenous pigments because they include hemoglobin, the cytochromes, and a variety of enzymes. Central to an understanding of disorders involving these pigments is a knowledge of the uptake, metabolism, excretion, and storage of iron. A normal adult male requires approximately 1 mg of iron per day to balance the average net loss each day through bile, sweat, minute episodic blood loss in the gut, and cell turnover in the gastrointestinal tract and skin. During periods of rapid body growth (infancy and puberty), menstrual years of women, and the last two trimesters of pregnancy, daily iron requirements are increased. Iron in food, which is in the ferric state, is reduced to the ferrous form by reducing substances present in food and is absorbed across the duodenal and jejunal mucosa. The sites of absorption merit mention because of their important function of closely regulating the uptake of iron into the body. Clinical and experimental studies suggest that some of the iron entering the mucosal cell is complexed to amino acids and transferred directly and rapidly (within 8 hours after ingestion) into the plasma. The remainder of iron is oxidized back to the ferric form and unites with a β-globulin called apoferritin to form ferritin, a compound containing about 17% to 23% iron. Ferritin is then slowly absorbed into the blood, taking several days; since it is in equilibrium with ferrous iron in the cell, its slow removal tends to maintain ferrous iron at a high saturated level. Such intracellular levels of ferrous iron inhibit further uptake of iron from the lumen of the intestine and enhance the movement of ferritin from the cell into the blood. Iron absorption is also regulated by the level of plasma iron, being increased when plasma iron is low, as in individuals with sustained blood loss or anemia. A variety of dietary factors affect iron absorption; alcohol, ascorbic acid, and fructose tend to enhance absorption, whereas phytates (plant salts), phosphates, fats, and calcium impair it. Conditions such as achlorhydria (very low levels of gastric acid) and the altered gastric mucosa associated with it also tend to diminish absorption.

Excess storage of tissue iron. Before beginning a discussion of excess iron storage in tissues, we should briefly review the transport of iron in the plasma and its relation to distribution of iron in the three types of iron-containing cells in the blood and in the plasma and tissue stores. Iron enters the plasma from tissue stores, from the intestinal mucosa as just described, and from reticuloendothelial cells, which remove and destroy effete and damaged red cells. Plasma iron then enters the bone marrow where it is used for synthesis of hemoglobin. The levels of plasma iron also depend on the synthesis, entry, and removal (turnover) of transferrin, a β-globulin that is the major iron transport protein. Iron is stored in tissues in essentially two forms: ferritin, which is not apparent with light microscopy but is visualized with electron microscopy as a tetrad aggregation of intensely electron-dense particles, and hemosiderin, which is composed of large, irregular aggregates of ferritin that are insoluble and appear as coarse, brown, cytoplasmic granules. The granules can be demonstrated to contain ferric iron because they form a deep blue product, ferric ferrocyanide, on reaction of tissue with an acid solution of potassium ferrocyanide (Prussian blue reaction). The equilibrium between storage and plasma iron depends on the degree of transferrin saturation by iron. Low plasma iron levels and reduced saturation shift the equilibrium so that iron is mobilized from stores to the plasma; when the converse is true, iron moves from plasma to tissue stores.

Hemosiderin and hemosiderosis. Local accumulations of hemosiderin (hemosiderosis) occur regularly around areas of bruising and hemorrhage and in lungs and spleen subjected to the protracted congestion that accompanies recurrent heart failure. In each instance the pigment is localized in cells of the reticuloendothelial system. In the lungs hemosiderin-laden macrophages are appropriately referred to as "heart failure cells." The pigment imparts a deep brown color to tissues and organs when it is present in high concentrations. The generalized form of this condition is most commonly encountered in patients who have received repeated blood transfusions or more rarely after prolonged parenteral administration of iron; it can also occur in patients with chronic ineffective erythropoiesis (for example, thalassemia major), presumably from increased absorption of dietary iron across the duodenal mucosa. Alcohol ingestion when carried to extremes can lead to hemosiderosis (Fig. 3-19) because of the augmentation of iron uptake by alcohol; wines, which are rich in iron, place the alcoholic in double jeopardy. In the South African Bantu there is an added interesting facet in that the alcoholic beverages are conventionally prepared in iron pots, which probably serve as an abundant source of additional dietary iron (estimated to be as high as 100 mg per day). Although iron deposition in hemosiderosis is initially limited to the reticuloendothelial system, with time the parenchymal cells of the liver, kidney, and heart are also affected and the condition becomes clinically and pathologically indistinguishable from primary hemochromatosis.

Hemochromatosis. The rare disease hemochromatosis is genetically determined by a locus on chromosome 6 with variable penetrance, the full clinical disorder having autosomal recessive inheritance. A linkage to HLA types A3, B7, and B14 has been found in kindreds. Hemochromatosis is a disorder of iron metabolism that appears in middle life (80% of cases appear after the age of 40). It is characterized clinically by the triad of pigment cirrhosis of liver, diabetes mellitus, and slate gray to bronze-colored pigmentation of the skin, which interestingly enough is caused by increased melanin deposition rather than iron. In some instances heart failure is added to the triad, attributable presumably to injury of heart muscle cells resulting from intracellular accumulation of iron. Hemochromatosis is more common in men; women presumably are protected by their periodic loss of blood by menstruation, and therefore the disease is usually manifest during the postmenopausal years. The average woman may lose between 10 and 35 g of iron through menstruation, pregnancy, and lactation during her lifetime. Approximately 50% of women with hemochromatosis have a history of scant or absent menses. The protective effect of menstruation on the development of this genetic disease is an excellent example of sex-determined modification of gene expression. Since normal function of the X chromosome is responsible for normal menses, its abnormal function, as would be expected, allows the autosomal dominant gene defect to be expressed.

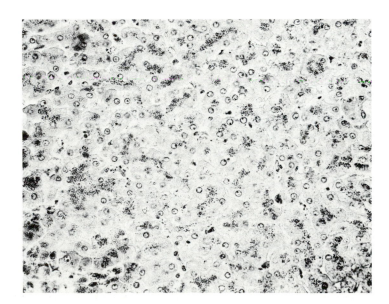

Fig. 3-19. Hemosiderosis of liver in patient with severe hemolytic anemia who required numerous blood transfusions. Note fine granular deposits of hemosiderin in cytoplasm of hepatocytes.

Liver, pancreas, spleen, heart, and in fact all other tissues contain increased amounts of iron and are brown to chocolate brown in color. Affected organs are enlarged and firm. The liver is cirrhotic with numerous nodules measuring from several millimeters to 1 cm in diameter and may contain more than 50 g of iron. Granular deposits of hemosiderin are present in the cytoplasm of affected cells; in the liver, granules are present in both hepatocytes and Kupffer cells. The basic metabolic defect in this disease is still not clear; however, results of careful clinical studies suggest some interesting possibilities. A significant abnormality that has been identified is a 10- to 20-fold increase in movement of iron from plasma to intracellular storage sites. This movement may be quantitatively as high as 20 g of iron. This finding suggests that there may be a pronounced increase in the avidity of tissues for iron.[76] A second defect in patients with hemochromatosis, which may be relevant, is the absence of the iron-binding protein gastroferrin, which has been found in gastric juice.[21] This protein has been implicated in the regulation of iron absorption from the gut. Both of these defects may have a genetic basis and may ultimately fit into the probably complex pathogenetic mechanism responsible for this disease.

Iron accumulation in tissues is common in chronic alcoholics, but alcohol consumption may occasionally help to unmask a genetic predisposition to primary hemochromatosis. In general, iron accumulation in alcoholism remains confined to the reticuloendothelial system and hepatic scarring is more prominent than tissue accumulation of iron, whereas in primary hemochromatosis the reverse is true. Occasionally, however, a precise diagnosis is difficult.

Hematin. Hematin is a brown-black pigment derived from hemoglobin. Although its precise composition has not yet been determined, it is known to contain heme iron in the ferric form. The pigment is associated most commonly with chronic malaria or a severe hemolytic crisis after transfusion of incompatible blood. It is usually found in the cytoplasm of reticuloendothelial cells. This pigment is not stained by Prussian blue despite the presence of ferric iron; this anomaly is believed to be attributable to the presence of an as yet unknown material, perhaps a protein that has formed a complex with the iron so that it is unable to react.

Bilirubin. Bilirubin is a non-iron-containing yellow pigment derived from the porphyrin ring of the heme moiety of hemoglobin as a result of red cell destruction by cells of the reticuloendothelial system. Bilirubin is essentially water insoluble and is kept in solution in blood plasma by its binding to albumin. Since it is formed normally as a result of the turnover of red cells, there is an efficient pathway in the body for its metabolic conversion and ultimate excretion.

Circulating bilirubin in plasma (normal levels range between 0.1 and 0.8 mg/dl) is removed from albumin at the surface of the hepatocyte and subsequently bound by two cytoplasmic proteins, ligandin (formerly called Y protein) and Z protein. Z protein is a fatty acid–binding protein also found in the mucosa of the small intestine. The amount of ligandin is increased by administration of phenobarbital. In the hepatocyte, bilirubin is conjugated to glucuronic acid to form the water-soluble diglucuronide. This reaction is catalyzed by glucuronyl transferase, an enzyme that is localized in the smooth endoplasmic reticulum and is one of a group of enzymes capable of modifying foreign toxic compounds by conjugation. All of these enzymes, interestingly enough, are also induced by phenobarbital. Thus the liver handles bilirubin as a potentially toxic compound. In this regard, it is significant to note that phenobarbital is used to treat patients with low levels of glucuronyl transferase enzyme attributable to a defective gene (Gilbert's disease and the Crigler-Najjar type of congenital jaundice). If, however, the defect is so severe that the enzyme is totally absent, such treatment is fruitless. Conjugated bilirubin is excreted through the biliary tract into the intestine as bile, a micellar complex of cholesterol, phospholipid, bilirubin diglucuronide, and bile salts. In the small intestine, bilirubin is changed to urobilinogen, a small amount of which is reabsorbed into the portal circulation. Most of it is excreted by the kidneys or is reduced to stercobilin in the large bowel and excreted as a brown pigment in the feces.

Jaundice is a condition in which the level of bilirubin in plasma is greater than 2 mg/dl and the skin and scleras are yellow. Clinically, jaundice is classified into three major types: hemolytic, obstructive, and hepatocellular.

Hemolytic jaundice results from an excessive breakdown of red cells in conditions such as a genetically determined primary red cell membrane defect, an immune reaction, a severe infection, circulating intravascular toxic substances causing red cell destruction (snake venoms), or transfusion of incompatible blood. Because of the amount and rapid rate of formation of bilirubin in hemolytic crises, the liver's capacity to conjugate it is exceeded, and the level of unconjugated bilirubin rises in the plasma. However, since the liver's capacity is much greater than is normally required, even massive red cell destruction does not lead to bilirubin levels in plasma higher than 5 mg/dl. Since unconjugated bilirubin is not water soluble, its concentration in plasma cannot be measured by chemical means until alcohol is added; alcohol, a lipid solvent that is miscible with water, allows the bilirubin to react with diazotized sulfanilic acid to form the red compound azobilirubin, which is then measured spectrophotometrically. This is the indirect van den Bergh test, which should be distinguished from the direct van den Bergh test in which water-soluble conjugate reacts directly with the reagent. As one would expect, in patients with hemolytic jaundice the level of unconjugated bilirubin is elevated and bilirubin-uria is not present.

Obstructive jaundice results from an obstruction of the passage of conjugated bilirubin from hepatocytes to the intestine. Clinically, this is broadly classified on the basis of the location of obstruction as (1) extrahepatic because of obstruction of the common bile duct by gallstones, carcinomas of the pancreas and the common duct, and extrinsic masses, or (2) intrahepatic because of obstruction of normal bile flow through the bile canaliculi, most commonly caused by adverse reactions to drugs such as chlorpromazine and other phenothiazine derivatives, estrogenic hormones, and the anesthetic halothane. Ultrastructural studies have demonstrated dilatation of bile canaliculi with a sharp diminution of microvilli on the secretory surface. In obstructive jaundice, bilirubin in the plasma is predominantly the conjugated diglucuronide and results in a direct van den Bergh reaction.

Hepatocellular jaundice results from failure both of hepatocytes to conjugate bilirubin and of bilirubin to pass through the liver into the intestine. Failure to conjugate may involve a primary defect in the hepatocyte because of the absence or very low levels of glucuronyl transferase, the enzyme responsible for catalyzing the reaction of uridinediphosphoglucuronic acid with bilirubin to form the diglucuronide. Jaundice in a newborn infant, after postnatal physiologic hemolysis of red cells, is attributable to functional immaturity of the infant, who has had little or no need for conjugation of foreign compounds during its intrauterine existence. Enzyme levels rise a few days after birth, and the jaundice begins to subside. In severe cases of jaundice, as in prematurity, Rh incompatibility, or infection, very high levels of bilirubin can exert a toxic effect on neurons in the basal ganglia (kernicterus). This occurs because the blood-brain barrier in newborn infants, unlike that in adults, is permeable to bilirubin. Such injury can lead to mental retardation, motor dysfunction, and muscle atrophy. Low to absent levels of glucuronyl transferase resulting from a gene defect are a much rarer occurrence. The obstructive element in hepatocellular jaundice is characterized by intrahepatic cholestasis with fine structural alterations of bile canaliculi and ductules described earlier. The dual features of impaired cell function and obstruction are reflected in the fact that high levels of both indirect- and direct-reacting bilirubin are present in the plasma, a pattern often referred to as biphasic.

The organs of patients with jaundice are deeply stained, being yellow early and becoming dark green in more protracted cases. Bilirubin is present in cells as dark mahogany brown to green droplets; in liver, bile fills the sinusoids, canaliculi, and ductules.

Because of its lipid solubility and structure, bilirubin has the potential for inducing cell injury, a fact that has been documented clinically especially in the case of ker-nicterus. However, the precise mechanism or mechanisms by which cytotoxicity occurs have not been elucidated. In the body, albumin has a significant protective effect by binding free bilirubin, a fact amply supported by experimental studies in which it was shown that albumin-bound bilirubin is nontoxic to tissue-culture cells and that albumin is capable of extracting significant amounts of cell-bound bilirubin from such cells.[16] Free bilirubin exerts two effects—uncoupling of oxidative phosphorylation and a loss of cell proteins—suggesting a primary effect on the inner membrane of mitochondria and other cell membranes, including the plasma membrane. Clearly, that one does not encounter evidence of significant cell injury in most cases of jaundice is probably the result of the protective effects of serum albumin and conjugation.

Lipofuscin. Lipofuscin is an insoluble lipid pigment present in cells of elderly individuals and those with malnutrition or a chronic wasting disease. It is a brown intracellular pigment found in hepatocytes, cardiocytes, and neurons (Fig. 3-20). It represents the accumulation of indigestible material in lysosomes after autophagy. Ingested material may accumulate when the rate of autophagy exceeds the capacity for digestion or when the membranous material that has been ingested has been chemically altered, for example, by lipid peroxidation, which would render it more difficult or impossible to degrade. Organs containing large amounts of lipofuscin are deep brown; in the heart this is referred to as brown atrophy. This condition appears to correlate directly with age[96]; however, since such pigment can also accumulate rapidly with extensive wasting, it seems prudent not to attribute its presence strictly to aging.

Mineral dusts. The presence of considerable amounts of inhaled pigmented particulate materials in the lungs of the majority of individuals, especially those in urban centers, attests to the state of the environment. The most common condition, anthracosis, is seen in the lungs of almost every adult and is most marked in smokers. Black pigment is localized subpleurally in irregular patches, in the hilar lymph nodes, and around bronchi and intrapulmonic vasculature. Microscopically, the pigment consists of coal-like dust in lymph nodes and alveolar macrophages and around capillaries and larger vessels (Fig. 3-21). Such material is apparently quite bland, since it does not appear to incite either inflammation or scarring. However, it may be accompanied by toxic substances, including polycyclic hydrocarbons, which are cytoxic and account for the deleterious effects of cigarette smoking.

Pneumoconiosis of coal workers is a serious condition encountered in anthracite coal miners. It develops over a period of years and leads to excessive deposition of black pigment in the lung. The impairment of respiratory function after the development of emphysema suggests that

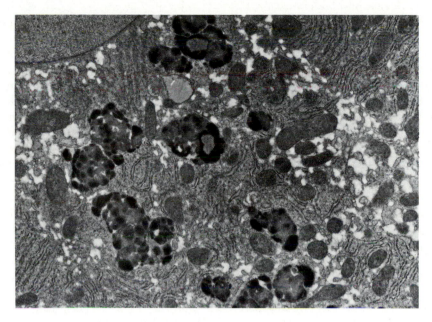

Fig. 3-20. Lipofuscin granules in liver biopsy specimens from patient with a history of drug abuse and acute hepatitis. Lipofuscin granules are the result of protracted autophagy and are synonymous with residual bodies. (Courtesy Dr. Itaru Watanabe, Kansas City, Mo.)

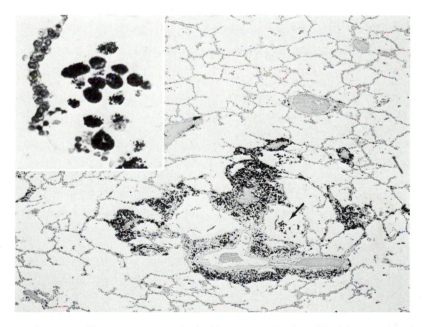

Fig. 3-21. Anthracosis of lung in a patient who had been a city dweller all his life. Particles of inhaled carbon are phagocytized by macrophages in perivascular connective tissue and desquamated pneumocytes *(arrow). Inset,* These are shown at higher magnification; carbon particles fill the entire cytoplasm and obscure nuclear detail.

the dusts causing pneumoconiosis are not identical to the common dusts responsible for anthracosis. This is a major health problem today, and much effort is being directed to elucidating the cause and understanding the pathogenetic mechanism or mechanisms responsible for this disease (see also p. 227).

Silica. Silicosis, also encountered in coal miners, is caused by fine (10 μm or smaller) silica dust particles, which after inhalation are phagocytized and carried through lymphatics to lymphoid tissues in the lung and hilar lymph nodes. Fibrosis develops in areas of tissue injury and inflammation wherever the silica particles reside. The fibrosis is quite extensive, leading to rippling pulmonary failure and right-sided heart failure. The persistence of fibrosis even when the patient has left the dust-laden environment responsible for this disease suggests that the silica already present perpetuates the development of fibrosis. The most popular theory concerning pathogenesis is based on an immune mechanism. Presumably silica dust particles react with serum proteins to form complexes, which in turn act as antigens. Although this has not been confirmed in humans, silica coated with homologous serum proteins is capable of inciting antibody formation in rabbits.[85] Furthermore, patients with silicosis have increased levels of gamma globulin (see also p. 227).[102]

Heavy metals. Long-term use of silver and gold salts for therapeutic purposes leads to their deposition in the basement membranes of skin and other tissues, causing pigmentation. At one time when silver nitrate was widely used as a disinfectant, argyria, a slate gray pigmentation of skin, was not uncommon.

Long-standing exposure to lead, usually through ingestion, gives rise to a line of black pigment on teeth at the gum line, presumably because of the formation of lead sulfide owing to the presence of hydrogen sulfide–forming bacteria.

Calcium

Abnormal deposits of calcium in injured and dead tissue are a common finding in human pathologic conditions (Fig. 3-22). Earlier, we dealt with one important mechanism for the accumulation of calcium in injured tissues: rapid influx across damaged plasma membranes and calcium uptake by injured mitochondria. Another mechanism explaining the predilection of calcium salts to localize on the walls of alveoli in lungs, basilar cytoplasm, and basement membrane of renal tubules and gastric epithelium is the secretion of acid at each of these sites, leading to local increases in hydroxyl ions, which subsequently result in precipitation of calcium ions that form calcium hydroxide $(Ca[OH]_2)$ and the mixed salt hydroxyapatite $(3\ Ca_3[PO_4]_2 \cdot Ca[OH]_2)$.

Pathologic calcification is classified into two types: dystrophic and metastatic. "Dystrophic" denotes the calcifi-

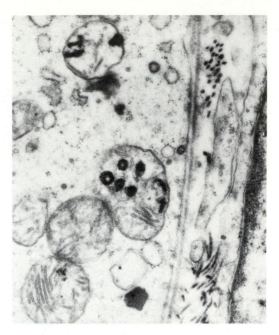

Fig. 3-22. Accumulation of calcium salt (hydroxyapatite) in mitochondria of an epithelial cell of proximal convoluted tubule in kidney of rat in which hypercalcemia was induced by high doses of vitamin D. Dense circular structures represent deposits of calcium phosphate. *Left,* Linear deposits are aligned along a crista. (From Scarpelli, D., and Trump, B.F.: Cell injury, Bethesda, Md., 1974, Universities Associated for Research and Education in Pathology, Inc.)

cation of severely injured and dead tissues. It is frequently localized in necrotic tissues. The mechanism for calcification in such instances is unclear, but it is suggested that denatured proteins preferentially bind phosphate ions, which in turn react with calcium ions to form a precipitate of calcium phosphate. "Metastatic calcification" is a term used for a condition in which mineral deposits occur in essentially normal tissues, most commonly because of persistent hypercalcemia such as that encountered in hyperparathyroidism, hypervitaminosis D, or the rapid and extensive demineralization of bone that results from the spread of cancer to bone (Fig. 3-23). Experimental studies of hypervitaminosis D in rats indicate that excessive levels of calcium accumulate in kidney only after the oxidative phosphorylative capacity of kidney mitochondria is impaired and furthermore that pathologic calcification can be accelerated by the administration of 2,4-dinitrophenol, a potent uncoupler of phosphorylation. These findings suggest that, even in so-called metastatic calcification, cell injury precedes the morphologic appearance of calcium.[83]

Urate

In mammals the purine moieties of nucleic acids and nucleotides are catabolized and appear in urine as uric acid or allantoin. In humans and other primates, uric acid

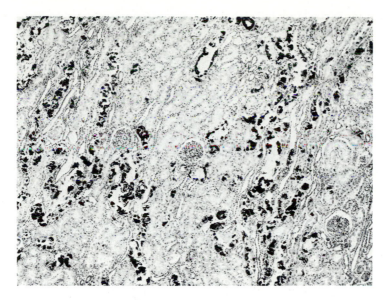

Fig. 3-23. Calcification in kidney of a patient with breast cancer that has metastasized widely to the bony skeleton. Hypercalcemia resulting from lytic bone lesions led to numerous deposits of calcium salts in epithelial cells of renal tubules.

is the major end product of purine catabolism because of the absence of urate oxidase (uricase). Other mammals have urate oxidase in the liver and excrete allantoin as the end product. Dalmation dogs, although possessing urate oxidase, excrete uric acid because of a defect in the renal tubular reabsorption of uric acid.

In humans, uric acid is present as the monosodium salt in plasma at pH 7.4. The solubility of monosodium urate in body fluid is approximately 6.4 mg/dl. The serum urate concentration is in general quite stable, the average being approximately 5 mg/dl in postpubertal males and 4.1 mg/dl in postpubertal females. Although the intake of foods rich in nucleoprotein, such as liver, thymus, pancreas, and certain fish, tends to increase the serum urate concentration and the restriction of such foods tends to reduce it, the influence of exogenous purine on the serum urate concentration is considered minor. There is a complex interrelated balance among the production of purine nucleotides, catabolism of purine-containing compounds to produce free purine, oxidation of purine to uric acid by xanthine oxidase, tubular reabsorption of urate, and finally tubular secretion of urate. Disturbances of this balance can result in hyperuricemia and deposition of sodium urate crystals in the tissues, leading to painful acute arthritis, chronic gouty arthritis, tophus formation, and nephritis.[49] Hyperuricemia is the cardinal biochemical feature of the group of clinical disorders collectively referred to as gout. Ninety-five percent of the cases occur in males.

In primary gout, hyperuricemia is attributable to gene defects leading to repeated overproduction of uric acid through increased purine biosynthesis[48] or undersecretion of uric acid by the proximal renal tubules,[80] or in some cases both. Some of these are associated with specific genetic metabolic diseases, such as type I glycogen storage disease and the Lesch-Nyhan syndrome.[55]

In secondary gout, hyperuricemia occurs as a complication of other diseases, of the administration of certain drugs, and in some instances of both. In leukemia and lymphoma, particularly after their treatment with cytotoxic antineoplastic agents, accelerated catabolism of nucleic acids after cell death results in overproduction of uric acid. Hyperuricemia is a common feature of eclampsia. Although hyperuricemia in this condition is attributable to the frequent occurrence of tissue injury and necrosis, there are probably other mechanisms involved, especially the secretion of uric acid by the kidney. Indeed, uric acid secretion is often impaired in diseased kidneys regardless of etiology. The mechanism of uric acid secretion by renal tubules is a sensitive one. It is impaired by a variety of disease states and therapeutic agents, such as the accumulation of the keto acids acetoacetate and β-hydroxybutyrate in diabetic ketoacidosis and starvation[33]; the lactic acidemia that accompanies excessive ethanol ingestion[57]; and the thiazide diuretics used in the treatment of edema in cardiac and renal failure. In some cases of secondary gout, particularly those induced by the use of diuretics, there may be a preexisting genetically determined disposition toward hyperuricemia.

Persistent hyperuricemia results in the deposition of urate in tissues, cell injury, and an inflammatory reaction. Microcrystals of monosodium urate are phagocytized by leukocytes and eventually enter lysosomes. This is followed by increased permeability of the lysosomal membrane, which leads to leakage of hydrolytic

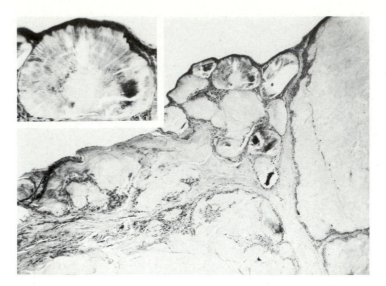

Fig. 3-24. Deposits of urate crystals in connective tissue of skin in patient with gout. Large nodular deposits are surrounded by thin strands of connective tissue with inflammatory foci. *Inset,* Higher magnification of a deposit shows radial arrays of urate crystals.

enzymes.[90,108] Since urate crystals are not degradable by lysosomal enzymes, they remain in the face of the digestion of dead cells and cellular debris. Labilization of lysosomes may play an important pathogenetic role in chronic gout, particularly in the severe damage that occurs in the joint space and articular surfaces of joints. The crystals of monosodium urate initiate an inflammatory reaction by virtue of their physical presence in the interstitial fluid and tissues. Urate crystals activate Hageman factor,[47] which in turn leads to activation of the kallikreinogen-kininogen system and ultimately increased capillary permeability. Urate crystals cause the emigration of inflammatory cells to crystalline deposits in tissues and tissue spaces by activating the complement system. The combination of these events precipitates the clinically well-known severe inflammatory reaction seen in acute bouts of gout. These are characterized by the development of hot, swollen, and very painful joints, especially those of the great toe. The most effective drug for treatment of an acute attack of gout is the plant alkaloid colchicine, which is a potent stabilizer of the lysosomal membrane and, furthermore, inhibits leukocyte motility and function by interfering with microtubules in the cytoplasm.

Continued deposition of urate results in the formation of characteristic tophi; these are firm, nodular, subcutaneous deposits of urate crystals surrounded by foreign body giant cells and fibrosis (Fig. 3-24). When such deposits are preserved by fixation of tissue in absolute alcohol, urate crystals can be demonstrated as brilliantly double refractile crystals by polarized light (birefringence). They can also be demonstrated by a silver-containing stain as brown-black crystals. Urate deposition tends to occur in relatively avascular tissues, such as cartilage, epiphyseal bone, and periarticular structures. In chronic gouty arthritis, both cartilage and subchondral bone are destroyed. Proliferation of fibrous tissue and marginal bone tissue leads finally to crippling immobilization of the joint. Urate deposits also occur in the kidney, leading to severe renal damage. Crystals of monosodium urate monohydrate are needle shaped and arranged radially in small, sheaflike clusters. Calcific material may be deposited in the matrix, rendering such deposits radiopaque. The tissues in which urate deposits commonly occur are those rich in mucopolysaccharides. Some authorities have suggested that the release of lysosomal enzymes from leukocytes may alter protein-mucopolysaccharide conjugates in connective tissues so that urates are preferentially deposited in this matrix.

Amyloid

Amyloidosis is associated with advanced aging and with a variety of chronic diseases, especially those accompanied by chronic infection and inflammation, disturbances of immune and autoimmune reactions, excessive tissue breakdown and wasting, and certain neoplasms.[70] These include chronic tuberculosis, osteomyelitis, lupus erythematosus, rheumatoid arthritis, Hodgkin's disease, multiple myeloma, and medullary carcinoma of the thyroid. More rarely amyloidosis is encountered as a primary disease that in some cases appears to have a genetic background and is familial. The most common form of this disease is the secondary type, which is systemic with involvement of multiple organs including the kidney, liver, spleen, adrenals, pancreas, and lymph nodes. Occasionally more widespread involvement including the heart, gastrointestinal tract, and blood vessels is encountered. Amyloid accumulation may in some

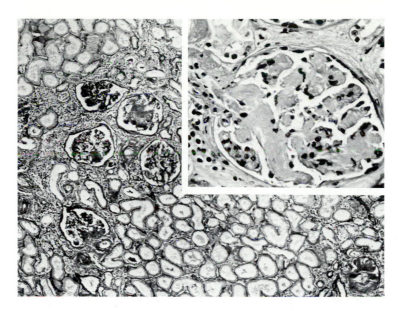

Fig. 3-25. Amyloidosis of kidney in a patient with severe long-standing infection of bone (osteo-myelitis) occurring after trauma. Amyloid deposits obliterate normal structure of glomeruli. *Inset*, Higher magnification of glomerulus shows amyloid deposited along the course of capillaries. There is a reduction in the number of nuclei and patency of capillary lumina.

cases be limited to one organ such as the heart, tongue, brain, or, in association with diabetes mellitus, the islets of Langerhans in the pancreas.

Amyloid is an amorphous, insoluble, pink-staining material deposited between cells; involved organs are pale and enlarged and have the consistency of hard rubber. More rarely, the kidney may be smaller than normal because of atrophy resulting from vascular narrowing by intramural deposits of amyloid. In the kidney, amyloid is present as homogeneous eosinophilic deposits in the mesangium of the glomerulus, the basement membrane of interstitial arteries and arterioles, and, in advanced cases, the basement membrane and peritubular tissue of renal tubules (Fig. 3-25). In the liver, deposits begin in the space of Disse between the endothelium of the sinusoids and the hepatocytes and ultimately extend to involve the entire liver lobule. Deposits in spleen are localized either to the splenic follicles where amyloid accumulates between and around individual or small groups of lymphoid cells or to the pulp where it is deposited along the basement membrane of the sinuses and between the connective tissue cells and fibers that surround them. In other organs the same general pattern of extracellular deposits pertains. As the condition worsens, the deposits enlarge to the point that entrapped cells become atrophic and ultimately die. When cell loss is excessive and the vascular supply to an organ is severely diminished, its function is compromised. Thus renal or cardiac failure is not uncommon in patients with advanced amyloidosis. Amyloid can be further identified in tissue sections by its staining reaction with the metachromatic dyes crystal violet and toluidine blue, which

impart a rose-pink coloration to the deposits, and its avid binding of Congo red dye, which stains it orange and has an intense green birefringence when viewed with polarized light. Congo red has been used clinically for the diagnosis of amyloidosis in living patients by virtue of its rapid disappearance from the blood after injection, presumably because it is bound by amyloid deposits. High-resolution electron microscopy has established that the homogeneous-appearing deposits in tissues actually consist of a meshwork of nonbranching fibrils each measuring 7.5 nm in diameter; each fiber in turn appears to be composed of a pentagonal array of protofibrils that measure 2.5 to 3.5 nm in diameter and are twisted in a plait-like fashion so that they impart periodicity to the fibril.[89] A second component contained in such deposits consists of short, ringlike structures with a pentagonal profile (P component),[6] which appears to be identical to a 9.5S α-glycoprotein normally present in serum. P component constitutes about 10% of the protein in all amyloid proteins and is periodic acid–Schiff positive. The presence of substances such as immunoglobulins, complement, and mucopolysaccharides demonstrated by immunofluorescence and histochemical staining methods, although interesting, has been interpreted by most simply as substances secondarily bound to the surface of the amyloid deposits rather than as integral components. Large masses of amyloid in glomeruli or the follicles of the spleen can be seen with the unassisted eye as pinhead-sized gray bodies.

After its initial description in 1842 by Rokitansky and subsequent studies by Virchow[103] that led to its naming a few years later, the nature of amyloid until recent years

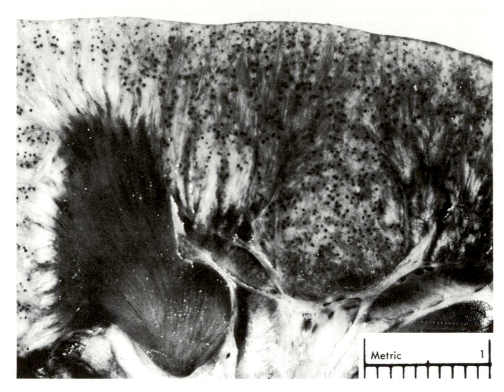

Fig. 3-26. Amyloidosis of kidney, showing glomeruli deeply stained with Lugol's solution. (Courtesy Dr. Joseph H. Davis, Miami, Fla. From Rezek, P.R., and Millard, M.: Autopsy pathology, Springfield, Ill., 1963, Charles C Thomas, Publisher.)

was a matter of considerable controversy. On the basis of its mahogany-brown staining reaction with an aqueous solution of iodine and violet coloration after subsequent exposure to dilute sulfuric acid (Fig. 3-26), Virchow was convinced that such deposits consist of a starchlike carbohydrate, hence its name. Subsequent studies a few years later by Friederich and Kekule suggested rather that amyloid was a protein. Despite these findings, it was generally accepted for many years that amyloid was a carbohydrate, although in more recent years the view was modified and some considered it a glycoprotein.

The clinical association of amyloid with diseases characterized by chronic antigenic stimulation, plasma cell proliferation, and frequently the presence of abnormal immunoglobulins in the blood and urine has long suggested that the condition is related to a protracted immune response that has gone awry.[6] Amyloid is frequently encountered in horses that have been used for 20 years or so for the commercial production of antitoxin by the pharmaceutical industry. Although the idea of an immune mechanism was supported by experimental studies showing that splenectomy prevented the development of amyloid in mice after the injection of casein[75] and that it could be induced in normal syngeneic hosts by transfer of splenic cells from animals with amyloidosis,[35] it remained largely a point of speculation rather than fact.

A major feature of amyloid that proved to be a hurdle to its definitive chemical characterization was its insolubility. The finding that amyloid could be readily solubilized in a 6 M solution of guanidine hydrochloride allowed a detailed analysis of its amino acid sequence. Solubilized amyloid fibrils have an amino acid sequence identical to that found in the amino terminal variable segment of the light chains of immunoglobulin, usually of the λ type.[32] The current view is that amyloid is a fibrillar protein with a β-pleated structure and a molecular weight ranging from 5000 to 18,000.[30] Furthermore, it was found that in contrast to native amyloid, which is nonimmunogenic, solubilized denatured amyloid is immunogenic. The resulting antisera have been used in a variety of immunochemical studies that have further established that a close relationship exists between light chains of immunoglobulin and amyloid. A feature of plasma cell myeloma that has been of assistance in furthering our knowledge of the nature of amyloid is the synthesis and secretion of immunoglobulins and their light chain subunits (Bence Jones proteins) by this tumor. On proteolytic digestion the fraction of Bence Jones protein that contains the variable portion of the light chain molecule forms fibrils with properties similar to those of amyloid.[30]

On the basis of detailed studies of the sequence of amino acids in solubilized amyloid "protein," it has become clear that amyloid is a heterogeneous spectrum of proteins.[31] At least five clearly distinct types have been identified:

1. *AL type*. The major protein component is derived from immunoglobulin.
2. *AA type*. This type is encountered in rheumatoid arthritis, tuberculosis, malaria, and familial Mediterranean fever. The major protein component has an *N*-terminal amino acid sequence differing from that of the AL type. In some cases a light chain protein of λ type has been demonstrated as well, suggesting that the immunoglobulin light chain may also be involved.
3. *Variant of AA type*. This has been found in patients with Mediterranean fever.
4. *AF₄ type*. The major protein is a polypeptide with an amino acid sequence identical to part of the hormone thyrocalcitonin and thought to represent calcitonin precursor protein.
5. *ASc type*. The major protein appears to be both chemically and immunochemically unique. This type is seen in amyloid that occasionally accumulates in the heart of patients in the eighth and ninth decades of life, giving rise to so-called senile amyloid heart disease.

It may well be that amyloid can arise from any protein that is converted to β-pleated fibrils. If this is the case, the catalog of amyloid proteins will surely increase as more cases of this disease complex are studied. Although the pathogenesis of amyloid is far from understood, it appears that one facet involves the proteolytic alteration of protein to β-pleated fibrils. Presumably, amyloid fibrils could be derived from intracellular proteolysis of either endogenous protein synthesized by β-lymphocytes or exogenous circulating protein that has undergone endocytosis by phagocytic cells. In both instances the "insoluble" fibrils would be released into the extracellular space by exocytosis. Such a scheme would be consonant with the two popularly accepted major pathogenetic mechanisms: (1) that amyloid is secreted by cells of the immune system or (2) that an amyloid precursor substance is rendered insoluble and accumulates in the extracellular compartment as a consequence of local cellular activity.

Hyaline change

The term "hyaline," derived from *hyalos*, the Greek word for glass, is used to describe a morphologic change frequently encountered within cells or in the extracellular space of diseased tissues. Hyaline is a homogeneous glasslike alteration that is stained a pale pink with the hematoxylin-eosin stain. Careful ultrastructural and chemical studies have established that hyaline change can result from the accumulation of a variety of different substances and in some instances cellular organelles. The

following types of intracellular hyaline change have been clearly established:

1. Mallory bodies are intracytoplasmic accumulations of intermediate filaments. Although their pathogenesis is not understood, the current view is that they result from a dysfunction of the cytoskeleton.[64] Mallory bodies are frequently encountered in hepatocytes injured by chronic alcohol abuse, and until recently their presence was thought to be specific for alcohol-induced injury. However, they are also seen in a wide variety of chronic diseases of the liver and must be regarded simply as a general cellular reaction to injury.
2. Hyaline droplets in the cytoplasm of epithelial cells lining the proximal portion of renal tubules represent phagolysosomes containing protein reabsorbed from the urinary fibrate. They occur in cases of excessive loss of protein in the urine (proteinuria).
3. In certain virus infections intracellular accumulations of virus particles (inclusion bodies) often appear as hyaline inclusions.
4. Russell bodies represent homogeneous deposits of immunoglobulin in the endoplasmic reticulum.

Extracellular hyaline is encountered in connective tissues in chronic diseases such as diabetes mellitus, hypertension, and rheumatoid arthritis, in foci of chronic infection, in atrophy, and in aging. Foci of hyaline change seen between connective tissue cells and collagen fibers probably represent accumulation of proteins that remain to be identified. In arterioles and medium-sized arteries of patients with diabetes mellitus, hyaline change appears to be due to excessive basement membrane material, whereas in severe hypertension such change appears to be largely the result of accumulations of plasma proteins, including fibrinogen and fibrin, which have passed across injured endothelium into the blood vessel wall. Hyaline in chronically injured renal glomeruli contains excessive basement membrane material and plasma proteins. Although some authors include amyloid as an example of hyaline change, it has been so well studied and characterized, and appears to lead to such well-defined clinical conditions, that we have described it as a separate entity.

ADAPTIVE CELL REACTIONS
Hypertrophy

The heart and kidneys respond to an increased demand for work by undergoing hypertrophic growth and have served as excellent experimental models for the study of this condition. Any sustained abnormality of the heart such as a malfunctioning valve or increased resistance of the peripheral arterial system will lead to its enlargement. Experimental studies indicate that initially the enlargement is caused by dilatation of the cardiac chambers but that this is relatively short lived and is followed by augmented synthesis of cardiac muscle proteins and subsequent physical enlargement of the muscle fibers, enabling them to perform more work. The synthetic events are apparently triggered by the stretch of muscle fibers induced by cardiac dilatation. When muscle fibers are stretched, the uptake of amino acids increases within a matter of minutes, mediated by an augmentation of transport enzymes localized in the plasma membrane.[54] (Currently this is believed to involve the sodium-potassium ATPase pump.) Shortly after this, protein and lipid synthesis is activated, followed by new formation of all the cytoplasmic components of the muscle cell, such as mitochondria, sarcoplasmic reticulum, and myofibrils.[78] Although most studies have concentrated on the pattern of augmented protein and phospholipid synthesis, the synthesis of other cellular macromolecules must also be increased.

In cardiac hypertrophy in humans, the nucleus is also hypertrophic and there appears to be augmented synthesis of DNA. Thus, even though differentiated heart muscle cells are unable to undergo mitosis, they are capable of increased DNA synthesis when appropriately stimulated. The role if any that redundant genetic material plays in the hypertrophic response is not clear. Cardiac hypertrophy is limited by the vascular supply for the delivery of substrates required for increased synthetic metabolism. Since the interstitial capillary bed does not proliferate significantly in hypertrophy, especially when it is in response to an increased work demand imposed as a consequence of a cardiovascular pathologic condition, the hypertrophic muscle fibers eventually outstrip the capillaries' capacity to supply them adequately and their growth stops. Furthermore, since hypertrophic muscle fibers have increased oxygen consumption, a marginal vascular supply dooms them to a tenuous and often short-lived existence.

Hypertrophy of the kidney after removal of the contralateral kidney deserves mention because in this situation the adaptive response to increased demand for work involves not only an increase in the size of cells of the renal tubules but also an increase in the number of cells.[62] The proliferative phase of the response consists of a brief burst of mitosis leading to about a 7% increase in the number of epithelial cells. However, since this accounts for only 25% of the increase in kidney cell mass, it represents only a minor part of the response. The major contribution to renal enlargement is hypertrophy (Fig. 3-27). The hyperplastic phase begins within an hour or so after removal of the contralateral kidney, the initial event being an increased synthesis of RNA followed rapidly by an increase in protein synthesis that plateaus at 3 hours and is sustained at this level. Synthesis of DNA does not begin until about 9 to 10 hours after nephrectomy (Fig. 3-28). Although the factors that initiate and control compensatory renal growth are not clearly

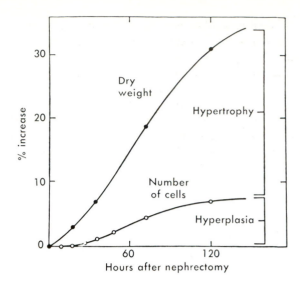

Fig. 3-27. Compensatory renal enlargement after unilateral nephrectomy is caused by hypertrophy and hyperplasia; this graph shows relative contributions of both cellular reactions. (From Johnson, H.A., and Vera-Roman, J.M.: Am. J. Pathol. 49:1, 1966.)

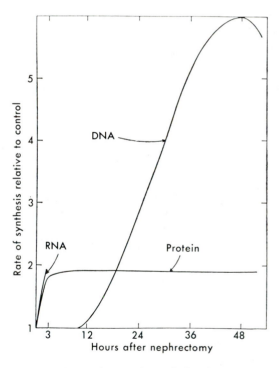

Fig. 3-28. Sequence and rate of metabolic alterations in RNA, DNA, and protein synthesis during compensatory renal enlargement after unilateral nephrectomy. (From Johnson, H.A., and Vera-Roman, J.M.: Am. J. Pathol. 49:1, 1966.)

defined, the nutritional state and age of the animal appear to be important.

At the beginning of this section, mention was made of demands on certain organs for increased work that are part of normal living and therefore must be considered as physiologic. A case in point is the augmented growth of the uterus and mammary glands in response to pregnancy. Numerous studies have established that the growth of these organs is triggered and maintained by hormones. In the uterus, smooth muscle cells bind estrogen, a receptor in the cytosol that transports the hormone into the nucleus where it interacts with nuclear DNA, ultimately activating specific genes responsible for the synthesis of smooth muscle proteins as well as other cytoplasmic components. The uterine muscle mass increases many fold so that the organ is eventually transformed into a large, saclike structure with a thick muscular wall capable of the contractions necessary to expel the fetus at the time of birth. The mammary glands also grow during pregnancy as a result of high levels of estrogen, progesterone, and prolactin. These hormones stimulate both proliferative and hypertrophic growth of the terminal ends of the mammary ducts. In addition, prolactin induces the synthesis of milk proteins. The synthesis and secretion of milk continue as long as suckling is permitted; if milk is not removed, the mammary glands become greatly distended and milk production ceases quickly.

Atrophy

In both instances just mentioned, regression of augmented physiologic growth occurs when the need for increased function is over. The degree of involution is remarkable; the term uterus with a weight of 1000 g and a wall 5 cm thick returns to its nongravid state of 100 g and a muscular wall only 0.4 cm thick in a period of 5 to 6 weeks. Changes of a similar magnitude occur in the mammary glands. Regression is characterized by macrophages that infiltrate the tissues and ingest and digest some of the augmented cell mass, an increased rate of focal self-digestion by muscle cells (autophagy),[2] and a rapid diminution of cell growth caused by an absence of the stimulating hormones as well as a decrease in the local blood supply. There is an increase in the activity of various hydrolytic enzymes in involution of the mammary gland after weaning (Fig. 3-29).[38] Secondary sex characteristics diminish as a consequence of aging or surgical ablation of the gonads. Regression of a tissue or organ because of a decrease in the size and number of cells is commonly referred to as atrophy. Atrophy also occurs in other organs such as skeletal muscle, the heart, and the central nervous system as an adaptation to a decrease in workload, use, nutrition, denervation, or blood supply. Experimental studies of muscle atrophy after denervation illustrate that a sharp lowering of oxygen consumption, amino acid uptake, and protein synthesis occurs within 15 to 24 hours. This is ultimately reflected in decreased synthesis of sarcoplasmic components such as mitochondria and myofibrillar proteins. Muscle fibers decrease in size and within several weeks are reduced to thin, ribbonlike cells. In such cells there seems to be an increased turnover of proteins. Thus denervation atrophy appears to be the net result of diminished synthesis

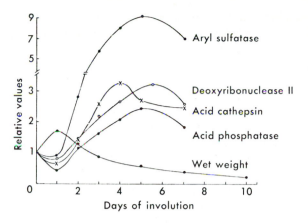

Fig. 3-29. Activity of various hydrolytic enzymes during atrophy of mammary gland after cessation of weaning. (From Woessner, F.J., Jr. In Dingle, J.T., and Fell, H.B., editors: Lysosomes in biology and medicine, vol. 1, Amsterdam, 1969, Elsevier/North-Holland Biomedical Press.)

amplified by increased breakdown of muscle protein. Since denervation of a muscle also quickly leads to a diminution of its blood supply, it is difficult to separate general effects from local cellular ones. This model is of interest to students of aging because it closely resembles the pattern of muscle atrophy in animals of advanced age.

In heart muscle and liver cells of animals that have lost considerable body weight as a result of either extended malnutrition or a debilitating chronic disease, the cytoplasm contains numerous, refractile, yellow-brown granules that are highly insoluble pigments termed "lipofuscin" or "aging pigments," the latter because they are seen with greater frequency in old individuals.[96] Ultrastructural and biochemical studies suggest that the pigment granules represent cytoplasmic foci of self-digestion, or autophagy. Focal autophagy is a common cellular reaction to sublethal injury and is a major mechanism for decremental modulation of cell size in response to an adverse environment.[2] Autophagic vacuoles arise in the cytoplasm apparently around a focus that is to be digested. Such vacuoles frequently contain mitochondria and endoplasmic reticulum and presumably are responsible for their removal by virtue of a full complement of acid hydrolases. Lipfuscin pigment is believed to arise from the presence of lipid debris that has been rendered indigestible by oxidation. Whether this is oxidation that occurs after internalization in the vacuole or lipid peroxidation as a consequence of an injurious chemical insult, or both, is not clear. In individuals with debilitating diseases, such pigment arises in part as a result of the rapid tissue breakdown that accompanies wasting.

Hyperplasia

As mentioned previously, organ growth can also be the result of an increase in the number of cells, a process called "hyperplasia." In the context of this discussion, hyperplasia as a response to injury occurs when the injury has been sufficiently severe and prolonged to have caused cell death. The loss of cells in epithelial surfaces and in liver and kidney triggers DNA synthesis, which is followed by mitosis. The means by which a loss of cells is transduced into a series of synthetic activities that culminate in cell division is not clear, but it is generally accepted that the initial event involves the plasma membrane. The phenomenon is probably closely akin to the return of proliferative growth in contact-inhibited tissue culture cells when they are trypsinized and a dilute suspension of cells is explanted to a new culture dish. Regeneration of the renal tubules after injury with mercuric chloride has shown that the proliferative response leads to an increase in the rate of DNA synthesis reflected by a shortening of the synthetic (S) phase of the cell cycle of tubular epithelial cells from the normal 12 hours to 9 hours. Increased mitoses become apparent about 20 hours after the administration of mercuric chloride and reach a peak on the third day. Proliferating epithelial cells rapidly reline the renal tubules and largely complete this stage by the fifth day. By the ninth day the mitotic index has returned to its normal preinjury level. The glomerular filtration rate drops to a low level by the fifth day and returns to normal by the ninth day. Tubular reabsorption does not return to normal levels until the twentieth day after the initial injury, indicating that considerable differentiation of the epithelial cells must occur before they are capable of effective transport.

The liver has an even greater capacity for regeneration than does the kidney and because of the greater homogeneity of its cell population has been the model of choice for studies of hyperplastic growth. Surgical removal of 75% of the liver mass leads to mitosis of hepatocytes, which peaks at about 25 to 30 hours and begins a gradual decline at 44 hours. This is followed by a second and small wave of mitosis that reaches a maximum at 56 hours and ceases at 65 hours. DNA synthesis begins 12 hours after hepatectomy and peaks at 27 hours. The mass of liver excised is totally restored by the twelfth day. In contrast to the kidney, the liver rapidly regains its normal capacity for function, suggesting that newly formed hepatocytes do not have to undergo an extensive period of differentiation to carry on the numerous synthetic, catabolic, and transport functions characteristic of the liver in adults. The extent to which liver cells respond to the perturbation of hepatectomy can be emphasized by recalling that in the normal liver in an adult less than 1% of the liver is synthesizing DNA at any one time, whereas at the peak of regeneration about 10% of the cells are in the S phase of the mitotic cycle. Epithelial cells of the kidney tubules and hepatocytes are examples of differentiated cells that are in the G_0, or resting, phase of the mitotic cycle but are capable of reentering the mitotic cycle when stimulated appropriately (Fig. 3-30).

Thus far we have limited our discussion of hyperplasia to instances of repair and regeneration. Neoplasia is a major condition in which hyperplastic growth plays a central role. Hyperplasia associated with neoplasia differs from that just described in that growth-regulatory mechanisms are lost because of a change in cellular heredity. The growth advantage of neoplastic cells operates to the disadvantage of the host because it is often accompanied by either loss or abnormality of cell func-

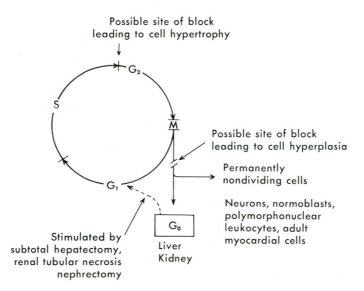

Fig. 3-30. Cell cycle showing possible sites of blocks in G_2, the period between completion of DNA synthesis and initiation of mitosis (M). Blocks in this phase lead to hypertrophy. Blocks after mitosis prevent cells from entering G_0, which leads to hyperplasia. (From Scarpelli, D., and Trump, B.F.: Cell injury, Bethesda, Md., 1974, Universities Associated for Research and Education in Pathology, Inc.)

tion and in the case of malignant tumors leads ultimately to death. In view of the previous discussion of the modes by which cell proliferation is controlled, it is of interest that both physical and chemical alterations of the cell surface have been encountered in neoplastic cells. This has been found with such regularity in a variety of both induced experimental tumors in animals and spontaneous ones in humans that such changes are believed to be an important basic characteristic of the neoplastic transformation.

ERRORS OF METABOLISM
Role of genetic factors in cell injury

Disease develops through interaction of the genetic constitution of the organism with the environment. A unique and important environment is that given the fetus by its mother. This may be unfavorably altered by the genetic constitution of the mother. For example, pregnant women with phenylketonuria may have mentally retarded offspring who are heterozygous. In these cases the fetus has suffered from exposure to the high concentration of phenylalanine, not because of its genetic constitution but because of its mother's. The role played by the genetic constitution of the individual varies from disease to disease and from patient to patient having the same disease. At one extreme the development of a disease is dependent on the patient's genetic constitution alone. At the other extreme, environmental factors solely determine the development of disease. Within this spectrum one can select the diseases in whose development genetic constitution is of major importance. Cell injury from genetic causes is similar or identical to that caused by environmental factors. Exceptions to this are diseases in which the proximate genetic expression, for example, synthesis of a specific protein, can lead to a specific alteration of cells such as sickling of red cells.

Cell injury on a genetic basis, either nonspecific or specific, is mediated by genetic effects producing disturbances in one or more of the three major components of cell homeostasis: extracellular fluid, plasma membrane, and intracellular membrane structure and metabolism. These disturbances are considered in the following.

Chromosomal abnormalities

Changes in the body associated with chromosomal abnormalities are often gross congenital malformations that have occurred during fetal development. If these were caused by cell injury, they would have occurred during the first trimester of gestation. Thus individuals with chromosomal abnormalities are unlikely to show either conspicuous or specific cell injury. Compared with diseases caused by a single gene mutation, in which a protein or enzyme abnormality occurs and about which much is known, chromosomal abnormalities are not well

understood. This is no doubt attributable to our current primitive understanding of the molecular anatomy of the chromosome and its genes and of the molecular events involved in gene expression. Similarly, it is not known how a chromosomal abnormality disturbs cell homeostasis.

Manifestations of genetic diseases and levels of biologic organization

Changes involving many genes in chromosomal abnormalities may be termed mutations, for occasionally a person with a chromosomal abnormality survives and transmits the abnormal chromosome to future generations. However, mutations affecting a single gene, which are more amenable to precise study, have been studied more extensively, and their inheritance and genetic expression are far better known. Therefore the knowledge derived from studies of single-gene mutations is more useful in the study of genetically induced cell injury, and some salient points are summarized briefly here. The manifestations (phenotype) of a genetic abnormality (genotype) can be observed at different levels of biologic organization ranging from the molecule to the population. Depending on the level of biologic organization at which the observation is made, manifestations of different genetic diseases may be indistinguishable (genocopy), or genetic effects may be indistinguishable from environmental ones (phenocopy). Observations at different levels of biologic organization modify the interpretation of inheritance. Many recessive traits that are not clinically obvious in heterozygotes are detectable when one studies the characteristics of specific proteins, for example, enzyme activity or electrophoretic mobility of a protein. Therefore, in considering cell injury, one must keep in mind various levels of phenotypic organization. These are the inheritance pattern arising from mating; clinical signs and symptoms expressed at the organismal level; classical pathologic changes at the organ, tissue, and cell levels; metabolic disturbances reflected by metabolites; abnormal proteins and enzymes; and finally abnormal genetic information at the nucleic acid level.

One gene–one enzyme concept

The pioneering effort of Sir Archibald Garrod, culminating in his monograph *Inborn Errors of Metabolism*,[29] laid the foundation for the present-day understanding of genetic diseases of humans, particularly the applicability of Mendelian genetics and the one gene–one enzyme concept, which is now modified to the one cistron–one polypeptide concept. Mutation involving a gene may be mediated by the loss of the gene and the loss of the specific protein coded for by this gene. Alternatively, mutation of a gene may result in the production of a structurally altered protein. Such proteins may have different characteristics compared with their normal counterparts.

In this event the absence of protein activity is not an indication of absence of a gene or its expression, but rather an example of expression of an altered gene. One can envision the potential ability of single-gene mutations to produce different yet related proteins. Such relatedness may be documented by various characteristics such as catalytic activity and antigenicity of an enzyme protein. For example, Lesch-Nyhan syndrome is an X-linked recessive disease in which hypoxanthine-guanine phosphoribosyltransferase activity is nearly absent (about 0.1% of normal), which may be attributable to an extreme instability of the mutant enzyme.[28] Recently a clinical disease identical to the Lesch-Nyhan syndrome was encountered in which the enzyme activity was about 10% of normal, a level at which clinical disease should not develop. However, since the enzyme in this case had a Michaelis-Menten constant (K_m) 10 times higher than that of the enzyme in normal individuals, its substrate affinity was so low that clinical disease developed.[66] This case may be considered a variant of Lesch-Nyhan syndrome in which a single-gene mutation produced yet another altered enzyme. In α-1-antitrypsin deficiency, an autosomal recessive disease, an antigenically related protein accumulates and appears as cytoplasmic globules in the hepatic cell[88] (see Chapter 27). Presumably a single-gene mutation has produced an abnormal α-1-antitrypsin molecule (substitution of a glutamic acid residue with lysine[46] or valine[71]) with a reduced sialic acid content that prevents its normal export and results in cytoplasmic accumulation in the liver cell. Thus there must be a variety of protein alterations underlying the 2811 Mendelian genetic diseases cataloged by McKusick.[67]

Genetic alterations of protein and their consequences

Alterations of protein on a genetic basis involve both structural proteins, such as collagen and elastin, and proteins with transport and catalytic functions. McKusick[67] proposed the useful thesis that structural protein alteration is found in dominant diseases and enzyme alteration is seen in recessive diseases. In both cases the alteration of protein is presumably caused by a change in the amino acid sequence as determined by gene mutation.

After their synthesis, some proteins require secondary chemical modification before becoming completely functional. If the enzyme or enzymes responsible for this modification are defective, the protein, which is essentially a normal one, will be unable to function normally. A case in point is Ehlers-Danlos syndrome, a group of diseases that for the most part have an autosomal dominant pattern of inheritance and defective collagen. However, in the variant Ehlers-Danlos syndrome type VI, a genocopy, the abnormality is not attributable to a defect in the primary structure (amino acid sequence) but rather to a deficiency of lysyl hydroxylase, an enzyme that catalyzes the hydroxylation of the lysine residues in col-

lagen. The foregoing emphasizes the fact that a single protein, in this case collagen, can in effect be under the control of more than one gene. The pattern of inheritance in this disease is autosomal recessive.[74,97]

This example indicates the usefulness of McKusick's thesis and the necessity of differentiating protein alterations attributable to a change in amino acid sequence (primary structure) from those attributable to faulty secondary modification of the polypeptide chain to bring the protein to full functional capacity. The concept of abnormalities of macromolecules owing to faulty secondary modification can be expanded to involve macromolecules other than proteins (see the discussion of type IV glycogen storage disease later in the chapter).

Genetic alteration in the quality and quantity of functional protein may result in various types of metabolic disturbances. One of them occurs because of the abnormal capacity of certain circulating proteins to transport specific molecules, as occurs in hemoglobinopathies such as sickle cell disease. A second type is related to the probable protein alteration involved in membrane transport. The third and most common type is the metabolic disturbances resulting from an enzyme alteration. In this situation the products of the defective enzyme reaction may be reduced, absent, or altered, or the substrate, its precursors, or their derivatives may accumulate. These metabolic disturbances may in turn be related to cell injury as discussed in a subsequent section.

The apparent metabolite abnormality in an enzyme deficiency does not necessarily involve the metabolite directly related to the defective enzyme reaction. An example of this is hyperuricemia in Lesch-Nyhan syndrome. Uric acid is not the substrate of the deficient enzyme hypoxanthine-guanine phosphoribosyltransferase. However, because of the enzyme-deficiency levels of its substrate, phosphoribosyl pyrophosphate increases and is readily available as substrate to other reactions. One of these is phosphoribosylamine synthesis, which is increased. Since this reaction is the initial step in purine biosynthesis, overall purine synthesis is also increased. The deficiency of hypoxanthine-guanine phosphoribosyltransferase also results in the reduced production of purine nucleotides, which in turn releases the allosteric inhibition of phosphoribosylamine synthetase. Thus purine biosynthesis is doubly stimulated by the deficiency of an enzyme that is not directly involved in its synthesis. The enhanced purine biosynthesis leads to increased production of uric acid, the end product of purine catabolism.

Heterozygotes

Most patients with diseases of dominant inheritance are heterozygous. In diseases of recessive inheritance, the heterozygotes are usually clinically normal, although in an increasing number of diseases some abnormality has been identified, such as 50% galactose-1-phosphate uridyltransferase activity in the hemolysate of the heterozygotes with a galactosemic gene.[24] Since heterozygotes of a given recessive disease greatly outnumber homozygotes (affected individuals), an effort to identify the heterozygotes is important. The frequency of heterozygotes can be estimated by using the Hardy-Weinberg law,[36,106] which in its simplest form can be expressed as follows:

$$(p + q)^2 = p^2 + 2pq + q^2$$

Suppose that the frequencies of a pair of allelomorphic genes are p and q, and p + q = 1. Therefore the frequency of individuals with two p genes is p^2, with two q genes q^2, and one gene of each 2 pq. If p is the normal gene and q is the abnormal gene, p^2 is the frequency of the normal homozygotes, q^2 that of the abnormal homozygotes, and 2 pq the frequency of the heterozygotes. This law depends on random mating and has worked well in human genetics. From the preceding formula it is apparent that heterozygotes of recessive diseases are much more frequent than are homozygotes. For instance, if the frequency of a recessive disease is one in 10,000, that of heterozygotes is as follows:

$$2 \times \left(1 - \frac{1}{100}\right) \times \frac{1}{100} \approx \frac{1}{50}$$

Such heterozygotes contribute to the persistence of the severe recessive diseases, which are usually fatal before puberty. Consideration of heterozygotes has further importance, since the majority of severe genetic diseases have either autosomal recessive or X-linked recessive inheritance. By contrast, autosomal dominant diseases and rare X-linked dominant diseases (such as familial vitamin D–resistant rickets with hypophosphatemia) are clinically less severe. Y-linked traits cause no disease of clinical significance.

When heterozygotes possessing an abnormal gene enjoy an advantage over the normal homozygotes in a given environment, the frequency of the abnormal gene becomes high and consequently a high frequency of the homozygotes of the disease results. The heterozygotes of sickle cell anemia are resistant to malignant tertian malaria in infancy and early childhood. Thus in large parts of Africa the frequency of sickle cell anemia is very high.

Women who are heterozygous for X-linked traits have provided information substantiating Lyon's hypothesis that one of the two X chromosomes of each cell is inactivated early in embryonic life.[61] The fibroblasts cultured from such women have two populations for X trait. For instance, the heterozygous mothers of individuals with Hunter's disease (X-linked recessive mucopolysaccharidosis) carry the phenotype in about half of their fibroblasts, as shown by the detection of cellular mucopolysaccharide accumulation.[10]

Studies of genetic diseases using cultured cells have proved particularly successful and are gaining increased application. One of the benefits is the prenatal diagnosis of genetic disease based on examination of exfoliated fetal cells obtained by amniocentesis.

Mutation and immune deficiency

There are many forms of immune deficiencies in man. Most of these occur as hereditary disorders with fairly well-defined inheritance patterns. Aplasia, or hypoplasia of the thymus and lymphoid follicles, and agammaglobulinemia (or hypogammaglobulinemia) are often associated with these diseases. However, the mechanism for the development of these changes attributable to the function of a mutant gene is unknown. Furthermore, such changes may occur because of external environmental factors such as radiation and immunosuppressive agents. Cell injury commonly present in patients with these diseases is often caused by infectious agents.

Mutation without cell injury

Mutations that have occurred through phylogeny and ontogeny and that are indifferent to the preservation of the human species can persist in the population. Therefore there is probably a much greater degree of genetic heterogeneity than the frequencies of genetic diseases imply. For instance, interest in the amino acid sequence of hemoglobin has uncovered hemoglobin variants that are not accompanied by functional abnormalities. This is a clear indication that there probably are many mutations that do not cause cell abnormalities. Sometimes such an indifferent gene mutation can produce a clinical problem in an unusual environment. For example, pseudocholinesterase deficiency can produce prolonged apnea in an individual given succinylcholine, a muscle relaxant. Except for this problem, the individual manifests no clinical abnormalities.[51]

Genetically determined alterations in composition of extracellular fluid

Examples of alterations of this type include genetic endocrine diseases such as familial cretinism and adrenogenital syndrome. In the former, thyroxine synthesis is impaired on a genetic basis and a variety of cells in the body do not receive the necessary supply of thyroxine through the extracellular fluid. Because of this there is generalized hypoplasia and presumably impeded maturation of various cell types. Mental and physical retardation at the organismal level is evident (see also p. 1400). In adrenogenital syndrome, certain enzyme deficiencies in the adrenal cortex lead to defective cortisol formation, which is reflected by a compensatory increase in ACTH secretion and excessive androgen production. There is conspicuous virilization of the female, with clitoral hypertrophy. In terms of cellular change there is an adrenal cortical hyperplasia (see also p. 1431).

Although these two examples involve hormones, other

metabolites may also be involved in this type of disturbance. In the genetic disorder Lesch-Nyhan syndrome, the elevated concentration of uric acid in the extracellular fluid results in the deposition of sodium urate crystals in tissue (gouty tophus), which leads to cell injury as previously discussed.

In some instances disturbed homeostasis of the extracellular fluid caused by a genetic defect in one type of cell results in the intracellular accumulation of a chemical substance in other types of cells, resulting in cell injury. For instance, the inability of hepatic cells to produce normal α-apolipoprotein in the genetic abnormality (Tangier disease) results in anomalous lipid transport in the blood and presumably in extracellular fluid so that cholesteryl esters accumulate in reticuloendothelial cells in various organs, most notably the tonsils, which are large, lobulated, and orange.[39]

Genetically determined alterations of plasma membrane

Recent advances have elucidated many important functions of the plasma membrane and its specialized structures. Ascribed to it are specialized ion-transport functions, hormone receptors often associated with adenylate cyclase, acetylcholine receptors with adjacent acetylcholine esterase in the excitable cell membrane, and special concentrations of enzymes in the brush border of the intestinal epithelium that facilitate transport of carbohydrates, to name but a few. These specialized functions of the plasma membrane are presumably altered in certain genetic diseases, which are manifest primarily as receptor and transport disorders. At present, alterations of the plasma membrane in these diseases are deduced only functionally and no structural abnormality has as yet been ascertained. Also, there is little morphologic abnormality in cells whose plasma membrane is functionally abnormal. However, in these diseases pathologic changes may become evident elsewhere in the body. For instance, familial hypercholesterolemia and its consequence, atherosclerosis, may result from a defective cell-surface receptor for low-density lipoprotein.[8] In cystinuria, the functional impairment of the renal tubular and intestinal epithelia is expressed as cystine stones (calculi) in the urinary tract.[99]

Cell injury from intracellular accumulation of metabolites

Thus far, several possible disturbances of cell homeostasis on a genetic basis have been considered in which the cells that have a genetically altered metabolism do not show evidence of cell injury. However, there are distinct situations in which cells with inborn errors of metabolism are eventually injured. Some of these may be caused by the cell's inability to synthesize a metabolite it requires, as in the rare genetic disorder orotic aciduria.[92] In this condition the bone marrow contains meg-aloblasts because of unbalanced macromolecular synthesis consisting of diminished synthesis of nucleic acids. Diminished nucleic acid synthesis is mediated by the inability to synthesize pyrimidine nucleotide because of deficiencies of orotidine-5′-phosphate pyrophosphorylase and orotidine-5′-phosphate decarboxylase.

When genetically abnormal cells show evidence of cell injury, it is usually because of an intracellular accumulation of metabolites. Such accumulation may be caused by the alteration of either anabolism or catabolism, the latter being the more prevalent. Cell injury resulting from faulty anabolism is rare. An example of this is type IV glycogen storage disease (Andersen's disease).[41] The deficiency of branching enzyme results in the formation of an amylopectin-like glycogen that is less soluble than normal glycogen. Hepatosplenomegaly and hepatic cirrhosis occur. Because of the presence of anomalous glycogen, hepatic parenchymal cells suffer cell injury, die, and are removed with concomitant fibrosis.

Cell injury caused by faulty catabolism is more common. A number of genetic diseases, particularly those called "storage diseases," fall in this category. Deficiency of an enzyme in a catabolic pathway results in the accumulation of substrate, its precursor, or their derivatives. Storage of the same metabolite can be caused by different enzyme deficiencies (genocopy). Tissue distribution of the deficient enzyme, its substrate, and its precursors will often determine the pattern of tissues involved by a storage disease. For example, in type I glycogen storage disease, the deficient enzyme is glucose-6-phosphatase, which is present in liver and kidney. Thus glycogen accumulation occurs in these organs. Glycogen is not the substrate of the deficient enzyme in this instance, but it is the major precursor of glucose-6-phosphate, the substrate of the deficient enzyme. In some cases the accumulated substance has been synthesized in the same cell, as in type I glycogen storage disease. In others, metabolite accumulation results from the inability of the cell to degrade the metabolite after its engulfment.

Cell injury resulting from faulty catabolism includes a subgroup of inborn errors of metabolism in which the defect is localized in lysosomes.[40] Overloading of lysosomes is the morphologic characteristic of this group of diseases.

Accumulated substances in lysosomes may have been synthesized by the cell, which develops lysosomal overloading as a result of autophagy, or they may have been taken into the cell by endocytosis and subsequently into lysosomes by heterophagy.

Genetically determined adverse reactions to foreign substances

A small number of people are adversely affected by drugs and other foreign substances to the extent that cell injury ensues. Various foreign substances become biologically inactive or active after being transformed in the liver by the drug-metabolizing enzyme system. Genetic variations involving this system may be responsible for the individual variation in response to drugs and other foreign substances. These are the subject of pharmacogenetics, a relatively new field in medicine.[52] In addition to pseudocholinesterase deficiency, which has already been cited, there are other well-known examples of adverse response to drugs. These include hemolysis caused by the antimalarial drug primaquine in cases of glucose-6-phosphate dehydrogenase deficiency (X-linked recessive), isoniazid neuropathy in individuals who slowly inactivate the antituberculous chemotherapeutic agent isoniazid (autosomal recessive, slow-reacting N-acetyltransferase), and cumulative toxicity of phenytoin in individuals with slow-reacting liver microsomal hydroxylase. Further examples of pharmacogenetic disorders may be found in textbooks of pharmacology.

Polygenic (multifactorial) disease

There are many diseases that suggest involvement of a genetic element although they do not show either a chromosomal abnormality or a distinct single-gene mutation. Some of these may be attributable to lowered penetrance of a single-gene mutation. However, at present these diseases are considered to involve polygenic inheritance. Presumably there are alleles at an unspecified number of different loci, and their combined action predisposes the individual to disease. The incidence of such diseases is higher among first-degree relatives (parents, sibs, and children) than in the general population, and it falls off rapidly in more distant relatives. The rate of fall is more rapid than would be the case if such diseases were attributable to single-gene mutations. These diseases include common congenital malformations such as harelip, infantile pyloric stenosis, some congenital heart diseases, anencephaly, spina bifida, and hydrocephalus and such common diseases as duodenal ulcer, hypertension, and diabetes mellitus. The pathologic condition in these instances is attributable to distant genetic effects comparable to those described in the foregoing section on intracellular accumulation of metabolites because of single-gene defects. Although glycogen is present in the kidney in both type I glycogen storage disease and some cases of uncontrolled diabetes mellitus, in the former case it is caused by an enzyme deficiency in the tubular cells but in the latter case it is a reflection of hyperglycemia, which has an as yet unelucidated genetic basis.

Metabolic disturbances in selected genetic diseases

As discussed thus far, only some of the expressions of genetic diseases may eventuate in cell injury. Traditionally cell injury has been related to disturbances in carbohydrate, lipid, or protein metabolism. By use of this classification, some of the genetic metabolic disturbances are discussed below and summarized in Table 3-3.

Table 3-3. Certain characteristics of selected genetic diseases

Disease	Inheritance	Protein defect	Metabolites involved (or deficient)	Organs involved	Lysosomal disease
GLYCOGEN STORAGE DISEASES					
Type I (von Gierke's disease)	AR	Glucose-6-phosphatase	Glycogen	Liver, kidney	No
Type II (Pompe's disease)	AR	Acid-α-1,4-glucosidase	Glycogen	Muscle, liver, heart, brain	Yes
Type III (Forbes' disease, Cori's disease)	AR	Amylo-1,6-glucosidase (debrancher)	Limit dextrin–like	Muscle, liver, heart	No
Type IV (Andersen's disease)	AR	Amylo-(1,4 to 1,6)-transglucosidase (brancher)	Amylopectin-like	Liver	No
Type V (McArdle's disease)	AR	Myophosphorylase	Glycogen	Muscle	No
Type VI (Hers' disease)	AR	Phosphorylase	Glycogen	Liver	No
Type VII	AR	Phosphofructokinase	Glycogen	Muscle	No
Type VIII	XR	Phosphorylase kinase	Glycogen	Liver, leukocyte	No
GLYCOGEN SYNTHETASE DEFICIENCY	AR	Glycogen synthetase	(Glycogen deficient)	Liver	No
MUCOPOLYSACCHARIDOSES					
Type I (Hurler's syndrome)	AR	α-L-Iduronidase	Dermatan sulfate and heparan sulfate	Connective tissue, liver, spleen, kidney, brain	Yes
Type I (Scheie's syndrome)	AR	α-L-Iduronidase	Dermatan sulfate	Connective tissue, liver, spleen, kidney, brain	Yes

AR, Autosomal recessive; XR, X-linked recessive.

Continued.

Table 3-3. Certain characteristics of selected genetic diseases—cont'd

Disease	Inheritance	Protein defect	Metabolites involved (or deficient)	Organs involved	Lysosomal disease
MUCOPOLYSACCHARIDOSES—cont'd					
Type II (Hunter's syndrome)	XR	L-Iduronosulfate sulfatase	Dermatan sulfate and heparan sulfate	Connective tissue, liver, spleen, kidney, brain	Yes
Type III (Sanfilippo's syndrome)	AR	Heparan sulfate sulfatase, N-acetyle-α-D-glucosaminidase	Heparan sulfate	Connective tissue, liver, spleen, kidney, brain	Yes
Type IV (Morquio's syndrome)	AR	N-Acetylhexosaminidase 6-sulfate sulfatase	Keratan sulfate	Connective tissue, liver, spleen, kidney, brain	Yes
Type VI (Maroteaux-Lamy syndrome)	AR	N-Acetylhexosaminidase 4-sulfate sulfatase	Dermatan sulfate	Connective tissue, liver, spleen, kidney, brain	Yes
MUCOPOLYSACCHARIDE-LIPID STORAGE MUCOLIPIDOSIS					
Type II	AR	Multiple hydrolases	Mucopolysaccharide and lipid	Liver, connective tissue	Yes
Type III	AR	Multiple hydrolases	Mucopolysaccharide and lipid	Liver, kidney, connective tissue, nervous tissue	Yes
Type IV	AR	?	?	Cornea	?
Sialidosis	AR	Neuraminidase	Sialic acid–containing material	Connective tissue	?
Fucosidosis	AR	α-L-Fucosidase	Fucose containing polysaccharide and glycolipid	Liver, spleen, brain, and many others	Yes
GM$_1$ gangliosidosis (Landing's pseudo-Hurler's disease)	AR	β-Galactosidase	Keratan sulfate GM$_1$ ganglioside	Liver, kidney, spleen, heart, brain	Yes
GLYCOLIPID STORAGE					
Tay-Sachs disease	AR	Hexosaminidase A	GM$_2$ ganglioside	Brain, retina	Yes
Fabry's disease (diffuse angiokeratoma)	XR	α-Galactosidase	Ceramide trihexoside, digalactosyl ceramide	Skin, kidney, heart, spleen, all other tissues	Yes
Gaucher's disease	AR	Glucocerebroside β-glucosidase	Glucocerebroside	Spleen, liver, bone marrow	Yes
Globoid cell leukodystrophy (Krabbe's disease)	AR	Galactocerebroside β-galactosidase	Galactocerebroside	Nervous system, central and peripheral, kidney	Yes
Metachromatic leukodystrophy		Cerebroside sulfatase (arylsulfatase A)	Cerebroside sulfate	Brain, liver, spleen, heart, kidney	Yes
PHOSPHOLIPID STORAGE					
Niemann-Pick disease	AR	Sphingomyelinase	Sphingomyelin	Spleen, bone marrow, liver, lung, lymph node	Yes
CHOLESTEROL ESTER AND TRIGLYCERIDE STORAGE					
Wolman's disease	AR	Acid esterase	Triglycerides, cholesteryl esters	Liver, spleen, adrenal kidney, all other tissues	Yes
GLYCOPROTEIN-DERIVATIVE STORAGE					
Aspartylglycosaminuria	AR	Aspartylglycosylamine amidase	Aspartylglycosylamine-containing components	Liver, brain, connective tissue	Yes

Glycogen storage diseases

The glycogen storage diseases are rare genetic diseases usually occurring in infancy. There are a number of types, defined by the deficient enzymes. The marker substance in these diseases is glycogen except in types III and IV.

Type I is characterized by massive hepatomegaly, failure to thrive, severe hypoglycemia, ketosis, and increased plasma lactic acid and lipid. Administration of epinephrine or glucagon causes a smaller than normal rise in the blood glucose level but a greater elevation in the lactic acid level, which is a useful diagnostic aid. Hyperuricemia is also commonly present, presumably because of the reduced tubular urate secretion resulting from lactic acid and ketone elevations in the blood. Hyperuricemia leads to gouty tophi, arthritis, and nephropathy. This disease was first described by von Gierke[104] in 1929, was elucidated with respect to its enzyme deficiency by Cori and Cori[14] in 1952, and became the prototype of the glycogen storage diseases.

Type II is the prototype of genetic lysosomal disease. The enzyme acid α-1,4-glucosidase (acid maltase) is normally present in almost all types of cells. Therefore a deficiency affects many tissues, a reason why this disease is also referred to as generalized glycogenosis. However, functional disturbances are focused in heart and skeletal muscle because of massive cardiomegaly and hypotonia without muscle wasting. In some instances the central nervous system is also severely affected. Death from cardiac failure usually occurs before 2 years of age. Electron micrographs show a predominant segregation of glycogen in vacuoles surrounded by a single membrane with a lesser amount of glycogen freely dispersed in the cytoplasm. The intravacuolar glycogen is predominantly of the α-particulate type, which is aggregated in the form of rosettes (Fig. 3-31). In postmortem tissue intravacuolar glycogen is unaltered, whereas free glycogen is rapidly depolymerized. This is further evidence that the defective enzyme is a lysosomal one.

Type III is characterized clinically by massive hepatomegaly. Hypoglycemia and responses to epinephrine and glucagon are variable. Type IV is characterized by progressive cirrhosis, hepatosplenomegaly, and ascites. Death is caused by hepatic failure and usually occurs before 2 years of age. Individuals with type V have painful cramps on strenuous exercise. The symptoms do not usually appear until about 20 years of age, and myoglobinuria is a common occurrence after strenuous exercise because of myocytolysis. In this glycogen storage disease there is no hypoglycemia. Type VI includes a heterogeneous group of patients who have increased liver glycogen and do not clearly fit into any of the other defined types. Some of these patients have reduced liver phosphorylase activity. Type VII is clinically identical to type V in that exercise causes cramping pain in peripheral skeletal muscles, accompanied by myoglobinuria. Type VIII is characterized by mild hepatomegaly, increased levels of liver glycogen, and moderate hypoglycemia.

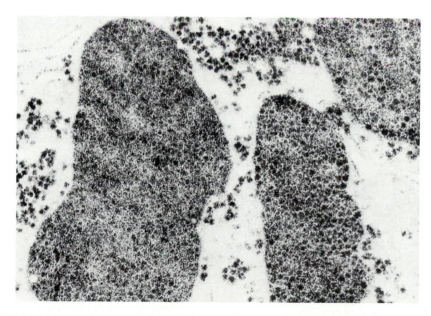

Fig. 3-31. Intralysosomal accumulations of glycogen in the cytoplasm of a hepatocyte from patient with glycogen storage disease resulting from deficiency of α-1,4-glucosidase (acid maltase), a lysosomal enzyme responsible for degradation of glycogen. This variant of glycogen storage disease, also referred to as Pompe's disease, led to pathologic enlargement of heart, liver, and kidney because of excessive accumulation of glycogen. Death in this infant was attributable to heart failure. (Courtesy Dr. Itaru Watanabe, Kansas City, Mo.)

From a metabolic point of view, liver glycogen synthetase deficiency, a disease manifested as hypoglycemia in infants, is the opposite of glycogen storage disease.[56]

Mucopolysaccharidoses

Description of multiple deformities by Hunter[42] in 1917 and Hurler[43] in 1918 intitiated the characterization of what is now an impressive group of diseases classified as the mucopolysaccharidoses.[25] During the intervening years, similar diseases have been reported under various names, such as osteochondrodystrophy, dysostosis multiplex, and gargoylism. Some of the clinical features of these diseases are moderate dwarfism, a broad thorax with short and thickened long bones, a protuberant abdomen with hepatosplenomegaly often accompanied by hernia, gargoylelike facial features, coarse dry skin, and mental retardation. Cardiac valvular disease is often present because of excessive accumulation of mucopolysaccharides in the connective tissue of the valves.

Important observations have been made pertaining to the mucopolysaccharidic nature of the deposits in visceral tissues (Fig. 3-32), lipid accumulation in the neurons of the brain, excessive excretion of mucopolysaccharides in urine, and intralysosomal accumulation of mucopolysaccharide in affected tissues and in fibroblasts cultured from patients (Fig. 3-33). These have established the mucopolysaccharidoses as a group of lysosomal diseases resulting from a genetic defect of a variety of lysosomal hydrolases capable of hydrolyzing carbohydrates.

Mucopolysaccharides are long-chain polyanionic carbohydrates with disaccharide repeating units, one component of which consists of D-glucosamine or D-galactosamine and the other of either D-glucuronic or L-iduronic acid. Because of these units, mucopolysaccharides have now been renamed glycosaminoglycans. The amino group and the fourth or sixth carbon of hexosamine are often either acetylated or sulfated. Depending on the major consituents, six different acidic glycosaminoglycans are recognized. These are hyaluronic acid, chondroitin 4- and 6-sulfate, keratan sulfate (formerly called keratosulfate), dermatan sulfate (formerly called chondroitin sulfate B), heparin, and heparan sulfate (formerly called heparitin sulfate). These glycosaminoglycans are present largely as structural constituents of extracellular connective tissue. They are also present in mast cells, granulocytes, and platelets. Glycosaminoglycans normally occur covalently attached to proteins, in which case they are called proteoglycans. In pathologic states, intracellular glycosaminoglycans are free and readily soluble in water or aqueous fixatives.

Mucopolysaccharide-synthesizing cells such as fibroblasts, endothelial cells, and leukocytes secrete proteoglycan. The portion that is not secreted enters lysosomes and is degraded by various lysosomal hydrolases including proteases. When there is a deficiency of an enzyme necessary for mucopolysaccharide catabolism, mucopolysaccharide accumulates within the lysosomes. The proteoglycan or mucopolysaccharide (or both) secreted by the mucopolysaccharide-synthesizing cells is taken up by endocytic cells and enters lysosomes (heterophagy). The same enzyme deficiency then results in lysosomal overloading in the non-mucopolysaccharide-synthesizing cells such as those in the liver, spleen, and kidney. Overloading and subsequent dysfunction of fibroblasts, chondrocytes, and osteocytes causes multiple skeletal deformities, corneal clouding, and hepatosplenomegaly. Free mucopolysaccharide secreted by the mucopolysaccharide-synthesizing cells or released after death of severely affected cells appears in the urine.

Glycolipid (see the discussion of glycolipidases for more detail) accumulation in neurons may be caused by autophagy; since mucopolysaccharide and glycolipid can contain the same glycosidic bond, a hydrolase deficiency could lead to lysosomal accumulation of glycolipid in neurons while mucopolysaccharide accumulates in other cells.

In extraneural tissues fixed in aqueous fixative, affected cells show some cytoplasmic vacuolization and cell ballooning (swelling). On electron microscopic examination the vacuoles contain fine granular material and, like lysosomes, are limited by a single membrane. As mentioned previously, accumulated mucopolysaccharides are water soluble and are leached during fixation and processing. When tissue is fixed in mucopolysaccharide-insoluble fixatives such as alcohol, the accumulated material shows intense metachromasia (purple-blue staining) with toluidine blue; it also stains intensely with Alcian blue, stains weakly with periodic acid–Schiff (PAS), and is impregnated with colloidal iron.

In the neuron the material distending the cytoplasm shows PAS reactivity that is amylase resistant (which means that the substance is not glycogen), metachromasia with toluidine blue, and staining with Sudan black B, Nile blue, or Alcian blue. The material can be extracted with a chloroform-methanol mixture. These characteristics indicate the glycolipid nature of the accumulated material. Ultrastructurally, the lysosomes are filled with parallel lamellae, usually perpendicular to the limiting membrane, which are appropriately called zebra bodies.

A classification of mucopolysaccharidoses based on the specific nature of the protein deficiency is shown in Table 3-3. As mentioned previously, classification of these disorders has been significantly advanced by study of the patients' fibroblasts in tissue culture. These cells not only develop mucopolysaccharide accumulation in culture but also show the ability to exchange macromolecules, including the missing enzymes. This unique phenomenon allows in vitro correction of mucopolysaccharide accumulation of affected cells by mixed culture with nor-

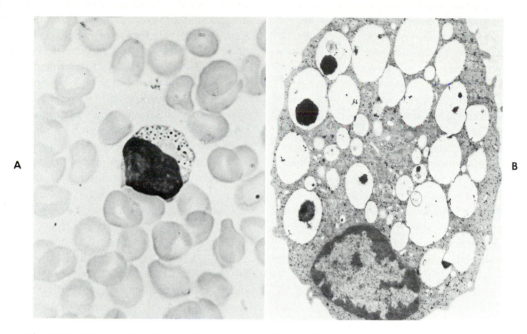

Fig. 3-32. Cytoplasmic inclusions in lymphocytes in peripheral blood from patient with Hunter's syndrome or mucopolysaccharidosis type II, a condition clinically and biochemically very similar to, although less severe than, Hurler's syndrome. **A,** Cytoplasmic inclusions (Alder bodies) are stained dark bluish red with Giemsa-Wright stain. **B,** Electron micrograph of lymphocyte shows these bodies to consist of vacuoles containing dense amorphous material chemically identified as a mixture of the mucopolysaccharides dermatan sulfate and heparan sulfate. (Courtesy Dr. Itaru Watanabe, Kansas City, Mo.)

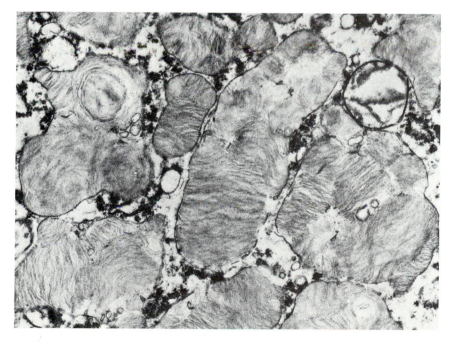

Fig. 3-33. Lamellar inclusions in lysosomes in cytoplasm of a neuron from patient with Hurler's syndrome. Lysosomes are filled with lamellated material, probably ganglioside, in which the lamellae are oriented perpendicular to the lysosomal membrane, giving rise to structures referred to as zebra bodies. (Courtesy Dr. Itaru Watanabe, Kansas City, Mo.)

mal fibroblasts. It appears that some substance supplied by the normal cells prevents mucopolysaccharide accumulation in the abnormal ones. Such substances were initially called corrective factor because their precise nature was unknown. In several instances the factor has been identified as the missing enzyme.

Since mucopolysaccharide binds strongly with such dyes as Alcian blue, a simple spot test on filter paper can provide a rough estimation of mucopolysaccharide excreted in the urine. Intracellular mucopolysaccharide accumulation can also be found in some other, clinically quite different diseases such as Fabry's disease (a lipid storage disease), Marfan's syndrome (a heritable disorder of connective tissue), and mucoviscidosis (cystic fibrosis of the pancreas, a membrane transport disorder involving exocrine glands). The reason or reasons for mucopolysaccharide accumulation in these diseases remain to be elucidated.

Disturbances of carbohydrate and lipid metabolism

It has already been mentioned that even in well-established mucopolysaccharidoses there is an additional lipid accumulation in neurons. In certain other diseases the accumulation of both mucopolysaccharide and lipid is significant, and for such diseases the category of mucopolysaccharide-lipid storage has been created. Mucolipidosis type II (I-cell disease) and type III (pseudo-Hurler polydystrophy) have clinical features resembling those of Hurler's disease, including facial and skeletal deformities.[68] However, the urinary excretion of mucopolysaccharide is normal. Morphologically affected cells, such as hepatocytes, show considerably less vacuolization than is seen in the mucopolysaccharidoses; in addition, the lysosomes have a more polymorphic content, consisting of membrane lamellae, probably representing glycolipid-rich material. In these diseases there are multiple lysosomal hydrolase deficiencies. The clinical features of mucolipidosis type IV are corneal clouding and psychomotor retardation.[58] The term "sialidosis" has replaced the old term "mucolipidosis I"; this group of diseases is characterized by neurodegeneration with Hurler-like features, skeletal dysplasia, and a cherry-red spot in the macula. The material that accumulates in affected cells is rich in sialic acid.[60] Fucosidosis and GM_1 gangliosidosis are additional examples of diseases in which both a polysaccharide and a glycolipid accumulate. The former is manifested by progressive neurologic deterioration with some features resembling Hurler's disease. Ultrastructural changes consist of lysosomal accumulation of polysaccharide and glycolipid, as evidenced by vacuoles containing fine tubular elements. In these diseases the absence of a single lysosomal enzyme that is required for the cleavage of the same glycosidic bond in both mucopolysaccharide and glycolipid results in lysosomal overloading.

Glycosphingolipidoses. Lipids are substances extractable with fat solvents. Among these substances, sphingolipids, which are primarily membrane components of eukaryotic cells, are singularly involved in many classical genetic diseases.[7] Glycolipids are lipids containing one or more carbohydrate residues. Whereas the phosphatidylinositol-containing lipids appear to be uninvolved in genetic disorders, glycosphingolipid accumulation occurs in many well-known genetic diseases. In addition to the well-established glycosphingolipid storage disorders, the mucopolysaccharidoses are accompanied by some accumulation of glycosphingolipid, as has been mentioned. Glycosphingolipids have one or more hexose or hexosamine moieties linked to N-acylsphingosine (ceramide). When one or more sialic acids are present, the glycosphingolipid is called a ganglioside.

In Tay-Sachs disease, in which there is a deficiency of β-N-acetylhexosaminidase, neurons accumulate GM_2 ganglioside, whose structure is as follows:

$$\text{Ceramide-Glucose-Galactose-}N\text{-Acetylgalactosamine}$$
$$|$$
$$N\text{-Acetylneuraminic acid}$$

By contrast, in GM_1 gangliosidosis, a disease caused by a deficiency of β-galactosidase, the structure of the accumulated substance is as follows:

$$\text{Ceramide-Glucose-Galactose-}$$
$$N\text{-Acetylgalactosamine-Galactose}$$
$$|$$
$$N\text{-Acetylneuraminic acid}$$

Tay-Sachs disease is manifested clinically by the startle reaction, motor weakness beginning between 3 and 6 months of age, rapid mental and motor deterioration after 1 year of age, progressive deafness, blindness, convulsions, and spasticity. Affected individuals usually die before 3 years of age. Ophthalmoscopy discloses a characteristic cherry-red spot in the fovea centralis surrounded by an area of paleness caused by ganglion cells swollen with ganglioside. Morphologic changes include accumulation of PAS-positive glycolipid in neurons. Electron microscopic studies reveal the presence of numerous concentric membranous bodies with lamellae 50 Å thick in the cytoplasm (Fig. 3-34).

In Fabry's disease, affected cells are filled with ceramide trihexoside (ceramide-glucose-galactose-galactose) and digalactosyl ceramide. In this disease lysosomes lack α-galactosidase. Lipid accumulation occurs in most tissues, and a characteristic skin eruption develops that is bright red to bluish black and angiectatic. The eruption is not associated with itching or bleeding and is usually found in the area between the umbilicus and the knees. There is generalized vascular and renal involvement; cardiovascular and cerebrovascular accidents and renal failure are common causes of death. Affected cells are filled with doubly refractile lipidic material that is intensely osmiophilic and lamellated in a myelin-like form.

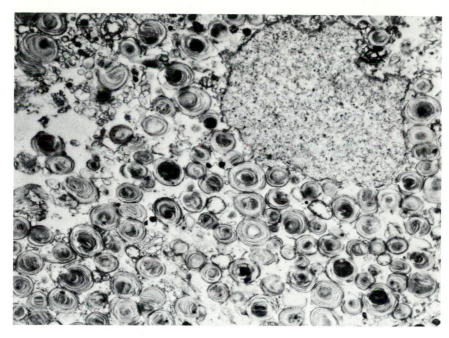

Fig. 3-34. Whorled membranous bodies in a neuron from patient with GM$_2$ gangliosidosis, or Tay-Sachs disease. (Courtesy Dr. Itaru Watanabe, Kansas City, Mo.)

In Gaucher's disease the accumulated substance is cerebroside or ceramide monosaccharide (ceramide-glucose), and the deficient lysosomal enzyme is cerebroside β-glucosidase. Lysosomal overloading in Gaucher's disease is unique in that heterophagy appears to be the major mechanism of cellular uptake. The major precursor of the accumulated glucocerebroside is derived from membrane glycolipids of old erythrocytes and leukocytes, particularly ceramide lactoside (ceramide-glucose-galactose) of leukocytes. The foamy cytoplasm of reticuloendothelial cells in Gaucher's disease is filled with PAS-positive, autofluorescent, Prussian blue–positive, and oil red O–positive material, indicating that the accumulated substances are a mixture of glycolipid with hemosiderin (Fig. 3-35). These cells often show erythrophagocytosis and are strongly positive for acid phosphatase. The cytoplasm contains rod-shaped, membrane-bound bodies 0.6 to 4 μm in diameter, which, in turn, consist of sheaves of small tubules about 130 to 750 Å in diameter. Clinically, Gaucher's disease is characterized by hepatosplenomegaly, cortical erosion of long bones, anemia, leukopenia, and thrombocytopenia.

In Krabbe's disease the deficient enzyme and the metabolite that accumulates are chemically similar to those in Gaucher's disease. The deficient enzyme in Krabbe's disease is cerebroside β-galactosidase, and galactosyl ceramide accumulates in certain cells. The cytoplasm contains tubules about 100 Å in diameter, which closely resemble those observed in Gaucher's disease. Since galactocerebroside is a membrane component limited largely to myelin, involvement in Krabbe's disease is localized to the nervous system. Clinical features of this disease are hyperirritability, stiffness of limbs, and episodic fever beginning at the age of 3 to 6 months. Rapid mental and motor deterioration with pronounced hypertonicity ensues. The patients become blind and decerebrate. There is also an increase in cerebrospinal fluid protein with a normal cell count. In the brain, the white matter is primarily involved and the lesion is characterized by the presence of unique globoid cells, demyelination, and severe astrocytic gliosis. The pathogenesis of demyelination is unclear. Globoid cells, which are presumably of nonneural mesodermal origin, contain the aforementioned cytoplasmic tubular structures. Although a lysosomal enzyme deficiency is clearly present, thus far there is no evidence of lysosomal overloading in this disease. Since oligodendroglia are the seat of myelin synthesis, one would expect that these cells would show also increased storage of galactocerebroside. However, this is not the case. In the brain of a patient with Krabbe's disease, there is in fact a profound loss of oligodendroglia. These findings set Krabbe's disease apart from the other lysosomal diseases we have considered thus far.

Galactocerebroside in which the C-3 of galactose is sulfated is called sulfatide. A disease characterized by the accumulation of sulfatide because of the deficiency of cerebroside sulfatase has been described. Because of the negative charge imparted by the sulfuric acid ester group, sulfatide stains reddish brown (spectrum shift toward red, or metachromasia) with certain blue cationic dyes such as toluidine blue. Since sulfatide is localized in myelin, which is the major component of the white matter of the brain, this condition is appropriately referred

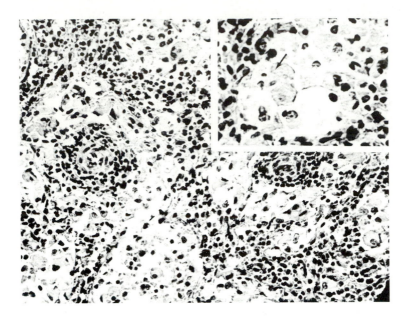

Fig. 3-35. Spleen from 23-year-old man with glucosyl ceramide lipoidosis (Gaucher's disease). Spleen and liver were greatly enlarged. Foamy cells are present in the spleen and largely obliterate the structure of lymphoid follicles. *Inset,* Higher magnification shows striated appearance of cytoplasm of Gaucher cells *(arrow),* which is attributed to the fact that glucosyl ceramides form elongate tubular structures packed in elongate lysosomes. Ultrastructural studies of Gaucher cells have shown that the cytoplasm and lysosomes are filled with membrane-bound tubules measuring up to 5 μm in length.

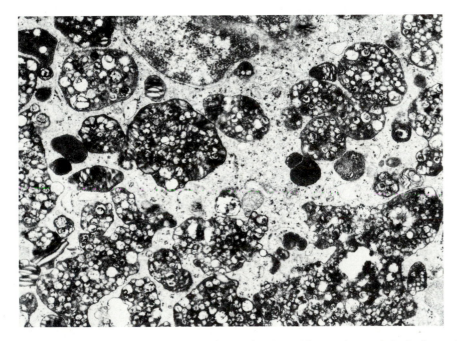

Fig. 3-36. Cytoplasm of an oligodendrocyte in brain of patient with metachromatic leukodystrophy, showing numerous secondary lysosomes or residual bodies filled with dense membranous material and small vacuoles. This is the result of a deficiency of arylsulfatase A and cerebroside sulfatase enzymes in lysosomes; the membranous material in lysosomes is myelin sulfatides. (Courtesy Dr. Itaru Watanabe, Kansas City, Mo.)

to as metachromatic leukodystrophy. Although this disease can manifest itself clinically at any age, most cases begin in late infancy. The affected infant has muscular weakness, hypotonia, and reduced reflexes. Involvement of upper motor neurons, quadriparesis, and dementia occur. The brain is atrophic, and oligodendroglia and phagocytes are distended by PAS-positive, metachromatic material in the cytoplasm. The material is enclosed within single membrane–limited bodies with structural and enzymatic properties consistent with those of lysosomes (Fig. 3-36). There is extensive demyelination, the mechanism of which is unclear. In the visceral organs, intracellular metachromatic deposits are also present. In addition to the deposits of cerebroside sulfate, sulfated mucopolysaccharide and steroid sulfate can also accumulate, since all of these compounds contain the chemical bond that requires sulfatase for its cleavage. In this sense, metachromatic leukodystrophy fits into the category of mucopolysaccharide-lipid storage diseases. Indeed, some patients with neurologically typical metachromatic leukodystrophy may also show signs resembling those of Hurler's disease, such as facial and bone deformities, vacuolated cells in the peripheral blood and bone marrow, and elevated urinary excretion of mucopolysaccharide.

Phosphosphingolipidosis. Niemann-Pick disease is characterized chemically by the accumulation of sphingomyelin, which is the only major sphingolipid containing phosphorus. Sphingomyelin is found in virtually all tissues and is more abundant than the glycosphingolipids. Sphingomyelin accumulates in this disease because of a deficiency of sphingomyelinase, an enzyme that hydrolyzes sphingomyelin into phosphorylcholine and ceramide. Niemann-Pick disease is characterized clinically by physical and mental underdevelopment and hepatosplenomegaly. Some 30% of the affected infants have a cherry-red spot in the macula. Cells of the reticuloendothelial system are large and lipid laden and are found in the spleen, liver, bone marrow, lung, and lymph nodes. Hepatic and ganglion cells may also be involved. Affected cells contain cytoplasmic lipid inclusions measuring 2 to 3 μm in diameter. These are concentrically laminated, myelin-like figures with a periodicity of approximately 50 Å.

Cholesterol ester and triglyceride storage

Deposition of cholesterol, cholesterol ester, and triglyceride in tissue in the form of lipid-laden macrophages is common in many pathologic conditions, such as atherosclerosis, xanthoma, and cholesterolosis of the gallbladder. Some of these disorders, such as familial hypercholesterolemia[8] and Tangier disease,[39] have a genetic basis. In these cases alterations in the proteins responsible for lipid transport in the blood result in the intracellular deposition of lipids, which may ultimately lead to cell injury and death.

Wolman's disease[1] becomes clinically manifest in the first weeks of life and is characterized by vomiting, diarrhea, steatorrhea, failure to thrive, hepatosplenomegaly, and adrenal enlargement and calcification. It is usually fatal by the age of 6 months. Nearly all organs are filled with lipid-laden cells. Lipid droplets are also present in lymphocytes, neutrophils, and monocytes in the peripheral blood. The lipid is strongly stainable with the Sudan dyes. Lipid accumulation is attributable to a deficiency of acid esterase, a lysosomal enzyme responsible for hydrolysis of cholesterol esters and triglycerides.

Disturbances of protein metabolism

As discussed previously in the section on genetic alterations of protein and their consequences, alteration of structural proteins such as collagen and elastin is involved in the genetic connective tissue diseases. These include Ehlers-Danlos syndrome, Marfan's syndrome, and osteogenesis imperfecta. Genetically determined alterations of protein are well documented in the hemoglobinopathies and functional defects involving plasma proteins, and these conditions can in a broad sense be classified as metabolic disturbances. However, since they are discussed in sections dealing with diseases of connective tissue, the hemoglobinopathies and dysproteinemias, they will not be included here.

One example of faulty catabolism of protein seems worth emphasizing. Mucopolysaccharides normally exist covalently bound to proteins, the so-called proteoglycans. Proteoglycans may also be classified as glycoproteins or mucoproteins depending on their relative polysaccharide content. The term "glycoprotein" may be limited to proteins that contain less than 4% carbohydrate, whereas mucoproteins contain a larger amount of polysaccharide. Proteoglycans are constantly synthesized and degraded; degradation requires cleavage of the covalent bond between the protein and carbohydrate moieties. The amino acid residues involved in this type of bond are asparagine, serine, threonine, and hydroxylysine. One common compound constituting this connecting point between protein and carbohydrate is 2-acetamido-1-N-(4-L-aspartyl)-2-deoxy-β-D-glucopyranosylamine (GlcNAcoAsn). In this compound asparagine is attached through its amide group to the reducing end of N-acetylglucosamine. This compound is excreted in large quantities, approximately 300 mg per day, in the genetic disease aspartylglycosylaminuria.[65] This disease can be considered an example of disturbed glycoprotein catabolism. It is characterized clinically by psychomotor retardation and bone and connective tissue deformities including sagging cheeks, broad nose, short neck, cranial asymmetry, and scoliosis. Cytoplasmic vacuolation of lymphocytes is a common finding. There is a deficiency of amidase, an enzyme that splits aspartylglycosylamine into aspartate, ammonia, and N-acetylglucosamine and that is normally present in plasma and many tissues. In patients with this disease intralysosomal degradation of glycoprotein proceeds normally through the action of cathepsins and glycosidases to form smaller molecules containing aspartylglycosylamine. In the absence of the amidase, further degradation does not occur and aspartylglycosylamine does not readily diffuse out of lysosomes, leading to overloading. Morphologically, glial cells, neurons, and hepatocytes contain many large cytoplasmic vacuoles filled with flocculent material, which probably represents the stored metabolite. Although catabolic errors involving amino acids are well known in such diseases as phenylketonuria, homocystinuria, cystathioninuria, and alkaptonuria, catabolic errors involving proteins are less well known at present. In time, no doubt, more genetic defects involving catabolism of proteins and conjugated proteins will be identified.

Summary

In the foregoing a limited number of genetic diseases have been presented and discussed briefly. These were selected on the basis of a known error of catabolism that frequently causes accumulation of metabolites, which in turn leads to cell injury. Whether the accumulating metabolite is a carbohydrate or a lipid, the majority of the enzyme deficiencies described are deficiencies of glycosidases. Inasmuch as carbohydrate is present in complex lipid, protein, and polysaccharide molecules, and as a large variety of glycosyl bonds are found in nature, it is not surprising that many of the genetic disorders accompanied by intracellular storage are diseases of glycosidase deficiency.

It is also striking that the tissue distribution of the enzymes affected and their substrates and precursors causes a great diversity of clinical and pathologic manifestations in the storage diseases. Thus, even when the involved enzymes are ubiquitous, as are the lysosomal hydrolases, the localization of lesions can be surprisingly limited by the distribution of substrates and their precursors.

Although there are hundreds of known genetic diseases in which the lack or modification of enzyme and protein has been established in the tradition of the one gene—one enzyme concept originated by Beadle and Tatum, the bulk of these are not included here because of space limitations. They include faulty metabolism of low—molecular weight metabolites such as monosaccharides, oligosaccharides, amino acids, and structural and circulating proteins.

REFERENCES

1. Abramov, A., Schorr, S., and Wolman, M.: Generalized xanthomatosis with calcified adrenals, AMA J. Dis. Child. **91:**282, 1956.
2. Arstila, A.U., and Trump, B.F.: Studies on cellular autophagocytosis: the formation of autophagic vacuoles in the liver after glucagon administration, Am. J. Pathol. **53:**687, 1968.
3. Atkinson, D.E.: Regulation of enzyme activity, Annu. Rev. Biochem. **35:**85, 1966.
4. Bacq, Z.M., and Alexander, P.: Fundamentals of radiobiology, New York, 1955, Academic Press, Inc.,
5. Bessis, M.: Studies on cell agony and death: an attempt at classification. In De Reuck, A.V.S., and Knight, J., editors: Cellular injury, Boston, 1964, Little, Brown & Co.
6. Bladen, H.A., Nylen, M.U., and Glenner, G.G.: The ultrastructure of human amyloid as revealed by the negative staining technique, J. Ultrastruct. Res. **14:**449, 1966.
7. Brady, R.O.: Heritable catabolic and anabolic disorders of lipid metabolism, Metabolism **26:**329, 1979.
8. Brown, M.S., and Goldstein, J.L.: Familial hypercholesterolemia: model for genetic receptor disease, Harvey Lect. **73:**163, 1979.
9. Burke, J.P., and Rubin, E.: The effects of ethanol and acetaldehyde on the products of protein synthesis by liver mitochondria, Lab. Invest. **41:**393, 1979.
10. Capobianchi, M.R., and Romeo, G.: Mosaicism for sulfoiduronate sulfatase deficiency in carriers of Hunter's syndrome, Experientia **32:**459, 1976.
11. Chien, K.R., et al.: Accelerated phospholipid turnover and associated membrane dysfunction in irreversible ischemic liver cell injury, J. Biol. Chem. **253:**4809, 1978.
12. Cleaver, J.E.: DNA repair and radiation sensitivity in human (xeroderma pigmentosum) cells, Int. J. Radiat. Biol. **18:**557, 1970.
13. Cole, G.A., et al.: Lymphocytic choriomeningitis virus: pathogenesis of acute central nervous system disease, Fed. Proc. **30:**1831, 1971.
14. Cori, G.T., and Cori, C.F.: Glucose-6-phosphatase of the liver in glycogen storage disease, J. Biol. Chem. **199:**661, 1952.
15. Cormack, D.V., and Johns, H.E.: Electron energies and ion densities in water irradiated with 200 keV, 1 MeV and 25 meV radiation, Br. J. Radiol. **25:**369, 1952.
16. Cowger, M.L.: Mechanism of bilirubin toxicity on tissue culture cells: factors that affect toxicity, reversibility by albumin, and comparison with other respiratory poisons and surfactants, Biochem. Med. **5:**1, 1971.
17. Dal Canto, M.C., and Rabinowitz, S.G.: Experimental models of virus-induced demyelination of the central nervous system, Ann. Neurol. **11:**109, 1982.
18. Dale, W.M., Davies, J.V., and Gilbert, C.W.: The kinetics and specificities of deamination of nitrogenous compounds by X-radiation, Biochem. J. **45:**93, 1949.
19. Dales, S.: Penetration of animal viruses into cells, Prog. Med. Virol. **7:**1, 1965.
20. Daniels, F., Jr.: Physiological effects of sunlight, J. Invest. Dermatol. **32:**147, 1959.
21. Davis, P.S., Luke, C.G., and Deller, D.J.: Reduction of gastric iron-binding protein in haemochromatosis: a previously unrecognized metabolic defect, Lancet **2:**1431, 1966.
22. de Duve, C., and Wattiaux, R.: Functions of lysosomes, Annu. Rev. Physiol. **28:**435, 1966.
23. Dingle, J.T., and Fell, H.B., editors: Lysosomes in biology and pathology (in two parts), Amsterdam, 1969, North Holland Publishing Co.
24. Donnell, G.N., et al.: The enzymatic expression of heterozygosity in families of children with galactosemia, Pediatrics **25:**572, 1960.
25. Dorfman, A., and Matalon, R.: The mucopolysaccharidoses (a review), Proc. Natl. Acad. Sci. **73:**630, 1976.
26. Duryee, W.R.: The nature of radiation injury to amphibian cell nuclei, J. Natl. Cancer Inst. **10:**735, 1949.
27. Franklin, R.M., and Baltimore, D.: Patterns of macromolecular synthesis in normal and virus-infected mammalian cells, Cold Spring Harbor Symp. Quant. Biol. **27:**175, 1962.
28. Fujimoto, W.Y., and Seegmiller, J.E.: Hypoxanthine-guanine phosphoribosyl-transferase deficiency: activity in normal mutant, and heterozygotes-cultured human skin fibroblasts, Proc. Natl. Acad. Sci. **65:**577, 1970.
29. Garrod, A.E.: Inborn errors of metabolism, London, 1909, Oxford Press.
30. Glenner, G.G.: The creation of "amyloid" fibrils from Bence Jones proteins in vitro, Science **174:**712, 1971.

31. Glenner, G.G.: Amyloid deposits and amyloidosis: the β-fibrilloses, N. Engl. J. Med. **302**:1283, 1980.

32. Glenner, G.G., Ein, D., and Terry, W.D.: The immunoglobulin origin of amyloid, Am. J. Med. **52**:141, 1972.

33. Goldfinger, S., Klinenberg, J.R., and Seegmiller, J.E.: Renal retention of uric acid induced by infusion of beta-hydroxybutyrate and acetoacetate, N. Engl. J. Med. **272**:351, 1965.

34. Good, R.A., and Campbell, B.: The precipitation of latent herpes simplex and encephalitis by anaphylactic shock, Proc. Soc. Exp. Biol. Med. **68**:82, 1948.

35. Hardt, F.: Transfer amyloidosis. I. Studies on the transfer of various lymphoid cells from amyloidotic mice to syngeneic nonamyloidotic recipients. II. Induction of amyloidosis in mice with spleen, thymus and lymph node tissue from casein-sensitized donors, Am. J. Pathol. **65**:411, 1971.

36. Hardy, G.H.: Mendelian proportions in a mixed population, Science **28**:49, 1908.

37. Hasumura, Y., Teschke, R., and Lieber, C.S.: Characteristics of acetaldehyde oxidation in rat liver mitochondria, J. Biol. Chem. **251**:4908, 1976.

38. Helminen, H.J., Ericsson, J.L.E., and Orrenius, S.: Studies on mammary gland involution. IV. Histochemical and biochemical observations on alterations in lysosomes and lysosomal enzymes, J. Ultrastruct. Res. **25**:240, 1968.

39. Herbert, P.N., Gotto, A.N., and Fredrickson, D.S.: Familial lipoprotein deficiency (abetalipoproteinemia, hypobetalipoproteinemia, and Tangier disease). In Stanbury, J.B., Wyngaarden, J.B., and Fredrickson, D.S., editors: The metabolic basis of inherited diseases, ed. 4, New York, 1980, McGraw-Hill Book Co.

40. Hers, H.B., and Van Hoof, F., editors: Lysosomes and storage diseases, New York, 1973, Academic Press, Inc.

41. Huijing, F.: Glycogen metabolism and glycogen-storage diseases, Physiol. Rev. **55**:609, 1975.

42. Hunter, C.: A rare disease in two brothers, Proc. R. Soc. Med. (Section for the study of disease in children) **10**:104, 1916-1917.

43. Hurler, G.: Uber einen Typ multipler Abartungen, vorwiegend am Skellett-system, Z. Kinderheilkd. **24**:220, 1919.

44. Jennings, R.B., and Reimer, K.A.: Lethal myocardial ischemic injury, Am. J. Pathol. **102**:241, 1981.

45. Jennings, R.B., et al.: Ischemic injury of myocardium, Ann. N.Y. Acad. Sci. **156**:61, 1969.

46. Jeppsson, J.O.: Amino acid substitution Glu leads to Lys alpha 1-antitrypsin PiZ, FEBS Lett. **65**:195, 1976.

47. Kellenmeyer, R.W.: Hageman factor and acute gouty arthritis, Arthritis Rheum. **11**:452, 1968.

48. Kelley, W.N., and Wyngaarden, J.B.: Enzymology of gout, Adv. Enzymol. **41**:1, 1974.

49. Klinenberg, J.R., editor: Proceedings of the second conference on gout and purine metabolism, Arthritis Rheum. **18**(suppl. 6), 1975.

50. Kohn, A., and Fuchs, P.: Initial effects of viral infection in bacterial and animal host cells, Adv. Virus Res. **18**:159, 1973.

51. La Du, B.N.: Isoniazid and pseudocholinesterase polymorphism, Fed. Proc. **31**:1276, 1972.

52. La Du, B.N.: Pharmacogenetics: defective enzymes in relation to reactions to drugs, Annu. Rev. Med. **23**:453, 1972.

53. Lea, D.E.: Actions of radiations on living cells, Cambridge, 1946, Cambridge University Press.

54. Lesch, M., Gorlin, F., and Sonnenblick, E.H.: Myocardial amino acid transport in the isolated rabbit right ventricular papillary muscle: general characteristics and effects of passive stretch, Circ. Res. **27**:445, 1970.

55. Lesch, M., and Nyhan, W.L.: A familial disorder of uric acid metabolism and central nervous system function, Am. J. Med. **36**:561, 1964.

56. Lewis, G.M., Spencer-Peet, J., and Stewart, K.M.: Infantile hypoglycemia due to inherited deficiency of glycogen synthetase in liver, Arch. Dis. Child. **38**:40, 1963.

57. Lieber, C.S., et al.: Interrelation of uric acid and ethanol metabolism in man, J. Clin. Invest. **41**:1863, 1962.

58. Livini, N., and Merin, S.: Mucoplipidosis. IV. Ultrastructural diagnosis of a recently defined genetic disorder, Arch. Pathol. Lab. Med. **102**:600, 1978.

59. Lombardi, B.: Considerations on the pathogenesis of fatty liver, Lab. Invest. **15**:1, 1966.

60. Lowden, J.A., and O'Brien, J.S.: Sialidosis: a review of human neuraminidase deficiency, Am. J. Hum. Genet. **31**:1, 1979.

61. Lyon, M.F.: Sex chromatin and gene action in the mammalian X-chromosome, Am. J. Hum. Genet. **14**:135, 1962.

62. Malt, R.A.: Compensatory growth of the kidney, N. Engl. J. Med. **280**:1446, 1969.

63. Mason, H.S., Ingram, D.J.E., and Allen, B.: Free radical property of melanins, Arch. Biochem. Biophys. **86**:226, 1960.

64. Matsud, Y.I., et al.: Effects of ethanol on liver microtubules and Golgi apparatus: possible role in altered hepatic secretion of plasma proteins, Lab. Invest. **41**:455, 1979.

65. Maury, P.: Accumulation of two glycoasparagines in the liver in aspartylglycosaminuria, J. Biol. Chem. **254**:1513, 1979.

66. McDonald, J.A., and Kelley, W.N.: Lesch-Nyhan syndrome: altered kinetic properties of mutant enzyme, Science **171**:689, 1971.

67. McKusick, V.A.: Mendelian inheritance in man, ed. 5, Baltimore, 1978, Johns Hopkins University Press.

68. McKusick, V.A., Neufeld, E.F., and Kelly, T.E.: The mucopolysaccharide storage diseases. In Stanbury, J.B., Wyngaarden, J.B., and Fredrickson, D.S., editors: The metabolic basis of inherited diseases, ed. 4, New York, 1978, McGraw-Hill Book Co.

69. Monod, J., Changeux, J.-P., and Jacob, F.: Allosteric proteins and cellular systems, J. Mol. Biol. **6**:306, 1963.

70. Osserman, E.F.: Plasma-cell myeloma. II. Clinical aspects, N. Engl. J. Med. **261**:952, 1959.

71. Owen, M.C., and Carrel, R.W.: Alpha-1-antitrypsin: molecular abnormality of S variant, Br. Med. J. **1**:130, 1976.

72. Penttila, A., and Trump, B.: Studies on the modification of the cellular response to injury. II. Electron microscopic studies on the protective effect of acidosis on anoxic injury of Ehrlich ascites tumor cells, Virchows Archiv. (Cell Pathol.) **18**:1, 1975.

73. Pereira, H.G.: The cytopathic effect of animal viruses, Adv. Virus Res. **8**:245, 1961.

74. Pinnel, S.R., et al.: A heritable disorder of connective tissue, hydroxylysine-deficient collagen disease, N. Engl. J. Med. **286**:1013, 1972.

75. Pirani, C.L., Catchpole, H.R., and Moore, O.: Prevention of casein-induced amyloidosis by splenectomy, Fed. Proc. **18**:500, 1959.

76. Pollycove, M.: Hemochromatosis. In Stanbury, J.B., Wyngaarden, J.B., and Fredrickson, D.S., editors: The metabolic basis of inherited disease, ed. 3, New York, 1972, McGraw-Hill Book Co.

77. Puck, T.T., and Marcus, P.I.: Action of x-rays on mammalian cells, J. Exp. Med. **103**:653, 1956.

78. Rabinowitz, M., et al.: Synthesis and turnover of heart mitochondria in normal hypertrophied and hypoxic rat. In Alpert, N.R., editor: Cardiac hypertrophy, New York, 1971, Academic Press, Inc.

79. Reynolds, E.S., Thiers, R.E., and Vallee, B.L.: Mitochondrial function and metal content in carbon tetrachloride poisoning, J. Biol. Chem. **237**:35, 1962.

80. Rieselback, R.W., et al.: Diminished renal urate secretion per nephron as a basis for primary gout, Ann. Intern. Med. **73**:359, 1970.

81. Rosa, J., and Rubin, E.: Effects of ethanol on amino acid uptake by rat liver cells, Lab. Invest. **43**:366, 1980.

82. Rottenberg, H., Robertson, D.E., and Rubin, E.: The effect of ethanol on the temperature dependence of respiration and ATPase activities of rat liver mitochondria, Lab. Invest. **42**:318, 1980.

83. Scarpelli, D.G.: Experimental nephrocalcinosis: a biochemical and morphologic study, Lab. Invest. **14**:123, 1965.

84. Schanne, F.A.X., et al.: Calcium dependence of toxic cell death: a final common pathway, Science **206**:700, 1979.

85. Scheel, L.D., et al.: Toxicity of silica. II. Characteristics of protein films absorbed by quartz, Arch. Industr. Hyg. **9**:29, 1954.

86. Scholes, G., and Weiss, J.: Chemical action of x-rays on nucleic acids and related substances in aqueous systems. II. The mecha-

nism of the action of x-rays on nucleic acids in aqueous systems, Biochem. J. **56**:65, 1954.

87. Scrutton, M.C., and Utter, M.F.: Regulation of glycolysis and gluconeogenesis in animal tissues, Annu. Rev. Biochem. **37**:249, 1968.

88. Sharp, H.L.: Alpha$_1$-antitrypsin deficiency, Hosp. Pract. **6**:83, 1971.

89. Shirahama, T., and Cohen, A.S.: High resolution electron microscopic analysis of the amyloid fibril, J. Cell Biol. **33**:679, 1967.

90. Shirahama, T., and Cohen, A.S.: Ultrastructural evidence for leakage of lysosomal contents after phagocytosis of monosodium urate crystals, Am. J. Pathol. **76**:501, 1974.

91. Siekevitz, P.: On the meaning of intracellular structure for metabolic regulation. In Wolstenholme, G.E.W., and O'Connor, C.A., editors: Regulation of cell metabolism, London, 1959, J. & A. Churchill.

92. Smith, L.H., Jr., Sullivan, M., and Huguley, C.M., Jr.: Pyrimidine metabolism in man. IV. The enzymatic defect of orotic aciduria, J. Clin. Invest. **40**:656, 1981.

93. Smith, M.T., Thor, H., and Orrenius, S.: Toxic injury to isolated hepatocytes is not dependent on extracellular calcium, Science **213**:1257, 1981.

94. Smuckler, E.A., and Benditt, E.P.: Studies on CCl$_4$ intoxication. III. A subcellular defect in protein synthesis, Biochemistry **4**:671, 1965.

95. Smuckler, E.A., Iseri, O.A., and Benditt, E.P.: A defect in protein synthesis induced by carbon tetrachloride, J. Exp. Med. **116**:55, 1962.

96. Strehler, B.L., et al.: Rate and magnitude of age pigment accumulation in the human myocardium, J. Gerontol. **14**:430, 1959.

97. Sussman, M., et al.: Hydroxylysine-deficient skin collagen in a patient with a form of Ehlers-Danlos syndrome, J. Bone Joint Surg. **56**:1228, 1974.

98. Tanaka, T., et al.: Two types of pyruvate kinase from rat tissues, J. Biochem. (Tokyo) **62**:71, 1967.

99. Thier, S.O., and Segal, S.: Cystinuria. In Stanbury, J.B., Wyngaarden, J.B., and Fredrickson, D.S., editors: The metabolic basis of inherited diseases, ed. 4, New York, 1978, McGraw-Hill Book Co.

100. Thomson, M.L.: Relative efficiency of pigment and horny layer thickness in protecting the skin of Europeans and Africans against solar ultraviolet radiation, J. Physiol. **127**:236, 1955.

101. Trump, B.F., Croker, B.P., Jr., and Mergner, W.J.: The role of energy metabolism, ion, and water shifts in the pathogenesis of cell injury. In Richter, G.W., and Scarpelli, D.G., editors: Cell membranes: biological and pathological aspects, Baltimore, 1971, The Williams & Wilkins Co.

102. Vigliani, E.C., Boselli, A., and Pecchiai, L.: Studi sulla compnente emoplasmopatica della silicosi, Med. Lav. **41**:33, 1950.

103. Virchow, R.: Die Cellularpathologie in ihrer Begründung auf physiologische und pathologische Gewebelehre, Berlin, 1858, A. Hirschwald.

104. von Gierke, E.: Hepato-nephromegalia glykogenica (Glykogenspeicherkrankheit der Leber und Nieren), Beitr. Pathol. **82**:4971, 1929.

105. Weber, G., Singhal, R.L., and Srivastava, S.K.: Regulation of biosynthesis of hepatic gluconeogenetic enzymes. In Weber, G., editor: Advances in enzyme regulation, vol. 3, Oxford, 1965, Pergamon Press, Inc.

106. Weinberg, W.: Uber den Nachweis der Verbung beim Menschen, Jahreshefte Verein f. vaterl, Naturk in Württemberg **64**:368, 1908.

107. Weissler, A.M., et al.: Role of anaerobic metabolism in the preservation of functional capacity and structure of anoxic myocardium, J. Clin. Invest. **47**:403, 1968.

108. Weissman, G.: Crystals, lysosomes and gout, Adv. Intern. Med. **19**:239, 1974.

CHAPTER 4   Injuries Caused by Physical Agents

CHARLES S. HIRSCH
ROSS E. ZUMWALT

Physical injuries include those caused by mechanical trauma, increases or decreases of atmospheric pressure, sound waves, heat (local and systemic), cold (local and systemic), and electricity. In terms of morbidity and mortality, mechanical trauma is more important by an order of magnitude than all other modalities of physical injury combined. Therefore, more than half of this chapter is devoted to mechanical trauma.

MECHANICAL TRAUMA

Force or mechanical energy is that which changes the state of rest or uniform motion of matter. When force applied to any part of the body results in a harmful disturbance in function or structure, a mechanical injury is said to have been sustained.

The most common manifestation of such an injury is a disruption in the continuity of tissue, or a wound. The force responsible for wound production is usually liberated incident to a collision between the body and some external mass and may be derived from the motion of the body itself, from the motion of the other participant in the collision, or from both.

Wounding by mechanical trauma is governed by (1) the amount of force transmitted to the tissues, (2) the rate of application of force to the tissues, (3) the surface area involved in energy transfer, and (4) the characteristics of the target area.

Physical principles
Amount of force

The kinetic energy or wound-producing capacity that an object has in consequence of its motion is determined by its weight and velocity. In the case of simple forward motion, this force may be computed by the formula $MV^2/2g$, in which M = weight, V = velocity, and g = the acceleration of gravity. It is important to note that the kinetic energy of a moving object increases arithmetical-ly in relation to its weight and geometrically in relation to its velocity. If two objects, one weighing twice as much as the other, are traveling at the same velocity, the kinetic energy of the former will be twice that of the latter; however, if they weigh the same but one is traveling twice as fast as the other, the energy will be four times as great. Wounding by bullets provides an important application of this principle to an understanding of the resulting injuries. Bullets fired from military and hunting rifles commonly have muzzle velocities three to four times as great as those fired from handguns. Consequently, such high-velocity bullets have kinetic energies nine to 16 times greater than their low-velocity counterparts.

One should not infer that the kinetic energy and the wound-producing force of a mass in motion are necessarily identical. Only that part of the total energy of motion actually utilized in changing the state of rest or uniform motion of the tissues is capable of contributing to injury production. Unexpended force, possessed by the source of energy after the impulse of collision, is still capable of doing work and has not contributed to injury production. Force of impact utilized to induce uniform motion of the tissues or to displace or deform the object that has struck the tissue is likewise noninjurious, since it has been expended for work other than disturbing the uniform state of rest or motion of the tissues.

In addition to the kinetic energy of forward motion, an object may possess energy by reason of the fact that it is rotating on its own axis. Such energy frequently is possessed by a flying missile and adds to the wound-producing capacity of bullets. The extra energy possessed by a spinning object may be calculated from the formula $IW^2/2g$, in which I = the rotary inertia or $Mr^2/2g$ (r = radius of cross section and M = weight), W = the angular velocity in radians per second or $2\pi \times$ number of rotations/second, and g = the acceleration of gravity.

Rate of energy transfer

The duration of impulse or period of energy transfer is an important factor in determining how much of the force of an impact will be expended in the causation of uniform or noninjurious motion and how much in the causation of nonuniform or potentially injurious movement of the tissues. Athletes are aware of the desirability of prolonging the duration of impulse. To diminish the amount of force likely to be expended in the production of nonuniform or disruptive movement of tissues, the tumbler rolls with his fall, the ballplayer moves his gloved hand with the caught ball, and the fighter endeavors to move with his opponent's blow. Protracted deceleration probably accounts in large measure for the occasional and seemingly miraculous survival of people who have fallen from great heights.

Surface area

Another important factor in determining the wound-producing capacity of an impact is the size of the surface area to which the force is applied. The larger the area through which a given amount of impact force is transmitted, the less will be its intensity. Thus, an impulse of a certain number of foot-pounds might cause uniform tissue displacement without injury when acting over a large area and yet be capable of causing severe disruption of tissue when acting through an area comparable to the edge or point of a knife.

Target area

Many other factors may modify the disruptive effects of impacts even when they are similar in respect to the amount of energy expended, the duration of impulse, and the area of collision contact. Among these is the extent to which the force may be intensified by lever action or by hydrostatic effect. A small force applied near the end of a lever will be greatly intensified as the fulcrum is approached. This phenomenon is particularly important in relation to the production of fractures of long bones. Similarly, a relatively small compression of a large hollow viscus may displace a sufficient volume of fluid to rupture the wall of a less voluminous communicating structure. Differences in the elasticity, plasticity, or inertia of tissues are of great importance in respect to whether a given force will produce disruptive change. Liver is ordinarily more friable and more readily disrupted by distortion than is lung or muscle. A hyperplastic and friable spleen may be torn to pieces by an impact that would be harmless to a normal spleen. The capillary fragility of persons with certain vitamin deficiencies is often greater than that of the normal individual.

The foregoing discussion of the mechanics of injury production by the energy of motion has concerned disruption of tissue or wound production. Although a wound is the most common manifestation of injury caused by the energy of motion, it is by no means the only one. Force has been defined as that which changes the state of rest or uniform motion of matter. The application of force to the surface of the body may alter subsurface relationships sufficiently to cause severe functional disturbance even though no cutaneous wound is produced. In fact, many victims of fatal blunt trauma have no externally visible wound. This pertains especially to persons with head injuries whose scalp is shielded by thick hair or a hat and to persons who sustain chest and abdominal impacts over a broad area.

Also, the application of pressure in many situations may cause harmful interference with the function of the compressed or displaced tissue even though the force is insufficient to produce a wound. Mechanical obstruction of the air passages for more than a few minutes is likely to cause death from systemic anoxia. A tight tourniquet applied for 30 minutes may result in ischemic necrosis of a limb. Furthermore, as in many other areas of pathology, traumatically induced functional disturbances can be profound, or even lethal, yet not structurally demonstrable. For example, the term *instantaneous physiologic death* can be used to describe the rapidly fatal outcome of a blunt impact to the chest that fails to mark the skin, causes no fractures of the sternum or ribs, and does not produce a cardiac contusion.[2] Such deaths probably result from ventricular fibrillation, a structurally traceless lethal mechanism.

Local effects of mechanical violence
Wounds

As previously indicated, a wound is a mechanically produced interruption in the continuity of tissue. There are several anatomic types of such disruptive lesions, for which distinctive terms are used.

Abrasion. An abrasion (scratch or scrape) represents the tearing away of epidermal cells by friction or crushing. Such a defect may or may not penetrate to the corium. Although an abrasion may provide a portal of entry for infection, such a wound is ordinarily of little pathologic significance beyond the fact that it provides objective evidence that force has been applied to the surface of the body. The direction of motion responsible for an abrasion can frequently be recognized by the manner in which the partially detached sheets of epidermis have been rolled on themselves at the distal end of the defect (Fig. 4-1). In some instances the nature of the abrading object can be recognized by the distribution and configuration of the epidermal defects.

Laceration. The word "laceration" is commonly *misused* as a synonym for a cut (or incised wound). A laceration is a split or tear and represents the effect of excessive stretching of tissue. Although any tissue may be disrupted in this manner, such injuries most commonly involve the integument, particularly where it is

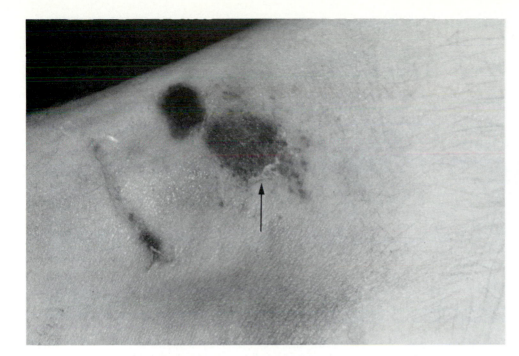

Fig. 4-1. Abrasion of left medial malleolus of a pedestrian who was "knocked out of his shoes" when struck by auto. Force acting on ankle as it exited the shoe was directed distally and nearly parallel to the surface. Heaping of epidermis (arrow) on lower margin of injury reflects direction and orientation of abrading force.

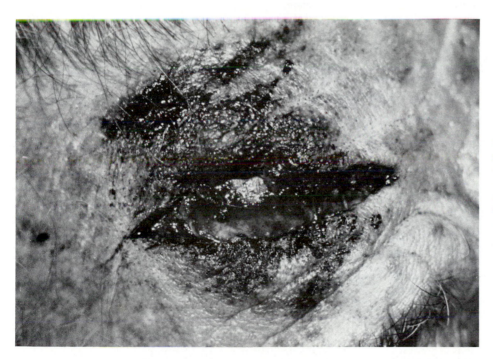

Fig. 4-2. Abraded laceration of forehead caused by impact of circumscribed object with force directed perpendicular to the skin. Abrasion resulted from crushing of epidermis, and laceration was due to stretching of skin over subjacent bone.

stretched over bone, as in the hands or over the skull. Lacerations of skin caused by the unidirectional displacement and stretching that occur incident to the impact of an obliquely directed force are likely to be linear or curved, whereas those produced by the multidirectional radial displacement of a crushing impact oriented at a right angle to the skin may be linear or stellate. The latter commonly have crushed, abraded margins; such an injury is an *abraded laceration* (Fig. 4-2). Linear lacera-

tions may be so cleanly disrupted as to resemble an incised wound. In such a circumstance it may be necessary to identify the attenuated strands of tissue that bridge the margins of the defect in order to recognize it as a laceration (Fig. 4-3). In the case of curved or angular lacerations of the skin, the apex of the angle or the convexity of the curve will face the direction from which the force was applied.

The force of an external impact may lacerate internal

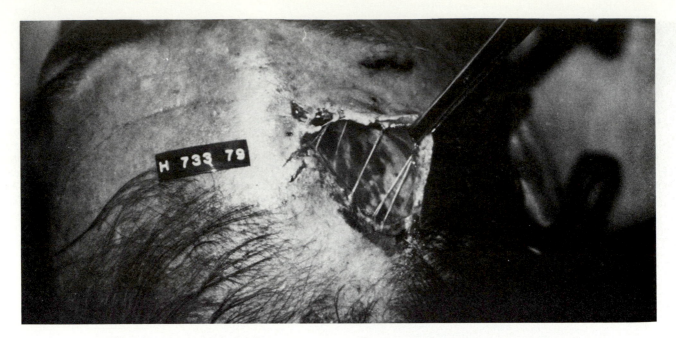

Fig. 4-3. Linear laceration of forehead with undermining of distal margin. Strands of tissue bridging defect indicate that injury is a laceration rather than an incised wound, because a cutting instrument cannot leave intact tissue above its deepest penetration.

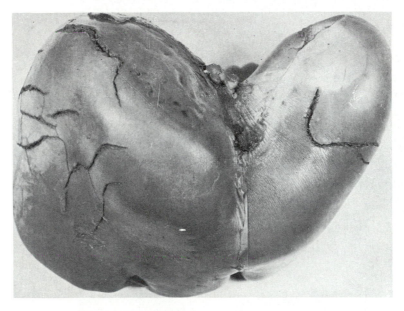

Fig. 4-4. Multiple lacerations of liver caused by lateral compression of thorax. There were no external wounds or fractures. Death resulted from hemoperitoneum.

structures without damage to the skin or subcutaneous tissue (Fig. 4-4). Thus ligaments, muscles, or blood vessels are frequently lacerated by excessive stretching with or without superficial injury. Compression of fluid or gas in hollow viscera may cause laceration and perforation of their walls (Fig. 4-5). Soft tissues adjacent to the site of a fracture are usually lacerated by the broken ends of the bone.

Contusion. A contusion or bruise is an injury in which the force of an impact is transmitted through the skin to the underlying tissues with sufficient intensity to disrupt the walls of small blood vessels and to cause interstitial bleeding without disruption of the epidermis (Fig. 4-6).

Usually the interstitial bleeding is so superficial as to be almost immediately visible through the skin. Howev-

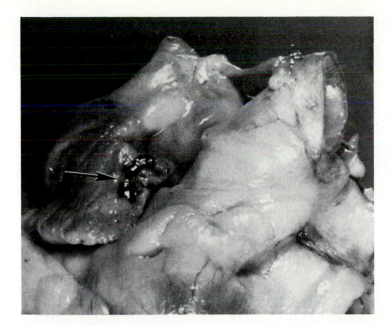

Fig. 4-5. "Blowout" laceration of right atrial appendage *(arrow),* the sole cardiac injury in young woman who fell from a height and landed on her chest. Compression of right atrium during diastole caused hydrostatic transmission of pressure into atrial appendage with laceration of its tip. Death resulted from hemopericardium with tamponade.

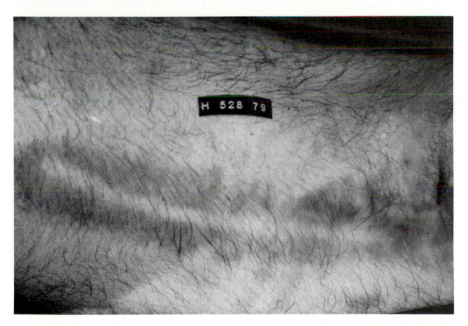

Fig. 4-6. Contusions caused by one impact with cylindrical object on posterior thigh. Linear pale mark indicates point of impact, which was subjected to uniform compressive stress. Adjacent, parallel, linear contusions correspond to areas of maximal shearing stress along edges of striking object.

er, a bruise may be so deep that either hours elapse before the extravasated blood becomes superficial enough to be visible or it is never seen from the surface. An external impact may cause extensive bruising of internal viscera without damage to the skin or subcutaneous tissue.

Individuals vary enormously in their susceptibility to mechanical disruption of small blood vessels. Persons with certain dietary deficiencies or blood dyscrasias are likely to sustain remarkably extensive contusions as a result of relatively mild impacts.

Incision. An *incised wound* (or cut) is one produced by the pressure and friction against skin or other tissues by an instrument having a sharp edge. By definition an incised wound is longer than it is deep. *Stab wounds* are deeper than they are long. In these types of injury the tissues are uniformly displaced to either side of the cutting edge with the result that the primary damage is limited largely to the immediate vicinity of the defect.

Penetrating injury. The impact of any appropriately shaped resistant object against the skin may produce a defect so deep and of such relatively small diameter that its outstanding characteristic is penetration. Slender sharp objects and flying missiles are the most common causes of such injuries. Although the majority of penetrating wounds involve the skin and subcutaneous tissue, the broken end of a bone often causes penetrating injury without involving the integument.

Fracture. Any force that tends to change the state of uniform motion or rest of the body is likely to disrupt its least plastic tissue, the bony skeleton. A fracture is a mechanically produced disruption in the continuity of bone. Such osseous defects vary from a simple linear break, caused by excessive bending, to an explosive comminution caused by the impact of a high-velocity projectile. Of particular importance in the mechanics of fracture production is the transmission of force from the site of external application and its intensification at a distant point through lever action. One should not assume that the stress responsible for a fracture is necessarily of unusual magnitude or of external origin. A relatively minor stress may cause *pathologic fractures* of diseased bones.

Traffic injuries

Because traffic injuries are so common and exemplify the physical principles involved in blunt wound production, they deserve separate consideration.[38]

Injuries to vehicle occupants. The most straightforward situation with respect to the fate of vehicle occupants is a head-on crash without ejection. Such a collision with another vehicle or fixed object (such as a bridge abutment) causes the car to decelerate rapidly or come to a dead stop. The occupants are, of course, moving at the same speed and in the same direction as the vehicle at the instant of its crash. However, because they are not riveted to the vehicular frame, they do not decelerate and stop with it. Instead, they continue on their forward course as masses in motion until they meet an opposing force. The latter force is exerted by their impact against the vehicle interior. To recapitulate, the first collision involves the vehicle and some other object; the second collision involves the occupant and the interior of the vehicle, and this is the injury-producing energy transfer. Other types of vehicular crash (such as side impacts) add a complicating factor in that the initial collision changes the vehicle's direction as well as its speed. In these more complex situations, the occupants move toward the point of vehicular crash en route to their decelerating impact with the car's interior.

The extent and severity of resulting injuries are determined by the initial velocity of the occupant, the rate of the occupant's deceleration, the nature and distribution of the opposing force that causes occupant deceleration, and the part of the body involved in energy transfer. As with other modalities of mechanical violence, rapid energy transfer and concentration of force over a small area produce more injurious, nonuniform displacement of tissues than does slowly applied, widely distributed force. All types of occupant safety systems, whether some form of restraining belt or an air bag, a collapsible steering column, padded interior panels, or recessed knobs and buttons, are designed to prolong the energy transfer of deceleration, to distribute the decelerating force over the broadest or sturdiest possible area of the occupant's body, and to prevent unrestrained movement (and ejection) of the occupant after the vehicular crash.

Injuries to the head and neck commonly result from impacts against the windshield, side windows, or upper part of the vehicular frame. Trunk injuries are caused by decelerating impacts against the steering wheel (Fig. 4-7) or column, dashboard, or back of the front seat in the case of rear-seat passengers. Injuries of the lower limbs are frequently produced by impacts against the dashboard, foot compression against the floor, or entanglement of the feet in pedals or beneath the seats. Arm fractures can be produced when an occupant braces for a front-end collision by gripping the steering wheel or the dashboard.

Improperly worn safety belts can cause or contribute to patterns of injury.[12,49] Lap belts should be worn over the pelvic area so that the sturdy iliac crests absorb the stress of deceleration. If they are worn loosely or high, the force thereby transmitted to the abdomen can injure virtually any structure between the diaphragm and pelvis (Fig. 4-8). Likewise, an improperly worn shoulder strap, resting against the side of the neck rather than the upper chest, can cause severe cervical injury.

Occupant ejection from the vehicle allows for second or additional impacts with the road and other objects, greatly increasing the likelihood of serious injury or death. A crash that causes such severe deformity of the vehicle interior that the occupants are crushed is a nonsurvivable accident.

Injuries to pedestrians. Pedestrian fatalities are of three general types, with an approximately equal incidence. One third are children who carelessly dart into the path of a moving vehicle; one third are elderly persons who may have defective vision or hearing, which usually is coupled with diminished agility; and one third are healthy adults who commonly are under the influence of ethanol. Pedestrians sustain injuries when they are run over, "run under," or violently slammed aside.

A person is run over in one of two circumstances; either he is lying in the path of a moving vehicle or his center of gravity lies below the point of impact with the vehicle. The latter situation arises with children and crouching adults or when the involved vehicle is a bus or truck whose front end is high and broad. Tire tread marks on the victim's skin or clothing can be conspicuous or subtle, but the injured area almost invariably shows underlying avulsions of subcutaneous fat and severe crushing. An exception to the foregoing sometimes occurs when the victim is lying on a surface that yields, such as soft dirt or grass.

It is far more common for pedestrians to be *run under* than *run over*.[38] This occurs when an upright adult is struck by a moving vehicle below his center of gravity.

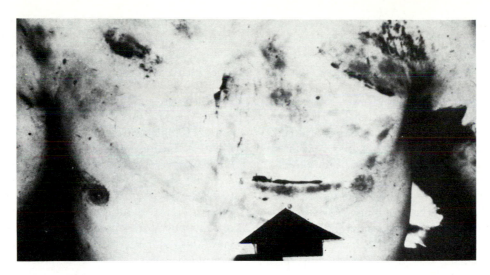

Fig. 4-7. Multiple contusions and abrasions on chest of driver killed in head-on collision. Curved abrasion *(arrow)* resulted from impact against steering wheel. (Courtesy Office of the Chief Medical Examiner, Baltimore, Md.)

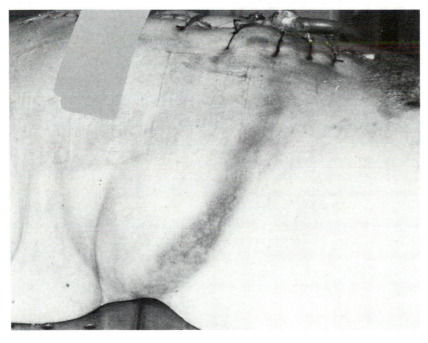

Fig. 4-8. Bandlike contusion extending across right flank and lower abdomen of driver who sustained mesenteric and small intestinal lacerations in a head-on collision. Patterned bruise and visceral injuries probably resulted from force applied to trunk by way of improperly worn lap belt.

Compound ("bumper") fractures of the lower legs are the classic stigmas of such impacts, but the thighs, hips, and low back are other common areas of initial impact.[46] As a result of the primary impact, the pedestrian's legs are thrown forward and elevated. His next impact usually occurs when he strikes the automobile hood or roof, after which he bounces to the pavement. The point or points of secondary impact with the vehicle are determined by the victim's height and weight and the speed and config-

uration of the moving vehicle. If the auto is moving rapidly, it may pass completely beneath the victim, who is tossed high into the air and comes down on the road. The majority of pedestrian fatalities result from head injuries.

Victims who walk or run into the side of a moving vehicle usually are hurled aside. They may impact against a wide variety of nearby objects before hitting the ground and generally sustain head injuries.

Injuries to cyclists. Cyclists sustain injuries when they are struck by motor vehicles, when they drive into a vehicle or some other object, or when they lose their balance and fall. The cyclist who is hit by a moving vehicle is the mechanical equivalent of a "sitting pedestrian," and the principles governing injury in this circumstance are similar to those mentioned previously. The cyclist who hits another object is the mechanical equivalent of an unrestrained, open-vehicle occupant who is "launched" when he continues in forward motion after his cycle is stopped by its decelerating impact. As with pedestrians, the vulnerability of cyclists allows for multiple severe injuries of more than one body area, although craniocerebral trauma is the leading cause of cyclist fatalities.

Common medicolegal problems associated with traffic injuries

Toxicology. Blood ethanol determinations should be done on all teenage and adult victims of traffic accidents who survive their injuries for less than 24 hours. Tests for carboxyhemoglobin are indicated when vehicles catch fire or when there is a possibility that the car had a defective exhaust system or extensive rusting of its undersurface. On the latter basis, we have seen fatal asphyxia by carbon monoxide in occupants of a car parked in an open area with its engine running.

The slightest suspicion of drug involvement in any victim of a fatal traffic incident should prompt the pathologist to save at least 50 ml of blood and urine, all available bile, stomach content, and generous samples of liver, kidney, and brain. Toxicologists have adequate means to dispose of samples they do not need, but none can retrieve a specimen that went down the drain or into an incinerator. Nothing frustrates the toxicologist more than a 5 to 10 ml sample of blood accompanied by an all-encompassing request that it be analyzed for "drugs."

Identity of driver. When all vehicle occupants are ejected, important medicolegal questions may arise concerning the identity of the driver. Patterns of injury may provide the answer, and comparison of the victims' blood groups with the location of blood stains in the car may be helpful. Hair samples should be plucked from any hair-bearing area that is injured. The victims' clothing should be preserved carefully for evidentiary evaluation by trained personnel. In this regard, smooth-soled shoes should be examined, since they may show patterned imprints imparted by forces transmitted through the brake or accelerator pedals or the floor mats.

Hit-skip (hit and run) pedestrians. Samples of blood and hair should be saved as mentioned previously. In addition, fragments of metal, glass, or paint are usually present on the victim's clothing and may be on or in the victim's body. Reconstruction of the accident situation may hinge on correlation of the victim's impact areas with damage to the suspected vehicle. It should be standard practice to measure the height of impact areas on the lower limbs above the level of the heels. The presence of cataracts or optic atrophy occasionally helps to explain why an elderly pedestrian walked into the path of an oncoming vehicle, thereby exonerating an innocent driver.

Firearm injuries

Guns and bullets. Pulling the trigger of a loaded gun causes the firing pin to strike the cartridge base, detonating the primer. The latter event causes ignition of gunpowder in the cartridge. Gunpowder combustion produces rapidly expanding gas, the pressure of which propels the bullet.

A bullet's diameter, or caliber, can be expressed in hundreths of an inch or in millimeters. Fig. 4-9 shows representative handgun bullets of commonly available calibers. The .25- and .45-caliber bullets have full copper jackets, and the .38-caliber bullet on the right has a partial copper jacket. The .22-caliber bullet has been coated with a thin film of copper ("copper wash"), which is not a discrete jacket. The specimens arranged on the bottom row of Fig. 4-9 are bullets that have been deformed and

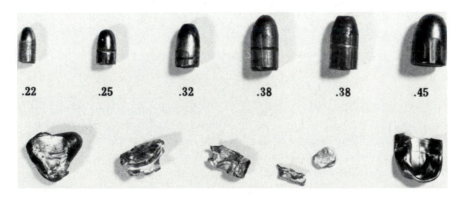

Fig. 4-9. *Top row,* Bullets of commonly available calibers for handguns. *Bottom row,* Deformed bullets, misshapen bullet fragments, and a deformed partial jacket (see text).

fragmented as a result of their passage through a hard object such as bone. A misshapen partial jacket, which has been separated from the bullet core after contact with a hard object, is shown at the far right of the bottom row. Deformed bullets and fragments such as these present irregular surfaces to the tissues in their path. Consequently, they are likely to expend all of their energy in wound production. From the standpoint of "wounding efficiency," the residual kinetic energy possessed by a bullet as it exits from the victim is wasted because it has not been utilized in injury production.

During the manufacture of handgun and rifle barrels, a rifling tool cuts a series of spiral grooves in their interiors. The elevated surfaces between the grooves are called "lands." Because the internal diameter of the barrel is slightly smaller than the bullets intended for use in the gun, the fired bullet entering the breech end of the barrel is gripped by the lands, which impart a spin to it as it passes through the barrel. This spin about its long axis produces the bullet's gyroscopic stability while it is in flight and is responsible for some of the important characteristics of cutaneous wounds to be described presently.

In addition to the bullet, a variety of particulate matter emerges from the muzzle of a fired gun. The smallest particles are the residue of completely burned gunpowder and take the form of a black, dustlike material. These particles are so light that they generally travel only 6 to 8 inches from the gun muzzle. As a result, targets shot at ranges closer than 6 to 8 inches usually show a zone of black *fouling* or *smudging* surrounding the bullet perforation (Fig. 4-10). Larger particles emerging with or behind the bullet consist of partially burned or unburned gunpowder, metal shavings, and other debris or lubricant from the barrel interior or bullet surface. Since these particles are larger and heavier than the dustlike

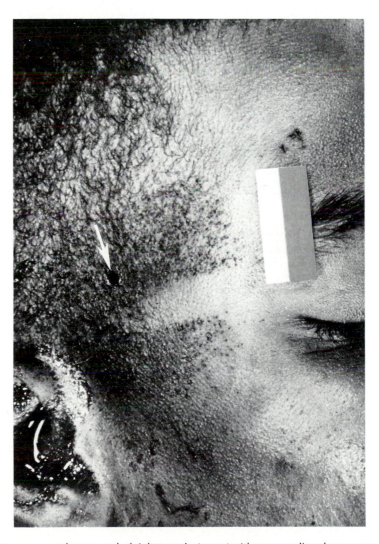

Fig. 4-10. Entrance gunshot wound of right temple *(arrow)* with surrounding dense zone of fouling. Skin adjacent to lateral aspect of eyebrow has been shielded by frame of decedent's eyeglasses. (Courtesy Office of the Chief Medical Examiner, Baltimore, Md.)

residue of completely burned powder, they travel farther. In flight they take the form of tiny individual missiles, each creating a punctate impression on or in the target. Collectively, these individual marks are referred to as *stippling* or *tattooing* (Fig. 4-11). Most handguns produce stippling up to ranges of 1½ to 3 feet.

Cutaneous entrance wounds. In reference to muzzle-target distance, we use the following classification for handgun and rifle wounds. *Contact* shots are those in which the muzzle of the gun touches the target. When the muzzle is pressed firmly against the skin that all of the powder residue is blasted *into* the tissue, the wound is classified as *tight contact* (Fig. 4-12). If the seal between muzzle and skin is imperfect, a *loose contact* wound results in which powder residue is deposited *on* the cutaneous surface as well as being blasted *into* the wound track (Fig. 4-13). In either instance the expanding gas that follows the bullet augments the severity of the injury. When the muzzle does not touch the target but is sufficiently close to produce fouling, the wound is *close*

range. Wounds having stippling but no fouling are *intermediate range*, and those beyond the range of stippling are *distant*. In reference to cutaneous wounds, the foregoing criteria are inappropriate when the skin is not the primary target. Passage of a bullet through thick hair, clothing, or some other object before it strikes the skin may filter some or all of the powder residue, shielding the skin from fouling and stippling (Figs. 4-10 and 4-11).

The appearance of a contact-range gunshot wound is determined by the amount of gunpowder in the cartridge (load), the characteristics of the firearm, the firmness of the seal between muzzle and skin, and the part of the body that is shot. If sufficient expanding gas is blasted into an area with underlying firm bony support (such as the head), the skin is torn loose from its attachment and lacerated (Fig. 4-12, *A*). Such wounds are commonplace with contact-range wounds produced by handguns of .32 caliber or greater. Smaller-caliber handgun ammunition often does not produce sufficient gas to lacerate the skin.

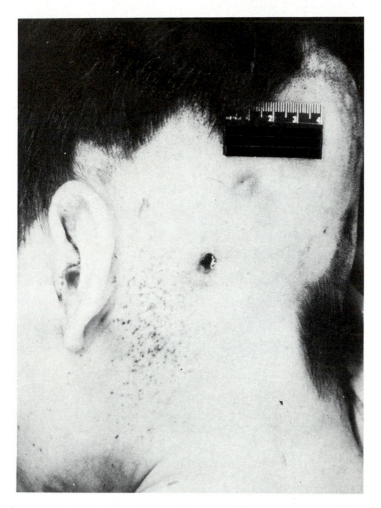

Fig. 4-11. Left occipital entrance gunshot wound with stippling visible in left mastoid area and on decedent's left cheek. The scalp, exposed by postmortem shaving, shows no stippling because it was shielded by hair. Fouling is absent. (Courtesy Office of the Chief Medical Examiner, Baltimore, Md.)

Instead it may elevate the skin from its support and press it back against the face of the gun, imparting a "muzzle stamp" to the skin surrounding the gunshot perforation (Fig. 4-12, *B*). If the arrangement of the tissues is such that the explosive force can be decompressed *internally*, as is likely with contact wounds of the chest or abdomen, the external characteristics of the cutaneous wound may resemble those of a distant wound.

Typical distant cutaneous entrance wounds are abraded perforations whose central defect is slightly smaller than the bullet diameter. This characteristic appearance is the combined result of the bullet's spin about its long axis (see the preceding) and the skin's elasticity. In the process of perforating the skin, the bullet initially indents and stretches it. The epidermis in contact with the margin of the spinning bullet is scraped away, creating a rim of abrasion about the perforation. The outer circumference of the abrasion collar may be soiled by lubricant or dirt ("gray ring"), which must not be misinterpreted as fouling. Bullets striking the skin at right angles usually produce a uniform margin of abrasion (Figs. 4-14 and 4-15), whereas those that strike at an angle of less than 90 degrees leave asymmetric abrasions whose widest margin indicates the direction from which

A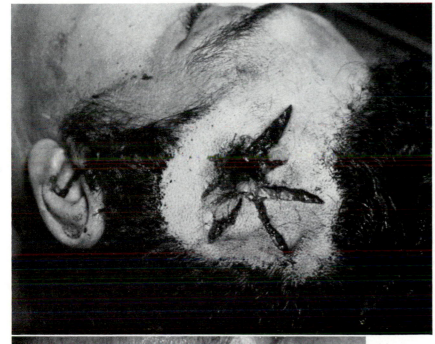

B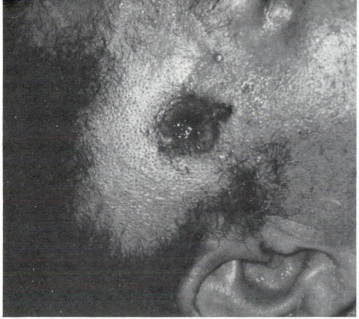

Fig. 4-12. Typical, tight contact-range gunshot wounds with no escape of powder residue onto cutaneous surface adjacent to perforations. Expanding gas blasted into wound in **A** caused extensive lacerations, whereas in **B**, gas elevated scalp and pressed it against gun, producing "muzzle stamp" abrasion that includes impression of the gun site in 3 o'clock position. In **B**, quantity of gas was insufficient to lacerate skin. Internally both wounds contain abundant powder residue.

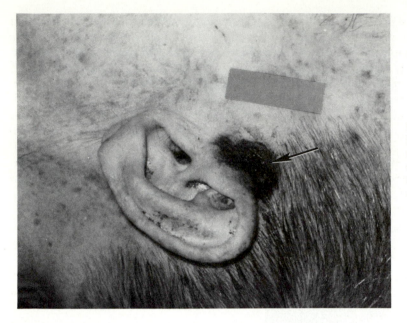

Fig. 4-13. Loose contact-range gunshot wound with imperfect seal between muzzle and skin, allowing escape of gas and powder residue onto cutaneous surface adjacent to perforation. Arrow indicates centrally located perforation. Internally, tracks of such wounds contain powder residue.

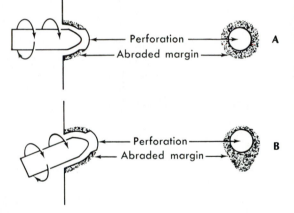

Fig. 4-14. Schematic representation of mechanism whereby spinning bullets cause abraded defects when they perforate an elastic structure such as skin. Bullet striking at a right angle, **A,** creates a uniform margin of abrasion, whereas bullet approaching at an acute angle, **B,** leaves asymmetric abrasion that is widest on the side from which the bullet approached.

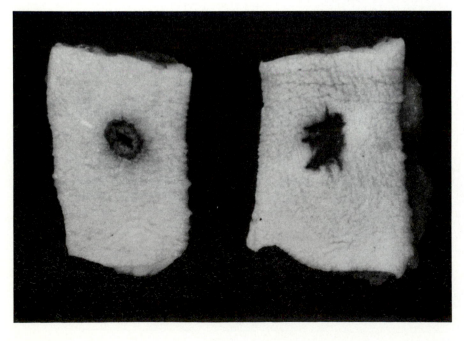

Fig. 4-15. Cutaneous entrance *(left)* and exit wounds made by same bullet. Symmetric, uniform margin of abrasion surrounding entrance perforation indicates that bullet approached at a nearly right angle. Exit wound is a lacerated, nonabraded perforation.

the bullet approached the skin (Figs. 4-14 and 4-16).

Atypical entrance gunshot wounds are those having unusual configurations, which commonly include lacerated margins and alteration of the typical abrasion collar described previously. Such anomalies occur in a variety of circumstances. Alterations of a bullet's normal gyroscopic spin and exaggerations of its yaw may be produced by defective guns or faulty ammunition, ricochet off a solid object, or passage of a bullet through some other target before it strikes the skin. In the last instance, if the primary target is close to the victim or is a personal item, such as spectacles or jewelry, fragments of the article may act as secondary missiles, which complicate the bullet perforation. In like fashion, primary perforation of a victim's hand or arm may render a wound of reentrance on his trunk or face decidedly atypical (Fig. 4-17). Finally, when the skin of the target area has a texture or contour different from that of ordinary skin, its wound (of entrance or exit) may have a totally different appearance. Examples of such areas include the eyelids, nose, lips, external ears, penis, scrotum, and fingertips.

Rifle wounds usually differ from those inflicted by handguns because the former typically are caused by bullets with much greater kinetic energy. Commonly available handguns loaded with standard ammunition generally fire bullets with an initial muzzle velocity of 600 to 1000 feet per second, whereas rifle bullets frequently are in the range of 2000 to 3000 feet per second. Since a bullet's kinetic energy varies with the square of its velocity, a tripling of velocity increases its energy by a factor of 9.

Contact-range wounding with military and powerful civilian rifles causes massively destructive or explosive injuries. Distant wounding with these weapons will, in many instances, produce cutaneous wounds of entrance and exit that are atypical and larger than those inflicted by handguns (Fig. 4-18). Although distant rifle wounds may resemble handgun injuries externally, they generally inflict far more visceral trauma than do handgun bullets (Fig. 4-19). Small-caliber, low-velocity civilian rifle wounds may be similar to those produced by handguns.

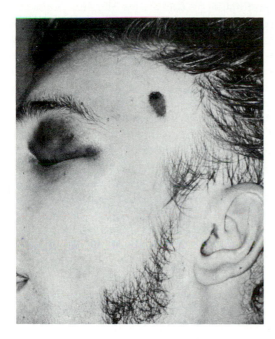

Fig. 4-16. Entrance gunshot wound of left side of forehead. Bullet approached victim at acute angle from his lower left, creating asymmetric margin of abrasion that is widest at lower left side of perforation. Ecchymosis and swelling of his left upper eyelid were produced by fracture of orbital roof as a result of gunshot wound rather than by direct facial trauma.

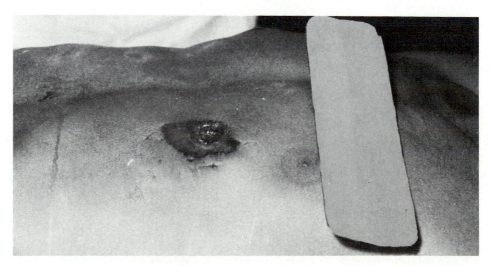

Fig. 4-17. Gunshot wound of reentrance in left inframammary area. Before striking decedent's chest, bullet perforated his right hand, passing from dorsum to palm, with exit defect on thenar eminence. At instant of wounding, palmar surface of his hand was resting against the chest. Oval abrasion, asymmetrically surrounding perforation, reflects configuration of his thenar eminence.

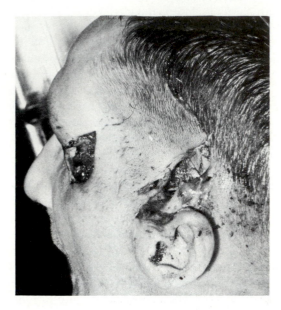

Fig. 4-18. Instantly fatal, distant-range, high-velocity (.30-caliber rifle) bullet wound of head. Entrance defect is adjacent to lateral aspect of left eyebrow, and exit defect is located above superior attachment of auricle. Skin between entrance and exit wounds has been torn loose from its attachments and shows tiny, stretch-type lacerations. (Dark spots on and behind ear are dry blood rather than stippling.) Subjacent skull was shattered, and multiple bone fragments ("secondary missiles") penetrated brain.

Cutaneous exit wounds. When a bullet leaves the body, it is traveling at a slower speed and is frequently deformed. It normally produces an irregularly lacerated wound with everted edges (Fig. 4-15). A slowly moving bullet may leave only a small, easily overlooked slit in the skin. The surface of an exit wound lacks the marginal epidermal abrasion that characterizes an entrance wound unless the skin was somehow supported at the moment it was perforated by the exiting missile. Support of this type can be provided by elastic bands of undergarments, belts, articles in pockets, or a firm external surface, such as a wall or the floor, against which the cutaneous surface was resting when perforated. With high-velocity bullets, the exit wound is usually larger than the entrance wound.

Internal injuries. Internal injuries produced by gunfire have peculiar and important characteristics caused by the velocity of the wounding missile. The extent of the injury is characteristically much greater than would be expected from the diameter of the bullet. The force of the impulse is projected radially from the path of the bullet (Figs. 4-19 and 4-20) with such intensity that it causes a cylindrical zone of disruptive change in the tissues that surround the main track of the wound.[10] Thus blood vessels may be lacerated or bones fractured at considerable distances from the path of a bullet. One of the more commonly encountered manifestations of radially transmitted forces from bullets is comminution of the orbital plates, which occurs frequently in association with transcerebral passage of projectiles (Fig. 4-16). Bul-

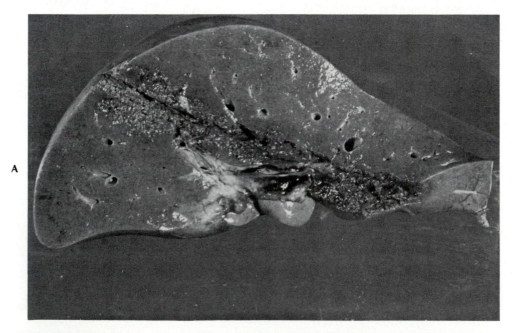

Fig. 4-19. A, Wound track through liver caused by low-velocity, .38-caliber bullet fired from revolver. Zone of tissue damage is larger than diameter of bullet, but the injury is far less destructive than that shown in **B.**

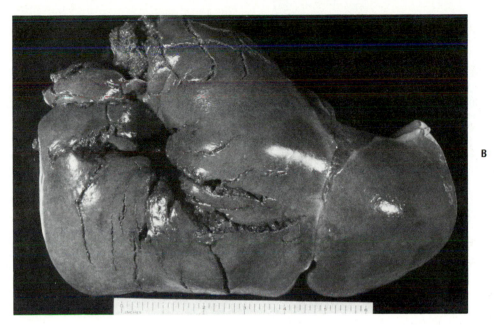

Fig. 4-19, cont'd. B, Injury caused by high-velocity, .30-caliber rifle bullet. Extensive splits of Glisson's capsule reflect radial transmission of energy. Striking contrast between the two specimens exemplifies the dominance of velocity over weight in determining wounding potential, because the .38-caliber handgun bullet was slightly heavier than the .30-caliber rifle bullet.

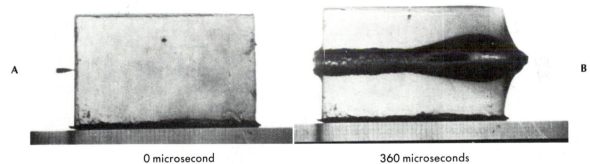

0 microsecond

360 microseconds

2160 microseconds

Fig. 4-20. Temporary cavity formation in gelatin block. **A,** A 7.62 mm rifle bullet approaching from left at velocity of 2800 feet/second. **B,** At 360 microseconds, bullet is approximately two thirds through the block and temporary cavitation has started. **C,** At 2160 microseconds, maximum formation of temporary cavity after bullet has exited the block. In living tissue the entire area of temporary cavitation is devitalized, and damage extends even beyond limits of temporary cavity. (Courtesy Armed Forces Institute of Pathology.)

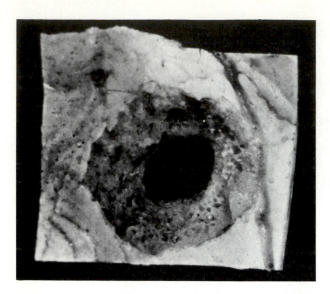

Fig. 4-21. Entrance perforation of skull made by .38-caliber bullet, viewed from the inner table, showing bone beveling in direction of flight and exemplifying principle that fractures dissipate forces acting on bone. In entrance wound of skull, bullet first strikes and fractures outer table. Force is dissipated as it is transmitted through bony trabeculae and therefore is exerted over larger area on inner table, causing larger perforation of the latter. Beveling is reversed in exit wounds, with the larger defect on outer table of skull. Most bones develop morphologically similar defects when perforated by bullets.

let perforations in bones are characteristically conical, with the entrance defect being smaller than the corresponding exit (Fig. 4-21).

Medicolegal evidence in death by gunfire. Frequently, the only opportunity to acquire reliable evidence as to the circumstances in which the injury occurred or to establish the identifying characteristics of the responsible weapon is provided by the autopsy. Such evidence may be readily lost or destroyed unless it is looked for and preserved. Loss or destruction of such medical and paramedical evidence can be disastrous. Thus failure to recognize powder residue in the interior of a wound may lead to the exclusion of suicide and give support to the erroneous suspicion that murder has been committed. Failure to distinguish an entrance wound from an exit wound may seriously distort the official investigation of a homicidal incident.

General considerations. A detailed examination and description of all skin wounds, all associated holes in the clothing, and such changes in either as might have resulted from powder residue should be routine practice in all cases of death by gunfire. It is common for a bullet that has passed through the body to be found in the clothing. The dimensions and precise location of each wound, each hole in clothing, and each area of fouling or stippling should be recorded with their locations related to standard anatomic landmarks as well as to the standing height of the victim. Color photographs are an indispensable supplement to the descriptive text.

Bullets or fragments of bullets. Any bullet or fragment of a bullet (sufficiently large to be recovered) in the body should be retrieved, even though no reason for preserving the bullet is anticipated at the time of operation or autopsy. Each bullet should be placed in its own properly labeled container and saved. In cases where more than one bullet or fragment of bullet are recovered, each should be identified in relation to the entrance wound with which it is associated.

Although the need for exercising care in the handling of projectiles and projectile fragments recovered from a victim should be common knowledge, many surgeons and some pathologists still make the mistake of extracting and handling such objects in the unprotected jaws of metal instruments or of scratching identifying initials across rifling marks on the sides of the bullet. Fig. 4-22 shows two bullets, each of which has been inscribed with the victim's initials, J.D.H. The specimen on the left is improperly marked because the initials obliterate some of the rifling striations. The correctly initialed specimen on the right has been marked on its base.

Because bullets often migrate or travel considerable distances from their entrance sites, autopsies of persons who have died from gunfire should be performed in locales where x-ray facilities are available. In the case of a perforating wound, where the bullet has emerged from the victim and has been lost, it may be extremely important to collect bullet fragments that have been sheared off in passing through a bone or deposited along the track of the wound. X-ray examination is often essential to locate such metallic debris. Subsequent identification of the chemical composition of the fragment or fragments may establish that it could or could not represent a certain type or brand of ammunition.

Direction of fire. In a case of death by gunfire, it is necessary to verify the direction from which the bullet came. If there is only one surface wound (that is, entrance defect) and the bullet is still in the victim, the problem is simplified. With low-power handguns, the bullet is frequently palpable beneath the skin of the side of the body opposite to the site of entrance. Skin offers greater resistance to perforation than any tissue other than bone or tooth.

If more than one hole is present in the skin, entrance must be distinguished from exit. The gross appearances of typical and atypical entrance and exit wounds have been described already; Adelson[1] has reported the histopathologic characteristics of cutaneous gunshot wounds. Also, one should be aware that bullet defects in clothing are frequently easier to orient as entrance or exit wounds than are the corresponding perforations of the victim's skin.

If bullet wounds in the skin (entrance or exit) have been altered or destroyed as a result of putrefaction or other postmortem change or surgery, it may still be possible to recognize the direction in which the bullet was

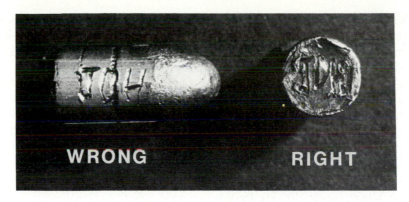

Fig. 4-22. Two nonjacketed .38-caliber bullets, each bearing initials J.D.H. Specimen on left is marked improperly because initials obscure rifling striations ("autograph" of gun from which it was fired). Specimen on right has been properly marked on its base.

traveling by the manner in which bones have been fractured. In passing through a bone, a bullet characteristically produces a larger defect at the site of exit than at the site of entrance (Fig. 4-21). It also displaces fragments of bone in the direction of its flight.

Range of fire. The evidence needed to establish the distance between the gun and the target when the shot was fired has been mentioned in connection with entrance wounds. Gray-black powder residue beneath the periosteum of the outer table of the skull or on the underlying dural margins is often seen with contact gunshot wounds of the head. Blotting of the wound with paper towels may help demonstrate powder soiling by removing excess blood. Removal of blood by this means must be done with care because contact or near-contact wounds produced by some ammunition may result in minimal surface fouling that is easily overlooked. The potential importance of such evidence for reconstructing the fatal incident is so great that the decedent should be examined by the pathologist before clothing has been removed and before the skin has been washed. If the clothing is dark, it may need to be photographed with infrared technique or tested chemically to disclose the presence or absence of combustion residues. When gunshot wounds are sustained through clothing, range of fire determinations rest on an evaluation of the garments rather than the person's skin. The effectiveness with which clothing shields the skin from powder residue is determined by the range of fire, the characteristics of the gunpowder, the number of layers of cloth perforated, and the tightness of weave of the fabric.

Contact wounds in areas with underlying skeletal muscle (such as the chest) commonly show a zone of pink discoloration in muscle surrounding the wound track. This is attributable to an uptake of carbon monoxide by myoglobin and probably also to a staining of muscle by nitrites in powder residue. The pink discoloration fades when the muscle is exposed to air.

Number and sequence of shots fired. The number of entrance wounds may not coincide with the number of bullets that have been fired into the body. Since the *number* of shots fired is often a matter of critical medicolegal importance, the causes of such "discrepancies" deserve investigation. The most common circumstance in which there may be a disparity between the number of bullets fired and the number of entrance wounds occurs when a bullet passes through an arm or hand before entering the trunk or head (Fig. 4-17). In such circumstances it is obvious that a single bullet can produce two or more entrances. Another type of discrepancy arises when a bullet strikes a compact bone and splits into two or more pieces. In such circumstances there may be more than one exit wound for a single hole of entrance. In rare instances, two bullets enter the same cutaneous perforation. This can occur with tandem or "piggyback" bullets or in contact-range wounding when the muzzle of the gun is pressed against a previous site of entrance. Bullets can be coughed up, expectorated, vomited, or defecated when their tracks terminate in an air passage or the gastrointestinal tract, explaining the occasional situation in which there is an entrance wound without a corresponding exit defect and no bullet in the body.

Time and degree of disability after gunshot injury. Great caution should be exercised in estimating the immediate disabling effects of a bullet wound. Through-and-through wounds of the heart commonly fail to cause immediate disability. Only when there is massive destruction of the motor area of the central nervous system or of the brainstem or cervical cord, or when the heart or aorta has been extensively damaged can it be said "with reasonable medical certainty" that the injury was immediately and totally disabling.

Shotgun wounds. Shotguns are smooth-bore weapons that fire a charge composed of one or more projectiles plus wadding. The single projectile shotgun ammunition, called a rifled slug, is encountered rarely in human wounding and will not be considered further. Pellets in shotgun shells vary in size from 0.36 inch (000 buckshot) to 0.05 inch (number 12 shot). In our jurisdiction, the most frequently encountered sizes of shot in civilian wounding are from 0.10 to 0.15 inch in diameter, and average loads contain 100 to 250 such pellets. Police "riot guns" usually are loaded with large-sized buckshot.

Shotgun *gauge* formerly was defined as the number of spherical lead balls, each of the same diameter as the bore, required to weigh 1 pound. In actual measure a 12-gauge shotgun has a bore diameter of 0.729 inch and a 16-gauge bore is 0.662 inch in diameter. Bore diameter also can be expressed in thousandths of an inch—for example, .410 ("four-ten").

Choke refers to constriction of the muzzle end of the barrel and is designed to reduce pellet dispersion. The amount of choke varies from "full" to none. It is measured functionally by the percentage of shot falling in a 30-inch circle when the weapon is fired at a distance of 40 yards and ranges from 65% to 75% for full choke to 25% to 35% in the case of an unchoked cylinder bore. Choke either is added to the barrel during the manufacturing process or can be controlled with a variable choke adapter.

Contact-range shotgun wounds of the trunk are round or oval, smoothly marginated defects that may or may not contain an abundance of powder residue. Contact wounds in the interior of the mouth or against the scalp frequently produce explosive semidecapitation. The appearance of shotgun wounds beyond contact range is determined by the muzzle-target distance, barrel choke and length, shot size, and presence or absence of clothing or other intermediate objects in the path of the charge. Consequently, an estimate of range of fire in a given case is made with considerable latitude unless appropriate experimental test firings have been done. Generally speaking, at ranges beyond 3 to 6 feet the charge begins to separate, producing a skin defect with ragged margins, often referred to as a "rat hole." Next, a few pellets create individual satellite perforations adjacent to the major defect. As the distance lengthens, the main defect becomes smaller, more satellite perforations appear, and the spread of satellite perforations increases. Beyond approximately 5 yards, the wound pattern consists mainly of individual perforations with or without wad injuries in the form of circular, nonpenetrating abrasions.

Passage of the shotgun charge through clothing or any intermediate object, no matter how flimsy, accelerates the pellet spread and renders the skin pattern inappropriate for estimating range of fire. An x-ray film of the victim showing the spread of pellets cannot be utilized to estimate range of fire because the final distribution of pellets may be identical in contact and distant wounds.

Shotgun pellets usually do not exit from the body except for the following situations: contact wounds of the head that cause virtual explosions; tangentially oriented wounds, either close or distant, where part or all of the charge follows a short track through the body; wounding of a thin part of the body, such as the neck or a limb; and wounding by large-sized buckshot.

Local sequelae of mechanical injury

The mechanical disruption of living tissue is attended and followed by various local disturbances, the nature of which depends in part on the site and severity of the disruptive lesion and in part on the organism's capacity to react.

Hemorrhage. Hemorrhage is an immediate and inevitable sequel to mechanical disruption of living vascularized tissue. Blood continues to flow from the damaged vessels until prevented from doing so by thrombosis, vasoconstriction, or equalization of intravascular and extravascular pressures (through a drop in the former or a rise in the latter).

In the case of damage to the small vessels (capillaries, arterioles, venules), vasoconstriction is a more important mechanism than thrombosis in the induction of hemostasis. This is also true when vessels, whether large or small, are lacerated or crushed. When a vessel is incised or injured in such a manner that the disturbance is limited to the site of the defect, hemostasis is more dependent on the occurrence of thrombosis.

In noncommunicating injuries such as may occur with fracture or other forms of internal laceration, the opposition offered by the surrounding intact tissue to the accumulating mass of extravascular blood is an important mechanism of hemostasis. When injury has caused a state of shock, the fall in systemic blood pressure contributes to other factors in preventing further loss of blood.

Mechanical disturbances resulting from an extravascular accumulation of blood may be caused by distension, compression, or obstruction. Pain is an outstanding manifestation of distension of tissue by hemorrhage. It may be the first evidence of the accumulation of a relatively small amount of blood beneath the periosteum or immediately below the peritoneum. The most important compressive effects of extravasated blood are those seen in relation to intracranial and intrapericardial hemorrhage. The rapid accumulation of as little as 50 ml in the former situation or 150 ml in the latter may be fatal by its compressive effect. The importance of the rate of hemorrhage in determining such a mechanical effect is revealed by the fact that a considerably larger amount of blood can be tolerated in either situation if it has accumulated slowly. In the case of a slowly developing subdural hemorrhage, more than 100 ml may accumulate before signs of increased intracranial pressure become apparent. If the pericardium is distended slowly, a liter or more of fluid may be tolerated without the occurrence of fatal cardiac tamponade.

One of the best examples of obstructive disturbance

caused by extravasated blood may occur when blood is aspirated into the lower air passages. The foam created by mixing blood and air in such a situation may be sufficiently obstructive to cause asphyxiation, although the lungs need not be heavier than normal.

The preceding paragraphs have been concerned with early mechanical disturbances caused by the extravascular accumulation of blood. The possibility of late mechanical disturbances attributable to secondary edema incident to the presence of blood in tissue spaces should not be ignored. One of the best examples of this phenomenon is the progressive expansion of a subdural hematoma. Although the space originally consumed by such a hemorrhage may fail to cause a significant amount of cerebral compression, the subsequent imbibition of fluid by the hematoma or secondary spontaneous bleeding from capillaries contained in newly formed granulation tissue sometimes gives rise to a progressively incapacitating or even fatal rise in intracranial pressure.

Pigmentary changes are a striking feature of the deterioration of blood at the site of hemorrhage. As the oxyhemoglobin is reduced, the color of the injured tissue changes from red through purple to blue. In the case of small extravasations, either the erythrocytes are ingested by phagocytes and transported from the site of injury or the products of their disintegration in situ are carried away by the lymph so rapidly that secondary pigmentary changes are inconspicuous. If the mass of extravasated blood is large or its disposal is delayed by inadequate lymph flow, the iron is separated from the globin after hemolysis in situ and the pigment is subsequently converted to bilirubin and biliverdin, with chromatic changes ranging through brown, green, and yellow. In addition to these color changes, two types of crystalline derivatives of hemoglobin may be identified on microscopic examination: hematoidin and hemosiderin. (For further discussion of hemoglobin pigments, see p. 1107.)

Chronologic changes in the gross and microscopic appearances of contusions can provide the basis for important medicolegal interpretations. However, caution is in order when making such interpretations because of variability in temporal evolution of the gross appearances of bruises and of the histopathologic inflammatory responses. Such variability is governed by the vascularity of the injured locus, the quantity of blood accumulating in the tissues, the integrity of the overlying skin, and the factors that combine to define the host response to injury.

Aseptic inflammation. Unless immediately fatal, a mechanical injury of living tissue is almost invariably followed by a series of local reactive changes comprising the phenomenon of aseptic inflammation. The extent to which the inflammatory reaction progresses or eventually disturbs the tissue usually depends on the severity and location of the injury that elicited it. The inflammatory cycle in such instances is probably set in motion and maintained by a variety of chemical and physical alterations. (Inflammation and wound healing are discussed in detail in Chapter 2.)

Other local circulatory disturbances. Attention has already been directed to the circulatory disturbances that may be induced by an expanding hematoma and to those that occur incident to vascular participation in the phenomenon of inflammation. Various other factors may contribute to local disturbances in circulation following a mechanical injury.

One of these is the occurrence of regional vascular spasm of sufficient extent and severity that the original injury is enlarged by the occurrence of secondary ischemic necrosis. Generalized ischemia of a limb may result from reactive spasm of large and apparently unwounded arteries after the occurrence of an injury whose disruptive effects were local. Nonthrombotic ischemia apparently from vasospasm is sometimes responsible for the progressive enlargement, by infarction, of relatively small primary injuries of the brain or kidney.

Similar enlargement of the original scope of injury may result from the propagation of a thrombus from the site of a disruptive vascular injury or from stasis and thrombosis caused by posttraumatic vascular compression by edema or interstitial hemorrhage. In the case of disabling injuries, the inactivity imposed by disability is an additional cause of stasis and may be responsible for thrombosis in the region of injury or in the lower extremities.

Intravascular stasis may be sufficient to cause thrombosis independent of preceding injury to the affected vessel. Although it is unlikely that thrombosis will occur in a normal vessel, the lining of a vessel does not remain normal for long after the blood within it has ceased to flow. Degeneration of the lining endothelium and edema of the intima occur concomitantly with stasis. Platelets adhere to the damaged lining. In larger vessels, clot formation begins at the periphery of the stream and progresses toward the center until the obstruction is complete. In small vessels, much or most of the fluid elements of the blood diffuse through the vascular wall, leaving the distended lumen occluded by a solid, sausagelike mass of closely packed erythrocytes.

Local infection. Any injury that disturbs the continuity of the protective and especially adapted layer of cells that stands between the organism and its external environment, whether it be the integument or the mucous membrane lining an internal passage, may create a portal of entry for infection. The infective agent may be carried into the tissues on the surface of the instrument that was responsible for the wound, or it may subsequently gain access to the tissues because of the existence of a wound.

Under nonsurgical conditions, any instrument responsible for the production of a mechanical injury is likely to be contaminated with pathogenic organisms. Soil is an important source of such contamination, and *Clostridium tetani* and *Clostridium welchii* are among the more important pathogenic inhabitants of soil. Streptococci, staphylococci, *Proteus vulgaris*, *Pseudomonas aeruginosa*, and *Escherichia coli* are commonly present on the skin. Pathogenic organisms that may be present on mucous membranes of the body include streptococci, pneumococci, meningococci, *Haemophilus influenzae*, *Klebsiella pneumoniae*, *E. coli*, *Corynebacterium diphtheriae*, and *C. welchii*.

The creation of an external portal of entry is by no means the only mechanism by which mechanical violence may render the site of an injury vulnerable to infection. Even though primary wound infection does not take place, a locus of diminished resistance may be established. Delayed infection of the injured tissue by way of the bloodstream may occur because of the creation of conditions favorable to bacterial growth at the wound site.

Systemic effects of mechanical injury

Almost immediately incapacitating systemic anoxia may be the direct consequence of an injury if its primary effect is such as to interfere with respiration or systemic circulation. Certain types of disruptive injury of the brain or heart may thus be the direct and immediate cause of fatal systemic disturbance. One should not conclude, however, that wounds of these structures are invariably fatal. As long as the brainstem escapes damage, extensive and disruptive cerebral injury may be survived. Through-and-through stab or bullet wounds of the heart are sometimes survived, and even those that eventually cause death may not be immediately incapacitating.

It is a fact, however, that even though the function of the damaged tissue is not normally concerned with such basic physiologic processes as respiration, circulation, nutrition, or elimination, such an injury may be responsible for systemic disturbances by any of several mechanisms.

Although the cause and nature of such disturbances are described in detail in various other places in this book, it is not unduly repetitive to bring them to the reader's attention at this time.

Primary shock

A mechanical injury to any part of the body may elicit a reflex vasodilatation and a fall in blood pressure of sufficient severity to cause collapse, loss of consciousness, and in some instances death. This type of posttraumatic circulatory disturbance constitutes the syndrome of primary or neurogenic shock. Pressure on the carotid sinuses, a blow to the epigastrium or a testicle, puncture

of the pleura, or dilatation of the rectum may lead to sufficient fall in blood pressure to result in unconsciousness and occasionally in death. The reduction in blood pressure in such circumstances is caused by vasodilatation rather than by heart failure or a reduction in blood volume.

Secondary shock

Secondary shock is the state of circulatory failure that results from an excessive reduction in blood volume. It occurs whenever the amount of blood or plasma that has escaped from damaged vessels exceeds the limits of physiologic compensation. The vascular damage responsible for the escape of blood or plasma may be local and attributable to the direct effects of trauma or may be generalized and attributable to infection or some other systemic complication of what was originally a local injury.

Vasoconstriction is the initial homeostatic reaction to reduced blood volume. This may or may not be sufficient to maintain blood pressure, depending on the amount of blood lost. The secondary compensation is a movement of extravascular fluid into the vascular system, with hemodilution that may or may not be compensated by the mobilization of the erythrocyte reserves from the bone marrow and spleen. In its initial stages, shock is reversible. Severe and uncompensated shock may become irreversible as a result of widespread hypoxic parenchymatous injury. If bleeding or plasma loss continues, compensation fails and the volume of circulating blood decreases. When the pressure falls below a certain critical level, the vasomotor centers become anoxic and the resulting vasodilatation leads to rapid circulatory collapse and death.

The amount of hemorrhage necessary to produce circulatory collapse is governed by the rate of blood loss, the individual's general cardiovascular condition, and the presence or absence of other factors, such as alcohol or drug intoxication, that may predispose to hypotension. In otherwise healthy persons, rapid loss of one third of the blood volume causes hemorrhagic shock, and death ensues when half of the blood volume is lost rapidly. Slow bleeding permits the occurrence of previously mentioned physiologic compensations and allows larger volumes of blood to be lost without causing shock or death.

In cases of death from acute massive hemorrhage, the most significant postmortem changes are gross rather than microscopic and consist of generalized pallor of tissue, collapse of the great veins, and a flabby, shrunken, gray spleen.

Shock kidney

Irreversible renal injury leading to anuria and death as a complication of secondary shock first attracted general attention during World War II. It did so because of the frequency with which persons who had sustained severe crushing injuries as a result of being caught in buildings demolished by air raids subsequently became anuric and died of renal insufficiency. Examination disclosed segmental obstruction of the renal tubules by pigmented casts, which were particularly conspicuous in the lower portions of the nephrons. It was first believed that the extensive crushing of skeletal muscle was responsible for the renal lesion. Subsequent studies, however, indicated that the essential damage to the kidney in such circumstances was probably attributable primarily to the renal ischemia that occurs during, and that may be prolonged beyond, the posttraumatic episode of systemic hypotension. Any injury that is followed by secondary shock is capable of causing renal damage if the state of shock is sufficiently severe or protracted. If the original injury is associated with extensive muscle injury or intravascular hemolysis, the renal casts tend to be conspicuous by reason of their brown pigment. The injury is not confined to the lower reaches of the nephrons, and the casts represent the result rather than the cause of renal injury (p. 758).

Shock lung

The term "shock lung" is probably a misnomer because shock alone fails to explain the pathogenesis of a variety of nonspecific pulmonary abnormalities that occur in injured persons. Lung injury from shock can be regarded as one of the local and systemic causes of the adult respiratory distress syndrome. In addition to chest wall and lung injuries, such patients may have aspiration of gastric content with pneumonia and/or lung abscess, bronchopneumonia, septicemia, fat embolism, large or small thromboemboli, embolism of cellular aggregates in massive blood transfusions, cardiac failure, fluid overloads, retained secretions, abdominal distension, atelectasis, and all of the complications of prolonged mechanical ventilation.

Pulmonary pathologic changes are understandably variable and include alveolar and interstitial edema, thickening and fibrosis of alveolar septa, interstitial lymphocytic infiltrates, and alveolar hyaline membranes in various stages of organization. Obliterative changes in the pulmonary microvasculature, owing to fibrin and platelet thromboemboli, commonly complicate disseminated intravascular coagulation and multiple transfusions. Bacterial, fungal, and viral pulmonary infections are common complications of trauma associated with coma, burns, debility, or inactivity.

General adaptation syndrome

The frequent occurrence of a posttraumatic neuroendocrine disturbance in the form of an evanescent hyperglycemia has long been recognized. That the neuroendocrine reaction to an injury may be such as to modify significantly the injury's total effect on the organism was not fully appreciated before the investigations of Selye.[43,44]

It is postulated that a wide variety of damaging stimuli may cause the pituitary gland to discharge an excessive amount of corticotropic hormone, which in turn leads to an outpouring of cortical hormones from the adrenal glands. Pathologic evidence of this effect on the adrenal glands is partial or complete depletion of lipid from the cortical cells within the first few days after an injury. That the reaction is part of a defense mechanism can be inferred from the fact that cortical hormone may cause a rapid release of antibodies from lymphoid tissue. The pathologic evidence of this effect is the rapid involution of thymus and lymphoid tissue.

Embolism

Fat droplets of sufficient size to obstruct capillaries may be found in the blood after almost any kind of disruptive injury involving adipose tissue and particularly after fractures of long bones. Unless the number and size of the emboli are such that fat-distended arterioles and capillaries are seen in every low-power field of lung, their lethality is doubtful. For many years the importance of pulmonary fat embolism as a cause of death has been controversial. A relatively enormous amount of fat is required to produce fatal embolism in an animal. Scully[42] found that only when the cerebral vessels are obstructed are fat emboli capable of causing death. Usually when droplets and cylinders of fat are numerous in the pulmonary capillaries, emboli will also be found in the brain and kidneys (Fig. 4-23).

Controversy also exists regarding the origin of the fat. Originally it was believed that fat released from the damaged adipose tissue (or bone marrow) at the site of injury was forced or aspirated into the central ends of the lacerated veins. That this does happen is indicated by the occasional finding of organized masses of myeloid tissue in the pulmonary vessels of persons who have died after fractures. However, the amount of fat found in the pulmonary vascular bed in some instances is far in excess of what might plausibly be derived from the site of injury.

Lehman and Moore[19] were among the first researchers to suggest that the phenomenon of posttraumatic fat embolism was the result of a change in the droplet size of the endogenous plasma lipids. Support for this point of view has been provided by the work of LeQuire and associates,[20] who found that the cholesterol content (10% to 30%) of the embolic fat in nine cases they studied was much higher than that of adipose tissue (about 1%). Pulmonary fat embolism occurring independent of mechanical violence may be encountered in association with such diverse conditions as diabetes

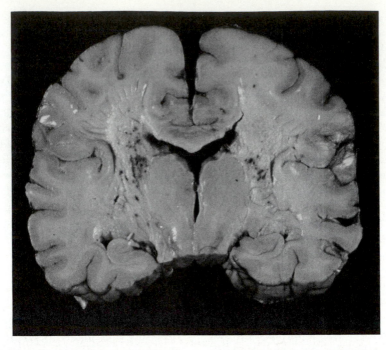

Fig. 4-23. Cerebral fat embolism. Small hemorrhagic infarcts caused by fat emboli produce gross appearance of white matter petechiae.

mellitus, extensive cutaneous burns, and decompression sickness.[45]

A detached blood clot is another type of embolism frequently caused by mechanical injury. Venous thrombosis may occur as a direct result of trauma to a vein or as a result of stasis caused by edema or inactivity. Thus the thrombus may form at the site of injury or at some remote place in the body. The spontaneous detachment of such a thrombus frequently results in fatal pulmonary embolism.

A third type of embolism that may be caused by mechanical injury results from the entrance of air into the circulating blood. The most common portals of entry for fatal air embolism are the dilated veins of the gravid uterus. Large amounts of air may be sucked into the uterine veins during an attempt to empty the uterus by instrumentation or by irrigation. Air embolism may result from tubal insufflation, from the insufflation of a nongravid uterus, from the injection of air into the peritoneal cavity, or from incision or laceration of veins anywhere in the body. Small amounts of air may enter the veins and be carried to the lungs without causing significant disturbance. If the amount of air is large, however, the right side of the heart and the pulmonary arteries become occluded by foam, and death results from acute circulatory failure. As a result of penetrating injuries of the lungs, air may be carried to the left side of the heart and thence to the systemic circulation, where it causes death as the result of cerebral or coronary air embolism.

INJURIES CAUSED BY CHANGES IN ATMOSPHERIC PRESSURE

The biologic consequences of changes in atmospheric pressure are dependent on two physical properties of gases:

1. The volume of gas contained in an elastic membrane increases in size as the surrounding barometric pressure is reduced.
2. The solubility of a gas in a liquid solvent (such as blood) is proportional to the partial pressure of that gas in the ambient atmosphere.

These two characteristics of gases in general are responsible for the signs and symptoms created by *trapped* and *evolved* gases that are observed with sudden changes in barometric pressure.

Gases may be trapped in body cavities that are usually in free communication with the ambient atmosphere if ready passage of air into and out of the cavity is blocked. Thus, in the presence of acute upper respiratory tract inflammation with resultant edema and swelling of the mucous membrane, the sinus orifices and eustachian tubes may be blocked or narrowed so that equalization of pressures within the paranasal air sinuses or middle ear cavities and the outside atmosphere is delayed or prevented. The clinical consequences may be severe.

Sufficient decrease in atmospheric pressure leads to expansion of gastric and intestinal gases with resultant abdominal distension. Expansion progresses until deflation occurs as a result of gaseous eructations or the passage of flatus or both.

Injuries associated with changes in atmospheric pressure may be seen in underwater use of a caisson, in high-altitude climbing or flight, or most commonly in diving with *self*-contained *underwater* *breathing* *apparatus* (scuba). The three characteristics of an episode of abnormal atmospheric pressure that determine its injurious effects on humans are as follows:

1. Direction and magnitude of change
2. Rate of change
3. Duration of change

Decreased atmospheric pressure

The human organism tolerates an increase in atmospheric pressure better than a decrease of equal magnitude. Thus the atmospheric pressure of the human environment can be tripled without harm, and yet a lowering of the pressure by as little as 50% incident to elevation to an altitude of 20,000 feet results in severe systemic hypoxia and may cause death.

Rapid accentuation of hypoxia as a result of diminished barometric pressure is followed by strong peripheral vasoconstriction with consequent shifting of a large portion of the blood volume to the pulmonary circuit. This hemodynamic disturbance leads to pulmonary arterial hypertension associated with anoxic damage to pulmonary capillary endothelium and alveolar pneumocytes. The result of the combined action of these two responses to the abnormal physical environment is the so-called pulmonary edema of high altitudes.[16,37]

Acute high-altitude pulmonary edema usually occurs between 3 and 48 hours after exposure to altitudes above 2600 m, especially if severe physical exertion has taken place in the unaccustomed environment. This illness poses a particular hazard to those who climb or ski at high altitudes. Therefore most instances occur in athletic young adults who are otherwise healthy. The condition is also a threat to those who live and work permanently at high altitudes, especially if they are faced with repeated reentry into the hypoxic environment after trips to lower altitudes. Fatalities can be indistinguishable clinically from fulminant pneumonia. At autopsy the lungs are congested and have interstitial and alveolar edema. Hyaline membranes may be present.[15]

In addition to decreased barometric pressure and decreased partial oxygen pressure encountered at high altitudes, there is often a simultaneous exposure to decreased environmental temperature and increased ultraviolet irradiation. A further source of physiologic stress is the decreasing humidity of air at high altitudes. This factor in concert with the hyperventilation that accompanies even moderate physical exertion can lead to rapid dehydration with resultant extreme thirst. The combination of hyperventilation and profuse diaphoresis can bring about a moderate degree of hypokalemic alkalosis. These multiple physical and biochemical assaults may give rise to acute mountain sickness, a syndrome characterized by headache, palpitations, nausea, anorexia, weakness, and insomnia.

Exposure to increasing altitudes activates various adaptive mechanisms that permit the body to tolerate the changes. The types and degrees of adaptation depend on many factors, including duration of exposure, level of physical activity, age, and general physical condition. Persons with limited cardiorespiratory reserve may experience dyspnea, nausea, and insomnia at altitudes as low as 1500 m above sea level. On the other hand, persons who are well acclimatized and in good physical condition can tolerate exposure to extreme altitude while climbing the highest Himalayan peaks.

Increased atmospheric pressure

The effects of an increase in atmospheric pressure are far less injurious than those of decompression. Therefore injuries associated with increased atmospheric pressure usually occur during the return from elevated to normal barometric pressure. The rate at which the atmospheric pressure changes—more particularly, the rate at which it is decreased—is an exceedingly important factor in injury production. Unless barometric pressure is lowered slowly to normal, decompression sickness (also known as dysbarism, caisson disease, the bends, the staggers, or the chokes) may occur. A very rapid change from normal to subnormal pressure, as may occur during rapid ascent in supersonic aircraft, may also cause decompression sickness.

An increase in atmospheric pressure results in a net flow of nitrogen, which makes up four fifths of the inspired air, from the alveoli, via the blood in which the gas dissolves, to tissue. When the return to normal pressure is slow, the loss of gas from tissue is analogous to gas uptake. However, if the return to normal pressure is rapid, gas bubbles form in tissue and blood because nitrogen evolves faster than it can be transported to the lungs and expired.[48]

Some degree of microscopic bubble formation probably occurs whenever the tissue partial pressure of nitrogen even moderately exceeds that in the surrounding atmosphere. However, symptom-producing bubbles (decompression sickness) will not occur until the partial pressure of nitrogen is more than twice that of the surrounding atmosphere.[33] (At the ocean's surface a diver and his viscera are under a pressure of 1 atmosphere [760 mm Hg], and 1 additional atmosphere of pressure is added for each 33 feet he descends.[47])

The nature and severity of decompression sickness are determined by the rate and location of nitrogen release. Disability and death may supervene within minutes or hours after decompression. Pulmonary and central nervous system involvement dominate in the causation of sudden fatalities. Subacute or chronic effects of decompression are characterized by lower limb, bladder, and rectal paralysis from demyelination of the dorsal and lateral columns of the inferior thoracic spinal cord rather than the upper cord or brain.[13] In divers and tunnelers with a history of the bends and persistent joint symptoms, foci of aseptic necrosis have usually developed in bones. Venous gas embolism with resultant vascular obstruction is the most likely basis for the localized areas of osseous destruction. Because of the solubility of nitrogen in fat, obesity predisposes to the development of decompression sickness.[54]

With the acute decompression seen in rapid ascent of a scuba diver who fails to exhale, mediastinal interstitial emphysema, subcutaneous emphysema, pneumothorax, and *arterial* air embolism may follow rupture of distended pulmonary alveoli from expanding intrapulmonary air. The air embolism is the most serious consequence because of the possibility of cerebrovascular involvement with the production of such phenomena as hemiplegia, confusion, blindness, unconsciousness, and death. Inasmuch as the incident occurs in an aquatic environment, the victim may drown. It is of interest that this series of catastrophic events can occur during rapid ascent in water from a depth of only 10 feet.

Rapid descent in an aircraft or rapid ascent during a scuba dive can lead to sinus barotrauma, so-called *aero-sinusitis* and *aero–otitis media* with rupture of the tympanum. As the air in the intracranial spaces expands during ascent (1 volume of air at sea level becomes 2 volumes at 18,000 feet and 4 volumes at 33,000 feet), it passes easily through the natural ostia of the sinuses to equilibrate with the ambient barometric pressure. During *descent*, air must enter the sinuses through the ostia to equalize the intrasinus pressure with the *increasing* atmospheric tension. When sinus ostia and nasal mucosa are normal, the air exchange occurs efficiently and promptly. (Similar dynamic changes occur in all the hollow body structures that communicate with the exterior.)

However, if a sinus ostium is obstructed by tenacious mucus (a "mucus plug"), edematous mucosa, or a bony structural deformity, the defect may act as a cork during descent, effectively occluding the orifice, which is now under negative pressure. The negative pressure in the sealed-off sinus cavity is resolved by the sinus's filling with fluid transudate or blood. Indeed, if the pressure changes are especially rapid or severe, the mucous membrane may be stripped from the sinus wall with formation of a hematoma. The frontal sinus is most vulnerable to barotrauma because of the long, narrow bony nasofrontal defect with its dependent position on the floor of the sinus and the lack of accessory ostia.[53]

Although most cases of sinus barotrauma occur with compression (rapid descent in an aircraft or in diving), a considerable pressure disequilibrium can occur during ascent if the same type of interference exists with the passage of air *out* of the sinus.[18]

Explosions

The term *blast injury* designates the disruptive effects of the sudden changes in pressure that result from an explosion. If the force of the explosion is transmitted through the air, the term *air blast* is employed; if through water, *immersion blast*, and if through more or less rigid structures, *solid blast*.[7]

The shock wave of an air blast is a sound wave of very high pressure that emanates radially from an explosive source at the speed of sound. The air pressure is highest in the region of the explosion and falls rapidly, almost exponentially, as the distance from the blast increases. The amount of injury inflicted depends on the peak pressure and to a lesser degree on the duration of the shock wave.[35] In the case of an air blast the compression tends to be unilateral, and its principal effect is on the side of the body that faces the explosion. Here, much of the energy is reflected, but at least part is transmitted through the tissues and strikes the subjacent organs during the succeeding millisecond or less. Solid organs are virtually incompressible and consequently undergo little or no internal displacement. They vibrate as a whole and so escape serious injury. However, organs that contain air or gas respond differently because they *are* compressible and contain gas-liquid interfaces. Compression generates displacement, and whenever tissues of different density exist side by side, the amount of displacement varies from point to point, causing distension and tearing. An air blast also gives rise to surface phenomena such as epithelial shredding. Lesions tend to be most severe at tissue junctions. When loose, poorly supported tissues attached to dense unyielding tissues are displaced beyond their elastic limits, they are lacerated or otherwise damaged. Differences in fixation, cohesion, compressibility, and inertia on the part of the various components of the body result in nonuniform response to the displacing force and in widespread disruptive change. Thus the walls or compartments of hollow viscera are particularly susceptible to blast injury.

The lungs are especially vulnerable to blast injury. Alveolar septa are torn, permitting neighboring alveoli to coalesce, with ensuing emphysema. Alveolar parenchyma shears away from vascular structures, and alveolar epithelium is shredded. At the same time, bronchiolar epithelium is stripped from its basement membrane. These lesions lead to destruction of the fluid-air barrier. Blood and edema fluid escape into the alveoli, and air is forced into pulmonary vessels as a result of the formation of alveolar-venous fistulas. Cerebral air embolism attributable to the aspiration of air by disrupted pulmonary veins may be an important component of such an injury. Visible damage ranges from petechiae to massive hemorrhages and extensive areas of hemorrhagic edema. The hemorrhages tend to be more severe in the pulmonary parenchyma underlying the intercostal spaces, with the lung tissue beneath the protecting ribs being comparatively only slightly damaged. At autopsy, the pleural surfaces show alternating light and dark bands, the former corresponding to the ribs ("rib markings") and the latter to the intercostal spaces. Diffuse injuries of both the thoracic and the abdominal viscera may occur and may be sustained with little or no external evidence of trauma. Hemorrhage may occur in the gastric wall and elsewhere. The greater the degree of distension of the viscus when the shock waves strike, the more severe the injury.[9]

Since a blast wave is a sound wave of high intensity, it is obvious that the ear, built specifically for the reception of sound, is likely to be damaged by explosions. The pressure pulse approaching the human ear is concentrated as it passes down the external auditory canal so that the pressure on the tympanic membrane is approximately 20% higher than that just outside the ear. Injuries to the ears range from hyperemia and punctate bruising of the intact tympanic membrane to laceration of the membrane and damage to the cochlea. Membrane laceration usually occurs when the pressure rises to 15 psi and typically is associated with bleeding into the middle ear.[17]

In the case of an immersion blast, a shock wave is propagated at approximately the speed of sound in water (1450 m/second). Since water is much less compressible than air, corresponding pressures are much higher in a water shock wave than in those produced in air. Injury can occur from the shock wave or from the subsidiary pulse when the shock wave is reflected, for example, from the surface or from the bottom. The sequel of the pressure pulse injury is hemorrhage and laceration of air-containing organs. Lung damage of the type already described under air blast is a constant feature in fatalities. Small perforations of the gut, especially of the cecum, may occur, and there may be subperitoneal contusions.[35]

In the case of solid blast, the disruptive force of the explosion is transmitted to the body through those parts that are in contact with an agitated rigid structure, such as the deck of a ship or the wall of an air raid shelter. Most solid blast injuries involve fractures of the lower extremities with marked soft tissue damage.[4]

One should bear in mind that proximity to either air or immersion blast may result in virtual destruction of the body by the extreme air or water turbulence induced by the blast. Flying missiles may add an infinite variety of wounds to those induced by turbulence and compression. These lesions are called *secondary blast* injuries; they result from missiles energized by blast pressures and winds and are distinguished from the *primary blast* injuries caused by the blast per se. In civilian explosions, including terrorist bombings, most fatalities are caused by injuries from high-velocity fragments and falling debris (secondary blast injuries).[27]

Blast injuries sustained incident to atomic bomb explosion may be complicated by exposure to excessive heat and ionizing radiation. The cutaneous burns incurred in this manner are often unique by reason of the extremely high intensity and short duration of the hyperthermic episode. The injurious effects of ionizing radiation frequently require weeks to years for the development of signs and symptoms (p. 256).

INJURIES CAUSED BY SOUND WAVES
Noise

Permanent hearing loss resulting from excessive exposure to noise has long been recognized as an occupational hazard in industry. Such hearing defects develop with chronic exposure when the "work noise" exceeds the critical level of 80 to 90 decibels (dB).[41] It is less well known that many noise levels encountered in the community exceed standards found injurious in industry. For example, animals exposed to live rock music for 2½ hours in a discotheque had loss of sensory cells in the organ of Corti. The average sound pressure level measured in the discotheque was 107 dB.[5]

Chemical and structural changes in the spiral ganglion and hair cells have been demonstrated during exposure to sound, and exposure to sound levels of the degree produced by home food blenders causes noticeable changes in the hair cells, which characteristically show cytoplasmic vacuolization and swelling with compression of their nuclei and changes in their shape.[11]

In human autopsy studies no clear histologic picture has been identified in which morbid anatomic changes can be correlated with clinical hearing loss. Postmortem changes in the organ of Corti are the rule and complicate attempts to find such relationships.

Studies of persons subjected to high noise levels have revealed that long-term exposure to acoustic insult first affects hearing in the range between 3000 and 6000 Hertz (Hz, cycles per second), whereas hearing for frequencies below 3000 Hz and above 8000 Hz remains essentially normal for long periods of time. High-frequency receptors deteriorate with age, and the burden of extra noise increases the wear.[39]

Ultrasound

Ultrasonic vibrations are those above limits of hearing of the human ear. Although ultrasound can be generated at frequencies exceeding 1000 megahertz (MHz), in current medical practice the useful range is generally from 900 kilohertz (KHz) to 6 MHz. The medical literature has been almost unanimous in suggesting that there is little or no danger associated with diagnostic or therapeutic exposure of current levels.[3] Reports that diagnostic levels of ultrasound produced chromosomal damage in vitro and retarded rapidly growing tissue have not been confirmed in human cells.[24] However, since the use of diagnostic ultrasound has increased rapidly during the past several years, particularly in obstetrics, continued monitoring of possible effects of ultrasound is warranted.[21]

High-frequency ultrasound producing intensities many times that used in diagnostic or therapeutic procedures may cause biologic changes by increasing tissue temperature or producing tissue microcavitation. Wittenzellner[55] carried out self-experiments by irradiating both thighs in the frequency range of 20 to 800 KHz. Postirradiation changes in the skin receiving 800 KHz for 25 minutes included an acute inflammatory infiltrate and intraepidermal vesicles. Twenty-five years later the irradiated skin showed no significant signs.

INJURIES FROM HEAT AND COLD

Despite humans' ability to survive wide variations in environmental temperature, internal temperature must be maintained within a narrow range to avoid thermal injury. Cellular injury or death occurs if tissue temperature is maintained at a level more than 5° C above or more than 15° C below that which is normal for the blood. The severity of injury caused at any given temperature tends to be proportional to the duration of the hypothermal or hyperthermal episode. The somatic function of circulation is more susceptible to irreversible disturbance by dysthermia than are the individual cells of the body, and hence somatic death may result from a systemic alteration in temperature that would not cause cellular death if it were localized.

The skin is the principal site of heat loss during exposure to a cold environment or of heat gain during exposure to a hot environment. The respiratory membranes are rarely injured by heat or cold—and then only when the alteration of air temperature is so extreme that the skin is burned or frozen.[30,31]

Local hypothermia

Chilling of tissue retards the metabolic activity of the cells and may cause irreversible cellular change attributable to intracellular ice formation. This is not to imply, however, that hypothermal injury is dependent on the occurrence of congelation. The most important injurious effects of chilling are alterations in the walls and contents of the small blood vessels. A brief period of severe tissue hypothermia or a protracted period of mild tissue hypothermia may injure capillary endothelium sufficiently to cause transudation of fluid and edema. Superficially, such edema may lead to extensive vesication. The threshold for edema formation incident to chilling varies greatly among individuals.

If chilling is rapid and severe, the tissue may be rendered ischemic so quickly that evidence of vascular injury does not become apparent until the temperature rises and circulation is reestablished. Intense hyperemia is usually the immediate response to restitution of circulation after hypothermia. The hyperemia is followed by edema as soon as sufficient time has elapsed for plasma to diffuse through the walls of the injured vessels.

During a protracted episode of nonfreezing hypothermia such as that causing immersion or trench foot or after a brief episode of freezing hypothermia such as that causing frostbite, the local vascular injury may be so severe that the capillaries and even the larger vessels become plugged by tightly packed masses of erythrocytes. The nature and severity of the subsequent changes are determined by the extent and permanence of the ensuing ischemia. If the vascular occlusion is extensive, complete infarction in the form of moist or dry gangrene takes place. If the necrotic tissue becomes moist and dark colored, one can infer that infarction was preceded or accompanied by some degree of vascular patency. If the necrotic tissue becomes dry and mummified, one can infer that vascular occlusion was complete from the beginning.

Most if not all of the residual injury from protracted nonfreezing hypothermia can be attributed to the ischemia that results from the vascular occlusion. Atrophic and degenerative changes are seen in the epidermis, sweat glands, nerves, subcutaneous fat, and skeletal muscle, with proliferation of fibrous connective tissue in all situations.

Systemic hypothermia

If the area exposed to cold is relatively small, a severe local injury may be sustained without significant lowering of the blood temperature. If the area of exposure is large, the body temperature may be lowered sufficiently to cause death from circulatory failure even though no local injury has been sustained. Circulation fails when the temperature of the blood is reduced to approximately 20° C. Immersion in cold water or exposure to a rapidly moving current of cold air may lower the body temperature to a fatal level in a remarkably short time. There are no histologic or anatomic changes that can be regarded as pathognomonic of death from systemic hypothermia. Postmortem examination of persons who have died from exposure to cold usually discloses nothing more than moderate, right-sided cardiac dilatation and pulmonary edema. However, autopsy examinations of some persons who have died after accidental hypothermia have demonstrated widespread thromboses and visceral infarction along with acute, necrotizing pancreatitis (Fig. 4-24).

Circulatory stasis and ischemia are probably responsible for the vascular phenomena and for the acute pancre-

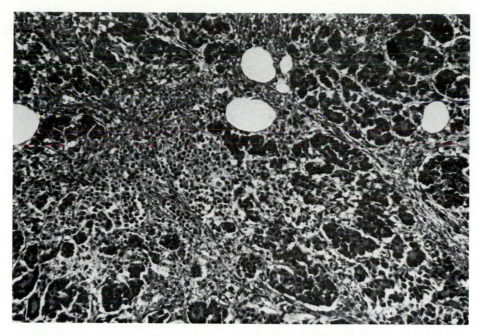

Fig. 4-24. Pancreas from 85-year-old man who died approximately 24 hours after being found in a snowbank and who suffered from exposure. Parenchyma is abundantly infiltrated with acute inflammatory cells. (150x.)

atitis that has been observed in experimental and clinical situations. In accidental hypothermia the pancreatitis usually occurs when exposure to cold is prolonged, with coma preceding death.[36,40]

Local hyperthermia

Humans are far more susceptible to injury from an increase in tissue temperature than from a corresponding decrease.

Cutaneous burns

An elevation of tissue temperature by even a few degrees above that which is normal for the blood may be injurious. At any given temperature the nature and extent of the resulting injury are determined by the duration of the hyperthermal episode. During episodes of low intensity (40° to 45° C), injury is the result of accelerated metabolism of the hyperthermal tissue, and ordinarily many hours are required before irreversible changes have occurred. The higher the temperature, the shorter the time required to cause cell death.[28,29] Transepidermal necrosis occurs if the epidermal temperature is brought to and maintained at 70° C or higher for a second or less, whereas transepidermal temperature elevation to 50° C for periods as long as 10 minutes may or may not destroy the epidermis.

The earliest evidence of hyperthermal injury is functional rather than structural. Capillaries and small blood vessels become dilated as the tissue temperature is raised, the permeability of the capillary walls is increased, and the fluid components of the blood leave the vessel and enter the interstitial spaces, with resulting edema. When thermal edema occurs in the superficial portion of the skin, the fluid may collect beneath the epidermis, with resulting vesiculation.

The earliest cytologic evidence of hyperthermal injury is a redistribution of the fluid and solid components of the nuclei, followed by nuclear swelling attributable to the imbibition of fluid, rupture of the nuclear membranes, and finally pyknosis. Since the rise in tissue temperature incident to exposure of the surface of the skin to excessive heat is greatest at the surface and becomes progressively less as the distance from the surface is increased, it is apparent that any given burn will include a wide range of thermal effects. The cytoplasm of thermally injured cells becomes at first granular and later homogeneously coagulated. The collagen tends to lose its fibrillar character and to take on the appearance of a more or less homogeneous gel. The pH of the thermally denatured cells falls, as indicated by their increased affinity for basic stains.

Cutaneous burns may be designated as first, second, or third degree. First-degree burns are manifested by erythema without significant alteration of the epidermis. Second-degree burns are those in which the epidermis has been destroyed without significant irreversible injury to the dermis (Figs. 4-25 and 4-26). Such burns are characteristically vesicated, but because there is little or

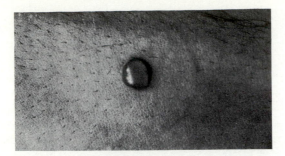

Fig. 4-25. Experimentally produced second-degree burn of human skin caused by maintaining surface temperature at 45° C for 3 hours. There is transepidermal necrosis with vesication. Irreversible dermal injury was minimal, and epidermal regeneration was complete in 10 days.

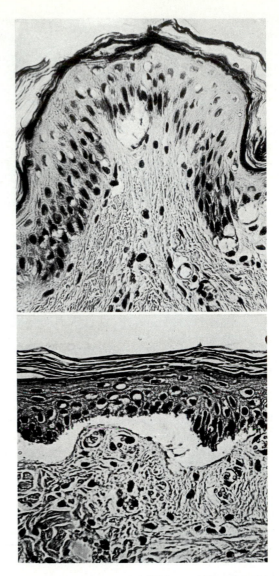

Fig. 4-26. Cutaneous burns. **A,** Mild burn. Although epidermis is damaged, it is not completely destroyed. Many nuclei are swollen and show eccentric displacement of chromatin. Minute vesicles have formed at junction of dermis and epidermis. **B,** Second-degree burn. Vesication is complete. Entire thickness of epidermis is necrotic and detached from relatively uninjured dermis. (400×.)

no permanent damage to the dermis, healing by epithelial regeneration is ordinarily rapid. The new epithelium in cases of second-degree burns is derived in part from the margin of the burned area and in part from the underlying hair follicles. Third-degree burns are those in which there has been sufficient damage to the dermis to interfere with epithelial regeneration. The irreversibly injured dermis must be disposed of before a new layer of epithelium can be regenerated. The organization and repair of the damaged dermis are accomplished by growth of new fibrous connective tissue and often result in extensive scar formation.

The flash burn resulting from exposure to the tremendous caloric flux of the first 0.6 second of the fireball of the atomic bomb explosion differs from the ordinary relatively low temperature burn in several respects.[22,34] Despite carbonization of the epidermis and subjacent dermis, the zone of injury may be shallow and sharply demarcated.

Vascular reaction with hyperemia and edema is inevitable if the tissue hyperthermia has been sufficient to be injurious, and this reaction frequently occurs before the duration or the intensity of the exposure has been great enough to cause other perceptible evidence of injury.

In the case of exposure to intense heat, the superficial vessels may become so rapidly fixed in a state of contraction that neither edema nor hyperemia is visible from the surface. In such an event, the reactive vascular changes will occur at a lower level but with no less severity. One of the most important systemic effects of extensive cutaneous burning is secondary shock brought on by hemoconcentration from loss of plasma at the site of injury.

Thermally denatured tissue elicits an aseptic inflammatory reaction, represents a foreign body, and must undergo lysis and organization or be sloughed off as a sequestrum. Prior to organization or sequestration, it provides a favorable medium for bacterial growth and predisposes the adjacent tissue to infection.

Systemic disturbances caused by cutaneous burns. Burning of the surface of the body may result in a wide variety of secondary disturbances. Such an injury may precipitate the development of primary or neurogenic shock with rapid peripheral circulatory collapse leading to syncope or death. The progressive loss of plasma from the burned surface or into the damaged tissue beneath it may result in hemoconcentration and secondary shock.

Patients with third-degree burns experience an average water loss of 0.35 ml/sq cm of burned area per day during the first week.[8] It is a reasonable inference that the hemoconcentration, low blood pressure, and systemic anoxia of secondary shock predispose not only to phlebothrombosis, particularly in immobilized limbs, but also to the occurrence of the degenerative changes so commonly observed in the kidneys, liver, and adrenal glands of burned persons.

Although the precise cause of the ulcers that sometimes develop in the proximal portion of the small intestine of severely burned persons is not known, local mesenteric thrombosis and mucosal infarction would appear to constitute a plausible explanation. The degenerative changes frequently observed in the cortical cells of the adrenal glands of persons who have died several days after severe cutaneous burning result from a systemic stress or adaptation reaction.[43]

Erythrocytes break down rapidly in vitro at temperatures over 50° C and in vivo at temperatures over 42.5° C, and intravascular hemolysis usually takes place if the hyperthermal episode has been of sufficient intensity or duration to destroy the epidermis. Free plasma hemoglobin is excreted rapidly by the kidneys, where it may be precipitated in the lower segments of the nephrons to form obstructive casts similar to those formed as a result of a mismatched transfusion.

The combined effects of these pigmented casts and the irreversible tubular damage caused by prolonged shock result in the renal failure so often associated with severe burns.[23]

Systemic hyperthermia

The temperature of the body may be raised to an injurious level either by the inflow of heat from without or by the body's failure to eliminate the heat developed by metabolic processes. A general rise in the temperature of the circulating blood to a level higher than 42.5° C leads to profound functional disturbances, including the following:

1. Generalized vasodilatation with resulting reduction in effective blood volume as a consequence of the disparity between the newly expanded capacity of the circulatory apparatus and the unchanged quantity of the fluid (blood) available to fill it
2. Rapid pulse and dilatation of the heart with impairment of cardiac efficiency
3. Stimulation of the respiratory centers, manifested first by tachypnea, later by irregularity, and finally by suspension of respiratory activity[32]

It is difficult to determine which of these several physiologic effects of systemic hyperthermia may contribute most to somatic deterioration and death. It is of interest in this connection that a heart-lung preparation fails when the temperature of the perfusate reaches approximately 42.5° C .

Heatstroke is the result of uncontrolled overproduction of body heat or impairment of the body's ability to lose heat; it occurs most frequently in susceptible persons exposed to unusually hot conditions. Heat is dissipated principally by evaporative cooling through sweating and by cutaneous vasodilatation with increased cardiac output. The more labile thermoregulatory mechanism of small children and, particularly, the elderly renders them vulnerable to heatstroke; heatstroke rates are 10 to 12 times higher in persons older than 65 years than in younger adults. Other factors that predispose individuals to heatstroke include alcoholism, any skin disease or injury that impairs or prevents sweating, cardiovascular disease, general debility, coexistence of a febrile disorder, dehydration, obesity, anticholinergic drugs, and some medications that are used to treat psychiatric disorders (such as chlorpromazine, fluphenazine, promazine, and haloperidol). Environmental risk factors include hot temperature, high humidity, and the entire complex of living conditions in poorly insulated urban housing, especially the multistory buildings of slums.

Heatstroke also can occur in healthy individuals who exert themselves with such intensity that the heat produced by skeletal muscles cannot be dissipated quickly enough to cool the body. This exertional heatstroke occurs in unacclimated athletes, such as football players during spring training, or in military recruits who undergo basic training in summer. Athletes wearing heavy equipment or impervious plastic sweatsuits increase their risk. Autopsy findings in heatstroke fatalities are nonspecific and are governed by the survival interval, treatment, and previous condition of the victim.

Delayed systemic disturbances from systemic hyperthermia include widely distributed degenerative changes in the parenchymatous viscera and particularly in the brain. For a complete account of the delayed pathologic changes caused by systemic hyperthermia, the reader is referred to the extensive studies by Malamud, Haymaker, and Custer.[25]

ELECTRICAL INJURY

Electrical injury does not occur unless some part of the body completes the circuit between two conductors. An electrician supported by an insulated boom may safely handle a high-tension conductor because he is isolated from the ground.

The path of a current through the body tends to follow the most direct route between the contact points. The current may cause injury or death by altering the function of a vital organ (for example, throwing the heart into ventricular fibrillation or paralyzing the respiratory center), by stimulating strong (and occasionally tetanic) muscular contractions, or by creating large quantities of heat (electrothermal effect).

When conditions (contacts) are appropriate for the flow of current through the body (or tissues), the occurrence and nature of the harmful effects created by its passage depend on the following:

1. The kind of current (direct or alternating)
2. The amount of current (amperage)
3. The electromotive force (voltage)
4. The amount of resistance offered by the tissues in the path of the current
5. The actual path of the current from the site of entrance to the point of exit
6. The duration of current flow
7. The surface area of contact

An alternating current is more effective in the production of physiologic disturbances than is a direct current, and some alternating frequencies are more disturbing than others. The 60-cycle alternating current commonly available for domestic and industrial use lies in the frequency range that is particularly disturbing to the respiratory centers of the brain and to the heart. One of the major dangers of alternating current is its tetanizing effect, so that a person becomes "locked" to the contact until the circuit is broken. He may thus succumb to a current that would otherwise not be lethal.

The amount of current that will flow through the body when it becomes part of a circuit is determined by the formula $C = V/R$, in which C is the current in amperes, V is potential in volts, and R is the resistance in ohms with which the body opposes the flow of the current. Thus the higher the voltage or the lower the resistance, the greater the flow of current. The usual currents available for domestic use have a potential of either 110 volts or 220 volts.

A 60-cycle alternating current as small as 100 milliamperes is sufficient to cause ventricular fibrillation. Since the resistance of the human body may be reduced to less than 40 ohms under particularly favorable circumstances (large areas of electrode contact against a moist skin surface), it is possible that currents of even less than 100 milliamperes may be dangerous. Mant[26] reported the fatality of a masochist who inserted needles into the skin of his chest and connected them to a 20-volt electric train transformer. For such small currents to produce fatal shock, it is probably necessary that they pass directly through the heart or brainstem with minimum scatter. That the path taken by the current is of critical importance in determining whether a fatal shock will occur is indicated by the fact that, in electroshock therapy, transcranial current flow as great as 1 ampere may be survived without injury.

In general, the severity of the disturbance caused by the flow of a given amount of current between similar external contacts is proportional to the duration of flow. Certainly the generation of heat bears a linear relationship to time. Physiologic disturbances that are evanescent after a momentary shock may be rendered irreversible by a longer period of electrical exposure.

Electrical burns

The amount and place of heat formation incident to the flow of a given amount of electricity through the body are determined by the resistance that the tissue offers to the current. Most of the resistance offered by the human body to an electrical current is that of the skin and the interface between skin and external conductor. Thus electrothermal injuries are ordinarily limited to the skin and the immediately subjacent tissue.

Thin skin is less resistant to the flow of electricity than is thick skin, and moist skin offers less resistance than does dry skin. Heavily callused dry skin may provide a resistance-protection of several hundred thousand ohms. Because of this fact, persons with callused hands often handle with impunity live wires that would be exceedingly dangerous if brought into contact with a less-resistant portion of the body surface.

If the contact between the skin and an external conductor is large, the generation of heat in terms of calories per square centimeter of surface per second may be too low to produce a burn, and yet the amperage may be more than enough to paralyze respiration or circulation. On the other hand, if the skin contact is a small one such as may occur by touching the end of a live wire, the amount of heat generated in a few cubic millimeters of epidermis may be sufficient to produce a burn even though the total amperage has been insufficient to cause a significant degree of physiologic disturbance. The significance of the surface area of contact is best exemplified by what is observed in low-voltage incidents. A child sucking on a live cord may sustain deep labial burns without suffering systemic effects, whereas a person lying in a bathtub who touches an ungrounded electrical element of identical voltage may well be killed immediately without the production of any localized injuries.

In a recent study of 108 electrocutions by low voltage (less than 1000 volts), electrical burns were absent in over 40% of the cases.[56]

Typical low-voltage cutaneous electrical burns are small, circumscribed, indurated lesions that have a central, depressed, gray or black focus of charring surrounded by a zone of grayish white discoloration (Fig. 4-27). The latter change represents coagulation necrosis of the skin and often is surrounded by a narrow areola of erythema. Microscopically there is an abrupt transition from normal to burned skin. The burn commonly shows microvesicles in the epidermis, separation of the lower epidermis, and transcutaneous coagulation extending into the dermis. Epidermal nuclei are pyknotic, elongated, and aligned in a parallel or palisading fashion, often referred to as "nuclear streaming" (Fig. 4-28). High-voltage burns usually have large areas of contact and generate sufficient heat to produce extensive, deep charring that may amputate extremities (Fig. 4-29). Ignition of clothing is a frequent concomitant of contact with high-

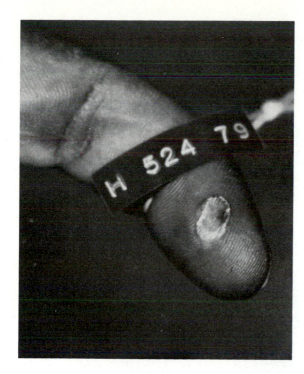

Fig. 4-27. Typical low-voltage electrical burn of index finger.

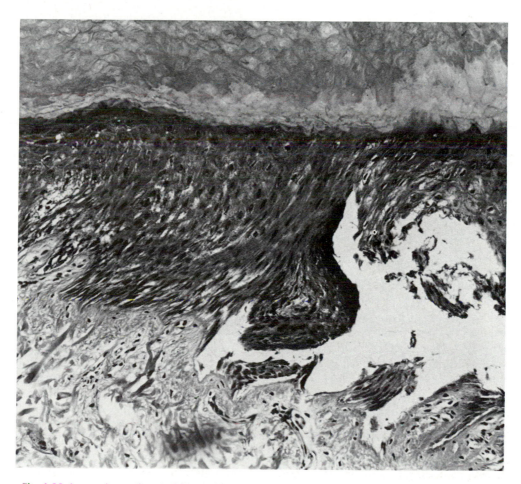

Fig. 4-28. Low-voltage electrical burn of hand. Epidermal separation *(right)* and nuclear streaming *(left).*

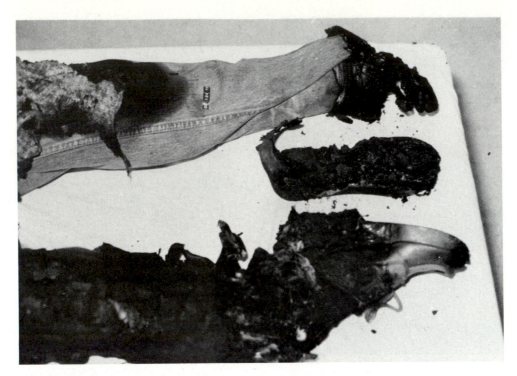

Fig. 4-29. High-voltage electrical burns of lower extremities in young woman who came in contact with downed 13,000-volt power line. There is extensive charring, with partial amputation of left foot and heat fractures of right tibia and fibula. Shoes and clothing were ignited, with superimposed thermal trauma.

voltage electrical current and results in the superimposition of ordinary burning on the electrical injury.

Arcing of the current may produce pitlike defects on the surface of hair or epidermis that are rarely, if ever, produced by other forms of heat. Metallic constituents of the external conductor may be deposited in or on the surface of an electrical burn, and their presence may help to establish the kind of electrode with which the skin was in contact. In the case of alternating current, such metallic deposits may be present at both sites of contact. With direct current the deposits will occur only at the site of contact with the negative electrode.

In persons who survive high-voltage electrical injury, the size of the primary burn does not change, but a surrounding zone of secondary ischemic necrosis may enlarge progressively in the days or weeks after the incident. Such ischemic progression results primarily from thrombosis of arterioles and arteries whose intima was damaged when they served as conduits for the transmission of electricity. These arterial sequelae may necessitate repeated debridement or amputations before the circulatory state is stabilized.

Electrothermal injuries should not be confused with the burns caused by contact with an object that has been rendered hot by a short circuit. If a short circuit occurs through a metallic conductor, the flow of current through it may be so great that even with a potential of 110 volts its temperature is raised almost immediately to the melting point. Contact with such a superheated conductor will cause severe and instantaneous burning even though no electricity flows through the skin. When a current of 110 volts flows through the skin, the resistance is ordinarily so great that there is insufficient amperage for rapid elaboration of heat. Rarely does a current of 110 volts produce a large electrothermal injury of the skin unless the contact is maintained for a considerable period of time.

Apart from injuries caused by heat production and the explosive effects of currents of extremely high voltage, there are no tissue changes that can be regarded as consistently pathognomonic of electricity. Attention has already been directed to the facts that an electrical current flowing through the brainstem may cause death by inhibition of the respiratory centers and that electricity flowing through the heart may cause death by central circulatory failure. Victims of fatal accidental electrocution resulting from a transthoracic current pathway have spoken rationally and continued breathing up to 15 seconds after contact with the electrical circuit was broken. During this interval, they complained of such symptoms as "tightness" in the chest, difficulty in breathing, a sensation of "strangulation," and a feeling of the heart pounding fiercely against the chest wall.[51]

Whether death results from ventricular fibrillation or

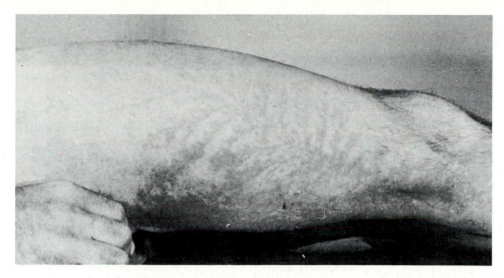

Fig. 4-30. Arborescent pattern of injury marking site of passage of lightning on surface of skin.

from respiratory paralysis is immaterial from the standpoint of the production of characteristic gross or microscopic alterations in the viscera. In neither instance are there internal organic lesions that indicate the cause or mechanism of death. In both circumstances, somatic death is likely to be preceded by a brief period of intense systemic anoxemia, which may lead to the occurrence of petechiae in the serous membranes and central nervous system.

Myoglobinuria of the type that occurs after muscle injury from crushing force or excessive exercise is occasionally encountered in survivors of electric shock. It is a consequence of tissue damage caused by heat generation and coagulation necrosis, both of which are functions of current intensity (amperage), duration and pathway of current flow, tissue resistance, and grounding of the victim.

The myoglobinuria is usually associated with renal tubular necrosis with resulting oliguria or even anuria. The extremely high voltage and amperage characteristics of lightning (see the following) render the survivor of a lightning stroke a likely candidate for this life-threatening, posttraumatic sequel.[57]

Lightning

When a bolt of lightning approaches the earth or a grounded conductor, it tends to break up into many paths of varying intensity. In such circumstances a person struck by lightning may become the conductor of a current so small that his injury is superficial and inconsequential or so large as to be fatal with or without extensive burning. In some instances the current produces an arborescent cutaneous hyperemia that resembles a fern (Fig. 4-30). That some of the electrical energy of a bolt of lightning has produced a superficial injury does not preclude the simultaneous passage of a fatal current through the body with severe burning at the sites of entrance, exit, or both.

In addition to skin burns of varying degrees of severity, victims of lightning may suffer fractures and ruptures of blood vessels and abdominal viscera. The enormous energy (as much as 1×10^9 volts) of a lightning bolt may cause injury by direct effect of the current or by the expanded (and returning) air resulting in blastlike injuries.[6] Current passing through the body may cause either ventricular fibrillation or respiratory paralysis. Instances of fetal electrocution with maternal survival have been reported in which the path of electrical current passed through the gravid uterus following a lightning strike.[14,52]

A broad variety of ocular injuries can develop in survivors of lightning strikes. These include cataracts, corneal ulcers (occasionally going on to perforation), iridocyclitis, hyphema, and vitreous hemorrhage. In rare instances, choroidal ruptures, chorioretinitis, macular tears, retinal detachments, and even optic nerve injury have been recorded.[50]

REFERENCES

1. Adelson, L.: A microscopic study of dermal gunshot wounds, Am. J. Clin. Pathol. **35:**393, 1961.
2. Adelson, L., and Hirsch, C.S.: Sudden and unexpected death from natural causes in adults. In Spitz, W.U., and Fisher, R.S., editors: Medicolegal investigation of death, ed. 2, Springfield, Ill., 1980, Charles C Thomas, Publisher.
3. Baker, M.L., and Dalrymple, G.V.: Biological effects of diagnostic ultrasound: a review, Radiology **126:**479, 1978.
4. Barr, J.S., Draeger, R.H., and Sager, W.W.: Solid blast personnel injury: a clinical study, Milit. Surg. **98:**1, 1946.
5. Bohne, B.A., Ward, P.H., and Fernandez, C.: Rock music and inner ear damage, Am. Fam. Physician **15:**117, 1979.
6. Brown, K.L.: Electrical injuries, J. Trauma **4:**608, 1964.
7. Cohen, J., and Biskind, G.R.: Pathologic aspects of atmospheric blast injuries in man, Arch. Pathol. **42:**12, 1946.

8. Davies, J.W.L., Lamke, L.O., and Liljedahl, S.O.: A guide to the rate of non-renal water loss from patients with burns, Br. J. Plast. Surg. **27**:325, 1974.

9. DeCandole, C.A.: Blast injury, Can. Med. Assoc. J. **96**:207, 1967.

10. Department of the Army: Wound ballistics, Washington, D.C., 1962, Superintendent of Documents.

11. Dougherty, J.D., and Welsh, O.L.: Community noise and hearing loss, N. Engl. J. Med. **275**:759, 1966.

12. Fletcher, B.D., and Brogdon, B.G.: Seat-belt fractures of the spine and sternum, J.A.M.A. **200**:167, 1967.

13. Fryer, D.I.: Pathological findings in fatal sub-atmospheric decompression sickness, Med. Sci. Law **2**:110, 1962.

14. Guha-Ray, D.K.: Fetal death at term due to lightning, Am. J. Obstet. Gynecol. **134**:103, 1979.

15. Heath, D., and Williams, D.R.: Man at high altitude, Edinburgh, 1977, Churchill Livingstone.

16. Heath, D., and Williams, D.R.: The lung at high altitude, Invest. Cell Pathol. **2**:147, 1979.

17. Hill, J.F.: Blast injury with particular reference to recent terrorist bombing incidents, Ann. R. Coll. Surg. Engl. **61**:4, 1979.

18. Idicula, J.: Perplexing case of maxillary sinus barotrauma, Aerospace Med. **43**:891, 1972.

19. Lehman, E.P., and Moore, R.M.: Fat embolism including experimental production without trauma, Arch. Surg. **14**:621, 1927.

20. LeQuire, V.S., et al.: A study of the pathogenesis of fat embolism based on human necropsy material and animal experiments, Am. J. Pathol. **35**:999, 1959.

21. Liebeskind, D., et al.: Diagnostic ultrasound: effects on the DNA and growth patterns of animal cells, Radiology **131**:177, 1979.

22. Liebow, A.A., Warren, S., and DeCoursey, E.: Pathology of atomic bomb casualties, Am. J. Pathol. **25**:853, 1949.

23. Lucké, B.: Lower nephron nephrosis, Milit. Surg. **99**:371, 1946.

24. Lyon, M.F., and Simpson, G.M.: An investigation into the possible genetic hazards of ultrasound, Br. J. Radiol. **47**:712, 1974.

25. Malamud, N., Haymaker, W., and Custer, R.P.: Heat stroke: clinico-pathologic study of 125 fatal cases, Milit. Surg. **99**:397, 1946.

26. Mant, A.K.: Forensic medicine, Chicago, 1960, Year Book Medical Publications, Inc.

27. Marshall, T.K.: Explosion injuries in forensic medicine. In Tedeschi, C.G., Eckert, W.G., and Tedeschi, L.G., editors: Forensic medicine, Philadelphia, 1977, W.B. Saunders Co.

28. Moritz, A.R.: Studies of thermal injury: pathology and pathogenesis of cutaneous burns; experimental study, Am. J. Pathol. **23**:915, 1947.

29. Moritz, A.R., and Henriques, F.C., Jr.: Studies of thermal injury: relative importance of time and surface temperature in causation of cutaneous burns, Am. J. Pathol. **23**:695, 1947.

30. Moritz, A.R., Henriques, F.C., Jr., and McLean, R.: Effects of inhaled heat on air passages and lungs, Am. J. Pathol. **21**:311, 1945.

31. Moritz, A.R., and Weisiger, J.R.: Effects of cold air on air passages and lungs: experimental investigation, Arch. Intern. Med. **75**:233, 1945.

32. Moritz, A.R., et al.: Studies of thermal injury: exploration of causality-producing attributes of conflagrations; local and systemic effects of general cutaneous exposure to excessive circumambient (air) and circumradiant heat of varying duration and intensity, Arch. Pathol. **43**:466, 1947.

33. Neuman, T.S., et al.: Cardiopulmonary consequences of decompression stress, Respir. Physiol. **41**:143, 1980.

34. Pearse, H.E., and Kingsley, H.D.: Thermal burns from atomic bombs, Surg. Gynecol. Obstet. **98**:385, 1954.

35. Rawlins, J.S.P.: Physical and pathophysiological effects of blast, Injury **9**:313, 1978.

36. Read, A.E., et al.: Pancreatitis and accidental hypothermia, Lancet **2**:1219, 1961.

37. Roy, S.B., et al.: Haemodynamic studies in high altitude pulmonary oedema, Br. Heart J. **31**:52, 1969.

38. Ryan, G.A.: Injuries in traffic accidents, N. Engl. J. Med. **276**:1066, 1967.

39. Sataloff, J., Vassallo, J. and Menduke, H.: Occupational hearing loss and high frequency thresholds, Arch. Environ. Health **14**:832, 1967.

40. Savides, E.P., and Huffband, B.I.: Hypothermia, thrombosis and acute pancreatitis, Br. Med. J. **1**:614, 1974.

41. Schwetz, F.: The critical intensity for occupational noise, Acta Otolaryngol. **89**:358, 1980.

42. Scully, R.E.: Fat embolism in Korean battle casualties: its incidence, clinical significance and pathologic aspects, Am. J. Pathol. **32**:379, 1956.

43. Selye, H.: The general adaptation syndrome and the diseases of adaptation, J. Clin. Endocrinol. **6**:117, 1946.

44. Selye, H.: Stress and disease, Science **122**:625, 1955.

45. Sevitt, S.: Fat embolism, London, 1962, Butterworth & Co.

46. Spitz, W.U.: Essential postmortem findings in the traffic accident victim, Arch. Pathol. **90**:451, 1970.

47. Strauss, R.H., and Prockop, L.D.: Decompression sickness among scuba divers, J.A.M.A. **223**:637, 1973.

48. Strauss, R.H., and Yount, D.E.: Decompression sickness, Am. Sci. **65**:598, 1977.

49. Sube, J., Ziperman, H.H., and McIver, W.J.: Seat belt trauma to the abdomen, Am. J. Surg. **133**:346, 1967.

50. Taussig, H.B.: "Death" from lightning—and the possibility of living again, Ann. Intern. Med. **68**:1345, 1968.

51. Walter, C.W.: Is death from accidental electric shock instantaneous? J.A.M.A. **221**:922, 1972.

52. Weinstein, L.: Lightning: a rare cause of intrauterine death with maternal survival, South. Med. J. **72**:103, 1979.

53. Weissman, B., Green, R.S., and Roberts, P.T.: Frontal sinus barotrauma, Laryngoscope **82**:2160, 1972.

54. Whitcraft, D.D., III, and Karas, S.: Air embolism and decompression sickness in scuba divers, J.A.C.E.P. **5**:355, 1976.

55. Wittenzellner, R.: Tissue damaging effects of ultrasound, Ultrasonics **14**:281, 1976.

56. Wright, R.K., and Davis, J.H.: The investigation of electrical deaths: a report of 220 fatalities, J. Forensic Sci. **25**:514, 1980.

57. Yost, J.W., and Olmes, F.F.: Myoglobinuria following lightning stroke, J.A.M.A. **228**:1147, 1974.

CHAPTER 5

Drug and Chemical Injury—Environmental Pathology

GORDON R. HENNIGAR
PAUL GROSS

DRUG INJURY AND IATROGENIC DISEASES
Adverse medicinal drug reactions

An adverse drug reaction (ADR) is defined as any response to a drug that is noxious and unintended and that occurs at dosage used in humans for prophylaxis, diagnosis, or therapy, excluding failure to acomplish the intended purpose.

Incidence

It is frequently stated that 5% of patients are admitted to the hospital as a result of drug reactions. One study suggested that, during their hospital stay, 20% of all patients had suffered from the complications of diagnostic or therapeutic procedures utilizing drugs. Adverse effects from drug therapy may account for 1 in 40 consultations in general practice. They are obviously important in terms of morbidity and may affect the physician-patient relationship and cause noncompliance in the future. One group is heard to cry, "Bad prescriptions kill thousands a year," and to assert that 30,000 Americans die as a direct result of the drugs their physicians prescribe. A second group holds an altogether different view and considers the seriousness of drug toxicity to be overemphasized; they are quick to point out that a drug-related fatality of 2.4:1000 patients admitted to the hospital medical services represents a small risk and that drugs, compared with many daily hazards to which we all are exposed, are in general remarkably benign. A third group considers the debate useless on the grounds that valid data on the prevalence and incidence of adverse drug reactions are unavailable.

Considering the number of prescription and over-the-counter preparations (approximately 1500 generic types) that are dispensed to the public, the number of toxic and allergic reactions is small. Physicians, and the public as well, should not be concerned about all adverse reactions but rather about the number of *unwarranted* adverse reactions. A patient who appears to be dying of advanced congestive failure and is not responding to conventional doses of digitalis may be given larger doses of this drug in a desperate attempt that is recognized as heroic. Signs of digitalis intoxication may supervene, and if the patient dies, he may well be classified as having a toxic drug reaction contributing to his death. But the use of additional digitalis in this instance was a well-considered and warranted intervention. The death may be classified for statistical purposes as drug related, but this statistic has no bearing on the quality of medical practice. This kind of warranted drug reaction is part of the risk any physician and patient must assume when treatment, whether medical or surgical, is instituted. The crucial parameter is the one that will indicate whether the quality of drug use is good or bad, and this will be governed by the number of unwarranted adverse reactions noted.

Consider the instance in which diarrhea develops in a patient receiving clindamycin. The pathologist interprets biopsy results as indicative of early ulcerative colitis when actually the patient has a clindamycin-associated lesion. A state of toxic megacolon develops and the patient dies. The cause of death is recorded as complications of *Clostridium difficile* toxic colitis associated with the administration of clindamycin. In this instance the compound is blamed for the death, although the clinician and pathologist using their gross and microscopic findings should not have rendered the diagnosis of ulcerative colitis in the first place. Ulcerative colitis is a diffuse disease, whereas antibiotic-associated colitis is focal, becoming diffuse only in fatal or nearly fatal incidences.

Causative components of adverse drug reactions

Drugs as toxins. The term *toxin* is frequently used loosely to encompass all injurious substances, whatever the means by which injury is induced. We use it here in a more restricted sense to refer to chemical agents producing a direct, predictable, dose-related injury to cells and organs, thus excluding a large group of ADRs related to immunologic responses.

Although most toxic ADRs result from overdose or prolonged high-dose therapy, in some instances an ADR may occur from normal dosage. This may be the result of (1) preexisting kidney or liver disease, with limited ability to excrete or detoxify the drug, producing high concentrations in tissues or circulation in the face of normal dosage; (2) interaction with other drugs, producing synergistic effects; or (3) quantitative alterations in pharmacokinetics, that is, absorption, distribution, and elimination.

Toxic reactions in cells and organs are predictable and dose related, occur within a specific time after administration of the drug, and can be consistently reproduced in animals. All of these characteristics are also true of the desired pharmacologic effect; thus toxic ADRs may simply be a magnification of the pharmacologic effect or may include new, unrelated responses (Table 5-1). The dose-response curves for the two may overlap, as in the case of digoxin: a dose of digoxin sufficient to ensure fully therapeutic levels for 100% of patients will also cause vomiting, an ADR, in 15%.

Drugs as antigens. Drugs, chemical structures with potent pharmacologic activity, are foreign to the body's immunologic system. They are also, in general, treated by the body as undesirable substances and are excreted as soon as possible. There is hardly a drug that is excreted in the form in which it is taken; this implies that the drug is chemically transformed by metabolic processes, with the ultimate effect of facilitating excretion. Hepatic microsomal enzymes are capable of hydroxylating, conjugating, reducing, or oxidizing drugs to make them more polar. Metabolites that are more polar than the original compound are more water soluble and are therefore easier to excrete via the urine or feces.

The possibility of a drug metabolite becoming immunologically significant rests with its ability to react with proteins or other macromolecule structures, since drug molecules, for the most part, are of low molecular weight and are by themselves unable to act as complete antigens. A supply of susceptible carrier molecules is essential for antigen formation. The proteins synthesized locally within the liver are ideally suited to combine with newly formed reactive drug metabolites. It is known that very few individuals develop altered immune (hypersensitivity) reactions to drugs, although reactive metabolic products are formed; this implies that factors *unique to the host* play a considerable part in the development of the allergic state.

Under appropriate conditions, then, altered immune responses of the humoral or cellular type may occur, characterized by the appearance of specific circulating antibody or skin sensitivity or both. However, attempts to demonstrate such evidence of sensitization may be unsuccessful in many patients with drug-induced hypersensitivities. For instance, the finding of so-called markers of autoimmunity, such as L.E. cell phenomenon, antinuclear factor, antimitochondrial antibody, rheumatoid factor, and positive Coombs' test results, indicates an altered immunologic response but may not be accompanied by *direct evidence* of humoral or cell-mediated drug sensitization and should not imply that such a reaction is responsible for the accompanying lesions.

Drugs are not generally reactive enough to form the irreversible complexes with proteins that are necessary for sensitization, but the metabolic or oxidative products of many common drugs are sufficiently reactive to form stable immunogenic complexes. Some of the minor metabolites, formed in minute quantities, can be responsible for the most severe reactions. The major metabolite responsible for sensitization with penicillin, for example, has been identified as the minor benzylpenicilloyl group, which combines irreversibly with proteins. With quinine or quinidine, it has been suggested that sensitization results from the drugs being metabolized to a more reactive molecule; antibodies from 20% of sensitized patients do not react with quinine and quinidine isomers but with quininone, an oxidative derivative of both drugs. Thus it is apparent that metabolic products of drugs, rather than native drugs, are frequently responsible for sensitization, even though the antibodies elicited by the metabolite, as a rule, react with the native drug.

In contrast to direct toxic action, altered immune responses are not necessarily dose related. Withdrawal of the drug leads in most instances to prompt recovery, and the hypersensitivity or immunologic reaction is variable and not target organ specific. Not infrequently, the clinical manifestations may be comprised of any one or more of the following: blood eosinophilia, mucocutaneous lesions, fleeting joint pains, hepatosplenomegaly, generalized lymphadenopathy, and (most important) fever.

Table 5-1. Comparison of immunologic and "toxic" medicinal drug reactions

Immunologic	Toxic
Usually more than one exposure	Frequently only one exposure
Not necessarily dose related	Cellular severity of reaction related to amount of dose or cumulative dosage
Withdrawal of drug leads, in most cases, to prompt recovery	Permanent damage to cells and tissues depends on organ site and total amount of drug administered
Hypersensitivity or immunologic reactions variable and not target organ specific	Target organ specific

A definitive diagnosis of an allergic drug reaction is often impossible to make. One frequently ends up with a diagnosis of "probable" or "possible," rather than "definitive." In attempting to demonstrate a causal relationship between the observed clinical manifestations and the drug, the investigator must recognize that the signs and symptoms that develop are those that are usually associated with the natural history of disease or that can be accounted for by a complication of the disease process. This was recently well illustrated when jaundice developed in a patient who had for several months been taking the phenothiazine chlorpromazine. A liver biopsy was performed. Within the bile canaliculi were observed bile "thrombi," accompanied by eosinophils and lymphocytes in the portal tracts. A diagnosis of chlorpromazine cholestatic hepatitis was made, and the drug was stopped. The direct-reacting serum bilirubin level continued to rise, and it was discovered that the patient had a small bile duct carcinoma at the bifurcation of the common bile duct!

Eosinophils are frequently suggestive of a drug reaction, but there are many other causes of tissue eosinophilia. One of the earliest signs of an ADR is the development of mild fever, but of course this is very nonspecific. However, careful and frequent scrutiny of the temperature chart should be routine during any drug treatment, especially with multiple drugs or if the drugs are known to be potential antigens. For example, one of the main causes of postsurgical fever, 4 to 7 days after an operation, is a hypersensitivity reaction to the anesthetic halothane. Therefore, if the surgeon is not satisfied that the fever is related directly to the surgical procedure, the anesthetic should be suspect.

The syndrome of fever, arthritis and myalgia, eosinophilia, lymphadenopathy, and hepatosplenomegaly is not uncommon in patients admitted to the hospital. Frequently the referring physician is thinking of diagnoses such as sarcoidosis, tuberculosis, and malignant lymphoma. A careful history, however, may reveal that the patient has been taking one or more medicinal compounds, and within a few days after withdrawal of these drugs, the fever subsides. Such a patient was a 45-year-old woman who was quite ill when admitted to the hospital, with fever, malaise, recent weight loss, and a mild leukocytosis. A bone marrow biopsy revealed the presence of several noncaseating granulomas, and similar granulomas were found during a liver biopsy. When attempts to identify organisms within the granulomas failed, it was decided that the granulomas could be drug induced. A survey of the woman's drug regimen revealed that she had been, and was at the time of her hospital admission, taking some 18 different medicinal compounds for such varied problems as headache, pain, cardiac arrhythmia, and edema. All drugs except the antiarrhythmic were discontinued for 3 days. The patient's fever disappeared, her leukocyte count reverted to normal, and she was talking about leaving the hospital.

A classification of the mechanisms of immunologic-induced adverse tissue reactions to drugs is as follows:
1. Anaphylactic (IgE-mediated) response
2. Circulating antigen-antibody complexes (the antigen being the drug or metabolite)
3. Cell-mediated response
4. Autoimmune response
   a. L.E. phenomenon (antinuclear antibodies)
   b. Cytotoxic (for example, hemolytic anemia, agranulocytosis, thrombocytopenia)

It should be appreciated that *more than one* of these mechanisms may be operative in any immunologic reaction to a drug or its metabolite (Table 5-2).

Table 5-2. Classification of altered immune reactions to medicinal drugs

Type	Antibody	Disease state	Cellular reaction	Drugs*
Anaphylactic	Essentially IgE	Acute anaphylactic shock; status asthmaticus; laryngeal edema	Basophil and mast cell degeneration; eosinophils	Penicillins and cephalosporins; iodinated contrast media; vaccines and antisera
Cytotoxic	IgG or IgM	Hemolytic reactions; autoimmune reactions (e.g., L.E. phenomena)	Lysed red cells; lymphocytes, plasma cells, and macrophages; vasculitis	Penicillins; sulfonylureas; phenothiazines; hydralazine and procainamide; rifampin
Acute immune complex disease (antigen-antibody complement)	IgG	Serum sickness	Eosinophils, lymphocytes, plasma cells, macrophages; acute vasculitis	Antisera; penicillins
		Membranous glomerulonephritis	No inflammatory cells	Gold salts; penicillamine; cimetidine; aspirin; phenytoin
Cell-mediated reactions	Sensitized T lymphocytes	Contact dermatitis	Lymphocytes; edema and necrosis of epidermal cells	Ethylene diamine; antibiotics (e.g., neomycin); benzocaine; procaine
		Organic and systemic granulomas	Focal collection of macrophages	Nonsteroid analgesics (e.g., phenylbutazone)

*Commonly implicated as prototypes of hypersensitivity reactions.

Genetically related adverse drug reactions (pharmacogenetics)

Genetic factors may predispose an individual to ADRs, and in some cases there may be inheritance of abnormal receptors and enzymes. Examples include drug-induced hemolysis in glucose-6-phosphate dehydrogenase deficiency, prolonged paralysis following administration of succinylcholine to patients with atypical pseudocholinesterase, susceptibility to malignant hyperthermia during anesthesia, drug-induced exacerbation of porphyria, and the link between ABO blood group and thromboembolic disease caused by oral contraceptives. Polymorphic hydroxylation and acetylation of drugs may also predispose individuals to toxicity. Thus drug-induced lupus erythematosus, hemolysis, and peripheral neuropathy are related to polymorphic acetylation of procainamide and sulfasalazine, as well as isoniazid. There is an association between the HLA-DR antigen phenotype and adverse reactions to gold and penicillamine.

In the context of ADRs, the term *idiosyncrasy* has been used extensively as a label for bizarre responses that were assumed to result from some qualitative abnormality in the patient. Until recently, drug idiosyncrasies were a catchall classification for ADRs that could not be classified under any other heading. This situation is now changing slowly as the mechanisms of ADRs have become clearer and it has become apparent that the majority have a genetic basis.

Age and sex. The incidence of ADRs is greatest in the very young and the very old. The newborn are particularly vulnerable, especially if they are premature, and the responsiveness of the tissues to a given drug concentration may not be the same as in adults. Very young children are said to be particularly sensitive to narcotics, anticholinergics, diazepam, salicylates, and agents that cause methemoglobinemia (fetal hemoglobin is more easily oxidized to methemoglobin than is the adult form). In addition, the metabolism and renal excretion of drugs may be abnormally slow in neonates and infants, resulting in exaggerated and prolonged effects. Thus the maternal use of diazepam is associated with apneic spells, hypotonia, poor feeding, and hypothermia lasting for several days in the newborn—the "floppy baby syndrome."

The elderly are also vulnerable to ADRs. Not only are the functional reserves of many organs reduced and compensatory mechanisms impaired, but the capacity to metabolize and eliminate drugs is reduced. Central nervous system (CNS) depressants are a particular problem for the elderly, in whom they readily cause confusion, disorientation, dementia, depression, incontinence, ataxia, and falls resulting in fractures. In most surveys the incidence of ADRs has been higher in women than in men, possibly because women take more drugs and make up a higher proportion of the vulnerable geriatric population.

Renal disease. ADRs are more common in patients with renal disease. Contributory factors include decreased renal clearance of drugs and their metabolites, increased receptor responsiveness, decreased plasma protein binding, changes in drug distribution, impaired drug metabolism, and the effects of acid-base and electrolyte disturbances. Many drugs are excreted in the urine largely unchanged, and the half-life increases disproportionately as the creatinine clearance falls below 20 to 30 ml/minute. Drug metabolites that normally have little or no activity may accumulate to a remarkable degree and cause toxicity. Use of nephrotoxic combinations such as gentamicin plus cephalothin should obviously be avoided, and preexisting renal disease may potentiate the nephrotoxicity of drugs such as tetracycline, sulfamethoxazole (Septra), phenylbutazone, and aspirin.

Morphologic aspects

Immunologic reactions. Generalized necrotizing vasculitis, especially polyarteritis, is one of the most common allergic drug reactions. For years the sulfonamides were the most common cause of this reaction, but more recently penicillin has assumed this role. The reaction is similar to the Arthus phenomenon and to polyarteritis nodosa, with complement and IgG demonstrable in the inflammatory necrotizing lesions of small vessels. The cellular reactions in drug-induced states show wide variability (Table 5-2).

Immunologic reactions to drugs are frequently characterized by disproportionate numbers of eosinophils and "immunoblasts." These cells are prominent in other conditions as well, but when they are seen in tissue sections, it is important to entertain the diagnosis of allergic drug reaction. Immunoblastic lymphadenopathy, which occurs occasionally in patients taking phenytoin (Dilantin) and other drugs, has been mistaken for malignant lymphoma.

Noncaseous granulomatous inflammation is also seen occasionally as a marker of allergic drug reaction, particularly in the skin, liver, and bone marrow.

Toxic reactions. The tissue(s) or organ(s) involved and the nature of the reactions in a toxic response depend on the chemical and pharmacologic nature of the drug. There is thus a bewildering array of such reactions. The brain, kidneys, lungs, heart, liver, or gastrointestinal tract may be most seriously involved, and the lesion may be acute, inflammatory, necrotizing, fibrotic, metabolic, neoblastic, or thrombotic, to mention a few. A drug such as acetaminophen may appear to selectively involve a single organ—the liver—whereas the toxic manifestations of phenytoin include acute epithelial necrolysis of the skin, megaloblastic anemia, hepatitis, teratogenesis, and gingival hyperplasia, in addition to immunologic responses such as vasculitis, immunoblastic lymphadenopathy, and granulomatous reactions.

Table 5-3. Toxic hepatic injury

Lesion	Prototype
Fatty infiltration (steatosis)	Tetracycline
Hepatic cell necrosis	Acetaminophen
Cholangionecrosis	Chlorpromazine
Cirrhosis	Methotrexate
Cholestasis	Methyltestosterone
Cholestatic hepatitis	Chlorpropamide
Vascular thrombosis	Oral contraceptives
Peliosis hepatis	Methyltestosterone
Hyperplasia and adenoma	Oral contraceptives
Malignant neoplasia	Thorotrast

From Hennigar, G.R.: Adverse drug reactions. In Hill, R.B., and Terzian, J.A., editors: Environmental pathology: an evolving field, New York, 1982, Alan R. Liss, Inc.

Table 5-3 presents a list of reactions in the liver, thought to be toxic, to illustrate the large variety of such reactions. The toxic reactions to each of the drugs listed may be more complex than is implied by this table, and the prototype drug listed is not the only one that can produce each of these lesions. Several reactions that appear to be allergic, such as granulomatous inflammation, chronic active hepatitis, and necrotizing vasculitis, are not included.

Medicinal hazards of therapy
Antibiotics

Tetracycline. The tetracyclines, when administered intravenously, particularly in the presence of renal dysfunction, may lead to fat accumulation in the liver cells. This may be accompanied by acute tubular necrosis, characterized by swelling, hydropic change, and fatty accumulations within the cells of the proximal convoluted tubules. Other changes such as focal hemorrhagic pancreatitis and ulceration of the esophagus, stomach, and proximal portion of the small intestine have been noted.

Both in humans and in some laboratory animals, fatty degeneration (steatosis) of the liver is produced by the intravenous injection of tetracycline. Grossly, the liver is of normal size or slightly enlarged. Sectioning reveals it to be bulging, yellow, and greasy. This is not associated with inflammation or necrosis. Studies with tritium-labeled tetracycline show that this antibiotic accumulates in the spleen, lymph nodes, and skeleton, with the highest concentration in the liver. It is quickly excreted into the bile and within the liver acinus or lobule, where there tends to be a centrilobular localization. Microscopically, tetracycline localizes within mitochondria as demonstrated by fluorescence. The degree of involvement seems to depend on the dosage. At the cellular level, in contrast to the alcoholic type of fatty liver, the nuclei are in the center of the cell rather than "squeezed over" to the margin by a single large globule of intracellular fat (Fig. 5-1). The appearance is reminiscent of the liver in

"obstetric yellow atrophy," or fatty liver of pregnancy. In that condition the fatty accumulation in the liver cell assumes the same cytologic configuration as in tetracycline toxicity, but, in addition, inflammatory changes and necrosis are frequently seen, whereas they are rare in tetracycline toxicity. There is no direct evidence that the liver of a pregnant woman is especially susceptible to tetracycline hepatotoxicity. Ultrastructurally, evidence of tetracycline toxicity is manifested by the finding of cytoplasmic collections of lipid closely associated with lipofuscins (Fig. 5-1, *A*). All of this swims in a sea of glycogen.

The centrilobular localization is not surprising, since these cells contain the highest levels of esterase and β-hydroxybutyric dehydrogenase. Such enzyme localization points to the central part of the liver as the location where most of the lipids are metabolized, and interference with such metabolism would allow changes to be visible initially in this portion of the lobule. Physiologically, intracellular lipids are believed to be in the form of laminar micelles, which in turn are incorporated into the membranous structures of the cell and are not identifiable as lipid by light microscopy. The stability of this lipid dispersion depends on protein and abundant phospholipid as an emulsifier or stabilizer. When there is a deficiency of these substances as well as choline and inositol, a low oxygen supply, or an excess of cholesterol, one may expect to find interference with this form of cellular lipid dispersion. The exact mechanism whereby tetracycline interferes with one or more of these factors is not clear. It is known, however, that the tetracyclines inhibit protein synthesis, so that an antianabolic effect is produced. If there is interference with the normal membrane localization of intracellular lipids, globules of fat that can be stained by the usual fat-staining methods appear. The fatty change in the liver in tetracycline toxicity is reversible.

The formation of lipoprotein-tetracycline complexes in the blood of patients may partially explain why tetracyclines sometimes have anticoagulant properties. They apparently impair the conversion of prothrombin to thrombin and the generation of thromboplastin. Both of these reactions require phospholipid for activation. The bleeding phenomenon noted clinically may be related in part to this property, but the hypoprothrombinemia that is observed probably also constitutes an important factor.

Renal tubular necrosis, when it occurs, is caused largely by the toxic degradation products of tetracycline metabolism, the most important of which is anhydrotetracycline. This substance has been responsible for producing the renal Fanconi syndrome (glucoaminophosphate diabetes). The syndrome, when related to tetracycline administration, is reversible.

All compounds of tetracycline may cause tooth discoloration, with oxytetracycline being the most innocuous.

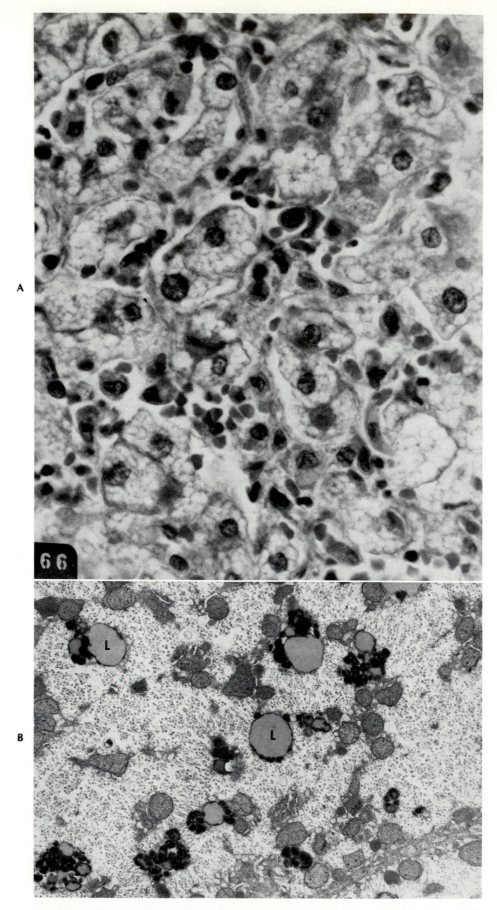

Fig. 5-1. Effects of tetracycline therapy on liver. **A,** There is steatosis of liver cells with centrally placed nuclei. Cytoplasm has a foamy, vacuolated appearance. Oil red O stain for neutral fat was positive. **B,** Lipid droplets, *L,* are closely associated with lipofuscins (dark pigment). (**A,** Hematoxylin and eosin; 400×.)

The mechanism of discoloration is that tetracyclines form chelation complexes with calcium at a physiologic pH and become incorporated into bone and teeth. Since teeth do not undergo a constant remodeling as does bone, they can be stained only during their calcification stage. Both deciduous and permanent teeth can be stained. Tetracycline passes the placental barrier and therefore stains teeth in the process of calcification in utero.

Amphotericin B. Amphotericin B is produced by the streptomycete *Streptomyces nodosus*. It is available in either the crystalline or the colloidal form. The crystalline form is useful only through oral administration and has been effective, for the most part, in the treatment of infections caused by *Candida albicans*. Very few signs or symptoms of toxicity are noted with oral administration. Colloidal amphotericin B that is solubilized with desoxycholate is used either intravenously or intrathecally. Signs of toxicity are associated mainly with these routes of administration. The toxic manifestations of intravenous administration consist of phlebitis, hypokalemia, abnormal renal function, and anemia, whereas those of intrathecal administration are pain at the site of injection or along the lumbar nerve roots, headache, paresthesias, nerve palsies, difficulty in voiding, and chemical meningitis.

The colloidal form of amphotericin B has been successful in the treatment of a wide spectrum of mycotic diseases. The two major toxic problems are related to abnormal renal function and anemia. Morphologically, in both humans and dogs, numerous renal lesions have been noted after amphotericin treatment. These predominantly involve the proximal and distal convoluted tubules and consist of hydropic degeneration or necrosis with tubulorrhexis and amorphous material containing calcium and phosphate in the lumen and interstitium. The effects of amphotericin B on the tubules are probably the result of vasospasm of the afferent arterioles leading to acute hypoxic nephrosis or tubular necrosis with renal shutdown. The glomerular lesions have included basement membrane thickening with increased lobulation and ischemic glomerular loops and infraglomerular epithelial reflux.

These renal changes are believed to be reversible, with the exception of the nephrocalcinosis. The anemia is independent of the azotemia and occurs after a relatively small amount of the drug has been administered. The anemia is usually not incapacitating and is of the normocytic normochromic type. There is usually no reticulocytosis. Bone marrow examinations have shown no consistent histologic findings. There is, however, suppression of erythropoiesis without correlation between the total dose and duration of the drug and the degree of the anemia. In vitro studies using exceedingly high levels of amphotericin have shown damage to tissue culture cells and human red blood cells.

Clindamycin. Clindamycin (Cleocin) is an effective antibiotic against gram-positive bacteria. Recommend-

ed, and particularly excessive, doses may result in diarrhea, abdominal pain, and a shocklike state. These findings are highly suggestive of clindamycin-induced pseudomembranous colitis. Grossly, the initial lesion is white or gray plaques that extend from the ileocecal valve to the rectum (Fig. 5-2, A). More advanced lesions of antibiotic-associated colitis involve the mucosa, being manifested as a diffuse necrosis of the superficial layers of epithelium. The result is a sheetlike, gray, diffuse pseudomembrane. The underlying mucosa is red-brown, granular, and superficially denuded (Fig. 5-2, B).

Histologically, the earliest focal lesions are characterized by necrosis of the surface epithelium with exudation of mucus, fibrin, leukocytes, and necrotic glandular epithelium (Fig. 5-2, C). Advanced lesions appear as a diffuse pseudomembrane (Fig. 5-2, C). Superficially, the underlying mucosa is denuded and replaced by necrotic debris, inflammatory cells, fibrin, and "streamers" of mucus emanating from the overdistended, ruptured mucous glands (Fig. 5-2, D and E). The appearance is reminiscent of lava spewing from an activated volcanic crater. The underlying muscularis is not involved by the inflammatory process.

The microscopic appearance of early antibiotic-associated colitis has been confused with that of idiopathic ulcerative colitis. This confusion has led to continued use of clindamycin with fatal outcome. Interestingly, *C. difficile* toxin leads to aggravation of idiopathic ulcerative colitis. The necrosis of the mucosa is due to toxins of the *Clostridium* class, most notably *C. difficile* and in some cases *C. perfringens*. Antibiotic-associated colitis has also followed the administration of ampicillin and tetracycline. Recently, rifampin and metronidazole, an effective combination against *Bacteroides*, and other antibiotics have been documented as causes of the condition. Some years ago, vigorous antibiotic therapy before intestinal surgery was routine. Pseudomembranous enterocolitis developed in these patients and was attributed to antibiotic-resistant staphylococcal toxins. It should be noted that this is different from the current antibiotic-associated colitis that is confined to the colon, since the staphylococcal cases involved the small intestine as well. During the past several decades, stool cultures have failed to reveal the presence of staphylococci in cases of antibiotic-associated pseudomembranous colitis. The toxins of *C. difficile* can be identified by a tissue culture cell assay technique, both during life and at autopsy.

Chloramphenicol. The most serious complication after the administration of chloramphenicol is the development of aplastic anemia. Since there is no hemolysis, as one would expect to find as a manifestation of an autoimmune reaction, the development of the anemia probably represents specific idiosyncrasy of the individual. The reaction is not necessarily related to dosage but is more common with prolonged use.

Selective depression of bone marrow does occur in

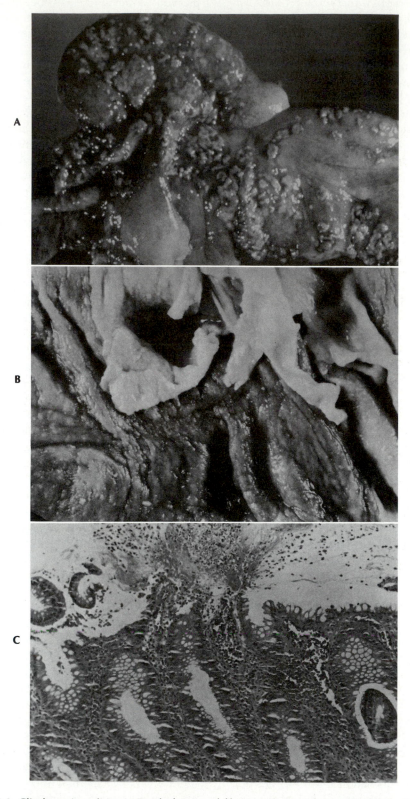

Fig. 5-2. Clindamycin colitis. **A,** Focal plaques of fibrin, mucus, and necrotic debris. **B,** Diffuse pseudomembrane reflected to demonstrate underlying red-brown, granular, superficially denuded mucosa. **C,** Early lesion showing focal necrosis of superficial epithelium and mucosa with outpouring of mucus, fibrin, and nuclear fragments.   *Continued.*

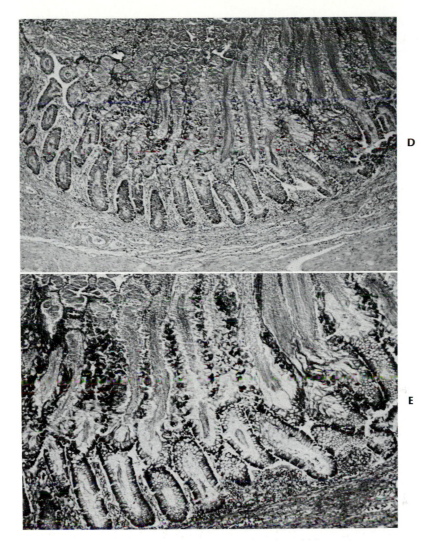

Fig. 5-2, cont'd. D, Necrosis and inflammatory infiltrate extends through mucosa and minimally involves submucosa. Muscularis is spared. Note necrotic glands, hyperactive goblet cells, and "streamers" of mucus. The luminal side of lesions is composed of necrotic debris. **E,** Higher magnification of micrograph in **D.**

mild cases of toxicity, but this usually involves the granulocytes or platelets and spares erythropoiesis. Evidence for the direct toxic reaction is the observation of greatly vacuolated nucleated red cells in the marrow. The toxic action of chloramphenicol is believed to be attributable to the nitrobenzene ring within its structure. It is not clear why aplasia occurs in some patients after the administration of small doses, whereas other patients can receive very high doses without apparent permanent effect on the marrow.

Chloramphenicol is normally detoxified by conjugation with glucuronic acid in the liver and is excreted in the urine as inert nitro compounds. The idiosyncrasy may be related to the inability to metabolize chloramphenicol or may be the result of some other genetically determined defect in the marrow cells themselves. The possibility exists, as it does with virtually all drugs, that some form of hypersensitivity mechanism is at work. At autopsy the marrow has a pale or fatty appearance. There is no lymphadenopathy or splenomegaly. Microscopically, in patients with aplasia, the bone marrow takes on the appearance of vascularized adipose tissue. Hemosiderosis throughout the reticuloendothelial system is observed in patients who have received a number of blood transfusions. Focal myocardial hemorrhages sometimes occur. As is the case with many antibiotics, infection by opportunistic fungi is common.

Newborn infants are devoid of an effective glucuronic acid conjugation mechanism for degradation and detoxification of the antibiotic. Consequently, when such infants are given chloramphenicol in doses of 75 or more mg/kg body weight/day, the drug may accumulate, resulting in the "gray syndrome" with hyperthermia, acidity, gray color, shock, and collapse. This mechanism is also applicable to the neonatal hyperbilirubinemia occurring after the administration of streptomycin.

Penicillins. For many years the short-acting sulfonamides were the outstanding culprit that brought about hypersensitivity angiitis and polyarteritis nodosa, but penicillin has now assumed this role. Medium-sized and small vessels, as well as capillaries, may be the target of penicillin hypersensitivity. The metabolite benzylpenicilloyl serves as the antigen or hapten for the induction of humoral and cell-mediated responses. The semisynthetic penicillins such as methicillin, ampicillin, oxacillin, and carbenicillin have been clearly pinpointed as etiologic agents of acute interstitial nephritis of hypersensitivity etiology. The cephalosporins (prototype cephalothin), which have a cross-sensitivity with the penicillins, and the aminoglycosides (prototypes streptomycin, kanamycin, and gentamicin) also cause this hypersensitivity nephritis. Drug-induced acute interstitial nephritis is characterized by acute renal failure accompanied by marked hematuria, proteinuria, and the presence of tubular epithelial cells and eosinophils in the urine. Concomitantly, clinical manifestations of allergy, such as fever, skin rash, and joint pains, and blood eosinophilia

are observed. It is estimated that acute interstitial nephritis may cause between 7% and 10% of cases of clinically obscure acute renal failure. Unexpected death, occurring within minutes after parenteral injection of penicillin, has been recorded numerous times. The mechanism is anaphylactic shock manifested by pulmonary arteriolar and bronchiolar spasm, leading to acute dilatation of the right side of the heart with pooling of blood in the vena caval system. Pulmonary alveolar congestion and edema are consistent findings (Fig. 5-3). Petechial hemorrhages of the conjunctiva and serosal surfaces of visceral organs are noted. Patients may complain of chest pain, which is followed by dyspnea, cyanosis, generalized convulsions, and frothing at the mouth. The manifestations are reminiscent of those seen after fatal bee sting, accidental parenteral injection or overdosage in clinical hyposensitization procedures, and anaphylaxis in experimental animals.

A syndrome characterized by transient eosinophilic pulmonary infiltrates and vasculitis may be the result of acute immune complex disease occurring after penicillin therapy. The syndrome is almost identical to that seen in patients who manifest hypersensitivity reactions to infec-

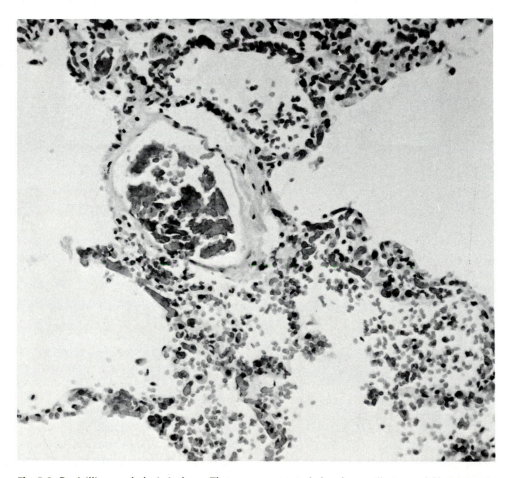

Fig. 5-3. Penicillin anaphylaxis in lung. There are congested alveolar capillaries and fibrinogen in vessel.

tion with the *Ascaris* parasite. In this instance the condition is referred to as Löffler's syndrome.

Cephalosporins. Cephalothin, a prototype of the cephalosporins, may produce immune hemolytic anemia. This effect is shared with the penicillins, with which there is cross-sensitivity. Antibiotic-associated colitis may follow the administration of cephalothin and/or penicillin. Cephalothin therapy occasionally leads to a "toxic effect" on the proximal convoluted tubular epithelial cells, which may result in necrosis and subsequent acute renal failure. The hypersensitivity reaction in the kidney to cephalothin is characterized by the appearance of acute interstitial nephritis (see discussion of penicillins, opposite).

Aminoglycosides. Gentamicin and polymyxin B, like neomycin and kanamycin, are aminoglycosides that cause degeneration of the proximal convoluted tubules. On occasion, tubular necrosis supervenes. Gentamicin is concentrated in the renal cortex and excreted slowly. It is the most nephrotoxic of the aminoglycosides, causing nephrotoxicity in 2% to 14% of patients treated. The incidence is lowest in those who do not have preexisting renal disease. The evidence points to a direct cellular toxic damage to the proximal tubular epithelium and is characterized by a granular type of necrosis, with the lumina being filled by an amorphous eosinophilic material. The basement membranes are intact. Electron microscopic examination shows a group of changes that are associated with toxic damage to the cell, including numerous phagosomes with myeloid bodies and swelling of the mitochondria. The newer aminoglycoside antibiotics tobramycin and amikacin produce renal lesions similar to those caused by gentamicin but are less nephrotoxic.

Neomycin and kanamycin. Orally administered neomycin in doses of 3 to 12 g/day produces moderate malabsorption of a variety of substances, including fat, protein and amino acids, cholesterol, glucose, sodium, calcium, vitamin B_{12}, iron, and penicillin. A lesser degree of malabsorption may occur after the administration of tetracycline, kanamycin, polymyxin, or bacitracin.

Neomycin has a cholesterol-lowering effect. The morphologic changes consist of shortening of the fingerlike villi of the small intestine, accompanied by an infiltration of the lamina propria by round cells and macrophages. The latter frequently contain cellular debris and bacteria-like structures. Dense bodies that may represent aggregated neomycin are seen within the crypt cells. Since there is evidence that cholesterol synthesis takes place within intestinal crypt cells, these changes may explain the sharp cholesterol-lowering effect of neomycin. In addition to the disturbances in the structure and villi of the mucosa of the small intestine, there is evidence of defective reabsorption by the proximal convoluted tubules of the kidney after neomycin administra-

tion. Amino acid levels may be greatly increased in the urine, as well as the feces, because of this dual toxicity to the intestinal villi and the tubular epithelium (Fig. 5-4).

Kanamycin belongs to the same group as neomycin but is far less toxic. Acute swelling and hydropic degeneration of the proximal convoluted tubules may occur after dosage with either drug (Fig. 5-4).

Streptomycin. An effect on the eighth nerve, leading to vestibular impairment and sometimes hearing loss, is one of the toxicologic manifestations of streptomycin therapy. Streptomycin, like kanamycin, is autotoxic and is capable of bringing about swelling and hydropic degeneration of the proximal convoluted tubules, accompanied by mild proteinuria. The tubular changes are reversible when treatment is discontinued. This compound has been reported to cause polyarteritis nodosa. It is the least nephrotoxic of all the aminoglycosides.

Analgesics and antipyretics

Salicylates. Aspirin and methyl salicylate (wintergreen oil) are salicylates that together constitute the most common cause of accidental poisoning in children. Death has occurred in infants, children, and adults after an intake of 2 to 5 g of aspirin.

In acute salicylate poisoning the primary effect of salicylate overdosage is direct stimulation of the respiratory center. This provokes a respiratory alkalosis that at first is compensated by increased renal excretion of bicarbonate and retention of hydrogen ions. Disturbance of the intermediate metabolism of carbohydrate and fat leads to a superimposed metabolic acidosis, possibly from the accumulation of lactate and pyruvate. Hypokalemia then develops, partly because of the loss of potassium in the urine in the early stages, but probably mainly because the alkalosis causes a shift of potassium into the cells. Hypokalemia is known to impair renal excretion of bicarbonate and may increase renal excretion of hydrogen ions, both factors tending to increase the alkalosis.

In fatal cases of overdosage in children or adults, the gross anatomic finding is hemorrhagic gastroenteritis, sometimes with superficial ulceration. One may find necrosis of the germinal centers of the lymphoid tissue of the body, which is probably caused by lympholysis as a result of sudden sharp elevations in the serum corticosteroid level. The elevation is a manifestation of the "stress reaction" that acetylsalicylic acid readily produces in human and experimental animals. Acute ulceration of the stomach may be attributed in part to this phenomenon. The hemorrhagic gastrointestinal mucosa and the petechial hemorrhages in the meninges and serosal surfaces of the viscus may be attributed to the anticoagulant property of acetylsalicylic acid. This drug interferes with the production of factor IV by the platelets. Factor IV neutralizes heparin, so that a deficiency would lead to an

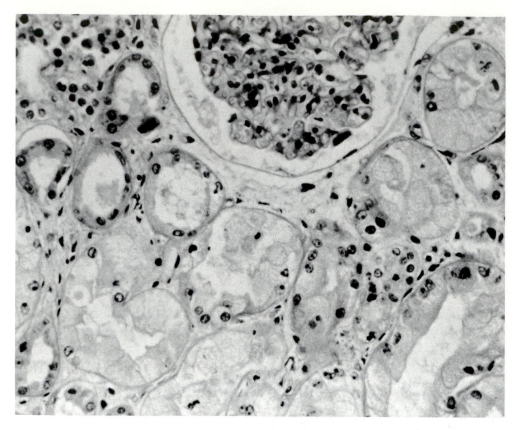

Fig. 5-4. Neomycin-kanamycin nephrosis in kidney. Cells of proximal convoluted tubules are swollen and hydropic with nuclei in various stages of degeneration.

increased serum heparin level. Salicylate depression of the formation of prothrombin by the liver accentuates the hemorrhagic diathesis. Aspirin added to platelet-rich plasma inhibits "second-phase" platelet aggregation, as well as release of platelet adenosine diphosphate (ADP), serotonin, and platelet factor IV after the addition of collagen, ADP, or epinephrine. The effect of aspirin on platelet function tests is not clear. In fact, the mechanism by which aspirin acts on platelets is incompletely understood. There remains enormous interest in the possibility of preventing thrombosis by inhibiting the platelet-release reaction.

The probable cause of death in most cases of fatal salicylate intoxication may be attributed to the metabolic and electrolyte disturbances. The shock resulting from loss of gastrointestinal fluids is also an important factor. Salicylates given to hypersensitive patients with bronchial asthma may precipitate serious systemic reactions within 30 minutes. The acute fatal event may be manifested by an uncontrollable attack of bronchial asthma. There is a high incidence of chronic peptic ulcer in patients who abuse analgesics.

Of the salicylic acid group of compounds, methyl salicylate is the most potent toxin. One teaspoon of methyl salicylate equals 12 ordinary aspirin tablets in content of salicylate. Metabolic acidosis is a more prominent feature of poisoning by the methyl ester than with other common derivatives of salicylic acid.

Aminophenols. Acetaminophen (Tylenol) is a metabolite of phenacetin and acetanilid. It is an analgesic that has certain advantages over salicylates (aspirin). It does not initiate or aggravate hyperacidic states and gastroduodenitis. Chronic ethanol abusers frequently have chronic gastroduodenitis and varying degrees of malabsorption; acetaminophen is therefore a preferred compound for these individuals. A further advantage of acetaminophen is that it does not give rise to hypersensitivity reactions. On the other hand, acetaminophen is a dangerous drug when consumed in excess of therapeutic doses. It is rapidly and almost completely absorbed from the gastrointestinal tract. It is metabolized in the liver, and about 3% is excreted in the urine unchanged; the remainder is comprised of 60% glucuronide conjugates, 30% sulfate conjugates, and 5% cystine conjugates. Acetaminophen is a hepatotoxin, and this action is mediated through the formation of active toxic metabolites that are normally detoxified in the liver by conjugation with glutathione. Overdosage of acetaminophen leads to depletion of liver cell glutathione and subsequent failure of the glutathione protective mechanism. The toxic metabolites then bind

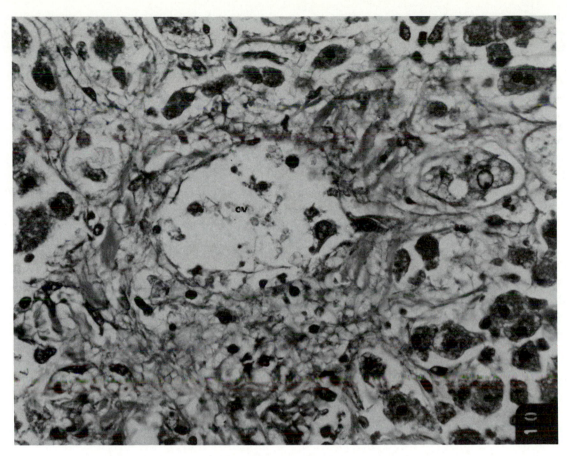

Fig. 5-5. Acetaminophen hepatotoxicity. Hepatocytolysis is visible around the central vein (cv). Collagen-reticulin remains. Coagulative hepatocellular necrosis is displayed by the cells with intact cellular outlines and shrunken, pyknotic nuclei. An identical microscopic picture follows hepatic injury by acute ischemia, severe shock, or heatstroke.

to macromolecules of hepatocellular protein. Through a mechanism that is not clear, there is a loss of vital cellular function, which leads to death of the hepatocytes. The central portion of the hepatic lobule is specifically involved (Fig. 5-5). The necrosis is characteristically of the coagulative type and is not preceded by the centrilobular fatty change that is characteristic of hepatocellular toxins in general. Early damage to the centrilobular hepatocytes is evidenced by the loss of glycogen from the cytoplasm of these cells. The functional and morphologic effects of long-standing acetaminophen therapy (greater than 2 g/day) have not been documented.

Phenacetin (acetophenetidin) also belongs to the group of aminophenol analgesics. It is rapidly absorbed after oral administration, reaching a maximum concentration in the blood at the end of 2 hours. One hour after administration to humans, the greater part of phenacetin has been converted to N-acetyl-p-aminophenol (acetaminophen), which is assumed to be the active ingredient and analgesic agent. A small part, less than 1%, is converted to p-phenitidin. Elimination is rapid, and only 0.2% is excreted in the urine as unconverted phenacetin.

The greater part is eliminated in the urine within the first 22 hours as N-acetyl-p-aminophenol after conjugation in the liver with glucuronic acid, approximately 3% as free N-acetyl-p-aminophenal and less than 1% as p-phenetidin. Phenacetin is generally used in drug combinations with other antipyretics such as acetanilid and acetylsalicylic acid, as well as with barbiturates and caffeine. In the United States there is only the occasional over-the-counter preparation containing phenacetin. Although phenacetin is characterized by low toxicity in humans, during the past 25 years there have been an increasing number of reports of syndromes caused by persistent intake of prolonged high doses. Most of these reports have been from Switzerland, Australia, and the Scandinavian countries, where the consumption of phenacetin has increased multifold, and from areas where there has been severe abuse of phenacetin-containing compounds. The effect of such abuse is described mainly as an effect on the blood (hemolytic anemia, methemoglobinemia) and kidneys (chronic interstitial nephritis, papillitis necroticans).

The pathogenesis of chronic interstitial nephritis, with

or without papillitis necroticans, following chronic analgesic abuse has not been clarified. Experimental studies suggest that the initial damage is located in the medulla with subsequent cortical changes. Papillitis necroticans is believed to develop during the course of tubular epithelial necrosis caused by acetaminophen (phenacetin metabolite) and aspirin, both of which attain a high concentration in the papillae. However, another theory invokes an ischemic mechanism as the cause of papillitis necroticans. Aspirin inhibits prostaglandin PGE_2 synthesis, resulting in a reduction of medullary blood flow. The observation in experimental animals that phenacetin and aspirin, when administered together, cause papillitis necroticans is in contrast to a diminished incidence when the drugs are used separately. This synergistic effect has not been explained. Compared with the general population, phenacetin abusers in Scandinavia and Australia are more prone to transitional cell carcinoma of the renal pelvis and bladder. This experience has rarely been documented in the United States and Canada.

Acute hemolytic anemia may follow short- or long-term intake of small therapeutic doses of phenacetin. It is likely that acute hemolytic anemia more often represents a hypersensitivity reaction, with the phenacetin playing the role of hapten. The more prolonged chronic type of anemia, after continuous high levels of phenacetin intake, probably represents a direct toxic effect on the erythropoietic tissues, leading to disturbance in hemoglobin synthesis with the accumulation of abnormal blood pigments (methemoglobin and sulfhemoglobin). In such instances, Heinz bodies are often demonstrable after careful staining, the results of direct and indirect Coombs' tests are negative, and the reticulocyte count is elevated, while white cell and platelet counts are normal. Moderate elevations of serum iron and serum bilirubin levels and splenomegaly may occur. Examination of the bone marrow reveals increased erythropoiesis and an increased deposition of iron.

The occurrence of unknown primary aromatic amines in the urine of patients receiving acetophenetidin (phenacetin) and acetaminophen (Tylenol) is recorded. Humans excrete only traces in their urine. It is of interest that the extent of excretion of these diazotizable amines parallels the ability of acetophenetidin to cause methemoglobinemia. There is also an indication of a direct relationship between the extent of the excretion of the diazotizable amines (2-hydroxyphenetidin sulfate and 2-hydroxyphenetidin glucuronide) and the concentration of methemoglobin. A stimulating observation is a significant reduction in erythrocyte survival after the administration of acetophenetidin to individuals who have phenacetin-induced kidney damage. When similar dosage of phenacetin is given to patients with renal insufficiency of other origin, no decrease in the red cell life span is observed.

The individual variation in drug metabolism as a cause of drug toxicity is well known. Individual variation in the metabolism of phenacetin is obviously another example. Phenacetin-induced kidney damage in two or more members of the same family has been reported on several occasions. Time may clarify whether individuals who show adverse hematologic reaction to phenacetin are candidates for interstitial nephritis.

Corticosteroids

The role of corticosteroids as anti-inflammatory and immunosuppressive agents is established. Only some of the mechanisms involved in cortisone action at the cellular level are understood. The compounds inhibit the release of lysosomes (neutrophilic granules) from the polymorphonuclear leukocytes. Cortisone and its analogs are capable of slowing down the proliferation of many types of cells (fibroblasts, histiocytes, and lymphocytes). The "lytic" effect on lymphocytes, particularly thymic-dependent lymphocytes, is of interest. With high concentrations, nuclear fragmentation of the lymphocytes is profound. Large lymphocytes and cells of the germinal centers of lymph follicles become pyknotic and karyorrhectic under the influence of these compounds. On the other hand, plasma cells are unaffected by adrenal hormones.

Cortisone may be considered an immunosuppressive drug by virtue of its ability to inhibit nucleoprotein synthesis and mitosis of lymphocytes. This effect on small lymphocytes is more readily demonstrable in animals than in humans, in whom there is some resistance to depletion by corticosteroids. The question of whether a steroid-induced mechanism affects the processing of antigen and transfer to lymphocytes has not been solved. Cortisone may inhibit or enhance an animal's ability to produce circulating antibodies, depending on the dose and time of administration. The maximum effect for suppression is obtained when treatment is started approximately 12 hours before the antigen administration. Steroid suppression of antibody synthesis in humans requires a great deal of new investigation. By virtue of its effect on cellular immunity, cortisone prolongs the survival of normal tissue allografts in many animals. It has been used to suppress tumor immunity and to increase the survival of tumor allografts and xenografts. Administration of steroids may facilitate metastases from tumors.

In graft rejection the union and interaction of antigen and antibody elicit a violent acute inflammatory reaction. There is a strong possibility that corticosteroids may enhance the likelihood of graft acceptance by suppressing inflammation and thereby improving the host environment for the graft. On the other hand, prolonged and continued use of steroids after the cessation of "graft rejection inflammation" may prove to be deleterious.

As opposed to the anti-inflammatory action, it should be kept in mind that patients with chronic recurring disease states (such as rheumatoid arthritis and lupus erythematosus) who are receiving continuous cortisone therapy may have reactivation of tuberculous foci or may die as a result of other disseminated bacterial or fungal infections. Under such circumstances, fever, leukocytosis, and constitutional signs and symptoms are masked by the steroid therapy. Necropsies on such patients may reveal adrenal atrophy of the zona fasciculata and reticularis with preservation of the glomerulosa zone. The beta cells of the pancreatic islets reveal glycogen infiltration, Crooke's changes develop in the mucoid cells of the pituitary gland (Fig. 5-6), and fatty infiltration of the liver is observed.

Widespread necrosis of muscle fibers in experimental animals after the administration of large amounts of ACTH or cortisone has been demonstrated. Similar lesions in humans with Cushing's syndrome or after corticosteroid therapy are debatable.

It is well known that changes in carbohydrate metabolism are produced by steroids derived from the adrenal cortex. The term *steroid diabetes* therefore has usually been applied to the syndrome resulting from the administration of steroids. The diabetogenic action of adrenal corticosteroids was first suspected in 1925, when it was reported that patients with adrenocortical insufficiency exhibited pronounced sensitivity to insulin. After adrenalectomy there is a noticeable improvement in the diabetic state and a diminished insulin requirement. It is well known that patients with Cushing's syndrome have an abnormal glucose tolerance and that diabetic patients with Addison's disease require higher doses of insulin after cortisone treatment.

However, not all adrenal corticosteroids are diabetogenic. It seems that the steroids principally concerned with this action are those with an 11-oxy group. These glucocorticoids have an opposing action to insulin in the regulation of carbohydrate, protein, and lipid metabolism in that they stimulate glucose production, protein breakdown, and fatty acid mobilization. Some of the most potent and frequently administered drugs (such as cortisol and prednisone) belong to this type.

The mechanism of action of the 11-oxy steroids on metabolic processes is still insufficiently understood. They do not destroy insulin or accelerate insulin break-

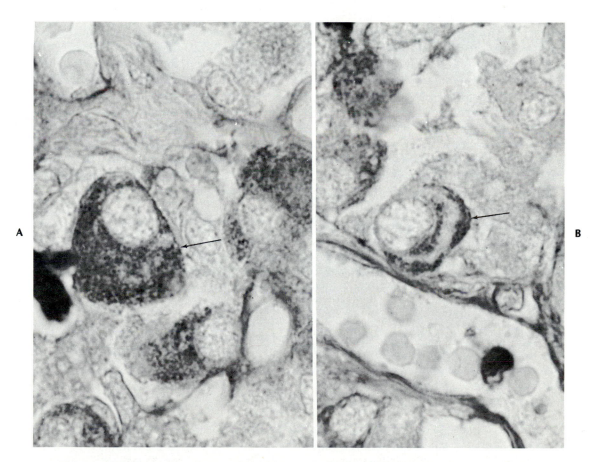

Fig. 5-6. Prednisone therapy (30 mg/day for 6 years). Human hypophyseal ACTH cells. **A,** Dark granules are periodic acid–Schiff positive *(arrow)*. **B,** Crooke's hyaline "degeneration"; degranulation of cytoplasm *(arrow)*. (Alcian blue at pH 2.5; periodic acid–Schiff; orange G; 1500×.)

down. The glucocorticoids enhance glucose production primarily by increasing hepatic glucose production. The catabolic action on proteins contributes by increasing the level of plasma amino acids, some of which are converted into glucose. The administration of 11-oxy steroids increases fatty acid release from tissue stores, and there is evidence that the intermediate metabolism of lipids is modified by steroid therapy, resulting in an increased production of glucose. From these facts it would appear that glucocorticoids interfere with the normal disposal of glucose, while at the same time the glucose concentration is increased by gluconeogenesis, mainly from amino acids.

Clinical observations lead us to believe that latent diabetes may become manifest and the severity of existing diabetes may be increased after the administration of these drugs. Whether treatment with corticosteroids induces diabetes in previously nondiabetic patients is not clear. There is no definite evidence that these drugs can induce diabetes in normal individuals without a hereditary predisposition.

Early in the administration of steroids to rabbits, the pancreas shows glycogen accumulation in the small duct cells. After prolonged administration, the beta cells of the islets, as well as the ductules, contain increasing amounts of glycogen. The beta cells become degranulated, and proliferating ductules become filled with inspissated secretion. This results in leakage of pancreatic enzymes from increased hydrostatic pressure in the ductal lumina with separation of acinar cells, bringing about focal pancreatitis. Similar changes have been described in humans with chronically elevated corticosteroid levels.

In partially depancreatized dogs, permanent diabetes may result after termination of steroid treatment. Whether these findings can be extrapolated to humans receiving steroids is problematic.

The pathognomonic diabetic lesions of nodular glomerulosclerosis in the kidney and hyalinization of the islets have not been observed in patients treated with steroids in the absence of known hereditary diabetes. Likewise, the findings of these lesions in patients with Cushing's syndrome (endogenous steroid production), if they occur, are rare.

In recent years an impressive body of circumstantial evidence has accumulated suggesting that primary adult aseptic bone necrosis is linked in some way to the use of corticosteroid drugs. The bones usually involved are the head of the femur and humerus, and in some cases concomitant involvement of the hip and shoulder joints has occurred. The osteolytic and necrotic process involves the trabeculae of the epiphyses and causes extreme joint pain (Fig. 5-7, A). There are disturbing indications that cessation of corticosteroid therapy once joint necrosis has begun may be of no benefit in altering the course of joint disorganization. The pathogenic mechanisms whereby corticosteroids predispose individuals to bone necrosis are not known. The possibility that the corticosteroids may produce a vasculitis in small vessels supplying the hip and shoulder joints has not been borne out by histologic examination of surgically removed specimens.

Suggestions that aseptic bone necrosis may result from fat embolism are intriguing. Patients with alcoholic (nutritional) fatty livers have been observed to have an increased incidence of the disease, and fatty metamorphosis in the normal liver after corticosteroid administration has been observed. Some workers have speculated that corticosteroid-induced fatty livers may be the source of embolus-sized fat globules that occlude the terminal interosseous capillaries and produce microinfarcts (Fig. 5-7, B).

Sclerosing retroperitonitis and sclerosing mediastinitis after the use of the corticosteroid dexamethasone have frequently been reported. Similar reactions after the ingestion of halogen compounds (for example, bromides or iodides) have been described. Administration of the corticosteroid prednisone to patients with rheumatic fever or leukemia has also resulted in the development of these lesions.

One of the best-known functions of the corticosteroids is their ability to retard the inflammatory process. Phagocytic activity is depressed, capillary permeability is decreased, the number of leukocytes and monocytes is reduced, and the exudate is less rich in fibrin. The inhibitory effect of the corticosteroids on the accumulation of ground substance and fibroblastic proliferation results in a diminution of the formation of granulation tissue. Once granulation tissue and fibrosis have appeared, the corticosteroids have no retarding influence on further development, nor will they lyse existing granulation of fibrous tissue elements.

Androgenic-anabolic steroids

Methyltestosterone. Methyltestosterone norethandrolone may, in the upper limits of dosage, give rise to one or more of the following adverse cellular reactions in the liver: (1) cholestatic hepatitis, (2) peliosis hepatis, and (3) biliary cirrhosis, indistinguishable from the entity described as primary biliary cirrhosis. The mechanism of action whereby the compound causes the characteristic destruction of the bile ductules and elicits a profound plasma cell response is not clear. In drug-induced hepatitis and biliary cirrhosis the patient's serum may contain macroglobulins, circulating antinuclear antibodies, and antibodies to bile ductules. The presence of nonspecific antimitochondrial antibodies may be observed. These immunologic findings tempt the observer to speculate that the drug or its metabolite acting on liver or bile duct protein has given rise to prolonged antigenic stimulation. This mechanism, referred

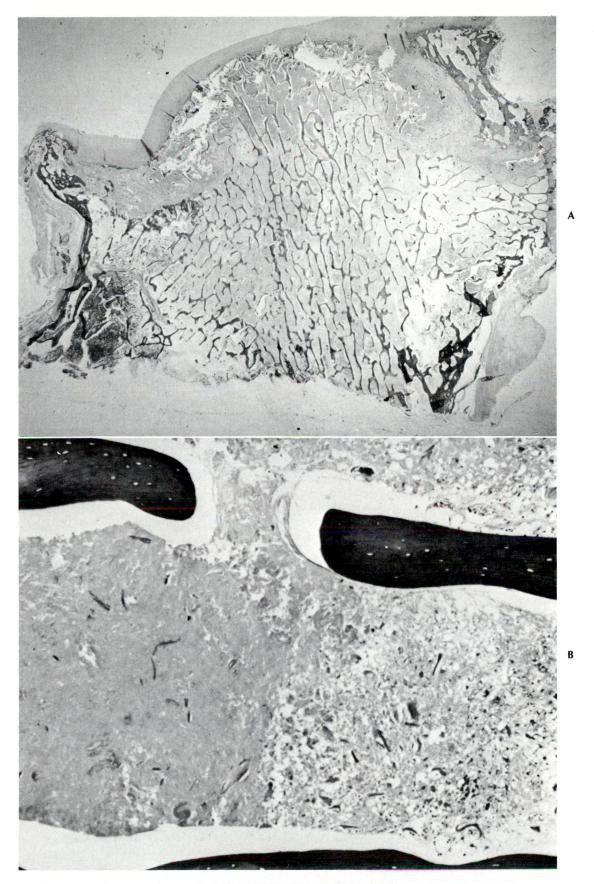

Fig. 5-7. Cortisone therapy. **A,** Aseptic necrosis of head of femur. Note cyst formation beneath articular cartilage and necrosis of adjacent bony trabeculae and marrow. **B,** Same specimen shown in **A.** "Infarctlike" area of necrosis may be seen on left. Necrotic bone spicules are in evidence.

to as autoimmunity, is veiled in mystery. With the passage of time many cases that are now referred to as primary biliary cirrhosis may be discovered to have resulted from medicinal drug therapy.

Oral contraceptives (the "pill")

Histologic changes in both arteries and veins of women receiving antiovulants have been described. The change may occur over a period of a week to months after initiation of the medication. Most individuals in whom vascular changes have developed received a combination type of preparation of estrogens and progestins. There is no absolute evidence that the type of oral contraceptive taken is responsible for the appearance of the vascular lesions.

Irey, Manion, and Taylor[84] have drawn attention to the involvement of pulmonary, systemic, and portal circulations. Arteries and veins of large, medium, and small caliber show changes throughout the vessel wall, frequently accompanied by thrombosis. Most spectacular are the intimal fibrosis and profound endothelial proliferation frequently found in small pulmonary arteries. This latter finding is interpreted by Irey and associates as a primary effect of the drugs on the vascular wall and can be distinguished from the secondary intimal changes occurring after thromboembolism in persons not taking the "pill."

Endothelial hyperplasia has been noted in blood vessels in the endometrium of women taking oral contraceptives. Other evidence of the hyperplastic effect of steroids is the hyperplasia of endocervical glandular epithelium and increased cellularity in uterine leiomyomas noted in women using oral contraceptives.

Substantiation of a direct cause-and-effect association between the administration of oral contraceptives and the development of vascular thrombosis and thromboembolism is fraught with conflicting statistical evidence. The increasing number of cases of the Budd-Chiari syndrome (hepatic vein thrombosis) that occur in women taking the "pill" may point to its implication in thrombus formation (Fig. 5-8). Despite an increasing number of reports in the literature suggesting the cause-and-effect relationship between oral contraceptives and cerebral artery occlusion, this relationship requires further scrutiny. Evidence strongly suggests that some type of thromboembolic disorder is associated with the use of oral contraceptives, particularly in the group of women with no known medical condition predisposing to thrombosis. The evidence is strongest for venous thrombosis (superficial and deep).

How oral contraceptives would contribute to the factors that could bring about thrombosis seems to be entirely obscure, and the many in vitro coagulation studies have not shed much light on the problem. In evaluating the thromboembolic phenomena, one must also take into consideration that thrombosis may strike the young and healthy without previous warning.

The ovaries of women taking oral contraceptives are devoid of corpora lutea with a paucity of developing graafian follicles. Follicular cysts are not uncommon. There are conflicting reports as to the presence or absence of stromal hyperplasia and fibrosis of the tunica albuginea. It is possible that FSH and LH activity may persist despite inhibition of ovulation. The gonadotropic function of the pituitary gland under such circumstances is in need of clarification. It has been suggested that the

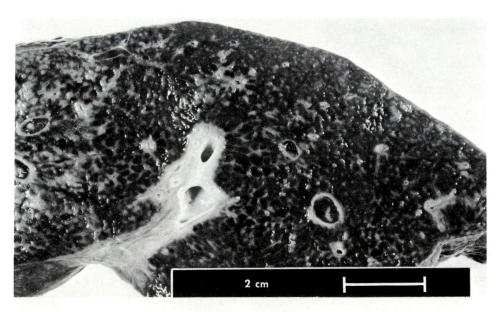

Fig. 5-8. The "pill" and Budd-Chiari syndrome. Large hepatic veins are filled with thrombus, and there is pronounced centrilobular congestion.

Stein-Leventhal syndrome may develop after prolonged usage of ovulation inhibitors. If and when ovarian fibrosis occurs, it is believed to be reversible in most instances. The role of these hormones as possible inducers of malignant neoplasia in humans will be established or refuted after a longer time interval of usage has been established.

The incidence of jaundice in women using oral contraceptive tablets has been estimated to be 1 in 10,000. This event may occur during the first cycle of therapy or appear after several months. The laboratory findings reveal elevations in direct-reacting (conjugated) bilirubin and alkaline phosphatase and, frequently, a moderate rise in SGOT and SGPT. There is invariably an increase in BSP retention. No abnormal levels in the flocculation tests have been observed. These findings are consistent with the morphologic features observed in liver biopsy specimens. The architectural pattern is normal and not associated with hepatocellular necrosis. A pronounced portal triad inflammatory reaction is usually present, and no bile duct hyperplasia is observed.

On the other hand, the microscopic picture is characterized by slightly swollen liver cells accompanied by pronounced intracanalicular bile stasis confined to the centrilobular area. Occasionally a mild portal inflammatory reaction composed of lymphocytes, plasma cells, and eosinophils is noted. The clinical, biochemical, and histologic findings are strikingly similar to those in intrahepatic cholestasis of pregnancy, suggesting that hormonal effect is the common denominator. Whether the estrogen or progesterone component of the oral contraceptive is the culprit is not clear. Likewise, the mechanism of interference with intracellular bile metabolism in these cases has not been elucidated by histochemical, light microscopic, and electron microscopic methods. In patients manifesting inflammatory reaction with a pronounced eosinophil infiltrate, the possibility of anaphylactic (immediate) type of hypersensitivity may be considered. In the majority of cases the contraceptive steroids probably exert a toxic effect on the hepatocytes. Generally, when the patient discontinues the "pill," there is complete reversal of the cholestatic state within 1 week to 2 months. A clinicopathologic picture similar to that induced by the oral contraceptives may be observed after the administration of methyltestosterone and norethandrolone.

Experiments in laboratory rodents suggest that estrogenic compounds may be responsible for the development of focal nodular hyperplasia and liver cell adenomas. Adenomas of the liver are more often found in younger women in contrast to their infrequent appearance in older women and men. It is now clear that the appearance and regression of hepatic cell adenomas show a cause-and-effect relationship in young women taking the "pill." That focal nodular hyperplasia is caused by estrogenic and progestin components of the "pill" is not proved at this time. Whereas significant epidemiologic data point to the involvement of androgenic steroids in the development of hepatocellular carcinoma, this does not appear true of estrogenic stimulation in the form of Premarin or oral contraceptive steroids. In recent years it has been customary to associate development of intralobular vascular dilatation (peliosis hepatis) with the administration of androgenic anabolic steroids; it now seems clear that estrogen likewise can be realistically implicated. Since the induction of hepatogenic tumors seems to be related to the dosage and length of time of hormonal contraceptive use, a reduction of the tumor risk is likely if the organism is less exposed to these preparations. The initiation, cellular multiplication, and resolution of hepatic cell adenoma are clearly dose dependent.

Benign cholestatic jaundice associated with oral contraceptive use is similar to that of pregnancy. Some women apparently cannot metabolize increased secretions of estrogen and progesterone during pregnancy. Conjugated bilirubin and alkaline phosphatase accumulate in the bloodstream, and jaundice develops. However, the hepatic parenchymal cells remain normal, results of flocculation tests are normal, and serum transaminase levels are normal or slightly increased. Liver biopsy shows cholestasis in the liver cells and the bile canaliculi. There usually is a slight to moderate lymphocytic and eosinophilic cell response in the portal triads. Epidemiologic studies strongly suggest the increased incidence of inflammatory gallbladder disease after prolonged use of oral contraceptives.

Estrogens

Estrogen preparations came into use in the United States in the 1930s and were looked on by many menopausal women as the long-awaited "fountain of youth." Having drunk from the fountain, a number of these women have had their enthusiasm dampened by the possibility of promotion of carcinoma of the endometrium. In predisposed women, the unopposed action of estrogenic substances, exogenous or endogenous, results in adenomatous hyperplasia, atypical hyperplasia, and adenocarinoma of the endometrium. In menopausal and postmenopausal women, conjugated estrogenic preparations are effective in modifying menopausal symptoms including vasomotor instability (hot flashes, hot flushes), atrophy of the reproductive tract, and immediate postmenopausal osteoporosis.

Characteristic vaginal or cervical neoplasms designated as clear cell carcinoma may develop in women who have been exposed to diethylstilbestrol (DES) in utero. More commonly observed changes are cervical erosion, transverse ridges of the uterine cervix and upper vagina that may constitute the cervical or vaginal hood, a pseudopolypoid appearance of the uterine cervix, the so-called cockscomb cervix, and the changes that are designated as adenosis. The cellular detection of vaginal adenosis consists of the demonstration of columnar cells resembling those of the endocervix and metaplastic squamous cells. Cytologic examination of young girls or women with vaginal adenosis does not demonstrate sufficient atypicalities to suggest adenosis as a premalignant lesion. From 1948 to 1970, DES was used for threatened abortion. It was estimated that 10,000 to 16,000 females born between 1960 and 1970 are now at risk. In 85% of cases of vaginal and clear cell adenocarcinoma there is a history of maternal estrogen ingestion before the fourth month of pregnancy. Some 30% of young women whose mothers had estrogen during pregnancy have some vaginal lesion—partial strictures, firm ridges, or histologically confirmed adenosis. The investigation of these lesions and the relationship to adenocarcinoma of the vagina is a matter of urgency (see also p. 1470).

Tranquilizers

Chlorpromazine (Thorazine) is a phenothiazine that may produce intrahepatic cholestasis with or without accompanying changes of hepatitis. Various reports estimate that the incidence of cholestatic jaundice in patients receiving chlorpromazine ranges from less than 0.2% to 4%. The basic disorder of centrilobular cholestasis is postulated to be a disturbance of the biliary secretion of the micelles of bile salts, mixed with other biliary solids. Bile canaliculi and ductules are dilated and contain precipitated bile, referred to as bile plugs or thrombi. Bile canalicular microvilli are absent, distorted, or bleblike. The Golgi apparatus is enlarged, and conspicuous hypertrophic smooth endoplasmic reticulum is observed.

Chlorpromazine and other amine salts cause precipitation of bile salts, thus interfering with micelle formation and bile secretion. The cholestasis may persist for weeks or months. This may depend, in part, on the fact that retained bile salts interfere with the transformation of cholesterol to bile salts because of reduced hydroxylation. Subsequently, secretion of bile salt micelles is blocked, and this further leads to centrilobular cholestasis, creating a vicious circle. Severe and prolonged intrahepatic cholestasis results in more pronounced cellular changes and the appearance of inflammation. The hepatocytes become swollen, vacuolated, and feathery, as observed with the light microscope. Some liver cells have disappeared, and focal inflammatory exudate is seen in the vicinity of cellular disruption. Kupffer cells become prominent because of "stuffing" with bile pigment. This reactive cholestatic hepatitis is accompanied by cellular inflammation in the portal tracts. The cellular response is frequently composed of lymphocytes, plasma cells, and varying numbers of eosinophilic granulocytes.

The observation of numerous eosinophilic leukocytes in the portal areas suggests a hypersensitivity mechanism. This is particularly significant when coupled with the clinical triad of blood eosinophilia, allergic rashes, and joint pains.

It appears that prolonged intraductal cholestasis per se may initiate the presence of lymphocytes in the portal areas, as well as ductular proliferation. The histopathologic distinction from mild viral hepatitis, with or without jaundice, may be impossible without relying on clinical information (for example, epidemiologic history) or the results of a diagnostic virologic procedure. Although mild portal fibrosis may develop, clinical cirrhosis probably does not appear. From the laboratory standpoint, there is a serum increase in direct-reacting and indirect-reacting bilirubin. A rise in blood cholesterol, bile acids, and alpha and beta lipoproteins, as well as the activity of alkaline phosphatase enzymes, is the rule. Some believe that the drug or its metabolites acting in the role of hapten bring about the formation of antibodies, which are then believed to remain attached to the hepatocytes. On further administration of the drug, an antigen-antibody reaction occurs on the surface of the cells, leading to cytotoxic damage. Interestingly, a prolonged increase in the serum alkaline phosphatase level may be the only laboratory indication of hepatotoxicity.

Morphologic evidence of myocardial damage characterized by myofibrillar degeneration and some instances of necrosis has been found after chlorpromazine therapy. Focal interstitial myocarditis in association with chlorpromazine therapy is also documented.

Phenothiazines, notably chlorpromazine, may cause gynecomastia and galactorrhea. A number of other medicinal compounds are likewise responsible for these findings, namely, spironolactone, reserpine, isoniazid, and those used in carcinoma of the prostate and in prolonged digitalis therapy and estrogen administration.

Antihypertensive drugs

Methyldopa (Aldomet) evokes an acute hypersensitivity reaction in approximately 3% of patients. Manifestations of this include acute colitis and granulocytopenia with thrombocytopenia. An autoimmune hemolytic anemia may occur. This is accompanied by the presence of antinuclear antibodies and L.E. phenomena, positive results of a rheumatoid arthritis test, and a not infrequent elevation of the serum immunoglobin levels. Hypersensitivity myocarditis, rich in eosinophils, has been documented. One of the most notable adverse tissue reactions to methyldopa is acute diffuse and spotty hepatitis that is indistinguishable clinically and histologically from the usual viral hepatitis. Most of these reactions are mild and reversible. Occasionally, however, an autoimmune phenomenon appears to supervene so that chronic active hepatitis is observed. In this situation various degrees of hepatocellular necrosis may occur, and the eventuality is a mixed macronodular and micronodular cirrhosis. Granulomatous hepatitis characterized by fever, eosinophilia, and a slight elevation of serum alkaline phosphatase levels may be detected. The granulomas in this instance are similar to those of other drug-induced granulomatous hepatitis in that they are noncaseous and may be situated in both the portal and the lobular areas of the liver. On discontinuation of the drug, the lesions rapidly disappear, leaving no residua.

Hydralazine (Apresoline) is a monoamine oxidase (MAO) inhibitor. The mechanism of its hypotensive action is intensification of beta-sympathomimetic effects rather than sympathoplegic. Hydralazine is not a powerful hypotensive agent. In some instances, indiscriminate administration of this compound gives rise to an end-stage chronic interstitial pulmonary fibrosis similar to that produced by the ganglion-blocking agents. The pathogenesis of the lesion is still unsettled. It is probable that the fibrosis is the terminal event in a series of episodes of hypersensitivity alveolitis with necrosis of bronchioloalveolar epithelium and intra-alveolar capillary thrombosis of the septa. In approximately 10% of patients receiving hydralazine, symptoms of peripheral neuritis that are responsive to pyridoxine develop.

Hydralazine is known to cause a clinical syndrome identical to that of classic systemic lupus erythematosus. The manifestations are protean and include arthritis, fever, skin rashes, and myalgia. The L.E. phenomenon is observed in the blood. The pathologic findings are the same as those of classic systemic lupus erythematosus in which there has been no history of causative medication. One difference, however, is the reversibility of the hydralazine syndrome when the inciting drug is discontinued.

Epidemiologic studies have implicated reserpine (*Rauwolfia* alkaloids) in the development of human mammary carcinoma. Whether the mechanism is mediated by causing elevation of the serum prolactin level is not certain.

Diuretics

Among the most effective of the diuretic drugs are the thiazides, with chlorothiazide serving as a prototype of the group. Pharmacologic adverse reactions include hypokalemia, hyperuricemia, and hyperglycemia. Toxic and hypersensitivity responses are manifested by skin rashes, agranulocytosis, and acute pancreatitis. Acute diffuse and spotty hepatitis and cholestatic hepatitis are uncommonly observed.

Furosemide possesses a structural configuration similar to that of chlorothiazide; therefore it is no surprise to learn that it likewise causes acute pancreatitis. At postmortem examination, inspissated mucous secretion is observed in the ductular lumina.

Hypersensitivity reaction to diuretics, if indeed they do occur, are of minimal importance. The potassium-sparing diuretic spironolactone may induce gynecomastia in males. There is no hard evidence incriminating spironolactone as a tumor-inducing agent.

Antithyroid drugs

Thiouracil and iodine compounds are frequently noted as a cause of hypersensitivity vasculitis (angiitis). As with many other drugs, notably penicillin, sulfonamides, and phenylbutazone, an acute or chronic vasculitis may emerge after therapy. If, after removal of the compound, the vasculitis persists for a long period of time, the drug should not be implicated as the source of the antigenic stimulus. Experimental findings do not point to any evidence that a brief exposure to an antigen can produce a chronic vasculitis in which fresh (acute) lesions appear many months after the immunologic stimulus is removed. Although not clear cut, it is feasible that a medicinal drug may bring about an autoimmune vasculitis of protracted nature.

Antidiabetic drugs—oral hypoglycemic agents

Prominent among the oral hypoglycemic compounds in general use are tolbutamide (Orinase), chlorpropamide (Diabinese), and phenformin (DPI). Of these, chlorpropamide evokes reactions with a frequency of approximately 5%. The reactions are mainly cholestatic hepatitis similar to the changes occurring after hypersensitivity reactions to the tranquilizers. Phenformin therapy has been associated with irreversible lactic acidosis in individuals with histories of renal disease and infection.

Patients receiving sulfonylurea therapy respond with a number of interesting islet cell changes. The maturity-onset diabetic subject usually has an increase in the number and size of the islets. Cytologically, the most striking finding is hyperplasia and new formation of the islets of Langerhans with a reduction in the percentage of beta cells and an increase in alpha cells. A further observation in this group of patients is the appearance of islet cell adenomas. Morphologic changes in the islets in patients treated with sulfonylureas are in need of further observation.

H₂ receptor antagonists

Cimetidine (Tagamet) is a potent antagonist of the H_2 receptors that exist in many cell types. Cimetidine is used to inhibit gastric acid secretion in diseases such as duodenal ulcer (short-term and maintenance therapy), Zollinger-Ellison syndrome, and other gastric hypersecretory states. The incidence of serious adverse tissue reactions to cimetidine is far less than 1%. A bothersome complication of the therapy is the appearance of gynecomastia, which is usually florid and which disappears following cessation of therapy in most cases. The gyneco-mastia is commonly bilateral, and the causative mechanism is unknown. In rare cases, renal adverse tissue reactions may occur in the form of acute interstitial nephritis. The renal biopsy reveals interstitial foci of lymphocytes, plasma cells, and abundant eosinophils. Destruction of the tubular basement membranes may occur as part of this hypersensitivity reaction. No chronic renal disease has resulted from the acute insult. Acute diffuse hepatitis is an additional hypersensitivity reaction to cimetidine. No instances of "chronic active" hepatitis or cirrhosis have been documented. Currently there is no convincing evidence that cimetidine is carcinogenic.

Antitubercular drugs

Isoniazid and rifampin are agents widely used in the prophylaxis and treatment of tuberculosis. Para-amino-salicylic acid is not as widely used, and it is associated with a greater incidence of hepatitis and hepatic necrosis than are the other antitubercular agents (Fig. 5-9).

Isoniazid. Isoniazid (INH, Rimifon) is metabolized by the liver via an acetylation pathway, producing innocuous metabolites. As a result of arylating and acrylating pathways, however, a metabolite known as acetylhydrazine is formed. It is this metabolite that probably brings about damage of the hepatocytes in the small percentage (1% to 2%) of people who are genetically predisposed to this damage. It may be postulated that, following the

damage, a hypersensitivity state ensues that is responsible for the hepatitis and, in rare instances, necrosis of the liver. Fifty percent of whites are slow acetylaters, and this group is prone to the development of autoimmune reactions characterized by the L.E. phenomenon. Following cessation of the drug, all of the clinical and serologic features of this phenomenon usually disappear rapidly, but in a few instances the time interval is prolonged over months. Whether it is advantageous to be a slow or a fast acetylater is controversial.

Isoniazid is similar to methyldopa, chlorpromazine, and halothane in that an increasing number of reports point to the occurrence of chronic active hepatitis, in some instances leading to cirrhosis. It is noteworthy that the morphologic changes induced by isoniazid may be identical to those of viral acute spotty hepatitis, as well as viral-initiated chronic active hepatitis and massive necrosis. Any drug- or viral-induced chronic active hepatitis may lead to cirrhosis. In INH-associated chronic active hepatitis the portal areas may contain numerous plasma cells, particularly in patients showing the concomitant L.E. phenomenon. The onset of clinical signs and symptoms of INH hepatitis usually occurs in the first 2 months of prophylactic or preventive therapy. Onset after 8 to 10 weeks is usually more severe. The hepatitis is also more severe in the older age groups and in black women, again suggesting a genetic influence.

Rifampin. Rifampin (Rifadin, Rimactane), a semisyn-

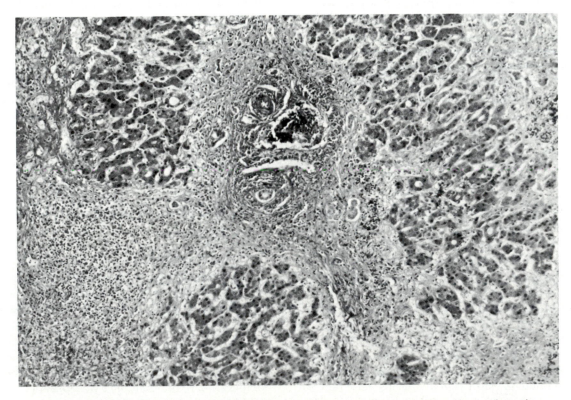

Fig. 5-9. INH hepatitis. Cells of peripheral lobules have disappeared and are replaced by condensed reticulum and lymphocytes. This may be impossible to distinguish from viral hepatitis.

thetic antibiotic that is derived from *Streptomyces mediterranei* and is similar to isoniazid, may cause transient abnormalities in liver function test results and, rarely, fatal hepatitis. It reduces or abolishes the tuberculin reaction in guinea pigs infected with tubercle bacilli. Likewise, in humans there is a strong suggestion that rifampin may suppress cell-mediated immunity as manifested by delayed cutaneous hypersensitivity to purified protein derivative of *Mycobacterium tuberculosis*. It also inhibits in vitro lymphoblast transformation in both phytohemagglutinin and purified protein derivative. Rifampin or its metabolite desacetylrifampicin may elicit a type II cytotoxic allergic reaction, based on the observation that in some cases antigen-antibody complexes are formed in the serum and attach to the cell surface of the erythrocyte, resulting in lysis. In patients demonstrating this hemolytic reaction, indirect Coombs' test results are positive in the presence of the drug. As in isoniazid therapy, acute spotty hepatitis with a portal inflammatory infiltrate, rich in eosinophils, lymphocytes, and a few macrophages, and accompanied by focal intralobular necrosis, may be observed. In combined tuberculostatic therapy with rifampin and isoniazid, liver injuries are more severe than in monotherapy with either isoniazid or rifampin. Rifampin, being an enzyme inductor, results in a high level of the cytotoxic metabolite isoniazid acetylhydrazine. Although its exact mechanism of action has not been defined, rifampin is known to inhibit DNA-directed RNA synthesis, probably by interfering with the activity of RNA polymerase. Unlike isoniazid, rifampin is a powerful stimulator of the activity of drug-metabolizing enzymes of the human liver microsomes. Acute interstitial nephritis characterized by oliguria and rising BUN levels has been attributed to rifampin as an altered immune response to the drug or its metabolites. On cessation of the drug, the signs and symptoms disappear rapidly, and there is no evidence that irreversible damage to the interstitium of the kidney or the tubules has occurred.

Anesthetics

Halothane. There is little question that halothane is capable of causing a variety of morphologic types of hepatitis, including (1) acute diffuse and spotty hepatitis, (2) persistent hepatitis, (3) chronic active hepatitis, and (4) acute and subacute massive necrosis. The majority of hepatic reactions to halothane are either acute diffuse spotty hepatitis or persistent hepatitis. Massive necrosis is rare. These reactions depend on the appearance of the altered immune response in the patient, who has almost invariably received more than one dose of this quite safe anesthetic. Clinical and laboratory evidence of the altered immune reaction includes blood eosinophilia, low-grade fever, arthralgia, and rash. Recrudescence of halothane hypersensitivity follows rechallenge with the drug. The appearance of antimitochondrial antibodies

and positive results of a lymphocyte transformation test have been observed in a significant number of cases. The exact location of halothane's effect on the hepatocyte remains unclear. Centrilobular fat accumulation, which commonly occurs in other direct toxic reactions, may be observed. The toxic reaction may bring about denatured proteins, to which the body now reacts unfavorably, and brings about many of the well-known altered immune reactions. Both the toxic reactions (if indeed they exist) and the hypersensitivity reactions are probably mediated at the hepatocyte cell membrane level. Histologically, the hepatic lesions are indistinguishable from those occurring in the many morphologic variations of viral hepatitis. Not infrequently, a plethora of eosinophils and noncaseous granuloma formations in the portal tracts and the lobules is the morphologic indicator of the hypersensitivity mechanism. The ultrastructural changes following halothane administration are nonspecific and include swelling of the mitochondria with crystalline inclusions and abnormal cristae and marked dilatation of both smooth and rough endoplasmic reticulum.

Methoxyflurane. Methoxyflurane, an excellent, non-explosive, fluorinated anesthetic agent, has occasionally been reported to produce liver injury. It may give rise to hepatitis identical to that caused by halothane, probably through the same mechanisms of action. Cross-sensitivity between the two agents has been observed. In addition to liver involvement, nephrotoxicity aimed primarily at the proximal convoluted tubules may develop. The degree of tubular dysfunction can be correlated with the dose of the anesthetic agent and its metabolites, inorganic fluoride and oxalic acid. Metabolically, methoxyflurane is readily defluorinated. The acute polyuria resulting from methoxyflurane administration is attributed to the effect of inorganic fluoride on the tubule. The amount of oxalic acid found in the kidney is probably not a significant factor in the development of the tubular lesion. In human cases of nephrotoxicity, light microscopic examination of the proximal convoluted tubules is unimpressive. It is characterized by some dilatation of the tubular lumen and flattening of the epithelium. Ultrastructurally, the mitochondria are swollen with disruption of their cristae, and they contain dense bodies (probably fluoride proteinate). The mechanism may be similar to the disturbance in oxidative phosphorylation observed in lead poisoning.

Anticonvulsants

Phenytoin. Of the anticonvulsants, phenytoin (Dilantin) appears to be the major compound eliciting adverse tissue reactions. Direct dose-related cytotoxicity has not been ascribed to phenytoin, nor has any toxic metabolite been identified. On the other hand, the altered hypersensitivity or altered immunologic responses of a human organism to phenytoin, although uncommon, are protean. Foremost among these are the dermatologic reactions, which consist mainly of erythema multiforme and toxic epidermal necrolysis. Both of these are severe adverse reactions to the drug, and the mortality of toxic epidermal necrolysis has been reported to be approximately 25%. The histologic features of the epidermal form of erythema multiforme and toxic epidermal necrolysis reveal many similarities. There are eosinophilic necrosis of keratinocytes and hydropic degeneration of basal cells. Cleft formation at the dermal-epidermal junction follows necrosis of the basal cells. Pericapillary minimal infiltrates with lymphocytes are the rule. Occasionally thrombosis of the capillaries is observed. It is assumed that these two phenytoin-induced skin disorders are mediated through an immunologic cytotoxic mechanism.

Less frequently, hypersensitivity reactions are directed toward the kidney as acute interstitial nephritis accompanied by renal failure and peripheral eosinophilia. Renal dysfunction is promptly reversed after discontinuation of phenytoin administration. An interesting observation is the presentation of phenytoin-induced lymphadenopathy as clinical malignant lymphoma. The haptenic action of phenytoin may elicit any of the common immunologic responses known to exist. Circulating antibodies to phenytoin have been demonstrated. A lymph node may show a distortion of the architecture with lymphocyte hyperplasia, eosinophils, plasma cells, and necrosis. Large so-called histiocytic or reticulin cells are in evidence (Fig. 5-10). In other instances the enlarged lymph nodes may be characterized by the presence of numerous immunoblasts and endothelial proliferation of small blood vessels. This is referred to as angioimmunoblastic lymphadenopathy, and in some instances, it proceeds to the more serious condition of immunoblastic sarcoma. Finally, noncaseous granulomas, frequently accompanied by numerous eosinophils, may be noted.

Phenytoin is one of the drugs that has been identified as causing systemic hypersensitivity necrotizing angiitis. In fatal cases of phenytoin allergic reactions, morphologic reflections of several of the basic altered immune responses may be present. On occasion, phenytoin may fire off an autoimmune response characterized by the L.E. phenomenon in the blood, hemolytic anemia, positive results of the indirect Coombs' test, antinuclear antibodies, and skin lesions, all of which are reminiscent of clinical disseminated lupus erythematosus. Withdrawal of the drug results in disappearance of the clinical and serologic manifestations. Phenytoin may invoke a microscopic appearance suggesting Hodgkin's disease (Fig. 5-10). However, the Reed-Sternberg cells characteristic of Hodgkin's disease are not identified and, unlike Hodg-

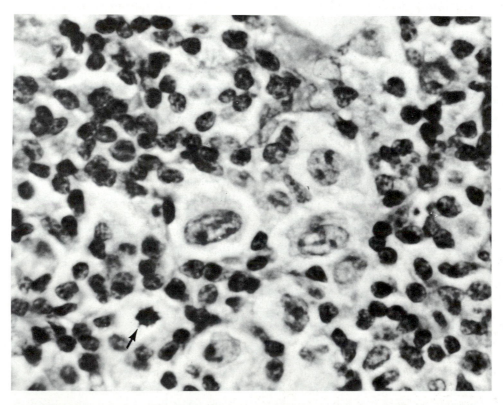

Fig. 5-10. Phenytoin (Dilantin) lymphadenopathy. Distortion of the normal cellular topography with replacement by numerous large cells (histiocytes, immunoblasts) with prominent nucleoli and mitoses *(arrow)* may lead to misdiagnosis of malignant lymphoma.

kin's disease, the lymphadenopathy recedes following discontinuation of the drug. Nevertheless, an increasing number of reports suggest that long-term administration of phenytoin may give rise to Hodgkin's disease or non-Hodgkin's malignant lymphoma. Hepatic injury associated with phenytoin therapy reflects literally all the histologic features seen in viral hepatitis. The most common acute reaction is hepatocellular degeneration or necrosis, or both, with panlobular "spotty" reaction. Hepatocellular and cholestatic injury may be displayed. Rarely, submassive and massive necrosis supervenes. Granulomatous hepatitis, with or without vasculitis, is one of the forms of hepatic injury. Phenytoin can cause megaloblastic anemia associated with low folate levels in the serum,

red cells, and cerebrospinal fluid. There is a disturbance of cell utilization of folate by an as yet undetermined mechanism.

Gingival hyperplasia may promptly appear after phenytoin therapy is begun. Following painless enlargement of the interdental papillae, the gingival surface becomes pebbled and lobulated (Fig. 5-11, A). Microscopically, the squamous epithelium projects down into the avascular hyperplastic connective tissue as prominent rete pegs (Fig. 5-11, B and C). Careful oral hygiene slows the hyperplastic process, but recurrence is common. A number of anticonvulsants, including phenytoin, when administered to the mother during the first trimester of pregnancy, may result in congenital anomalies. These include cleft lip and palate and the fetal hydantoin syndrome. The latter shares with the fetal alcohol syndrome a number of anomalies including ptosis, epicanthal folds, and flat nasal bridge.

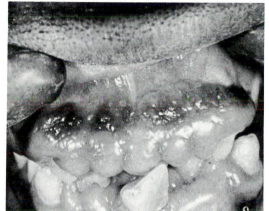

A

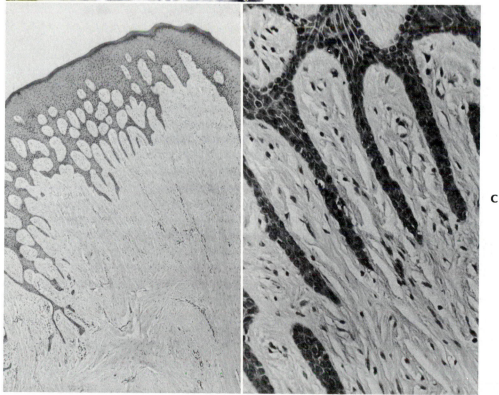

B   C

Fig. 5-11. A, Phenytoin (Dilantin) gingival hypertrophy. Prominent interdental papillae obscure teeth. **B** and **C,** Phenytoin gingival hypertrophy and hyperplasia characterized by penetrating rete pegs and fibrosis of submucosa. Relatively avascular connective tissue proliferation.

Anti-infective agents

Nitrofurantoin. Nitrofurantoin (Furadantin, Macrodantin) is a synthetic antimicrobial agent used to treat urinary infections. It is primarily excreted by the kidney. This drug is a cause of acute pulmonary eosinophilia (Löffler's syndrome), which is characterized by blood eosinophilia and a variety of radiographic findings consisting of segmental fan-shaped infiltrations or, less commonly, a diffuse, small, nodular pattern. Microscopically, the alveolar walls are widened and the airspaces are filled with a fibrinous, nonhemorrhagic exudate containing macrophages, lymphocytes, and plasma cells. However, the preponderant cell in the inflammatory picture is the eosinophilic polymorphonuclear leukocyte. If the condition is recognized early and administration of the drug is discontinued, recovery is complete. If, however, the pulmonary damage is allowed to progress, a chronic eosinophilic pneumonia and a nonreversible, diffuse interstitial fibrosis may develop (Fig. 5-12). Nitrofurantoin-induced acute spotty and diffuse hepatitis has occurred concomitantly with eosinophilic pneumonia. Thus the single compound is focused on two target organs, and a patient with either organ involved should be tested for dysfunction of the other. In some instances, persistent therapy will bring about chronic active hepatitis.

Nitrofurantoin has been implicated in producing the clinical syndrome of lupus nephritis and the full-blown picture identical to disseminated lupus erythematosus. In the presence of chronic renal impairment, nitrofurantoin therapy may lead to peripheral axon degeneration, with resultant numbness and tingling of the extremities. Remyelination resulting from revision of the Schwann cells takes place after cessation of therapy.

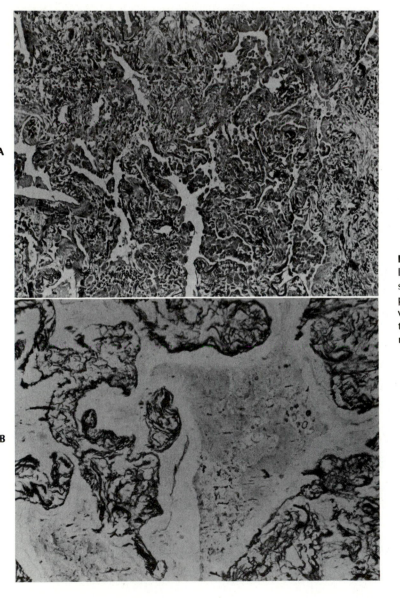

Fig. 5-12. A, Nitrofurantoin. Broad alveolar walls filled with lymphocytes, macrophages, and collagen severely constrict airspaces, which contain fibrin, desquamated macrophages, and pneumocytes. **B,** Reticulin stain emphasizes widened alveolar walls. Fibrin and cellular debris occupy terminal airspaces. (**A,** Hematoxylin and eosin, 250×; **B,** reticulin stain; 330×.)

Antiarrhythmics

Digitalis. Mixtures of steroid glycosides, all having the same effects on the heart, are present in at least 39 genera of the plant kingdom. The genus *Digitalis* is the common commercial source for the crude product, digitalis, as well as for the specific glycosides digoxin and digitoxin. Although the cardiac glycosides, in therapeutic doses, are valuable in the treatment of several heart diseases, in higher doses these agents are potent cardiac poisons. The immediate danger with digitalis poisoning is the production of fatal ventricular fibrillation.

Prolonged sublethal concentrations of the glycosides produce myocardial lesions, which have been described in humans and experimental animals. The histologic findings consist of focal necrosis, cellular infiltration, interstitial edema, fibrosis, and hyaline degeneration, these changes being especially prominent in the subendocardial region of the myocardium. Affected cardiac cells commonly show a loss of striations, fibrillar fraying, and pyknosis of nuclei. The coronary vessels remain patent. In dogs, ultrastructural changes become obvious in some cells within 2 hours after a toxic infusion of digoxin. These early changes consist of a degeneration of myofibrillar banding patterns and contracture band formation, intracellular edema, and clumping and margination of nuclear chromatin. The cardiac glycosides probably exert their beneficial effect on cardiac contractility by "facilitating" the handling of calcium by the sarcoplasmic reticulum, whereas the arrhythmic toxic effect is attributable to their inhibitory effect on sarcolemmal Na-, K-activated ATPase (the sodium pump). The latter action produces potassium depletion, a situation frequently correlated with edema and myofibrillar degeneration. A severe interference with the normal cycle of intracellular flux of calcium between the sarcoplasmic reticulum and the myofilaments may also account for some of the lesions.

Gazes and associates[143] have drawn attention to profound venous engorgement of the small intestine with areas of mucosal hemorrhage in patients receiving high or toxic doses of digitalis (Fig. 5-13). This finding appeared particularly significant in patients who showed no evidence of congestive failure. The syndrome can be suspected when abdominal pain develops in a patient receiving large amounts of digitalis; unnecessary surgery thus may be avoided. Gazes and associates speculate that hepatic vein or sinusoid sphincter constriction with resultant portal splanchnic venous congestion is a possible mechanism by which digitalization produces this syndrome.

Digitalis therapy is occasionally associated with gynecomastia, the mechanism of which is not well understood. However, it may be attributed to the basic steroid structure of the digitalis glycosides. There is no accepted evidence of a relationship between digitalis therapy and breast cancer.

Oxygen

Respiratory therapy, using increased partial pressures of oxygen at sea level, as well as under hyperbaric conditions, is a vital constituent of modern medicine. Higher than normal atmospheric oxygen tensions at ambient as well as hyperbaric pressures are employed therapeutically in humans primarily in hypoxic states. However, oxygen must be employed with an understanding of its potential adverse effects. In humans these are primarily

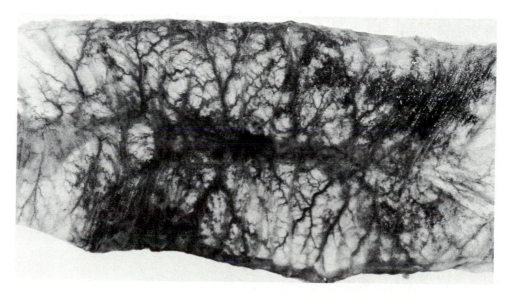

Fig. 5-13. Digitalization effect. Transilluminated segment of small intestine showing profound venous engorgement with areas of mucosal hemorrhage. (From Gazes, P.C., et al.: Circulation 23:358, 1961; by permission of the American Heart Association, Inc.)

changes in the eyes of premature infants and in the lungs; however, experimental studies reveal that all organ systems, including the brain, heart, kidney, and liver, are at risk.

Biochemical data have shown that excessive oxygen inhibits many enzymes, including those involved in the Embden-Meyerhof pathway, the conversion of pyruvate to acetyl-CoA, the tricarboxylic acid cycle, electron transport, synthesis of neurotransmitters, proteolysis, and membrane transport. Enzymes with essential sulfhydryl (SH) groups seem to be especially vulnerable. The biochemical mechanisms of oxygen toxicity are related to the metabolism of oxygen through free radical and hydroperoxide intermediates, a process that normally occurs in the cells and is accelerated on exposure to high oxygen tensions. This hypothesis is summarized in Fig. 5-14, *F*. The intermediate reactions in oxygen metabolism, through unknown mechanisms, induce lipid peroxidation. Lipid peroxides may disrupt membranes directly, oxidize SH groups, and shift the redox state of glutathione toward oxidation. The last results in the oxidation of pyridine nucleotides, which impairs energy production, leading, as does enzyme inhibition or disruption of membranes, to cell injury and eventual cell death. Hyperoxia may also directly inhibit RNA, DNA, and protein synthesis via free radical and hydroperoxide intermediates.

Pulmonary oxygen toxicity in the mature human lung is one of the many causes of diffuse alveolar damage (DAD), which begins with an exudative phase characterized by necrosis of epithelial and endothelial components of the alveolar wall, associated with pulmonary edema, congestion, fibrin deposition, and hemorrhage. The fibrin-rich inflammatory exudate leads to the formation of fibrin caps and, later, hyaline membranes (Fig. 5-14, *A*). The exudative changes are rapidly followed by proliferative alterations consisting of interstitial fibrosis, hyperplasia of the alveolar type II cells (granular pneumocytes), and organization and collagenosis (Fig. 5-14, *B*). Studies in a variety of experimental animals, as well as in humans, have shown that the exudative changes begin within 2 to 3 days of exposure to approximately 1 atmosphere absolute (ATA) of oxygen, and the proliferative changes are observed shortly thereafter. In human cases, interstitial fibrosis may appear after 3 days of oxygen therapy and become diffuse and severe by 1 to 2 weeks. Ultrastructural studies reveal that the initial changes in the lung consist of focal interstitial edema followed by swelling of endothelial and epithelial cells. Following this, both endothelial and type I epithelial alveolar cells (membranous) become necrotic. The endothelial cells are more vulnerable than the alveolar pneumocytes. The sequence of events is summarized in Fig. 5-14, *C* to *E*.

With regard to the immature human lung, oxygen has

been considered in the pathogenesis of the pathologic changes (hyaline membrane disease) associated with the idiopathic respiratory distress syndrome (IRDS) of premature infants. The IRDS begins before oxygen therapy, however, and it is clearly associated with biochemical immaturity of surfactant and morphologic immaturity of the lung. The IRDS is a disease entity related solely to factors involving the epithelial component of the air-blood barrier. Atelectasis is a prominent feature of the IRDS. Bronchopulmonary dysplasia is a chronic lung disease characterized by DAD and obliterative bronchiolitis, attributed to prolonged oxygen therapy for the IRDS.

Acute central nervous system oxygen toxicity is manifested by grand mal epileptic convulsions in humans. In experimental adult animals, repeated exposure to hyperbaric oxygen results in paralysis and selective necrosis of neurons and gray matter. Prolonged exposure of neonatal animals to oxygen at or near 1 ATA inhibits RNA, DNA, and protein synthesis in the brain. Recent reports suggest that certain types of neuropathologic lesions (such as periventricular leukomalacia and pontosubicular necrosis) occurring in the brains of premature human infants suffering from hypoxia may be the result of oxygen therapy.

It has been established in humans and experimental animals that, during hyperoxic exposure, immature developing retinal vessels become necrotic and obliterated. This is followed by a proliferative reparative response resulting in the growth of new blood vessels, mesenchymal and glial cells from the inner retina extending into the vitreous. As the growth of this regenerative tissue progresses, the retina is detached, leading to blindness. The retinal response to hyperoxic exposure that occurs in premature infants is known as retrolental fibroplasia and was formerly referred to as the retinopathy of prematurity.

Antineoplastic and immunosuppressive agents

Alkylating agents. The more commonly used alkylating agents include the nitrogen mustards, chlorambucil, cyclophosphamide (Cytoxan), busulfan (Myleran), triethylenethiophosphoramide (Thio-TEPA), triethylenemelamine (TEM), and mitomycin C. Although they differ in action, all have the capacity of replacing hydrogen atom with alkyl radicals (aliphatic hydrocarbons deprived of an H atom). They inhibit DNA synthesis, but the effect on RNA synthesis is less pronounced. The alkylating agents readily penetrate the cell walls and interfere with a number of enzymatic reactions, inhibit phosphorylation of ATP, glycolysis, respiration, protein synthesis, and mitosis, and, in addition to producing mutations, cause breaks in chromosomes and irregular accumulation of chromatin in proliferating cells (Fig. 5-15). A striking clinical improvement in patients with Burkitt's lympho-

Text continued on p. 180.

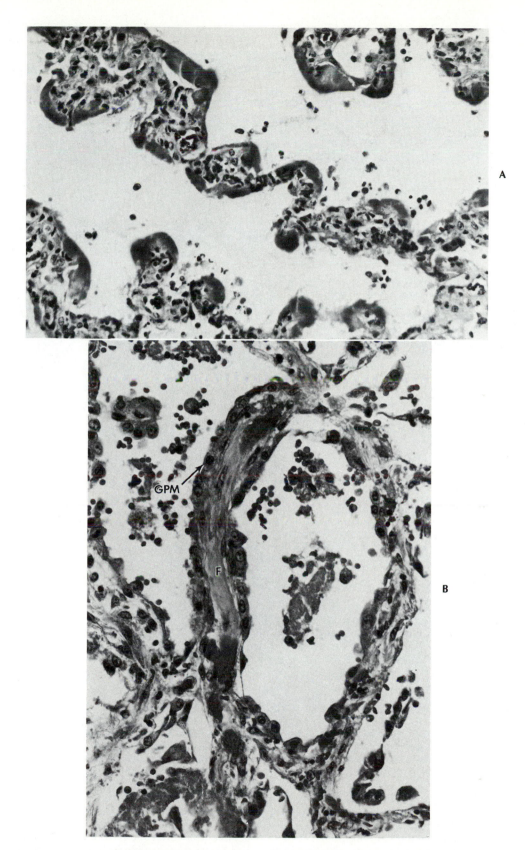

Fig. 5-14. A, Oxygen toxicity—early lesion. Fibrin "caps" adhere to surface of alveolar lining of epithelial cells. Alveolar capillaries show acute inflammatory reaction. **B,** Later lesion consists of thickened alveolar walls with fibrosis *(F)* and proliferative changes manifested by granular pneumocyte metaplasia *(GPM).*

Continued.

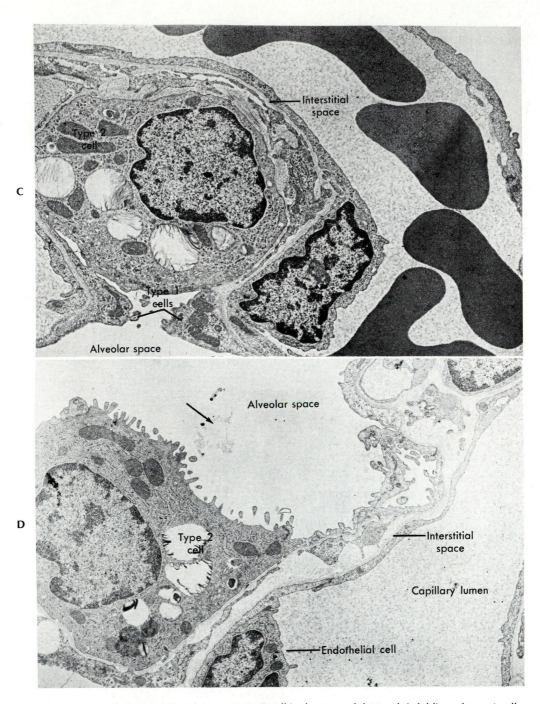

Fig. 5-14, cont'd. C, Normal rat lung—a type 2 cell is shown sunk beneath infolding of type 1 cells lining the alveolar space. Interstitial space is normal, is reduced in width, and contains some collagen bundles and fibroblasts. Fragments of fibroblasts appear in this section. **D,** Oxygen exposure (900 mm Hg), 24 hours—type 2 cell shown here is typically last affected by oxygen and remains so in a reversible lesion. Interstitial space is beginning to expand because of accumulation of edema fluid. Endothelial cell shows increased numbers of pinocytic vesicles but, as shown here, tight junctions remain intact. To right of type 2 cell (note junction between the two) is a type 1 cell. This cell type responds to increased oxygen tension by surface blebbing and infolding prior to its death. The picture seen here continues to become more severe over the next 12 hours. *Arrow,* Tubular myelin fragments, possibly representing type 2 cell secretory material.

Continued.

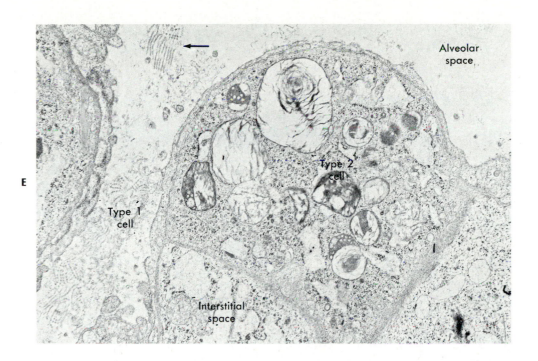

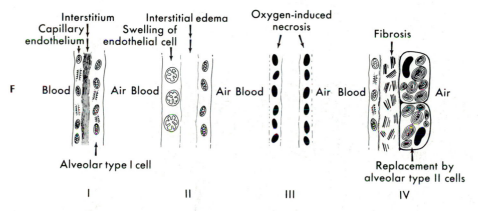

Fig. 5-14, cont'd. **E,** Oxygen exposure (900 mm Hg), 48 hours—this is an irreversible lesion caused by oxygen. Type 2 cell is relatively intact, but it contains numerous multivesicular bodies, many of which are closely associated with lamellar bodies. Under conditions of toxic Po_2 exposure these cells often hypersecrete. In alveolar space, numerous tubular myelin figures *(arrow)* offer additional evidence of such hypersecretion. In addition, alveolar space contains flocculent protein attributable presumably to capillary leakage. Remnants of endothelial cell on far left also have associated regions of fibrin accumulation. Several type 1 cells surround the central type 2 cell and, though they appear intact, show surface discontinuities and infolding indicative of early degenerative changes. The interstitial space is completely disrupted and contains cellular debris. **F,** Diagrammatic illustration of the changes occurring in experimentally induced hyperoxic DAD, progressing from the exudative *(II, III)* to the proliferative *(IV)*. The drawings represent a composite interpretation concerning the essential events in pulmonary oxygen toxicity. Initially *(II),* there is swelling of the interstitial space and capillary endothelium, emphasizing that the initial changes are related to the endothelial component of the air-blood barrier. Both membranous epithelial and capillary endothelial necrosis *(III)* ensue, however. The granular pneumocyte is a reserved repair cell and is relatively resistant to oxygen toxicity. The proliferative or reparative phase *(IV)* consists of interstitial fibrosis and replacement of the alveolar epithelium by alveolar type 2 cells (granular pneumocytes). (**A,** 250×; **B,** hematoxylin and eosin, 300×; C to E, 2400×; **A, C,** and **E,** courtesy Dr. Robert M. Rosenbaum, Bronx, N.Y.; **B** and **F,** from Balentine, J.D.: Pathology of oxygen toxicity, New York, 1982, Academic Press, Inc.)

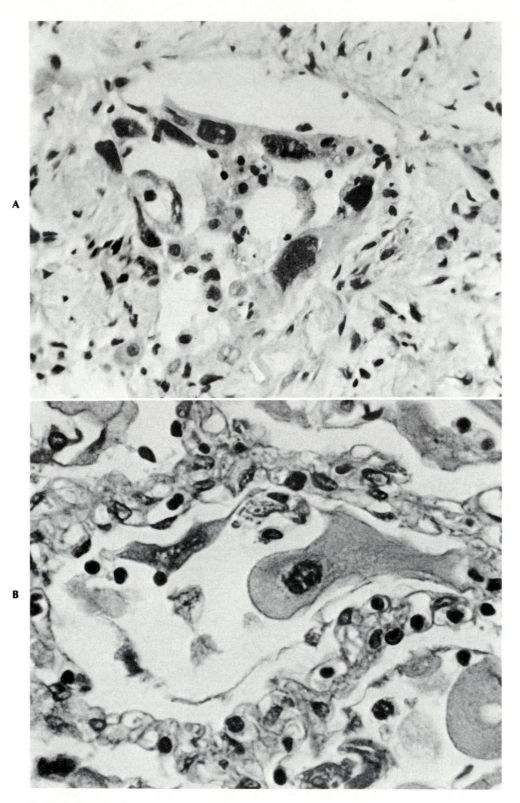

Fig. 5-15. Busulfan therapy. **A,** Bronchiolar epithelium showing hyperchromatic nuclei composed of condensed chromatin leading to bizarre nuclear contours. Nuclear fragments in evidence. **B,** This cytologic picture is reminiscent of radiation effect. Several large bronchioloalveolar cells have desquamated into air sac. Nuclear membrane of largest cell is fragmented.

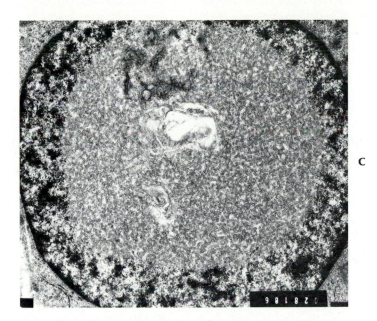

Fig. 5-15, cont'd. C, Type 2 pneumocyte from busulfan lung. Large numbers of curved, interwoven tubular structures, devoid of chromatinic DNA, fill the nucleus (**C,** 32,500×; from Gyorky, F., Gyorky, P. and Sinkovics, J.G.: Ultrastruct. Pathol. **1:**217, 1980.)

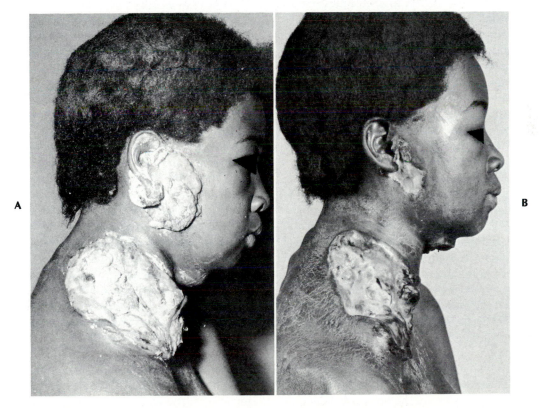

Fig. 5-16. Cyclophosphamide (Cytoxan) therapy. Large cell non-Hodgkin's lymphoma. **A,** Before therapy. **B,** After single dose of Cytoxan.

ma and some forms of large cell non-Hodgkin's lympho-ma may follow a single dose of cyclophosphamide (Fig. 5-16).

The alkylating agents can initiate and enhance malignant tumor growth and suppress immune responses. The latter effect is characteristic of many antitumor agents. Of the group of alkylating agents, cyclophosphamide is the most widely used for immune response suppression. In experimental animals, particularly guinea pigs, suppression of antibody production is most evident if the agent is administered just before and immediately after introduction of the antigen. There is extensive lysis of small and large lymphocytes, but the cells of the reticuloendothelial system are not particularly affected.

Alkylating agents and antifolates cause epithelial atypias of the urogenital tract. The extent of the atypia correlates with the total dosage and duration of therapy. The epithelial abnormalities may persist for a long period following cessation of therapy. Cyclophosphamide, busulfan, Thio-TEPA, and chlorambucil cause epithelial atypia and cytomegaly in a variety of epithelial surfaces, but particularly in the lungs, urinary tract, and cervix (Fig. 5-15, A). Type 2 alveolar cells develop strongly acidophilic cytoplasm, which is increased in amount (Fig. 5-15, B). The nuclei are arrested during the process of DNA synthesis and are converted to grotesque, shapeless masses of condensed chromatin. Mitoses are absent (Fig. 5-15, A). Ultrastructurally, an interesting observation is the finding of abundant intranuclear tubular structures in type 2 alveolar pneumocytes. This is probably the result of interaction of the drug with perichromatin (Fig. 5-15, C). Severe lung damage by the alkylating agent leads to diffuse interstitial fibrosis, with all of the gross and microscopic characteristics of the "honeycomb" lung. Recent observations raise the possibility that the alkylating agents may actually generate the development of malignancies.

Bleomycin, unlike other antibiotic members of its class, seldom causes stem cell suppression of bone marrow elements. Like busulfan, it causes degeneration and necrosis of type 1 pulmonary alveolar and endothelial cells, with subsequent exudative alveolitis and eventual alveolar fibrosis. Regeneration by type 2 pneumocytes is reminiscent of that seen in the lung affected by busulfan (Fig. 5-15, A and B). Bleomycin does not affect as wide a variety of epithelial tissues as busulfan. For example, the uroepithelium is not affected.

Cyclophosphamide gives rise to acute myocardial changes, particularly if high dose levels are attained. The cardiac damage occurs in a matter of 2 to 5 days. The gross and microscopic features of the myocardial damage are shared by cyclophosphamide, the anthracycline antibiotics (see the following discussion), and the sympathetic catecholamines (norepinephrine). The endocardium, myocardium, and epicardium of the left ventricle, inter-ventricular septum, and papillary muscles reveal toxic myocarditis as shown by the presence of myocytolysis and myocyte necrosis. Focal necrosis or mini-infarcts are observed throughout the myocardium of the left side. The mini-infarcts result from capillary microthrombosis. Examination of the left ventricle also reveals small, focal subendocardial and intramyocardial hemorrhages. Ultrastructural studies of the lesions reveal endothelial damage with prominent thick and thin filaments in both the myocyte and the endothelial cell nuclei.

Nitrogen mustard was one of the early antitumor agents to be given extensive clinical trial, specifically for the treatment of Hodgkin's disease. It quickly became apparent to pathologists that the cellular effects of the compound were bizarre and profound. The familiar and classic histologic features of Hodgkin's granuloma (Reed-Sternberg cells, "owls-eye," reticulum cells, eosinophils, and lymphocyte hyperplasia) were converted to a bizarre conglomeration of cells with large, hyperchromatic pyknotic nuclei and increased chromatin content. In other words, the cellular pattern became more pleomorphic and malignant in cytologic appearance. These changes are reminiscent of cellular radiation effect. With the development of additional alkylating agents, cellular changes similar to those observed after nitrogen mustard therapy became apparent. The pathologist interpreting a "treated node" may be misled if he or she is unaware of this fact. The histologic appearance of a Hodgkin's granuloma may be converted into a false appearance of Hodgkin's sarcoma (reticulum cell sarcoma), a lesion of more serious prognostic import.

The role of nitrogen mustard therapy as a cause of the elaboration and deposition of amyloid in patients with malignant lymphoma is a controversial issue. Certainly, in untreated persons with malignant lymphoma, particularly Hodgkin's disease, generalized amyloidosis has been observed. In mice receiving casein injections with nitrogen mustard, there appears to be an acceleration in the deposition of amyloid. Whether the latter result can be extrapolated to humans is problematic.

Anthracycline antibiotics. Two important members of the anthracycline antibiotics group are daunorubicin (Daunomycin) and doxorubicin (Adriamycin), antineoplastic antibiotics that are effective in the treatment of acute leukemias in humans. The cardiotoxic effects of long-term therapy with daunorubicin and doxorubicin comprise a variety of histopathologic lesions consisting of myocytes characterized by the development of myeloid bodies, which is frequently observed in toxic cell damage. There is myofibril loss within the myocyte; the nucleus is frequently intact, and the mitochondria contain their compact cristae. With a high cumulative dose, one may observe myocyte necrosis, which progresses to interstitial fibrosis. Inflammatory cells are not a feature of chronic anthracycline cardiotoxicity. Reactive vascular lesions have not been described following therapeutic doses. The earliest lesions are to be found predominantly in the subendocardium and the ventricular trabeculae.

Antimetabolites. The antimetabolites include compounds that are folic acid and purine antagonists. Methotrexate (Amethopterin) acts by inhibition of folic acid reductase. The inhibition of dihydrofolate reductase blocks the conversion of folic acid to tetrahydrofolic acid, which is essential for the synthesis of DNA, RNA, and purine-containing coenzymes. The folic acid antagonists exert profound mitotic arrest. 6-Mercaptopurine acts by inhibition of de novo purine synthesis. Azathioprine (Imuran) is 6-mercaptopurine modified by the addition of an imidazole ring. This compound enjoys current clinical popularity. The synthesis of IgG is inhibited more readily by 6-mercaptopurine than is the synthesis of IgM. Both 6-mercaptopurine and azathioprine may prolong allograft survival and "stunt" the delayed hypersensitivity reaction.

Prolonged administration of azathioprine in renal transplant recipients has led to the appearance of large cell non-Hodgkin's lymphoma involving a number of organs of the body, including the lungs and meninges. The appearance of peliosis hepatis ("livid spots") in these patients is well documented (Fig. 5-17). Peliosis hepatis gives rise to hepatic dysfunction and, if extensive, even to portal hypertension and ascites. Bone marrow depression, usually leukopenia, has been the most common manifestation of azathioprine therapy.

Methotrexate is a derivative of aminopterin and circulates in the blood bound to plasma albumin. Approximately 80% is excreted unchanged in the urine within 12 hours after administration. Its use in patients with any degree of renal impairment is contraindicated, and this precludes its employment as an immunosuppressant in kidney transplant procedures. Most cancer chemotherapists agree that it is essential to administer doses that produce some degree of measurable host effect (toxicity) to achieve maximum response. The major toxic manifestations of methotrexate relate to cells with a high mitotic index, such as are found in the bone marrow, intestinal crypts, and hair follicles. Anemia, granulocytopenia, and thrombocytopenia may occur after long-term administration.

The extreme responsiveness of erythropoiesis to methotrexate probably depends on the observation that the turnover of erythroid precursors is more rapid than that of granulocytic elements. Bone marrow megaloblastosis of the red blood cell series may appear in patients receiving methotrexate. When given to patients with certain deficiency states, antimetabolites bring about selective decrease of DNA biosynthesis. Hence, the morphologic change may be attributed to continued protein and RNA synthesis in the face of arrested DNA synthesis. Methotrexate causes a decrease in the mitotic activity of immature proliferating granulocytes, which results in granulocytopenia. The danger of the development of severe infections and septicemia is obvious. By a similar mechanism, thrombocytopenia may develop, giving rise to severe hemorrhages. Ulcerations of the buccal mucosa and gastrointestinal tract are common signs of methotrexate toxicity.

One of the dangers of prolonged methotrexate therapy for psoriasis is the appearance of liver damage, predominantly a cirrhosis that is mixed macronodular and micronodular with the septal bands of connective tissue being frequently narrow. Fat is usually seen scattered through the regenerative nodules. At no time is there appreciable microscopic evidence of hepatocyte degeneration or regeneration. The nuclei are frequently characteristically vacuolated, but unlike the nuclei of poorly controlled

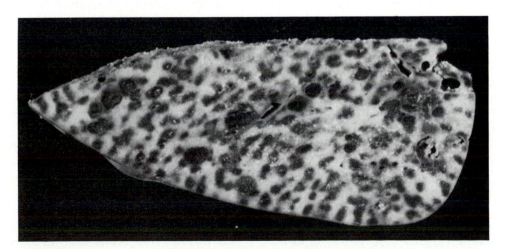

Fig. 5-17. Azathioprine. Peliosis hepatis. Livid spots characterized by dilated sinusoids and vascular channels.

diabetes mellitus, they do not stain for soluble or partly soluble glycogen. It is unusual to find any sustained elevation of serum transaminase, alkaline phosphatase, or serum bilirubin levels. These data suggest that liver biopsies are mandatory every 6 to 12 months for patients undergoing prolonged therapy for severe psoriasis. The incidence of cirrhosis is calculated to be between 4% and 7%. The consensus is that the cirrhosis might well be accelerated if there is concomitant chronic ethanol toxicity. Chronic active hepatitis followed by cirrhosis has been observed after prolonged methotrexate therapy. There is no evidence that methotrexate predisposes patients directly to the development of hepatocellular carcinoma.

The severity of liver damage is related to the duration of therapy. Methotrexate may be responsible for diffuse interstitial pneumonia (DIP), which may progress to extensive interstitial fibrosis. Occasionally, widespread noncaseating granulomas may be induced by methotrexate; these are characterized by focal collections of macrophages, frequently accompanied by eosinophils and plasma cells.

The lung may also be affected. The hypersensitivity response in the lung is usually that of a noncaseating, granulomatous reaction.

The folic acid antagonists affect both cellular and humoral immunity, but greater influence is on the cellular type. The antineoplastic agents affect the cell at various stages of the mitotic cycle. Methotrexate and cytosine arabinoside attack cell division during the DNA synthesis stage of the mitotic cycle. They are not aggressive when in contact with nonproliferating cells. The periwinkle alkaloids, vincristine and vinblastine, are also active only against proliferating cells in metaphase. The alkylating agents can inhibit cells exposed during any stage of their mitotic cycle.

The majority of cytotoxic drugs bring about an elevation in the levels of serum hepatic cell enzymes, as well as alkaline phosphatase enzymes, accompanied by increased bromsulphalein retention and a rise in the serum bilirubin level. Findings reminiscent of viral hepatitis can be produced by many of these cytotoxic drugs, including 6-mercaptopurine and 5-fluorodeoxyuridine.

Azathioprine is therapeutically employed for the treatment of acute myeloid leukemia and immunosuppressive therapy, commonly in patients undergoing transplantation of organs. Among the adverse tissue reactions is the development of cholestatic hepatitis, which is possibly the result of a direct toxic action of the compound. Tumors, in particular large cell (histiocytic non-Hodgkin's) malignant lymphoma and Kaposi's sarcoma, are frequently observed. Other malignancies, involving the bladder, breast, and endometrium, are also being found. Bone marrow suppression as a result of direct toxic action is to be expected, accompanying higher doses. Hyper-

sensitivity reactions such as fever, skin rashes, and abdominal pain occasionally occur. In recent years, development of acute pancreatitis associated with long-term azathioprine therapy has been documented. The long-term therapy has usually been in patients being treated for rheumatoid arthritis, systemic lupus erythematosus, or Crohn's disease.

Other agents

Methysergide. Used in the therapy for migraine, methysergide (Sansert) possesses antiserotonin activity and is a powerful vasoconstrictor agent. The basic structure of the compound is similar to that of the ergot alkaloids, for example, ergotamine tartrate. In addition to endomyocardial fibrosis, both methysergide and ergotamine tartrate bring about mitral, aortic, and tricuspid fibrosis resulting in valvular incompetence. The patchy endocardial fibrosis is reminiscent of that observed in carcinoid disease in which serotonin levels are elevated. The fibrous plaque covers, if it does not invade, the leaflets so the underlying valve architecture is normal, but it may extend to the chordae tendineae and papillary muscles. The major difference between the drug-induced cardiac changes and the carcinoid syndrome is the preponderance of right ventricular involvement in the latter, compared with a predominantly left-sided disease in methysergide. The drug may give rise to brawny edema and inflammatory fibrosis affecting retroperitoneal and pleuropulmonary tissues, endocardium, and large vessels. The mechanism of action has some similarities to serotonin activity but is not clearly understood.

The drug-induced fibrosis is microscopically identical to that found in the idiopathic forms. There is a distinct possibility that vasoconstriction and vasculitis may play some part in the causation of these drug-induced localized collagenoses. In most instances the disease process is reversible after discontinuation of the compound. Histologically, accompanying the fibrosis, the cellular component of the inflammatory reaction is composed primarily of lymphocytes in clumps and with the formation of germinal centers, frequently surrounded by plasma cells. As in the idiopathic variety, eosinophils may be prominent. Since the disease process is usually well advanced before clinical discovery, the nature of the earliest inflammatory lesion has not been delineated.

Thorotrast. Thorotrast is a colloidal solution containing 20% thorium (^{232}Th) dioxide and 20% dextran with 0.15% methyl-*p*-hydrobenzoate as a preservative. It was first used clinically in 1928. During the period from 1930 to 1945, it was used primarily in diagnostic radiology for visualization of the liver, spleen, and cerebral arteries. It was not until 1947 that this chemically inert and presumed innocuous compound was found to give rise to neoplasia. ^{232}Th, present in Thorotrast, is the parent of a series of radioactive daughter elements, including two

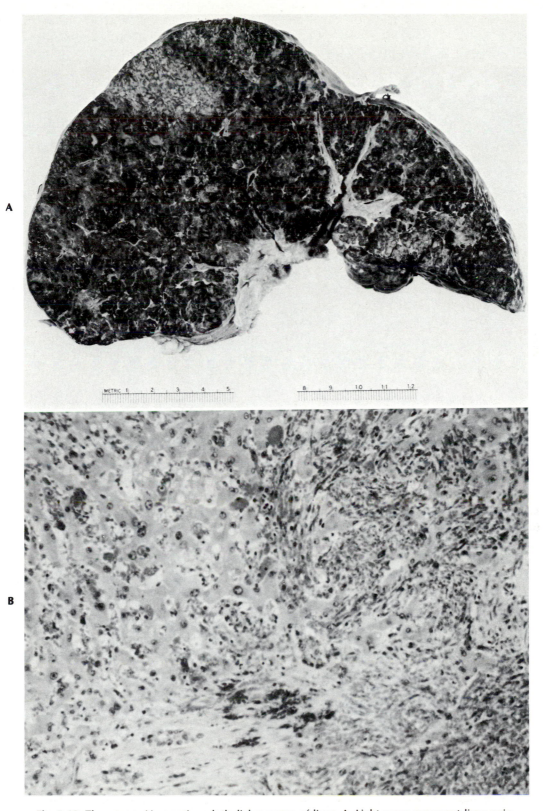

Fig. 5-18. Thorotrast. Hemangioendothelial sarcoma of liver. **A,** Light areas represent liver uninvolved by tumor. **B,** Liver biopsy. Aggregates (dark granules) of Thorotrast are embedded in connective tissue. Spindle areas are composed of neoplastic endothelial cells.

Continued.

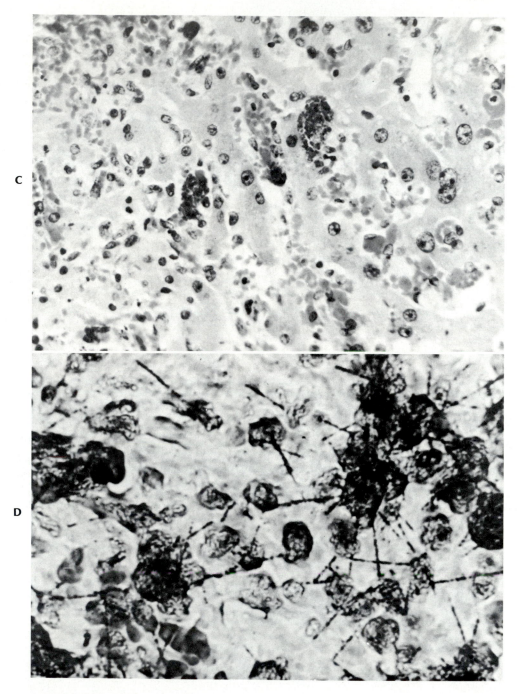

Fig. 5-18, cont'd. C, Clumps of Thorotrast surrounded by dilated sinusoids. **D,** Autoradiograph. Alpha-particle tracks "shoot out" from Thorotrast-laden Kupffer cells. Thorotrast was introduced 20 years earlier for demonstration of suspected amebic abscess of liver.

long-lived daughters, mesothorium (^{228}Ra) and radiothorium (^{228}Th). The unstable thorium nucleus goes through a chain of reactions, giving off alpha and beta particles and gamma rays until it reaches the stable element lead (^{208}Pb). ^{232}Th has a half-life of 1.4×10^{10} years and a biologic half-life of more than 400 years. Estimates by different investigators of the percentage of injected amounts of thorium retained in the organs of greatest Thorotrast deposition are as follows: liver, 71% to 73%; spleen, 7% to 17%; and bone marrow, 6% to 10%. More than 90% of ^{232}Th introduced into the body is deposited in the reticuloendothelial system.

The number and variety of malignant tumors that have been described and attributed to Thorotrast in humans are protean. Hemangioendothelioma of the liver was the neoplasm first associated with Thorotrast, and for some years it was believed to be the prevalent type (Fig. 5-18). Recently an increasing number of reports of hepatocarcinoma and cholangiocarcinoma have appeared. The time interval from the introduction of the compound to appearance of the tumor is greater than 20 years. Sarcomas and carcinomas may occur at injection sites and in body cavities into which Thorotrast has been instilled. Leukemia and carcinoma of the maxillary sinus have occurred after the introduction of Thorotrast into the body. Both Thorotrast sarcomas and carcinomas have been produced in experimental animals. There is a remarkable resemblance between the angiosarcoma produced by Thorotrast and that occurring after use of polyvinyl chloride in plastic workers. In each instance the earliest lesion appears to be sinusoid dilatation and hyperplasia of the endothelial and Kupffer cells.

Potassium chloride. The need for potassium chloride as replacement therapy in patients receiving thiazide-type drugs has resulted in the development of focal ulceration of the distal portion of the jejunum and of the ileum. Thiazide drugs deplete the body stores of potassium chloride, and the unpalatability of potassium chloride necessitated incorporation of the drug in an enteric-coated tablet or capsule form. Experiments on monkeys have shown that neither the coatings nor the thiazide itself is responsible for the development of the ulcer. The ileum and distal portion of the jejunum are highly susceptible to chemical trauma, since they lack mucous glands for protection. Chronic stenosing ulcers appear to be the result of repeated chemical irritation by localized potassium chloride released in the small bowel (Fig. 5-19). A segment of previous irritation, spasm, and ulceration could block subsequent tablets, which would prevent healing and perpetuate the ulcerogenic process. Ulcers can apparently develop following an intake of very few tablets, but the individual susceptibility to the potassium-induced ulcers is not understood.

Grossly, the ulcers are acute or chronic and may be punctate or annular. They have a "punched-out" appear-

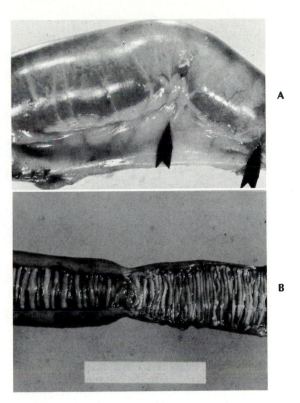

Fig. 5-19. Potassium chloride ulcer in small intestine. **A**, Constricted areas *(arrows)*. **B**, Focal, superficial ulcer and annular constriction of bowel. (Courtesy Dr. H. Rawling Pratt-Thomas, Charleston, S.C.)

ance. Proximal dilatation of the bowel occurs as a result of obstruction, in which case there is a tendency to perforation. Microscopically, the pathologic changes are confined to the mucosal and submucosal layers. There is an abrupt interruption of the normal mucosa, and the submucosa shows varying degrees of acute and chronic inflammatory infiltrate composed of neutrophils, eosinophils, and plasma cells. Extension of the inflammatory process through the muscle of the small bowel is not frequently seen. Occasionally the mucosa may regenerate and regain an intact appearance. This is accompanied by disappearance of the inflammatory infiltrate in the submucosa with replacement fibrosis leading to a circumferential "napkin ring–like" stricture.

Milk and alkali. After the prolonged ingestion of milk and absorbable alkali in the treatment of peptic ulcer, the milk-alkali syndrome, characterized by hypercalcemia followed by calcium deposition in the kidneys, resulting in renal insufficiency, may occur. This renal calcification predisposes the patient to repeated attacks of acute pyelonephritis, resulting in a scarred, nonfunctional kidney. The syndrome must be distinguished from the calcification of hypervitaminosis D and primary pulmonary alveolar calcinosis. Other causes of hypercalcemia, such as hyperparathyroidism with the common complication

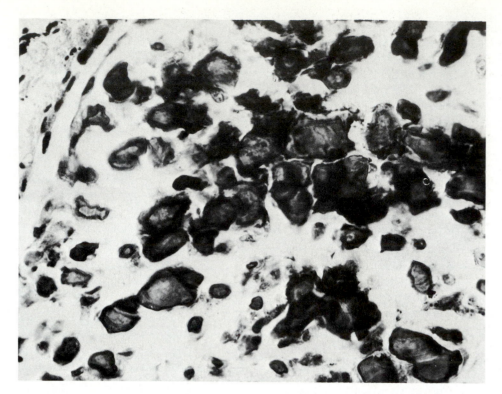

Fig. 5-20. Milk-alkali syndrome. Pulmonary alveolar microlithiasis associated with milk-alkali syndrome. Calcified desquamated alveolar cells occupy alveolar sac. (Hematoxylin and eosin; 350×.)

of renal calcification, also may be complicated by peptic ulcer, thereby confusing the issue.

The association of pulmonary alveolar microlithiasis with the milk-alkali syndrome has been observed. In one case we observed, the alveoli were dilated throughout the lung and literally filled with calcified, desquamated bronchioloalveolar epithelial cells and macrophages. The conversion of the clumps of cells to microliths by their mineralization with calcium phosphate was extensive throughout all lobules (Fig. 5-20). The septa, although fibrosed in part, were free of mineral deposits. Cut sections of the lungs had the appearance and feel of grains of sand.

Mineral oil. At necropsy, the pathologist may find numerous lipogranulomas caused by mineral oil in such organs as the spleen, lymph nodes, and portal tracts of the liver. The source of the mineral oil in such cases is frequently foods, such as bread, that are prepared on stainless steel tables that are rubbed down daily with mineral oil. In many food-processing plants, rust is kept off the machinery by applying this substance. Thus, over many years, a considerable amount of mineral oil may be ingested in contaminated foods. Furthermore, mineral oil has been a common form of self-medication for such conditions as peptic ulcer, diarrhea, and constipation.

Since this petrolatum oil does not elicit the cough reflex, the oily substances may reach the dependent portions of the lungs. Unlike fish and animal oils, which contain varied amounts of unsaturated fatty acids that produce an acute hemorrhagic or necrotizing reaction, mineral oil produces a mild foreign body type of reaction. It elicits macrophages, which then phagocytose the foreign material (Fig. 5-21). Giant cells are abundant, depending on the amount and duration of the oil dosage (Fig. 5-22). Over a long period of time, the small globules of mineral oil coalesce to form large vacuoles, and the process is accompanied by a chronic inflammatory reaction rich in lymphocytes and plasma cells. The eventuality is a diffuse lobar interstitial pneumonia and fibrosis or a localized reaction referred to as a paraffinoma (Fig. 5-23). These lesions radiologically have simulated pneumonia and localized or diffuse tumor (p. 896).

Skin cancer caused by mineral oil was first noted during the latter part of the nineteenth century among mule spinners in the cotton industry. Between 1920 and 1943, no fewer than 1400 cases of skin cancer attributable to industrial exposure to mineral oil were reported. Of these, the scrotum was affected in 885 patients, nearly all of whom were cotton workers. Only 50 of the patients worked in the engineering industry. Mineral oils consist of three types of compounds—paraffins, naphthenic compounds, and aromatic compounds. It is believed that

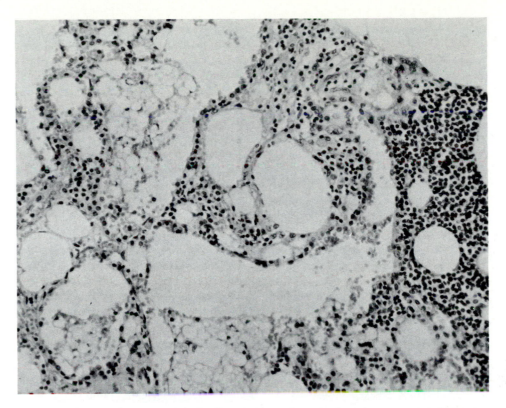

Fig. 5-21. Mineral oil pneumonitis. Small vacuoles coalesce to form larger ones. Inflammatory response is predominantly lymphocytic.

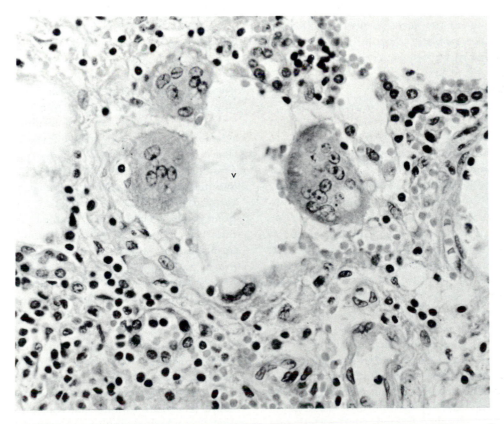

Fig. 5-22. Mineral oil granuloma in lung. Foreign body giant cells containing mineral oil surround large vacuole *(v)*. Lymphocytes and plasma cells are prominent.

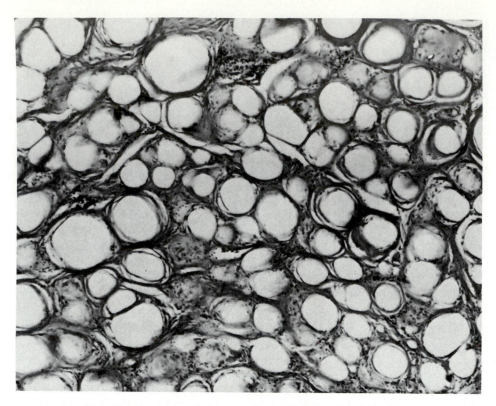

Fig. 5-23. Lung of patient who used mineral oil as laxative for 30 years. X-ray film suggested malignancy of right lower lobe. Large vacuoles of mineral oil are demarcated by bands of fibrous tissue.

most of the carcinogenicity of cutting oils is attributable to compounds in the aromatic fraction, particularly the polycyclic aromatics containing four to six condensed benzene rings.

TOXICOLOGIC ASPECTS OF FORENSIC PATHOLOGY
Alcohols and glycols

Alcohol continues to be the most frequently abused chemical compound among adults in the United States. More socioeconomic problems are created by alcohol abuse than all other medicinal and illicit drugs combined. Alcoholism is the nation's leading public health problem. In a significant proportion of sudden unexpected deaths among adults, alcohol has been implicated as either a direct or a contributory cause. This statement holds true not only for natural deaths but also for those classified as homicide, accident, or suicide. What may be interpreted at first glance as sudden unexpected death in a chronic alcoholic on a spree may prove to be otherwise, for example, asphyxia by aspiration of a meat bolus. In such cases there is a rapid onset of dyspnea, gasping for breath, and choking. This series of events has been referred to as a "café coronary," a term that is misleading and should be discarded. A postmortem examination reveals that large chunks of food, undigested and unchewed, are present in the larynx. This is invariably accompanied by high blood-alcohol levels. It is mandatory that the student of chronic alcoholism realize that an alcoholic undergoing sudden or rapid death may have a background of numerous diseases that develop as a result of many years of recurrent alcohol-poisoning episodes.

Pathophysiologic effects of alcohol include interference with normal metabolic effects (hypoglycemia, acidosis) and suppression of phagocytosis and of normal immunologic responses. Common findings at autopsy are subdural hematoma and hemorrhage resulting from ruptured viscera, fatty and cirrhotic liver changes, acute hemorrhagic pancreatitis, anemia, and miscellaneous infections, notably Friedländer's pneumonia. Toxicologic studies may reveal that contaminants in alcoholic beverages may have contributed to the patient's demise; among these are lead, propyl alcohol, ethylene glycol, methanol, and cobalt. At autopsy the finding in alcoholics of dangerous levels of barbituric acid derivatives, and in recent years such compounds as amphetamines and tranquilizers, is not unusual. Well over 95% of the deaths attributed to alcohol may be classified as accidental and resulted from overdose unrelated to suicidal intent.

Acute subdural hematomas are not uncommon in alcoholics. There are innumerable documented cases of "jail death" in which alcoholics are moved to the jail cell and told to "sleep it off." Some hours later they are discovered dead, and autopsy reveals an acute subdural hematoma that has caused fatal supratentorial pressure on the brainstem. Interestingly, the blood-alcohol level may be very low as a result of the metabolic oxidation that occurred while the deceased was in the jail cell. However, the pathologist can closely estimate the alcohol level at the time of injury by analyzing the blood in the subdural hematoma for alcohol content. This portion of blood has not been recirculated through the liver for its metabolism and therefore reflects a more accurate blood-alcohol level at the time of injury. The hopeless alcohol addict may envision himself or herself as an inspired bartender and may devise a fatal concoction by adding such toxic substances as antifreeze, ethylene glycol, and rubbing alcohol (isopropyl alcohol) to the alcoholic drink. The addition of a touch of Sterno and paint thinner may prove to be the "straw that broke the camel's back."

Ethanol

A not uncommon set of circumstances associated with acute ethanol (alcohol) intoxication is that of an individual who, after a heavy bout of drinking, retires and is found dead in bed the next morning with a blood-alcohol level that is well below the lethal level (Table 5-4). At autopsy, various changes may be found in the liver ranging from a large fatty liver to various stages of Laënnec's (alcoholic or nutritional) cirrhosis. The mechanism of death with central nervous system depression is not clearly understood. In other instances, unexpected deaths occur in chronic alcoholics, and the pathologist finds only a large fatty liver at autopsy. Again, the level of blood alcohol may be less than the levels associated with acute fatal poisoning.

Incidents of alcoholics who have consumed over a pint a day for several weeks without eating are commonly encountered. In these cases clinical manifestations are vomiting, jaundice, fever, and leukocytosis, with pneumonia and delirium tremens frequently complicating the picture. Death occurs in approximately 66% of the cases with this clinical setting. The pathologist usually finds evidence of hepatocellular necrosis and bile stasis superimposed on a fatty or cirrhotic liver, but occasionally the morphologic features of complicating acute viral hepatitis are observed. Indeed, the alcoholic liver may well have an increased susceptibility to acute and chronic viral hepatitis. Acute alcoholic hepatitis is an appropriate morphologic designation when focal scattered necrotic liver cells are observed among the fat cells. When the alcohol intake has been excessive (over a pint a day) for a long period of time in the presence of dietary lack, one not infrequently observes intracytoplasmic hyaline bodies that first appear in a perinuclear location and are known as Mallory's alcoholic hyaline bodies. When they are found abundantly in fatty livers, they are characteristic of an acute and severe alcoholic insult. The hyaline bodies may be observed in smaller numbers in conditions other than acute toxic alcoholic damage, namely morbid obesity (twice normal weight) and acute viral hepatitis. Individuals with large fatty livers may suffer fat embolism after traumatic injury to the liver. Examination of the brain will reveal the telltale petechial hemorrhages caused by the embolic fatty material. Microscopically, the liver cells are so engorged with fat that the cell boundaries may rupture and form microcysts.

Some cases of sudden or unexpected death in acute alcohol poisoning have been attributed to alcoholic myocardiosis (alcoholic myopathy). It has been presumed that the mechanism of death in these cases is cardiac arrhythmia. An association between alcohol use and cardiac arrhythmias, particularly atrial fibrillation, has long been suspected, but the specific etiologic role of alcohol is difficult to establish. In an emergency room setting, one encounters patients who drink heavily and habitually, and examination shows that many have arrhythmias that return rather rapidly to sinus rhythm. Regan and Haider[193] point to this situation as a rather typical weekend or holiday presentation and refer to it as "holiday heart syndrome." They define this as an acute disturbance of cardiac rhythm or conduction, or both, that follows heavy ethanol consumption in a person without other clinical evidence of heart disease and that disappears, without evident residua, with abstinence.

Clinically, electrocardiographic changes indicate myocardial dysfunction in alcoholics, but the morphologist has not been able to characterize any pathognomonic lesions by light and electron microscopy. Of the morphologic observations on the myocardium of the chronic alcoholic, probably the most significant is the presence of myocytes containing numbers of irregularly deposited intramyocardial lipid droplets, which are composed of triglycerides. The action of alcohol on the myocytes results in the loss of some Krebs' cycle enzymes and electrolytes from the cell, thereby interfering with the utilization of fatty acids for energy production and leading to the accumulation of triglycerides. If, indeed, toxic alcoholic cardiomyopathy exists as a separate entity, its morphologic manifestations are shared in patients who demonstrate nutritional cardiomyopathy such as thiamine deficiency (beriberi heart disease).

Ethanol is a drug that has been classified as a food yielding 7 "empty" calories per gram. In excess amounts it behaves as a toxin. It supports growth, has a protein-sparing effect, is well absorbed from the gastrointestinal tract even in patients with malabsorption, and increases the smooth endoplasmic reticulum of the hepatocyte and the rate of hepatic drug metabolism, including its own oxidation. In general the fundamental cytologic differences between patients with alcoholic hepatitis who live and those who die lie in the amount of hepatic cell necro-

Table 5-4. Levels of common and uncommon chemicals and drugs found in body tissue at necropsy of accidental, suicidal, and homicidal poisoning victims (all values in mg/dl)

Chemical	Blood	Urine	Brain	Liver	Kidney	Other
COMMON						
Acetaminophen	150	—	—	—	—	—
Alcohols	84	—	—	—	—	—
Butanol						
Ethanol	360-544	—	—	—	—	—
Methanol	20-630	—	—	10-180	20-230	—
Propanol	150-200	—	—	—	—	—
Amphetamine	0.05-4.1	2.5-70	0.28-0.3	0.43-7.4	0.32-5.2	—
Aromatics	0.5-33	—	—	0.7-125	1.4-3	—
Barbiturates	2.9-6.8	0.7-9.8	17.2	10.6-58	21	—
Amobarbital						
Amobarbital and secobarbital (Tuinal)	0.6-8.5	0.3-12.1	—	3.8-26	—	—
Barbital	10-38	114	6.3	10-93	—	—
Barbiturates and alcohol (20-260 mg/dl)	0.8-5.3	0.1-17	3.4-4.8	3-16	1.7	—
Butabarbital	3-8.8	—	—	5.1-25	—	—
Pentobarbital	0.5-11.2	1.4-18	1.2	2.3-55	1.8	—
Phenobarbital	8-15	—	—	8.9-26.6	—	—
Carbon monoxide	10%, may be significant; 20%, chronic; 40%+, acute					
Cyanide	0.11-5.3	0.005-0.11	0.06-1.6	0.07-2.3	0.02-8.4	—
Glutethimide (Doriden)	1-9.7	2.8	1.1	6.3-14.1	0.4-1.6	—
Meprobamate	1.4-34.6	—	140	5.8-41.2	50	—
Morphine	0.02-0.23	1.4-8.1	0.002-0.75	0.04-1.8	0.02-0.15	Bile, 0.2-5.7
Nicotine	1.1-6.3	1.7-5.8	—	10-500	0.3-5.3	—
Propoxyphene (Darvon)	0.1-1.7	0.25-3.5	0.88-4	0.73-11.9	0.1-6.4	—
UNCOMMON						
Acetone	55	90	—	—	—	—
Amitriptyline (Elavil)	0.27-0.47	0.04-0.79	2.6-1.8	1.3-32	1.2-31	—
Arsenic	0.06-0.93	—	0.02-0.4	0.2-120	0.02-70	Bile, 14.1; stomach contents, 30.6
Benzene	0.09	0.06	3.9	1.6	1.8	—
Boron	8-296	—	—	—	—	—
Bromide	200	—	—	—	—	—
Brompheniramine	0.02	0.51	0.10	0.2	—	—
Caffeine	7.9-15.9	11.4-54.2	7.5-10.8	9.2-32.9	10.4-23	—
Chloral hydrate (trichloroethanol)	10-64	59	—	0.9-17	—	—
Chlordiazepoxide (Librium)	2	—	—	2	—	—
Chloroform	1-4.8	0-6	5.5-31	0.6-13	1.6-2.7	—
Chlorpromazine	0.3-3.5	—	—	5.4-211	—	—
Codeine	0.1-0.88	2.9-22.9	0	0.06-4.49	0.23-3.63	—
Desipramine	0.3	—	—	—	—	—
Diazepam (Valium)	2	—	—	—	—	—
2,4-Dichlorophenoxyacetic acid (2,4-D)	66.9-82.6	26.4	1.3	2.1-18.3	6.3	—
Dieldrin	5 (IV)	—	—	—	—	—

Data from Sunshine, I., editor: Handbook of analytical toxicology, Akron, Ohio, The Chemical Rubber Co.

Table 5-4. Levels of common and uncommon chemicals and drugs found in body tissue at necropsy of accidental, suicidal, and homicidal poisoning victims (all values in mg/dl)—cont'd

Chemical	Blood	Urine	Brain	Liver	Kidney	Other
UNCOMMON—cont'd						
Ethchlorvynol (Placidyl)	15	3.1-5.4	1.3-5.7	1.8-7.2	1.8-6.3	Adipose, 6-104
Ethylene glycol	200-400	200-1130	30-390	20-1510	20-1130	—
Fluoride	0.2-0.3	—	—	—	—	—
Hydroxychloro-quine (Plaquenil)	4.8-6.1	97	—	7.1	—	—
Imipramine (Tofranil)	0.28-0.7	0.69-6.4	3-7.4	8.6-25	3.8-5.6	—
Iron	1.9-5	—	—	—	—	—
Lead	0.11-0.35	—	—	—	—	—
Mebumate	1	—	—	—	—	—
Meperidine	3	177	7	11	11.4	—
Mercury	—	—	0	0.9	1.2	—
Methamphetamine	4	—	—	—	—	—
Methapyrilene	0.4-3	—	—	2.5-16	0.6	—
Methaqualone	3	—	—	—	—	—
Methyprylon (Noludar)	8.9-10	—	—	22	1.1	—
Nortriptyline	0.1-3	2.5-12	—	0.78-22	0.7-9.4	—
Paraldehyde	11.5-48	13	15-37	20-60	50-260	—
Pentachlorophenol	4.6-17.3	2.8-5.2	1.4-3.5	5.9-22.5	4.1-12.3	—
Phenytoin	10	—	7.8	27	11	—
Quinine	1.2	—	—	—	—	—
Strychnine	0.05-0.61	0.1-3.3	0.05-2.6	0.5-25.7	0.007-10.6	—
Thioridazine	2-8	—	—	2.5-51.3	—	—
Trichloroethane	0.15-72	0.1-0.3	0.32-59	0.49-22	0.26-12	—
Trichloroethylene	0.3-11	0.2-7.3	0.7-27	0.5-25	1.1-11.2	—

sis and the individual capability for hepatocellular regeneration. In acute alcoholic hepatitis, one observes, in addition to steatotic hepatic cells, the presence of non-fatty "balloon cells." The balloon cells contain deformed mitochondria, some being of giant configuration while others appear shrunken and are closely approximated into groups. The cristae frequently have a grotesque and bizarre pattern. Among the numerous nonspecific mitochondrial alterations, the most conspicuous are crystal-like inclusions resembling myelin degeneration. The smooth endoplasmic reticulum is diffusely hypertrophied and vacuolated. The changes in the endoplasmic reticulum reflect the fact that ethanol can influence microsomal drug metabolism in humans. Alcoholics metabolize tolbutamide more rapidly than do nonalcoholics, and this should be considered when alcoholics are given tolbutamide for the treatment of diabetes. People who ingest alcohol chronically have an increased level of the hepatic enzyme that metabolizes pentobarbital, whereas the activity of this enzyme system is inhibited by the in vitro addition of alcohol to the incubation mixture. These observations may explain the increased tolerance of alcoholics to barbiturates and other sedatives when sober and the enhanced sensitivity of these individuals to sedatives when inebriated. The ergastoplasm is vacuolated, and dispersion of the ribosomes is observed. The giant mitochondrial forms and altered endoplasmic reticulum probably form the morphologic basis for the alcoholic hyaline bodies of Mallory.

The oral and intravenous administration (25% and 20% ml, respectively, of absolute alcohol in 100 ml of water) of lethal and sublethal doses of alcohol (12 and 8 ml, respectively, of absolute alcohol per kilogram) to unanesthetized dogs produces changes in the lymphatic tissues. These changes consist of necrosis of germinal follicles throughout the entire lymphatic system (Fig. 5-24). Hemorrhagic gastritis and superficial ulceration, particularly of the distal part of the stomach, were noted after oral administration (Fig. 5-25). Occasionally, loss of lipid in the deeper layers of the adrenal zona fasciculata was observed. Continuous intravenous infusion of epinephrine or norepinephrine to alcoholized dogs did not appear to intensify this reaction. These changes did not occur in adrenalectomized dogs. The lympholysis and germinal center necrosis were probably a reflection of adrenal stimulation with acutely elevated serum corticosteroid level.

It is of interest that these changes, particularly those in

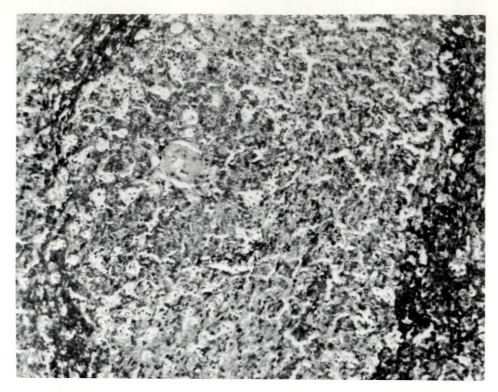

Fig. 5-24. Sublethal dose of ethyl alcohol (oral) in spleen of dog. Germinal follicles of all lymphatic tissues show necrosis of germinal follicles with presence of "nuclear dust" (lympholysis), which probably represents cortisone effect. Similar lesions are seen in humans after fatal salicylate poisoning and burns.

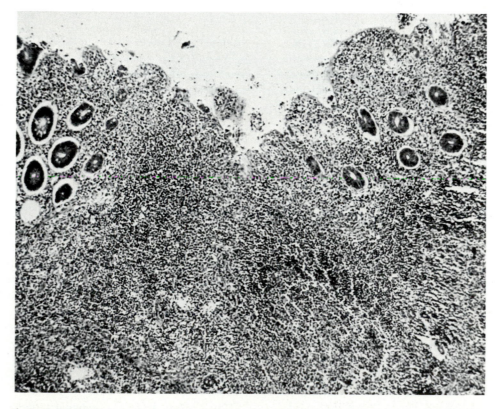

Fig. 5-25. Sublethal dose of ethyl alcohol (oral) in dog stomach. Superficial ulceration and gastritis 4 days after dosage.

the mitochondria, probably occur only in individuals who have a very excessive alcohol intake in the presence of adequate food consumption or in individuals who consume lesser quantities of alcohol in the absence of adequate diet. In addition to the effect on the liver cell, ethanol may have a direct "toxic" effect on the bone marrow. This is reflected in the observation of vacuolation of primitive erythroblasts. The action appears independent of nutritional deficiencies or other toxins.

The occurrence of pancreatitis and pancreatic lithiasis in alcoholics is well known. Whether this can be accounted for by duct and ductule blockage by inspissated pancreatic secretion during a period of dehydration is unresolved. On the other hand, there may be a direct "toxic" effect on the pancreatic acinar cell (see discussion of methyl alcohol). Although alcohol administration regularly induces mild hyperlipemia, pronounced hyperlipemia develops in some individuals at intoxicating levels. The explanation for this unusual response to alcohol is not clear. It is possible that pancreatitis is incriminated, or possibly the low plasma lipoprotein lipase, which often is decreased in patients with liver disease, is at fault. Zieve[200] reported hyperlipemia in association with jaundice, fatty liver, and hemolytic anemia, and this association of signs and symptoms is now known as Zieve's syndrome.

The congeners (which include fusel oil, aldehydes, furfural, esters, solids, tannins, and many uncharacterized compounds) are necessary for the taste, bouquet, and color of whiskey. Some workers believe that their presence in large amounts enhances the possibility of toxic reactions. The evidence suggests that small quantities of congeners in proper balance, such as found in some types of blended whiskies, may lessen undesirable physiologic effects through interaction with ethanol and other constituents of the beverage. A consideration of these factors points to the desirability of further biochemical and toxicologic investigations, with emphasis on the fundamental mechanisms.

Methyl alcohol

In Atlanta, Georgia, in 1951, more than 300 patients who had ingested bootleg whiskey containing 35% methyl alcohol were treated at the Grady Memorial Hospital. They presented the classic symptoms of wood alcohol poisoning—visual disturbances from mild blurring to total blindness, severe abdominal pain, nausea, headache, and central nervous system manifestations ranging from dizziness and convulsions to coma. Many patients manifested severe acidosis as evidenced by reduction in plasma carbon dioxide combining power. The mechanism of the acidosis is incompletely understood, although it is well known that the breakdown of methyl to formic acid and possibly formaldehyde may have some role in bringing it about. A number of patients had initial

serum amylase levels exceeding 300 units, and at autopsy the lesions varied from scattered areas of pancreatic acinar destruction with edema of the stroma to a pronounced hemorrhagic necrosis that was easily visualized in the gross examination. The mildest, and possibly earliest, changes were degranulation and increased basophilism of the acinar cells with pooling of secretion in the ducts accompanied by edema of the connective tissue of the lobules. More conspicuous changes consisted of necrosis of both arterial and venous walls with extravasation of blood through the parenchyma. Histologic examination of the eyes from fatal cases showed retinal ganglion cell degeneration with sparing of the optic nerve and tract.

Methanol is easily absorbed through the skin, respiratory tract, or gastrointestinal tract, and human poisoning is possible by any of these routes. According to several authorities, 200 parts of methanol per million parts of air is the maximum limit of safety in industry. In the Atlanta incident the smallest amount that produced a fatal result was about 15 ml of 40% methyl alcohol. The highest dose recorded in a survivor was 500 ml of the same concentration. This unusual variation in susceptibility constitutes one of the unusual features of this type of poisoning and has not been fully explained. The oxidation rate of methyl alcohol in the body is less than one-fifth that of ethyl—hence its long persistence. A small proportion is excreted unchanged in the urine, but a much larger amount is lost in expired air. As stated previously, methanol poisoning is attributed partially to the acidosis caused by formic acid and partially to the local toxic effects of formaldehyde, both compounds resulting from metabolism of methanol. Both methanol and ethanol are converted by the enzymes alcohol dehydrogenase and aldehyde dehydrogenase. The consequence is that high doses of ethanol compete with methanol, delaying and reducing its toxification. Ethanol inhibits the bioactivation—in this case a toxification—of methanol.

Isopropyl alcohol

Fatal isopropanol poisoning is much less common than that from methanol. Isopropyl alcohol has many important uses in industries, where it has been substituted for ethyl alcohol in a number of processes. At a concentration of 70%, it is readily available to the public as "rubbing alcohol." Adelson[179] points out that no specific organic lesions are found in individuals who die within a few hours after ingestion of isopropyl alcohol. Death, which occurs rapidly after absorption, is the result of profound depression of the central nervous system with ultimate respiratory paralysis. In this respect isopropanol acts in the same manner as other respiratory depressants (ethyl alcohol, anesthetics, and barbiturates). The acute tubular nephrosis in cases of fatal poisoning probably is due to the circulatory effect of existing shock in the victims. Since 15% of isopropyl alcohol is metabolized to acetone, the patient in coma could be subject to an erroneous diagnosis of diabetic coma, except that glycosuria is absent.

Gadsden and associates[185] reported 50 cases of isopropyl alcohol intoxication after ingestion of what has been referred to as "scrap iron." The drink is made by using cracked corn, yeast, and sugar. The mixture is fermented for 48 hours, with Clorox used as a catalyst. Isopropyl alcohol and mothballs (naphthalene) are added at the end of the fermentation period. After distillation, the drink tastes like the galvanized steel drum in which it was made, hence the name "scrap iron." Gadsden and associates conclude that this drink is for high voltage and not vintage.

Glycols

Ethylene glycol, a hygroscopic secondary alcohol, is best known as a constituent of antifreeze. In the body it is metabolized to oxalic acid. The importance of this chemical in accidental, and sometimes suicidal, death cannot be overemphasized. It appears as an intentional contaminant in moonshine whiskey. Fatal accidental ingestion of numerous compounds containing oxalic acid and ethylene glycol has been recorded. Household cleaners such as brass polish and ink spot and iron stain removers are sometimes the culprits. Glycols are excellent industrial solvents; in the navy they are used for cleaning torpedoes and are known under names such as "torpedo juice," "pink lady," or "hen wine." These chemicals also are used by shoemakers, bookbinders, and straw hat manufacturers.

Shortly after the ingestion of as little as 100 ml of ethylene glycol, evidence of drunkenness ensues, followed rapidly by headache, convulsions, coma, and death. If the individual survives for 1 to 3 days, the initial central nervous system depressant effect lightens and cardiopulmonary manifestations appear with the development of pulmonary edema. By the second day there is evidence of azotemia and uremia. Depending on the dosage and the initiation of therapy, shock may appear at any time during the first 24 hours. At necropsy the kidneys are swollen and tense, and on cut section the pale cortex stands out in contrast to the dark color because of vascular stasis that occupies the medullary zone. If shock has been severe and prolonged, cortical necrosis may be evident. Microscopically, the cellular features of acute tubular nephrosis or necrosis accompanied by jamming of the lumina of the tubules by sheaf-shaped, semiopaque calcium oxylate crystals are observed (Fig. 5-26). The crystals are strongly birefringent. Lesser numbers of calcium oxalate crystals are to be found in the distal nephron. Tubulovenous anastomoses and red cell casts are part of the histologic picture. Other findings consist of chemical meningitis and pericapillary calcification of

the meninges. Oxalate crystals may be demonstrated within the intrameningeal and intracerebral blood vessels and, less frequently, localized within the white matter of the brain. Gross hydropic degeneration of the hepatocytes of the centrilobular region is usual.

Diethylene glycol, also an occasional constituent of antifreeze and a one-time vehicle for drugs, is twice as toxic as ethylene glycol. It is not metabolized to oxalic acid, and crystals of calcium oxalate are not to be found in the tissues. Like ethylene glycol, the diethylene compound may bring about centrilobular hydropic or "ballooning" hepatocyte changes. Necrosis of the liver has been documented. Renal cortical necrosis is prone to develop and is probably more closely related to the tubular hypoxia of shock than to toxic nephropathy. In the majority of cases, remarkable swelling and hydropic degeneration occur in the proximal convoluted tubules. Ethylene glycol dinitrate produces methemoglobin formation that may be a direct cause of the renal injury found after ingestion of this compound. Propylene glycol, on the other hand, induces hemolysis and tubular necrosis.

Among the various ethylene glycol derivatives of low molecular weight (such as diethylene glycol, dipropylene glycol, and dioxane), the presence of an ether linkage appears to cause a more intense renal damage.

Dioxane

Dioxane is a powerful dehydrating agent often used as a substitute for alcohol in tissue preparation and stains. In poorly ventilated areas, dangerous concentrations may develop in the air. Dioxane, like other nephrotoxins, causes cytoplasmic vacuolation, rarefaction, and loss of the brush border. Like mercuric chloride, this agent induces proliferation of the smooth endoplasmic reticulum; in contrast to mercuric chloride, it does not cause dissociation of polysomes. Mitochondria are severely damaged and undergo swelling, and amorphous intramatrical deposits develop. With established necrosis, spicular crystals, believed to be calcium salts, appear on the cristae and eventually fill up most of the mitochondrion.

Metals and metallic salts
Mercury

Mercury and its compounds enter the body by absorption through the skin, by ingestion, and by inhalation. However, the chemical form of mercury has a significant effect on its disposition. Practically, there are three general forms of mercury: elemental mercury (Hg^0); inorganic mercury—mercurous (HG^{+1}) and mercuric (Hg^{+2}); and organic mercury, which is usually limited to methyl, ethyl, and phenyl mercury salts and the family of alkoxyalkyl mercury diuretics.

Inhalation is the most important route of absorption from the industrial point of view and is responsible for

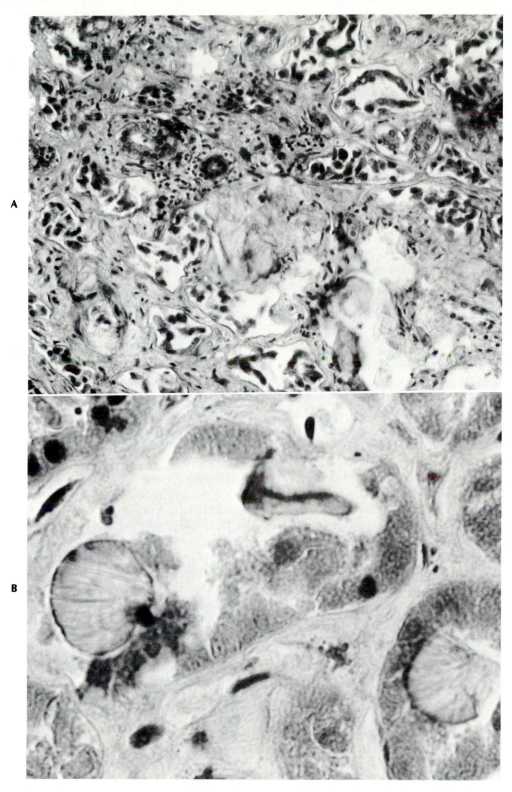

Fig. 5-26. Ethylene glycol poisoning resulting from ingestion of antifreeze. Acute tubular necrosis with "stuffing" of tubular lumens by calcium oxalate crystals. Focal chronic interstitial nephritis is evident. **A,** Characteristic calcium oxalate crystals. **B,** Nuclei at upper left pyknotic. Remainder of tubules reveal loss of nuclear staining, swelling, and necrosis of tubular cells.

many cases of mercury poisoning. Elemental mercury and monoalkyl mercurials (such as methyl mercury) are important in this route of entry because both have high vapor pressures and high lipid solubility. Oral intake of mercury does occur but usually only in cases of suicide or as a result of accidental contamination of food and drink with mercury compounds. Elemental mercury is very poorly absorbed from the gastrointestinal tract (<0.01%), and organic mercury compounds are much better absorbed than inorganic compounds. Systemic absorption of all alkyl mercury compounds probably is substantial because there are cases of poisoning from the dermal application of methyl mercury ointments.

The distribution of mercury varies considerably depending on the chemical form and, to a lesser extent, on the route of administration. Mercurous compounds and metallic mercury are oxidized to mercuric mercury, whereas the organic mercury compounds are variably metabolized to the mercuric form. The mercuric salts form soluble compounds with proteins, sodium chloride, blood, and tissue fluid alkalis. The accumulation of mercury is independent of the mode of administration—mercury entering the body as a vapor behaves no differently than mercury injected into the body. However, the chemical form of administration significantly affects the disposition. For example, whereas both mercuric mercury and organic mercury (methyl mercury) are distributed preferentially to the kidneys, the amount of mercury in other tissues is much higher with methyl mercury. Mercuric chloride has a more toxic effect on parenchymal cells than the organic mercurials such as methyl mercury chloride and methyl mercury dicyanamide. Organic mercury is more firmly bound to the tissues than is inorganic mercury and possesses greater power of penetration of the blood-brain barrier. Mercury, regardless of form, moves readily across the placenta and may be concentrated in fetal tissue. The concentration of mercury in the blood has been used as a biologic indicator of exposure. In general, the distribution within the blood depends on the chemical form; organic mercury is carried mainly by erythrocytes and inorganic mercury by the plasma.

Absorbed mercury leaves the blood rapidly, with the greater part excreted in the urine and feces; some, however, is also excreted in bile, sweat, saliva, and milk. The relative contribution of urine and feces to the total elimination of mercury also depends on the chemical form of mercury present. With prolonged administration of metallic and mercuric mercury, urinary excretion somewhat exceeds the fecal route; however, methyl mercury is excreted mainly by the fecal route. After any short exposure in both animals and humans, excretion is normally greater in feces than in urine. The mechanism of renal excretion is poorly understood, but glomerular filtration is not thought to play a major role. There is also

urinary reabsorption in the renal proximal tubules primarily, with some by distal tubules. During exposure of short duration, excretion is rapid; hence the tissue concentration is lowered within a week after cessation of exposure. After prolonged exposure, mercury accumulates in the brain, and the gradual buildup in the kidneys results in slow excretion. After termination of the exposure, the amount in the urine is approximately proportional to the mercury content of the kidneys. With prolonged low exposure, excretion approximately equals absorption so that the tissue levels of mercury remain the same. Interestingly, the administration of mercury, zinc, or cadmium stimulates the synthesis in the kidney of metallothionein, a low–molecular weight protein rich in sulfhydryl groups, with a high affinity by mercury for the sulfhydryl moiety. The renal concentration of metallothionein is increased as much as sixfold by administration of inorganic mercury, which may serve a protective role for the kidney by sequestering mercury, since the minimal concentration of mercury in kidney associated with toxic effects is considerably greater with long-term administration than with acute administration.

A significant local inflammatory reaction to metallic mercury and its compounds in the body tissues depends on the presence of, or the oxidation of such compounds to, the mercuric ion. The mercuric ion, when present in large amounts, will cause protein precipitation. Mercury also inhibits multiple enzyme systems such as oxidative mitochondrial phosphorylation and cytochrome C oxidase. Mercury decreases the activity of the liver microsomal detoxification systems and thus indirectly potentiates the harmful effects of other toxicants. It has been found that mercury combines with both sulfhydryl and phosphoryl groups in the cell membrane, particularly the former. The exact mechanism entailed in the diuretic action of mercuric chloride and organic mercurial compounds is not completely understood, but the result is a diminution in the reabsorption of sodium and chloride by the kidney tubules, particularly the straight portion of the loop of Henle.

The toxic effects of mercury involve numerous organs and systems, but the major target organs are the central nervous system and the kidney. Although the kidney contains the highest concentration of mercury regardless of the chemical form absorbed, it is the primary target organ only for inorganic mercury. In acute mercury poisoning, mercuric chloride is usually identified as causing the massive damage to proximal convoluted tubules that results in acute renal failure. The ingestion of this material is usually associated with suicide or accidental death. Autopsy findings reveal enlarged kidneys with pale and swollen cortices and dark and congested pyramids. When death does not ensue until a period of 3 or 4 days has passed, the proximal convoluted tubules undergo extensive cellular necrosis, with the lumina becoming

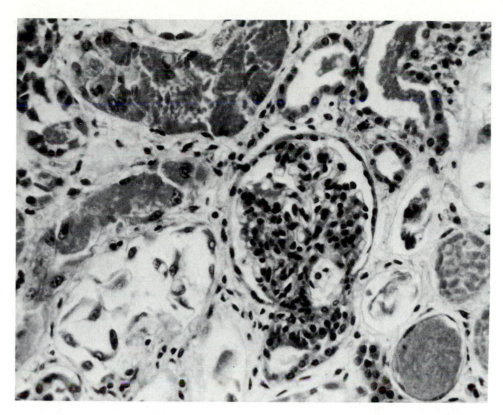

Fig. 5-27. Mercury poisoning. Death occurred 4 days after ingestion of several tablespoonfuls of bichloride of mercury. Coagulative necrosis of proximal convoluted tubules is characteristic.

filled with eosinophilic granular cytoplasmic debris (Fig. 5-27). The basement membrane of the nephron is intact. The ascending limbs, distal convoluted tubules, and collecting tubules contain casts, and there is only slight epithelial loss in the distal convoluted tubules. At approximately 8 days the necrotic debris has disappeared from the tubular lumina. The proximal convoluted tubules are dilated, and the epithelium shows signs of regeneration as evidenced by the presence of mitotic figures (Fig. 5-28, *A*). By approximately 14 days the epithelium of the proximal convoluted tubules has returned to the normal configuration. Healing of the lesion is characterized by reabsorption of the interstitial edema fluid and repair of the tubular epithelium along the intact basement membrane, thereby reestablishing tubular integrity.

This is in contrast to pure ischemic changes in which the basement membrane is fragmented and ruptured, with complete disintegration of the tubular structure and leakage of the tubular contents into the renal interstitium. The latter lesion is referred to as tubulorrhexis. In severe acute tubular nephrosis or necrosis resulting from inorganic mercurial salt ingestion, ischemia, as well as direct toxic action of the insulting agent, may have its effect on the tubules. For example, in cases of severe mercury poisoning, there is considerable ulceration of the colonic mucosa, with severe diarrhea and fluid loss leading to hypovolemic shock with its accompanying

peripheral circulatory failure. This set of circumstances results in tubular damage as a result of the ischemia of hypovolemic shock, as well as the direct toxic action of the mercury. Calcification, particularly of the proximal convoluted tubules, may occur in a matter of a few days (Fig. 5-28, *B*). Ultrastructural observations suggest that initially the intracellular calcification is in the mitochondria.

It is known that detectable glomerular damage does not take place in acute poisoning, but in clinical cases of chronic exposure there is documentation of thickening of the glomerular basement membrane leading to proteinuria. An additional mechanism in the development of proteinuria in such cases is tubular damage leading to inability of the tubule to resorb protein, which results in minor degrees of the nephrotic syndrome. Chronic poisoning usually develops in workers in the mercury industry who handle mainly mercuric oxide and calomel (mercurous chloride).

Electron microscopic examination of tubular epithelium of the pars recta of the rat kidney following subcutaneous injection of 4 to 16 mg of mercuric chloride per kilogram of body weight reveals tubular necrosis. The following changes are observed: fragmentation and disruption of the plasma membrane and its appendages, vesiculation and disruption of endoplasmic reticulum, dissociation of polysomes and loss of ribosomes, vesicu-

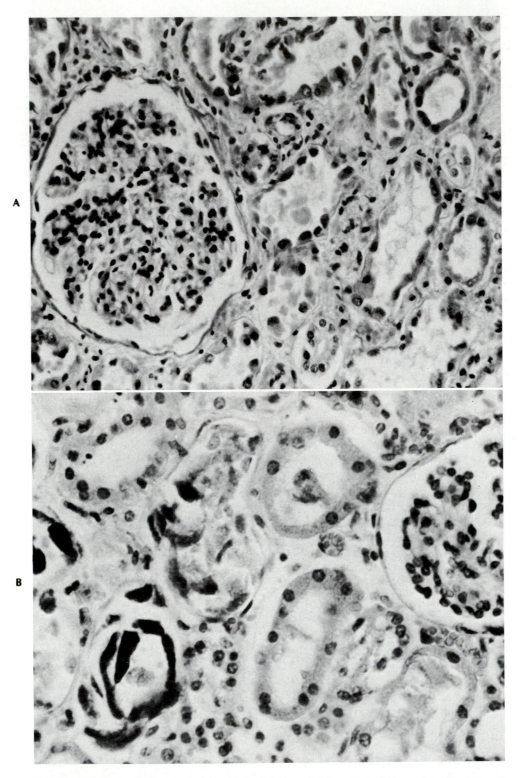

Fig. 5-28. A, Mercury poisoning. Death occurred 7 days after ingestion of mercurial salts. Attempts at regeneration of proximal tubular epithelial cells are observed. However, regeneration was not sufficient to prevent death from renal insufficiency. **B,** Calcification of renal tubules.

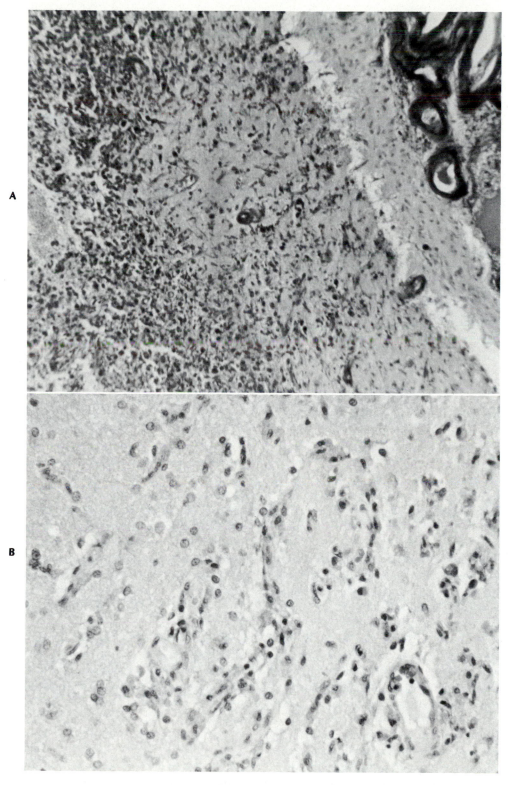

Fig. 5-29. Acute mercury poisoning (10 days' duration). **A,** Necrosis of occipital cortex and "fibrinoid necrosis of pia vessels." **B,** Capillary proliferation and necrosis. (Courtesy Dr. W.D. Hiers, Spartanburg, S.C.)

Continued.

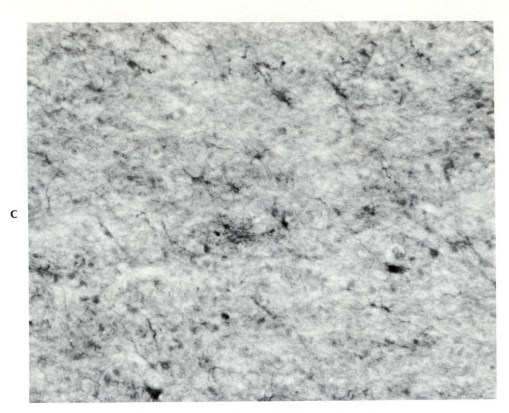

C

Fig. 5-29, cont'd. C, Astrocytic proliferation.

lation of Golgi apparatus, mitochondrial swelling with loss of mitochondrium-dense granules, and condensation of the nuclear chromatin.

In acute mercury poisoning the brain is characterized by necrosis of gray matter, hyalinization of vessels, proliferation of capillaries, and astrocytic proliferation (Fig. 5-29). As stated previously, exposure to both elemental mercury vapor and short-chain alkyl mercury compounds exerts a pronounced effect on the central nervous system. There are similarities and striking differences between these two forms. Mercury vapor effects are neuropsychiatric in nature and occur at relatively low levels. Symptoms include excessive shyness, insomnia, and emotional instability with depression and irritability.

Intention tremors occur with both forms of mercury toxicity. In contrast to mercury vapor toxicity, methyl mercury effects are largely sensorimotor in nature and include paresthesias, constriction of the visual field, loss of hearing, loss of sense of smell and taste, incoordination, paralysis, and abnormal reflexes. In addition, spontaneous fits of laughing and crying and intellectual deterioration occur only in methyl mercury poisoning. Morphologically, in both forms of poisoning degenerative changes are widespread and include degeneration of both exoplasm and the myelin sheath.

In addition to its role as a cytoplasmic toxin, mercury may assume the role of a hapten by virtue of its ability to

denature protein. Uncommonly, mercurial diuretics have been implicated in the pathogenesis of the clinical nephrotic syndrome. In these instances there is a chronic transmembranous glomerulonephritis with dense deposits (presumably immune complexes) located between the visceral epithelial cells and the basement membrane of the glomeruli. Immunostaining has in some instances demonstrated immunoglobulin deposits at these sites. Other heavy metals such as gold have been implicated in the production of transmembranous glomerulonephritis, resulting in the nephrotic syndrome.

Lead

The lead content of some exterior paints and a few interior paints, as well as that of glazing putty, offers a very serious and potential hazard for the development of lead poisoning in children. It is estimated that some 5% to 10% of children between the ages of 1 and 6 years have abnormally high blood levels of lead so that in the United States the projected figure may be as high as 200,000. The habit of eating nonfood objects such as peeling paint and slivers of glazed putty from window frames is known as pica (a reference to the omnivorous magpie). During the past 30 years there has been an increasing effort on the part of public health authorities to urge paint and putty manufacturers to discontinue the use of lead, substituting compounds such as titanium dioxide as an opa-

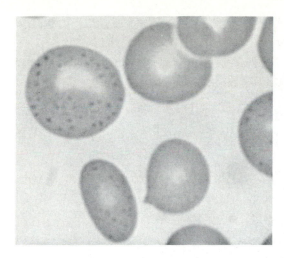

Fig. 5-30. Lead poisoning. Basophilic stippling of red blood cells.

cifier. Consumers of moonshine liquor also risk lead intoxication because metallic lead may be used in the construction of the still.

The diagnosis of lead poisoning encompasses such findings as high blood content of lead, increased free erythrocyte protoporphyrin (**FEP**) content, decreased erythrocyte δ-aminolevulinate dehydrase (**ALAD**) activity, convulsions, intestinal cramps, vomiting, anemia, and basophilic stippling of red blood cells (Fig. 5-30).

Lead inhibits several enzymes, notably ALAD, ferrochelatase, and nucleotidase. Inhibition of the first two enzymes blocks synthesis of hemoglobin. Inhibition of the nucleotidase is the probable cause for basophilic stippling and an associated increase in red cell fragility. Both effects contribute to anemia.

Feeding lead to rats for several weeks causes swelling of kidney mitochondria in vivo and inhibition of the phosphorylating system in vitro. Dense particles are found in both mitochondria and lysosomes of dogs fed lead at high levels for long periods of time. In part, they are composed of magnesium, calcium, and protein (Fig. 5-31, A). Electron-dense, lead-containing intranuclear inclusions are a common finding. The nuclear inclusions also contain other metals and are bound to a highly anionic protein. In humans and experimental animals they appear to be present only in acute lead intoxication and are acid fast when stained with carbol fuchsin (Fig. 5-31, B). Many of the morphologic and functional sequelae of lead poisoning are believed to be secondary results of a primary inhibition of mitochondrial activity by lead.

In acute cases of lead poisoning, the brain is extremely edematous and, microscopically, necrosis of the cerebral and cerebellar white matter may occur, followed by diffuse astrocytic proliferation (Fig. 5-32). This is probably due in part to the role of lead as a mitochondrial poison. Similar to mercurial encephalopathy, there is endothelial proliferation of small capillaries of the white matter and

thickening of small intercerebral arteries. Characteristically, protein droplets accumulate in perivascular spaces (Fig. 5-33). Experimentally, toxic levels of lead acetate may bring about liver necrosis in rats that are fed a diet containing 40% fat. Lipotropic agents, such as the sulfur-containing amino acid methionine, prevent this necrosis. In humans, necrosis of the liver is not observed in acute and chronic lead poisoning.

Cytochrome P450 serum levels are diminished, suggesting some hepatocyte dysfunction. The kidney lesions are restricted to the proximal convoluted tubule, where there is some interference with function, resulting in aminoaciduria. Changes in the mitochondria of the proximal convoluted tubules are observed. In children with chronic lead poisoning, lesions of the myocardium, consisting of edema and fibroblastic activation in the interstitial tissue accompanied by a lymphocytic inflammatory infiltrate, have been described. Similar lesions have not been described in chronic lead poisoning in adults. However, lead has been implicated as an etiologic factor in the production of premature atherosclerosis and of nephrosclerosis with hypertension and cardiac hypertrophy. Experimentally, such factors as vitamin D administration, ultraviolet radiation, increasing body temperatures, and acidosis have been shown to mobilize lead salts from the bony skeleton, thereby increasing the serum levels. The gingival dental margin is pigmented as a result of the deposition of lead sulfite—the so-called lead line of the gums.

Arsenic

Arsenic is a metalloid, exhibiting variable valences −3, +3, +5; it is capable of forming both cationic and anionic salts. It is ubiquitous in distribution in soil, occurring mainly in the pentavalent state, whereas arsenic added to the environment is trivalent. Arsenic trioxide (As_2O_3) is used as the initial reactant in the manufacture of most arsenic compounds. Major uses of white arsenic and other arsenic compounds are as active ingredients of rodenticides, insecticides, fungicides, wood preservatives, soil sterilants, defoliants, feed additives, and weed killers. They are also used in the textile, tanning, and glass industries, as well as in the manufacture of pigments and in antifouling paints. Arsenic has been used therapeutically for 2000 years.

Compounds of arsenic may be absorbed after ingestion or by inhalation. It is generally true that trivalent forms of arsenic are more toxic than pentavalent forms and that most poisoning results from inorganic arsenicals. Arsenate in the valence form is most prevalent in nature and probably does not accumulate in the body, being rapidly excreted by the kidneys. Arsenites, however, bind easily to tissue proteins and accumulate primarily in liver, muscles, hair, nails, and skin. Acute arsenic poisoning has its major manifestation in the stomach, nervous system, and

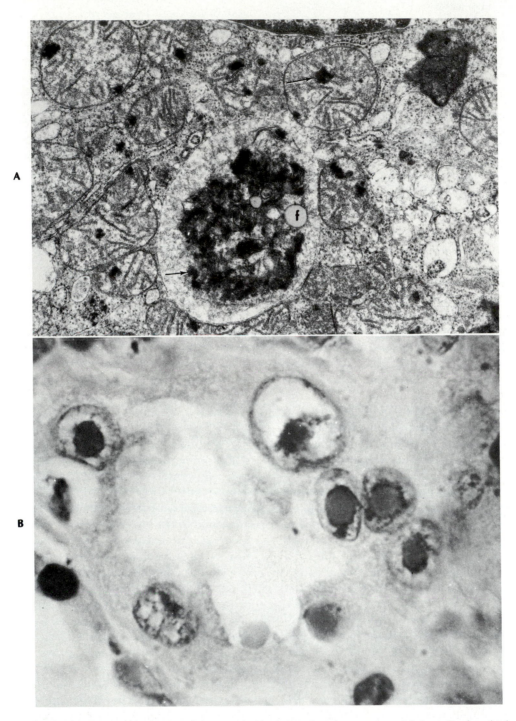

Fig. 5-31. A, Center of micrograph is occupied by large phagolysosome containing mitochondrial fragments, lipofuscin pigment, and fat (*f*). Dense particles are observed in the mitochondria and phagolysosome *(arrows)*. **B,** Lead poisoning. Intranuclear inclusions in cells of proximal convoluted tubules. (37,500×; courtesy William B. Greene, Bakersfield, Calif.)

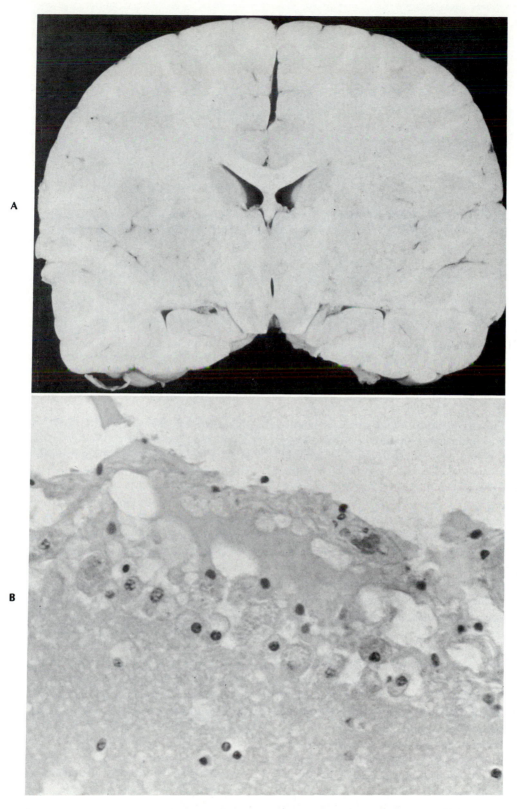

Fig. 5-32. Acute lead poisoning. Patient, 2½-year-old child, died a few hours after admission with diagnosis of brain tumor. **A,** Brain noticeably swollen. Samples of both gray and white matter yielded toxic content of lead. **B,** Subpial vesicles filled with proteinaceous fluid and macrophages. (Courtesy Dr. Stanley M. Aronson, Providence, R.I.)

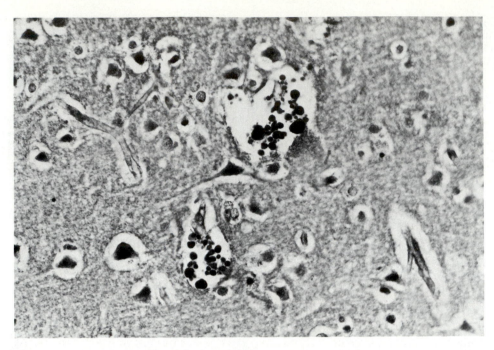

Fig. 5-33. Adult male, a "moonshiner" who was admitted to hospital with convulsions and died from pneumonia. Lead serum level was 140 µg/dl (normal 0 to 50). Note protein globules, prominent astrocyte *(center)*, and perinuclear and perivascular edema. (Phosphotungstic acid and hematoxylin stains; 270×.)

vascular endothelium. Symptoms include nausea; vomiting; diarrhea; acute and severe irritation of the nose, throat, and conjunctiva; severe abdominal pain; and inflammation. Total toxic effects may be produced by the gaseous form of arseniureted hydrogen (arsine, AsH_3). A 30-minute exposure to 250 ppm in air is lethal to humans and animals, the maximum concentration inhalable for 1 hour without toxicity being 5 to 20 ppm. The intensity of the acute toxic reaction depends to a great extent on the physical state of the subject and quantity of the arsenic ingested or inhaled. Shock may cause early death, in which case no striking anatomic changes are evident.

In suspected acute poisoning, obtaining an alkaline reaction with litmus on the vomitus may be helpful. Most common poisons are acid in reaction.

In acute as well as chronic poisoning, significant amounts of arsenic may be identified in clippings of hair, fingernails, and toenails. Contamination of fingernails from vomitus or other external sources must always be kept in mind. Arsenic binds rapidly and firmly with sulfhydryl (SH) groups in nails, hair, and skin. In fact, this ability to combine with SH groups probably explains the lethal action of high concentrations of arsenic by inhibition of respiratory SH enzymes. At necropsy, particles of yellow sulfide of arsenous oxide may be seen attached to the stomach mucosa. These crystals are readily identifiable on chemical and microscopic examination. In patients surviving a few days, there will be congestion, edema, and hemorrhage in the gastric mucosa and

degenerative changes in the heart, liver, and kidneys. There may also be purpuric hemorrhages in various tissues, a striking feature being the discovery of extensive subendocardial splashes of hemorrhage in the left ventricle.

Chronic arsenic poisoning from repeated exposure results in a highly suggestive group of signs and symptoms: loss of weight, nausea, alternating constipation and diarrhea, paresthesia and numbness (frequently in a symmetric stocking-glove distribution), and muscle weakness of the limbs caused by peripheral neuritis. In addition, perforation of the nasal septum, ulceration of the alimentary tract, and tremors may occur. Dermatologic manifestations are protean: loss of hair, increased melanin pigmentation, maculopapular rash, "arsenical dermatitis," and hyperkeratosis of the palms and soles. Reported hepatic damage includes noncirrhotic portal hypertension, cirrhosis, and hemangiosarcoma of the liver. Arsenicals are readily excreted in the sweat, but the main route of elimination is the urine. Moderate anemia resulting from hemolysis and erythropoietic depression may be manifest. Basophilic stippling also occurs frequently. The diagnosis is substantiated by examination of the urine (over 0.2 mg of arsenic per liter is significant), sweat, hair, or nails.

Arsenous acid (arsenous oxide, white arsenic) is the substance most commonly employed in homicidal arsenical poisoning. It is manufactured as a gritty white material in the form of powder or cakes. It is quite insoluble in cold water. It dissolves in hot water, but three fourths of the particles settle out as the water cools. Solubility in caustic soda is easily accomplished. Exhumed bodies testify to the preservative action of arsenic on body tissues. As is the case with fluoride, gross and microscopic examinations are facilitated by prior tissue exposure.

Involvement of arsenic in carcinogenesis is not unequivocally established, since the epidemiologic and experimental findings are in contradiction. Epidemiologic evidence indicates that industrial and agricultural exposure to arsenic is implicated in cancer of the skin and respiratory tract. The individuals at greatest risk are smelter workers, although there is some evidence that women residing near such operations incur a greater incidence of respiratory cancer. Also, studies have implicated arsenic ingestion as goitrogenic, and this possible effect has been confirmed in animals. Epithelial carcinomas of the skin develop with chronic arsenicalism, with latent periods of 3 to 40 or more years. Sound experimental evidence for the carcinogenic activity of inorganic arsenic compounds appears to be nonexistent.

Ferrous sulfate

Accidental ferrous sulfate intoxication is a relatively common and frequently fatal poisoning in childhood. Approximately 2000 cases of acute poisoning occur annually, with only acute intoxications from aspirin, other unknown medications, and phenobarbital occurring more frequently.

After ingestion of ferrous sulfate in toxic doses, there are five clinical phases of subsequent toxicity. The first phase, lasting 30 minutes to 2 hours, is characterized by lethargy, restlessness, hematemesis, abdominal pain, and bloody diarrhea. The direct corrosive effect of iron initiates necrosis of the gastrointestinal mucosa and may result in severe hemorrhagic necrosis and subsequent shock. Shock may also in part be attributed to vasodepressor activity of ferritin resulting from rapid iron absorption through the intact mucosa. "Shock lesions" (centrilobular necrosis of liver cells, acute tubular nephrosis, and brain and pulmonary congestion and edema) are observed. Experimentally, ferrous sulfate–induced liver damage is reminiscent of that seen in humans. At the lethal dose level, severe hepatic necrosis develops by 8 hours. Ultrastructural studies demonstrate mitochondrial damage in parenchymal cells within 2 hours after ingestion. Within 4 hours there is extensive mitochondrial alteration with the accumulation of iron particles between the cristae. As is common after the ingestion of numerous hepatocellular toxins, there is hypertrophy of the smooth endoplasmic reticulum.

The second phase represents apparent recovery, which progresses into the third phase 2 to 12 hours after the first phase. The third phase is heralded by the appearance of shock, cyanosis, fever, and acidoses. The

last results from conversion of ferric $^{(+3)}$ to ferrous$^{(+2)}$ ions with concomitant release of hydrogen ions, as well as accumulation of lactic and citric acids. Signs of pneumonitis and convulsions may occur. The fourth phase occurs 2 to 4 days after ingestion and is characterized by the development of hepatic necrosis, again owing to direct toxic action of iron on mitochondria. Recovery is generally rapid if survival is 3 to 4 days. The fifth phase, 2 to 4 weeks after ingestion, is characterized by gastrointestinal obstruction resulting from gastric or pyloric scarring.

Pertinent autopsy findings are confined to the gastroduodenal mucosa and liver. The mucosa is brown from staining with iron chloride and reveals focal or diffuse superficial necrosis with petechial hemorrhages. Stainable iron is easily identifiable in the mucosal lamina propria and connective tissue of the submucosa. This probably represents diffusion. Iron is readily demonstrated in the endothelium of the submucosal veins and lymphatics, as well as the intrahepatic portal vein branches and Kupffer cells. Staining of the reticulin fibers in the portal areas is easily visualized. The periportal hepatocytes are swollen and contain stainable finely dispersed fat, and loss of glycogen and necrosis may be evident.

Whereas acute overload studies strongly suggest the toxic role of iron for mitochondria, there may not be an analogous situation in chronic iron overload. Fig. 5-34, A, demonstrates hemosiderin-laden hepatocytes prepared from a man who ingested 5000 mixed vitamin and iron pills per annum for several years. He was in "good health," a nutritional faddist, and hepatosplenomegaly was discovered on a routine physical examination. Light and electron microscope examination revealed iron impregnation of collagen and reticulin fibers. The hepatocytes contained large aggregates of membrane-bound hemosiderin and intact mitochondria (Fig. 5-34, B).

Chronic excessive intake of iron may lead to hemosiderosis or hemochromatosis. Hemosiderosis refers to generalized increased iron content in body tissues, particularly the liver and reticuloendothelial system. Hemochromatosis indicates histologic hemosiderosis with diffuse fibrosis of the affected organ.

Cobalt

Cobalt is an essential micronutrient for mammals, but its function is unknown except as a component of vitamin B_{12}. Cobalt salts are generally well absorbed in normal dietary amounts, but larger doses are more poorly absorbed. It is not sequestered easily, since it is stored in intestinal mucosa and lost through desquamation of the epithelium. Cobalt salts are retained primarily in the heart, liver, bone marrow, pancreas, kidneys, and spleen. Excretion is mainly urinary. Poisoning can occur from inhalation of cobalt alloy vapors in industrial settings and from the therapeutic use of cobalt-containing

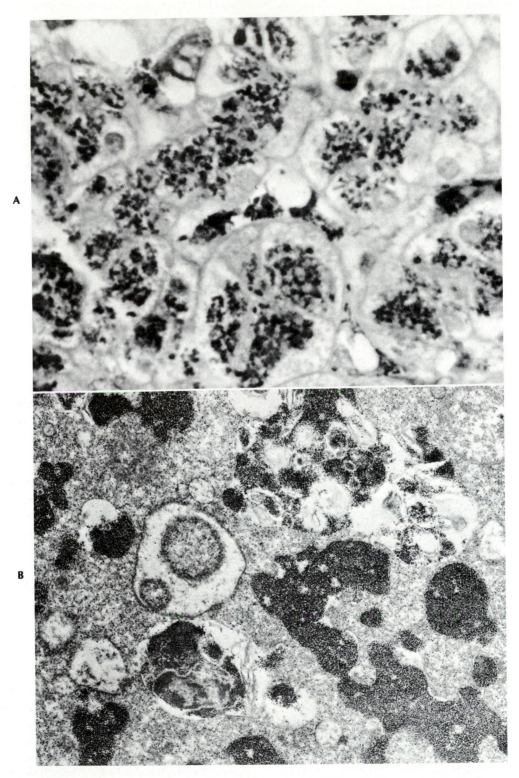

Fig. 5-34. Excessive iron intake. **A,** Food faddist consumed 5000 mixed iron and vitamin pills per annum for several years. Enlarged liver was an incidental finding on routine physical examination. Hepatocytes are loaded with hemosiderin. **B,** Normal amount of glycogen and dense intracellular aggregates of hemosiderin. No mitochondrial damage is noted. (34,000×.)

compounds in treatment of anemia and radioactive cobalt in cancer treatment.

Polycythemia characteristically occurs with ingestion of excessive amounts of cobalt. Acute toxicity following ingestion has been reported to lead to vomiting, paralysis, lowering of blood pressure, liver and adrenal hemorrhages, alveolar thickening, and renal and pancreatic degeneration. Inhalation causes acute lung inflammation, edema, and hemorrhages; massive pericardial effusions; and peritoneal effusions.

Before the banning of cobalt in proprietary preparations, it was not uncommon to see diffuse thyroid hyperplasia primarily in children treated for anemia with Roncovite, an enteric-coated, ferrous-cobaltous chloride preparation. This goitrogenic compound did not give rise to thyrotoxicosis. Experimentally, the role of cobalt in stimulating erythrocytosis is well known.

A decade ago, beer manufacturers in the United States and Belgium added excessive amounts of cobalt acetate to their products so that the froth would stick to the sides of the glass to produce a good "head." However, the levels of ingestion were lower than doses tolerated in other conditions, such as for treatment of anemia. Many of the beer drinkers were in a state of thiamine and nutritional deficiency, and it has been shown that thiamine and protein deficiencies enhance the cardiotoxicity of cobalt. In addition, ethanol sensitizes animals to cobalt toxicity. The situation is comparable to so-called alcoholic cardiomyopathy, making it impossible to characterize the entities of cobalt and alcoholic myocardiosis.

Grossly, the hearts of persons who have died of what has been referred to as beer drinkers' heart disease have shown cardiac dilatation and hypertrophy. Signs and symptoms were those of congestive heart failure. Histologically, in cases in which cobalt was a suspected factor in the death of the patient, the myocardium revealed vacuole formation and accumulation of sudanophilic material that appeared as fine droplets in all parts of the sarcoplasm. A slight and fine focal fibrosis was observed that is interpreted as a condensation fibrosis occurring after myocytolysis. Although pyknotic nuclei may be observed, there is no extensive overt necrosis.

Experimentally, structural changes in animal myofibrils and mitochondria have been produced by cobalt administration alone. Cobalt ions are known to depress oxygen uptake in heart mitochondria by inhibiting the enzymes α-ketoglutarate dehydrogenase and pyruvate dehydrogenase.

Mild cobalt toxicity has been reported to cause hyperglycemia in dogs and rats because of transient and reversible damage to alpha cells of the pancreas.

Although no evidence for carcinogenicity of dietary cobalt is known, it has been shown experimentally that oxides and sulfides of cobalt cause cancer in animals. Tumors reported include fibrosarcomas, liposarcomas, and tumors in the thyroid gland and at injection sites.

Cadmium

Acute inhalation of relatively large concentrations of cadmium vapors produces acute cadmium pneumonia approximately 8 to 10 hours after inhalation of the vapors. Histologically, the lung is characterized by diffuse alveolar damage, with striking congestion and edema of the alveolar capillaries. Death occurs in approximately 16% of those exposed to high concentration of the vapors. Chronic inhalation of smaller amounts of cadmium vapors can result in interstitial fibrosis of the lungs. This eventuates in the honeycomb lung that is the result of repeated attacks of acute bronchiolitis and interstitial pneumonia with reparative scarring (Fig. 5-35).

There are several reports of an increased incidence of emphysema in persons exposed to low concentrations of cadmium fumes over a long period of time. The maximum permissible level of cadmium vapors in the air, in both England and the United States, is 100 μg/cubic meter. According to Nandi and associates,[223a] the cadmium contained in cigarettes is transmitted to the lungs during smoking. One pack of 20 cigarettes contains 30 μg of cadmium. One must conclude therefore that cadmium accumulates in the tissues of heavy smokers and could theoretically cause lung, liver, and kidney disease. However, if *all* the cadmium in two packs of cigarettes were inhaled, this would still be less cadmium than would be inspired in 2 hours of normal breathing at maximum safe levels of atmospheric cadmium. There is no unchallenged evidence that cigarette smoking causes emphysema. There is no question, on the other hand, that cigarette smoking results in acute and chronic bronchitis and worsens the state of emphysema. Emphysema may develop in cadmium workers in the alkaline battery industry as a result of exposure to low concentrations of cadmium fumes over a long period of time. To properly assess the significance of the relationship of cadmium to the development of emphysema, further epidemiologic and other studies are required. At the present time there is no information available as to the type and degree of emphysema seen at autopsy in such individuals.

Nickel

Nickel and its compounds have been implicated in producing a contact type of dermatitis, carcinoma of the lung and nasal passages, and various soft tissue malignancies in experimental animals. Nickel dermatitis has been noted to be a rather common occurrence. Nickel workers in Great Britain, Germany, Norway, Russia, Japan, and Canada have been noted to have an increased incidence of respiratory cancer, particularly of the nasal passages.

Experimental studies with nickel carbonyl, $Ni(CO)_4$, have produced carcinomas in rats by inhalation of the vapor and by parenteral administration. It is interesting to note that, even with intravenous administration of nickel carbonyl, the lungs are the target of the acute reaction. There is also an increased mitotic index of the

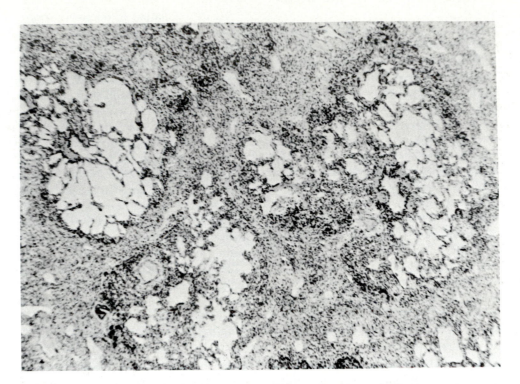

Fig. 5-35. Cadmium inhalation—dog lung. Interstitial fibrosis, lymphocyte infiltration, and expanded alveolar sacs. (Courtesy Dr. Charles B. Carrington, Stanford, Calif.)

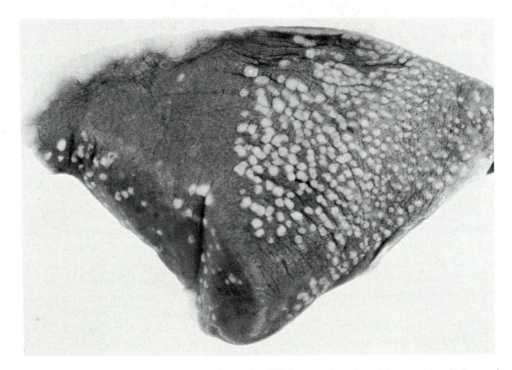

Fig. 5-36. Chronic nickel sulfate poisoning in dog. White subpleural nodules contain cholesterol macrophages. Edge of lung is pale after air trapping attributable to chronic bronchiolitis with mucus plugging.

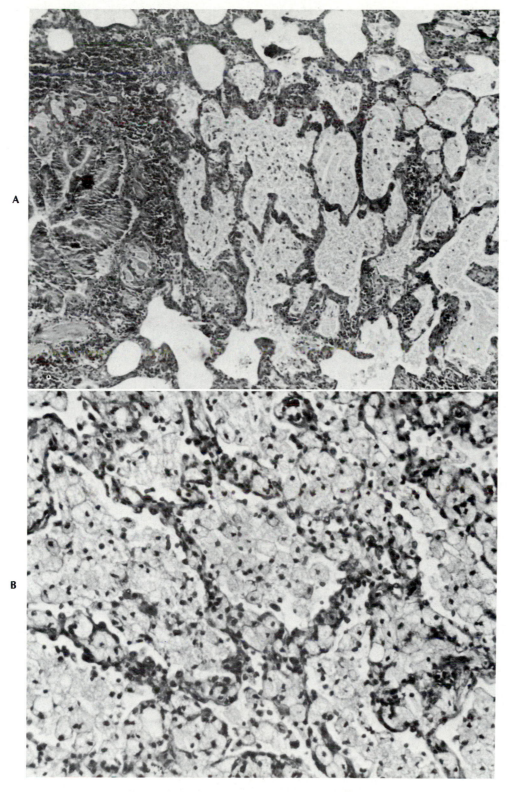

Fig. 5-37. Nickel sulfate. **A,** Bronchiolitis with narrowing of bronchial lumen has led to accumulation of cholesterol macrophages in alveolar sacs—often called "golden pneumonia." **B,** Higher magnification of section shown in **A.**

bronchiolar and alveolar epithelial cells. To a lesser extent the liver shows loss of glycogen, the kidney shows sporadic vacuolization of the proximal convoluted tubules without necrosis, and the adrenal glands reveal intense congestion of the cortical sinusoids. When viewed by electron microscopy, the proliferative reaction of the alveolar epithelium appears to involve both the granular and membranous pneumocytes. Discharge of cytoplasmic inclusions and granular pneumocytes is noted. The membranous pneumocytes develop large nucleoli, nuclei, and cytoplasm and have a distinct increase in cytoplasmic organelles, including free ribosomes, endoplasmic reticulum, and Golgi zones.

There are a few studies concerning the long-range effects of continued oral ingestion of nickel in mammals. Dogs fed nickel sulfate orally for a period of 2 years show a remarkable reaction in the lungs. Grossly there are pale subpleural collections of cholesterol macrophages that are associated with the peripheral chronic bronchiolitis observed (Figs. 5-36 and 5-37). This may be the result of irritative qualities of the nickel ion being secreted by the bronchial mucosa. Whereas nickel carbonyl has been implicated in the production of respiratory neoplasia, it is not known if nickel salts (sulfate, chloride) consumed orally over a long period of time cause tissue damage or serve as carcinogens.

Thallium

The etiologic agent of thallotoxicosis is a heavy metal. Thallium sulfate or acetate appears in rat poisons and common insecticides. Because it is one of the most toxic metals, it has been used as a homicidal poison and for suicidal purposes. As a medicinal agent, the compound has enjoyed its greatest popularity through the years in the topical treatment of ringworm. It also has been used as a depilatory agent. In fact, some cases of accidental poisoning have occurred when the use of the agent in this manner resulted in rapid absorption. The metal is dispersed widely throughout all the body tissues and is excreted slowly. It interferes with the telogen phase of hair follicle growth, and because of its delayed excretion, alopecia may occur approximately 2 weeks after ingestion. Interestingly, axillary and facial hair and the inner one third of the eyebrows are spared, a feature of diagnostic importance.

Children are particularly susceptible to the effects of thallium compounds, with ingestion of 10 mg being responsible for fatal outcome. The lethal dose of thallium acetate in adults is approximately 1 g. Acute poisoning appears 12 to 36 hours after ingestion of a toxic amount. The signs and symptoms are abdominal pain, vomiting, and varied neurologic findings such as ataxia and other manifestations of toxic encephalopathy. Morphologically, neurons, nerve fibers, and glial elements throughout the central nervous system reveal various degenerative and even necrotic changes. More than 40 products con-

taining 1% to 3% thallium salts are available in retail stores in the United States today. Reed and associates[240] point out that the ingestion of 1 ounce of a pesticide containing 1% thallium could be fatal to a small child. The actual mode of toxicity remains unclear.

Uranium

After the administration of uranyl nitrate to rats, renal tubular lesions become manifest. There is loss of the brush borders, dispersion of mitochondrial matrix, fragmentation and vesiculation of endoplasmic reticulum, and disruption of cytoplasmic membrane with whorl formation. The earliest observable changes after the administration of this compound appear to be clumping and margination of chromatin accompanied by nuclear shrinkage. This observation may indicate that uranyl nitrate attacks the nucleus before attacking cytoplasmic organelles, the intactness of which is responsible for the resorptive mechanism.

Platinum

For many years chemical injury from platinum was confined to the syndrome of platinosis, characterized by excessive histamine release and the concomitant hypersensitivity manifestations, in industrial platinum workers. In 1969, however, the compound cis-dichlorodiammine-platinum (II) was shown to be active against a transplantable rodent tumor. Following extensive clinical evaluation, this compound was marketed as cisplatin in 1979. It is active against squamous cell carcinoma, lymphosarcoma, pancreatic carcinoma, and fibrosarcoma. It is particularly effective against metastatic ovarian tumors when combined with doxorubicin and cyclophosphamide and against metastatic testicular tumors when combined with vinblastine and bleomycin.

Following intravenous administration, the first side effects noted in most patients are severe nausea and vomiting, occurring within a period of a few minutes to a few hours. This common reaction is so severe and long lasting that some patients refuse a second course of treatment. The mechanism of this effect is unknown.

The principal dose-limiting toxic action of cisplatin is nephrotoxicity; histologically similar renal lesions have been observed in rats, dogs, and humans after administration of the drug. The earliest marker of proximal tubular damage is an increased rate of excretion of $beta_2$ microglobulins; this is followed by increases in BUN and serum creatinine levels, as well as hyperuricemia. The damage is considered mild when BUN and serum creatinine values are 25 to 35 mg/dl and 1.5 to 2 mg/dl, respectively, and severe when the BUN value increases to greater than 50 mg/dl or the serum creatinine level reaches more than 2.5 mg/dl, or both.

Histologically, the proximal tubular necrosis resembles that observed following administration of certain other heavy metals. Necrosis and desquamation of tubular epithelium are accompanied by the presence of intraluminal granular material and cellular debris. Cisplatin inactivates mitochondrial ATPase activity, thus inhibiting the energy-dependent functions of the tubular cells. Co-administration of cisplatin with large fluid volumes and mannitol to promote diuresis can ameliorate renal toxicity to some extent, but once incurred, damage is frequently irreversible.

Ototoxicity is observed in almost 30% of patients treated with a single dose of cisplatin at 50 mg/m². This is manifested by tinnitus or hearing loss in the high-frequency range, or both, and is more severe in children than in adults. Additional toxic effects of cisplatin include leukopenia, thrombocytopenia, a normocytic anemia, and marrow hypoplasia. Noted less often is neurotoxicity, characterized by peripheral neuropathies. Anaphylactic-like reactions have also been reported.

Catecholamines

The vasopressor amines are commonly used to treat clinical states of shock and myocardial infarction. As early as 1906, experiments using multiple intravenous injections in rabbits were found to result in the appearance of hyaline necrosis with granular change, loss of muscle striation, and mononuclear leukocyte infiltration of the cardiac muscle fibers. The myocardial damage was not the result of arterial lesions, since no vascular change was demonstrated. Healing was characterized by interstitial edema and fibrosis of the myocardium.

Since that time, experimental cardiac lesions have been produced with epinephrine, isoproterenol, norepinephrine, and ephedrine. The most severe lesions are produced by isoproterenol, and the severity of the lesions can be correlated with increasing dosage. In cats, electrical stimulation of the midbrain reticular formation, the stellate ganglion, or the lateral hypothalamus can produce demonstrable myofibrillar degeneration. The degeneration is attributable to the rising concentration of catecholamines that have been induced by stimulation of the central nervous system pathways. The buildup and release of catecholamine in granular vesicles in close apposition to the sympathetic nervous system have been well demonstrated by Reichenbach and Benditt[251] after midbrain stimulation and the administration of isoproterenol. Histologically, by the end of the first day after the administration of norepinephrine or isoproterenol, the myocardial fibers are the "seat" of cytoplasmic banding, pyknosis of myocardial nuclei, loss of myocardial nuclear staining, and mononuclear proliferation (Fig. 5-38). At this stage there is disorganization of the cardiac myofi-

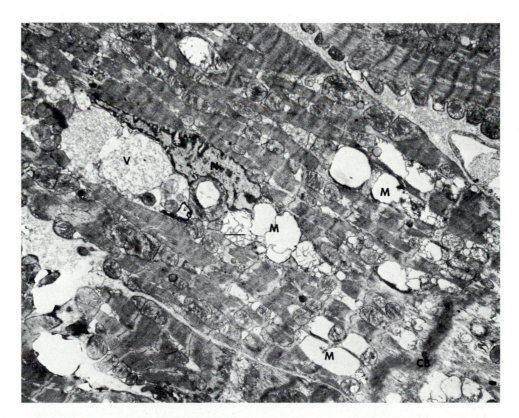

Fig. 5-38. Experimental isoproterenol hydrochloride in dog myocardium. After administration of 8 μg/kg body weight/minute for 2 hours, alterations include swelling of many mitochondria *(M)* with cristolysis and myofibrillar disruption with formation of contracture bands *(CB)*. Clumping and margination of nuclear chromatin *(N)* and vacuolization *(V)* of extracellular space. (4000×; courtesy Dr. David W. Hiott, Walterboro, S.C.)

brils, and by the end of 3 days mineralization of mitochondria is evident. After 9 days, myocytolysis and fibrosis appear.

Factors capable of potentiating catecholamine induction of myofibrillar degeneration include sodium excess, desoxycorticosterone acetate (Doca) administration to animals deficient in dietary potassium, and low potassium content of the myocardial cells. Myofibrillar degeneration has been reported in patients dying of pheochromocytoma. Histologic findings in these patients were cytoplasmic band formation and mononuclear cell infiltration. Myofibrillar degeneration is not associated solely with endogenous or exogenous catecholamine states. On the other hand, it does explain the focal subendocardial patches of necrosis sometimes found after a variety of intracranial spontaneous and traumatic hemorrhages. It would seem logical that the cytotoxic effects of catecholamine may be the mechanism responsible for cardiac injury in a number of exogenous and endogenous disease states. From the standpoint of the pathologist, the recent enlightening literature concerning catecholamine damage may go a long way toward explaining early myofibrillar degeneration that was previously attributed to agonal or postmortem alterations. In addition, some cases of idiopathic myocardial fibrosis may in the future be discovered to be attributable to catecholamine myofibril toxicity.

Barbiturates

The barbiturates are similar in action to alcohol in that they are central nervous system depressants. The severity of the depression depends on the barbiturate used, mode of administration, degree of tolerance, presence or absence of other drugs in the body, and state of excitability of the individual. The potentially fatal oral doses of barbiturates are 5 g (long-acting) or 3 g (short-acting). Potentially fatal blood levels are 8 mg/dl of a long-acting or 3.5 mg/dl of a short-acting barbiturate, indicating that short-acting barbiturates are more toxic. However, it is generally accepted that considerable individual variation exists. Recovery after the ingestion of 33 g of phenobarbital has been observed.

Barbiturates (goof balls, redbirds, yellow jackets, blue heavens), like innumerable other drugs, may play the role of a hapten and give rise to a wide spectrum of hypersensitivity tissue reactions. Notable among these is the development of polyarteritis nodosa lesions indistinguishable from the acute lesions of the spontaneous disease. Barbiturates are a leading cause of dermatitis medicamentosa, challenging penicillin for first place. Furthermore, the compounds may cause severe skin reactions such as those seen in exfoliative dermatitis and the Stevens-Johnson syndrome. Clinicians and pathologists are familiar with the large bullous lesions of the skin that develop in approximately 6% to 9% of patients with acute barbiturate intoxication. They are often referred to as the barbiturate blister (Fig. 5-39). Clinically, they are adequately characteristic to be valuable in the differential diagnosis of coma. The lesions are probably caused by a pressure phenomenon and are not the result of a specific toxic effect. In support of this is the common finding of the lesions on the inner aspects of the knees and ankles. The presence of lesions in other sites may be explained if the precise position of the patient when found is known.

Microscopically, the lesions are characterized by

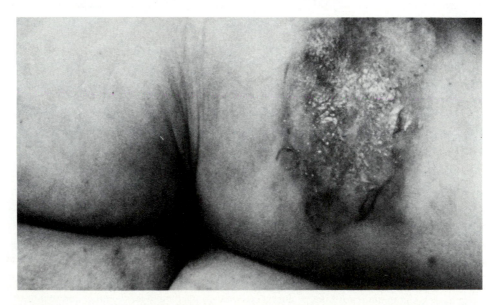

Fig. 5-39. Acute barbiturate intoxication. Patient died in coma 10 days after ingestion of pills. Irregularly outlined lesion of thigh is characterized by vesicles and excoriated epidermis with a dark coloration at periphery. (Courtesy Dr. Sandra E. Conradi, Charleston, S.C.)

intraepidermal and subepidermal vesicles and bullae. Necrosis of eccrine sweat gland epithelia is a common observation. The absence of abundant lymphocytes, plasma cells, macrophages, vasculitis, and granulomas leads the morphologist away from considering hypersensitivity-immunologic reactions as causative mechanisms for the production of the skin lesions. Clear-cut zones of hemorrhagic infarction are found in the subcutaneous fat. The barbiturates, like chloral hydrate, DDT isomers, and alcohol, generate hyperplasia of the smooth endoplasmic reticulum in the hepatocyte. This is the morphologic reflection of "enzyme induction," resulting in accelerated enzymatic action in the liver microsomes. This mechanism explains the depression of anticoagulant response in patients receiving both barbiturate derivatives and bishydroxycoumarin (dicumarol). The increased enzyme activity stimulated by barbiturates and chloral hydrate rapidly metabolizes the coumarin drug. In contrast, phenylbutazone and thyroxine inhibit the breakdown of coumarin, leading to an accentuated prolongation of the prothrombin time. Failure to recognize these effects may result in serious hemorrhagic complications.

Barbiturates should be administered with caution to patients who have hepatocellular damage such as fatty liver, alcoholic hepatitis, viral hepatitis, or severe generalized circulatory failure. The alcoholic with cirrhosis may show a prolonged peak of blood barbiturate after therapeutic dosage. The investigation of apparently natural deaths that actually resulted from alcohol-barbiturate intake is of immense importance to the medical examiner, the coroner, and the public. The *manner* of death determined from such investigations appears on the death certificate as accident, suicide, or undetermined. At the same time the probable *cause* of death may be clearly attributed to alcohol-barbiturate intake. The finding of a suicide note aids the investigator. On the other hand, a history of alcoholic and barbiturate intake is of little help in determining whether fatal consumption was intentional or accidental. What appears on the death certificate is important, since relatives are frequently emotionally upset when proved suicide occurs and rightfully resent a designation of suicide on suspicious grounds only. An understanding of the additive effect of alcohol and barbiturate is essential in determining the probable cause of death in such cases.

Currently, barbiturates are being used increasingly for nonmedicinal purposes and have outstripped alcohol in popularity in many age and socioeconomic groups. The question of accuracy of postmortem blood examinations is often raised. In a refrigerated room the blood-alcohol level remains stable for several days, but it is not known whether this is true of barbiturate. As mentioned previously, an estimation of the amount of barbiturate consumed, from postmortem chemical examination of the blood, depends on such factors as the varying speed of action of the compound and individual variation in metabolism, physical activity, and functional integrity of the liver cells. Obviously, in many accidental deaths caused by alcohol-barbiturate poisoning, some degree of liver damage exists. In his series of barbiturate suicides, Teare notes that "over 90% of cases were found dead of were dead on arrival at the hospital—suggesting that death was rapid, though of course, many suicides choose circumstances and places for their final act where they are unlikely to be disturbed."[261] It is noteworthy that decomposition will raise the postmortem blood level of alcohol, whereas the opposite is true for barbiturates. In the analysis of suspected alcohol-barbiturate deaths, it is mandatory to observe the stomach contents, when present, and to submit a specimen for barbiturate content. Sometimes the contents are "loaded" with barbiturate but no barbiturate is found in the blood. A finding of this nature may be attributed to death from acute coma and aspiration after alcohol intake before sufficient time had elapsed for barbiturate absorption.

Narcotics

Complications of intravenous administration of narcotics (heroin and morphine) by addicts are arteritis and thrombosis of pulmonary arteries, arterioles, and capillaries ("mainline lesions") with the result of pulmonary hypertension and cor pulmonale. Addicts injecting a mixture known as "blue velvet" (concentrated paregoric and a tripelennamine hydrochloride tablet) and "red devil" (contents of a Seconal capsule) have shown these lesions. The offending agent was found to be the talc contained in the tripelennamine hydrochloride tablet and the starch granules in the Seconal capsule. Kranier, Berman, and Wishnick[262] reported a similar case in a meperidine (Demerol) addict, in whom granulomatous lesions were found in the lungs. Again, the offending agent was talc, which was used as a filler in the Demerol oral tablet. Both starch and talc have been shown experimentally to produce these lesions. Multiple scars on the skin may be observed. Frequently the addict does not heed the principles of asepsis, so that pitted scars result from healed abscesses at the site of injection. Recent lesions have an ecchymotic appearance.

Homicidal death may follow the forced administration of a "hot shot," consisting of a narcotic plus strychnine. Accidental or homicidal death may result from the addict's administering a purer blend than he or she has been accustomed to receiving. Therefore the addict accidentally takes an overdose of the narcotic, not knowing of the increased potency at the same dose level. Heroin "cut" with lactose can be detected by tasting the sweet flavor. Quinine reestablishes the bitter taste of the narcotic. Some addicts have died as a result of hypersensitivity reaction to quinine.

Morphine may play a role in the death of patients receiving oxygen therapy. Because of its depressant action, morphine predisposes such patients to oxygen toxicity. Likewise, this characteristic of morphine makes it contraindicated in alcohol poisoning. Since morphine is detoxified by the liver, patients with hepatocellular damage should not receive the morphine group of narcotics. Morphine causes vasoconstriction of the bronchial smooth musculature. The administration of morphine to an individual in a state of status asthmaticus (bronchiolar spasm, mucus plugging, and air trapping with oxygen retention) may rapidly bring on death. The postmortem appearance in cases of morphine poisoning is not particularly striking. Frequently the appearance is that of asphyxia. Cyanosis, congestion of the viscera, and abundant, dark, fluid blood may be observed. If an addict has taken morphine plus quinine, the latter may be identified in the urine. This finding, particularly with the fluorescent demonstration of quinine sulfate in a fresh skin puncture wound, is significant. Sulfuric acid is applied to the skin, and it rapidly penetrates the dermis to combine with quinine, forming quinine sulfur that is fluorescent under Wood's light. Congested lungs are commonly "beefy red" in fatal cases, probably attributable, in part, to the alveolar capillary damage from quinine.

The student should keep in mind that morphine may influence laboratory tests. Elevation of serum amylase levels after constriction of the sphincter of Oddi, leading to increased intraductular pressure, may occur after morphine administration. The increased intraluminal pressure "drives" amylase into the periacinar venular network. Morphine can cause BSP retention; elevation of transaminase levels in certain patients can precipitate attacks of acute intermittent porphyria.

Other agents
Carbon monoxide

The incidence of carbon monoxide intoxication is increasing at a faster rate than population growth and hence is of even greater significance than in the past. Although the popularity of carbon monoxide as a suicide agent has been superseded by the barbiturates, this form of intoxication has taken on greater significance in view of space and underwater conquests where confinement in enclosed space is necessary.

The medicolegal aspects of carbon monoxide intoxication are of great importance when related to the public interest and safety. Dangerous levels of carbon monoxide may accumulate when almost any heating device is defective from incomplete combustion of any carbon fuel. If negligence on the part of manufacturer leads to illness or death from carbon monoxide intoxication, the medicolegal importance of suits and compensation insurance becomes obvious. The proper investigation of a case of suspected suicide carries with it great responsibility. At first glance it is often impossible to determine whether the death of a victim of carbon monoxide poisoning is attributable to suicide, accident, or homicide. An exhaustive history at the scene by persons acting in the public interest (medical examiners, coroners, law enforcement officers, pathologists) is mandatory. The importance of the classification of death as homicide or accident is obvious. On the other hand, to glibly designate a death as suicide from carbon monoxide intoxication may lead to considerable psychologic trauma to the victim's family and friends.

From the purely medical standpoint, it should be appreciated that carbon monoxide intoxication may be responsible for coma. If recognition is not prompt and therapy is not quickly instituted, irreparable damage to the brain may ensue with eventual death. In the investigation of medical coma, blood is usually drawn and a reserve sample is placed in the refrigerator. This sample may be used to detect the stable carboxyhemoglobin hours or days after the specimen has been drawn. In interpreting the level of carbon monoxide, a number of factors must be taken into consideration. Many smokers and some industrial workers normally carry a level of 10% carbon monoxide saturation in the blood. The functional integrity of the cardiovascular and pulmonary systems, the rate of blood flow in the vascular system, the number of red cells and total amount of hemoglobin available, and the age, physical activity at the time of exposure, and metabolic rate of the individual will affect the response to a given level of carbon monoxide. It is apparent that survival depends on the amount and length of exposure, as well as all of those factors that normally govern the optimum exchange of oxygen between the red cells and the parenchymal cells of the body. The presence of drugs such as alcohol and barbiturates in depressant doses will enhance the effects of carbon monoxide.

Means of detection include sampling of carbon monoxide by air-sampling devices and the rapid detection of carboxyhemoglobin in the blood. Recording spectrophotometry allows the rapid identification of carbon monoxide using as little as two drops of blood. Gas chromatographic demonstration of small quantities of carbon monoxide is used in practically all toxicology laboratories. An exact determination of blood carbon monoxide can be made by infrared spectrophotometry.

Carbon monoxide is odorless and tasteless. It unites with hemoglobin to form a compound, carboxyhemoglobin, which is over 200% more stable than oxyhemoglobin. Carbon monoxide displaces normal oxyhemoglobin and interferes with the exchange of oxygen between the red cells and the extravascular tissue. In fatal cases there is a cherry-red livor of the skin from the color of the carboxyhemoglobin that is present in the superficial capillaries. One can observe the blanching or lack of cherry-red color over the pressure areas because of mechanical obliteration of the skin capillaries. In cases of death not related to carbon monoxide poisoning, there is a blue

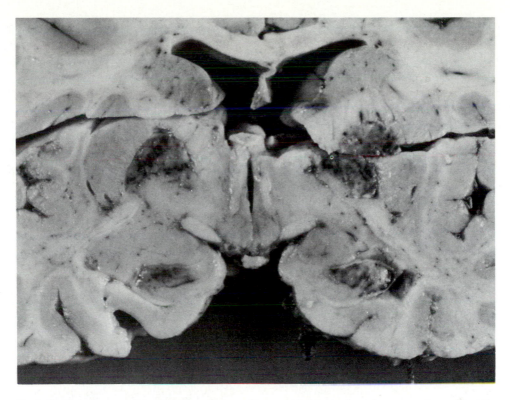

Fig. 5-40. Carbon monoxide poisoning. Patient, 15-year-old girl, was found comatose in automobile with motor running. She remained in coma for 5 days. Distribution of hemorrhagic necrosis is typical. Cross section of cerebral hemisphere at level of lenticular nuclei shows bilateral hemorrhage and necrosis of globus pallidus and hippocampus. (Courtesy Dr. Stanley M. Aronson, Providence, R.I.)

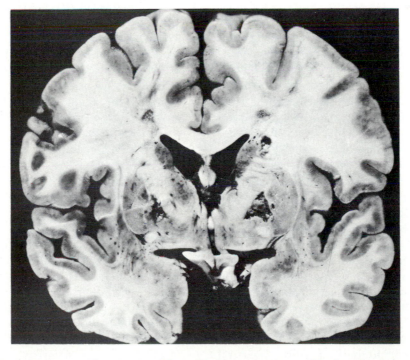

Fig. 5-41. Carbon monoxide poisoning. Bilateral necrosis of globus pallidus in patient who died 41 days after exposure. Also, necrosis of centrum semiovale, which may be caused by secondary vascular changes. Cystic transformation is evident. (From Finck, P.A.: Milit. Med. **131:**1513, 1966; AFIP.)

discoloration of the skin (livor mortis) after somatic death. In this instance the blue color is caused by reduced hemoglobin. A cherry livor also may be caused by fluoroacetate or cyanide poisoning or by freezing. Fluoroacetate and cyanide are cellular toxins that paralyze the metabolism of the cells so that utilization of the freed oxygen from oxyhemoglobin cannot be incorporated into the cytoplasm.

In the acute, rapidly fatal type of carbon monoxide poisoning, anatomic findings may be limited to the observation of small petechial hemorrhages of serosal surfaces and white matter of the cerebral hemispheres. However, if the individual survives 4 to 5 days or more, gross lesions become evident and are characterized by striking hemorrhagic necrosis of the basal ganglia and lamellar necrosis of the cortical gray matter (Fig. 5-40). If there is longer survival, cystic areas develop in these regions (Fig. 5-41). The subendocardial layer of the myocardium is characterized by minute foci of necrosis. The findings in the brain and heart are not pathognomonic for carbon monoxide poisoning and may be seen in other conditions in which acute severe hypoxia develops.

Carbon tetrachloride

Shortly after the ingestion of as little as 5 ml to as much as 100 ml of carbon tetrachloride (a halogenated hydrocarbon) and depending on the resistance of the individual (high-fat diet increases the susceptibility to the toxicity), swelling and hydropic degeneration of the centrilobular hepatic cells develop. These changes progress to a diffuse fatty degeneration and necrosis in the centrilobular parenchyma with collapse of the reticulum network, followed shortly by hemorrhage and leukocytic infiltration. The relative specificity of this agent for the centrilobular areas appears to be related not to ischemia but to a direct effect of the agent on the cells in the centrilobular area. Autoradiographic studies have shown a rapid uptake of carbon tetrachloride by the cytoplasm and nuclei of the cells of the centrilobular areas (Fig. 5-42). There is moderate uptake in the midzonal areas and very little uptake in the periportal areas. Autoradiographic evidence shows that radioactive ^{14}C and carbon tetrachloride remain in the centrilobular areas as long as 2 days after ingestion. Regeneration of liver parenchyma begins on approximately the third day and is often completed by 2½ weeks.

The initial intracellular structure to be involved is the endoplasmic reticulum, which is damaged within 30 minutes of the administration of carbon tetrachloride, whereas the mitochondria survive unaltered for several hours. Experimentally, protein synthesis is reduced within 2 hours of poisoning. Fatty acids are mobilized from peripheral fat depots to the liver. In the liver cell they are oxidized to triglyceride. The latter is conjugated with globulin to form lipoproteins, which are secreted.

This mechanism is believed to be responsible for the formation of plasma lipoproteins. If protein synthesis (carrier protein) is blocked, lipoprotein is not formed and fat accumulates in the liver cell. This explains the steatosis resulting from the inhibition of protein synthesis by carbon tetrachloride. At the same time, it must be realized that diminution of protein synthesis plays no major role in the pathogenesis of liver cell necrosis. Ultrastructurally, an early observation is the direct "toxic" attack on the endoplasmic reticulum, leading to the detachment of ribosomes.

Renal lesions in acute carbon tetrachloride poisoning consist of acute tubular nephrosis or necrosis. Microscopically, tubulovenous communications and calcified necrotic tubular cells, the latter reminiscent of acute mercurial nephrosis, are observed.

Boric acid

Boric acid (boron) is a white crystalline powder used as a weak antiseptic, a food preservative, and a buffering and fungistatic agent in talcum powder. Fatalities have resulted from the accidental ingestion of boron or in some cases from the therapeutic use of the compound. Accidental ingestion has involved children almost entirely. Many of the accidents have resulted from boric acid powder being mistaken for an infant formula, from borate powders or solutions being left in places accessible to small children, and from the ingestion of sodium perborate as a mouthwash. In some instances the application of boric acid to large areas of denuded burned skin or excoriated dermatitis has resulted in boric acid poisoning.

A lethal dose of boric acid is estimated to be between 5 and 15 g. After ingestion a gastroenteritis develops and results in severe diarrhea. Autopsy findings consist of cerebral edema, petechial hemorrhages in the white matter of the brain, and acute tubular nephrosis or necrosis of the proximal convoluted tubules of the kidney. In the majority of cases a hemorrhagic cystitis is found. The skin manifestations in children are fairly constant and typical. Erythema is usually intense and may cover the entire body. The subject presents a characteristic "boiled lobster" appearance.

Hexachlorophene

Hexachlorophene is a chlorinated bisphenol. Hexachlorophene liquid soap is bactericidal and to some extent fungicidal. It has wide topical application, and many surgical and germicidal soaps contain this compound in a concentration of approximately 3%. Bathing of infants with detergents containing hexachlorophene has been shown to reduce greatly the incidence of staphylococcal infection. However, frequent bathing of premature infants may lead to a pronounced disturbance of myelin in the white matter of the reticular formation of

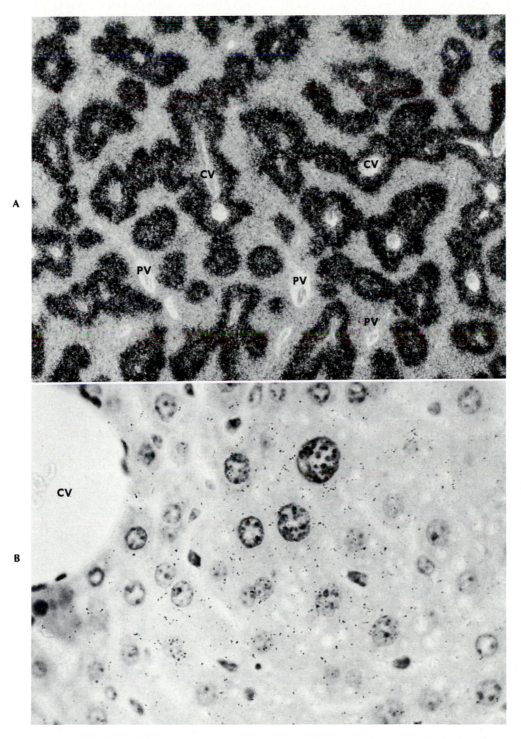

Fig. 5-42. Experimental carbon tetrachloride poisoning. **A,** Topographic autoradiography 1 hour after injection of ^{14}C-CCl$_4$. Localization of radioactive material concentrated around centrilobular veins *(CV)*, with periportal veins *(PV)* spared. **B,** Higher resolution showing ^{14}C-CCl$_4$ "grains." (Courtesy Dr. Augustine Roque, Morehead City, N.C.)

the medulla, resulting in fatal respiratory distress. Premature infants under the weight of 1400 g are particularly susceptible. Hexachlorophene, when applied to large exposed areas of the skin that are the site of burns or skin diseases allowing rapid absorption, may also lead to splitting of the myelin and demyelination of the white matter of the cerebral hemispheres, brainstem, and medulla. The central nervous system damage in adults, however, is for the most part reversible.

Elemental phosphorus

The majority of cases of phosphorus poisoning in the United States in recent years have been attributable to the ingestion of certain rat poisons or roach pastes. In the past, yellow phosphorus matches were the primary source for such intoxication.

Phosphorus is a general protoplasmic poison, but it exerts its most profound effects on the liver and kidneys. After ingestion of as little as 15 mg of yellow phosphorus, immediate, mostly nonspecific gastrointestinal symptoms attributable to the local effect of this poison are usually noted. Clinical and pathologic evidence of hepatic damage usually is noted after a variable interval. Electron microscopic studies show that, after the initial ingestion, a decrease in the hepatocyte cytoplasmic basophilia, reflecting alterations of the ergastoplasm, is observable within 12 hours and that mitochondrial swelling is detectable by 24 hours. Abnormal accumulations of hemosiderin granules in the hepatocytes have been observed in experimental phosphorus poisoning. Steatosis of the hepatic cells usually begins approximately 15 hours after experimental injection of phosphorus. Uncoupling of oxidative phosphorylation is one reflection of enzymatic derangement in phosphorus poisoning. Perilobular necrosis is characteristic of phosphorus intoxication. Liver enlargement with extensive fatty degeneration, principally periportal, possibly with a mild inflammatory infiltrate in the portal triads, is usually found at autopsy. Only rarely is massive necrosis observed.

The liver lesions of Reye's syndrome may morphologically resemble phosphorus poisoning. In these fatty livers, necrosis when present is frequently situated in the periphery of the lobule.

Plant poisons

"Bush tea." The pyrrolizidine chemical series constitutes a group of some 50 alkaloids, many of which are known to be highly toxic to man and animals. These poisonous substances occur in all parts of the world. At least 2000 common plants contain pyrrolizidine.

Bras and associates[273] incriminated the pyrrolizidine alkaloid fulvine as being the hepatotoxic agent responsible for the occurrence of veno-occlusive disease of the liver among the natives of Jamaica. Many people in the West Indies are addicted to the ingestion of "bush teas."

These aqueous infusions of plant material are imbibed in the belief that they are herbal remedies for a wide variety of common complaints. *Crotalaria fulva* (which contains the pyrrolizidine alkaloid fulvine) is used for one "bush tea." The consumption of an extract of *C. fulva* is now definitely linked with the high incidence of liver disease in the Caribbean ("veno-occlusive disease of the liver"). The disease, unlike Chiari's syndrome, does not affect the larger hepatic veins. The toxin exerts a dual attack on the liver—on the centrilobular hepatocytes, causing necrosis, and on the hepatic veins, leading to endothelial damage and thrombosis (Fig. 5-43).

Mushrooms. Mushroom poisoning is primarily caused by *Amanita phalloides* and *A. muscaria*. Of the 80 species of mushrooms known to be toxic for many individuals, only one, *A. phalloides*, affects the liver. Two types of toxins isolated from *A. phalloides* are phallin, a thermolabile glucoside with hemolytic properties, and amanita toxin, a thermostable mixture of cyclic polypeptides. The former is readily destroyed by cooking and ingestion and probably plays little role in human poisoning.

The toxin causes a cholera-like gastroenteritis, followed in several days by tender hepatomegaly and jaundice. In fatal cases death occurs within 10 days. There is a 50% mortality. At autopsy the liver is small because of the massive hemorrhagic hepatocellular necrosis. Persistent, peripherally located fatty liver cells are observed. An acute inflammatory exudate is found throughout the organ. The morphologic findings in other organs—kidney, brain, and heart—are of lesser severity and consist mainly of fatty changes and hydropic degeneration in the proximal convoluted tubules of the kidney, nonspecific neuronal reactions widely scattered throughout the brain, and fatty myocardial fibrils. In nonfatal cases, periportal hepatic fibrosis has been reported in several instances. The alkaloid muscarine is the toxin derived from *A. muscaria* and exhibits cholinergic effects.

ENVIRONMENTAL PATHOLOGY
Insecticides and pesticides
Organophosphates

Organophosphates, a large class of compounds, were originally prepared as nerve gases for warfare. Fortunately they were not released in this role, and it was discovered that they could be used in agriculture. The most widely used are parathion and malathion. Their action is based on the inhibition of cholinesterase. This leads to accumulation of acetylcholine, consequent blockade of the intercostal muscles, and respiratory failure resulting in brain anoxia. Although all of the compounds are anticholinesterases, only a small group leads to the development of demyelination of peripheral nerves. The mechanism of the demyelination is unknown. At necropsy, no specific pathologic changes are noted.

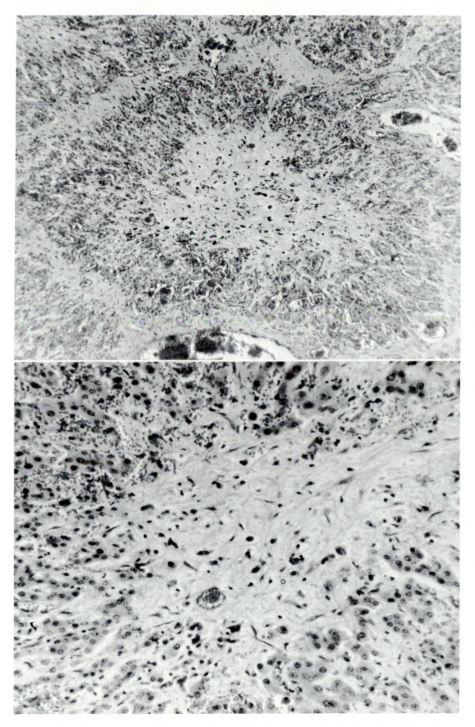

Fig. 5-43. "Bush tea" poisoning. Liver of pig after intraperitoneal dose of monocrotaline. Hepatic lobule with centrilobular disappearance of hepatic parenchymal cells and condensation of connective tissue supporting framework.

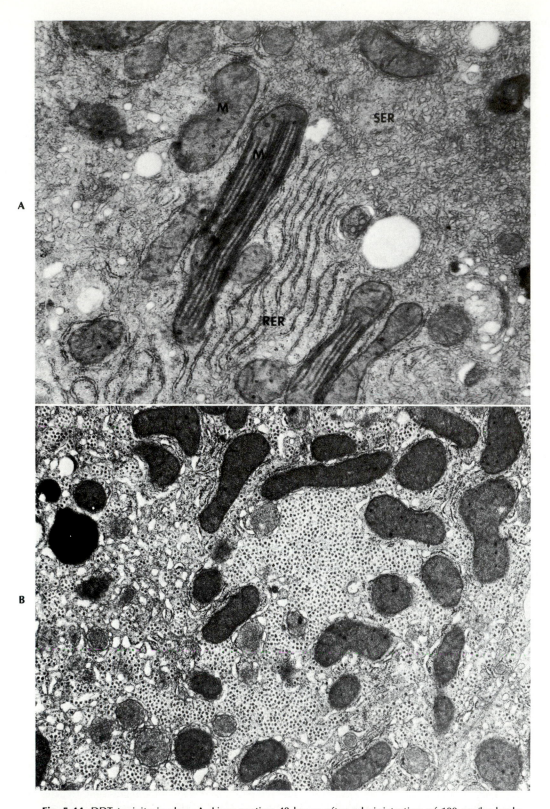

Fig. 5-44. DDT toxicity in dog. **A,** Liver section 48 hours after administration of 100 mg/kg body weight. Proliferation of smooth endoplasmic reticulum *(SER)* from rough endoplasmic reticulum *(RER)* may be seen. *M,* Mitochondria. **B,** Animal was sacrificed 56 hours after 200 mg/kg body weight was administered. Proliferation and dilatation of smooth endoplasmic reticulum in hepatocyte. Cell is rich in glycogen, and mitochondria are not abnormal. Dark globules at top left corner are fat. (**A,** 50,000×; **B,** 35,000×.)

There have been two instances of widespread poisoning of humans. One occurred in the 1930s in the United States, when a contaminated cargo of ginger, which was used primarily for preparing illicit alcoholic drinks in prohibition days, left several thousand people with nerve damage to the lower limbs. The resultant irregular motion of the victims became known as "ginger Jake paralysis." Another episode occurred in Morocco in the 1950s, when contaminated motor oil was sold for cooking purposes. In many parts of the world, parathion is sold over the counter as a pesticide. In Puerto Rico, for example, parathion poisoning leads acute alcoholism as a cause of accidental death.

Organic chlorinated hydrocarbons

DDT is an abbreviation of the earlier chemical name p,p'-dichlorodiphenyltrichloroethane. The present designation is 1,1,1-trichloro-2,2-bis (p-chlorophenyl) ethane. DDT is the most widely used insecticide, but since 1962 the volume has decreased because of a number of factors: (1) increased insect resistance, (2) storage in plants and animals, which has led to environmental contamination, and (3) lack of understanding of its mode of action after deposition in the adipose tissue of humans.

Disturbing also has been the observation of its possible role as a carcinogen, teratogen, and antifertility agent, as demonstrated in experimental animals.

Vertebrate animals receiving fatal doses of DDT manifest a myriad of neurologic signs and symptoms including tremors, hyperexcitability, ataxia, and paralysis. The severity of the reaction is in proportion to the dose administered. The clinical response of acute poisoning in humans is similar to that in animals. At necropsy, no dramatic evidence of neurologic damage is appreciated. Minimal adrenolytic changes are evident in the inner fasciculata and reticularis zones. Ultrastructurally, the hepatocytes show hypertrophy of the smooth endoplasmic reticulum, probably representing an intracellular adaptive change (Fig. 5-44). It thus appears that DDT and its analogs are capable of increasing microsomal activity. In chronic DDT poisoning, animals respond with a variety of changes. Fatty degeneration occurs in the myocardium and in the centrilobular portions of the liver and the proximal convoluted tubules of the kidney. Pyknosis and shrinkage of neurons, including those of the cerebral cortex, dentate nucleus, and spinal cord, are observed.

In humans, chronic or recurrent deposition of DDT in

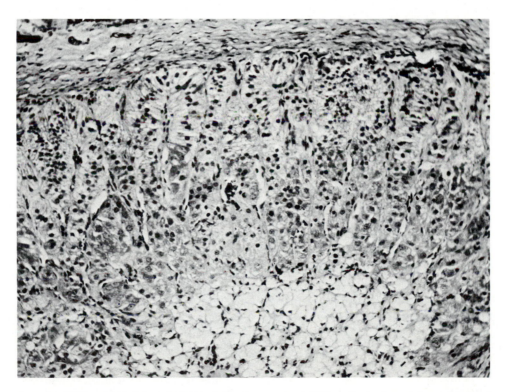

Fig. 5-45. DDT toxicity. Adrenal gland of dog that received 1800 mg/kg body weight over 3-week period. Capsule is thickened because of loss of underlying zona fasciculata cells. Zona glomerulosa is remarkably preserved (normally, 12 to 15 cell layers thick). Zona fasciculata adjacent to zona reticularis has undergone atrophy and replacement by adipose-appearing tissue. Remainder of zona fasciculata reveals granular cells in various stages of degeneration. Minor changes with these characteristics are found in humans with Cushing's syndrome who have been treated with o-p'-DDD.

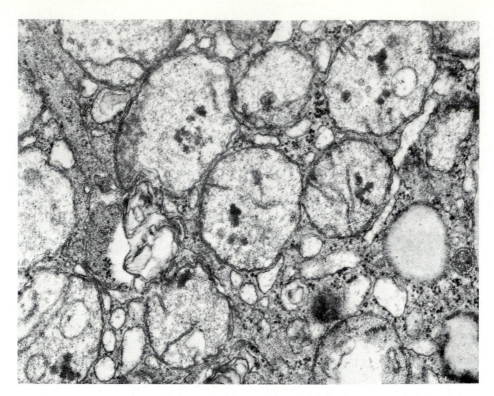

Fig. 5-46. DDT toxicity. Zona fasciculata cells in adrenal gland of dog 56 hours after administration of 200 mg/kg body weight. Mitochondria are swollen. Loss of cristae and normal contour and precipitation of electron-dense material in mitochondrial matrix. (40,000×.)

adipose tissue, brain, liver, and adrenal zona fasciculata leads to no cellular changes observable by light microscopy. A remarkable change in the adrenal zona fasciculata and zona reticularis after the administration of DDT to dogs is of interest. After a total cumulative dose of approximately 1800 mg/kg body weight, the adrenal gland undergoes considerable atrophy, leaving little more than a fairly intact zona glomerulosa and medulla (Fig. 5-45). There is pronounced mitochondrial enlargement (Fig. 5-46). Correspondingly, serum corticosteroid levels fall. Regeneration occurs in approximately 90 days after withdrawal of the compound. Unfortunately, this antisteroid effect is seen to a strong degree only in dogs and should be considered a species-specific phenomenon.

Isomers of DDT, o,p'-DDD and m,p'-DDD, have been used to treat humans with Cushing's syndrome and functioning adrenocortical carcinoma. The compounds are especially useful as palliative agents if surgical procedures are not indicated.

Polychlorinated biphenyls

Polychlorinated biphenyls (PCBs) are a group of chlorinated aromatic compounds that are structurally similar to DDT but are more resistant to environmental degradation. DDT contains between its two phenyl rings an ethane portion, which serves as the site of its oxidative breakdown in the environment, whereas PCBs contain no ethane structure and are thus more stable in the ecosystem.

PCBs were introduced into commerce in 1929 and have been used as plasticizers, extenders for pesticides, heat exchangers, dielectric fluids, and nonflammable hydraulic and lubricating fluids and as an ingredient in caulking compounds, adhesive paints, printing inks, and carbonless duplicating paper. It is estimated that 25,000 tons of PCBs are lost into the environment each year. Recent studies strongly suggest that DDT vapor can be converted to PCBs by ultraviolet sunlight in the lower atmosphere.

Toxic findings in animals reveal liver lesions (fatty infiltration, centrilobular atrophy, necrosis, hyaline bodies), kidney and intestinal damage (especially in birds), hydropericardium and ascites (birds), immunosuppressive effects (chickens), and detrimental reproductive effects (rats). Toxic effects in exposed PCB workers are chiefly chloracne with dermal cysts and comedos developing after a latent period of about 7 months after the time of most recent exposure and lasting for periods ranging from several months to 4 years after removal from the source of exposure. The main sources in the human diet are believed to be fish, shellfish, and poultry.

Carbamates

Carbamates are derivatives of carbamic acid. Physostigmine (eserine) was identified from the beans of a poisonous plant, *Physostigma venenosum,* and neostigmine (Prostigmin) is a synthetic analog medically. The best known of the carbamate insecticides is carbaryl (arylam, Sevin). As with the organophosphates, the mode of action is cholinesterase inhibition. On the other hand, none of the carbamates causes demyelination.

Insects do not utilize cholinesterase in their neuromuscular junctions, and their vital cholinesterase is all central and protected by a barrier system that hinders penetration by ionized molecules. All the medicinal carbamates are ionized or ionizable and therefore have little effect on insects.

Fluorine compounds

The fluoro-organic compound known as fluoroacetate is an insecticide but is most widely used as a rodenticide. It is sold under the name "1080." Lethal doses cause symptoms in 20 to 60 minutes, at which time convulsions herald rapidly approaching death. Elevated citrate levels are found, particularly in the heart and kidney. Fluoroacetate is metabolically converted to fluorocitric acid, which is an acetate-activating enzyme. In the presence of this enzyme, there is formation of the coenzyme A derivative, fluoroacetyl CoA, followed by condensation with oxaloacetate to give fluorocitrate. It is possible that death results from "jamming" of the Krebs citric acid cycle, with resulting disruption of energy-producing reactions.

Sodium fluoride has long been used as a bait for cockroaches and ants. The findings in acute fluoride poisoning in humans and animals are analogous. Acute gastrointestinal disturbances develop, rapidly followed by respiratory or cardiac failure. Two teaspoons of fluoride may kill a human in 2 hours. Rapid absorption with high concentration of fluoride ion throughout the body is the rule. At the same time, rapid deposition in the skeleton and excretion in the urine occur. Depending on the circumstances, a patient surviving toxic levels for 4 or more hours may be expected to live. Fluoride is a powerful metabolic inhibitor. It forms complexes with and inhibits a large number of metal-containing enzymes. The magnesium-containing enzymes, especially acid phosphatase and ATPase, are inhibited. Other metal-containing enzymes such as succinic dehydrogenase, cytochrome oxidase, peroxidase, and catalase are likewise affected. Considering this wide spectrum of enzyme paralysis, it is not difficult to understand why the finger cannot be pointed at a specific mechanism responsible for the death of the organism. Superimposed on the enzyme effects is the old knowledge of the calcium-precipitating role of fluoride. Indeed, the myocardial effects

of fluoride resemble those brought about by excess of calcium ion. It is probable, then, that calcium fluoride becomes deposited on the cell membrane, yielding a local excess of calcium. At necropsy the epithelial mucosa of the stomach and small intestine is desquamated, and widespread superficial ulceration is demonstrated. Rigor mortis appears rapidly, and preservation of the tissues is prolonged. A usual finding is unclotted blood, probably the result of calcium binding by fluoride. The microscopic examination of the myocardium, liver, and nephrons reveals no specific pathologic change.

Chronic fluorosis was first described as an industrial disease. A "poker back" hypermineralization of the skeleton and broad ligaments developed in cryolite powder workers. Exostoses evolved from both long and flat bones. Lipping of the vertebral bodies led to nerve root compression, with weakness and atrophy of leg muscles. Microscopically, distorted architecture of bony trabeculae, accompanied by poorly developed haversian canals, is suggestive of chronic fluorosis. Fluorine, unlike iodine, is not taken up preferentially by the thyroid gland, nor is there substitution of iodine by fluorine in the gland. These facts contradict an old concept that repeated large doses of fluorine could lead to the development of colloid goiter. Fluorine, at the recommended concentration level in fluoridated water supplies, has no proved deleterious effect on growth of teeth and bones in children. However, excessive fluoride intake may lead to brown staining and mottled tooth enamel. Mottled enamel develops during tooth formation, before eruption. The report of Dean[283] that caries resistance may be facilitated by fluoridation of drinking water (1 to 3 ppm) has been a notable advance in this area.

Herbicides

Paraquat dichloride, diquat dibromide, and morfamquat dichloride are weed killers. Paraquat is the one most commonly used. Animals may be poisoned by paraquat given parenterally, orally, or by aerosol spray. If death supervenes shortly after the initial dose, the lungs are the seat of severe pulmonary congestion and edema. If death occurs several days after dosage, proliferative alveolitis, hyaline membranes, and terminal bronchiolitis are observed. With longer survival, pulmonary fibrosis and subsequent cor pulmonale occur.

Paraquat toxicity in humans may occur after the oral ingestion of only a few milliliters of the compound. Absorption from the skin is also a method of introduction. Depending on the dosage, symptoms may appear within a few days or weeks. By the same token, death may occur within the first 24 hours or 3 to 4 weeks after imbibition of the paraquat solution. With smaller doses, gingival and oropharyngeal pseudomembranous ulcers (diphtheria-like membranes) are the initial signs. X-ray examination of the chest shows the basilar linear infiltration, which becomes progressively diffuse with time. Grossly, the lungs are dark and rubbery and have a "meaty" consistency during the first 5 days. What appears to be cystic change is the result of hemorrhage into the terminal airspaces (Fig. 5-47). The histologic findings in the first 6 days consist of hemorrhagic edema with bleeding into the airspaces. In the first few days, hyaline membranes are in evidence. From 6 to 30 days there is progressive buildup of a fibrous alveolitis leading eventually to interstitial fibrosis and the classic "honeycomb lung." During the later stages, bronchioloalveolar hyperplasia with squamous metaplasia is a prominent feature of honeycomb lung. Changes in hepatocytes and interlobular bile ducts vary with the amount of paraquat ingested and the survival time. Centrilobular necrosis, fatty changes in the lobular hepatocytes, acute cholangitis, and necrosis of the interlobular bile ducts have all been described as morphologic reflections of paraquat injury. With few exceptions, such as allopurinol and

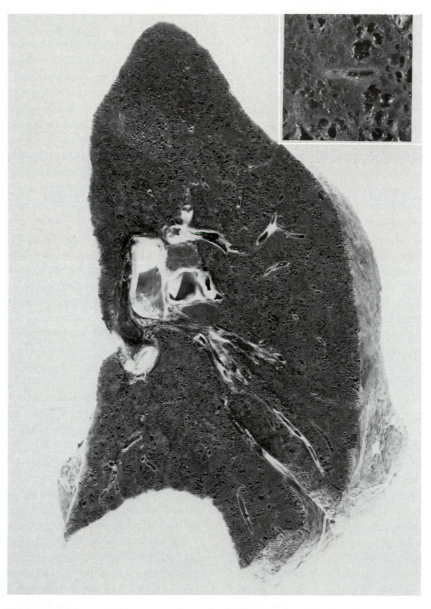

Fig. 5-47. Fatal paraquat poisoning. Lung is markedly congested, rubbery, and nonaerated. Inset shows what appear to be cysts but proved to be distended terminal airways filled with blood. Patient was admitted with acute glossitis and pharyngitis 5 days after ingestion of paraquat and died on the sixth hospital day as a result of respiratory, hepatic, and renal failure. (Courtesy Dr. Sandra E. Conradi, Charleston, S.C.)

methotrexate, one does not associate these changes of acute cholangitis or bile duct injury with medicinal drugs. On the contrary, intrahepatic cholestasis is the most common morphologic adverse reaction to therapeutic compounds. Proximal renal tubular dysfunction as manifested by glycosuria and aminoaciduria, as well as acute tubular necrosis, has been recorded following paraquat ingestion. It is probable that the toxicity mediated by paraquat induces the production of a superoxide ion (through electron transfer) that, via an intermediate, reacts with lipids to form fatty acid hydroperoxides, which in turn interfere with pulmonary surfactant function. The formation of the toxic superoxide radical is more rapid under higher oxygen tension, which may explain why the lung is the preferential site of paraquat toxicity.

Diquat does not produce the same pulmonary changes as paraquat but results in gastrointestinal erosion. In severe toxicity, acute tubular necrosis of the kidneys and centrilobular hepatic necrosis may occur. Morfamquat primarily affects the kidneys, leading to necrosis of the proximal convoluted tubules. The mechanism of the toxic damage resulting from paraquat is the subject of disagreement among investigators.

Air pollutants

As long-term exposure to increasing levels of air pollution is experienced by larger segments of the population, the results in terms of human pathology will become increasingly obvious. The role of air pollution in the development of emphysema and other chronic respiratory conditions is generally recognized. Epidemiologic data indicate that the same causal relationship exists in conditions affecting the cardiovascular system. In the United States alone, approximately 150 million tons of air pollutants are emitted each year, with 60% of this amount resulting from vehicular emissions, including automobiles, trucks, and buses; 31% from industrial processes; 6% from the heating of homes and offices; and 3% from the burning of trash and refuse. Although the sources are varied, approximately 85% of all air pollution results from the burning of fossil fuels. Industrial pollutants are as varied as the types of industries, and many may be harmful to animal and plant life. The damage from acid emissions such as HCl, H_2SO_4, HNO_3, or HF can be readily recognized, but the relationship between some other emissions and human pathologic conditions is not yet clearly established.

Of increasing concern is the widespread and often indiscriminate use of toxic chemical compounds, especially pesticides and herbicides. Compounds such as DDT have reportedly caused massive bird kills and adversely affected reproduction in songbirds. Although specific human effects have not been noted as a result of minimal exposures, the compound is being found in increasing concentrations in human tissues. The main cause of concern with DDT and all the chlorinated hydrocarbons is that they remain in the environment for an indefinite period of time without loss of potency. We have no idea what the results of long-term exposure will be.

Ozone is a form of oxygen. Under ordinary circumstances it is a colorless or pale blue gas with a characteristic pungent odor. In high concentrations it is extremely flammable, and in liquid form it becomes a dangerous explosive. There are two general sources of exposure to ozone: (1) the discharge of high-voltage electrical equipment, welding operations, and ultraviolet light spectrographic equipment and (2) emanations from ozone generators used in industrial processes (such as those involved in the production of ozone for use as a disinfecting germicide or for controlling growth of fungi, molds, and bacteria in food processing).

As pointed out by Deichmann and Gerarde, "The danger of undesirable health effects far outweigh any benefits presumed to be derived from the industrial or institutional use of ozone for the control of odors or bacteria in air."[290] Ozone, like many other chemical agents, including phosgene, chlorine, irritating smoke gases, ammonia, nitrogen dioxide, and cadmium fumes, may damage the alveolar capillaries, rendering them exceptionally permeable. Continued exposure to the irritating gases will lead to permanent damage manifested by alveolar septal derangement, desquamative bronchioloalveolitis, and eventual interstitial fibrosis.

A classic example of such a mechanism occurs in silo-filler's disease. In this condition the culprits are nitric oxide and nitrogen dioxide. Nitric acid is used extensively in industry for copper, brass, and silver dipping, the preparation of nitrocellulose, collodion, and methyl nitrate, and the production of sulfuric, chromic, and picric acids. It is used as an oxidizer in rocket fuel. Nitrous fumes are expelled from silos filled with cattle forage collected during times of partial drought. Under these circumstances the forage (corn) is often harvested before it is fully grown, and the young plants contain a high nitrate content. Later, during storage, anaerobic fermentation of potassium nitrate liberates nitrates, which, as the temperature rises with fermentation, liberate various oxides of nitrogen. The reaction to high concentrations of nitrogen dioxide is profound. Desquamation of bronchial and bronchioalveolar epithelium is prompt. The alveolar capillaries become rapidly dilated, and edema fluid flows into the alveoli. Within a matter of days, a well-developed bronchiolitis obliterans, accompanied by interstitial lymphocytic infiltration and slight fibrosis of the alveolar septa, appears (Fig. 5-48). If the pathologic process has been one primarily of edema with very little alveolar

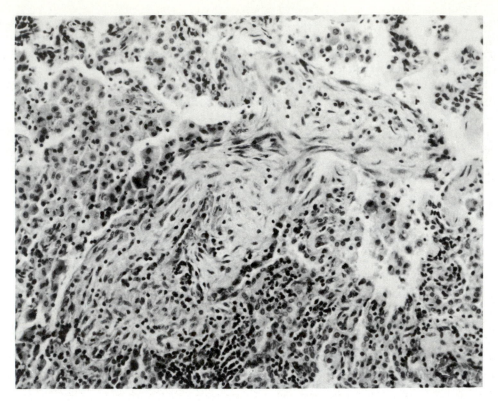

Fig. 5-48. Silo-filler's disease of lung. Bronchiolitis obliterans attributable to connective tissue proliferation. Lymphocytes and desquamative granulocytes complete microscopic picture.

septal destruction, reversible changes may be expected within a period of 6 months. Severe cases result in the persistence of interstitial fibrosis, and centrilobular emphysema follows the bronchiolitic destruction.

Occupational chest diseases

As a result of acute or chronic occupational exposure to harmful aerosols or gases, any one or several of the following diseases may develop in the lower respiratory tract: pneumoconiosis, pneumonitis, pulmonary edema, bronchitis, bronchial constriction, pleural inflammation, or cancer. To a considerable degree, whether an aerosol will produce disease, or where the disease will be initiated in the respiratory tract, may be governed largely by the size of the suspended particles. Particles less than 7 μm are generally considered respirable. Small particles are deposited in the airspaces to a greater degree than a dust with a significantly larger average particle size. Larger particles tend to be trapped on the tracheobronchial mucous membrane by a combination of inertial and gravitational deposition. Deposition in the airspaces, on the other hand, occurs largely by diffusion—a process that is caused by collisions of gas molecules with the particles. It is dependent on the near absence of air flow that is the rule in the alveoli.

Dust particles that are deposited on the tracheobronchial mucous membrane are transported toward the pharynx by the mucociliary mechanism. The motive force is supplied by cilia that beat 20 times per second with a rapid, whiplike cephalad stroke requiring one third of the cycle, followed by a slower recovery stroke occupying the remaining time of the cycle. In the trachea the mucous film or blanket, normally about 5 μm thick, is thereby propelled proximally with its embedded macrophages and dust particles at a rate of about 1 cm per minute. It is apparent that at this rate the tracheobronchial tree is capable of cleansing itself within 24 hours of particles that have been deposited on its surface.

There is also an alveolar clearance mechanism. This consists of a film of fluid about 0.2 μm thick that moves from the most peripheral alveoli toward the terminal bronchiole where it merges with the mucous blanket and becomes its nethermost layer. Because the respiratory bronchiole has a surface area that is only 1/500 of the surface area of the structures draining into it, the respiratory bronchiole becomes the locus where stagnation of the alveolar clearance mechanism first becomes manifest. In effect, the respiratory bronchiole is the narrow end of a large funnel. Thus, when the clearance mechanism is overwhelmed by excessive dust deposition, dust macules form in the lungs. In the center of each macule is a respiratory bronchiole, the evaginating alveoli of which are filled with dust and dust-filled macrophages. As the exposure continues and more dust accumulates, alveoli situated peripheral to the respiratory bronchiole become filled and the macule thereby becomes larger and tends to fuse with adjacent macules.

Pneumoconiosis

Pneumoconiosis is defined as an accumulation of dust in the lungs and the tissue reaction to its presence. Pneumoconiosis occurs most often in people who have resided many years in highly industrialized smoky cities. The lungs of these people often accumulate enough soot and fly ash to give the lungs a mottled black appearance. These people have pneumoconiosis, but they are in no manner handicapped by it. There is no demonstrable departure from health because of the presence of this dust. Their pneumoconiosis is merely a condition, *not a disease.*

The pneumoconiosis-producing dusts have been divided into two main categories: those that are fibrogenic and those that are nonfibrogenic. The latter are also called nuisance dusts. A nonfibrogenic dust is defined as one whose tissue reaction has the following three characteristics: (1) the alveolar architecture remains intact, (2) the stromal proliferation is minimal and consists of reticulin fibers, and (3) the reaction is potentially reversible. In contrast, a fibrogenic dust is one that provokes a tissue reaction having the following features: (1) the alveolar architecture is destroyed, (2) the stromal proliferation is significant and tends to be collagenous, and (3) the reaction is irreversible.

Nonfibrogenic dusts. Examples of nonfibrogenic dusts include soot, kaolin, stannic oxide, barium sulfate, aluminum oxide, iron oxide, and coal, as well as many other dusts. These dusts, when deposited in the airspaces, evoke a macrophage reaction associated with very little stromal proliferation. The latter consists of delicate reticulin fibers that course between the dust-filled macrophages. The airspaces containing the dust generally are alelectatic, thereby sequestering the dust-containing cells. Because tin oxide, iron oxide, and barium sulfate dusts are radiopaque, the chest x-ray films of the workers who have inhaled these dusts may demonstrate alarming shadows even though there are no symptoms of disease.

Coal workers' pneumoconiosis. Coal workers' pneumoconiosis can be presumed to be present in all coal miners who have inhaled the dust. However, it has been found that only 10% of working coal miners have x-ray evidence of pneumoconiosis.

Simple coal workers' pneumoconiosis consists of coal dust macules scattered throughout the lungs. In the center of each macule is a respiratory bronchiole. This bronchiole is often greatly enlarged, a condition termed focal emphysema. Focal emphysema is not productive of symptoms and must not be confused with the centrilobular emphysema (see Chapter 22) caused by cigarette smoking that affects many coal miners. Simple pneumoconiosis is asymptomatic and causes no disability, although it has been associated with a slight reduction in lung function values in some miners.

Complicated coal workers' pneumoconiosis, or progressive massive fibrosis (PMF), is characterized by black, dense, stony-hard masses in an anthracotic lung. The masses may be so small as to cast a shadow on the x-ray film only 1 cm in diameter, or they may be so large as to involve a major portion of one or both lungs and undergo cavitation. Only 3% of working coal miners have PMF (one third of the 10% that have x-ray evidence of pneumoconiosis). Many coal miners who have x-ray evidence of PMF are not incapacitated.

It has been possible to produce PMF experimentally in sensitized guinea pigs that have a large lung burden of coal dust by means of various kinds of living acid-fast bacilli, dead acid-fast organisms, and even tuberculin alone injected intratracheally. It is probable that an immunologically determined alteration in tissue reactivity is a requisite to the conversion of simple pneumoconiosis to PMF.

The development of PMF in coal miners may be associated with severe sclerosis of pulmonary vessels, resulting in pulmonary hypertension and cor pulmonale. The latter is a common immediate cause of death in cases of PMF in which the disease is far advanced.

Fibrogenic dusts

Silicosis. Silicosis has been recognized for centuries as a debilitating and often fatal disease. However, in more recent times, studies have demonstrated that, except for exposure to extremely heavy dosage of very fine dust of crystalline silica, the debility and fatal outcome of silicosis are usually attributable to an associated complicating tuberculosis. Of the crystalline forms of silica (SiO_2), quartz dust is the most common cause of silicosis. Silica particles ingested by macrophages cause death of the latter by dissolution of lysosomal membranes, thereby spilling autolytic enzymes into the macrophagic cytoplasm. An unidentified substance from the dead macrophages stimulates the production of fibrous tissue.

As with nonfibrogenic dusts, the respiratory bronchiole with its evaginating alveoli is the locus of silica dust accumulation and therefore the site of the initial lesion. Within a very few days after the dust accumulation, the macrophages become associated with fibroblasts and reticulin fibers. This inflammatory tissue occludes the lumina of the respiratory bronchiole and the evaginating alveoli; thus the tissue is solidified. A silicotic nodule is formed by a cluster of involved respiratory bronchioles situated circumferentially around a central blood vessel

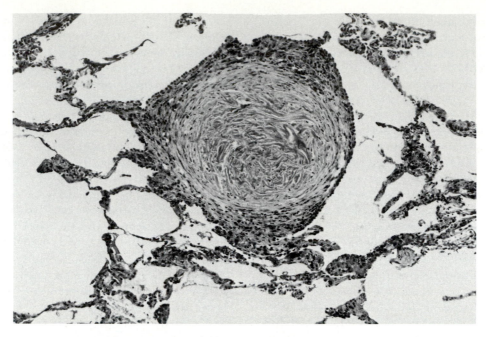

Fig. 5-49. Silicotic nodule, composed of acellular, hyaline collagenous tissue. Focal septal thickening and emphysema in area of nodule are frequent findings. (250×.)

that becomes obliterated as the nodule matures. Maturation of the inflammatory tissue in the nodule to the acellular, hyaline collagenous tissue characteristic of the mature silicotic nodule requires many months or even years (Fig. 5-49).

The number and size of the nodules in the lungs of an individual depend on the amount of silica dust deposited in the lung tissue over a lifetime. They may vary from very few widely scattered nodules no larger than 1 to 2 mm to hundreds of nodules, still widely separated but usually not more than 4 to 5 mm in diameter. Except for some paracicatricial types of emphysema, the alveolar tissue around and between silicotic nodules is normal. This is simple silicosis.

Simple silicosis, like the simple pneumoconiosis of coal miners, is asymptomatic. It is the abundance of normal lung tissue between the nodules in simple silicosis that is responsible for its asymptomatic character. Although not handicapped, for reasons still unknown the worker with simple silicosis is highly susceptible to tuberculosis. The resultant silicotuberculosis is much more serious than tuberculosis alone and is more difficult to treat. Fifty years ago it was estimated that 75% of the deaths among silicotic workers were attributable to an associated tuberculosis. With the great reduction in the incidence of tuberculosis, this cause of death among silicotic workers has likewise decreased.

Another form of silicosis, diatomaceous-earth pneumoconiosis, is caused by a dust created when natural diatomaceous earth is heated to a high temperature in the presence of lime (flux-calcined) and a significant portion of the amorphous silica becomes crystalline. Usually this dust exposure is associated with exposure to the unaltered natural diatomaceous earth as well, the net result of this being a mixed-dust pneumoconiosis. Many of the airspaces not destroyed by scars are plugged with macrophages containing amorphous silica. Natural diatomaceous earth, without quartz admixture, does not cause silicosis. Amorphous silica, if it is prepared by precipitation from aqueous sodium silicate solution with acid, likewise does not cause silicosis. However, amorphous silica, prepared by heating silica above its boiling point, producing silica fumes, or by burning organic silicates, is fibrogenic and capable of causing pulmonary fibrosis. This fibrosis may be diffuse and interstitial in character rather than nodular.

Acute silicosis is caused by the inhalation of very high concentrations of extremely fine crystalline silica (less than 1 μm in diameter). The tissue reaction is different from that usually seen. Although silicotic nodules form, they are few and remain cellular in character, as well as microscopic in size. There is a diffuse alveolar lipoproteinosis that is the predominant aspect of the reaction and that, by extensive plugging of the airspaces, has been responsible for the early deaths of the afflicted workers.

Whether silicosis is responsible for an increased incidence of lung cancer is a question that is raised occasionally. Epidemiologic studies that have taken the tobacco-smoking history into account indicated that there was no increased risk of lung cancer production in silicotic lungs. Because silicotic nodules are scars, and cancers are known to arise in tuberculous and other scars of lungs, it would be logical to expect some lung cancers to arise in silicotic nodules. This expectation is nullified by the fact that, unlike other scars, silicotic nodules do not contain epithelial parenchymal remnants from which cancers might arise (see also p. 907).

Asbestos-related diseases. The mechanism by which asbestos dust induces tissue damage is not known at present, nor is there an explanation for the difference in biologic activity of the different kinds of asbestos. This biologic activity includes pulmonary and pleural inflammation as well as neoplastic involvement of the lungs, pleura, and peritoneum. The different kinds of asbestos include chrysotile, amosite, crocidolite, and anthophyllite. Of these, chrysotile, which is mined in Canada, constitutes more than 95% of the asbestos used in America. Amosite and crocidolite are imports from South Africa and have limited use. Anthophyllite is extensively mined in Finland and the Soviet Union but is not used in America. Another type of asbestos, tremolite, is not used as such, but it is associated with most talc deposits and may constitute as much as 25% of the weight of commercial talc.

Inasmuch as serpentine rock, the mother ore of chrysotile, as well as other mineral fiber–containing rocks are common geologic outcroppings, they are subject to erosion by streams and winds. As a result of this erosion, mineral fibers are ubiquitous in ambient air. However, because of a greatly increased industrial consumption of asbestos and other mineral fibers over the past 50 years, the ambient air of cities has a significantly greater mineral fiber content than that of rural communities. This is consonant with the discovery that the lungs of all adult city dwellers contain mineral fibers ranging from 140,000 to almost 7 million per gram of dry lung tissue. Of these fibers, about 6%, on the average, have been identified morphologically as chrysotile. The presence of mineral fibers in the lungs is not always accompanied by demonstrable pulmonary disease. This suggests that there is a level of pulmonary asbestos deposition below which no demonstrable disease occurs.

The initial reaction to asbestos dust, similar to that of other dusts, involves the repiratory bronchioles and their evaginating alveoli. As with silicosis, there is a rapid proliferation of reticulin upon the alveolar surfaces that obliterates these alveoli. However, in contrast to silicosis, the bronchiole and alveolar ducts remain patent. Months and years later the reticulin is converted to collagen. With increased deposition of asbestos, the involvement extends peripherally, thereby causing confluence of neighboring lesions. In this process, some alveoli remain patent but their walls are thickened. There is thickening of the walls of respiratory bronchioles and alveolar ducts caused, in part, by the fibrous obliteration of their evaginating alveoli and, in part, by

newly deposited fibrous tissue. The end result is a relatively diffuse but nonuniform fibrosis that is most severe in the basal portions of the lower lobes and is more pronounced around bronchi and vessels and in the central portions of the primary lobule than in the peripheral portions.

Some alveolar septa are devoid of patent capillaries because of the fibrosis, and some that remain patent are covered by inflammatory tissue. The net result in advanced asbestosis is that some alveoli that are capable of being ventilated are poorly perfused or unperfused. Because of the fibrosis, some perfused alveoli are not ventilated. The interposition of inflammatory tissue between the capillary and the alveolar wall causes impairment in gaseous diffusion. All these deficiencies contribute to the dyspnea seen in advanced asbestosis. The collagenization and subsequent contraction of the scar tissue increase the stiffness of the lungs, decrease their compliance, restrict the respiratory excursions, and increase the cost of respiration in terms of the effort and work involved.

Some of the asbestos fibers become incorporated in the inflammatory tissue and are thereby sequestered. Other asbestos fibers remain in the airspaces and become covered by an iron-containing protein. Because of the characteristic high iron component, these coated fibers are called "ferruginous bodies." The ferruginous bodies are red-brown or golden structures, often segmented and clubbed, and straight or curved. Their length and thickness are variable, dependent on the length and diameter of the central fiber. Because inhaled fibers composed of materials other than asbestos may also be converted into ferruginous bodies, the latter are not specific for asbestos. Only if the central fiber of a ferruginous body is composed of asbestos may the latter be termed an asbestos body.

The nature of the pulmonary fibrosis caused by the inhalation of asbestos dust is not distinctive or diagnostic of asbestosis. It is usually most severe in the basal portions of the lung. However, fibrosis together with the presence of ferruginous bodies would constitute a fairly secure base upon which the diagnosis of asbestosis can rest.

Excessive lung carcinomas among asbestos workers occur in those most heavily exposed to dust; that is, asbestotic lung cancer occurs in association with severe asbestosis. The implication of this finding is that there is a dose-effect relationship between asbestos dust exposure and lung cancer development, so that there is a level of asbestos dust exposure below which lung cancer is not likely to develop. Support for this conclusion is found in the published statistics from a large English asbestos factory in which the lung cancer incidence prior to 1932 was about 10 times that of the general population. After the institution of "good-housekeeping" measures in the factory, another survey indicated that the risk of developing lung cancer in that factory was no higher than in the general population.

In a study of asbestos insulation workers it was found that, among the nonsmokers, the risk of lung cancer was relatively slight. But compared with a cigarette smoker not exposed to asbestos, the risk of lung cancer in a cigarette-smoking asbestos insulation worker was eight times greater, and about 90 times greater than that of a nonsmoking worker not exposed to asbestos.

Many asbestos-related lung cancers are bronchogenic in character—squamous, or undifferentiated carcinomas—but some are adenocarcinomas of peripheral origin. Although much of the inhaled dust inclusive of asbestos is cleared from the lungs via the bronchial mucosa, it is difficult to explain the genesis of bronchogenic cancers on the basis of asbestos dust alone. The adenocarcinomas of peripheral origin are more readily explained inasmuch as all experimentally produced asbestotic lung cancers originated peripherally within asbestotic scars.

Mesotheliomas of the pleura and of the peritoneum have been reported not only in people occupationally exposed to asbestos dust, but also in people exposed to this dust nonoccupationally. Among the latter are the wives of workers who washed work clothes heavily impregnated with very fine asbestos fibers that tended to remain suspended in air indefinitely. Another type of nonoccupational exposure included in these reports was living within one-half mile of a factory or shipyard fabricating or applying asbestos.

A satisfactory explanation for the occurrence of peritoneal mesotheliomas does not exist. This occurrence is particularly perplexing in those workers who have no asbestotic involvement of the lungs. Even more puzzling is the occurrence of mesotheliomas in Karain, Turkey, where mesothelioma deaths are endemic and asbestos exposure is nonexistent. Here exposure to aluminum silicate fibers of volcanic origin and classified as zeolite minerals is suspected as the cause.

The ability to cause mesothelioma is not shared equally by all types of asbestos. In South Africa, the excess of mesotheliomas was almost limited to the crocidolite-producing area. Very few mesotheliomas were reported from areas where amosite was mined and none from chrysotile mines. Among 380 deaths of New York asbestos-insulation workers who had been exposed to various types of asbestos dusts, 6% were attributed to mesothelioma. Of 436 British asbestos workers, also exposed to more than one kind of asbestos, 5% had died of mesotheliomas. On the other hand, of 2413 deaths among Canadian chrysotile mine and mill workers, only three, or 0.1%, died of mesothelioma.

Talcosis is a pneumoconiosis that closely resembles asbestosis. This resemblance is probably related to the tremolite asbestos content of the dust to which talc miners are exposed. As in exposure to other forms of asbestos dust, talc miners suffer from an increased incidence of lung cancer. However, mesotheliomas have not been reported associated with talc-dust exposure.

Another type of pneumoconiosis, although rarely encountered and inadequately studied, has been reported among some workers exposed to dust from hard metals such as tungsten carbide. Cobalt has been incriminated as the responsible agent in these cases. The disease takes the form of a diffuse pulmonary fibrosis with granulomatous features.

Pneumonitis

The occupationally induced pneumonitides are of two types: hypersensitivity and toxic. The hypersensitivity type is caused exclusively by certain dusts, whereas the toxic type may be caused by dust, vapor, or gas—any inhaled material that is chemically irritating to the lung parenchyma.

A dust-related hypersensitivity pneumonitis differs from a pneumoconiosis in that although the inflammation in the former is unquestionably caused by the inhaled dust, there is no demonstrable dust accumulation. Most of the dusts causing these pneumonitides are organic in character, consisting of the spores of fungi, but one dust is inorganic—beryllium.

The inhalation of beryllium, either as a metallic dust or as a dust of its chemical compounds, may result in serious disease, berylliosis. There is, however, one notable exception. Miners exposed to beryl ore dust (beryllium aluminum silicate) have not been affected by this disease.

Berylliosis may occur as an acute pneumonitis in which alveoli are filled with fluid containing macrophages and few lymphocytes. Alveolar walls are swollen and infiltrated by lymphocytes, monocytes, and scattered plasma cells. With persistence of the inflammation, fibroblastic proliferation and multiplication of reticulin fibers upon the alveolar walls usher in the subacute stage of the disease. The chronic form of berylliosis is characterized by a granulomatous inflammation that so closely resembles sarcoidosis in all of its histologic aspects that it is often difficult to differentiate these two diseases microscopically. As is true for sarcoidosis, the inflammatory stroma of berylliosis retains its reticulin character over periods of months and years. It is this delay in collagenization of the stroma that allows for successful therapy with steroid drugs.

Because lung cancers have been readily produced experimentally with beryllium compounds by intratracheal injection in rats and, after many years of inhalation, also in monkeys, beryllium-caused cancers have been anticipated in people exposed to these materials. However, no evidence of cancer production by occupational exposure to beryllium or its compounds has been forth-coming.

The other hypersensitivity pneumonitides of occupational origin are caused by aerosolized components of different kinds of fungi that are characteristic of particular occupational settings. The thermophilic organisms that grow on bagasse and cause bagassosis, or the organism growing on moldy hay, causing farmer's lung, the mold growing on the bark of maples, causing maple bark–stripper's disease, and the spores of mushrooms causing mushroom-grower's disease are but a few examples. The diseases named are pathologically identical, having similar pathogenic backgrounds and histopathologic features.

The pneumonitis is both proliferative and exudative. There is thickening of septal walls by fibroblastic proliferation associated with multiplication of reticulin fibers and infiltration of these tissues by lymphocytes and plasma cells. In addition, there is also a granulomatous component in the inflammation. This takes the form of scattered foci of foreign body giant cells surrounded by reticulin fibers, lymphocytes, monocytes, plasma cells, and fibroblasts.

The irritants responsible for the production of the chemical or toxic pneumonitides or pneumonias of occupational origin are generally agents that would cause death from pulmonary edema at higher dose levels. As a matter of fact, the first reaction to a sublethal dose of such inhaled irritant is the development of pulmonary edema. If the victim does not "drown" in his alveolar fluid and if he survives 24 hours or longer, exudation of leukocytes occurs in the airspaces. The chemical pneumonia may be complicated by infection and conversion to a bacterial pneumonia.

Manganese oxide has been reported to cause chemical pneumonia in workers inhaling this dust. Mercury vapor and nickel carbonyl vapor have caused chemical pneumonia and pneumonitis among workmen, ranging from the acute form to the chronic variety and pulmonary fibrosis. More frequent causes of chemical pneumonias are gases in common industrial use such as nitrogen dioxide, sulfur dioxide, chlorine, and ammonia. Nitrogen oxides are also produced by decomposition of silage and are responsible for the acute edema or chronic pneumonitis and bronchiolitis termed "silo-filler's disease."

Pulmonary edema

As indicated above, all inhaled irritants that cause chemical pneumonia initially traumatize the alveolar capillary endothelium and produce pulmonary edema. If the dose level of the inhaled irritant is sufficiently high, the amount of capillary endothelial damage may be so extensive that death occurs before much cellular exudation can take place. Because there is usually a latent period of some hours after exposure before the pulmonary edema becomes clinically manifest, an erroneous concept of the mechanism of the edema is often held, namely, that the inhaled irritant is continuing its pathogenic action over this period of time. Actually, the damaging action of the irritant upon the capillary endothelium is completed within minutes of the inhalation and leakage of fluid into the airspaces occurs promptly. If a major portion of the alveolar capillary bed has been injured, the development of pulmonary edema can be explosive. With only a minor portion of the capillary bed affected, hours may be required to fill a sufficient amount of lung tissue with fluid to become clinically apparent.

To the irritants that cause pulmonary edema by virtue of causing chemical pneumonia, cadmium fumes (CdO) and phosgene (COCl$_2$) should be added as potent producers of pulmonary edema in occupational settings. Workers welding cadmium-coated steel under conditions of inadequate ventilation are often victims of pulmonary edema. Phosgene is manufactured as an intermediate for the production of other chemicals. It is a hermitized process, situated outside of buildings. However, accidents such as leakages do occasionally occur.

Irritant gases can be divided into two general categories: those with a high solubility in water and those with a low solubility in aqueous solutions. Gases in the first category are considered upper respiratory irritants because in the concentrations usually encountered and from which people can escape the lungs are generally not involved. These gases are removed from the airstream prior to reaching the airspaces by the moisture of the tracheobronchial mucosa. Included in this category are sulfur dioxide, chlorine, and ammonia. Nitrogen dioxide and phosgene belong in the class of gases with low solubility in water. They are deep lung irritants and are known to produce pulmonary edema even in low concentrations. It is to be noted that gases that are upper respiratory irritants may also cause severe pulmonary damage and death if they are inhaled at high dose levels.

Bronchitis

Chemically active gases that have a high solubility in water, inclusive of sulfur dioxide, chlorine, and ammonia, tend to cause acute bronchitis if inhaled in sufficiently high concentrations.

Industrial bronchitis

Occupationally caused chronic bronchitis has been a somewhat controversial subject because in the United Kingdom, where this illness was most intensively studied, it was difficult to determine whether an increased risk of this disease was caused by occupational factors or the more evident causes so prevalent in the general population. There now appears to be adequate evidence that soft-coal miners, foundry men, and byssinotic workers described below do have an increased risk of developing chronic bronchitis even after allowances are made for genetic factors and cigarette smoking. Evidence for an increased risk of chronic bronchitis in other dusty occupations is lacking.

Bronchial constriction

Byssinosis is an occupational bronchial constriction affecting cotton-mill workers as well as those working with flax and hemp. In the former, it is caused by the inhalation of cotton dust. Some of the workers develop a hypersensitivity to an as yet unknown but heat-labile component of bracts of cotton. Subsequent inhalation of this dust results in the local release of histamine followed by the development of bronchial constriction with a feeling of chest tightness. Investigators who have studied cotton-mill workers believe that some of the workers, after many years of exposure to cotton dust, develop chronic obstructive lung disease and cor pulmonale. It has been difficult to sort out the other more common causes of chronic obstructive lung disease in cotton-mill workers to be certain that the obstructive changes were indeed caused by the inhalation of cotton dust. Prior to the development of chronic obstructive lung disease, no morphologic changes in the bronchi or lung tissue that could be identified with the clinical symptoms of byssinosis are known.

Toluene 2,4-diisocyanate, or TDI ($CH_3C_6H_3[NCO]_2$), is also known to sensitize workers. As with byssinosis, the sensitization that occurs has not been shown to have an immunologic basis. Exposure of sensitized workers to this vapor results in bronchial constriction and attendant symptoms. No morphologic changes have been documented as a result of such exposure, although concentrations of 1 to 2 ppm cause tracheobronchitis in rats and a concentration of 12 ppm is lethal to this animal. Related diisocyanates may have similar effects.

Pleural fibrosis

Except for the development of pleural hyaline plaques from exposure to asbestos dust, the role played by inhaled dust in the pathogenesis of pleural inflammation is uncertain. The inconstancy of pleural inflammation in the presence of substantial subpleural dust deposition raises the question of requisite factors additional to the inhaled dust for the production of pleural fibrosis. The occurrence of parietal pleural hyaline plaques in the absence of asbestos dust exposure would seem to support the assumption that factors other than dust also participate in the production of the pleural fibrosis encountered in some pneumoconiotic lungs.

Emphysema

Sporadic case reports have claimed that debilitating emphysema developed after a massive one-time exposure to nitrogen dioxide, phosgene, or cadmium oxide fumes. Emphysema has also been claimed to be the result of exposure to such dusts as coal, asbestos, silica, and cement. These claims rest upon very insecure bases. Most of the reports and claims neglected to consider cigarette smoking, recognized as the most common cause of emphysema, in the evaluation of causative factors. Nevertheless, it has been possible to produce emphysema in rats by long-term exposure to low concentrations of nitrogen dioxide (also present but in relatively high concentrations in cigarette smoke).

Oncogenesis

Two kinds of occupational cancers involving thoracic tissues are recognized today. The more common one is lung cancer and the other, mesothelioma. The most widespread occupational lung cancer is caused by excessive exposure to asbestos dust. The asbestotic lung cancer and the asbestos-related mesothelioma have already been discussed.

Other occupationally caused lung cancers include those caused by exposures in the refining of nickel and in the production of chromates and exposures to coke-oven emissions, inorganic arsenic compounds, and radioactive material in mines.

Nickel. The specific dusts involved as possible carcinogens include the subsulfide and oxide of nickel as well as the metal itself. However, nickel furnace workers are also exposed to polycyclic hydrocarbons that may be factors in the cancer production. Lung cancer rates among nickel workers have been reported to be as much as 10 times greater than expected, but are generally much lower.

Inasmuch as nickel carbonyl vapor exposure has produced lung cancers in rats, this material has been suspected of being responsible for human lung cancer production. Because the increase in risk of lung cancer production in a Wales nickel refinery disappeared despite the continued use of nickel carbonyl, it now appears unlikely that this chemical was the only or the main factor in the lung cancer production.

Coke-oven emissions. Coke-oven emissions contain particulate polycyclic organic matter (POM) and workers exposed to them suffer an increased risk of developing lung cancer. Which of the many components of POM is responsible for this increased risk is not known, although benzo[a]pyrene (BAP) is often selected.

Chromates. The number of deaths from respiratory tract cancers in chromate-producing plants between 1940 and 1948 in the United States was 29 times the expected number according to a 1953 report, but in a 1966 study the number had dropped ninefold. The lung cancers occurred in workers exposed mainly to hexavalent chromium, particularly lead and zinc chromate. The carcinogenicity of chromates has been confirmed experimentally by the production of lung cancer in rats that had pellets of calcium as well as zinc chromate in cholesterol embedded in their bronchi.

Radioactive materials. Uranium mines in Colorado and fluorspar mines in Nova Scotia contain radioactive materials consisting of radon gas and its radioactive decomposition products—the radon daughters. The radon daughters differ from each other physically. Some consist of submicronic solid particles. An investigation of 249 deaths among white underground uranium miners disclosed a lung cancer incidence that was four times the expected one.

REFERENCES
General

1. Baselt, R.C.: Disposition of toxic drugs and chemicals in man, Canton, Ohio, 1978, Biomedical Publications.
2. Baselt, R.C., and Cravey, R.H.: A compendium of therapeutic and toxic concentrations of toxicologically significant drugs in human biofluids, J. Anal. Toxicol. **1:**81, 1977.
3. Biava, C.: Fine structure of hepatocellular and canalicular bile pigment, Lab. Invest. **13:**1099, 1964.
4. Browning, E.: Toxicity of industrial metals, ed. 2, New York, 1969, Appleton-Century-Crofts.
5. Camps, F., editor: Gradwohl's legal medicine, ed. 2, Baltimore, 1968, The Williams & Wilkins Co.
6. Davies, D.M.: Textbook of adverse drug reactions, ed. 2, New York, 1981, Oxford Medical Publications.
7. Deichmann, W.B., and Gerarde, H.W.: Toxicology of drugs and chemicals, ed. 4, New York, 1969, Academic Press, Inc.
8. Gonzales, T.A., et al.: Legal medicine: pathology and toxicology, ed. 2, New York, 1954, Appleton-Century-Crofts.
9. Grundemann, E.: Drug-induced pathology. In the series Current topics in pathology, vol. 69, New York, 1980, Springer-Verlag.
10. Hennigar, G.R., and Gross, P.: Drug and chemical injury—environmental pathology. In Anderson, W.A.D., and Kissane, J.M., editors: Pathology, ed. 7, St. Louis, 1977, The C.V. Mosby Co.
11. Herrold, K.M., Rabson, A.S., and Smith, R.: Liver in generalized hypersensitivity, Arch. Pathol. **66:**306, 1958.
12. Inglefinger, F.J.: Counting adverse drug reactions that count, N. Engl. J. Med. **294:**1003, 1976.
13. Irey, N.S.: Tissue reactions to drugs, Am. J. Pathol. **82:**617, 1976.
14. Landsteiner, K., and Jacobs, J.: Studies on the sensitization of animals with simple chemical compounds, J. Exp. Med. **61:**643, 1935.
15. McLean, A.E.M., and Judah, E.: Cellular necrosis in the liver induced and modified by drugs, Int. Rev. Exp. Pathol. **4:**127, 1965.
16. McMaster, K.R., III, and Hennigar, G.R.: Drug-induced granulomatous hepatitis, Lab. Invest. **44:**61, 1981.
17. Meyler, L. In Dukes, M.N.G., editor: Meyler's side effects of drugs, ed. 9, Princeton, N.J., 1980, Excerpta Medica.
18. Meyler, L., and Peck, H.M.: Drug-induced diseases, vol. 4, Amsterdam, 1972, Excerpta Medica Foundation.
19. Meyler, L., and Peck, H.M. In Bristow, M.R., editor: Meyler and Peck's drug-induced diseases, vol. 5, New York, 1980, Elsevier/North-Holland Biomedical Press.
20. Moser, R.H.: Disease of medical progress: a study of iatrogenic disease, ed. 3, Springfield, Ill., 1969, Charles C Thomas, Publisher.
21. Parker, C.W.: Mechanisms of drug allergy, N. Engl. J. Med. **292:**511, 1975.
22. Popper, H., and Schaffner, F.: Pathophysiology of cholestasis, Hum. Pathol. **1:**1, 1970.
23. Riddell, R.H.: Pathology of drug-induced and toxic diseases, New York, 1982, Churchill Livingstone.
24. Schimmel, M.E.: The hazards of hospitalization, Ann. Intern. Med. **60:**100, 1964.
25. Spain, D.M.: The complications of modern medical practices, New York, 1963, Grune & Stratton, Inc.
26. Sunderman, F.W., and Sunderman, F.W., Jr.: Laboratory diagnosis of diseases caused by toxic agents, St. Louis, 1970, Warren H. Green, Inc.
27. Zaki, F.G.: Ultrastructure of hepatic cholestasis, Medicine **45:**537, 1966.

Drug injury and iatrogenic diseases
Drug-induced systemic lupus erythematosus

28. Bodman, S.F., Hoffman, M.J., and Condemi, J.J.: Procainamide-induced lupus erythematosus, Arthritis Rheum. **10:**269, 1967.
29. Dammin, G.J., Nora, J.R., and Reardan, J.B.: Hydralazine reactions—case with lupus erythematosus, J. Lab. Clin. Med. **46:**806, 1955.
30. Fakhro, A.M., Ritchie, R.F., and Lown, B.: Lupus-like syndrome induced by procainamide, Am. J. Cardiol. **20:**367, 1967.
31. Ladd, A.T.: Procainamide-induced lupus erythematosus, N. Engl. J. Med. **267:**1357, 1962.
32. Lee, S.L., Rivero, I., and Siegel, M.: Activation of systemic lupus erythematosus by drugs, Arch. Intern. Med. **117:**620, 1966.
33. Shulman, L.E., and Harvey, A.M.: Nature of drug-induced systemic lupus erythematosus, Arthritis Rheum. **3:**464, 1960.
34. Siegel, M., Lee, S.L., and Peress, N.S.: Epidemiology of drug-induced systemic lupus erythematosus, Arthritis Rheum. **10:**407, 1967.

Medicinal hazards of therapy
Antimicrobial agents

35. Andres, G.A., and McCluskey, R.T.: Tubular and interstitial renal disease due to immunologic mechanisms, Kidney Int. **7:**271, 1975.
36. Andres, G.A., et al.: Histology of human tubulo-interstitial nephritis associated with antibodies to renal basement membranes, Kidney Int. **13:**480, 1978.
37. Bartlett, J.G., et al.: Antibiotic-associated pseudomembranous colitis due to toxin-producing clostridia, N. Engl. J. Med. **298:**531, 1978.
38. George, R.H., et al.: Identification of *Clostridium difficile* as a cause of pseudomembranous colitis, Br. Med. J. **1:**695, 1978.
39. Heptinstall, R.H.: Interstitial nephritis: a brief review, Am. J. Pathol. **83:**214, 1976.
40. Linton, A.L., et al.: Acute interstitial nephritis due to drugs: a review of the literature with a report of nine cases, Ann. Intern. Med. **93:**735, 1980.
41. Mayaud, C., et al.: Interstitial nephritis after methicillin, N. Engl. J. Med. **292:**1132, 1975.
42. Medline, A., Shin, D.H., and Medline, N.M.: Pseudomembranous colitis associated with antibiotics, Hum. Pathol. **7:**693, 1976.
43. Mery, J., and Morel-Maroger, L.: Acute interstitial nephritis: a hypersensitivity reaction to drugs. In Grovannetti, S., and Bonomini, V. editors: Proceedings of the 6th International Congress of Nephrology, Florence, June 8-12, 1975, Basel, 1976, S. Karger.
44. Ooi, B.S., et al.: Acute interstitial nephritis: a clinical and pathologic study based on renal disease, Am. J. Med. **59:**614, 1975.
45. Pittman, F.E.: Antibiotic-associated colitis—an update, Adverse Drug Reaction Bull. **75:**268, 1979.
46. Price, A.B., and Davies, D.R.: Pseudomembranous colitis, J. Clin. Pathol. **30:**1, 1977.

Tetracycline

47. Andre, T.: Studies on the distribution of tritium-labelled dehydro-streptomycin and tetracycline in the body, Acta Radiol. **142** (suppl.):1, 1957.
48. Davis, J.S.: Drug-induced diseases, vol. 3, New York, 1968, Excerpta Medica Foundation.
49. Davis, J.S., and Kaufman, R.H.: Tetracycline toxicity, Am. J. Obstet. Gynecol. **95:**523, 1966.

50. Dowling, H.F., and Lepper, M.H.: Hepatic reactions to tetracycline, J.A.M.A. **188**:307, 1964.
51. Gale, E.F., and Folkes, J.P.: The assimilation of amino-acids by bacteria, Biochem. J. **53**:493, 1953.
52. Schultz, J.C., et al.: Fatal liver disease after intravenous administration of tetracycline in high dosage, N. Engl. J. Med. **269**:999, 1963.
53. Sheehan, H.L.: The pathology of acute yellow atrophy and delayed chloroform poisoning, J. Obstet. Gynecol. Br. Emp. **47**:49, 1940.

Amphotericin B

54. Hill, G.J., II: Amphotericin nephrotoxicity, Ann. Intern. Med. **61**:349, 1964.
55. Kinsky, S.C., et al.: Amphotericin and erythrocytes, Biochem. Biophys. Res. Commun. **9**:503, 1962.
56. Perlman, D., Giuffre, N.A., and Brindle, S.A.: Amphotericin and tissue culture cells, Proc. Soc. Exp. Biol. Med. **106**:880, 1961.
57. Sanford, W.G., Rasch, J.R., and Stonehill, R.B.: The treatment of disseminated coccidioidomycosis with amphotericin B, Ann. Intern. Med. **56**:554, 1962.
58. Utz, J.P., et al.: Amphotericin B toxicity, Ann. Intern. Med. **61**:334, 1964.

Aminoglycosides: neomycin, chloramphenicol, gentamicin

59. Dobbins, W.O., III, Herrero, B.A., and Mansbach, C.M.: Morphologic alterations associated with neomycin-induced malabsorption, Am. J. Med. Sci. **255**:63, 1968.
60. Faloon, W.W., et al.: Effect of neomycin and kanamycin upon intestinal absorption, Ann. N.Y. Acad. Sci. **132**:879, 1966.
61. Kosek, J.C., Mazze, R.I., and Cousins, M.J.: Nephrotoxicity of gentamicin, Lab. Med. **30**:48, 1974.
62. McCurdy, P.R.: Action of chloramphenicol, Blood **21**:363, 1963.
63. Schentag, J.J., et al.: Gentamicin tissue accumulation and nephrotoxic reactions, J.A.M.A. **240**:2067, 1978.

Analgesics and antipyretics
Salicylates

64. Done, A.K.: Salicylamide toxicity, Pediatrics **23**:774, 1959.
65. Eichenholz, A., Mulhausen, R.O., and Redleaf, P.S.: Salicylate effect on respiratory center, Metabolism **12**:164, 1963.
66. Lawson, A.A.H., et al.: Acute salicylate intoxication in adults, Q. J. Med. **38**:31, 1969.
67. Maher, J.F., and Schreiner, G.E.: Death in acute salicylate poisoning, Trans. Am. Soc. Artif. Intern. Organs **11**:349, 1965.
68. Smith, M.J.H., and Smith, P.K.: The salicylates, New York, 1966, Interscience Publishers, Inc.
69. Tobin, J.A., and Hennigar, G.R.: Salicylate intoxication, V. Med. Monthly **79**:486, 1952.

Acetaminophen

70. Jollow, D.J., et al.: Acetaminophen-induced hepatic necrosis. IV. Protective role of glutathione, J. Pharm. Exp. Ther. **187**:211, 1973.

Aminophenols

71. Black, M.: Acetaminophen hepatotoxicity, Gastroenterology **78**:382, 1980.
72. Brodie, B.B., and Axelrod, J.: Fate of phenacetin in man, Pharmacol. Exp. Ther. **97**:58, 1949.
73. Burry, A.F.: Pathology of analgesic nephropathy: Australian experience, Kidney Int. **13**:34, 1978.
74. Gloor, F.J.: Changing concepts in pathogenesis and morphology of analgesic nephropathy as seen in Europe, Kidney Int. **13**:27, 1978.
75. Gonwa, T.A., et al.: Analgesic-associated nephropathy in transitional cell carcinoma of the urinary tract, Ann. Intern. Med. **93**:249, 1980.
76. Grimlund, K.: Kidney damage in members of same family, Acta Med. Scand. **174**(suppl. 405):3, 1963.
77. Kincaid-Smith, P.: Analgesic nephropathy: a common form of renal disease in Australia, Med. J. Aust. **2**:1131, 1969.
78. MacGibbon, B.H., et al.: Autoimmune hemolytic anemia, Lancet **1**:7, 1960.

79. Mitchell, J.R., and Jollow, D.J.: Metabolic activation of drugs to toxic substances, Gastroenterology **68**:392, 1975.
80. Nissen, N.I., and Friis, T.: Phenacetin anuria and interstitial nephritis, Acta Med. Scand. **171**:125, 1962.
81. Shadidi, N.T.: Phenacetin methemoglobinemia, Ann. N.Y. Acad. Sci. **151**:822, 1968.

Androgenic-anabolic steroids

82. Antunes, C.M.F., et al.: Endometrial cancer and estrogen use: report of a large case-control study, N. Engl. J. Med. **300**:9, 1979.
83. Glover, G.A., and Wilkerson, J.A.: Biliary cirrhosis following the administration of methyltestosterone, J.A.M.A. **204**:168, 1968.

Oral contraceptive (the "pill")

84. Irey, N.S., Manion, W.C., and Taylor, H.B.: Vascular lesions in women taking oral contraceptives, Arch. Pathol. **89**:1, 1970.
85. Mann, J.I., et al.: Myocardial infarction in young women with special reference to oral contraceptive practice, Br. Med. J. **2**:241, 1975.
86. Tausk, M.: Drug-induced diseases, vol. 3, New York, 1968, Excerpta Medica Foundation.

Estrogens

87. Herbst, A.L., Kurman, R.J., and Scully, R.E.: Vaginal and cervical abnormalities after exposure to stilbestrol in utero, Obstet. Gynecol. **40**:287, 1972.
88. Herbst, A.L., and Scully, R.E.: Adenocarcinoma of vagina in adolescence, Cancer **25**:745, 1970.
89. Ng, A.B.P., et al.: Cellular detection of vaginal adenosis, Obstet. Gynecol. **46**:323, 1975.

Tranquilizers

90. Alexander, C.S., and Nino, A.: Cardiovascular complications—phenothiazines, Am. Heart J. **78**:757, 1969.
91. Campbell, J.E.: Myocardial lesions—chlorpromazine, Am. J. Clin. Pathol. **34**:133, 1960.
92. Margolis, I.B., and Gross, C.G.: Gynecomastia during phenothiazine therapy, J.A.M.A. **199**:942, 1967.
93. Walker, C.O., and Combes, B.: Biliary cirrhosis induced by chlorpromazine, Gastroenterology **51**:631, 1966.

Antihypertensive drugs

94. Alarcon-Segovia, D., Fishbein, E., and Betancourt, V.M.: Antibodies to nucleoprotein and to hydrazide-altered soluble nucleoprotein in TB patients receiving isoniazid, Clin. Exp. Immunol. **5**:429, 1969.
95. Graham, C.F., Gallagher, K., and Jones, J.K.: Acute colitis with methyldopa, N. Engl. J. Med. **304**:1044, 1981.
96. Maddrey, W.C., and Boitnott, J.K.: Severe hepatitis from methyldopa, Gastroenterology **68**:351, 1975.
97. Maddrey, W.C., and Boitnott, J.K.: Drug-induced chronic liver disease, Gastroenterology **72**:1348, 1977.
98. Perry, H.M., O'Neal, R.M., and Thomas, W.A.: Hexamethonium pneumonia, Am. J. Med. **22**:37, 1957.
99. Refshauge, W.D.: Hydralazine polyneuritis, Med. J. Aust. **1**:58, 1963.
100. Seeverens, H., DeBruin, C.D., and Jordans, J.G.: Myocarditis and methyldopa, Acta Med. Scand. **211**:233, 1982.

Antithyroid drugs

101. Griswold, W.R., et al.: Vasculitis associated with propylthiouracil: evidence for immune complex pathogenesis and response to therapy, West. J. Med. **128**:543, 1978.
102. Houston, B.D., et al.: Apparent vasculitis associated with propylthiouracil use, Arthritis Rheum. **22**:925, 1979.

Antidiabetic drugs

103. Balodimos, M.C., et al.: Pathologic findings after sulfonylurea, Diabetes **17**:503, 1968.
104. Bloodworth, J.M.B., Jr.: Morphologic changes associated with sulfonylurea, Metabolism **12**:287, 1963.
105. Sackner, M.A., and Balian, L.: Sulfonylurea-induced hypoglycemia, Am. J. Med. **28**:135, 1960.

H_2 receptor antagonists

106. Freston, J.W.: Cimetidine. II. Adverse reactions and patterns of use, Ann. Intern. Med. **97**:728, 1982.
107. McGowan, W.R., and Vermillion, S.E.: Acute interstitial nephritis related to cimetidine therapy, Gastroenterology **79**:746, 1980.
108. Sawyer, D., Conner, C.S., and Scalley, R.: Cimetidine: adverse reaction and acute toxicity, Am. J. Hosp. Pharm. **38**:188, 1981.

Antitubercular drugs

109. Bellamy, W.E., Jr., et al.: Jaundice associated with the administration of sodium P-aminosalicylic acid, Ann. Intern. Med. **44**:764, 1956.
110. Elmendorf, D.F., Jr., et al.: INH toxicity, Am. Rev. Tuberc. **65**:429, 1952.
111. Lichtenstein, M.R., and Cannemeyer, W.: PAS hypersensitivity, J.A.M.A. **152**:606, 1953.
112. Paine, D.: Fatal hepatic necrosis associated with aminosalicylic acid, J.A.M.A. **167**:285, 1958.
113. Reynolds, E.: INH jaundice, Tubercle **43**:375, 1962.
114. Warring, F.C., Jr., and Howlett, K.S.: Allergic reactions to PAS, Am. Rev. Tuberc. **65**:235, 1952.

Anesthetics
Halothane

115. Paronetto, F., and Popper, H.: Lymphocyte-stimulation test, N. Engl. J. Med. **283**:277, 1970.
116. Peters, R.L., et al.: Hepatic necrosis associated with halothane, Am. J. Med. **47**:748, 1969.
117. Touloukian, J., and Kaplowitz, N.: Halothane-induced hepatic disease, Semin. Liver Dis. **1**:134, 1981.

Methoxyflurane

118. Cousins, M.J., et al.: Etiology of methoxyflurane nephrotoxicity, J. Pharmacol. Exp. Ther. **190**:530, 1975.
119. Frascino, J.A., Venemee, P., and Rosen, P.P.: Renal oxalosis and azotemia after methoxyflurane, N. Engl. J. Med. **283**:676, 1970.
120. Powell, H.C., et al.: Methoxyflurane nephropathy, Hum. Pathol. **5**:359, 1974.

Anticonvulsants

121. Carrington, C.B., et al.: Eosinophilic pneumonia, N. Engl. J. Med. **280**:787, 1969.
122. Crofton, J.W., et al.: Pulmonary eosinophilia, Thorax **7**:1, 1952.
123. Gams, R.A., Neal, J.A., and Conrad, F.G.: Hydantoin-induced pseudo-pseudolymphoma, Ann. Intern. Med. **69**:557, 1968.
124. Gately, L.E., III, and Lam, M.A.: Phenytoin-induced toxic epidermal necrolysis, Ann. Intern. Med. **91**:59, 1979.
125. Hansen, J.W., Jones, K.L., and Smith, D.W.: Fetal alcohol syndrome, J.A.M.A. **235**:1458, 1976.
126. Hepner, G.W., et al.: Inhibition of intestinal ATPaSE by diphenylhydantoin and acetazolamide, Clin. Res. **18**:382, 1970.
127. Kleckner, H.B., Yakulis, V., and Heller, P.: Severe hypersensitivity to diphenylhydantoin with circulating antibodies to the drug, Ann. Intern. Med. **83**:522, 1975.
128. Larmas, L.: A comparative enzyme histochemical study of hydantoin-induced hyperplastic and normal human gingiva, Proc. Finn. Dent. Soc. **73** (suppl. 1): 1, 1977.
129. Li, F.P., et al.: Malignant lymphoma after diphenylhydantoin (Dilantin) therapy, Cancer **36**:1359, 1975.
130. McMaster, K.R., III, and Hennigar, G.R.: Drug-induced granulomatous hepatitis, Lab. Invest. **44**:61, 1981.
131. Meadow, S.R.: Harelip and cleft palate, Lancet **2**:1296, 1968.
132. Meynell, M.J.: Megaloblastic anemia in anticonvulsant therapy, Lancet **1**:487, 1966.
133. Monson, R.R., et al.: Congenital malformations and teratogenesis, N. Engl. J. Med. **289**:1049, 1973.
134. Mullick, F.G., and Ishak, D.G.: Hepatic injury associated with diphenylhydantoin therapy: a clinicopathologic study of 20 cases, Am. J. Clin. Pathol. **74**:442, 1980.
135. Rausing, A.: Hydantoin-induced lymphadenopathies and lymphomas, Rec. Res. Cancer Res. **64**:263, 1978.

136. Reynolds, E.H.: Diphenylhydantoin hematologic aspects of toxicity. In Woodbury, D.M., Penry, J.K., and Schmidt, R.P., editors: Antiepileptic drugs, New York, 1972, Raven Press.
137. Saltzstein, S.L., and Ackerman, L.V.: Dilantin-induced lymphadenopathy, Cancer **12**:164, 1959.
138. Sheth, K.J., Casper, J.T., and Good, T.A.: Interstitial nephritis due to phenytoin hypersensitivity, J. Pediatr. **91**:438, 1977.
139. Smith, D.W.: Fetal alcohol syndrome. In Schaffer, A.J., consulting editor: Recognizable patterns of human malformation, ed. 2, Philadelphia, 1976, W.B. Saunders Co.
140. Yermakov, V.M., Hitti, I.F., and Sutton, A.L.: Necrotizing vasculitis associated with diphenylhydantoin: two fatal cases, Hum. Pathol. **14**:182, 1983.

Digitalis

141. Caldwell, J.L., and Thompson, C.T.: Intestinal hemorrhagic necrosis as a complication of digitalis intoxication, J. Okla. State Med. Assoc. **61**:487, 1968.
142. Dearing, W.H., Barnes, A.R., and Essex, H.E.: Experimental myocardial damage, Am. Heart J. **25**:648, 1943.
143. Gazes, P.C., et al.: Acute hemorrhage and necrosis of the intestines associated with digitalization, Circulation **23**:358, 1961.
144. Hiott, D.W.: Early ultrastructural changes in heart muscle produced by digoxin and emetine, Fed. Proc. **27**:347, 1968.
145. Molnar, Z., Larsen, K., and Spargo, B.: Cardiac changes in potassium-depleted rat, Arch. Pathol. **74**:339, 1962.
146. Reichenbach, D.D., and Benditt, E.P.: Catecholamines and cardiomyopathy: the pathogenesis and potential importance of myofibrillar degeneration, Hum. Pathol. **1**:125, 1970.
147. Walton, R.P., and Gazes, P.C.: Cardiac glycosides II—pharmacology and clinical use. In DiPalma, J.P., editor: Drill's pharmacology in medicine, ed. 3, New York, 1965, McGraw-Hill Book Co.
148. Wenzel, D.G.: Myocardial lesions, J. Pharm. Sci. **56**:1209, 1967.

Oxygen

149. Balentine, J.D.: Pathology of oxygen toxicity, New York, 1982, Academic Press, Inc.
150. Chance, B., and Boveris, A.: Hyperoxia and hydroperoxide metabolism. In Robin, E.D., editor: Extrapulmonary manifestations of respiratory disease, New York, 1978, Marcel Dekker.
151. Yamamoto, E., Wittner, M., and Rosenbaum, R.M.: Resistance and susceptibility to oxygen toxicity by cell types of the gas-blood barrier of the rat lung, Am. J. Pathol. **59**:409, 1970.

Antineoplastic and immunosuppressive drugs

152. Billingham, M.E.: Morphologic changes in drug-induced heart disease. In Bristow, M.R., editor: Meyler and Peck's drug-induced diseases. Vol. 5. Drug-induced heart disease, New York, 1980, Elsevier/North-Holland Biomedical Press.
153. Buja, L.M., and Ferrans, V.J.: Myocardial injury produced by antineoplastic drugs: pathophysiology and morphology of myocardial cell alterations, In Fleckenstein, A., and Rona, G., editors: Recent advances in the studies on cardiac structure and metabolism, vol. 6, Baltimore 1975, University Park Press.
154. Buja, I.M., et al.: Cardiac ultrastructural changes induced by daunorubicin therapy, Cancer **32**:771, 1973.
155. Bulkley, B.H., and Roberts, W.C.: The heart in systemic lupus erythematosus and the changes induced in it by corticosteroid therapy, Am. J. Med. **58**:243, 1975.
156. Castlemen, B., Schull, R.E., and McNeely, B.U.: Case records of the Massachusetts General Hospital, Case 6, N. Engl. J. Med. **290**:390, 1974.
157. Gyorkey, F., Gyorkey, B., and Sinkovics, J.G.: Origin and significance of intranuclear tubular inclusions in Type II pulmonary alveolar epithelial cells of patients with bleomycin and busulfan toxicity, Ultrastruc. Pathol. **1**:211, 1980.
158. Jones, A.W.: Bleomycin lung damage: the pathology and nature of the lesion, Br. J. Dis. Chest **72**:321, 1978.
159. Kirschner, R.H., and Esterly, J.R.: Pulmonary lesions associated with busulfan therapy of chronic myelogenous leukemia, Cancer **27**:1074, 1971.

160. Koss, L.G.: The respiratory tract in the absence of cancer. In Koss, L.G., editor: Diagnostic cytology and its histopathologic basis, ed. 3, vol. 2, Philadelphia, 1979, J.B. Lippincott Co.
161. Kraus, H., et al.: Cytologic findings in vaginal smears from patients under treatment with cyclophosphamide, Acta Cytol. **21**:726, 1977.
162. Kreis, H., et al.: Peliosis hepatis in recipients of renal transplants, Gut **19**:748, 1978.
163. Mallory, A., and Kern, F., Jr.: Drug-induced pancreatitis: a critical review, Gastroenterology **78**:813, 1980.
164. Reimer, R.R., et al.: Acute leukemia after alkylating-agent therapy of ovarian cancer, N. Engl. J. Med. **297**:177, 1977.
165. Seiber, S.M., and Adamson, R.H.: Toxicity of antineoplastic agents in man: chromosomal aberrations, antifertility effects, congenital malformations and carcinogenic potential, Adv. Cancer Res. **22**:57, 1975.
166. Weiss, B.R., and Muggia, F.M.: Cytotoxic drug-induced pulmonary disease: update 1980, Am. J. Med. **68**:259, 1980.

Other agents

167. Bana, D.S., et al.: Cardiac murmurs and endocardial fibrosis associated with methysergide therapy, Am. Heart J. **88**:640, 1974.
168. Graham, J.R., et al.: Fibrotic disorders associated with methysergide therapy for headache, N. Engl. J. Med. **274**:359, 1966.
169. Hache, L., Utz, D.C., and Woolner, L.B.: Methysergide and idiopathic fibrous retroperitonitis, Surg. Gynecol. Obstet. **115**:737, 1962.
170. Hursh, J.B., et al.: Thorotrast excretion, Acta Radiol. (Stockholm) **47**:481, 1957.
171. Looney, W.B.: Thorotrast—late clinical findings, Am. J. Roentgenol. **83**:163, 1960.
172. Mason, J.W., Billingham, M.E., and Friedman, J.P.: Methysergide-induced heart disease: a case of multivalvular and myocardial fibrosis, Circulation **56**:889, 1977.
173. Reeves, D.L., and Stuck, R.M.: Thorotrast—clinical and experimental, Medicine **17**:37, 1938.

Potassium chloride, milk and alkali, mineral oil

174. Baker, D.R., Schrader, W.H., and Hitchcock, C.R.: Small-bowel ulceration apparently associated with thiazide and potassium therapy, J.A.M.A. **190**:586, 1964.
175. Bingham, E., Horton, A.W., and Tye, R.: Cancer from mineral oil, Arch. Environ. Health **10**:449, 1965.
176. Diener, R.M., Shoffstall, D.H., and Earl, A.E.: Experimental potassium-induced ulcer in monkeys, Toxicol. Appl. Pharmacol. **7**:746, 1965.
177. Pinkerton, H.: Reaction to oils and fats in lung, Arch. Pathol. **5**:380, 1928.
178. Portnoy, L.M., Amadeo, B., and Hennigar, G.R.: Pulmonary alveolar microlithasis, Am. J. Clin. Pathol. **41**:194, 1964.

Toxicologic aspects of forensic pathology
Alcohols and glycols

179. Adelson, L.: Fatal intoxication with isopropyl alcohol (rubbing alcohol), Am. J. Clin. Pathol. **38**:144, 1962.
180. Bennett, I.L., Jr., Nation, T.C., and Olley, J.F.: Pancreatitis—methyl alcohol, J. Lab. Clin. Med. **40**:405, 1952.
181. Biava, C.: Mallory alcoholic hyalin, Lab. Invest. **13**:301, 1964.
182. Factor, S.M.: Intramyocardial small-vessel disease in chronic alcoholism, Am. Heart J. **92**:561, 1976.
183. Ferrans, V.J., et al.: Alcoholic cardiomyopathy: a histochemical study, Am. Heart J. **69**:748, 1965.
184. Flax, M.H., and Tisdale, W.A.: Electron microscopy of alcoholic hyalin, Am. J. Pathol. **44**:441, 1964.
185. Gadsden, R.H., Mellette, R.R., and Miller, W.C., Jr.: Scrap-iron intoxication, J.A.M.A. **168**:1220, 1958.
186. Hourihane, D.O., and Weir, D.G.: Suppression of erythropoiesis, Br. Med. J. **1**:86, 1970.
187. Lieber, C.S.: Hepatic and metabolic effects of alcohol, Gastroenterology **50**:119, 1966.
188. MacDonald, R.A., and Baumslag, N.: Iron in alcoholic beverages, Am. J. Med. Sci. **247**:649, 1964.

189. Makar, A.B., Tephly, T.R., and Mannering, G.J.: Ethanol inhibition of bile activation and toxification by methanol, Mol. Pharmacol. **4**:471, 1968.
190. McCord, W.M., Switzer, P.K., and Brill, H.H., Jr.: Isopropyl alcohol intoxication, South. Med. J. **41**:639, 1948.
191. McKennis, H., Jr., and Haag, H.B.: On the congeners of whiskey, J. Am. Geriatr. Soc. **7**:848, 1959.
192. Popper, H., et al.: Drug-induced liver disease, Arch. Intern. Med. **115**:128, 1965.
193. Regan, T.J., and Haider, B.: Pathophysiologic effects of ethanol on cardiac tissue. In Bristow, M.R., editor: Meyler and Peck's drug-induced diseases, vol. 5, New York, 1980, Elsevier/North-Holland Biomedical Press.
194. Reppart, J.T., et al.: Alcoholic hyalin bodies, Lab. Invest. **12**:1138, 1963.
195. Rubin, E., and Lieber, C.S.: Early fine structural changes in the human liver induced by alcohol, Gastroenterology **52**:1, 1967.
196. Rubin, E., and Lieber, C.S.: Induction and inhibition of hepatic microsomal enzymes by ethanol, Science **162**:690, 1968.
197. Schaffner, F., et al.: Hepatocellular cytoplasmic changes in acute alcoholic hepatitis, J.A.M.A. **183**:343, 1963.
198. Svoboda, J.D., and Manning, R.T.: Mitochondrial alterations, Am. J. Pathol. **44**:645, 1964.
199. Wendt, V.E., et al.: Hemodynamic and metabolic effects of chronic alcoholism in man, Am. J. Cardiol. **15**:175, 1965.
200. Zieve, L.: Jaundice, hyperlipemia and hemolytic anemia: a heretofore unrecognized syndrome associated with alcoholic fatty liver and cirrhosis, Ann. Intern. Med. **48**:471, 1958.

Metals and metallic salts
Mercury

201. Becker, C.G., et al.: Nephrotic syndrome, Arch. Intern. Med. **110**:178, 1962.
202. Brown, J.R., and Kulkarni, M.V.: Toxicity and metabolism of mercury—a review, Med. Serv. J. Canada **23**:786, 1967.
203. Cameron, J.S., and Trounce, J.R.: Membranous glomerulonephritis and the nephrotic syndrome, Guy's Hosp. Rep. **114**:101, 1965.
204. Gage, J.C.: Distribution and excretion of inhaled mercury vapor, Br. J. Ind. Med. **18**:287, 1961.
205. Gritzka, T.L., and Trump, B.F.: Renal tubular lesions caused by mercuric chloride, Am. J. Pathol. **52**:1225, 1968.
206. Oliver, J., MacDowell, M., and Tracy, A.: Pathogenesis of acute renal failure, J. Clin. Invest. **30**:1307, 1951.

Lead

207. Aronson, S.M.: Lead encephalopathy. In Carter, C.H., editor: Medical aspects of mental retardation, Springfield, Ill., 1965, Charles C Thomas, Publisher.
208. Blackman, S.S., Jr.: Inclusions in lead poisoning, Bull. Johns Hopkins Hosp. **58**:384, 1936.
209. Blackman, S.S., Jr.: Lead encephalitis, Bull. Johns Hopkins Hosp. **61**:1, 1937.
210. Chiodi, H., and Cardeza, A.F.: Experimental hepatic lesions caused by lead, Arch. Pathol. **48**:395, 1949.
211. Cramer, K., et al.: Variation in morphology and function of kidney in humans with increased length of exposure to lead, Br. J. Ind. Med. **31**:113, 1974.
212. Goyer, R.A.: The renal tubule in lead poisoning, Lab. Invest. **19**:71, 1968.
213. Goyer, R.A., and Krall, A.: Ultrastructural transformation in mitochondria isolated from kidneys of normal and lead-intoxicated rats, J. Cell. Biol. **41**:393, 1969.
214. Goyer, R.A., Krall, R.A., and Kimball, J.P.: The renal tubule in lead poisoning, Lab. Invest. **19**:78, 1968.
215. Goyer, R.A., and Rhyne, B.C.: A general review of pathology of lead, Int. Rev. Exp. Pathol. **12**:1, 1973.
216. Landing, B.H., and Nakai, H.: Histochemistry of lead inclusions, Am. J. Clin. Pathol. **31**:499, 1959.
217. Moore, J.F., Goyer, R.A., and Wilson, M.: Lead inclusion bodies, Lab. Invest. **29**:488, 1973.
218. Paglia, D.E., Valentine, W.N., and Dahlgren, J.C.: Inhibition of pyrimidine 5-nucleotidase in workers chronically exposed to lead, J. Clin. Invest. **56**:1164, 1975.

219. Piomelli, S., et al.: Free erythrocyte protoporphyrin (FEP) in blood as an indicator of lead intoxication, Pediatrics **51**:254, 1973.

Arsenic, cobalt, cadmium

220. Axelson, O.: Arsenic compounds and cancer, J. Toxicol. Environ. Health **6**:1229, 1980.
221. Grice, H.C., Munro, I.C., and Wiberg, G.S.: Experimentally induced cobalt cardiomyopathies: comparison with beer drinker's cardiomyopathy, Clin. Toxic. **2**:273, 1969.
222. Ivankovic, S., Eisenbrand, G., and Preussmann, R.: Lung carcinoma induction in BD rats after a single intratracheal instillation of an arsenic-containing pesticide mixture formerly used in vineyards, Int. J. Cancer **24**:786, 1979.
223. Lander, H., Hodge, P.R., and Crisp, C.S.: Arsenic in the hair and nails, J. Forensic Med. **12**:52, 1965.
223a. Nandi, M., et al.: Cadmium content of cigarettes, Lancet **2**:1329, 1969.
224. Newman, J.A., et al.: Histologic types of bronchogenic carcinoma among members of copper-mining and smelting communities, Ann. N.Y. Acad. Sci. **271**:260, 1976.
225. Pryce, D.M., and Ross, C.F.: Ross's post-mortem appearances, ed. 6, London, 1963, Oxford University Press.
226. Rona, G., and Chappel, C.I.: Pathogenesis and pathology of cobalt cardiomyopathy: recent advances in studies on cardiac structure and metabolism. In the series Cardiomyopathies, vol. 2, Baltimore, 1973, University Park Press.
227. Sandusky, G.E., Henk, W.G., and Roberts, E.D.: Histochemistry and ultrastructure of the heart in experimental cobalt cardiomyopathy in the dog, Toxicol. Appl. Pharmacol. **61**:89, 1981.
228. Schroeder, H.A., Nason, A.P., and Tipton, I.H.: Essential trace metals in man: cobalt, J. Chronic Dis. **20**:869, 1967.
229. Szuler, I.M., et al.: Massive variceal hemorrhage secondary to presinusoidal portal hypertension due to arsenic poisoning, Can. Med. Assoc. J. **120**:168, 1979.
230. Venugopal, B., and Luckey, T.D.: Metal toxicity in mammals, vol. 2, New York, 1977, Plenum Press.
231. Webb, J.L.: Enzyme and metabolic inhibitors, vol. 3, New York, 1966, Academic Press, Inc.
232. Wiberg, G.S., et al.: Factors affecting cardiotoxic potential of cobalt, Clin. Toxicol. **2**:257, 1969.

Nickel, thallium, uranium, platinum, and other group VIIIb transition complexes

233. Bencosme, S.A., et al.: Acute tubular and glomerular lesions in rat kidneys after uranium injury, Arch. Pathol. **69**:470, 1960.
234. Committee On Medical and Biologic Effects of Environmental Pollutants, Division of Medical Sciences, National Research Council: Nickel, Washington, 1975, National Academy of Sciences.
235. Gale, G.R.: Platinum compounds. In Sartorelli, A.C., and Johns, D.G., editors: Hanbuch der experimentellen Pharmakologie. Vol. 38. Antineoplastic and immunosuppressive agents, Berlin, 1975, Springer-Verlag.
236. Hackett, R.L., and Sunderman, F.W., Jr: Acute pathologic reactions to administration of nickel carbonyl, Arch. Environ. Health **14**:604, 1967.
237. Hackett, R.L., and Sunderman, F.W., Jr.: Nickel carbonyl and nickel compounds, Arch. Environ. Health **16**:349, 1968.
238. Hardaker, W.T., Stone, R.A., and McCoy, R.: Platinum nephrotoxicity, Cancer **34**:1030, 1974.
239. Prestayko, A.W., Crooke, S.T., and Carter, S.K.: Cisplatin: current status and new developments, New York, 1980, Academic Press, Inc.
240. Reed, D., et al.: Thallitoxicosis, J.A.M.A. **183**:516, 1963.
241. Rosenberg, B., Van Camp, L., and Krigas, T.: Inhibition of cell division in *Escherichia coli* by electrolysis products from platinum electrode, Nature **205**:698, 1965.
242. Stone, R.S., et al.: Renal tubular fine structure studied during reaction to acute uranium injury, Arch. Pathol. **71**:160, 1961.
243. Watt, T.L., and Baumann, R.R.: Nickel dermatitis, Arch. Dermatol. **98**:155, 1968.

Catecholamines

244. Bloom, S., and Cancill, P.A.: Myocytolysis and mitochondrial calcification in rat myocardium after low doses of isoproterenol, Am. J. Pathol. **54**:373, 1969.
245. Ferrans, V.J., et al.: Isoproterenol-induced myocardial necrosis, Am. Heart J. **68**:71, 1964.
246. Greenhoot, J.H., and Reichenbach, D.D.: Cardiac injury and subarachnoid hemorrhage, Neurosurgery **30**:521, 1969.
247. Hiott, D.W.: Heart muscle—experimental use of isoproterenol, Arch. Int. Pharmacodyn. Ther. **180**:206, 1969.
248. Kline, I.K.: Myocardial alterations associated with pheochromocytomas, Am. J. Pathol. **38**:539, 1961.
249. Lillehei, R.C., et al.: Plasma catecholamines in open heart surgery, Surg. Forum **14**:269, 1963.
250. Pearce, R.M.: Epinephrine myocarditis, J. Exp. Med. **8**:400, 1906.
251. Reichenbach, D.D., and Benditt, E.P.: Catecholamines and cardiomyopathy, Hum. Pathol. **1**:125, 1970.
252. Sode, J., Getzen, L.C., and Osborne, D.P.: Cardiac arrhythmias and cardiomyopathy associated with pheochromocytomas, Am. J. Surg. **114**:927, 1967.
253. Wiswell, J.G., and Crazo, R.M.: Cardiomyopathy and pheochromocytoma, Trans. Am. Clin. Climatol. Assoc. **80**:185, 1969.

Barbiturates

254. Beveridge, G.W., and Lawson, A.A.: Bullous lesions in acute barbiturate intoxication, Br. Med. J. **1**:835, 1965.
255. Cucinell, S.A., et al.: The effect of chloral hydrate on bishydroxycoumarin metabolism, J.A.M.A. **197**:366, 1966.
256. Dayton, P.G., et al.: Barbiturates and prothrombin response, J. Clin. Invest. **40**:1797, 1961.
257. Matte, M.L., Winer, L.H., and Wright, E.T.: Dermatitis medicamentosa, Arch. Dermatol. **82**:56, 1960.
258. Meyler, L., et al.: Barbiturates—arteritis, Acta Med. Scand. **167**:95, 1960.
259. Rostenberg, A., Jr., and Fagelson, H.J.: Life threatening drug eruptions, J.A.M.A. **194**:660, 1965.
260. Sorensen, B.F.: Barbiturate blister, Dan. Med. Bull. **10**:130, 1963.
261. Teare, R.D.: Alcohol-barbiturate deaths. In Meyler, L., and Peck, H.M., editors: Drug-induced diseases, Amsterdam, 1965, Excerpta Medica Foundation.

Narcotics

262. Kranier, L., Berman, E., and Wishnick, S.C.: Parenteral talcum granulomatosis—complication in narcotic addicts, Lab. Invest. **11**:671, 1962.
263. Puro, H.E., et al.: Experimental production of human "blue velvet" and "red devil" lesions, J.A.M.A. **197**:1100, 1966.

Other agents
Carbon monoxide

264. Finck, P.A.: Exposure to carbon monoxide: review of the literature and 567 autopsies, Milit. Med. **131**:1513, 1966.

Carbon tetrachloride

265. Judah, J.D.: Mechanisms in acute carbon tetrachloride poisoning, N.Z. Med. J. **67**(suppl.):73, 1968.
266. Magee, P.N.: Toxic liver necrosis, Lab. Invest. **15**:111, 1966.
267. Recknagel, R.O.: Carbon tetrachloride effect on ribosomes, Pharmacol. Rev. **19**:145, 1967.
268. Smuckler, E.A., Iseri, O.A., and Benditt, E.P.: Carbon tetrachloride poisoning and protein synthesis, J. Exp. Med. **116**:55, 1962.

Boric acid

269. Fisher, R.S., et al.: Boron absorption from borated talc, J.A.M.A. **157**:503, 1955.
270. Goldbloom, R.B., and Goldbloom, A.: Boric acid poisoning, J. Pediatr. **43**:631, 1953.

Hexachlorophene

271. Schuman, R.M.: Hexachlorophene spongiosus myelinopathy, Arch. Neurol. **32**:320, 1975.

Plant poisons
"Bush tea"

272. Allen, J.R., Carstens, L.A., and Katagiri, G.J.: Hepatic veins of monkeys with veno-occlusive disease: sequential ultrastructural changes, Arch. Pathol. **87:**279, 1969.
273. Bras, G., Jelliffe, D.B., and Stuart, K.L.: Veno-occlusive disease of liver in Jamaica, Arch. Pathol. **57:**285, 1954.

Mushrooms

274. Abul-Haj, S.K., Ewald, R.A., and Kazyak, L.: Fatal mushroom poisoning, N. Engl. J. Med. **269:**223, 1963.
275. Dubash, J., and Teare, D.: Poisoning by *Amanita phalloides*, Br. Med. J. **1:**45, 1946.
276. Grossman, C.M., and Malbin, B.: Mushroom poisoning: a review of the literature and report of two cases caused by a previously described species, Ann. Intern Med. **40:**249, 1954.
277. Himsworth, H.P.: Mushroom poisoning—hepatic fibrosis. In Himsworth, H.P., editor: Lectures on the liver and its diseases, Cambridge, Mass., 1947, Harvard University Press.

Environmental pathology
Insecticides and pesticides

278. Nichols, J., and Hennigar, G.R.: Studies on DDD,2,2-bis(parachlorphenyl)-1,1,1-dichloroethane, Exp. Med. Surg. **15:**310, 1957.
279. Temple, T.E., Jr., et al.: Treatment of Cushing's disease, N. Engl. J. Med. **281:**801, 1969.

Polychlorinated biphenyls

280. Greene, W.B., et al.: PCB-DDT toxicity on mouse liver cells: an electron microscopic study. In Deichmann, W.B., editor: Pesticides and the environment: a continuing controversy, vol. II, New York, 1973, Intercontinental Medical Book Corp., Publisher.

281. Moilanen, K.W., and Crosby, D.G.: DDT: an unrecognized source of polychlorinated biphenyls, Science **180:**578, 1973.

Fluorine compounds

282. David, W.A.L., and Gardiner, B.O.A.: Fluoracetamide as a systemic insecticide, Nature **181:**1810, 1958.
283. Dean, H.T.: Endemic fluorosis and its relation to dental caries, Public Health Rep. **53:**1443, 1938.
284. Hodge, H.C.: Highlights of fluoride toxicology, J. Occup. Med. **10:**273, 1968.
285. Hodge, H.C., and Smith, F.A.: Fluorides and man, Annu. Rev. Pharmacol. **8:**395, 1968.
286. Loewi, O.: On the mechanism of the positive inotropic action of fluoride, oleate, and calcium on the frog's heart, J. Pharmacol. Exp. Ther. **114:**90, 1955.

Herbicides

287. Conning, D.M., Fletcher, K., and Swan, A.A.B.: Paraquat and related bipyridyls, Br. Med. Bull. **25:**245, 1969.
288. Parkinson, C.: The changing pattern of paraquat poisoning in man, Histopathology **4:**171, 1980.
289. Vaziri, N.E., et al.: Nephrotoxicity of paraquat in man, Arch. Intern. Med. **139:**172, 1979.

Air pollutants

290. Deichmann, W.B., and Gerarde, H.W.: Toxicology of drugs and chemicals, ed. 4, New York, 1969, Academic Press, Inc.

Ocupational chest diseases

291. Morgan, W.K.C., and Seaton, A.: Occupational lung diseases, Philadelphia, 1975, W.B. Saunders Co.

CHAPTER 6 Radiation Injury

ROBERT E. ANDERSON

Under appropriate circumstances, all forms of radiation are injurious. The purpose of this chapter is to describe some of the consequences of exposure of individual cells and groups of cells to ionizing and nonionizing radiation. The primary emphasis, however, will be on injury to human tissues, and much of the background information will be drawn from the accidental and therapeutic exposure of human populations to ionizing radiation.

Basic to an understanding of radiation-induced tissue injury is an appreciation of the physics of radiation and the effects of radiation on individual cells and their subcellular components. Much of our knowledge in this regard has been derived from normal and abnormal cells grown in tissue culture. A discussion of these general concepts will be followed by a description of the morphologic and clinical features of radiation injury involving cells and tissues in situ with particular reference to the acute and delayed effects of whole-body or partial-body exposure of humans.

This chapter is written with the conviction that radiation will continue to increase in importance in the diagnosis and treatment of disease. For this reason, considerable emphasis will be placed on the use of radiation in the treatment of persons with malignant tumors and on the biologic consequences of radioisotopes administered therapeutically or diagnostically.

RADIATION SPECTRUM

Radiation is the emission, transmission, and absorption of radiant energy. Such energy may be characterized in terms of the mode by which the energy is emitted, propagated, and absorbed. With respect to propagation, radiation is classified as electromagnetic or particulate.

Electromagnetic radiation

Electromagnetic radiation can be visualized conceptually as bundles of energy. This form of energy is propagated by means of wave motion and is subclassified on the basis of the length and frequency of the waves. The penetrating power varies greatly depending on the wavelength. In a vacuum, electromagnetic radiation travels at the speed of light.

As shown in Fig. 6-1, electromagnetic radiation forms a continuous spectrum covering a wide range of wavelengths and frequencies. Microwaves and radio waves exhibit long wavelengths (up to several miles), but the number of waves per unit of time is small. At the other end of the spectrum are cosmic, gamma, and roentgen (x) rays, which exhibit short wavelengths and high frequencies. Intermediate between these extremes are ultraviolet, visible light, and infrared rays.

Those forms of electromagnetic radiation characterized by short wavelengths and high frequencies carry sufficient energy to produce ionization in the materials that absorb them. *Ionizing* refers to the capacity to produce ions, that is, atoms or molecules that possess an electrical charge, on passage through matter.

In terms of physical characteristics, gamma rays and x rays are essentially identical. By convention, however, a distinction is made between the electromagnetic radiation produced artificially by a roentgen-ray tube (x rays) and that emitted spontaneously by a radioactive substance (gamma rays). Gamma rays have defined energies characteristic of the nuclide that emits them and ionize matter indirectly by the ejection of high-speed electrons from the molecules that form the absorbing material. X rays ionize matter in an identical fashion, and the energies involved depend on the energy characteristics of the source of the x rays.

Particulate radiation

Radiation related to the movement of discrete particles is known as particulate radiation. This form of radiation may be generated either (1) directly by accelerating electrons, deuterons, protons, or other atomic particles to high speeds in a device such as a cyclotron or a linear accelerator, or (2) indirectly by the decay of naturally

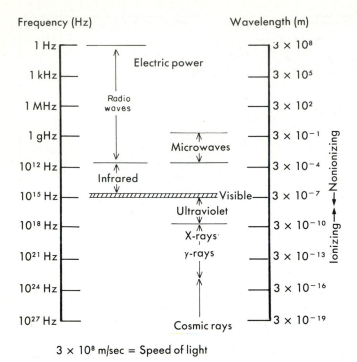

Frequency (Hz) — Wavelength (m)

occurring or artificially produced radioactive substances.

Particulate radiation may be subclassified on the basis of the type of particles involved. The biologically important particles are alpha and beta rays, protons, neutrons, deuterons, and mesons. These particles differ primarily in terms of mass, charge, and angular momentum.

Alpha and beta rays are particles emitted by the nuclei of certain radioactive nuclides, such as radium, thorium, and actinium. Alpha particles are helium nuclei and thus possess a mass of 4 and a positive charge. Beta particles are high-speed positrons or electrons and have an extremely small mass ($1/1836$) and either a positive or a negative charge. These particles travel at speeds less than that of light, and like other moving bodies, their energy depends on their rest mass and their velocity. The energies of these particles are measured in electron volts or, more commonly, in million electron volts (MeV).

Protons and neutrons are constituents of the nuclei of atoms. Each has a mass of 1. Protons possess a positive charge equal to that of an electron, but opposite in sign. Neutrons have no charge.

Deuterons represent nuclei of deuterium, a stable isotope of hydrogen. Considerable interest has been devoted to a relatively new particle, the negative pi meson, as a potentially effective tool in the radiotherapeutic treatment of malignant tumors. One type of meson, the pion,

has a mass 273 times the mass of an electron. An accelerator to produce these particles is in operation at the Los Alamos National Laboratory in New Mexico. The particular therapeutic advantage of this particle is that, when it is captured by a molecule of oxygen, the mass of the meson is converted into energy with the consequent violent disruption of the oxygen nucleus. This disruption produces neutrons, protons, and alpha particles, which in turn produce dense ionizations along their tracks. Alpha particles are particularly significant in this regard because they transmit large amounts of energy over short distances so that the damage they induce can be confined or localized to a small volume of tissue such as a tumor.

RADIOACTIVE SUBSTANCES

Radioactivity refers to disintegration of the nucleus of an unstable atom with the release of energy. This disintegration may involve naturally occurring substances, such as radium or thorium, or substances rendered radioactive by artificial means. Both natural and artificially produced radioactive substances are termed *radioisotopes*. These radioactive nuclides give off radiations as a result of the disintegration or decay of individual atoms. During radioactive decay, unstable daughter nuclei are often formed and in turn undergo disintegration.

Types of decay

There are three common modes of decay: alpha emission, beta emission, and electron capture. Many nuclei with high atomic numbers decay by alpha emission and thus are known as alpha (α) emitters. For example, radium, with an atomic number of 88 and a mass number of 226, decays to radon ($^{222}_{86}$Rn) as follows:

$$^{226}_{88}\text{Ra} \rightarrow\ ^{222}_{86}\text{Rn} + ^{4}_{2}\text{He} + \text{Gamma radiation}$$

During decay, energy is released as kinetic energy of the alpha particles. Alpha particles (helium nuclei) from a specific nuclide are ejected with discrete energies. Additional energy may also be released as gamma radiation, such as that just shown. The total energy released during the radioactive decay of a nucleus is termed the *transition energy*.

Beta (β) emitters are the most numerous of the radioactive isotopes. β^- decay, or negatron decay, involves the transformation of a neutron into a proton with the release of a neutrino and energetic electrons (beta particles). β^+ decay, or positron decay, is somewhat more complicated but involves the transformation of a proton to a neutron followed by a variable series of steps that include the release of a neutrino and a positron. β^+ decay may also be accompanied by electron capture.

In beta decay, the transition energy exceeds the sum of the energies contributed by gamma radiation and the kinetic energy of the ejected electrons. The energy unaccounted for during such a transition is possessed by an additional particle known as the neutrino (υ). Neutrinos are uncharged particles with zero rest mass.

The movement of an electron, usually from the innermost shell to the nucleus, with the release of a neutrino is known as electron capture. Holes or vacancies in electron shells are promptly filled by electrons cascading from energy levels farther away from the nucleus. As these vacancies are filled, energy is released, usually in the form of a photon of electromagnetic radiation.

Gamma rays are often formed during the transition from the excited state to a stable energy level. However, no radioactive substance decays solely by gamma emission. Gamma transition is always preceded by either electron capture or emission of an alpha or a beta particle.

Measurement of decay

The rate of decay of a radioactive substance is referred to as the activity of the sample. The unit of measurement in this regard is the Curie (Ci).

$$1 \text{ Ci} = 3.7 \times 10^{10} \text{ disintegrations per second}$$
$$1 \text{ mCi} = 3.7 \times 10^{7} \text{ disintegrations per second}$$
$$1 \text{ } \mu\text{Ci} = 3.7 \times 10^{4} \text{ disintegrations per second}$$

The specific activity of a radioactive sample refers to the activity per unit mass.

The radioactive decay of substance is expressed as follows:

$$\frac{N}{N_o} = e^{\lambda t}$$

N_o is the initial number of radioactive atoms at zero time. N is the number of radioactive atoms left after a defined period of time (t). Lambda (λ) is the decay constant. It is the fraction of the radioactive nuclei present that decays in unit time and is characteristic for each radionuclide.

The character of the preceding equation suggests that radioactive substances take an infinitely long time to decay totally. For this reason, it is customary to express the activity in terms of half-life ($T_{1/2}$) or the time necessary to reduce the activity to one half of the initial value. The half-life periods of the known radioactive isotopes range from a fraction of a second to many centuries.

It is important to note that the Curie is not a measure of energy. In characterizing a radionuclide in terms of disintegrations per second, no indication is given as to the character of the radiation emitted of the energy involved. In addition to the specific activity and the physical characteristics of the radiation emitted, the biologic consequences of exposure to a radionuclide depend on at least two other factors: (1) the distribution of the isotope within the host and the rate of excretion and (2) the half-life of the substance involved. The internal deposition of radium in humans illustrates the importance of these factors. Radium has a very long half-life

(1638 years), is concentrated in the skeleton, and, together with its poorly soluble decay products, subjects the involved tissues to a continuous bombardment of alpha, beta, and gamma particles throughout the life span of the host. Thus as little as 0.1 to 0.3 μCi of radium deposited in the human body is dangerous to the health of the recipient.

RADIATION UNITS

Several units are employed to measure levels of ionizing radiation. The oldest unit, the roentgen, is used for x and gamma (γ) rays to measure the quantity of ionization per unit volume of air. Thus the roentgen is a unit of exposure and not absorption (see below). Furthermore, to indicate intensity, a time frame must also be indicated (for example, roentgens per minute).

To represent particulate radiation in terms that can be related to x and gamma rays, two other units—the rad and the Gray—have been devised. These units are based on absorbed dose. One rad is the dose of radiation that will result in the absorption of 100 ergs of energy per gram of the absorbing substance. The energy absorbed by 1 g of most tissues on exposure to one γ of roentgen rays is about 93 ergs or almost the same as 1 rad. Therefore, in many discussions involving radiobiology, rads and roentgens are employed almost interchangeably. As with roentgens, the rad is a measure of quantity and, to convey intensity, an indication of dose rate must also be introduced.

Recently there has been a move toward the use of Système Intèrnationale (SI) units in radiobiology and nuclear medicine. SI units are based on fundamental units of mass (kilograms), length (meters), and time (seconds). SI units have not yet achieved widespread use in the United States but may do so during the next several years. Therefore familiarity with both SI and traditional units is necessary.

The Gray is the accepted SI unit to measure absorbed dose. One Gray is defined as that dose of any form of radiation resulting in the absorption of 1 joule of energy per kilogram of the absorbing material. Thus 1 Gray corresponds to 100 rad.

One rad of particulate radiation generally causes more damage to cells and tissues than 1 rad of x or gamma rays. For this reason, the rem was introduced to normalize the effects produced by different types of radiation. One rem can be defined loosely as that dose of any radiation that produces a biologic effect equivalent to 1 rad of x or gamma rays. In situations where the rem is an inconveniently large unit of measure, the millirem (mrem), which is $\frac{1}{1000}$ of a rem, is employed. The sievert is the accepted SI unit of dose equivalence. One sievert is that dose that produces a biologic effect equivalent to 1 Gray of x or gamma rays. One sievert thus corresponds to 100 rem.

The traditional unit to measure the activity of a radioactive substance is the Curie. The corresponding SI unit

Table 6-1. Sources and average exposure levels to radiation in the environment

Category	Source	Average dose rate (mrem/yr)*
Natural	Cosmic radiation	44
	Terrestrial radiation	40
	Internally deposited radioactive isotopes	18
	Subtotal	102
Man made	Medical diagnosis and treatment	73
	Technologically enhanced sources	4
	Global fallout	4
	Nuclear power	0.003
	Occupational	0.8
	Miscellaneous	2
	Subtotal	84
	TOTAL	186

From Advisory Committee on the Biological Effects of Ionizing Radiation: The effects on populations of exposure to low levels of ionizing radiation (BEIR Report), Washington, D.C., 1980, National Academy of Sciences–National Research Council; Klement, A.W., et al.: Estimates of ionizing radiation doses in the United States, 1960-2000, U.S. Environmental Protection Agency, 1972; and Interagency Task Force on the Health Effects of Ionizing Radiation: Report of the Work Group on Exposure Reduction, Department of Health Education and Welfare, June 1979.
*Data for 1970 in the United States. Dose rates for cosmic and terrestrial radiation vary greatly with altitude and geographic region, respectively. Also, estimates for nuclear power may be high owing to improved technology.

Table 6-2. Biologic significance of single whole-body exposures to various levels of ionizing radiation

Dose (roentgens)	Biologic response
0.001	3 times daily natural background
0.01	No detectable somatic effects
0.1	No detectable somatic effects
1.0	No detectable somatic effects
10	Detectable morphologic and functional alterations in specific subpopulations of lymphocytes
100	Mild radiation sickness in some persons, with nausea and vomiting; decrease in mitotic index of bone marrow and transient leukopenia
1000	Extensive damage to bone marrow with leukopenia, thrombocytopenia, and anemia; necrosis of gastrointestinal mucosa; severe radiation sickness; death within 30 days
10,000	Immediate disorientation or coma; death within hours
100,000	Death of some microorganisms
1,000,000	Death of some bacteria
10,000,000	Death of all living organisms; some denaturation of proteins

From Warren, S.: The pathology of ionizing radiation, Springfield, Ill., 1961, Charles C Thomas, Publisher.

is the becquerel. One becquerel corresponds to a decay rate of one disintegration per second. Since 1 Curie equals 3.7×10^{10} disintegrations per second, 1 Curie represents 3.7×10^{10} becquerels.

BACKGROUND RADIATION

Life on earth has evolved in the presence of ionizing radiation from several sources. This natural background radiation is derived from three major sources: cosmic rays from the sun and outer space, radium and other radioactive elements contained in the earth's crust, and potassium 40 and other naturally occurring radionuclides that are normally present in the body. Cosmic radiation varies with altitude, and residents of Albuquerque, New Mexico, for example, receive approximately twice the dose as do the inhabitants of Boston, Massachusetts. Airline personnel and astronauts are also exposed to above average doses of cosmic rays. Similarly, the radiation emitted by the earth's crust varies markedly by geographic region depending on variations in the content of radioactive materials in the soil and subterranean rock. Terrestrial radiation is of particular importance to miners who may be exposed to radioactive components of the earth's crust in aerosol form in the atmosphere of mines. Inhalation of these substances, when they are of appropriate size and shape, results in their deposition in the terminal ramifications of the lungs where they may emit

radioactivity for a long time to the detriment of the host.

In addition to natural background radiation, humans are exposed to radiation from man-made sources. The largest component of man-made background radiation relates to exposures associated with medical diagnosis and treatment. Lesser contributions come from "technologically enhanced" sources (such as the use of radionuclide-containing minerals in phosphate fertilizers and building materials), fallout from atomic weapons, nuclear power production, and consumer products (color television sets, smoke detectors, luminescent instrument and clock dials, and so on).

Table 6-1 shows the estimated annual exposure to various types of man-made and natural background radiation. Table 6-2 shows how these doses compare with other whole-body exposures. In Table 6-2 some of the biologic effects of single exposures to 10-fold increments of radiation are summarized. Only somatic effects are included, since the dose levels at which an increased incidence of genetic abnormalities may be expected in humans are unknown.

CELLULAR AND MOLECULAR RADIATION BIOLOGY

Much of our understanding of the effects of ionizing radiation in humans relates to studies that involve the exposure of cells grown in tissue culture. Such cells can be analyzed for evidence of (1) overt injury such as cell death or loss of the ability to undergo cell division and (2) occult injury such as nonlethal alterations of plasma membranes, enzymes, specific macromolecules, and even specific molecules. In this section a portion of these data will be discussed with particular reference to the mechanisms by which radiation injures and kills cells.

Reproductive death

A reduction in reproductive capacity constitutes one of the most important effects of radiation on mammalian cells. After irradiation of a population of cells, a variable number become pyknotic, undergo lysis, or otherwise exhibit evidence of cell death. The residual cells remain viable and are indistinguishable morphologically from their nonirradiated counterparts. However, despite this absence of recognizable morphologic alterations, many of the irradiated cells have lost their capacity to divide and are therefore sterile. Loss of a cell's ability to divide in unlimited fashion is referred to as reproductive death. On occasion, irradiated cells may continue to replicate and grow without actual physical separation. The result is the formation of multinucleated giant cells, which represents one of the morphologic hallmarks of radiation injury.

In order to document reproductive death, one needs to quantitate the loss of the ability of irradiated cells to proliferate indefinitely. This may be accomplished in vivo or in vitro. The ability of hemopoietic stem cells to form macroscopic colonies in the spleen after intravenous transfer to lethally irradiated mice of the same inbred strain is a frequently employed in vivo method to quantitate the reproductive death of stem cells. Since each colony is derived from a single stem cell that has divided innumerable times, one may develop a dose-response curve, which relates radiation dose to the capacity of the irradiated cells to reproduce in a compatible environment. Results from such an experiment are shown in Fig. 6-2.

Alternatively, the irradiated cells may be grown in tissue culture and colony formation determined in vitro. In this setting, it is also known that each colony arises from a single cell. Abortive colonies, containing subnormal numbers of cells, are not included in the calculation of the survival curves. Results from an experiment that employs this type of approach are shown in Fig. 6-3. Survival curves determined in vitro closely approximate those obtained in vivo for the same cell population.

The sequence of events that leads to reproductive death is not totally understood. There is general agreement that the initial event is the absorption of energy by the involved cells with the subsequent disruption of individual molecules or sequences of molecules. Damage of this type is believed to be initiated randomly in cells as a result of a series of ionizations and excitations, which are known to occur along the tracks of charged particles moving with a high velocity. The mechanisms by which radi-

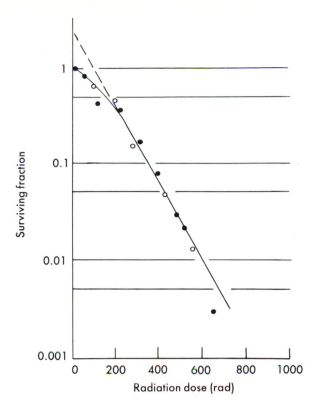

Fig. 6-2. Survival of reproductive capacity of normal mouse bone marrow stem cells as function of radiation dose. Open and closed circles represent two experiments. (From Till, J.E., and McCullock, E.A.: Radiat. Res. **14**:213, 1961.)

ation-induced alterations of individual molecules are translated into a loss of sustained reproductive capacity are poorly understood. Two broad theories have been postulated and are referred to as the target theory and the indirect effects theory.

Target theory

The target theory predicts that a biologic unit (such as a cell, cell membrane or molecule) will respond in adverse fashion after a minimum number of radiation "hits" or absorption events. Fig. 6-4 shows a hypothetical dose-response curve to illustrate this hypothesis. Note that the dose-response curve of Fig. 6-4, A, becomes a straight line in Fig. 6-4, B, when the surviving fraction is plotted on a logarithmic scale against the dose on a linear scale. Thus the number of surviving cells is an exponential function of dose. Even at low dose levels, there is a corresponding decrease in the number of survivors with each incremental increase in radiation dose. This type of dose-response curve is referred to as a "single-hit" curve because only one "hit" (ionization) is required for the inactivation of a definable number of cells. The results are unaffected by the time over which the radiation is administered (dose rate) or whether it is administered on one or several occasions (fractionated).

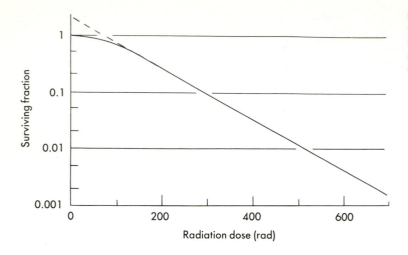

Fig. 6-3. Survival of reproductive capacity of HeLa cells as function of radiation dose. (From Puck, T.T., and Marcus, P.I. Reproduced from The Journal of Experimental Medicine, 1956, vol. 103, pp. 653-666, by copyright permission of The Rockefeller University Press.)

Fig. 6-4. A, Idealized dose-response curve in which fraction of surviving cells is plotted as function of radiation dose. Note absence of shoulder. **B,** Semilog plot of curve from **A.** Dose is linearly related to logarithm of surviving fraction.

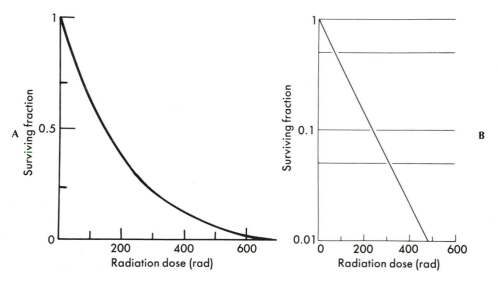

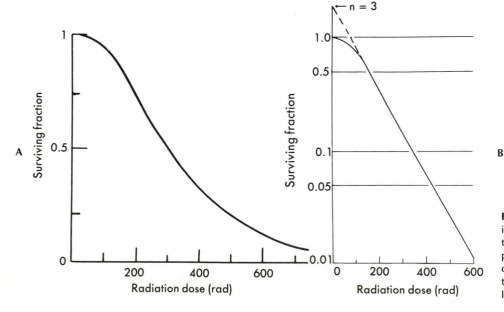

Fig. 6-5. A, Idealized dose-response curve in which fraction of surviving cells is plotted as function of radiation dose. Note presence of shoulder. **B,** Semilog plot of curve from **A.** Dose is not linearly related to logarithm of surviving fraction, particularly at low dose levels.

Indirect effects theory

Fig. 6-5 shows a second type of dose-response curve, which is not exponential at low dose levels. The nonlinear region in Fig. 6-5, *B*, is referred to as the shoulder or the threshold region of the curve. At least two explanations exist for this threshold effect: (1) each target must sustain more than one "hit" or related deleterious event in order to be inactivated, and, at low dose levels, the probability of several such random events occurring to one cell, or perhaps even to a specific region of the cell, approaches zero; and (2) the damage sustained by individual cells at low dose levels is minimal and therefore susceptible to repair by intracellular enzymes.

With the exception of the shoulder region, Figs. 6-4, *B*, and 6-5, *B*, are identical. Therefore in order to describe and compare survival curves, two pieces of information are generally included:

1. The slope of the linear portion of the curve or, more commonly, the dose that results in a 37% survival; this value is referred to as the D_{37}, the mean lethal dose, or the D_o; it is important to reemphasize that these calculations must be made on the straight portion of the curve
2. The intercept of the straight portion of the curve extrapolated to zero dose (dotted line in Fig. 6-5, *B*); this number is the extrapolation number and in the example given is 3

Dose-survival experiments utilizing the approaches outlined above have established D_{37} values of 80 to 200 rad for most mammalian cells exposed in vitro to x or gamma rays. These figures stand in contrast to similar data for microorganisms, such as *Escherichia coli*, yeast, and viruses, which often exhibit D_{37} values in excess of several thousand rad.

Radiation-related formation of free radicals has been suggested as a mechanism to explain the inactivation of target molecules in an indirect manner. Free radicals are known to be produced by ionizing radiation. Since water is an important constituent of all cells, it is postulated that many of these indirect effects are related to the interaction of radiation with water. In this situation, hydrogen and hydroxyl free radicals are formed. Free radicals are extremely strong oxidizing or reducing agents. As such they can (1) react with water to form peroxides, (2) form cross linkages with critical molecules such as DNA and RNA, which may result in inactivation of the parent molecule, or (3) attach directly to key structures, such as plasma membranes, to render them incapable of discharging their normal functions.

Factors affecting radiation response

Radiation produces injury in biologic systems by both direct and indirect effects. The relative contribution of each mechanism depends on the system involved and a variety of other factors, especially the character of the radiation and the presence or absence of agents known to protect against the effects of radiation. We will now move to a consideration of some of these factors.

The important factors that influence the radiosensitivity of mammalian cells can be divided into three groups: physical, chemical, and biologic. These factors will be considered separately although their contributions usually overlap in both the experimental and the therapeutic setting.

Physical factors

The most important physical factors that affect the magnitude of a biologic response to radiation are the character of the radiation, the total amount administered, and the time within which this dose is given. The term *relative biologic effectiveness* (RBE) is used to compare the effectiveness (in terms of absorbed dose) of two forms of radiation in producing the same biologic effect. The generally accepted reference standard for this type of comparison is x rays generated at 150 to 300 kiloelectron volts (keV) with filtration provided by 1 mm of copper. In general, fast neutrons are more effective than x rays in producing most of the late somatic effects associated with radiation injury. Therefore with respect to these effects, fast neutrons have an RBE of greater than 1.

The RBE of a particle relates primarily to how it distributes energy along its track. This sequence of events is known as *linear energy transfer* (LET), which is a measure of the average rate at which an ionizing particle loses energy along its path. LET therefore depends on the mass, the charge, and the velocity of the particle. A particle with a relatively large mass and charge but a low velocity will in general exhibit a higher LET than a small noncharged particle with a high velocity. Heavy particles, such as atomic nuclei, which are given velocity (or accelerated) by a machine (a generator) constructed for this purpose, produce dense paths of ionization over short tracks and are referred to as *densely ionizing particles*. X and gamma rays, as well as energetic electrons produced by an accelerator, are referred to as *sparsely ionizing* because they lose small amounts of energy to the absorbing substance over a long path until finally all of the energy is spent and they come to a halt.

Also important in energy transfer is the Bragg effect. This effect, shown schematically in Fig. 6-6, relates to a change from a relatively constant rate of energy release to a more rapid one near the end of the particle range. The result is a localized effect in tissue at the point of the more rapid release of energy (Bragg peak).

Dose rate also influences cell survival, especially for low LET radiation. With low LET radiations, a greater total dose is required to produce the same effect when the radiation is (1) delivered in multiple small doses known as fractions or (2) given continuously over a pro-

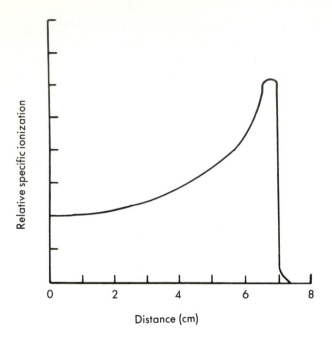

Fig. 6-6. Schematic representation of Bragg effect.

longed period of time. The basis of these observations is believed to relate to the repair of sublethal radiation damage that occurs during the actual time of exposure at low dose rates or between exposures with fractionalization.

Chemical factors

Chemical factors may either exert a protective effect or potentiate the effects of ionizing radiation. Perhaps the most important substance in this regard is molecular oxygen. The ability of oxygen to potentiate many of the effects of ionizing radiation is known as the oxygen effect. This effect is especially pronounced with low LET radiations such as x and gamma rays. The involved mechanisms have not been completely defined but may relate to the observation that oxygen increases the production of free radicals by radiation. The oxygen effect is especially important in the treatment of malignant tumors with ionizing radiation. Most tumors exhibit considerable variability in oxygen tension, presumably because of the nonuniform distribution of blood vessels within the neoplasm. When the discrepancy between local requirements and available oxygen becomes critical, necrosis results. Adjacent to areas of necrosis are hypoxic but still viable tumor cells. Such hypoxic foci are less sensitive to many types of ionizing radiation than are the surrounding, well-oxygenated tissues, and they may give rise to local recurrence of tumor following radiotherapy. Considerable effort has been devoted to attempts to increase the oxygen tension in tumors prior to radiotherapy.

Another group of agents that have been used chemically to increase the radiosensitivity of cells is the halo-

genated pyrimidines. These analogs of DNA bases can increase several fold the radiosensitivity of cells in culture. The mechanism involved is not known.

A second class of chemical agents serves to protect against radiation-induced cell injury. The best-known examples of these radioprotective agents are the sulfhydryl amines such as cysteine and cystamine. Several hypotheses exist to explain the mechanisms of action of these compounds. One well-accepted theory postulates that sulfhydryl groups compete effectively with biologically important compounds, such as DNA, for free radicals formed by the interaction of radiation and water. Oxidation of the sulfhydryl amines to relatively stable compounds may serve to protect more complex molecules known to be critical to the viability of the cell.

Biologic factors

Although exceedingly complex and poorly understood, a variety of biologic factors are known to influence the response of individual cells to radiation. Two of the most important factors are the repair of nonlethal injury and the timing of the radiation exposure with respect to the cell cycle. The radiosensitivity of synchronized cell populations grown in tissue culture is related to the generation cycle. For most tissue culture lines, cells are most sensitive to radiation during G_2 and mitosis, less sensitive in G_1, and least sensitive toward the end of the S period.

Repair of sublethal radiation injury appears to begin immediately after the damage is incurred. Under optimal conditions, such repair proceeds rapidly. It is important to note that repair is much more prominent with respect to low LET radiations (x rays, gamma rays) than with high LET radiations (alpha particles). The point is illustrated in the hypothetical dose-response curves shown in Figs. 6-4, *B*, and 6-5, *B*. Fig. 6-5, *B*, with a well-defined shoulder, represents the situation that would be encountered experimentally utilizing low LET radiations. The breadth of the shoulder is thought to relate roughly to the magnitude of repair. In contrast to Fig. 6-5, *B*, the dose-response curve of Fig. 6-4, *B*, demonstrates no shoulder and would be typical of high LET radiation. From this and related evidence it appears that cells exposed to high LET radiation either die or escape unscathed. In either case there is no sublethal damage to repair. Repair will be discussed in greater detail when we consider radiation-induced injury to DNA.

Radiation effects involving macromolecules

In the past several years a large body of information has developed with respect to the effects of radiation upon DNA, RNA, and proteins. Much of the currently available evidence points to DNA as the "target" of greatest radiobiologic importance. For example, in experiments utilizing microbeams of radiation, the nucleus of the cell was found to be more radiosensitive than the cytoplasm. In addition, the sensitivity of cells from different species to reproductive death is directly proportional to their DNA content. Finally, DNA alterations are implicated in many of the delayed effects of radiation exposure.

The effect of radiation on DNA is dependent on the dose, the quality or type of particle involved, and the stage of the cell cycle during which the event occurs. In vitro, radiation of DNA in solution results in (1) breaking of hydrogen bonds, (2) formation of cross linkages between adjacent strands or closely apposed regions of the same strand, (3) base damage, (4) disruption to the sugar-phosphate backbone of the molecule, and (5) impairment of the ability of DNA to act as a template for the synthesis of a new DNA strand. The latter observation has received particular attention recently.

Experiments show that radiation can result in breaks of one or both DNA strands. The effect may result directly from a strategically located ionization or indirectly by means of the activation of specific nucleases. The majority of single-stranded breaks are believed to be rapidly repaired, with the intact strand serving as a template to direct the rejoining process. The intact strand apparently holds the broken strand in place while repair occurs and may also provide a coding function for the involved enzymes. The rejoining process proceeds extremely rapidly. In contradistinction to single-strand breaks, the majority of double-strand breaks are believed to be irreparable. The total loss of local structure, and the formation of DNA fragments that quickly become separated, produce a situation in which restoration of normal structure is extremely unlikely.

The exposure of rapidly dividing mammalian cells to intermediate doses of radiation generally results in a phenomenon known as division delay. Typically, irradiated cells immediately cease division for a period of time proportional to the absorbed dose. After this delay, the cells resume their normal growth patterns for one or more generations. Cell death, when it occurs, usually takes place during the first postirradiation division although damaged cells occasionally undergo several divisions prior to death. Less commonly, radiation can induce DNA synthesis outside the period of normal synthesis in the cell cycle. This phenomenon, which involves all phases of the cell cycle, is referred to as *unscheduled* DNA synthesis. Unscheduled synthesis can also be induced by ultraviolet rays and alkylating agents. The biologic implications of unscheduled synthesis are not entirely known, but the phenomenon is probably related to DNA repair.

Experiments designed to evaluate the effects of radiation on RNA have in general been concerned with RNA synthesis in toto and have not included species analysis (messenger RNA, transfer RNA, ribosomal RNA). In addition, RNA synthesis is dependent on DNA integrity, and the relative contribution of these two effects upon radiation-induced cell injury has been difficult to differentiate experimentally. Despite these technical problems, however, RNA synthesis is believed to be less radiosensitive than is DNA synthesis.

Large doses of radiation are required to destroy the function of most proteins. Several enzymes have been carefully investigated in this regard. The apparent radioresistance of most proteins may relate to their relatively small size, particularly in comparison with such molecules as DNA and RNA.

GENERAL MORPHOLOGIC FEATURES OF RADIATION INJURY

Before a discussion of the effects of radiation on select cell types and tissues is begun, it is important to emphasize that none of the morphologic events that result from injury is unique. Each of the alterations encountered in irradiated cells may be found in association with other forms of injury, such as that caused by ischemia, heat, cold, microbiologic agents, or toxic substances. In fact, the effects of some alkylating agents so closely mimic those associated with ionizing radiation that they are often referred to as radiomimetic drugs.

Cells injured by radiation show changes in both the nucleus and the cytoplasm. As noted previously, the nucleus of most cells appears to be more radiosensitive than the cytoplasm. At low dose levels, the nuclear chromatin becomes somewhat more clumped, and the nucleus appears swollen and presumably is edematous. At moderate and high dose levels, the nucleus is often pyknotic and may show karyorrhexis. Swelling and focal loss of the nuclear membrane and fragmentation of the chromatin may be observed by electron microscopy. The cytoplasmic changes after irradiation include swelling, vacuolization, and alterations in the various components of the plasma membrane. Variable degrees of disintegration of the endoplasmic reticulum are apparent. Mitochondria have been noted to be enlarged and distorted forms are readily apparent, but these changes may be secondary to metabolic and membrane alterations, since several studies have shown that mitochondria themselves are relatively radioresistant.

Although all mammalian cells are affected by ionizing radiation, moderate variability exists among different cell types and tissues with respect to susceptibility to a specific effect such as cell death. In general, rapidly dividing cells are more radiosensitive than are slowly dividing cells. This difference presumably relates to radiation-induced inhibition of DNA synthesis and interference with normal cell division. The morphologic consequences of these changes are a variety of chromosomal abnormalities including translocations, breaks, deletions, and the formation of fragments and rings. Such

Table 6-3. Relative radiosensitivity of normal cells and select tumors

Radiosensitivity	Normal cells	Tumors
Very high	Lymphocytes Immature hemopoietic cells Intestinal epithelium Spermatogonia Ovarian follicular cells	Most forms of lymphoma Leukemia Seminoma, dysgerminoma Granulosa cell tumor
High	Urinary bladder epithelium Esophageal epithelium Gastric mucosa Mucous membranes of mouth and pharynx Epidermal epithelium (including hair follicles and sebaceous glands) Epithelium of optic lens	Transitional cell carcinoma of bladder Adenocarcinoma of stomach Epidermoid carcinoma of skin, oropharynx, esophagus, cervix
Intermediate	Endothelium Growing bone and cartilage Fibroblasts Glial cells Glandular epithelium of breast Pulmonary epithelium Renal epithelium Hepatic epithelium Pancreatic epithelium Thyroid epithelium Adrenal epithelium	Vascular and connective tissue component of most tumors Osteogenic sarcoma Astrocytoma Chondrosarcoma Epidermoid carcinoma of lung Liposarcoma Adenocarcinoma of breast, kidney, thyroid, colon, liver, pancreas
Low	Mature hemopoietic cells Muscle cells Mature connective tissue Mature bone and cartilage Ganglion cells	Rhabdomyosarcoma Leiomyosarcoma Ganglioneuroma

alterations are best appreciated by chromosome analysis. However, abnormal mitotic figures may be seen in tissue sections, often in association with multinucleated giant cells.

The relationship between radiosensitivity and mitotic activity was first appreciated in 1906 by Bergonié and Tribondeau, and their names have been applied to what has become a key concept in radiobiology. They stated that:

X rays are more effective on cells which have greater reproductive activity; the effectiveness is greater on those cells which have a longer dividing future ahead, on those cells the morphology and the function of which are least fixed. From this law, it is easy to understand that roentgen radiation destroys tumors without destroying healthy tissues.*

These relationships, semiquantitated in Table 6-3, have been paraphrased as follows: radiosensitive tissues are those with the greatest mitotic activity and the least degree of differentiation.

Vascular changes are an extremely important consequence of the irradiation of several tissues and may be responsible for some of the acute and delayed effects of such exposure. Vascular abnormalities are seen after irra-

diation of both normal and neoplastic tissues. As shown in Table 6-3, endothelial cells are not especially radiosensitive, but degenerative vascular abnormalities are almost always seen in association with a neoplasm that has been irradiated optimally. Furthermore, degenerative changes are not confined to the tumor but also involve the adjacent normal parenchyma of the affected organ and other tissues that may be interposed between the source of the radiation and the tumor.

Vascular dilatation is responsible for the erythema of the skin frequently noted in the immediate postirradiation period. Similar dilatation of the blood vessels probably occurs in a variety of sites and may account for the transient increase in function documented in some organs after exposure. Somewhat later, and generally in association with high dose levels, regressive changes appear, including swelling and vacuolization of the endothelium, focal necrosis of the vessel wall with hemorrhage, or, on occasion, rupture. Months or years after exposure various degenerative abnormalities are apparent. They include (1) fibrous and hyaline sclerosis of the subintimal region and media of small arteries and arterioles, which results in focal narrowing, and endothelial cell proliferation, which may partially obliterate the lumen, and (2) decreased numbers of capillaries with considerable ectasia of those that persist.

From the above description it is not difficult to visual-

---

*From Bergonie, J., and Tribondeau, L.: Interpretation de quelques resultats de la radiotherapie et essai de fixation d'une technique rationnelle, Compt. Rend. Acad. Sci. **143**:983, 1906.

ize some of the alterations that might be expected in a structure irradiated several years previously. Grossly, the organ will be somewhat smaller than normal because of necrosis and loss of radiosensitive parenchymal cells and subsequent ischemia of less radiosensitive cells by a compromised circulation. Microscopically, atrophic or absent parenchymal cells will have been replaced by dense hyalinized connective tissue, which may contain pleomorphic, often very large, fibroblasts. Multinucleated giant cells may be present except in organs populated by fixed postmitotic cells. Small arteries and arterioles will be lined by increased numbers of very prominent endothelial cells. Focally, the walls of these vessels will be thick and sclerotic and the lumen small or obliterated.

The functional consequences of these morphologic abnormalities are significant. Loss of parenchymal cells may result in impairment of function. Diffusion across thick basement membranes may be impeded. Structures may be distorted or compressed by the dense fibrous connective tissue referred to above. For example, obstruction of the ureter is a not uncommon complication of pelvic irradiation administered to eradicate or impede the growth of a malignant tumor of the urinary bladder. Surgical procedures are often more difficult in areas that have been irradiated months or years previously. Increased amounts of dense connective tissue make dissection of vital structures more difficult than usual. Postoperatively, hypoperfusion of the area by abnormal blood vessels predisposes to poor wound healing and increases the likelihood of the breakdown of anastomotic sites. Impaired circulation also compromises the defense mechanisms needed to deal with untoward complications such as infection. Poor healing and an increased incidence of infection are not confined to the postoperative state but may be associated with any form of trauma.

RADIATION INJURY IN HUMANS
General effects

Radiation effects can be divided into two general categories: somatic effects and genetic effects. Somatic effects are those manifested by the recipient. In contrast, genetic effects do not show up directly in the irradiated organism but rather in its progeny. Somatic effects may be further divided into (1) acute or early and (2) delayed or late.

Acute effects are those that produce signs and symptoms of radiation damage from within minutes to 30 to 60 days subsequent to exposure. Clinical manifestations of acute effects occur only after relatively high doses (above about 50 rad) delivered over a short period of time. Symptoms increase in severity with increasing dose. Although all tissues probably are involved to a varying degree, the symptoms during the acute phase generally

relate to malfunction of rapidly proliferating tissues, the integrity of which is vital to homeostasis. Rapid renewal systems such as the bone marrow, lymphoid organs, testes, and the epithelium of the gastrointestinal tract are particularly susceptible to such injury.

Late or delayed effects are those that manifest themselves many months or, more commonly, years after exposure. They tend to be probabilistic functions of the total accumulated dose. Radiation carcinogenesis is perhaps the best known of the delayed effects. Other life-threatening delayed effects involve the kidney (radiation nephritis), gastrointestinal tract (stricture, chronic ulcer), lung (radiation pneumonitis), bladder (ulcer and fistula formation), spinal cord (transverse myelitis), and the heart (constrictive pericarditis). Life-threatening delayed effects may be associated with repeated (fractionated) local exposures or are the sequelae of a single whole-body exposure.

The effects of radiation injury can also be classified as stochastic or nonstochastic. A stochastic effect varies in frequency but not in severity with dose and fails to exhibit a threshold, a dose below which no effect is seen. Examples of stochastic effects are heritable effects on germ cells, teratogenic effects on the developing embryo, and many types of radiation-induced tumors. Nonstochastic effects vary in severity but not in frequency with dose and often exhibit a threshold. Many of the acute effects of radiation injury are stochastic in nature. Stochastic and nonstochastic effects will be discussed in more detail in subsequent sections of this chapter.

In this section, both genetic and somatic effects in humans will be considered. Acute and delayed effects will be considered as will be the consequences of both local and whole-body exposures. By way of introduction, the human populations that have been exposed to significant amounts of ionizing radiation will be reviewed briefly because much of the subsequent information has been obtained from this experience.

Exposed populations

A significant number of persons have been accidentally or therapeutically exposed to biologically significant amounts of ionizing radiation. However, evaluation of many cases is not possible because of incomplete follow-up data or insufficient demographic data. Thus much current knowledge with respect to radiation injury in humans has been obtained from an evaluation of the populations summarized in Table 6-4. Even among these groups, direct comparisons are often complicated by differences in age, variability in the conditions of exposure (extent, magnitude, time frame, external versus internal emitters, and so on), and the presence or absence of known preexisting disease. In reviewing the exposed human populations, specific mention will be made of some of these variables.

Table 6-4. Summary of irradiated human populations

Population	Primary type of radiation	Region primarily irradiated	Sample size	Comments
British adults irradiated for ankylosing spondylitis	X rays	Spine	13,352	Increased frequency of malignant tumors
Children irradiated for suspected enlarged thymus and other benign lesions of head and neck	X rays	Mediastinum	24,604*†	Increased frequency of benign and malignant tumors, especially of thyroid
American radiologists	X rays, radium	Partial to whole body	425-82,441*	Increased frequency of malignant tumors, decreased life span
Radium dial painters and related workers; adults treated with radium	Gamma, alpha, and beta particles (^{226}Ra, ^{228}Ra)	Skeleton	760+	Increased frequency of malignant tumors, especially of bone, and blood dyscrasias
Thorium dioxide	Alpha particles	Predominantly liver, spleen, bone marrow	16,074*	Increased frequency of hepatic and other neoplasms, cirrhosis, blood dyscrasias, and local granulomas at site of injection
Children irradiated in utero during diagnostic or therapeutic procedures involving the mother	X ray	Whole body	7346	Increased frequency of congenital abnormalities, mental retardation
Rongelapese	Gamma plus internally deposited radionuclides	Whole body but with disproportional irradiation of thyroid	334*	Retardation of growth and development, benign and malignant thyroid tumors, chromosomal abnormalities, possible increased frequency of miscarriages and stillbirths
Japanese atomic bomb survivors	Gamma plus neutrons	Whole body	120,000*	Increased frequency of developmental abnormalities, benign and malignant tumors, and degenerative changes

*Includes comparable group of nonexposed ("control") individuals.
†May be some overlap in reported persons.

During the period 1935 to 1954, a significant number of individuals were irradiated, primarily to the spine, for the relief of symptoms associated with ankylosing spondylitis. Subsequent evaluation of a group of British males treated in this fashion has revealed an increased frequency of malignant disease, especially leukemia, and persistent chromosome abnormalities. In the context of this discussion it is important to note that these people were afflicted with a preexisting disease of significant magnitude. Although symptoms relate primarily to the spine, ankylosing spondylitis is currently thought to be a systemic disease with features common to the collagen disorders. In addition, these individuals' exposures were restricted to one region of the body, and animal experiments have demonstrated that a standard dose administered to part of the body produces less pronounced acute and delayed effects than it would if administered to the whole body.

Similarly, infants treated with x rays for so-called status thymolymphaticus were exposed in a regional manner. These treatments were given to shrink a supposedly enlarged thymus gland, a procedure formerly believed to alleviate respiratory distress or, is some instances, to protect against the sudden infant death syndrome. An increased incidence of benign and malignant thyroid tumors has been documented in this population as well as a probable increase in lymphoma and leukemia and perhaps other types of tumors. In addition, thymic irradiation early in life may alter permanently the immunologic responsiveness of the recipient. In this connection, an apparent increased incidence of asthma and a constellation of uncommon diseases with immunologic features has been noted among people irradiated for "status thymolymphaticus." Other groups of children were irradiated for cervical lymphadenitis or prominent pharyngeal tonsils, but the follow-up study of these individuals has been less sucessful than with the "status thymolymphaticus" group.

An unknown number of early American radiologists were exposed to considerable radiation as a result of the poor shielding of their equipment. The magnitude of exposure in these persons is unknown. An increased prevalence of leukemia and skin tumors, with a probable decrease in life span, has been documented in this population.

Internally deposited radionuclides can also cause

severe radiation injury. One of the first reports in this regard concerned the early radium-dial painters. These workers, principally young women, applied luminescent radium-containing paint to watch and clock dials with fine camel's hair brushes, which they pointed with their tongue and lips. A significant portion of these radium compounds was ingested, absorbed from the gastrointestinal tract, and deposited in bone. In this location continuous decay led to bone necrosis, infection, and irradiation of adjacent structures. Of particular significance in this regard was the exposure of the respiratory epithelium in the nasal sinuses and air sacs from radium concentrated in the adjacent skull bones.

It is important to note that the paint used by the dial painters contained a relatively low concentration of radium. However, this substance localizes very efficiently in teeth and bone, especially in those regions where new mineral is being formed. In addition, the radium incorporated in this fashion remains in the involved tissues for a long period of time. Thus the long-term consequences represent the cumulative effects of a relatively low initial dose and include malignant tumors of bone, the epithelial lining of the paranasal sinuses, and colon as well as a probable increased incidence of leukemia and blood dyscrasias.

Because of its radiopacity, colloidal thorium dioxide (Thorotrast) was widely employed as a contrast medium from 1930 to 1945 by diagnostic radiologists. When administered intravenously, this radioactive substance localizes primarily in the liver, spleen, and bone marrow. Unfortunately, thorium dioxide is chemically inert, is poorly eliminated from the body, and has a long physical half-life and a biologic half-life in the liver of 200 to 400 years. It is phagocytosed by reticuloendothelial cells and remains there until the cell dies, whereupon it is often rephagocytosed by a neighboring cell. A variety of malignant tumors of the liver have been associated with thorium dioxide administration including hepatomas, cholangiocarcinomas, and hemangioendotheliomas; such tumors develop after an average latent period of approximately 20 years. Thorotrast is an alpha emitter and serves to illustrate the importance of the relationship between the way in which a radioactive substance is presented to the host and the probability of subsequent deleterious effects. Harmless externally because of a limited capacity to penetrate surface tissues, alpha particles, which are highly destructive when located within cells, may be responsible for the death of the host when they are deposited internally. In addition, evidence exists to suggest that Thorotrast and related colloids are chemically carcinogenic.

Radiation of the embryo or fetus in utero has long been recognized as injurious. After such exposure small head circumference and mental retardation have been documented among the offspring of mothers irradiated therapeutically and of mothers exposed, particularly during the first trimester, to the atomic bombs. More recently, in utero exposure has also been implicated in the subsequent development of leukemia and other tumors in human offspring.

Eighty-two inhabitants of Rongelap and Ailingnae in the Marshall Islands were accidentally exposed in 1954 to varying amounts of fallout released during the testing of a nuclear weapon on Bikini Atoll. A significant portion of the radiation absorbed by these islanders resulted from the deposition of radionuclides. The maximum whole-body exposure from external radiation was estimated to be 175 rad. Localized deposition of the various isotopes of iodine produced mean thyroid exposures of 1000 rad in young children, proportionately less in older children and adults. Subsequent follow-up examination has been extremely careful, and the population under evaluation now includes a control group and totals 334 people. Problems thus far encountered by the exposed Rongelapese have involved primarily the thyroid gland, although disturbances of growth and development and increased numbers of chromosome abnormalities have also been noted. To date, irradiation of the thyroid gland has been manifest by an increased prevalence of benign thyroid nodules, frequently multiple and often associated with hypothyroidism, as well as an increase in carcinoma. The growth retardation noted in these children probably relates to hypothyroidism.

The estimated civilian populations of Hiroshima and Nagasaki in August, 1945, were 225,000 and 174,000, respectively. Of the total civilian population of both cities, approximately 106,200 died within the initial 12 weeks after exposure. Dosimetry is now available for almost all of the survivors. The magnitude of possible exposure of an unshielded individual, as a function of his or her distance from the hypocenter, is shown in Fig. 6-7. The hypocenter is the point on the ground immediately beneath the center of the explosion. The intercity discrepancies in Fig. 6-7 are primarily attributable to differences between the two bombs. The fissionable material in the Hiroshima bomb was uranium 235, and the resultant radiation spectrum contained a mixture of gamma rays and neutrons. The Nagasaki bomb contained plutonium 238 and released primarily gamma rays admixed with relatively few neutrons. In this connection, it is important to reemphasize the observation that fast neutrons are more effective than gamma rays in producing most of the delayed effects thus far studied.

Early deaths were caused by acute radiation sickness, flash burns, and mechanical injuries from falling buildings. Most victims and survivors sustained more than one type of injury. Table 6-5 shows the estimated distribution of the types of injury among the survivors.

Mechanical injuries were mostly of the "indirect" blast type; that is, they were produced by falling beams, flying glass, or other debris. Most of these injuries were contu-

Hiroshima

Nagasaki

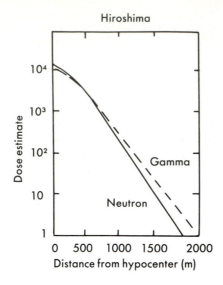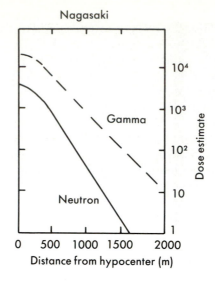

Fig. 6-7. Air dose estimates for both neutrons and gamma rays, Hiroshima and Nagasaki.

Table 6-5. Types of injury among atomic bomb survivors

Type of injury	Etiologic factor	Percent of survivors with injury*	Farthest distance injury reported (meters)
Mechanical trauma	Blast	70	4000
Burn	Heat	65	4000
Radiation sickness	Ionizing radiation	30	1500

Modified from Key, C.R.: Hum. Pathol. **2:**475, 1971.
*Total exceeds 100% because many persons have multiple injuries.

sions or lacerations; only a small number of the injured survivors sustained fractures. Examples of trauma occurred at least as far as 4000 meters from the hypocenter.

More than 90% of the survivors with burns had "flash" or "profile" types of burns on the exposed areas of the skin that were in the direct path of the bomb's intense heat rays. An example of such injury is shown in Fig. 6-8. In some cases a person's clothing was ignited and produced coexisting "flame" burns, which were present in about 15% of the burned survivors.

An indication of the intensity of the heat is reflected in the bubbling or blistering of the exposed portions of roof tiles, a phenomenon observed up to 1200 meters from the hypocenter in Hiroshima and even farther in Nagasaki. The radiant thermal energy was about 40 calories per square centimeter at that distance, and it has been estimated that the damaged tiles had to attain a temperature above 1800° C to exhibit this effect.

Roughly 20% to 30% of the acute fatalities were caused by flash burns. Apart from other injuries, flash burns would have been fatal to all unshielded persons at distances up to 2000 meters from the hypocenter. Even

beyond 4000 meters there were instances of burns severe enough to require treatment.

The direct effects of ionizing radiation were outlined by a local physician, Dr. Hachiya, for the Hiroshima newspaper on September 1, 1945.*

1. Those who were exposed within 500 meters out-of-doors were killed instantly or died within four or five days.
2. Some who were within 500 meters were protected by buildings and hence not burned. Within a period of two to 15 days many of these people developed a so-called "radiation sickness" and died. This sickness was manifested by anorexia, vomiting, hematemesis, and hemoptysis.
3. Those exposed in the 500 to 1000 meter zone have shown symptoms similar to those who were exposed within 500 meters but the onset of symptoms was later and insidious. The death rate in this group has been high.
4. I have studied the location of the in-patients and a great number of the out-patients and found most of them were exposed between 1000 and 3000 meters. Those in this group who were closest to the center became critically ill and some have died but the majority are in stable condition or well.
5. A great number of patients have complained of falling hair that began as late as two weeks following the explosion. Some of these patients have had an uneventful course while others have had a bad one.
6. The most serious clinical sign of radiation sickness is a decrease in white blood cells and pathologically great changes were found in the hematopoietic system, especially in the bone marrow. Those who received fatal injuries have died within the past month. Patients with low white blood counts who survived this period are now stable or convalescing. Within the past week the hospital has become very cheerful.

*From Hachiya, M.: Hiroshima diary—the journal of a Japanese physician, August 6–September 30, 1945, Chapel Hill, 1955, The University of North Carolina Press.

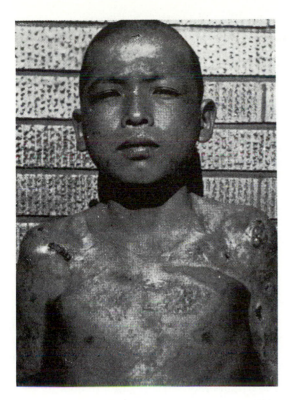

Fig. 6-8. Flash burns from atomic bomb. This 15-year-old boy was standing in the open, 5250 feet from hypocenter, bare to waist, watching the planes. Flash burns on his chest have partially healed, but several areas of excess granulation tissue persist. (Courtesy Medical Division, The U.S. Strategic Bombing Survey.)

Dr. Hachiya's failure to mention decreased platelets, petechiae, and purpura was an oversight that he noted in a later entry in his diary.

Approximately 30% of those who died received lethal doses of radiation, although this was not always the immediate cause of death. Most of those who developed severe signs and symptoms of acute radiation sickness were within 1500 meters of the hypocenter.

Additional irradiated human populations include the following:

1. An unknown number of young women who received variable doses of radiation to one or both breasts for postpartum mastitis, unilateral hypertrophy, or fibrocystic disease; these individuals have developed excessive numbers of malignant breast tumors
2. Women with pulmonary tuberculosis treated with pneumothorax to collapse the affected lung and then monitored with repeated chest fluoroscopies to ascertain the degree of collapse; these patients also developed increased numbers of malignant breast tumors
3. Children with tinea capitis treated with x ray to cause epilation; these people showed an increased incidence of leukemia
4. Women with menometrorrhagia treated with radi-

ation to cause an artificial menopause; these women also showed an increased incidence of leukemia

Genetic effects

Ionizing radiation was the first mutagenic agent discovered. In common with spontaneous mutations, radiation-induced mutations may involve either somatic cells, in which case the effects are limited to the irradiated individual, or germinal tissues, in which case the consequences may affect future generations. Mutations may also be classified as point mutations or chromosomal aberrations. Point mutations generally involve small alterations in the sequence or composition of the DNA bases and are not evident by standard karyotyping. Most radiation-induced mutations of this type are recessive and therefore do not become expressed unless carried by both members of homologous chromosomes. Hence most of the available information relating to point mutations is derived from large numbers of carefully controlled breeding experiments on *Drosophila* and mice.

Chromosomal aberrations generally refer to changes that are evident by standard karyotyping with light microscopy. Although chromosomal and point mutations may occur simultaneously within the same cell, it is convenient to discuss them as separate entities.

Point mutations. Point mutations occur spontaneously but, at least in recognizable form, at a low natural rate. It is estimated that approximately 10% of spontaneous mutations are attributable to the background radiation, which has always been a part of our environment; the remainder are believed to be caused by either mutagenic chemicals or the thermal movement of molecules.

Although they may be dominant, most of the mutations induced by radiation are recessive and a high percentage of them are lethal. The frequency of radiation-induced point mutations is dose dependent in the low and midlethal dose range. Although still a matter of controversy, it is believed that the type and frequency of point mutations are dependent on the time interval between exposure and mating. If mating occurs soon after exposure (within about 60 days in humans), fertilization may involve irradiated mature germ cells (spermatocytes, spermatids, and spermatozoa). The mutation rate for recessive genes in these cells is believed to be roughly twice that associated with irradiated immature germ cells (spermatogonia and stem cells).

On the basis of the above information, individuals should be advised to avoid procreation during the initial few months after the exposure of unshielded gonads to radiation incurred either accidentally or for therapeutic purposes. After this initial period, fewer radiation-induced mutations are transmitted to the offspring by the female than by the male. This observation probably reflects either a more efficient repair mechanism or a difference in the relative radiosensitivity of oocytes and male germ cells.

Chromosomal aberrations. Chromosomal aberrations arise when radiation breaks a chromosome or a chromatid at one or more points along its length. Such an interruption may result in an alteration in the number of genes in the cell or in the linear sequence of the genes or both. The broken ends of a chromosome may (1) rejoin with no resultant lesion, (2) heal without rejoining, (3) join with the broken ends of other chromosomes, or (4) fail to heal. It is estimated that 90% of individual chromosome breaks rejoin with no demonstrable lesion.

As might be expected, the frequency of nonviable chromosomal aberrations is greater than the frequency of nonviable gene mutations. Chromosomes also exhibit increased stickiness when irradiated with doses of 100 rad or more just before or during metaphase. This poorly understood phenomenon often causes individual chromosomes to stick together and form loosely adherent clumps. At anaphase such clumps do not separate properly and such separation results in an unequal distribution of genes to the daughter cells.

Dose-response effects. In general, the number of detectable point mutations increases in linear fashion with increasing dose. There is no evidence of a threshold effect. Even very low doses, doses in the 1 rad range, may be associated with a small increase in the number of mutations. In the mouse an exposure of 30 to 40 rad would be expected to produce about as many point mutations in a generation as are believed to occur from all natural causes. This is known as the doubling dose.

Single chromosome breaks, also known as single-hit aberrations, also bear a linear relationship to dose. Two-hit chromosome breaks are the result of two single aberrations that must occur in proximity. As might be expected, two-hit breaks increase in frequency at a rate greater than a single power of the dose, and they demonstrate an apparent threshold.

Geneticists are appropriately concerned about the hazards of the exposure of human beings to ionizing radiation, particularly with respect to the implications for future generations. Most radiation-induced mutations, however, are transmitted as recessive traits. As such, they can be transmitted, in concealed fashion, to many offspring until matings between carriers begin to occur. For this reason, deleterious recessive mutations, although not evident immediately, are more dangerous to a population than are harmful dominant mutations, particularly when the latter are damaging enough to prevent carriers from reproducing. Since the majority of detectable mutations are indeed deleterious, an artificially increased mutation rate could result in a general decline in the genetic health of human beings unless balanced by an increased selection against such mutations. Although selection against mutant genes occurs exten-sively in most natural situations, improving standards of medical practice may increasingly tend to reduce selection against deleterious traits in many human populations.

With respect to radiation exposure, geneticists are particularly concerned about the following categories of people:

1. *Radiology personnel.* The unfortunate experience of the pioneer American radiologists focused attention on some of the hazards in this regard and resulted in stringent safety precautions. Despite these precautions, however, lymphocytes from the peripheral blood of radiologists and radiotherapy nurses occasionally demonstrate a significant increase in the frequency of chromosomal aberrations.

2. *Patients receiving radioactive isotopes.* Isotopes may be potentially hazardous depending on the distribution of the substance in the patient. For example, an individual with thyrotoxicosis who is treated with an average therapeutic dose of iodine 131 will receive the following average tissue exposures: 4000 to 10,000 rad to the thyroid gland; 2 to 5 rad to the hemopoietic tissues; 1 rad to the testes or 2 rad to the ovary. The dose estimates for the testes and ovary are particularly significant to future generations.

3. *Workers in nuclear installations.* Studies on radiation workers in a nuclear installation have demonstrated that low levels of exposure over a prolonged period of time can significantly increase the number of chromosomal aberrations in peripheral blood lymphocytes.

4. *Patients exposed to x rays during diagnostic radiologic examinations.* At present, medical-dental radiation is the most significant source of iatrogenic radiation effects. Of particular importance are diagnostic procedures that involve repeated exposures or simultaneous fluoroscopic examinations. Many of these procedures involve exposures to the gonads that are two to 20 times the average natural background. The scope of the problem is evident from the following figures collected in the United States from a survey made in 1964: 600,000 patients received radiation therapy; 7.8 million were given fluoroscopic examinations; 46 million received dental x-ray examinations; 66 million were exposed during diagnostic medical radiographic examinations, this in a total population of approximately 181 million at that time. More recent data are not available.

Diagnostic radiology is an indispensable part of medical practice, but physicians must be aware of the genetic effects of radiation in order to balance the benefits of a specific procedure against the possible hazards.

Experience with Japanese atomic bomb survivors.
Residual chromosomal aberrations have been documented in 61% of heavily exposed atomic bomb survivors. In addition, a variety of complex chromosomal aberrations (rings, dicentrics, acentric fragments, and translocations) were documented among 39% of the individuals exposed in utero as compared with 1% of the controls. In contrast to the cytogenetic defects observed after intrauterine (postconception) exposure, no such effects have been associated thus far with preconception irradiation. Specific observations include the following:

1. No significant relationship could be documented between the frequency of congenital malformations and either maternal or paternal exposure.
2. Similarly, no consistent effect could be documented between maternal or paternal exposure and the frequency of stillbirths or neonatal deaths.
3. To date, no clear evidence exists for an increased death rate among children born to exposed parents.
4. Cytogenetic examination of the children of heavily exposed survivors has as yet failed to reveal any aberrations ascribable to radiation injury.

It is important, however, to introduce a note of caution in the interpretation of these four observations. Even with high doses to the reproductive tissues of the parents, the expected risk to an individual offspring is exceedingly small. Very large numbers of offspring must therefore be studied to detect any effect. In addition, both congenital abnormalities and stillbirths occur primarily on nongenetic bases, and therefore the effects of an alteration in the genetic component that influences these two phenomena would tend to be masked by a large number of "spontaneous" events.

Somatic effects

As noted before, the majority of radiation-induced chromosome breaks apparently rejoin immediately so that no lesion results. Permanent chromosomal alterations are generally of little significance to the host when they occur in an organ with a stable cell population such as adult liver cells. The lethal aspects of chromosomal aberrations become manifest at the time of cell division when one or more sets of genes are lost to a cell. This line of reasoning forms the basis of the law of Bergonié and Tribondeau, which states that dividing cells are more radiosensitive than nondividing cells. Thus hemopoietic cells and gastrointestinal epithelium are more radiosensitive than are neurons or cardiac muscle, and the embryo and fetus are more susceptible than the adult to radiation injury.

Somatic effects of radiation injury may be divided into acute or delayed. With respect to acute effects, early lethality is of prime concern. Among the important delayed effects are carcinogenesis, abnormalities of growth and development, alterations in life span, and a variety of injuries to individual organs.

Early lethality

Key to an understanding of early lethality is an appreciation of the concept of $LD_{50(30)}$. In toxicology, the lethal dose 50 or LD_{50} is the amount of an agent that causes a 50% mortality in the experimental group. The same approach has been applied to radiation injury, especially injury associated with whole-body exposure. However, death after whole-body exposure is often delayed for days or even weeks, depending on the magnitude of exposure. Therefore, with respect to radiation exposure, mortality is expressed in terms of a specific period of time, generally 30 days. The $LD_{50(30)}$ is defined as the dose associated with a 50% mortality within 30 days of exposure.

In humans the sequence of events after radiation injury is slower than for experimental animals. Therefore the frame of reference generally employed is the $LD_{50(60)}$ or the amount of radiation that would be expected to kill 50% of a population within 60 days of exposure.

A quantitative dose-response relationship for early lethality in humans is not known. Several investigators have derived hypothetical dose-response curves based upon animal experiments integrated with the available human experience. Most of the latter data are derived from reactor accidents and the acute mortality associated with the atomic explosions in Japan. On these bases, the $LD_{50(60)}$ for humans exposed to a single dose of highly penetrating electromagnetic radiation (x or gamma rays) delivered over a period of less than 24 hours is believed to be in the 225 to 270 rad range.

Within a given population, many host factors are known to influence the response of the individual to whole-body irradiation. In general, males are more sensitive than females. Middle-aged persons appear to exhibit a greater degree of tolerance to radiation than do the young and old. Environmental factors are of particular importance. The presence of infection sharply increases the mortality from whole-body exposure. The microorganisms implicated in these infections appear to be of both exogenous and endogenous origin. The latter are the normal flora of the body, especially of the gastrointestinal tract, which gain entry through denuded mucosal surfaces. Dissemination of these opportunistic offenders is facilitated by the accompanying leukopenia. Finally, people appear to vary considerably in their individual susceptibility to irradiation.

Of greater magnitude than the individual differences just outlined are the strong discrepancies among species. For example, the $LD_{50(30)}$ of sheep is about 150 rad and of one inbred strain of female mice is 689 rad. Even

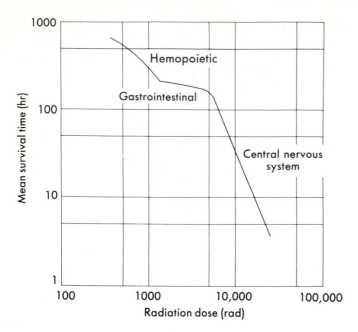

Fig. 6-9. Relationship among mean survival time, magnitude of whole-body exposure, and primary mode of death in humans. (After Langham, W.H., et al.: Aerospace Med. **36:**1, 1965.)

among the various inbred strains of mice there is a remarkable variation in radiosensitivity as expressed by the $LD_{50(30)}$. The basis for these intraspecies and interspecies differences is not known.

If an area of the body is shielded, the effects of a constant amount of radiation are decreased. Partial-body shielding can protect an individual from an otherwise lethal exposure to ionizing radiation. Shielding of the bone marrow, spleen, and gastrointestinal tract is especially beneficial.

The relationship between survival time and magnitude of whole-body exposure of humans is illustrated in Fig. 6-9. The purpose of showing these data is not to predict survival time, radiation dose, and mode of death. The dose-response curve in Fig. 6-9 shows three distinct components. The first region covers the dose range of 400 to 1200 rad over which survival time decreases exponentially with increasing dose. This range is generally referred to as the region of *hemopoietic death* because bone marrow damage is the most prominent finding, both clinically and at autopsy. Designation of this component of the dose-response curve as the region of hemopoietic death should not, however, be interpreted as an indication that damage is confined to the bone marrow. Injury to hemopoietic cells is the most conspicuous finding, but destruction involving other organs also contributes to the death of the patient. In particular, signs and symptoms attributable to necrosis of the mucosa of the gastrointestinal tract are often prominent in the 400 to 1200 rad dose range. Bacteremia contributes greatly to lethality in the hemopoietic range. It often results from

ulceration of the gastrointestinal tract and the invasion of opportunistic microorganisms, which quickly become widely disseminated because of the associated leukopenia. The increasing importance of gastrointestinal damage in the death of the patient is in part responsible for the exponential decrease in the mean survival time with increasing dose over this portion of the dose-response curve in Fig. 6-9.

Throughout the dose range of 1200 to 5000 rad there is a pronounced plateau in the mean survival curve (Fig. 6-9). The range associated with exposures of 1200 to 5000 rad is generally referred to as the region of *gastrointestinal death*. Again, this distinction is based on the most prominent clinical and morphologic findings. Morphologically, there is a progressive loss of gastrointestinal mucosa secondary to impaired proliferation of the stem cell or renewal population. Necrosis of mucosal cells leads to ulceration, bacteremia, hemorrhage, and loss of fluids and electrolytes. In this dose range the bone marrow is totally aplastic and numerous other tissues also show severe damage. However, it appears clear that damage to the gastrointestinal tract is the primary limiting factor with respect to survival in the 1200 to 5000 rad dose range.

Above about 5000 rad mean survival time again begins to decrease exponentially with increasing dose (Fig. 6-9), and death is characterized by a variety of central nervous system signs and symptoms. For this reason, the region of the survival curve associated with exposures in excess of 5000 rad is referred to as the region of *central nervous system death*. Incapacitation occurs relatively rapidly and is characterized by confusion, convulsions, apathy, and coma, followed by death.

Late somatic effects

Various somatic effects have been attributed to radiation injury; of these, the most important are carcinogenesis, abnormalities of growth and development, and changes in life span.

Carcinogenesis (see also Chapter 15). The carcinogenic effects of ionizing radiation have been recognized for more than half a century. A significant number of the pioneer radiation workers developed epidermoid and basal cell carcinomas of the hands. Such tumors generally arose in areas of radiation dermatitis caused by repeated exposures with massive accumulated doses, which often totaled several thousand rad. For example, many of the early workers focused their equipment on the bones of their hands. They were also accustomed to positioning their patients with their unshielded hands while their equipment was in operation.

Despite the early recognition of this untoward effect of ionizing radiation, even today the mechanisms involved in radiation-induced neoplasia remain poorly understood. Some of the problems involved in obtaining these kinds of data include poorly documented dosimetry and the small size and inadequate follow-up studies of many of the exposed populations. In view of these limitations, only tentative dose-incidence conclusions are warranted in humans at present for most radiation-related neoplasms. Furthermore, any such conclusions, and related inferences about possible mechanisms of radiation carcinogenesis, must also take into consideration the relevant experimental observations on laboratory animals. Such observations will be noted in the subsequent discussion.

Despite the inadequacy of existing information, several generalizations with respect to radiation carcinogenesis appear warranted. First, all forms of ionizing radiation are carcinogenic. Second, multiple doses are more tumorigenic than is a single exposure of the same total magnitude. Third, tumors of almost any type may be induced by irradiation under appropriate conditions in susceptible subjects. Fourth, susceptibility to the carcinogenic action of radiation appears to be widely shared by many different species of animals including human beings. Fifth, indirect effects of radiation on the host are responsible for some types of neoplasms, indicating that radiation need not always be absorbed at the site of the subsequent tumor in order to be carcinogenic. Sixth, the incidence of some neoplasms is greatly increased by relatively small amounts of radiation. In most instances the incidence of these neoplasms is correlated with the absorbed dose, dose rate, volume of tissue exposed, and the LET of the radiation.

Possible mechanisms. Current available evidence from both human and animal studies suggests that multiple factors influence the evolution of most neoplasms. In addition, the relative importance of these various genetic and environmental influences must vary as a function of the biologic experience of the host and the individual characteristics of specific tumors. An extension of this line of reasoning suggests that radiation may influence tumorigenesis in a variety of ways and that the dose-response relationship may be expected to vary from organ to organ and according to (1) the age and sex of the individual, (2) possible occupational or other exposure to cocarcinogens, (3) the genetic predisposition of the host, (4) diet, (5) socioeconomic factors, and (6) numerous other variables, the action of which is not yet understood. Depending upon the circumstances, radiation may act as an initiator, a promoter, or, most commonly, a complete carcinogenic agent.

The character of the primary subcellular events induced by radiation that ultimately result in a tumor is not known. Two prime suspects are the activation of latent oncogenic viruses and permanent DNA aberrations. A considerable amount of experimental evidence exists to support both of these hypotheses, which are not mutually exclusive. Viruses have been shown to induce tumors in experimental animals, and carcinogens often cause permanent DNA aberrations. Radiation is known to alter gene expression in susceptible cells, which could facilitate the penetration of opportunistic latent viral genomes. However, it is important to note that in humans no direct relationships between the induction of cancer by radiation and the activation of latent oncogenic viruses or the induction of somatic mutations have been demonstrated.

Radiation-induced somatic mutations have long been postulated to play an etiologic role in radiation carcinogenesis. Radiation is a potent mutagen, and many tumors are associated with chromosome abnormalities. Proponents of the somatic mutation theory suggest that these two observations are causally related. An extension of this line of reasoning is the single-hit hypothesis. The theoretical basis of this hypothesis is the concept that neoplastic transformation follows the passage of a single ionizing particle through a susceptible cell. This approach postulates a linear relationship between radiation dose and the incidence of cancer in a uniform population. However, because neoplasms appear to evolve stepwise through a succession of alterations, it appears unlikely that tumors arise from a single mutation. If this were the case, for example, age at exposure would not be expected to be a significant factor in radiation carcinogenesis. A mutation would be expected to result in a neoplasm irrespective of the age of the person involved. Such is not the case. With respect to several neoplasms thus far evaluated, the number of tumors induced by irradiation varies in relation to the age at exposure. Nevertheless, if tumors arise as the result of a series of alterations, some of which may involve mutations, it is conceivable that a single radiation-induced mutation might act as a promoter in a suitably conditioned host.

A variety of indirect effects of radiation upon the induction of neoplasms has been well documented experimentally. For example, thymic lymphomas occur in susceptible strains of mice when nonirradiated thymus is transplanted into irradiated recipients. The mechanism involved has only been partially defined but is believed to involve activation of a tumorigenic virus that is released from a nonthymic site by the action of radiation. Released virus is presumably widely disseminated throughout the host but has a predilection for regenerating thymus. In this example, the thymus is regenerating from mechanical injuries sustained at the time of transplantation. In similar fashion, the induction of pituitary tumors in irradiated mice is believed to relate in part to hormonal disturbances caused by radiation-related injury to target organs such as the thyroid. The resultant hypothyroidism activates the pituitary by well-characterized feedback mechanisms, and hyperfunction ensues. Hyperfunction results in hyperplasia and in some cases neoplasia eventually occurs. More recently, radiation-

258 ANDERSON'S PATHOLOGY

induced impairment of normal immunologic surveillance mechanisms has been implicated in select tumors.

To summarize, a variety of diverse effects must be contemplated in a consideration of the mechanisms involved in radiation carcinogenesis. Direct and indirect effects must be considered, the nature and relative importance of which probably vary with respect to the type of neoplasm in question as well as the conditions of irradiation. In a growing number of instances, however, carcinogenesis appears to involve interactions among the effects of radiation, viruses, chemicals, and a variety of host factors.

Dose-response relationships. Considerable effort has been given to an attempt to define in mathematical terms the relationships between dose of irradiation and tumor incidence especially at low dose levels. The latter are of particular importance in defining maximum permissible exposure levels for radiation workers. Unfortunately, the available data are insufficient to establish with confidence the shape of the dose-incidence curve at low doses. Hence efforts to estimate the possible risks of low level irradiation involve extrapolation from observations made at higher dose levels. These extrapolations, based upon unproved assumptions, yield three types of curves: linear nonthreshold, linear threshold, and linear-quadratic. These curves are represented schematically in Fig. 6-10.

The concept of threshold is of critical importance in a consideration of the carcinogenic effects of radiation. As depicted in Fig. 6-10, threshold implies "safe" dose of radiation below which there is no increased incidence of the disease in question. At present the available evidence does not support the concept of a threshold with respect to the carcinogenic effects of radiation. For this

reason most authorities have recommended that the linear, nonthreshold dose-incidence model (Fig. 6-10) be employed to derive risk estimates for carcinogenesis among people exposed to low doses of radiation. This conservative approach assumes that any level of exposure is associated with some risk of harm. Corollaries to this axiom include (1) no exposure to radiation is justifiable if it is avoidable or fails to provide a benefit commensurate with the presumed risk and (2) every exposure, even when amply justified, must be kept as low as possible. In contrast with low dose effects, considerable data are available concerning the characteristics of the dose-incidence curve at intermediate and high exposure levels. The linear-quadratic model (Fig. 6-10) appears in many instances to best describe stochastic effects at these dose levels.

Abnormalities of growth and development. Radiation is known to be especially injurious to rapidly dividing tissues. For this reason the developing embryo and the preadolescent child are particularly susceptible to radiation-induced disorders of growth and development. In general, the character of the defect reflects those tissues that are undergoing the most rapid growth and differentiation at the time of exposure. From this standpoint it is convenient to divide radiation-related disorders of growth and development into four phases: the preimplantation period, the period of major organogenesis, the fetal period, and the postnatal period.

Preimplantation period. Irradiation shortly after conception is associated with one of two extremes: it is likely to be either lethal or of no apparent significance to the preimplantation embryo, which therefore survives without evidence of abnormality. When the organism consists of only a few cells, radiation-induced damage to only

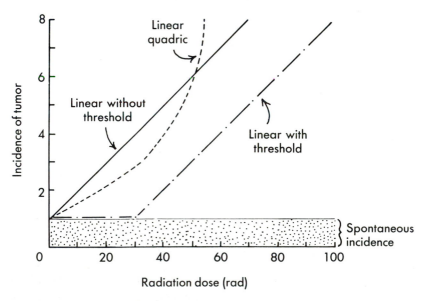

Fig. 6-10. Hypothetical dose-response curves for radiation carcinogenesis.

one cell is likely to be fatal to the embryo. Under such circumstances, the mother is generally unaware that she has conceived.

Period of major organogenesis. This period, which begins at the time of implantation (day 8 or 9) and extends through the initial 6 weeks of gestation, is the time when the developing fetus is maximally radiosensitive. Exposure during this period of remarkable growth and differentiation is associated with one or more of a vast number of possible congenital malformations. Susceptibility to the induction of specific types of developmental anomalies is sharply pinpointed in time, apparently as a function of the organ or organs that are undergoing major differentiation at the time of exposure. Thus the developing fetus is a mosaic of constantly changing, organ-specific radiosensitivities.

Fetal period. From the sixth week of gestation until the time of parturition, susceptibility to recognizable morphologic anomalies decreases. Most of the organ systems are structurally differentiated, and therefore exposure of the fetus would not be expected to result in gross congenital abnormalities. However, susceptibility to radiation-induced functional disabilities persists during this period. Such disturbances, which involve particularly the central nervous system and the gonads, are difficult to recognize and identify, especially since development continues until well after birth. Radiation during the fetal period apparently depletes the total number of functional nerve and reproductive cells. With respect to the central nervous system, such depletion may be manifest by a reduced IQ. Thus identification of the defect may be postponed until the child reaches school age. Even then the deficit may not be related by the parents or the teacher to previous radiation exposure. And if the loss is slight, the reduced IQ may fall within the normal range and thus never be recognized as abnormal for the particular child.

Postnatal period. Radiation-induced abnormalities, especially of bone, are associated with the exposure of infants and children before the cessation of physical growth and development. With respect to bone, the magnitude of impairment appears to relate to the rate of growth at the time of exposure. Other tissues that continue to develop in the postnatal period, such as the eye, the central nervous system, and the teeth, are also susceptible to radiation-induced abnormalities in growth and development.

• • •

Additional radiation-induced defects that result from exposure of the developing fetus and the preadolescent child include (1) growth retardation, (2) neurologic effects, and (3) neoplasia. In this connection it is important to note that much of our information with respect to the consequences of in utero irradiation in humans is derived from two populations: (1) persons whose mothers in the late 1920s received pelvic radiotherapy during early pregnancy and (2) individuals born of mothers who were located close to the site of the atomic bomb explosion in Hiroshima. The findings in these two groups of people are in accord with the results from a large number of animal experiments.

Exposure during the period of major organogenesis, the fetal period, or the postnatal period can result in a diffuse retardation of normal growth. When exposure occurs in utero, this retardation is manifested by subnormal head circumference, body height, and weight. The maximum effect appears to occur when the fetus is exposed between the third and twentieth weeks of gestation. Radiation-related retardation of growth induced during the postnatal period is almost always a consequence of local exposure and involves only the irradiated region, often a limb.

With respect to neurologic defects, it has been estimated that 80% of malformed children with a history of irradiation in utero have a subnormal head circumference. As might be expected, mental retardation is also a sequela of fetal irradiation, with or without reduced head size. This combination of a small head circumference and mental retardation represents the only congenital malformation thus far described as a result of exposure to the atomic bombs. This effect was noted primarily among women who were within 15 weeks of their last menstrual period at the time of exposure and who were located in the proximity. A variety of other central nervous system defects can be produced by irradiation throughout the fetal period in experimental animals. The character of the malformation is determined by the stage of gestation at the time of exposure. Malformations after low doses of radiation have also been reported, but the significance and the putative reversibility of these lesions are not known. In this connection it is important to note that the fetal nervous system is capable of significant repair of radiation-induced injury.

Moderate to high doses of radiation administered to the fetus are carcinogenic. With respect to low dose radiation, most investigators believe that in utero exposure during diagnostic radiographic procedures performed during pregnancy increases the risk of leukemia and other malignancies in human offspring. One study has implicated doses as low as 2 rad. However, other observers question this association, and the issue probably will not be resolved until more is known about the mechanisms involved in leukemia induction.

On the basis of some of the above observations, however, many institutions have adopted a policy that limits elective diagnostic medical radiographic examinations among women of childbearing age to the first 10 days after the start of the last menses to prevent exposure of an unsuspected conceptus.

Finally, it should be emphasized that the discussion in this section has focused especially upon exposure from external sources. Fetal irradiation may also occur when radioactive isotopes are administered to the mother. Radioactive iodine, strontium, tritium, phosphorus, and plutonium are among the many isotopes that can cross the placenta to become incorporated into and injure fetal tissues. For example, radioactive iodine administered late in pregnancy for maternal hyperthyroidism can be concentrated in the thyroid of the developing fetus and result in cretinism.

Life span. Whole-body irradiation of rodents results in shortened life span. This life shortening results from an increase in age-specific mortality and persists even when appropriate corrections are made for the early mortality associated with radiation sickness and late deaths caused by radiation-induced neoplasms.

To date, however, experimental studies have not shown unequivocally that radiation truly accelerates the aging process. The possibility remains that radiation reduces life span by some other mechanism. Autopsies of irradiated animals reveal that death is generally caused by the same diseases that kill their nonexposed contemporaries. In particular, radiation hastens the development of a variety of degenerative and neoplastic diseases as well as autoimmune phenomena. Not all age-dependent alterations, however, are temporally advanced by irradiation, and even for those that are advanced, the magnitude of change is not necessarily uniform.

Comparable data pertinent to humans are fragmentary. One of the first suggestions of a similar life-shortening effect came from the observation that pioneer American radiologists experienced a higher age-specific death rate than did other specialists. The increase in mortality was not attributable to a specific lesion and was interpreted as a nonspecific shortening of life span from occupational exposure. Interestingly, the excess mortality has progressively decreased in all but the oldest age groups, possibly because of improved shielding and other radiologic safety procedures.

ACUTE RADIATION SYNDROME
General effects

The clinical signs and symptoms produced by intensive exposure of the entire body to penetrating radiation are referred to as the acute radiation syndrome or radiation sickness. This syndrome is characterized by three successive phases.

1. *A transient prodromal phase, which develops within a few hours of exposure to as little as 75 to 100 rad.* In humans this phase is characterized by apathy, anorexia, nausea, and vomiting. As shown in Fig. 6-11, the incidence and duration of prodromal symptoms are dose dependent and therefore provide a rough indication of the degree of irradiation in persons accidentally exposed to a dose of unknown magnitude. The prodromal phase rarely exceeds 24 hours except in very severe cases.

2. *An ensuing asymptomatic latent period, which reflects the time required for the development of disturbances in specific organs.* As will be seen subsequently, this period generally reflects the time required for the depletion of cells in mitotically active tissues through interference with normal renewal mechanisms. As such, the duration of the latent period is dose dependent.

3. *The principal phase of the illness.* As noted previously, the acute radiation syndrome can be divided into three major categories on the basis of the organ system most conspicuously involved; they are the

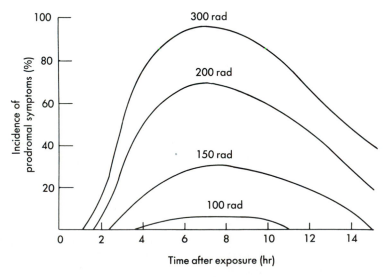

Fig. 6-11. Incidence and duration of prodromal symptoms as function of dose. (From Langham, W.H., et al.: Aerospace Med. **36**:1, 1965.)

hemopoietic, gastrointestinal, and central nervous system syndromes. In varying degrees each syndrome is associated with death, and much of our understanding of the acute radiation syndrome has been gained from an evaluation of persons accidentally exposed during reactor accidents.

Some of the clinical and morphologic characteristics of the individual components of the acute radiation syndrome are summarized in Table 6-6. The most sensitive organ is the bone marrow, and symptoms relating to hemopoietic dysfunction are apparent after exposure to as little as 50 to 100 rad. Maximum expression of symptoms referable to the bone marrow is generally delayed until 2 to 3 weeks after exposure. At the other end of the spectrum is the central nervous system (CNS) syndrome, which follows very large doses (1000 rad or more) and where the clinical manifestations are often apparent within minutes of exposure. Intermediate between these extremes is the gastrointestinal syndrome.

Pathogenesis

The pathogenesis of the CNS component of the acute radiation syndrome is not known. Current evidence suggests that injury to small blood vessels may be the initiating event. Vacuolization of capillary endothelial cells, perivascular foci of hemorrhage, and perivascular collections of inflammatory cells have been described. Vascular permeability is increased, and cerebral edema is uniformly present, among both individuals exposed accidentally and animals exposed experimentally. It may well be that significant edema of other organs is associated with the high doses responsible for the CNS syndrome but that the rigid confines of the adult skull dictate that CNS symptoms precede those attributable to other organs. At extremely high dose levels, death may be caused by direct neuronal damage; the estimated intracerebral dose associated with this phenomenon is in excess of 100,000 rad for humans.

The cellular basis of the gastrointestinal and hemopoietic syndromes is directly related to the rate of cell turnover in these organs. The epithelial cells lining the digestive tract and the circulating leukocytes are short lived and therefore must be renewed at a rapid rate. In both instances renewal depends on a population of rapidly dividing stem cells that undergo a series of maturational steps to differentiate into the mature components that characterize these organs. Irradiation interferes with the proliferation of the stem cell population. Therefore replacements are not available after irradiation when normal biologic attrition causes the progressive loss of mature cells.

In the gastrointestinal tract, the stem cell population is located in the crypts of Lieberkühn. Irradiation of these cells inhibits division or, if the dose is sufficiently large, kills them outright. The mature cells at the tips of the villi undergo spontaneous aging at the usual rate and are sloughed into the lumen of the intestine. Meanwhile, partially mature cells continue to migrate toward the tips of the villi to replace these senescent cells, thus depleting the crypts even further. In the absence of appropriate replacements, the villi become denuded and vital functions are compromised. In particular, loss of the normal mucosa permits fluid and electrolytes to escape from exposed tissue spaces and allows microorganisms, especially the normal intestinal flora, easy access to the bloodstream. Hemorrhage from exposed blood vessels may further complicate the clinical situation. If recovery is to occur, small foci of regenerating epithelium are generally evident by the end of the first week. This sequence of events is shown diagrammatically in Fig. 6-12.

Table 6-6. Important features of the acute radiation syndrome in humans

Subcategory	Clinical threshold dose*	Latent period	Primary morphologic manifestations	Characteristic signs and symptoms	Cause of death	Time of death after exposure (mean)
Hemopoietic syndrome	100	2-3 weeks	Hypoplasia of bone marrow with leukopenia, thrombocytopenia, and (occasionally) anemia	Petechia, purpura, hemorrhage, infection	Infection	3 weeks
Gastrointestinal syndrome	500	3-5 days	Depletion of epithelium of small intestine with ulceration	Fever, diarrhea, fluid-electrolyte disturbances, infection	Dehydration, infection, electrolyte loss	10-14 days
Central nervous system syndrome	2000	15 minutes–3 hours	Edema, necrosis of neurons, vasculitis	Confusion, apathy, somnolence, tremor, ataxia, convulsions, coma	Increased central nervous system pressure	14-36 hours

*Air dose in roentgens.

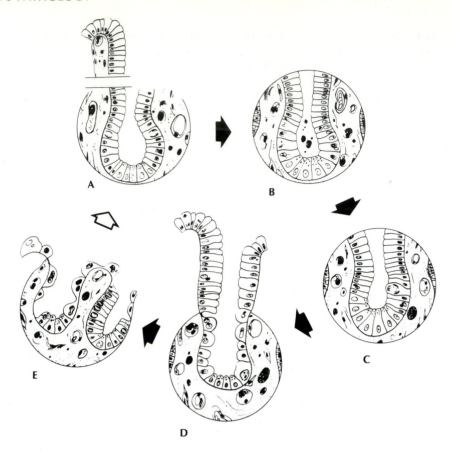

Fig. 6-12. Acute radiation injury to epithelium of small intestine. **A,** Normal state. Crypt area consists of basally situated Paneth cells, zone of proliferating cells, and narrow band of differentiating cells immediately beneath gland neck. Villus is lined by mature, epithelial cells, which undergo continuous migration to cell-extrusion zone at villus tip. **B,** Six hours after irradiation. Note inhibition of mitosis and marked necrosis of immature cells in proliferative zone. **C,** Twelve to 24 hours after irradiation. Inhibition of mitosis ceases with large number of abortive cell divisions, many of which are abnormal and result in death of involved cells or abnormal daughter cells. **D,** One to 6 days after irradiation. In absence of effective cell division, epithelial cell population continues to diminish and many of residual cells are abnormally large and pleomorphic. Villi become progressively shortened, and residual abnormal cells spread out, possibly to preserve in part the integrity of the epithelial barrier. **E,** Six to 8 days after irradiation. If regeneration is to occur, small foci of regenerating epithelium are evident by end of first week. (After White, D.C.: Atlas of radiation histopathology, ERDA Report TID-26676.)

The acute response of the stomach, colon, and rectum is similar to that of the small intestine. However, because cell turnover is highest in the small intestine, cell depletion occurs earlier there than elsewhere.

The pathogenesis of the events associated with the hemopoietic syndrome is very similar. With the exception of lymphocytes, the mature elements of the peripheral blood are remarkably resistant to the effects of radiation. However, they have a finite life span and cannot reproduce themselves. After whole-body exposure of sufficient magnitude, the majority of bone marrow stem cells are damaged or dead and therefore are not available for division and maturation in order to replace those cells lost by natural attrition. The consequences of this situation, in order of appearance, are lymphopenia, thrombocytopenia, neutropenia, and anemia.

The severity of the acute radiation syndrome depends primarily on the number of surviving stem cells in mitotically active tissues. These cells constitute the only available source of the cells required for the restoration of tissue integrity.

Repair and regeneration

After whole-body exposure, recovery of damaged cell populations occurs by two primary mechanisms: (1) repair of nonlethal injuries in individual cells and (2) proliferation of radioresistant or otherwise spared stem cells. The latter mechanism is of prime importance in the recovery of the bone marrow and the gastrointestinal tract after whole-body exposure. Stem cell proliferation begins almost immediately following irradiation, generally within 24 to 48 hours. In the bone marrow, recruitment of previously nondividing stem cells, which appear to serve as a reserve component for just such occasions, accelerates the process. Production of additional stem cells appears to have preference over the maturational phases. Some 2 to 3 weeks after exposure the absolute number of bone marrow stem cells and other nucleated hemopoietic precursors exceeds preexposure levels. Over the subsequent several weeks this situation is reversed, and normal steady-state dynamics ensues.

RADIATION INJURY IN SELECT TISSUES

In general, the effects of radiation in most tissues are quantitatively related to dose. The magnitude of the resultant loss of function reflects a balance among many factors but especially the number of cells irreparably damaged, the capacity of uninjured cells to undergo hypertrophy and thereby increase function, and the regenerative capability and reserve capacity of the irradiated tissue.

Highly differentiated and complex tissues have poorly developed regenerative capacities. Therefore radiation injury generally results in a dose-dependent loss of functional mass. As with other forms of necrosis, connective tissue proliferation often ensues and, when the involved organ is examined roentgenographically or at autopsy, may serve to mask the magnitude of the atrophy. Compensatory hypertrophy and hyperplasia are particularly apparent with respect to the kidney where destruction of one kidney is accompanied by remarkable hypertrophy and hyperplasia of the nonirradiated, contralateral organ.

In some organs radiation injury is transiently associated with enhanced function. An increase in diffusion capacity after extensive exposure of the lung in humans has often been noted clinically. A transient increase in glomerular filtration rate has also been noted under similar circumstances. The basis of these unexpected observations is not clear, but radiation-related vasodilatation has been strongly implicated.

Finally, most organs are composed of a variety of interdependent cell types, each of which responds in a somewhat different fashion to the effects of radiation. Therefore instead of referring to radiation pneumonitis, for example, one would be more precise in speaking of radiation injury to the bronchial mucosa, type I alveolar lining cells, or capillary endothelial cells. Unfortunately, our knowledge of the response to radiation of these individual components is very limited. Therefore despite the inherent oversimplications, much of the subsequent discussion is focused upon the response of an entire organ rather than the effects on individual components.

Skin

Radiation injury of the skin is the best known and most carefully studied of all radiation-induced responses in humans. During accidental or therapeutic exposures to most kinds of radiation, the skin generally receives the largest dose. The skin is also a good biologic dosimeter because of the great predictability of its response to various doses.

The first sign of radiation damage to the skin is the development of an erythema, which resembles sunburn. After sufficiently large exposures, there occurs a series of reactions, which often overlap. In chronological order, these are erythema, epilation, bleb formation, necrosis often accompanied by ulceration, and repair, which is generally associated with hyperpigmentation.

Erythema occurs in 50% of persons who receive more than 600 rad to the skin. A dose of as little as 200 rad of soft radiation may produce temporary epilation. The scalp and face are especially sensitive. Regrowth of hair is usually complete in 3 to 6 months. Dry desquamation and wet desquamation (ulceration) occur after approximately 1000 and 2000 rad, respectively. These effects are reliable and points for study as well as potential undesirable side effects for the radiotherapist to keep in mind.

Chronic radiodermatitis manifests itself in several ways: (1) an atrophic, thin, parchmentlike tissue that exhibits hyperkeratosis with telangiectasia and increased pigmentation, (2) an unusual susceptibility to injury with poor healing capabilities and a propensity for ulcer formation, and (3) an increased incidence of malignant tumors.

Shortly after the discovery of x rays, radiation "burns" became an occupational and therapeutic problem. In 1902 the first neoplasm attributed to radiation injury was reported. The tumor was an epidermoid carcinoma of the hand; the patient was an x-ray tube maker. Within the next decade more than 90 similar cases were reported among physicians and others exposed occupationally to ionizing radiation. The tumors generally involved the hands and arose in sites of antecedent radiodermatitis. The majority of the neoplasms were epidermoid carcinomas and were associated with a long latent period. With respect to neoplasia, latent period refers to the interval between irradiation and the appearance of the tumor. The peak incidence of radiation-induced skin tumors occurred approximately 8 years after the initial exposure.

With the advent of adequate protective measures, epidermoid carcinoma is no longer an occupational hazard among radiologists. More recently, however, there have been reports of radiodermatitis and radiation carcinogenesis among dentists and others who have used radiation equipment without strict adherence to protective guidelines.

The acute dose required to induce skin cancer is believed to be in excess of 1000 roentgens, which greatly exceeds the $LD_{50(60)}$ dose for humans. This discrepancy accounts for the fact that, to date, the prevalence of skin cancer is not increased among the atomic bomb survivors, most of whom were exposed in whole-body fashion.

The mechanisms involved in radiation carcinogenesis of the skin are reasonably well known. A high incidence of neoplasia is associated with doses of radiation that result in ulcers with residual local vascular damage and scarring. Permanent damage to hair follicles also appears to be important. The subsequent neoplasms appear to arise from proliferating epithelial cells at the margin of ulcers or in association with irreparably damaged hair follicles. In approximately 30% of cases, multiple tumors are present.

Cardiovascular system

For a long time the heart was believed to be extremely radioresistant. Recently reexamination of this supposition has been prompted by a remarkable increase in cardiac complications among persons who have received large amounts of curative therapeutic radiation to the mediastinum for Hodgkin's disease and other neoplasms.

Radiation-induced heart disease has been reported in 5.8% of patients irradiated to the mediastinum for malignant lymphoma and 3.4% of individuals irradiated prophylactically after a simple or a radical mastectomy for carcinoma of the breast. The most common abnormality is fibrous pericarditis, often accompanied by effusion, which may organize, constrict the heart, and necessitate

pericardectomy. Diffuse interstitial fibrosis of the myocardium is also a not infrequent finding. Although important, these abnormalities are rarely life threatening.

In contradistinction to the heart and major vessels, the smaller components of the vascular system have been known for some time to be extremely susceptible to both the acute and delayed effects of ionizing radiation. Erythema of the skin is an early response to radiation injury and is believed to relate to vasodilatation and increased vascular permeability, probably secondary to endothelial injury. Endothelium is moderately radiosensitive, and injury is manifest morphologically by swelling and necrosis. Such changes are particularly pronounced with respect to the nucleus. Endothelial injury is often accompanied by subintimal edema. Although the endothelium is the most radiosensitive component, no element of the vessel wall is immune to the effects of irradiation. Pronounced changes that involve each element of the vessel wall are shown in Fig. 6-13. The functional consequences of vascular injury probably relate to varying degrees of interstitial edema and, less commonly, perivascular hemorrhage and thrombosis.

Chronic vascular changes associated with radiation injury are most conspicuous in arterioles and capillaries. They consist of segmental sclerosis and thickening of the wall, narrowing of the lumen, and reduplication of the endothelial cells, which may also be increased in size. Some of these changes are shown in Fig. 6-14.

Animal experiments have demonstrated the arterial

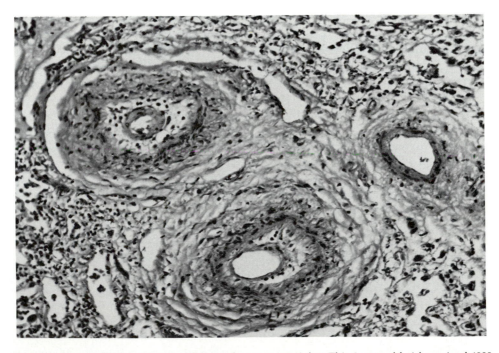

Fig. 6-13. Acute radiation injury involving pulmonary arterioles. This 2-year-old girl received 4000 rad of ionizing radiation for metastatic undifferentiated carcinoma 9 weeks before death. Arterioles show necrosis of endothelial cells, edema of subintimal region, edema and focal necrosis of media, and edema of adventitia. Acute and chronic inflammatory cells are present throughout vessel wall.

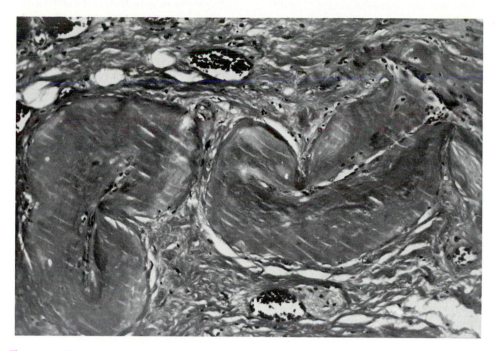

Fig. 6-14. Chronic radiation injury involving small artery of rectum of 66-year-old woman who received 4500 rad to uterus 22 years before death. Vessel shows thickening of wall with accumulation of hyaline-like substance and near complete occlusion of lumen.

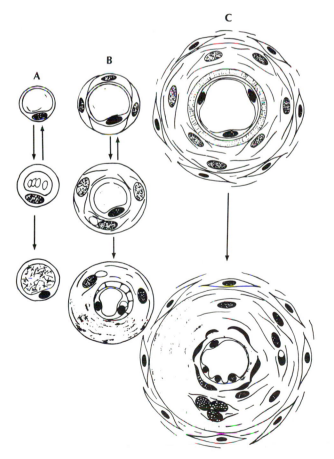

Fig. 6-15. Radiation injury involving capillary, arteriole, and small artery. **A,** Capillary. Acute response of capillary is dilatation accompanied by increased permeability. This is followed by narrowing of lumen from swelling of endothelial cells and sclerosis of vessel wall. Later a thrombus may form and occlude lumen completely. **B,** Arteriole. Changes in arteriole are similar to those noted in capillary. Initial vasodilatation is followed by endothelial swelling and edema of smooth muscle, both of which serve to narrow lumen. Subsequent degenerative changes include endothelial proliferation, subendothelial deposition of hyaline-like substance, and thickening of vessel wall with focal destruction of smooth muscle cells. **C,** Small artery. Because small arteries are fairly rigid structures, early changes are less pronounced. With passage of time, however, progressive damage to endothelium and media becomes evident. There are fragmentation and discontinuity of internal elastic lamella, degenerative changes in smooth muscle of media with large accumulations of hyaline-like substance, and fibrosis of the adventitia. (After Kligerman, M.M.: Principles of radiation therapy, In Holland, J.F., and Frei, E., editors: Cancer medicine, Philadelphia, 1973, Lea & Febiger.)

system to be more radiosensitive than the venous system and have also shown that arterioles and capillaries are more sensitive than arteries. Injury to arterioles and capillaries, with resultant relative ischemia, involves virtually every tissue and may be responsible for many of the delayed effects of radiation.

Some of the acute and chronic changes associated with radiation injury of blood vessels are summarized diagrammatically in Fig. 6-15.

Lung

Radiation injury to the lung is primarily associated with inhalation of radioactive substances or a consequence of radiotherapy for carcinoma of the lung, esophagus, or breast or mediastinal tumors. The magnitude of injury appears to depend on a number of factors but especially the total dose, the dose rate, and the presence or absence of preexisting lung disease such as one of the pneumoconioses.

Little is known about the acute effects of radiation injury to the human lung. Persons who die shortly after whole-body exposure generally exhibit significant alveolar damage, in part related to systemic disturbances such as septicemia, fluid and electrolyte abnormalities, and shock. Experimentally, the primary acute alterations in the lung consist of interstitial and intra-alveolar edema with hyaline membrane formation. The latter changes are associated with swelling of the endothelial cells of small blood vessels and are probably related to increased capillary permeability. Direct injury to type I alveolar

lining cells is manifested by necrosis. Organization and repair of the acute changes lead to interstitial fibrosis and vascular sclerosis. At autopsy such lungs are pale, rubbery, and less crepitant than normal.

The morphologic abnormalities described above are summarized diagrammatically in Fig. 6-16. They are referred to as acute and chronic radiation pneumonitis, although they are associated with surprisingly little in the way of an inflammatory response. The functional correlates of these changes in structure include a deterioration of most of the measurements of pulmonary function, especially when reserve capacity is evaluated during exercise. Because the pathologic changes are distributed irregularly, the normal ventilation-perfusion relationships are altered, and impaired gas exchange results. A reduction in the compliance of the whole lung occurs as well. When severe, these functional abnormalities are associated with dyspnea, especially on exertion. As with any interstitial pulmonary inflammatory process, a nonproductive chronic cough is also a prominent feature of severe radiation pneumonitis.

External irradiation of the thorax is associated with a moderate increase in the incidence of carcinoma of the lung in humans, especially when combined with other carcinogenic effects such as smoking. Inhalation of radioactive particles of a size and configuration known to reach the gas-exchange zone distal to the terminal bronchioles results in a high incidence of pulmonary neoplasms. In this connection carcinoma of the lung has been recognized for some time to be an occupational disability

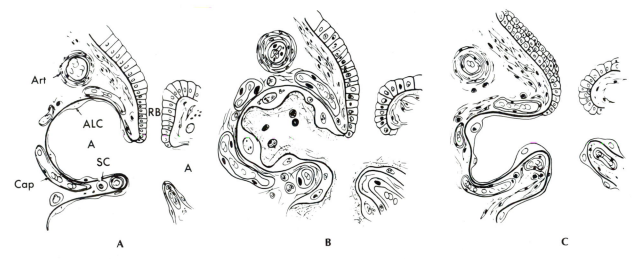

Fig. 6-16. Radiation injury to pulmonary parenchyma. **A,** Normal parenchyma. *A,* Alveolus; *ALC,* alveolar lining cell; *Art,* arteriole; *Cap,* capillary; *RB,* respiratory bronchiole; *SC,* septal cell. **B,** Acute radiation pneumonitis. Note capillary dilatation and swelling of endothelial cells. This may result in interstitial edema and loss of proteinaceous fluid into alveoli with formation of hyaline membranes. Septal cells respond to pulmonary edema by migrating into alveoli. Note also prominent enlargement and pleomorphism of alveolar lining cells and ciliated columnar epithelium that lines terminal bronchioles. **C,** Chronic radiation pneumonitis. Pronounced arteriolar sclerosis is associated with severe septal fibrosis. Bronchiolar epithelium is metaplastic. (After White, D.C.: Atlas of radiation histopathology, ERDA Report TID-26676.)

among certain groups of miners. For example, in the period 1921 to 1926, 50% of the deaths among the miners in the Schneeberg region of Saxony were attributable to carcinoma of the lung. An increased mortality from lung cancer has also been reported among fluorspar miners in Newfoundland, iron ore miners in Britain, uranium miners of the Colorado Plateau of the United States, and tungsten, fluorspar, and lithium miners in Czechoslovakia. Only recently, however, has it been shown that the excessive number of deaths from carcinoma of the lung is attributable to radiation. Underground mines, and especially uranium mines, contain variable amounts of the gaseous radionuclide radon. Radon 222 and its radioactive daughters attach to aerosol products in the environment. When inhaled, the aerosols are distributed throughout the tracheobronchial tree primarily on the basis of size. The smaller particles, particularly those between 0.1 and 1 μm in diameter, reach the bronchioles and alveoli where they remain trapped to deliver high LET radiation to the surrounding lung parenchyma.

Determination of dose-incidence relationships among various groups of miners is complicated by uncertainties about the circumstances of irradiation. In addition to the usual demographic considerations, corrections need to be made for cigarette consumption and the relative proportions of individual radon daughters in the atmosphere. Therefore estimates of the cumulative dose received by an individual over a prolonged period of time have until recently been fraught with uncertainty.

In miners who develop carcinoma of the lung the average duration of exposure is 15 to 20 years. Small cell undifferentiated carcinoma is the most frequent type of tumor. Among the uranium miners, and perhaps other mining populations as well, cigarette smoking appears to be a potent cocarcinogen.

Cigarette smoke is known to contain a number of chemical carcinogens. Recently it has been suggested that one or more radionuclides may act as a synergistic agent in the cigarette-related carcinoma of the lung. Two radionuclides implicated in this regard are polonium 210 and lead 210. The former is an alpha emitter of the uranium series, which is present in trace amounts in most plants and foodstuffs. Lead 210 is also present in cigarette smoke in the form of insoluble particles of high specific activity that are derived from the combustion of trichromes in the tobacco leaf. The insoluble lead 210 particle, which is retained in the lung and has a physical half-life of 22 years, decays by beta emission to polonium 210.

Gastrointestinal tract

The sequence of radiation-induced alterations in the mucous membranes of the mouth and upper digestive tract is similar to that seen in the skin, but clinical evidence of injury appears much more quickly in the former sites. Salivary gland exposure results in noticeable swelling of the gland, which may be associated with an elevation in serum amylase levels and dryness of the mouth (xerostomia). The response of the oral mucosa and salivary glands is of particular interest because radiotherapy appears to be the treatment of choice in many tumors of the head and neck, and these structures often must be included in the treatment field.

Some aspects of radiation damage to the alimentary tract have been discussed previously under the acute radiation syndrome. The onset of acute esophagitis, gastritis, enteritis, colitis, and proctitis occurs 1 to 3 weeks after exposure, depending primarily on how much of the gastrointestinal tract is irradiated and on the exposure level. The morphologic consequences of such exposure relate to a loss of the regenerative capacity of stem cells, which are the precursors of the epithelial lining cells. The attendant symptoms resemble those associated with other inflammatory disorders.

The delayed sequelae of gastrointestinal exposure include strictures, ulcers, and malignant tumors. Strictures are responsible for varying degrees of obstruction, whereas ulcers predispose to perforation and hemorrhage. Ulcers may involve any part of the alimentary tract, but the colon, rectum, and stomach are particularly susceptible. As shown in Fig. 6-17, radiation-induced injury to small blood vessels, and especially small arteries and arterioles, appears to be responsible for most of these late sequelae. The resultant vascular insufficiency causes atrophy of the mucosa and reactive fibrosis. The atrophic mucosa is especially prone to ulcer formation. Corrective surgery is difficult because of vascular insufficiency and poor healing of anastomotic sites. Carcinogenesis has been implicated as a delayed effect of exposure of the gastrointestinal tract in humans. Primary sites include the colon, esophagus, stomach, and possibly the pancreas.

Liver

The liver is moderately radioresistant. However, well-defined morphologic alterations are associated with radiation doses employed clinically. Thus a significant number of patients who receive 4000 rad or more to the entire liver develop radiation hepatitis. Although still the subject of some controversy, the pathogenesis of this disorder appears to relate to occlusion of the small hepatic veins. The characteristic morphologic alterations include dilatation of the central veins, centrilobular congestion with focal hemorrhage, and variable degrees of necrosis and atrophy of parenchymal cells. Children are more susceptible than adults to radiation hepatitis. The nutritional status of the host also appears to influence the magnitude of the necrosis. Portal fibrosis may be a late sequela of radiation-induced necrosis.

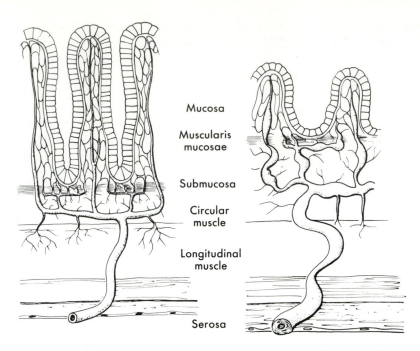

Fig. 6-17. Delayed effects of radiation injury to intestine. Majority of effects are related to abnormalities of vascular supply. Segmental sclerosis is most pronounced in small arteries and arterioles with secondary ectasia and loss of capillaries. Resultant relative tissue ischemia causes loss of the more differentiated cell populations, especially epithelial cells, and reactive fibrosis. Atrophic mucosa is particularly prone to ulceration. (After White, D.C.: Atlas of radiation histopathology, ERDA Report TID-26676.)

Evidence suggests that external irradiation of the liver is rarely associated with delayed sequelae. On the other hand, administration of thorium dioxide (Thorotrast) for diagnostic imaging purposes with subsequent localization and retention in the Kupffer cells has been associated with cirrhosis, hepatic cell carcinoma, cholangiocarcinoma, and hemangioendothelioma.

Bone marrow

The bone marrow is extremely sensitive to both the acute and the delayed effects of ionizing radiation. Acute necrosis of hematopoietic stem cells is primarily responsible for the panhypoplasia of the bone marrow and the cytopenias noted in the peripheral blood that are associated with whole-body exposure in the 200 to 1000 rad range. In terms of delayed effects, leukemia and related disorders are among the most frequently encountered malignancies after partial- or whole-body exposure. Degenerative changes, such as marrow fibrosis, are an infrequent complication of whole-body exposure but are not unusual after regional or local irradiation.

The leukemogenic action of radiation was initially recognized in 1911 in a report that dealt with five instances of leukemia among radiation workers. The authors of the report suggested that occupational exposure may have been a significant factor in the development of the disease. Since 1911, well over 500 cases of leukemia have been attributed to occupational, therapeutic, or accidental exposure. These cases involve most of the irradiated human populations. The type of leukemia depends primarily on the age at the time of exposure and the conditions of irradiation. In this connection, whole-body exposure is more leukemogenic than local irradiation, fractionated doses are more leukemogenic than single exposures, and irradiation increases primarily those types of leukemia that are most likely to occur in the age group at risk. Thus acute and chronic myelogenous leukemias are associated with irradiation in adult life, whereas acute lymphatic leukemia is more characteristic of the exposure of children. To date, no evidence exists to suggest that the incidence of chronic lymphocytic leukemia is influenced by irradiation.

In individuals irradiated for ankylosing spondylitis and in the atomic bomb survivors an increased incidence of leukemia first became evident 1 to 2 years after exposure, reached a peak after 3 to 7 years, and then declined to background levels over the subsequent 15 to 35 years.

An increased rate of occurrence of malignant lymphoma has also been reported among the pioneer American radiologists, persons irradiated for ankylosing spondylitis, and possibly the Hiroshima atomic bomb survivors. Multiple myeloma is also increased in prevalence among atomic bomb survivors, radium dial painters, workers in the nuclear industry, the early American radiologists, persons irradiated for ankylosing spondylitis, and patients given thorium dioxide. The magnitude of increase with respect to radiation-related lymphoma and multiple myeloma is much less than that noted for leukemia.

Genitourinary system

The kidney is moderately radiosensitive. Controversy exists with respect to the radiosensitivity of the various components of the kidney and thus the pathogenesis of the acute and chronic effects. Injury to the convoluted tubules and small blood vessels has been most strongly implicated in this regard.

Acute radiation injury is generally accompanied by tubular necrosis, vasodilatation, interstitial edema, and proteinuria. After a variable asymptomatic latent period, progressive vascular and tubular changes develop quite regularly in people and experimental animals exposed to large doses. In most cases, the sclerosis of the small blood vessels proceeds slowly, often accompanied by varying degrees of hypertension. The vascular lesions result in ischemia of nephrons with consequent hyalinization of glomeruli. Tubular injury is manifest by marked atrophy. Grossly, the kidney of chronic radiation nephritis is small with a thin cortex and a finely irregular surface.

Clinically, most instances of radiation nephritis terminate in renal failure with uremia, hypervolemia, dyspnea, headache, and vomiting. Rapid acceleration of the process with pronounced hypertension, evidence of increased intracranial pressure, and abnormalities of the optic fundus suggest malignant hypertension. Recovery from radiation nephritis is possible only when the damage is unilateral and the involved kidney is removed.

Effects reminiscent of those described above have been documented experimentally with radioisotopes known to localize in the kidney; however, to date, this has not been a significant problem in humans. Similarly, although rodents develop renal tumors as a consequence of whole-body or local exposure, radiation-induced tumors have not been reported in human beings with the possible exception of a few cases associated with the administration of thorium dioxide.

In contrast with the kidney, where chronic effects are of paramount importance, the urinary bladder is highly susceptible to acute radiation injury. This is to be expected because the bladder mucosa undergoes constant replacement. The response of the urinary bladder to such injury is similar to that noted for skin. Initial hyperemia is often followed by suppression of normal cell division, loss of mucosal cells, and ulceration. Contracture, infection, and carcinogenesis are other important complications of radiation injury to the bladder.

The germinal epithelium of the testes is extremely radiosensitive. Even after exposures at low dose levels, recovery is very slow and may never be complete. Acute-

ly, radiation produces an immediate suppression of mitosis followed by necrosis of the germinal epithelial cells. Spermatogonia are more sensitive than spermatocytes and spermatids. Persistent effects include sclerosis of seminiferous tubules and hyalinization of blood vessels. In more severe cases there may be total tubular atrophy with hyalinization. Sertoli cells and interstitial cells are radioresistant.

The ovary is also very radiosensitive. Within several days after exposure to 300 rad, the human ovary shows a sharp increase in atretic follicles. However, a few primary primordial oocytes and their follicular epithelium are spared. Thus, about 6 months later, the cortex contains a few maturing follicles in an otherwise atrophic fibrous parenchyma.

Cartilage and bone

With respect to radiation-induced injury of cartilage and bone, it is important to distinguish between growing and mature tissues. Growing cartilage and bone are relatively radiosensitive, and exposure often results in growth abnormalities. Abnormal growth of the spine resulting in scoliosis is of particular importance because of the not infrequent exposure of this structure during the irradiation of abdominal tumors in children. The effect of externally applied radiation upon developing bone and cartilage is predictable: a reduction in the numbers of mitoses and disorderly maturation followed by the asymptomatic degeneration and necrosis of less mature elements. Proliferating chondroblasts are more sensitive than osteoblasts. Recovery is possible by a more radioresistant population of nondividing reserve cells unless there is also severe damage to the small blood vessels that supply the area. However, subtle abnormalities often persist in the form of a disoriented microstructure, which may be associated with a loss of normal tensile strength. In addition, even temporary interruption of normal growth results in a stunted bone.

In contradistinction to this, mature cartilage and bone are among the most radioresistant tissues of the body. Radionecrosis of mature bone and cartilage is unusual and when present appears to be related to injury to the arterioles and capillaries that supply these tissues. The resultant ischemia causes degeneration and necrosis of parenchymal cells and loss of tensile strength. Another consequence of such injury is an increased susceptibility to infection.

Bone-seeking radionuclides induce injury in a fashion similar to that described for external irradiation. Thus "radium jaw" among the early luminous dial painters was first described in 1924 by Beum, a New York dentist. The changes in the maxilla and mandible of these patients consisted of arrested maturation of bone among young patients, localized regions of bone resorption,

resorption of teeth, and foci of sclerosis, bone necrosis, and pathologic fractures. The abnormalities seen in the facial bones of these people were mirrored by comparable changes elsewhere in the skeleton. However, because of the frequent association of tooth decay and infection, the oral manifestations of osteoradionecrosis tended to become evident clinically while similar lesions elsewhere remained asymptomatic. In addition to these degenerative changes, a variety of malignant tumors have been documented among the radium dial painters. The first reports, which concerned the development of osteogenic sarcoma, began to appear some 10 years after the initial exposure to this bone-seeking radionuclide.

Definition of a dose-incidence relationship for bone tumors induced by internal emitters such as radium is complicated by several factors. In the first place, the isotope is not distributed uniformly within the skeleton. Regions of intense localization result in "hot spots," which contain more radioactivity than does the surrounding bone, often by a factor of 10 or more. Second, changes occur with time in the distribution of the radioelement and its decay daughters. Such shifts result from the metabolic turnover of the bone constituents and the redistribution and excretion of the internal emitters. Last, the magnitude of exposure is influence by the progressive diminution in the dose rate of the emitted radiation because of the physical decay of the isotope. Despite these problems in determining dose-response relationships, the incidence of bone tumors is believed to vary approximately as the square of the terminal concentration of radium in the skeleton. Such a relationship is consistent with comparable observations in experimental animals.

Tumors other than osteogenic sarcomas have been reported after radium exposure. They include not only fibrosarcomas but also carcinomas of the epithelial cells that line the paranasal sinuses, the mastoid air cells, the gingival tissues, and the nasopharynx. These epithelial cells, because of their proximity to the bones of the skull, were also exposed to significant amounts of radiation. Recently, an apparent increase in the prevalence of blood dyscrasias, multiple myeloma, and malignant tumors of the central nervous system has also been noted in this group.

Lesions similar to those described have developed among patients treated with "radium water" and the inhabitants of regions of the world where the drinking water contains significant amounts of radium. Benign tumors, principally exostoses, have also been noted in children treated with radium.

Rare instances of osteosarcoma have been reported in association with therapeutic irradiation utilizing an external source. The doses have been extremely large, ranging from 3000 to more than 15,000 rad with an average latent period of 9 years.

Thyroid

An increased incidence of thyroid tumors has been noted among Japanese atomic bomb survivors, the Marshallese who were accidently exposed to nuclear fallout, and children irradiated therapeutically for "status thymolymphaticus" or tinea capitis. Jewish individuals, females, and children less than 10 years of age at the time of exposure appear to be particularly susceptible. An increased prevalence has also been noted among adult Japanese atomic bomb survivors, principally women, who were exposed to 50 rad or more. Papillary adenocarcinomas, adenomas, and hyperplastic nodules have been associated with exposure. The majority of the carcinomas noted among the Hiroshima and Nagasaki survivors were noted initially at autopsy and did not apparently contribute to the patient's death. Some of the adenomas documented among the Marshall Islanders were associated with hypothyroidism.

The incidence of carcinoma of the thyroid appears to be increasing in the United States, perhaps as a result of earlier irradiation of children for benign conditions of the head and neck. For this reason individuals with a history of prior exposure to this region should be carefully followed medically with particular attention to the thyroid. Conversely, patients with suspected thyroid tumors should be questioned about prior irradiation of the head and neck region.

A relationship between iodine 131 administration for thyrotoxicosis and carcinoma of the thyroid has been postulated but not confirmed. If such a relationship exists, it must be rare. The reason for this may relate to the severe local destructive effect of the doses employed (5000 to 50,000 rad or more to the thyroid), which probably destroys entirely the epithelial component of the gland.

Breast

An increased incidence of carcinoma of the breast has been documented among several populations of women exposed to ionizing radiation: the Japanese atomic bomb survivors, tuberculous patients who received multiple chest fluoroscopies to monitor pneumothorax therapy, and individuals in whom one or both breasts were irradiated for a variety of benign conditions including acute postpartum mastitis, unilateral hypertrophy, and fibroadenomatosis. Analysis of these data shows that the female breast is extremely sensitive to radiation carcinogenesis with the risk of developing such tumors increasing approximately linearly with increasing dose. Risk is also heavily dependent upon age at exposure, with women below 40 years particularly vulnerable. For this reason, mammographic screening of women below 40 is generally limited to persons with a personal history of breast cancer. Similarly, routine mammography for women ages 40 to 49 years is recommended only if they have a personal history of breast cancer or if a mother or a sister has breast cancer. In this context, a distinction must be made between screening and evaluation. Mammography is an important diagnostic tool in a woman with suspected breast cancer, irrespective of age.

Among irradiated individuals, an increased incidence of carcinoma of the breast begins within 10 years of exposure and persists for at least 30 years. The mean latent period is approximately 25 years. The vast majority of tumors are infiltrating ductal adenocarcinomas.

Central nervous system

As noted previously, the development of the brain may be severely disturbed by exposure to relatively small amounts of radiation during early embryonic development. Mature nervous tissue is relatively resistant to acute morphologic changes although functional abnormalities are often encountered, especially after whole-body exposure to doses in excess of 5000 rad (see under central nervous system syndrome). Late morphologic abnormalities of the brain are not uncommon, however, especially after local exposure. Focal necrosis, often associated with demyelination, is a frequent manifestation. The white matter is more susceptible than the gray matter to focal necrosis, perhaps because of its less abundant vasculature.

Irradiation of the spinal cord can also lead to acute necrosis. In such a situation, the cord usually has been unavoidably included in the treatment field of a thoracic or abdominal tumor. Vascular injury and thrombosis of small blood vessels are believed to be responsible for the necrosis of the spinal cord, which in its most severe form may result in permanent paraplegia and a syndrome known as transverse myelitis.

Eyes

Either single or multiple exposures of the optic lens can result in the formation of opacities, which may progress to clinically significant cataracts. Cataract formation depends upon the magnitude of the dose and the character of the radiation; densely ionizing radiations are especially cataractogenic. A single acute exposure is more injurious and produces opacities sooner than the same dose administered in divided exposures.

Other tumors

Such a wide variety of neoplasms has been reported in exposed animals that radiation must be considered to be potentially carcinogenic for almost all tissues under the proper conditions of dose, shielding, host responsiveness, and exposure to the relevant cocarcinogens. Although most tissues may be potentially susceptible to radiation-induced carcinogenesis, individual organs vary greatly with respect to their relative susceptibility. Quantitation of relative susceptibility is not yet possible in humans because most of the irradiated populations have not been followed until the death of all members. However, Fig. 6-18 shows the relative risk for the development of specific malignant tumors among atomic bomb survivors. In this population, as in others, malignancies of the hemopoietic system show the greatest relative increase in frequency.

RADIOTHERAPY

Late in the nineteenth century, Wilhelm Konrad Roentgen's discovery of a "new kind of ray," coupled with the discovery of radium by Marie and Pierre Curie, launched a new era in medicine. Physicians quickly began to use x rays and radium diagnostically and thera-

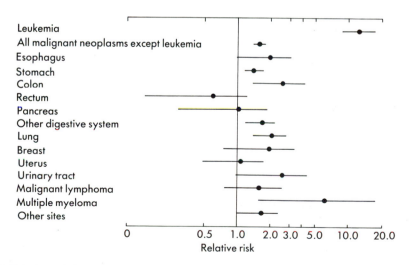

Fig. 6-18. Relative risk for specific types of tumors among atomic bomb survivors. Results are based on comparison between 200+ rad groups and 0 rad group. Therefore value of 1.0 indicates no increase in risk. Horizontal bars on either side of data points indicate 90% confidence limits. (After Kato, H., and Schull, W.J.: Radiat. Res. **90:**395, 1982.)

peutically. X rays and radium became the treatment of choice for almost every type of illness imaginable. As a result, many tragic examples of radiation injury, of both patients and physicians, occurred and were subsequently documented. Unfortunately, the untoward effects often were not manifest until many years later, and only recently have stringent controls been adopted to protect patients, physicians, and technical personnel.

On the positive side, the therapeutic value of radiation was quickly recognized, and the complete eradication of otherwise fatal tumors was reported. A new discipline of medicine was soon launched, and today radiotherapy, singly or in conjunction with surgery and chemotherapy, represents the treatment of choice for a variety of neoplasms. Before presenting a more detailed consideration of radiation as a therapeutic modality, it is important to review a few aspects of the radiobiology of tumors.

Tumor radiobiology

Fig. 6-19 shows a hypothetical dose-response curve for tumor cells grown in tissue culture. The narrow shoulder indicates that these cells are relatively poorly equipped to repair sublethal damage. The steep slope of the linear portion of the curve indicates that the tumor cells are relatively radiosensitive. The exponential character of the curve indicates that the vast majority of cells are killed by small amounts of radiation but that a large dose is required to kill the last viable malignant cell. Put another way, it requires the same dose to reduce the number of viable cells from 10^7 to 10^6 (a reduction of 9 million cells) as from 10^2 to 10^1 (a reduction of 90 cells). The critical task of the radiotherapist in attempting to eradicate a malignant tumor is either to kill all tumor cells or to reduce the number to such a level that host defense mechanisms can complete the task. The radiotherapist must accomplish this without undue injury to adjacent normal tissues and intervening vital structures. In reaching this goal the radiotherapist is greatly assisted by the difference between normal and abnormal cells with respect to repair of radiation-induced injury. This relationship is shown schematically in Fig. 6-20. The injury created among the normal and abnormal cells by each individual exposure dose, or fraction, is the same. However, the time interval (24 to 72 hours) between the completion of one radiation exposure and the start of the next provides a period for both the normal and abnormal cells to repair radiation-induced lesions. Since normal tissues generally possess a greater capability for repair than do neoplastic cells, a larger fraction of the former is present at the beginning of each subsequent treatment. For this reason, most radiation treatments are fractioned and protracted over a period of several weeks or months.

Fig. 6-21 depicts the effect of treatment, as a function of radiation dose, on normal and malignant cells. The

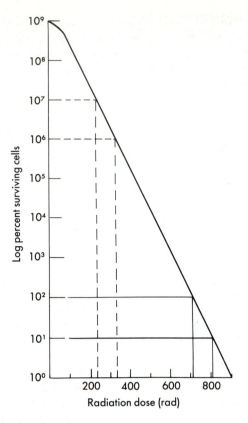

Fig. 6-19. Hypothetical survival curve for tumor cells.

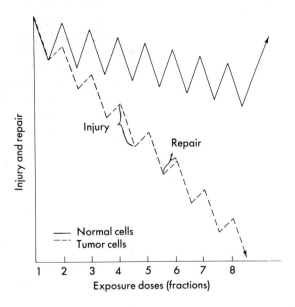

Fig. 6-20. Effect of fractionation on response of normal and neoplastic cells to radiation-induced injury. Although magnitude of injury is the same for most normal and neoplastic tissues, as illustrated by identical down segments of two curves, normal tissues generally have greater recovery ability, represented by up segments of curves. Therefore, with fractionation, normal tissue survives radiation injury more effectively than does tumor. (Modified from Kligerman, M.M.: Principles of radiation therapy. In Holland, J.F., and Frei, E., editors: Cancer medicine, Philadelphia, 1973, Lea & Febiger.).

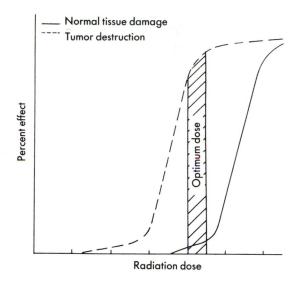

Fig. 6-21. Effect of treatment as function of dose with respect to normal and abnormal cells. Optimal dose for specific tumor-host system is amount of radiation that will cause greatest number of tumor cells to be destroyed in exchange for minimal amount of normal tissue damage. (After Kligerman, M.M.: Principles of radiation therapy. In Holland, J.F., and Frei, E., editors: Cancer medicine, Philadelphia, 1973, Lea & Febiger.)

optimal dose is that amount of radiation that will kill the greatest number of tumor cells while injuring only a small number of normal cells. It is important to note that, although a small amount of normal tissue destruction is acceptable, the dose must not be so large as to approach the linear portion of the "normal tissue damage" curve in Fig. 6-21.

Types of radiation generators

X and gamma rays cover a broad range of wavelengths. Within this range, the shorter the wavelength, the greater the energy and penetrating power of the rays. For this reason, long wavelengths generated at 30 to 80 keV are used for routine diagnostic procedures in radiology. Although most of the radiation is absorbed by the skin, enough energy reaches the underlying structures to provide a satisfactory roentgenographic or fluoroscopic image. In radiation therapy, shorter wavelengths are generally employed in order to deliver a greater proportion of the energy to deeper structures. Hence, x-ray machines designed for diagnostic purposes are not used for radiotherapy. It also follows that a given dose of x rays from a diagnostic machine will produce greater skin damage and less injury to underlying tissues than the same dose delivered by a therapy machine.

On the basis of the foregoing discussion, it is evident that a variety of radiation energies is required to treat patients with dissimilar tumors in optimal fashion. For example, energies in the lower ranges, 50 to 100 keV, are employed to treat superficial lesions such as the majority of skin tumors. On the other hand, energies in the ortho-

voltage range, 200 to 400 keV, are used to treat larger or more aggressive skin tumors such as carcinomas of the lower lip, whereas energies in the supervoltage range, 2 MeV or greater, are important in the treatment of most deep-seated tumors.

X rays are usually produced by accelerating electrons to a variable degree and then permitting them to strike a tungsten target. Absorption of the energy by the target results in the production of electromagnetic radiation and heat. Depending upon the energy imparted to the electrons, x rays in the superficial orthovoltage or supervoltage range are produced. The Van de Graaff generator and the linear accelerator are two machines used to accelerate electrons. The latter is the most common supervoltage machine in use today.

Currently there is considerable interest in the use of neutrons and other high LET particles in radiotherapy because of their ability to kill anoxic tumor cells. So much ionization is produced when heavy particles pass through tissues that little recovery is possible regardless of the presence or absence of oxygen. Therefore the relative advantage enjoyed by tumor cells, which are generally less well oxygenated than the surrounding normal tissues, is largely abolished. Although neutrons were first employed to treat malignant tumors in the late 1930s, the initial experience was marred by significant injury to adjacent normal tissues. At that time, the concept of relative biologic effectiveness and the inhibition of normal tissue repair by heavy-particle irradiation had not yet been appreciated. Because of extensive injury to normal tissues and a variety of unfortunate complications, neutron therapy lost favor among radiotherapists until the past several years when interest again developed based upon a better understanding of the biologic effects of this particle.

Palliative and curative therapy

Radiation therapy may be employed to relieve symptoms caused by an inoperable tumor or to eradicate totally a malignant neoplasm. In many medical centers radiation represents the treatment of choice for stage I and stage II malignant lymphomas, select epidermoid carcinomas of the uterine cervix, invasive epidermoid carcinomas of the laryngeal glottis, epidermoid carcinomas of the skin and lip, invasive epidermoid carcinomas of the pharynx, most carcinomas of the mouth, and select transitional cell carcinomas of the urinary bladder. Curative radiotherapy is also often employed in conjunction with surgery in one of two ways: (1) prophylactically, when the surgeon thinks that the tumor has been completely removed but cannot discount the possible presence of tumor cells in areas adjacent to the primary neoplasm such as the draining lymphatics or regional lymph nodes, and (2) therapeutically, when the surgeon is unable to totally resect the tumor because of adjacent vital structures.

Palliative radiotherapy is often employed to relieve symptoms or to abort impending complications. An example of the latter is the irradiation of a tumor metastasis in the neck of the femur or other weight-bearing bone, which if left untreated might be expected to result in a pathologic fracture. Palliative radiotherapy is also used to relieve pain, which often occurs in association with bone tumor metastases, to relieve compression of a vital structure, such as the spinal cord, or to prevent ulceration by a subcutaneous or submucosal metastasis.

As with surgery, injury to normal tissues is an inevitable consequence of radiation therapy. A margin of normal tissue adjacent to a treatable tumor must be included in the treatment field in order to anticipate possible microscopic extension. Regional lymph nodes are often irradiated to eradicate possible metastases. Intervening tissues and structures are also injured by ionizations. The morphologic consequences of such injury in specific organs were discussed in the previous section.

Radiation therapy can also cause radiation sickness and depress the number of circulating platelets and leukocytes. Radiation sickness is associated with treatment of the thorax or abdomen, most frequently the latter. The symptoms of radiation sickness (fatigue, anorexia, vomiting) are short lived and are usually controlled by small reductions in the daily dose. Leukopenia and thrombocytopenia can occur when large portions of the bone marrow are included in the treatment field and may dictate temporary interruption of treatment.

A small risk of inducing a new malignant tumor exists among irradiated patients. Other complications of radiotherapy include actinic conjunctivitis; cataract formation, especially in children; sterility; transverse myelitis; asymmetric growth retardation in children after exposure of long bones; radiation pneumonitis; radiation pericarditis; and constriction of a hollow viscus (especially the intestine) by fibrous connective tissue.

Radioisotopes

It was noted in the previous discussion that certain naturally occurring substances such as radium, thorium, and actinium give off radiant energy spontaneously. In addition, unstable isotopes of most known elements can be produced artificially. Since the radioactive isotope of an element is essentially identical chemically to the nonradioactive form, these substances have found widespread diagnostic and therapeutic application.

Diagnostic advantage is taken of the known propensity of organs to concentrate specific elements. For example, the thyroid gland concentrates iodine. By the administration of radioactive iodine, the physician can determine, with appropriate counting techniques, the capacity of this gland to concentrate iodine normally. More important, however, the organ can be scanned and the relative distribution of the isotope throughout the gland

can be quantitated. Failure of the radioactive iodine to be distributed evenly throughout the gland suggests the displacement of normal thyroid by nonfunctioning tissue, for example, a cyst, an abscess, a nonfunctioning adenoma, or a carcinoma. Similar methods are used with other organs.

Radioisotopes are also used therapeutically. The administration of large doses of an isotope such as iodine 131, with a known propensity to concentrate in a specific organ, ensures the release of a significant amount of radioactivity within that organ. This approach may be employed to damage or destroy a malignant tumor or suppress a hyperfunctioning gland. In this connection, it is important to note that the selective concentration of most elements is not complete and therefore other tissues may be exposed, albeit to much smaller doses. This latter observation is of primary concern only with respect to the gonads and possible radiation-induced genetic effects.

Finally, it is important to remember that radiation may also be received by the fetus when a radioactive isotope is administered to the mother, who may or may not be aware that she is pregnant. Radioactive strontium, plutonium, phosphorus, tritium, iodine, and many other isotopes cross the placenta and can become incorporated into the fetus. Perhaps the most striking example is radioactive iodine, which, when administered to the mother late in pregnancy, is also concentrated in the fetal thyroid where the resultant radiation-induced injury can result in cretinism. Other examples have been documented experimentally in rodents and have been associated with malformations, neoplasms, and decreased life span in the fetus.

INJURY FROM NONIONIZING RADIATION

Thus far tissue injury caused by ionizing radiation has represented the primary focus of this chapter. In the past several years it has been recognized that tissues may also be injured by nonionizing forms of radiation. Table 6-7 lists some of the known deleterious effects of exposure to various types of nonionizing radiation. The industrial and medical applications of these forms of energy continue to increase dramatically. Therefore the potential for human injury from nonionizing radiation will also increase.

Numerous electronic devices represent potential sources of injury from nonionizing radiation. Currently, popular devices of this type include radar units, microwave ovens, and lasers. Despite the increasing use of these devices, surprisingly little attention has been paid to possible deleterious effects.

Microwaves represent a form of electromagnetic radiation in the frequency range between ultra-high frequency television and the infrared region of the spectrum. Potential sources of exposure to microwaves include microwave ovens and the high output radar devices used

Table 6-7. Types of injury caused by types of nonionizing radiations

Type of radiation	Sources	Populations at particular risk	Effects
Ultraviolet	Sun; sunlamps; welder's arcs; industrial and medical applications	All mankind; sun worshippers; occupational groups	Burns of skin and eye; malignant melanoma; benign skin tumors; senile keratoses
Visible light	Sun; artificial lights; lasers; communications, industrial, and medical applications	All mankind; occupational groups	Burns of retina; photosensitization
Infrared	Sun; industrial and military applications	All mankind; occupational groups	Cataracts
Microwaves; radiowaves	Ovens; radar and other communications; industrial, military, and medical applications	Much of mankind; occupational groups	Thermal effects at high power levels; cataracts; possible behavioral effects and blood dyscrasias

From DHEW Pub. No. NIH 77-1277, U.S. Department of Health, Education and Welfare, Washington, D.C., U.S. Government Printing Office, p. 135.

in navigation and weather systems as well as burglar alarms. Animal experiments have shown that lens opacities and hematologic, endocrine, and possibly genetic effects can be caused by microwave radiations.

Microwave ovens appear to represent a particular health hazard for several reasons. In the first place, these ovens are becoming increasingly popular. Second, several surveys have documented detectable leakage around the door. And last, most owners and operators appear to be unaware of any radiation hazard.

The laser also represents a potential source of injury of nonionizing radiation. Because of the focusing characteristics of the lens of the eye, the retina is especially vulnerable to laser radiation. Even reflected beams represent a potential hazard. Pulsed lasers, which operate at very high power levels, can cause retina burns in 1 microsecond or less. The medical and industrial applications of lasers have increased dramatically in the past several years. Unfortunately, until recently, occupational safety measures lagged behind the foregoing technologic advancements.

RADIATION PROTECTION STANDARDS AND THE CONCEPT OF RELATIVE RISK

Recognition of some of the untoward effects of radiation occurred within months of Roentgen's discovery of x rays in 1895. Beginning soon thereafter various national and international committees have developed radiation protection standards. The efforts of these groups received significant impetus during the 1950s when large-scale testing of nuclear weapons led to widespread concern about the possible hazards of global contamination by radioactive fallout. More recently, the development of nuclear power as an energy source, in conjunction with our increasing knowledge of the risks associated with low-level exposure, has prompted a continuing assessment of radiation safety standards. Viewed in historical perspective, the evolution of these standards represents a movement toward progressively more cautious

exposure limits both for the general public and for radiation workers.

As shown in Table 6-1, the average dose of radiation to the general public from medical and dental uses in medically advanced countries currently approaches that from natural background. Approaches for reducing the exposure of the patient include using radiography in preference to fluoroscopy whenever practical; proper installation and use of equipment; shielding tissues outside the area of interest, especially the gonads; using fast film to reduce the duration and intensity of exposure per radiograph; reducing the number of radiographs per patient; limiting the size of the field to regions of prime interest; and proper education of personnel working in the field.

Possible risks related to the nuclear power industry deserve special mention, especially in light of the accident at Three Mile Island in 1979. Table 6-8 summarizes some of the key features of the accident. On the basis of very careful dosimetry, it is estimated that two adverse health effects will occur in the general population at risk. Other activities associated with a one-in-a-million risk of death include: 1.5 weeks of typical factory work (death owing to a job-related accident), 1 hour of coal mining (black lung disease), 3 hours of coal mining (accident), smoking three cigarettes (cancer, heart disease), 2 months of living with a cigarette smoker (cancer, heart disease), 2 days of living in New York (air pollution), a 2-month visit to Denver, Colorado (cancer caused by cosmic rays), 2 months living in a stone or brick building (cancer caused by natural background), and traveling 60 miles by automobile. Risk estimates, as well as risk/benefit ratios, become of immense importance. Imagine what would have happened if the governor of Pennsylvania had followed the advice of some well-meaning public officials and evacuated the area. Two million people traveling, for example, an average of 120 miles under reasonable traffic conditions would be expected to result in four fatalities.

Table 6-8. Key aspects of Three Mile Island accident

Date	March 28, 1979
Population at risk	2 million within 50-mile radius
Radionuclides released	Xenon 133 (5.3 days) Xenon 135 (9.2 hours) Iodine 131 (8.0 days) Krypton isotopes
Maximum dose	<100 mrem
Average dose	1.5 mrem (within 50 miles) 8.0 mrem (within 10 miles)
Risk estimates	1 fatal neoplasm (vs. 325,000 "spontaneous" neoplasms expected in population at risk) 2 adverse health effects (fatal and nonfatal neoplasms, genetic effects)

REFERENCES
General

1. Behrens, C.F., King, E.R., and Carpender, J.W.J., editors: Atomic medicine, ed. 5, Baltimore, 1969, The Williams & Wilkins Co. (Selective review with timely references.)
2. Dalrymple, G.V., et al., editors: Medical radiation biology, Philadelphia, 1973, W.B. Saunders Co. (Excellent review, particularly with respect to molecular and cellular radiobiology.)
3. Hollaender, A., editor: Radiation biology, vols. 1-4, New York, 1954–1956, McGraw-Hill Book Co. (Extremely comprehensive review.)
4. Rubin, P., and Casarett, G.W., editors: Clinical radiation pathology, Philadelphia, 1968, W.B. Saunders Co. (General review with particular emphasis on clinical-morphologic correlations.)
5. Upton, A.C.: Radiation injury: effects, principles and perspectives, Chicago, 1969, The University of Chicago Press. (Concise review of radiation pathology.)

Radiation spectrum; radioactive substances; radiation units

6. Hendee, W.R.: Medical radiation physics, ed. 2, Chicago, 1979, Year Book Medical Publishers.
7. Hendee, W.R.: Radiation therapy physics, Chicago, 1981, Year Book Medical Publishers.
8. Johns, H.E., and Cunningham, J.R.: Physics of radiology, ed. 4, Springfield, Ill., 1982, Charles C Thomas, Publisher.

Cellular and molecular radiobiology

9. Altman, K.I., Gerber, G.B., and Okada, S.: Radiation biochemistry, vol. I, New York, 1970, Academic Press, Inc. (Broad discussion of biochemical effects.)
10. Bacq, Z.M., and Alexander, P.: Fundamentals of radiobiology, ed. 2, New York, 1971, Pergamon Press.
11. Casarett, A.P.: Radiation biology, Englewood Cliffs, N.J., 1968, Prentice-Hall, Inc. (Broad review of radiobiology.)
12. Elkind, M.M., and Whitmore, G.F.: Radiobiology of cultured mammalian cells, New York, 1967, Gordon & Breach. (Classic reference on cellular radiobiology.)
13. Puck, T.T.: Effect of radiation on mammalian cells. In Puck, T.T., editor: The mammalian cell as a microorganism, San Francisco, 1972, Holden-Day Inc., p. 102.
14. Puck, T.T., and Marcus, P.I.: Action of X-rays on mammalian cells, J. Exp. Med. **103**:653, 1956.
15. Sinclair, W.K.: Cyclic X-ray responses in mammalian cells in vitro, Radiat. Res. **33**:620, 1968.
16. Smith, K.C., and Hanawalt, P.C.: Molecular photobiology: inactivation and recovery, New York, 1969, Academic Press, Inc. (DNA damage and repair.)
17. Till, J.E., and McCullock, E.A.: A direct measurement of the radiation sensitivity of normal mouse bone marrow cells, Radiat. Res. **14**:213, 1961.

General morphologic features of radiation injury

18. Bergonie, J., and Tribondeau, L.: Interpretation de quelques resultats de la radiotherapie et essai de fixation d'une technique rationnelle, Compt. Rend. Acad. Sci. **143**:983, 1906. (Radiosensitivity of tissues.)
19. Upton, A.C., and Lushbaugh, C.C.: The pathological anatomy of total-body irradiation. In Behrens, D.F., King, E.R., and Carpender, J.W.J., editors: Atomic medicine, ed. 5, Baltimore, 1969, The Williams & Wilkins Co., p. 154.
20. Warren, S.: Effects of radiation on normal tissues. Arch. Path. **34**:443, 562, 749, 917, 1070, 1942; **35**:121, 304, 1943. (A series of articles on the effects of radiation on normal tissues.)
21. Warren, S.: Histopathology of radiation lesions, Physiol. Rev **24**:225, 1944.

Radiation injury in humans

22. Advisory Committee on the Biological Effects of Ionizing Radiation: The effects on populations of exposure to low levels of ionizing radiation (BEIR Report), Washington, D.C., 1980, National Academy of Sciences–National Research Council.
23. Anderson, R.E.: The delayed consequences of exposure to ionizing radiation: pathology studies at the Atomic Bomb Casualty Commission, Hiroshima and Nagasaki, 1945-1970, Hum. Pathol. **2**:469, 1971.
24. Andrews, G.A.: Criticality accidents in Vinca, Yugoslavia, and Oak Ridge, Tennessee, J.A.M.A. **179**:191, 1962.
25. Bender, M.A., and Gooch, P.C.: Somatic chromosome aberrations in normal and irradiated humans, Radiat. Res. **14**:451, 1961.
26. Borek, C., and Hall, E.J.: Effect of split doses of x-rays on neoplastic transformation of single cells, Nature **252**:499, 1974.
27. Brent, R.L.: Effects of radiation on the fetus, newborn and child. In Fry, R.J.M., et al., editors: Late effects of radiation, London, 1970, Taylor & Francis, p. 23.
28. Cole, L.J., and Nowell, P.C.: Radiation carcinogenesis: the sequence of events, Science **150**:1782, 1965.
29. Conard, R.A., et al.: Review of medical findings in a Marshallese population twenty-six years after accidental exposure to radioactive fallout, Springfield, Va., 1980, National Technical Information Service, U.S. Department of Commerce.
30. Court Brown, W.M., and Doll, R.: Mortality from cancer and other causes after radiotherapy for ankylosing spondylitis, Br. Med. J. **2**:1327, 1965.
31. Evans, R.D.: The effect of skeletally deposited alpha-ray emitters in man, Br. J. Radiol. **39**:881, 1966.
32. Gaulden, M.E.: Genetic effects of radiation. In Dalrymple, G.V., et al., editors: Medical radiation biology, Philadelphia, 1973, W.B. Saunders Co., p. 52.
33. Hachiya, M.: Hiroshima diary—the journal of a Japanese physician, August 6–September 30, 1945, Chapel Hill, 1955, The University of North Carolina Press.
34. Hempelmann, L.H., and Grossman, J.: The association of illnesses with abnormal immunologic features with irradiation of the thymic gland in infancy: a preliminary report, Radiat. Res. **58**:122, 1974.
35. Hempelmann, L.H., et al.: Neoplasms in persons treated with X-rays in infancy: fourth survey in 20 years, J. Nat. Cancer Inst. **55**:519, 1975. (Children irradiated for allegedly enlarged thymus.)
36. Kato, H., and Schull, W.J.: Studies of the mortality of A-bomb survivors. VII. Mortality, 1950-78. Part I, Cancer Mortal. Radiat. Res. **90**:395-432, 1982.
37. Langham, W.H., Brooks, P.M., and Grahn, D.: Radiation biology and space environmental parameters in manned spacecraft design and operations, Aerospace Med. **36**:1, 1965.
38. Lewis, E.B.: Ionizing radiation and tumor production. In Genetic concepts and neoplasia, 23rd Symposium and Fundamental Cancer Research, M.D. Anderson Hospital and Tumor Institute, 1969, Baltimore, 1970, The Williams & Wilkins Co.
39. Lindop, P.J., and Sacher, G.A., editors: Radiation and aging: a colloquium held in Semmering, Austria, London, 1966, Taylor & Francis. (Radiation-induced life shortening.)

40. Looney, W.B.: Radiation genetics. In Behrens, C.F., King, E.R., and Carpender, J.W.J., editors: Atomic medicine, ed. 5, Baltimore, 1969, The Williams & Wilkins Co., p. 350.

41. Martland, H.S.: Occupational poisoning in manufacture of luminous watch dials, J.A.M.A. **92:**466, 1929.

42. Miller, R.W.: Delayed radiation effects in atomic-bomb survivors, Science **166:**569, 1969.

43. Neel, J.V., Kato, H., and Schull, W.J.: Mortality in the children of atomic bomb survivors and controls, Genetics **76:**311, 1974.

44. Neel, J.V., and Schull, W.J.: The effect of exposure to the atomic bomb on pregnancy termination in Hiroshima and Nagasaki, National Research Council Pub. No. 461, Washington, D.C., 1961, National Academy of Sciences.

45. Oughterson, A.W., and Warren, S.: Medical effects of the atomic bomb in Japan, New York, 1956, McGraw-Hill Book Co.

46. Polednak, A.P., Stehney, A.F., and Rowland, R.E.: Mortality among women first employed before 1930 in the U.S. radium dial-painting industry, J. Epidemiol. **107:**179, 1978.

47. Report of the United Nations Scientific Committe on the effects of atomic radiation, New York, 1964, United Nations (General Assembly, Official Records: Nineteenth Session, Suppl. No. 14 [A/5814]), p. 1. (Radiation carcinogenesis.)

48. Rubin, P., and Casarett, G.W.: Clinical radiation pathology, Philadelphia, 1968, W.B. Saunders Co. (General review.)

49. Russell, W.L., and Russell, L.B.: Radiation-induced genetic damage. In Proceedings of the Second U.N. International Conference on the Peaceful Uses of Atomic Energy, 1958, United Nations, Geneva **22:**362. (Point mutations in the mouse.)

50. Russell, W.L., Russell, L.B., and Oakberg, E.F.: Radiation genetics of mammals. In Claus, W.D., editor: Radiation biology and medicine, Reading, Mass., 1958, Addison-Wesley Publishing Co., p. 189.

51. Seltser, R., and Sartwell, P.E.: The influence of occupational exposure to radiation on the mortality of American radiologists and other medical specialists, Am. J. Epidemiol. **81:**2, 1965.

52. Setlow, R.B., and Carrier, W.L.: The disappearance of thymine dimers from D.N.A.: an error-correcting mechanism, Proc. Natl. Acad. Sci. **51:**226, 1964.

53. United States Department of Health, Education and Welfare: Review of the use of ionizing radiation for treatment of benign diseases, Washington, D.C., 1977, U.S. Government Printing Office.

54. Upton, A.C.: The dose response relation in radiation-induced cancer, Cancer Res. **21:**717, 1961.

55. Upton, A.C.: Physical carcinogenesis: radiation history and sources. In Becker, F.F., editor: Cancer, a comprehensive treatise, vol. 1, New York, 1975, Plenum Press, p. 387.

56. Warren, S., and Lombard, O.M.: New data on the effects of ionizing radiation on radiologists, Arch. Environ. Health **13:**415, 1966. (Aging among radiologists.)

Acute radiation syndrome

57. Bond, V.P., Cronkite, E.P., and Conard, R.A.: Acute whole body radiation injury: pathogenesis, pre- and postradiation protection. In Behrens, C.F., King, E.R., and Carpender, J.W.J., editors: Atomic medicine, ed. 5, Baltimore, 1969, The Williams & Wilkins Co., p. 221.

58. Bond, V.P., Fliedner, T.M., and Archambeau, J.O., editors: Mammalian radiation lethality: a disturbance in cellular kinetics, New York, 1965, Academic Press, Inc. (Cell turnover and acute radiation injury.)

59. Gerstner, H.B.: Acute clinical effects of penetrating nuclear radiation, J.A.M.A. **168:**381, 1958.

60. Hempelmann, L.H., Lisco, H., and Hoffman, J.G.: The acute radiation syndrome: a study of nine cases and a review of the problem, Ann. Intern. Med. **36:**279, 1952.

Radiation injury of select tissues

61. Anderson, R.E., et al.: Pathogenesis of radiation-related leukemia and lymphoma, Lancet **1:**1060, 1972.

62. Archambeau, J.O., et al.: The response of the skin of swine to increasing single exposures of 250-KVp X-rays, Radiat. Res. **36:**299, 1968.

63. Cuzick, J.: Radiation-induced myelomatosis, N. Engl. J. Med. **304:**204, 1981. (Multiple myeloma in irradiated populations.)

64. DeGroot, L., and Paloyan, E.: Thyroid carcinoma and radiation: a Chicago endemic, J.A.M.A. **225:**487, 1973.

65. Haley, T.J., and Snider, R.S.: Response of the nervous system to ionizing radiation, New York, 1962, Academic Press, Inc.

66. Hempelmann, L.H.: Risk of thyroid neoplasms after irradiations in childhood, Science **160:**159, 1968.

67. Ishimaru, M., Ishimaru, T., and Belsky, J.L.: Incidence of leukemia in atomic bomb survivors belonging to a fixed cohort in Hiroshima and Nagasaki, 1950-71, J. Radiat. Res. **19:**262, 1978.

68. Kato, H., and Schull, W.J.: Studies of the mortality of A-bomb survivors. VII. Mortality, 1950-78. Part I. Cancer mortality, Radiat. Res. **90:**395-432, 1982.

69. Knowlton, N.P., Jr., et al.: Beta ray burns of human skin, J.A.M.A. **141:**239, 1949.

70. MacMahon, B.: Prenatal X ray exposure in childhood cancer, J. Natl. Cancer Inst. **28:**1173, 1962.

71. Nishiyama, H., et al.: The incidence of malignant lymphoma and multiple myeloma in Hiroshima and Nagasaki atomic bomb survivors, Cancer **32:**1301, 1973.

72. Puck, T.T.: Cellular aspects of the mammalian radiation syndrome, Radiat. Res. **27:**272, 1966.

73. Saccomanno, G., et al.: Histologic types of lung cancer among uranium miners, Cancer **27:**515, 1971.

74. Stewart, A., Webb, J., and Hewitt, D.: A survey of childhood malignancies, Br. Med. J. **1:**1495, 1958. (In utero irradiation.)

Injury from nonionizing radiation

75. Brill, A.B., and Johnston, R.E.: Exposure of man to radiation. In Fry, R.J.M., et al., editors: Late effects of radiation, proceedings of a colloquium, University of Chicago, 1969, London, 1970, Taylor & Francis, Ltd.

76. Microwave hazards (editorial), Lancet **2:**694, 1975.

77. Peyton, M.F., editor: Biological effects of microwave radiation, New York, 1961, Plenum Press.

CHAPTER 7 Bacterial Diseases

JOHN M. KISSANE

Most bacteria are harmless; indeed, many are beneficial to humans. The essential preoccupation of medicine with disease tends to obscure the fact that microorganisms are ubiquitous and that interaction between humans and microorganisms is only a particular aspect in the complex interrelationship among all living things. Abnormal circumstances in which this interrelationship leads to disease in the human host must be examined for the circumstances related to both the host and the microorganism, whereby the more usual balance between host and parasite becomes disturbed. In this broad view, opportunism is merely an isolated component of the diverse patterns of parasitism.

INFECTION VERSUS DISEASE

Two terms, *pathogenicity* and *virulence*, are used to describe the relationship between a microorganism (for our purposes a bacterium) and disease in its host (for our purposes a human). Although the terms are often used synonymously, it is useful to distinguish their connotations.[14] *Pathogenicity* implies the ability of the organism to produce disease and is usually presented as an absolute. In point of fact, however, a cause-and-effect relationship between infection and disease is rarely inevitable. *Virulence* embodies the concept of degree and expresses the ability of an organism to produce disease in some circumstances but not in others, in some levels or routes of exposure but not in others, and in some species of host or even individuals within a species but not in others. The relationship between host and infecting microorganism is often symbiotic (*sym-*, "together" + *bios*, "life"), and disease results only when one or another component of the equilibrium is disturbed.

DISTINCTION BETWEEN INFECTION AND DISEASE

Several circumstances can be distinguished in which microbial infection remains inapparent or subclinical and is not accompanied by functional or clinical abnormalities recognizable as constituting a disease.

Incubation period

The interval between the lodgment of a pathogenic microorganism on or in its host and the appearance of signs or symptoms of disease is known as the incubation period. If appropriate cultures are made during the incubation period, often fortuitously the organisms may be detected. The individual who is incubating the microorganism may be infectious to others.

Three processes can be considered as occurring during the incubation period: (1) organisms are invading the body of the host from their site of lodgment through a portal of entry ultimately to reach tissue suitable for their proliferation or subject to damage by the organisms, (2) the infecting organisms are proliferating to a quantitative level that overwhelms factors in the resistance of the host, and (3) reactions are occurring in the host, most importantly immunologic, that require the passage of time. These host responses contribute to both the clinical aspects of the disease and the morphologic features of the lesions.

Carrier state

Relatively resistant individuals may harbor pathogenic organisms for an indefinitely prolonged period without manifesting symptoms or signs and without morphologic alterations. Such a prolonged period, in contrast to the relatively brief and less variable incubation period, is described as a carrier state.

Carrier states are of great importance in control of many diseases by public health measures. The carrier may, because of fluctuations in resistance, develop disease. Asymptomatic and mobile, this person may become a soure of infection to others. An individual recovering from a disease may harbor organisms for varying periods as a "convalescent carrier." Often a convalescent carrier is demonstrably immune to the relevant microorganisms, but there may be morphologic factors in the failure of this person's defense mechanisms to eradicate the organisms (such as their lodgment in structures relatively inaccessible to immunologic or other defenses). A patient convalescing from typhoid fever, for example, may harbor typhoid bacilli in a chronically inflamed gallbladder.

DISTINCTION BETWEEN DISEASE AND LESION

Disease is a composite phenomenon—the collective deviations from normal of the patient, however manifested and however perceived. Lesions are morphologic abnormalities, which may be silent or clinical, to which signs and symptoms can be attributed.

Some infectious diseases are highly characteristic in the features by which they are recognized clinically. Meningitis, for example, is a relatively homogeneous clinical entity. Recognition of the disease "meningitis," however, does not have specific implications as to the etiologic agent. Many different microorganisms or even sterile irritants can produce meningitis if they gain access to the subarachnoid space. *Meningitis* therefore designates both the disease and the lesion. Many lesions are morphologically so nonspecific as to etiology that the morphologic designation of the lesion serves as the name of the disease—bronchopneumonia, acute appendicitis, acute cholecystitis.

Scarlet fever, on the other hand, not only is a quite specific clinical entity but also is almost always caused by specific erythrogenic strains of *Streptococcus pyogenes*. Even here, however, occasional cases of scarlet fever appear to be related to toxigenic strains of *Micrococcus pyogenes* var. *aureus* (staphylococcus).

FACTORS IMPORTANT IN PATHOGENESIS OF INFECTIOUS DISEASES (LESIONS)

Many factors enter into the equilibrium between host and bacterial parasite, which may be disturbed, resulting in disease. Among these are (1) access of the organism to the host, (2) portal of entry, (3) infectious dose, (4) host factors, and (5) factors intrinsic to the microorganism.

Access. In strictly "infectious" diseases the infecting organism must reach the body of the host before it can produce disease. Exceptions to this generality are the pure exotoxicoses (p. 281). Often the infecting organism is an invariable or at least frequent parasite on or in the human body. In other instances access of the organism to the potential host requires contact with contaminated objects (fomites) or transmission by vectors, often arthropods.

Portal of entry. The anatomic point at which a parasitic organism gains access to the body is referred to as the portal of entry. Rarely, highly virulent microorganisms may penetrate the intact skin. More frequently, organisms that normally subsist innocuously on the skin gain access to susceptible tissues through sites of injury either trivial and unrecognized or clinically significant and grossly obvious. Ingestion of infectious agents provides an alimentary portal of entry. Inhalation, usually of organisms colonizing microaerosols, provides a portal of entry to the respiratory tract. Instrumentation of the lower urinary tract may introduce organisms from the urethra into the bladder. The depth or extent of invasion by organisms beyond the portal of entry depends in turn on many factors: nature or size of the inoculum in which the organisms are introduced and propulsion of the inoculum as by peristalsis, the periodic flushing effect of the urinary voiding, or (more subtly) the mobility of the mucociliary blanket of the respiratory tract.

In some diseases the portal of entry defines the anatomic distribution of lesions. In others it is nonspecific, and organisms reach and produce lesions in susceptible tissues unrelated to the portal of entry. In still other diseases lesions may occur both at the portal of entry and systemically.

Infectious dose. The size of the infectious inoculum bears importantly, but variably, on the fluctuating equilibrium between host and parasite. Often host defenses can eradicate or at least counterpose considerable numbers of microorganisms before disease results. Alteration of the microbiologic population at a given site, often iatrogenically as by the administration of broad-spectrum antibiotics, may allow normally symbiotic species to proliferate to the extent that they become pathogenic.

Host factors. Almost innumerable factors in the host, many of them poorly understood, influence the pathogenicity of infecting organisms. These factors may be very specific and readily identifiable (such as species, previous experience with the microorganism, or immunologic competence) or quite nonspecific (such as age, general health, nutrition, or the presence of other diseases).

Organismic factors. The explication of mechanisms is particularly the province of pathology. Unfortunately the mechanisms whereby particular infections give rise to particular diseases (or lesions) is much less well understood than microbial metabolism, on the one hand, or the host's immune response, on the other. No doubt the reason is that such mechanisms are exceedingly complex and represent the result of the interplay among many factors, some related to the infecting organism, others to the host.

Mechanical factors. Simple massive proliferation of microorganisms is rarely a factor in the production of lesions. Yet proliferation of *Bacillus anthracis* in bronchopulmonary lymph nodes has been assigned a mechanical role in the production of the pulmonary edema so characteristic of pulmonary anthrax. That lesion now seems, however, to result from the action of the exotoxin elaborated by *B. anthracis*.

Metabolic factors. Early in the twentieth century the discovery of the importance of trace nutrients, notably vitamins, raised the possibility that some features of infectious diseases might result from consumption of significant quantities of critical nutrients by the infecting agents. Although highly artificial animal models of such a mechanism have been devised, nutritional deficiency on this basis has been convincingly demonstrated only in cases of infestation by the fish tapeworm, *Diphyllobothrium latum*, and in abnormal circumstances of consumption by organisms of vitamin B_{12} in blind loops of the intestine. This is not to say, of course, that infectious diseases may not interfere with nutrition by other means.

Toxins. Bacterial toxins are products of bacterial metabolism that exert deleterious effects on cells of the host. It is at least didactically useful to recognize exotoxins, endotoxins, and other toxic bacterial products. *Exotoxins* are soluble products secreted by certain bacteria into the surrounding medium. Most are complex proteins secreted by gram-positive bacteria. Exotoxins mediate major specific features associated with certain bacterial diseases. Strongly antigenic, exotoxins or their nontoxic derivatives, toxoids, excite the production of humoral antibodies, antitoxins, which are strongly protective.

Endotoxins are either proteins or complex polymolecular aggregates of proteins, polysaccharides, and phospholipids. They are believed to be associated with the cell walls of many gram-negative bacteria. In contrast to the highly specific actions of exotoxins, the toxic effects of endotoxins are nonspecific, largely involving the host's cardiovascular system. Antibodies to endotoxins are generally not protective.

Other products of certain bacteria have been ascribed roles in pathogenicity. Many of these substances are chemically incompletely characterized and are identified chiefly by the procedures that isolate them or by their empirically observed effects on living cells on other assay systems. Among these are the staphylococcal and streptococcal leukocidins (enzymes that lyse certain human and other mammalian leukocytes) and hemolysins (which lyse erythrocytes). Pathogenic staphylococci elaborate a coagulase that, acting on a thermolabile factor in either human or rabbit plasma, converts fibrinogen to fibrin. A bound form of coagulase, clumping factor, is found on the surface of most coagulase-positive staphylococci. Coagulase and clumping factor are believed to contribute to the tendency of staphylococci to produce localized abscesses.

Many gram-positive organisms form hyaluronidases, enzymes that are capable of depolymerizing the hyaluronic acid polysaccharide, which contributes to viscosity of extracellular tissue fluid. It is suggested that these agents facilitate the spread of infectious organisms such as streptococci through tissue spaces (Fig. 7-1).

Streptococci and staphylococci produce fibrinolytic agents known respectively as streptokinase and staphylokinase. The role of these agents in infections by the appropriate organisms is not known.

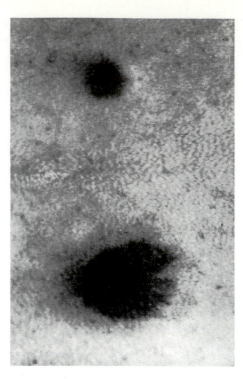

Fig. 7-1. Effect of hyaluronidase on spread of particulate carbon (india ink) of size comparable to staphylococci. Photograph taken 30 minutes after intradermal injections of 0.1 ml of carbon suspension into rabbit. Larger lesion represents increased spread of india ink because of added hyaluronidase.

Many bacteria produce proteolytic enzymes. Several gas-forming clostridia produce a potent collagenase, which liquefies collagen while leaving other components of connective tissue intact. Although collagenase might be considered as contributing to the tendency of certain clostridial infections to liquefy connective tissue, specific anticollagenase is not protective against experimental gas gangrene.

As implied in the foregoing summary, attribution of either the occurrence of a specific bacterial disease or the morphologic features of its lesions to specific biochemical activities of one or more bacterial products is largely conjectural. There has been little progress in this area since the assignment of several morphologic features of tuberculous infection to specific chemically defined fractions of tubercle bacilli.

Certain products of bacterial metabolism exert essentially mechanical effects on pathogenicity and virulence. Among these products are the polysaccharide capsules elaborated, for example, by pathogenic types of *Diplococcus pneumoniae*. Pathogenic and nonpathogenic strains of *Haemophilus influenzae* differ only in production by the former of a capsule that appears to interfere with phagocytosis by host leukocytes. Waxy components of the cell wall of *Mycobacterium tuberculosis* enable that organism to survive in an intracellular habitat after phagocytosis.

Table 7-1. General correlates of infectious processes with degree of parasitism

Degree of parasitism	Site of infection	Classification of disease	Tissue response	Organ/tissue specificity	Infectious processes
None	External	Exotoxicoses	Functional	None	Botulism Food poisoning Tetanus
Slight	Surface	Noninvasive infections	Surface exudation	Portal of entry	Diphtheria Gas gangrene Anthrax Pertussis Cholera Bacillary dysentery

Intermediate	Extracellular	Pyogenic infections	Necrosis	Portal of entry + systemic	Infections by
					  Staphylococcus
					  Streptococcus
					  Pneumococcus
					  Neisseria
					  Enteric opportunists
					    etc.
					Glanders
					Melioidosis

Intimate	Intracellular	Systemic infections (often species specific)	Proliferation (including granulomas)	Reticuloendothelial	Typhoid fever Brucellosis Tularemia Plague Tuberculosis
Obligatory	Intranuclear	Viral infections (viral tumors)	Neoplasia	Cell specific	Verrucae Papillomas Animal tumors
	Ultrastructural	None (organelles, e.g., mitochondria?)			Mitochondria?

DISEASES AND LESIONS ASSOCIATED WITH INFECTIONS BY SPECIFIC BACTERIA

In the discussions that follow, results of infections by specific bacteria will be described. Bacteriologic, serologic, epidemiologic, and clinical features will be touched on only briefly and descriptively, since details of these aspects are more appropriate to works devoted to microbiology, immunology, public health, and clinical medicine. In contrast to the familiar presentation of these disorders in systems of classification based on microbiologic or clinical features, this presentation will be, insofar as possible, along lines of similarity of pathogenic mechanism. Where possible, there is developed a system of classification that relates pathogenic mechanism and morphologic response of the host to the level of parasitism established by the infecting microorganisms (Table 7-1)

Exotoxicoses

There are several diseases in which bacterial toxins lead to profound systemic effects. In these diseases minimal parasitic interrelationships or even none at all exist between the causative microorganisms and the host. Most of the microorganisms responsible for diseases of this type are gram-positive cocci, usually spore bearing. Species, organ, and tissue specificities cannot really be described because there is such a minimal parasitic relationship. This is not to say, however, that the respective exotoxins do not have considerable species and organ specificities in their pharmacologic actions.

Botulism

Botulism results from the ingestion of the potent exotoxin produced by *Clostridium botulinum*—a soil anaerobe common throughout the world, particularly in the western United States. Contamination of foodstuffs, especially vegetables, by the organism is therefore relatively common. Spores of *C. botulinum* withstand dry heat as high as 180° C for as long as 15 minutes. If proper precautions are not taken in the preservation of food, conditions favorable to germination, proliferation, and toxin production by the organism may be established. Inadequate heating during processing, in fact, favors the growth of this organism by killing other bacteria that are less heat resistant and that cannot therefore overgrow and inhibit *C. botulinum*. Destruction of other organisms also prevents obvious warning features of spoilage such as bad odor and color. Most cases of botulism in the United States result from the ingestion of home-processed vegetables, especially nonacid ones such as beans or corn. In Europe most cases result from contamination of preserved meat such as ham and sausage (Latin *botu-*

lus, "sausage"). Five to 10 sporadic cases of botulism occur annually in the United States. Cases in young infants have been attributed to germination of spores of *C. botulinum*, with toxin production in the immature intestine. Rarely, systemic botulism follows infections of wounds by *C. botulinum*.

Botulinus toxin is the most potent of all bacterial toxins. Because it resists destruction by proteolytic enzyme, it remains effective when ingested. Six types of botulinus toxin have been identified. Four are responsible for human disease. Type A, the most potent, carries a mortality of approximately 75%, and type B a mortality of approximately 20%. The promptness of onset of the symptoms depends on dose, usually beginning between 12 and 36 hours after ingestion, rarely as little as 3 to 4 hours. Nausea and vomiting, sometimes with a sense of abdominal distress but no real pain, are observed early. Diplopia and difficulty swallowing are usually the first features of the characteristic paralyses produced by the toxin. Paralysis of pharyngeal muscles leads to regurgitation of ingested food and liquids through the nose. This often causes aspiration pneumonia. The patient may be unable to hold the head erect because of involvement of the neck muscles. Death, if it occurs, usually results from respiratory failure. Specific antitoxin is the only therapeutic measure available and is of value only early. The toxin is bound to neural tissues once the disease becomes established and in those sites can no longer be neutralized by specific antitoxin.

Botulinus toxin acts something like curare, affecting principally the end-plates of nerves and specifically the myoneural junctions of the motor apparatus. No morphologic changes occur that are specific for botulism. There may be petechiae and ecchymoses on serous surfaces and in the central nervous system as secondary effects of anoxia. The specific diagnosis depends on the demonstration of an antitoxin-neutralizable paralysis in rodents injected with the suspected food material or even with a sample of the patient's blood.

Staphylococcal food poisoning

Food poisoning that results from the ingestion of a potent exotoxin produced by certain strains of *Micrococcus pyogenes* (*Staphylococcus pyogenes*) is a common public health problem. Since the disease is not reportable, however, its frequency is unknown. In contrast to botulism, symptoms appear rapidly and are of short duration; recovery is usually prompt and complete. Excessive salivation is often the first sign of intoxication, followed shortly by nausea and vomiting, abdominal cramps, and diarrhea. Toxigenic strains of staphylococci produce toxin during their growth phase at temperatures above 40° F. Circumstances favorable for toxin production are most commonly encountered in cream-filled bakery goods or other foodstuffs with an approximately

neutral reaction. Staphylococcal enterotoxin is extremely heat resistant and is also stable during prolonged refrigeration. Clinical and epidemiologic features of staphylococcal food poisoning are sufficiently characteristic to establish the diagnosis in most cases. Formal laboratory confirmation is difficult to achieve. Morphologic changes have not been described.

A prostrating illness with an appreciable mortality has been designated the toxic shock syndrome (TSS). The disorder usually occurs in menstruating women and is characterized by shock, features of disseminated intravascular coagulation, hepatorenal failure, and an erythematous desquamative cutaneous eruption. TSS has been attributed to a staphylococcal toxin A. Almost all patients with it have staphylococci in their vaginal exudates whereas few controls do. A role for occlusive vaginal tampons has been suggested.[20]

Salmonellal food poisoning

Contamination of foods by any of the strains of *Salmonella* produces a self-limited nonspecific gastroenteritis often clinically and epidemiologically confused with staphylococcal food poisoning.

Tetanus

Tetanus (lockjaw) results from the absorption of the potent exotoxin produced by *Clostridium tetani*. This free-living saprophyte, widespread in nature, especially in cultivated soil, is commonly found in the feces of cattle and horses and less commonly of humans. It therefore tends to colonize manured areas of cultivation. Once introduced into an area, spores of *C. tetani* persist almost indefinitely. Tetanus is therefore particularly a hazard in intensively cultivated rural areas.

Tetanus results from the introduction of spores of *C. tetani* into tissue, where anaerobic conditions favorable to germination and toxin production may be present. Puncture wounds as from a nail or splinter are particularly dangerous. Tetanus was once a frequent complication of abortion and was also commonly seen in infants as *tetanus neonatorum*, which resulted from infection of the umbilical stump. Active immunization has contributed to a decline in the occurrence of tetanus, but 150 or so cases are reported annually in the United States.

Tetanus toxin is absorbed from the local site of production and is transmitted into the central nervous system along the axons of neurons. Tetanus toxin is a potent neurostimulatory agent. Clinical features of tetanus may appear several weeks or even months after the responsible injury, and in a considerable number of cases no injury can be demonstrated or recalled. Symptoms begin with headache, followed shortly by difficulty in swallowing and stiffness of the jaw. Muscle stiffness or spasm may initially be confined to the region of the local infection (*local tetanus*). Spasm of the muscles of the trunk may lead to opisthotonos. Contraction of facial muscles produces the characteristic *risus sardonicus*. Consciousness is undisturbed, and perception of pain is undiminished. Death results from inanition or secondary complications such as bronchopneumonia. Specific morphologic changes have not been described. A reliable diagnostic procedure is the demonstration of muscle spasms in guinea pigs injected with wound scrapings suspended in a saline solution. The presence of tetanus bacilli established by culture is not diagnostic, since spores of *C. tetani* frequently contaminate wounds.

Infections of surfaces of the body

A small group of bacterial diseases results from infection of body surfaces by indigenous bacterial flora that may occasionally be introduced into deeper tissues and cause disease. The diseases discussed here result from infection of the surface per se. The systematically heterogeneous organisms responsible for this group of infections have little or no inherent capacity to invade deeper tissues and manifest a degree of parasitism with their human host only slightly more intimate than that manifested by organisms responsible for the exotoxicoses just described. Included in this group of diseases are diphtheria, gas gangrene, pertussis, bacillary dysentery, and Asiatic cholera.

Diphtheria

Diphtheria is amenable to virtually complete eradication by routine immunization with diphtheria toxoid. Even in medically advanced countries, however, diphtheria may occur when immunization procedures break down because of war, complacency, or cultism. An important epidemic occurred in Texas in 1970.[24]

The low-grade endemicity of diphtheria depends on the occurrence of toxigenic *Corynebacterium diphtheriae* in the nasopharynges of a small number (fewer than 1%) of asymptomatic human carriers. Transmission to nonimmune individuals usually occurs by the respiratory route.

In diphtheria, unlike food poisoning or tetanus, a parasitic relationship exists between the causative microorganism, *C. diphtheriae*, and its host. Diphtheria is a composite of a local inflammation and a systemic intoxication. Toxic produced locally by toxigenic strains of *C. diphtheriae* is responsible for an inflammatory reaction on body surfaces at the site of infection (usually the oral pharynx, from which the process often extends to the nose or larynx). Occasionally the tracheal, esophageal, or gastric mucosa is involved as well. Less commonly, but particularly in the tropics, cutaneous trauma or burns may be the site of diphtheria. The umbilical cord (in diphtheria neonatorum), the genital tract, and the conjunctivae are rare sites. Unlike streptococcal tonsillitis, diphtheria is often insidious in onset and may be preced-

ed by 2 or 3 days of listlessness, malaise, and headache before local symptoms occur. Cervical adenopathy seems out of proportion to the pharyngeal lesion. Soon small gray or white patches of exudate appear on the pharyngeal mucosa, usually over the tonsils. These enlarge and coalesce and, with the accumulation of blood, become gray or black. This exudate constitutes the characteristic diphtheritic membrane, which consists of leukocytes and numerous bacteria enmeshed in a dense network of fibrin (Fig. 7-2). The epithelial surface becomes necrotic and densely adherent to the overlying membrane; this adherency explains why raw bleeding points are exposed when the membrane is forcibly removed. If particularly extensive, the local process may produce mechanical respiratory obstruction, stridor, and even asphyxiation.

The local inflammatory process and its mechanical consequences are less important in the evolution of diphtheria than is the profound toxemia that characterizes the infection. Diphtheria toxin, produced by *C. diphtheriae* in response to infection of that organism by a specific bacteriophage, is a potent inhibitor of cellular protein

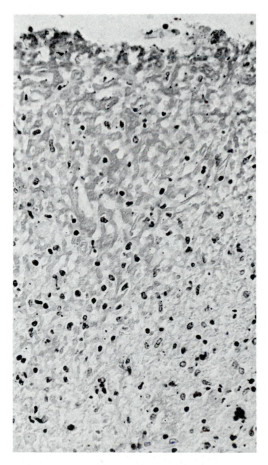

Fig. 7-2. Diphtheria. Membrane that overlies tonsil consists of feltwork of fibrin, necrotic debris, and sparse leukocytes. (From Kissane, J.M.: Pathology of infancy and childhood, ed. 2, St. Louis, 1975, The C.V. Mosby Co.)

synthesis. It is readily absorbed from the point of production into the bloodstream, and its effects are noted in many organs and systems throughout the body. The lymphoid tissues both in regional lymph nodes and systemically (as in the spleen) undergo hyperplasia with the development of prominent germinal centers that are often centrally necrotic.

Diphtheria toxin is particularly toxic to myocardium. In the early stages interstitial edema, cloudy swelling of myocardial fibers, and the accumulation of fine cytoplasmic granules of lipid are seen microscopically. Later these changes become widespread and more severe. Myocardial fibers eventually undergo necrosis, and a focal interstitial myocarditis with exudation of mononuclear cells occurs. Cardiac involvement, either acutely in the form of cardiovascular collapse or as an arrhythmia or more chronically in the form of congestive heart failure, is the most comon threat to life in diphtheria.

A nonspecific, nonsuppurative interstitial nephritis is frequent in diphtheria and is believed to be responsible for the proteinuria often observed. The renal lesion usually resolves completely in patients who recover. The liver is characteristically enlarged; hepatocytes exhibit cloudy swelling and less commonly focal necrosis.

Diphtherial toxin has a special affinity for peripheral nerves. Toxic effects are manifested in degeneration or even destruction of myelin sheaths. Axis cylinders undergo swelling and rarely necrosis. The paralytic effects of diphtheritic neuropathy are often sharply localized. Paralysis of the voluntary muscles of the palate may produce a peculiar nasal quality of the voice and a tendency to regurgitate fluids through the nose. Hypopharyngeal involvement may lead to aspiration pneumonia. Involvement of extraocular muscles may produce diplopia, and involvement of the ciliary body may result in defective visual accommodation. Clinically apparent weakness or paralysis of limbs is rare. Neuropathic manifestations of diphtheria are usually temporary and disappear within 2 or 3 months if the patient survives.

Gas gangrene

Three members of the genus *Clostridium*, *C. welchii* (*perfringens*), *C. novyi* (*oedematiens*), and *C. septicum*, may produce gas gangrene; at least three other members of this genus may contribute to such a process although incapable of producing it themselves. Infections associated with gas gangrene are often mixed and include various anaerobic organisms as well as toxicogenic clostridia. Gas-forming clostridia are strictly anaerobic, gram-positive, sporulating bacilli widely distributed in nature. Gas-forming clostridia may be introduced into wounds as spores that, devoid of toxin, are incapable of producing disease. Conditions that seem to favor germination of spores and subsequent toxin production include exten-

sive necrosis (such as that produced by crushing injuries) or the presence of foreign particulate matter (especially that containing calcium salts or silicic acid).

A curious and interesting disease, known locally as *pig-bel*, occurs in the highlands of central New Guinea. In that locality pig-bel is the most common cause of acute abdominal emergencies. Anatomic lesions include enteritis with deep, often perforating, peculiarly serpiginous ulcers. Epidemiologic studies are ambiguous, but some emphasize the association of pig-bel with ritual feasts on putrid pork carcasses. Gas-forming clostridia have been cited as etiologically important.

The various toxins produced by gas-forming clostridia are locally toxic and perpetuate the local process while being available for absorption and systemic effects as well. Appropriate surgical management, particularly debridement of all devitalized tissue from wounds subject to gas gangrene, and prompt initiation of antibiotic therapy have drastically reduced the incidence and morbidity of this bacterial disease. Hyperbaric oxygen has both advocates and skeptics.[22]

In peacetime, sporadic cases of gas gangrene are occasionally observed, particularly among agricultural workers. Features of gas gangrene usually appear within hours to days after the relevant injury. Tissues about the wound become swollen, edematous, and painful as a result of increased tension. Once established, the process often advances with great rapidity. The injured member becomes tense and crepitant because of the accumulation of gas bubbles within the tissues. A scanty serosanguineous fluid exudes from the wound. Rarely the fluid may be effervescent. Soon the wounded tissue becomes grayish black and extremely foul smelling. This local process, called clostridial cellulitis, may in itself occasionally threaten life. The syndrome, gas gangrene, however, includes the systemic toxic effects of several clostridial toxins and, once it develops, has a significant mortality.

The most conspicuous local effects involve muscle. The muscle fibers undergo coagulative necrosis and occasionally liquefy (Fig. 7-3). Large gram-positive bacilli are present in great numbers. In later cases a zone of intense leukocytic reaction and hyperemia confines the area of infection. In severe cases there is practically no leukocytic response about the region of frank necrosis but a wide zone of edema and congestion. Capillary and venous thrombi are common.

There are at least 12 immunologically distinct toxins produced by gas-forming clostridia. The most important of these are the potent lecithinase (alpha toxin) and another necrotizing toxin (sigma toxin). Potent hemolytic toxins may produce a precipitous drop in the number of circulating erythrocytes. Terminally, bacilli invade the bloodstream and are distributed widely throughout the

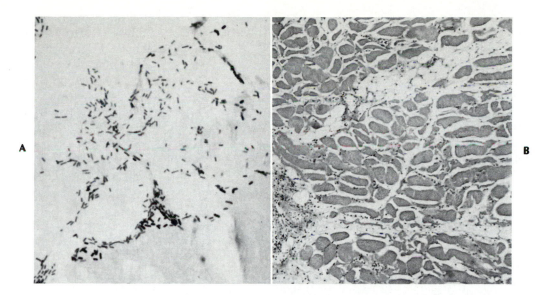

Fig. 7-3. Gas gangrene. **A,** Numerous *Clostridium welchii* and necrosis of muscle fiber. **B,** Large gas-filled spaces and separation of individual muscle fibers from their sarcolemmal sheaths.

body. Pulmonary edema and hyperemia are usually pronounced. If postmortem examination is delayed even a few hours, gas formation occurs in virtually any organ of the body.

Anthrax

The inclusion of anthrax among these diseases resulting from a minimal parasitic relationship between organism and host may seem inappropriate. In fact, anthrax organisms are found in great profusion in tissues of infected animals or humans. They excite almost no inflammatory response, however, and the hemorrhagic edema so characteristic of the lesions is now attributed to a very potent exotoxin.

A disease known since antiquity, anthrax was described in Homer's *Iliad*. It is of great historical interest, for it was the first human disease of proved bacterial origin. Although numerous, large, rod-shaped organisms had been observed in the blood of animals dying of anthrax in 1850, it remained for Robert Koch to prove that these organisms were actually the cause of anthrax. This he did in 1876, at the same time formulating what we now accept as Koch's postulates. In 1881 Pasteur succeeded in attenuating the organism and produced an effective vaccine, the first successful practical application of active immunization in the control of disease.

Bacillus anthracis is a long (4.5 to 10 μm), square-ended, gram-positive rod that often grows in short chains. It is capable of forming very resistant spores, but spore forms do not occur in animals or humans with the disease. A great variety of animals are susceptible to infection, but grazing animals are most commonly affected, especially sheep and cattle. The disease in animals

almost invariably results in septicemia and death. In the so-called apoplectic form, death may occur within an hour or two after symptoms are first noticed. Animals, in contrast to humans, usually become infected by ingesting the spores. These pass unharmed through the stomach and invade the intestinal mucosa. The spore forms are so resistant that pastures once seeded with *B. anthracis* remain a source of infection indefinitely.

The disease is uncommon in the United States, with an average of four or five cases per year having been reported during the past 5 years. However, it is interesting to note that during this period the number of cases of anthrax considerably exceeded that of smallpox. Among humans in the United States, most infections are occupational, appearing in textile workers and stevedores who handle wool, hides, or hair. Agricultural anthrax is very rare in the United States. Human gastrointestinal anthrax, unknown in the United States, occurs when unenlightened or impoverished people eat the carcasses of animals dead of anthrax. Farmers, butchers, and veterinarians are occasionally infected, and a small number of cases have been reported in which the disease followed the use of a shaving brush or hairbrush with contaminated bristles. Infection also occurs from the biting of flies (family Tabanidae).

Most commonly the disease occurs in the form of the malignant pustule (Fig. 7-4), as a result of entry of *B. anthracis* into an abrasion or scratch of the skin. In the majority of instances, the primary infection is of the head or neck. The lesion first appears as a papule, soon surrounded by a zone of edema and hyperemia. Vesiculation occurs, and on rupture of the small blister an eschar forms. Soon there is central necrosis, and a small ragged

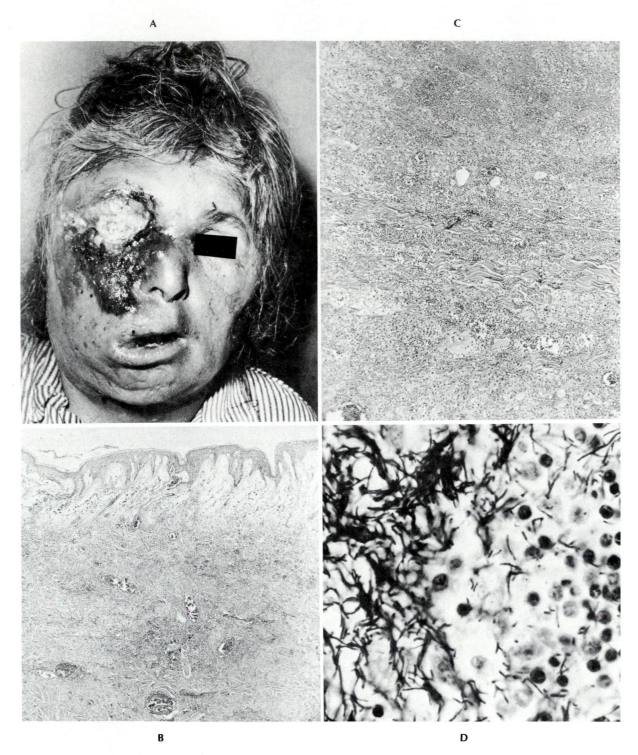

Fig. 7-4. Anthrax. **A,** Severe malignant pustule. **B** and **C,** Histopathologic appearance of skin. **D,** Bacilli. (**B** and **C,** , Hematoxylin and eosin; **B,** 35×; AFIP 66-13163; **C,** 77×; AFIP 66-13164; **D,** Gram stain of tissue section; 800×; AFIP 66-13179; **A** to **D,** from Dutz, W.: Int. Pathol. **8:**38, 1967.)

black ulcer develops. This may be surrounded by minute vesicles or pustules. Sometimes the local lesion involves a large area. The lesion is not particularly painful, although characteristically there is intense itching. Regional lymph nodes are somewhat swollen and tender, but involvement is not comparable to that seen in tularemia or plague. In the majority of instances the disease remains localized, and in a week or two the small ulcer heals. The eschar may separate from the underlying tissue, leaving a suppurating slough. Especially if lymphadenopathy is a prominent feature, forces of localization may be overcome and septicemia may result. This is accompanied by profound systemic manifestations, and death is the usual consequence. Occasionally no ulcer forms at the site of initial infection, but rather an area of malignant edema. This may or may not be associated with acute hyperemia and other signs of acute inflammation. Generalization of the infection (septicemia) is more likely to occur here than in the case of the malignant pustule. Next in frequency is the pneumonic form (woolsorter's disease), which occurs from inhalation of the spores. In this case the malignant pustule forms in a bronchus, and this soon leads to an extensive hemorrhagic consolidation of the involved lobe or lobes. There are striking systemic manifestations, progressive dyspnea, and cough productive of bloody sputum. Before antibiotic therapy was available, septicemia and death occurred in the majority of those affected. Rarely, in humans there is a third form—quite similar to that seen in cattle—the intestinal type. In this infection, also, septicemia and death usually result.

Morphologic changes are characterized principally by a bloody mucinous edema that affects many tissues and is found in most serous cavities. Meningitis may be a prominent feature. The damage wrought by *B. anthracis* in the septicemic form of anthrax is so overwhelming that there is relatively little cellular reaction, principally necrosis with massive bloody edema. In the acute septicemic forms death occurs in over 90% of the patients unless they are treated promptly with specific antiserum or sulfonamides.

Curiously, until recently anthrax—so extensively studied and the first bacterial disease for which an effective vaccine was produced—has resisted analyses to determine its lethal mechanism of action. Of the many toxins elaborated by *B. anthracis*, the "lethal factor" is an exotoxin, its concentration varying with the number of organisms present in the blood. This is an edema-producing toxin, affecting capillary permeability, that is mainly responsible for the secondary shock, which in turn is the usual precipitating cause of death.

In persons with typical skin manifestations, the diagnosis is not difficult. Large numbers of the characteristic organisms can be seen in smears made from the pustule or from sputum in the pulmonic form. The organisms also should be cultured and their virulence ascertained by inoculation into guinea pigs or mice.

Pertussis (whooping cough)

Pertussis is traditionally attributed to superficial infection of the distal airway by *Bordetella pertussis* (formerly *Haemophilus pertussis*). *B. pertussis* is a short, gram-negative bacillus that produces both an endotoxin and an exotoxin. A clinically indistinguishable disorder can be produced by numerous viruses. Some authorities have even challenged any etiologic role of *B. pertussis* in whooping cough. Formerly the most important acute infectious disease of childhood, pertussis has in the last few decades diminished in both frequency and severity. Only 2000 to 3000 cases are reported annually in the United States, with only five deaths in 1973.

Morphologic changes, in the uncomplicated case, are mostly limited to the air passages and lungs (Fig. 7-5). Findings include laryngitis, tracheitis, bronchitis, and bronchiolitis; however, changes are most noticeable in the bronchi. Bacterial stains reveal many of the specific organisms contained within the mucopurulent exudate that overlies the mucosa and is intertwined and tangled with the cilia of the columnar epithelium. Occasionally areas of superficial necrosis and erosion are evident. Hyperemia and excessive production of mucus occur. The smaller bronchi may contain dense plugs of mucus, and these will include a few inflammatory cells and many organisms. Peribronchitis and interstitial pneumonitis, especially around small bronchi, are characteristic findings but are not by any means pathognomonic since they are seen also in other diseases (for instance, atypical pneumonia). Little exudate is to be found in alveoli unless there is secondary bronchopneumonia. Emphysema is almost always evident microscopically. Peribronchial lymph nodes are hyperemic and exhibit moderate hyperplasia.

Diseases caused by vibrios

Members of the genus *Vibrio* are responsible for Asiatic cholera and also for a form of food poisoning relatively prevalent in Japan. One of the great historical pestilences, Asiatic cholera has apparently been perennially endemic in the Indian subcontinent. Escaping from this homeland early in the nineteenth century, cholera has occurred in six pandemics elsewhere in the world—including the classic one in London, traced to the contamination of the Broad Street pump by John Snow. Cholera occurred in eastern Europe until 1923. Epidemics also occurred in the United States during the nineteenth century, but there have been only three rigorously identified cases during the twentieth century, a fatal case in a longshoreman in New Orleans in 1941 and two laboratory infections in 1964.

In India, cholera has traditionally been caused by clas-

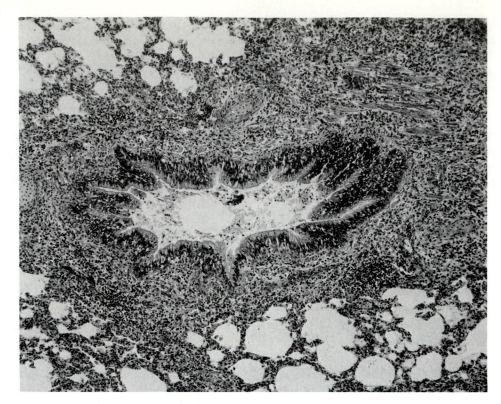

Fig. 7-5. Pertussis. Tenacious exudate clings to side of bronchus. Bronchitis, peribronchitis, and focal areas of emphysema are present. (From Kissane, J.M.: Pathology of infancy and childhood, ed. 2, St. Louis, 1975, The C.V. Mosby Co.)

sic *Vibrio cholerae*. Infection by the El Tor biotype identified in Suez in 1906 was not considered "cholera" until 1961. In 1964 the disease produced by the El Tor organism essentially replaced that attributable to classic *V cholerae* in India, but not in Bangladesh. Since 1968 the El Tor biotype has predominated there as well.

The most recent sizable outbreak of cholera outside India occurred in Italy in 1972. The epidemiology of that contagion has not been firmly established, but contamination of shellfish imported from North Africa has been suggested.

The only significant natural reservoir of cholera appears to be humans, and the only clinically significant portal of entry is the alimentary tract by the fecal-oral route. *V. cholerae* are appreciably sensitive to normal gastric acidity. Oral infection can be produced by 10^8 ingested organisms, but that figure drops to 10^4 if gastric acidity is neutralized. Interestingly, a disproportionate number of patients afflicted in an outbreak in Israel had undergone surgical procedures (vagotomy, pyloroplasty, or gastrectomy), which tend to vitiate the protective effect of gastric acidity.[29]

The incubation period is usually 1 to 5 days, after which a profuse watery diarrhea occurs usually without tenesmus or abdominal distress. Fluid loss can exceed 10 liters per day. Prostration is therefore rapid and profound. The disease is ordinarily self-limited, with death or recovery occurring within a few days. An asymptomatic convalescent carrier state is uncommon but can occur.

Cholera can be reproduced in all essentials by cell-free extracts of cultures of *V. cholerae*. Manifestations of the disease are attributable to a very potent enterotoxin, choleragen, which has been highly purified as a protein with a molecular weight of about 90,000. Choleragen acts on the mucosal cells of isolated loops of rabbit intestine by reversing the normal direction of ion transport, thereby causing fluid to accumulate in the lumen. This action appears to be mediated by adenosine-3,5-cyclic monophosphate (cyclic AMP). Either choleragen or cyclic AMP stimulates secretion of chloride by intestinal mucosal cells and inhibits absorption of sodium. *V. cholerae* ordinarily does not invade beyond the intestinal mucosal surface, although infection of bile and the presence of organisms in the liver at least at autopsy have been reported.

Intestinal biopsies from living patients with severe cholera have shown the mucosa of the intestine to be intact with only slight edema and hypercellularity of the lamina propria. Parenchymatous degeneration of solid viscera, traditionally described among findings at autopsy, appears to be a nonspecific feature of fluid and electrolyte loss.

Noncholera vibrios. The genus *Campylobacter* has recently been designated to include motile gram-negative curved organisms other than *V. cholerae*. There are two biotypes, *C. fetus* (var. *intestinalis*) and *C. fetus* (var. *jejuni*), both pathogenic for humans.

Initially recognized in the tropics, representatives of the genus *Campylobacter* are now known to be distributed throughout the world. Animal reservoirs are suspected, but the mode of transmission to humans has not been established. Human infections by *Campylobacter* are associated with three clinical syndromes: (1) *C. fetus* (usually var. *jejuni*) is responsible for about 6% of cases of infantile enteritis (enterocolitis) in the United States, and as much as 30% in the tropics. Most often self-limited, the disease may be severe and prostrating, even fatal. Morphologically *C. fetus* produces a nonspecific acute enterocolitis, occasionally hemorrhagic or necrotizing. (2) *C. fetus* (especially var. *intestinalis*) is responsible for occasional examples of localized infections in elderly adults debilitated by other diseases. Septicemia, meningoencephalitis, and infectious arthritis have been described. (3) *C. fetus* (especially var. *intestinalis*) causes some perinatal infections, presumably acquired by the infant from an asymptomatic carrier mother.

Diseases caused by shigellae

Members of the genus *Shigella* cause a readily communicable infectious colitis, bacillary dysentery, that has historically afflicted troops in the field, prisoners of war, victims of natural disasters, and those subject to unsanitary overcrowded conditions (as in orphanages or mental hospitals). The disease was distinguished from amebic dysentery in 1896 by Shiga, who recognized the first representative of the genus now known as *Shigella dysenteriae*.

The four species of *Shigella* (*S. dysenteriae*, *S. flexneri*, *S. boydii*, and *S. sonnei*) are nonmotile gram-negative bacilli distinguished from other Enterobacteriaceae by means of biochemical reactions and from each other by their biochemical and antigenic characteristics. All known species are pathogenic for humans.*

The natural disease occurs only in primates, and shigellae are found only in the intestinal tracts of humans, subhuman primates, and rarely dogs.

Early in the twentieth century *S. dysenteriae* was the most common cause of bacillary dysentery. Since then, *S. sonnei* and *S. flexneri* have become more commonly recognized as causes of dysentery. *S. sonnei* now pre-

*Doubtful pathogens formerly designated *S. alkalescens* and *S. dispar* are now classified as *Escherichia coli*.

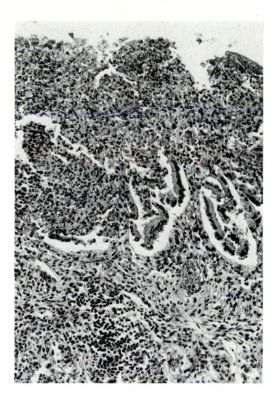

Fig. 7-6. Colon in bacillary dysentery. Acute inflammation of mucosal surface is in response to infection by essentially noninvasive organism *Shigella dysenteriae*.

dominates in medically more advanced countries, and *S. flexneri* in the less advanced. *S. boydii* is rarely isolated. *S. dysenteriae* had nearly disappeared from most parts of the world until the late 1960s, when epidemics caused by this agent appeared in Central America and subsequently spread to Mexico. Since 1968 bacillary dysentery from *S. dysenteriae* has occurred in tourists returning to the United States from Central America and Mexico and in their contacts. The disease has remained a major public health problem in Central America. In the United States, bacillary dysentery develops most often in children younger than 10 years of age, often from socioeconomically deprived segments of the population.

Transmission occurs by the fecal-oral route. Although shigellae compete poorly with other intestinal bacteria both in vitro and in vivo, as few as several hundred bacilli can produce disease in healthy volunteers. Factors responsible for pathogenicity are poorly understood. *S. dysenteriae* produces a heat-labile neurotoxin and an enterotoxin (possibly the same product) that, like the enterotoxins of *E. coli* and *V. cholerae*, induce fluid accumulation in isolated segments of rabbit ileum.

Lesions of the natural disease are confined to the terminal ileum and colon and consist of shallow ulcers, usually transversely arrayed, with serpiginous borders and coated by a delicate filmy membrane of fibrin, polymorphonuclear leukocytes, cell debris, and bacteria (Fig. 7-6). The ulcers probably result from entry of the bacilli into the lamina propria, where release of endotoxin causes death of host cells and an acute inflammatory response. Further invasion is almost unknown. In some patients, almost always those with *S. dysenteriae*, encephalopathic manifestations that are usually transitory develop.

Extracellular infections

Most human bacterial infections are attributable to organisms to which the host response is acute inflammation characterized by the formation of pus. These organisms are therefore appropriately designated *pyogenic bacteria*. The most typical members of this group are gram-positive cocci, although gram-negative cocci of *Neisseria* species and *Haemophilus influenzae* also evoke typically purulent responses. Furthermore, many genera of gram-negative bacilli, particularly those whose normal habitat is the gastrointestinal tract, evoke a purulent response when they gain access to tissues of the host beyond their usual habitat. Morphologic features of lesions produced by pyogenic organisms include predominantly the polymorphonuclear leukocyte plus local necrosis and its consequences. These responses constitute acute inflammations, described elsewhere (p. 41). The degree of parasitism manifested by agents that produce a purulent response is expressed by an almost entirely extracellular habitat, pathogenic aspects of the relationship being largely neutralized when organisms are phagocytosed and come to reside intracellularly. Although there is some variability in the response of different species to infections by members of this group of microorganisms, species specificity is not pronounced. Susceptibility of various organs and tissues within a given species to infection by organisms of this category is not highly specific and is usually related to the portal of entry or point of lodgment. Mechanisms by which these organisms produce lesions, although incompletely understood, seem to be related to the production of cell death—necrosis—both of migratory phagocytic cells of the host and of fixed cellular elements of the host's tissues. In general, the host's immunologic response to infections in this category is humoral. Endogenous humoral antibodies produced during these infections are often important in limiting the course of the disease. Humoral antibodies in the form of antisera have played important roles in therapy directed against certain of these diseases (for example, pneumococcal pneumonia and meningococcal meningitis), although in these roles they have largely been superseded by antibiotics.

Many, perhaps technically all, pyogenic infections represent expressions of virulence by organisms that are at least occasionally avirulent commensals in one or another compartment of the host's environment. This category of infections therefore introduces the concept of *opportunism* (that is, of diseases or lesions resulting when one set of circumstances leads to a given host's being parasitized by microorganisms of a given category).

Infections caused by staphylococci

Bacteria of the genus *Micrococcus (Staphylococcus)* are gram-positive, nonencapsulated, non-spore-forming cocci that grow in grapelike clusters. Natural habitats of staphylococci include the human skin and nasopharynx. Smith[9] has estimated that 80% of people have a staphylococcal infection sometime during their lives and that a staphylococcal lesion develops in 5% in any one year. Staphylococci, especially the *aureus* variety, are the most common cause of purulent infections of the skin and subcutaneous tissues—lesions collectively designated *pyodermas*. These lesions bear such designations as *furuncle, carbuncle, impetigo, acne, paronychia, felon, phlegmon,* and *abscess*. The characteristic feature of dermal infection by staphylococci is necrosis of skin. Recent evidence suggests that this results largely from ischemia, which in turn is a consequence of vasoconstrictive action of a toxin product of the staphylococcus. Other important toxins elaborated by this group of organisms, named according to their activities, include leukocidin, necrotoxin, hyaluronidase, and coagulase. Other features of staphylococci that contribute to virulence are (1) a surface constituent that enables the organism to resist phagocytosis and (2) the ability of certain strains of the organism to survive within leukocytes. Some strains of staphylococci elaborate an enterotoxic exotoxin, clinicopathologic aspects of which are described on p. 281.

Besides its primary, although in the broad sense opportunistic, role as a causative agent in pyodermas, *Staphylococcus*, especially the variant *aureus*, is a major cause of bacterial wound infections. *S. aureus* may complicate or contribute to chronicity of otherwise primary infections such as pneumonia, measles, pertussis, and scarlet fever. The staphylococcus is frequently responsible for otitis media or paranasal sinusitis. From these loci related to the respiratory tract, the staphylococcus may secondarily cause meningitis or brain abscess. The organism may infect serous surfaces, producing purulent peritonitis, pericarditis (Fig. 7-7), or pleuritis (empyema). In infants and young children, primary staphylococcal pneumonia is a characteristic clinicopathologic entity with a relatively high mortality (see p. 848). Staphylococci may lodge in the kidney and cause hematogenous pyelonephritis. Staphylococci are the most common cause of purulent osteomyelitis.

Impetigo contagiosa is an infectious and communicable disease largely restricted to children. Epidemic out-

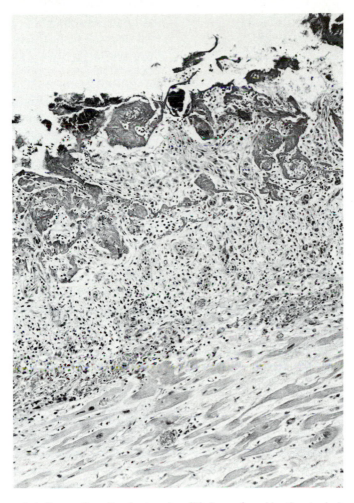

Fig. 7-7. Pyrogenic inflammation. Purulent pericarditis is produced by the staphylococcus *(Micrococcus pyogenes* var. *aureus).*

breaks occur in institutions such as nurseries or orphanages. Traditionally ascribed to infection by staphylococci, impetigo may also result from streptococcal infection of the skin. Impetigo consists of the sequential development of pustules, vesicles, and crusted lesions (Fig. 7-8). Sometimes large confluent bullae occur. In newborn or debilitated infants, impetigo is occasionally fatal. The streptococcal form may be associated with glomerulonephritis.

Infections caused by streptococci

Streptococci are gram-positive organisms that grow in chains. Pathogenic varieties produce either alpha or beta hemolysis when cultured on blood agar. Alpha hemolysis results from incomplete lysis of blood cells in the culture medium and produces a green discoloration around the colony. Organisms that produce alpha hemolysis are customarily designated alpha-hemolytic streptococci (formerly *Streptococcus viridans)*. This organism is a commensal in the mouth but gains clinical significance as the

most common cause of subacute bacterial endocarditis (see p. 800).

Bacteria that produce beta hemolysis (complete hemolysis, with a clear, colorless halo about growing colonies) tend to be more invasive than alpha streptococci. Nonhemolytic (delta) streptococci only exceptionally produce human disease.

In contrast to staphylococcal lesions, wherein thick purulent exudation is characteristic, streptococcal infections usually produce thin watery exudate, a reaction that has been attributed to the fact that streptococci elaborate streptokinase. This is by no means a rule, however. Pronounced diversity of reaction is an outstanding characteristic of streptococcal infection, and streptococci often produce pyogenic reactions. Examples of focal lesions include otitis media, appendicitis, impetigo, wound infections, tonsillitis, and pharyngitis. More generalized diseases are puerperal sepsis, bronchopneumonia, meningitis, erysipelas, scarlet fever, and septicemia. In addition to these, streptococcal infection is undoubt-

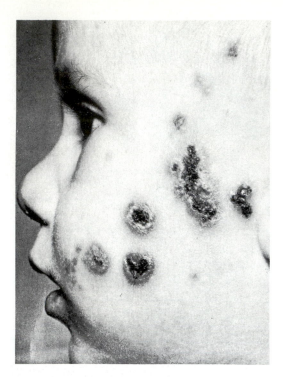

Fig. 7-8. Impetigo. Older lesions are dark and encrusted. (From Wehrle, P.F., and Top, F.H.: Communicable and infectious diseases, ed. 9, St. Louis, 1981, The C.V. Mosby Co.)

edly concerned in (although not the immediate cause of) rheumatic fever and glomerulonephritis. It appears that allergic reaction to the products of bacterial growth and the infectious process are direct causative mechanisms, although much remains to be explained (p. 736). The variation in reaction to streptococcal infection often pertains to the host, and age is an important factor, as has been emphasized by Powers and Boisvert.[54] In adults, streptococcal infections tend to be of a more spreading nature and produce less suppuration.

The high incidence of streptococcal infection is attributable not only to the pathogenicity of the streptococcus but also to its wide distribution in nature. *Streptococcus pyogenes* is found in the throat of 5% to 10% of the healthy adult population. Occurrence of this organism in the nose is a much more serious matter. Nasal carriers scatter large numbers of these organisms in the air and are also much more likely to infect their hands, clothing, and so on than are oral carriers. Alpha-hemolytic streptococci are found almost invariably in the nasopharynx of healthy individuals and are normal inhabitants of the small intestine.

Sore throat. Sore throat, when of infectious etiology, is more properly termed nasopharyngitis. Beta-hemolytic streptococci (*S. pyogenes*) are one of the most frequent causes and certainly the most important. As a rule the infection is superficial and characterized by a swollen, velvety, red pharyngeal mucosa, with swollen tonsils

whose crypts exude purulent exudate. In addition to local pain, swelling, and tenderness, usually a generalized discomfort, headache, and malaise provide clinical evidence of toxemia. The process may extend further. Local extension may produce peritonsillar abscess (quinsy). With suppuration in or around the tonsil, there may be such swelling as to cause pronounced interference with eating and breathing. As a consequence of peritonsillar abscess, there may be wide dissemination of the infection through the soft tissues of the neck, resulting in cellulitis (Ludwig's angina). Before the advent of chemotherapy and antibiotics, such a complication caused death in the majority of patients. Considerable regional extension may come about also as the result of suppuration with cervical lymph nodes, with spread along fascial planes to cause retropharyngeal or lateral pharyngeal abscess. Extension to tissues of other regions may occur as well, and both otitis media and sinusitis are frequent complications of streptococcal pharyngitis. Epidemic forms of streptococcal nasopharyngitis have occurred as a result of the ingestion of milk contaminated with *S. pyogenes*. In such cases the source of infection may be traced either directly or indirectly to humans. In the latter case the cow contracts streptococcal mastitis (group A) as a result of contact with a dairy worker who is infected with, or is a carrier of, this organism. Septicemia is a complication especially feared. Finally, in considering complications of streptococcal nasopharyngitis and tonsillitis, one can hardly overemphasize the relationship these infections bear to rheumatic fever and glomerulonephritis.

Bronchopneumonia. Bronchopneumonia of streptococcal etiology is almost always the result of streptococcal pharyngitis or of infection superimposed on pertussis, measles, influenza, or other viral pneumonitis. As a rule, signs and symptoms of streptococcal pneumonia are severe, and the condition is often complicated by pleural empyema. In the great influenza epidemic that occurred during World War I, most deaths were actually the result of streptococcal pneumonia. In these cases, tracheitis and bronchitis were striking features. The pneumonia was largely interstitial, tending to involve mostly the regions around bronchioles, and this was manifested grossly by small white areas of nodular induration. Aveolar exudate was predominantly serous.

Erysipelas. Erysipelas, a specific form of cellulitis caused by beta-hemolytic streptococci, illustrates the diffusely spreading nature of many streptococcal infections. It usually begins without obvious portal of entry, although occasionally a primary injury or defect can be demonstrated. The lesion is most often self-limited except in the very young or very old. The tissue involved is the subcutaneous, usually of the face but occasionally of the trunk or limbs. There is pronounced interstitial edema of subcutaneous tissues, and this exudate contains fibrin, some extravasated erythrocytes, and moderate

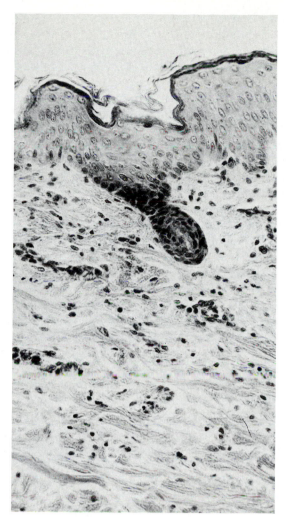

Fig. 7-9. Cellulitis in erysipelas. Cells of inflammation extending through loose, edematous, hyperemic, subcutaneous tissue.

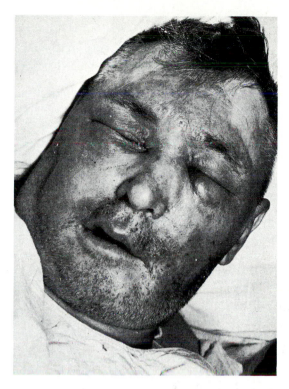

Fig. 7-10. Facial erysipelas Note sharp demarcation of discolored edematous area. (From Wehrle, P.F., and Top, F.H.: Communicable and infectious diseases, ed. 9, St. Louis, 1981, The C.V. Mosby Co.)

numbers of inflammatory cells, mostly monocytes and lymphocytes (Fig. 7-9). Streptococcal organisms are present in great quantities in this fluid, especially in the zone of subepidermal tissue just ahead of the spreading lesion. Despite this, there is little evidence of necrosis. Suppuration does not occur except as a complication. The noticeable reddish discoloration that characterizes the lesion, and from which the name erysipelas ("red skin") is derived, is an effect of great congestion. Direct injury to blood vessels is evident also in the hemorrhage that occurs through diapedesis. It is by this means that erythrocytes are contributed to the exudate and that blood pigment accumulates within macrophages. Usually within a week or 10 days there is spontaneous remission, and shortly thereafter complete healing occurs. Clinically, although the sharply circumscribed brawny edematous area discolored a fiery red (Fig. 7-10) is dramatic, the outstanding feature is profound toxemia.

Scarlet fever (scarlatina). The precise etiology and pathogenesis of scarlet fever were not evident until the Dicks demonstrated in 1924 that an erythrogenic toxin obtained from broth filtrate of certain beta-hemolytic streptococci would, on injection into a susceptible individual, produce a typical erythematous reaction. As a result of widespread application of the Dick test, it became apparent that only a minority of adults were susceptible to scarlet fever and that the number who were "immune" was far greater than the number who had actually had the disease previously. Thus some of the difficulties in earlier experiments were explained. It appears that repeated experiences with S. pyogenes may confer immunity to scarlet fever even though the individual has not been exposed to the disease per se. Further evidence of the significance of erythrogenic toxin in the production of scarlet fever is furnished by the Schultz-Charlton phenomenon, and this is used also as a diagnostic test. When a patient with scarlet fever is given an intradermal injection of a small amount of specific antiserum (convalescent serum), blanching of the characteristic erythematous rash soon occurs in the immediate area of the injection. Since the specific effect of such an injection is neutralization of the streptococcic toxin, it follows that the generalized skin reaction must be an effect of toxemia. The importance of individual variation in the host is illustrated by the fact that streptococcal pharyngitis may develop from the same strain of organism in several or all members of a family, yet scarlet fever may develop in only one of the group, the others manifesting only nasopharyngitis. It is apparent from this that scarlet fever may be contracted from an individual who has only streptococcal pharyngitis.

In the early stages there are rather severe pharyngitis and tonsillitis. These, combined with fever, vomiting, and headache, make up the cardinal prodromal symptoms of scarlet fever. Because there is no specific strain of beta-hemolytic streptococci responsible for scarlet fever, bacteriologic studies do not provide a means for early diagnosis; in other words, a diagnosis of throat infection caused by *S. pyogenes* is not a diagnosis of scarlet fever. The diagnosis cannot be positively made until the second stage of the disease, which is reached 1 to 5 days after the onset. This is characterized by erythematous rash, and it is this skin reaction, more than any other feature, that defines scarlet fever as a distinct disease entity. The hyperemia and resultant red coloration of skin are manifestations of toxic injury (atony and dilatation) of vascular endothelium. This hyperemia blanches on pressure and disappears on death; thus little of the characteristic skin reaction is evident at autopsy. The skin is edematous, and particularly around hair follicles there are focal aggregations of lymphocytes and monocytes. In the middle layers of the epidermis an inflammatory exudate accumulates, and there is an accelerated keratinization at this level—pseudokeratosis. It is because of this that desquamation occurs sometime between the fifth and twenty-fifth days. The outer layers of skin separate from the intermediate zone, which has become keratinized. The tongue usually participates in this reaction too. During the first few days, it presents a "strawberry" appearance because of the erythematous papillae that project from a gray-coated background. When peeling occurs, the tongue becomes beefy red and glistening. Complications are divisible into three major categories:

1. The results of bacterial dissemination locally—otitis media, sinusitis, cervical adenitis, acute suppurative mastoiditis, and retropharyngeal abscess
2. The result of bacterial dissemination generally—metastatic foci of infection throughout the body, or frank septicemia
3. The manifestation of extraordinary reactions to toxins (this may be brought about by hypersensitivity)—interstitial nephritis or myocarditis, pericarditis, nonsuppurative arthritis, and glomerulonephritis

Puerperal sepsis. In the days before antiseptic surgery, puerperal sepsis was an important cause of death. In the maternity hospitals of that day, as many as one woman out of six died of septicemia. The very efforts that were exerted to determine the cause of this dread "childbed fever" served only to spread the disease, since the careful dissection and study of the dead women by their

accoucheurs made gross contamination a certainty and increased the likelihood that the next patient would also be infected. Semmelweis, through his painstaking studies, and Oliver Wendell Holmes, by his brilliant writings, convinced the physicians and midwives of that day that childbed fever was the result of infection and that the etiologic agent was introduced by "unclean hands." Today, many of the cases of puerperal sepsis occur after criminal abortions performed by unskilled and unclean persons.

The inevitable trauma incident to separation of the placenta from its site of implantation and to passage of the fetus through the cervical os and birth canal provides an opportunity for bacterial invasion comparable to that offered by an open wound. *S. pyogenes* is the organism responsible for most cases of puerperal sepsis. Since "natural" incidence of *S. pyogenes* in the vaginal flora is very low during and immediately after the puerperium, it follows that infection is usually of extrinsic origin. Colebrook and Hare [44] reviewed 63 cases of puerperal sepsis of which approximately one third were shown to be the result of infection by *S. pyogenes* antigenically identical to that obtained from the patient's throat or nose. In slightly over half the cases, hemolytic streptococci of identical strain were isolated from the nose or throat of the physician in attendance or from other persons who had been in close contact with the patient. Anaerobic streptococci are frequently responsible for puerperal sepsis. *Clostridium welchii*, especially after abortion, is an occasional cause.

Clinical signs of puerperal endometritis usually appear 3 or 4 days after labor but may be delayed for as long as 2 or 3 weeks. Symptoms are predominantly those of septicemia and include a septic type of fever, often with chills. Infection of the uterus as such does not ordinarily cause much discomfort, although this organ may be somewhat enlarged and tender to palpation. The vaginal discharge (lochia) may be either scanty or abundant but usually has a foul odor. Within the uterus, the inflammatory process is rather superficial and tends to be unimpressive. Thrombophlebitis is the really significant local change, since this is the means by which wide dissemination of the infection is accomplished. Uterine, pelvic, and ovarian veins may all be involved. Septic thrombosis of the femoral vein also may occur. A second route by which infection often spreads is the lymphatic channels, extending along the broad ligaments and other attachments to the celiac lymphatic cistern and then to the thoracic duct and subclavian vein. Peritonitis is a frequent accompaniment of septic endometritis.

Endocarditis. Acute endocarditis, as a complication of septicemia, has been mentioned previously. Often this is caused by *S. pyogenes*, but it also commonly results from pneumococci, staphylococci, gonococci, and influenzal bacilli. Any organism that can cause septicemia may produce acute bacterial endocarditis. Subacute bacterial endocarditis (endocarditis lenta) is much more important, since the endocarditis in this instance represents the primary lesion and is a cause of bloodstream infection rather than a result. *Streptococcus viridans* is the organism responsible in approximately 95% of the cases and *Haemophilus influenzae* in approximately 3%. Infection of the heart valves results from bacteremia. Usually the cause of this bacteremia is not apparent. Often, however, it is a direct result of tooth extraction. Normal heart valves are practically never subject to the type of "chronic" infection (extending over months) that characterizes subacute bacterial endocarditis. Previous injury by rheumatic fever is by far the most common predisposing cause, although such congenital anomalies as bicuspid aortic valve, septal defects, and patent ductus arteriosus are also predisposing factors.

Infections caused by pneumococci

Diplococcus pneumoniae is responsible for most cases of lobar pneumonia (Fig. 7-11) and many cases of bronchopneumonia. Since the portal of entry for pneumococci is the respiratory tract, it is understandable that they are often responsible for otitis media and paranasal sinusitis. Brain abscess may follow septic thrombosis of venous sinuses of the brain. The pneumococcus is an important cause of meningitis in both adults and children. In adults about half the cases occur without clinical evidence of a primary focus. In children, meningeal involvement is usually the result of an upper respiratory infection or otitis media. Pneumococcal meningitis is occasionally seen without antecedent pneumococcal infection, although most often it is caused by an upper respiratory process. Its manifestations are similar to those of other pyogenic meningitides. Suppurative arthritis, acute bacterial endocarditis, and peritonitis are complications of bacteremia or septicemia.

Pneumococci have an antiphagocytic factor in their capsule, and they elaborate a hemolytic toxin, pneumolysin. However, neither of these, nor any other toxin that they produce, is known to be related to the virulence. Thus, the pathogenesis of pneumococcal infection is not understood.

D. pneumoniae resembles alpha-hemolytic streptococci in many morphologic characteristics. However, its bile solubility and special antigenic properties serve to differentiate this oval- or lance-shaped encapsulated gram-positive coccus. The organism usually occurs in diploform but may exist in short chains. Serologic studies have been concerned mostly with pneumococci isolated from patients with lobar pneumonia. Systematic studies have led to the establishment of specific types 1, 2, and 3, leaving a large residual group of unclassified types (group IV). Extension of these observations has separated from group IV 80 additional types. Approximately half of human infections result from types 1 through 8. There is an important practical aspect of this work, since these serologic differences—the result of specific capsular polysaccharides—determine antigenic behavior and are responsible for the fact that antibodies produced against one type are effective only for that type. Before chemotherapy and antibiotics proved so effective, serum therapy was extensively used in the treatment of pneumococcal pneumonia, and it was essential that the type of

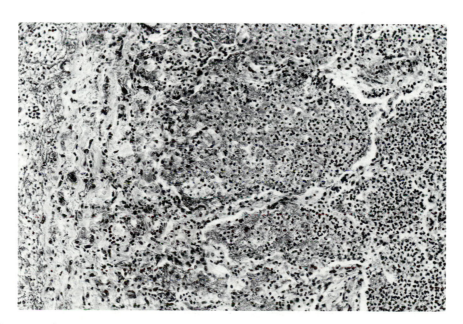

Fig. 7-11. Lobar pneumonia *(right)* and fibrinopurulent pleurisy *(left)*. Purulent inflammation is in response to infection by pneumococcus.

organism be known so that type-specific antiserum could be given promptly. The determination of type is easily accomplished by mixing the organism (from sputum or the peritoneal exudate of an infected mouse) with type-specific antiserum. When the type of organism and antiserum correspond, pronounced swelling ("quellung") of the capsule becomes readily apparent (Neufeld reaction). Before World War I, lobar pneumonia was believed to be primarily of endogenous origin, since it could be demonstrated that many apparently healthy individuals carried pneumococci in the throat. It was observed, however, that frequently when lobar pneumonia developed among a large group of men closely associated, as in a barracks, the majority of cases were caused by organisms of the same serologic type and that this type was foreign to the person infected. Nearly all persons harbor pneumococci in their nasopharynx, although, from a single bacteriologic examination, the incidence would appear to be only 40% to 50%. As many as seven different types have been reported in a single carrier at one time. It is these same types that are frequently responsible for postoperative or postinfectious pneumococcal pneumonia, the result of lowered resistance. This form of infection usually results in bronchopneumonia.

The investigations of Hamburger and Robertson[52] leave little doubt that lobar pneumonia results from bacterial entry and invasion by the bronchial route and that the infection spreads through the respiratory passageways rather than by hematogenous or lymphogenous means. The presence of mucin has been shown experimentally to promote invasion of the pneumococcus as well as certain other organisms. This has been variously explained to have an inhibitory effect on phagocytosis or intracellular digestion and to interfere with bactericidal properties of the blood. Thus aspiration of pneumococcal organisms incorporated within mucus would favor development of the disease, which explains in part why lobar pneumonia frequently follows a cold. For a detailed discussion of this disease, see p. 845.

Infections caused by meningococci

Neisseria meningitidis, a small, oval- or bean-shaped, gram-negative coccus, usually occurs in pairs and occasionally in tetrads. It closely resembles the gonococcus morphologically. A capsule may be demonstrated but is not usually apparent. As in the case of pneumococcus, types based on antigenic differences are of practical importance, since immunity is largely type specific. Four serologic types have been described. The phenomenon of capsular swelling (quellung reaction) occurs when the organisms are mixed with type-specific serum, and it is similar to that described for pneumococci. This reaction is often helpful in immediate diagnosis (for example, in specimens of spinal fluid) in that it allows sharp differentiation from the morphologically similar pneumococcus and *H. influenzae*.

In addition to an antiphagocytic factor contained in the capsule, meningococci produce considerable endotoxin, and this is probably most important in the pathogenesis of meningococcal disease. The two major diseases resulting from meningococcal infection are meningitis and a fulminating form of septicemia.

Meningococcal meningitis. Meningococcal meningitis (cerebrospinal fever, epidemic cerebrospinal meningitis, spotted fever) may be sporadic, endemic, or epidemic. It affects children and young adults most often. The source of infection is usually a healthy carrier or a person recently recovered from the disease. Ordinarily the population at large will include 2% to 5% of healthy individuals who harbor meningococci in the nasopharynx. When this figure approaches 20%, there is danger of an epidemic. During the height of an epidemic the carrier rate may reach 70%. Obviously the virulence of the prevailing strain of organisms will be of at least equal importance to the number of carriers. The disease is not highly contagious, and the infection rate rarely exceeds 1 in 1000, even during epidemics. Under conditions of crowding and poor sanitation, however, as occurred in some army camps during World War I, the attack rate may be as high as 1 in 20.

Meningococcal meningitis is conveniently considered under three stages. *Stage 1* consists of a local infection in the area of the portal of entry—the nasopharynx. This initial reaction is rarely given significance by the patient and may escape notice. *Stage 2* is characterized by septicemia (in approximately 25%, organisms are readily demonstrable in venous blood), and symptoms do not point toward any specific organ. There is fever, often associated with slight chills. The patient complains of generalized aching and prefers to lie still and quiet. The most striking feature is the rash, which has led to the term *spotted fever*. These "spots" begin as small areas of erythema. Soon, however, hemorrhage is evident as a result of thrombosis of arterioles and capillaries. Most of these are petechial in form (less than 2 mm), but there may be confluent areas as large as 1 cm in diameter. Fulminant forms often present massive purpuric hemorrhages, and the regions so involved may become gangrenous. At this time, should a spinal puncture be made, the fluid would appear essentially normal.

Stage 3 is the period of metastatic localization, principally to the cerebral meninges. Intense headache, vomiting, and prostration are followed by drowsiness or irritability and later by delirium or stupor, which may progress to coma. There are stiffness of the neck and, especially in children, a rigid posterior curvature of the back (opisthotonos). Another manifestation of muscle spasm prevents extension of the knee when the thigh is flexed to a right angle with the body—Kernig's sign. At this time examination of the spinal fluid is diagnostic. There is increased pressure, often over 300 mm H_2O, and the fluid is cloudy or turbid because of its high content of leukocytes, mostly neutrophils. Glucose is usually greatly reduced or absent altogether. Smears of this fluid (sediment obtained by centrifugation) frequently reveal the characteristic diplococci. The ratio between intracellular and extracellular organisms is of prognostic value. Sometimes the fluid must be cultured so the meningococci can be detected. Within the brain the first changes occur in the blood vessels of the leptomeninx (pia and arachnoid): hyperemia, slight serous exudation, and minute areas of hemorrhage. These progress, and soon cellular exudate becomes apparent. The pathologic picture varies depending on the duration and severity of the disease. In an advanced stage thick purulent exudate is present, most prominently over the base of brain, filling in around vessels and sulci and often obscuring cranial nerves. The vessels of the pia are engorged. The ventricles contain no great excess of fluid, but the fluid is turbid and filled with pus cells. Careful microscopic examination usually demonstrates the considerable efficiency of the pia as a mechanical barrier in preventing the spread of organisms into the brain substance. Degenerative changes are present in the superficial layers, however, as a result of the diffusion of toxins. The inflammatory exudate is composed principally of polymorphonuclear leukocytes enmeshed in numerous strands of fibrin (Fig. 7-12). Exudate is densest around blood vessels and may follow the vessels for some distance within the substance of the brain. These morphologic changes are similar to those occurring in most types of purulent meningitis.

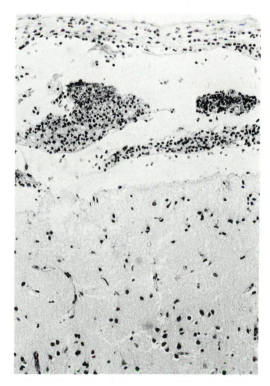

Fig. 7-12. Acute purulent meningitis caused by *Neisseria meningitidis.*

There is often focal encephalitis, evident as minute aggregations of leukocytes and, perhaps, tiny hemorrhages. In patients who die within the first few days, cerebrospinal fluid is increased in amount but there is no evidence of hydrocephalus. In chronic forms internal hydrocephalus is often striking. Before specific therapy was developed, the mortality averaged 60% to 70%. Today the expected mortality is 5% to 10%.

Meningitis may be complicated by blindness or deafness from direct involvement of cranial nerves. Strabismus and facial weakness or spasm may occur after injury to cranial nerves III and VII. Otitis media is common. Other organs are not immune to metastatic infection. Endocarditis and, occasionally, purulent monarthritis occur. The latter is to be differentiated from the transient polyarthritis that frequently occurs, probably as an effect of hemorrhage within the joint. Pneumonia often complicates severe forms of the disease. When this occurs, there may be meningococcal infection of pulmonic tissues. However, the infection is usually of mixed type, and bacteria such as staphylococci and streptococci exert the major effect.

Rarely, there occurs a chronic meningococcemia that may persist as long as several months, often resolving spontaneously.

Fulminant meningococcemia. In fulminant meningococcemia the onset of symptoms is precipitous and the disease runs a violent and rapid course. Moritz and Zamcheck,[53] in their comprehensive study, found that meningococcemia was responsible for 110 of approximately 750 sudden and unexpected deaths in young soldiers. This figure represented roughly one third of the total reported deaths (army) from meningococcal infection. More than half the patients died within 6 hours after coming under medical observation. In all instances death occurred within 24 hours after onset of incapacitating symptoms, although approximately 70% of the patients had had prodromal signs in the form of a mild upper respiratory infection or subnormal feeling. Clinically the predominant manifestation was peripheral vascular collapse and shock; cyanosis was often a prominent feature, and cutaneous hemorrhages were observed in the majority (Fig. 7-13). This picture is essentially similar to that seen in infants and children. Clinical evidence of meningitis is not common because the rapid course of the disease usually leads to death before opportunity for noticeable involvement. Even though meningeal involvement does occur, symptoms are frequently masked by the shocklike state of collapse. The term *Waterhouse-Friderichsen syndrome* is applied to this condition when, in addition to cutaneous hemorrhages, there is hemorrhage (usually massive and bilateral) into the adrenal glands. Some authorities have considered the state of collapse, which is so prominent in this condition, to be a manifestation of acute adrenocortical deficiency. However, complete cessation of adrenocortical function does

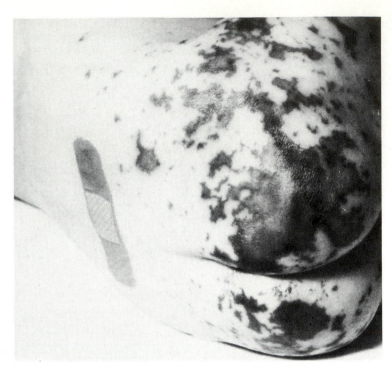

Fig. 7-13. Purpura in fulminating meningococcemia.

not produce peripheral vascular collapse within so short a time. The action of bacterial toxins seems sufficient to explain the clinical picture in the majority of cases.

A presumptive diagnosis of meningococcemia should be made in any fulminating septic state, especially when accompanied by purpuric hemorrhages, so that decisive treatment can be instituted at once. The time required to secure positive blood cultures is not compatible with prompt action. Repeated examinations of blood smears may disclose meningococci. A more reliable method is to examine smears obtained from areas of petechial or purpuric hemorrhage.

Infections caused by gonococci

Neisseria gonorrhoeae is the other important member of the group *Neisseria* and was the first to be described. Its detection by Neisser, in 1879, in inflammatory exudate from gonorrheal lesions settled the long controversy as to the true nature of this disease. The organism is very similar to the meningococcus. It is gram negative and most often occurs in diploform. There has been some question as to the character of toxins produced by this organism, but toxic action in experimental animals seems largely, if not entirely, a result of endotoxins, as is also the case with the meningococcus. Studies of serologic types have yielded very irregular results. Since the organism is fastidious in its growth requirements and dies quickly under unfavorable conditions, infection is almost always the result of direct personal contact. The gonococcus is quite restricted in its portal of entry. In human experiments, large quantities of virulent organisms have been injected subcutaneously without resultant disease.

Differences in colonial morphology correlate with pathogenicity in human volunteers, chimpanzees, or chick embryos. Organisms from colonies of types 1 and 2 retain virulence and are piliated; that is, they possess slender elongated filaments arising from their surface.[38] A possible antiphagocytic role has been attributed to the pili. The gonococcus elaborates a factor that damages ciliated epithelium of cultured human fallopian tubes.[41] Both gonococci and meningococci produce a soluble protease that cleaves the heavy chain of IgA1, with loss of its antimicrobial activity. It is reasonable to suppose that this property correlates with the surface pathogenicity of *Neisseria*.

The only natural host of *N. gonorrhoeae* is humans, and the usual mode of transmission is sexual contact. Gonorrhea is the most common venereal disease. Approximately 1 million cases are reported in the United States annually, but because of underreporting and asymptomatic infections the annual occurrence of new cases may be nearer 3 million. The highest frequency is in men and women between 20 and 24 years of age, and the second highest is in the age group 15 to 19 years. Homosexuality and juvenile sexuality have recently become more important than prostitution in perpetuating gonorrhea in medically advanced societies.

The incubation period of genital gonorrhea is between 2 and 7 days depending, at least in part, on the number of infecting organisms. Gonorrhea is an acute purulent inflammation largely confined to mucus-secreting surfaces. Deep or systemic pyogenic infections are likewise pathologically nonspecific.

In males the earliest manifestation is an acute urethritis manifested by dysuria, frequency, and a purulent urethral discharge. Seminal vesiculitis and acute prostatitis are now uncommon. In untreated cases an acute epididymitis, usually exquisitely painful, may occur. Late complications in males include periurethritis with urethral strictures, prostatic abscesses, and chronic epididymitis. Sterility may result.

In females the most common site of infection is the cervix. Urethritis and infection of accessory glands (Bartholin's and Skene's) may occur. At least half the infected women are asymptomatic. Gonococcal endometritis is virtually unknown, but infection of the mucosal surface of the uterine tubes is common. In many cases, fimbriae coalesce and purulent inflammation of the obstructed tube (pyosalpinx) results. In others, adherence of fimbriae to the ovary is followed by the development of an inflammatory mass (tubo-ovarian abscess). This constellation of clinicopathologic syndromes, of which gonorrhea is the major etiologic factor, is clinically designated *pelvic inflammatory disease* (PID).

Although usually confined to mucus-secreting surfaces, infection by gonococci may rarely spread as disseminated gonococcal infection (DGI) to joints, the endocardium, or the meninges. The gonococcus is the most common agent identified in acute monarticular purulent arthritis. A variety of cutaneous and renal lesions, some of them probably immunologically mediated, have been described.

Acute pelvic peritonitis may occur from leakage of exudate from tubal orifices. Rarely a general peritonitis or perihepatic peritoneal inflammation is seen.

Gonococcal infection of the rectum occurs in women and homosexual men by penoanal intercourse with an infected partner and by secondary spread from the endocervix in women. Stratified squamous anal epithelium is resistant to infection, but the columnar rectal mucosa is susceptible. Most cases of rectal gonorrhea are asymptomatic with minimal or nonspecific histologic features, but an acute mucopurulent or hemorrhagic proctitis may occur.

Gonococcal pharyngitis occurs in women and homosexual men who practice fellatio. Most cases are asymptomatic, but histologically nonspecific pharyngitis, tonsillitis, and gingivitis have been described.

Gonococcal infection of the conjunctiva and an acute purulent conjunctivitis may occur in newborn infants during passage through the infected birth canal. Historically an important cause of blindness, gonococcal conjunctivitis has been largely prevented by such procedures as routine conjunctival instillation of silver nitrate solution at delivery.

Acute purulent gonococcal vulvovaginitis occurs in young girls in whom nonkeratinized epithelium of the reproductive tract is susceptible to invasion of gonococci. Although fomites such as contaminated underclothes or bed linens may occasionally be implicated, most cases result from sexual contact with adults.

Infections caused by Haemophilus

Haemophilus influenzae (Pfeiffer's bacillus), a minute gram-negative rod so short as to be almost coccal, often occurs in chains. It frequently exhibits pleomorphism, and pathogenic strains are almost always encapsulated. It is indistinguishable morphologically from *Bordetella pertussis*. The species name, *influenzae*, was suggested by Pfeiffer in 1892 as a result of observations that led him to conclude, erroneously, that this was the causative organism of influenza. It is now established that influenza is caused by a virus and that the frequent association of *H. influenzae* with this disease is evidence of secondary infection. The genus name, *Haemophilus*, refers to the hemophilic nature of this group of organisms. Blood is a necessary part of their nutriment because it furnishes a coenzyme and also an iron-containing pigment from which the organism may synthesize cytochrome and related compounds.

H. influenzae normally inhabits the nasopharynx and tonsillar region of approximately 50% of individuals, and infections with this organism are usually secondary to some other disease. After a "cold" or other upper respiratory infection it commonly produces sinusitis or otitis media. *H. influenzae*, although a frequent cause of primary pneumonia in children, rarely causes pneumonia in adults except as a complication of influenza or primary atypical pneumonia. Pneumonia produced by the influenzal bacillus is characterized by bronchitis, bronchiolitis, and patchy bronchopneumonia. Purulent exudate may fill the bronchioles and lead to bronchiectasis. This picture contrasts sharply with that of interstitial pneumonia caused by *S. pyogenes*, which may also complicate influenza (see p. 347). In infants and young children, *H. influenzae* infection of the respiratory passages may cause pronounced edema, obstructive laryngitis or acute epiglottitis, and death within a few hours.

No exotoxin has been recovered from *H. influenzae*, and it appears that the serious effects of infection result from endotoxins. Most pathogenic strains have a capsule, and this is believed to offer protection against phagocytosis by leukocytes.

H. influenzae is responsible for approximately 3% of cases of subacute bacterial endocarditis. After bacteremia it may on occasion produce a variety of pyogenic infections (such as cholecystitis, pyelitis, arthritis, or osteomyelitis). Especially in children, this organism causes a particularly destructive meningitis.

One of the most common causes of acute infectious conjunctivitis is the so-called Koch-Weeks bacillus (*Haemophilus aegyptius*), an organism closely related to or identical with *H. influenzae*.

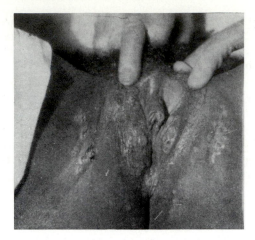

Fig. 7-14. Multiple chancroidal ulcers on vulva, perineum, and thighs.

A more recently recognized variety of *Haemophilus* has been termed *Haemophilus vaginalis* because of its frequent occurrence in the vagina and its production of what was formerly considered nonspecific vaginitis.

Chancroid is an infection by *Haemophilus ducreyi*. Now uncommon in medically advanced countries, it occurs in socioeconomically deprived societies in emerging cultures. The disease is almost always venereally transmitted.

Chancroid begins as a nonspecific papule in the genitourethral epithelium of either sex and progresses to ulceration and purulent inflammation on the penile corona of males or the genital vestibule of females. It then progresses to a purulent destructive lesion in the inguinal region. Ragged, often excavated, local genital ulcers occur (Fig. 7-14). Spontaneous resolution is accompanied by considerable fibroblastic distortion. During the evolution of the genital lesions, reactive hyperplasia of inguinal lymph nodes results in the production of buboes, which with purulent necrosis and the formation of abscesses become painful. Many inguinal swellings in chancroid are actually subcutaneous areas of inflammation (pseudobuboes) independent of regional lymph nodes.

Microscopically the genital lesions of chancroid present three zones: (1) a zone of ulceration and acute inflammation consisting of fibrin, pyknotic nuclear fragments, erythrocytes, and polymorphonuclear cells, (2) a deeper and peripherally spreading zone of actively inflamed granulation tissue, and (3) a zone of perivascular lymphocytic and plasmacytic infiltration. Tissue is rarely made available for microscopic examination but is occasionally examined when the clinical question of malignancy is raised.

Infections caused by Proteus

Highly pleomorphic gram-negative bacilli that are actively motile, *Proteus* organisms are widely dispersed in nature, especially in relation to decaying meat and manure. They are commonly found in the feces of humans but in small numbers as a rule.

As far as disease production is concerned, there are two main species: *P. vulgaris* and *P. morganii*. These organisms are principally saprophytes. However, *P. vulgaris* often produces cystitis. Frequently it can be recovered from the urine in pure culture. Because this organism produces ammonia from urea, infection is characterized by very alkaline urine. This may precipitate calcium, magnesium, and ammonium salts from the urine, resulting in alkaline-encrusted cystitis. Otitis media is occasionally produced by *P. vulgaris* and is characterized by rather widespread necrosis of both osseous and soft tissues. *Proteus* organisms can be recovered in approximately 10% of cases of appendicitis. These organisms often occur in abscesses, infected wounds, and burns as one component of a mixed infection, and their effects are obscured by the other, more predominant organisms. This fact is of considerable significance in these days of antibiotic therapy, since *Proteus* organisms are resistant to most antibiotics and what was originally a mixed infection may, by antibiotic therapy, be converted into a pure *Proteus* infection.

P. morganii was originally isolated from the stools of infants with summer diarrhea and ever since that time (1906) has been considered one of the etiologic agents of summer diarrhea. Many careful studies would indicate that there is no single specific bacterial etiology for this clinical entity.

Infections caused by Pseudomonas aeruginosa

Pseudomonas aeruginosa is a slender, gram-negative rod that varies considerably in length. It is a common cause of wound infection, and the nature of the infection is often recognized clinically by the greenish blue color imparted to the purulent exudate. It was formerly called *Bacillus pyocyaneus* because of this property. Particularly in the case of burns, infection with *P. aeruginosa* is often associated with delayed wound healing. Cruickshank and Lowbury[45] have shown that pyocanin, the principal blue-green pigment elaborated by *P. aeruginosa*, has a relatively high toxicity for human skin and human leukocytes in vitro. The level of concentration of this material, as measured in a series of infected human burns, was sufficient to account for such toxic effects. Infections of the nasal fossae, middle ear, and external ear are occasionally produced by this organism, especially in children. These tissues may undergo extensive necrosis, leading to meningitis. Especially in infants and small children, a serious form of pneumonia may be produced. Infection of the skin can lead to patchy areas of necrosis and ulceration sometimes referred to as *ecthyma gangrenosum* (Fig. 7-13). The organism is occasionally responsible for pyelonephritis and also infection of the eye and of joints.

As with *Proteus* infections, the frequency and importance of *P. aeruginosa* in mixed infections have been more fully appreciated since antibiotics have become widely used. Frequently the presence of *P. aeruginosa*, masked by other, antibiotic-sensitive organisms, is apparent only when these other organisms are destroyed. Particularly in debilitated persons (treated with antibiotics), *P. aeruginosa* is becoming a common cause of septicemia and death. In these cases there are many foci of necrosis, resembling the Shwartzman phenomenon, with exudation being minimal. Walls of small arteries and veins are necrotic and thrombosed, and large numbers of organisms are evident within the vessels. In one series of 23 cases reported by Forkner and associates,[49] abnormal neurologic manifestations occurred in more than half. In all, peripheral vascular collapse occurred as a terminal event.

As in the case of *Proteus* organisms, *P. aeruginosa* has been recovered frequently from the stools of those with summer diarrhea and is considered to be one of the etiologic agents of this disease.

Pseudomonas pseudomallei infection (that is, melioidosis) is discussed on p. 312.

Infections caused by Legionella

Legionella pneumophila is a fastidious gram-negative bacillus demonstrated with difficulty in diseased tissue. The organism causes Legionnaires' disease (a sporadic pneumonic infection with an appreciable mortality) and Pontiac fever (a febrile, flulike illness with minimal mortality and nonpneumonic clinical features).

Infections caused by Escherichia coli

Escherichia coli (Bacillus coli) is a gram-negative bacillus, varying in form from a short coccobacillus to a long slender rod, indistinguishable from the typhoid, dysentery, and paratyphoid group of organisms except by cultural or serologic characteristics. It is a normal inhabitant of feces, and the infections it produces are largely on the basis of opportunism (except in infants, in whom *E. coli*, particularly serogroups O 111 and O 55, may produce severe diarrhea—often of epidemic proportions and occasionally causing death, with minimal or no anatomic lesions). This organism frequently is considered together with *Pseudomonas aeruginosa* and bacilli of the *Proteus* group, since it produces pyogenic infections of similar type. Resultant purulent exudate is ordinarily grayish green, in contrast to the blue-green color that characterizes infection by *P. aeruginosa*.

E. coli is of great importance as a cause of infections of the urinary tract, where it ranks first in frequency. It often acts alone and may be recovered in pure culture. Frequently, however, there is a mixed infection, and an important component is *Streptococcus faecalis* (group D hemolytic streptococcus). As in all ascending infections of the urinary tract, obstruction to the outflow of urine is an important predisposing factor. First, there is infection of the bladder, and cystitis may represent the total extent of bacterial involvement. Often, however, this is followed by ureteritis and pyelonephritis (p. 760).

Since *E. coli* normally inhabits the intestinal tract, fecal peritonitis invariably includes this organism as a part of the infectious mixture. Where there is mechanical injury, local injury from interference with blood supply (volvulus, obstructive appendicitis, diverticulitis, infarction of the bowel), or preliminary injury resulting from a primary hematogenous infection, *E. coli* avails itself of the opportunity provided and causes or contributes to infection.

In cholecystitis and cholangitis, *E. coli* is frequently demonstrable on culture. However, there is evidence that cholecystitis is usually of hematogenous origin and that streptococci most often initiate the disease. The failure to find streptococci more often may be because bile inhibits the growth of this organism, and culture of the bile fails to indicate the nature of infection within the wall of the gallbladder.

E. coli is an important cause of wound infection, especially in the region of the buttocks or thighs.

Toxemia from local infections with *E. coli* occurs most frequently in association with acute infections of the urinary tract, and as a result of this there may be a strong febrile reaction, malaise, and the like. Septicemia very rarely occurs except in newborn infants. This condition, sometimes termed Winckel's disease, often runs a rapidly fatal course.

Infections caused by Klebsiella and Enterobacter aerogenes

Klebsiella pneumoniae (Friedländer's bacillus) is a short, gram-negative, encapsulated bacillus that often occurs in diploform, in which case it resembles the pneumococcus in appearance. As with the pneumococcus, the capsule contains an antigenic polysaccharide that is responsible for type specificity; nucleoprotein contained within the body of the organism (somatic antigen) confers species specificity. Three principal strains have been isolated and defined—A, B, and C. A large group (group X) remains unclassified. Type B of *K. pneumoniae* is similar immunologically to type 2 pneumococcus. Protective antibodies are type specific. The organism inhabits the nasopharynx of 5% to 25% of individuals.

Enterobacter aerogenes (an uncommon organism) is virtually identical to *K. pneumoniae*. Consequently, these organisms often are referred to as the *Klebsiella-Enterobacter* group. Traditionally *E. aerogenes* is considered to occur normally in the intestinal tract, whereas *K. pneumoniae* is found in the nasopharynx. Actually differentiation between the two often cannot be made on morphologic or antigenic grounds.

Pneumonia. Pneumonia caused by *K. pneumoniae* (Friedländer's pneumonia) probably accounts for 2% or

3% of all pneumonias, although estimates of frequency range from 0.4% to 18%. It most often affects those in the older age group, and its occurrence is favored by any condition of general debility, including chronic alcoholism. The early course of the disease, with its acute onset, resembles that of pneumococcal pneumonia, but prostration is usually more striking and is often associated with pronounced dyspnea and cyanosis. The sputum usually contains more blood than in the case of pneumococcal pneumonia and appears mucinous. There may be frank hematemesis. Organisms are readily seen in the sputum and are there in great abundance. Characteristically the lung presents an area of massive consolidation that may exceed the limits of a single lobe. Grossly, the picture is similar to the one seen with pneumococcal lobar pneumonia except that cut surfaces of the lung appear slimy and the lung parenchyma is friable. Histologically the major point of difference between this and ordinary lobar pneumonia is necrosis of the alveolar walls (Fig. 7-15). It is this effect that makes the lung friable and greatly predisposes to such serious complications as lung abcess and organization. Fibrinous pleuritis is a characteristic feature of the disease, and empyema is another complication to be feared. Bacteremia is readily detectable in over half the cases and may lead to metastatic involvement of the meninges or joints. Septicemia with endocarditis has been observed. This may occur independent of pneumonia, and often the source of infection is obscure. The mortality of Friedländer's pneumonia was formerly very high, averaging 70% to 80%, and the majority of those who survived had major complications. Although antibiotics are effective in treatment, the mortality from Friedländer's pneumonia is still 20% to 25%.

Chronic pulmonic infections. Chronic pulmonic infections with Friedländer's bacillus often arise in patients with chronic bronchitis or bronchiectasis, tuberculosis, influenza, or pneumonia. Occasionally, acute pneumonia caused by this organism continues as a persistent chronic disease, leading to chronic abscesses, bronchiectasis, cavity formation, and extensive fibrosis. The condition often closely simulates pulmonary tuberculosis.

K. pneumoniae has been isolated from a wide variety of focal suppurative lesions (otitis media, salpingitis, subphrenic abscess, and cholecystitis). An epidemic of infectious diarrhea in infants, with high mortality, has been ascribed to this organism.

Rhinoscleroma. Rhinoscleroma, a chronic and progressive granulomatous infection of the mucosa of the nose and pharynx, has been attributed to *Klebsiella rhinoscleromatis,* but more recent studies suggest that this organism is identical to type C of *K. pneumoniae.*

Atrophic rhinitis. A persistent atrophic rhinitis, characterized by abundant encrusted purulent discharge and a foul odor, is apparently caused by *Klebsiella ozaenae.* This organism shares the somatic antigen of *K. pneumoniae* but has a different capsular antigen from A, B, or C.

Listeria and Erysipelothrix

Members of the genera *Listeria* and *Erysipelothrix* are small gram-positive rods that are nonsporulating, aerobic, facultative anaerobes of the family Corynebacteriaceae.

Infections caused by Listeria. *Listeria monocytogenes* is easily confused with diphtheroids and has often mistakenly been considered a contaminant. Although the importance of listeriosis as a disease of animals (especially cattle, sheep, goats, and rabbits) has been long recognized, the role of *L. monocytogenes* as a human pathogen has been appreciated only recently. In humans there are four principal forms that the infection may take. In order of decreasing importance these are as follows:

1. Listeria meningitis, an acute purulent meningitis that cannot be differentiated morphologically from several other purulent meningitides
2. Granulomatosis infantiseptica, resulting from intrauterine infection complicating bacteremia or mild septicemia in the mother; usually causes death of the fetus or newborn infant; petechial hemorrhages of the skin often occur, progressing to purpura—a

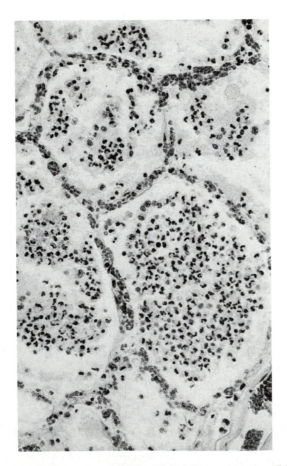

Fig. 7-15. Pneumonia caused by *Klebsiella pneumoniae* (Friedländer's bacillus).

picture similar to the one seen with meningococcemia; most characteristic are the numerous and widely disseminated focal necroses that occur throughout organs and tissues

3. Listeria septicemia, which may resemble septicemia produced by numerous other organisms, including *Salmonella typhosa*, and requires isolation of the organism for specific diagnosis

4. Oculoglandular listeriosis

Infections caused by Erysipelothrix. In humans, *Erysipelothrix rhusiopathiae* causes erysipeloid, a skin infection that usually occurs on the hands and appears somewhat like erysipelas. The infection is ordinarily localized, but occasionally lymphadenitis develops. In approximately 6% of cases, arthritis occurs in the joints adjacent to the area of primary infection. Rarely the infection becomes generalized, producing septicemia. *E. rhusiopathiae* principally affects animals. When human infection occurs, it is usually an occupational disease, developing in workers who pack meat (particularly swine), dress poultry (particularly turkeys), or process seafood (including crabs).

Infections caused by Mycoplasma

Mycoplasma is a genus of bacteria (PPLO organisms) that has only recently come to be recognized as pathogenic for humans, although for many years species have been known to produce disease in a variety of animals, some of which are of economic importance. These organisms are the smallest free-living cells yet recognized. They have no cell walls and are quite pleomorphic. Their range of size is considerable. Many are 0.2 to 0.5 μm, although the smallest infective unit is less than 0.2 μm, and colonies of organisms cluster together to form bodies larger than 0.5 μm. Obviously, these organisms are beyond the resolution of light microscopy. They behave as intracellular parasites but grow on a variety of artificial (including solid) media. Individual colonies are too small to be seen without magnification, although when grown on blood agar, the zone of hemolysis (produced by some species) is visible to the naked eye.

A causal relationship between *Mycoplasma pneumoniae* and primary atypical pneumonia has been proved. Although *Mycoplasma* organisms frequently have been recovered from affected tissues in several of the arthritides and certain ill-defined urogenital diseases, causal relationship has not been proved.

L (Lister Institute) forms of a variety of bacteria somewhat resemble *Mycoplasma* morphologically and in cultural characteristics. The role of L forms in human pathogenesis is controversial.

Intracellular infections

A limited number of bacterially mediated diseases constitute the next step of parasitic intimacy. In this group of bacterial infections a relatively close relationship between parasite and host is reflected by considerable species specificity, a relatively circumscribed habitat of microorganisms within their host (largely within cells of the reticuloendothelial system), and a tendency for these infections to be associated with proliferation of parasitized cells rather than necrosis of host cells. This group of bacterial infections constitutes the zoonoses—phenomenologically defined infectious diseases of defined animal species, including humans. Among these infections are the characteristic human zoonoses *Salmonella typhosa* typhoid fever and *Mycobacterium tuberculosis* (var. *hominis*) tuberculosis. Also included would be the inadvertent interposition of a human host along the chain of infectivity, for example, in the almost innumerable species-characteristic (if not species-specific) salmonelloses, tularemia, and plague.

Occurrence of many of these diseases in the human host requires the interposition of geographic, occupational, or other environmental exposures that make possible contact with infected fomites. Uncommon and exotic infections such as glanders and melioidosis may present features of either an acute septicopyemia or a disseminated reticuloendothelial granulomatous disease depending on a variety of factors, most important among which is probably the dose of infecting microorganisms.

The tendency of many diseases in this category to exist in nature as overt (epizootic) or latent (enzootic) zoonoses reflects considerable species specificity. It is perhaps worth reemphasis that this level of species specificity may recognize humans as in the case of typhoid fever or tuberculosis. In the category of infections under discussion, organ and tissue specificity is much less related to portal of entry than in the infections by pyogenic bacteria described previously. Infections in the category under discussion tend to produce systemic manifestations and are accompanied by lesions, particularly in components of the reticuloendothelial system, almost irrespective of or at least in concurrence with lesions at the portal of entry. Bacteria responsible for this group of diseases promptly tend to be phagocytosed by fixed phagocytic cells of the reticuloendothelial system and to stimulate responses by mononuclear cells, an inflammatory reaction characterized by infiltration and proliferation of fixed mononuclear cells and designated granulomatous. Many infectious lesions attributable to microorganisms in the category of this discussion therefore fall into the group of granulomatous inflammations.

The immunologic response of the host to infections of this class of microorganisms tends increasingly to be mediated by the cellular limb of the immune response and also to be less than completely protective. Often, however, immunologic aspects of these infections assume diagnostic importance, particularly inasmuch as formal isolation and identification of these organisms may be less easy than in the case of pyogenic infections.

Infections caused by salmonellae

The genus *Salmonella* contains species pathogenic for both animals and humans. Originally salmonellae were classified by the human diseases they caused, the species from which they were isolated, or the geographic location in which they were first isolated. Recent usage recognizes only three species: *S. choleraesuis, S. typhosa,* and *S. enteritidis.* The first two are serologically homogeneous. *S. enteritidis* is not, consisting of more than 1000 strains conventionally designated with nonitalicized characterizations, for example, *S. enteritidis* (serotype paratyphi A).

With respect to host preference, salmonellae fall into three groups: (1) *S. typhosa,* which is more or less strongly adapted to humans, (2) *S. choleraesuis,* of which the primary host is swine but which also occurs in other animals including humans, and (3) a very large number of salmonellae that produce disease in humans and other animals with equal facility.

Salmonellae cause three types of human disease: specific enteric fevers, septicemic diseases without specific organ-system localization, and gastroenteritis.

Enteric (typhoid and paratyphoid) fevers. In 1926 the death rate from typhoid fever in the United States was 20.54 per 100,000 population. In 1973 only 680 cases of typhoid fever were reported, with only 7 deaths. At present only a few hundred cases occur annually in the United States. Epidemics such as the one in Zermatt, Switzerland,[62] continue to occur, however, even in medically advanced countries. As our vigilance relaxes, new and large epidemics may be expected as a reminder that *S. typhosa* is a highly pathogenic organism.

S. typhosa is a short, plump, gram-negative rod that is flagellated and actively motile. It is indistinguishable morphologically from other members of the enteric group. Its relative lack of resistance to common antiseptics, drying, sunlight, and heat is one reason why sanitary measures have been so effective in controlling the disease. Infection occurs directly or indirectly from an individual afflicted with or convalescing from the disease or from a healthy carrier. Contaminated food or water is the common medium of contagion. The "five F's" most concerned with spread of this disease are food, fingers, flies, fomites, and feces. Urine is often a more important source of infection than feces, since contamination of the hands is more likely to occur after urination, and the urine is more likely to be "deposited" in an unsuitable container or on the ground. Then, too, in those whose typhoid fever is complicated by pyeloureteritis, the number of organisms passed in the urine is greatly in excess of those commonly found in the feces.

S. typhosa is, for all practical purposes, restricted in portal of entry to the gastrointestinal tract. In human volunteers, 10^5 to 10^7 ingested bacilli are required to induce the disease. Typhoid bacilli have been injected subcutaneously without harm and, in fact, some vaccines have contained viable organisms. On penetrating the intestinal mucosa, the organisms quickly enter lymphatic vessels and mesenteric nodes, whence they reach the liver and then, by the thoracic duct, the bloodstream. All this occurs in the incubation period, usually 10 to 14 days. This is the first stage of the disease, in which generalization of the infection occurs before localizing lesions draw attention to the intestine.

In the second stage there are severe headaches; generalized aching, especially of the arms and legs; malaise; and fatigue. Shortly thereafter the picture changes to one of frank septicemia, with chills, fever, prostration, splenic enlargement, and the characteristic rose spots. The last usually occur during the second week of the disease and at first glance resemble petechial hemorrhages. The fact that they blanch on pressure reveals them to be an effect of severe hyperemia (capillary atony). Aggregations of macrophages and edema in these focal areas indicate that they represent sites of bacterial localization (embolization) and resultant local toxic injury. They disappear after a few days.

The third stage, after a week to 10 days, is dominated by effects of local bacterial injury, especially in the intestinal tract, mesenteric lymph nodes, spleen, and liver.

Last is the stage of lysis, in which the infectious process is gradually overcome. Symptoms slowly disappear and the temperature gradually returns to normal.

The four stages of the disease and their significance are illustrated in Fig. 7-16.

Although septicemia dominates the early stages of typhoid fever, significant local changes begin to occur during the third stage—7 to 10 days after clinical onset—first in the lymphoid tissue of the intestinal tract. Peyer's patches of the ileum and the solitary lymph follicles in the region of the cecum become hyperplastic and so swollen as to produce almost buttonlike protrusions (Fig. 7-17). The mesenteric lymph nodes become hyperplastic too, as a result of infection through the lymphatics, and *S. typhosa* can usually be recovered in pure culture from these nodes. Along with this, the reticuloendothelial system as a whole is responding to septicemia, and there is hyperplasia of other lymph nodes, the spleen, reticular elements of the bone marrow, and the Kupffer cells of the liver. After 7 to 10 days, the picture in the intestine is complicated by necrosis and ulceration of areas that formerly exhibited lymphoid hyperplasia. Long oval ulcers in the ileum parallel the long axis of the bowel and correspond in shape and arrangement to Peyer's patches (Fig. 7-17). In the colon, ulcers are smaller and punctate, corresponding to the smaller lymphoid follicles there.

Microscopically an outstanding characteristic is the lack of polymorphonuclear leukocytes. The predominant cell of reaction is a large monocyte (macrophage) that somewhat resembles the blood monocyte. These are

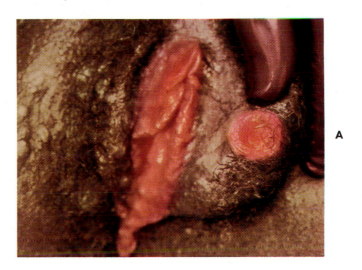

A

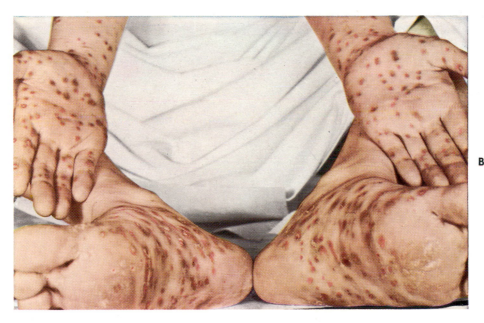

B

Plate 1. Syphilis. **A,** Primary lesion of vulva (chancre).**B,** Papulos-
quamous secondary lesions. (Reprinted from *Therapeutic Notes;*
courtesy Parke, Davis & Co.)

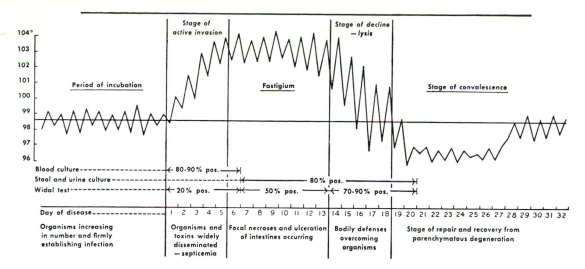

Fig. 7-16. Typhoid fever. Clinicopathologic correlation.

present in abundance in the base and margins of the ulcer. Lymphocytes and plasma cells are seen too. Lymph nodes exhibit foci of necrosis that may be as large as several millimeters in diameter. There is gross proliferation of the sinusoidal cells, and sinusoids are filled with macrophages similar to those observed in the intestinal ulcers. This picture is almost pathognomonic of typhoid fever. The lack of participation by polymorphonuclear leukocytes is reflected by the absence of leukocytosis. Leukopenia is characteristic and an important clinical sign, since very few bacterial infections are associated with a low white blood cell count.

Among other organs, most changes occur in the spleen and liver. The spleen is greatly enlarged, frequently weighing 500 g or more. Its capsule is tense, and the parenchyma is soft. The organ is so soft and swollen that occasionally it ruptures during removal at autopsy (splenic rupture rarely occurs "spontaneously" during life). The striking cherry-red color is reflected microscopically by hyperemia. There is hyperplasia, especially of the red pulp. Areas of focal necrosis are seen, similar to those observed in mesenteric lymph nodes.

The liver also is enlarged and swollen, as evidenced by the tense capsule and rounded edges. It presents the picture of gross cloudy swelling. Parenchymatous degeneration is evident microscopically, and focal necrosis is a characteristic finding. The distribution of these minute foci bears no constant relation to the architecture of the hepatic lobule; some will be found perilobularly, others adjacent to the central vein, and still others midway between. This is in striking contrast to the zonal necrosis of yellow fever, eclampsia, chloroform poisoning, and so on. Formerly these areas were considered analogous to tiny infarcts, a result of embolization by agglutinated bacilli. This has been disproved, however, and it appears that the primary reaction is not a degeneration but an

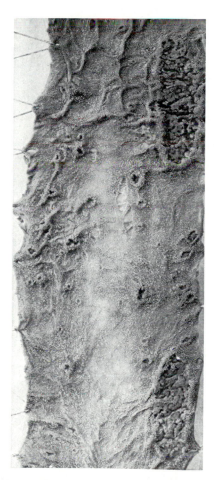

Fig. 7-17. Typhoid fever. Ulceration of ileum. Ulcerative lesions of ileum correspond in location to lymphoid follicles and Peyer's patches. Where they occur in Peyer's patches *(on right),* their oval shape with long axis is parallel to that of intestine. (AFIP 2803.)

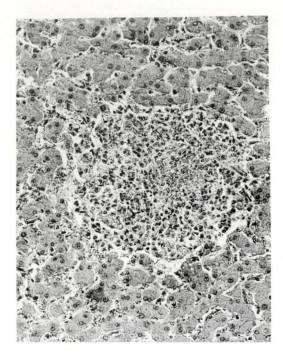

Fig. 7-18. Typhoid nodule in liver.

aggregation of macrophages that have come from the intestine (portal vein). As these continue to accumulate, the capillaries are distended and liver cords compressed. After this some necrosis of hepatic cells may occur, perhaps from a combination of injuries—pressure, toxic effect, and ischemia. It would seem better to term this lesion the typhoid nodule, since necrosis is neither the primary nor the outstanding feature. This is a characteristic reaction of typhoid fever and occurs in lymph nodes, spleen, and bone marrow, as well as the liver (Fig. 7-18).

The heart and kidneys show cloudy swelling as a manifestation of toxemia. This change in the heart is reflected by a persistent bradycardia (an important diagnostic sign) that appears out of place alongside the patient's fever.

Skeletal muscles are particularly susceptible to these toxins and exhibit a pronounced degree of Zenker's (waxy) degeneration. As is the usual case, this nonspecific degenerative change affects principally the skeletal muscles that are most active when the patient is at rest—intercostals, diaphragm, and rectus abdominis. The damage is occasionally so severe as to lead to rupture of the rectus muscles, with pain, hemorrhage, and the like. This may simulate "acute surgical abdomen" and lead to surgical exploration.

There are many other complications from this disease. Most feared is massive intestinal hemorrhage, which occurs in 5% to 10% of the patients. Next in importance is peritonitis resulting from perforation of the bowel. The most common site is the terminal ileum, and the most common time is during the second or third week. When perforation of the intestine occurs, the resultant fecal peritonitis is usually fatal. Rupture of a mesenteric lymph node will produce a specific *Salmonella typhosa* peritonitis, which is less severe and from which the patient often recovers. Intestinal obstruction as a sequel to ulceration rarely occurs because there is relatively little scar formation on healing. Since typhoid fever is a septicemic disease, focal metastatic infections can develop in a variety of places and may be responsible for osteomyelitis, meningitis, endocarditis, or nephritis. In approximately 5% to 10% of cases, thrombophlebitis of the femoral or saphenous veins occurs. This rarely develops before the fourth week and comes at a time when the patient appears well on the road to recovery. Infection of the gallbladder occurs almost invariably. This poses a special problem if the resultant cholecystitis becomes chronic, leading to a persistent carrier state. Focal paralysis sometimes occurs and seems to be an effect of toxemia. Relapses occur in 5% to 10% of the cases.

Death may result from one of the complications previously described but often simply from typhoid fever per se. The terminal phase is one of severe debility and wasting, but most characteristic are the mental signs and symptoms. The individual is semistuporous and yet very restless, nervously plucking at the bedclothes and groaning. The mortality, formerly 10% to 20%, has been greatly reduced by use of chloramphenicol.

Typhoid fever is one of the most protean of all bacterial diseases, and often the diagnosis does not become apparent until late in the course—or perhaps until autopsy. For this reason laboratory procedures are usually depended on to confirm or disprove a suspicion of typhoid fever. The place of blood culture, serologic studies, and bacteriologic examination of feces and urine in establishing the diagnosis is shown in Fig. 7-16. Agglutination tests (Widal) for typhoid fever deserve a further word of explanation. The serum of most individuals has the capacity of agglutinating typhoid organisms at a dilution of at least 1:50. If a person has been immunized against the disease, the serum antibody titer may be considerably higher. Therefore interpretation must be made on a quantitative rather than a qualitative basis. In addition, because of the close antigenic relationship that exists between *S. typhosa* and organisms that cause paratyphoid fever, it may be difficult to differentiate between these diseases by serologic means. A determination of antibody response against different antigenic fractions of the organisms—O (somatic) antigen, H (flagellar) antigen, and Vi antigen—is of considerable value. Some individuals with typhoid or paratyphoid fever develop antibodies against O antigen only, and, furthermore, titers of O antigen disappear more quickly and usually do not reach the height of H titers as a result of active immunization. It thus follows that antibodies against O antigen (above 1:50) are most significant in establishing the diagnosis of infection. On the other hand, the titer against H antigen is more helpful in determining which of the typhoid-paratyphoid group of organisms is responsible for the infection.[14] Agglutination titers against Vi antigen are always low, but specific. They are diagnostic if it is known that the patient is not a typhoid carrier.

Septicemia. *Salmonella* septicemias produce high remittent fevers ordinarily without gastrointestinal manifestations. Foci of suppuration may occur in almost any organ—kidneys, biliary tract, heart, meninges, bones, joints, or lungs. Predisposing factors include sickle cell disease, the hemolytic anemia of bartonellosis, and treatment of other conditions with broad-spectrum antibodies, which disturb the normal flora of the intestine.

Enteric fevers (paratyphoid fever) caused by salmonellae other than *S. typhosa* are milder than classic typhoid fever and usually have a shorter incubation period.

Gastroenteritis. Any of a very wide group of salmonellae can cause acute gastroenteritis. The source of infection is ingestion of organisms contained in contaminated food or drink, often meat or eggs. *Salmonella* gastroenteritis is one bacterial disease that is not decreasing in incidence in the United States. Annually 15,000 to 20,000 cases are reported. The incubation period is somewhat longer than in staphylococcal food poisoning, with which *Salmonella* gastroenteritis may be easily confused. Headache, chills, and abdominal pain are followed by nausea, vomiting, and diarrhea. The diagnosis depends on isolating the organism from stool or from the suspected food.

Brucellosis (undulant fever, Mediterranean fever, Malta fever)

The serious aspects of brucellosis, as it exists in the United States, have been generally appreciated only recently. Despite its high incidence, brucellosis long escaped proper notice because of its protean nature and because of the many diseases that it commonly simulates—notably typhoid fever, tuberculosis, malaria, influenza or other viral disease, infectious mononucleosis, some hidden focus of pyogenic infection, appendicitis, and cholecystitis. Often it has paraded under the name "neurasthenia."

Three different members of the genus *Brucella* may cause the disease, and each has a different animal reservoir. The caprine (goat) strain, *B. melitensis*, is prevalent in the Maltese islands and the Mediterranean area, whence came the original name of Malta fever or Mediterranean fever. It is the least common cause of brucellosis in the United States, occurring principally in the southwestern part. The bovine (cow) strain, *B. abortus*, is widespread among the dairy herds of the United States and produces in cattle what is commonly known as Bang's disease, or contagious abortion. *B. abortus* is responsible for the majority of human infections in the United States. The porcine (pig) strain, *B. suis*, is also an important cause of human disease in the United States, especially in swine-raising areas. Two species relatively

recently described, the canine (dog) strain, *B. canis*, and the ovine (sheep) strain, *B. ovis*, rarely cause human infections.

In each of these animals, symptoms commonly result from infection by *Brucella*. The predominant effect is abortion, but there may also be mastitis, lameness, and (especially in swine) vertebral abscesses. Sheep, horses, dogs, rats, guinea pigs, cats, and birds may be infected by and harbor *Brucella*.

These organisms are small, gram-negative coccobacilli that are difficult to cultivate on artificial media and are slow to grow. The natural host of each of the organisms is a common domestic animal, and humans contract brucellosis as a result of contact with these animals or their products. It has been demonstrated that the organisms may pass through the unbroken epidermis; thus the disease is a serious occupational hazard to meat packers, farmers who raise hogs and cows, and laboratory workers who handle the organisms. The respiratory route is a possibility too; the disease has been produced experimentally by inhalation of the organisms suspended in aerosol. Ingestion of infected milk, once an important means of contracting the disease, is now responsible for less than 10% of the cases in the United States.[108]

Brucella organisms elaborate no exotoxins but produce a potent endotoxin. An important factor in virulence is their ability to survive intracellularly—within polymorphonuclear leukocytes and monocytes.

Because of the many variations of the disease, it is almost impossible to describe all the forms it may assume. One clinical classification is according to acute, subacute, or chronic form. In another classification, based on clinical course, differences in temperature curves are characteristic: *malignant* (fulminant type), *undulant* (intermediate in severity), and *intermittent* (persistent, chronic form).

The malignant type of disease, which fortunately is quite uncommon, is most likely to be produced by *B. melitensis*, the most aggressive strain. After sudden onset, there is high fever with severe prostration. The mortality is high, and this form of the disease may terminate in death in 1 to 3 weeks.

The undulant type, caused almost always by *B. melitensis*, is less common in the United States than in other countries. It is characterized by an undulating fever, gradually reaching its peak in 4 to 7 days, persisting thus for a week or so, and then in a few days gradually subsiding. These periods of fever, 2 to 3 weeks in duration, alternating with a week or two of relatively normal temperature, may continue for 3 months to a year. *B. suis* ordinarily produces less serious disease than *B. melitensis*, and *B. abortus*, in turn, less serious disease than *B. suis*.

The incubation period for the intermittent form of the disease, usually 1 to 3 weeks, may extend several months. Typically, *B. abortus* infection leads to this form. Often the patient is unaware of any specific time of onset, complaining rather of progressive tiredness and malaise and inability to work effectively. Along with this, there develops mental depression, with generalized aching, especially of the head and back. Frequently there are rheumatic-type pains, often in the sacroiliac region or taking the form of sciatic neuritis. The patient usually complains also of constipation and insomnia. After a while, fever with night sweats may be a distressing feature. Temperature, usually near normal in the morning, rises to 101° to 104° F in the late afternoon or evening. In infection with *B. abortus*, the leukocyte count is normal or less than normal, although this is not true in infection with *B. melitensis*.

Since there are no pathognomonic signs or symptoms of brucellosis, diagnosis rests primarily on bacteriologic or serologic studies. The simplest procedure is the skin test, in which 0.1 ml of protein nucleate fraction, Brucellergen, is injected intradermally. As with the tuberculin test, however, a positive reaction does not necessarily mean active disease, since this tests only the person's sensitivity to the infecting agent and may simply reflect an infection of long ago—one that may have been subclinical and thus unrecognized. Demonstration of a significantly high serum agglutination titer is probably the most helpful laboratory procedure, although many patients with brucellosis have no demonstrable serum agglutinins. The opsonocytophagic index is difficult to perform properly and is not suited to routine use. The surest laboratory finding on which to base a diagnosis of

brucellosis is demonstration of the organism in the blood, urine, or feces. This is a dangerous, difficult, and time-consuming procedure. Although the cultures may exhibit growth after a week, one cannot properly consider them to be negative until 3 or 4 weeks have elapsed. Furthermore, repeated samplings of the blood may be necessary before the organisms are demonstrated. Since the guinea pig is quite susceptible to these organisms, subcutaneous or intraperitoneal injection of the material in question may substitute for in vitro culture. This requires a period of 6 weeks or so for the disease to develop in unmistakable form.

In the United States the majority of affected persons (81% in Spink's series[107]) acquire their infection directly through contact with diseased animals. After initial localization, usually in the skin, there is extension along lymphatics and involvement of regional lymph nodes. The organisms, phagocytosed first by granulocytes and, subsequently, by monocytes and macrophages, produce focal granulomatous reaction, often with minute areas of necrosis. Assuming that there is progressive infection, the organisms proliferate and spread from lymph nodes to the bloodstream, an event that can occur within hours or may require days depending on the virulence, dose of the organism, and resistance of the host. Once in the bloodstream, the organisms are widely disseminated, but with preferential localization to reticuloendothelial tissues such as bone marrow, spleen, and liver and to the kidneys. In these organs, as in the lymph nodes, multiple minute granulomas form (Fig. 7-19). These may provide

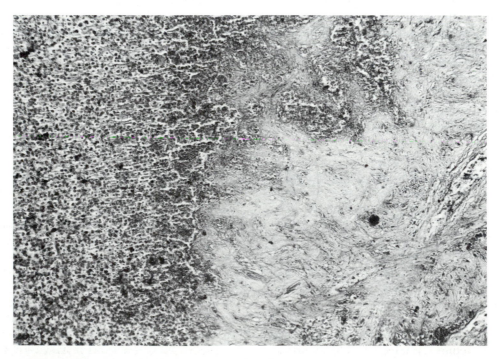

Fig. 7-19. Granulomatous inflammation produced by a bacillus, *Brucella abortus*, in bone.

a basis for diagnosing the disease, since they are sometimes apparent on histologic study of bone marrow aspirate or needle biopsy specimens of the liver or spleen. Since brucellosis is a septicemic disease, focal lesions may occur in almost any organ or tissue, producing meningitis, osteomyelitis, orchitis, vegetative endocarditis, or empyema. The spleen is often considerably enlarged, and splenomegaly is a characteristic physical finding. There may be hepatomegaly also, and lymph nodes (particularly those of the mesentery) are usually considerably enlarged, soft, and diffluent. Most epithelial tissues show parenchymatous degeneration.

Tularemia (rabbit fever)

Tularemia is a relatively recently recognized disease entity. McCoy and Chapin of the U.S. Public Health Service first identified the causative organism in 1911 and named it tularensis after Tulare County, California. Shortly after this, Wherry recognized, and for the first time proved, infection in a human. The bulk of our knowledge and understanding of this disease we owe to the long and efficient work of Edward Francis. Tularemia is caused by *Francisella tularensis* (formerly *Pasteurella tularensis*), a small gram-negative bacillus that is pleomorphic, sometimes appearing in coccal form. It grows only on special culture media. Plague and tularemia have much in common. A variety of wild animals forms a natural reservoir for *F. tularensis*. Especially important in human infection are wild rabbits (cottontails), hares (jackrabbits), and ground squirrels. The disease is rapidly fatal in these animals. Francis has estimated that 1% of wild rabbits are infected. In Russia, outbreaks of the disease have occurred in those who obtain and prepare the skins of water rats for the fur industry. Infection will occur from direct contact with infected animals, and thus the disease is especially likely to occur among trappers, hunters, butchers, and laboratory workers. *F. tularensis* is capable of passing readily through the unbroken skin, and it is said to be the most dangerous of all infectious agents from the standpoint of the laboratory worker. The second most common method of infection is by the bite of insects, especially ticks (*Dermacentor andersoni, D. variabilis, D. occidentalis,* and *Haemaphysalis leporis palustris*), horseflies, or deerflies (*Chrysops discalis*). Ingestion of the poorly cooked meat of infected animals has also produced the disease. In at least one instance a small epidemic of tularemia occurred from drinking contaminated water. On the average, around 180 cases are reported in the United States each year.

According to Francis and Callender,[77] the mortality is nearly 4%, with slow convalescence in many cases. The occurrence of suppurative or granulomatous late lesions with attendant prostration and debility emphasized the seriousness of contracting this infection. The incubation period is ordinarily 3 to 5 days, after which there suddenly develop headache, chills, and high fever, along with generalized aching and the severe prostration characteristic of septicemia. Not until 36 to 48 hours later does the patient usually notice painful swollen lymph nodes, most often in an axilla. This may direct attention for the first time to the focus of primary infection, an area drained by the involved lymph nodes. Usually the lesion is on the finger or hand. It begins as a tender red papule. Soon there is central necrosis, and a "punched-out" ulcer develops. Over three fourths of the cases are associated with such a primary ulcerating lesion, which is slow to heal and persists, on the average, a month or so. Regional lymph nodes enlarge to a pronounced degree and resemble somewhat the buboes of plague. In about one fourth of the cases these enlarged lymph nodes suppurate and may spontaneously rupture and drain cheesy purulent material. This is the so-called ulceroglandular type of the disease, and approximately 75% of cases fall within this category.

Next in frequency, accounting for 10% or less of cases, is the oculoglandular type, essentially similar to the ulceroglandular type just described except that the focus of inoculation is the conjunctiva. Edema, severe hyperemia, itching, and pain are present. Multiple, small, discrete, yellowish nodules may be seen on the mucous membrane. These signs are accompanied by cervical lymphadenopathy. Corneal scarring and blindness are occasional sequelae.

Less common are the glandular and typhoidal forms, in which there is no evident site of initial infection. Pneumonic tularemia is rare.

Tularemia is a septicemic disease, and signs and symptoms often point to a variety of organs. Involvement of the lung, when it occurs, is usually quite evident clinically. Pulmonic lesions may be discrete and nodular, closely resembling those of tuberculosis, or they may occur in the form of confluent bronchopneumonia or lobar pneumonia.

Morphologic changes are essentially similar, regardless of which of the four clinical forms the disease has taken. Often there is a close resemblance to miliary tuberculosis, and minute (2 to 3 mm) hard "tubercles" may be found in the liver (Fig. 7-20), spleen, kidneys, lungs, and other organs. If the tularemic nodules are of larger size, central necrosis is quite evident, and the lesions may be mistaken for abscesses. Tissue changes depend largely on the stage of the disease. Early in its course the predominant change is focal necrosis. If there has been time for reaction to this, the granulomatous nature of the disease is readily evident. The predominant cell of reaction is the macrophage, and these cells often are arranged in a radial manner around a central area of caseous necrosis, the whole enclosed within a fibrous capsule. Occasional giant cells of the Langhans type are seen. Organisms cannot be demonstrated in histologic

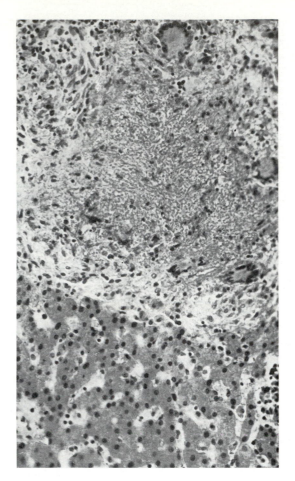

Fig. 7-20. Tularemia. Granulomatous reaction in liver closely simulates tuberculosis.

preparations of human tissues. In addition, there is generalized hyperplasia of the reticuloendothelial system. The spleen may be enlarged to 400 or 500 g and is often palpable on physical examination. Parenchymatous degeneration is found in many organs.

Sensitivity to bacterial proteins is a prominent feature of tularemia, and a small percentage of patients have spectacular cutaneous eruptions during the second or third week. The Foshay intradermal test is useful in establishing the diagnosis, as is the demonstration of specific agglutinins. A disadvantage of this latter test is that the disease must be a week or so old before antibodies can be demonstrated in the blood. Cross agglutination occurs between *F. tularensis* and organisms of the genus *Brucella*, and if either disease is suspected, agglutination titers should be determined against both; the specific titer will be much higher in one than the other. The organism may be cultured from the local external lesion, from the blood, or—in cases of tularemic pneumonia—from the sputum. In the absence of specific media, a guinea pig may be injected and will die of the disease within 5 to 7 days. Although the handling of infected patients is apparently without much hazard, anyone who attempts to culture the organisms is in serious danger of contracting the disease.

Infections caused by Yersinia

Plague (bubonic plague, black death, pest). This most dreaded of medieval diseases has ravaged Europe and Asia in numerous pandemics. One of the most serious of these began in China in 1374, killing 13 million people there and spreading to involve all of Europe. An estimated 25 million lives were lost to the disease within a 3-year period, approximately one fourth of the total population of Europe at that time. There have been recent pandemics, the most serious of which raged intermittently for 30 years, affecting principally India and costing 12 million lives there.

The causative organism is *Yersinia pestis*, a pleomorphic, gram-negative coccobacillus that presents bipolar bodies; it is often encapsulated. Depending on the animal reservoir, two forms of the disease are recognized. In murine plague, rats (most commonly the gray sewer rat) serve as the primary source of infection. As the rodent succumbs to the disease, it often enters some human dwelling to die. Infected fleas leave its body, and an acceptable host is found in the common black house rat. In sylvatic plague, rodents of nondomestic habits are the source of infection. In the United States the ground squirrel is most dangerous, but infection has been reported in at least 72 different animal species.

The disease is endemic in India, China, East Africa, and South America. In the United States, an endemic focus of wild rodent plague exists, and several outbreaks of human plague have been reported, all of them west of the 100th meridian. According to Holmes,[5] in 1907 to 1908, within a 12-month period, 37 deaths from plague occurred in the San Francisco–Oakland area, and there have been cases in New Orleans, Beaumont and Galveston, Texas, and Pensacola, Florida. Infections also have been reported in New Mexico, southwestern Oregon, Idaho, Utah, and Nevada.[85]

The disease is transmitted to humans in two principal ways. More commonly, infection results from the bite of an infected flea (especially *Xenopsylla cheopis* and *Pulex irritans*). The body louse and bedbug also may serve as vectors of infection. Less common is the pneumonic form of the disease, spread directly from person to person by droplets. Occasionally, especially in children who may handle dead rodents, there is direct infection of wounds or other lesions. The incubation period averages 2 to 4 days. Although there may be prodromal symptoms such as malaise and headache, more often the individual first responds with a sudden chill, fever, and other symptoms of severe toxemia or septicemia, including nausea and vomiting. As in the case of tularemia, it may be a day or two before onset of the obvious lymphadenitis. This occurs most commonly in the inguinal lymph nodes, less often in the axillary nodes, and only occasionally in the cervical nodes. The buboes (bubonic plague) are very painful and may attain great size, up to 4 or 5 cm in diameter. Within a day or two, organisms find their way into the bloodstream, by entering blood vessels directly or in infected thoracic duct lymph, and the septicemic stage of the disease develops. Profound systemic manifestations progress, and the patient, at first very nervous and apprehensive, may sink into coma and die within a few days. There are three clinical forms of the disease. That just described represents the bubonic type, which is the most common. Death occurs in 60% to 90% of the patients. In the primary septicemic type there may or may not be buboes. This form of the disease is almost always quickly fatal, as is the highly infectious pneumonic type, in which death may occur within a few hours after first symptoms. A much milder form of the disease, pestis minor, is occasionally seen. In this type the organisms remain localized and septicemia does not occur.

Morphologic changes in those dying of plague represent the effects of overwhelming infection by bacteria that produce potent necrotizing toxins coupled with disseminated intravascular coagulation (DIC). The picture is much the same everywhere. Large areas of necrotic tissue are seen, and these tissues are teeming with organisms. In the fulminant forms of the disease, lesions include relatively little inflammatory exudate but much hemorrhage. When the infection is not so overwhelming, exudation of inflammatory cells may be prominent, even to the point of suppuration. For instance, in the pneumonic form of the disease, only severe hyperemia and sanguineous edema may be found in the lungs of persons dying quickly. If the process continues longer, lobular pneumonia develops and may progress to confluence, giving the picture of lobar pneumonia.

In involved lymph nodes (buboes), the gland is almost replaced by hemorrhagic necrotic tissue. This reaction spreads beyond the confines of the capsule, and in the surrounding tissues, necrosis, hemorrhage, and cellulitis also are evident (Fig. 7-21).

The disease may simulate tularemia, but its course is so fulminating that its true nature is usually soon evident. Smears may be made from contents of buboes and will usually reveal *Y. pestis* in great numbers. The organisms may be cultured or an animal (guinea pig or white rat) inoculated. The latter is accomplished by rubbing some of the infected material into the shaved skin of the anterior abdominal wall. If the material contains *Y. pestis*, the animal will die within 3 to 5 days, presenting typical findings. Blood cultures are positive in approximately 50% of cases. Extreme caution must be taken in all such procedures and with the infected person to prevent direct infection of the person or an insect vector. Tetracycline and chloramphenicol are effective in early cases. Active

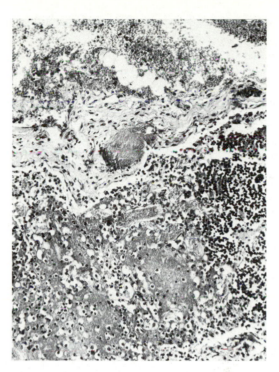

Fig. 7-21. Lymph node in plague. Hemorrhagic edematous cellulitis *(top)* extends from infected lymph node. Despite obvious acuteness of process, cellular reaction is almost exclusively mononuclear. Gray myxoid interstitial haze *(bottom)* is produced by profusion of microorganisms.

immunization provides only relative temporary protection.

Other Yersinia infections. The genus *Yersinia* includes two human pathogens, *Y. entercolitica* and *Y. pseudotuberculosis,* other than the plague bacillus. Although the distribution of these organisms is worldwide, early reports were predominantly from Europe, particularly Scandinavia. The early reports of human cases emphasized contact with household pets or exotic species, but those reservoirs have recently been less emphasized although animal reservoirs are assumed.

Y. enterocolitica causes a usually self-limited, anatomically nonspecific enterocolitis, particularly in infants and young children. *Y. pseudotuberculosis* is more frequently incriminated in cases of mesenteric adenitis in older children and adolescents, in whom the disease may mimic acute appendicitis.

Infections caused by Pasteurella

Members of the genus *Pasteurella* are frequent commensals of the oral cavity of animals (cats, dogs, and rodents). *P. multocida* causes occasional human infection in three circumstances: (1) victims of animal bites, (2) patients with chronic pulmonary disease, often with animal contacts but without a history of animal bites, and (3) patients with chronic gastrointestinal (especially hepatic) disease without a history of animal bites. Three categories of lesion are associated with infections by *P. multocida:* (1) an acute cellulitis or abscess at the site of a bite or scratch by a pet animal, (2) pulmonary suppuration complicating preexisting chronic pulmonary disease, or (3) peritonitis or sepsis in a patient with chronic hepatic disease, often with a history of animal contact.

Glanders

Glanders is another example of a disease that affects animals primarily; humans are rarely involved and then, it would seem, by accident. This is a disease of horses and mules principally, and in these animals it may assume either of two forms. *Glanders* is a relatively acute disease affecting principally the lungs and bringing death in the majority of cases, within 4 to 6 weeks. *Farcy* is a relatively chronic condition that involves primarily the skin, subcutaneous tissues, and their lymphatic vessels. The disease is caused by *Actinobacillus (Malleomyces) mallei*, a rather pleomorphic, usually slender, gram-negative rod. It does not produce an exotoxin. The disease is uncommon in humans and is almost always confined to those who work closely with horses and mules or to laboratory workers who cultivate the organism. Therefore its incidence has dropped sharply in recent years. *A. mallei* ranks with *Francisella tularensis* in the hazard it presents to laboratory workers. Although the organism can penetrate intact epithelium, the site of infection is usually an abrasion or other minor injury to the skin, after which there develops a small nodule that usually ulcerates. Regional lymph nodes become swollen and tender. Shortly thereafter, fever and frequently a mucopurulent nasal discharge occur. An important characteristic at this stage of the process is the exceptional prostration, disproportionate to other signs and symptoms. In many patients a generalized pustular rash develops involving skin and mucous membranes—not unlike that of smallpox. Focal areas of suppuration or nodular granulomas occur in many organs, the joints, and especially the subcutaneous tissues (farcy buds), where they ulcerate and discharge a thick, tenacious, bloody pus.

Morphologically the disease resembles pyemia, with abscesses to be found in many organs. Often, if it is chronic, a granulomatous reaction may predominate. This chronic form particularly may simulate other infectious diseases, and the condition may persist, with frequent remissions, for years. Formerly the disease in its acute form was almost always fatal; in its chronic form the mortality was 50% to 70%. The use of sulfonamides has reduced this figure somewhat.

Diagnosis rests on demonstration of complement-fixing antibodies, recovery of the organism from a subcutaneous lesion (preferably a recent one), or guinea pig inoculation (Straus reaction). Skin tests (mallein) become positive in 3 to 4 weeks and resemble a positive tuberculin test.

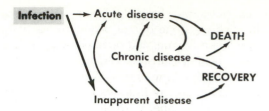

Fig. 7-22. Interrelationships among various forms of melioidosis.

Melioidosis

Until a few years ago melioidosis was considered to be an uncommon, usually fatal, disease limited to Southeast Asia. Now it is recognized that the infection is much more common than the clinically apparent disease (7% to 10% of persons living in highly endemic areas have demonstrable antibodies) and that it occurs also in Australia, Africa, Malagasy, the Caribbean, and tropical America. For a long time the causative agent was known as *Malleomyces pseudomallei* because it was believed to be of the same genus as the organism that causes glanders. Recently, however, its name has been changed to *Pseudomonas pseudomallei*. The organism is a small (0.5 × 1.5 to 2 μm), motile, pleomorphic, gram-negative rod with bipolar staining properties. It has no capsule, nor does it form spores. In the early 1900s, Whitmore collected and described some 38 cases of the disease in Rangoon (Whitmore's disease). Thirty-one of these cases had occurred in drug addicts, and for a while the disease was called morphine addict's septicemia. Shortly after this time the disease virtually disappeared, except for rare sporadic cases. Interest was reawakened in connection with the experience of French troops in Indochina from 1948 to 1954, during which time approximately 100 cases of the disease were recognized. The experience of soldiers in Vietnam has stimulated further interest and extensive clinical and laboratory studies from which much new information has emerged.

Melioidosis presents a broad clinical spectrum, varying from inapparent infection on the one extreme to fulminant septicemia on the other. Interrelationships among the various forms of the disease are shown diagrammatically in Fig. 7-22.

The precise mechanism by which infection occurs is not known. It has been hypothesized that the organism enters through a minute break in the skin or as a wound infection. The possibility of entry by inhalation and ingestion has also been considered. *P. pseudomallei* is widely dispersed in water and soil in endemic areas and also may be found in a variety of infected animals (reservoirs?), including domestic ones, where it often produces serious disease, sometimes occurring as epizootics.

Although the manifestations of melioidosis vary enormously, particular forms of the disease are recognized.

The acute pulmonary form of infection is most common, and the picture is one of pronounced sepsis with high fever, profound fatigue, and often chest pain. Leukocytosis is variable in occurrence and degree, with the number of cells ranging from normal to around 20,000. X-ray findings include patchy infiltrations or even consolidation of a pulmonary lobe. With progression of the disease (without treatment), cavitation may develop within several days. The radiologic changes often simulate those of tuberculosis, and this is an important differential diagnostic consideration. The acute septicemic form of the disease usually begins as a pulmonary infection and may run a rapid course, terminating in death within several days. A form of chronic septicemia, which requires several months to run its course, is occasionally seen. The chronic condition is similar to glanders in that many abscesses occur, involving most tissues of the body. Still another form of the disease is characterized by localized suppurative infections, and almost any organ or tissue may be involved.

Pathologic changes cover as wide a range as clinical manifestations, their form depending in large measure on whether the disease is rapidly progressive, subacute, or chronic. In the acute progressive cases the characteristic lesion is a well-defined abscess that is usually small, firm, and yellow or yellowish. The exudate is composed primarily of neutrophils with lesser numbers of histiocytes and considerable fibrin. The abscesses are usually multiple and may affect virtually any organ, especially the lungs, lymph nodes (Fig. 7-23), liver, and spleen. In the less rapidly progressive disease the lesions are again focal but are granulomatous. Often the granulomas present central areas of caseous necrosis and contain Langhans' (or foreign body–type) giant cells. It may be impossible on histopathologic grounds alone to differentiate these lesions from those caused by tuberculosis. The larger granulomas frequently present extensive central necrosis, associated with purulent exudate, forming stellate abscesses—a response that closely simulates the lesions produced by tularemia, cat-scratch disease, lymphogranuloma venereum, and sporotrichosis. Unfortunately, in the granulomatous lesions the causative organisms can rarely be demonstrated—in contrast to the acute suppurative lesions.

One of the treacherous aspects of the disease, which has earned it the name "Vietnamese time bomb," is that an isolated focus of the disease, often producing few if any signs or symptoms, may lie dormant for as long as several years and then, for no evident reason, suddenly become active to produce serious disease.

Positive diagnosis can be made only by demonstration of the organism, although serologic studies (especially hemagglutination) may be helpful. Chloramphenicol, in combination with other drugs, and tetracyclines are useful in treating the disease, but the more fulminant forms still carry a mortality of 90% and persistent chronic melioidosis may lead to death in 30% to 50% of the cases.

Granuloma inguinale (donovanosis)

Uncommon in medically advanced countries, granuloma inguinale is caused by a minute negative coccobacillus now designated *Calymmatobacterium granulomatus*. This organism, which has been cultivated only on embryonated eggs or on media that contain egg yolk, is antigenically related to *Klebsiella* species, but its taxonomy remains unclear.

Granuloma inguinale is very rare in the United States but is endemic in socioeconomically deprived tropical and subtropical populations, particularly in South America, the West Indies, India, Africa, and Southeast Asia.

Although the role of sexual transmission of granuloma inguinale has been debated, recent epidemiologic and clinical experience suggests that the disease is usually venereally transmitted. The earliest lesion is an indurated papule that over several days to a few weeks ulcerates. Three types of lesions then may result: (1) virtually painless hyperplastic granulomatous lesions, (2) a chronically ulcerating form, often very painful (Fig. 7-24), or (3) a hypertrophic form that, by chronic obstruction of lymphatic vessels, may lead to genital elephantiasis. Extragenital lesions, such as a multifocal osteomyelitis, are very rare. Microscopically lesions of granuloma inguinale are nonspecific except for the demonstration of minute coccobacillary forms with bipolar hyperchromatic staining in large macrophages (Fig. 7-25).

Diseases caused by spirochetes

The order Spirochaetales includes three genera pathogenic for humans. The genus *Treponema* includes *T. pallidum*, *T. pertenue*, and *T. carateum*, which cause syphilis, yaws, and pinta, respectively. The genus *Borrelia* includes many species or strains that cause relapsing fever. The genus *Leptospira* consists of a large number of immunologically heterogeneous organisms. A single species, *L. interrogans*, is systematically recognized, but the serology is complex, variously recognizing serotypes pathogenic for humans (among other mammals) and groups nonpathogenic for mammals.

Many representatives of this order are not readily cultured on artificial media. They are, moreover, not identifiable in routine stains of sectioned material but require special histologic techniques such as darkfield examination of fresh material or demonstration of organisms by immunofluorescence.

Mechanisms whereby spirochetes damage tissues of the host are not clearly established. Some, such as *Borrelia* or *Leptospira*, are thought to produce hemolysins, to which the destruction of erythrocytes in the appropriate diseases is attributed. No direct toxic mechanism has

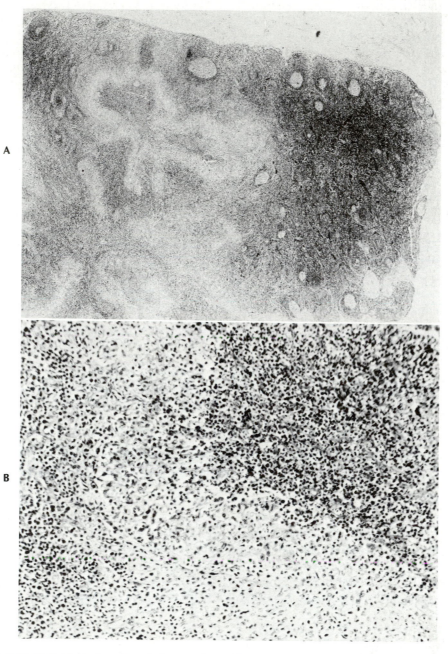

Fig. 7-23. Melioidosis. Lymph node from patient with progressive chronic melioidosis of 15 months' duration. **A,** Irregular "stellate" areas of necrosis. **B,** Small areas of necrosis with borders of epithelioid cells (lymphoid follicle to right). (Hematoxylin and eosin; **A,** 11×; AFIP 68-796; **B,** 67×; AFIP 68-3516.)

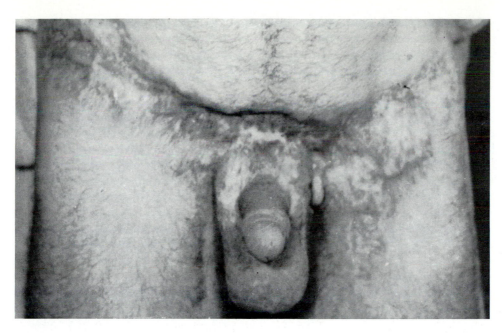

Fig. 7-24. Granuloma inguinale. Bilateral serpiginous ulcers with involvement of inguinal regions and scrotum.

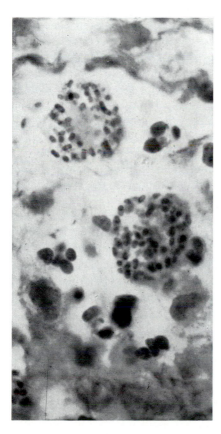

Fig. 7-25. Granuloma inguinale. Donovan bodies within macrophages stain with silver. Because of bipolar staining, "closed safety pin" appearance is observed in many. With this stain, cysts are not easily seen. (Dieterle's silver stain; 1900×; from Torpin, R., Greenblatt, R.B., and Pund, E.R.: Am. J. Surg. **44:**551, 1939.)

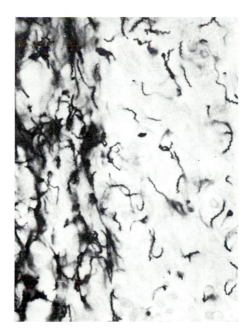

Fig. 7-26. Spirochetes *(Treponema pallidum)* in section from mucous patch of vulva.

been incriminated in diseases produced by *Treponema*. Immunologic response by the host is a major mechanism of tissue injury in this group of diseases.

Syphilis. Syphilis, the archetypal spirochetal disease, is of relatively recent occurrence in humans. Clinical features or lesions attributable to it were not clearly described in Western medicine until the late fifteenth and early sixteenth centuries. The Renaissance epidemiologist and poet Fracastoro left us the name of the disease as that of a shepherd, the protagonist in one of his narrative poems. This systematic designation abjures, or nearly so, ethnic attributions (*morbus gallicus*) as well as many that are more specific ("the great pox" as opposed to smallpox, then a less fearful disease) or euphemistic (*lues*, "plague").

Many historically renowned medical scientists are associated with studies of syphilis: John Hunter, for his autoinoculation experiment, which he misinterpreted as establishing identity between syphilis and gonorrhea; the French physician Villemin, who recognized the unity of the many clinical expressions of syphilis and promulgated the clinical classification, variations of which are basic to discussions of the disease even today; Schaudinn and associates, who first identified the spirochete in syphilitic lesions; and Wasserman and co-workers, who established an immunologic diagnostic procedure based on nonspecific antibodies elaborated during treponemal infection.

T. pallidum, the causative agent of syphilis, is a tightly coiled, regularly spiraling organism 6 to 15 μm in length that moves with a distinctive rhythmicity as viewed in darkfield illumination. It is best demonstrated in sectioned material by silver impregnation (Fig. 7-26). Although *T. pallidium* may preserve viability and infectivity in artificial media for a few days and there is some evidence of replication under these conditions, the organism is regarded as noncultivable by routine methods in artificial media. Experimental infection can be produced in primates and a few other species, but humans are the only natural reservoir. No endotoxin or exotoxin has been attributed to *T. pallidum*. The mechanisms of its pathogenicity are not known; however, the host's immunologic responses appear to be a major factor. Two broad groups of antigens are associated with treponemal infection: (1) a nonspecific group known as reagins and (2) a specific group known as antigen antibodies that immobilize treponemes (treponemal immobilization antibody) and that can be located by immunofluorescence studies. Although *T. pallidum* (the cause of syphilis), *T. pertenue* (the cause of yaws), and *T. carateum* (the cause of pinta) are given species designations, no morphologic or immunologic differences exist among these organisms, however geographically, epidemiologically, or clinically distinctive the respective diseases are.

Except for congenital syphilis, an epidemiologic and clinically distinct problem, and for currently uncommon events such as transfusion of infected blood, syphilis is transmitted by intimate person-to-person contact, usually sexual. The organisms are thought to gain entry into the host through minute subclinical breaks in an epithelial surface, such as that of the glans penis, vulva, vagina, or cervix.

Fourteen to 21 days after infection a painless papule develops at the site of inoculation. This expands peripherally while it ulcerates centrally, producing a circular or ovoid indurated lesion with a clean central ulceration (unless secondarily infected), the chancre of primary syphilis (Plate 1). Hyperplasia of regional lymph nodes reflects lymphatic dissemination of spirochetes in the formation of usually inguinal buboes. One or more bouts of spirochetemia may disseminate organisms throughout the body and precede acquisition of host immunity. Lesions remote from the chancre and regional lymph nodes constitute the outward manifestations of secondary syphilis. It must be emphasized that some of these manifestations may appear before the primary chancre has healed. Within weeks, however, the chancre heals, usually without scarring.

Secondary syphilis produces lesions most conspicuously on mucocutaneous surfaces of the body, especially the skin and oropharynx. At this stage, too, systemic manifestations, generalized lymphadenopathy, and slight fever may occur. Grossly the lesions of secondary syphilis are highly variable and include maculopapular, usually nonpruritic, cutaneous patches characteristically involving the palms and soles (Plate 1). Epithelial proliferation may predominate on moist intertriginous locations, such as about the anus or on the perineum. The result is a lesion known as the condyloma latum (Fig. 7-27).

Microscopically both primary chancres and mucocutaneous secondary lesions manifest distinctly perivascular aggregates of mononuclear cells, particularly plasma cells. Hyperplastic lymph nodes in the secondary stage show marked proliferation of sinus histiocytes and infiltration of mononuclear cells, especially plasma cells about afferent and efferent lymphatics. Treponemes can usually be demonstrated in primary or secondary lesions either by silver impregnation of sectioned material or, more important, by darkfield examination of wet mounted specimens.

Although one or more mucocutaneous relapses may occur during "early syphilis," after 2 years beyond the primary infection such relapses no longer occur (if treatment has been adequate) and the patient enters the clinical stage referred to as late syphilis. Many of these patients remain asymptomatic (although pathologically recognizable lesions may develop) through the rest of their lives and are designated as having late latent syph-

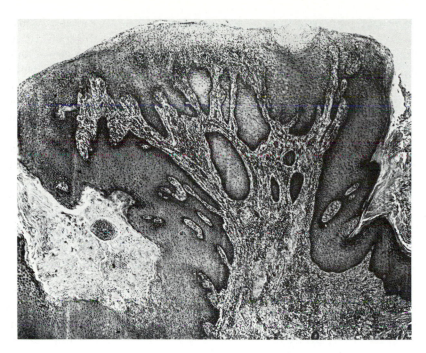

Fig. 7-27. Section from condyloma latum.

ilis. Clinically recognizable manifestations constitute tertiary syphilis, which in turn is classified as benign late syphilis, late cardiovascular syphilis, and late neurosyphilis; the incidence of these tertiary forms among untreated patients observed for many years is 15%, 10%, and 7%, respectively.

Benign late (gummatous) syphilis is characterized by the occurrence of solitary or (more commonly) multiple syphilitic granulomas, known as gummas, in bone or solid viscera, most commonly the liver, brain, or testis. Gummas are circumscribed, rubbery, opalescent, spherical lesions from a few millimeters to several centimeters in diameter. Microscopically the major part of a gumma consists of coagulative necrosis surrounded by a veil of epithelioid cells, lymphocytes, and plasma cells. Treponemes are occasionally demonstrable in gummas, unlike the lesions of late cardiovascular syphilis or late neurosyphilis, in which organisms are rarely identifiable.

Congenital syphilis. Congenital syphilis may develop in the fetus exposed in utero to an episode of maternal spirochetemia. Conventional teaching is that the fetus is subject to congenital syphilis only after about 16 weeks of gestation, when the Langhans layer of the placenta has disappeared. Treponemes have been identified in abortuses as early as 10 to 12 weeks of gestation, so it appears that absence of lesions recognizable as congenital syphilis is a consequence of fetal immunologic nonreactivity rather than exclusion of organisms.

Fetuses with congenital syphilis may die in utero, be born prematurely, or be born alive but with features of congenital infection. Hepatosplenomegaly and lymphad-enopathy are common, as are mucocutaneous lesions, often concentrated about the mouth (rhagades) or anus. Skeletal lesions (periostitis and osteochondritis) are common and account for such clinical features as saber shins and saddle nose. Disturbed dentition (Hutchinson's teeth and peg-shaped, screwdriver-shaped, or pumpkin seed–shaped incisors) is evident when eruption of deciduous teeth occurs.

In solid viscera, histologic maturation is retarded and there is a distinctive, poorly collagenized, interstitial stromal expansion in such organs as the liver, heart, kidney, and pancreas. Treponemes are usually readily identified in fetal tissues and in the placenta. Without treatment, growth failure and marasmus lead to death after a few months to a few years. Long-term survivors may manifest the tertiary signs of acquired syphilis.

Nonvenereal treponematosis. Treponemes are the etiologic agents of a variety of infectious diseases besides venereal (or congenital) syphilis. Although there are no morphologic or immunologic features that distinguish the agents of these diseases from *T. pallidum*, these agents are given specific designations on the basis of epidemiologic features. Thus the agent of yaws is designated *T. pertenue*, that of pinta *T. carateum*, and that of nonvenereal syphilis (bejel) *T. pallidum*. There are diseases of regional, especially tropical, significance with distinctive epidemiologic, geographic, and clinical features but no rigorous microbiologic, serologic, or morphologic distinctions from syphilis. (Salient features are compared with those of syphilis in Table 7-2.) Public health measures have markedly diminished the occurrence of yaws

Table 7-2. Comparative features of treponematoses

	Pinta	Yaws	Nonvenereal syphilis	Venereal syphilis
Usual mode of transmission	Personal contact, arthropods (?)	Personal contact, arthropods (?)	Personal contact, fomites	Venereal
Congenital transmission	No	No	No	Yes
Primary	Yes, skin	Yes, skin	Rare	Skin or mucous membrane
Regional lymphadenopathy	Yes	Yes	Yes	Yes
Secondary lesions	Skin only	Skin, mucous membrane, rare	Skin, mucous membrane	Skin, mucous membrane
Latency	Probably	Yes	Yes	Yes
Tertiary lesions	Yes, but may resemble secondary lesions	Yes	Yes	Yes, visceral
Osseous lesions	No	Yes	Yes	Yes
Nasopharyngeal gummas	No	Yes	Yes	Yes
Aortitis and CNS disease	Undocumented	Undocumented	Undocumented	Yes
Visceral gummas	No	No	No	Yes
Juxta-articular nodules	Questionable	Yes	Yes	Yes
Ocular lesions	Undocumented	Undocumented	Undocumented	Yes

From Binford, C.H., and Connor, D.H., editors: Pathology of tropical and extraordinary diseases, Washington, D.C., 1976, Armed Forces Institute of Pathology. Reproduced with permission.

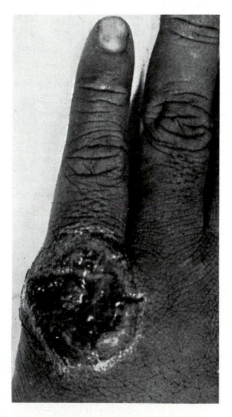

Fig. 7-28. Yaws. Primary lesion (mother yaw or chancre). (Courtesy Dr. Herbert S. Alden, Atlanta, Ga., and Dr. P.D. Gutierrez.)

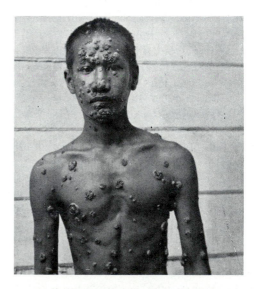

Fig. 7-29. Yaws. Secondary frambesiform lesions. (AFIP 39201.)

and pinta. The specialized literature should be consulted for clinicopathologic details.

Yaws. This disease of the arid tropics usually begins in childhood and progresses to chronic dermatologic and/or orthopedic manifestations in later life (Figs. 7-28 and 7-29).

Pinta. This chronic dermatologic disorder of the tropical Western Hemisphere features areas of cutaneous depigmentation.

Nonvenereal syphilis. This disease goes by a host of local vernacular designations, the most familiar of which is bejel in Arabia, Syria, and Iraq. Cutaneous and osseous lesions resemble those of syphilis.

Diseases caused by Leptospira. Leptospiras are helicoid organisms 6 to 20 μm in length with hooked ends. Some representatives are straight or have single hooks. Leptospiral infections are zoonoses widely distributed throughout the world. At least 180 mammalian species have been described as harboring leptospiras, the most important being rats, swine, dogs, and cattle. Currently a single species, *L. interrogans*, is recognized, of which there are many serologically distinctive variants.

Human leptospirosis results from contact of humans with infected animal products, usually urine with which the human subject comes in contact. In developed societies, therefore, most cases occur among dock workers, sewer workers, slaughterers, and so on. It is not clinically useful to distinguish epidemiologically characteristic leptospiroses by such designations as "Weil's disease," "swineherd's disease," and "swamp disease," since different biovars may be identified in identical epidemiologic situations.

Human leptospirosis is characterized by involvement of many organ systems in an acute febrile illness. Myalgia, focal meningoencephalitis, cutaneous purpura, and hepatic and renal failure may occur. Degenerative lesions in solid viscera (the liver, kidney, myocardium, and skeletal muscle) have been described. Organisms can be demonstrated in infected tissues, especially by silver impregnation techniques.

Diseases caused by Borrelia. Representatives of the genus *Borrelia* are coarsely and irregularly helical gram-negative organisms 10 to 20 μm in length. Some 18 species are distinguished, partially serologically but more importantly by the arthropod vectors (lice or ticks) responsible for their transmission from a primary rodent reservoir to humans. *Borrelia* causes relapsing fever, a clinically nonspecific recurring febrile illness distributed throughout the world but uncommon in the United States or Western Europe. In rare fatal cases foci of necrosis in the liver and kidneys have been described in which organisms can be demonstrated. Splenic microabscesses are typical.

Diseases caused by Spirillum minor and Streptobacillus moniliformis. *Spirillum minor* and *Streptobacillus moniliformis* are unrelated organisms that cause clinically similar diseases. Many cases follow bites of rats, other rodents, or species that eat rodents. *S. minor* is associated with sodoku, a disease chiefly in Japan. *S. moniliformis* causes rat-bite fever, a febrile illness that is accompanied by generalized lymphadenopathy and is distributed throughout the world. Cases lacking histories of rodent bites are designated Haverhill fever, after an outbreak in Haverhill, Massachusetts, attributed to drinking contaminated raw milk. Infections by both organisms are accompanied by rashes. Toxic changes and nonspecific inflammatory lesions in various solid viscera have been described in rare fatal cases.

Synergistic fusospirochetosis. In a variety of synergistic infections occurring in several organ systems, one component is a spirochete variously designated *Treponema* or *Borrelia vincentii*. These infections feature dirty indolent ulcerative processes, which are painful if they occur on mucocutaneous surfaces. Infections are usually found in circumstances of suboptimal local hygiene or other secondary predisposing factors. Examples are genital fusospirochetosis, oropharyngeal fusospirochetosis (trench mouth, Vincent's infection), orofacial gangrene (noma, cancrum oris), and fusospirochetal complications of chronic sinopulmonary infection.

REFERENCES
General

1. Ash, J.E., and Spitz, S.: Pathology of tropical diseases, Philadelphia, 1945, W.B. Saunders Co.
2. Binford, C.H., and Connor, P.H.: Pathology of tropical and extraordinary diseases, Washington, D.C., 1976, Armed Forces Institute of Pathology.
3. Braude, A.I., editor: Medical microbiology and infectious diseases, Philadelphia, 1981, W.B. Saunders Co.
4. Burnett, M.: The natural history of infectious disease, London, 1953, Cambridge University Press.
5. Holmes, W.H.: Bacillary and rickettsial infections, New York, 1940, The Macmillan Co.
6. Mackoweak, P.A.: Microbial synergism in human infections, N. Engl. J. Med. **298:**24, 1978,
7. Mandell, G.L., Douglas, G., Jr., and Bennett, J.E.: Principles and practice of infectious diseases, New York, 1979, John Wiley & Sons, Inc.
8. Margaretten, W., and McAdams, A.J.: An appraisal of fulminant meningococcemia with reference to the Shwartzman phenomenon, Am. J. Med. **25:**868, 1958.
9. Smith, H.: Biochemical challenge of microbial pathogenicity, Bacteriol. Rev. **32:**164, 1968.
10. Symmers, W.S.: Opportunistic infections: the concept of opportunistic infections, Proc. R. Soc. Med. **58:**341, 1965.
11. van Heyningen, W.E., and Arseculeratne, S.N.: Extotoxins, Annu. Rev. Microbiol. **18:**195, 1964.
12. Wehrle, P.F., and Top, F.H., Sr., editors: Communicable and infectious diseases, ed. 9, St. Louis, 1981, The C.V. Mosby Co.
13. Weinstein, L., and Dalton, A.C.: Host determinants of response to antimicrobial agents (concluded), N. Engl. J. Med. **277:**580, 1968.
14. Wilson, G.S., and Miles, A.A.: Topley and Wilson's principles of bacteriology and immunology, ed. 6, Baltimore, 1975, The Williams & Wilkins Co.

Intoxications

15. Brooks, G.F., Bennett, J.V., and Feldman, R.A.: Diphtheria in the United States, 1959-1970, J. Infect. Dis. **129:**173, 1974.
16. Christee, A.B.: The chemical aspects of anthrax, Postgrad. Med. J. **49:**565, 1973.

17. Elder, J.M., and Miles, A.A.: The action of the lethal toxins of gas gangrene clostridia on capillary permeability, J. Pathol. Bacteriol. **74:**133, 1957.
18. Fox, M.D., et al.: Anthrax in Louisiana 1971: epizootiologic study, J. Am. Vet. Med. Assoc. **163:**446, 1974.
19. Marcuse, E.K., and Grand, M.G.: Epidemiology of diphtheria in San Antonio, Texas, 1970, J.A.M.A. **224:**305, 1973.
20. McKenna, V., et al.: Toxic shock syndrome, a newly recognized entity, Mayo Clin. Proc. **55:**63, 1980.
21. Pappenheimer, A.M., Jr., and Gill, D.M.: Diphtheria, Science **182:**353, 1973.
22. Roding, B., Groenveld, P.H.A., and Boerema, I.: Ten years of experience in the treatment of gas gangrene with hyperbaric oxygen, Surg. Gynecol. Obstet. **134:**579, 1972.
23. Schlievert, P., Schoettle, D., and Watson, D.: Purification and physicochemical and biological characterization of a staphylococcal pyrogenic exotoxin, Infect. Immun. **23:**609, 1979.
24. Zalma, V.M., Older, J.J., and Brooks, G.F.: The Austin, Texas, diphtheria outbreak: clinical and epidemiological aspects, J.A.M.A. **211:**2125, 1970.

Noninvasive infections

25. Dupont, H.L., et al.: Immunity in shigellosis (in two parts), J. Infect. Dis. **125:**5, 12, 1972.
26. Dutz, W., and Kohout, E.: Anthrax. In Sommers, S.C., editor: Pathology annual, vol. 6, New York, 1971, Appleton-Century-Crofts.
27. Field, M.: Intestinal secretion: effect of cyclic AMP and its role in cholera, N. Engl. J. Med. **284:**1137, 1971.
28. Finkelstein, R.A.: Cholera, C.R.C. Crit. Rev. Microbiol. **2:**553, 1973.
29. Gitelson, S.: Gastrectomy, achlorhydria, and cholera, Isr. J. Med. Sci. **7:**663, 1971.
30. Goette, D.K.: Gonococcal arthritis, Cutis **11:**337, 1973.
31. Hornick, R.B., et al.: The Broad Street pump revisited: response of volunteers to ingested cholera vibrios, Bull. N.Y. Acad. Med. **47:**1181, 1971.
32. Keusch, G.T., et al.: The pathogenesis of *Shigella* diarrhea. I. Enterotoxin production by *Shigella dysenteriae 1*, J. Clin. Invest. **51:**1212, 1972.
33. Klein, E.J., et al.: Anorectal gonococcal infection, Ann. Intern. Med. **86:**340, 1977.
34. Levine, M.M., et al.: Pathogenicity of *Shigella dysenteriae 1* (Shiga) dysentery, J. Infect. Dis. **127:**261, 1973.
35. Macumber, H.H.: Acute bacillary dysentery: clinico-pathologic study of 263 consecutive cases, Arch. Intern. Med. **69:**624, 1942.
36. McCormack, W.M., et al.: Clinical spectrum of gonococcal infection in women, Lancet **1:**1182, 1977.
37. McMillan, A., et al.: Histology of rectal gonorrhea in men, with a note on anorectal infection with Neisseria meningitis, J. Clin. Pathol. **36:**511, 1983.
38. Penn, C.W., Veale, D.R., and Smith, H.: Selection from gonococci grown *in vitro* of a colony type with some virulence properties of organisms adapted *in vivo*, J. Gen. Microbiol. **100:**147, 1977.
39. Pierce, N.F., Greenough, W.B., and Carpenter, C.C.J., Jr.: *Vibrio cholerae* enterotoxin and its mode of action, Bacteriol. Rev. **35:**1, 1971.
40. Smith, L.W.: Pathologic anatomy of pertussis with special reference to pneumonia caused by pertussis bacillus, Arch. Pathol. **4:**732, 1927.
41. Ward, M.E., Watt, P.J., and Robertson, J.N.: The human fallopian tube: a laboratory model for gonococcal infection, J. Infect. Dis. **129:**650, 1979.
42. Weisner, P.J., et al.: Clinical spectrum of pharyngeal gonococcal infection, N. Engl. J. Med. **288:**181, 1973.
43. Weissman, J.B., et al.: Impact in the United States of the *Shiga* dysentery pandemic of Central America and Mexico: a review of surveillance data through 1972, J. Infect. Dis. **129:**218, 1974.

Pyogenic infections

44. Colebrook, L., and Hare, R.: Anaerobic streptococci associated with puerperal fever, J. Obstet. Gynaecol. Br. Emp. **40:**609, 1933.
45. Cruickshank, C.N.D., and Lowbury, E.J.L.: The effect of pyocyanin on human skin cells and leucocytes, Br. J. Exp. Pathol. **34:**583, 1953.
46. DuPont, H.L., et al.: Pathogenesis of *E. coli* diarrhea, N. Engl. J. Med. **285:**1, 1971.
47. Felner, J.M., and Dowell, V.R.: "Bacteroides" bacteremia, Am. J. Med. **50:**787, 1971.
48. Fetzer, A.E., Werner, A.S., and Hagstrom, J.W.C.: Pathologic features of pseudomonal pneumonia, Am. Rev. Respir. Dis. **96:**1121, 1967.
49. Forkner, C.E., Jr., et al.: *Pseudomonas* septicemia: observations on twenty-three cases, Am. J. Med. **25:**877, 1958.
50. Gaisin, A., and Heaton, C.L.: Chancroid: alias the soft chancre, Int. J. Dermatol. **14:**188, 1975.
51. Gardner, H.L., and Dukes, C.D.: *Haemophilus vaginalis* vaginitis, Am. J. Obstet. Gynecol. **69:**962, 1955.
52. Hamburger, M., and Robertson, O.H.: Studies on pathogenesis of experimental pneumococcus pneumonia in the dog: secondary pulmonary lesions; relationship of bronchial obstruction and distribution of pneumococci to their inception, J. Exp. Med. **72:**261, 1940.
53. Moritz, A.R., and Zamcheck, N.: Sudden and unexpected deaths of young soldiers: diseases responsible for such deaths during World War II, Arch. Pathol. **42:**459, 1946.
54. Powers, G.F., and Boisvert, P.L.: Age as a factor in streptococcosis, J. Pediatr. **25:**481, 1944.
55. Rho, Y.M., and Josephson, J.E.: Epidemic enteropathogenic *Escherichia coli*, Newfoundland, 1963: autopsy study of 16 cases, Can. Med. Assoc. J. **96:**392, 1967.
56. Schaffer, A.J., and Oppenheim, E.H.: *Pseudomonas (pyocyanea)* infection of the gastrointestinal tract in infants and children, South. Med. J. **41:**440, 1948.
57. Wollenman, O.J., Jr., and Finland, M.: Pathology of staphylococcal pneumonia complicating clinical influenza, Am. J. Pathol. **19:**23, 1943.
58. Zinserberg, A.: Dysentery and colienterocolitis: some aspects of pathogenesis and pathological anatomy, Virchows Arch. (Pathol. Anat.) **361:**19, 1973.

Bacillary infections

59. Annotations: listerial infection of the nervous system, Lancet **1:**362, 1968.
60. Balows, A., and Fraser, D.W., editors: International symposium on legionaire's disease, Ann. Intern. Med. **90:**491, 1979.
61. Barber, M., Nellen, M., and Zoob, M.: Erysipeloid of Rosenbach: response to penicillin, Lancet **1:**125, 1946.
62. Bernard, R.P.: The Zermatt typhoid outbreak in 1963, J. Hyg. **63:**537, 1965.
63. Beyt. B.E., et al.: Human pulmonary pasteurellosis, J.A.M.A. **242:**1647, 1979.
64. Bondy, P.K., and Barnwell, C.H.: Chronic typhoid pyonephrosis: report of a case, J. Urol. **57:**642, 1947.
65. Buchner, L.H., and Schneierson, S.S.: Clinical and laboratory aspects of *Listeria monocytogenes* infections: with a report of ten cases, Am. J. Med. **45:**904, 1968.
66. Busch, L.A.: Human listeriosis in the United States, J. Infect. Dis. **123:**328, 1971.
67. Butler, T., et al.: *Yersinia pestis* infection in Vietnam. I. Clinical and hematological aspects, J. Infect. Dis. **129:**578, 1974.
68. Chuttani, H.K., Jain, K., and Misra, R.C.: Small bowel in typhoid fever, Gut **12:**709, 1971.
69. Clasener, H.: Pathogenicity of the L-phase of bacteria, Annu. Rev. Microbiol. **26:**55, 1972.
70. Collins, R.N.: The 1964 epidemic of typhoid fever in Atlanta: clinical and epidemiologic observations, J.A.M.A. **197:**179, 1966.
71. Cox, C.D., and Arbogast, J.L.: Melioidosis, Am. J. Clin. Pathol. **15:**567, 1945.
72. Dannenberg, A.M., Jr., and Scott, E.M.: Melioidosis: pathogenesis and immunity to mice and hamsters. I. Studies with virulent strains of *Malleomyces pseudomallei*, J. Exp. Med. **107:**153, 1958.
73. Delorme, J., et al.: Yersiniosis in children, Can. Med. Assoc. J. **110:**281, 1979.

74. Evans, A.C.: Brucellosis in the United States, Am. J. Public Health **37**:139, 1947.

75. Finegold, M.J.: Pathogenesis of plague: a review of plague deaths in the United States during the last decade, Am. J. Med. **45**:549, 1968.

76. Francis, D.P., Holmes, M.A., and Brandon, G.: *Pasteurella multocida* infections after domestic animal bites and scratches, J.A.M.A. **233**:42, 1975.

77. Francis, E., and Callender, G.R.: Tularemia: microscopic changes of lesions in man, Arch. Pathol. **3**:577, 1927.

78. Gerding, D.N., et al.: *Pasteurella multocida* peritonitis in hepatic cirrhosis with ascites, Gastroenterology **70**:413, 1976.

79. Glick, T.M., et al.: Pontiac fever, an epidemic of unknown etiology in a health department. I. Clinical and epidemiologic aspects, Am. J. Epidemiol. **107**:149, 1978.

80. Goodpasture, E.W., and House, S.J.: Pathologic anatomy of tularemia in man, Am. J. Pathol. **4**:213, 1928.

81. Gray, M.L., and Killinger, A.H.: *Listeria monocytogenes* and listeric infections, Bacteriol. Rev. **30**:309, 1966.

82. Greenwald, G.A., Nash, G., and Foley, F.D.: Acute systemic melioidosis: autopsy findings in four patients, Am. J. Clin. Pathol. **52**:188, 1969.

83. Grieco, M.H., and Sheldon, C.: *Erysipelothrix rhusiopathiae*, Ann. N.Y. Acad. Sci. **174**:523, 1970.

84. Hayfick, L., and Chanock, R.M.: *Mycoplasma* species of man, Bacteriol. Rev. **29**:185, 1965.

85. Hoekenga, M.T.: Plague in Americas, J. Trop. Med. **50**:190, 1947.

86. Hornick, R.B., et al.: Typhoid fever: pathogenesis and immunologic control, N. Engl. J. Med. **283**:686, 1970.

87. Howe, C., and Miller, W.R.: Human glanders: report of 6 cases, Ann. Intern. Med. **26**:93, 1947.

88. Howe, C., Sampath, A., and Spotnitz, M.: The pseudomallei group: a review, J. Infect. Dis. **124**:598, 1971.

89. Hunt, A.C., and Bothwell, P.W.: Histological findings in human brucellosis, J. Clin. Pathol. **20**:267, 1967.

90. Klauder, J.V.: Erysipeloid as an occupational disease, J.A.M.A. **111**:1345, 1938.

91. Kohn, L.A.: Experimental typhoid in man, N. Engl. J. Med. **278**:739, 1968.

92. Lavetter, A., et al.: Meningitis due to *Listeria monocytogenes*: a review of 25 cases, N. Engl. J. Med. **285**:598, 1971.

93. Leino, R., and Kalliomaki, J.L.: Yersiniosis as an internal disease, Ann. Intern. Med. **81**:458, 1974.

94. Mair, I.W., Natuig, K., and Johannessen, T.A.: Otolaryngological manifestations of tularemia, Arch. Otolaryngol. **98**:156, 1973.

95. McDiarmid, A.: Some veterinary aspects of the eradication of brucellosis, Postgrad. Med. J. **49**:526, 1973.

96. Medoff, G., Kunz, L.J., and Weinberg, A.N.: Listeriosis in humans: an evaluation, J. Infect. Dis. **123**:247, 1971.

97. Meyer, K.F.: The natural history of plague and psittacosis, Public Health Rep. **72**:705, 1957.

98. Mollaret, H.H.: Un domaine pathologique nouveau: l'infection à *Yersinia enterocolitica*, Ann. Biol. Clin. **30**:1, 1972.

99. Piggott, J.A.: Demonstration for diagnosis: melioidosis, Int. Pathol. **9**:34, 1968.

100. Pollitzer, R.: Plague, WHO Monogr. Ser., No. 22, 1954.

101. Prost, E., and Riemann, H.: Food-borne salmonellosis, Annu. Rev. Microbiol. **21**:495, 1967.

102. Pullen, R.L., and Stuart, B.M.: Tularemia: analysis of 225 cases, J.A.M.A. **129**:495, 1945.

103. Rubin, H.L., Alexander, A.D., and Yager, R.H.: Melioidosis—a military medical problem, Milit. Med. **128**:538, 1963.

104. Schultz, M.G.: A history of bartonellosis (Carrion's disease), Am. J. Trop. Med. Hyg. **17**:503, 1968.

105. Sheehy, T.W., Deller, J.J., Jr., and Weber, D.R.: Melioidosis, Ann. Intern. Med. **67**:897, 1967.

106. Smith, P.F.: The biology of mycoplasmas, New York, 1971, Academic Press, Inc.

107. Spink, W.W.: The nature of brucellosis, Minneapolis, 1956, University of Minnesota Press.

108. Stuart, B.M., and Pullen, R.L.: Tularemia pneumonia: review of American literature and report of 15 additional cases, Am. J. Med. Sci. **210**:223, 1945.

109. Stuart, B.M., and Pullen, R.L.: Typhoid: clinical analysis of 360 cases, Arch. Intern. Med. **78**:629, 1946.

110. Takeuchi, A.: Electron microscopic studies of experimental *Salmonella* infection. I. Penetration into the intestinal epithelium by *Salmonella typhimurium*, Am. J. Pathol. **50**:109, 1967.

111. Torin, D.E.: A typhoid fever outbreak on a university campus, Arch. Intern. Med. **129**:606, 1969.

112. Typhoid fever (editorial), Lancet **2**:416, 1972.

113. Weber, J., Finlayson, N.B., and Mark, N.B.D.: Mesenteric lymphadenitis and terminal ileitis due to *Yersinia pseudotuberculosis*, N. Engl. J. Med. **283**:172, 1970.

114. White, P.C., Jr.: Brucellosis in a Virginia meat packing plant, Arch. Environ. Health **28**:263, 1974.

115. Zucker-Franklin, D., Davidson, M., and Thomas, L.: The interaction of mycoplasmas with mammalian cells. I. HeLa cells, neutrophils, and eosinophils, J. Exp. Med. **124**:521, 1966.

116. Zucker-Franklin, D., Davidson, M., and Thomas, L.: The interaction of mycoplasmas with mammalian cells. II. Monocytes and lymphocytes, J. Exp. Med. **124**:533, 1966.

Donovanosis

117. Davis, C.M.: Granuloma inguinale: a clinical, histological, and ultrastructural study, J.A.M.A. **211**:632, 1970.

118. Kuberski, T.: Granuloma inguinale (donovanosis), Sex. Transm. Dis. **7**:29, 1980.

119. Stewart, D.B.: Ulcerative and hypertrophic lesions of the vulva, Proc. R. Soc. Med. **61**:363, 1968.

Spirochetal diseases

120. Arean, V.M.: The pathologic anatomy and pathogenesis of fatal human leptospirosis (Weil's disease), Am. J. Pathol. **40**:393, 1962.

121. Beeman, H., et al.: Syphilis: review of the recent literature, 1959-1960, Arch. Intern. Med. **107**:121, 1961.

122. Benirschke, K.: Syphilis—the placenta and the fetus, Am. J. Dis. Child. **128**:142, 1974.

123. Clark, E.G., and Danbolt, N.: The Oslo study of the natural course of untreated syphilis: an epidemiologic investigation based on a restudy of the Boeck-Brussgard material, Med. Clin. North Am. **48**:613, 1964.

124. Guthe, T.: The treponematoses as a world problem, Br. J. Vener. Dis. **36**:67, 1960.

125. Hager, W.D.: Transplacental transmission of spirochetes in congenital syphilis: a new perspective, Sex. Transm. Dis. **5**:122, 1978.

126. Harter, C.A., and Benirschke, K.: Fetal syphilis in the first trimester, Am. J. Obstet. Gynecol. **124**:705, 1976.

127. Hume, J.C.: Worldwide problems in the diagnosis of syphilis and other treponematoses, Med. Clin. North Am. **48**:721, 1964.

128. Jeerapaet, P., and Ackerman, A.B.: Histologic patterns in secondary syphilis, Arch. Dermatol. **107**:373, 1973.

129. Judge, D.M.: Louse-borne relapsing fever in man, Arch. Pathol. **97**:136, 1974.

130. Lees, R.E.M.: A selective approach to yaws control, Can. J. Public Health **64**(suppl. 2): 52, 1973.

131. Marshall, A., and Brown, J.: An unusual case of Vincent's infection of the penis, Br. J. Surg. **48**:340, 1960.

132. Mendelson, R.W.: Pulmonary spirochetosis, J.A.M.A. **146**:727, 1951.

133. Willcox, R.R.: "Epidemiological" treatment in non-venereal and in treponemal diseases, Br. J. Vener. Dis. **49**:107, 1973.

134. Willcox, R.R.: The American perspective, Br. J. Vener. Dis. **50**:404, 1974.

135. Willcox, R.R.: Changing patterns of treponemal disease, Br. J. Vener. Dis. **50**:169, 1974.

CHAPTER 8

Leprosy

CHAPMAN H. BINFORD

DEFINITION, HISTORY, AND PREVALENCE

Leprosy is a chronic infectious disease of humans caused by *Mycobacterium leprae* and affecting chiefly the cooler parts of the body—skin, upper respiratory tract, anterior part of eyes, certain peripheral nerves, and testes.

Although it is probable that leprosy existed at the time of Moses, the description of the lesions recorded in Leviticus does not fit leprosy as it is known today. The Hebrew word *sāra'ath*, which has been translated as "leprosy," probably referred to various severe skin lesions of the nomadic Israelites. Leprosy was widely prevalent in Europe during a period of approximately 1000 years, dating roughly from the fall of the Roman Empire to the fifteenth century.

In 1965 the World Health Organization (WHO) placed the estimated number of cases of leprosy in the world at 10,758,000 (Fig. 8-1). In 1970 WHO stated that 500,000 cases had been registered since the 1965 report. The highest recorded prevalence rates are now in tropical Africa, South America, India, Southeast Asia, the Philippines, and the South Pacific islands. Although most cases at the present time occur in the warm climates, the experience in Europe and Norway has shown that leprosy is not a tropical disease. The spread of leprosy is probably related to living conditions rather than climate. In the United States indigenous cases occur in southeastern Texas, Louisiana, southern Florida, California, and Hawaii. The National Hansen's Disease Center, Carville, Louisiana, has approximately 250 patients under treatment. There is no evidence on which to base valid conclusions on differences in susceptibility among races. In lepromatous leprosy the ratio of males to females affected is generally reported as being around 2:1. In the tuberculoid type no sex differentiation has been found. In areas of high prevalence the greatest number of cases is discovered in the second decade of life. In the United States the greatest number of patients represents those

not showing signs of the disease before adulthood.

During the period 1967 to 1980, 2356 new patients were reported from the continental United States and Hawaii.[22] Approximately 80% were foreign born. Six states reported the majority of cases: California (758), Texas (385), Hawaii (382), New York, principally New York City (227), Florida (71), and Louisiana (59). The influx of refugees from countries with endemic leprosy caused the reported number of cases in the United States to increase from 151 in 1976 to 223 in 1980.

LEPROSY BACILLUS

The leprosy bacillus, *Mycobacterium leprae*, resembles *M. tuberculosis* in morphology and staining, but it can be decolorized more easily by acids. It is stained well by the Fite-Faraco[9] procedure but only poorly by the usual Ziehl-Neelsen technique. *M. leprae* in old lesions may be arranged in compact rounded masses (globi) or may be grouped in a parallel fashion in bundles comparable to the arrangement of cigarettes in a pack. In 1874 Hansen[11] reported the discovery of bacillary bodies in skin lesions, but the cultivation of *M. leprae* in vitro has not yet been acceptably demonstrated.

TRANSMISSION

Traditionally, leprosy is believed to be spread by contact of an infected person with a healthy person without aid of an insect vector or animal host. Indirect contact with recently contaminated objects may play a role. The prevailing opinion is that transmission of the bacilli is through the skin or mucous membrane of the mouth or nose. Patients with moderately advanced or advanced lepromatous leprosy shed numerous bacilli from even minor skin abrasions and in the discharges of the mouth or nose. *M. leprae* in nasal secretions are viable by the mouse footpad test (see below) up to 9 days after drying in open petri dishes.[5] In unbroken skin, bacilli may escape by the hair follicles. Patients with tuberculoid

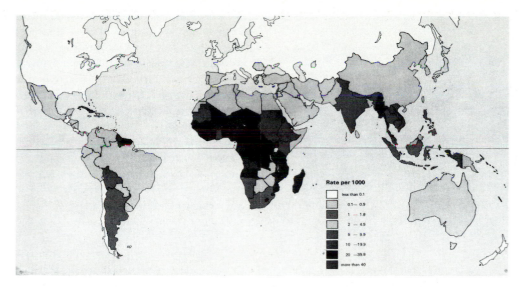

Fig. 8-1. Leprosy throughout the world. (AFIP 75-4786; courtesy Drs. Luiz Bechelli and Dominguez Martinez; from WHO Bulletin, **34:**811, 1966. Reprinted in WHO World Health, October 1971.)

leprosy in reaction also may release many bacilli from skin cuts or abrasions. The attack rate among healthy spouses living with infected mates is usually given as approximately 6%. The prevalence of leprosy in spouses corresponds in general with the belief that approximately only 5% of people the world over are susceptible to leprosy.

The period between exposure and the first signs of the disease is generally believed to be about 3 years. In some patients the disease has not been diagnosed until 10 to 20 years after alleged exposure. In such cases, however, mild lesions may have been overlooked.

Beginning shortly after Hansen discovered the leprosy bacillus, numerous animal transmission experiments were made, but only in recent years, after investigators realized that in humans the leprosy bacillus grew best in the cooler tissues, has success been achieved. Shepard[21] succeeded in establishing multiplication of *M. leprae* in the footpads of mice and thereby provided a valuable method for determining the viability of *M. leprae* in biopsy specimens.

Mild infection with *M. leprae* has been obtained in several species of normal rodents.[1-3] Severe lepromatous infections have been achieved in immunosuppressed[8,19] and in immunodeficient[4] rodents.

The nine-banded armadillo *(Dasypus novemcinctus) is* an excellent laboratory model for lepromatous leprosy. In a large percentage of inoculated animals, a disseminated disease histopathologically resembling human leprosy, including nerve infection, develops. Presumably because of the body temperature, 32° to 35° C, viscera in the armadillo are more severely involved than occurs in human leprosy.

LEPROSY AS A ZOONOSIS[24]

An indigenous leprosy-like disease was found in armadillos captured in Louisiana. The disease cannot be distinguished histopathologically, bacteriologically, or immunologically from that seen in armadillos inoculated with *M. leprae* from lepromatous patients. In a survey of 451 wild armadillos in Texas, Smith[21a] found that 4.66% had lepromatous leprosy. Armadillos, being highly susceptible to leprosy, may have become infected from discarded dressings of patients who lived at home before effective sulfone therapy was used. There was one report of a patient with lepromatous leprosy in the United States who, many years before the diagnosis, had captured and dressed many armadillos for cooking at home.[10] This patient had no known contact with leprosy patients.

Two primates from Africa used in U.S. laboratories have developed lepromatous leprosy, possibly from exposure to untreated leprosy patients before being sold to dealers. Leininger and co-workers[16] at the University of Iowa discovered that a chimpanzee from Sierra Leone had advanced lepromatous leprosy. Unfortunately, this animal died following anesthesia for blood collection. At the Delta Regional Primate Research Center in Covington, Louisiana, a mangabey monkey from Africa with advanced lepromatous leprosy is being studied (Fig. 8-2).[17] Before beginning antileprosy treatment to prevent death, transmission of the infection to several other mangabey monkeys has been successful.

While the presence of many indigenously infected armadillos in Louisiana establishes leprosy as an endemic zoonotic disease in that state, there is insufficient information on leprosy in wild primates to consider them as a reservoir for leprosy at this time.

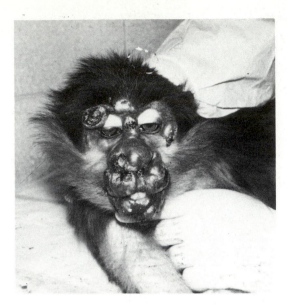

Fig. 8-2. Numerous ulcerated lesions on face of mangabey monkey with lepromatous leprosy. (AFIP 80-9993-2.)

CLASSIFICATION

The Sixth International Congress of Leprosy in 1953 classified leprosy into two principal types: *lepromatous* and *tuberculoid*. Cases not falling into these principal types were classified into two groups: *indeterminate* and *borderline*. Subsequent congresses, the last in 1978, have not changed the classification.

The lepromatous and tuberculoid types represent the opposite poles of lack of resistance and resistance in the host, respectively. In lesions of lepromatous leprosy, great numbers of bacilli occupy histiocytes (Fig. 8-5, *C*). In advanced cases almost the entire skin area is affected. In tuberculoid leprosy, a few bacilli, or products of bacilli, excite severe tissue reaction of the epithelioid cell granulomatous type (Fig. 8-7, *D*).

Ridley and Jopling[19a] divided the spectrum of leprosy into five groups based on the patient's ability to mount cellular resistance to *M. leprae*. These are tuberculoid (TT), borderline tuberculoid (BT), borderline (BB), borderline lepromatous (BL), and lepromatous (LL). The tuberculoid and lepromatous groups are stable both clinically and histopathologically. The borderline groups, being unstable, may shift toward either pole during the course of the disease.

Indeterminate leprosy (Fig. 8-9) is an early stage of the disease in which neither the clinical nor the histopathologic features have become well established.

The first responsibility of the pathologist is to make or rule out a diagnosis of leprosy, but because each type of leprosy requires a different treatment and management, the specific classification is important. If assistance is needed, the pathologist should consult with a colleague experienced in the recognition and treatment of leprosy.

Lepromin test. In 1919 Mitsuda introduced a skin test employing an antigen of heat-treated lepromatous tissue.[12] This test is very useful in classifying the types of disease in patients with known leprosy, but *it is not a diagnostic test* because it is positive in many people who have never been exposed to leprosy. It is considered an indication of host resistance to *M. leprae*. The lepromin test is negative in patients with lepromatous leprosy, but in patients with tuberculoid leprosy there is an early erythematous reaction in 24 to 28 hours (Fernández test[7]) and a delayed nodular epithelioid cell granulomatous reaction after 3 to 4 weeks (Mitsuda test). Lepromin is not available commercially.

CLINICAL FEATURES

The patient with *lepromatous* leprosy may have a variety of lesions ranging from slightly erythematous macules to papules, nodules, plaques, or diffuse infiltrations (Fig. 8-3, *B* and *D*). Typically, the borders of lepromatous lesions are not sharply defined. Lesions tend to become confluent, and as the disease progresses, almost the entire skin becomes involved. The lesions of lepromatous leprosy are hypesthetic, and old lesions may be anesthetic. Sensory disturbance, however, is not so distinct as in tuberculoid leprosy. In *tuberculoid* leprosy (Fig. 8-4, *B*), depending on skin color, the mild lesions are sharply defined, hypopigmented or slightly erythematous macules in which there is distinct impairment of sensation. During increased activity, the borders of these lesions may become elevated and erythematous, while the centers remain flat and hypopigmented. In some patients, plaquelike lesions may occur during increased activity.

A *borderline lesion* begins as a macule that develops into a plaque with an elevated center and sloping periphery. Later the central area flattens and becomes hypesthetic or anesthesic, and the circinate or serpiginous borders become elevated and slope into the adjacent normal skin. Borderline lesions with predominant tuberculoid features are called borderline tuberculoid (BT). Those with predominantly lepromatous changes are classified borderline lepromatous (BL). The lepromin test may be weakly positive. Indeterminate leprosy may first present as a nonelevated disc-shaped pink or hypopigmented skin area as small as 1 cm in diameter but usually 2 or 3 cm. In some patients indeterminate lesions may be hypesthetic or anesthetic. The lepromin test may be negative or positive.

Lucio or *spotted leprosy* is an interesting variety of lepromatous leprosy first reported in 1852 by Lucio and Alvarado.[16a] Latapi and Chevez Zamora[15] described its clinical and histologic features. This form, occurring principally in patients of Mexican origin, is characterized by diffuse involvement of the skin without discrete lesions. In some of these patients, a necrotizing vasculitis causes multiple small ulcers.

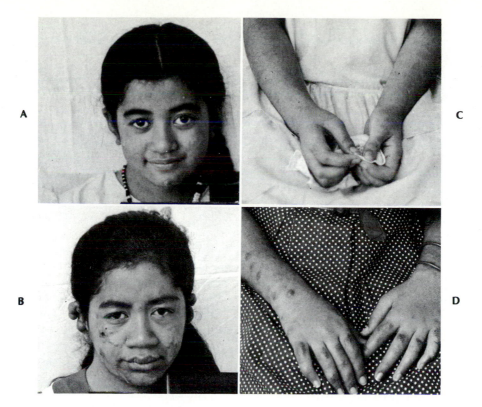

Fig. 8-3. Lepromatous leprosy. **A,** Hawaiian girl, 11 years of age, with early lepromatous leprosy. Hypopigmented, inconspicuous lesions can be seen on cheeks and chin. **B,** Same girl at 13 years of age. Observe nodular thickening of right ear, lesions of cheeks and chin, and conspicuous change in facial appearance. Diffuse infiltration of skin by lepra cells caused thickening of skin that distorted face. **C,** Forearms and hands when patient was 11 years of age. No lesions are definitely evident. **D,** Hands when patient was 13 years of age. In 2-year period, nodular lesions have developed in skin of right forearm and fingers. In addition, there is diffuse thickening of entire skin of forearm resulting from infiltration by lepra cells.

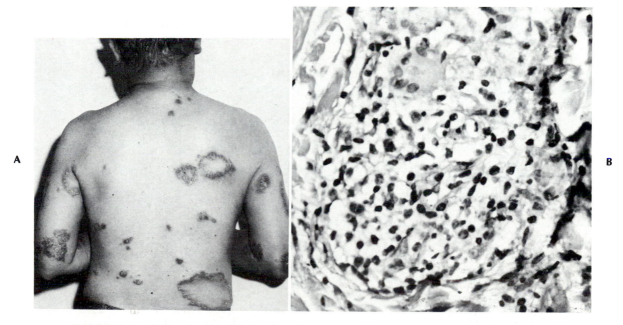

Fig. 8-4. A, Borderline leprosy. Lesions have hypopigmented and hypesthetic centers. Elevated borders are erythematous. Inner margins of ring lesions are sharp, whereas outer margins slope into normal skin. Exacerbation of these lesions appeared shortly after this Filipino man arrived in United States to attend school. **B,** Borderline leprosy, midzone, with tuberculoid features. Nerves in this section showed mild round cell infiltrate and many phagocytes with bacilli. (440×; AFIP 72-12458.)

Erythema nodosum. A common and disabling complication of lepromatous leprosy, especially in patients receiving sulfone therapy, is erythema nodosum, which in leprosy patients is called erythema nodosum leprosum (ENL). An ENL episode is characterized by a simultaneous outcropping of erythematous, deep, tender nodules, sometimes covering the entire body, that disappear in a week or two. Multiple or recurrent attacks are not uncommon. Histopathologically, the lesions are located in the lower dermis and adjacent subcutis and consist of focal infiltration of neutrophils and other inflammatory cells in older preexisting lepromatous tissue. There are vascular changes such as edema, endothelial swelling, and, in many lesions, an allergic type of vasculitis. ENL resembles the Arthus reaction and is thought to result from antigen released from dead *M. leprae* organisms. Even after lesions become bacteriologically negative by acid-fast techniques, the persisting intracellular dead bacilli may cause ENL to continue.

Amyloidosis. Before effective sulfone treatment was used, amyloidosis was a serious complication of lepromatous leprosy in some countries. Powell and Swan,[18] in reviewing 50 consecutive autopsies of patients dying at the U.S. Public Health Service Hospital, Carville, from September 1948 through April 1954, found secondary amyloidosis in 23 patients. Renal insufficiency secondary to amyloidosis was the cause of death in 38%. Although sulfone therapy was being used at Carville during this period, in many patients the disease was well advanced before effective treatment was started.

In 103 autopsies at the Palo Seco Leprosarium in the Canal Zone, Kean and Childress[13] found amyloidosis of the kidneys in four cases. They stressed the high incidence of glomerulonephritis.

HISTOPATHOLOGY

The two principal types of leprosy and the two remaining groups have characteristic histopathologic features.

Lepromatous type. Skin lesions in lepromatous leprosy result from the proliferation of histiocytes (macrophages) that first form small infiltrations around blood vessels, nerves, and dermal glands and, in more advanced cases, replace almost the entire dermis (Fig. 8-5, *A*). The infiltrate of lepromatous leprosy, although so prolific that nodules may result, characteristically does not encroach on the basal layer of the epidermis but is separated from it by a thin band of sparsely cellular stroma (clear zone). In advanced lesions the epidermis is thinned over nodular lesions, rete ridges are absent, and papillae are flattened. The thinned, stretched epithelium over nodules

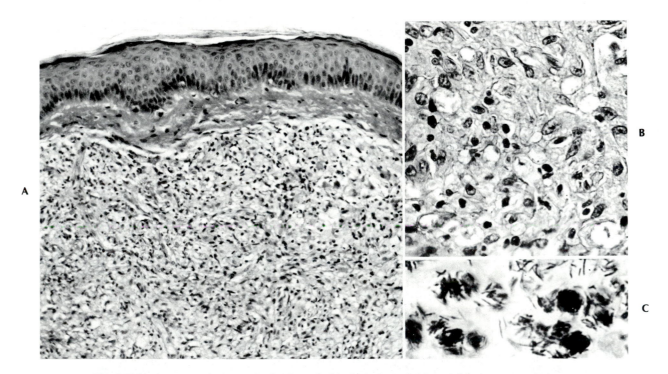

Fig. 8-5. Lepromatous leprosy. **A,** Section of skin in lesion of advanced lepromatous leprosy. Observe nearly total replacement of entire dermis by massive infiltrate but no encroachment on basal part of epidermis. **B,** Lepromatous infiltrate. Cells are histiocytes (lepra cells); many show no vacuolization, but in **C** observe cells filled with bacilli. **C,** Lepromatous infiltrate stained by Fite-Faraco acid-fast technique. Green filter was used. Jet black structures are bacilli, nearly all within cells. (**A** and **B,** Hematoxylin and eosin; **A,** 145×; AFIP 65-1653; **B,** 400×; **C,** 1600×; AFIP 54-17674.)

may break, resulting in ulceration. The histiocytes offer almost no resistance to the growth of the bacilli, so that eventually as the disease progresses, the entire skin bed may become infiltrated by macrophages, which serve to accommodate the multiplying bacilli (Fig. 8-5, *B*). The histiocytes are supported by a delicate stroma vascularized by a rich network of capillaries. Other inflammatory cells are not prominent in these lesions.

"Aging" histiocytes contain many bacilli and exhibit lipid vacuolization. The name *Virchow lepra cell* is commonly applied to these old, foamy histiocytes. Acid fast–stained slides, if a satisfactory method is used, in the moderately advanced and advanced lesions demonstrate numerous bacilli within the histiocytes (lepra cells) (Fig. 8-5, *C*). Characteristically, as previously mentioned, bacilli are frequently arranged in parallel ("cigarette packs") and in the older lesions are seen in compact globular masses (globi) that eventually replace the entire intracellular structures. When the cell walls are destroyed, the freed bacilli may coalesce to form large, compact, rounded masses that frequently are found in foreign body giant cells (giant globi). In lepromatous leprosy the bacilli generally are present in large numbers within the small skin nerves. The infected nerves may show very little histopathologic change other than the increased number of histiocytes and Schwann cells in which the bacilli are found. Bacilli may be seen in macrophages in the walls and endothelial cells of blood vessels, and in the epithelial cells of hair follicles, but are rarely observed within the cells of sweat or sebaceous glands.

In effectively treated lepromatous leprosy the intracellular bacilli lose acid fastness but may be well demonstrated by Gomori methenamine-silver stain (GMS) if the time in the silver solution is slightly prolonged. The persistence for long periods of these dead bacilli and their fragments accounts for the slow resolution of lepromatous lesions.

Tuberculoid type. In contrast to the lack of host resistance that distinguishes lepromatous leprosy, the skin lesion in tuberculoid leprosy exhibits much cellular evidence of intense host resistance (Fig. 8-6). The characteristic reaction is that of the production of epithelioid cells, which usually are arranged in clusters or cords and may or may not contain Langhans' giant cells. Tuberculoid leprosy of the skin histopathologically resembles Boeck's sarcoid (Fig. 8-7, *D*), tuberculosis without caseation, and other diseases in which the host reaction is that of epithelioid granulomas with Langhans' giant cells. The infiltrate of tuberculoid leprosy extends into the papillary stroma up to the basal cells of the epidermis (Fig. 8-8, *A*). Thus, in contrast to lepromatous lesions, there is no "clear zone" between the infiltrate and the overlying epidermis. Lymphocytes in considerable numbers may border the epithelioid cell granulomas.

In this form of the disease, small dermal nerves generally show severe histopathologic involvement (Fig. 8-8, *B*). The infiltrate of the small nerves may consist of epithelioid cells or cells indistinguishable from lymphocytes. In tuberculoid lesions of the skin, nerve destruction occurs early. Therefore in more advanced lesions no nerves may be seen in the histopathologic sections. The absence of nerves in a granulomatous skin lesion should

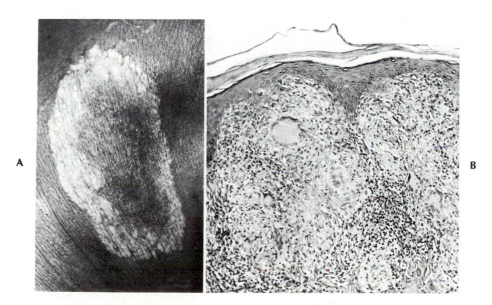

Fig. 8-6. A, Tuberculoid leprosy on back of Zairian woman. Margins are distinct and papillary. Lesion is anesthetic. **B,** Tuberculoid leprosy. Compact infiltrate is composed of epithelioid cells, Langhans' giant cells, and lymphocytes. There is no clear zone as in lepromatous leprosy, but infiltrate extends to and erodes basal layer of epidermis. (84×; AFIP 72-12465.)

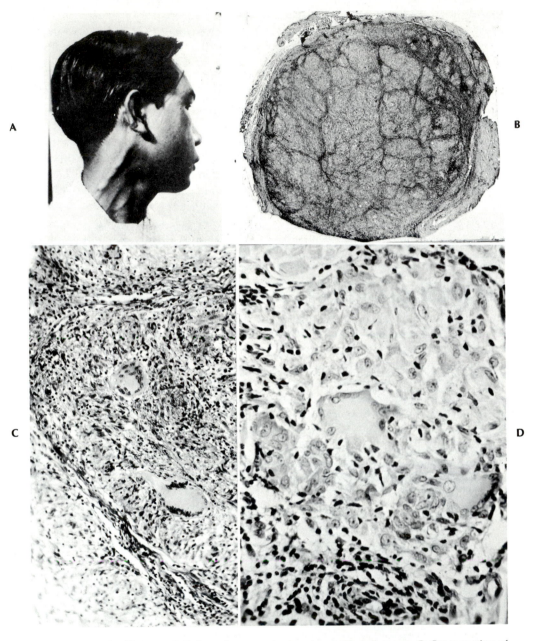

Fig. 8-7. Tuberculoid leprosy. **A,** Enlarged great auricular nerve in Hawaiian man. **B,** Cross section of enlarged nerve in tuberculoid leprosy. Almost entire nerve is replaced by epithelioid cell granulomatous infiltration. Few bacilli are seen. **C,** High magnification of section of nerve in tuberculoid leprosy showing epithelioid cells, Langhans' giant cells, and lymphocytes. **D,** Epithelioid cell granuloma with Langhans' giant cells in skin lesion of tuberculoid leprosy. Observe similarity to nodular granulomas seen in Boeck's sarcoid. (Hematoxylin and eosin; **B,** 9½×; AFIP 55-10845; **C,** approximately 100×; **D,** approximately 200×.)

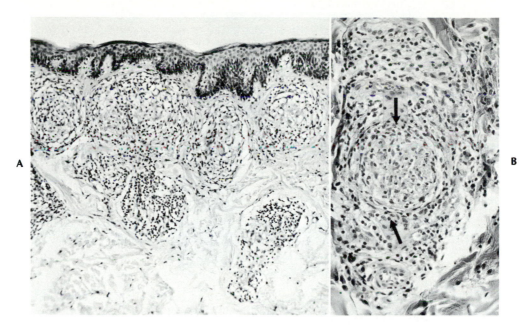

Fig. 8-8. Tuberculoid leprosy. **A,** Section of skin showing early tuberculoid leprosy. Observe small epithelioid cell granulomas, one with giant cell, and lymphocytes surrounding granulomas. Infiltrate extending into papillae. **B,** Small nerve in tuberculoid leprosy *(between arrows)* enveloped and almost completely infiltrated by epithelioid cells. Bacilli are usually absent on single section, but searching many sections stained by Fite-Faraco method reveals occasional bacillus. (Hematoxylin and eosin; **A,** 210×; AFIP 56-19556; **B,** approximately 200×; AFIP 658941.)

cause a pathologist to suspect leprosy. In the chronic tuberculoid lesion, even with prolonged search, bacilli are found with great difficulty or not at all. Bacilli, if present, are usually within small nerves, and then only two or three bacilli may be found in an entire section. In reactive tuberculoid leprosy, however, a fairly large number of bacilli may be observed in the edematous epithelioid cell infiltrate as well as in the nerves.

Indeterminate group. The histopathologic features in lesions of the indeterminate group are nonspecific. The pathologist may make the diagnosis of mild, nonspecific, chronic dermatitis (Figs. 8-9 and 8-10, *A*). The lack of characteristic changes in the lesions of the indeterminate group is probably attributable to the fact that the process is too early for development of the features on which types are based. The usual finding is that of a mild degree of round cell infiltration located around the small vessels of skin appendages. Small nerves, although generally intact, may show infiltration by round cells. In the indeterminate group, bacilli may be found in nerves that otherwise appear normal (Fig. 8-10, *B*). The demonstration of acid-fast bacilli in a lesion of this group enables the pathologist to make a diagnosis of leprosy (Fig. 8-10, *C*).

Borderline group. In the borderline or dimorphous group, a single slide may contain infiltrates of macrophages containing many bacilli and focal aggregates of epithelioid cells with few, if any, bacilli. The nerves may reveal varying degrees of cellular involvement and usually contain bacilli.

HISTOID VARIETY OF LEPROMATOUS LEPROSY

In 1963 Wade[23] described in patients with relapsed lepromatous leprosy sharply circumscribed nodules that clinically and histopathologically resembled dermatofibromas. They frequently protruded upward to produce dome-shaped or pedunculated tumors elevated 0.5 cm or more above the surface of the surrounding skin (Fig. 8-11, *A*). Simulating fibromas, they were composed of whorls and fascicles of spindle cells (Fig. 8-11, *B*). Characteristically, the spindle cells were crowded with long, well-stained, acid-fast bacilli that frequently were arranged parallel to the long axis of the cell (Fig. 8-11, *C*). Rodriguez,[20] who observed histoid lesions in 28 of 72 patients with relapsed lepromatous leprosy, theorized that the bacilli in the lesions were mutants of *M. leprae* that had become resistant to diaminodiphenylsulfone (DDS), the drug now universally used in the treatment of leprosy.

NERVE INVOLVEMENT

A salient feature of *M. leprae* is its predilection for peripheral nerves. It appears to be the only bacterium causing human disease that regularly invades nerves. Nerve involvement occurs in all patients with leprosy of any form. In the skin lesions of all types small nerves are regularly infected. The large peripheral nerves that lie nearest to the skin surface are common sites of involvement. These are the ulnar at or near the elbow, the great auricular over the neck (Fig. 8-7, *A* and *B*), the peroneal,

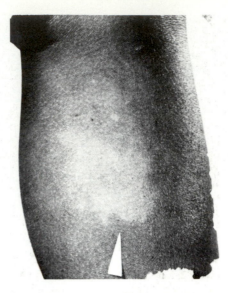

Fig. 8-9. Lesion of indeterminate leprosy on leg of Filipino patient. Lesion is now flat and hypopigmented but earlier was probably erythematous. (AFIP 74-9029-1.)

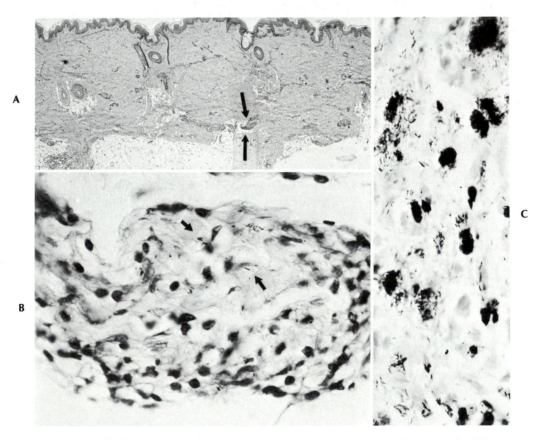

Fig. 8-10. Indeterminate leprosy, unrecognized. **A,** Skin of boy 6 years of age. Histopathologic diagnosis was chronic, mild dermatitis. At 14 years of age, condition was diagnosed as advanced lepromatous leprosy, at which time study of slides made 8 years before revealed several acid-fast bacilli in small dermal nerve *(arrows)*. **B,** Nerve is that shown in **A** but stained for acid-fast bacilli. Observe increased number of nuclei within nerves. *Arrows,* Well-defined bacilli. **C,** Section of skin lesion of patient at 14 years of age when diagnosis of advanced lepromatous leprosy was made. Photograph taken with green filter. All black material represents acid-fast bacilli, usually in globular masses. (**A,** Hematoxylin and eosin, 16×; AFIP 63-2022; **B** and **C,** Fite-Faraco stain; **B,** 650×; AFIP 32-0211; **C,** 1100×; AFIP 59-255.)

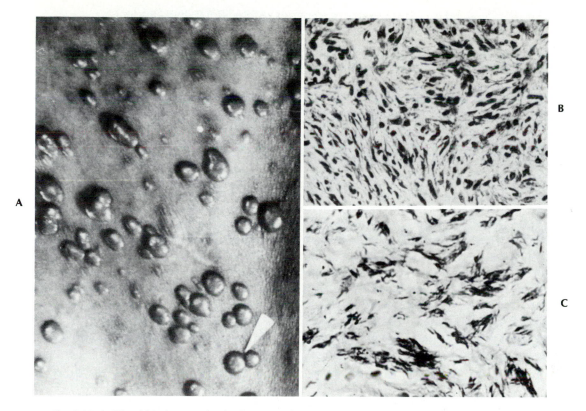

Fig. 8-11. A, Histoid lesions on back of 35-year-old Filipino patient with lepromatous leprosy who had received sulfone therapy regularly for 4 years and intermittently for following 5 years. *Arrow,* Lesion on which biopsy was performed. **B,** Hematoxylin and eosin–stained section of typical histoid lesion. Observe fascicular arrangement of spindle cells that cause lesion to resemble dermatofibroma. **C,** Fite-Faraco- and acid-fast-stained section showing presence of large numbers of *Mycobacterium leprae* in spindle cells that compose lesion. Note that bacilli usually are arranged parallel to long axis of spindle cells. (**A,** From Rodriguez, J.N.: Int. J. Leprosy 37:1, 1969; **B,** 175×; **C,** 530×.)

and small branches of the radial and ulnar nerves around the wrist. In the less advanced cases of either type, nerve involvement may be seen only on microscopic examination. However, generally in moderate and in advanced cases, nerves may be visibly and palpably enlarged.

The clinical examination of any patient suspected of having leprosy must include the palpation of the superficial nerves to determine if there is an enlargement. The histopathologic changes observed in the larger nerves follow those of the skin lesions for that corresponding type. In lepromatous leprosy histiocytes containing bacilli may replace a part of the nerve trunk and involve the perineural stroma. In the tuberculoid form, epithelioid cell granulomas may replace the intraneural structures (Fig. 8-7, *C*). The result of the involvement of either type may be total anesthesia of the skin and paresis or paralysis of the muscles supplied by the nerves. Especially in India, nerve abscesses of the caseous type involving peripheral nerves may resemble caseous abscesses caused by *M. tuberculosis*.

In some individuals, there may be no evident skin lesions, the manifestations of disease being confined entirely to one or more peripheral nerves.

Nerve involvement is responsible for many of the severe deformities that occur in leprosy and therefore may have been largely responsible for the great fear of this disease. Paralysis, caused by neural destruction, results in the masklike face, inability to close the eyes, claw-hand, and drop-foot. Because of anesthesia, patients may be unaware of cuts, puncture wounds, bruises, and burns of the skin of the feet or hands. Secondary infection from wounds in the anesthetic skin may extend into the underlying soft tissues and bone. Also probably caused by nerve involvement is the so-called concentric atrophy that results in the digits becoming narrowed and shortened and, in advanced cases, finally absorbed.

TEMPERATURE SELECTIVITY

M. leprae appears to grow best in parts of the body that are relatively cool. These are the prominences of the skin, the ears, the nose, the mucous membrane of the upper respiratory tract, especially that of the turbinates and septum of the nose, the anterior part of the eye, the testes, the lymph nodes draining the skin, and the nerve trunks that are near the skin surface. Although leprosy bacilli are readily demonstrated in monocytes of the blood of patients with advanced lepromatous leprosy, visceral lesions are never prominent. The reticuloendothelial cells of the liver, spleen, and adrenal gland phagocytose circulating bacilli; therefore microscopic aggregates of lepra cells are found in these organs. However, these lesions generally appear nonprogressive and rarely can be seen with the naked eye. Reticuloendothelial cells of lymph nodes draining the liver may contain many bacilli. In active, advanced lepromatous leprosy biopsy or autopsy specimens of various organs may show leprosy bacilli in a few histiocytes, but there is no evidence of progressive lesions in these viscera. Although the larynx may be severely involved in untreated advanced cases, leprosy does not involve the lower trachea and lungs. There has not been definite proof that leprosy involves the gastrointestinal tract, brain, or spinal cord. Orchitis caused by *M. leprae* is regularly seen in moderately advanced and advanced cases of lepromatous leprosy. The end results of leprosy of the testes are hyalinization of the seminiferous tubules and replacement of the lumina of the tubules and interstitial tissues by lepromatous infiltrates. This testicular involvement is in sharp contrast to the absence of lesions in the ovary, in which definite disease has not been observed, although in an ovary removed from a patient during an acute exacerbation of lepromatous leprosy, foci of a few lepra cells were seen.

In lepromatous leprosy destructive cystic osteitis caused by *M. leprae* is occasionally observed in the bones of the hand and foot but not in the larger bones. Bone marrow aspirated from patients with advanced lepromatous leprosy usually contains bacilli in small groups of lepra cells, but larger lesions have not been reported.

Involvement of the relatively cooler parts of the upper respiratory tract is regularly seen in patients with lepromatous leprosy in whom the nose is affected, and in those with more advanced disease in whom the mouth and larynx are involved. The histopathologic picture of these lesions is that of a profuse development of histiocytes containing bacilli (lepra cells) immediately beneath the transitional epithelium. Because of the loose structure of this epithelium, even when gross ulceration has not occurred, there is a constant shedding of bacilli that contaminate the nasal discharge and sputum, thereby providing one method for spreading bacilli from a person with active leprosy to healthy people.

In untreated lepromatous patients severe lesions may occur in the cornea, iris, and ciliary body, with resulting impairment or loss of sight. The affected parts are relatively cooler than the retina and optic nerve, which have not been definitely shown to be infected with *M. leprae*.

LYMPH NODE INVOLVEMENT

Lymph nodes draining cutaneous lesions of lepromatous leprosy histopathologically may be largely replaced by foamy histiocytes filled with bacilli, but enlargement is only moderate.

In tuberculoid leprosy epithelioid cell granulomatous lesions may be seen in the lymph nodes draining the affected skin. The histopathologic reaction in these nodes resembles that seen in sarcoidosis.

IMMUNOLOGY

Cell-mediated immune responses are now receiving much attention in leprosy research. Apparently the clinical type of leprosy with its histopathologic counterpart is dependent on the capacity of host cells to resist the leprosy bacillus by the proliferation of lymphocytes and epithelioid cells. The failure of these cells to respond when challenged by the leprosy bacillus enables the bacillus to proliferate freely in the macrophages of the patient, and clinical lepromatous leprosy results.

In lepromatous leprosy, in addition to the negative lepromin reaction, the patients show other defects in their ability to respond to certain antigens. Approximately only 50% of lepromatous patients can be sensitized to dinitrochlorobenzene (DNCB). There are several reports that lepromatous patients reject heterologous skin grafts more slowly than do normal people. Experiments designed to enhance resistance in lepromatous patients by the administration of transfer factor from tuberculoid or from normal, lepromin-positive individuals have been undertaken but as yet results are inconclusive.

In lepromatous leprosy there is no depression in the development of humoral antibodies. Hyperglobulinemia is a common finding, and some patients have immunologic features similar to those occurring with autoimmune diseases such as rheumatoid arthritis or lupus erythematosus.

Total numbers of T lymphocytes are decreased in lepromatous leprosy, and the defect in cell-mediated immunity to *M. leprae* seems to be in the area of T lymphocyte formation.

LABORATORY DIAGNOSIS

The finding of acid-fast bacilli in packets or in globular masses in smears of skin lesions will confirm a clinical diagnosis of leprosy. At the Armed Forces Institute of Pathology (AFIP) indeterminate leprosy is diagnosed histopathologically *only* if acid-fast bacilli are seen *within nerves*. Because of the possibility of obtaining other acid-fast bacilli from the nasal mucosa, nasal scrapings should not be used in a primary diagnostic procedure.

The moderately advanced or advanced lepromatous skin lesion can be diagnosed histopathologically if the infiltrate contains lepra cells with bacilli characteristically arranged in packets or globi and if persisting nerves contain bacilli. The diagnosis of borderline and tuberculoid leprosy must be based on typical histopathologic patterns plus nerve involvement. In all types of leprosy the finding of acid-fast bacilli in nerves is pathognomonic.

Skin smears, obtained by splitting the skin and scraping the cut edges of the dermis, may be successfully stained by the techniques used for *M. tuberculosis* on sputum smears. Special techniques such as the Fite-Faraco[9] stain must be used for adequate staining of tissue sections. A clinical diagnosis should be confirmed by histopathologic examination, if practical. Especially in non-endemic areas, biopsy examination should be done for medicolegal documentation, even in patients with advanced disease.

The fear of leprosy, irrespective of geographic location or race, is so deeply ingrained that a diagnosis of leprosy even in its mildest form may stigmatize a patient to such a degree that he or she can never again lead a normal life. A histopathologist uncertain of the diagnosis or inexperienced in the recognition and treatment of leprosy should obtain help from more experienced colleagues. Diagnoses "compatible with" or "consistent with" leprosy should *not be made* because of the stigmatizing potential of such a diagnosis for a person without leprosy and also to prevent possible malpractice action.

DIFFERENTIAL DIAGNOSIS

As was emphasized with syphilis in earlier years, leprosy lesions clinically and histopathologically may mimic many other diseases. At the AFIP, when establishing a diagnosis of leprosy histopathologically in any form in either humans or animals, *intraneural cellular and/or bacterial involvement must be demonstrated.* This is especially needed when sarcoidosis is considered and when skin lesions caused by atypical or anonymous mycobacteria must be distinguished from leprosy.

LEPROSY CONTROL

After the administration of effective therapy with dapsone (DDS), chlorfazamine, or rifampin, *M. leprae* in suspensions obtained from patients with lepromatous leprosy who are under treatment will no longer reproduce in mouse footpads and therefore these patients are not considered infectious. In most countries leprosy patients are no longer subject to compulsory segregation and are treated as outpatients. In the United States physicians responsible for treatment of a newly diagnosed patient should consult the municipal or state health authorities for advice on management. Physicians needing advice on recognition, management, and treatment of leprosy should call the Medical Officer in Charge, National Hansen's Disease Center (formerly U.S. Public Health Service Hospital), Carville, LA 70721, telephone (504) 642-7771.

Consultation on histopathologic diagnosis may be obtained from the Armed Forces Institute of Pathology, Washington, DC 20306, Attention: Leprosy Registry, or from the National Hansen's Disease Center, Carville, LA 70721.

With requests for histopathologic consultation, the pathologist should send (to either institution) full name and age of patient, description of lesion and history, one hematoxylin and eosin–stained slide of each specimen, and four unstained slides or blocks of each specimen.

REFERENCES

1. Binford, C.H.: The problem of transmission of *M. leprae* to animals, Transactions of the Leonard Wood Memorial–Johns Hopkins University Symposium on Research in Leprosy, Baltimore, 1961.
2. Binford, C.H.: Studies on a mycobacterium obtained from the golden hamster (*Cricetus auratus*) after inoculation with lepromatous tissue, Lab. Invest. **11**:942, 1962.
3. Binford, C.H.: The transmission of *M. leprae* to animals: attempts to find an experimental model (abstract), Int. J. Lepr. **36**:599, 1968.
4. Colston, M.J., and Hilson, G.R.F.: Growth of *Mycobacterium leprae* and *M. marinum* in congenitally athymic (nude) mice, Nature **262**:399, 1976.
5. Desikan, K.V.: Viability of *Mycobacterium leprae* outside the human body, Lepr. Rev. **48**:231, 1977.
6. Feldman, R.A., and Hershfield, E.: Mycobacterial skin infection by an unidentified species: a report of 29 patients, Ann. Intern. Med. **80**:445, 1974.
7. Fernández, J.M.M.: The early reaction induced by lepromin, Int. J. Lepr. **8**:1, 1940.
8. Fieldsteel, A.H., and Levy, L.: Dapsone chemotherapy of *Mycobacterium leprae* infection of the neonatally thymectomized Lewis rat, Am. J. Trop. Med. Hyg. **25**:854, 1976.
9. Fite, G.L., Cambre, P.J., and Turner, M.H.: Procedure for demonstrating lepra bacilli in paraffin sections, Arch. Pathol. **43**:624, 1947.
10. Freiberger, H.F., and Fudenberg, H.: An appetite for armadillo, Hosp. Pract., **16**:137, 1981.
11. Hansen, G.A.: Spedalskhedens arsager, Norsk Mag. Laegevidensk. **4**:76, 1874; reprinted in part, in English translation, as Causes of leprosy, Int. J. Lepr. **23**:307, 1955.
12. Hayashi, F.: Mitsuda's skin reaction in leprosy, Int. J. Lepr. **1**:31, 1933.
13. Kean, B.H., and Childress, M.E.: A summary of 103 autopsies on leprosy patients on the Isthmus of Panama, Int. J. Lepr. **10**:51, 1942.
14. Kirchheimer, W.F., and Storrs, E.E.: Attempts to establish the armadillo (*Dasypus novemcinctus* Linn.) as a model for the study of leprosy. I. Report of lepromatoid leprosy in an experimentally infected armadillo, Int. J. Lepr. **39**:693, 1971.
15. Latapí, F., and Chevez Zamora, A.: The "spotted" leprosy of Lucio (La lepra "manchada" de Lucio): an introduction to its clinical and histological study, Int. J. Lepr. **16**:421, 1948.
16. Leininger, J.R., Donham, K.J., and Meyers, W.M.: Leprosy in a chimpanzee: postmortem lesions, Int. J. Lepr. **48**:414, 1980.
16a. Lucio and Alvarado: Opusculo sobre el mal de San Lázaro o elefancíasis de los griegos, México, 1852, M. Murguía y Cia.
17. Meyers, W.M., et al.: Naturally-acquired leprosy in a mangabey monkey (*Cercocebus* sp.), Int. J. Lepr. **48**:495, 1980.
18. Powell, C.S., and Swann, L.L.: Leprosy: pathologic changes observed in fifty consecutive necropsies, Am. J. Pathol. **37**:1131, 1955.
19. Rees, R.J.W., et al.: Experimental lepromatous leprosy, Nature **215**:599, 1967.
19a. Ridley, D.S., and Jopling, W.H.: Classification of leprosy according to immunity: a five group system, Int. J. Lepr. **34**:255, 1966.

20. Rodriguez, J.N.: The histoid leproma: its characteristics and significance, Int. J. Lepr. **37**:1, 1969.

21. Shepard, C.C.: The experimental disease that follows the injection of human leprosy bacilli into footpads of mice, J. Exp. Med. **112**:445, 1960.

21a. Smith, J.H., et al.: Leprosy in wild armadillos (*Dasypus novemcinctus*) of the Texas Gulf Coast: epidemiology and mycobacteriology, J. Reticuloendothel. Soc. **34**:75, 1983.

22. Trautman, J.R.: Personal communication.

23. Wade, H.W.: The histoid variety of lepromatous leprosy, Int. J. Lepr. **31**:129, 1963.

24. Walsh, G.P., et al.: Leprosy—a zoonosis, Lepr. Rev. **52**(suppl. 1):77, 1981. (In Press.)

CHAPTER 9

Rickettsial and Chlamydial Diseases

DAVID H. WALKER

Obligate intracellular bacteria, members of the genera *Rickettsia*, *Coxiella*, and *Chlamydia*, comprise a unique group of infectious agents of human disease.[7,79,80] These microorganisms have never been cultivated outside of eukaryotic cells and thus occupy an interesting ecologic niche. Intracellular parasitism is necessary for their survival in nature. It should be recognized that bacterial interactions with human cells form a spectrum from free-living bacteria such as *Pseudomonas aeruginosa* to obligate intracellular rickettsiae and chlamydiae. Intermediate positions in the spectrum of bacterium–host cell interaction include facultative intracellular bacteria (for example, *Mycobacterium*, *Brucella*, *Listeria*, and *Salmonella*), which may grow within or outside of host cells, and extracellular organisms, such as *Bartonella*, which appear to grow best attached to the outside of the host cell. Other extracellular bacteria, such as *Escherichia coli*, have attachment mechanisms that anchor the bacteria in their ecologic niche with less chance of removal by the mechanical current of the local cleansing mechanism. Because rickettsiae and chlamydiae are in part defined by the negative characteristic of being unable to proliferate extracellularly, their members are constantly liable to being expelled by a scientist who discovers conditions permitting their cultivation in a cell-free environment. An example of this reclassification is *Rochalimaea quintana*, the etiologic agent of trench fever, which was considered a louse-borne rickettsial disease until successful cell-free cultivation of the bacterium.[5]

Many of these obligate intracellular bacteria cause zoonoses. A *zoonosis* is a disease that is spread to humans from a reservoir in other animals. *Chlamydia psittaci* is spread to poultry workers from infected turkeys and other fowl and to those who own and sell infected pet birds. *Coxiella burnetii* is spread mainly via aerosol from infected ruminants, especially from the placentas of infected sheep and cattle. Rickettsiae are transmitted to humans from infected ticks, mites, lice, and fleas.[1] As a group the zoonoses exist independent of humans, who are infected only accidentally and usually as a dead end from the point of view of the microorganism, which is rarely shed or transmitted from humans back into nature. *Chlamydia trachomatis* is the only obligate intracellular bacterium that is usually transmitted directly from one person to another.

Rickettsia, *Coxiella*, and *Chlamydia* were all considered viruses before elucidation of their bacterial characteristics. At one time the term *virus* was used to mean "infectious agent." Subsequently, "virus" was often used to refer to an infectious agent that passed through a Berkefeld filter or required living host cells such as cell culture, embryonated eggs, or animals for its propagation. Except for intracellular proliferation, rickettsiae and chlamydiae share the properties of bacteria rather than viruses. They differ from viruses in that they contain DNA and RNA, ribosomes, and metabolic enzymes, have a gram-negative type of bacterial cell wall, replicate by binary fission, and are susceptible to antimicrobial agents. Because these microorganisms are cultivated with much more difficulty[31] and, in some instances, more danger than other bacteria, diagnosis of rickettsial and chlamydial infection is seldom documented by isolation of the agent.[2,28] More often a tentative diagnosis is made on clinical grounds, and later acute and convalescent sera are tested to demonstrate the appearance or rise in titer of specific antibodies.[30] In the last decade rapid, clinically useful diagnostic tools have been developed that demonstrate specific microbial antigens in specimens from the patient.[36,42]

RICKETTSIAL DISEASES

Rickettsiae are small, obligate, intracellular coccobacilli measuring 0.3×1 to $2\ \mu m$ that spend all or a portion of their life cycle in an arthropod host and contain antigens of the spotted fever, typhus, or scrub typhus group. *Coxiella burnetii*, which on occasion has been isolated from ticks and had traditionally been considered closely related to the genus *Rickettsia*, has major differences,

Table 9-1. Rickettsial diseases of humans

Disease	Etiologic agent	Transmission	Pathologic lesion	Geographic distribution
SPOTTED FEVER GROUP				
Rocky Mountain spotted fever	*Rickettsia rickettsii*	Tick bite	Microvascular injury involving skin, brain, lungs, and other organs	North and South America
Rickettsialpox	*Rickettsia akari*	Mite bite	Microvascular injury with rash and eschar	U.S.A., U.S.S.R., Korea
Boutonneuse fever	*Rickettsia conorii*	Tick bite	Microvascular injury with rash and eschar	Mediterranean basin, Africa, Indian subcontinent
North Asian tick typhus	*Rickettsia sibirica*	Tick bite	Microvascular injury with rash and eschar	Asiatic U.S.S.R., Mongolia
Queensland tick typhus	*Rickettsia australis*	Tick bite	Microvascular injury with rash and eschar	Australia
Central European tick typhus	*Rickettsia slovaca*	Tick bite	Microvascular injury	Central Europe, Armenia
TYPHUS GROUP				
Epidemic typhus	*Rickettsia prowazekii*	Louse feces	Microvascular injury involving skin, brain, and other organs	Potentially worldwide, recently in Africa, South America, Central America, Mexico
Brill-Zinsser disease	*Rickettsia prowazekii*	See text	Microvascular injury involving skin, brain, and other organs	Potentially worldwide including U.S.A., U.S.S.R., Canada, and eastern Europe
Flying squirrel typhus	*Rickettsia prowazekii*	Ectoparasite of flying squirrel	Microvascular injury involving skin, brain, and other organs	Southeastern U.S.A.
Murine typhus	*Ricksettsia mooseri (typhi)*	Rat flea feces	Microvascular injury involving skin, brain, and other organs	Worldwide
SCRUB TYPHUS GROUP	*Rickettsia tsutsugamushi*	Mite bite	Microvascular injury involving skin, brain, lungs, and other organs	Southern Asia, Japan, western Pacific, Indonesia
Q FEVER	*Coxiella burnetii*	Inhalation of aerosol from infected animals	Pneumonia, granulomas of liver and bone marrow, endocarditis	Worldwide

including a spore form[71] and intraphagolysosomal location[68] as well as unrelated antigens and different pathologic lesions.[4] Organisms of *Rickettsia* and *Coxiella* cause the infectious diseases of humans shown in Table 9-1.

Spotted fever group infections
Rocky Mountain spotted fever

Rocky Mountain spotted fever (RMSF) is one of the severest infectious diseases, with a mortality in previously healthy persons of 20% prior to the advent of antimicrobial therapy. RMSF is the most important rickettsiosis in the United States from the aspects of morbidity and mortality.[10,20,21] However, contrary to its name, the majority of cases occur in the southeastern states. *R. rickettsii* are released from the salivary glands of a feeding *Dermacentor variabilis*, *D. andersoni*, or *Rhipicephalus sanguineus* tick and are regurgitated into the feeding blood pool of the host's skin. After an incubation period of 2 to 12 days, the patient develops severe headache and fever. A maculopapular rash, which may become petechial, appears on the wrists and ankles 2 to 5 days later and usually spreads to involve the trunk, palms, and soles.[18,25] In severe cases the patient may manifest signs of encephalitis, noncardiogenic pulmonary edema, skin necrosis, coagulopathy with bleeding, acute renal failure, jaundice, and hypovolemic

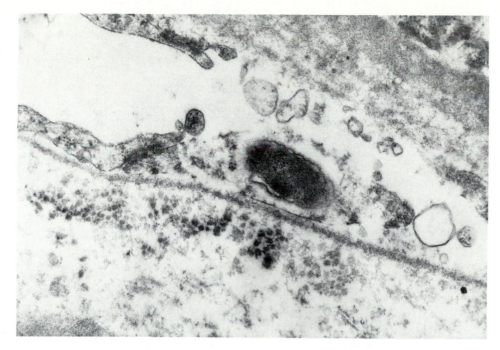

Fig. 9-1. Electron photomicrograph of *Rickettsia rickettsii* in cytoplasm of endothelial cell from patient with Rocky Mountain spotted fever. (From Walker, D.H.: Rickettsial diseases: an update. In Majno, G., and Cotran, R., editors: The inflammatory process and infectious diseases, Baltimore, 1981, The Williams & Wilkins Co.)

shock.[22,23] In fatal cases death usually ensues 8 to 15 days after onset. There is a fulminant form of RMSF in which the patient may die before the fifth day of illness.[29] Early treatment with tetracycline or chloramphenicol cures most patients; however, late diagnosis and inappropriate treatment result in an overall mortality of 3% to 8%.[17]

Pathologic lesions. Rickettsiae spread via the bloodstream, penetrate endothelial cells, proliferate within the cytoplasm and nuclei of endothelial and vascular smooth muscle cells of the microcirculation of virtually all organs (Fig. 9-1), and directly injure the foci of infected cells. The consequence is a systemic vasculitis that is the pathologic basis for the rash, interstitial pneumonia, interstitial myocarditis, meningoencephalomyelitis, hepatic portal triaditis, and interstitial nephritis. Microscopically, the vasculitis consists of swollen or necrotic endothelial cells; intramural and perivascular infiltration, predominantly by macrophages and lymphocytes with few polymorphonuclear (PMN) leukocytes; focal extravasation of erythrocytes; and occasional, usually nonocclusive, eccentric thrombi in the foci of rickettsial infection (Fig. 9-2).[24,41] In the skin these foci are located principally in the dermis. In the brain the lesions assume a characteristic appearance, so-called typhus nodules, found most frequently in the brainstem (Fig. 9-3).[3] These perivascular accumulations of mononuclear cells, which measure 100 to 180 μm in diameter, suggest a rickettsial infection although they are not pathogno-

monic. Other neuropathologic lesions include microinfarcts of white matter and a mild mononuclear leptomeningitis. Lungs are congested and heavy.[37] Microscopic pulmonary lesions include mononuclear interstitial pneumonia and interstitial and alveolar edema and hemorrhages (Fig. 9-4).

The heart is grossly normal except for epicardial petechiae, but it usually manifests a mild mononuclear interstitial myocarditis on microscopic examination (Fig. 9-5).[12,24,40] The hepatic portal triaditis and multifocal perivascular interstitial nephritis correspond to foci of infection of hepatic portal blood vessels and the renal microcirculation near the corticomedullary junction, respectively.[9,39] Erythrophagocytosis occurs in Kupffer cells and macrophages within sinuses of lymph nodes. In fulminant RMSF there are more thrombi and fewer intramural and perivascular leukocytes in foci of vascular injury.[34]

Clinicopathologic correlations. Disseminated vascular foci of rickettsial infection and microvascular injury result in leakage of intravascular fluid into the interstitial space with consequent edema and hypovolemia.[19] Consumption of platelets and coagulation factors in thrombi at the sites of injury can cause thrombocytopenia and in very severe cases more severe coagulopathy. Focal lesions in the skin are the cause of the rash. Vasodilatation and petechiae are the basis of the cutaneous erythematous macules and central "spots," respectively.

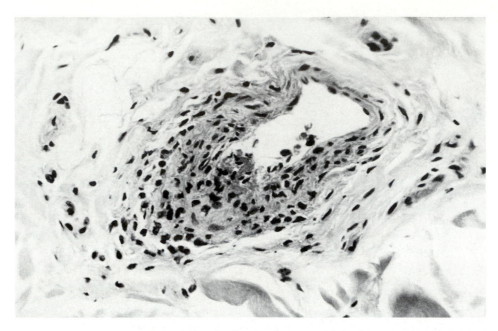

Fig. 9-2. Blood vessel from hemorrhagic skin lesion of patient with Rocky Mountain spotted fever shows characteristic rickettsial vasculitis with infiltration of blood vessel wall and perivascular tissue by mononuclear cells and with small, focal, nonocclusive thrombus. (From Green, W.R., Walker, D.H., and Cain, B.G.: Am. J. Med. **64:**523, 1978.)

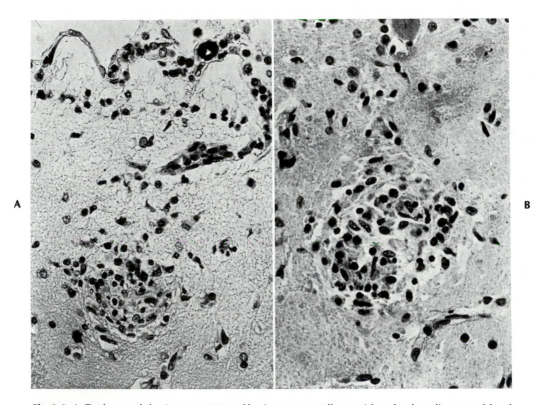

Fig. 9-3. A, Typhus nodules in gray matter of brain are generally considered to be adjacent to blood vessel, although vessel may not always be visible. **B,** Histologic components of these inflammatory foci are predominantly macrophages and lymphocytes. (AFIP 77543 and 78556; from Ash, J.E., and Spitz, S.: The rickettsial diseases. In Ash, J.E., and Spitz, S.: Pathology of tropical diseases, Philadelphia, 1945, W.B. Saunders Co.)

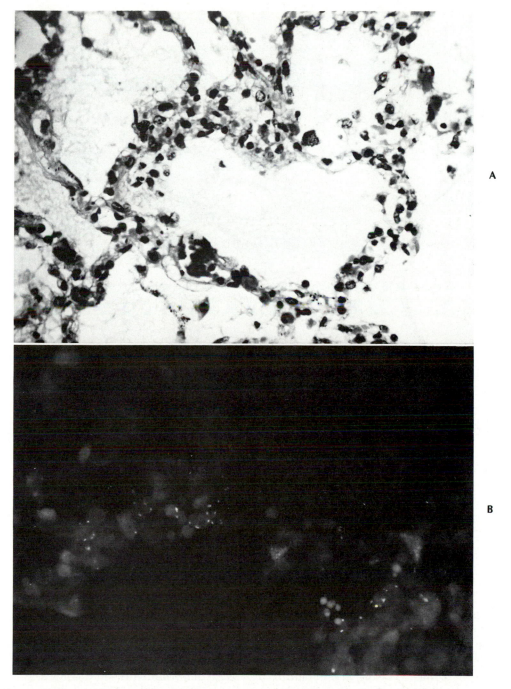

Fig. 9-4. A, Interstitial pneumonia of Rocky Mountain spotted fever with mononuclear infiltration of alveolar septa and proteinaceous edema fluid in alveolar spaces. **B,** Immunofluorescent *Rickettsia rickettsii* in thickened alveolar septum are cause of noncardiogenic pulmonary edema in Rocky Mountain spotted fever. (From Walker, D.H., and Mattern, W.D.: Am. Heart J. **100:**896, 1980.)

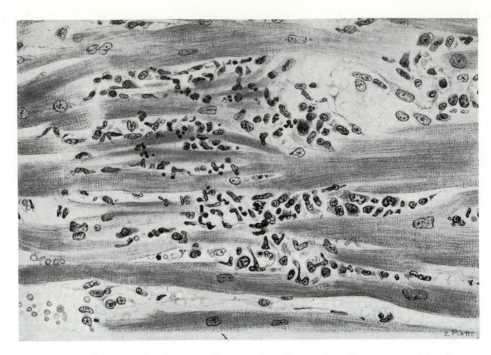

Fig. 9-5. Myocarditis in typhus fever. Infiltration of mononuclear cells and neutrophils between muscle fibers. (From Wolbach, S.B., Todd, J.L., and Palfrey, F.W.: The etiology and pathology of typhus, Cambridge, Mass., 1922, Harvard University Press.)

Increased vascular permeability of the infected pulmonary microcirculation may result in noncardiogenic pulmonary edema.[6,37] Central nervous system lesions are the cause of coma, seizures, multifocal neurologic signs, and probably cardiorespiratory arrest. Jaundice correlates with hemolysis and portal triadal inflammation.[9] Acute renal failure results from hypovolemic prerenal azotemia or, in more severe cases, acute tubular necrosis.[39]

Pathogenesis. Immunopathology, coagulation, and inflammation have not been demonstrated experimentally as primary pathologic mechanisms in RMSF, although thrombosis and activation of the kallikrein-kinin pathways may exacerbate the disease.[26,27,33,38,43] Moreover, *R. rickettsii* has not been shown to produce a toxin. On the other hand, direct injury of infected cells by rickettsiae has been documented. The pathogenic mechanisms of the host cell injury have not been elucidated.

Other spotted fever group infections

Boutonneuse fever,[13] North Asian tick typhus,[14] Queensland tick typhus,[11] and rickettsialpox[16,32] are milder rickettsioses with similar clinical and pathologic features. In contrast to RMSF, these diseases are frequently associated with an eschar, a focus of skin necrosis at the original site of feeding by the arthropod vector. Interestingly, several apparently nonpathogenic rickettsiae have been identified in a substantial proportion of ticks in the United States.[15] Their role in the ecology of *R. rickettsii* and possibly in human infections is currently unknown.

Typhus group infections
Typhus

Epidemic louse-borne typhus fever is one of the classic scourges of mankind. In times of war, famine, and other disasters, louse infestation, crowding, and malnutrition join forces with *R. prowazekii* to cause explosive epidemics of typhus. It has been postulated that more wars have been lost as a result of epidemic typhus than have been won by battlefield victories.[8] During and just after World War I, 15 million persons suffered from typhus and more than 3 million died. Infections by *R. prowazekii* occur in the southeastern United States as a zoonosis with a reservoir in flying squirrels.[46,49] A milder clinical type of typhus fever known as Brill-Zinsser disease occurs as recrudescence of an infection with *R. prowazekii* that has remained latent following acute typhus fever many years previously.[50,51,60] The reason for the recrudescence is not known.

Organisms of *R. prowazekii* proliferate in the intestinal epithelial cells of the human louse, are shed in its feces, and eventually kill the louse. After entry through human skin, the pathogenic events of typhus parallel those of RMSF and the other rickettsioses with spread via the bloodstream to skin, brain, and other organs. In contrast to RMSF, rickettsial infection involves only endothelial cells, and the rash begins on the trunk between days 4 and 8 of illness and spreads centrifugally to involve the arms and legs.[57] Pathologic lesions comprise disseminated mononuclear vasculitis of skin, typhus nodules of brain (Fig. 9-3), interstitial myocarditis, mild interstitial pneumonia, perivascular interstitial nephritis, and portal triaditis. Biopsies of skin of patients with epidemic typhus in Poland during World War I were examined by Wolbach, thus providing a sequence of pathologic lesions. The earliest lesion was swelling of endothelial cells parasitized by rickettsiae. Subsequently, leukocytic infiltration of the vessel wall was observed. The pathophysiology of typhus fever is similar to that of RMSF.[58,59]

Typhus rickettsiae contain a lipopolysaccharide that is relatively nontoxic.[52,53] In vitro experiments have shown that cell membrane injury is associated with phospholipase activity.[55,56] The so-called mouse toxin phenomenon is unlikely to be caused by a toxin. Intravenous injection of nonviable typhus rickettsiae does not cause a toxic death in mice.[44] Moreover, no toxin has been identified that reproduces this phenomenon. Some other mechanism, such as massive rickettsial penetration involving phospholipase activity, may explain the mouse toxicity.

Murine typhus

Another typhus group rickettsia that causes human disease is *R. mooseri* (*R. typhi*).[47,48] Murine typhus is transmitted from rats to humans by the infected rat flea, which excretes rickettsiae in feces. Murine typhus is very rarely fatal, although it resembles the other rickettsial diseases clinically.[45,54] As with epidemic typhus an eschar does not occur in murine typhus.

Scrub typhus group

Organisms of *R. tsutsugamushi* are transmitted to humans by the bite of a larval trombiculid mite.[62-64] Like the tick with *R. rickettsii*, transovarial infection of mites may account for the maintenance of *R. tsutsugamushi* in nature, although feral rodents do become infected and appear to amplify the distribution of rickettsiae. These rickettsiae have great diversity with many antigenically distinct strains that do not necessarily confer cross-protection. Scrub typhus occurs in southern and eastern Asia, Japan, Indonesia, northern Australia, and the islands of the western Pacific. The disease was of military importance during World War II with loss of manpower to the morbidity of the infection. The characteristic, but not uniformly present, eschar marks the site of feeding by the mite. Regional lymph nodes draining the site of localized cutaneous necrosis and ulceration are swollen and inflamed. Diagnosis is facilitated by detection of the eschar. The pathologic lesions in blood vessels of skin, brain, lung, heart, and kidney resemble those of spotted fever and typhus except there are fewer capillary thrombi.[61,65,66]

Q fever

Q fever refers to the disease caused by *Coxiella burnetii*. The letter Q is for *query*, designating the unknown etiology during the early days of recognition of the ill-ness. Derrick[67] first described Q fever in 1937 as an occupational disease among slaughterhouse workers and dairy farmers in Australia. *C. burnetii* differs remarkably from organisms of genus *Rickettsia* in its capability to generate spores and in its cellular location within phagolysosomes, where it functions most efficiently in the acid milieu. In contrast, members of genus *Rickettsia* are usually found in cytosol, with spotted fever group organisms occasionally in nucleoplasm. Moreover, Q fever may have a chronic as well as an acute form, and pneumonia with no vascular infection or rash contrasts with the disseminated vasculitis and microvascular injury of the rickettsioses. Chronic Q fever is a systemic granulomatous disease that may also include infective endocarditis.[76]

Pathologic lesions. Because Q fever is rarely fatal, few tissues have been examined from the acute stage of the illness. Those cases have shown bronchopneumonia with a component of interstitial pneumonia also.[69,74] Alveolar, bronchiolar, and bronchial exudates contain many macrophages with variable quantities of lymphocytes, erythrocytes, and polymorphonuclear leukocytes. Alveolar septa are slightly to moderately thickened by mononuclear cell infiltration. Some patients develop granulomas of the liver or bone marrow.[72,73] The hepatic granulomas often have a characteristic doughnut appearance with a central clear zone surrounded concentrically by layers of fibrinoid material and epithelioid macrophages (Fig. 9-6). Chronic Q fever may manifest chronic infective endocarditis, hepatic involvement, and thrombocytopenia.[70,75,76]

Pathogenesis. Humans acquire Q fever via inhalation of spores or aerosols of *C. burnetii*, usually from sources such as highly infectious placentas of infected sheep. Presumably the organisms proliferate inside the phagolysosomes of pulmonary macrophages. The mechanisms of cell and tissue injury are unclear, although endotoxin and delayed hypersensitivity have been suggested as hypotheses. Spread may occur via the bloodstream to liver, bone marrow, and previously abnormal cardiac valves.

CHLAMYDIAL DISEASES

Chlamydiae are 0.2 to 1 μm coccoid, obligate, intracellular bacteria that reside within a cytoplasmic vacuole.[79,80] They differ from rickettsiae in that they have two morphologic and functional forms and are unable to synthesize ATP. The elementary body, with a diameter of 0.2 to 0.4 μm and a rigid cell wall, survives extracellularly without metabolic activity or replication. Moreover, this form is equipped for infectivity by its capability to induce its phagocytosis and to inhibit fusion of phagosome and lysosome. The reticulate particle has a diameter of 0.6 to 1 μm, and although unsuited for extracellular survival or infectivity, it is the metabolically active, replicative form of the organism. The chlamydial diseases of humans are shown in Table 9-2.

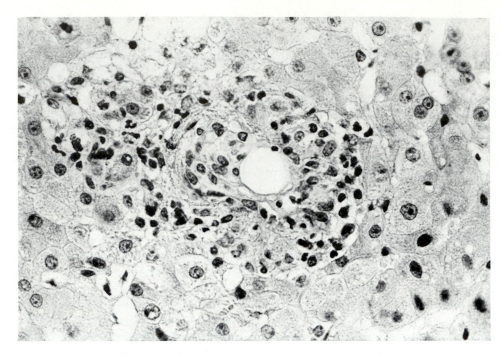

Fig. 9-6. Hepatic granuloma of Q fever with peripheral epithelioid macrophages and lymphocytes and characteristic central "doughnut" hole.

Table 9-2. Chlamydial diseases of humans

Etiologic agent	Disease	Pathologic lesion	Transmission
Chlamydia psittaci	Psittacosis	Pneumonia	Aerosol from infected birds
Chlamydia trachomatis			
Serotypes A, B, Ba, and C	Trachoma	Chronic conjunctivitis	Contact
Serotypes L-1, L-2, and L-3	Lymphogranuloma venereum	Inguinal lymph node abscesses and granulomas	Sexual contact
Serotypes D-K	Various genital infections	Urethritis, epididymitis, proctitis, cervicitis, salpingitis, bartholinitis, perihepatitis	Sexual contact
	Neonatal infections	Conjunctivitis, pneumonia	Contact with infection in birth canal

Psittacosis

Psittacosis occurs in humans as pneumonia; a toxic nonrespiratory illness with fever, myalgia, and headache; or a subclinical infection. The mortality is low. The pathologic lesions are interstitial, predominantly mononuclear pneumonia with gelatinous, sparsely cellular, mononuclear, alveolar exudates and focal hepatic and splenic necrosis.[82] Infection follows inhalation of infected dust or aerosols from infected birds. Penetration of host cells including macrophages by infective elementary bodies is followed by their reorganization into reticulate particles, which replicate by binary fission and eventually change again into elementary bodies before release from the host cell.

Trachoma

Trachoma, a major cause of blindness particularly in Africa, the Middle East, and southeastern Asia, is a chronic conjunctivitis caused by certain serotypes (A, B, Ba, and C) of *Chlamydia trachomatis*. Person-to-person spread occurs especially among children within families, and persons are frequently reinfected. Intracellular chlamydial infection of conjunctival epithelium is associated with epithelial proliferation and necrosis. Chronic inflammation of the conjunctiva leads to conjunctival scarring and distortion of the eyelid such that inturned lashes continually traumatize the cornea. Corneal injury with secondary bacterial infections causes corneal opacification by scarring.

Lymphogranuloma venereum

Serologically distinct, more invasive serogroups (L-1, L-2, and L-3) of *C. trachomatis* are the cause of lymphogranuloma venereum (LGV), a venereal disease. LGV occurs more often in males and is characterized by inguinal lymph node enlargement (buboes) and fever in men and by rectal strictures in women. The pathologic lesions in the inguinal lymph nodes are stellate abscesses surrounded by a granulomatous reaction of epithelioid macrophages.

Genital and neonatal infections

Another set of serogroups (D-K) of *C. trachomatis* are the etiologic agents of a variety of sexually transmitted infections of the male and female genitalia and of neonatal infections acquired during passage through the birth canal. A large portion of cases of nongonococcal urethritis[81] and epididymitis[77] in males is caused by *C. trachomatis*. Females with this infection may manifest cervicitis, urethritis, acute nongonococcal salpingitis,[78] or inflammation of Bartholin's glands. Neonatal inclusion conjunctivitis occurs in 25% to 50% of infants of infected mothers, with onset 1 to 2 weeks after birth. This frequent infection is generally benign. Neonatal chlamydial pneumonia usually occurs at 1 to 3 months of age and is characterized by tachypnea, cough, and lack of fever. Pneumonia is observed in 10% to 20% of infants of infected mothers. Chlamydiae infect the mucosal epithelial cells of the genital and respiratory tracts in these diseases. After intracellular proliferation, they are shed onto the mucosal surface and may be spread by direct contact such as sexual intercourse. Thus these obligate intracellular bacteria are able to spread to the appropriate ecologic niche in another host and to survive.

• • •

It is likely that the future holds a great expansion of knowledge about chlamydial and rickettsial diseases as techniques for their detection are refined and come into more general use. The final chapter on diseases of the obligate intracellular bacteria will not be written soon.

REFERENCES
General

1. Burgdorfer, W.: Tick-borne diseases in the United States: Rocky Mountain spotted fever and Colorado tick fever; a review, Acta Tropica **34**:103, 1977.
2. Elisberg, B.L., and Bozeman, F.M.: Rickettsieae. In Diagnostic procedures for viral and rickettsial infections, ed. 4, New York, 1969, American Public Health Association.
3. Manuelidis, E.E., and Krigman, M.R.: Rickettsial encephalitides. In Minckler, J., editor: Pathology of the nervous system, vol. 3, New York, 1972, McGraw-Hill Book Co.
4. Moulton, F.R., editor: Rickettsial diseases of man, Washington, D.C., 1948, American Association for the Advancement of Science.
5. Vinson, J.W.: Etiology of trench fever in Mexico. In Industry and tropical health. V. Boston, 1964, Harvard School of Public Health.
6. Walker, D.H., and Mattern, W.D.: Rickettsial vasculitis, Am. Heart J. **100**:896, 1980.
7. Weiss, E.: Growth and physiology of rickettsiae, Bacteriol. Rev. **37**:259, 1973.
8. Zinsser, H.: Rats, lice, and history, New York, 1935, Little, Brown & Co.

Spotted fever group infections

9. Adams, J.S., and Walker, D.H.: The liver in Rocky Mountain spotted fever, Am. J. Clin. Pathol. **75**:156, 1981.
10. Aikawa, J.: Rocky Mountain spotted fever, Springfield, Ill., 1966, Charles C Thomas, Publisher.
11. Andrew, R., Bonnin, J.M., and Williams, S.: Tick typhus in North Queensland, Med. J. Australia **2**:255, 1946.
12. Bradford, W.D., and Hackel, D.B.: Myocardial involvement in Rocky Mountain spotted fever, Arch. Pathol. Lab. Med. **102**:357, 1978.
13. Burgdorfer, W.: Boutonneuse fever (Marseilles fever, Kenya tick typhus, South African tick bite fever, Indian tick typhus). In Hubbert, W.T., McCulloch, W.F., and Schnurrenberger, P.R., editors: Diseases transmitted from animals to man, ed. 6, Springfield, Ill., 1975, Charles C Thomas, Publisher.
14. Burgdorfer, W.: North Asian tick typhus. In Hubbert, W.T., McCulloch, W.F., and Schnurrenberger, P.R., editors: Diseases transmitted from animals to man, ed. 6, Springfield, Ill., 1975, Charles C Thomas, Publisher.
15. Burgdorfer, W., et al.: *Rhipicephalus sanguineus:* vector of a new spotted fever group rickettsia in the United States, Infect. Immun. **12**:205, 1975.
16. Dolgopol, V.B.: Histologic changes in rickettsialpox, Am. J. Pathol. **24**:119, 1948.
17. Fegin, R.D., et al.: Rocky Mountain spotted fever: successful application of new insights into physiologic changes during acute infections to successful management of a severely-ill patient, Clin. Pediatr. **8**:331, 1969.
18. Harrell, G.T.: Rocky Mountain spotted fever, Medicine **28**:333, 1949.
19. Harrell, G.T., and Aikawa, J.K.: Pathogenesis of circulatory failure in Rocky Mountain spotted fever, Arch. Intern. Med. **83**:331, 1949.
20. Hattwick, M.A.W., O'Brien, R.J., and Hanson, B.F.: Rocky Mountain spotted fever: epidemiology of an increasing problem, Ann. Intern. Med. **84**:732, 1976.
21. Hattwick, M.A.W., et al.: Fatal Rocky Mountain spotted fever, J.A.M.A. **240**:1499, 1978.
22. Haynes, R.E., Sanders, D.Y., and Cramblett, H.G.: Rocky Mountain spotted fever in children, J. Pediatr. **76**:685, 1970.
23. Kaplowitz, L.G., Fischer, J.J., and Sparling, P.F.: Rocky Mountain spotted fever—a clinical dilemma. In Remington, J.S., and Swartrz, M.N., editors: Current clinical topics in infectious diseases, vol. 2, New York, 1980, McGraw-Hill Book Co.
24. Lillie, R.D.: The pathology of Rocky Mountain spotted fever, Nat. Inst. Health Bull. **177**:1, 1941.
25. Maxey, E.E.: Some observations on the so-called spotted fever of Idaho, Med. Sentinel **7**:433, 1899.
26. Moe, J.B., et al.: Functional and morphologic changes during experimental Rocky Mountain spotted fever in guinea pigs, Lab. Invest. **35**:235, 1976.
27. Mosher, D.F., et al.: Studies of the coagulation and complement systems during experimental Rocky Mountain spotted fever in rhesus monkeys, J. Infect. Dis. **135**:985, 1977.
28. Oster, C.N., et al.: Laboratory-acquired Rocky Mountain spotted fever, N. Engl. J. Med. **297**:859, 1977.
29. Parker, R.R.: Rocky Mountain spotted fever, J.A.M.A. **110**:1185, 1273, 1938.
30. Philip, R.N., et al.: A comparison of serologic methods for diagnosis of Rocky Mountain spotted fever, Am. J. Epidemiol. **105**:56, 1977.
31. Ricketts, H.T.: The study of "Rocky Mountain spotted fever" (tick fever?) by means of animal inoculations, J.A.M.A. **47**:33, 1906.
32. Rose, H.M.: The clinical manifestations and laboratory diagnosis of rickettsialpox, Ann. Intern. Med. **31**:871, 1949.
33. Walker, D.H.: Rickettsial diseases: an update. In Majno, G., Cotran, R., and Kaufman, N., editors: The inflammatory process and infectious diseases, Baltimore, 1981, The Williams & Wilkins Co.
34. Walker, D.H., and Bradford, W.D.: Rocky Mountain spotted fever in childhood, Perspect. Pediatr. Pathol. **6**:35, 1981.
35. Walker, D.H., and Cain, B.G.: The rickettsial plaque: evidence for direct cytopathic effect of *Rickettsia rickettsii*, Lab. Invest. **43**:388, 1980.
36. Walker, D.H., Cain, B.G., and Olmstead, P.M.: Laboratory diagnosis of Rocky Mountain spotted fever by immunofluorescent demonstration of *Rickettsia rickettsii* in cutaneous lesions, Am. J. Clin. Pathol. **69**:619, 1978.

37. Walker, D.H., Crawford, C.G., and Cain, B.G.: Rickettsial infection of the pulmonary microcirculation, the basis of interstitial pneumonitis of Rocky Mountain spotted fever, Hum. Pathol. 11:263, 1980.
38. Walker, D.H., and Henderson, F.W.: Effect of immunosuppression on *Rickettsia rickettsii* infection in guinea pigs, Infect. Immun. 20:221, 1978.
39. Walker, D.H., and Mattern, W.D.: Acute renal failure in Rocky Mountain spotted fever, Arch. Intern. Med. 139:443, 1979.
40. Walker, D.H., Paletta, C.E., and Cain, B.G.: Pathogenesis of myocarditis in Rocky Mountain spotted fever, Arch. Pathol. Lab. Med. 104:171, 1980.
41. Wolbach, S.B.: Studies on Rocky Mountain spotted fever, J. Med. Res. 41:2, 1919.
42. Woodward, T.E., et al.: Prompt confirmation of Rocky Mountain spotted fever: identification of rickettsiae in skin tissues, J. Infect. Dis. 134:297, 1976.
43. Yamada, T., et al.: Activation of the kallikrein-kinin system in Rocky Mountain spotted fever, Ann. Intern. Med. 88:764, 1978.

Typhus group infections

44. Allen, E.G., Bovarnick, M.R., and Snyder, J.C.: The effect of irradiation with ultraviolet light on various properties of typhus rickettsiae, J. Bacteriol. 67:718, 1954.
45. Binford, C.H., and Ecker, H.D.: Endemic (murine) typhus: report of autopsy findings in three cases, Am. J. Clin. Pathol. 17:797, 1947.
46. Bozeman, F.M., et al.: Epidemic typhus rickettsiae isolated from flying squirrels, Nature 255:545, 1975.
47. Dyer, R.E., Rumreich, A., and Badger, L.F.: Typhus fever: a virus of the typhus type derived from fleas collected from wild rats, Pub. Health Rep. 46:334, 1931.
48. Maxcy, K.F.: An epidemiological study of endemic typhus (Brill's disease) in the southeastern United States: with special reference to its mode of transmission, Pub. Health Rep. 41:2967, 1926.
49. McDade, J.E., et al.: Evidence of *Rickettsia prowazeki* infections in the United States, Am. J. Trop. Med. Hyg. 29:277, 1980.
50. Murray, E.S., et al.: Brill's disease, J.A.M.A. 142: 1059, 1950.
51. Murray, E.S., et al.: Brill's disease. IV. Study of 26 cases in Yugoslavia, Am. J. Pub. Health 41:1359, 1951.
52. Schramek, S., Brezina, R., and Kazar, J.: Some biological properties of an endotoxic lipopolysaccharide from the typhus group rickettsiae, Acta Virol. 21:439, 1977.
53. Schramek, S., Brezina, R., and Tarasevich, I.V.: Isolation of a lipopolysaccharide antigen from *Rickettsia* species, Acta Virol. 20:270, 1976.
54. Stuart, B.M., and Pullen, R.L.: Endemic (murine) typhus fever: clinical observations of one hundred and eighty cases, Ann. Intern. Med. 23:520, 1945.
55. Winkler, H.H.: Immediate cytotoxicity and phospholipase A. In Burgdorfer, W., and Anacker, R., editors: Rickettsia and rickettsial diseases, New York, 1981, Academic Press, Inc.
56. Winkler, H.H., and Miller, E.T.: Phospholipase A activity in the hemolysis of sheep and human erythrocytes by *Rickettsia prowazeki*, Infect. Immun. 29:316, 1980.
57. Wolbach, S.B., Todd, J.L., and Palfrey, F.W.: The etiology and pathology of typhus, Cambridge, Mass., 1922, Harvard University Press.
58. Woodward, T.E., and Bland, E.F.: Clinical observations in typhus fever; with special reference to the cardiovascular system, J.A.M.A. 126:287, 1944.
59. Yeomans, A., et al.: Azotemia in typhus fever, Ann. Intern. Med. 23:711, 1945.
60. Zinsser, H.: Varieties of typhus virus and the epidemiology of the American form of European typhus fever (Brill's disease), Am. J. Hyg. 20:513, 1934.

Scrub typhus group infections

61. Allen, A.C., and Spitz, S.: A comparative study of the pathology of scrub typhus (Tsutsugamushi disease) and other rickettsial diseases, Am. J. Pathol. 21:603, 1945.
62. Berman, S.J., and Kundin, W.D.: Scrub typhus in South Vietnam: a study of 87 cases, Ann. Intern. Med. 79:26, 1973.
63. Blake, F.G., et al.: Studies on tsutsugamushi disease (scrub typhus, mite-borne typhus) in New Guinea and adjacent islands; epidemiology, clinical observations, and etiology in the Dobadura area, Am. J. Hyg. 41:243, 1945.
64. Brown, G.W., et al.: Scrub typhus: a common cause of illness in indigenous populations, Trans. R. Soc. Trop. Med. Hyg. 70:444, 1976.
65. Levine, D.H.: Pathologic study of thirty-one cases of scrub typhus fever with especial reference to the cardiovascular system, Am. Heart J. 31:314, 1946.
66. Settle, E.B., Pinkerton, H., and Corbett, A.J.: A pathologic study of tsutsugamushi disease (scrub typhus) with notes on clinicopathologic correlation, J. Lab. Clin. Med. 30:639, 1945.

Q fever group

67. Derrick, E.H.: "Q" fever, a new fever entity: clinical features, diagnosis and laboratory investigation, Med. J. Aust. 2:281, 1937.
68. Hackstadt, T., and Williams, J.C.: Biochemical stratagem for obligate parasitism of eukaryotic cells by *Coxiella burnetii*, Proc. Natl. Acad. Sci. U.S.A. 78:3240, 1981.
69. Lillie, R.D., Perrin, T.L., and Armstrong, C.: An institutional outbreak of pneumonitis. III. Histopathology in man and rhesus monkeys in the pneumonitis due to the virus of "Q" fever, Pub. Health Rep. 56:149, 1941.
70. Marmion, B.P., et al.: A case of subacute rickettsial endocarditis; with a survey of cardiac patients for this infection, Br. J. Med. 2:1264, 1960.
71. McCaul, T.F., and Williams, J.C.: Developmental cycle of *Coxiella burnetii* structure and morphogenesis of vegetative and sporogenic differentiations, J. Bacteriol. 147:1063, 1981.
72. Okun, D.B., Sun, N.C.J., and Tanaka, K.R.: Bone marrow granulomas in Q fever, Am. J. Clin. Pathol. 71:117, 1979.
73. Pellegrin, M., et al.: Granulomatous hepatitis in Q fever, Hum. Pathol. 11:51, 1980.
74. Perrin, T.L.: Histopathologic observations in a fatal case of Q fever, Arch. Pathol. 47:361, 1949.
75. Picchi, J., et al.: Q fever associated with granulomatous hepatitis, Ann. Intern. Med. 53:1065, 1960.
76. Turck, W.P.G., et al.: Chronic Q fever, Q. J. Med. 178:193, 1976.

Chlamydial diseases

77. Berger, R.E., et al.: *Chlamydia trachomatis* as a cause of acute "idiopathic" epididymitis, N. Engl. J. Med. 298:301, 1978.
78. Moller, B.R., et al.: *Chlamydia trachomatis* infection of the Fallopian tubes, Br. J. Vener. Dis. 55:422, 1979.
79. Schaechter, J.: Chlamydial infections, N. Engl. J. Med. 298:428, 490, 540, 1978.
80. Schaechter, J., and Caldwell, H.D.: Chlamydiae, Annu. Rev. Microbiol. 34:285, 1980.
81. Swartz, S.L., et al.: Diagnosis and etiology of nongonococcal urethritis, J. Infect. Dis. 138:445, 1978.
82. Yow, E.M., et al.: The pathology of psittacosis, Am. J. Med. 27:739, 1959.

CHAPTER 10   # Viral Diseases

JOSE COSTA
ALAN S. RABSON

Illnesses now known to be caused by viruses have been recognized since antiquity. However, major advances in the study of viruses have only been possible in the twentieth century because of the development of tissue culture, electron microscopy, and immunologic techniques. In recent years molecular biology has given us a detailed understanding of the genetics and life cycles of some viruses.

To prove that a disease is caused by a specific viral agent, the postulates of Rivers (modified Koch's postulates) must be fulfilled. These are (1) isolation of a virus from diseased hosts, (2) cultivation of the agent in experimental host or host cells, (3) proof of filterability of the pathogen, (4) production of a similar disease in the original host species or an animal model, and (5) reisolation of the virus from the experimentally inoculated diseased host. In some instances these postulates have not been fulfilled because there is no known experimental host or no system in the laboratory to culture the virus. However, when sera from patients suffering from a particular clinical syndrome show a definite increase in antibodies reacting with a particular virus, an etiologic relationship of the virus to the syndrome is assumed. If, in addition, morphologic evidence of viral infection (such as inclusion bodies or visualization of capsids with the electron microscope) is found in the lesions that are characteristic of the disease, the etiologic relationship of the agent with a specific syndrome is reinforced.

Viruses are organisms that can be characterized as having two distinct phases in their life cycle—an intracellular and an extracellular phase. The intracellular phase is the replicative phase during which the virus multiplies in the infected cell. There it borrows the metabolic machinery of the cell to direct the synthesis of proteins coded by the viral genome. The structural and nonstructural virion components are synthesized independently, and the structural proteins are assembled into whole virions during the final stages of reproduction. When virions leave the cell they are particles of uniform size, shape, and chemical composition that in some cases can crystallize. This is the extracellular phase of the virus. The viral particles can initiate the infectious process of new cells, and hence they constitute the infectious form of the virus.

The morphology of the virions provides a good basis for their classification. Information about the morphology of viruses is gained through study of purified populations of particles with the electron microscope. The basic component of the virions is the capsid, which contains in its interior the genome of the virus. According to the structural characteristics of the capsid, viruses are divided into two major groups, viruses with helical symmetry and those with icosahedral symmetry. Some viruses also acquire an envelope as they bud through the cell membrane of the infected cells.

The genome of a virus can be either RNA or DNA, and the type of nucleic acid is one of the most important characteristics of any virus. Other characteristics of the genome, such as the size or the fact that in some RNA viruses the genome can be segmented, are also very important in the understanding of the life cycles and properties of the viruses (see influenza virus).

Most taxonomic systems for viruses rely on the morphology of the particles and the nucleic acid–type genome. Groups are thus established that reveal evolutionary and phylogenetic relationships among the members of the group.

Many of the disturbances that we recognize as symptoms and signs of viral diseases result from the direct effects of viruses on cells. There are three types of virus–host cell interaction: (1) cytocidal infection, (2) steady-state infection, and (3) transformation.

In *cytocidal infection* the virus kills the cells in which it reproduces. During viral replication different morphologic alterations of the cell can be shown to progress as the viral cycle proceeds. One of the best-known morphologic results of cytocidal infection is the formation of inclusion bodies. These inclusions are located either in the nucleus or in the cytoplasm and are seen in infections

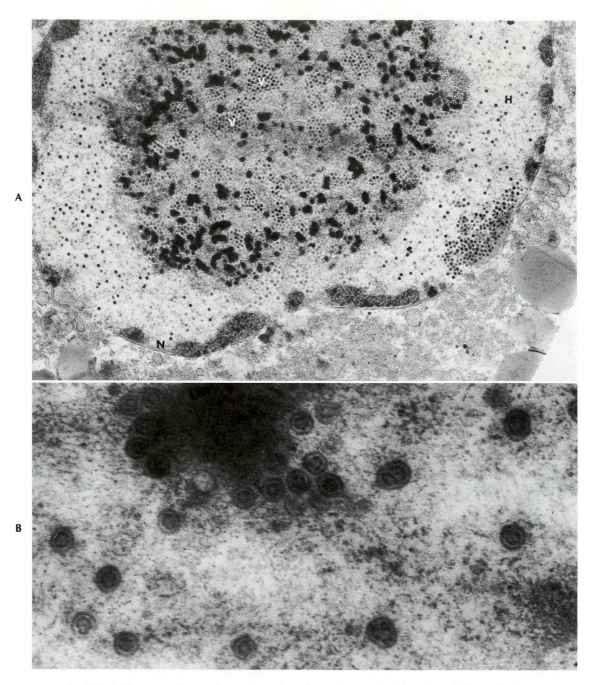

Fig. 10-1. A, Electron micrograph showing adenovirus inclusion body in cultured KB cell. Inclusion is composed of virions *(V)*, chromatin, and dense bodies of unknown nature. Between inclusion body and nuclear membrane *(N)* is halo *(H)*. **B,** Human cytomegalovirions within nuclear inclusion in cultured human fibroblast line. Diameter is 100 nm; addition of lipid envelope from nuclear membrane gives complete virion diameter of 220 nm. (**A,** 10,000×; **B,** 50,000×.)

caused by the herpes simplex virus, cytomegalovirus, rabies, vaccinia, adenovirus, measles, and papovaviruses (Fig. 10-1).

In *steady-state infection* the infected cells continuously produce virus without a drastic alteration of the cellular metabolism. In many cases of steady-state infection the progeny virions are released by budding through the cell membrane, and the cells can continue to divide and function.

The third type of virus cell interaction and perhaps one of the best studied is *transformation*. It is seen when oncogenic viruses (viruses capable of causing tumors when inoculated into laboratory animals) infect a cell. The main properties acquired by the transformed cell after infection are (1) the cell becomes immortalized (can be passaged in vitro indefinitely) and (2) the cells are capable of producing a tumor when injected into the animal of origin. Because many of the transforming viruses cause tumors when injected into animals, transformation of cultured cells provides an in vitro model for the study of carcinogenesis and has been extensively studied.

Viral disease is not only the result of the cellular alterations caused by the virus but also it is in most instances the result of the interplay of host defense mechanisms with the infected cell. The effects of human antibody on virus particles or virally infected cells are quite variable. Humoral immunity helps limit the infection when interaction of the antibody with the virus blocks the attachment of virus to susceptible cells, decreases the intracellular initiation of replication by interfering with uncoating of the genome, or damages the virus coat by activating complement. Lysis of infected cells by antibody and complement can result in clearance of cells supporting viral replication. Cell-mediated immunity is a very important determinant of host resistance to many virus infections. Different subsets of lymphocytes may be capable of killing virus-infected cells, may produce chemotactic factors that attract mononuclear phagocytes, or may produce interferon. The importance of the immune mechanism in viral disease is easily understood by keeping in mind two observations: (1) most viral infections are asymptomatic, indicating that the host defense mechanisms are capable of limiting the infection with little consequence for the host, and (2) viral infections in naturally or iatrogenically immunosuppressed individuals are often devastating.

RNA VIRUSES
Orthomyxoviruses

Influenza is a disease characterized by abrupt onset, fever, sore throat, headache, muscle pains, and acute toxic state. Dry cough and nasal discharge are present but usually are overshadowed by systemic symptoms. In uncomplicated cases the illness lasts a few days, but pulmonary complications such as influenza pneumonia and

secondary bacterial infection of the lung may complicate and prolong the course. Epidemics of influenza have been recorded for the past 400 years. Between 1173 and 1875 there were at least 299 outbreaks of the disease at an average interval of 2.4 years. When epidemics are of worldwide scope they are referred to as pandemics. The greatest pandemic occurred in 1918 and caused 21 million deaths.[19] Influenza A virus was first isolated in ferrets by Smith and co-workers[106] in 1933. Influenza B virus was isolated by Francis[35] in 1936, and Taylor[113] isolated influenza C virus in 1950. The first vaccines for influenza were developed in the 1950s and have since been used in various parts of the world to protect selected segments of the population.

Influenza virus is a filamentous or spherical particle measuring from 80 to 100 nm in diameter when spherical. It exhibits projections or spikes at the surface of the envelope. The filamentous particles may measure up to 400 nm in length.[25] The surface spikes are glycoproteins with two biologic properties: a hemagglutinin and a neuraminidase.[101] The hemagglutinin is the molecule that mediates attachment of the virus to the susceptible host cell and also to erythrocytes. If the hemagglutinin spikes are removed by chymotrypsin, the infectivity is reduced to one thousandth of the original activity.[91] The neuraminidase spike may function to remove sialic acid from the mucins present at the surface of the cells lining the respiratory tract. It also is thought to play an important role in the release of mature virions from the infected cell.

Influenza virus has eight different segments of RNA in its genome. The genome shows high levels of recombination between genes located in different segments. The segmented nature of the influenza virus genome explains the antigenic variations observed among the isolates made in different epidemics. Minor changes in antigenicity are referred to as *antigenic drift*, and they occur frequently within a given influenza subtype. Major antigenic shifts usually herald pandemics and are likely to result from genetic recombination of viruses that have replicated in nonhuman reservoirs. Continual shifting of RNA segments between animal and human influenza viruses allows for the emergence of new antigenic types that infect the human population.[122] Thus new strains of influenza A, for example, can arise in nature by genetic reassortment in animal hosts. Once a new strain emerges it may be at selective advantage, since there is a high level of immunity in the human population to the old strain but a lack of immunity to the new strain.

Infection in the human is usually acquired by transfer of virus-containing respiratory secretions from an infected to a susceptible person. Biopsies of patients with acute influenza reveal desquamation of the ciliated and columnar epithelium of the nasopharynx, nasal cavity, and bronchi. Individual cells show pyknosis of the nuclei

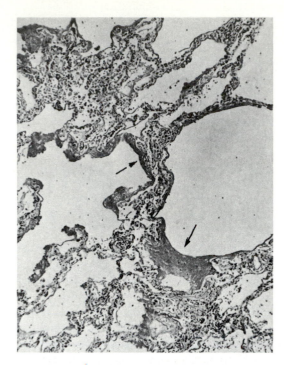

Fig. 10-2. Asian influenza. Pure viral lesion with interstitial pneumonia and hyaline membrane *(arrows)* lining air sacs.

and loss of cilia. If influenza pneumonia complicates the case, the lungs are dark red and firm with interstitial emphysema that may extend into the mediastinal tissue. Microscopically there is marked sloughing of the bronchial epithelial cells into the bronchial lumina. Intra-alveolar hemorrhage and hyaline membrane formation can be seen in such cases (Fig. 10-2). The inflammatory infiltrate is sparse. If bacterial superinfection occurs, the picture is indistinguishable from that of ordinary bronchopneumonia or lobar pneumonia. Superinfection with hemolytic streptococci or *Haemophilus influenzae* results in a diffuse hemorrhagic consolidation. Myocarditis and pericarditis, as well as encephalitis, might be found at postmortem examination of fatal cases but they are uncommon.

Paramyxoviruses

Paramyxoviruses are spherical enveloped particles with a diameter ranging from 100 to 800 nm containing a nucleocapsid with an RNA genome. In common with the influenza viruses (orthomyxoviruses) they have spikes in the envelope with hemagglutinin activity and in some cases also with neuraminidase activity. In contrast, however, to influenza viruses they are antigenically stable and genetic recombination does not occur. The paramyxoviruses that infect humans include the parainfluenza viruses 1, 2, 3, 4A, and 4B; the mumps virus; the measles virus; and the respiratory syncytial virus. Newcastle disease virus, which is a pathogen for chickens, may accidentally infect humans.

The *parainfluenza viruses* are important causes of respiratory disease in infants and young children. They are indeed the most common identifiable agents in the croup syndrome and are second only to respiratory syncytial virus as a cause of lower respiratory disease requiring hospitalization in infants.[76] The parainfluenza viruses are distributed worldwide, and the best evidence of infection is a fourfold rise of antibody titer in convalescent serum collected 3 to 4 weeks after infection. The clinical manifestations vary from no illness or a very minor cold episode to life-threatening croup and bronchiolitis. The most common symptom associated with parainfluenza is a "cold." The viruses are transmitted from person to person by transfer of respiratory tract secretions. The virus infects the cells of the upper respiratory tract mucosa, and multiplication of the viruses in those cells is probably the pathogenic substrate of the most common clinical manifestation. Parainfluenza virus antigens have been demonstrated by immunofluorescence in the ciliated columnar epithelial cells in the nasal secretions of ill children.[38] When the lung is involved, the pathologic changes are indistinguishable from those produced by other viral pneumonias.[128]

Mumps is an acute generalized benign and self-limited infection that occurs primarily in school-aged children and young adolescents. When it occurs in the postpubertal person, it is a more severe illness and more commonly leads to extrasalivary gland involvement. The complete mumps virion has an irregular spherical shape with a diameter ranging from 90 to 300 nm. The viral envelope exhibits glycoprotein spikes that possess hemagglutinin and neuraminidase activity. In addition, it also has a cell fusion activity. The genome of the virus consists of a continuous linear molecule of single-stranded RNA surrounded by symmetric repetitions of protein subunits.

Mumps is an endemic disease throughout the world. Humans are the only known natural host, but monkeys and other laboratory animals can be experimentally infected. The disease is naturally transmitted through direct contact, respiratory droplets, or fomites, which enter through the nose or mouth. Experimental infection in monkeys has been produced by direct instillation of the virus into Stensen's duct.[56]

The most common clinical manifestion of mumps is bilateral or unilateral parotiditis. It is preceded by nonspecific prodromal symptoms. Involvement of the submaxillary, submandibular, and sublingual glands is uncommon but might occur. Meningitis and encephalitis are the most common extrasalivary gland manifestations of mumps in the preadolescent, whereas in the adult male epididymitis and orchitis are the most commonly encountered. Oophoritis, arthritis, and pancreatitis have also been reported. Many case reports can be found in the literature relating maternal mumps infection to a wide variety of congenital anomalies. However, there is no convincing evidence that mumps virus is a fetal pathogen. Manson and co-workers[68] in their classic study observed no significant difference in fetal complications between 501 cases of maternal mumps and a control group irrespective of the stage in which infection occurred. These results have also been confirmed in Siegel's studies.[102] St. Geme and others[109] have suggested that intrauterine mumps infection may be linked to endocardial fibroelastosis. Hutchins and Vie[54] suggest that endocardial fibroelastosis may be the result of interstitial myocarditis with persistent left ventricular dilatation, relative mitral valvular insufficiency, and increased endocardial tension leading to compensatory hypertrophy. This in turn causes the accumulation of the thick layer of collagen and elastic tissue beneath the endocardial lining resulting in the classic picture of endocardial fibroelastosis. This mechanism could be operative in myocarditis caused by a variety of viral agents.

The lesions of the salivary glands have been best characterized in experimentally infected monkeys. The affected glands are swollen, edematous, and show minute capsular hemorrhages. Microscopically there is marked interstitial edema with inflammatory infiltrate in the ducts and degenerative changes of the ductal epithelium. The glandular cells are spared but may be focally affected by the inflammatory reaction present in the interstitial tissue. Multinucleated cells are not seen in vivo.

In *orchitis* focal hemorrhages and necrosis are frequently seen. There are also microscopic areas of infarction and a conspicuous polymorphonuclear infiltrate. Healing is associated with focal testicular atrophy. *Encephalitis* is uncommon, and when it is of early onset in the disease it usually represents damage to the neurons caused by viral replication in the neuronal cells.[112] Late-onset encephalitis is usually a postinfectious demyelinating process or perivenular postinfectious encephalitis (Fig. 10-3).

Respiratory syncytial virus (RSV) was first isolated in 1956 by Morris and co-workers[78] who named it "chimpanzee coryza agent." Shortly thereafter, Chanock and co-workers[13] confirmed that the agent was able to cause respiratory illness in humans. Respiratory syncytial virus measures from 121 to 300 nm. It has an RNA genome, and like all members of the paramyxovirus family, the envelope exhibits spokes of glycoprotein.[8] RSV is of worldwide distribution, and primary infection occurs in the very young.[92]

In the initial pulmonary infection there is a lymphocytic peribronchiolar infiltrate with some edema of the bronchial walls. Necrosis of the cells lining the bronchioles can be seen. Subsequently there is a proliferative response of the bronchial epithelium. The lumen of the small airways becomes narrowed because of sloughing of

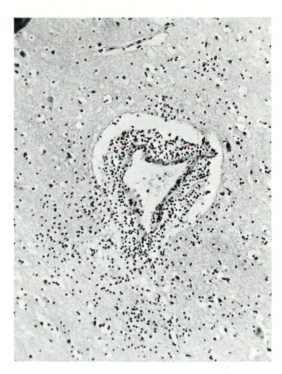

Fig. 10-3. Mumps encephalitis. Perivascular cuffing and spillage of phagocytic microglial cells into area of incipient demyelinization.

necrotic epithelium and an increase in mucin secretion. Obstruction of airflow occurs, resulting in hyperinflation and trapping of air. Complete bronchiolar obstruction may lead to atelectasis. In severe cases there is a prominent interstitial alveolar infiltrate accompanied by edema.[33,118] Other manifestations of RSV infection include otitis media, meningitis, myelitis, and myocarditis.

Measles (rubeola) is a highly communicable disease characterized by fever, cough, coryza, conjunctivitis, and an erythematous cutaneous eruption. The rash is composed of small, reddish, macular papules. It appears first on the face and spreads rapidly to the abdomen and limbs. Koplik spots are practically pathognomonic of the disease and consist of blue-gray specks with a red base that appear in the mucosa. They are most often seen opposite the second molar but in severe cases they can involve the entire mucous membrane of the mouth. These persist for several days and begin to disappear as the cutaneous rash appears. Involvement of the respiratory tract is common. Complications include involvement of the central nervous system. Measles virus is a pleomorphic agent but is usually spherical, ranging from 120 to 250 nm with hemagglutinin glycoprotein on the surface of the envelope but no neuraminidase.[28,55,83] The nuclear capsid contains an RNA genome with a molecular weight of 6.2×10^6 daltons. When grown in epithelial cells in tissue culture, measles virus produces two types of cytopathic effects. The first is the production of multinucleate giant cells with intranuclear and intra-

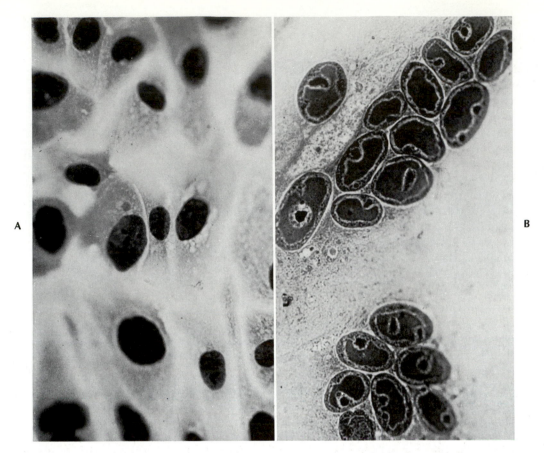

Fig. 10-4. Culture of human renal cells. **A,** Control. **B,** Cytopathogenic effect of measles giant cell pneumonia virus (strain 1) 12 days after inoculation, with giant cell formation and nuclear inclusions. (Hematoxylin and eosin; 500×; from Enders, J.F., et al.: N. Engl. J. Med. **261**:875, 1959.)

cytoplasmic inclusions (Fig. 10-4). These cells are similar to giant cells seen in the lymphoid tissue of patients with the disease and are characteristic of the virus. The other type of cytopathic effect is the so-called spindle cell transformation; it is typically produced by the vaccine strains of the virus.

Humans are the only natural host for wild-type measles virus, but monkeys may be experimentally infected. It is an endemic virus throughout the world, but the widespread use of measles vaccine has led to a marked decrease in the incidence of the disease. The infection is spread by direct contact with droplets from the respiratory tract of infected individuals.

Measles virus first infects the upper respiratory tract of the patients. After multiplying locally there is a primary viremia with spread of the virus to the reticuloendothelial system and circulating lymphocytes, especially T lymphocytes. The selective infection of T lymphocytes may be responsible for the immune defects observed in patients with measles. When the virus replicates in the lymphoid tissue of the body, it gives rise to the Warthin-Finkeldey giant cells.[34,121] After replication of the virus in the lymphoid tissue, a secondary viremic phase

occurs, and within a few days the Koplik spots appear followed by the development of the rash.

Pathologically the cutaneous lesions show vascular congestion, edema of the dermis, and perivascular lymphocytic infiltrate. The endothelial cells are swollen. Mitotic figures can be seen, and vascular thrombosis with extravasation of erythrocytes may occur. There is hyperkeratosis and vacuolization of the epidermal cells. The Koplik spots show a similar histologic picture but with more prominent necrosis of the epithelial mucosal cells and a more neutrophilic exudate.[62,63,99,107] Bronchopneumonia is the most common fatal complication of the disease. The histopathologic picture varies from almost pure interstitial pneumonitis to bacterial pneumonia. The diagnosis can be made if Warthin-Finkeldey cells are seen, although this is unusual. *Encephalitis* following measles may be acute or chronic[73] (see subacute sclerosing panencephalitis, below). The acute form is a result of viral infection of the central nervous system; mortality is estimated to be between 10% and 30%.

Measles giant cell pneumonia[29] is a characteristic pulmonary lesion observed in hosts unable to mount an antibody response to the virus. The disease usually occurs as

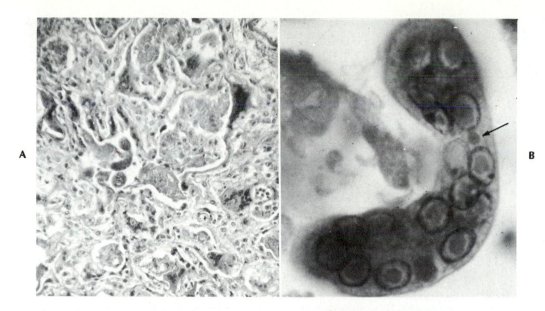

Fig. 10-5. Measles giant cell pneumonia. A, Low power showing syncytial giant cells lining alveoli and thickening of alveolar walls. B, High power of one giant cell seen in A showing many nuclear inclusions and one cytoplasmic inclusion (arrow).

a massive pneumonia in children. Histologically the pulmonary parenchyma shows marked consolidation with massive formation of syncytial giant cells showing the characteristic intranuclear eosinophilic inclusions surrounded by a halo, and intracytoplasmic inclusion bodies (Fig. 10-5). This picture was described under the term "giant cell pneumonia of infants" before the pathogenesis of the lesion was understood.

Subacute sclerosing panencephalitis (SSPE) is a progressive inflammatory brain disease of children and young adults first described by Dawson in 1934. Dawson suspected that it was a viral disease because of the inflammatory character of the lesions and the presence of intranuclear inclusion bodies in the cells about the lesion. These inclusion bodies are mainly found in neuroglial cells but also can be seen in neurons (Fig. 10-6). Cytoplasmic inclusions are less numerous but can be found. The virus recovered from cerebral biopsies and lymph node biopsies of patients with SSPE[6,52] is closely related to measles virus and probably represents a defective measles virus with a biochemical lesion that interferes with completion of the viral maturation process in the infected cell. The pathologic findings in SSPE are those of a subacute encephalitis involving both the white and gray matter of the cerebral hemispheres and the brainstem. There are perivascular lymphocytic infiltrates, and there is evidence of neuronal loss. In later stages diffuse proliferation of glial cells and degeneration of myelin occur. By electron microscopy the inclusions are seen to contain tubular paramyxovirus-like nucleocapsids. Measles virus antigen can be demonstrated in the nuclei and cytoplasm of infected neurons and glial cells.[42,114]

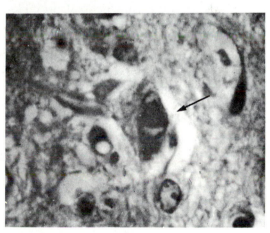

Fig. 10-6. Subacute sclerosing panencephalitis. *Arrow,* Neuron containing homogeneous eosinophilic nuclear inclusion with halo.

Coronaviridae

Coronaviruses cause disease in a variety of animals such as rats, mice, chickens, turkeys, cats, and pigs. In humans they were first isolated from patients with the common cold by inoculating respiratory tract secretions into human embryonic tracheal organ cultures.[117] The viral particles have a diameter ranging from 60 to 200 nm. They are enveloped virions with widely spaced, petal-shaped projections 20 nm in length that give a crownlike appearance to the virion, hence the name coronavirus.[116] The genome is a single-stranded RNA molecule with a molecular weight of about 6×10^6 daltons. Coronavirus infections have been found throughout the world.

The human coronaviruses cause upper respiratory

tract disease,[71] and several strains have been recovered from adults suffering from the common cold.

Rhabdoviridae

The rhabdoviruses are RNA viruses with a single-stranded RNA genome of 4 million daltons in molecular weight. The nuclear capsid is enclosed within a bullet-shaped capsid that measures approximately 175×75 nm. Rhabdoviruses infect vertebrates, insects, and plants. The most important rhabdovirus in humans is rabies virus. Other rhabdoviruses are vesicular stomatitis virus, the Mokola virus, the Lagos bat virus, the Obodhiang virus, and the Katonkan virus.

Rabies is one of the oldest known and most feared of human diseases.[5] It is primarily a disease of animals, and the epidemiology of human rabies closely parallels the epizoology of animal rabies. Where domestic animal rabies has not been controlled, dog or cat bites account for 90% of the reported human cases. In areas where the domestic animal rabies is well controlled, the majority of exposures are the consequence of wild animal bites such as bat, skunk, wolf, coyote, and raccoon bites. It is likely that rabies maintains itself as an endemic illness in each of these species. Rabies is transmitted to humans practically always as a result of a bite from a rabid domestic or wild animal. The disease has also rarely been transmitted through corneal transplants. Clinically the initial symptoms of the disease are nonspecific, such as malaise, fatigue, and headache, followed by a period of acute neurologic symptomatology including hyperactivity, disorientation, hallucinations, seizures, and bizarre behavior, followed by coma and death. Combined immune serum and vaccine are the recommended postexposure prophylaxis of the disease in the United States. Specific chemotherapy for clinical rabies is not available, and treatment consists of intensive supportive care.

The rabies virus multiplies at the site of the local bite and travels to the central nervous system through the peripheral nerves. Once in the central nervous system it replicates within the neurons.[80] Grossly the brain and spinal cord show edema and petechial hemorrhages. Involvement of the spinal cord is most conspicuous when the portal of entry is on the lower part of the body. Microscopically the predominant inflammatory lesion consists of lymphocytic perivascular cuffing within the parenchyma of the nervous system. Little meningeal reaction is seen. Nodules of glial cells termed Babès' nodes are often seen and consist of nonspecific glial aggregates. In about 75% of cases Negri bodies can be seen on hematoxylin and eosin–stained sections. These cytoplasmic inclusion bodies in the neurons are pathognomonic for rabies and are an important diagnostic finding (Fig. 10-7). They are most consistently present in the Purkinje cells of the cerebellum and in the large neurons of the hippocampus. They are found in intact neurons as round to oval eosinophilic bodies measuring 2 to 10 μm

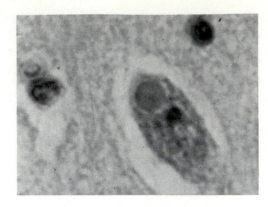

Fig. 10-7. Negri bodies of rabies.

in diameter.[27,84] Ultrastructural studies have shown that the Negri body consists of a mass of nucleocapsids surrounded by viral particles budding from intracytoplasmic membranes.[111] Those bodies can be seen in axons, and it is in this way that the virus spreads from the central nervous system to many organs of the body. Because Negri bodies are usually seen in intact neurons, they are found away from the inflammatory, nonspecific lesions. Rabies viral antigens can be demonstrated in infected cells by means of fluorescent antibody techniques.[80] Antigens can be shown to be present in cells in the absence of Negri bodies, and hence this technique is much more sensitive than the search of sections of brain for the pathognomonic cytoplasmic inclusions.

Bunyaviridae

The *Bunyavirus* genus consists of over 80 antigenically related viruses of which the California encephalitis group is the most important.[94] The virions are enveloped spherical particles approximately 100 nm in diameter, and they contain a three-part segmented genome of single-stranded RNA segments. This allows for genetic recombination or reassortment to occur in doubly infected cells. The principal member of the California encephalitis virus group in the United States is the La Crosse (LAC) virus. It is transmitted to humans by *Aedes triseriatus*, a forest-dwelling mosquito of the north central and northeastern United States. Infection of humans may result in a mild febrile illness or sometimes a severe encephalitis or meningoencephalitis.[59] Most patients appear to recover completely, although personality changes and learning disorders have been reported as sequelae.

Togaviridae

Many viruses have been classified in the past based on their mode of transmission. The viruses transmitted from person to person or from animal to human by means of arthropods were classified as arthropod-borne animal viruses or arboviruses.[12] Information accumulated on the physical and biochemical properties of the viruses grouped under arboviruses indicates that several different virus families were included and that some members of those families were not transmitted by arthropod vectors. Viruses that are transmitted by arthropod vectors are now classified under one of the following families: Bunyaviridae, Togaviridae, Reoviridae, and Rhabdoviridae. Togaviridae are spherical, enveloped virions measuring 40 to 90 nm in diameter with a nuclear capsid that exhibits cubic symmetry.[32] There are two genera of Togaviridae that contain viruses transmitted by arthropod vectors, the alphaviruses and the flaviviruses.

Rubella virus (German measles) is a spherical, enveloped virus measuring approximately 60 nm in diameter. It has an RNA genome, and it replicates in the cell cytoplasm maturing by budding from the cell membrane.[79] The virus is classified in the togavirus family as a separate genus, *Rubivirus*, based on the RNA genome, icosahedral capsule, and lipoprotein envelope. The virus is spread by droplets that are shed from respiratory secretions of infected persons. Infants born with congenital rubella shed large quantities of virus from body secretions for many months.

Infection with rubella virus leads to very different diseases depending on the age at which the virus interacts with the host. Postnatally acquired rubella is generally an innocuous infection. Probably most cases are subclinical, and the patients who are symptomatic do not experience a prodromal phase. The major symptoms of infection by rubella virus in the adult are adenopathy, especially in the occipital and posterior cervical region, fever, malaise, leukopenia, and relative lymphocytosis. The picture is accompanied by a mild, generalized, macular eruption that is probably related to the antibody response. Rubella virus has been detected in leukocytes of patients during the viremic phase and has been recovered also from skin lesions at the time of the rash.[51] Contrasting with the benign, self-limited course of the postnatal infection, the fetus is at high risk for developing severe disease with long-standing sequelae if infected transplacentally.[15] In some cases infection will be incompatible with fetal life. Not all the consequences of fetal infection are evident at birth, and some lesions resulting from the viral infection become apparent years after birth. The effects of the virus on the fetus are in part dependent on the time of infection. The younger the fetus, the more severe the effects. During the first 2 months of fetal life, the fetus has a 40% to 60% chance of being affected with an outcome of either multiple congenital defects or spontaneous abortion. During the third month of the fetal life, rubella has been associated with 30% to 35% chance of developing a single defect such as deafness or congenital heart disease. Fetal infection during the fourth month carries a 10% risk of a single congenital defect.

The results of rubella infection are varied and multiple and involve the cardiovascular system, the ocular and auditory systems, the liver, the reticuloendothelial system, and (predominantly) the central nervous system.[26,30] To explain such varied lesions a number of mechanisms have been proposed. They include inhibition of cellular growth after infection, fetal vasculitis and placental angiopathy, and tissue necrosis. Human fibroblasts infected with rubella virus produce a growth inhibition factor, which could perhaps be related to retardation of fetal growth.

Alphaviruses

The *Alphavirus* genus includes 20 viruses. They are antigenically related and correspond to the group A arboviruses in Casals' serologic classification. There are enveloped spherical virions containing a single-stranded RNA genome of 4×10^6 daltons. Eastern, western, and Venezuelan equine encephalitis are the three significant diseases caused by these viruses in humans.[50] They are initiated by inoculation of the virus by a mosquito bite. In the laboratory alphaviruses can be transmitted by aerosol and have caused numerous infections in laboratory workers by this route. After inoculation the virus multiplies in the nonneuronal tissues causing a febrile illness. The infection may be eliminated by the host defense mechanisms after a subclinical infection or a benign febrile illness, or the virus may invade the central nervous system giving rise to an encephalitis. Alphaviruses replicate in the central nervous system causing cell destruction and a severe inflammatory response. The fatality rate for western equine encephalitis is approximately 10% and for eastern equine encephalitis 70%. Total recovery is uncommon, and patients are left with sequelae that include mental retardation, behavioral changes, and convulsive disorders. The mortality resulting from Venezuelan equine encephalitis is in general low, although a more severe form of the disease has been recognized and is probably caused by the lymphocytolytic effect of the virus.

Gross examination of the brain in fatal cases of *eastern equine encephalitis* shows edema. Microscopically, there is a marked meningoencephalitis with a conspicuous, acute, neutrophilic infiltrate and an acute vasculitis with fibrinoid necrosis of the vessel wall. Neuronal necrosis and neuronophagia are very common. At later stages glial nodules and perivascular cuffing become prominent. The lesions involve all regions of the brain, but the brainstem and basal ganglia may be the most severely involved regions.

In *western equine encephalitis* the inflammatory response is less intense and composed of mononuclear cells. The greatest damage is seen in the basal ganglia and in the white matter of the cerebral hemispheres. Cystic degeneration of the white matter has been described in patients under 1 year of age.

Little is known about the pathology of *Venezuelan equine encephalitis* since the mortality is low. The encephalomyelitis is milder than the other types and morphologically consists mostly of perivascular cuffing and microglial nodules. The inflammatory lesions may be most prominent in the putamen and cerebral white matter.

Establishing the diagnosis of alphavirus infection depends on clinical and epidemiologic information and obtaining the appropriate specimens for biologic and serologic tests. In fatal cases of encephalitis the virus may be isolated from the central nervous system tissues obtained at autopsy. As a rule, virus is not present in the cerebrospinal fluid.

Flaviviruses

Flaviviruses are immunologically distinguishable from alphaviruses. They are enveloped, spherical, and slightly smaller than alphaviruses, measuring 40 to 50 nm. All flaviviruses with the exception of dengue have complex primary cycles of transmission involving arthropod vectors, wild birds, and mammals. In many cases humans are an accidental end host because the levels of viremia produced are insufficient to infect vectors. Flaviviruses cause the following diseases in humans: dengue (breakbone fever), St. Louis encephalitis, Japanese B encephalitis, tick-borne encephalitis, and yellow fever. Dengue virus has a human-mosquito-human cycle.

Dengue virus infection causes a syndrome characterized by fever, rash, and muscle and joint pains. It also can cause a severe hemorrhagic disease (dengue hemorrhagic fever, which is now recognized as an epidemic disease in Southeast Asia). Biopsy studies of the rash seen in nonfatal dengue fever show a lymphocytic vasculitis in the dermis. In cases of fatal dengue hemorrhagic fever, the gross findings are petechial hemorrhages in the skin and hemorrhagic effusions in the pleural, pericardial, and abdominal cavities. Hemorrhage and congestion are seen in many organs. Histologic studies show hemorrhage, perivascular edema, and focal necrosis but no vasculitic or endothelial lesions. It is believed that most of the morphologic abnormalities seen result from disseminated intravascular coagulation and shock.[123]

St. Louis encephalitis was recognized in 1933 when an epidemic occurred in southern Illinois and in the area of St. Louis, Missouri. The virus was recovered from brain tissue at autopsy from persons who died of the disease during the 1933 epidemic. The St. Louis encephalitis virus replicates at the site of inoculation and probably gains access to the central nervous system through viremia. In fatal cases of St. Louis encephalitis the brain may appear normal at gross examination. The histologic features are those of a meningoencephalitis, with leptomeningeal mononuclear cell infiltration and parenchymal lesions consisting of perivascular cuffing and reactive microglial nodules. The lesions are more intense in the substantia nigra and thalamic nuclei.[87]

Severe epidemics of encephalitis have occurred in Japan since 1871. The mortality in acute cases is between 30% and 40%, and epidemics are caused by the *Japanese encephalitis* virus transmitted by an arthropod. Cases have been reported in Japan, Korea, China, Southeast Asia, and India. Pathologically the meningoencephalitis involves especially the subcortical zone of the white matter. In patients surviving for a long time the lesions may become heavily calcified. Neuronophagia is commonly seen in the ventral horns of the spinal cord.

Tick-borne encephalitis virus is responsible for epidemics of *Russian spring-summer encephalitis*. The disease occurs in the U.S.S.R., central Europe, and Finland. The virus is maintained between ticks and various warm-blooded mammals. Most clinical cases occur in people exposed to infections in forests or in the laboratory. The clinical disease ranges from meningeal irritation to frank meningoencephalitis with paralysis. In fatal cases there is congestion of the brain; microscopically lesions are found in the gray matter of the precentral cortex, basal ganglia, brainstem, cerebellum, and spinal cord. In the spinal cord the lesions are more severe in the cervical and lower lumbar segments.

Yellow fever is an acute illness manifested by abrupt onset of chills and fever, conjunctival injection, leukopenia, a brief period of remission, and then reappearance of fever with jaundice, punctate hemorrhages of the soft palate, epistaxis, and gingival and gastrointestinal bleeding (black vomit). Approximately 50% of the patients develop relative bradycardia in relation to the degree of fever. The yellow fever virus is viscerotropic, causing the most damage in the liver, kidney, heart, and gastrointestinal tract. The gross features in fatal cases are not specific. The heart when involved is flabby and pale with scattered pericardial and petechial hemorrhages. Microscopically there are degeneration of myocardial fibers and accumulation of fat. The kidneys may show edema; microscopically the features are those seen in cases of acute tubular necrosis. Hemoglobin casts may be seen. The most characteristic pathologic changes are seen in the liver.[11,103] The appearance of the lesions is typical between the seventh and ninth day of the illness. The liver is grossly normal in size, pale, and yellow because of fatty metamorphosis. Microscopically there is extensive midzonal necrosis, which in severe cases may extend to become panlobular (Fig. 10-8). Intracellular condensations of cytoplasm that appear as round to oval, well-demarcated, eosinophilic inclusions are termed *Councilman bodies*. These are also found in the cytoplasm of Kupffer cells. These inclusions are not composed of virus particles and are nonspecific for the disease. They are periodic acid–Schiff (PAS) positive. A hallmark of the hepatitis caused by yellow fever virus is the absence of an inflammatory component. Also distinctive of the lesion is the fact that despite massive necrosis, the reticulin

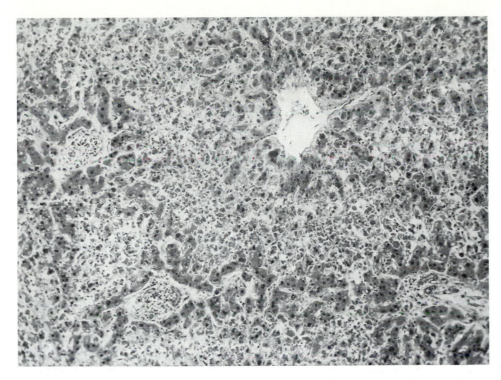

Fig. 10-8. Yellow fever. Liver lesion characterized by midzonal necrosis as shown here. However, damage may involve other portions of lobule or even entire lobule. Early degeneration and necrosis of hepatic cells are attended by relatively little inflammatory reaction. (AFIP 68426; from Ash, J.E., and Spitz, S.: Pathology of tropical diseases, Philadelphia, 1945, W.B. Saunders Co.)

framework of the hepatic lobule is preserved. Fatty metamorphosis of the microvacuolar type is invariably seen.

Arenaviridae

Arenaviruses are round, oval, or pleomorphic with a range in size between 100 and 130 nm. They are enveloped particles, and the envelope contains club-shaped projections at its surface. Electron-dense granules are found in variable numbers in the interior of the virions. These granules are 20 to 25 nm in diameter and represent host ribosomes. The sandlike granules gave the name to this group of viruses (*arena*, Latin for sand).[81] The genome of arenaviruses consists of four pieces of single-stranded RNA and several small pieces of RNA, some of which may be of host origin. Rodents are the natural host of arenaviruses, and humans are accidentally infected when they come in contact with infected urine. Person-to-person spread is unusual except for Lassa virus. The relevant members of the Arenaviridae family are lymphocytic choriomeningitis virus, Lassa virus, Junin virus, and Machupo virus.

Lymphocytic choriomeningitis (LCM) virus infection is probably widespread throughout the world, although it has been rigorously documented only in North America and Europe.[65] The mode of spread of LCM virus in most sporadic human cases is unknown, but studies suggest direct contact with rodents or spread by infected aerosols. The clinical disease produced by LCM is a meningitis, a meningoencephalitis, or a self-limited febrile illness. Arthritis, parotiditis, orchitis, and myopericarditis have also been reported. Fatal cases in humans are extremely rare. In monkeys infected by inhalation, virus can be recovered from the lungs and hilar lymph nodes 2 days after infection. Lymphocytic meningitis is often the most conspicuous lesion, but hemorrhagic necrosis may also be seen in liver, kidney, heart, adrenal gland, and other organs. The spleen and the lymph nodes show hyperplasia.

Lassa fever is a disease that ranges in severity from mild and perhaps even subclinical infection to an inexorably progressive, multisystem illness with a mortality of over 45%. The early symptoms of Lassa fever are nonspecific. The diagnosis may be made serologically or by isolation of the virus from serum, throat washings, pleural or ascitic fluid, or urine. Attempts to isolate the virus should be made only in a maximum containment laboratory.

Junin and Machupo viruses are the etiologic agents of the Argentine and Bolivian hemorrhagic fevers. These fevers have similar clinical features, which result from involvement of the hemopoietic, cardiovascular, and central nervous systems. Mortality averages 10% to 20%. The illness begins with fever, malaise, marked myalgia, retro-orbital headache, and cutaneous hyperesthesia. As the illness progresses there are hypertension, diaphoresis, and neurologic manifestations ranging from irritability to seizures. The diagnosis is established by isolation of the virus or by demonstration of significant rises in neutralizing antibody in the serum of the patient. Virus can be recovered from blood, throat, and less commonly urine.

The pathology of hemorrhagic fevers caused by arenaviruses (Lassa, Argentine, and Bolivian hemorrhagic fevers) varies.[14,119,125,129] Interstitial pneumonitis sometimes with hyaline membrane disease is prominent. Morphologic evidence of encephalitis is unusual and inconspicuous when present even though the clinical picture may include encephalopathy and other central nervous system symptoms. The reticuloendothelial system appears activated, and phagocytic activity in Kupffer cells is a common finding. In all three diseases there are focal areas of central and pericentral hepatic necrosis. Eosinophilic or acidophilic bodies similar to Councilman bodies are present in hepatocytes and Kupffer cells. The fatty metamorphosis observed in almost all cases of yellow fever is not present in Lassa fever.

Picornaviridae

The picornaviruses are characterized by nonenveloped virions with icosahedral capsids 20 to 30 nm in diameter. They contain a single-stranded RNA genome with a molecular weight of 2.6×10^6 daltons. Two genera of picornaviruses that commonly infect humans are the enteroviruses, which have at least 67 recognized immunologic types, and the rhinoviruses, with more than 100 types infecting the human. Enteroviruses have been subdivided on the basis of antigenic relationships and differences in host range into polioviruses, coxsackieviruses groups A and B, and echoviruses.

Coxsackieviruses were first isolated in suckling mice from the feces of two children suffering from a poliomyelitis-like syndrome in the town of Coxsackie, New York.[127] When additional agents of the same group were isolated, it was recognized that some, called group A, produced generalized myositis and flaccid paralysis in the mice used for isolation. Others, classified as group B, produced a focal myositis but also affected the myocardium, brown fat, pancreas, and central nervous system. Damage to the central nervous system results in spastic paralysis. Coxsackieviruses, like most members of the enterovirus group, are transmitted predominantly by the fecal-oral route rather than by respiratory secretions. They have been associated with the following diseases of children: aseptic meningitis, encephalitis, herpangina, pleurodynia, hand-foot-mouth syndrome, pericarditis, lymphonodular pharyngitis, epidemic conjunctivitis, and myocarditis.

The *echoviruses* (enteric cytopathogenic human or-

phan viruses) were isolated from fecal specimens of healthy children.[127] They produce cytopathic effects in primate cell cultures, but at isolation they were nonpathogenic for suckling mice or primates. They are immunologically distinct from polioviruses and have been associated with a variety of diseases including nonspecific febrile illnesses with or without respiratory symptoms, aseptic meningitis, paralysis and encephalitis, exanthem, generalized disease of newborn, and neonatal diarrhea. They also have been associated with chronic meningoencephalitis in agammaglobulinemic patients.

Three immunotypes of *polioviruses* can be distinguished on the basis of neutralization tests. Most paralytic disease in the prevaccine era was caused by type 1. Humans are the only natural host and reservoir of polioviruses, although in the laboratory polioviruses infect other primates. Early after infection in humans the virus replicates in the gut and adjacent lymphoid tissues, spreading to the regional lymph nodes. From there, there is a minor viremia that disseminates the virus to all susceptible reticuloendothelial tissues. At this point, in many patients, there is an antibody response that limits the infection, which remains subclinical. In some, however, extensive viral replication in the reticuloendothelial system gives rise to a second major viremia, which corresponds with the clinical minor illness or abortive poliomyelitis. These viremias may result in meningitis. It is probably through viremia—although spread via the nervous system has not been ruled out—that the viruses reach the central nervous system and replicate in the neurons of the gray matter, destroying them.

Before the late 1800s poliomyelitis was predominantly sporadic. Early in the nineteenth century epidemics were recognized in Scandinavia and western Europe, and in the first half of the twentieth century epidemics of the disease occurred in developed countries. In the early 1950s around 20,000 cases of paralytic disease were being reported annually in the United States. The introduction of inactivated vaccines in 1955 and attenuated oral vaccines in 1962 brought a dramatic reduction in incidence of paralytic poliomyelitis in the developed countries of the world. In the postvaccine era an increasing proportion of cases of paralytic poliomyelitis in the United States are associated with the use of oral poliovaccines. This vaccine-associated disease is seen not only in the recipients of the vaccine but occasionally in their contacts. The estimated risk of vaccine-associated disease is one recipient case and two contact cases per 10 million doses of trivalent oral polioviruses distributed.[86]

The manifestations of infection by polioviruses are extremely variable. The varieties of illness are inapparent infection; abortive, nonparalytic, spinal paralytic, or bulbar poliomyelitis; and encephalitis. A number of risk factors are known to influence the likelihood that an individual will develop paralysis once infected with poliovirus. Boys are more commonly paralyzed than girls, and exercise, trauma, tonsillectomy, and pregnancy all increase the risk of paralytic forms of the disease. Tonsillectomized persons have a risk of acquiring bulbar poliomyelitis that is approximately eight times that in those with intact tonsils. The risk is true not only for those with onset of infection shortly before or after tonsillectomy but also when tonsillectomy is remote.

The gross pathology in both acute and chronic cases of poliomyelitis infection may be inconspicuous. The most severe lesions are usually found in the anterior two thirds of the gray matter of the spinal cord.[1,9] They vary from level to level and might be asymmetric in the same section of spinal cord. The ventral horns and the base of the dorsal horns are infiltrated by lymphocytes and hypertrophied microglial cells. Polymorphonuclear leukocytes are often numerous in the neuronophagic nodules that are seen in the early stages of the disease (Fig. 10-9). The leptomeninges show a varying degree of infiltration with inflammatory cells. The earliest lesion in neurons is loss of Nissl substance in the cytoplasm. There is subsequent progression to eosinophilic necrosis with presence of type B intranuclear inclusions. Death of the neuron is followed by neuronophagia. The perivascular infiltration with lymphocytes and plasma cells in the leptomeninges and parenchyma may persist for weeks or even months.

In cases that come to autopsy long after onset of paralysis the most obvious change is loss of neurons in the ventral horns. The axons of the neurons that have been destroyed undergo wallerian degeneration, and the affected muscle shows the typical features of denervation atrophy. Lesions outside the nervous system are less striking. In patients dying in the acute stage of the disease there is generalized lymph node enlargement with disseminated petechial hemorrhages.

Rhinoviruses

Rhinoviruses share many of the properties of the picornavirus group.[46] Human rhinoviruses will infect only humans and higher primates, and epidemiologic studies have shown that rhinoviruses are the major cause of the common cold. They have also been implicated in acute paranasal sinus infection. Currently over 90 types of rhinoviruses have been identified. The identification of new types of rhinoviruses may continue, since it is possible that antigenic drift occurs in this virus. Rhinovirus colds are one of the most common infections in humans, with a rate of 1.2 infections per person per year in children under the age of 1 year and 0.7 infections per year in young adults. The major site for rhinovirus transmission is the home, and the infection is often introduced by a child of school age. Efficient transmission of the rhinoviruses probably depends on close contact.

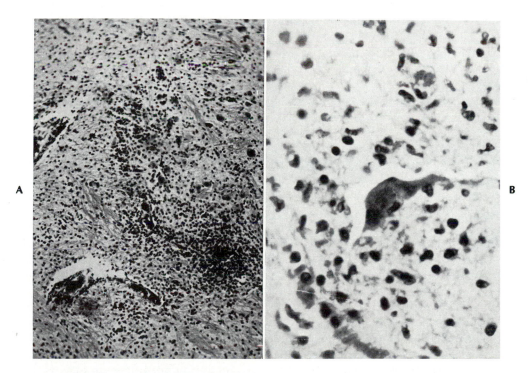

Fig. 10-9. Poliomyelitis. **A,** Focal and diffuse inflammatory cell infiltration in anterior horn of spinal cord. **B,** Degenerating neuron in anterior horn, surrounded by inflammatory cells, some of which are neutrophils. (**A,** From Anderson, W.A.D., and Scotti, T.M.: Synopsis of pathology, ed. 7, St. Louis, 1968, The C.V. Mosby Co.)

Other RNA viruses

Marburg and *Ebola viruses* are pleomorphic RNA viruses that are distinct from all other viruses and from each other serologically. Their natural reservoir remains undetermined. The initial Marburg virus outbreak in 1967 resulted in 31 infections in Marburg and Frankfurt, Germany, and in Yugoslavia. All patients had contact with infected monkey kidneys. The source of the virus was African green monkey cells imported from Uganda for use in the preparation of vaccines. Additional cases of Marburg virus disease were reported from Johannesburg, South Africa, in 1975. The epidemiology and epizootiology of Ebola virus are unclear. The only reported outbreaks of the disease occurred in Sudan and Zaire in 1976. Both Marburg and Ebola viruses produce hemorrhagic fevers.[58,69] Death usually results from hemorrhagic complications, renal failure, or shock. Epidemics have been controlled by strict isolation procedures.

Orbiviruses belong to the family of Reoviridae. The genus *Orbivirus* was created to classify a group of about 25 arthropod-borne viruses with distinctive physical, chemical, and serologic properties. Three viruses in this genus are known to cause disease in humans. They are the *Colorado tick fever virus*, the *Kemerovo virus*, and the *Orungo virus*. The Colorado tick and Kemerovo viruses are transmitted by ticks, while the Orungo virus is mosquito borne. Colorado tick fever is a self-limited disease characterized by fever, chills, lethargy, and prostration.[108] The duration of the acute illness is 7 to 10 days, and the fever is characteristically biphasic in about 15% of the cases. Encephalitis, meningoencephalitis, and meningitis are possible complications in children. Kemerovo and Orungo viruses produce myalgias, headache, and febrile illnesses.

Electron microscopy and immune electron microscopy of stool filtrates from patients suffering from viral gastroenteritis have identified two classes of agents, the Norwalk group of viruses and the rotavirus group. The *rotavirus group* is very likely a major etiologic agent of infantile gastroenteritis in many parts of the world. It has been associated with about 50% of acute diarrheal illnesses in hospitalized pediatric patients.[61,62] Rotaviruses are nonlipid-containing RNA viruses with a double-stranded RNA genome composed of 11 segments. The human rotavirus induces a diarrheal illness in various newborn animals. In the few cases that have been pathologically studied the changes observed include infiltration of the lamina propria of the small intestine with mononuclear cells and shortening of the mucosal villi.[100] Ultrastructurally, mitochondrial swelling, irregularities in the microvilli, and dilatation of the endoplasmic reticulum have also been observed.

The term *Norwalk-like agents* refers to a group of viruses detected in stools from patients with acute gastroenteritis. These agents are named in most instances for the location of the outbreak of illness from which they have been identified. The Norwalk-like agents have not been cultivated in vitro but are identified by electron microscopy and immune electron microscopy. They appear as nonenveloped particles 25 to 27 nm in diameter with cubic symmetry. Gastrointestinal illness has been transmitted to normal volunteers after oral administration of Norwalk and Hawaii agents. Infection with the Norwalk and Hawaii agents results in jejunal lesions characterized by blunting of the villi and inflammatory cell infiltrate in the lamina propria.[24]

Hepatitis A virus

The visualization by Feinston and co-workers[31] in 1973 of a viral particle by immune electron microscopy in the acute phase of experimentally and naturally infected individuals indicated that infectious hepatitis had at least two etiologic agents: the hepatitis A virus, a spherical particle 27 to 29 nm in diameter with icosahedral symmetry, and the hepatitis B virus (see p. 367).

Hepatitis A virus purified from stool has been found to be infectious in the chimpanzee and has been used as an immunogen for production of monospecific antibodies in rabbits.[10] Using this antibody, researchers can detect hepatitis A antigen in hepatocytes of experimentally infected chimpanzees. The staining is finely granular, which is localized in cytoplasm and not in the nucleus. Examination of other tissues including small and large bowel mucosa reveals no evidence of antigen synthesis.

The hepatitis A virus is usually transmitted by close person-to-person contact, probably almost always by the fecal-oral route. Patients are probably most infectious in the late incubation period or about the time symptoms begin. No cases of chronic hepatitis A virus shedding have been documented. The histopathology of acute viral hepatitis is discussed in Chapter 27.

DNA VIRUSES
Adenoviruses

Adenoviruses were first isolated in 1953 by Rowe and co-workers[97] from human adenoids removed at surgery. At present more than 30 human serotypes have been described. Many serotypes are not linked to a specific disease. Human adenoviruses have a capsid with icosahedral symmetry. Rodlike structures with knobs at the ends protrude from the capsid. The genome of the virus is a double-stranded DNA linear molecule with a weight of 23×10^6 daltons. When infecting cells in vitro, adenoviruses are capable of lytic infection, latent infection, and transformation. Because of the ability to transform cells and to produce tumors in rodents, they have been considered possible human tumor viruses, but to date there is no evidence that links adenoviruses to human tumors. Adenoviruses are associated with the following diseases:

coryza and pharyngitis in infants; upper respiratory disease, pharyngoconjunctival fever, and hemorrhagic cystitis in children; acute respiratory disease and pneumonia in young adults; and epidemic keratoconjunctivitis and pneumonia in immunocompromised and normal adults.

The histopathology of *adenovirus pneumonia* was described by Goodpasture and co-workers[44] in a paper reporting five cases of pneumonia in infants up to 2½ years of age. Goodpasture postulated the viral etiology of the disease based on the presence of intranuclear inclusion bodies. Adenovirus pneumonia is characterized by a necrotizing bronchitis and bronchiolitis. There is intense necrosis and desquamation of the respiratory epithelium into the bronchial lumina.[110,126] These foci of bronchiolitis are surrounded by areas of consolidation, hemorrhage, and atelectasis. At low power the appearance may be confused with bacterial bronchopneumonia. In the areas of consolidation and among the necrotizing bronchiolar epithelial lesions, cells with intranuclear inclusion bodies may be found. In the early stages cytopathic effects are manifested by granular, slightly enlarged nuclei containing eosinophilic bodies intermixed with clumped basophilic chromatin (Fig. 10-10). The eosinophilic bodies coalesce, forming larger masses to end as a central, granular, ill-defined mass surrounded by a halo.

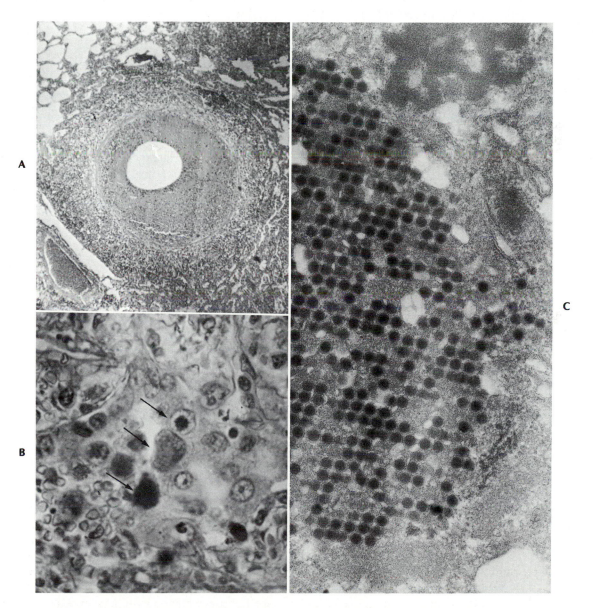

Fig. 10-10. Adenovirus pneumonia. **A,** Necrotizing bronchiolitis with inspissated secretion. **B,** *Arrows from above downward,* Nuclear inclusion of rosette type, hypertrophied nucleus, and smudge cell, with fusion of nucleus and cytoplasm. **C,** Electron micrograph of smudge cell, showing spillage of adenovirions and other nuclear components into cytoplasm. (**A,** AFIP 971609; **C,** 36,000×.)

The second type of inclusion, which is more common and probably corresponds to a late-stage infected cell, is designated the "smudge cell." The nucleus is rounded or ovoid, large, and completely occupied by a granular amphophilic to deeply basophilic mass. There is no halo, and the nuclear membrane and nucleus are indistinct. Electron microscopy of the lung demonstrates viral particles in the bronchiolar and alveolar lining cells.

Herpesviruses

The family of herpesviruses consists of a large group of enveloped DNA viruses measuring approximately 120 nm in diameter. Inside the capsid there is a nucleoprotein core that contains a linear, double-stranded DNA molecule with a molecular weight of 100 million daltons. Herpesviruses multiply in the nucleus of the host cell and mature by budding from the cell membranes. The members of the herpesvirus family of relevance to human disease are herpes simplex virus, cytomegalovirus, varicella-zoster virus, Epstein-Barr virus, and herpes simiae virus (B virus). The first four viruses have humans as their natural host; herpes simiae virus infects humans only as a laboratory accident. One pathogenetic property of importance that is shared by all human herpesviruses is the ability to produce latent infections. Following a primary infection, infectious virus can no longer be recovered from the host tissues, but the virus resides in an inactive form in cells from which it can be reactivated at a later time. The exact nature of the latent state and the factors triggering reactivation are not clear.

Herpes simplex virus can be divided into two types on the basis of antigenicity, pathogenicity, and genetic properties. Herpes simplex type II is the major cause of urogenital infections whereas type I is more often isolated from nongenital infections. Herpes simplex viruses have a worldwide distribution, and direct contact with infected secretions is the principal mode of spread. Herpes simplex causes diseases of the skin and mucosa such as acute gingivostomatitis, recurrent stomatitis, oral ulcers (cold sores), herpetic keratoconjunctivitis, herpetic esophagitis, and genital herpes. It also causes systemic disease as in disseminated herpetic infection of infants, acute necrotizing encephalitis of the adult, and infections in the immunodeficient host.

The two types of cytopathology seen in herpes simplex infections are rounding and degeneration of the cells with inclusion body formation and cell fusion with formation of syncytia. The intranuclear inclusion is the characteristic cellular lesion, and it consists of a single, eosinophilic, well-demarcated inclusion body surrounded by a halo and marginated chromatin. By electron microscopy the inclusion body consists of paracrystalline arrays of viral capsids and electron-dense glycoprotein.

Herpetic infection of skin and mucosa is manifested by the appearance of red papules that quickly become vesic-

ulated. Histologically there is degeneration of the cells in the stratum malpighii and the stratified squamous epithelium. In early stages one observes ballooning of the epidermal cells and clearing of the nuclear chromatin. There is acantholysis and formation of a unilocular vesicle. The typical inclusion bodies (Cowdry type A) can be seen in epidermal cells. The upper dermis or submucosal portions of the affected regions show an inflammatory infiltrate around capillaries. The histologic lesion of herpes simplex in the skin and mucosa is practically indistinguishable from that caused by herpes zoster. Immunohistochemistry using fluorescent antibodies or immunoperoxidase can, however, make the distinction between these viruses and even allows typing of the herpesvirus.[89]

Disseminated herpetic infection of the newborn affects neonates in the first 4 weeks of life as well as an older group of infants in whom it causes hepatoadrenal necrosis.[82] Autopsies of infants dying from disseminated herpetic disease show multiple miliary foci of necrosis surrounded by hemorrhagic borders in the liver, adrenal gland, and brain (Fig. 10-11). Microscopically these foci consist of a zone of central coagulative necrosis surrounded by an area of hyperemia with a sparse mononuclear inflammatory reaction. Inclusion bodies characteristic of the herpetic infection are found in nuclei of the parenchymal cells surrounding the necrotic zone. The pathology may be complicated by the presence of gram-negative septicemia.[66,115] Morphologic manifestations of disseminated intravascular coagulation (DIC) may be also prominent. The virus can be easily demonstrated in the lesions by electron microscopic examination.[96]

Herpes simplex virus has been shown to be a cause of *acute necrotizing encephalitis of the adult*.[48] Patients with this syndrome may display a picture of encephalitis or a clinical picture of an expanding lesion, often of the temporal lobe. In fatal cases the brain shows asymmetric necrosis particularly prominent in the temporal lobes but also involving the hippocampus and the posterior occipital cortex. Hemorrhage may be prominent. In the early stages of the disease the histopathologic picture is that of acute necrosis associated with a diffuse meningoencephalitis. Inclusion bodies within the nuclei of neurons and glial cells can be seen but on occasion are difficult to find (Fig. 10-12).

Reactivation and dissemination of herpetic lesions are not uncommon in immunocompromised hosts. Esophageal and upper respiratory tract lesions are commonly found at autopsy in patients who have undergone intense chemotherapy. Dissemination occasionally occurs, and a picture similar to the disseminated disease in newborns can be seen. Dissemination with a fatal outcome also occurs in some severely burned patients.

Cytomegaloviruses are a group of species-specific agents capable of causing asymptomatic infections to severe or fatal illnesses in mammalian species. In vivo and in vitro infection with human cytomegalovirus is characterized by a specific cytopathic effect consisting of distinctly enlarged cells (cytomegaly), 25 to 40 μm in diameter, containing an intranuclear reniform or ovoid inclusion body that measures 8 to 10 μm (Fig. 10-13). The inclusion body is often surrounded by a clear halo and is Feulgen positive. Punctate amphophilic, PAS-positive, cytoplasmic inclusions can also be found in the cytomegalic cells. Ultrastructural studies of both in vivo and in vitro infected cells show herpesvirus capsids forming the inclusion body in the nucleus. The cytoplasmic inclusions are formed by aggregates of dense osmiophilic material surrounding enveloped virions.

Cytomegalovirus (CMV) is a ubiquitous infection and, depending on the socioeconomic condition of the population, the prevalence of antibodies in the adult ranges from 40% to 100%. CMV is usually transmitted by close

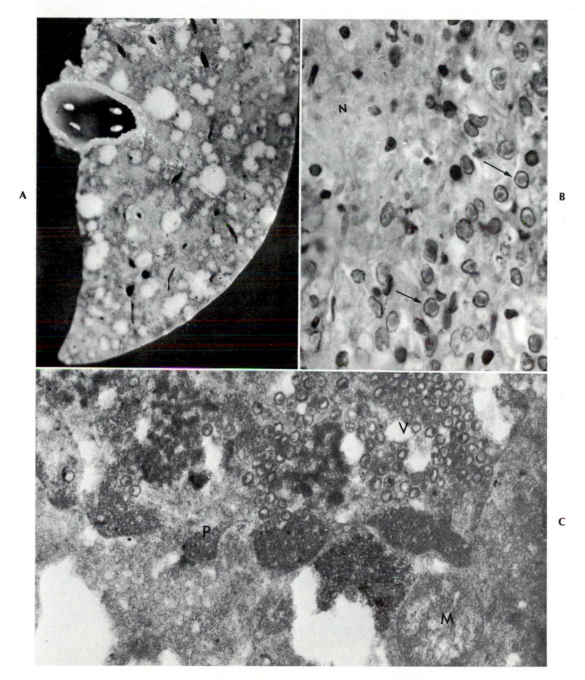

Fig. 10-11. Herpes neonatorum. **A,** Focal necroses in liver. **B,** Nuclear inclusions *(arrows)* at edge of necrotic lesion. **C,** Electron micrograph of inclusion-bearing cell. *M,* Mitochondrion; *P,* peripheral nuclear chromatin; *V,* herpes virions, probably type 2, in nuclear inclusion. Some contain nucleoids, but enveloped forms are not seen. (**A,** 4×; AFIP 997583; **B,** 800×; **C,** 30,000×.)

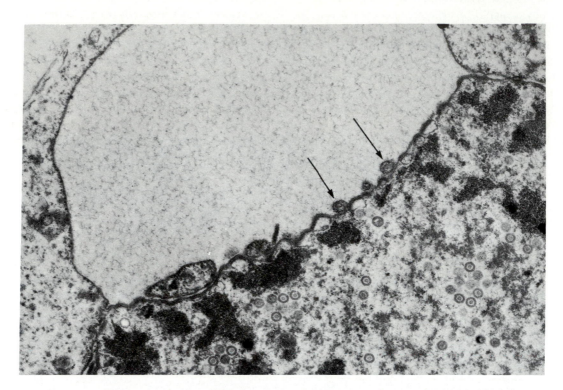

Fig. 10-12. Fatal herpes simplex encephalitis in 18-year-old person. Electron micrograph of formalin-fixed brain tissue showing intranuclear herpes virions, separation of outer and inner nuclear membranes, and acquisition of envelope from latter *(arrows)*. (32,000×; courtesy Drs. Vincent G. Palermo and J.R. Taylor, St. Louis, Mo.)

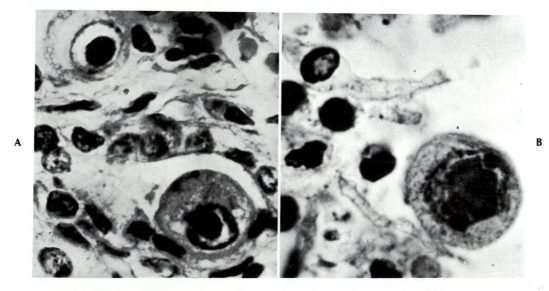

Fig. 10-13. Cytomegalovirus infection of kidney. **A,** Section showing two huge nuclear inclusions in tubular epithelium. **B,** Diagnostic cell in hematoxylin and eosin–stained urinary sediment *(lower right)*. Compare with normal-appearing tubular epithelial cell *(upper left)*.

contact. It may be venereally transmitted and is one of the agents that can be transmitted by blood transfusions.

Infection of the fetus in utero or of the newborn produces a disease that may vary from asymptomatic to a serious and often fatal syndrome. The clinical manifestations of congenital cytomegalovirus infection appear to be a reflection of the duration of the infection in utero.[47,][75] Cytomegalic inclusion disease of the newborn is manifested by jaundice, petechiae, chorioretinitis, microcephaly, thrombocytopenia, diarrhea, and central nervous system disease. The pathologic changes in newborn infants with cytomegalic inclusion disease are usually severe in the liver, kidneys, lungs, and brain. In the liver one observes persistence of hemopoietic tissue and periportal necrosis of hepatocytes with a dense mononuclear inflammatory cell infiltrate. In some cases the histologic picture is that of giant cell hepatitis. Inclusion bodies are difficult to find. The classic lesion in the cerebral nervous system is destruction with subsequent calcification of the cerebral tissue beneath the ependyma of the ventricles. In most cases gross and microscopic evidence of interference with the normal brain development is manifested by abnormal patterns of development of cerebral convolutions. Other organs such as adrenal glands, pancreas, thyroid, pituitary, bone marrow, and myocardium may be found to have cells with the characteristic inclusion bodies.

Cytomegalovirus in the adult is most often associated with *gastrointestinal tract disease*[22] or as an opportunistic agent in the immunosuppressed patient. Recent studies suggest that cytomegalovirus may be a common latent infection of the human gastrointestinal tract. Overt infection with viral replication is most often associated with ulcerative diseases such as Crohn's disease and ulcerative colitis. In those cases viral inclusions can be found in cells at the ulcer bed and in the endothelial cells underlying the ulcerated area. Occasionally the inclusion bodies are found in cells lining the mucosa surrounding the ulcer.

CMV pneumonitis is seen in the debilitated adult and in patients who are immunosuppressed.[70] It may be evident on chest radiographs as a reticular nodular density; the diagnosis is established through lung biopsy. The histopathologic picture is that of an interstitial pneumonitis in which the alveolar lining cells show the features of cytomegalovirus infection. It is often associated with a combined infection of the lungs with other organisms such as *Candida, Aspergillus, Nocardia, Mycobacterium tuberculosis,* and quite often *Pneumocystis carinii.* In patients dying with neoplasms, CMV was isolated in 8.8% of 502 unselected autopsy cases at the Mayo Clinic.[105] CMV inclusion bodies in this series with or without associated inflammation were found in descending order of frequency in the lung, kidney, liver, pancreas, adre-

nal, esophagus, prostate, testes, thyroid gland, parathyroid, stomach, small intestine, and heart.

Varicella-zoster virus (VZ virus) is the etiologic agent of two clinically distinct entities in the human. Chickenpox (varicella) is an acute infectious disease of childhood characterized by crops of vesicles on the face and tongue. Herpes zoster (shingles) is typified by a painful vesicular eruption restricted to one or more segmental dermatomes in adults. It is often seen in debilitated patients or in immunosuppressed patients. Initial infection with VZ virus at a young age results in the acute disease and dissemination of the agent. It is thought that during the viremic phase the virus infects the neurons of the dorsal root ganglia and is capable of remaining there in a latent state.[7] Zoster (shingles) is the manifestation of the reactivation of the latent infection in the ganglion cells in a partially immune host.

The cutaneous lesion of *varicella* is characterized by crops of vesicles, which may become confluent in severe cases. Microscopically the vesicles of varicella are indistinguishable from the lesions caused by herpes simplex. In fatal cases the predominant lesion is pneumonia.[57,88] It usually occurs within 1 to 5 days after the appearance of rash, with chest pain, cyanosis, and hemoptysis. Radiologically it is characterized by nodular densities throughout the lung fields. Clinical resolution might occur in 2 to 3 weeks, but if the case is fatal, autopsy will demonstrate heavy edematous lungs with dark color and pale areas throughout the parenchyma resembling foci of consolidation. The bronchi are usually filled with hemorrhagic mucus. Microscopically there is hemorrhagic intra-alveolar exudate with hyaline membrane formation and desquamation of alveolar epithelial cells. The desquamated cells may contain inclusion bodies (Fig. 10-14). Nodular calcification has been described as a late sequela to lung necrosis. Varicella is particularly severe in neonates who have acquired infection in utero. Babies dying from the disease usually show disseminated visceral lesions that grossly resemble miliary tuberculosis or disseminated herpes simplex.

The pathology of the *zoster* cutaneous lesion is similar to that of varicella and herpes simplex.[72] The virus may be identified specifically as zoster by means of immunofluorescence or immunohistochemical techniques. In the acute stage the dorsal root ganglion affected by the virus is swollen and hemorrhagic. Microscopically there is an intense inflammation composed of round cells, and the neurons show chromatolysis, with eosinophilia of the cytoplasm. Neuronophagia may also be observed. Inclusion bodies may be seen in the neurons, but as a rule they are hard to demonstrate. Disseminated forms of zoster may be seen in severely immunocompromised patients.[21]

The *Epstein-Barr virus* (EBV) was discovered by Epstein, Achong, and Barr in the course of ultrastructur-

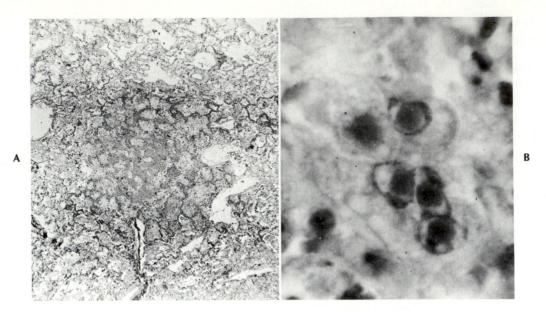

Fig. 10-14. Varicella pneumonia. **A,** Focal hemorrhagic lesion in lung. **B,** Four cells from lesion shown in **A,** each containing inclusion body that partially fills nucleus. Giant cells, although present in cutaneous lesions, are seen only very rarely in varicella pneumonia. (**A,** 30×.)

al examination of cell lines derived from Burkitt's lymphoma patients. Epstein-Barr virus has the characteristic morphology of the herpes group of viruses. The host range is limited, and in nature EBV infects only humans. In vitro cultivation of the virus can be carried out only in human B lymphocytes. Following infection some of the lymphocytes are "immortalized" (that is, they acquire the ability to grow continuously and indefinitely in culture). Cells infected with Epstein-Barr virus express a variety of antigens that can be detected by sera of different specificity. These antigens are a nuclear antigen (EBNA), early viral antigens (EA), viral capsid antigens (VCA), and antigens present on the membrane of infected and immortalized cells (MA). Antibodies to Epstein-Barr virus have been found in all population groups studied. In the United States and Great Britain EBV seroconversion occurs before the age of 5 years in about 50% of the population. A second wave of seroconversion occurs midway through the second decade of life. Lower socioeconomic groups have a higher EBV antibody prevalence than do more affluent matched controls. The immune response to Epstein-Barr virus infected or immortalized lymphocytes is complex and involves both humoral and cell-mediated immune mechanisms.

EBV induces a broad spectrum of illness. Classic *infectious mononucleosis* is an acute disease characterized by sore throat, fever, lymphadenopathy, transient heterophil antibodies, and leukocytosis, which consists in part of atypical lymphocytes. The age of the patient has a profound influence on the clinical expression of EBV expression. However, EBV infection in the young is often asymptomatic.

The atypical lymphocytes seen in peripheral blood of patients with EBV mononucleosis are slightly larger than normal lymphocytes with a pale blue vacuolated cytoplasm and scalloped border (Dutch skirt appearance). The oval nucleus contains a coarse chromatin network. The atypical lymphocytes are heterogeneous in morphologic appearance as opposed to those malignant diseases such as leukemia or lymphosarcoma. It is now known that the atypical cells that circulate in patients with infectious mononucleosis represent activated T cells that are mounting a cell-mediated immune response against infected B lymphocytes.[93] Lymph node biopsies in patients with mononucleosis and a clinically typical course usually show marked follicular hyperplasia with atypical lymphocytes in the sinuses. Foci of necrosis may be observed. Atypical cells may be prominent and together with architectural effacement may mislead pathologists into a diagnosis of malignancy.[98] Cells indistinguishable from Reed-Sternberg cells have been noted.

One of the complications of mononucleosis can be a ruptured spleen resulting from minor trauma.[104] In such a case gross examination reveals a capsular tear with a subcapsular hematoma. Histologic examination shows the red pulp and the capsule to be infiltrated by atypical lymphocytes. The autopsy findings of a patient dying of mononucleosis have been described by Custer and Smith.[19] Liver biopsies in patients with mononucleosis are almost always abnormal. Microscopically Kupffer cell activation is prominent as is infiltration of the portal triads with mononuclear cells.[85] Occasionally small foci of necrosis with eosinophilic bodies can be observed. Bone marrow granulomas have been reported in patients with infectious mononucleosis.[53]

Epstein-Barr virus reactivation can be detected serologically in immunosuppressed allograft recipients. Lack of control of cellular proliferation induced by Epstein-Barr virus may result in lymphoproliferative disorders. This has been best documented in patients with the X-linked recessive lymphoproliferative syndrome.[95]

Papovaviruses

The name *papova* is an acronym derived from papilloma, polyoma, and simian vacuolating virus. This family of viruses can be divided in two genera, *Polyomavirus* and *Papillomavirus*. Viruses of the polyoma genus have been studied the most because they have been known to cause tumors in experimental animals. Polyomaviruses can also transform cells in vitro, rendering them oncogenic. The polyomavirus of mouse and the SV40 virus of monkeys have been intensely studied by molecular biologists. The genomes of SV40 and polyoma (3×10^6 daltons) have been completely sequenced. The relevant human members of the family are JC and BK virus in the polyoma genus and human papillomavirus or human wart virus. All members replicate in the nuclei of mammalian cells and form nonenveloped nucleocapsids, 30 to 50 nm in diameter, containing the DNA genome.

Progressive multifocal leukoencephalopathy (PML) is a rare neurologic disease primarily affecting adults between the ages of 50 and 70. The neurologic manifestations of the disease indicate diffuse asymmetric involvement of the cerebral hemispheres. The duration from onset of symptoms to death is usually less then 6 months. PML is most often seen in immunocompromised hosts, especially in patients with leukemia, lymphoma, Hodgkin's disease, diffuse carcinomatosis, sarcoidosis, or tuberculosis. It has also been reported in patients with congenital immunodeficiencies. The incidence of PML is low; of 3000 consecutive autopsy cases studied by Del Duca and Morningstar,[21a] PML was diagnosed in only two instances. The pathologic diagnosis of PML is usually established at postmortem examination, but it can be made on a brain biopsy. At autopsy the lesions appear most often in the cerebrum, beneath the cortical ribbon, and look like small necrotic areas.[4] They tend to coalesce to form larger foci of demyelination. When several months old, the lesions appear as retracted foci grossly resembling a cerebral infarct. The distribution in the central nervous system is variable, the cerebrum being the most frequently affected site.

Histopathologically the hallmark of the disease is the presence of oligodendrocytes with enlarged nuclei containing basophilic intranuclear inclusion bodies. Reactive hypertrophic astrocytes with giant hyperchromatic nuclei that often contain a cytoplasmic invagination are also typical, especially of the late stage of the lesion. No cytologic abnormalities are seen in neurons, ependymal cells, endothelial cells, or macrophages. Ultrastructural examination reveals the presence of viral capsids in the nuclei of the oligodendrocytes.[130] They are seldom seen in the giant astrocytes. A polyomavirus, named *JC virus*, has been consistently isolated in PML cases from brain tissue at biopsy or at autopsy.[90] Viral antigens can be shown to be present in the abnormal oligodendrocytes by immunohistochemical techniques. The disease has not been transmitted to experimental animals, but monkeys have a pathologic lesion identical to PML that has been shown to be caused by the SV40 virus, the polyomavirus of the monkey. Inoculation of JC virus into newborn hamsters causes a variety of tumors, often in the nervous system.[120]

BK virus, the other human polyomavirus, was first isolated by Gardner and co-workers[39] from the urine of a renal allograft recipient on immunosuppressive therapy. It has also been isolated from the urine of patients with Wiskott-Aldrich syndrome and from a biopsy of a cerebral lymphoma in a child with Wiskott-Aldrich syndrome. Recent studies suggest that BK virus may be latent in the kidney and may be reactivated during the immunosuppressed state. BK virus, like JC virus, is capable of inducing tumors in the newborn hamster and transforming cells in vitro. No specific clinical syndrome has been unequivocally linked to BK infection. In kidney transplant patients urinary cytology may show cells with intranuclear inclusions very similar to those seen in the oligodendrocytes infected with JC virus. Similar inclusions have been observed in the urothelium of the renal pelvis and have been shown by electron microscopy to contain papovavirus capsids. Both BK and JC viruses are found throughout the world, and, judging by the levels of antibody in sera, the prevalence of infection is high.

Papillomaviruses are distinguished from the polyoma group by the size of their capsid (55 nm in diameter) and the molecular weight of their genome—5×10^6 daltons compared with 3×10^6 daltons in the polyoma genus. Papillomaviruses are highly species specific and tissue specific. They are capable of inducing epithelial and mesenchymal proliferative lesions in a variety of animals. It has now been proved that papillomaviruses in some animals play an etiologic role in some tumors. Human papillomaviruses (HPV) cause a variety of epithelial tumors with distinct clinicopathologic characteristics. Different strains of the virus are responsible or more often associated with specific types of lesions. HPV type 1 is the usual etiologic agent of common skin cutaneous warts. HPV 2 is the etiologic agent of plantar warts. HPV type 3 and 4 are associated with lesions in a rare genetic disease called *epidermodysplasia verruciformis*.

The viruses associated with *condyloma accuminata*, *oral focal epithelial hyperplasia*, and *juvenile laryngeal papilloma* are not yet characterized. *Cutaneous warts* (verruca vulgaris) are found anywhere on the skin. They are circumscribed nodular growths having a hyperkeratotic surface. Histologically, there is thickening of the epidermis caused by proliferation of epidermal cells. In some of the cells the nuclei are deeply basophilic, surrounded by a clear halo, and can be shown by electron microscopy and immunocytochemistry to contain HPV particles or antigens.[2] Warts also often contain cells with vacuolated clear cytoplasm called koilocytes. Skin warts may regress spontaneously, and at least two thirds of the cases do so. There is a high incidence of warts in immunosuppressed patients or patients with congenital immune deficiencies. Malignant transformation does not occur except in some patients with epidermodysplasia verruciformis.

Condyloma accuminata are verruciform anogenital lesions that are venereally transmitted.[77] They occur in young adults and are not associated with skin warts. Some of the condylomas may become very large (giant condyloma of Buschke-Löwenstein). Verrucous carcinoma may also be seen in large condylomatous lesions.

Papillomaviruses have been also implicated in cervical dysplasia, and they are often the cause of well-known cytologic alterations such as koilocytosis. The koilocytic cells have been shown by electron microscopy to contain papilloma particles in their nuclei.

Multiple *laryngeal papillomas* occurring during infancy and childhood have been also linked epidemiologically and by means of immunocytochemistry to papillomaviruses.[16] The lesions appear grossly as thin, whitish nodules, either sessile or pedunculated. Histologically they are composed of a fibrovascular core covered by thick, stratified, squamous epithelium. The lesions may exhibit malignant potential if irradiated.

Poxviridae

The poxviruses of mammals are a complex group of agents that produce vesicular skin lesions. They are the largest animal viruses, containing a double-stranded DNA genome of 200 million daltons. They are brick shaped, measuring 390 × 260 nm, and are very resistant to chemical and physical inactivation. They multiply in the cytoplasm of cells, and the virions mature in cytoplasmic foci or "viral factories." Some of the important poxviruses are the etiologic agents for vaccinia, variola, ectromelia, monkeypox, and molluscum contagiosum.

As a result of the successful campaign sponsored by the World Health Organization (WHO), *smallpox* (variola) has been practically eradicated worldwide.[23,124] Variola infection is limited to humans, and study of the virus has been somewhat limited because of the laboratory hazards. There are at least two strains of variola virus; the most virulent causes variola major with a mortality of 20% to 50%. Variola minor or alastrim has a mortality of less than 1%. The two strains can be differentiated by

their temperature-sensitive growth characteristics on chorioallantoic membrane. Variola virus is transmitted by close contact and is spread through the air, gaining entrance to the respiratory tract where it multiplies in the epithelium and regional lymph nodes. This first replicative period is followed by viremia with dissemination of the virus to the reticuloendothelial system. A second replicative phase follows in which a second viremia spreads to the skin, lymphatics, and internal organs. This secondary viremia marks the beginning of clinical symptoms. Clinically smallpox is characterized by fever followed a few days later by a centrifugal papular rash that appears first on the face and the skull and spreads to the back, chest, arms, and legs. The macules become papules, vesicles, and finally pustules (Fig. 10-15). The pustules dry up, forming scabs during the second week of the rash. The clinical disease produced by smallpox has a spectrum of severity that ranges from the very mild to the very severe and often fatal form. WHO describes four clinical types of smallpox: ordinary, modified, flat, and hemorrhagic. The third and fourth are the most severe.

The cutaneous lesions in the papular stage have a diameter of 2 to 4 mm and are partially buried in the skin. Microscopically the cutaneous lesions first show vascular congestion with mononuclear cell infiltrate in the dermis. The epidermal cells show ballooning degeneration with formation of an intraepidermal vesicle.[74] There is involvement of the adnexal elements. Cells with

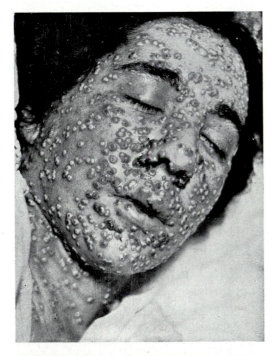

Fig. 10-15. Smallpox in unvaccinated woman. (Courtesy Dr. Samuel Sweitzer; from Sutton, R.I., Jr.: Diseases of the skin, ed. 11, St. Louis, 1956, The C.V. Mosby Co.)

cytoplasmic inclusion bodies (Guarnieri bodies) can be found in early vesicles and disappear with healing. These inclusion bodies are variable in size, granular, eosinophilic, round to oval, and surrounded by a halo. Electron microscopic examination of the epidermal lesions demonstrates the presence of "viral factories" in the cytoplasm of the infected cells.[18] In fatal cases pneumonia of the interstitial type is often seen. The viral lesions are often obscured by superimposed bacterial infection.

The present *vaccinia virus* is probably derived from the cowpox virus by the process of person-to-person vaccination. Jenner was the first to observe in 1798 that pustular material from the lesions of cowpox protected humans from infection with smallpox. Jenner's observations form the basis for vaccination. Vaccination results in a modified swelling at the site of vaccination and regional lymphadenopathy. Primary vaccination sites develop a vesicle within 3 to 5 days that will become pustular and reach maximum size after approximately 9 days. The lesion will form a scab and leave a small circular scar approximately 1 cm in diameter. Complications that result from vaccination are postvaccination encephalitis, vaccinia necrosum seen in patients with T cell immune deficiencies, eczema vaccinatum seen in patients with atopic dermatitis, generalized vaccinia, and erythematous urticarial lesions.

Molluscum contagiosum is a benign skin disease of worldwide distribution characterized by the occurrence of raised, umbilicated, waxy, cutaneous nodules. The lesions may be multiple or solitary. Histologically molluscum contagiosum is a proliferative lesion of the epidermal cells, which form a lobulated mass. The infected cells contain large intracytoplasmic eosinophilic inclusion bodies (Fig. 10-16).[49,67]

Two additional poxviruses that cause disease in humans are the paravaccinia virus of cattle, which produces milkers' nodules, and orf virus of sheep, which causes contagious pustular dermatitis.

Hepatitis B virus

Hepatitis B virus infection is widespread throughout the world. Infection often occurs at very young ages. It is one of the most common persistent viral infections of humans. The hepatitis B virion is a complex structure measuring approximately 42 nm in diameter, possessing in its surface the hepatitis B surface antigen (HBsAg), an envelope, and an electron-dense 28 nm internal core or nucleocapsid containing a small DNA genome. Hepatitis B virus is a most unusual virus, and one of its unique properties is the configuration of the small circular DNA within the core of the virion (Dane particle). The circular DNA molecule is double stranded for about two thirds of its length and single stranded for the remainder. The DNA polymerase enzyme present in the core is probably responsible for closing the single-stranded gap upon infection and making a double-stranded circular DNA molecule of approximately 3200 nucleotide pairs. Present in the blood of infected patients are small spherical particles, 16 to 25 nm in diameter, that bear surface antigenic activity. Two additional antigenic activities are found associated with hepatitis B. One is the hepatitis B core antigen found associated with the dense nucleoprotein core of the viral particles (Dane particles).[20] Structures with the morphology of the viral cores can be seen by electron microscopy in nuclei of hepatocytes infected with hepatitis B virus.[3,40] Another is the activity of the e antigen, which exists in serum as a large protein of approximately 300,000 daltons. Immunofluorescence staining of tissue sections for viral antigens suggests that hepatocytes are the only cell type infected with hepatitis B virus during the persistent infection. During the acute phase of disease the majority of the hepatocytes appear to be infected.[45]

Blood and blood products are the best-documented vehicles for transmission of hepatitis B virus. In addition to serum, saliva and semen have been also shown to contain infectious virus in experimental transmission studies. Before screening of blood donors for hepatitis B antigen was introduced, from 1% to 10% of transfused patients acquired hepatitis. The pathology of hepatitis B is discussed in Chapter 27.

UNNAMED VIRAL-LIKE AGENTS PRODUCING DISEASE OF THE CENTRAL NERVOUS SYSTEM

The *spongiform encephalopathies* (kuru, Jakob-Creutzfeldt disease, scrapie, and transmissible mink encephalopathy) are caused by transmissible agents of very small size and of great resistance to inactivation with chemical and physical agents. These transmissible agents lack a demonstrable nucleic acid.[41] They have been termed by Gajdusek[36] "unconventional viruses," but it is

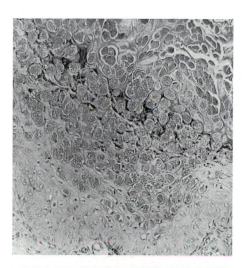

Fig. 10-16. Molluscum contagiosum.

still uncertain whether they should be considered viruses or members of a new group of microorganisms, perhaps similar to the viroids of plants.

Epidemiologically *kuru* has been confined to a primitive population in eastern New Guinea. The studies by Gajdusek suggested that kuru was transmitted by inoculation of infected tissue through skin cuts during participation of children and women in ritual cannibalism.[36] *Jakob-Creutzfeldt* disease is found throughout the world with a prevalence of approximately one case per million population. About 10% of the cases have an apparent inherited transmission but the pattern is equivocal. Jakob-Creutzfeldt disease has been transmitted from human to human by corneal transplant and by contaminated stereotactic brain electrodes. No cases have been diagnosed among virologists working with the disease or pathologists studying Jakob-Creutzfeldt cases. The unusual resistance of the agents to inactivation by physical and chemical agents necessitates special precautions in dealing with patients and pathologic specimens.[37]

Both kuru and Jakob-Creutzfeldt disease are spongiform encephalopathies[43,64] showing diffuse loss of neurons, marked gliosis with proliferation of astrocytes, and vacuolization of the neuronal and glial processes. The lesions in kuru are most frequent in the cerebellar, cortex, pons, thalamus, and basal nuclei. Electron microscopic study of the neurons demonstrates fragments of curled membranous material within the vacuoles of the cytoplasm. No viral organisms can be visualized.

REFERENCES

1. Adams, J.H.: Virus diseases of the nervous system. In Blackwood, W., and Corseless, J.A.N., editors: Greenfield's neuropathology, Chicago, 1976, Year Book Medical Publishers.
2. Almeida, J.D., Howartson, A.F., and Williams, M.G.: Electron microscope study of human wart: sites of virus production and nature of the inclusion bodies, J. Invest. Dermatol. 38:337, 1962.
3. Almeida, J.D., Waterson, A.P., and Trowell, J.M.: The findings of virus-like particles in two Australian antigen positive human livers, Microbiology 2:145, 1970.
4. Astrom, K.E., Mancall, E.L., and Richardson, E.P., Jr.: Progressive multifocal leukoencephalopathy, Brain 81:93, 1958.
5. Baer, G.M., editor: The natural history of rabies, vols. I and II, New York, 1975, Academic Press.
6. Barbosa, L.H., et al.: Subacute sclerosing panencephalitis: isolation of measles virus from a brain biopsy, Nature 221:974, 1969.
7. Bastian, F.O., et al.: Herpes virus varicellae: isolated from human dorsal root ganglia, Arch. Pathol. 97:331, 1974.
8. Berthiaume, L., Joncas, J., and Pavilanis, V.: Comparative structure, morphogenesis, and biological characteristics of the respiratory syncytial (RS) virus and the pneumonia virus of mice (PVM), Arch. Virol. 45:39, 1974.
9. Bodian, D.: Histopathologic basis of the clinical findings in poliomyelitis, Am. J. Med. 6:563, 1949.
10. Bradley, D.W.: Hepatitis A virus infection: pathogenesis and serodiagnosis of acute diseases, J. Virol. Meth. 2:31, 1980.
11. Camain, R., and Lambert, D.: Histopathologie des foies amarils preleves postmortem et par ponction-biopsie hepatique, Bull. WHO 36:129, 1967.
12. Casals, J., and Clarke, H.: Arboviruses group A. In Horsfall, F.L., and Tamm, I., editors: Viral and ricketsial infections of man, ed. 4, Philadelphia, 1965, J.B. Lippincott Co.
13. Chanuk, R., Roydsman, B., and Meyers, R.: Recovery from infants with respiratory illness of a virus related to chimpanzee coryza agent (CCA). I. Isolation: properties and characterization, Am. J. Hygiene 66:281, 1957.
14. Child, P.L., et al.: Bolivian hemorrhagic fever, Arch. Pathol. 83:434, 1967.
15. Cooper, L.Z.: Congenital rubella in the United States. In Krugman, S., and Gershon, A., editors: Infections of the fetus and the newborn infant, New York, 1975, Alan R. Liss.
16. Costa, J., et al.: Presence of human papilloma viral antigens in juvenile multiple laryngeal papilloma, Am. J. Clin. Pathol. 75:194, 1981.
17. Crosby, A.W.: Epidemic and peace, 1918, part IV, Westport, Conn., 1976, Greenwood Press.
18. Cruickshank, J.G., Bedson, H.S., and Watson, D.H.: Electron microscopy and the rapid diagnosis of smallpox, Lancet 2:527, 1966.
19. Custer, R.P., and Smith, E.B.: Pathology of infectious mononucleosis, Blood 3:830, 1948.
20. Dane, D.S., Cameron, C.H., and Briggs, M.: Virus-like particles in serum of patients with Australian antigen associated hepatitis, Lancet 1:695, 1970.
21. Dayan, A.D., et al.: Disseminated herpes zoster in the reticuloses, Am. J. Roentgenol. 92:116, 1964.
21a. Del Duca, V., and Morningstar, W.A.: Multiple myeloma associated with progressive multifocal leukoencephalopathy, J.A.M.A. 199:671, 1967.
22. Dent, D.M., et al.: Cytomegalic virus infection of bowel in adults, S. Afr. Med. J. 49:669, 1975.
23. Dickson, C.W.: Smallpox, London, 1962, Churchill.
24. Dolin, R., et al.: Viral gastroenteritis induced by the Hawaii agent: jejunal histopathology and serologic response, Am. J. Med. 59:768, 1975.
25. Dowdle, W.R., Noble, G.R., and Kendal, A.P.: Orthomyxovirus—influenza comparative diagnosis unifying concept. In Kurstak, E., and Kurstak, C.H., editors: Comparative diagnosis of viral diseases, New York, 1977, Academic Press.
26. Driscoll, S.G.: Histopathology of gestational rubella, Am. J. Dis. Child. 118:49, 1969.
27. Dupont, J.R., and Earle, K.M.: Human rabies encephalitis: a study of 49 fatal cases with a review of the literature, Neurology (Minneap) 15:1023, 1965.
28. Enders, J.F.: Measles virus historical review isolation and behavior in various systems, Am. J. Dis. Child. 103:282, 1962.
29. Enders, J.F., et al.: Isolation of measles virus at autopsy in cases of giant cell pneumonia without rash, N. Engl. J. Med. 261:875, 1959.
30. Esterley, J.R., and Oppenheimer, E.H.: Intrauterine rubella infection. In Rosenberg, H.S., and Bolande, R.P., editors: Perspective in pediatric pathology, vol. 1, Chicago, 1973, Year Book Medical Publishers.
31. Feinstone, S.M., Kapikian, A.Z., and Purcell, R.H.: Hepatitis A: detection by immune electron microscopy of a virus-like antigen associated with acute illness, Science 182:1026, 1973.
32. Fenner, F.: The classification and nomenclature of viruses. Summary of results of meetings of the International Committee on Taxonomy of Viruses in Madrid, Sept. 1975, Virology 71:371, 1976.
33. Ferris, J.A.J., et al.: Sudden and unexpected death in infants: histology and virology, Br. Med. J. 2:439, 1973.
34. Finkeldey, W.: Über Riesenzellebefunde in den Gaumenmandelu Zugleich ein Reitras zur Histopathologie der Maudelveranderungen im Maserninkubationsstadium, Virchows Arch. 281:323, 1931.
35. Frances, T., Jr.: A new type of virus from epidemic influenza, Science 92:405, 1914.
36. Gajdusek, D.C.: Unconventional viruses and the origin and disappearance of kuru, Science 197:943, 1977.
37. Gajdusek, D.C., et al.: Precautions in medical care of, and in handling materials from patients with transmissible virus dementia (Creutzfeldt-Jakob disease), N. Engl. J. Med. 297:1253, 1977.
38. Gardner, P.S., et al.: Observations on clinical and immunofluorescent diagnosis of parainfluenza virus infections, Br. Med. J. 2:1, 1971.

39. Gardner, S.D., et al.: New human papovavirus (BK) isolated from urine after renal transplantation, Lancet 1:1253, 1971.

40. Gerber, M.A., et al.: Electron microscopy and immune electron microscopy of cytoplasmic hepatitis B antigen in hepatocytes, Am. J. Pathol. 75:489, 1974.

41. Gibbs, C.J., and Gajdusek, D.C.: Studies on the viruses of acute spongiform encephalopathies using primates, the only available indicator, First Inter-American Conference on Conservation and Utilization of American Non-human Primates in Biomedical Research, P.A.H.O. Scientific Publication 317:831, 1976.

42. Gonatas, N.K.: Subacute sclerosing leukoencephalitis: electron microscopic and cytochemical observations in a cerebral biopsy, J. Neuropathol. Exp. Neurol. 25:177, 1966.

43. Gonates, N.K., Terry, F.D., and Vice, M.: Electron microscopic study in two cases of Jakob-Creutzfeldt disease, J. Neuropathol. Exp. Neurol. 25:575, 1965.

44. Goodpasture, E.W., et al.: Virus pneumonia of infants secondary to epidemic infections, Am. J. Dis. Child. 57:997, 1939.

45. Gudat, F., et al.: Pattern of core and surface expression in liver tissue reflects state of specific immune response in hepatitis B, Lab. Invest. 32:1, 1975.

46. Hamre, D.: Rhinoviruses. In Melnick, J.L., editor: Monographs in virology, 1, 1968, Basel, S. Karger.

47. Hanshaw, J.B.: Congenital cytomegalovirus infection, N. Engl. J. Med. 288:1406, 1973.

48. Harland, W.A., Adams, J.H., and McSweeney, D.: Herpes simplex virus in acute necrotizing encephalitis, Lancet 2:581, 1967.

49. Hasegawa, T., et al.: Further electron microscopic observation of molluscum contagiosum virus, Arch. Klin. Exp. Dermatol. 235:319, 1969.

50. Haymaker, W.: Mosquito borne encephalitides. In Van Bogaert, L., et al., editors: Encephalitides, Amsterdam, 1961, Elsevier.

51. Heggie, A.D.: Pathogenesis of rubella exanthem: isolation of rubella virus from skin, N. Engl. J. Med. 285:664, 1971.

52. Horta-Barbosa, L., et al.: Subacute sclerosing panencephalitis: isolation of suppressed measles virus from lymph node biopsies, Science 173:840, 1971.

53. Hovder, F., and Sundberg, R.D.: Granulomatous lesions in the bone marrow in infectious mononucleosis, Blood 5:209, 1950.

54. Hutchins, G.M., and Vie, S.A.: The progression of interstitial myocarditis to idiopathic endocardial fibroelastosis, Am. J. Pathol. 66:483, 1972.

55. Imagaba, D.T.: Relationships among measles, canine distemper and rinderpest virus, Prog. Med. Virol. 10:116, 1968.

56. Johnson, C.B., and Goodpasture, E.W.: An investigation of the etiology of mumps, J. Exp. Med. 59:1, 1934.

57. Johnson, H.N.: Visceral lesions associated with varicella, Arch. Pathol. 30:292, 1944.

58. Johnson, K.M., et al.: Isolation and partial characterization of a new virus causing acute hemorrhagic fever in Zaire, Lancet 1:569, 1977.

59. Johnson, K.P., Lepov, M.L., and Johnson, R.T.: California encephalitis. I. Clinical and epidemiological studies, Neurology 8:250, 1968.

60. Kapikian, A.Z., et al.: Human reovirus-like agent as the major pathogen associated with winter gastroenteritis and hospitalized infants and young children, N. Engl. J. Med. 294:965, 1976.

61. Kapikian, A.Z., et al.: Visualization by immune electron microscopy of a 27 nm. particle associated with acute infectious non-bacterial gastroenteritis, J. Virol. 10:1075, 1972.

62. Kimora, A., Tosaka, K., and Nakow, T.: An immunofluorescence and electron microscopic study of measles skin eruptions, Tohuku J. Exp. Med.: 117:245, 1975.

63. Kimora, A., Tosaka, K., and Nakow, T.: Measles rash. I. Light and electron microscopic study of skin eruptions, Arch. Virol. 47:95, 1975.

64. Klatzo, I., Gajdusek, D.C., and Zigas, V.: Pathology of kuru, Lab. Invest. 8:799, 1959.

65. Lehmann-Grube, F.: Lymphocytic choriomeningitis virus, New York, 1971, Springer-Verlag.

66. Ling, J.A., et al.: Disseminated neonatal herpes simplex virus infection, N.Y. State J. Med. 75:608, 1975.

67. Lutzner, M.A.: Molluscum contagiosum, vermica and viruses, Arch. Dermatol. 87:436, 1963.

68. McIntosh, K., et al.: Diagnosis of human coronavirus infection by immune fluorescence: method and application to respiratory disease in hospitalized children, J. Med. Virol. 2:341, 1978.

69. McSorley, J., et al.: Herpes simplex and varicella zoster: comparative histopathology of 77 cases, Int. J. Dermatol. 13:69, 1974.

70. Manson, M.M., and Logan, W.P.D.: Rubella and other virus infections in pregnancy: reports on public health and medical subjects, No. 101, London, 1960, Ministry of Health.

71. Martini, G.A.: Marburg virus disease: the clinical syndrome. In Martini, G.A., and Siegert, R., editors: Marburg virus disease, Berlin, 1971, Springer-Verlag.

72. Mayers, J.D., et al.: Cytomegalovirus pneumonia after human marrow transplantation, Ann. Intern. Med. 82:181, 1975.

73. Meulen, V.T., et al.: Isolation of infectious measles virus in measles encephalitis, Lancet 2:1172, 1972.

74. Michaelson, H.E., and Ikeda, K.: Microscopic changes in variola, Arch. Belg. Dermatol. Syphiligr. 15:138, 1927.

75. Moniff, G.R.G., et al.: The correlation of maternal cytomegalovirus infection during varying stages in gestation with neonatal involvement, J. Pediatr. 80:17, 1972.

76. Monto, A.S.: The Tecumseh study of respiratory illness. V. Patterns of infection with the parainfluenza viruses, Am. J. Epidemiol. 97:338, 1973.

77. Morin, C., et al.: Confirmation of the papilloma virus etiology of condylomatous cervix lesions by the peroxidase antiperoxidase technique, J. Natl. Canc. Inst. 66:831, 1981.

78. Morris, J.A., Blunt, R.E., and Savage, R.E.: Recovery of cytopathogenic agent from chimpanzees with coryza, Proc. Soc. Exp. Biol. Med. 92:544, 1956.

79. Murphy, F.A., Halomen, P.E., and Harrison, A.K.: Electron microscopy of the development of rubella virus in BHK-21 cells, J. Virol. 2:1223, 1968.

80. Murphy, F.A., and Whitfield, S.G.: Morphology and morphogenesis of arenaviruses, Bull. WHO 52:408, 1975.

81. Murphy, F.A., et al.: Comparative pathogenesis of rabies and rabies-like viruses, Lab. Invest. 29:1, 1973.

82. Nahmias, J.A.: Disseminated herpes simplex infection, N. Engl. J. Med. 282:684, 1970.

83. Nakai, M., and Imagaba, D.T.: Electron microscopy of measles virus replication, J. Virol. 3:187, 1969.

84. Negri, A.: Beitrag zum Studium der Aetiologie der Tollwith, Z. Hys. Infektionskr. 43:507, 1903.

85. Nelson, R.S., and Darragh, J.H.: Infectious mononucleosis hepatitis: a clinicopathological study, Am. J. Med. 21:26, 1956.

86. Neurotropic diseases surveillance, Poliomyelitis Summary 1974-1976, Atlanta, 1977, Center for Disease Control.

87. Nieberg, K.C., and Blumberg, J.M.: Viral encephalitides. In Minckler, J., editor: Pathology of the nervous system, vol. 3, New York, 1972, McGraw-Hill Book Co.

88. Nisenbaum, C., Wallis, K., and Henzey, E.: Varicella pneumonia in children, Helv. Paed. Acta 24:212, 1969.

89. Olding-Stenkvist, E., and Grandien, M.: Early diagnosis of virus caused vesicular rashes by immunofluorescence on skin biopsy. I. Varicella zoster and herpes simplex virus, Scand. J. Infect. Dis. 8:27, 1976.

90. Padgett, B.L., et al.: Cultivation of papova-like virus from human brain with progressive multifocal leukoencephalopathy, Lancet 1:1257, 1971.

91. Palese, P., et al.: Characterization of temperature sensitive influenza virus mutants defective in neuroaminidase, Virology 61:397-410, 1974.

92. Parrot, R.H., et al.: Immunology of respiratory syncytial virus infection in Washington, D.C. II. Infection and disease with respect to age, immunological status, race and sex, Am. J. Epidemiol. p. 98, 1973.

93. Pattengale, P.K., Smith, R.W., and Perlin, E.: Atypical lymphocytes in acute infectious mononucleosis identification by multiple T and B lymphocyte markers, N. Engl. J. Med. 291:1145, 1974.

94. Portefield, J.S., et al.: Bunyaviruses and Bunyaviridae, Intervirology 2:270, 1974.

95. Purtillo, D.T., et al.: Hematopathology and pathogenesis of the x-linked recessive lymphoproliferative syndrome, Am. J. Med. **62:**219, 1977.

96. Rose, A.G., and Becker, W.B.: Disseminated herpes simplex infection: retrospective study by light microscopy and electron microscopy of paraffin embedded tissues, J. Clin. Pathol. **25:**79, 1972.

97. Row, W.P., et al.: Isolation of a cytopathogenic agent from human adenoids undergoing spontaneous degeneration in tissue culture, Proc. Soc. Exp. Biol. Med. **84:**570, 1953.

98. St. Geme, J.W., et al.: Experimental gestational mumps virus infection and endocardial fibroelastosis, Pediatrics **48:**821, 1971.

99. Salvador, A.H., Harrison, E.G., and Kyle, R.A.: Lymphadenopathy due to infectious mononucleosis: its confusion with malignant lymphoma, Cancer **27:**1029, 1971.

100. Schellmann, J., and Samson, J.G.: Prodromal stages of measles diagnosed at autopsy, J. Pediatr. **67**,39, 1965.

101. Schreiber, D.S., Blacklow, N.R., and Trier, G.S.: Mucosa lesion of the proximal small intestine in acute infectious non-bacterial gastroenteritis, N. Engl. J. Med. **228:**1318, 1973.

102. Schulze, I.T.: The structure of influenza virus. I. The polypeptides of the virion, Virology **42:**890, 1970.

102. Siegel, M.S.: Congenital malformations following chicken pox, measles, mumps and hepatitis: results of a cohort study, J.A.M.A. **226:**1521, 1973.

104. Smetana, H.F.: The histopathology of experimental yellow fever, Virchows Arch. (Pathol. Anat.) **335:**411, 1962.

105. Smith, E.B., and Custer, R.P.: Rupture of spleen in infectious mononucleosis: clinical pathological report of seven cases, Blood **1:**317, 1946.

106. Smith, T.F., et al.: Cytomegalovirus studies of autopsy tissue. I. Virus isolation, Am. J. Clin. Pathol. **63:** 854, 1975.

107. Smith, W., Andrewese, H., and Laidlaw, P.P.: A virus obtained from influenza patients, Lancet **2:**66, 1933.

108. Solinga, D.W.R., Bang, L.J., and Ackerman, A.B.: Role of measles virus in skin lesions and Koplick spot, N. Engl. J. Med. **83:**1139, 1970.

109. Spurance, S.L., and Bailey, A.: Colorado tick fever: a review of 115 laboratory confirmed cases, Arch. Int. Med. **131:**228, 1973.

110. Strano, A.J., and Henson, D.E.: Fatal adenovirus pneumonia: a study of 17 cases (abstract), Lab. Invest. **31:**346, 1975.

111. Sung, J.H., et al.: A case of human rabies and ultrastructure of the negri body, J. Neuropathol. Exp. Neurol. **35:**541, 1976.

112. Taylor, F.B., and Torenson, W.E.: Primary mumps meningeal encephalitis, Arch. Int. Med. **112:**216, 1963.

113. Taylor, R.M.: A further note on 1233 (influenza C) virus, Arch. Gesamte Virusforshung. **4:**485, 1951.

114. Telle, Z., Nagol, J., and Harter, D.H.: Subacute sclerosing leukoencephalitis: ultrastructure of intranuclear and intracytoplasmic inclusions, Science **154:**899, 1966.

115. Tucker, E.S., and Scofield, G.E.: Hepatoadrenal necrosis: fatal systemic herpes simplex virus infection: review of the literature and report of two cases, Arch. Pathol. **71,**538, 1961.

116. Tyrrell, D.A.J., and Bynoe, M.L.: Cultivation of a novel type of common cold virus in organ cultures, Br. Med. J. **1:**1467, 1965.

117. Tyrrell, D.A.J., et al.: Coronaviruses, Nature **220:**650, 1968.

118. Waherene, W., et al.: Pathological changes in virus infections of the lower respiratory tract in children, J. Clin. Pathol. **23:**7, 1970.

119. Walker, D.H., et al.: Comparative pathology of lassa virus infection in monkeys, guinea pigs, and *Mastomys natalensis*, Bull. WHO **52:**523, 1975.

120. Walker, D.L., et al.: Human papovavirus (JC): induction of brain tumors in hamsters, Science **187,**674, 1973.

121. Warthin, A.S.: Occurrence of numerous large giant cells in tonsils and pharyngeal mucosa in prodromal stage of measles: report of four cases, Arch. Pathol. **11:**864, 1931.

122. Webster, R.G., Campbell, C.H., and Granoff, A.: In vivo production of new influenza A viruses. I. Genetic recombination between avian and mammalian influenza viruses, Virology **44:**317, 1971.

123. WHO Memorandum: Pathogenic mechanism in dengue hemorrhagic fever: report of an international collaborative study, Bull. WHO **48:**117, 1973.

124. WHO Technical Report, Series No. 493, WHO Expert Committee on Smallpox Irradication, second report, Geneva, 1972, WHO.

125. Wind, W.C., Jr., and Walker, D.H.: Pathology of human lassa fever, Bull. WHO **52:**535, 1975.

126. Wright, H.D., Jr., Beckwith, J.B., and Guinn, J.L.: A fatal case of inclusion body pneumonia in an infant infected with adenovirus type III, Gen. Pediatr. **64:**528, 1964.

127. Young, N.: Coxsackievirus and echovirus. In Mandell, G.L., Douglas, G., and Bennett, J.E., editors: Principles and practice of infectious diseases. New York, 1979, John Wiley & Sons.

128. Zingerling, A.: Peculiarities of lesions in viral and mycoplasma infections of the respiratory tract, Virchows Arch. (Pathol. Anat.) **356:**259, 1972.

129. Zimmerman, L.E., and Binford, C.H.: Pathology of epidemic hemorrhagic fever, AFIP Syllabus, October, 1953.

130. Zu Rhein, G.M., and Aron, J.M.: Particles resembling papovaviruses in human cerebral demyelinating disease, Science **148:**1477, 1965.

CHAPTER 11 Mycotic, Actinomycotic, and Algal Infections

FRANCIS W. CHANDLER
JOHN C. WATTS

Fungi are eukaryotic, unicellular, or filamentous organisms that are ubiquitous in nature. Most are saprophytes that live in organic debris or in soil enriched with organic matter. Of more than 100,000 fungal species, only about 150 are pathogenic for humans. Their ability to cause disease depends on the virulence and dose of the agent, the route of infection, and the immunologic status of the host. Fungal diseases can be grouped arbitrarily into three broad categories based on the predominant location of infection within the body: superficial and cutaneous, subcutaneous, or systemic. The histopathologic features of the more common mycoses (fungal diseases) in each of these categories are summarized in Table 11-1.

The *superficial and cutaneous mycoses* are those in which the fungus is usually confined to the keratinized layer of the skin and its appendages. Because fungal growth is superficial, there is little or no inflammatory response. These infections are the most common of the mycoses; they cause minor discomfort and are primarily of cosmetic importance. They are rarely encountered by the histopathologist. The *subcutaneous mycoses* are a polymorphic group of diseases caused by a wide variety of fungi. These fungi enter the skin and subcutaneous tissues as a result of traumatic implantation or contamination of open wounds. Although infections usually remain localized, they occasionally spread via the lymphatics to involve other sites. The *systemic mycoses* usually have a pulmonary inception from which they may disseminate to other organs. The gastrointestinal tract is occasionally a primary focus of infection, and primary cutaneous forms of the systemic mycoses occur rarely as a result of direct inoculation of an agent following injury. In some patients systemic infections are asymptomatic; in others they produce severe disease, which can be fatal if not promptly diagnosed and treated.

Traditionally, actinomycosis and nocardiosis have fallen within the province of medical mycology and are therefore included in this chapter, even though their eti-

ologic agents are filamentous bacteria in the order Actinomycetales and are not true fungi. Diseases caused by the *Prototheca* spp. are also included, although most taxonomists consider these agents to be achloric mutants of green algae. For further information on the taxonomy of the fungi and classification of mycotic and actinomycotic diseases, several references are recommended.[4,6,9]

With the exception of tinea versicolor, the dermatophytoses, and candidiasis in the newborn, there is no clear-cut evidence that the mycoses are communicable. Most mycoses are contracted by exposure to environmental sources. A few, such as actinomycosis and candidiasis, are endogenous. The agents of these endogenous infections occur as commensals on the skin and mucous membranes and in the gastrointestinal tract.

Although some of the systemic mycoses, such as coccidioidomycosis and histoplasmosis, are caused by fungi that are familiar pathogens, many others are caused by opportunistic fungi. These opportunists are saprophytes that are usually innocuous and assume the role of pathogens only under conditions that render a host abnormally susceptible to infection.[2,7] They rarely infect the noncompromised, healthy individual. During the past two decades there has been an alarming increase in the incidence of opportunistic infections, particularly candidiasis, aspergillosis, cryptococcosis, zygomycosis, and nocardiosis. Contributing to this increased incidence is the widespread use of modern medical treatments that predispose patients to infection, such as cancer chemotherapeutic agents, irradiation, immunosuppressive agents, hyperalimentation, and the prolonged and frequent use of broad-spectrum antibiotics. Individuals who have malignancies (especially leukemia and lymphoma), burns, organ transplants, metabolic diseases, malnutrition, or inborn immunologic deficiencies; who have undergone abdominal or cardiac surgery; or who have received repeated intravenous injections are at special risk for mycotic infections. Some of the basic alterations thought to be responsible for this increased susceptibility

Table 11-1. Histologic features of the more common mycoses

Disease	Etiologic agent(s)	Typical morphology in tissue	Usual tissue reaction
SUPERFICIAL AND CUTANEOUS MYCOSES			
Black piedra	*Piedraia hortai*	Pigmented, closely septate hyphae, 4-6 μm diameter (D), organized as nodules surrounding hair shaft; asci containing ascospores may also be present	None; involves the hair exclusively
Tinea nigra	*Exophiala werneckii, Stenella araguata*	Pigmented, branched, septate hyphae, 1.5-3 μm D, and elongated budding cells, 1.5-5 μm D	Mild to moderate hyperkeratosis; little or no dermatitis
Tinea versicolor	*Malassezia furfur*	Short, curved and bent, hyaline hyphae, 2.5-4 μm D, and clusters of oval or round, thick-walled cells (phialospores), 3-8 μm D	Like tinea nigra
White piedra	*Trichosporon beigelii*	Hyaline hyphae, 2-4 μm D, arthrospores and blastospores organized as nodules surrounding hair shaft; invades and destroys hair	Like black piedra
Dermatophytoses	Pathogenic members of the genera *Epidermophyton, Microsporum,* and *Trichophyton*	Hyaline, septate hyphae that break up into chains of arthrospores	Hyperkeratosis, acanthosis, and mild mononuclear infiltrate in dermis; rarely suppurative or granulomatous
SUBCUTANEOUS MYCOSES			
Chromoblastomycosis	*Cladosporium carrionii, Fonsecaea compacta, F. pedrosoi, Phialophora verrucosa,* and others	Large, 6-12 μm D, round to polyhedral, thick-walled, dark brown muriform cells (sclerotic bodies) with septations along one or two planes; pigmented hyphae sometimes present	Mixed suppurative and granulomatous
Lobomycosis	*Loboa loboi*	Spherical, budding yeasts, 5-12 μm D, that form chains of cells	Granulomatous
Mycetoma (actinomycotic)	*Actinomadura madurae, A. pelletieri, Streptomyces somaliensis, Nocardia* spp., and others	Granules, 0.1 mm to several millimeters D, composed of delicate filaments (≤1 μm D) that are often branched and beaded	Like actinomycosis
Mycetoma (eumycotic)	*Pseudallescheria (Petriellidium) boydii, Madurella grisea, M. mycetomatis, Curvularia geniculata, Exophiala jeanselmei, Leptosphaeria senegalensis,* and others	Granules, 0.2 mm to several millimeters D, composed of broad (2-6 μm), hyaline (white to yellow granules) or dematiaceous (black granules) septate hyphae that often branch and form chlamydospores	Like actinomycosis
Protothecosis	*Prototheca wickerhamii, P. zopfii*	Spherical, oval, or polyhedral spherules, 2-25 μm D, that, when mature, contain 2-20 endospores	Varies from little or no reaction to granulomatous
Rhinosporidiosis	*Rhinosporidium seeberi*	Large sporangia, 100-350 μm D, with thin walls (3-5 μm) that enclose numerous endospores, 6-8 μm D	Nonspecific chronic inflammatory or granulomatous
Sporotrichosis	*Sporothrix schenckii*	Pleomorphic, spherical to oval and, at times, cigar-shaped yeasts, 2-10 μm D, that produce single and, rarely, multiple buds	Mixed suppurative and granulomatous; Splendore-Hoeppli material surrounds fungus in some cases (asteroid body)
Subcutaneous phaeohyphomycosis	*Exophiala jeanselmei, Phialophora parasitica, P. richardsiae, Wangiella dermatitidis,* and others	Pigmented (brown) hyphae, 2-6 μm D, branched or unbranched, and often constricted at their frequent and prominent septations; yeast forms and chlamydospores sometimes present	Subcutaneous cystic or solid granulomas; overlying epidermis rarely affected
Subcutaneous zygomycosis	*Basidiobolus haptosporus, Conidiobolus coronatus*	Short, poorly stained hyphal fragments; 6-25 μm D, with nonparallel sides and random branches	Eosinophilic abscesses and granulation tissue; hyphal fragments bordered by prominent Splendore-Hoeppli material

Table 11-1. Histologic features of the more common mycoses—cont'd

Disease	Etiologic agent(s)	Typical morphology in tissue	Usual tissue reaction
SYSTEMIC MYCOSES			
Actinomycosis	*Actinomyces israelii, A. naeslundii, A. viscosus, Arachnia propionica, Rothia dentocariosa,* and others	Organized aggregates (granules) composed of delicate, branched filaments ≤ 1 μm D; entire granules 30-3000 μm D	Suppurative, with multiple abscesses, extensive fibrosis and formation of sinus tracts; Splendore-Hoeppli material usually borders granules
Adiaspiromycosis	*Chrysosporium (Emmonsia) parvum* var. *crescens*	Large adiaspores, 200-400 μm D, with thick (20-70 μm) cell walls	Granulomatous, noncaseating
Aspergillosis	*Aspergillus fumigatus* group, *A. flavus* group, *A. niger* group, and other aspergilli	Septate, dichotomously branching hyphae of uniform width (3-6 μm); conidial heads may be present in cavitary lesions	Suppurative necrosis; sometimes granulomatous; tendency for angioinvasion
Blastomycosis	*Blastomyces dermatitidis*	Spherical, multinucleated yeasts, 8-15 μm D, with thick walls and single, broad-based buds	Mixed suppurative and granulomatous
Candidiasis	*Candida albicans* and other *Candida* spp.	Oval, budding yeasts, 2-6 μm D, and pseudohyphae; septate hyphae may also be present	Suppurative, less commonly granulomatous; minimal inflammation in preterminal infections
Coccidioidomycosis	*Coccidioides immitis*	Spherical, thick-walled, endosporulating spherules, 20-200 μm D; mature spherules contain small, 2-5 μm D, uninucleate endospores	Mixed suppurative and granulomatous
Cryptococcosis	*Cryptococcus neoformans*	Pleomorphic yeasts, 2-20 μm D, with gelatinous, carminophilic capsules and single or multiple narrow-based buds; some strains lightly encapsulated and may not be carminophilic	Varies from minimal response ("cystic" or "mucoid" lesion) to granulomatous response
Histoplasmosis capsulati	*Histoplasma capsulatum* var. *capsulatum*	Round to oval budding yeasts, 2-4 μm D; often clustered because of growth within mononuclear phagocytes	Granulomatous, caseating or noncaseating; proliferation of histiocytes (reticuloendothelial mycosis) may cause bland necrosis
Histoplasmosis duboisii	*Histoplasma capsulatum* var. *duboisii*	Round to oval, uninucleate, thick-walled yeasts, 8-15 μm D, that bud by a narrow base, creating typical hourglass or figure-eight forms	Granulomatous; many fungi in cytoplasm of huge multinucleated giant cells
Nocardiosis	*Nocardia asteroides, N. brasiliensis, N. caviae*	Long, delicate (≤1 μm D), branching filaments that are gram positive, weakly acid fast, and often beaded	Suppurative
Paracoccidioidomycosis	*Paracoccidioides brasiliensis*	Large spherical yeasts, 10-60 μm D, with multiple buds attached by narrow necks ("steering wheel" forms)	Mixed suppurative and granulomatous; like blastomycosis
Systemic phaeohyphomycosis	*Cladosporium bantianum (trichoides), Drechslera hawaiiensis,* and others	Pigmented (brown) hyphae, 2-6 μm wide, that may be branched or unbranched and are often constricted at their frequent and prominent septations	Mixed suppurative and granulomatous; large abscesses surrounded by giant cells
Torulopsosis	*Candida (Torulopsis) glabrata*	Oval yeast cells, 2-4 μm D	Varies from minimal response to suppurative and granulomatous
Zygomycosis	*Absidia corymbifera, Mucor ramosissimus, Rhizomucor pusillus, Rhizopus oryzae,* and others	Broad, thin-walled, infrequently septate hyphae, 6-25 μm wide, with nonparallel sides and random branches	Suppurative necrosis, less commonly granulomatous; tendency for angioinvasion

are leukopenia, suppression of humoral and cellular immunity, suppression of the acute inflammatory response, neutrophil or mononuclear phagocyte dysfunction, disruption of mucosal and cutaneous barriers, and reduction of the bacterial flora of the body that normally inhibit fungal overgrowth. Other factors contributing to the increased incidence of certain mycoses include migration of susceptible persons into highly endemic areas, aging of the population, and greater awareness of fungal infections in compromised hosts. In the future, "new" opportunists will surely be recognized as agents of disease in the abnormal host.

There are four basic approaches to the diagnosis of mycotic diseases: (1) clinical, (2) mycologic, (3) immunologic, and (4) pathologic.[1,5,6,9] Diseases caused by fungi may be difficult to distinguish, both clinically and pathologically, from those caused by other microbial agents. Because serologic tests have certain limitations and have not been developed for some fungal diseases, a definitive diagnosis of a mycotic disease often rests on direct microscopic demonstration of a fungus in tissues and exudates or on isolating and identifying it in culture. Histopathology should not be a substitute for cultural techniques, but rather the two should complement each other whenever possible. When cultural studies are not possible, as when only fixed tissues are available, a histopathologist can nevertheless provide a presumptive or specific diagnosis of a mycotic disease if the agent can be detected in a tissue section and accurately identified. The agents of some mycoses, such as lobomycosis and rhinosporidiosis, have not yet been isolated in culture, and the only means of establishing a diagnosis is by direct microscopic examination of tissue or exudate. Although certain inflammatory patterns suggest the presence of a fungus, the diagnosis of a mycotic infection can never be based on the tissue reaction alone.[1,3,4]

Histologic evaluation provides indisputable evidence of tissue invasion and therefore can confirm the pathogenic significance of a cultural isolate that belongs to the normal body flora or that is usually encountered as an environmental contaminant in culture. Histopathology can also confirm the presence of coexisting infections by other fungi, bacteria, viruses, and protozoa, thus guiding the clinician in selecting the most appropriate therapy and management for the patient. No other diagnostic approach can assess whether the host response signifies tissue invasion or a purely allergic reaction (for example, invasive versus allergic pulmonary aspergillosis).

Even though most fungi can be isolated from clinical materials, the cultivation and characterization of an isolate may take weeks, and the clinician usually cannot wait to begin therapy. Because the management of one mycosis may be entirely different from that of another, the pathologist must often play a key role in recognizing mycoses and identifying their etiologic agents. In attempting to identify fungi using conventional histologic methods, it is helpful to remember that these microbes appear in tissue as hyphae, yeastlike cells, endosporulating spherules, or a combination of these forms. Based on the morphologic distinctiveness of their etiologic agents in tissue, the mycoses can be grouped as follows[4]:

1. *Those caused by fungi that can be identified because they have a distinctive morphology in tissue.* If typical forms are observed, a specific diagnosis can be made (for example, adiaspiromycosis, blastomycosis, coccidioidomycosis, cryptococcosis, histoplasmosis capsulati, histoplasmosis duboisii, lobomycosis, paracoccidioidomycosis, protothecosis, rhinosporidiosis, sporotrichosis).

2. *Those caused by any one of several species of a genus that are so similar morphologically that they can be identified only to the genus level.* Nevertheless, the diseases that they cause can be diagnosed generically (for example, aspergillosis, candidiasis, nocardiosis).

3. *Those caused by any of a number of fungi belonging to various genera that appear similar if not identical to one another in tissue.* Although the agent cannot be specifically identified, the mycosis can still be named (for example, actinomycosis, chromoblastomycosis, dermatophytosis, phaeohyphomycosis, zygomycosis).

4. *Mycetomas, which are special cases that constitute a group by themselves.* Because most agents of mycetoma form their own distinctive type of granule, the experienced microscopist can often identify the etiologic agent by observing the size, shape, architecture (morphology of mycelial elements and their arrangement), and color of a granule. It is possible to determine if the granule is composed of an actinomycete (filamentous bacterium) or a eumycete (true fungus), and whether it is hyaline (white grain) or dematiaceous (black grain).

Although some fungi can be detected in hematoxylin and eosin–stained tissue sections, special histologic stains are usually necessary to demonstrate their morphology in detail. These stains and their diagnostic applications are listed in Table 11-2.

Direct fluorescent antibody (DFA) staining of tissue sections is a valuable adjunctive procedure that can be used to confirm a presumptive histologic diagnosis.[8] Formalin-fixed, paraffin-embedded tissues are adequate for DFA studies of fungi because the polysaccharide antigens in fungal cell walls are not altered by formalin fixation. Because of the added dimension of serologic specificity, DFA can greatly increase the accuracy of conventional histologic evaluation, especially when only atypical forms of a fungus are present. A broad battery of sensitive and specific fluorescent antibody (FA) reagents is available for detecting and identifying many of the com-

Table 11-2. Useful stains for demonstrating fungi and actinomycetes in tissue sections

Stains	Diagnostic applications
Hematoxylin-eosin (H&E)	Demonstrates tissue response and some fungi, including those that are naturally pigmented; stains nuclei of some yeast-form cells
Special fungal stains Gomori methenamine-silver (GMS) Periodic acid–Schiff (PAS) Gridley fungus (GF) GMS with H&E counterstain (GMS-H&E)	Excellent for detecting fungi and studying their morphology in detail; GMS is best for screening and also stains the actinomycetes; GMS-H&E demonstrates fungi and tissue components simultaneously
Mucopolysaccharide stains Mayer's mucicarmine Southgate's mucicarmine Alcian blue	Demonstrate mucoid capsule of *Cryptococcus neoformans,* thus differentiating this fungus from others of similar morphology
Modified Gram stains Brown and Brenn (B&B) Brown-Hopps (Humberstone) MacCallum-Goodpasture	Demonstrate gram-positive filaments of the actinomycetes and nonfilamentous bacteria of botryomycosis; some fungi, especially *Candida* spp., are gram positive
Modified acid-fast stains Fite-Faraco Kinyoun's	Demonstrate filaments of the *Nocardia* spp., most of which are weakly acid fast; fungal cell walls and the agents of actinomycosis are not acid fast
Giemsa stains May-Grünwald Wolbach's	Demonstrate kinetoplast of leishmanial forms and intracystic sporozoites of *Pneumocystis* spp.; both are protozoans that may be mistaken for fungi

mon pathogenic fungi, actinomycetes, and protothecae in tissue sections.[4,8] At present only a few medical mycologic diagnostic centers can perform these tests. In the future, however, specific FA reagents should become readily available to most hospital and public health laboratories.

Because mycologic terminology is highly specialized and essential for a discussion of fungi, actinomycetes, and algae in tissue, the following terms that pertain to these agents are defined:

arthrospore Asexual spore formed by mycelial disarticulation.

bud (blastospore) Asexual spore produced by lateral outgrowth from a parent cell; buds may be single or multiple.

chlamydospore Thick-walled, rounded, resistant spore formed by direct differentiation of the mycelium.

conidiophore Specialized hypha that produces and bears conidia.

conidium Asexual spore formed on but easily detached from a conidiophore.

dematiaceous Naturally pigmented, usually brown or black.

dimorphic Applied to fungi that grow as hyphae in vitro at 25° C and as budding yeasts or spherules in infected tissues or in vitro at 37° C on special media.

endospore Asexual spore formed within a closed structure such as a spherule.

germ tube Tubelike process that is produced by a germinating spore and eventually develops into a hypha.

granule Compact mass of organized mycelium that may be embedded in a cementlike substance; formed in actinomycosis and in actinomycotic and eumycotic mycetomas; also formed by nonfilamentous bacteria in botryomycosis.

hypha Filament that forms the thallus or body of most fungi.

mycelium Mass of intertwined and branched hyphae.

pseudohypha Short hyphal-like filament produced by the successive buds of a yeast that elongate and fail to separate.

septate Having cross walls.

spherule Closed, thick-walled, spherical structure within which asexual endospores are produced by progressive cytoplasmic cleavage.

Splendore-Hoeppli material Eosinophilic, refractile substance that surrounds some fungi and represents a localized antigen-antibody reaction in the hypersensitized host.

yeast Round to oval unicellular fungus that reproduces by budding.

SUPERFICIAL AND CUTANEOUS MYCOSES

The superficial mycoses comprise a group of fungal diseases that are confined to the outermost layers of the skin or its appendages.[10,11] Two of these diseases, black piedra and white piedra, involve the hair exclusively, and histopathology is not used for their diagnosis. The agents of tinea nigra and tinea versicolor grow in the stratum corneum and rarely invade the deeper skin layers. The histopathologist seldom encounters these infections unless the lesions are atypical and the clinician suspects another disease (tinea nigra has been mistaken for junctional nevus and malignant melanoma). The histologic features of these mycoses are summarized in Table 11-1. For more detailed information, several texts are recommended.[6,9-11]

The cutaneous mycoses involve the skin, hair, and nails to a greater degree than do the superficial mycoses. The most important disease in this group is dermatophytosis, a clinical entity caused by any of 31 recognized species of pathogenic and taxonomically related fungi (dermatophytes) of the genera *Epidermophyton, Microsporum,* and *Trichophyton.*[12] Diseases produced by the dermatophytes occur worldwide and are known as tineas or ringworm. The more common tineas include (1) tinea capitis of the scalp, eyebrows, and eyelashes (Fig. 11-1, A); (2) tinea corporis of the body; (3) tinea cruris of the groin (Fig. 11-2); (4) tinea pedis of the feet; and (5) tinea unguium of the nails (onychomycosis). Tineas of the hairy skin often appear as circular or ring-shaped patches of alopecia with erythema and scaling or as more diffusely distributed papules, pustules, vesicles, and kerions. Ringworm of the glabrous skin also commonly appears as erythematous and scaling patches, but more severe forms of tinea corporis may resemble other dermatologic disorders. Tinea unguium is manifested as thickening, discoloration, and deformity of the nails (Fig. 11-3).

Histologic features of the dermatophytoses are sum-marized in Table 11-1. Tissue forms of the dermatophytes are similar to one another. They usually stain with hematoxylin and eosin but are best demonstrated by special fungal stains. Hyphae and arthrospores invade the stratum corneum, hair follicles, and hairs (Fig. 11-1, B). The pattern of hair invasion is ectothrix, endothrix, endoectothrix, or favic, depending on the etiologic agent.[10,11] Occasionally, rupture of a hair follicle and

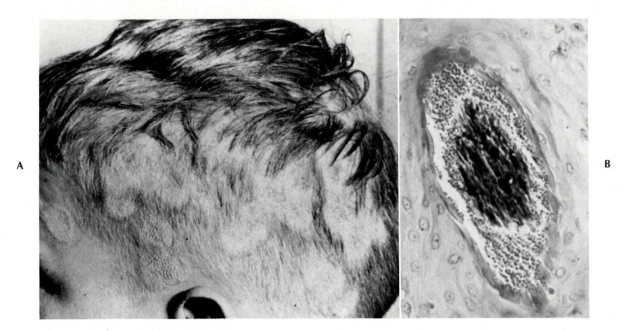

Fig. 11-1. A, Tinea capitis caused by *Microsporum canis*. **B,** Arthrospores of *M. canis* surrounding a partially degenerated hair. (Hematoxylin and eosin; 600×; **A,** courtesy Dr. William Kaplan, Centers for Disease Control, Atlanta.)

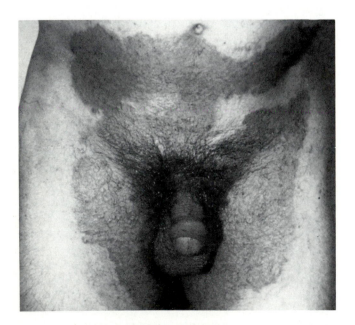

Fig. 11-2. Tinea cruris and tinea corporis caused by *Trichophyton rubrum*. (Courtesy Dr. Libero Ajello, Centers for Disease Control, Atlanta.)

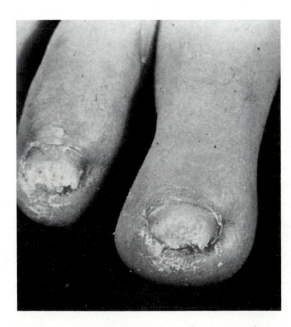

Fig. 11-3. Tinea unguium caused by *Trichophyton rubrum* in an adult male. Note thickening and discoloration of the nails.

release of fungal elements into the dermis elicit acute suppurative inflammation that eventually becomes granulomatous. The term *Majocchi's granuloma* refers to nodular, granulomatous lesions in the dermis that contain individual dermatophyte hyphae.

Agents of both the superficial and cutaneous mycoses are routinely demonstrated by direct microscopic examination of skin scrapings or hair in 10% potassium hydroxide. Cultural studies are required for their definitive identification.[12]

Certain fungi that commonly infect internal organs may also involve the skin and mucous membranes. The cutaneous manifestations of these mycoses are discussed separately under the respective disease headings.

SUBCUTANEOUS MYCOSES
Chromoblastomycosis

Chromoblastomycosis is an indolent cutaneous infection caused by any of several related dematiaceous (pigmented) fungi. The most common etiologic agents are *Fonsecaea pedrosoi*, *F. compacta*, *Phialophora verrucosa*, and *Cladosporium carrionii*.[14,15] The disease is cosmopolitan, but most cases are encountered in tropical regions. A locally spreading verrucous plaque or nodule develops in the skin at the site of implantation of the fungus, usually on an extremity. Satellite lesions may develop as a consequence of regional lymphatic spread or autoinoculation, but internal dissemination is rare.[14,15]

Although the agents of chromoblastomycosis can be distinguished from one another in culture, their tissue forms are identical. Round, thick-walled, dark brown muriform cells (sclerotic bodies), 5 to 12 μm in diameter, are grouped within the dermis where they elicit a granulomatous and suppurative inflammatory reaction.

These cells reproduce by septation in one or two planes (Fig. 11-4). Nonseptate cells and, rarely, septate hyphae are also observed in the lesions. Associated epidermal changes include hyperplasia and hyperkeratosis, and transepidermal elimination of the pigmented sclerotic bodies may be observed.[13]

Lobomycosis

Lobomycosis is a cutaneous mycosis that occurs in South America, especially Brazil and Surinam, and in parts of Central America. Natural infection occurs only in humans and dolphins[16] and produces locally enlarging cutaneous nodules that become verrucous.[17] These lesions are best treated by surgical excision. *Loboa loboi*, the etiologic agent, cannot be grown in culture.

Yeast-form cells of *L. loboi* are abundant in the dermis of the cutaneous nodules. These cells, 6 to 10 μm in diameter, are remarkably uniform. They reproduce by progressive budding in chains, three to eight cells in length, each of which resembles a string of pearls (Fig. 11-5). Adjacent cells are connected to one another by tubelike isthmuses, and secondary budding may be observed. Nonbudding and single-budding cells are also present. The surrounding dermis contains a dispersed epithelioid and giant cell granulomatous inflammatory reaction.

Mycetomas (Madura foot, maduromycosis)

Mycetomas are tumorous lesions of the subcutaneous tissues and bone caused by a wide variety of geophilic actinomycetes and fungi that form granules (compact mycelial aggregates) within tissue (Fig. 11-6). Patients

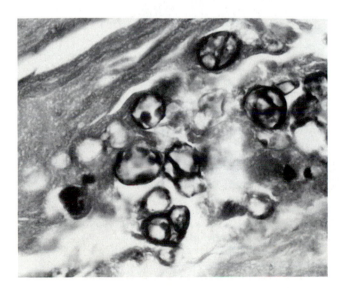

Fig. 11-4. Cutaneous chromoblastomycosis. Pigmented sclerotic bodies in keratin layer. Note septation in one or two planes. (Hematoxylin and eosin; 760×.)

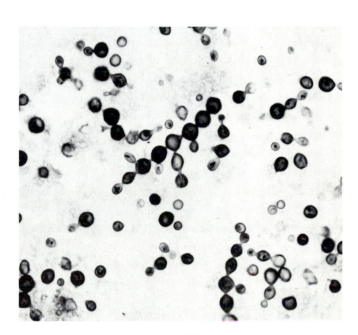

Fig. 11-5. Lobomycosis. Chains of budding cells with secondary budding are present, as well as nonbudding and single-budding cells. (Gridley stain; 480×.)

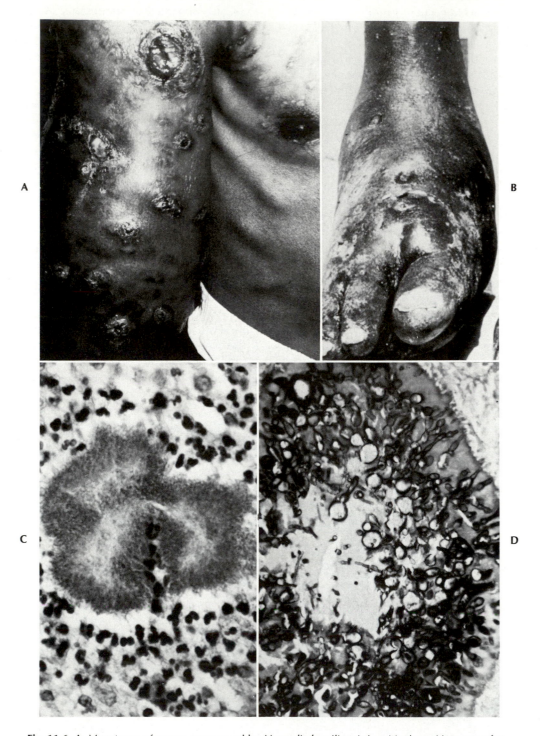

Fig. 11-6. A, Mycetoma of upper arm caused by *Nocardia brasiliensis* in a Mexican. Note tumefaction and multiple openings of draining sinuses. **B,** Mycetoma (Madura foot) in an Asiatic Indian. **C,** Granule of *N. brasiliensis* in biopsy of lesion shown in **A. D,** Granule of *Madurella mycetomatis* bordered by Splendore-Hoeppli material. Radially oriented hyphae and vesicular chlamydospores form the granule. (**C,** Hematoxylin and eosin; 600×; **D,** periodic acid–Schiff; 300×.)

are infected when these exogenous organisms are introduced into some part of the body, usually the lower extremities or the trunk, as the result of trauma. Most cases of mycetoma occur in tropical regions such as Asia, Africa, and Central and South America; the disease is rarely encountered in the United States.[19] There are two distinct types of mycetomas: actinomycotic and eumycotic. Their principal agents are listed in Table 11-1.[4]

Accurate histologic differentiation between the granules formed by actinomycetes and fungi is crucial in determining the form of treatment and the prognosis of mycetoma. Actinomycotic mycetomas usually respond to antibiotics or sulfonamides, but eumycotic mycetomas do not. Treatment of the latter is limited primarily to surgical excision and debridement.[20]

Special stains for bacteria and fungi (see Table 11-2) may be needed to determine if a granule is actinomycotic or eumycotic. Granules of actinomycotic mycetomas contain delicate, gram-positive, branched filaments, 1 μm or less in width, whereas those of eumycotic mycetomas contain broad, septate, fungal hyphae, 2 to 6 μm or more in width (Fig. 11-6, C and D).[18,21] Chlamydospores are sometimes found near the periphery of eumycotic granules. Granules may be pigmented (black grain) or hyaline (white grain) and may contain an amorphous cementlike substance, depending on the etiologic agent. Because many granules have a characteristic architecture, presumptive etiologic identification can often be made histologically. However, cultural studies are needed for definitive identification. FA conjugates are available for detecting *Pseudallescheria boydii*, the most common agent of eumycotic mycetoma in the United States.

The inflammatory reaction in mycetoma is similar regardless of the causative agent.[18,21] Lesions contain multiple sinus tracts, which usually discharge serosanguineous fluid, and, at times, grossly visible granules of various colors, sizes, and degrees of hardness depending on the agent involved. Histologically the dermis and subcutis contain localized abscesses, each of which usually has one or more granules in its center. Eosinophilic, clublike Splendore-Hoeppli material may border the granules (Fig. 11-6, C and D). Between abscesses there is extensive formation of granulation tissue, resulting in tumefaction and deformity often so severe as to be mistaken clinically for a neoplasm (Fig. 11-6, A and B). Mycetomas are insidious, localized infections, but they do not respect tissue planes. Infections often involve contiguous bone, resulting in destructive osteomyelitis. Lymphatic or hematogenous dissemination from the primary subcutaneous lesion rarely occurs.

Protothecosis

Protothecosis is an infection caused by achlorophyllous algae of the genus *Prototheca*. Although they do not contain chloroplasts, these saprophytic algae are believed to be related to green algae of the genus *Chlorella*.[27] Three species of protothecae are recognized, of which two, *P. wickerhamii* and *P. zopfii*, are known to cause disease. Human infections are cosmopolitan in distribution, and several have occurred in the United States.[26] The source of infection is often not apparent but can be related to penetrating injury in some cases.

Two clinically distinct forms of protothecosis are recognized: cutaneous infection and olecranon bursitis. Cutaneous protothecosis occurs as a spreading papulonodular or verrucous lesion, usually involving the distal extremities or head.[28] Infection may extend into the subcutaneous tissue and rarely spreads to regional lymph nodes.[24,28] Olecranon bursitis occurs as a subcutaneous nodule adjacent to the elbow.[26,28] Surgical excision is the treatment of choice. Chemotherapy alone has not effectively eradicated localized infection in most cases. The single reported case of disseminated human protothecosis occurred in a patient with transient depression of specific cell-mediated immunity to prototheca. He recovered after therapy with transfer factor and amphotericin B.[23]

The protothecae are found in tissue sections in the form of spherules, some of which contain endospores. Their asexual reproductive cycle in tissue is similar to that of the endosporulating fungi. Small, uninucleate, immature spherules undergo nuclear division accompanied or followed by progressive cytoplasmic cleavage to produce mature spherules that contain endospores. Characteristically, the endospores are polygonal or wedge shaped, fill the parent cell, and may be radially arranged around a central endospore, producing the distinctive "morula" form (Fig. 11-7, A). Spherules of the two pathogenic protothecae differ in size but are otherwise similar in morphology. Spherules of the small form, *P. wickerhamii*, measure 2 to 12 μm in diameter, whereas those of *P. zopfii* measure 10 to 25 μm in diameter. Morula forms are uncommon in infections caused by *P. zopfii*. Endosporulating cells of *P. zopfii* are oval, and their larger nuclei are more conspicuous than those of *P. wickerhamii* (Fig. 11-7, B).

The cell walls of both the spherules and the endospores are stained with the special fungal stains. With hematoxylin and eosin, these cells are hyaline, but their contents may be eosinophilic or basophilic. The two species are more reliably distinguished from one another in tissue sections by direct immunofluorescence and in culture by their patterns of carbohydrate assimilation.

Cutaneous lesions often show hyperkeratosis, parakeratosis, and acanthosis, and they may be ulcerated. Algal cells are abundant in the dermis and may also be found in the epidermis and keratin layer as a result of transepidermal elimination. The inflammatory reaction, when present, may be granulomatous or may consist of a mixture of acute and chronic inflammatory cells. Infection of

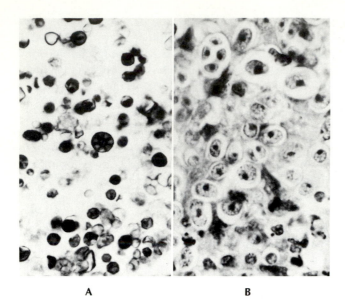

A   **B**

Fig. 11-7. Protothecosis. **A,** Distinctive endosporulating spherule ("morula form") of *Prototheca wickerhamii (center).* **B,** Oval cells of *P. zopfii.* Nuclei are visible in most cells. One endosporulating cell is present *(top left).* (**A,** Gridley stain; 760×; **B,** hematoxylin and eosin; 760×.)

the olecranon bursa produces a necrotic granuloma. The bursal lining contains a stellate zone of necrotic debris, neutrophils, and fibrin that is surrounded by palisaded epithelioid histiocytes and multinucleated giant cells. The adjacent soft tissue consists of granulation tissue that contains acute and chronic inflammatory cells and small granulomas. Prototheca cells are difficult to find in these lesions, which can be misinterpreted as rheumatoid nodules if special stains are not used to detect the algae. Endosporulating fungi such as *Coccidioides immitis* and *Rhinosporidium seeberi* are distinguished from the protothecae in tissue sections on the basis of their size and distinctive morphology (Table 11-1).

Green algae of the genus *Chlorella* cause cutaneous and systemic infections in animals, but human green algal infection has been recognized only recently.[25] In tissue the cells of *Chlorella*, 6 to 14 μm in diameter, are similar to those of *P. zopfii.* However, infections caused by the two algae can be differentiated by other criteria.[22] The protothecae can be distinguished from each other and from *Chlorella* in tissue sections by direct immunofluorescence.

Rhinosporidiosis

Rhinosporidiosis is a mucosal and cutaneous mycosis caused by *Rhinosporidium seeberi.* The disease is endemic in India, Sri Lanka, and parts of Africa, but sporadic cases occur in the Western Hemisphere, including the United States. Infection produces bulky, friable mucosal polyps in the nasal cavity and nasopharynx and on the palate. The conjunctiva, larynx, genitalia, rectum, and skin are involved less commonly.[32]

Since *R. seeberi* cannot be grown in culture, diagnosis of the disease depends on recognition of its distinctive morphology in tissue. The sporangia of *R. seeberi* are located predominantly in the stroma of the mucosal polyps. Spherical, uninucleate trophic forms (immature sporangia), 10 to 100 μm in diameter, develop into mature sporangia, 100 to 350 μm in diameter, by a process of progressive enlargement and endosporulation (Fig. 11-8).[31] Endospores are uninucleate and may contain several globular eosinophilic inclusions. Zonation of endospores within the sporangium is frequently observed.[29]

Cylindrical cell papillomas of the paranasal sinuses and nasal cavity that contain numerous intraepithelial mucous cysts can be mistaken for rhinosporidial polyps.[30]

Sporotrichosis

Sporotrichosis is a subacute or chronic disease caused by the dimorphic fungus *Sporothrix schenckii.* The disease occurs worldwide, but most reported cases have originated from the United States, South Africa, Mexico, and South America. Infection usually results from the traumatic implantation of the fungus, growing in soil or on plant materials, into the skin and subcutaneous tissue. In rare instances a primary cutaneous infection may disseminate to the bones, joints, lungs, and other organs.[37,38] Even more rarely, inhalation of the fungus results in primary pulmonary infection that may disseminate.[33] Sporotrichosis is not contagious, but infections can result from contamination of skin wounds with exudates from the lesions of humans or animals with sporotrichosis. There is no evidence that underlying disease or immunosuppression predisposes an individual to infection.

The most common form of sporotrichosis is lymphocutaneous.[34] Clinically, this form is manifested as a chain of subcutaneous nodules along the course of lymphatics draining a primary skin lesion that may be nodular and ulcerated. Lymphocutaneous lesions develop within 7 to 90 days or longer after penetrating injury to an exposed part of the body such as the hand, arm, neck, or foot. Eventually the subcutaneous nodules soften, ulcerate, and discharge pus. Solitary, ulcerated, and verrucous lesions of the skin without lymphatic involvement also occur. They are sometimes mistaken for a neoplasm and excised surgically. The treatment of choice for sporotrichosis is potassium iodide, especially in lymphocutaneous infections. Amphotericin B and other antifungals may also be useful in systemic infections.[37] If untreated, the infection may persist for years.

S. schenckii usually elicits a mixed suppurative and granulomatous inflammatory reaction accompanied by microabscess formation and fibrosis (Fig. 11-9, *A*).[34,36] This type of inflammation is typical of all forms of the disease, but it is not specific. In tissue, *S. schenckii* appears as round, oval, or elongated (cigar-shaped) yeast-

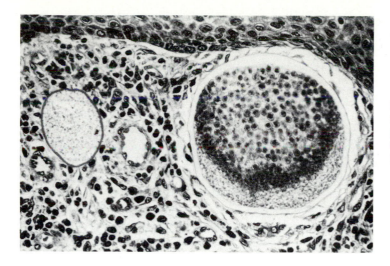

Fig. 11-8. Rhinosporidiosis. A trophic form and a mature sporangium of *Rhinosporidium seeberi* in the stroma of a nasal polyp. Note zonation of immature and mature endospores within sporangium. Mature endospores contain small, globular inclusions. (Hematoxylin and eosin; 300×.)

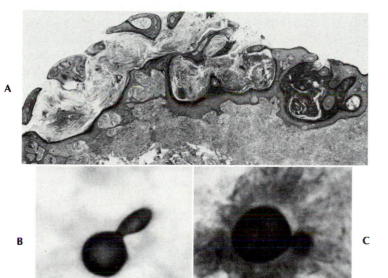

Fig. 11-9. Cutaneous sporotrichosis. **A,** Hyperplasia of epidermis and mixed suppurative and granulomatous inflammation in dermis. **B,** Single yeast-form cell of *Sporothrix schenckii* with elongated bud in dermal granuloma. **C,** Asteroid body composed of fungal cell surrounded by irregular spicules of Splendore-Hoeppli material. (**A,** Hematoxylin and eosin; 10×, **B,** Gomori methenamine-silver; 1500×; **C,** Gomori methenamine-silver/hematoxylin and eosin; 1500×.)

form cells, 2 to 6 μm or more in diameter. The fungal cells often bear elongated buds with narrow-based attachments to the parent cells (Fig. 11-9, *B*). Multiple budding is seen rarely. Although considered by some to be the classic tissue form of the fungus, cigar-shaped organisms are not commonly found. When present, they are most often observed in disseminated lesions. Hyphae are rarely formed in tissue.

The presence of asteroid bodies (fungal cells surrounded by Splendore-Hoeppli material) within microabscesses is helpful in making a presumptive histologic diagnosis of sporotrichosis (Fig. 11-9, *C*).[34,36] However, the asteroid body is not pathognomonic for this disease. Splendore-Hoeppli material may surround parasite ova, actinomycotic granules, eumycotic granules, foreign objects such as silk sutures, and other species of fungi, especially *Coccidioides immitis*, *Aspergillus* spp., *Candi-*

da spp., and the agents of entomophthoramycosis.[35] In many cases of sporotrichosis, asteroid bodies cannot be detected. Generally, few *S. schenckii* cells are found in cutaneous lesions, and special fungal stains, complemented by immunofluorescence staining, are needed to identify the fungus in fixed tissues. When immunofluorescence tests are not available, cultural examination or mouse inoculation is essential for an accurate diagnosis.

Subcutaneous and systemic phaeohyphomycosis

Phaeohyphomycosis comprises those subcutaneous and systemic diseases caused by opportunistic, naturally pigmented fungi that develop in tissue as dark-walled (brown), septate hyphae.[39] The inclusive name "phaeohyphomycosis" replaces the misleading and inappropriate term "phaeosporotrichosis" formerly applied to such infections. A wide variety of polymorphous fungi that are saprophytes of soil and wood can cause phaeohyphomycosis, for example, *Exophiala (Phialophora) jeanselmei*, *Phialophora* spp., *Cladosporium bantianum (trichoides)*, and *Drechslera* spp. Infections are encountered in healthy persons, but those who are immunosuppressed or chronically debilitated are at increased risk.

Phaeohyphomycosis has two clinical forms: subcutaneous and systemic. The subcutaneous form (phaeomycotic cyst) usually causes a single, firm to fluctuant, painless abscess, up to 7 cm in diameter, in the deep dermis or subcutaneous tissue.[42] Lesions occur on exposed parts of the body after penetrating injury by a wood splinter or other foreign object that acts as a vehicle of infection. Infection remains localized, and lymphangitis is uncommon. Microscopically the overlying skin is unaffected. The subcutis contains a large, cystic granuloma composed of compact multinucleated giant cells and histiocytes enclosed by granulation tissue or a well-defined fibrotic capsule. The centrally located abscess or cyst contains cellular debris, fibrin, polymorphonuclear leukocytes, and, at times, plant fibers or other foreign material. Short, closely septate hyphae, 2 to 6 μm in width, and chains of budding yeastlike cells are present in the wall of the abscess and amid the centrally located exudate. These moniliform fungi appear light brown when stained by hematoxylin and eosin and they are well demonstrated with special fungal stains. However, special stains mask their natural brown color, and a diagnosis of phaeohyphomycosis can be missed unless a replicate section stained by hematoxylin and eosin is examined. *Phialophora* and *Exophiala* spp. are most often found in cystic lesions, whereas other genera such as *Wangiella* and *Drechslera* are associated with solid granulomas that may contain small, stellate abscesses.[40]

In the systemic form (cerebral phaeohyphomycosis) the route of infection is generally via the respiratory tract, and the most commonly encountered agent is *Cladosporium bantianum*.[41] This fungus is extremely neurotropic, and most infections are confined to the brain and meninges; the lung and other organs are rarely involved. Brain lesions appear as encapsulated abscesses or generalized inflammatory infiltrates (Fig. 11-10, *A*). Symptoms include headache, nausea, vomiting, fever, and nuchal rigidity. The inflammatory reaction is similar to that seen in subcutaneous lesions.

The agents of phaeohyphomycosis are morphologically and tinctorially similar in tissue, where they cannot be differentiated from each other. However, a disease diagnosis can be based on the natural brown color of morphologically typical fungi (Fig. 11-10, *B*). Culture is needed for specific identification of the etiologic agents.

SYSTEMIC MYCOSES
Actinomycosis

Actinomycosis is a chronic suppurative disease caused by anaerobic, filamentous bacteria in the order Actinomycetales.[44,45] The disease occurs worldwide, and males

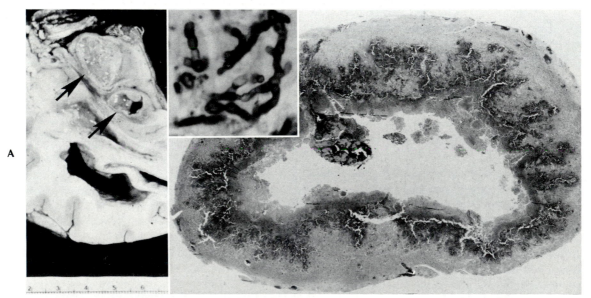

Fig. 11-10. Systemic (cerebral) phaeohyphomycosis. **A,** Two sharply circumscribed, encapsulated abscesses *(arrows)* caused by *Cladosporium bantianum* in brain of adult. **B,** Abscess caused by *C. bantianum* enucleated from left frontal lobe. The suppurative and necrotic center was lost during processing. (AFIP 62-5502; courtesy Dr. C.H. Binford, Armed Forces Institute of Pathology, Washington.) *Inset,* Dematiaceous hyphae in wall of abscess are branched and constricted at their prominent septations. (**B,** Hematoxylin and eosin; 10×; *inset,* 900×.)

are affected three times as frequently as females. The principal agent of actinomycosis in humans is *Actinomyces israelii*. This species and others listed in Table 11-1 have never been isolated from environmental sources. Rather, they occur as commensals in the mouth, and "sulfur" granules are commonly found in the tonsillar

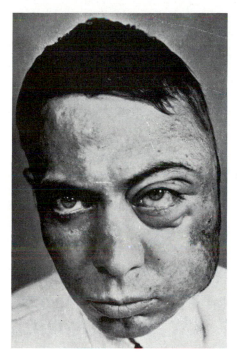

Fig. 11-11. Cervicofacial actinomycosis. Note swelling and openings of draining sinuses. (Courtesy Dr. Antonio González-Ochoa, Mexico City.)

crypts of healthy individuals. The actinomycetes are ordinarily of low pathogenicity. Underlying disease and interruption of mucocutaneous barriers predispose a person to actinomycosis by providing a medium in which these endogenous organisms can invade, proliferate, and disseminate. Unlike nocardiosis, actinomycosis does not occur preferentially in persons with defective immunity.[45]

Based on the anatomic site of the lesions, four clinical forms of actinomycosis are recognized: cervicofacial, thoracic, abdominal, and pelvic. Most commonly involved is the cervicofacial area, where the disease is often a sequela to dental caries, periodontal disease, or injury to the oral mucosa such as a tooth extraction. The localized lesion enlarges, abscesses form, and draining sinus tracts emerge (Fig. 11-11). If untreated, direct extension of the infection may involve the mandible, sinuses, orbit, cranial bones, and thorax, where it may then disseminate to the central nervous system, skin, and other bones. Thoracic infection may follow aspiration of infectious materials. Abdominal actinomycosis (Fig. 11-12) is frequently mistaken for advanced malignancy. It may result from direct extension of a thoracic infection but is more commonly seen as a consequence of a ruptured appendix or bowel perforation by swallowed foreign bodies such as toothpicks and needles. Pelvic actinomycosis is a well-recognized complication of intrauterine contraceptive devices.[43] Primary skin infections may develop after human bites.

The inflammatory reaction in actinomycosis is suppurative, with the formation of abscesses that contain one or more granules (organized aggregates of filaments), 30 to

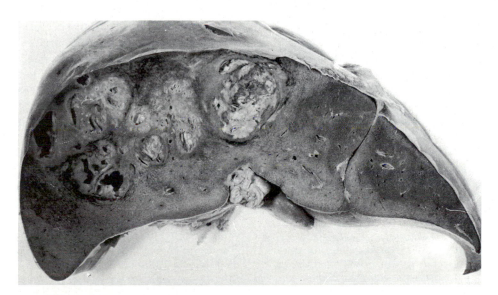

Fig. 11-12. Abdominal actinomycosis. Multiple abscesses in liver were caused by *Actinomyces israelii*. Primary infection in cecum or appendix resulted in retrocecal abscess that extended to skin surface in right inguinal region. (Courtesy Dr. Roger D. Baker, Silver Spring, Md.)

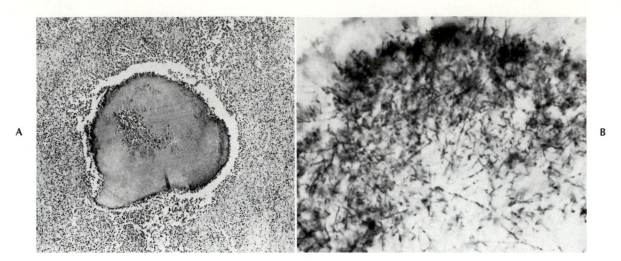

Fig. 11-13. A, Granule of *Actinomyces israelii* in hepatic abscess. **B,** Gram-positive, branched filaments and coccoid elements, 1 μm or less in diameter, in replicate section of granule in **A.** (**A,** Hematoxylin and eosin; 40×; **B,** Brown and Brenn; 480×.)

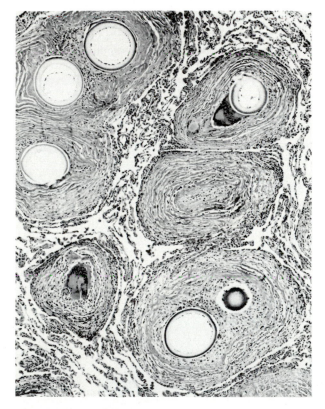

Fig. 11-14. Adiaspiromycosis. Fibrotic pulmonary granulomas contain large, thick-walled adiaspores of *Chrysosporium parvum* var. *crescens*. Outer portion of each adiaspore wall is eosinophilic; inner portion is hyaline. (Hematoxylin and eosin; 50×.)

3000 μm in diameter, that are bordered by eosinophilic, clublike, Splendore-Hoeppli material (Fig. 11-13, A).[44,46] Bacterial stains reveal that the granules are composed of delicate, branched, gram-positive filaments, 1 μm or less in diameter, haphazardly arranged in an amorphous matrix of uncertain composition (Fig. 11-13, B). The filaments may be fragmented and, unlike those of the *Nocardia* spp., are not acid fast.[46,47] Gomori methenamine-silver staining is also useful for demonstrating the filaments, which are not stained by the hematoxylin and eosin, periodic acid–Schiff, and Gridley stains. Specific identification requires culture or immunofluorescence staining because, in tissue, the agents of actinomycosis cannot be distinguished from each other. Both gram-positive and gram-negative bacilli and cocci may be found in close association with actinomycete filaments within a granule, but it is generally believed that these bacteria are secondary pathogens.

Penicillin is the drug of choice for treating actinomycosis.[45] It is speculated that fewer cases are seen today because of the widespread use of antibacterial antibiotics for treating minor, unrelated infections.

Adiaspiromycosis

Adiaspiromycosis is an uncommon pulmonary mycosis caused by *Chrysosporium parvum* var. *crescens* (*Emmonsia crescens*). Human infection is usually asymptomatic, self-limited, and confined to the lungs.[48] The inhaled conidia of *C. parvum* var. *crescens*, which are 2 to 4 μm in diameter, progressively enlarge within the lungs to a diameter of 200 to 400 μm at maturity, with chitinous walls 20 to 30 μm or more in width (Fig. 11-14).[48,49] No other fungus of medical importance has a wall this thick. Each mature adiaspore is enclosed within a fibrotic granuloma that compresses the surrounding

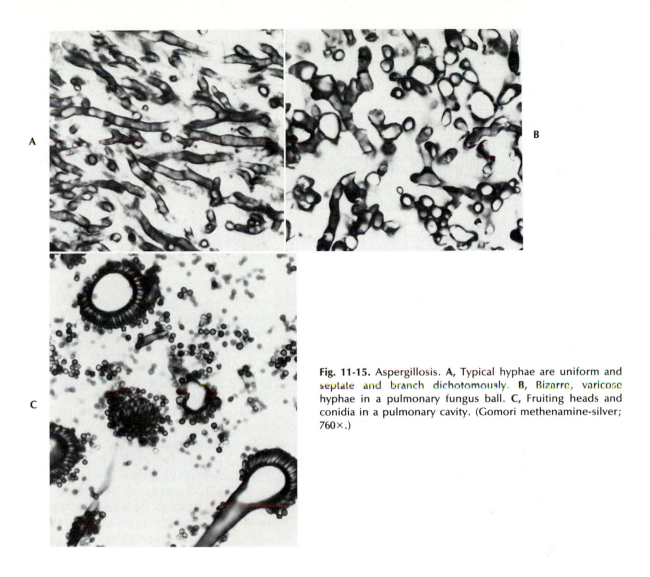

Fig. 11-15. Aspergillosis. **A**, Typical hyphae are uniform and septate and branch dichotomously. **B**, Bizarre, varicose hyphae in a pulmonary fungus ball. **C**, Fruiting heads and conidia in a pulmonary cavity. (Gomori methenamine-silver; 760×.)

lung tissue. Since *C. parvum* var. *crescens* does not replicate within the human host, the degree of impairment of pulmonary function is related to the number of spores inhaled and the frequency of exposure.[49]

Aspergillosis

The spectrum of disease produced by members of the genus *Aspergillus* includes indolent superficial infections, colonization of pulmonary cavities, allergic bronchopulmonary disease, and fulminant, invasive pulmonary and disseminated infections of immunocompromised patients. Aspergillosis is the second most common opportunistic mycosis among patients with malignant disease, accounting for 31% of fungal infections found at autopsy in these patients.[50] *A. fumigatus* is the species most frequently isolated from patients with invasive or disseminated infections,[59] but *A. flavus*, *A. niger*, and other species can also produce disease. Since the conidia of the aspergilli are ubiquitous in nature, recovery of an *Aspergillus* organism in culture must be interpreted cau-

tiously.[55] Proof of its etiologic role in infection requires microscopic demonstration of characteristic hyphae in tissue. A detailed account of the mycology of the aspergilli is provided by Raper and Fennell.[54]

Typical hyphae of *Aspergillus* have a characteristic appearance in tissue sections (Fig. 11-15, *A*). They are uniform, narrow (3 to 5 μm in width), and regularly septate. Branching is regular and dichotomous. Branches arise at acute angles from parent hyphae and radiate in similar directions. The contours of the hyphae are parallel. The hyphae may stain with hematoxylin but are demonstrated better with the special fungal stains.

The hyphae of the aspergilli occasionally exhibit several unusual features in tissue. Hyphae encountered in fungus balls and indolent granulomatous lesions may assume bizarre shapes with varicose dilatations and infrequent septa (Fig. 11-15, *B*). Such hyphae may be confused with those of the zygomycetes.[55] Conidial heads are produced in some lesions in contact with air, most frequently in intracavitary aspergillomas of the lung (Fig.

11-15, *C*). Calcium oxalate crystals may be deposited within the mycelium of fungus balls in the lungs or paranasal sinuses.[53] Hyphal fragments in chronic granulomatous lesions are sometimes surrounded by eosinophilic Splendore-Hoeppli material.

The immune status of the host and the site of infection largely determine the type of inflammatory reaction to *Aspergillus* infection. In the immunocompromised host, invasive pulmonary infection produces circumscribed or confluent abscesses that may be widely distributed throughout both lungs (Fig. 11-16). These may coexist with areas of infarction. Microscopically, abundant hyphae are found in areas of necrotizing and suppurative pneumonitis. In neutropenic patients mycelial colonies produce coagulative necrosis of tissue with little cellular reaction. Hyphal invasion of arteries and veins is conspicuous and results in vascular thrombosis, tissue infarction, and systemic dissemination.

The aspergilloma, or fungus ball, is a noninvasive compact mass of hyphae that forms within a preexisting pulmonary cavity. The mycelial ball measures up to 5 cm in diameter and is composed of tangled, often bizarre and distorted hyphae admixed with inflammatory exudate and tissue debris. Conidial heads are occasionally detected in these lesions. Allergic forms of pulmonary aspergillosis occur in sensitized individuals and include allergic bronchopulmonary aspergillosis, chronic eosinophilic pneumonia, mucoid impaction of large bronchi, asthmatic forms of bronchocentric granulomatosis, and microgranulomatous hypersensitivity pneumonitis.[52,57] It may be difficult to find hyphae in these lesions.

Disseminated aspergillosis is a disease of immunocompromised patients. The lungs are involved in almost all cases. The gastrointestinal tract, brain, kidneys, liver, esophagus, and heart are frequently involved, but lesions may be found in any organ.[60] Microscopically the systemic lesions are abscesses, granulomas, or infarcts that contain hyphal fragments.

Indolent, chronic granulomatous infections are occasionally encountered in the lungs, in subcutaneous tissue, and in the paranasal sinuses and orbit of diabetics and patients treated with corticosteroids. Cutaneous aspergillosis can be a manifestation of disseminated infection or can occur as a primary infection in burned patients. Aspergilli also cause superficial infections of the external ear canal and nails, as well as endocarditis involving previously damaged or prosthetic valves.[51]

Other pathogenic fungi that form branched, septate hyphae in tissue can be confused with the aspergilli. These fungi include *Pseudallescheria boydii*,[56] *Fusarium* spp.,[58] and, on occasion, *Candida* spp. Recognition of subtle differences in the morphology of these fungi may allow one to differentiate them from the aspergilli in tissue sections. However, unless typical conidial heads are observed in the lesion, a histologic diagnosis of aspergillosis should be considered presumptive until confirmed by direct immunofluorescence or isolation from the lesion of an *Aspergillus* sp. in pure culture.

Blastomycosis

Blastomycosis is a chronic granulomatous and suppurative infection caused by the dimorphic fungus, *Blastomyces dermatitidis*. This mycosis was long thought to be restricted to North America, but autochthonous cases are now known to occur in the Middle East and in several African countries. Although clinical and epidemiologic evidence indicates that individuals contract blastomycosis from sources in nature such as soil, the natural habitat of *B. dermatitidis* has not yet been discovered. Most infections result from inhalation of the spores of the saprophytic fungus, and thus the disease usually has a pulmonary inception.

Blastomycosis has two clinical forms: systemic and cutaneous.[62-65] In the systemic form the infection is often confined to the lungs but may spread via the bloodstream to other organs, especially the skin, bones, joints, male

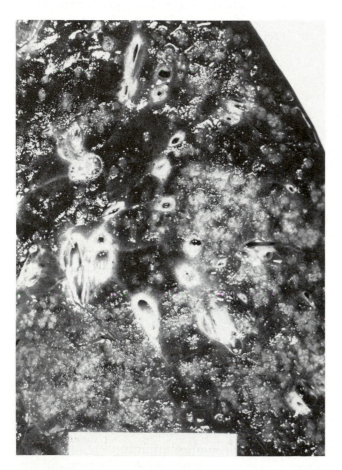

Fig. 11-16. Invasive pulmonary aspergillosis. Confluent, granular nodules occupy much of the sectioned surface. From a pancytopenic patient with disseminated aspergillosis that involved the lungs and brain and complicated chemotherapy for acute granulocytic leukemia.

genital tract, urinary bladder, brain, and spinal cord.[63-65] Pulmonary lesions are occasionally inapparent. Cutaneous blastomycosis appears as indolent, ulcerated or verrucous, granulomatous lesions that generally occur on exposed surfaces (Fig. 11-17, *A* and *B*). Both forms of the disease are best treated with amphotericin B; 2-hydroxystilbamidine has also been effective.[61]

In tissue *B. dermatitidis* appears as spherical, single-budding, yeast-form cells, 8 to 15 μm in diameter, with thick, double-contoured walls (Fig. 11-17, *C*). Several basophilic nuclei may be visible when optimally fixed tissues are stained by hematoxylin and eosin. The broad-based budding of this fungus is characteristic and aids in differentiating it from other yeast forms of similar size, such as *Histoplasma capsulatum* var. *duboisii* and *Cryptococcus neoformans*. These agents can also be distinguished from each other by direct immunofluorescence. Occasionally, small but morphologically typical forms of *B. dermatitidis* (2 to 4 μm in diameter) occur in tissue, but they are always present as part of a continuous series of sizes ranging from the unusually small to the larger forms characteristic of the fungus. This mixture of small and typical forms should not be mistaken for coexisting mycoses. Hyphae are rarely formed in tissue.

Blastomyces dermatitidis usually elicits a mixed sup-purative and granulomatous inflammatory reaction.[63,64] Early lesions are predominantly suppurative, whereas older ones tend to be granulomatous with abscess formation and caseation. Although diffuse fibrosis is common in chronic infections, solitary fibrocaseous nodules, as seen in histoplasmosis capsulati, are extremely rare in blastomycosis. Florid pseudoepitheliomatous hyperplasia of skin lesions can mimic squamous cell carcinoma (Fig. 11-17, *B*).

Botryomycosis (bacterial pseudomycosis)

Botryomycosis is a chronic, localized infection of the skin and subcutaneous tissues caused by nonfilamentous bacteria that form granules.[66] Disseminated infection is rare.[67] In hematoxylin and eosin–stained tissue sections, the granules may be mistaken for those of actinomycosis and actinomycotic mycetoma. Bacteria most commonly implicated include *Pseudomonas aeruginosa*, *Staphylococcus aureus*, *Escherichia coli*, and species of *Streptococcus* and *Proteus*. Botryomycotic granules and those of actinomycosis and mycetoma (see discussion of mycetomas) can be differentiated from each other if appropriate bacterial and fungal stains are used. Differentiation is important because each of these diseases is managed differently.

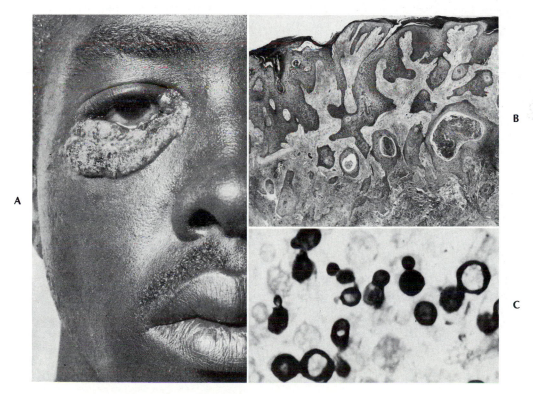

Fig. 11-17. Cutaneous blastomycosis. **A,** Elevated ulcer. B, Pseudoepitheliomatous hyperplasia of epidermis and mixed suppurative and granulomatous inflammation in dermis. C, Single and budding *Blastomyces dermatitidis* cells in dermal abscess. Note characteristic broad based budding of yeast-form cells. (**A** Courtesy Dr. Roger D. Baker, Silver Spring, Md.; **B,** hematoxylin and eosin; 10×; **C,** Gomori methenamine-silver; 600×.)

Candidiasis

Candidiasis is a mucocutaneous or systemic mycosis most often caused by the endogenous species *Candida albicans*. Occasional human infections are caused by other saprophytic *Candida* spp., including *C. guilliermondii*, *C. krusei*, *C. parapsilosis*, *C. pseudotropicalis*, and *C. tropicalis*. Infection by *Torulopsis glabrata*, recently reclassified in the genus *Candida*, is discussed separately.

C. albicans is found among the normal flora of the oral cavity, upper respiratory tract, digestive tract, and vagina. Infection may occur as a complication of mucosal ulceration, when the normal balance of endogenous flora is altered, or when cellular or humoral defense mechanisms are compromised by underlying disease or therapy. Thus factors that predispose to candidiasis include abdominal surgery, prolonged broad-spectrum antibiotic therapy, indwelling venous catheters, leukemia and lymphoma, granulocytopenia, cytotoxic chemotherapy, and corticosteroid therapy.[73,75] Candidiasis is the most common opportunistic mycosis in the United States.[50]

Superficial candidal infections involve the skin and the mucosal surfaces of the oral cavity and vagina. Intertriginous cutaneous infections occur in obese, diabetic, and alcoholic patients. Maceration of the skin owing to prolonged immersion in water may predispose a person to cutaneous candidiasis and to paronychia and infection of the nails. Vulvovaginal infection may occur in patients with diabetes mellitus and during pregnancy. Infection of the oral cavity (thrush) is encountered in newborns, in patients treated with broad-spectrum antibiotics, and as a complication of diabetes or other debilitating diseases. Thrush is manifested as soft, white, mucosal patches in the oral cavity that are composed of yeast forms, pseudohyphae, and hyphae. The organisms are restricted to the epithelium and incite a mild inflammatory reaction in the underlying tissues.

Chronic mucocutaneous candidiasis, a chronic superficial infection of the skin, nails, oral cavity, oropharynx, and vagina, usually afflicts patients with defective cell-mediated immunity.[68] Five clinically distinct forms are recognized, one of which is associated with endocrine abnormalities, most commonly hypoparathyroidism and adrenal failure.[70] Mucocutaneous infection begins early in life and is particularly resistant to topical or parenteral chemotherapy. The disease has responded in some cases to the administration of transfer factor with parenteral chemotherapy. About 25% of patients with chronic mucocutaneous candidiasis have no demonstrable abnormality of cell-mediated immunity. Some cases are associated with defective neutrophil chemotaxis.

Systemic candidiasis is an opportunistic mycosis that usually involves the gastrointestinal tract, kidneys, heart, and central nervous system but may involve almost any organ.[73,75] Within the gastrointestinal tract the distal esophagus and stomach are involved most frequently.[71] Gastrointestinal lesions consist of mucosal erosions or ulcers covered by friable pseudomembranes (Fig. 11-18, *A*) composed of yeast forms, pseudohyphae, and hyphae that extend into the submucosa and occasionally into submucosal blood vessels. In about 15% of immunocompromised patients with gastrointestinal candidiasis, the infection disseminates to other organs.[71] The *Candida* spp. may colonize preexisting ulcers without giving rise to disseminated infection.[72]

Cerebral candidiasis is the most common mycosis of the central nervous system, accounting for half of such infections in a recent series.[76] It is a late complication of disseminated candidiasis in patients with cardiac and renal involvement. Cerebral lesions consist of haphazardly distributed microabscesses, occasionally accompanied by noncaseating granulomas.[77] Meningeal involvement, when present, is usually localized.

Two patterns of pulmonary candidiasis are encoun-

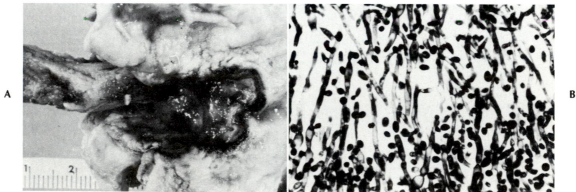

Fig. 11-18. Candidiasis. **A,** Ulcer at esophagogastric junction caused by *Candida albicans*. The 5-year-old patient was pancytopenic as a result of treatment for acute lymphocytic leukemia. At autopsy the lungs, liver, and spleen contained irregular, friable, yellow nodules. **B,** Yeast cells, pseudohyphae, and hyphae of *C. albicans*. (**B,** Gomori methenamine-silver; 480×.)

tered in immunosuppressed patients.[69] Endobronchial infection produces large nodular foci of bronchopneumonia in both lungs, predominantly in the lower lobes. Laryngeal and tracheal infection may be present, but disseminated infection is uncommon. Hematogenous pulmonary candidiasis produces round, hemorrhagic or gray nodules, 2 to 4 mm in diameter, distributed randomly but symmetrically throughout both lungs. Endobronchial and respiratory mucosal involvement is uncommon in this form of pulmonary infection, whereas extrapulmonary involvement is frequently found in the esophagus, stomach, liver, spleen, and kidneys.

Candida spp. are the most common cause of fungal infection of the heart.[79] Myocardial microabscesses are usually a sequela of disseminated infection and may be associated with endocardial vegetations.[74] The latter are bulky and friable and may give rise to arterial emboli. Preexisting deformities of the valves are not always found in candidal endocarditis; such infection may develop in immunosuppressed patients, drug addicts, and patients with central venous catheters. Candidal infection of prosthetic cardiac valves develops on neoendocardium that grows onto the sewing cloth and struts of the prostheses, and systemic arterial emboli are a frequent complication.[78]

Microscopically the lesions of invasive candidiasis contain yeast forms and pseudohyphae, either of which may predominate, and occasional hyphae (Fig. 11-18, *B*). The oval yeast cells, 2 to 6 μm in diameter, reproduce by budding. Pseudohyphae consist of chains of elongated yeast cells. Cells in the chain display constrictions at points of apposition to adjacent cells (Fig. 11-19, *A*). Septate, branched hyphae are slightly narrower than the pseudohyphae and do not have conspicuous constrictions at sites of septation (Fig. 11-19, *B*). The inflammatory response to infection is typically suppurative but may be both granulomatous and suppurative in chronic or indolent infections. Lesions in granulocytopenic patients or in patients whose infection is preterminal may lack cellular inflammatory reaction. Inflammatory cell infiltration is minimal at sites of mucosal ulcers and in mucocutaneous lesions where *Candida* is a colonist or does not deeply invade tissue. Mycelial and pseudomycelial invasion of small blood vessels is frequently found in disseminated candidiasis, but invasion of large vessels with parenchymal infarction, as seen in aspergillosis and zygomycosis, is not usually encountered. All *Candida* spp., with the exception of *C. glabrata*, are morphologically similar in tissue, and they cannot be distinguished from one another by direct immunofluorescence. However, the species can be differentiated by biochemical reactions in vitro.

Coccidioidomycosis

Coccidioidomycosis begins as a pulmonary infection. The disease, endemic in the southwestern United States, northern Mexico, and Central and South America,[83] is acquired by inhalation of the arthroconidia of *Coccidioides immitis*, a fungus that inhabits desert soil. The epidemiology and clinical aspects of the disease have been reviewed elsewhere.[80,84] In most patients primary pulmonary infection is asymptomatic and resolves spontaneously. Symptomatic patients usually have a self-limited febrile illness of brief duration. In approximately 5% of symptomatic patients, chronic or residual pulmonary infection develops. It can be detected as a solitary nodule or cavitary lesion on a chest roentgenogram. Disseminated infection develops in less than 1% of patients and involves the skin and subcutaneous tissue, bones, joints, lymph nodes, spleen, liver, kidneys, and meninges.[84] Disseminated infection, if untreated, may be fatal in up to 50% of cases. Primary cutaneous infection is exceedingly rare. The vast majority of patients with skin lesions have disseminated disease from a clinically inapparent pulmonary focus.

Acute suppurative pneumonitis characterizes the pri-

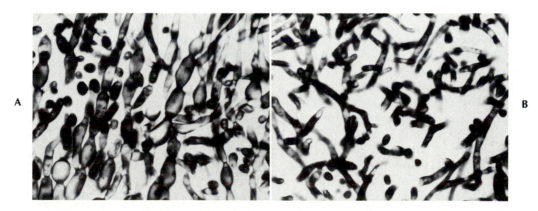

Fig. 11-19. A, Yeast cells and pseudohyphae of *Candida albicans*. Note constrictions between adjacent cells that form the pseudohyphae. **B,** Septate hyphae of *C. albicans* are uniform and narrow and lack prominent constrictions. (Gomori methenamine-silver, 760×.)

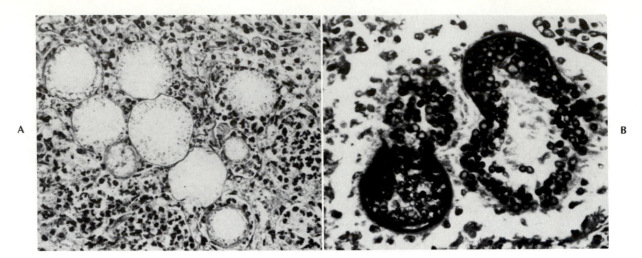

Fig. 11-20. Coccidioidomycosis. **A,** Endosporulating spherules in primary pulmonary coccidioido-mycosis. **B,** Endospores released following rupture of spherules. (**A,** Hematoxylin and eosin; 300×; **B,** Gomori methenamine-silver/hematoxylin and eosin; 480×.)

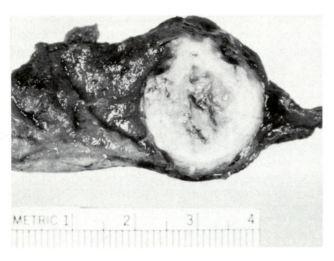

Fig. 11-21. Residual pulmonary coccidioidomycosis. Circumscribed subpleural fibrocaseous nodule is present.

mary pulmonary infection. Diagnostic tissue forms of *C. immitis*, usually abundant in active lesions, consist of mature spherules, 30 to 100 μm or more in diameter, that contain endospores, 2 to 5 μm in diameter (Fig. 11-20, *A*). Rupture of the spherules releases endospores into the surrounding tissue (Fig. 11-20, *B*). Released endospores enlarge to become immature spherules and, following endosporulation, mature spherules. Donnelly and Yunis[82] have studied the ultrastructure and developmental sequence of *C. immitis* in tissue.

The residual pulmonary lesion is a peripheral, sharply circumscribed, centrally necrotic granuloma (Fig. 11-21).[81] Diagnostic endosporulating spherules are scarce in these lesions, and a specific histologic diagnosis may require confirmation by direct immunofluorescence or culture. Septate hyphae and arthroconidia are occasionally found in cavitary lesions that communicate with the bronchial tree. Disseminated lesions are granulomatous or suppurative and granulomatous.

The "parent bodies" and "endobodies" found in myospherulosis, a pseudomycosis of the upper respiratory tract and middle ear,[85] are similar in size and morphology to the spherules and endospores of *C. immitis* but are readily distinguished by their inherent brown color. The structures of myospherulosis are derived from altered erythrocytes.[86]

Cryptococcosis

Cryptococcosis begins as a pulmonary disease that is usually acquired by inhalation of the soil-inhabiting yeast *Cryptococcus neoformans*.[90] This saprophytic fungus is ubiquitous in nature and worldwide in distribution. It is most abundant in habitats that are heavily contaminated by pigeon excreta. Cryptococcosis is not contagious. Although the disease occurs in apparently healthy individuals, those with defective immunity and severe underlying diseases such as hematologic malignancies are particularly at risk.

Clinically, two forms predominate: pulmonary cryptococcosis and, by hematogenous dissemination from a pulmonary focus, cerebromeningeal cryptococcosis. Dissemination from a primary pulmonary infection less often results in cutaneous, mucocutaneous, osseous, and visceral forms. In disseminated cryptococcosis, primary lung infection is frequently undetected, and the incubation period is unknown. A primary pulmonary lymph node complex develops in approximately 1% of the initial cases of cryptococcosis.[87] Rarely, cutaneous infection results from direct inoculation of the skin.[91]

For reasons that are poorly understood, *C. neofor-*

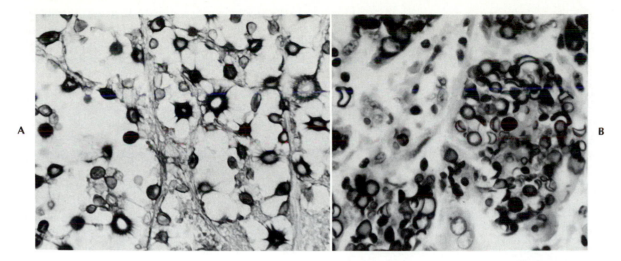

Fig. 11-22. A, Cerebromeningeal cryptococcosis. Numerous single and budding cryptococci have mucicarmine-positive capsules that have a spinous appearance because of shrinkage during processing of tissue. **B,** Granulomatous pneumonia caused by a poorly encapsulated strain of *Cryptococcus neoformans*. The pleomorphic yeast forms do not have conspicuous capsules. (**A,** Mayer's mucicarmine; 600×; **B,** Gomori methenamine-silver; 480×.)

mans is extremely neurotropic.[90] The clinical course of cerebromeningeal cryptococcosis varies from a few days to 20 years or more. However, it is usually fulminant and, if untreated, is almost invariably fatal. A diagnosis can be made by demonstrating *C. neoformans* cells in cerebrospinal fluid (CSF) or tissue, by isolating the fungus in culture, or by demonstrating cryptococcal polysaccharide antigen in the CSF by the latex agglutination test. About 25% of patients with cerebromeningeal infection undergo exploratory surgery before the disease is detected. These patients are usually afebrile and have an expanding intracranial lesion that mimics a brain tumor. Amphotericin B is the drug of choice for the treatment of cryptococcosis, and 5-fluorocytosine is effective in some cases.

In tissue *C. neoformans* is a round, oval, or elliptical yeastlike fungus that ranges from 5 to 20 μm in diameter. The cell walls of cryptococci are lightly basophilic when stained by hematoxylin and eosin, but they are demonstrated better by the special fungal stains. Typically, a clear zone of varying width surrounds each fungal cell, representing the space occupied by a mucoid capsule before fixation and processing of the tissue. When stained by mucicarmine, the clear zone contains carminophilic material that often has a spinous appearance resulting from irregular shrinkage of the mucopolysaccharide capsule during fixation (Fig. 11-22, A). Budding cells are numerous in lesions containing abundant, rapidly proliferating cryptococci. Cryptococci usually have single buds that are attached to parent cells by narrow bases; multiple buds are occasionally seen. Pseudohyphae are observed rarely, but true hyphae are rarely formed in tissue.

Because *C. neoformans* is unusually pleomorphic and its encapsulated forms are not always conspicuous, cryptococcosis should be considered in the differential histologic diagnosis of virtually any yeast infection.[89] When the capsules of typical cryptococci are carminophilic, a histologic diagnosis of cryptococcosis can be made with confidence. Unencapsulated cryptococci or those with small capsules produced by the so-called dry variants can be specifically identified by fluorescent antibody staining of tissue sections. In most instances, however, at least some cryptococci will have capsules that are detectable with the mucicarmine stain.

The spectrum of the inflammatory response to *C. neoformans* is broad and varies from little or no inflammation to a purely granulomatous reaction. At times, particularly in terminal or disseminated infections, cryptococci multiply profusely with no apparent host response (Fig. 11-22, A). Yeast cells displace normal parenchyma and form "cystic" lesions filled with myriad compact cryptococci whose wide mucoid capsules impart a glistening appearance and slimy consistency to lesions on gross examination. Generally, poorly encapsulated cryptococci elicit granulomatous inflammation in which numerous yeast cells without conspicuous capsules are seen within huge multinucleated giant cells and histiocytes (Fig. 11-22, B).[88]

Pulmonary infection by *C. neoformans* may occasionally result in solitary or multiple fibrocaseous granulomas (cryptococcomas) that, in hematoxylin and eosin–stained sections, are indistinguishable from those caused by infection with *Histoplasma capsulatum* var. *capsulatum* and *Coccidioides immitis* (Fig. 11-23). In these cryptococcomas the yeast cells are usually atypical, are frag-

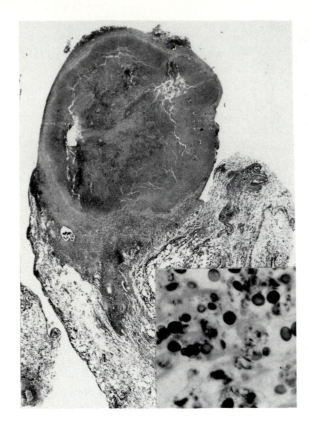

Fig. 11-23. Solitary fibrocaseous nodule (cryptococcoma) in lung of adult woman. *Inset,* Fragmented and unevenly stained cryptococci within central caseous material of nodule. (Hematoxylin and eosin; 10×; *inset,* Gomori methenamine-silver; 480×.)

mented, and stain poorly with the special fungal stains (Fig. 11-23, *inset*). Their capsules may not be carminophilic, and it is often difficult to culture cryptococci from these lesions. Immunofluorescence staining is a valuable diagnostic tool in these cases.

Histoplasmosis capsulati

Histoplasmosis capsulati, a systemic mycosis, is a respiratory disease contracted by inhalation of airborne infectious spores of the dimorphic fungus *Histoplasma capsulatum* var. *capsulatum*.[96,97] Spores and hyphae of the fungus are found in soil, where avian and chiropteran habitats such as blackbird roosts, chicken coops, caves, and attics favor their growth and multiplication. The disease occurs worldwide, but it is not contagious. In the United States highly endemic areas include the broad region of the Ohio and Mississippi river valleys. Other countries with high endemicity include Guatemala, Mexico, Peru, and Venezuela. Disease caused by *H. capsulatum* var. *duboisii* is discussed separately (see "Histoplasmosis duboisii") because it is a distinct clinical and pathological entity. It is confined to the African continent where both varieties of *H. capsulatum* exist. The two varieties can be distinguished only by the difference in size of their tissue forms.

Epidemiologists estimate that approximately 90% of human infections by *H. capsulatum* var. *capsulatum* are asymptomatic. Confirmation of either current or past infection is based on a positive reaction to the skin test antigen histoplasmin. In many asymptomatic individuals, multiple lung calcifications develop in time. Symptomatic infections in the remaining 10% fall into three clinical categories: (1) acute pulmonary,[97] (2) disseminated,[96] and (3) chronic pulmonary (cavitary).[95] About half of all patients with histoplasmosis capsulati have no apparent immune defects.

In patients who have the acute pulmonary disease, flu-like symptoms develop after an incubation period of about 15 days. With supportive therapy these infections either resolve or progress to solitary fibrocaseous nodules (histoplasmomas), and treatment with amphotericin B is only occasionally required. Hematogenous dissemination occurs in a small percentage of patients who have acute pulmonary infections. The yeastlike fungus disseminates by way of the mononuclear phagocyte system and infects various organs, particularly the lungs, lymph nodes, spleen, liver, bone marrow, gastrointestinal tract, and adrenals. It also tends to invade mucosal ulcers. Hepatomegaly and splenomegaly are common in this most severe and life-threatening form of the disease. Early diagnosis and antifungal therapy are imperative. The chronic cavitary form of histoplasmosis capsulati is seen primarily in adults, and it may become clinically apparent only after a long dormancy. Roentgenograms usually reveal unilateral cavities in the upper lung lobes that resemble those seen in tuberculosis. Sclerosing mediastinitis may complicate chronic infection.[94]

In tissue the yeast-form cells are round to oval, 2 to 4 μm in diameter, and reproduce by single budding.[4,93] In active lesions fungal cells are readily detected by hematoxylin and eosin. Their basophilic cytoplasm is retracted from the rigid but thin and poorly stained cell wall, creating a clear space or "halo" that gives the false impression of an unstained capsule (Fig. 11-24, *A*). Cell walls stain deeply with the special fungal stains, and the halo is not evident (Fig. 11-24, *B*). Pseudohyphae are occasionally seen, and hyphae have been rarely observed near the surface of valvular vegetations in patients with endocarditis.

Generally, in the disseminated form of the disease, numerous yeast-form cells replicate within mononuclear phagocytes in the nonimmune or compromised host, whereas the fungus elicits an epithelioid and giant cell granulomatous reaction in the immune host. Necrotic lesions may calcify, and epithelioid cell granulomas resemble those seen in sarcoidosis and tuberculosis.[93] Because of their intracellular confinement, fungal cells occur in prominent clusters.

Asymptomatic disease may not be detected until old fibrocaseous nodules are found incidentally at autopsy[92]

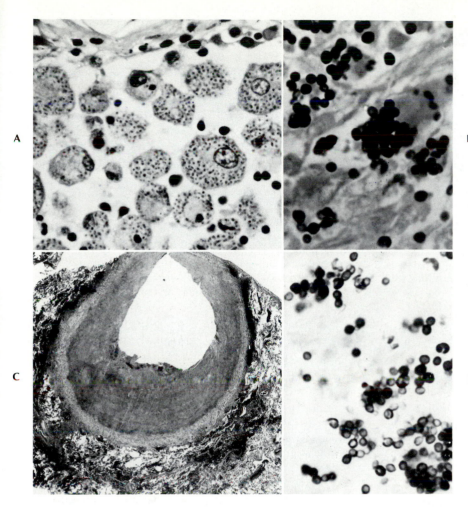

Fig. 11-24. Histoplasmosis capsulati. **A,** Acute pulmonary form. Alveolar macrophages are filled with small yeast forms, 2 to 4 μm in diameter, whose dark cytoplasm is retracted, creating a clear space or "halo." **B,** Disseminated form in adrenal gland. Note clustering of fungal cells. There is no "halo" effect when special fungal stains are used. **C,** Subpleural solitary nodule (histoplasmoma) in lung of adult man. **D,** Replicate section of nodule in **C** demonstrates distorted, poorly stained *Histoplasma* cells in central caseous material. (**A,** Hematoxylin and eosin; 480×; **B,** Gomori methenamine-silver; 600×; **C,** Hematoxylin and eosin, 10×; **D,** Gomori methenamine-silver; 600×.)

or are suspected of being neoplasms on the basis of chest roentgenograms and are resected. Microscopically these nodules (histoplasmomas) consist of a large central zone of caseous necrosis surrounded by a thick wall of dense collagenous connective tissue that may contain epithelioid and multinucleated giant cells (Fig. 11-24, *C*). In the caseous portion small numbers of distorted and unevenly stained yeast cells are usually demonstrated by Gomori methenamine-silver stain (Fig. 11-24, *D*). The Gridley, periodic acid–Schiff, and hematoxylin and eosin stains do not reliably stain the yeast cells in these lesions, and attempts to culture the fungus are usually unsuccessful. The organisms can be specifically identified by immunofluorescence staining.

Poorly encapsulated cryptococci and small tissue forms of *Blastomyces dermatitidis* can resemble yeast forms of *Histoplasma capsulatum* var. *capsulatum*. However, cryptococci are usually carminophilic, and *B. dermatitidis* cells are multinucleated, have a thick wall, and bud by a broad base. When these differentiating features are equivocal, immunofluorescence staining is invaluable. In hematoxylin and eosin–stained sections, intracellular forms of the *Leishmania* spp. mimic *Histoplasma*. The distinguishing bar-shaped kinetoplast of the *Leishmania* spp. can sometimes be seen under oil immersion but is best demonstrated by Giemsa and Wilder's reticulum stains. Cells of *Toxoplasma gondii*, which can also be confused with *Histoplasma*, are smaller, stain entirely by hematoxylin and eosin, and are usually not found within phagocytes. The *Leishmania* spp. and *T. gondii* are not reliably stained by the special stains for fungi.

Histoplasmosis duboisii (African histoplasmosis)

Histoplasmosis duboisii is a pulmonary disease with a marked tropism for bones and skin.[98-100] It is caused by the large-celled form or duboisii variety of *Histoplasma capsulatum*. When grown in vitro, mycelial and yeast forms of this fungus are indistinguishable from those of the classical, small-celled form or capsulatum variety of this species. The two can be distinguished from each other only by observing the size of the yeast-form cells that develop in tissue. Diseases caused by the two varieties of *Histoplasma capsulatum* are clinically and histologically distinct.

Other than one autochthonous case from Japan, natu-

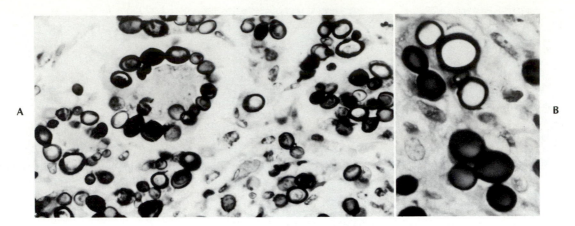

Fig. 11-25. Cutaneous histoplasmosis duboisii. **A,** Single and budding yeast forms within histiocytes and large multinucleated giant cells in dermis. **B,** Details of classical hourglass or double-cell yeast forms, 8 to 15 μm in diameter, with narrow-based buds and thick cell walls. (Gomori methenamine-silver/hematoxylin and eosin; **A,** 480×; **B,** 900×.)

ral infection from *H. capsulatum* var. *duboisii* has been reported only in humans and nonhuman primates from Africa. The disease is seen rarely in the United States in individuals who previously lived or traveled in Africa. Clinically, patients usually have one or more of the following: lymphadenopathy, mucocutaneous lesions that may be abscessed and ulcerated, and insidious osteolytic lesions, particularly of the ribs, long bones, and cranium. Disseminated disease may also involve the lungs, liver, spleen, and intestine. Amphotericin B and excision of isolated skin lesions are treatments of choice.

Lesions typically contain a dispersed granulomatous inflammatory reaction in which large numbers of yeast-form cells are seen within the cytoplasm of histiocytes and huge multinucleated giant cells (Fig. 11-25, *A*).[100] The round to oval fungal cells are uninucleate, 8 to 15 μm in diameter, and thick walled, and they bud by a relatively narrow base. Classical hourglass and double cell forms are created when budding daughter cells enlarge until they are equal in size to the parent cells, to which they remain connected by a narrow base (Fig. 11-25, *B*). Tissue forms of *H. capsulatum* var. *duboisii* and *Blastomyces dermatitidis* are of similar size and shape and thus may be mistaken for each other. However, the latter buds by a broader base and is multinucleated. Histoplasmosis capsulati also occurs in Africa, but its causative agent is much smaller (2 to 4 μm) in tissue than the large-celled duboisii variety.

Nocardiosis

Between 500 and 1000 new cases of nocardiosis, a subacute to chronic disease, are diagnosed annually in the United States. In about 85% of these cases infections are caused by *Nocardia asteroides*. The remaining 15% are caused by *N. brasiliensis* and *N. caviae*.[101] Infections by these filamentous bacteria of the order Actinomycetales

occur worldwide and are usually seen in individuals with underlying immunologic deficiency. Well-recognized conditions that predispose individuals to nocardial infection include lymphoma, Hodgkin's disease, chronic granulomatous disease of childhood, and pulmonary alveolar proteinosis. Unlike actinomycosis, nocardiosis is an exogenous disease, and infections are usually contracted by inhalation of nocardiae that live as saprophytes in nature. The disease is not contagious.

The clinical manifestations of nocardiosis are extremely variable.[101,102] All three *Nocardia* species may cause mycetomas, which are discussed elsewhere in this chapter. More commonly the disease is systemic with a pulmonary inception. Lung lesions may occur as large cavitating abscesses or as diffuse fibrinopurulent pneumonia similar to that caused by certain nonfilamentous bacteria. Fibrosis is usually minimal. There may be hematogenous dissemination to other body sites from a primary focus in the lungs. About 20% of patients with pulmonary nocardiosis have central nervous system involvement, usually in the form of cerebral abscesses.[101,104] Meningitis, a rare complication, results from rupture of an intracerebral abscess or direct extension of nocardial osteomyelitis. Nocardiosis may also occur as solitary or multiple subcutaneous lesions that result from either traumatic implantation or systemic infection. These localized lesions, with chains of nodules leading from a primary skin ulcer, can mimic those of cutaneous sporotrichosis.[101] This entity is known as the sporotrichoid form of nocardiosis. Sulfonamides are useful for treating all forms of the disease. Because of a strong tendency for relapse, prolonged therapy may be required.[101,103]

In systemic infections the *Nocardia* spp. almost never form granules. Rather, these organisms occur as individual, gram-positive, beaded filaments, 1 μm or less in width, that branch at approximately right angles (Fig.

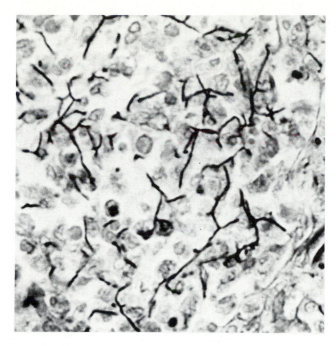

Fig. 11-26. Pulmonary nocardiosis. Delicate filaments that branch at approximately right angles are embedded in fibrinopurulent, alveolar exudate. (Gomori methenamine-silver/hematoxylin and eosin; 600×.)

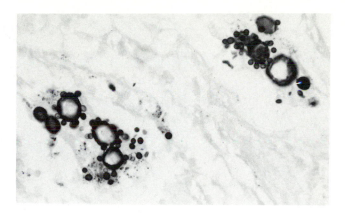

Fig. 11-27. Paracoccidioidomycosis. Several thick-walled cells have multiple surface buds. (Gomori methenamine-silver; 480×.)

11-26). The delicate filaments are not stained by hematoxylin and eosin, periodic acid–Schiff, or Gridley stains. However, they are readily demonstrated with the Gomori methenamine-silver and tissue Gram stains. All three *Nocardia* spp. are often partially acid fast in tissues when stained with modified acid-fast procedures using a weak decolorizing agent. They lose their acid fastness when cultured on artificial media. Usually the agents of actinomycosis are not acid fast.

Paracoccidioidomycosis (South American blastomycosis)

Paracoccidioidomycosis is endemic in South America, particularly Brazil, and in Central America and Mexico. Sporadic infections that occur in residents of the United States are acquired in these endemic areas.[106] The primary focus of infection is almost always pulmonary but may not be detectable clinically.[105] Dissemination from the lungs may lead to infection of the skin, mucous membranes of the oral cavity and upper respiratory tract, lymphoreticular system, liver, adrenal glands, and viscera.[105,107]

The etiologic agent, *Paracoccidioides brasiliensis*, is a dimorphic pathogen that occurs in tissue as yeast-form cells, 3 to 30 μm or more in diameter. These cells reproduce by budding. Histologic diagnosis depends on the identification of characteristic multiple-budding cells that resemble a ship's wheel (Fig. 11-27). Nonbudding and single-budding cells usually outnumber these diag-

nostic forms in lesions. Effete "mosaic" cells with fractured walls are characteristic but not diagnostic of the infection. Hyphae are rarely observed in tissue. The inflammatory reaction at sites of infection is both granulomatous and suppurative.[108] Verrucous cutaneous lesions display epidermal hyperplasia and intraepidermal microabscesses. Long-standing pulmonary infection results in progressive pulmonary fibrosis and cor pulmonale.

Torulopsosis

Torulopsosis is a rare opportunistic mycosis caused by the small (2 to 4 μm), budding, round to oval, yeastlike fungus *Torulopsis glabrata*.[109] This fungus, a dominant member of the body's natural flora, has been recently reclassified in the genus *Candida* as *C. glabrata*. It is the only species of *Candida* that occurs exclusively in a yeast form (see "Candidiasis"). Fungemia, the most common form of *C. glabrata* infection, has been associated with prolonged intravenous alimentation, severe abdominal trauma, and appendiceal abscesses.[110,111] Often the source of fungemia is unexplained. Tissue invasion by *C. glabrata* is uncommon. When it occurs, the endocardium, kidneys, lungs, and central nervous system are the sites most frequently involved with suppurative or, rarely, granulomatous inflammation. The tinctorial and morphologic features of *C. glabrata* are similar to those of *Histoplasma capsulatum* var. *capsulatum*, especially when cells of the former are clustered within histiocytes. Culture or immunofluorescence staining is needed for definitive identification.

Zygomycosis

Zygomycosis is a generic term that refers to infections caused by members of the class Zygomycetes (formerly Phycomycetes). Most of the human pathogens in this class belong to the orders Mucorales and Entomophtho-

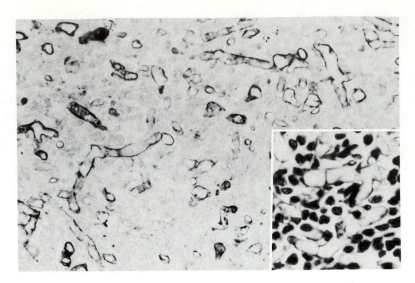

Fig. 11-28. Zygomycosis (mucormycosis). Broad, irregular hyphae of *Saksenaea vasiformis*. Note haphazard branching at right angles and absence of septa. Round and oval forms are hyphae sectioned transversely. *Inset,* Septa are occasionally present in some hyphae. (Gomori methenamine-silver; 300×; *inset,* periodic acid–Schiff; 480×.)

rales, and infections caused by these fungi are often referred to, respectively, as mucormycosis and entomophthoramycosis.

Mucormycosis

Mucormycosis is a sporadic opportunistic infection that occurs in patients with serious underlying diseases, such as diabetic acidosis and acute leukemia, and in patients treated with corticosteroids or cytotoxic drugs.[116] Well-authenticated agents of human mucormycosis include species within the genera *Rhizopus, Mucor, Absidia, Cunninghamella, Saksenaea,* and *Rhizomucor*.[4] These saprophytic fungi are widely distributed in nature, and infection is acquired by exposure to their sporangiospores. Mucormycosis is the third most common opportunistic mycosis among patients with malignant disease.[118]

Hyphae of the mucoraceous zygomycetes have a characteristic appearance in tissue (Fig. 11-28). They are broad (5 to 20 μm in width) and pleomorphic and have irregular, nonparallel contours. Branches arise haphazardly, often at right angles to the parent hyphae. The hyphae and their branches are randomly distributed in the lesions rather than aligned in similar directions as observed with the aspergilli. Septa may be found in some hyphae (Fig. 11-28, *inset*), although most of the hyphae are nonseptate (coenocytic). The hyphae often stain more deeply with hematoxylin than with the special fungal stains.

Infections caused by the mucoraceous zygomycetes

are characterized by tissue infarction and acute suppurative inflammation. Infarction is caused by thrombosis complicating hyphal invasion of arteries and veins. Vascular invasion by hyphae may also lead to hematogenous dissemination. Microscopically the lesions show coagulative necrosis and an infiltrate of neutrophils with abundant hyphae. Rarely, a granulomatous inflammatory reaction is observed in localized or partially treated chronic infections.

Several clinical forms of mucormycosis are recognized.[116,119] Rhinocerebral mucormycosis is a fulminant infection of the nasal cavity, paranasal sinuses, and soft tissues of the orbit (Fig. 11-29). The infection, often unilateral, may extend directly from these sites to involve the meninges and brain and may be complicated by thrombosis of the cavernous sinus and internal carotid artery. Patients with diabetic acidosis or leukemia are predisposed to rhinocerebral infection, usually caused by *Rhizopus oryzae*. Once established, this infection is difficult to treat and usually causes death within a few days.

Pulmonary mucormycosis occurs most commonly in patients with leukemia or lymphoma.[116,118] It is a progressive infection characterized by pulmonary vascular invasion, parenchymal infarction, and systemic dissemination. Gastrointestinal mucormycosis usually begins as a secondary infection of preexisting ulcers in malnourished patients,[116] but it may also be a manifestation of disseminated infection. The stomach is involved most commonly, followed by the colon and small intestine.

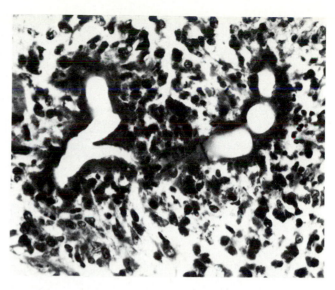

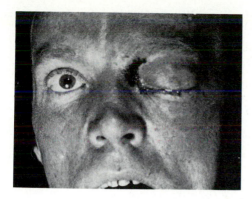

Fig. 11-29. Cellulitis of left orbit in a diabetic patient with rhino cerebral form of mucormycosis. (Courtesy Dr. Roger D. Baker, Silver Spring, Md.)

Infection results in ischemic necrosis of the ulcer base that may extend to involve adjacent segments of the stomach or intestine.

Cutaneous mucormycosis can be a manifestation of disseminated mucormycosis or may arise as a primary infection of burned patients[113] or patients whose surgical wounds are dressed with contaminated elastic bandages.[114,117] Bandage-associated infections have been caused by *Rhizopus rhizopodiformis*. The lesions are necrotic nodules of the skin and subcutaneous tissue that ulcerate and become covered with black exudate.[113] Disseminated mucormycosis can involve almost any organ. The lungs are involved in most cases and can serve as a source of hematogenous dissemination.

Successful treatment of mucormycosis depends on early recognition of the infection and control of the underlying disease. Devitalized tissue should be excised, and patients should be treated with antifungal chemotherapy.[116]

Entomophthoramycosis

Entomophthoramycosis is a sporadic infection that occurs most commonly in tropical areas of Africa, Asia, and South America.[112,120] Two clinical forms are recognized, neither of which occurs preferentially in patients with underlying disease or defective immunity.

Subcutaneous zygomycosis, caused by *Basidiobolus haptosporus*, is manifested as a firm, painless, disciform subcutaneous nodule of the trunk or extremities.[113] If untreated the nodule may enlarge and spread locally, but systemic dissemination is uncommon. The infection is probably initiated by penetrating trauma. Rhinofacial zygomycosis, caused by *Conidiobolus coronatus*, is a locally progressive infection of the nasal cavity, paranasal sinuses, and soft tissues of the face.[112] Involvement of the mediastinum has been reported.[115]

The microscopic findings are similar in both forms of

Fig. 11-30. Subcutaneous zygomycosis (entomophthoramycosis). Hyphal fragments of *Basidiobolus haptosporus*, surrounded by Splendore-Hoeppli material, are present within granulation tissue rich in eosinophils. (Hematoxylin and eosin; 480×.)

entomophthoramycosis.[115,120] A few broad, thin-walled, pauciseptate hyphal fragments are found in the lesions. Each hyphal fragment is enveloped by eosinophilic Splendore-Hoeppli material (Fig. 11-30). The inflammatory response immediately surrounding each hyphal fragment is either eosinophilic or granulomatous, and the adjacent stroma consists of granulation tissue with acute and chronic inflammatory cells, including many eosinophils. Unlike the agents of mucormycosis, those of entomophthoramycosis tend not to invade blood vessels, which accounts for the rarity of ischemic necrosis and systemic dissemination in this form of zygomycosis.

REFERENCES
General

1. Baker, R.D., editor: The pathologic anatomy of mycoses: human infection with fungi, actinomycetes and algae, New York, 1971, Springer-Verlag.
2. Baker, R.D., and Chick, E.W.: Proceedings of International Symposium on Opportunistic Fungus Infections, Lab. Invest. 11:1017, 1962.
3. Binford, C.H., and Connor, D.H., editors: Pathology of tropical and extraordinary diseases, Washington, D.C., 1976, Armed Forces Institute of Pathology.
4. Chandler, F.W., Kaplan, W., and Ajello, L.: Color atlas and text of the histopathology of mycotic diseases, Chicago, 1980, Year Book Medical Publishers, Inc.
5. Conant, N.F., et al.: Manual of clinical mycology, ed. 3, Philadelphia, 1971, W.B. Saunders Co.
6. Emmons, C.W., et al.: Medical mycology, ed. 3, Philadelphia, 1977, Lea & Febiger.
7. Grieco, M.H., editor: Infections in the abnormal host, New York, 1980, Yorke Medical Books.

8. Kaplan, W., and Kraft, D.E.: Demonstration of pathogenic fungi in formalin-fixed tissues by immunofluorescence, Am. J. Clin. Pathol. **52**:420, 1969.

9. Rippon, J.W.: Medical mycology: the pathogenic fungi and the pathogenic actinomycetes, Philadelphia, 1982, W.B. Saunders Co.

Superficial and cutaneous mycoses

10. Graham, J.H.: Superficial fungus infections. In Graham, J.H., Johnson, W.C., and Helwig, E.G., editors: Dermal pathology, Hagerstown, Md., 1972, Harper & Row, Publishers, Inc.

11. Graham, J.H., and Barroso-Tobila, C.: Dermal pathology of superficial fungus infections. In Baker, R.D., editor: Human infection with fungi, actinomycetes and algae, New York, 1971, Springer-Verlag.

12. Rebell, G., and Taplin, D.: Dermatophytes: their recognition and identification, Coral Gables, Fla., 1970, University of Miami Press.

Chromoblastomycosis

13. Batres, E., et al.: Transepithelial elimination of cutaneous chromomycosis, Arch. Dermatol. **114**:1231, 1978.

14. Carrion, A.L.: Chromoblastomycosis and related infections, Int. J. Dermatol. **14**:27, 1975.

15. Vollum, D.I.: Chromomycosis: a review, Br. J. Dermatol. **96**:454, 1977.

Lobomycosis

16. Caldwell, D.K., et al.: Lobomycosis as a disease of the Atlantic bottle-nosed dolphin, Am. J. Trop. Med. Hyg. **24**:105, 1975.

17. Wiersema, J.P.: Lobo's disease (keloidal blastomycosis). In Baker, R.D., editor: Human infection with fungi, actinomycetes and algae, New York, 1971, Springer-Verlag.

Mycetomas

18. Cameron, H.M., Gatei, D., and Bremmer, A.D.: The deep mycoses in Kenya: a histopathological study. I. Mycetoma, East Afr. Med. J. **50**:382, 1973.

19. Green, W.O., and Adams, T.E.: Mycetoma in the United States, Am. J. Clin. Pathol. **42**:75, 1964.

20. Mahgoub, E.S.: Medical management of mycetoma, Bull. WHO **54**:303, 1976.

21. Winslow, D.J., and Steen, F.G.: Considerations in the histologic diagnosis of mycetoma, Am. J. Clin. Pathol. **42**:164, 1964.

PrototLecosis

22. Chandler, F.W., Kaplan, W., and Callaway, C.S.: Differentiation between *Prototheca* and morphologically similar green algae in tissue, Arch. Pathol. Lab. Med. **102**:353, 1978.

23. Cox, G.E., Wilson, J.D., and Brown, P.: Protothecosis: a case of disseminated algal infection, Lancet **2**:379, 1974.

24. Davies, R.R., and Wilkinson, J.L.: Human protothecosis: supplementary studies, Ann. Trop. Med. Parasitol. **61**:112, 1967.

25. Jones, J.W., et al.: Green algal infection in a human, Am. J. Clin. Pathol. **80**:102, 1983.

26. Nosanchuk, J.S., and Greenberg, R.D.: Protothecosis of the olecranon bursa caused by achloric algae, Am. J. Clin. Pathol. **59**:567, 1973.

27. Sudman, M.S.: Protothecosis: a critical review, Am. J. Clin. Pathol. **61**:10, 1974.

28. Tindall, J.P., and Fetter, B.F.: Infections caused by achloric algae (protothecosis), Arch. Dermatol. **104**:490, 1971.

Rhinosporidiosis

29. Bader, G., and Grueber, H.L.E.: Histochemical studies of *Rhinosporidium seeberi*, Virchows Arch. (Pathol. Anat.) **350**:76, 1970.

30. Hyams, V.J.: Papillomas of the nasal cavity and paranasal sinuses, Ann. Otol. Rhinol. Laryngol. **80**:192, 1971.

31. Kannan-Kutty, M., and Teh, E.C.: *Rhinosporidium seeberi*: an electron microscopic study of its life cycle, Pathology **6**:63, 1974.

32. Karunaratne, W.A.E.: Rhinosporidiosis in man, London, 1964, Athlone Press.

Sporotrichosis

33. Berson, S.D., and Brandt, F.A.: Primary pulmonary sporotrichosis with unusual fungal morphology, Thorax **32**:505, 1977.

34. Bullpitt, P., and Weedon, D.: Sporotrichosis: a review of 39 cases, Pathology **10**:249, 1978.

35. Liber, A.F., and Choi, H.S.: Splendore-Hoeppli phenomenon about silk sutures in tissue, Arch. Pathol. **95**:217, 1973.

36. Lurie, H.I.: Histopathology of sporotrichosis, Arch. Pathol. **75**:92, 1963.

37. Lynch, P.J., Voorhees, J.J., and Harrell, E.R.: Systemic sporotrichosis, Ann. Intern. Med. **73**:23, 1970.

38. Marracco, G.R.: Granulomatous synovitis and osteitis caused by *Sporothrix schenckii*, Am. J. Clin. Pathol. **64**:345, 1975.

Phaeohyphomycosis

39. Ajello, L.: Phaeohyphomycosis: definition and etiology. In Mycoses, Scientific Publication No. 304:126, Washington, D.C., 1975, Pan American Health Organization.

40. Estes, S.A., Merz, W.G., and Maxwell, L.G.: Primary cutaneous phaeohyphomycosis caused by *Drechslera spicifera*, Arch. Dermatol. **113**:813, 1977.

41. Riley, O., Jr., and Mann, S.H.: Brain abscess caused by *Cladosporium trichoides*: review of three cases and report of fourth case, Am. J. Clin. Pathol. **33**:525, 1960.

42. Ziefer, A., and Connor, D.H.: Phaeomycotic cyst: a clinicopathologic study of twenty-five patients, Am. J. Trop. Med. Hyg. **29**:901, 1980.

Actinomycosis

43. Bhagavan, B.S., and Gupta, P.K.: Genital actinomycosis and intrauterine contraceptive devices, Hum. Pathol. **9**:567, 1978.

44. Brown, J.R.: Human actinomycosis: a study of 181 subjects, Hum. Pathol. **4**:319, 1973.

45. Causey, W.A.: Actinomycosis. In Handbook of clinical neurology, vol. 35, p. 383. Infections of the nervous system, part 3, Amsterdam, 1978, North Holland Publishing Co.

46. Hotchi, M., and Schwarz, J.: Characterization of actinomycotic granules by architecture and staining methods, Arch. Pathol. **93**:392, 1972.

47. Robboy, S.J., and Vickery, A.L.: Tinctorial and morphologic properties distinguishing actinomycosis and nocardiosis, N. Engl. J. Med. **282**:593, 1970.

Adiaspiromycosis

48. Schwarz, J.: Adiaspiromycosis, Pathol. Annu. **13**:41, 1978.

49. Watts, J.C., et al.: Human pulmonary adiaspiromycosis, Arch. Pathol. **99**:11, 1975.

Aspergillosis

50. Cho, S.Y., and Choi, H.Y.: Opportunistic fungal infection among cancer patients, Am. J. Clin. Pathol. **72**:617, 1979.

51. Kammer, R.B., and Utz, J.P.: *Aspergillus* species endocarditis, Am. J. Med. **56**:506, 1974.

52. Katzenstein, A.L., Liebow, A.A., and Friedman, P.J.: Bronchocentric granulomatosis, mucoid impaction, and hypersensitivity reactions to fungi, Am. Rev. Respir. Dis. **111**:497, 1975.

53. Nime, F.A., and Hutchins, G.M.: Oxalosis caused by aspergillus infection, Johns Hopkins Med. J. **133**:183, 1973.

54. Raper, K.B., and Fennell, D.I.: The genus *Aspergillus*, Baltimore, 1965, The Williams & Wilkins Co.

55. Schwarz, J.: Aspergillosis, Pathol. Annu. **8**:81, 1973.

56. Walker, D.H., Adamec, T., and Krigman, M.: Disseminated petriellidiosis (allescheriosis), Arch. Pathol. Lab. Med. **102**:158, 1978.

57. Warnock, M.L., Fennessy, J., and Rippon, J.: Chronic eosinophilic pneumonia, a manifestation of allergic aspergillosis, Am. J. Clin. Pathol. **62**:73, 1974.

58. Wheeler, M.S., et al.: *Fusarium* infection in burned patients, Am. J. Clin. Pathol. **75**:304, 1981.

59. Young, R.C., Jennings, A., and Bennett, J.E.: Species identification of invasive aspergillosis in man, Am. J. Clin. Pathol. 58:554, 1972.
60. Young, R.C., et al.: Aspergillosis: the spectrum of disease in 98 patients, Medicine 49:147, 1970.

Blastomycosis

61. Lockwood, W.R., et al.: The treatment of North American blastomycosis: ten years' experience, Am. Rev. Respir. Dis. 100:314, 1969.
62. Sarosi, G.A., and Davies, S.F.: Blastomycosis, Am. Rev. Respir. Dis. 120:911, 1979.
63. Schwarz, J., and Salfelder, K.: Blastomycosis: a review of 152 cases, Curr. Top. Pathol. 65:165, 1977.
64. Vanek, J., Schwarz, J., and Haken, S.: North American blastomycosis, Am. J. Clin. Pathol. 54:384, 1970.
65. Witorach, P., and Utz, J.P.: North American blastomycosis: a study of 40 patients, Medicine 47:169, 1968.

Botryomycosis

66. Winslow, D.J.: Botryomycosis, Am. J. Pathol. 35:153, 1959.
67. Winslow, D.J., and Chamblin, S.A.: Disseminated visceral botryomycosis: report of a fatal case probably caused by *Pseudomonas aeruginosa*, Am. J. Clin. Pathol. 33:43, 1960.

Candidiasis

68. Aronson, I.K., and Soltani, K.: Chronic mucocutaneous candidosis: a review, Mycopathologia 60:17, 1976.
69. Dubois, P.J., Myerowitz, R.L., and Allen, C.M.: Pathoradiologic correlation of pulmonary candidiasis in immunosuppressed patients, Cancer 40:1026, 1977.
70. Dwyer, J.M.: Chronic mucocutaneous candidiasis, Annu. Rev. Med. 32:491, 1981.
71. Eras, P., Goldstein, M.J., and Sherlock, P.: *Candida* infection of the gastrointestinal tract, Medicine 51:367, 1972.
72. Katzenstein, A.L.A., and Maksem, J.: Candidal infection of gastric ulcers, Am. J. Clin. Pathol. 71:137, 1979.
73. Myerowitz, R.L., Pazin, G.J., and Allen, C.M.: Disseminated candidiasis: changes in incidence, underlying diseases, and pathology, Am. J. Clin. Pathol. 68:29, 1977.
74. Parker, J.C.: The potentially lethal problem of cardiac candidosis, Am. J. Clin. Pathol. 73:356, 1980.
75. Parker, J.C., McCloskey, J.J., and Knauer, K.A.: Pathologic features of human candidiasis: a common deep mycosis of the brain, heart, and kidney in the altered host, Am. J. Clin. Pathol. 65:991, 1976.
76. Parker, J.C., McCloskey, J.J., and Lee, R.S.: The emergence of candidosis: the dominant postmortem cerebral mycosis, Am. J. Clin. Pathol. 70:31, 1978.
77. Parker, J.C., McCloskey, J.J., and Lee, R.S.: Human cerebral candidosis—a postmortem evaluation of 19 patients, Hum. Pathol. 2:23, 1981.
78. Robboy, S.J., and Kaiser, J.: Pathogenesis of fungal infection on heart valve prostheses, Hum. Pathol. 6:711, 1975.
79. Walsh, T.J., et al.: Fungal infections of the heart: analysis of 51 autopsy cases, Am. J. Cardiol. 45:357, 1980.

Coccidioidomycosis

80. Ajello, L., editor: Coccidioidomycosis, Tucson, 1967, University of Arizona Press.
81. Deppisch, L.M., and Donowho, E.M.: Pulmonary coccidioidomycosis, Am. J. Clin. Pathol. 58:489, 1972.
82. Donnelly, W.H., and Yunis, E.J.: The ultrastructure of *Coccidioides immitis*, Arch. Pathol. 98:227, 1974.
83. Drutz, D.J., and Catanzaro, A.: State of the art: coccidioidomycosis, part I, Am. Rev. Respir. Dis. 117:559, 1978.
84. Drutz, D.J., and Catanzaro, A.: State of the art: coccidioidomycosis, part II, Am. Rev. Respir. Dis. 117:727, 1978.
85. Kyriakos, M.: Myospherulosis of the paranasal sinuses, nose and middle ear, Am. J. Clin. Pathol. 67:118, 1977.
86. Rosai, J.: The nature of myospherulosis of the upper respiratory tract, Am. J. Clin. Pathol. 69:475, 1978.

Cryptococcosis

87. Baker, R.D.: The primary pulmonary lymph node complex of cryptococcosis, Am. J. Clin. Pathol. 65:83, 1976.
88. Farmer, S.G., and Komorowski, R.A.: Histologic response to capsule-deficient *Cryptococcus neoformans*, Arch. Pathol. 96:383, 1973.
89. Gutierrez, F., Fu, Y.S., and Lurie, H.I.: *Cryptococcus* histologically resembling histoplasmosis, Arch. Pathol. 99:347, 1975.
90. Littman, M.L., and Walter, J.E.: Cryptococcosis: current status, Am. J. Med. 45:922, 1968.
91. Noble, R.C., and Fajardo, L.F.: Primary cutaneous cryptococcosis: review and morphologic study, Am. J. Clin. Pathol. 57:13, 1972.

Histoplasmosis capsulati

92. Baker, R.D.: Histoplasmosis in routine autopsies, Am. J. Clin. Pathol. 41:457, 1964.
93. Binford, C.H.: Histoplasmosis: tissue reactions and morphologic variations of the fungus, Am. J. Clin. Pathol. 25:25, 1955.
94. Eggleston, J.C.: Sclerosing mediastinitis, Prog. Surg. Pathol. 2:1, 1980.
95. Goodwin, R.A., Jr., et al.: Chronic pulmonary histoplasmosis, Medicine 55:413, 1976.
96. Goodwin, R.A., Jr., et al.: Disseminated histoplasmosis: clinical and pathologic correlations, Medicine 59:1, 1980.
97. Vanek, J., and Schwarz, J.: The gamut of histoplasmosis, Am. J. Med. 50:89, 1971.

Histoplasmosis duboisii

98. Clark, B.M., and Greenwood, B.B.: Pulmonary lesions in African histoplasmosis, J. Trop. Med. Hyg. 71:4, 1968.
99. Lanceley, J.L., Lunn, N.F., and Wilson, A.M.A.: Histoplasmosis in an African child, J. Pediatr. 59:756, 1961.
100. Williams, A.O., Lawson, E.A., and Lucas, A.O.: African histoplasmosis due to *Histoplasma duboisii*, Arch. Pathol. 92:306, 1971.

Nocardiosis

101. Causey, W.A., and Lee, R.: Nocardiosis. In Vinken, P.J., and Bruyn, G.W., editors: Handbook of clinical neurology, Amsterdam, 1978, North Holland Publishing Co.
102. Frazier, A.R., Rosenow, E.C., III, and Roberts, G.D.: Nocardiosis: a review of 25 cases occurring during 24 months, Mayo Clin. Proc. 50:657, 1975.
103. Palmer, D.L., Harvey, R.L., and Wheeler, J.K.: Diagnostic and therapeutic considerations in *Nocardia asteroides* infection, Medicine 53:391, 1974.
104. Pizzolato, P., et al.: Nocardiosis of the brain: report of three cases, Am. J. Clin. Pathol. 36:151, 1961.

Paracoccidioidomycosis

105. Giraldo, R., et al.: Pathogenesis of paracoccidioidomycosis: a model based on the study of 46 patients, Mycopathologia 58:63, 1976.
106. Kroll, J.J., and Walzer, R.A.: Paracoccidioidomycosis in the United States, Arch. Dermatol. 106:543, 1972.
107. Restrepo, A., et al.: The gamut of paracoccidioidomycosis, Am. J. Med. 61:33, 1976.
108. Salfelder, K., Doehnert, G., and Doehnert, H.R.: Paracoccidioidomycosis: anatomic study with complete autopsies, Virchows Arch. (Pathol. Anat.) 348:51, 1969.

Torulopsosis

109. Grimley, P.M., Wright, L.D., and Jennings, A.E.: *Torulopsis glabrata* infection in man, Am. J. Clin. Pathol. 43:216, 1965.
110. Heffner, D.K., and Franklin, W.A.: Endocarditis caused by *Torulopsis glabrata*, Am. J. Clin. Pathol. 70:420, 1978.
111. Rodriguez, R., et al.: *Torulopsis glabrata* fungemia during prolonged intravenous alimentation, N. Engl. J. Med. 284:540, 1971.

Zygomycosis

112. Baker, R.D.: The phycomycoses, Ann. N.Y. Acad. Sci. **174**:592, 1970.
113. Baker, R.D., Seabury, J.H., and Schneidau, J.D.: Subcutaneous and cutaneous mucormycosis and subcutaneous phycomycosis, Lab. Invest. **11**:1091, 1962.
114. Gartenberg, G., et al.: Hospital acquired mucormycosis (*Rhizopus rhizopodiformis*) of skin and subcutaneous tissue: epidemiology, mycology, and treatment, N. Engl. J. Med. **299**:1115, 1978.
115. Gilbert, E.F., Khoury, G.H., and Pore, R.S.: Histopathological identification of *Entomophthora phycomycosis*, Arch. Pathol. **90**:583, 1970.

116. Lehrer, R.I., et al.: Mucormycosis, Ann. Intern. Med. **93**:93, 1980.
117. Marchevsky, A.M., et al.: The changing spectrum of disease, etiology, and diagnosis of mucormycosis, Hum. Pathol. **11**:457, 1980.
118. Rosen, P.P.: Opportunistic fungal infections in patients with neoplastic diseases, Pathol. Annu. **11**:255, 1976.
119. Straatsma, B.R., Zimmerman, L.E., and Gass, J.D.M.: Phycomycosis: a clinicopathologic study of 51 cases, Lab. Invest. **11**:963, 1962.
120. Williams, A.O.: Pathology of phycomycosis due to *Entomopthora* and *Basidiobolus* species, Arch. Pathol. **87**:13, 1969.

CHAPTER 12

Protozoal and Helminthic Diseases

MANUEL A. MARCIAL
RAÚL A. MARCIAL-ROJAS

PROTOZOAL DISEASES
Diseases caused by amebas
Amebiasis

Amebiasis is caused by *Entamoeba histolytica*. The life cycle of this protozoan is rather complex and involves several changes in structure. From the medical standpoint the most important of these are the cystic and the trophozoite or motile forms. The infection is acquired by the ingestion of food or water containing the cysts of *E. histolytica*. Homosexual practices[18] and colonic irrigation with contaminated water[19] have been identified as other modes of infection of amebiasis.

The cysts are spherical and have a refractile wall that protects them against the hazards of the environment. In humans the cyst wall is resistant to destruction by the acid content of the stomach; however, it is destroyed by the alkaline intestinal medium. When the alkaline content of the small intestine digests the wall of a cyst, a quadrinucleated parasite is liberated, which, after cytoplasmic division, gives rise to four amebulas. These develop into adult trophozoites. The trophozoites may be confined to the lumen of the intestine without giving rise to clinical disease, or they may penetrate the mucosa. The mucosa is damaged by membrane-bound cytolytic enzymes, which the ameba releases.[6,9] This cytolytic effect led to the name *E. histolytica*. A cytotoxin-enterotoxin has been isolated from cultures of *E. histolytica* and is thought to have a pathogenic role in the causation of diarrhea and mucosal damage.[12]

It is estimated that the prevalence of amebiasis in the United States is 2% to 5%,[9,10] but in the majority of cases the condition is asymptomatic. Persons with asymptomatic infection are carriers of the disease.

Infection with *E. histolytica* implies colonization. Colonization in the host occurs as a result of frequently repeated binary division. No sexual reproduction has been demonstrated for any species of ameba. The rapidity with which division occurs and the depth of penetration in the intestinal wall depend on the pathogenic capacity of the particular strain of *E. histolytica* at the time of exposure, whether the mucosal surface is intact, and host factors not yet identified. Only the trophozoites of *E. histolytica* affect the tissues. The trophozoites are passed in diarrheal stools, whereas the cysts are usually passed in well-formed stools. Viable cysts of *E. histolytica* in the external environment are soon killed by drying, bacterial putrefaction of the medium, hypertonicity, direct sunlight, and heat. The inflammatory reaction around these penetrations is minimal[16] and is mostly chemical in nature (Fig. 12-1). Occasionally, when there is secondary infection, there is a severe inflammatory response. The muscle coats of the intestine form a barrier to the penetrating trophozoites, which then extend along the surface of the muscle coat, producing a rather large, undermined, flask-shaped ulcer with a narrow neck. This ulcerative process may be very severe and diffuse (Fig. 12-2.) It is usually more prominent in the cecum and ascending colon, followed by the sigmoid and rectum in order of frequency. Only occasionally will one of these ulcers penetrate through the muscularis and produce perforation.

In the early stages the colonic ulcers have a narrow neck and thus appear as small nodules with a minute surface opening averaging 5 mm in diameter (Fig. 12-3). As the ulcers enlarge, they always retain their undermined base, but the ulcerated area of the mucosa becomes larger and covered by grayish white exudate. Only rarely do amebic ulcerations coalesce. There is always undenuded mucosa between the ulcers. Symptoms include abdominal pain and diarrhea, which may contain blood and mucus.[1]

In 40% of the cases of amebic colitis the trophozoites enter the circulation and are filtered in the liver, where they produce solitary or multiple abscesses (Fig. 12-4). The right lobe is involved in 50% to 68% of such cases, and the abscesses are multiple in 40% of cases. They are

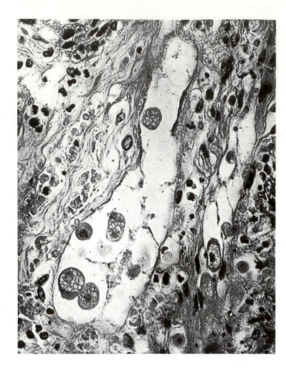

Fig. 12-1. Amebic colitis. Amebas are within lymphatic vessel and in tissues of submucosa; there is scant infiltration with neutrophils and lymphocytes. (360×.)

usually between 8 and 12 cm in diameter and are frequently located close to the dome of the right lobe of the liver or near its inferior surface, in proximity to the hepatic flexure of the colon. The outline of the abscesses is irregular. Abscesses compress the liver parenchyma around them, and a pseudocapsule of pale fibrous tissue is formed. The contents of the abscesses have been likened to anchovy sauce. The amebas are rarely demonstrable in the necrotic material. When demonstrable, they are found in the area near the capsule. These hepatic abscesses have been found to rupture[2,13] into the right pleural cavity in 37% of cases, into the right lung in 25%, and into the pericardial sac in 19%.[5] The abscesses usually appear 1 to 2 months after the onset of acute amebic colitis but may appear earlier or much later.

Hematogenous pulmonary abscesses may develop as a result of amebic emboli transported in the bloodstream. These emboli originate in the branches of the hepatic vein or in the colonic blood vessels. Direct extension of hepatic abscesses through the diaphragm into the right lobe of the lung is the most frequent mechanism in the production of pulmonary abscesses. Amebic abscesses of the brain are usually solitary and located in either cerebral hemisphere; the cerebellum is rarely involved. The amebas also reach the meninges and the cerebral substance, where they produce encephalomalacia. In the central nervous system they elicit very little inflammato-

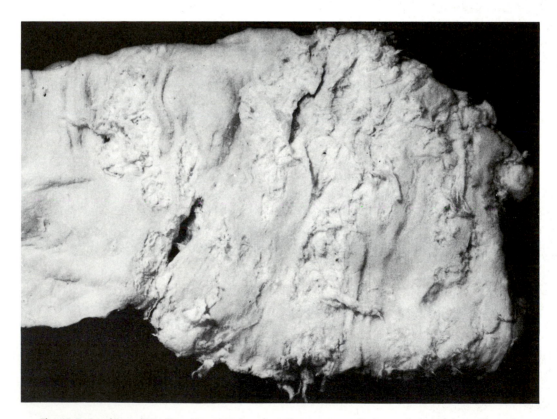

Fig. 12-2. Amebic colitis. Despite extensive ulcerations, mucosa in between remains unaffected. (Courtesy Dr. Gustavo A. Ramirez de Arellano, San Juan, Puerto Rico.)

ry response. Cerebral abscesses may reach a diameter of 10 cm. Patients with cerebral abscesses usually die 1 or 2 weeks after the clinical onset of the complication, and at autopsy concomitant amebic abscesses of the liver or lung are encountered.

E. histolytica may produce ulcers of the skin that discharge an anchovy sauce–like material. Cutaneous ulcers are usually secondarily infected and for this reason reveal severe polymorphonuclear infiltration. Amebas are present in the tissue at the base of the ulcer and in the exudate. The amebic skin ulcers develop more commonly in the subcutaneous tissue adjacent to a surgical incision for the drainage of an amebic abscess or in an appen-

dectomy scar in the case of amebiasis of the cecum and appendix. In children, especially girls, they may develop in the perianal or perivulvar region from self-contamination (Fig. 12-5.).

In rare instances a proliferative type of granulation tissue resulting from the amebic infection may produce an ulcerated area in the colon, with pronounced thickening of the wall. Such an area may be confused with carcinoma of the colon on roentgenographic study. The most commonly involved areas are the cecum, hepatic and splenic flexures, and sigmoid colon. The granulation tissue forming an amebic granuloma (ameboma) undergoes fibrosis, and the mass thus becomes firm.

It is important to remember that the presence of *E. histolytica* in the stools is not necessarily accompanied by clinical amebiasis.

Distinction of *E. histolytica* from *Entamoeba coli* and other amebas that are commensal inhabitants of the colon is important. The trophozoites of *E. histolytica* frequently phagocytose red blood cells and contain one to four nuclei in the encysted form, whereas the trophozoites of *E. coli* do not phagocytose erythrocytes and contain up to eight nuclei in the encysted form. *E. coli* does not penetrate the intestinal wall.

Sigmoidoscopic examination is useful to evaluate the mucosa[14] and to obtain fresh specimens in which hematophagous trophozoites can be identified.[15] It is also helpful in the differential diagnosis of other conditions, such as inflammatory bowel disease.

Because stool examination is difficult and can lead to both underdiagnosis and overdiagnosis, serodiagnosis has become very useful and important.[7,8,10]

Serologic diagnosis depends on the detection of antibodies that arise only as a result of invasive amebiasis. Methods available include indirect immunofluores-

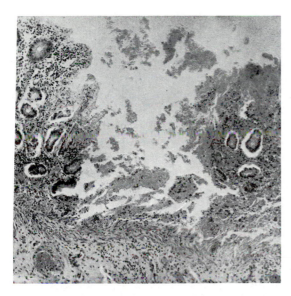

Fig. 12-3. Amebic colitis. This is very early ulcer with initial undermining shown at right. (800×.)

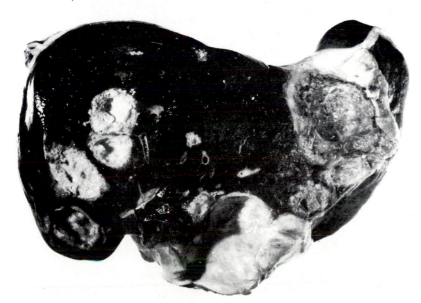

Fig. 12-4. Multiple amebic abscesses of liver. (AFIP 1058-3.)

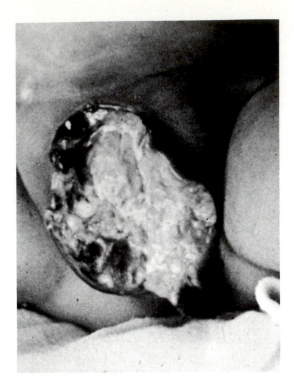

Fig. 12-5. Amebiasis of skin of vulva in child. (Courtesy Dr. Francisco Biaggi, Mexico City.)

cence,[21] indirect hemagglutination, enzyme-linked immunosorbent assay,[4,22] counterelectrophoresis,[3,11] and the gel diffusion precipitin test. The indirect hemagglutination (IHA) test is the most widely used, and it is the standard method performed at the Centers for Disease Control (CDC). Results are positive in 85% of patients with amebic colitis and in 95% of patients with amebic liver abscess.[23] Test results remain positive for a long period of time. The gel diffusion precipitin (GDP) test has an accuracy comparable to that of the IHA method,[15] and since its positivity correlates better with active disease, the IHA test should be used for epidemiologic studies and the GDP method as a test for symptomatic infection.[20] A recently described highly specific and sensitive solid-phase radioimmunoassay for *E. histolytica* antigens in human serum promises to be of great value in the diagnosis and monitoring of patients with colonic or hepatic amebiasis.[17]

Primary amebic meningoencephalitis

Amebic meningoencephalitis, caused by free-living amebas, has been recognized as a clinicopathologic entity only since the report of Fowler and Carter[27] in 1965. Butt[24] proposed the name "primary amebic meningoencephalitis," which has been adopted by most subsequent investigators. The disease has been recognized in many parts of the world.

The disease is caused by free-living amebas of the genera *Naegleria* and *Hartmannella-Acanthamoeba*. The clinicopathologic findings differ depending on the etiologic agent.[33]

The ameboflagellate *Naegleria fowleri* is the organism most commonly cultured from cerebrospinal fluid of patients with amebic meningoencephalitis. The route of entry is through the nasal mucosa via the cribriform plate, from which organisms can be cultured. Those affected are usually young, healthy individuals with a history of practicing aquatic sports in fresh water 3 to 7 days before the onset of symptoms. The possibility of acquiring the infectious organisms by washing the face with contaminated water[29] or inhaling contaminated dust[28] has been suggested. This disease resembles a fulminant bacterial meningitis with symptoms of headache, stiffness of the neck, fever, nausea, and vomiting.

The pathologic changes include a purulent exudate involving the base of the brain, the cerebellum, the frontal lobes, and the olfactory bulbs. Microscopically numerous trophozoites are seen in the fibrinopurulent exudate around the perivascular (Virchow-Robin) spaces. There is hemorrhagic necrosis, most prominent in the olfactory bulbs and in the cortical gray matter and occasionally also involving the spinal cord.[32] Histologic diagnosis of *Naegleria* can be confirmed by culture[35] and by either indirect immunofluorescence or immunoperoxidase studies of brain sections.

Amebic meningoencephalitis caused by the members of the genera *Hartmannella* and *Acanthamoeba*[34] is usually a disease of chronically ill or immunosuppressed patients.[31] *Hartmannella* and *Acanthamoeba* are grouped together because there is ongoing controversy concerning their classification.[26,30] The organisms have not been cultured,[25] but they have been identified both histologically and by immunologic techniques.[36]

The incubation period is longer and the route of entry unknown for *Hartmannella-Acanthamoeba* infections. There is no recent history of swimming in fresh water, and the clinical course is prolonged. The neuropathologic lesions can sometimes resemble those seen with *Naegleria* infections but more commonly are granulomatous with a slight chronic inflammatory reaction.

Balantidiasis

Balantidium coli, a parasite of cosmopolitan distribution, is found mostly in pigs but also may be found in monkeys and rats. The organism has two stages, trophozoite and cyst. The trophozoite is the largest of the protozoa parasitizing humans, with reported lengths up to 200 μm.[40] Their size, ciliary covering, and characteristic macronuclei and micronuclei (Fig. 12-6) make their recognition an easy task. The spherical cyst, which is about 50 μm in diameter, is the resting and transfer stage. Humans are infected by ingestion of the cyst forms in contaminated food or water. The human infection

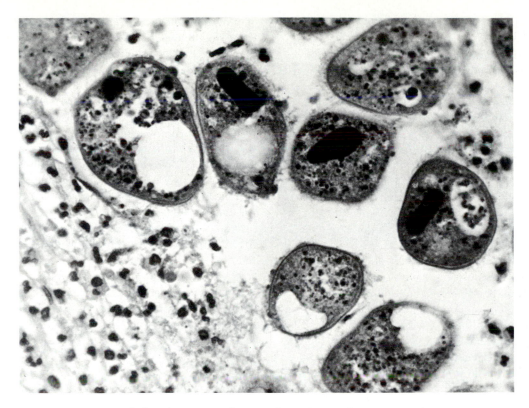

Fig. 12-6. Numerous balantidia in appendix. Note large characteristic macronuclei in some. (Hematoxylin and eosin; 430×.)

prevails in hot humid climates in persons who are on a high caloric diet and have multiple intestinal parasitoses.

The symptoms in balantidiasis vary from fulminating, sometimes fatal, dysentery to an essentially asymptomatic carrier state. The most severe cases in our experience were seen in hospitalized mental patients. These patients may also have fever, abdominal pain, nausea, and vomiting. Because of the presence of blood and mucus in the stools, balantidial infections must be differentiated from ulcerative colitis and amebic dysentery.[41] Intestinal ulcers may develop. Hemorrhage, perforation, and peritonitis[39] may complicate the picture.

B. coli usually inhabits the cecal level of the large intestine but can also occur at lower levels. The ulcerative lesions are encountered predominantly in the cecum, ascending colon, sigmoid colon, and rectum.[37,38] The ulcers resemble amebic ulcers morphologically, but because *B. coli* is a much larger, sturdier organism than *E. histolytica*, it produces a bigger opening in the intestinal mucosa as it enters the wall. The invasion seems to be facilitated by the production of proteolytic enzymes such as hyaluronidase. The parasites are readily identified in the mucosa and submucosa of the affected areas (Fig. 12-7). A zone of coagulation necrosis is evident at the base and margins of the ulcers. The adjacent submucosa is edematous and infiltrated with chronic inflamma-

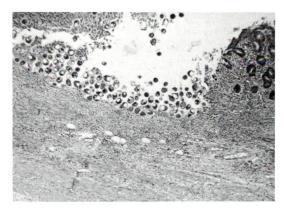

Fig. 12-7. Balantidiasis of appendix. Ulcer shows undermining borders. Wall of appendix discloses acute suppurative process. (Hematoxylin and eosin; 35×.)

tory cells. Neutrophilic infiltration is usually scanty or absent. Despite the fact that *B. coli* enters the venules, the occurrence of hepatic abscess has not been reported. In very unusual cases the organism has caused extraintestinal infections in the urinary tract and vagina.[42]

Diseases caused by flagellate protozoa

Some flagellates live in the human digestive tract,[49] others are found in the genital tract, and still others have become parasites in the blood and tissues.

Diseases caused by flagellates of the digestive tract and genital organs

Giardiasis. Giardiasis is caused by the ingestion of viable cysts of *Giardia lamblia* present in contaminated food or water.[45,57] Reports have identified oral-rectal sexual practice in homosexuals as a mode of transmission for both giardiasis[56] and amebiasis.[18]

G. lamblia has both trophozoite and cystic stages. Trophozoites inhabit the duodenum and jejunum, from which myriad organisms may be sampled either by duodenal aspiration or by small bowel biopsy. The stage commonly recovered in the feces is the cyst; trophozoites are seen only in frankly diarrheic stool. Since the passage of cysts in the feces is intermittent, the best diagnostic method is microscopic examination of small bowel fluid or mucosa. An immunofluorescence test[61] and an enzyme-linked immunosorbent assay[58] have been developed to detect antibodies to *G. lamblia*.

The changes in the mucosa of the small intestine can range from normal to total villous atrophy[47,50] with an increased mononuclear cellular infiltrate of the lamina propria. In our experience mucosal alterations are minimal; at the most a mild enteritis occurs with focal mild villus shortening, crypt hyperplasia, and focal epithelial damage. The organisms, although usually seen only in the lumen, have been noted to invade as deep as the lamina propria.[55] However, this finding has been questioned on the basis of alleged lack of convincing proof and the absence of tissue reaction. The question of invasion by the parasite remains moot.[62] Although some investigators believe that invasion is associated with a great number of parasites,[55] others do not find a good correlation between parasite load and either severity of symptoms or degree of mucosal damage.[64]

The most commonly reported symptoms are epigastric or right upper quadrant pain and persistent steatorrhea.[43] However, the infection is usually asymptomatic. Manifestation of symptoms or increase in their severity has been correlated with host factors such as achlorhydria and low secretory IgA levels.[63] The pathogenic mechanism by which *Giardia* causes malabsorption has not been elucidated. Theories include mechanical barrier to absorption, toxin production, competition for nutrients, damage to the microvilli, and bacterial overgrowth and bile salt deconjugation.*

Trichomoniasis. Of the several species of *Trichomonas* inhabiting humans, only *T. vaginalis* may become pathogenic to this host. This flagellate is found only in the trophozoite stage, and it multiplies by longitudinal binary fission. *T. vaginalis* is a common inhabitant of the vagina in females and the genital tract in males.[46] Transmission of the infection is accomplished principally through sexual intercourse.

In men the infection is usually asymptomatic but may occasionally produce a urethritis. In women *T. vaginalis* is an important contributor to a distinct type of vaginitis characterized by leukorrhea, pruritus and burning of the vagina and vulva, and chafing of the vulva. The disease is much more severe during certain hormonal states, such as pregnancy, the late luteal phase, and menstruation.[52] A definite diagnosis can be made by the identification of the trophozoite in a cervicovaginal smear. The organism can also be recovered from the urethra.[53]

Chronic infection with *Trichomonas*, particularly when the parasite settles in the endocervical canal, may produce certain atypical cellular changes that can be disturbing to the cytologist because they can be distinguished from true malignant change only with difficulty.

Cytohormonal evaluation of endocrine status is useless and misleading in the presence of *Trichomonas* because there is an alteration in the staining quality and karyopyknotic index, giving a falsely high estrogenic value.

Diseases caused by flagellates of blood and tissues

African trypanosomiasis. African trypanosomiasis, or sleeping sickness, is a disease caused by *Trypanosoma gambiense* or *T. rhodesiense*. It is transmitted by the bite of various species of *Glossina*, the tsetse fly. The trypanosomes give rise to two distinct clinical entities, Gambian trypanosomiasis and Rhodesian trypanosomiasis. African trypanosomiasis is limited to a wide belt of territory in the African continent between the latitudes of 10° north and 25° south. Cases seen in the United States have occurred in persons returning from trips to endemic areas.[75] The Gambian variety is much more widely distributed than the Rhodesian, which is limited to areas in East Africa. Neither type is present at elevations over 7000 feet above sea level. Humans are the main reservoir of both forms.

A firm, tender, reddened nodule may develop in a matter of a few days at the site of the bite. Trypanosomes may be identified in Giemsa-stained smears of fluid aspirated from the nodule. The ulcerated nodule, or "trypanosomal chancre," is accompanied by a regional lymphadenitis that lasts 1 or 2 weeks. The rapidity of the development of the chancre is related to the number of trypanosomes transmitted. The chancre precedes parasitemia. The hemoflagellates apparently reach the bloodstream via lymphatics.[67] This is followed within 1 to 5 weeks by the onset of fever, sweating, general malaise, and a generalized lymphadenitis often involving primarily the posterior cervical glands. Frequently there are transient skin eruptions characterized by erythema or edema. These symptoms and signs may progress to the phase of central nervous system involvement, or they may abate and then recur.

Numerous trypanosomes are found in the blood soon

---

*References 44, 48, 51, 54, 59, 60.

after the infection, especially after symptoms have developed. Other hematologic findings may include anemia, granulocytopenia, and thrombocytopenia.[72,75] There are an increase in sedimentation rate and a hypergammaglobulinemia especially of the IgM class. Patients have high levels of circulating immune complexes,[76] which are thought to lead to immune complex–mediated vasculitis.[68]

Lymph node enlargement, particularly of the posterior cervical lymph nodes (Winterbottom's sign), is a common clinical feature. The lymph nodes contain numerous parasites, and there is a generalized hyperplasia of lymphoid and reticular elements. Fibrosis of the lymph nodes develops later, with reduction in their size.

Trypanosomes evade the immunologic response of the host by the phenomenon of antigenic variation. The protozoan accomplishes this by presenting to the immune system progressively different surface glycoprotein constituents.[65,66,77] By the time the host mounts an immune response, the trypanosome has new surface antigens to which the formed antibodies are not specific. Trypanosomes also are known to cause immunosuppression by limiting specific antibody response, especially of the IgG type.[74] The host is left with nonspecific IgM production to combat the infection. This partially explains the rise in IgM levels in this chronic infection.

Although there is considerable overlap between the clinical manifestations of *T. gambiense* and *T. rhodesiense* infections, the latter usually follows a much more acute course. Untreated persons with *T. rhodesiense* infection frequently die within 6 to 9 months after onset of the disease. The systemic stage is often characterized by serous effusions and evidence of pancarditis. The parasites in the Rhodesian variety, after entering the lymph nodes, produce toxic substances that cause hyperplasia of the endothelial lining of the blood sinuses and perivascular infiltration of leukocytes. Only rarely does the victim survive long enough for the trypanosomes to invade the central nervous system and produce lesions characteristic of the third stage of *T. gambiense* infection. The neurologic symptoms and signs, when present, are similar to those of gambian trypanosomiasis. The latter is characteristically a chronic disease.

In the third stage the patient becomes indifferent, apathetic, and drowsy. Focal neurologic signs are uncommon, although athetosis, chorea, and sphincter disturbances may become apparent. The syndrome resulting from invasion of the central nervous system is commonly referred to as "sleeping sickness," but this designation suggests only one of the more advanced neurologic symptoms.

In the majority of cases there are no major macroscopic alterations in the brain substance other than edema and occasionally petechiae. Microscopically the picture is that of a diffuse meningoencephalitis. There is mononuclear infiltration of the superficial leptomeninges, sulci, and Virchow-Robin spaces. The cellular infiltrate, composed of lymphocytes and plasma cells in various proportions, may also infiltrate the white matter and to a lesser extent the gray matter.

The morular cell described by Mott[71] is a plasma cell whose cytoplasm contains numerous Russell bodies, which coalesce and partially or totally hide the nucleus of the cell. Although these cells are not pathognomonic of trypanosomiasis, their presence in large numbers is fairly characteristic of the disease.[69]

The simplest diagnostic test is the demonstration of the trypanosomes in the circulating blood during febrile episodes. Lymph node imprints may be useful for the identification of the parasite. Examination of the cerebrospinal fluid reveals trypanosomes as the disease progresses and may serve as an index of the course of the disease.

The great elevation of IgM in both the serum and cerebrospinal fluid can be used as a screening diagnostic test. Inoculation of blood into mice and blood culture are also reliable diagnostic methods. Serodiagnosis is available by indirect immunofluorescence, complement fixation, and enzyme-linked immunosorbent assay (ELISA).[70,73]

American trypanosomiasis (Chagas' disease). Existing as an acute or chronic disease, American trypanosomiasis, or Chagas' disease, is caused by *Trypanosoma cruzi*, a pleomorphic trypanosome. It occurs in the blood as a trypomastigote and in reticuloendothelial and other tissue cells typically as a leishmanial form, the amastigote. The amastigote form lacks flagella but retains the kinetoplast, which permits its differentiation from other intracellular organisms such as *Toxoplasma* and *Histoplasma*.

The disease occurs in North and South America, mostly in the area from Mexico to Argentina. It has never been reported outside the Western Hemisphere, although the vectors and the animal reservoirs are common to many parts of the world. The vectors are large biting insects of the genus *Triatoma*. These insects are found in areas where there are unhygienic conditions associated with poverty. They bite only at night. During the day they hide in cracks in the walls of primitive country dwellings.

The organism is sucked up by the triatomid bug as a free flagellate or as an intracellular leishmanial form within a macrophage. In the midgut of the insect the organism becomes flagellated, and binary multiplication occurs. It migrates to the hindgut, where it is transformed into the metacyclic trypanosome form infective for the vertebrate host. Since the *Triatoma* defecates at the time of biting, the infection is usually acquired by rubbing the feces containing the metacyclic trypanosome stage of the parasite into the tiny skin puncture or into other abrasions of the skin in the area. Infections through the intact mucous membranes occur most frequently in the lips or in the conjunctivae, when the eyes are rubbed with fingers soiled with the insect's feces.

T. cruzi enters macrophages by parasite-specified phagocytosis.[83,95] The protozoan does not remain within the phagocytic vacuole but escapes into the cytoplasm where it multiplies.[84] By leaving the parasitophorous vacuole, the organism escapes the action of microbicidal lysosomal enzymes. The circulating forms are susceptible to the trypanosomal activity of the lysosomal enzymes and major basic protein of eosinophils.[85]

Specific diagnosis of American trypanosomiasis may be accomplished by the finding of the typical trypanosome stage of *T. cruzi* in the blood during febrile episodes. Aspiration of spleen, liver, lymph nodes, or bone marrow will frequently reveal the leishmanial form of the organism in fixed macrophages. In reticuloendothelial cells *T. cruzi* cannot be easily distinguished from species of *Leishmania*, but only *T. cruzi* invades myocardial and neuroglial cells as a leishmanial type of organism. Xenodiagnosis can be performed, but it takes approximately 2 weeks to obtain the results. Serologic methods include complement fixation, indirect immunofluorescence, hemagglutination, enzyme-linked immunosorbent assay, and thin-layer immunoassay.[81,92,94]

Acute Chagas' disease. The acute form is the more common of the two types of Chagas' disease. It occurs predominantly in small children and is characterized by fever, slight generalized lymph node enlargement, moderate hepatosplenomegaly, facial edema, tachycardia, and the presence of *T. cruzi* in peripheral blood. In 50% of cases the primary site is the outer canthus of one eye, with unilateral palpebral edema and satellite preauricular lymph node enlargement (Romaña's sign) (Fig. 12-8, *A*). In 25% of cases the portal of entry is represented by a nodular or ulcerative skin lesion (chagoma), accompanied by enlargement of regional lymph nodes.[79]

Histologically the primary lesion is characterized by numerous histiocytes, chronic inflammatory cells, and areas of fat necrosis throughout which numerous leishmanial forms are encountered (Fig. 12-8, *B*). Multiplication of the organisms that have been engulfed by nearby macrophages is soon followed by the invasion of other structures such as smooth and striated muscle (including cardiac muscle), glial and nervous cells, and fat cells. Parasites are found in almost all organs, and their presence is accompanied by mononuclear cell infiltration, congestion, and edema and occasionally by granulomatous areas. Reticuloendothelial activity and increase in the number of fixed macrophage cells cause splenomegaly, hepatomegaly, adenopathy, and hyperplasia of bone marrow. The process is then a reticulopathy similar to kala-azar and histoplasmosis.

Death during the acute phase is caused by acute myocarditis with congestive cardiac failure, meningoencephalitis, or complications such as bronchopneumonia. A recent study showed that *T. cruzi* readily enters the central nervous system during the acute infection. Cerebrospinal fluid findings include pleocytosis and high protein levels.[82]

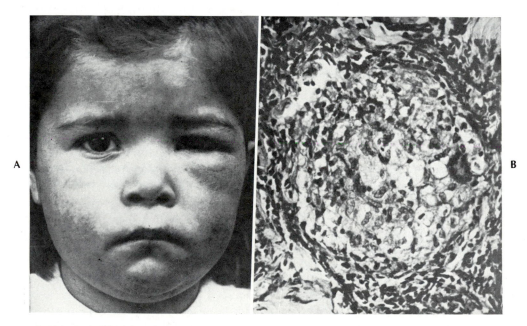

Fig. 12-8. Chagas' disease in child. **A,** Romaña's sign. Ophthalmoganglionary chagoma on left side, 16 days after insect bite. **B,** Initial lesion (chagoma) in arm. Focal histiocytic proliferation with formation of giant cells and peripheral infiltration with lymphocytes. (Courtesy Professor Mazza and the Misión de Estudios de Patología Regional del Norte, Argentina, Pub. 46.)

The heart is enlarged and flabby with pronounced dilatation of the left ventricle. The myocardium is pink and shows yellowish gray streaks. Microscopically the myocardium is diffusely involved but reveals only spotty cell destruction. The myocardial fibers are separated by intense edema, proliferation of histiocytes, and infiltration with chronic inflammatory cells and few polymorphonuclear cells. Within the muscle fibers are leishmanial forms either arranged in rows or in cystlike dilatations (Fig. 12-9). Cardiac fibers show degenerative changes,[87] the most important of which is hyaline necrosis of isolated fibers. Such fibers sometimes exhibit dark bars of clumped fibrils transversely arranged along the longitudinal axis of the fiber. This change, which is better observed in sections stained with iron-hematoxylin or in silver-impregnated sections, is known as the Magarinos Torres lesion[90] and is said to be specific for the acute myocarditis of Chagas' disease. Inflammatory changes in the myocardium also may involve the bundle of His and its ramifications.[80,91,93]

Chronic Chagas' disease. The dominant factor in the chronic stages of Chagas' disease is almost always some degree of myocardial fibrosis. Many patients report a previous acute attack. However, in a number of cases there is no history of a previous attack. The chronic cardiac form of Chagas' disease is a leading cause of cardiac failure and sudden death in endemic areas.

The heart is enlarged, with generalized hypertrophy and dilatation. Mural endocardial thromboses are usually present, most frequently in the right auricle and at the apex of the left ventricle. Apical thrombosis, with focal endomyocardial fibrosis at its base, represents the most important single gross finding suggestive of Chagas' myocarditis.[78] In the absence of thrombosis the myocardium at the apex frequently appears distended and thinned, sometimes even to the point of aneurysmal formation.[78,79] Embolic phenomena, both pulmonary and systemic, are present in about 75% of autopsied cases.[79] The main sources of emboli are intracardiac thrombi, which are also found at autopsy in approximately 75% of cases.

Microscopically the myocardium shows chronic, nonspecific, mononuclear inflammation. Hypertrophy of cardiac fibers, small focal areas of necrosis and granular degeneration of cardiac fibers, focal and diffuse fibrosis, vascular dilatation and congestion, and interstitial and interfibrillary edema are other common microscopic features. Parasites (leishmanial forms in pseudocysts) can be found within cardiac fibers in approximately 30% of cases.[79]

Digestive form of Chagas' disease. Megaesophagus and megacolon are manifestations of chronic Chagas' disease. Fibrosis and degeneration of autonomic ganglia in the heart have been demonstrated in individuals with megaesophagus,[96] as well as considerable diminution in the number of ganglionic cells in the Auerbach plexus of the esophagus and intestine.[86]

Congenital Chagas' disease. The transplacental transmission of *T. cruzi* infection has been well documented in both humans[88] and experimental animals, although its epidemiologic importance and frequency are not fully understood. Congenital Chagas' disease can lead to premature birth and fetal death. A chronic placentitis, similar in some respects to the syphilitic placenta, with bulky and ischemic villi, has been described.[88] Leishmanial forms are found within the cytoplasm of macrophages in variable numbers. Interstitial pneumonitis with a prominent mononuclear histiocytic infiltrate can develop in infants.[89]

Leishmaniasis. Leishmaniasis is a group of diseases caused by one or another of a number of species of protozoa belonging to the genus *Leishmania*. All of these protozoa are transmitted to humans by the bite of a small sand fly of the genera *Phlebotomus* in the Old World and *Lutzomya* in the New World. Each of the species of *Leishmania* is transmitted only by a certain sand fly species.

The protozoan exists in humans as an obligate intracellular parasite. It enters macrophages by phagocytosis[100] and multiplies in them by binary fission. The amastigote has developed mechanisms for survival within the phagolysosome.[110] These are thought to be inactivation of the microbicidal lysosomal enzymes[83] and the capacity for parasite-specified phagocytosis. Induced or facilitated phagocytosis is a mechanism of entry that leishmanias

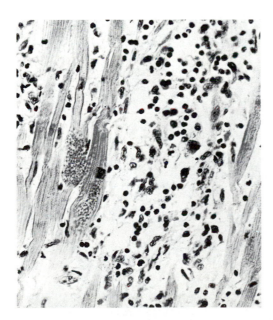

Fig. 12-9. Acute Chagas' disease. There is interstitial myocarditis, with loss of muscle fibers and dense infiltration with round cells and eosinophils. Colonies of *Leishmania* in two myocardial fibers appear at left of center. (360×.)

share with *Toxoplasma gondii* and *Trypanosoma cruzi*. They are able to parasitize nonactivated macrophages without triggering a respiratory burst. The activated phagocytes can produce toxic oxygen metabolites that are leishmanicidal.[99,108,109]

The diseases caused by the leishmanias are subdivided into two types—visceral, and cutaneous—based on the clinical picture. The organisms recovered from patients with these three diseases show differences in culture characteristics, in experimental animal inoculation, and especially in sensitivity or immunologic reactions.

Visceral leishmaniasis (kala-azar). Visceral leishmaniasis, or kala-azar, is a disease heralded by loss of weight, weakness, enlargement of the abdomen because of prominent splenomegaly and hepatomegaly, fever,[101] cough, and pain over the spleen. The onset is insidious, and the course is chronic.

Visceral leishmaniasis is caused by the species *Leishmania donovani, L. infantum,* and *L. chagasi.*[106] The latter two have been identified as the causative agents of Mediterranean and New World kala-azar, respectively.[115] The use of biochemical and immunologic methods has permitted this greater taxonomic accuracy. All three species have similar life cycles.

The sand fly ingests leishmanias with the blood of an infected person bitten. The promastigotes multiply rapidly in the midgut and then migrate to the pharynx and buccal cavity of the vector. When the fly attempts to obtain blood from a healthy individual, many of the flagellated promastigotes (leptomonads) are introduced into the outer dermis.

The incubation period varies from 2 weeks to 18 months. The onset may be sudden, with acute manifestations, but is usually insidious, and many patients have pronounced splenomegaly and hepatomegaly on examination.[116]

Kala-azar is endemic in many areas of India and in parts of China. It is also encountered in the countries bordering the Mediterranean and in parts of West Africa. It is sparsely distributed in South and Central America. In Mediterranean countries and China it is primarily a disease of infants and young children. In India and South America young adults are most frequently infected. In the Sudan a particularly fulminating type is observed commonly in young adults. The injected flagellates rapidly change to the oval-shaped amastigote form in the host, and after colonizing in the dermis, they gain access to the bloodstream or lymphatics and are transported to the viscera. The leishmanias parasitize reticuloendothelial cells in all parts of the body. The disease is manifested primarily in organs with reticuloendothelial tissue such as the spleen, liver, bone marrow, and lymph nodes.[116]

The outstanding characteristics of the parasitized reticuloendothelial cells are the distension of the cell membrane and the great multiplication of amastigotes (Leishman-Donovan bodies) within the cytoplasm.

The spleen is the most severely affected organ and may be involved to the point of losing all architectural detail, both grossly and microscopically (Fig. 12-10). The spleen may weigh several kilograms, and infarcts are not uncommon. In the liver there is marked Kupffer cell hyperplasia, and an inflammatory cell infiltrate may be found in the portal areas and in the sinusoids. The bone marrow is replaced by parasitized macrophages. The hematologic findings of anemia, leukopenia, and thrombocytopenia are thought to be the result of decreased production in the marrow and increased sequestration owing to hypersplenism.[113] Destruction by immunologic factors has also been proposed.

Severe secondary infections, especially cancrum oris or noma, develop terminally in patients with agranulocytosis. The presence of IgG hypergammaglobulinemia and hypoalbuminemia leads to an inverted albumin/globulin ratio. Most of this IgG is nonspecific and thus not protective.[98] Proteinuria and microhematuria associated with mesangial proliferation and immunoglobulin deposition have been reported.[114] Evidence of circulating immune complexes in kala-azar has recently been presented.[104] Skin macular and nodular lesions resembling those of leprosy may be a sequela to kala-azar. This

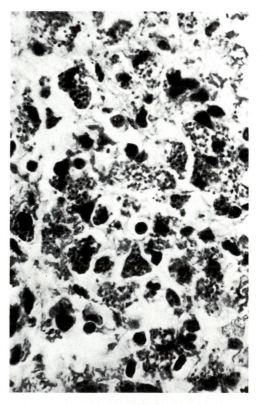

Fig. 12-10. Kala-azar. In this spleen of an Indian patient, reticuloendothelial cells of pulp and sinuses have become distended with *Leishmania*. (776×.)

is known as post-kala-azar dermal leishmaniasis.

The definite diagnosis of kala-azar is made by demonstrating the organism in Giemsa-stained tissue. Bone marrow biopsy is preferred to splenic or liver biopsy because it is safe and 90% sensitive.[112] Available methods of serodiagnosis[97,105,117] include complement fixation, indirect hemagglutination, indirect immunofluorescence, enzyme-linked immunosorbent assay,[103] and direct agglutination. The last is the preferred test because of its sensitivity[23] and lesser cross reactivity.

Cutaneous and mucocutaneous leishmaniasis. Cutaneous leishmaniasis is encountered in both the New and the Old World. The *Leishmania* organisms responsible for these related diseases cannot be differentiated morphologically or serologically. The differentiation among varieties of cutaneous leishmaniasis is based on clinical, epidemiologic, geographic, and immunologic grounds.

The primary lesion in all variants is usually an ulcer, which develops most frequently at the site of the bite of an infected sand fly (*Phlebotomus* or *Lutzomya*). It starts as a macule within 2 to 6 months after the bite and then becomes a papule, and finally the lesion breaks down in the center leaving an ulcer with sharply defined and elevated borders (Fig. 12-11). Biopsy of the lesion reveals a granulomatous reaction with lymphocytes, plasma cells, epithelioid histiocytes, and Langhans'-type giant cells. Numerous organisms are identifiable within macro-

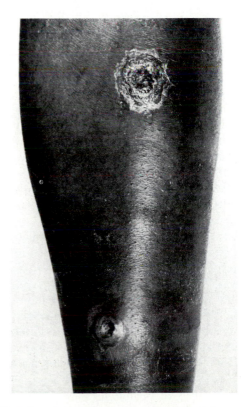

Fig. 12-11. Oriental sore. These two well-developed sores of lower leg have excavated centers and swollen borders. (AFIP 1440-1.)

phages. There are no systemic manifestations, and the symptoms in cutaneous leishmaniasis result from the primary skin lesion and from the metastatic lesions, if any. Characteristically there is only one ulcer for each infected sand fly bite, developing at or near the point of inoculation on the exposed skin. Two varieties of cutaneous leishmaniasis have been distinguished in the Old World, an urban or "dry" type and a rural or "wet" type. They are both known as "oriental sore." The wet type is caused by *L. tropica major* and the dry type by *L. tropica minor*. Lymphatic spread may rarely occur in the wet type, with the formation of metastatic nodules along the lymphatic vessel, and leishmanias can be found in the regional lymph nodes.

Cutaneous leishmaniasis in South and Central America is similar in many respects to the Old World disease, but metastatic spread is more frequent and the disease is mutilating, since frequently there is involvement of the nasal and mucosal surfaces of the mouth and upper respiratory tract. When this occurs, the disease is referred to as mucocutaneous leishmaniasis.

There are four clinical, epidemiologic, and geographic types in the New World. In Mexico, mainly in the Yucatán Peninsula, and in the jungles of Guatemala and Honduras, one encounters the *chiclero ulcer*. It is a self-limiting disease with no metastatic spread. The ulcer is most frequently found in the pinna of the ear but sometimes in the skin of the cheek, forehead, and less commonly other exposed areas of the body. It is ascribed to a separate species of leishmania, *L. tropica mexicana*.

The Andean or Peruvian lesion, known as *uta*, is similar to the chiclero ulcer, and metastases are uncommon. It is caused by *L. braziliensis*.

Pian bois, or forest yaws, may cause a single ulcerative lesion but often metastasizes along lymphatic channels, producing multiple cutaneous ulcers or nodules. Nasopharyngeal spread does not occur. It is also caused by *L. braziliensis*.

Another type of cutaneous leishmaniasis is found in Central America and the upper half of South America. It is known as *espundia* and is also caused by *L. braziliensis*. It is characterized by a high incidence of metastatic lesions, with migration of the organisms to secondary foci, mainly in mucocutaneous areas, particularly the nasal septum. Because of this mucosal tropism, this disease is referred to as the classical type of American mucocutaneous leishmaniasis. Extensive destruction of soft and underlying hard tissues of the nose and pharynx occurs, producing severe mutilation of the face. The organism's tropism for the nose cartilage is thought to result from the parasite's growth pattern, which is dependent on low skin temperature, and from the lack of a cellular immune response in the host tissue.[107]

A diffuse, chronic variant of cutaneous leishmaniasis with numerous nodular, fleshy swellings resembling lepromatous leprosy is known as *leishmaniasis tegmentaria diffusa*. It occurs mostly in Venezuela but is found in both the Old and the New World. Destructive mucocutaneous lesions do not occur. The lesions consist of organisms proliferating within macrophages.[94] There is no granulomatous response because of the host's depressed cell-mediated immunity.

Results of the leishmanin test are negative, hence the names *anergic* or *disseminated cutaneous leishmaniasis* occasionally used for this entity.

The patient's anergy is specific to the leishmanin skin test, since a delayed hypersensitivity reaction is elicited by other common skin test antigens. A lymphocyte proliferative response, although present for several mitogens, is not elicited by leishmanial antigens. This selective anergy could be modulated by an adherent suppressor cells mechanism.[111]

Diseases caused by sporozoans
Coccidiosis

Coccidia are parasites of the intestinal tract of many vertebrate species. They are usually transmitted by the ingestion of the sporulated oocyst in contaminated water or food. The life cycle of these sporozoans in humans has not been completely elucidated, but they have the distinguishing feature of undergoing both schizogony and gametogony in the small bowel epithelium.[119]

Two different genera of coccidia are known to parasitize humans. *Isospora belli* has been the most commonly identified *Isospora* species in the small bowel of patients with mucous diarrhea, fever, weight loss, abdominal pain, peripheral eosinophilia, and malabsorption.[133] The sporozoan formerly called *I. hominis* has been reclassified under the genus *Sarcocystis* because sexual and asexual reproduction takes place in different hosts.[122,123] *Sarcocystis* infections are asymptomatic. The cysts of *Sarcocystis* must be distinguished from those of other coccidia, that is, *Isospora* in the gastrointestinal tract and *Toxoplasma* in tissues.

Organisms of the genus *Cryptosporidia* have been encountered in several patients with diarrhea,[128] many of whom have been immunocompromised.[125-127,131,132] Although not occurring exclusively in this group,[118,124] *Cryptosporidia* is among the opportunistic pathogens recently described in patients with the acquired immune deficiency syndrome (AIDS).[120] Unlike *Isospora*, which invades and multiplies within the absorptive cells of the small intestine, *Cryptosporidia* inhabits the brush border exclusively. Light and electron microscopy of biopsy specimens from the small bowel is helpful in the diagnosis of coccidial infections.[121] The mucosal lesion is similar in both genera and consists of shortened villi, crypt lengthening, and a mononuclear infiltrate in the lamina propria.[129] In addition to the small intestinal mucosa, the stomach and large intestine have been found to contain cryptosporidial organisms.

Malaria

Malaria is a disease of worldwide distribution and is probably the most widespread of all diseases. It is caused by a protozoan parasite belonging to the genus *Plasmodium*. Humans are infected by four common species, the distribution of which is not uniform. *P. vivax* causes tertian malaria; *P. malariae*, quartan malaria; *P. ovale*, ovale malaria; and *P. falciparum*, the most severe form of the disease, known as pernicious, subtertian, malignant, or estivoautumnal malaria. The natural reservoir of the disease is humans. The vector is the female *Anopheles* mosquito. Recently the possibility of congenitally acquired malaria has been reported.[148] Plasmodia are found in great numbers in the intervillous spaces of the placenta of infected mothers. The disparity between the approximate 30% incidence of placental malaria in endemic areas[152] and the rarity of congenital malaria reports is thought to be related to an immunologically dependent placental barrier mechanism. The disease has been associated epidemiologically with many hematologic conditions. Inherited erythrocyte abnormalities, such as sickle hemoglobinopathy and glucose 6-phosphate dehydrogenase deficiency, are extremely common in malarial areas. Genetic selection for these conditions is thought to be the result of the abnormal RBC's resistance to infection, leading to a survival advantage for the heterozygous gene defect carrier. Studies have shown that sickle hemoglobin restricts both parasite invasion and growth.[146] The prevalence of Burkitt's lymphoma in malarious areas has led to the proposal that malaria may enhance the oncogenic potential of the Epstein-Barr virus.[141]

The life cycle of the malarial organism is divided into the asexual or endogenous cycle in the human (schizogony) and the sexual or exogenous cycle in the mosquito (sporogony). The asexual cycle begins with the introduction of the sporozoites by the bite of the infected mosquito. A preerythrocytic phase, which occurs within hepatic cells in the liver, antedates bloodstream invasion by the parasite. This takes from 7 to 10 days until finally the sporozoites invade the red blood cells. The sporozoites of *P. vivax* require for invasion the presence of specific blood group determinants on the surface of the erythrocyte.[144,145] Furthermore, *P. vivax* and *P. ovale* invade only reticulocytes, and *P. malariae* invades only senescent cells.[142] This explains the relatively benign course of infections with these organisms when compared with *P. falciparum*, which invades any erythrocyte and for which no requirement for invasion has been discovered.

The sporozoites grow and multiply within erythrocytes, passing through the successive developmental stages of trophozoite, schizont, and merozoite. The merozoites are set free in the circulation by rupture of the erythrocytes, ending the asexual cycle.

During the course of this asexual division, the parasite acts on the hemoglobin of the erythrocytes, producing a golden brown pigment known as malarial pigment, which accumulates in the red cells. When the erythrocytes rupture, malarial pigment is set free in the circulation and is phagocytosed by reticuloendothelial cells. As the number of parasites increases, the number of erythrocytes decreases with each successive schizogony.

The pathogenesis of the anemia in acute malaria is far from settled. Most investigators agree that rupture of parasitized cells and destruction of nonparasitized cells by activated reticuloendothelial cells of the spleen, liver, and bone marrow contribute to the anemia. The controversy concerns whether immunologic factors, such as complement-mediated hemolysis, have a role in the cause of anemia.[137,150,154]

The debris of the ruptured cells, together with the merozoites and their metabolic by-products, is set free in the bloodstream and acts as a pyrogen. When the pyrogen accumulates, it produces the characteristic chills and fever of a malarial attack.

Some of the trophozoites within red blood cells become differentiated into round or crescentic sexual forms called microgametocytes and macrogametocytes. These gametocytes are taken up by the *Anopheles* mosquito and undergo maturation in 7 to 12 days. The male microgamete then fertilizes the female macrogamete, producing a fertilized cell or zygote. The zygote penetrates the wall of the stomach and forms an oocyst. Large numbers of spores (sporozoites) develop within this cyst. The oocyst ruptures, and the sporozoites then reach the body cavity of the mosquito. From the body cavity the sporozoites invade other parts of the mosquito's body. Those reaching the salivary glands pass down the proboscis when the insect bites, thus infecting a human.

The clinical picture in the benign types of malaria is characterized by periodic paroxysms of shaking chills, followed by high fever and pronounced diaphoresis as the patient's body temperature falls. The paroxysms last from 4 to 10 hours and recur every third day in vivax and ovale infections and every fourth day in quartan malaria.

Our knowledge of the lesions of benign malaria is derived mainly from cases of death in the course of natural and therapeutic malarial infection. The main pathologic alterations are those of reticuloendothelial response to the malarial parasite and its pigment and a secondary anemia. The spleen is enlarged and is a slate gray as a result of deposition of malarial pigment. The latter is most abundant in the reticuloendothelial cells and in the macrophages of the red pulp. Parasites occasionally are demonstrable within some of the macrophages and reticuloendothelial cells. The liver is also enlarged and congested. The Kupffer cells show prominent phagocytic activity and contain abundant pigment and occasional parasites. The bone marrow discloses erythroid hyperplasia, mostly normoblastic. It also shows increased myeloid activity, but despite this, there is no leukocytosis in the peripheral blood.

Malignant pernicious malaria. Much more frequently than in the other types, falciparum malaria is accompanied by pernicious manifestations. The paroxysms in falciparum malaria are less regular than in other types. Severe parasitemia and multiple infection of red blood cells, although not diagnostic, are common in falciparum infections. The plasmodium evades the host's immune system by a combination of mechanisms that include antigenic variation, antigenic complexity, and intracellular development.[135,143]

The parasitized erythrocytes are less deformable and tend to adhere to endothelial walls, leading to prominent accumulation of parasitized red cells within the visceral capillaries. This phenomenon, known as the "visceral tide," explained why few or no parasites are found in peripheral blood samples from these patients.

The progressive decrease in circulating erythrocytes, the severe engorgement of small visceral capillaries with red cells, and the decrease in circulating blood volume are responsible for the severe anoxia of important organs in pernicious malaria. Although the red blood cells give the impression of being clumped, actual thrombosis is rare. Occasionally infarcts occur as the result of thrombosis of blood vessels. The accumulation of parasitized red cells is more common in the small vessels of the spleen, liver, bone marrow, brain, and lungs than in the kidneys, small intestine, pancreas, heart, and testes.

In the brain, perivascular "ring" hemorrhages and necrosis of surrounding parenchyma are seen (Fig. 12-12). These lesions, predominantly of the white matter, are thought to be the result of vascular damage by sludged, parasitized, red blood cells and antigen-antibody complexes.[151] The damage leads to a reactive gliosis with the formation of malarial granulomas, known as Dürck's glial nodes.

Abundant pigment and parasites are observed within reticuloendothelial cells and macrophages (Fig. 12-13). Pigmentation of the liver is not as noticeable as that in the spleen. The hepatic cells show cloudy swelling and fatty change. Kupffer cells are large and actively phagocytic. They contain parasites, erythrocytes, and malarial pigment (Fig. 12-13).

A disseminated intravascular coagulopathy may occasionally develop in patients with malaria.[138] This has been associated with the adult respiratory distress syn-

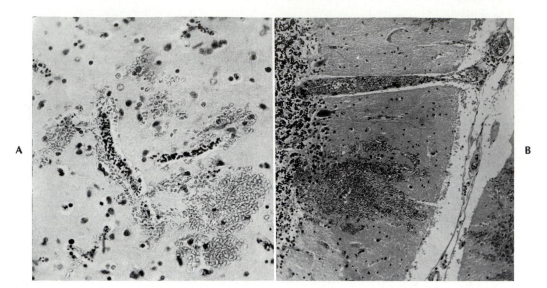

Fig. 12-12. Cerebral malaria. **A,** Multiple hemorrhages into brain. Capillaries are engorged with pigmented and parasitized erythrocytes. **B,** Hemorrhages may be as numerous in cerebellar cortex as in cerebrum. Smaller blood vessels are laden with parasitized erythrocytes. (80×.)

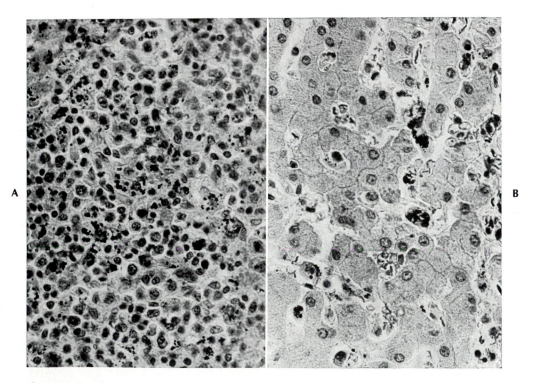

Fig. 12-13. Acute falciparum malaria. **A,** Spleen shows pronounced reticuloendothelial hyperplasia and loss of outline of sinuses. Finely divided malarial pigment appears within red blood cells and phagocytes. **B,** Liver shows cloudy swelling and some disarrangement of hepatic cords. Kupffer cells are swollen with malarial pigment and cellular debris. (360×.)

drome seen in some fatal cases of malaria. Recently an immune complex glomerulonephritis formed by *P. falciparum* antigen and corresponding antibodies has been documented by electron microscopy and immunofluorescence.[134]

Blackwater fever. Blackwater fever, or hemoglobinuric fever, is a very dangerous complication of malignant malaria. It occurs among persons previously infected with falciparum malaria or in individuals living in areas where this disease abounds. Within a few days of onset there are severe chills, with rigor, high fever, jaundice, vomiting, rapidly progressive anemia, and the passage of dark red or black urine.

The condition is more common in patients who have been subject to excessive fatigue, privation, exposure, exhaustion, shock, or injury; intercurrent infection; childbirth; or alcoholic excess; or who have received inadequate treatment with quinine.

The cause of the hemolytic crises that characterize the disease is unknown. There is rapid and massive destruction of red blood cells with the production of hemoglobinemia, hemoglobinuria, intense jaundice, anuria, and finally death in the majority of cases. The most probable explanation for blackwater fever is an autoimmune reaction. Grossly and microscopically the kidneys are similar to those of hemoglobinuric or tubular nephrosis as seen in other conditions such as the crush syndrome.

The diagnosis of malaria depends on the demonstration of the parasite in stained peripheral blood smears. Serologic tests are available. However, because of the time required to obtain the results, they are used mainly for epidemiologic studies and for the identification of infected donors in transfusion-related malaria. The tests available include complement fixation, indirect immunofluorescence, indirect hemagglutination,[140] and enzyme-linked immunosorbent assay.[136,149] The indirect immunofluorescent test, because of its specificity and sensitivity, is the preferred method for diagnosis of acute infections.[153]

Toxoplasmosis

Toxoplasmosis is caused by the obligate intracellular protozoan *Toxoplasma gondii* (Fig. 12-14). The parasite was originally identified in the small North African rodent *Ctenodactylus gundi*, hence its name. "Toxo-" refers to the curved or arcuate shape of the organism, not to a toxin. The organism's growth requirements are unknown, since it has not been grown extracellularly. It is widely distributed among domestic animals and humans throughout the world.

Toxoplasma is a tissue coccidia. Both coccidian stages, schizogonic and gametogonic, are found in the epithelium of the small intestine of cats. The *Toxoplasma* oocyst, similar in morphology to that of *Isospora belli*, is excreted in cat feces. The oocysts, millions of which may be

shed in a single stool of an infected cat, survive for months in moist environments, water, or soil.

In tissues the proliferative phase predominates during the acute infection. This phase leads to the production of trophozoites, called tachyzoites or bradyzoites depending on the speed of their development. Cysts containing hundreds and sometimes thousands of merozoites make their appearance in brain, skeletal muscles, and other tissues with the development of immunity.

Toxoplasma tachyzoites enter the cells by both phagocytosis and active invasion.[168] The latter mode of entry depends on specialized organelles, called rhoptries, and on "penetration-enhancing factor." During this infectious process an oxidative respiratory burst is not stimulated; thus no oxygen metabolites are formed to kill the protozoan. *T. gondii* also alters the membrane of the parasitophorous vacuole so that lysosomal fusion does not take place.[162]

Oocysts and cysts are the principal infective forms. Infection occurs when a person eats undercooked or raw meat of animals with chronic toxoplasmosis or ingests oocysts from the feces of cats. Recently an outbreak of acute toxoplasmosis associated with ingestion of contaminated water was reported.[155] Most of these primary infections are asymptomatic and result in a chronic carrier stage, again mostly symptomless.

Transplacental transmission occurs rarely but accounts for the majority of patients. Infection of the fetus is seen

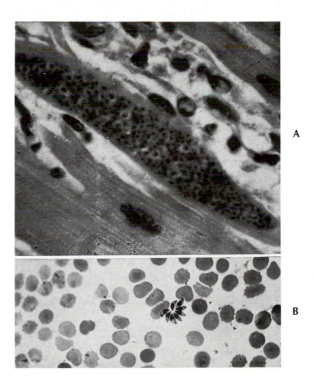

Fig. 12-14. Toxoplasmosis. **A,** *Toxoplasma* in human heart muscle. **B,** *Toxoplasma* in smear from omentum of guinea pig. (From Pinkerton, H., and Henderson, R.G.: J.A.M.A. **116:**807, 1941.)

in 30% to 40% of cases of acquired toxoplasmosis during pregnancy.[158] The yearly incidence of gestational infection in the United States is said to be two to six cases per 1000 pregnancies.[164]

Relatively few cases of human disease have been reported, but results of the skin test for *Toxoplasma* and the Sabin-Feldman dye test[170] have been positive in 10% to 50% of the adults tested, indicating that, although disease is rare, infection is common. Actually the prevalence can be less than 10% in dry areas such as Arizona and close to 100% in moist, lowland tropical areas such as Costa Rica and Guatemala. Prevalence increases with age. The majority of individuals infected with *Toxoplasma* have minimal or no symptoms. However, the disease, which is occasionally fatal, is of concern. The clinical picture varies according to the age of the patient. Two forms of the disease, congenital and adult, have been described.

Congenital toxoplasmosis. Congenital toxoplasmosis should be strongly suspected when the characteristic ocular lesions and the presence of cerebral calcifications in roentgenographic examinations are associated with hydrocephalus and pleocytosis of the cerebrospinal fluid. The pathologic lesions are those of hydrocephalus caused by necrotic foci in the brain, usually located in the periventricular areas. These lesions are microglial nodules surrounded by areas of vasculitis and necrosis. The vasculitis is thought to be immune complex mediated.[158] Calcium deposits in these focal lesions and bilateral chorioretinitis are evident. Focal areas of necrosis may be seen in viscera, leading to myocarditis, pneumonitis, and rarely hepatitis.

Adult toxoplasmosis. The clinical picture of adult toxoplasmosis is undoubtedly uncommon. It consists of lymphadenitis (usually posterior cervical), fever, and malaise. A biopsy of the firm, rubbery nodes is commonly done to rule out lymphoproliferative diseases, and it is the pathologist who first suggests the diagnosis of toxoplasmosis.[167] The architecture of the lymph node is preserved. There are marked follicular hyperplasia and clusters of histiocytes inside and surrounding the follicles. Organisms are rarely seen. Pathologic diagnosis is confirmed by the Sabin-Feldman dye test or by more recent serologic methods such as indirect immunofluorescence, indirect hemagglutination, complement fixation, and enzyme-linked immunosorbent assay.[172,173] Some of these serologic tests have been suggested as screening methods for toxoplasmosis in pregnancy.[156] Acute infection is diagnosed on the basis of a fourfold rise in antibody titer or detection of IgM antibodies by the indirect immunofluorescence method. A Paul-Bunell test for heterophil antibodies is usually done to rule out infectious mononucleosis. Immunoperoxidase methods have recently been developed for the diagnosis of toxoplasmosis in tissue sections.[157]

Other, less common manifestations of adult toxoplasmosis are interstitial pneumonitis, myocarditis, and hepatitis.[174] Chorioretinitis and uveitis sometimes occur.[161,165] Toxoplasmosis has been diagnosed serologically in patients with polymyositis.[160,163,171] The pathogenic interrelationship is unclear.

In immunosuppressed patients disseminated disease can occur.[169] Recently, several cases of immunoperoxidase-confirmed central nervous system toxoplasmosis have been described among Haitians[207] and homosexuals (see "Aquired immune deficiency syndrome [AIDS]"). Patients with disseminated disease have neurologic manifestations resulting from toxoplasmic meningoencephalitis or brain abscess.[159,166] The disease is usually fatal.

Pneumocystosis

Pneumocystosis (*Pneumocystis* pneumonia, interstitial plasma cell pneumonia) is an endemic or epidemic disease caused by the sporozoan *Pneumocystis carinii*. The development of tissue culture methods for this organism[191] has permitted a better understanding of the organism's life cycle and biologic behavior. The protozoan has trophozoite and cyst stages, and both are identified in the pulmonary lesions. The organisms, as confirmed in vitro, do not invade but remain extracellular, attached to the pulmonary alveolar epithelial cells by fine filaments or microtubules through which they obtain nutrients.[189] Occasionally they may be phagocytosed by alveolar cells.

The epidemic disease occurs chiefly in premature infants and debilitated children who are malnourished at a time when the immunologic mechanisms are incompletely developed. These patients have an interstitial plasma cell pneumonia, which was once thought to be characteristic of pneumocystosis. Since then, there have been many reports of endemic cases of pneumocystosis in immunosuppressed patients in which a plasma cell infiltrate is not prominent.

Any disease process or form of therapy that sharply reduces the immunologic defenses predisposes the patient to pulmonary pneumocystosis.* The disease is usually encountered in patients with congenital immunodeficiency states and in patients receiving corticosteroids or cytotoxic agents.[192] The incidence is high in transplant patients and in individuals receiving chemotherapy for malignancy. Concomitant infection with other opportunistic organisms such as *Aspergillus*, *Cryptococcus*,[175] *Candida*, and cytomegalovirus (CMV)[176,183,186,198] has been observed. The high rate of concurrent infection by CMV (10% to 20%) and the fact that it induces transient immunologic dysfunction raises the possibility of a pathogenic role of CMV in pneumocystosis.[182]

The transmission of pneumocystosis is thought to be

---

*References 177, 180, 181, 185, 193, 195, 197, 199.

airborne,[175] but a case of transplacental transmission has been reported.[190] Experimental evidence suggests that the disease occurs by activation of a latent infection.

The disease in marasmic children has an insidious onset[188] characterized by progressive dyspnea, weight loss, and failure to thrive. In immunosuppressed patients the onset of symptoms may be abrupt and fulminant. Symptoms include severe dyspnea, tachypnea, cough, fever, and cyanosis. The symptoms usually begin when the patient is in remission of the original disease and the immunosuppressive therapeutic agents have been withdrawn.

Despite the severity of the respiratory symptoms, physical findings are minimal. Dullness to percussion is practically never elicited. A few moist rales occasionally may be heard. Laboratory findings include leukocytosis, hypoxemia, and increase in the alveolar-arterial Po_2 gradient as a result of alveolocapillary diffusion abnormalities and ventilation-perfusion mismatches.

Roentgenographic examination early in the disease discloses ground glass–like infiltration of the pulmonary parenchyma, which is more conspicuous toward the hilar region and spreads peripherally in a butterfly pattern. Subsequently, the infiltrate assumes a nodular pattern, with intervening areas of radiolucency attributable to compensatory emphysema.

Pathologic changes are limited to the lungs, which are firm, rubbery, and noncrepitant. The cut surface is whitish or brownish and discloses several firm nodules with a granular mucinous appearance. These nodules may be separated from each other by spongy areas of emphysematous pulmonary parenchyma, but often they are confluent. On microscopy the respiratory bronchioles and alveoli are distended by a honeycombed foamy material that stains brightly eosinophilic (Fig. 12-15). On special stains the organisms are identified lining the alveolar walls. The cyst wall is best outlined with the methenamine-silver method, whereas the free trophozoites and cystic contents are best seen on Giemsa stains.[196] There is a minimal inflammatory reaction composed mainly of monocytes, occasional plasma cells, and histiocytes. Plasma cells are numerous only in cases of the "epidemic type" of disease. The disease seldom spreads to extrapulmonary sites.[179]

Diagnosis of pneumocystosis is established by examining tissue obtained by transbronchial, percutaneous, or open lung wedge biopsy,[194] the last being the preferred method. The organisms can occasionally be demonstrated on tracheobronchial secretions and gastric contents.[178,184,187] Open lung biopsy specimens should be cultured for bacteria, fungi, and viruses. Imprints should be done, and tissue should be processed for immunofluorescence and light and electron microscopy. This approach enhances the diagnosis of pneumocystosis and

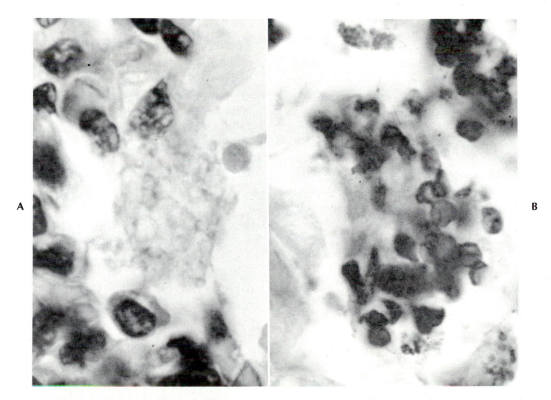

Fig. 12-15. A, Pneumocystosis. Foamy mass of organisms appears in alveolus of lung. **B,** Pneumocystosis. (**A,** Hematoxylin and eosin; **B,** Gomori methenamine-silver.)

other infectious and noninfectious diffuse processes commonly seen in patients undergoing chemotherapy, radiotherapy, or oxygen therapy. Serodiagnosis by an indirect immunofluorescence test is also available.

The mortality varies from 20% to 60% in malnourished and premature infants. In immunosuppressed adults the mortality is much higher.

Acquired immune deficiency syndrome (AIDS)

Recently a newly defined syndrome, the acquired immune deficiency syndrome (AIDS), has been described among homosexuals, intravenous drug abusers, Haitians,[207] and hemophiliacs.[208] This syndrome, which has high mortality and morbidity, is intimately associated with defective cell-mediated immunity, as determined by in vivo (delayed cutaneous hypersensitivity) and in vitro (T lymphocyte function) tests. Patients have clinical evidence of cutaneous anergy, lymphopenia, defective natural killer cell activity, diminished lymphocyte proliferative responses to mitogens, and decreased ratios of helper-inducer to suppressor-cytotoxic T lymphocyte subsets.[204]

AIDS victims are susceptible to infections by a multiplicity of agents, including viruses (CMV and herpes simplex), bacteria (*Mycobacterium tuberculosis* and *M. avium-intracellulare*), fungi (*Candida albicans* and *Cryptococcus neoformans*), and protozoa (*Pneumocystis carinii, Toxoplasma gondii, Cryptosporidia,* and *Entamoeba histolytica*).[200,201,203,205,206] The association of pneumocystosis with this syndrome, especially in the homosexual population, is extensively documented and has been widely studied. In most of these patients there is evidence of both a concomitant or past infection by CMV and a highly increased incidence of Kaposi's sarcoma.[202] The possible pathogenic role of CMV in these entities is being studied. As previously stated, there is a high concurrent rate of infection by both *Pneumocystis* and CMV even in the absence of AIDS. Furthermore, not only does CMV induce cellular immune function abnormalities,[209] but also the viral genome has been identified in several biopsy samples of Kaposi's sarcoma tumor.[200] Whether the immunodeficiency that seems to lead to opportunistic infections and Kaposi's sarcoma is the cause or the effect of CMV infection is at present unclear.

Babesiosis (piroplasmosis)

Babesiosis, formerly called piroplasmosis, is a serious hemolytic disease that affects cattle. Since the first case of human babesiosis was described by Skrabalo[223] in 1957, many other clinical and subclinical cases have been identified.[216,222]

The disease in humans is caused by three species of *Babesia* (family Babesiidae, order Piroplasmorida).[214] It is transmitted by the bite of ticks and rarely by transfusions.[219] In blood smears the *Babesia* species, mostly the young trophozoites, may be confused with *Plasmodium* species, leading to the misdiagnosis of malaria. The fundamental differential points are the lack of hemozoin pigment in the cytoplasm of *Babesia* and the absence of schizonts and gametocytes,[217] since *Babesia* divide by budding and not by schizogeny.[214]

The mechanism of penetration into the erythrocyte requires the presence of complement factors,[213,218,224] a requirement similar to the blood group determinant requirements of some plasmodia.[144,145]

The initial cases reported occurred in splenectomized individuals. The clinical course was hemoglobinuria, hemoglobinemia, jaundice, anemia, and renal failure frequently with a fatal outcome. Postmortem findings included bile staining of viscera and serosal membranes, hemoglobinuric nephrosis of the type seen in malarial blackwater fever, and a generalized reticuloendothelial response most prominent in the Kupffer cells.

Recent cases[210,221,225] in nonsplenectomized patients followed a milder course with a viral syndrome–like symptomatology. That the absence of the spleen leads to a more severe illness[212,220,226] has been confirmed in experimental animals. Older age also predisposes to clinical infection.[215]

The diagnosis of babesiosis can be confirmed by Romanowski stained blood smears and by an indirect immunofluorescence test. The presence of increased levels of circulating immune complexes has recently been recognized.[211] Their role if any in the pathogenesis of babesiosis is still an unanswered question.

HELMINTHIC DISEASES
Diseases caused by trematodes (flukes)
Distomiases

Hepatic distomiasis. Hepatic distomiasis is caused mainly by the trematodes of *Fasciola hepatica* (sheep liver fluke), *Chlonorchis sinensis* (Chinese liver fluke), *Opisthorchis felineus* (cat liver fluke), and *Opisthorchis viverrini*.

Fascioliasis. The trematode *Fasciola hepatica* is found most commonly in sheep- and cattle-raising countries, where it produces the disease known as liver rot. The operculated ova are passed in the feces. They mature in fresh water, after which they hatch a miracidium, which invades a freshwater snail. Cercariae are produced, which, instead of swimming freely as do those of the schistosomes, form cysts (metacercariae) that attach themselves to aquatic vegetation. Most infections are acquired by eating watercress. On ingestion metacercariae are liberated in the upper small intestine of humans or more frequently of sheep and cattle, and the parasites penetrate directly through the gut to the peritoneal cavity and into the hepatic parenchyma until they reach their usual habitat in the large biliary ducts. The disease is usually manifested by a pronounced leukocytosis and eosinophilia; eosinophils may reach a value of 70%.[242]

Hepatomegaly, splenomegaly, and lymphadenopathy are frequently encountered. In some cases the symptoms and signs are those of chronic cholecystitis or cholangitis. Intermittent jaundice may develop occasionally because of obstruction by the adult parasite. We have seen three cases in which the adult parasite or ova were incidental findings when tissue was studied after cholecystectomy (Fig. 12-16).

The adult parasites produce epithelial hyperplasia of the biliary epithelium, with periductal infiltration by eosinophils, lymphocytes, and plasma cells and eventual extensive fibrosis. Experimentally, the host's immunologic response to *Fasciola* is similar to that described for *Schistosoma* and *Trichinella* with eosinophil degranulation and release of toxic substances.[231]

It is extremely rare for cirrhosis to develop as the result of this parasitic infection. The diagnosis is established by finding the ova in the feces or in the duodenal contents. Serodiagnostic tests have been developed and include complement fixation, hemagglutination, and the enzyme-linked immunosorbent assay.[233,238,250]

Clonorchiasis. The liver fluke *Clonorchis sinensis* is parasitic in cats, dogs, and humans. Two intermediate hosts are required, a freshwater mollusk and one of several species of freshwater fish. The eggs passed in the feces do not hatch in fresh water but within the first host, a freshwater snail. The miracidium is transformed into a cercaria within the snail. The cercaria then leaves the snail and swims until it finally penetrates beneath the scales of the second host, a freshwater fish. Here it develops into a metacercaria. Humans are infected by eating raw fish. The liberated metacercariae adhere to the duodenal mucosa and migrate into the common duct and the intrahepatic ducts, where they develop into adult worms. When the parasites are numerous, they may block biliary flow.[232,246] Roentgenographic examination of the biliary tract sometimes leads to the diagnosis.[249]

Severe adenomatous hyperplasia of biliary duct epithelium is far more common in this disease than in fascioliasis (Fig. 12-17). Periductal inflammation with eosinophils and round cells also is seen. Severe portal fibrosis ensues, followed by cirrhosis with portal hypertension.

The clinical course is characterized by relative absence of symptoms. The symptoms and signs of cirrhosis are evident as late complications. Diagnosis is based on recovery of the ova in the feces or duodenal contents.

Carcinoma of the liver is often found in association with clonorchiasis. The hepatocellular form occurs frequently,[243] but the etiologic relationship of clonorchiasis in this malignancy is unclear.[241] On the other hand, clonorchiasis may play an etiologic role in cholangiocarcinoma as implied by both epidemiologic and animal studies.[229,234-237]

Opisthorchiasis. The cat liver fluke, *Opisthorchis felineus*, occurs endemically in Liberia, parts of the Orient, and Eastern Europe. *O. viverrini* is endemic in north-

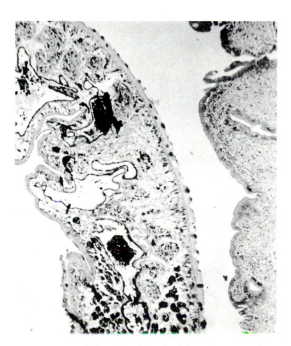

Fig. 12-16. *Fasciola hepatica* encountered accidentally in common bile duct in course of exploration for chronic cholecystitis. (Hematoxylin and eosin; 35×.)

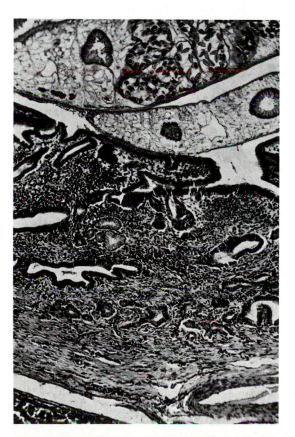

Fig. 12-17. *Clonorchis sinensis* with dilated intrahepatic bile duct. Wall of duct shows adenomatous proliferation and pronounced round cell infiltration. There is fibrosis of portal space. (80×.)

east Thailand, where 25% to 75% of the population is infected.[244,247]

As in clonorchiasis, the disease is acquired by eating raw fish. The adult parasite invades not only the bile ducts but also the pancreatic duct. The pathologic changes and symptomatology are similar to those of clonorchiasis.

Experimental data suggest that the host's immunologic response may be important in the development of portal fibrosis in a manner similar to schistosomiasis.[228] The same investigators have implied that the combined effect of nitrosamine compounds in the diet and of liver fluke infection may play an etiologic role in the pathogenesis of cholangiocarcinoma.[227,248] The diagnosis is based on finding the ova in the feces or duodenal contents.

Intestinal distomiasis. An infection limited to the Far East,[240] intestinal distomiasis is caused by the trematode *Fasciolopsis buski*. The adult fluke lives in the duodenum and upper jejunum and occasionally may be found in the colon. The ova are deposited in the stools. If the latter come in contact with fresh water, miracidia are liberated from the ova. These miracidia swim freely until they invade a freshwater snail and mature into infective cercariae. The cercariae, like those of *Fasciola hepatica*, leave the snail and become encysted on water plants. Humans acquire the disease by ingestion of aquatic vegetation. The metacercariae are liberated from the cyst wall by the gastric juice and then mature. The adult subsequently becomes attached to the mucosa of the duodenum.[239,245]

The main pathologic changes are ulceration in the intestinal mucosa and hemorrhages at the areas of attachment. Abscesses may develop occasionally. Both local tissue and peripheral eosinophilia may occur. The symptoms usually are limited to the gastrointestinal tract and include abdominal pain and diarrhea.

Pulmonary distomiasis (paragonimiasis). Paragonimiasis or endemic hemoptysis is caused by trematodes of the genus *Paragonimus*, mainly *P. westermani*. The disease occurs in the Far East, parts of Africa, the South Pacific, and the northern countries of South America. The operculated ova of the parasite pass to the outside with the sputum of the infected individual or in the feces if the sputum has been swallowed. As in all trematodes pathogenic to humans, the ova need a freshwater snail in which to mature to infective forms. The metacercariae liberated by action of gastric juice penetrate the wall of the duodenum and traverse the peritoneal cavity, diaphragm, pleural cavity, and pleura until they reach the lungs, where they mature. The parasite produces cystic spaces or cavities in the lungs, more numerous in the periphery. The adult worms are surrounded by a dense zone of eosinophilic, polymorphonuclear, and chronic inflammatory cell infiltration. A dense fibrous capsule envelops the area. The cavities produced by the presence of the worms contain brownish fluid that is rather viscid and resembles anchovy sauce. The fluid is composed of the inflammatory exudate, erythrocytes, eosinophils, and numerous ova.

Chronic cough productive of brownish sputum, thoracic discomfort, and recurring hemoptysis are the dominant clinical features of this disease. Other organs such as the brain, liver, intestine, and muscles may be affected. Secondary pulmonary infections, with consequent development of pneumonitis, pulmonary abscesses, and destruction of bronchi, occur rather frequently. In the later stages of the disease there are diffuse areas of focal fibrosis, which may adversely affect pulmonary function and produce chronic cor pulmonale. Pulmonary osteoarthropathy may be present in long-standing cases. The metacercariae that do not reach the lungs but remain in other organs produce small granulomas. These granulomas contain large numbers of eosinophils. Definite diagnosis of this condition rests on finding the characteristic ova in the sputum or the feces.[230] Immunologic tests have been developed for diagnosis.[251]

Schistosomiasis (bilharziasis)

Three different species of blood flukes or schistosomes are pathogenic to humans and are distributed in different regions of the globe. The urinary form of schistosomiasis, caused by *Schistosoma haematobium*, occurs mostly in Africa. In the Far East the responsible agent is *S. japonicum*. *S. mansoni* is seen in Africa, in parts of the Antilles, and in the northern part of South America. Blood flukes are known as schistosomes because of the "split body" on the ventral side of the male, in which the female is held during insemination and egg laying.

The ova of the different schistosomes are passed in the feces or urine of the infected mammal, usually a human. If they gain access to fresh water, free-swimming miracidia are hatched, and they penetrate certain species of freshwater snails. Numerous cercariae are liberated from the mollusk and enter the intact skin or mucosa of a person bathing in or wading through an infected pond, stream, or irrigation canal. Infection is far more frequent during the middle of the day when sunlight is very strong, for these cercariae are phototropic.

The fork-tailed cercariae lose their tails while entering the skin and thus become known as schistosomula. The latter enter through the lymphatics of the dermis and pass through the regional lymph nodes, apparently reaching the circulation through the thoracic duct. They pass through the pulmonary circuit, from the right to the left side of the heart, and finally enter the systemic circulation. The schistosomula, insofar as is known, can mature only in the intrahepatic portal veins, where each schistosomulum develops into an adult male or female worm. Apparently only those able to pass from the arterial to the venous side survive. This takes place for the most part in the abdominal organs drained by the portal system. The adult worms travel against the mesenteric circulation, where they copulate and where the females deposit their ova. Oviposition takes place in the urinary plexuses in the case of schistosomiasis haematobia and in the mesenteric and the hemorrhoidal plexuses in schistosomiasis japonica and mansoni. The ova are laid in narrow venules in the submucosa of the intestine or the urinary bladder, depending on the species. The ova are retained in these organs, swept back into the liver, or passed with the urine or feces.

Schistosomiasis has been referred to as an immunologic disease.[292] The pathogenesis of both acute and chronic schistosomiasis appears to involve immunologic mechanisms, either humoral or cell mediated. The major component of the host immune response against the schistosomula is the eosinophil.[291] Eosinophils have been shown to adhere to the surface of the schistosomula in the presence of antibody or complement. This is followed by degranulation and the release of granule contents, which include lysosomal hydrolytic enzymes, peroxidase, and major basic protein. Major basic protein is an arginine-rich cationic protein that seems to be the main effector of schistosomal damage.[253-255] The role of other effectors of eosinophil-mediated damage, such as the generation of the toxic oxygen metabolites superoxide and hydrogen peroxide, is uncertain.[268,282] Although neutrophils[266] and macrophages[252c] have been shown in vitro to be cytotoxic to schistosomula, their role as effector cells in schistosome immunity is unclear.[256]

The schistosomula attempt to evade the host's immune system by several mechanisms. They lose some of their surface antigens and mask others with a coat of host molecules[290] that include blood group and major histocompatibility antigens.[257,288] The schistosomula also develop an outer tegument or cytoplasmic syncytium comprised of two lipid bilayers, which is resistant to immune damage.[288]

The definitive diagnosis of schistosomiasis can be made only by finding schistosome eggs in urine or feces or in a proctoscopic mucosal biopsy. Serodiagnostic methods are available and include indirect immunofluorescence, circumoval precipitin test,[265] radioimmunoassay,[283,287] and enzyme-linked immunosorbent assay.[263,264,270,276] These tests are valuable in epidemiologic studies or in diagnosis of ectopic or central nervous system schistosomiasis where results of routine tests would be negative. Sonography has also been suggested as an adjunct in the diagnosis of schistosomal hepatic fibrosis and other schistosomal syndromes.[252]

Schistosomiasis mansoni

Acute schistosomiasis mansoni. The entrance of cercariae into the skin has been associated with immediate cutaneous manifestations. The pruritic papular rash or swimmer's itch is thought to be a hypersensitivity reaction, since it is uncommon among previously unexposed individuals. When present it is highly suggestive of reinfection.

Four to 8 weeks after infection a syndrome known as Katayama fever may develop, which includes fever, chills, sweating, headache, and cough. Hepatomegaly accompanied by pronounced eosinophilic infiltration of the portal areas has been encountered in the few cases in which liver biopsies have been performed. The spleen and lymph nodes are enlarged as a result of reticuloendothelial hyperplasia. The classic bilharzial pseudotubercles (Fig. 12-18) with centrally located ova are evident in biopsy specimens obtained 80 days after infection. The liver parenchyma is well preserved, and no biliary duct proliferation or portal fibrosis is evident.

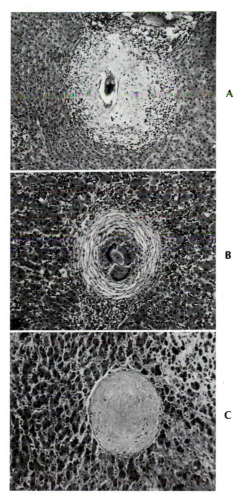

Fig. 12-18. Sequence of changes in pseudotubercles developing about eggs in Manson's schistosomiasis. **A,** Pseudotubercle at height of development is composed mainly of histiocytes (epithelioid cells). **B,** Peripheral capsule of concentric fibroblasts slowly replaces area previously occupied by epithelioid cells as foreign body giant cells digest egg shell. **C,** Ultimate result is fibrous nodule. (**A** and **B,** 80×; **C,** 100×; **A,** from Koppisch, E.: Puerto Rico J. Public Health **13:**1, 1937.)

This syndrome, which coincides with the beginning of oviposition, is more commonly seen in heavy infections. Although recovery is the rule, some fatal cases have occurred, especially with *S. japonicum* infections. This serum sickness–like syndrome is thought to be the result of immune complex formation that follows the antigenic challenge of oviposition.[271]

Chronic schistosomiasis mansoni

INTESTINAL SCHISTOSOMIASIS. The distal parts of the colon are more frequently and severely affected in intestinal schistosomiasis. In the vast majority of cases no gross changes are seen. To be grossly discernible, the infection has to be very severe, producing abundant fibroses or localized polypoid inflammatory lesions.

The lesions are composed of granulation tissue within which are innumerable ova of *S. mansoni* containing living embryos. Numerous chronic inflammatory cells, including moderate numbers of eosinophils, are encountered. These inflammatory polyps may reach 8 cm and may produce bleeding from their ulcerated surfaces. Occasionally a narrow segment of colon may be involved, with ulceration and dense fibrosis of the wall and a reduction in size of the intestinal lumen. The roentgenographic findings resemble those in segmental colitis or carcinoma. In the material available at the University of Puerto Rico School of Medicine, no etiologic relationship could be established between schistosomiasis mansoni and the development of adenocarcinoma of the colon.[273] The small intestine is rarely affected grossly.

HEPATOSPLENIC SCHISTOSOMIASIS. In the group of patients with hepatosplenic schistosomiasis the common denominator is the presence of portal hypertension. The chronic alterations in the liver are attributable to lodgement of the ova of *S. mansoni* in the small intrahepatic portal radicles. The ovum is surrounded by proliferating histiocytes, which give rise to a granulomatous type of reaction. The granulomatous response is a cell-mediated, delayed hypersensitivity–type reaction.[293]

The most frequently encountered vascular lesion is that in which the intrahepatic portal radicle is totally replaced by a granuloma that occludes the lumen (Fig. 12-19). Occasionally an acute endophlebitis of the intrahepatic radicles is encountered, which is probably most important in the final causation of the intrahepatic vascular block.[269] Inflammation and destruction of the coats of the vessels lead to thrombosis. The thrombi become recanalized, and the newly formed blood vessels communicate through the wall of the vein with adjacent vessels outside, forming telangiectasias in the portal areas.

Because of the prominent vascular and fibrotic changes in the portal areas, the latter are moderately broadened and lengthened and stand out in cross section, justifying the gross descriptive term of "pipestem" fibrosis (Fig. 12-20). The liver is enlarged, and the surface is smooth or only slightly nodular but not hobnailed.

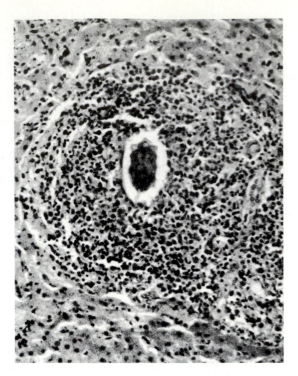

Fig. 12-19. Schistosomiasis mansoni. Granuloma with centrally located living ovum replaces radicle of portal vein. Portal branch of hepatic artery and common duct are visible to right of ovum. (Hematoxylin and eosin; 100×.)

Occasionally the surface is bosselated, forming so-called mountains separated by moderately deep valleys, which correspond to the areas of retraction in the fibrosed portal spaces. These pathologic changes in the liver lead to portal hypertension.

Findings in the adjacent liver parenchyma and the majority of the liver function tests in uncomplicated schistosomiasis mansoni are negative, contrary to the findings in classic liver cirrhosis.[284] The liver block in schistosomiasis mansoni is at the intrahepatic or presinusoidal level, whereas in Laennec's cirrhosis the blockage is at the suprahepatic circulation. We have not noted a parallelism between hepatic schistosomal involvement and liver cell carcinoma. Other workers have reached similar conclusions for both *S. mansoni*[275,286] and *S. japonica*.[279]

Massive congestive splenomegaly develops, with subsequent fibrosis of the pulp and formation of Gamna-Gandy bodies. Esophageal varices complicate the picture of portal hypertension. Death in patients with hepatosplenic involvement usually is attributable to rupture of these varices. Hepatic coma is unusual in the uncomplicated case.[260,261] The same can be said for liver cell necrosis and regeneration.

CARDIOPULMONARY SCHISTOSOMIASIS. Although ova may frequently be found in the lungs of patients with schistosomiasis, the finding of pulmonary obstructive arteriolitis leading to cor pulmonale is less common. This

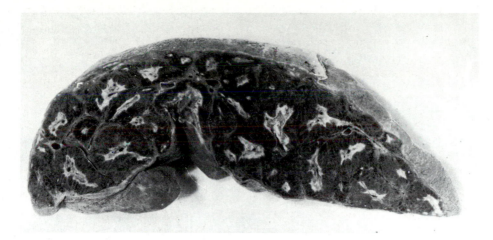

Fig. 12-20. Hepatic fibrosis of "pipestem" type in advanced schistosomiasis mansoni.

condition is rare, probably because considerable egg emboli must reach the lungs before the development of pulmonary arterial schistosomal disease. For sufficient numbers of ova to reach the lungs, portal hypertension with collateral venous channels must be present to allow direct passage of eggs to the right side of the heart and from there to the pulmonary arterial tree. For this reason cardiopulmonary bilharziasis almost always develops in patients with hepatosplenic schistosomiasis.

The wall of the artery is destroyed by an inflammatory process characterized by a granulomatous reaction, with chronic inflammatory cells and occasional eosinophils. This reaction surrounds the ova and extends toward the lumen of the vessel as well as through its wall. Finally it obliterates the lumen of the artery and, in the process of extending through its wall, pushes the fragmented elastic lamina ahead of it, producing a pseudoaneurysm. The result is a dumbbell type of granuloma formed by the intra-arterial and the para-arterial components, joined by a granulomatous isthmus in the destroyed arterial wall. Proliferation of endothelial cells with neoformation of blood vessels occurs in both the intra-arterial and the para-arterial granulomas. These blood vessels form communications among themselves and also with branches of the pulmonary veins destroyed by the para-arterial granulomas (Fig. 12-21). The newly formed blood vessels have been named "intra-arterial angiomatoids."[272] The newly formed blood vessels in the para-arterial granulomas, which form an anastomosis with the pulmonary veins and cause areas of dilatation because of their arteriovenous nature, are the classic angiomatoids considered characteristic of pulmonary schistosomal endarteritis. The occlusion of the arterioles by granulomatous tissue, the pseudoaneurysms, and the arteriovenous communications play a vital role in the causation of hypertension in the lesser circulation, with cor pulmonale and finally right-sided cardiac failure.[285]

A schistosomal glomerulopathy mediated by immune complex deposition has been described. The majority of cases have histopathologic findings consistent with a diffuse membranoproliferative glomerulonephritis in which immune complexes are detected by both immunofluorescent and electron microscopy.[252a]

ECTOPIC GRANULOMATOUS SCHISTOSOMIASIS. Isolated granulomas have been found in practically every organ,[267,294] including the heart. These granulomas do not give rise to clinical manifestations. The term "granulomatous schistosomiasis" is better reserved for those usually solitary lesions composed of numerous eggs, pseudotubercles, granulation tissue, and varying amounts of fibrous tissue that are always located in an ectopic site. These solitary lesions are usually large enough to produce replacement of normal tissues or protrusion into lumina or cavities, which accounts for their symptomatology. The lesions considered ectopic are those encountered outside the portocaval venous circulation, including the extension of the latter into the pulmonary arterioles.

Symptomatic ectopic granulomas in our experience have been most commonly localized to the spinal cord, producing a transverse myelitis.[274]

Schistosomiasis japonica. In the human host the habitat of *S. japonicum* is essentially the lower mesenteric venous system, although it often may be found in the veins of the small and large intestines. Occasionally it may limit itself to the veins of the small intestine. In general, schistosomiasis japonica is characterized by similar but more serious symptoms than those of schistosomiasis mansoni, probably because of the larger number of eggs produced by the parasite.[278]

The small intestine is far more frequently affected than in the mansoni type, and fibrotic stenotic lesions of the bowel are more common. Intestinal polyp formation is likewise more frequent and severe, as is involvement of the liver and lungs. The clinical signs and symptoms are

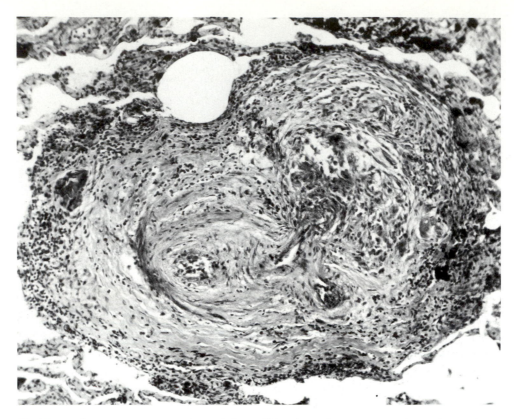

Fig. 12-21. Schistosomiasis mansoni. Newly formed blood vessels in para-arterial granuloma in lung communicate with original, partially destroyed pulmonary arteriole. (Hematoxylin and eosin; 100×.)

thus usually more pronounced than those of schistosomiasis mansoni. An association between schistosomiasis and colonic carcinoma has been reported from the People's Republic of China.[277] Since the investigators fail to show convincing evidence of dysplastic changes in the epithelium away from the carcinomas, we agree with others[280] that the proposed association is inadequately documented.

Schistosomiasis haematobia. S. haematobium is widely distributed throughout Africa. It is also encountered in the Middle East. The vesical and the pelvic venous plexuses constitute the final habitat of *S. haematobium*. Occasionally the parasites may be retained in the hemorrhoidal plexus of veins or in the terminal tributaries of the inferior mesenteric vein, producing lesions in the rectosigmoid as in other schistosomal infections.

The adult female parasite leaves the vesical and pelvic plexuses of veins and migrates into the venules, usually of the submucosa of the urinary bladder, where it lays its eggs. These eggs produce the classic bilharzial granulomas. The latter may coalesce and form larger "bilharzial nodules." These appear as polypoid or plateaulike elevations covered by granular or ulcerated mucosa. The adjacent mucosa becomes hyperplastic and undergoes glandular metaplasia, giving rise to the classic picture of cystitis glandularis. In other areas the mucosa may undergo squamous metaplasia, giving rise to a white patch known as "leukoplakic patch."[262]

The sharp reduction of blood supply caused by the granulomatous process and subsequent fibrosis may produce prominent ulcerations. The atrophy of the surface epithelium overlying plaques of calcified ova accounts for the formation of the "sandy patch." This process is followed by severe cicatrization, which may lead to obstruction. Obstruction is very prominent at the bladder neck and around the urethral orifices. Hydronephrosis[281] and hydroureter[289] may result. Calcifications may eventually occur.

In many of these patients carcinoma of the urinary bladder may develop.[258] The general consensus is that cancer of the bladder is related to urinary bilharziasis, but the exact relationship still remains obscure.[252b,259] The disease also may affect the prostate, seminal vesicles, spermatic cord, epididymis, testes, penis, penile urethra, and female urethra.

Diseases caused by cestodes (tapeworms)
Taeniasis saginata

Taenia saginata (beef tapeworm), a flatworm averaging 4 to 12 m (12 to 36 feet) in length, grows in the human intestinal tract; humans are the only definitive host. It attaches itself to the mucosa of the small intestine, usu-

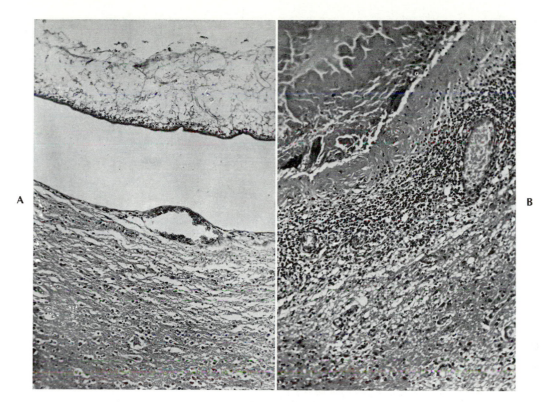

Fig. 12-22. Cerebral cysticercosis. **A,** Part of wall of larval cyst is included above. As long as cyst is alive, cerebral substance, below, shows only compression atrophy. **B,** When cyst dies, it is converted into formless debris that evokes granulomatous inflammatory reaction in surrounding cerebral tissues. (80×.)

ally in the jejunum, by four suckers. The worm contains from 1000 to 2000 proglottids. Ova develop in the distal half of the worm. The proglottids containing developing ova are cast off. Cattle ingest the liberated eggs or gravid proglottids occasionally released in the fecal stream. Within cattle the embryos hatch in the intestinal tract and finally migrate to skeletal muscle, where they develop to the next larval stage (cysticercus). Humans become infected by eating uncooked or poorly cooked meat harboring these larvae, which develop into adult worms in the intestine. Usually there is only one adult worm, but occasionally numerous adult worms are present. The symptoms are either allergic or nervous in nature, but in 72% of cases symptoms also are referable to the digestive system.[300]

Taeniasis solium

T. solium (pork tapeworm) ranges in length from 2 to 7 m (7 to 23 feet) and lives in the human small intestine. In contrast to *T. saginata*, it attaches itself to the mucosa of the small intestine by its head or scolex, which contains hooklets. In cases of taeniasis solium, generally only one worm is found, as the name implies, but occasionally there may be two or three. The ova or proglottids passed by humans in the feces are ingested by the intermediate host, the pig. The liberated embryos or oncospheres

penetrate the venules in the intestinal wall of the pig, enter the blood, and are carried to various organs and tissues. The embryo develops into the next larval stage, a cysticercus (formerly called *Cysticercus cellulosae*). A cysticercus consists of a small ovoid vesicle about 5 mm long and 10 mm wide, having an invagination on one side containing a small white spot that represents the scolex and its hooklets. Humans acquire the intestinal infection by the ingestion of viable cysticerci in undercooked pork. The cysticercus matures into the adult *T. solium* in the human intestine.

Cysticercosis. When an individual ingests food or water contaminated with the feces of a person harboring the eggs of *T. solium*, the cysticerci develop in the tissues. Individuals infected with *T. solium* may infect themselves when their fingers convey ova to the mouth. It is possible, although not probable, that in a few cases autoinfection may take place when ova or ripe proglottids are regurgitated into the stomach or duodenum. The larvae are liberated in the stomach or duodenum and penetrate through the wall, gaining access to the circulation. They travel in the bloodstream and subsequently develop into encysted larvae of cysticerci in tissue. In order of frequency, the tissues affected are the subcutaneous tissue, brain, muscles, heart, liver, lungs, and peritoneum. When the cysticerci are alive (Fig. 12-22, A), very slight

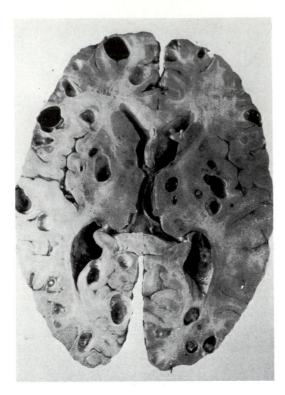

Fig. 12-23. Cerebral cysticercosis. Larval cysts may still be seen within some cavities, whereas they have dropped out of others. (From Ash, J.E., and Spitz, S.: Pathology of tropical diseases, Philadelphia, 1945, W.B. Saunders Co.; AFIP.)

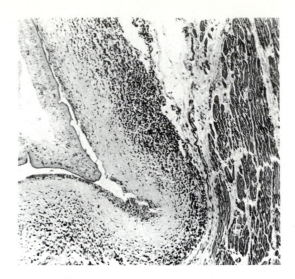

Fig. 12-24. Cysticercosis of myocardium. (Hematoxylin and eosin; 100×.)

inflammatory reaction, lymphocytic in type, is elicited. As soon as the larvae die, the cysticercus is surrounded by a dense infiltration composed of polymorphonuclear leukocytes, chronic inflammatory cells, epithelioid cells, and occasional foreign body giant cells (Fig. 12-22, *B*). Outside this zone is a zone of fibrosis and chronic inflammatory cell infiltration. Calcification is the result. In the subcutaneous tissue the larvae are palpable and firm. Roentgenograms of the soft tissues will disclose foci of calcification representing the end stage of the cysticerci. The average period of time for calcification to take place is 5 years.

Cysticerci do most damage to the brain and meninges. The larvae may project from the ependymal lining into the ventricles or may be located within the cerebral substance (Fig. 12-23). The symptoms produced by the cerebral cysticerci depend on the number of larvae present and their anatomic location. They may manifest themselves as space-occupying lesions, giving rise to symptoms of a cerebral neoplasm, or they may cause obstruction to the cerebrospinal fluid, with subsequent hydrocephalus.[297,309,317] There is glial proliferation around the larvae, and there also may be fibrosis of the leptomeninges. Occasionally cysticerci tend to grow as grapelike clusters and are then termed cysticercus racemosus. Epileptic seizures frequently are associated with cerebral

cysticercosis.[314] Occasionally cysticerci develop beneath the retina, and the subsequent inflammation leads to iridocyclitis and secondary glaucoma. When the heart is involved (Fig. 12-24), the cysticerci occur within the myocardium and valves. There may be cardiac arrhythmias.

Radiologic tests, including computed tomography scan[298,299] and arteriography, can be used for the diagnosis of cysticercosis. Serodiagnostic tests are useful in confirming the diagnosis.[306] Methods available include indirect hemagglutination, complement fixation,[308] indirect immunofluorescence,[313] and enzyme-linked immunosorbent assay.[301]

Diphyllobothriasis

Diphyllobothriasis is found principally among fish-eating people in the Scandinavian countries, in Russia, and in parts of Asia. In the United States it is found in northern Michigan,[312] Wisconsin, and Minnesota. The infection is extremely rare in tropical areas. The causative agent, *Diphyllobothrium latum* (fish tapeworm), measures between 3 and 10 m (10 and 33 feet) in length and is composed of 3000 or more proglottids. Humans and other mammals, especially dogs, acquire the infection by eating undercooked fish or fish products. The worm lives in the small intestine; the presence of multiple worms is not uncommon.

Infected individuals may be symptomless or may be asthenic and suffer from gastrointestinal disorders, especially abdominal pain. Occasionally a megaloblastic anemia (bothriocephalus anemia) is seen, especially when the worm is implanted high in the small intestine. The exact mechanism for the production of anemia has not been fully elucidated.[315] One explanation for the anemia is that the worm produces an enzyme that interferes with the association between vitamin B_{12} and the intrinsic factor.[319] The uncomplexed vitamin B_{12} is not absorbed in the ileum and is available for the tapeworm's utilization.[320] Megaloblastic hyperactivity of the bone marrow and even central nervous system degeneration may be encountered in some patients.

Differential diagnosis should be made primarily between tapeworm anemia and genuine pernicious anemia. Free hydrochloric acid in the gastric juice, remission after the worm cure without additional therapy, and a Schilling test value that becomes normal after the expulsion of the parasite constitute evidence of tapeworm anemia.[318]

Echinococcosis (echinococcal disease, hydatid disease)

Echinococcosis is caused by the adult tapeworm *Echinococcus granulosus*. The parasite is 3 to 6 mm in length. It attaches itself to the mucosa of the small intestine of its definitive hosts, the dog, wolf, and other carnivorous animals. The ova are discharged in the feces. These are ingested by intermediary hosts such as sheep, cattle, hogs, or humans. In humans the disease is usually acquired from an infected dog, frequently a sheep dog. The definitive host becomes infected by eating the entrails of the infected intermediary host.

The ova of *E. granulosus* are passed free as gravid proglottids in the dog feces. When swallowed by the intermediary host, the six-hooked embryo is liberated in the duodenum and penetrates the duodenal wall until it reaches the venules. Embryos that are not filtered by the liver may reach the lungs, and only a few go through the pulmonary circulation to the left side of the heart and then into the arterial circulation. The embryos that survive develop into hydatid cysts containing numerous scolices provided with hooklets. These scolices represent the future head of the adult tapeworm.

The cysts have an outer laminated, elastic layer and an inner germinal layer. They enlarge gradually for several months until they attain a diameter of 10 to 20 cm. Abundant clear fluid is contained within the cysts. The germinal layer develops numerous papillae, which become pedunculated vesicles (brood capsules) containing scolices (Fig. 12-25). The tapeworm *Echinococcus multilocularis* produces multilocular or alveolar cysts in the intermediate host (humans and other animals). Cysts of echinococcosis occur more frequently in the liver or in the lung. Approximately 70% of primary echinococcal cysts are found in the liver (Fig. 12-26), and four out of every five of these are in the right lobe.[296]

It has been estimated that approximately 25% of people infected with *Echinococcus* go through life without any symptoms referable to the tapeworm.[311] Symptoms may take a long time to develop, for the disease progresses slowly. The cysts may become secondarily infected, suppurate, and produce the clinical picture of hepatic abscess. Some of the cysts may collapse and

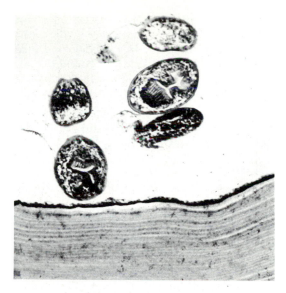

Fig. 12-25. Wall of echinococcal cyst disclosing numerous scolices, with hooklets evident in some. (Hematoxylin and eosin; $100\times$.)

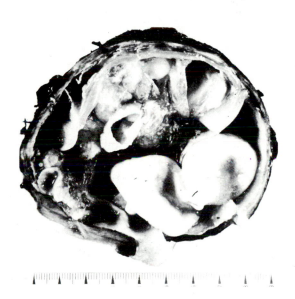

Fig. 12-26. Large echinococcal cyst of liver. (Courtesy Dr. Diego Ribas-Mujal; from Marcial-Rojas, R.A.: Parasitic diseases of the liver. In Schiff, L., editor: Diseases of the liver, Philadelphia, 1969, J.B. Lippincott Co.)

undergo fibrosis and, not infrequently, calcification. When the alveolar type of hydatid cyst develops in the liver, the gross appearance resembles that of a malignant tumor. The hydatid fluid, when liberated into the circulation, gives rise to pronounced eosinophilia. There may be allergic manifestations such as urticaria and angioneurotic edema. Diffuse implantation in the peritoneal or pleural cavities may develop after rupture of subpleural and subperitoneal cysts.

Eosinophilia is present in 25% of cases. The diagnosis of hepatic hydatid disease is suggested by the presence of an abdominal mass detected by palpation and confirmed by sonography,[303,310] liver scans, or computed tomography scans.[302] The diagnosis must then be confirmed serologically. Of the multiple methods available,[307,316] which include complement fixation, enzyme-linked immunosorbent assay,[304,305] and indirect hemagglutination, the last is the test of choice.[307]

Diseases caused by nematodes
Diseases caused by nematodes of the digestive tract

Ascariasis. Ascaris lumbricoides is a nematode of worldwide distribution, most prevalent in tropical and subtropical countries. The incidence and severity of the infection are closely related to hygienic levels. The incidence in some areas of Europe and the Orient is reported to be as high as 90% to 94%. One billion people are estimated to be infected by ascariasis.[401] Endemic regions exist in the United States, especially in the Southeast, where 30% to 40% of the rural population has been found to be infected.

The adult worms range from 15 to 30 cm in length and from 3 to 5 mm in diameter. The eggs are deposited in the soil, where they undergo a period of incubation. The infection is acquired by ingestion of the fully embryonated ova. The larvae are hatched in the small intestine and penetrate the wall, reaching the lungs by way of venules or lymphatics. They pass into the alveoli from the alveolar capillaries and migrate up the main bronchial tree and down the esophagus with the swallowed saliva. In the small intestine they grow into adult males or females. In severe infections, during the period of lung migration, the larvae produce areas of hemorrhage and inflammatory reaction characterized by the presence of neutrophils and eosinophils. A clinical picture resembling bronchial asthma and diffuse peribronchitis, with occasional hemoptysis, is sometimes encountered.[321,350,398]

Ascariasis is usually a benign and self-limited disease because of the short life span of the adult worm (6 to 12 months). The most frequent complications of ascariasis are caused by the adult parasite. Large masses of worms may produce intestinal obstruction[331] (Fig. 12-27) and rarely may lead to perforation[374] and peritonitis.[386] Although ascariasis has been shown to have an adverse effect on nutritional status,[330,332] there is little evidence that it can cause intestinal malabsorption.[333]

Ascaris worms have a tendency to wander into natural passages and may migrate into the biliary system, pancreatic duct, or lumen of the appendix. They may obstruct the extrahepatic biliary tree and produce jaundice, ascending cholangitis, or acute cholecystitis. Single or multiple abscesses of the liver are sometimes produced. Occasionally the adult worms migrate into the upper respiratory passages.

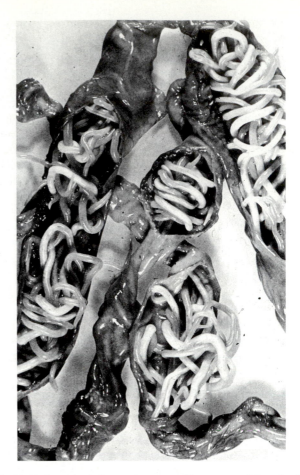

Fig. 12-27. Intestinal obstruction caused by masses of *Ascaris* adult worms in young child. (Courtesy Dr. Rafael Ramirez-Weiser, San Juan, Puerto Rico.)

Diagnosis is based on fecal examination. Serologic tests have been developed but are rarely used for diagnostic purposes.[368,397]

Trichuriasis (trichocephaliasis). One of the most common intestinal parasites of humans in tropical areas is *Trichuris trichiura*, formerly *Trichocephalus trichiurus*, also known as the whipworm. In some regions of the world (such as in some areas of Puerto Rico), more than 90% of the population is infected.[383]

The disease is contracted through the ingestion of food or water containing the ova. The larvae are released from the embryonated ova into the small intestine and become attached to the mucosa. Subsequently, they migrate downward to their usual habitat in the ileocecal region (Fig. 12-28). The anterior tip of the whipworm rarely penetrates below the muscularis mucosae, thus eliciting practically no reaction on the part of the tissues. In cases of massive infection with *T. trichiura*, prominent hyperemia and edema of the mucosa with occasional ulcerations may be produced, but in the majority of cases the infection does not produce symptoms. Although in severe cases blood-streaked stools are observed, there is controversy as to whether this amount

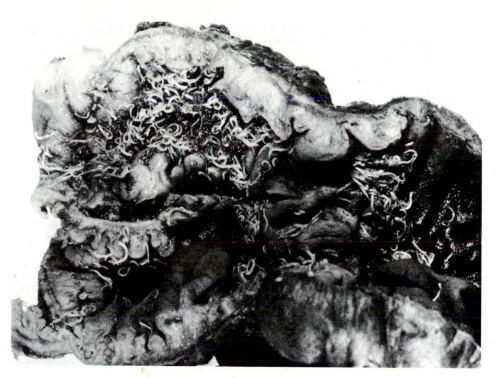

Fig. 12-28. Massive infestation with *Trichuris*, which produced severe hemorrhagic diarrhea and death in very young child.

of intestinal blood loss is enough to cause anemia.[353,362,364] In the most severe cases rectal prolapse may occur. Rapid, severe dehydration and concomitant electrolyte imbalance may cause death. Peripheral eosinophilia is practically never seen in pure *Trichuris* infection. Diagnosis is made by finding the characteristic ova on stool examination.

Ancylostomiasis (uncinariasis, hookworm disease). Hookworm disease is one of the most prevalent diseases in the world. It is not limited to tropical and subtropical areas but may be encountered in temperate climates. The disease is caused by *Ancylostoma duodenale*, the Old World hookworm, or by *Necator americanus*, the New World hookworm.[341]

From the ova deposited in the ground, rhabditiform larvae are hatched. These develop into the infective filariform larvae in about 5 to 8 days. The latter penetrate the skin, much like the filariform larvae of *Strongyloides*. The passage of the filariform larvae through the skin produces a sometimes severe irritation or dermatitis known as ground itch. This generally occurs in the feet, between and beneath the toes, since most people who acquire the infection live in impoverished and unsanitary areas and usually walk barefoot. The filariform larvae gain access to the lymphatics or the venules and finally reach the pulmonary circulation. From the interalveolar capillaries, they pass into the alveolar sacs, up the tracheobronchial tree, and eventually into the gastrointestinal tract. In the passage through the lungs, petechial

hemorrhages and areas of transient bronchopneumonia are produced. On reaching the small intestine, especially the duodenum and first portion of the jejunum, the adult parasites attach themselves to the mucosa by means of a well-developed buccal capsule (Fig. 12-29). In so doing, they damage small areas of the mucosa, producing punctate hemorrhages, and at the same time they draw blood from the mucosa. In heavy infections there is considerable blood loss as a result of both direct continuity between the oropharynx of the parasite and mucosal blood vessels and free bleeding from multiple points of attachment of the parasites, since they migrate from one area to another. The resulting classic picture of hookworm disease is characterized by severe, hypochromic microcytic anemia with deficiency of iron. The anemia usually is complicated by other nutritional deficiencies that are prevalent in economically poor, underdeveloped areas.

Although small intestinal mucosal changes of villous atrophy and crypt hyperplasia have been described,[369,407] the issue of whether ancylostomiasis can cause malabsorption is still unresolved.[333] When the severe sideropenic anemia occurs in young children, it retards growth as well as sexual and mental development. The presence of characteristic ova in the stools establishes the diagnosis. Serologic tests are available[379] but play little role in clinical diagnosis.[369]

Enterobiasis (oxyuriasis). Enterobiasis is a very common parasitic disease of cosmopolitan distribution. The

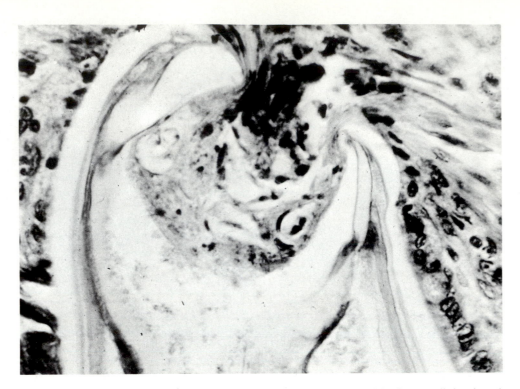

Fig. 12-29. *Ancylostoma caninum* attached to mucosa of small intestine of dog by its well-developed buccal capsule. (Hematoxylin and eosin; 430×.)

causative nematode is *E. vermicularis*, formerly known as *Oxyuris vermicularis* or commonly as the pinworm or threadworm. The disease is acquired by ingestion of the fully embryonated ova deposited by the female worm about the anus and transferred to other hosts by fecal contamination or to the same host to produce reinfection. The ova are very resistant to destruction, and the infection occasionally affects all persons in the same household. The life span of the worm is short (1½ to 2 months), and the chief problem is reinfection. The larvae are hatched from the fully embryonated ova in the region of the duodenum and then pass downward while they molt twice and mature, until they reach the ileocecal area. The adult worms attach themselves to the superficial portion of the mucosa of the terminal ileum, cecum, and appendix by their anterior end.

The pathologic changes produced by the adult worms in this area are minimal, and their role in the pathogenesis of appendicular symptoms in some cases is by no means settled.[372] It is our impression that, even when adult worms are present in acute appendicitis, they are not a significant cause of inflammation but merely represent a fortuitous association (Fig. 12-30).

The most important symptom of this disease is intense pruritus ani caused by the migration of the adult female worm to the perianal region, where she lays her eggs. The adult male worm is unimportant in the pathogenesis, since it dies after copulation.

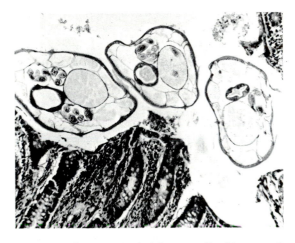

Fig. 12-30. *Enterobius vermicularis* in appendix. (Hematoxylin and eosin; 100×.)

Rarely, *E. vermicularis* can be seen in extraintestinal sites.[335] In females the nematode migrates up the uterus and fallopian tubes to produce a foreign body type of granulomatous inflammation most commonly seen in the surface of the ovaries,[327] omentum, and peritoneum. This parasite apparently cannot survive outside its natural habitat, and the granulomatous reaction described occurs after death of the worms.

Other less common ectopic sites include the urinary bladder, lung,[325] and liver.[363] An association has been reported between enterobiasis and lower urinary tract infections, with the nematode acting as a carrier of enteric bacteria when it migrates from the perianal region to the urinary bladder.[393] Diagnosis is made by identifying the ova by a cellophane-tape test.

Trichiniasis (trichinosis, trichinelliasis). A cosmopolitan disease, trichiniasis is most common in the temperate areas of the United States and Europe and is caused by *Trichinella spiralis*. The infection, although not as common as in the past, is still encountered in approximately 5% of the autopsies performed in the United States.[412] An average of 150 new cases are reported annually[399] to the Centers for Disease Control.

Humans usually become infected by eating raw or undercooked pork. Other sources of infection are walrus and bear meat.[389]

The larvae of the parasite become encysted in the muscles of the infected animal and are ingested by humans. During ingestion these larvae are liberated by proteolytic enzymes and pass on to the small intestine. The larvae attach themselves to the mucosa and attain sexual maturity within 2 days. Electron microscopic studies have identified the intracellular nature of both the enteric larvae and the adult worm.[409] The parasite inhabits the cytoplasm of either absorptive or goblet cells.

During its development the parasite expresses different surface antigenic constituents to which the host humoral and cellular immune system responds.[366,375] The multiple responses directed against the infectious larvae, the developing larvae, and the adult worm act synergistically to protect the host.[328]

The adult male worm dies soon after copulation, and the female adult dies after larviposition is completed.

Between 1000 and 1500 larvae may be produced by the female. Most of these larvae enter the lymphatics or the venules of the lamina propria. After traversing the pulmonary circulation, they enter the systemic circulation and are carried to all organs and tissues of the body.

The symptomatology during the period of invasion of the intestinal wall is the result of gastrointestinal irritation by the adult worm, which produces nausea, vomiting, diarrhea or constipation, and abdominal cramps. During the stage of hematogenous dissemination or migration, the symptoms are rather variable and are more frequently characterized by muscle aches, fever, chemosis of the conjunctivae, and occasionally prostration. Severe peripheral eosinophilia is frequently seen. The eosinophilic cell count may reach a value of 70% or more of the total white blood cell count.

The larvae become encysted only in striated voluntary muscles, although they also reach the heart, lungs, brain, and meninges. Once they penetrate individual

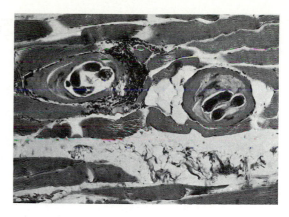

Fig. 12-31. Two *Trichinella* larvae encysted in voluntary muscle of rat infected experimentally. (180×.)

muscle fibers, they grow in size and then coil in corkscrew fashion and proceed to encyst.

The muscles most frequently affected are the diaphragmatic, gastrocnemius, intercostal, deltoid, gluteal, and pectoral. The parasitized muscle fiber becomes strongly basophilic. This process, once mislabeled "basophilic degeneration," is the result of increased muscle fiber endoplasmic reticulum and ribosomal RNA content.[342] The parasitized muscle fiber, called a "nurse cell," lives for extended periods. An inflammatory reaction in which lymphocytes and eosinophils predominate develops around the nurse cell–parasite unit. As in other helminthic infections, eosinophil leukocytes play a major role in the host immune response.[355] Elevated IgE levels are partially responsible for this level of eosinophilia.[344] Eosinophils adhere to the migrating parasite by an antibody-mediated process. Being unable to phagocytose the parasite, the eosinophil degranulates, releasing hydrolytic enzymes, cationic proteins such as major basic protein, and hydrogen peroxide, which destroy the larvae.[324,334,359,402]

The infected muscle fiber is destroyed by the inflammatory process, and adjacent muscle fibers undergo hyaline degeneration. A fibrous wall or capsule develops around the larvae, producing small cysts averaging 1 mm or less in diameter (Fig. 12-31). The wall of these cysts subsequently may calcify after 6 months to 2 years. The trichinae themselves also may undergo calcification.

Growth of larvae and encystation do not occur in cardiac muscles. In the cardiac muscle, acute inflammatory changes may be seen in the early stage of the infection, leading to a patchy or diffuse interstitial myocarditis. The larvae in the myocardium undergo necrosis and usually cannot be identified. Foci of necrosis in the muscle fibers of the myocardium and the nonspecific myocarditis are most noticeable in the area close to the epicardium.

The central nervous system usually reacts to invasion by the larvae with a diffuse leptomeningeal round cell type of infiltration.[376] Minute foci of gliosis around capillaries occasionally are seen. Renal involvement by an immune-mediated glomerulonephritis has been recently described.[394] Immune complex deposition in vessels has been suggested as a cause of vasculitis.[347]

The mortality in this disease is extremely low. Death may ensue in very severe, overwhelming infections as a result of involvement of the respiratory muscles, with secondary pulmonary complications. Involvement of the myocardium is the most common cause of death; massive involvement may lead to cardiac failure. A recent case report recognized trichiniasis as a possible fatal infection in the immunosuppressed host.[356]

The best method for diagnosis is muscle biopsy obtained from the tendinous insertions of the deltoid or gastrocnemius muscles. Serologic tests are available and usually show positive results after the third week of disease. Methods include the bentonite flocculation test, immunofluorescence, enzyme-linked immunosorbent assay, counterimmunoelectrophoresis, and gel diffusion.[343]

Capillariasis

Capillariasis hepatica. This disease is caused by the nematode *Capillaria (Hepaticola) hepatica.* This helminth is common in the liver of rats and, less frequently, in mice, hares, dogs, muskrats, beavers, and some species of monkeys. Human infections are rare; only about 25 authenticated cases have been reported in the world's literature.

The eggs are discharged in fecal matter or are released from the decaying carcasses of affected animals. The ova are nonembryonated and must attain maturity and infectivity when they reach the soil. They require certain conditions of humidity. Humans acquire the disease by ingesting food or dirt contaminated with embryonated ova. The ova hatch in the cecum; the free larvae penetrate venules of the portal system and ultimately reach the liver, where they mature. About 4 weeks after infection the adult worms disintegrate and release large numbers of ova in the liver substance.

Spurious infections are occasionally present in humans and are acquired by eating the undercooked or raw liver of a habitual host. In these instances the eggs are nonembryonated and are passed in the stools without undue harm to the individual.

The majority of cases occur in children or institutionalized mental patients. As would be expected from the life cycle of this organism, instances of the human disorder appear in persons who have dirt-eating habits or live in substandard sanitary conditions.

The clinical picture of an enlarged liver and a high-grade eosinophilia in a young patient must be differentiated from that of toxocariasis or visceral larva migrans. The diagnosis of this disease can be established only by liver biopsy, since ova are present only in the liver substance and are not detectable in intestinal content.[323]

The liver is enlarged with a smooth surface, and beneath the capsule are numerous grayish or yellowish white nodules measuring 0.1 to 0.2 cm. Many of these coalesce and form lesions 2 to 3 cm in diameter. The granulomas are composed of epithelioid cells and multinucleated giant cells surrounding parasites or ova. Occasionally necrosis is apparent with or without cuticular fragments of the disintegrated worms or ova. Peripheral portions of the granulomas exhibit a heavy infiltration of plama cells, eosinophils, and macrophages. The adjacent liver plates undergo degeneration and contain a similar inflammatory cell infiltration. Ultimately there may be extensive scarring in which ova may be preserved. Many eggs are engulfed by multinucleated giant cells. An experimental model has been developed in mice for a *C. hepatica* egg granuloma. The model suggests that granuloma formation has an immunologic basis in which both cell- and humoral-mediated immune responses participate.[384,385,395,396]

The ova of *C. hepatica* are barrel shaped, as are those of *Trichuris trichiura*, but possess a double shell containing visible radiations between the two layers.

Most cases reported in the literature have been fatal, since infections tend to be severe. In all probability, however, there are many unreported infections of lesser severity that remain clinically inapparent with mild and nonspecific manifestations.

Capillariasis philippinensis. *Capillaria philippinensis* has been held responsible for a severe form of protein-losing enteropathy associated with a malabsorption syndrome.[403] The disease may lead to death in 20% of cases, especially when severe bacterial infections supervene owing to the hypogammaglobulinemic state.[377] The disease may acquire epidemic proportions.[345,403,406]

It has been shown that the worm reproduces by internal autoinfection,[349] as the presence of larviparous female parasites in the lumen of the intestine has suggested.[345] The life cycle of *C. philippinensis* is still unknown. It is suggested by clinical evidence and animal experimentation that the disease is acquired by eating small uncooked fish.[338,406]

The parasites may penetrate the surface intestinal mucosa and that of the crypts but are not seen beyond the muscularis mucosae.[323] The parasite induces only a very mild inflammatory response, composed mostly of plasma cells and lymphocytes with some eosinophils. The exact mechanism by which the parasite produces the severe protein-losing enteropathy remains to be elucidated.[405] Roentgenographic examination reveals a classical malabsorption pattern in the small intestine.[377]

Diagnosis is based on the identification of the parasite in stool examination or mucosal biopsy of the small intestine.

Larva migrans

Cutaneous larva migrans. The localized or cutaneous form of larva migrans, also known as creeping eruption, results from infection with the canine or feline strains of *Ancylostoma braziliense* and less commonly with *A. caninum*. The disease is usually contracted at beaches or sandy playgrounds where cats or dogs have deposited their feces. The infective larvae penetrate the skin and migrate at a rate of about 2.5 cm daily, producing serpiginous tunnels between the stratum germinativum and the stratum spinosum.[346] The elevated tunnels frequently become vesicular, and the involved tissue is infiltrated by chronic inflammatory cells and numerous eosinophils. Because of severe pruritus and scratching, secondary infection frequently occurs.

Visceral larva migrans. Visceral larva migrans is a syndrome seen primarily in children under 4 years of age. It is characterized by pronounced and prolonged eosinophilia (in virtually 100% of cases), hepatomegaly (87%), pulmonary symptoms (50%), fever,[401] and other systemic manifestations. This condition was frequently referred to in the literature as tropical infiltrative eosinophilia, Löffler's syndrome, and even benign eosinophilic leukemia until the specific larvae of *Toxocara canis* were identified by Beaver and associates.[326]

In addition to high serum immunoglobulin levels, anti-A and anti-B titers are detected because the *Toxocara* larvae contain surface antigens that stimulate isohemagglutinins.[391]

This clinical syndrome can be produced by (1) human helminthic infections having an extraintestinal cycle but with localization in the intestine, (2) such infections but with localization outside the intestine, and (3) animal helminthic infections that occasionally affect humans. Examples of the first group are ascariasis, strongyloidiasis, and hookworm disease. Examples of the second are schistosomiasis and fascioliasis. The third group, diseases caused by larvae of nematodes normally parasitic in lower animals, is the most interesting one and the one to which the term *visceral larva migrans* is specifically applied. Secondary stage *T. canis* and *T. catis* larvae have been recognized as etiologic agents of visceral larva migrans.[326] The third-stage larva of *Ancylostoma caninum* is probably also an etiologic agent. *Capillaria hepatica* also may cause visceral larva migrans.

Only a few postmortem examinations of patients with visceral larva migrans have been performed.[322] The liver usually is enlarged with small gray-white nodules, 2 to 4 mm in diameter, scattered throughout the parenchyma (Fig. 12-32). Microscopically the nodules are composed of numerous eosinophils, Langhans' giant cells, and larvae. In patients with severe hyperergy, eosinophilic abscesses and adjacent hepatic necrosis are prominent. Other viscera may be affected. Massive fatal myocarditis has resulted from the presence of larvae within the myocardium.[322] Larvae also may localize in the eye, usually in the posterior chamber. They give rise to a granuloma that can cause detachment of the retina. The granuloma may simulate retinoblastoma clinically.[408] The granulo-

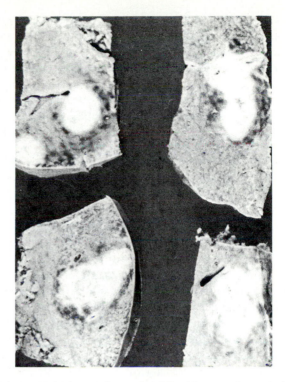

Fig. 12-32. Multiple, confluent, grayish white granulomas in liver of patient with visceral larva migrans. (Courtesy Dr. Manuel de Jesús; from Marcial-Rojas, R.A.: Parasitic diseases of the liver. In Schiff, L., editor: Diseases of the liver, Philadelphia, 1969, J.B. Lippincott Co.)

matous response, as in schistosomiasis, seems to be a cell-mediated process.[358]

The diagnosis of visceral larva migrans is difficult. We have been able to confirm the diagnosis by liver biopsy in several cases. In one case the larvae were seen in biopsy samples from a cervical lymph node. Of the serologic tests available, enzyme-linked immunosorbent assay[340,352] is sufficiently sensitive and specific to be clinically useful in the diagnosis of toxocariasis.

Strongyloidiasis (strongyloidosis). *Strongyloides stercoralis* is a parasite with a complicated life cycle. Strongyloidiasis occurs not only in tropical and subtropical areas but also in more northerly latitudes. It is not as common as ascariasis, trichuriasis, and ancylostomiasis.

The free-living, nonparasitic, rhabditiform larvae develop from ova in the intestine of humans and are passed in the stools to the soil, where they mature into adult males and females. After copulation of the adult worms, more ova are laid, and rhabditiform larvae hatch from them. This is known as the direct cycle. Under favorable conditions in the soil, the indirect cycle begins by the transformation of the rhabditiform larvae into infective filariform larvae. The infective filariform larvae penetrate the skin or oral mucosa of humans, gain access to venules, and finally reach the alveolar capillaries. In the lungs they mature into adult worms and pass into the alveoli, finally making their way through the tracheobronchial tree into the gastrointestinal tract.

The major anatomic changes are produced in the mucosa of the duodenum and jejunum by the female worms. The mucosa of the intestine becomes hyperemic and edematous. In severe infections, ulcerations are produced. The female worm deposits her eggs in the mucosa, where more rhabditiform larvae develop. Gastrointestinal symptoms include epigastric pain or tenderness, anorexia, nausea and vomiting, diarrhea, and malabsorption.[371,392]

Occasionally the noninfective rhabditiform larvae metamorphose into infective filariform larvae within the intestinal lumen and penetrate either the mucosa of the colon (endogenous autoinfection) or the perianal skin (exogenous autoinfection). The cycle of autoinfection can lead to clinical illness manifested many years after the patient has left an endemic area.[371]

The lungs are affected by the migratory phase of the maturing larvae through the alveoli. Areas of edema, congestion, and consolidation, not unlike those in the migratory phase of ascariasis, may develop.[367] Signs of bronchospasm or pneumonia and episodes of hemoptysis are sometimes seen.[382]

The inflammatory reaction at the site of entrance of the larvae into the skin is similar to that in the intestinal mucosa. It is characterized by a mixed leukocytic infiltration containing numerous eosinophils. The larvae may be seen migrating in the dermis as a type of cutaneous larva migrans.

In immunosuppressed patients the process of endogenous autoinfection can lead to disseminated disease known as hyperinfection.[339,382,387,388] In hyperinfection there are severe inflammatory changes in the intestinal mucosa (mostly of the distal parts of the sigmoid and rectum), and numerous larvae are seen within the mucosa and submucosa (Figs. 12-33 and 12-34). A massive inflammatory reaction develops, characterized by a predominantly eosinophilic infiltrate. These filariform larvae migrate through the systemic circulation and may produce an inflammatory reaction in other organs similar to that occurring in visceral larva migrans. The predominant feature is pulmonary involvement, which leads to respiratory failure and a 90% mortality.[329]

It is apparent that the alterations in the immune mechanism of the host brought about by diseases, such as lymphoma, leprosy, uremia, and severe malnutrition, or by drugs, such as steroids or cytotoxic agents, disturb the immunologic balance between the host and the parasite. This alteration in the immune mechanism of the host, especially of the cell-mediated responses, allows for increased pathogenicity and virulence of the parasite.

Diagnosis of the disease rests on the identification of the rhabditiform or the infective filariform larvae in the stools, duodenal aspirates, or small bowel biopsy specimens. Occasionally the diagnosis is made by demonstrating the larvae in the sputum.[360] Serologic methods of

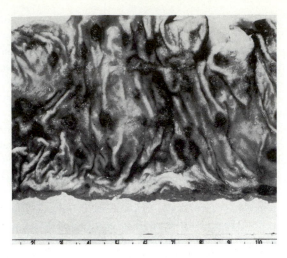

Fig. 12-33. Lesions of intestinal mucosa associated with *Strongyloides* infection. (From Anderson, W.A.D., and Scotti, T.M.: Synopsis of pathology, ed. 10, St. Louis, 1980, The C.V. Mosby Co.)

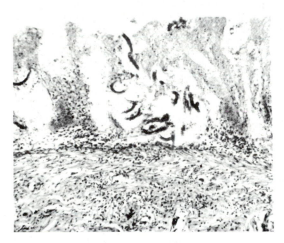

Fig. 12-34. Numerous strongyloidal larvae in mucosa and submucosa of intestine. Hemorrhage and inflammatory cells are evident. (Hematoxylin and eosin; 100×.)

diagnosis include indirect hemagglutination, complement fixation, and immunofluorescence.[354]

Angiostrongyliasis. Eosinophilic meningoencephalitis is acquired by eating land snails and slugs, which are the intermediate hosts of *Angiostrongylus cantonensis*, a lungworm of rats.[381] The first-stage larvae develop from eggs deposited in the lungs of rats by the adult worm living in the pulmonary arteries.[411] The larvae migrate up the trachea and are eventually passed in the feces. The intermediate molluskan hosts acquire the infection by ingesting the feces of infected rats. The third-stage infective larvae develop in mollusks in about 3 weeks.

When humans become infected, the third-stage larvae and the young adult worms usually die, most frequently in the brain (Fig. 12-35), spinal cord, and meninges.[361,378] Larvae sometimes migrate to the eye.[357]

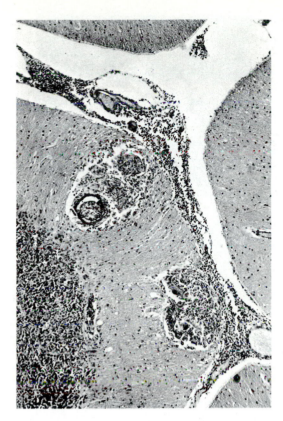

Fig. 12-35. Eosinophilic meningoencephalitis. Remnants of *Angiostrongylus cantonensis* may be seen in cerebellar fissure and cortex. Diffuse infiltration with eosinophils is evident in meninges. (Hematoxylin and eosin; 63×; from Rosen, L., et al.: J.A.M.A. **179:**620, 1962.)

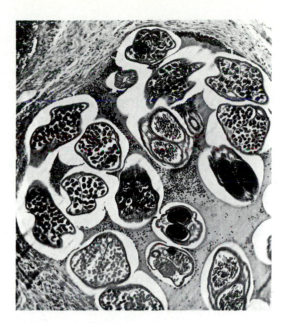

Fig. 12-36. Bancroftian filariasis. Living worms coiled in dilated afferent lymphatic vessel of greatly fibrosed inguinal node provoke only scant inflammatory reaction in wall of lymph vessel. (80×.)

The tissue reaction is characterized by severe eosinophilic infiltration, which is also frequently manifested in the peripheral blood and cerebrospinal fluid. The symptoms are those of a meningoencephalitis indistinguishable from that caused by cysticercosis, trichinosis, paragonimiasis, and schistosomiasis. Gastrointestinal symptoms are also seen.[410] Serodiagnostic methods include a complement fixation test and an indirect fluorescent antibody test[404]; the latter is the more sensitive.

A. costaricensis has been described in Costa Rica,[373] other Central and South American countries,[365] and the United States.[400] It lives as a parasite in the mesenteric arteries of wild rats. The life cycle is similar to that of *A. cantonensis*, although *A. costaricensis* larvae develop in the wall of the intestine. This species affects humans at the level of the wall of the intestine. It is seen usually in young children, who have acute abdominal symptoms, fever, and eosinophilia. Laparotomy reveals an inflammatory granulomatous mass in the appendix, cecum, or terminal ileum. The disease does not affect the central nervous system. Fecal examination is useless because neither eggs nor larvae appear in stools.[348] A precipitin test is available for serodiagnosis of chronic infection and for epidemiologic studies.[390]

Diseases caused by filarial nematodes (filariasis)

Bancroftian filariasis. Bancroftian filariasis is commonly referred to as filariasis. It is caused by *Wuchereria (Filaria) bancrofti*. The mature female worm measures up to 10 cm in length and 3 mm in width, whereas the male is only about one-third this size.

The microfilariae are taken up with the blood of humans by mosquitoes of the genus *Culex* and occasionally of the genera *Aedes* and *Anopheles*. The microfilariae penetrate the stomach wall of the mosquito and reach the thoracic muscles. They undergo multiple changes in the mosquito until they mature and are transmissible to humans. The larvae move down to the proboscis of the mosquito, migrate out of the labium, and are implanted on the human skin. They enter the dermal lymphatics and pass to the regional lymph nodes. Maturity occurs either within the lymph nodes or, more frequently, within the larger lymphatic trunks near the regional lymph nodes (Fig. 12-36). The adult worms copulate, and each female worm produces numerous microfilariae. The microfilariae are liberated into the lymphatics and eventually enter the bloodstream, producing a microfilaremia. In the bloodstream they are again available to complete their cycle if they are taken up by the mosquito.

There is a definite microfilarial periodicity, occurring toward midnight, in most endemic foci. This may be an adaptation to the feeding habits of the vector, which is a night-biting mosquito. A diurnal strain occurs in the South Pacific.

The most frequently involved lymphatic vessels are those of the lower limbs, retroperitoneal tissues, spermatic cord, epididymis, and mammary gland. The presence of worms in these areas, especially in the region of the spermatic cord, does not necessarily imply that the clinical symptoms fever, lymphadenitis, headache, and epididymitis will eventually develop.

In approximately 20% of necropsies on men in Puerto Rico, histopathologic evidence of filariasis is found in the spermatic cord even though there is no clinical history of the disease.[420,421] We have seen patients who have massive microfilaremia without the slightest symptom of the disease.

The pathologic changes in the lymphatics and lymph nodes are attributable to the presence of the adult worm.[435] While the worm is alive, there is minimal reaction on the part of the lymphatics, and the most frequent changes are those of polypoid endolymphangitis and distension of lymphatics. Death of the adult filarial worm is followed by a severe inflammatory reaction that is characterized by fibrinoid necrosis and pronounced eosinophilic infiltration (Fig. 12-37). The inflammatory reaction develops in nodular fashion around fragmented and necrotic worms. Epithelioid cells and foreign body giant cells appear subsequently. These filarial granulomas eventually undergo fibrosis, leaving a concentrically lamellated, hyalinized structure that frequently calcifies (Fig. 12-38). Numerous lymphocytes and plasma cells also are seen in the lesion, mostly in the periphery.

It is evident from the pathologic processes described that lymphatics will be obstructed and that the severity of this obstruction will depend on the number of worms present. When numerous lymphatics are obliterated by fibrosis, lymphedema results. The classical chronic edema of subcutaneous tissues and the consequent proliferation of fibrous connective tissue and thickening of the epidermis are characteristic of elephantiasis. The full-blown picture of elephantiasis usually develops after repeated episodes of lymphadenitis and ascending lymphangitis. In all probability, secondary streptococcal or other type of bacterial infection plays an important role in the pathogenesis of ascending lymphangitis and elephantiasis.[414] In tropical areas the frequency of hydrocele of the tunica vaginalis testis is at least partially related to the incidence of filariasis.[421,428,430]

The microfilariae only rarely produce visible damage. Occasionally small granulomas, measuring 1 to 2 cm in diameter, are discovered in lymph nodes or spleen, and they may contain microfilariae. The granulomas are composed of proliferating reticuloendothelial cells, fibroblasts, and eosinophils.

Malayan filariasis is caused by *Brugia malayi*, a species closely related to *W. bancrofti*. The clinical and pathologic findings are similar to those described for bancroftian filariasis.

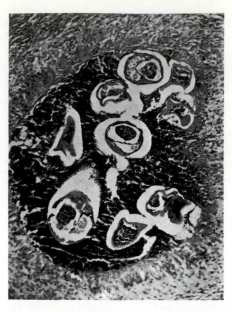

Fig. 12-37. Filarial funiculitis. Eosinophilic pseudoabscess and granulomatous reaction about dead filarial worm, with obliteration of lymphatic vessel. (80×.)

An immunosuppressive state, with altered cell- and humoral-mediated immune response, has been reported in patients infected with filariasis.[425,437,438] Since lymphatic obstruction is thought to be the result of allergic tissue reactions to the nematode, such immune unresponsiveness would be beneficial to the host[431] and would explain the lack of correlation between infestation and clinical symptomatology.

Tropical (filarial) eosinophilia is a syndrome characterized by coughing, wheezing, hypereosinophilia, and pulmonary infiltrates.[434] It is thought to be a form of occult filariasis that results from hypersensitivity to circulating microfilaria.[436]

The diagnosis of filariasis is made by identifying the microfilaria on Giemsa-stained blood smears. Serodiagnostic methods using antigens of the dog nematode *Dirofilaria immitis* have been developed and include a complement fixation and an enzyme-linked immunosorbent test.[429,433]

Onchocerciasis (onchocercosis). The filarial worm that causes onchocerciasis is known as *Onchocerca volvulus*. The disease is seen in west and central Africa and in circumscribed areas of Mexico, Guatemala, Venezuela, and Colombia.

Onchocerciasis is transmitted by small flies of the genus *Simulium* (gnat or black fly). These tiny flies ingest the microfilariae when they bite an infected person. After undergoing several transformations in the body of the fly, the microfilariae finally reach the thoracic muscles and develop into infective larvae. The larvae migrate into the proboscis and are introduced into the skin of a person who is bitten by the fly. The organisms travel

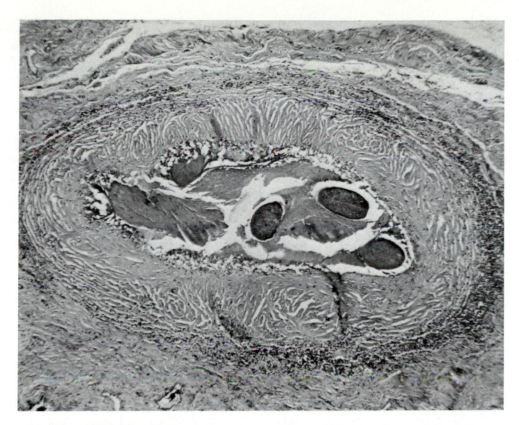

Fig. 12-38. Well-defined filarial granuloma in spermatic cord. Peripheral zone of dense fibrous tissue surrounds fragments of dead parasite. (Hematoxylin and eosin; 35×; courtesy Dr. Lorenzo Galindo, San Juan, Puerto Rico.)

freely along the dermis but appear only rarely in the blood or internal organs. They have been identified in the lungs, liver, spleen, and kidneys.[416,432]

The larvae mature in the dermis and produce solitary or multiple cutaneous nodules called onchocercomas, which are characteristic of this disease. In the African variant of the disease the nodules are limited to the skin over the pelvic bones and lower limbs, whereas in the Central American variant the nodules are usually located in the scalp (Fig. 12-39, *A*) and the skin of the face and neck. There is, however, considerable overlapping between these two variants of the disease.[415,426] The nodules (Fig. 12-39, *B*) represent an inflammatory reaction to the adult worms. Adult worms in small clefts are present in the onchocercomas, usually in a proportion of two or more males to each female. The worms may be living or dead. The inflammatory reaction is greater around dead worms.[419] Histiocytic proliferation and foreign body giant cell reaction are seen around many of the dead parasites. There is an accompanying pronounced leukocytic infiltration, mostly polymorphonuclear in type, but also chronic, with occasional eosinophils. Dense fibrosis ensues, so that the nodule is replaced by dense collagenous fibroconnective tissue. The nodules may even erode adjacent bone. Variable numbers of microfilariae are present in nearby areas. Migration of the microfilariae from the onchocercotic nodules to the adjacent dermis produces irritation of the skin. Small hemorrhages and an inflammatory reaction are seen microscopically. Edema and thickening of the skin and subcutaneous tissue develop after several months. Itching is occasionally present and in some cases may be severe. When the onchodermatosis is conspicuous in the facial region, leonine facies may develop (Fig. 12-40).

The most serious complication of the migratory phase of the microfilariae in onchocerciasis is the ocular involvement so frequently encountered in Central America. In 5% to 20% of cases in Guatemala and Mexico the microfilariae invade the eyeball.[417] A prominent horizontal punctate keratitis produced by the reaction of the corneal tissue to microfilariae is the most common finding. The keratitis does not appreciably reduce the visual acuity of these patients. When microfilariae reach the vitreous humor and penetrate the ciliary body, however, visual impairment develops. Photophobia, lacrimation, and finally blindness result. Secondary changes of a degenerative type develop in the crystalline lens; anterior synechiae are formed after exudation of fibrin and leukocytes into the anterior chamber. The posterior chamber and optic nerve also are occasionally affected. The outcome of all these processes is total blindness, with glaucoma and phthisis bulbi.

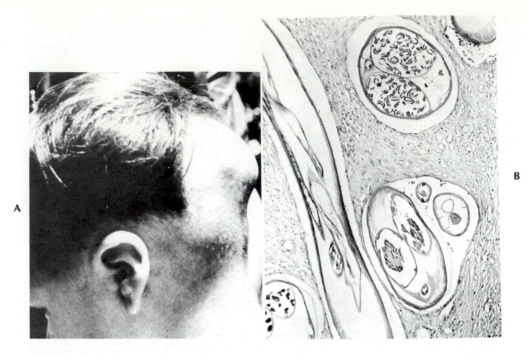

Fig. 12-39. Onchocercoma. **A,** Classic appearance in scalp of Guatemalan child. **B,** Microscopic section disclosing numerous *Onchocerca volvulus*. Interstitial tissue is fibrotic. (Hematoxylin and eosin; 100×; courtesy Dr. E. Pérez-Guisasola, Guatemala City, Guatemala.)

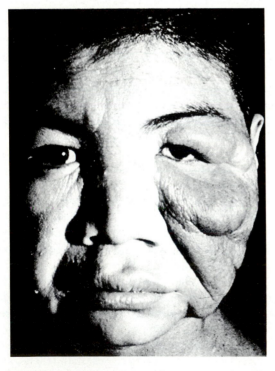

Fig. 12-40. Leonine facies in Guatemalan woman with onchocerciasis. (Courtesy Dr. E. Pérez Guisasola, Guatemala City, Guatemala.)

Lymphadenitis and rarely elephantiasis may develop in African patients. Obstructive lymphadenitis is thought to be the result of inflammation and fibrosis caused by immune complex deposition.[423]

Diagnosis is made by identifying the microfilariae in skin snips, in urine, or by slitlamp eye examination.[424] A skin test[427] and the serologic methods of complement fixation and enzyme immunoassay[413] are also available for diagnosis and epidemiologic studies.

Loaiasis (loiasis). Loaiasis is a form of filariasis limited to tropical West Africa. The causative organism, *Loa loa,* also known as the eye worm, travels through the subcutaneous tissue and occasionally in internal organs. The worms travel at the rate of about 1 cm per minute and produce serpiginous burrows that occasionally are evident externally. They sometimes migrate to the anterior chamber of the eye and appear beneath the ocular conjunctiva. The dead worms, as in other filarial diseases, cause a severe inflammatory response and eventually become calcified.

In contrast to bancroftian filariasis, the microfilariae in loaiasis appear in the peripheral bloodstream mostly during the daytime. The intermediate host and vector, the female *Chrysops* fly, bites during the day.

The so-called fugitive or Calabar swellings are subcutaneous nodules that develop suddenly in any part of the body in the course of this disease. They are painless, last for a few days, and disappear slowly. Occasionally they persist and become cystic. Calabar swellings are believed to represent an allergic manifestation to the parasite or its products.

A pronounced peripheral eosinophilia is frequently present during the course of the disease, the usual range being 30% to 40%.[441] The extensive fibrosis and obstruction of lymphatics commonly seen in bancroftian filariasis do not occur in loaiasis. Nodular areas of fibrosis are found in the spleen, together with eosinophilic infiltration. These are probably the result of rapid destruction of microfilariae.[440]

Dracunculiasis (dracunculosis, dracontiasis, guinea worm infection, Medina worm infection). Dracunculiasis affects an estimated 10 to 48 million persons in the Near East, western India, and some parts of northwestern Africa.[418] The parasite is *Dracunculus medinensis*, or the guinea worm. It is commonly referred to as a filaria, but it lacks a microfilarial stage and the adult worms are distinctly different from the true filariae.

The larvae are taken up by a freshwater crustacean of the genus *Cyclops*. They mature within the crustacean into elongated larvae infective for humans. These larvae are liberated by the gastric digestive juices when a person drinks water contaminated with infected *Cyclops*. The larvae migrate through the wall of the stomach or small intestine into the connective tissue of the abdominal wall. The male worm is small and probably dies after copulation. The female worm, which averages 1 m in length, wanders out to the subcutaneous tissue, especially that of the feet and legs. A small papule appears, which later becomes a vesicle with a small ulceration in the center through which the embryos are liberated. The latter usually are present in milky fluid contained in a segment of the worm's uterus that is extruded and breaks away from the body of the parasite.[439] On rare occasions the worms may be found in joints and serosal cavities.[422]

The signs and symptoms of dracunculiasis are limited to the period of liberation of embryos. Pruritus and moderate edema may be accompanied by low-grade fever and urticarial rash, caused by an anaphylactic reaction to the products of the worm. If the worm dies or if the embryos are liberated into the tissues, a severe inflammatory reaction with abscess formation ensues.

REFERENCES
Protozoal diseases
Amebiasis

1. Adams, E.B., and MacLeod, I.N.: Invasive amebiasis. I. Amebic dysentery and its complications, Medicine **56:**315-323, 1977.
2. Adams, E.B., and MacLeod, I.N.: Invasive amebiasis. II. Amebic liver abscess and its complications, Medicine **56:**325-334, 1977.
3. Alper, E.I., Littler, C., and Monroe, L.S.: Counterelectrophoresis in the diagnosis of amebiasis, Am. J. Gastroenterol. **65:**63-67, 1976.
4. Bos, H.J., Vander Eyk, A.A., and Streerenberg, P.A.: Application of ELISA in the serodiagnosis of amebiasis, Trans. R. Soc. Trop. Med. Hyg. **69:**440-446, 1975.
5. Craig, C.F.: The etiology, diagnosis and treatment of amebiasis, Baltimore, 1944, The Williams & Wilkins Co.
6. Deas, J.E., and Miller, J.H.: Plasmalemmal modifications of *Entamoeba histolytica* in vivo, J. Parasitol. **63:**25-31, 1977.
7. Elsdon-Dew, R.: Serodiagnosis of amoebiasis. In Cohen, S., and Sadun, E., editors: Immunology of parasitic infections, Oxford, 1976, Blackwell Scientific Publications.
8. Jones, T.C.: *Entamoeba histolytica* (amebiasis). In Mandell, G., Douglas, R.G., and Bennett, J.E., editors: Principles and practice of infectious diseases, New York, 1979, John Wiley & Sons, Inc.
9. Knight, R., and Wright, S.G.: Progress report: intestinal protozoa, Gut **19:**940-953, 1978.
10. Krogstad, D.J., et al.: Amebiasis: epidemiologic studies in the United States 1971-74, Ann. Intern. Med. **88:**89-97, 1978.
11. Krupp, I.M.: Comparison of counterimmunoelectrophoresis with other serologic tests in the diagnosis of amebiasis, Am. J. Trop. Med. Hyg. **23:**27-30, 1974.
12. Lushbaugh, W.B., et al.: Isolation of a cytotoxin-enterotoxin from *Entamoeba histolytica*, J. Infect. Dis. **139:**9-17, 1979.
13. Madanagopalan, N.: Amoebic liver disease, Trop. Gastroenterol. **1:**3-7, 1980.
14. Mahmoud, A.A.F., and Warren, K.S.: Algorithms in the diagnosis and management of exotic diseases. XVII. Amebiasis, J. Infect. Dis. **134:**639, 1976.
15. Patterson, M., Healy, G.R., and Shabot, J.M.: Serologic testing for amoebiasis, Gastroenterology **78:**136-141, 1980.
16. Pérez-Tamayo, R., and Brandt, H.: Amebiasis. In Marcial-Rojas, R.A., editor: Pathology of protozoal and helminthic diseases, Baltimore, 1971, The Williams & Wilkins Co.
17. Pillai, S., and Mohimen, A.: A solid-phase sandwich radioimmunoassay for *Entamoeba histolytica* proteins and the detection of circulating antigens in amoebiasis, Gastroenterology **83:**1210-1216, 1982.
18. Schmerin, M.J. Gelston, A., and Jones, T.C.: Amebiasis: an increasing problem among homosexuals in New York City, J.A.M.A. **238:**1386-1387, 1977.
19. Simmons, R., et al.: Amebiasis associated with colonic irrigation, Colorado, Morbid. Mortal. Weekly Rep. **30:**101-102, 1981.
20. Stamm, W.P.: The value of amebic serology in an area of low endemicity, Trans. R. Soc. Trop. Med. Hyg. **70:**49-53, 1976.
21. Thomas, V., Sinniah, B., and Leng, Y.P. Assessment of the sensitivity, specificity, and reproducibility of the indirect immunofluorescent technique for the diagnosis of amebiasis, Am. J. Trop. Med. Hyg. **30:**57-62, 1981.
22. Voller, A., Bartlett, A., and Bidwell, D.E.: Enzyme immunoassay for parasitic diseases, Trans. R. Soc. Trop. Med. Hyg. **70:**98-106, 1976.
23. Walls, K.W., and Smith, J.W.: Serology of parasitic infections, Lab. Med. **10:**329-336, 1979.

Primary amebic meningoencephalitis

24. Butt, C.G.: Primary amebic meningoencephalitis, N. Engl. J. Med. **274:**1473-1476, 1966.
25. Culbertson, C.G.: Amebic meningoencephalitides. In Binford, C.H., and Connor, D.H., Pathology of tropical and extraordinary diseases, Washington, D.C., 1976, Armed Forces Institute of Pathology.
26. Duma, R.J., Helwig, W.B., and Martínez, A.J.: Meningoencephalitis and brain abscess due to free-living amoeba, Ann. Intern. Med. **88:**468-473, 1978.
27. Fowler, M., and Carter, R.F.: Acute pyogenic meningitis probably due to *Acanthamoeba*, Br. Med. J. **2:**740-742, 1965.
28. Lawande, R.V., et al.: A case of primary amebic meningoencephalitis in Zaria, Nigeria, Am. J. Clin. Pathol. **71:**591-594, 1979.
29. Lawande, R.V., et al.: A case of primary amebic meningoencephalitis in a Nigerian farmer, Am. J. Trop. Med. Hyg. **29:**21-25, 1980.
30. Markell, E.K., and Voge, M.: Medical parasitology, Philadelphia, 1981, W.B. Saunders Co.
31. Martínez, A.J.: Is *Acanthamoeba* encephalitis an opportunistic infection? Neurology **30:**567-574, 1980.
32. Martínez, A.J., et al.: Primary amebic meningoencephalitis, Pathol. Annu. **12:**225-250, 1977.

33. Myerowitz, R.L.: Granulomatous amebic encephalitis and disseminated acanthamebiasis. In Myerowitz, R.L., editor: The pathology of opportunistic infections, New York, 1983, Raven Press.

34. Ringsted, J., Jager, B.V., and Visvesvara, G.S.: Probable *Acanthamoeba* meningoencephalitis in a Korean child, Am. J. Clin. Pathol. **66**:723-730, 1976.

35. Seidel, J.S., et al.: Successful treatment of primary amebic meningoencephalitis, N. Engl. J. Med. **306**:344-348, 1982.

36. Willaert, E., Stevens, A.R., and Healy, G.R.: Retrospective identification of *Acanthamoeba culbertsoni* in a case of amoebic meningoencephalitis, J. Clin. Pathol. **31**:717-720, 1978.

Balantidiasis

37. Areán, V.M., and Echevarría, R.: Balantidiasis. In Marcial-Rojas, R.A., editor: Pathology of protozoal and helminthic diseases, Baltimore, 1971, The Williams & Wilkins Co.

38. Areán, V.M., and Koppisch, E.: Balantidiasis: a review and report of cases, Am. J. Pathol. **32**:1089-1115, 1956.

39. Lahiri, V.L., Elhence, B.R., and Agarwal, B.M.: *Balantidium* peritonitis diagnosed on cytologic material, Acta Cytol. **21**:123-124, 1977.

40. Markell, E.K., and Voge, M.: Medical parasitology, Philadelphia, 1981, W.B. Saunders Co.

41. Marsden, P.D.: Balantidiasis. In Beeson, P.B., McDermott, W., and Wyngaarden, J.B., editors: Cecil-Loeb textbook of medicine, ed. 15, Philadelphia, 1979, W.B. Saunders Co.

42. Neafie, R.C.: Balantidiasis. In Binford, C.H., and Connor, D.H., editors: Pathology of tropical and extraordinary diseases, Washington, D.C., 1976, Armed Forces Institute of Pathology.

Flagellates of digestive tract and genital organs

43. Anand, B.S.: *Giardia lamblia*: clinical and immunological aspects, Trop. Gastroenterol. **1**:180-184, 1980.

44. Brasitus, T.A.: Parasites and malabsorption, Am. J. Med. **67**:1058-1065, 1979.

45. Dykes, A.C., et al.: Municipal waterborne giardiasis: an epidemiologic investigation; beavers implicated as a possible reservoir, Ann. Intern. Med. **92**:165-170, 1980.

46. Gallai, Z., and Sylvestre, L.: The present status of urogenital trichomoniasis: a general review of the literature, Appl. Therap. 773, 1976.

47. Hartong, W.A., Gourley, W.K., and Arvanitakis, C.: Giardiasis: clinical spectrum and functional-structural abnormalities of the small intestinal mucosa, Gastroenterology **77**:61-69, 1979.

48. Khosla, S.N., Sharma, S.V., and Strivastava, S.C.: Malabsorption in giardiasis, Am. J. Gastroenterol. **69**:694-700, 1978.

49. Knight, R., and Wright, S.G.: Progress report: intestinal protozoa, Gut **19**:940-953, 1978.

50. Levinson, J.D., and Nastro, L.J.: Giardiasis with total villous atrophy, Gastroenterology **74**:271-275, 1978.

51. Meyer, E.A., and Radulescu, S.: Giardia and giardiasis, Adv. Parasitol. **17**:1-47, 1979.

52. Novak, E.R., and Woodruff, J.D.: Novak's gynecologic and obstetric pathology with clinical and endocrine relations, Philadelphia, 1979, W.B. Saunders Co.

53. Rein, M.F., and Chapel, T.A.: Trichomoniasis, candidiasis and the minor venereal diseases, Clin. Obstet. Gynecol. **18**:73, 1975.

54. Rogers, A.I.: *Giardia* and steatorrhea, Gastroenterology **76**:224, 1979.

55. Saha, T.K., and Ghosh, T.K.: Invasion of small intestinal mucosa by *Giardia lamblia* in man, Gastroenterology **72**:402-405, 1977.

56. Schmerin, M.J., Jones, T.C., and Klein, H.: Giardiasis: association with homosexuality, Ann. Intern. Med. **88**:801-803, 1978.

57. Shaw, P.K., et al.: A communitywide outbreak of giardiasis with evidence of transmission by a municipal water supply, Ann. Intern. Med. **87**:426-432, 1977.

58. Smith, P.D., et al.: IgA antibody to *Giardia lamblia* detected by enzyme-linked immunosorbent assay, Gastroenterology **80**:1476-1480, 1981.

59. Smith, P.D., et al.: Chronic giardiasis: studies on drug sensitivity, toxin production, and host immune response, Gastroenterology **83**:797-803, 1982.

60. Tandon, B.N., et al.: Mechanism of malabsorption in giardiasis: a study of bacterial flora and bile salt deconjugation in upper jejunum, Gut **18**:176-181, 1977.

61. Vivesvara, G.S., et al.: An immunofluorescence test to detect antibodies to *Giardia lamblia*, Ann. Intern. Med. **93**:802-804, 1980.

62. Whitehead, R.: Mucosal biopsy of the gastrointestinal tract, Philadelphia, 1979, W.B. Saunders Co.

63. Wolfe, M.S.: Giardiasis, N. Engl. J. Med. **298**:319-321, 1978.

64. Yardley, J.H.: Giardiasis. In Binford, C.H., and Connor, D.H., editors: Pathology of tropical and extraordinary diseases, Washington, D.C., 1976, Armed Forces Institute of Pathology.

African trypanosomiasis

65. Borst, P., and Cross, G.A.M.: Molecular basis for trypanosome antigenic variation, Cell **29**:291-303, 1982.

66. Cross, G.A.M.: Antigenic variation in trypanosomes, Proc. R. Soc. Lond. (Biol.) **202**:55-72, 1978.

67. Emery, D.L., et al.: The chancre—early events in the pathogenesis of African trypanosomiasis in domestic livestock. In Van den Bossche, H., editor: The host invader interplay, Amsterdam, 1980, Elsevier/North-Holland.

68. Greenwood, B.M.: African trypanosomiasis. In Beeson, P.B., McDermott, W., and Wyngaarden, J.B., editors: Cecil-Loeb textbook of medicine, ed. 15, Philadelphia, 1979, W.B. Saunders Co.

69. Hutt, M.S.R., and Wilks, N.E.: African trypanosomiasis. In Marcial-Rojas, R.A., editor: Pathology of protozoal and helminthic diseases, Baltimore, 1971, The Williams & Wilkins Co.

70. Mahmoud, A.A.F., and Warren, K.S.: Algorithms in the diagnosis and management of exotic diseases. XI. African trypanosomiasis, J. Infect. Dis. **133**:487, 1976.

71. Mott, F.W.: Histological observations of sleeping sickness and other trypanosome infections, Reports of the Sleeping Sickness Commission, No. 7, 1906.

72. Robins-Browne, R.M., Schneider, J., and Metz, J.: Thrombocytopenia in trypanosomiasis, Am. J. Trop. Med. Hyg. **24**:226-231, 1975.

73. Ruitenberg, E.J., and Buys, J.: Application of the enzyme-linked immunosorbent assay (ELISA) for the serodiagnosis of human African trypanosomiasis (sleeping sickness), Am. J. Trop. Med. Hyg. **26**:31-36, 1977.

74. Sacks, D.L., Gross Kinsky, C.M., and Askonas, B.A.: Immune dysfunction caused by African trypanosomes: effect on parasite-specific responses and analysis of active fractions. In Van den Bossche, H., editor: The host invader interplay, Amsterdam, 1980, Elsevier/North Holland.

75. Spencer, H.C., et al.: Imported African trypanosomiasis in the United States, Ann. Intern. Med. **82**:633-638, 1975.

76. Van Marck, E.A.E., et al.: Renal disease in chronic experimental *Trypanosoma gambiense* infections, Am. J. Trop. Med. Hyg. **30**:780-789, 1981.

77. Vickerman, K., et al.: Antigenic variation in trypanosomes. In Van den Bossche, H., editor: The host invader interplay, Amsterdam, 1980, Elsevier/North Holland.

American trypanosomiasis (Chagas' disease)

78. Andrade, Z.A.: A lesato apical do corracão na miocardite crónica chagásica, Hospital (Rio) **50**:803, 1956.

79. Andrade, Z.A., and Andrade, S.G.: American trypanosomiasis. In Marcial-Rojas, R.A., editor: Pathology of protozoal and helminthic diseases, Baltimore, 1971, The Williams & Wilkins Co.

80. Andrade, Z.A., et al.: Histopathology of the conducting tissue of the heart in Chagas' myocarditis, Am. Heart J. **95**:316-324, 1978.

81. Beener, Z.: Immunity to *Trypanosoma cruzi*, Adv. Parasitol. **18**:247-292, 1980.

82. Hoff, R., et al.: *Trypanosoma cruzi* in the cerebrospinal fluid during the acute stage of Chagas' disease, N. Engl. J. Med. **298**:604-606, 1978.

83. Jones, T.C.: Interactions between murine macrophages and obligate intracellular protozoa, Am. J. Pathol., **102**:127-132, 1981.

84. Jones, T.C., and Masur, H.: Survival of *Toxoplasma gondii* and other microbes in cytoplasmic vacuoles. In Van den Bossche, H., editor: The host invader interplay, Amsterdam, 1980, Elsevier/North Holland.

85. Kierszenbaum, F., Ackerman, S.J., and Gleich, G.J.: Destruction of bloodstream forms of *Trypanosoma cruzi* by eosinophil granule major basic protein, Am. J. Trop. Med. Hyg. **30**:775-779, 1981.

86. Koeberle, F.: Patogenia do megaesôfago brasileiro e europeu, Rev. Goiana Med. **9**:79, 1963.

87. Laranja, F.S., et al.: Chagas' disease: a clinical, epidemiologic and pathologic study, Circulation **14**:1035, 1956.

88. Lisbôa, A.C.: Sobre a forma congênita da doença de Chagas: estudo anátomo-patológico de seis casos, Rev. Inst. Med. Trop. Sao Paulo **2**:319, 1960.

89. Lisboa Bittencourt, A., et al.: Pneumonitis in congenital Chagas' disease, Am. J. Trop. Med. Hyg. **30**:38-42, 1981.

90. Magarino Torres, C.: Estudo do miocardio na moléstia de Chagas (forma aguda), Mem. Inst. Cruz **9**:114, 1917.

91. Magarino Torres, C., and Duarte, E.: Lesôes do feixe de His-Tawara na cardiopatía chagásica aguda e crónica, Primeira Reunión Panamericana sobre enfermedad de Chagas **1**:23, 1950.

92. Mahmoud, A.A.F., and Warren, K.S.: Algorithms in the diagnosis and management of exotic diseases. IV. American trypanosomiasis, J. Infect. Dis. **132**:121, 1975.

93. Mott, K.E., and Hagstrom, J.W.C.: The pathologic lesions of the cardiac autonomic nervous system in chronic Chagas' myocarditis, Circulation **31**:273, 1965.

94. Nilsson, L.A., and Voller, A.: A comparison of thin layer immunoassay (TIA) and enzyme linked immunosorbent assay (ELISA) for the detection of antibodies to *Trypanosoma cruzi*, Trans. R. Soc. Trop. Med. Hyg. **76**:95-97, 1982.

95. Nogueira, N., and Cohn, Z.: *Trypanosoma cruzi*: mechanisms of entry and intracellular fate in mammalian cells, J. Exp. Med. **143**:1402-1420, 1976.

96. Oria, J., and Ramos, J. Alteracoes do metassimpático de coração nos portadores de megaesofago (cardiospasmo), Arq. Bras. Cardiol. **2**:311, 1949.

Leishmaniasis

97. Bray, R.S.: Immunodiagnosis of leishmaniasis. In Cohen, S., and Sadun, E., editors: Immunology of parasitic infections, Oxford, 1976, Blackwell Scientific Publications.

98. Bryceson, A.D.M.: Leishmaniasis. In Beeson, P.B., McDermott, W., and Wyngaarden, J.B., editors: Cecil-Loeb textbook of medicine, ed. 15, Philadelphia, 1979, W.B. Saunders Co.

99. Chang, K.P.: Leishmanicidal mechanisms of human polymorphonuclear phagocytes, Am. J. Trop. Med. Hyg. **30**:322-333, 1981.

100. Chang, K.P., and Dwyer, D.M.: *Leishmania donovani*: hamster macrophages interactions in vitro; cell entry, intracellular survival and multiplication of amastigotes, J. Exp. Med. **147**:515-530, 1978.

101. Geraci, J.E., Wilson, W.R., and Thompson, J.H.: Visceral leishmaniasis (kala-azar) as a cause of fever of unknown origin, Mayo Clin. Proc. **55**:455-458, 1980.

102. Haghighi, P., and Rezai, H.R.: Leishmaniasis: a review of selected topics, Pathol. Annu. **12**:63-89, 1977.

103. Hommel, M.: Enzymo-immunoassay in leishmaniasis, Trans. R. Soc. Trop. Med. Hyg. **70**:15-16, 1976.

104. Kharazmi, A., et al.: Evidence for the presence of circulating immune complexes in serum and C3b and C3d on red cells of kala-azar patients, Trans. Trop. Med. Hyg. **76**:793-796, 1982.

105. Mahmoud, A.A.F., and Warren, K.S.: Algorithms in the diagnosis and management of exotic diseases. XXIV. Leishmaniases, J. Infect. Dis. **136**:160-163, 1977.

106. Markell, E.K., and Voge, M.: Medical parasitology, Philadelphia, 1981, W.B. Saunders Co.

107. Marsden, P.D.: Leishmaniasis, N. Engl. J. Med. **300**:350-353, 1979.

108. Mavel, J.: The biology of the macrophage leishmania interaction. In Van den Bossche, H., editor: The host invader interplay, Amsterdam, 1980, Elsevier/North Holland.

109. Murray, H.W.: Susceptibility of leishmania to oxygen intermediates and killing by normal macrophages, J. Exp. Med. **153**:1302-1315, 1981.

110. Nathan, E.F., Murray, H.W., and Cohn, Z.A.: The macrophage as an effector cell, N. Engl. J. Med. **303**:622-626, 1980.

111. Petersen, E.A., et al.: Specific inhibition of lymphocyte-proliferation responses by adherent suppressor cells in diffuse cutaneous leishmaniasis, N. Engl. J. Med. **306**:387-391, 1982.

112. Rocha, H.: *Leishmania* species (kala-azar). In Mandell, G., Douglas, R.G., and Bennett, J.E., editors: Principles and practices of infectious diseases, New York, 1979, John Wiley & Sons, Inc.

113. Udani, P.M.: Leishmaniasis. In Vaughan, V.C., et al., editors: Nelson textbook of pediatrics, Philadelphia, 1979, W.B. Saunders Co.

114. Weisinger, J.R., et al.: Clinical and histological kidney involvement in human kala-azar, Am. J. Trop. Med. Hyg. **27**:357-359, 1978.

115. Werner, J.K., and Barreto, P.: Leishmaniasis in Colombia: a review, Am. J. Trop. Med. Hyg. **30**:751-761, 1981.

116. Winslow, D.J.: Kala-azar (visceral leishmaniasis). In Marcial-Rojas, R.A., editor: Pathology of protozoal and helminthic diseases, Baltimore, 1971, The Williams & Wilkins Co.

117. Zuckerman, A.: Current status of the immunology of blood and tissue protozoa, Exp. Parasitol. **42**:374-446, 1977.

Coccidiosis

118. Bobb, R.R., Differding, J.T., and Trollope, M.L.: Cryptosporidia enteritis in a healthy professional athlete, Am. J. Gastroenterol. **77**:833-834, 1982.

119. Brandborg, L.L., Goldberg, S.B., and Breindenbach, W.C.: Human coccidiosis, a possible cause of malabsorption, N. Engl. J. Med. **283**:1306-1313, 1970.

120. Cryptosporidiosis: assessment of chemotherapy of males with acquired immune deficiency syndrome (AIDS), Morbid. Mortal. Weekly Rep. **31**:589-592, 1982.

121. Dammin, G.J., and Dooley, J.R.: Coccidiosis. In Binford, C.H., and Connor, D.H., editors: Pathology of tropical and extraordinary diseases, Washington, D.C., 1976, Armed Forces Institute of Pathology.

122. Frenkel, J.K., et al.: Sarcocystinae: nominadubia and available names, Z. Parasitenkd. **58**:115-139, 1979.

123. Heydorn, A.O., et al.: Proposal for a new nomenclature of the sarcosporidia, Z. Parasitenkd. **48**:73-82, 1975.

124. Human cryptosporidiosis—Alabama, Morbid. Mortal. Weekly Rep. **31**:252-254, 1982.

125. Lasser, K.H., Lewin, K.J., and Tyning, F.W.: Cryptosporidial enteritis in a patient with congenital hypogammaglobulinemia, Hum. Pathol. **10**:234-240, 1979.

126. Meisel, J.L., et al.: Overwhelming watery diarrhea associated with a cryptosporidium in an immunosuppressed patient, Gastroenterology **70**:1156-1160, 1976.

127. Sloper, K.S., et al.: Chronic malabsorption due to cryptosporidiosis in a child with immunoglobulin deficiency, Gut **23**:80-82, 1982.

128. Stemmermann, G.N., et al.: Cryptosporidiosis: report of a fatal case complicated by disseminated toxoplasmosis, Am. J. Med. **69**:637-642, 1980.

129. Trier, J.S., et al.: Chronic intestinal coccidiosis in man: intestinal morphology and response to treatment, Gastroenterology **66**:923-935, 1974.

130. Tzipori, S., et al.: Experimental infection of lambs with *Cryptosporidium* isolated from a human patient with diarrhea, Gut **23**:71-74, 1982.

131. Weinstein, L., et al.: Intestinal cryptosporidiosis complicated by disseminated cytomegalovirus infection, Gastroenterology, **81**:584-591, 1981.

132. Weisburger, W.R., et al.: Cryptosporidiosis in an immunosuppressed renal transplant recipient with IgA deficiency, Am. J. Clin. Pathol. **72**:473-478, 1979.

133. Westerman, E.L., and Christensen, R.P.: Chronic *Isospora belli* infection treated with cotrimoxazole, Ann. Intern. Med. **91**:413-414, 1979.

Malaria

134. Boonpucknavig, V., and Sitprija, V.: Renal disease in acute *Plasmodium falciparum* infection in man, Kidney Int. **16**:44-52, 1979.
135. Cohen, S.: Plasmodium: mechanisms of survival. In Van den Bossche, H., editor: The host invader interplay, Amsterdam, 1980, Elsevier/North Holland.
136. Collins, W.E., Lunde, M.V., and Skinner, J.C.: Development of antibodies to *Plasmodium vivax* as measured by two different serologic techniques, Am. J. Trop. Med. Hyg. **24**:412-416, 1975.
137. Greenwood, B.M., Stratton, D., and Williamson, W.A.: A study of the role of immunological factors in the pathogenesis of the anemia of acute malaria, Trans. R. Soc. Trop. Med. Hyg. **72**:378-385, 1978.
138. Hall, A.P.: The treatment of severe falciparum malaria, Trans. R. Soc. Trop. Med. Hyg. **71**:367-379, 1977.
139. Jones, T.C.: Malaria. In Beeson, P.B., McDermott, W., and Wyngaarden, J.B., editors: Cecil-Loeb textbook of medicine, ed. 15, Philadelphia, 1979, W.B. Saunders Co.
140. Kagan, I.G.: Evaluation of indirect hemagglutination test as an epidemiologic technique for malaria, Am. J. Trop. Med. Hyg. **21**:683-698, 1972.
141. MacKowiak, P.A.: Microbial synergism in human infections. Part 1. N. Engl. J. Med. **298**:21-26, 1978.
142. Markell, E.K., and Voge, M.: Medical parasitology, Philadelphia, 1981, W.B. Saunders Co.
143. McBride, J.S., Walliker, D., and Morgan, G.: Antigenic diversity in the human malaria parasite *Plasmodium falciparum*, Science **217**:254-257, 1982.
144. Miller, L.H., et al.: Evidence for differences in erythrocyte surface receptors for the malarial parasites, *Plasmodium falciparum* and *Plasmodium knowlesi*, J. Exp. Med. **146**:277-280, 1977.
145. Miller, L.H., et al.: The Duffy blood group phenotype in American blacks infected with *Plasmodium vivax* in Vietnam, Am. J. Trop. Med. Hyg. **27**:1069-1072, 1978.
146. Pasvol, G.: The interaction between sickle hemoglobin and the malarial parasite *Plasmodium falciparum*, Trans. R. Soc. Trop. Med. Hyg. **74**:701-705, 1980.
147. Punyagupta, S., et al.: Acute pulmonary insufficiency in falciparum malaria: summary of 12 cases with evidence of disseminated intravascular coagulation, Am. J. Trop. Med. Hyg. **23**:551-559, 1974.
148. Quinn, T.C., et al.: Congenital malaria: A report of four cases and a review, J. Pediatr. **101**:229-232, 1982.
149. Spencer, H.C., et al.: The enzyme-linked immunosorbent assay (ELISA) for malaria. III. Antibody response in documented *Plasmodium falciparum* infections, Am. J. Trop. Med. Hyg. **30**:747-750, 1981.
150. Strickland, G.T., and Hunter, K.W.: Red cell antibodies in malaria: immunity or autoimmunity? In Van den Bossche, H., editor: The host invader interplay, Amsterdam, 1980, Elsevier/North Holland.
151. Toro, G., and Román, G.: Cerebral malaria: a disseminated vasculomyelinopathy, Arch. Neurol. **35**:271-275, 1978.
152. Walter, P.R., Garin, Y., and Blot, P.: Placental pathologic changes in malaria: a histologic and ultrastructural study, Am. J. Pathol. **109**:330-342, 1982.
153. Wilson, M., et al.: Comparison of complement fixation, indirect immunofluorescence and indirect hemagglutination test for malaria, Am. J. Trop. Med. Hyg. **24**:755-759, 1975.
154. Woodruff, A.W., Ansdell, V.E., and Pettiff, L.E.: Cause of anemia in malaria, Lancet **1**:1055-1057, 1979.

Toxoplasmosis

155. Benenson, M.W., et al.: Oocyst-transmitted toxoplasmosis associated with ingestion of contaminated water, N. Engl. J. Med. **307**:666-669, 1982.
156. Broadbent, E.J., Ross, R., and Hurley, R.: Screening for toxoplasmosis in pregnancy, J. Clin. Pathol. **34**:659-664, 1981.
157. Conley, F.K., Jenkins, K.A., and Remington, J.S.: *Toxoplasma gondii* infection of the central nervous system, Hum. Pathol. **12**:690-698, 1981.

158. Frenkel, J.K.: Toxoplasmosis. In Binford, C.H., and Connor, D.H., editors: Pathology of tropical and extraordinary diseases, Washington, D.C., 1976, Armed Forces Institute of Pathology.
159. Frenkel, J.K., Nelson, B.M., and Arias-Stella, J.: Immunosuppression and toxoplasmic encephalitis: clinical and experimental aspects, Hum. Pathol. **6**:97-111, 1975.
160. Greenlee, J.E., et al.: Adult toxoplasmosis presenting as polymyositis and cerebellar ataxia, Ann. Intern. Med. **82**:367, 1975.
161. Gump, D.W., and Holden, R.A.: Acquired chorioretinitis due to toxoplasmosis, Ann. Intern. Med. **90**:58-60, 1979.
162. Jones, T.C.: Interactions between murine macrophages and obligate intracellular protozoa, Am. J. Pathol. **102**:127-132, 1981.
163. Kagen, L.G., Kimball, A.C., and Christian, C.L.: Serologic evidence of toxoplasmosis among patients with polymyositis, Am. J. Med. **56**:186, 1974.
164. Krick, J.A., and Remington, J.S.: Toxoplasmosis in the adult: an overview, N. Engl. J. Med. **298**:550-553, 1978.
165. Masur, H., et al.: Outbreak of toxoplasmosis in a family and documentation of acquired retinochoroiditis, Am. J. Med. **64**:396-402, 1978.
166. McLeod, R., et al.: Toxoplasmosis presenting as brain abscess: diagnosis by computerized tomography and cytology of aspirated purulent material, Am. J. Med. **67**:711-714, 1979.
167. Miettinen, M.: Histological differential diagnosis between lymph node toxoplasmosis and other benign lymph node hyperplasia, Histopathology **5**:205-216, 1981.
168. Nichols, B.A., and O'Connor, G.R.: Penetration of mouse peritoneal macrophages by the protozoon *Toxoplasma gondii*: new evidence for active invasion and phagocytosis, Lab. Invest. **44**:324-335, 1981.
169. Ruskin, J., and Remington, J.S. Toxoplasmosis in the compromised host, Ann. Intern. Med. **84**:193-199, 1976.
170. Sabin, A.B., and Feldman, H.A.: Dyes as microchemical indicators of a new immunity phenomenon affecting a protozoon parasite (*Toxoplasma*), Science **108**:660-663, 1948.
171. Samuels, B.S., and Rietschel, R.L.: Polymyositis and toxoplasmosis, J.A.M.A. **235**:60-61, 1976.
172. Van Loon, A., and Van der Veen, J.: Enzyme-linked immunosorbent assay for quantitation of toxoplasma antibodies in human sera, J. Clin. Pathol. **33**:635-639, 1980.
173. Walls, K., Bullock, S., and English, D.: Use of the enzyme-linked immunosorbent assay (ELISA) and its microadaptation for the serodiagnosis of toxoplasmosis, J. Clin. Microbiol. **5**:273-277, 1977.
174. Weitberg, A.B., et al.: Acute granulomatous hepatitis in the course of acquired toxoplasmosis, N. Engl. J. Med. **300**:1093-1096, 1979.

Pneumocystosis

175. Areán, V.M.: Pulmonary pneumocystosis. In Marcial-Rojas, R.A., editor: Pathology of protozoal and helminthic diseases, Baltimore, 1971, The Williams & Wilkins Co.
176. Ariztia, A., et al.: Interstitial plasma cell pneumonia and *Pneumocystis carinii*, J. Pediatr. **51**:639-645, 1957.
177. Burke, B.A., and Good, R.A.: *Pneumocystis carinii* infection, Medicine **52**:23-51, 1973.
178. Erchul, J.W., Williams, L.P., and Meigham, P.P.: *Pneumocystis carinii* in hypopharyngeal material, N. Engl. J. Med. **267**:926-927, 1962.
179. Frenkel, J.K.: Pneumocystosis. In Binford, C.H., and Connor, D.H., editors: Pathology of tropical and extraordinary diseases, Washington, D.C., 1976, Armed Forces Institute of Pathology.
180. Frenkel, J.K., Good, J.T., and Shultz, J.A.: Latent *Pneumocystis carinii* in hypopharyngeal material, Lab. Invest. **15**:1559-1577, 1966.
181. Gilbert, C.F., Fordham, C.C., III, and Benson, W.R.: Death resulting from *Pneumocystis carinii* in an adult, Arch. Intern. Med. **112**:158-163, 1963.
182. Gottlieb, M.S., et al.: *Pneumocystis* pneumonia (editorial note), Morbid. Mortal. Weekly Rep. **30**:251, 1981.

183. Hamperl, H.: *Pneumocystis* infection and cytomegaly of lungs in newborn and adult, Am. J. Pathol. **32**:1-13, 1956.

184. Hendry, J., and Myers, R.F.: *Pneumocystis carinii* pneumonia: report of a case diagnosed during life, Can. Med. Assoc. J. **81**:831-834, 1959.

185. Kaftori, J.K., et al.: *Pneumocystis carinii* pneumonia in the adult: report of a primary case, Arch. Intern. Med. **109**:438-446, 1962.

186. Kramer, R.I., Cirone, V.C., and Moore, H.: Interstitial pneumonia due to *Pneumocystis carinii*, cytomegalic inclusion disease and hypogamma globulinemia occurring simultaneously in an infant, Pediatrics **29**:816-827, 1962.

187. Le Tan-Vinh, et al.: Diagnostic "in vivo" de la pneumonia a *Pneumocystis*, Arch. Fr. Pediatr. **20**:773-792, 1963.

188. Lunseth, J.H., Interstitial plasma cell pneumonia, J. Pediatr. **46**:137-155, 1955.

189. Murphy, M.J., Jr., Pifer, L.L., and Hughes, W.T.: *Pneumocystis carinii* in vitro: a study by scanning electron microscopy, Am. J. Pathol. **86**:387-394, 1977.

190. Pavlica, F.: The first observation of congenital pneumocystic pneumonia in a fully developed stillborn child, Ann. Paediatr. **198**:177-184, 1962.

191. Pifer, L.L., Hughes, W.T., and Murphy, M.J., Jr.: Propagation of *Pneumocystis carinii* in vitro, Pediatr. Res. **11**:305, 1977.

192. Robbins, J.B., De Vita, V.T., and Dutz, W.: Symposium on *Pneumocystis carinii* infection, National Cancer Institute Monograph 43, U.S. Department of Health, Education and Welfare, October 1976.

193. Robinson, J.J.: Two cases of pneumocystosis: observation in 203 adult autopsies, Arch. Pathol. **71**:156-159, 1961.

194. Rosen, P.P., Martini, N., and Armstrong, D.: *Pneumocystis carinii* pneumonia: diagnosis by lung biopsy, Am. J. Med. **58**:794-802, 1975.

195. Rubin, E., and Zak, F.G.: *Pneumocystis carinii* pneumonia in the adult, N. Engl. J. Med. **262**:1315-1317, 1960.

196. Smith, J.W., and Bartlett, M.S.: Diagnosis of *Pneumocystis* pneumonia, Lab. Med. **10**:430-434, 1979.

197. White, W.F., Saxton, H.M., and Dawson, I.M.P.: *Pneumocystis* pneumonia: report of three cases in adults and one in a child with a discussion of the radiological appearances and predisposing factors, Br. Med. J. **2**:1327-1331, 1961.

198. Williams, G., Stretton, T.B., and Leonard, J.C.: Cytomegalic inclusion disease and *Pneumocystis carinii* infection in an adult, Lancet **2**:951-955, 1960.

199. Woodward, S.C., and Sheldon, W.H.: Subclinical *Pneumocystis carinii* pneumonitis in adults, Bull. Johns Hopkins Hosp. **109**:148-159, 1961.

Acquired immune deficiency syndrome (AIDS)

200. Boldogh, I., et al.: Kaposi's sarcoma. IV. Detection of CMV DNA, CMV RNA and CMNA in tumor biopsies, Int. J. Cancer **28**:469-474, 1981.

201. Durack, D.T.: Opportunistic infection and Kaposi's sarcoma in homosexual men (editorial), N. Engl. J. Med. **305**:1465-1467, 1981.

202. Epidemiologic aspects of the current outbreak of Kaposi's sarcoma and opportunistic infections: report of the Centers for Disease Control Task Force on Kaposi's Sarcoma and Opportunistic Infections, N. Engl. J. Med. **306**:248-252, 1982.

203. Follansbee, S.E., et al.: An outbreak of *Pneumocystis carinii* pneumonia in homosexual men, Ann. Intern. Med. **96**:705-713, 1982.

204. Gottlieb, M.S., et al.: *Pneumocystis carinii* pneumonia and mucosal candidiasis in previously healthy homosexual men, N. Engl. J. Med. **305**:1425-1431, 1981.

205. Masur, H., et al: An outbreak of community-acquired *Pneumocystis carinii* pneumonia, N. Engl. J. Med. **305**:1431-1438, 1981.

206. Mildvan, D., et al.: Opportunistic infections and immune deficiency in homosexual men, Ann. Intern. Med. **96**:700-704, 1982.

207. Opportunistic infections and Kaposi's sarcoma among Haitians in the United States, Morbid. Mortal. Weekly Rep. **31**:353, 1982.

208. *Pneumocystis carinii* pneumonia among persons with hemophilia A, Morbid. Mortal. Weekly Rep. **31**:365-367, 1982.

209. Rinaldo, C.R., Jr., et al.: Mechanisms of immunosuppression in cytomegalovirus mononucleosis, J. Infect. Dis. **141**:488-495, 1980.

Babesiosis (piroplasmosis)

210. Anderson, A.E., Cassady, P.B., and Healy, G.R.: Babesiosis in man: sixth documented case, Am. J. Clin. Pathol. **62**:612-616, 1974.

211. Bonach, J.L., Habicht, G.S., and Hamburger, M.I.: Immunoresponsiveness in acute babesiosis in humans, J. Infect. Dis. **146**:369-380, 1982.

212. Bredt, A.B., Weinstein, W.M., and Cohen, S.: Treatment of babesiosis in asplenic patients, J.A.M.A. **245**:1938-1939, 1981.

213. Chapman, W.E., and Ward, P.A.: *Babesia rodhaini*: requirement of complement for penetration of human erythrocytes, Science **196**:67-70, 1977.

214. Dammin, G.J.: Babesiosis. In Weinstein, L., and Fields, B.N., editors: Seminars in infectious diseases, New York, Grune & Stratton, Inc.

215. Dammin, G.J.: Babesiosis, Infect. Dis. Pract. **4**:1-5, 1980.

216. Dammin, G.J., et al.: The rising incidence of clinical *Babesia microtic* infection, Hum. Pathol. **12**:398-400, 1981.

217. Healy, G.R., and Ruebush, T.K.: Morphology of *Babesia microti* in human blood smears, Am. J. Clin. Pathol. **73**:107-109, 1980.

218. Jack, R.M., and Ward, P.A.: *Babesia rhodaini* interactions with complement: relationship to parasitic entry into red cells, J. Immunol. **124**:1566-1573, 1980.

219. Jacoby, G.A., et al.: Treatment of transfusion transmitted babesiosis by exchange transfusion, N. Engl. J. Med. **303**:1098-1100, 1980.

220. Roebush, T.K., II, Collins, W.E., and Warren, M.: Experimental *Babesia microti* infections in *Macaca mulatta*: recurrent parasitemia before and after splenectomy, Am. J. Trop. Med. Hyg. **30**:304-307, 1981.

221. Roebush, T.K., II, et al.: Human babesiosis on Nantucket Island: clinical features, Ann. Intern. Med. **86**:6-14, 1977.

222. Roebush, T.K., II, et al.: Human babesiosis on Nantucket Island: evidence for self-limited and sub-clinical infections, N. Engl. J. Med. **297**:825-829, 1977.

223. Skrabalo, Z.: Babesiosis (piroplasmosis). In Marcial-Rojas, R.A., editor: Pathology of protozoal and helminthic diseases, Baltimore, 1971, The Williams & Wilkins Co.

224. Ward, P.A., and Jack, R.M.: The entry process of *Babesia* merozoites into red cells, Am. J. Pathol. **102**:109-113, 1981.

225. Western, K.A., et al.: Babesiosis in a Massachusetts resident, N. Engl. J. Med. **238**:854-857, 1970.

226. Zwart, D., and Brocklesby, D.W.: Babesiosis: non-specific resistance, immunological factors and pathogenesis, Adv. Parasitol. **17**:50-113, 1979.

Helminthic diseases

227. Bhamarapravati, N., and Thammavit, W.: Animal studies on liver fluke infestation, dimethyl nitrosamine and bile duct carcinoma, Lancet **1**:206-207, 1978.

228. Bhamarapravati, N., Thammavit, W., and Vajrasthira, S.: Liver changes in hamsters infected with liver fluke of man, *Opisthorchis viverrini*, Am. J. Trop. Med. Hyg. **27**:787-794, 1978.

229. Chin, K.Y., Lei, A.T., and Wang, T.Y.: Primary mucinous carcinoma of liver associated with *Clonorchis sinensis* infection, Chin. Med. J. **73**:26, 1955.

230. Chung, C.H.: In Marcial-Rojas, R.A., editor: Pathology of protozoal and helminthic diseases, Baltimore, 1971, The Williams & Wilkins Co.

231. Davies, C., and Goose, J.: Killing of newly encysted juveniles of *Fasciola hepatica* in sensitized rats, Parasite Immunol. **3**:81-86, 1981.

232. Gibson, J.B., and Sun, T.: Clonorchiasis. In Marcial-Rojas, R.A., editor: Pathology of protozoal and helminthic diseases, Baltimore, 1971, The Williams & Wilkins Co.

233. Hillyer, G.V.: Immunodiagnosis of fascioliasis in experimental animals and men, Fourth Intl. Congr. Parasitol. Short Communic. **C**:89, 1978.

234. Hou, P.C.: The relationship between primary carcinoma of the liver and infestation with *Clonorchis sinensis*, J. Pathol. Bacteriol. **72**:239, 1956.

235. Hou, P.C.: Primary carcinoma of bile duct of the liver of cat infested with *Clonorchis sinensis*, J. Pathol. Bacteriol. **87**:239, 1964.

236. Hou, P.C.: Pathological changes in the intrahepatic bile ducts of cats *(Felis catus)* infested with *Clonorchis sinensis*, J. Pathol. Bacteriol. **89**:357, 1965.

237. Hou, P.C.: Hepatic clonorchiasis and carcinoma of the bile duct in a dog, J. Pathol. Bacteriol. **89**:365, 1965.

238. Levine, D.M., Hillyer, G.V., and Floes, S.I.: Comparison of counter electrophoresis, the enzyme-linked immunosorbent assay and Kato fecal examination for the diagnosis of fascioliasis in infected mice and rabbits, Am. J. Trop. Med. Hyg. **29**:602-608, 1980.

239. Marcial-Rojas, R.A.: Fasciolopsiasis. In Marcial-Rojas, R.A., editor: Pathology of protozoal and helminthic diseases, Baltimore, 1971, The Williams & Wilkins Co.

240. Masihur Rahman, K., Idris, M.D., and Azad Khan, A.K.: A study of fasciolopsiasis in Bangladesh, J. Trop. Med. Hyg. **84**:81-86, 1981.

241. Nakashima, T., Sakamoto, K., and Okuda, K.: Hepatocellular carcinoma and clonorchiasis, Cancer **39**:1306-1311, 1977.

242. Náquira-Vildoso, F., and Marcial-Rojas, R.A.: Fascioliasis. In Marcial-Rojas, R.A., editor: Pathology of protozoal and helminthic diseases, Baltimore, 1971, The Williams & Wilkins Co.

243. Purtillo, D.T.: Clonorchiasis and hepatic neoplasms, Trop. Geogr. Med. **28**:21-27, 1976.

244. Sadun, E.H.: Studies on *Opisthorchis viverrini* in Thailand, Am. J. Hyg. **62**:81-115, 1955.

245. Sadun, E.H., and Maiphoom, C.: Studies on epidemiology of human intestinal fluke, *Fasciolopsis buski* (Lankester) in Central Thailand, Am. J. Trop. Med. Hyg. **2**:1070-1084, 1953.

246. Sullivan, W.G., and Koep, L.J.: Common bile-duct obstruction and cholangiohepatitis in clonorchiasis, J.A.M.A. **243**:2060-2061, 1980.

247. Tansurat, P.: Opisthorchiasis. In Marcial-Rojas, R., editor: Pathology of protozoal and helminthic diseases, Baltimore, 1971, The Williams & Wilkins Co.

248. Thammavit, W., et al.: Effects of dimethylnitrosamine on induction of cholangiocarcinoma in *Opisthorchis viverrini*–infected Syrian golden hamsters, Cancer Res. **38**:4634-4639, 1978.

249. Uflacker, R., et al.: Parasitic and mycotic causes of biliary obstruction, Gastrointest. Radiol. **7**:173-179, 1982.

250. Warren, K.S., and Mahmoud, A.A.F.: Algorithms in the diagnosis and management of exotic diseases. XXI. Liver, intestinal and lung flukes, J. Infect. Dis. **135**:692-696, 1977.

251. Yokogawa, M., et al.: Immunoglobulin E: raised levels in sera and pleural exudates of patients with paragonimiasis, Am. J. Trop. Med. Hyg. **25**:581-586, 1976.

Schistosomiasis (bilharziasis)

252. Abdel-Wahab, M., et al.: The use of ultrasonography in diagnosis of different schistosomal syndromes, Proceedings of the Third International Workshop on Diagnostic Ultrasound Imaging, Cairo, March 1978.

252a. Andrade, Z.A., and Rocha, H.: Schistosomal glomerulopathy, Kidney Int. **16**:23-29, 1979.

252b. Attah, E.B., and Kposong, E.O.: Schistosomiasis and carcinoma of the bladder: a critical appraisal of causal relationship, Trop. Geogr. Med. **28**:268-272, 1976.

252c. Bout, D.T., et al.: In vitro killing of *S. mansoni* schistosomula by lymphokine activated mouse macrophages, J. Immunol. **127**:1-5, 1981.

253. Butterworth, A.E.: Eosinophil-mediated damage to larval schistosomes in vitro. In Van den Bossche, H., editor: The host invader interplay, Amsterdam, 1980, Elsevier/North Holland.

254. Butterworth, A.E., and David, J.R.: Eosinophil function, N. Engl. J. Med **304**:154-156, 1981.

255. Butterworth, A.E., et al.: Damage to schistosomula of *Schistosoma mansoni* induced directly by eosinophil major basic protein, J. Immunol. **122**:221-229, 1979.

256. Butterworth, A.E., et al.: Interactions between human eosinophils and schistosomula of *Schistosoma mansoni*. II. The mechanism of irreversible eosinophil adherence, J. Exp. Med. **150**:1456-1471, 1979.

257. Capron, A., et al.: Schistosome mechanisms of evasion. In Van den Bossche, H., editor: The host invader interplay, Amsterdam, 1980, Elsevier/North Holland.

258. El-Bolkainy, M.N., et al.: The impact of schistosomiasis on the pathology of bladder carcinoma, Cancer **48**:2643-2648, 1981.

259. Elsebai, I.: Parasites in the etiology of cancer, CA **27**:100-106, 1977.

260. García-Palmieri, M.R., and Marcial-Rojas, R.A.: Portal hypertension due to schistosomiasis mansoni, Am. J. Med. 27:811-816, 1959.

261. García-Palmieri, M.R., and Marcial-Rojas, R.A.: The protean manifestations of schistosomiasis mansoni: a clinicopathological correlation, Ann. Intern. Med. **57**:763-775, 1962.

262. Gazayerli, M., Khalil, H.A., and Gazayerli, I.M.: Schistosomiasis hematobium (urogenic bilharziasis). In Marcial-Rojas, R.A., editor: Pathology of protozoal and helminthic diseases, Baltimore, 1971, The Williams & Wilkins Co.

263. Hillyer, G.V., and Gomez de Ríos, F.: The enzyme-linked immunosorbent assay for the immunodiagnosis of schistosomiasis, Am. J. Trop. Med. Hyg. **28**:237-241, 1979.

264. Hillyer, G.V., et al.: Immunodiagnosis of infection with *Schistosoma haematobium* and *S. mansoni* in man, Am. J. Trop. Med. Hyg. **29**:1254-1257, 1980.

265. Hillyer, G.V., et al.: The circumoval precipitin test for the serodiagnosis of human schistosomiasis mansoni and haematobia, Am. J. Trop. Med. Hyg. **30**:121-126, 1981.

266. Incani, R.N., and McLaren, D.J.: Neutrophil-mediated cytotoxicity to schistosomula of *Schistosoma mansoni* in vitro: studies on the kinetics of complement and/or antibody-dependent adherence and killing, Parasite Immunol. **3**:107-126, 1981.

267. Jakobiec, F.A., Gess, L., and Zimmerman, L.E.: Granulomatous dacryoadenitis caused by *Schistosoma haematobium*, Arch. Ophthalmol. **95**:278-280, 1977.

268. Jong, E.C., Mahmoud, A.A.F., and Klebahoff, S.J.: Peroxidase-mediated toxicity to schistosomula of *Schistosoma mansoni*, J. Immunol. **126**:468-471, 1981.

269. Lichtenberg, F.: Lesions of intrahepatic portal radicles in Manson's schistosomiasis, Am. J. Pathol. **31**:757-771, 1955.

270. Long, E.G., et al.: Comparison of ELISA, radioimmunoassay and stool examination for *Schistosoma mansoni* infection, Trans. R. Soc. Trop. Med. Hyg. **75**:365-371, 1981.

271. Mahmoud, A.A.F.: Trematodes (schistosomiasis, flukes). In Mandell, G., Douglas R.G., and Bennett, J.E., editors: Principles and practice of infectious diseases, New York, 1979, John Wiley & Sons, Inc.

272. Marchand, E.J., et al.: The pulmonary obstruction syndrome in *Schistosoma mansoni* pulmonary endarteritis, Arch. Intern. Med. **100**:965-980, 1957.

273. Marcial-Rojas, R.A.: Schistosomiasis mansoni. In Marcial-Rojas, R.A., editor: Pathology of protozoal and helminthic diseases, Baltimore, 1971, The Williams & Wilkins Co.

274. Marcial-Rojas, R.A., and Fiol, R.E.: Neurologic complications of schistosomiasis: review of the literature and report of two cases of transverse myelitis due to *S. mansoni*, Medicine **59**:215-230, 1963.

275. Martínez-Maldonado, M., et al.: Liver cell carcinoma (hepatoma) in Puerto Rico: a survey of 26 cases, Am. J. Dig. Dis. **10**:522, 1965.

276. McLaren, M.D., and Lillywhite, J.E.: Serodiagnosis of human *Schistosoma mansoni* infections: enhanced sensitivity and specificity in ELISA using a fraction containing *J. mansoni* egg antigens W₁ and L₁, Trans. R. Soc. Trop. Med. Hyg. **75**:72-79, 1981.

277. Ming-Chai, C., et al.: Evolution of colorectal cancer in schistosomiasis: transitional mucosal changes adjacent to large intestinal carcinoma in colectomy specimens, Cancer **46**:1661-1675, 1980.

278. Miyake, M.: Schistosomiasis japonicum. In Marcial-Rojas, R.A., editor: Pathology of protozoal and helminthic diseases, Baltimore, 1971, The Williams & Wilkins Co.

279. Nakashima, T., et al.: Primary liver cancer coincident with schistosomiasis japonica: a study of 24 necropsies, Cancer **36**:1483-1489, 1975.

280. Nash, T.E., et al.: Schistosome infections in humans: perspectives and recent findings, Ann. Intern. Med. **97**:740-754, 1982.

281. Oyediran, A.B.O.O.: Renal disease due to schistosomiasis of the lower urinary tract, Kidney Int. **16**:15-22, 1979.

282. Pincus, S.H., et al.: Antibody dependent eosinophil mediated damage to schistosomula of *Schistosoma mansoni:* lack of requirement for oxidative metabolism, J. Immunol. **126**:1794-1799, 1981.

283. Relley, R.P., Warren, K.S., and Jorden, P.: Purified antigen radio-immunoassay for the serological diagnosis of schistosomiasis mansoni, Lancet **2**:781-784, 1977.

284. Rodriguez, H.F., et al.: A comparative study of portal and bilharzial cirrhosis, Gastroenterology **29**:235-246, 1955.

285. Sadisgursky, M., and Andrade, Z.A.: Pulmonary changes in schistosomal cor pulmonale, Am. J. Trop. Med. Hyg. **31**:779-784, 1982.

286. Santana Filho, S.: Carcinoma primario do figado (estudo de 20 casos autopsiados) (thesis), 1964, University of Bahia, Brazil.

287. Schinski, V.D., Clutter, W.C., and Murell, K.D.: Enzyme and ^{125}I-labeled anti-immunoglobulin assay in the immunodiagnosis of schistosomiasis, Am. J. Trop. Med. Hyg. **26**:824-831, 1976.

288. Sher, A., and Moser, G.: Schistosomiasis: immunologic properties of developing schistosomula, Am. J. Pathol. **102**:121-126, 1981.

289. Smith, J.H., et al.: Surgical pathology of schistosomal obstructive uropathy: a clinicopathologic correlation, Am. J. Trop. Med. Hyg. **26**:96-108, 1977.

290. von Lichtenberg, F., Sher, A., and McIntyre, S.: A lung model of schistosome immunity in mice, Am. J. Pathol. **87**:105-124, 1977.

291. von Lichtenberg, F., et al.: Eosinophil enriched inflammatory response to schistosomula in the skin of mice immune to *Schistosoma mansoni,* Am. J. Pathol. **84**:479-500, 1976.

292. Warren, K.S.: Hepatosplenic schistosomiasis mansoni: an immunologic disease, Bull. N.Y. Acad. Med. **51**:545-550, 1975.

293. Warren, K.S.: The immunopathology of schistosomiasis. In Van den Bossche, editor: The host invader interplay, Amsterdam, 1980, Elsevier/North Holland.

294. Wright, E.D., Chiphangwi, J., and Hutt, M.S.R.: Schistosomiasis of the female genital tract: a histopathological study of 176 cases from Malawi, Trans. R. Soc. Trop. Med. Hyg. **76**:822-829, 1982.

Diseases caused by cestodes (tapeworms)

295. Abraham, J.L., Spore, W.W., and Benirschke, K.: Cysticercosis of the fallopian tube: histology and microanalysis, Hum. Pathol. **13**:665-670, 1982.

296. Barnett, L.: Hydatid cysts: their location in various organs and tissues of body, Aust. N.Z. J. Surg. **12**:240-248, 1943.

297. Berman, J.D., et al.: Cysticercus of 60 milliliter volume in human brain, Am. J. Trop. Med. Hyg. **30**:616-619, 1981.

298. Carbajal, J.R., et al.: Radiology of cysticercosis of the central nervous system including computed tomography, Radiology **125**:127-131, 1977.

299. Case records of the Massachusetts General Hospital 40-1977, N. Engl. J. Med. **297**:773-780, 1977.

300. Castillo, M.: Intestinal taeniasis. In Marcial-Rojas, R.A., editor: Pathology of protozoal and helminthic diseases, Baltimore, 1971, The Williams & Wilkins Co.

301. Diwan, A.R., et al.: Enzyme-linked immunosorbent assay (ELISA) for the detection of antibody to cysticerci of *Taenia solium,* Am. J. Trop. Med. Hyg. **31**:249-369, 1982.

302. Grabbe, E., Kern, P., and Heller, M.: Human echinococcosis: diagnostic value of computed tomography, Tropenmed. Parasit. **32**:35-38, 1981.

303. Hadidi, A.: Sonography of hepatic echnicoccal cysts, Gastrointest. Radiol. **7**:349-354, 1982.

304. Hillyier, G.V., and Kagan, I.G.: New advances in immunodiagnosis of parasitic infection. I. The enzyme-linked immuno-absorbent assay, Bol. Asoc. Med. P.R. **71**:366-377, 1979.

305. Iacona, A., Pini, C., and Vicari, G.: Enzyme-linked immunosorbent assay (ELISA) in the serodiagnosis of hydatid disease, Am. J. Trop. Med. Hyg. **29**:95-102, 1980.

306. Jones, T.C.: Cestodes (tapeworms). In Mandell, G., Douglas, R.G., and Bennett, J.E., editors: Principles and practice of infectious diseases, New York, 1979, John Wiley & Sons, Inc.

307. Kagan, I.G.: Serodiagnosis of hyatid disease. In Cohen, S., and Sadun, E., editors: Immunology of parasitic infections, Oxford, 1976, Blackwell Scientific Publications.

308. Mahajan, R.C., Chopra, J.S., and Chita Kara, N.L.: Comparative evaluation of indirect hemagglutination and complement fixation test in serodiagnosis of cysticercosis, Indian J. Med. Res. **63**:121-125, 1975.

309. Marquez-Monter, H.: Cystericercosis. In Marcial-Rojas, R.A., editor: Pathology of protozoal and helminthic diseases, Baltimore, 1971, The Williams & Wilkins Co.

310. Nakhla, N.B., et al.: Ultrasound and the monitoring of the medical treatment of hepatic hydatid disease, J. Trop. Med. Hyg. **84**:121-124, 1981.

311. Napier, L.E.: Principles and practice of tropical medicine, New York, 1946, Macmillan, Inc.

312. Peters, L., Cavis, D., and Robertson, J.: Is *Diphyllobothrium latum* currently present in Northern Michigan? J. Parasitol. **64**:947-949, 1978.

313. Rydzewski, A.K., Chisholm, E.S., and Kagan, J.G.: Comparison of serologic test for human cysticercosis by indirect hemagglutination, indirect fluorescent antibody and agar gel precipitating test, J. Parasitol. **61**:154-155, 1975.

314. Subianto, D.B., Tumada, L.R., and Margono, S.S.: Burns and epileptic fits associated with cysticercosis in mountain people of Irian Jaya, Trop. Geogr. Med. **30**:275-278, 1978.

315. Toskes, P.P., and Doren, J.J.: Vitamin B_{12} absorption and malabsorption, Gastroenterology **65**:662, 1973.

316. Varela-Díaz, V.M., et al: Evaluation of three immunodiagnostic tests for human hydatid disease, Am. J. Trop. Med. Hyg. **24**:312-319, 1975.

317. Vijayan, G.P., et al.: Neurological and related manifestations of cysticercosis, Trop. Geogr. Med. **29**:271-278, 1977.

318. Vik, R.: Diphyllobothriasis. In Marcial-Rojas, R.A., editor: Pathology of protozoal and helminthic diseases, Baltimore, 1971, The Williams & Wilkins Co.

319. von Bonsdorff, B.: *Diphyllobothrium latum* as a cause of pernicious anemia, Exp. Parasitol. **5**:207-230, 1956.

320. von Bonsdorff, B.: Diphyllobothriasis in man, London, 1977, Academic Press, Inc.

Diseases caused by nematodes of the digestive tract

321. Areán, V.M., and Crandall, C.A.: Ascariasis. In Marcial-Rojas, R.A., editor: Pathology of protozoal and helminthic diseases, Baltimore, 1971, The Williams & Wilkins Co.

322. Areán, V.M., and Crandall, C.A.: Toxocariasis. In Marcial-Rojas, R.A., editor: Pathology of protozoal and helminthic diseases, Baltimore, 1971, The Williams & Wilkins Co.

323. Areán, V.M.: Capillariasis. In Marcial-Rojas, R.A., editor: Pathology of protozoal and helminthic diseases, Baltimore, 1971, The Williams & Wilkins Co.

324. Bass, D.A., and Szejda, P.: Mechanisms of killing of newborn larvae of *Trichinella spiralis* by neutrophils and eosinophils: killing by generators of hydrogen peroxide in vitro, J. Clin. Invest. **64**:1558-1564, 1979.

325. Beaver, P.C., Kriz, J.J., and Lau, T.J.: Pulmonary nodule caused by *Enterobius vermicularis,* Am. J. Trop. Med. Hyg. **22**:711-713, 1973.

326. Beaver, P.C., et al.: Chronic eosinophilia due to visceral larva migrans: report of three cases, Pediatrics **9**:7-19, 1952.

327. Beckman, E.N., and Holland, J.B. Ovarian enterobiasis: a proposed pathogenesis, Am. J. Trop. Med. Hyg. **30**:74-76, 1981.

328. Bell, R.G., McGregor, D.D., and Despommier, D.D.: *Trichinella spiralis:* mediation of the intestinal component of protective immunity in the rat by multiple phase-specific antiparasitic responses, Exp. Parasitol. **47**:140-157, 1979.

329. Berger, R., Kraman, S., and Paciotti, M.: Pulmonary strongyloidiasis complicating therapy with corticosteroids, Am. J. Trop. Med. Hyg. **29**:31-34, 1980.

330. Blumenthal, D.S.: Intestinal nematodes in the United States, N. Engl. J. Med. **297**:1437-1439, 1977.

331. Blumenthal, D.S., and Schultz, M.G.: Incidence of intestinal obstruction in children infected with *Ascaris lumbricoides*, Am. J. Trop. Med. Hyg. **24**:801-805, 1975.

332. Blumenthal, D.S., and Schultz, M.G.: Effects on *Ascaris* infection on nutritional status in children, Am. J. Trop. Med. Hyg. **25**:682-690, 1976.

333. Brasitus, T.A.: Parasites and malabsorption, Am. J. Med. **67**:1058-1065, 1979.

334. Butterworth, A.E., and David, J.R.: Eosinophil function, N. Engl. J. Med. **304**:154-156, 1981.

335. Chandrasoma, P.T., and Mendis, K.N.: *Enterobius vermicularis* in ectopic sites, Am. J. Trop. Med. Hyg. **26**:644-649, 1977.

336. Chitwood, M.B., Valesquez, C., and Salazar, N.G.: *Capillaria philippinensis*, sp. n. (Nematoda: Trichinellida) from the intestine of man in the Philippines, J. Parasitol. **54**:368-371, 1972.

337. Cross, J.H.: Clinical manifestations and laboratory diagnosis of eosinophilic meningitis syndrome associated with angiostrongyliasis, Southeast Asian J. Trop. Med. Public Health **9**:161-170, 1978.

338. Cross, J.H., et al.: Studies on the experimental transmission of *Capillaria philippinensis* in monkeys, Trans. R. Soc. Trop. Med. **66**:819-827, 1972.

339. Cruz, T., Reboucas, G., and Rocha, H.: Fatal strongyloidiasis in patients receiving corticosteroids, N. Engl. J. Med. **275**:1093-1096, 1966.

340. Cypess, R.H., et al.: Larva specific antibodies in patients with visceral larva migrans, J. Infect. Dis. **135**:633-636, 1977.

341. De León, E., and Maldonado, J.F.: Uncinariasis (ancylostomiasis). In Marcial-Rojas, R.A., editor: Pathology of protozoal and helminthic diseases, Baltimore, 1971, The Williams & Wilkins Co.

342. Despommier, D.: Adaptive changes in muscle fibers infected with *Trichinella spiralis*, Am. J. Pathol. **78**:477-496, 1975.

343. Despommier, D., et al.: Immunodiagnosis of human trichinosis using counter-immunoelectrophoresis and agar gel diffusion techniques, Am. J. Trop. Med. Hyg. **23**:41-44, 1974.

344. Dessein, A.J., et al.: IgE antibody and resistance to infection. I. Selective suppression of the IgE antibody response in rats diminishes the resistance and the eosinophil response to *Trichinella spiralis* infection, J. Exp. Med. **153**:423-436, 1981.

345. Detels, R., et al.: An epidemic of intestinal capillariasis in man: a study in a barrio in northern Luzon, Am. J. Trop. Med. Hyg. **18**:676, 1969.

346. Editorial note: Centers for Disease Control, Morbid. Mortal. Weekly Rep. **30**:313, 1981.

347. Frayha, R.A.: Trichinosis-related polyarteritis nodosa, Am. J. Med. **71**:307-312, 1981.

348. Frenkel, J.K.: *Angiostrongylus costaricensis* infections. In Binford, C.H., and Connor, D.H., editors: Pathology of tropical and extraordinary diseases, Washington, D.C., 1976, Armed Forces Institute of Pathology.

349. Fresh, J.W., et al.: Necropsy findings in intestinal capillariasis, Am. J. Trop. Med. Hyg. **21**:169-173, 1972.

350. Gelpi, A.P., and Mustafa, A.: Seasonal pneumonitis with eosinophilia: a study of larval ascariasis in Saudi Arabia, Am. J. Trop. Med. Hyg. **16**:646-657, 1967.

351. Genta, R.M., and Ward, P.A.: The histopathology of experimental strongyloidiasis, Am. J. Pathol. **99**:207-220, 1980.

352. Glickman, L., et al.: Evaluation of serodiagnostic tests for visceral larva migrans, Am. J. Trop. Med. Hyg. **27**:492-498, 1978.

353. Greenberg, E.R., and Cline, B.L.: Is trichuriasis associated with iron deficiency anemia? Am. J. Trop. Med. Hyg. **28**:770-772, 1979.

354. Grove, D.I., and Blair, J.: Diagnosis of human strongyloidiasis by immunofluorescence, using *Strongyloides ratti* and *S. stercoralis* larvae, Am. J. Trop. Med. Hyg. **30**:344-349, 1981.

355. Grove, D.I., Mahmoud, A.A.F., and Warren, K.S.: Eosinophils and resistance to *Trichinella spiralis*, J. Exp. Med. **145**:755-759, 1977.

356. Jacobson, E.S., and Jacobson, H.G.: Trichinosis in an immunosuppressed human host, Am. J. Clin. Pathol. **68**:791-794, 1977.

357. Kanchanaranya, C., Prechanond, A., and Punyagupta, S.: Removal of living worm in retinal *Angiostrongylus cantonensis*, J. Ophthalmol. **74**:456-458, 1972.

358. Kayes, S.G., and Oaks, J.A.: Development of the granulomatous response in murine toxocariasis, Am. J. Pathol. **93**:277-294, 1978.

359. Kazura, J.W., and Aikawa, M.: Host defense mechanisms against *Trichinella spiralis* infection in the mouse: eosinophil-mediated destruction of larvae in vitro, J. Immunol. **124**:355-361, 1980.

360. Kenney, M., and Webber, C.A.: Diagnosis of strongyloidiasis in Papanicolaou-stained sputum smears, Acta Cytol. **18**:270-273, 1974.

361. Laqueur, G.L.: Eosinophilic meningitis (*Angiostrongylus cantonensis*). In Marcial-Rojas, R.A., editor: Pathology of protozoal and helminthic diseases, Baltimore, 1971, The Williams & Wilkins Co.

362. Layrisse, M., et al.: Blood loss due to infection with *Trichuris trichiura*, Am. J. Trop. Med. Hyg. **16**:613-619, 1967.

363. Little, M.D., Cuello, C.J., and D'Alessandro, A.: Granuloma of the liver due to *Enterobius vermicularis*, Am. J. Trop. Med. Hyg. **22**:567-569, 1973.

364. Lotero, H., Tripathy, K., and Bolaños, O.: Gastrointestinal blood loss in *Trichuris* infection, Am. J. Trop. Med. Hyg. **23**:1203-1204, 1974.

365. Malek, E.A.: Presence of *Angiostrongylus costaricensis Morera* and *Céspedes* 1971 in Colombia, Am. J. Trop. Med. Hyg. **30**:81-83, 1981.

366. Manson-Smith, D.F., Bruce, R.G., and Parrott, D.M.V.: Villous atrophy and expulsion of intestinal *Trichinella spiralis* are mediated by T cells, Cell. Immunol. **47**:285-292, 1979.

367. Marcial-Rojas, R.A.: Strongyloidiasis. In Marcial-Rojas, R.A., editor: Pathology of protozoal and helminthic diseases, Baltimore, 1971, The Williams & Wilkins Co.

368. Marsden, P.D.: Ascariasis. In Beeson, P.B., McDermott, W., and Wyngaarden, J.B., editors: Cecil textbook of medicine, ed. 15, Philadelphia 1979, W.B. Saunders Co.

369. Marsden, P.D.: Hookworm disease. In Beeson P.B., McDermott, W., and Wyngaarden, J.B., editors: Cecil-Loeb textbook of medicine, ed. 15, Philadelphia, 1979, W.B. Saunders Co.

370. Marsden, P.D.: Strongyloisiasis: a replicating human helminthic infection, Trop. Gastroenterol. **3**:9-14, 1982.

371. Milder, J.E., et al.: Clinical features of *Strongyloides stercoralis* infection in an endemic area of the United States, Gastroenterology **80**:1481-1488, 1981.

372. Moreno, E.: Enterobiasis (oxyuriasis, pinworm infection). In Marcial-Rojas, R.A., editor: Pathology of protozoal and helminthic diseases, Baltimore, 1971, The Williams & Wilkins Co.

373. Morera, P.: Life history and redescription of *Angiostrongylus costaricensis Morera* and *Céspedes*, Am. J. Trop. Med. Hyg. **22**:613-621, 1973.

374. Morgan, O., James, O., and Sahoy, R.: Intestinal perforation in ascariasis: case reports, Trans. R. Soc. Trop. Med. Hyg. **73**:183-184, 1979.

375. Most, H.: Trichinosis—preventable yet still with us, N. Engl. J. Med. **298**:1178-1180, 1978.

376. Most, H., and Abeles, M.M.: Trichiniasis involving nervous system: clinical and neuropathologic review with report of 2 cases, Arch. Neurol. **37**:589-616, 1937.

377. Neafie, R.C., Connor, D.H., and Cross, J.H.: Capillariasis. In Binford, C.H., and Connor, D.H., editors: Pathology of tropical and extraordinary diseases, Washington, D.C., 1976, Armed Forces Institute of Pathology.

378. Nye, S.W., et al.: Lesions of the brain in eosinophilic meningitis, Arch. Pathol. **89**:9-19, 1970.

379. Ogilvie, B.M., et al.: Antibody responses in self-infections with *Necator americanus*, Trans. R. Soc. Trop. Med. Hyg. **72**:66-71, 1978.

380. Paulino, G.B., Jr., and Wittenberg, J.: Intestinal capillariasis: a new cause of a malabsorption pattern, Am. J. Roentgenol. Radium Ther. Nucl. Med. **117**:340-345, 1973.

381. Punyagupta, S., Juttijudata, P., and Bunnag, T.: Eosinophilic meningitis in Thailand: clinical studies of 484 typical cases probably caused by *Angiostrongylus cantonensis*, Am. J. Trop. Med. Hyg. **24**:921, 1975.

382. Quiñones Soto, R.A., et al.: Estrongiloidiasis en el paciente immunocomprometido, Bol. Asoc. Méd. P.R. **72**:609-613, 1980.

383. Ramírez-Weiser, R.R.: Trichuriasis. In Marcial-Rojas, R.A., editor: Pathology of protozoal and helminthic diseases, Baltimore, 1971, The Williams & Wilkins Co.

384. Raybourne, R., and Solomon, G.B.: *Capillaria hepatica:* granuloma formation to eggs. III. Anti-immunoglobulin augmentation and reagin activity in mice, Exp. Parasitol. **38**:87-95, 1975.

385. Raybourne, R.B., Solomon, G.B., and Soulsby, E.J.L.: *Capillaria hepatica:* granuloma formation to eggs. II. Peripheral immunological responses, Exp. Parasitol. **36**:244-252, 1974.

386. Reddy, C.R.R., et al.: Granulomatous peritonitis due to *Ascaris lumbricoides* and its ova, J. Trop. Med. Hyg. **78**:146, 1975.

387. Rivera, E., et al.: Hyperinfection syndrome with *Strongyloides stercoralis*, Ann. Intern. Med. **72**:199, 1970.

388. Rogers, W.A., Jr., and Nelson, B.: Strongyloidosis and malignant lymphoma: opportunistic infection by a nematode, J.A.M.A. **195**:685-687, 1970.

389. Rosencrantz, M., et al.: Trichinosis associated with meat from a grizzly bear in Alaska, Morbid Mortal. Weekly Rep. **30**:115-116, 1981.

390. Sauerbrey, M.: A precipitin test for the diagnosis of human abdominal angiostrongyliasis, Am. J. Trop. Med. Hyg. **26**:1156-1158, 1977.

391. Schantz, P.M., and Glickman, L.T.: Toxocaral visceral larva migrans, N. Engl. J. Med. **298**:436-439, 1978.

392. Scowden, E.B., Schaffner, W., and Stone, W.J.: Overwhelming strongyloidiasis: an unappreciated opportunistic infection, Medicine **57**:527-544, 1978.

393. Simon, R.D.: Pinworm infestation and urinary tract infection in young girls, Am. J. Dis. Child. **128**:21-22, 1974.

394. Sitprija, V., et al.: Renal involvement in human trichinosis, Arch. Intern. Med. **140**:544-546, 1980.

395. Solomon, G.B., and Grigonis, G.J., Jr.: *Capillaria hepatica:* relation of structure and composition of egg shell to antigen release, Exp. Parasitol. **40**:298-307, 1976.

396. Solomon, G.B., and Soulsby, E.J.L.: Granuloma formation to *Capillaria hepatica* eggs. I. Descriptive definition, Exp. Parasitol. **33**:458-467, 1973.

397. Soulsby, E.J.L.: Serodiagnosis of other helminthic infections. In Cohen, S., and Sadun, E., editors: Immunology of parasitic infections, Oxford, 1976, Blackwell Scientific Publications.

398. Spillman, R.K.: Pulmonary ascariasis in tropical communities, Am. J. Trop. Med. Hyg. **24**: 791-800, 1975.

399. Trichinosis surveillance annual summary 1979, Atlanta, 1980, Center for Disease Control, U.S. Department of Health and Human Services.

400. Ubelaker, J.E., and Hall, N.M.: First report of *Angiostrongylus costaricensis Morera and Céspedes* 1971 in the United States, J. Parasitol. **65**:307, 1979.

401. Warren, K.S., and Mahmoud, A.A.F.: Algorithms in the diagnosis and management of exotic diseases. XXII. Ascariasis and toxocariasis, J. Infect. Dis. **135**:868-872, 1977.

402. Wassom, D.L., and Gleich, G.J.: Damage to *Trichinella spiralis* newborn larvae by eosinophil major basic protein, Am. J. Trop. Med. Hyg. **28**:860-863, 1979.

403. Watten, R.H., et al.: Clinical studies of capillariasis philippinensis, Trans. R. Soc. Trop. Med. Hyg. **66**:828-834, 1972.

404. Welch, J.S., Dobson, C., and Campbell, G.R.: Immunodiagnosis and seroepidemiology of *Angiostrongylus cantonensis* zoonoses in man, Trans. R. Soc. Trop. Med. Hyg. **74**:614-623, 1980.

405. Whalen, G.E., Rosenberg, E.B., and Strickland, G.T.: Circulating immunoglobulins, intestinal protein loss, and malabsorption in intestinal capillariasis, Ann. Intern. Med. **70**:1072, 1969.

406. Whalen, G.E., et al.: Intestinal capillariasis: a new disease in man, Lancet **1**:13, 1969.

407. Whitehead, R.: Mucosal biopsy of the gastrointestinal tract, Philadelphia, 1979, W.B. Saunders Co.

408. Wilder, H.C.: Nematode endophthalmitis, Trans. Am. Acad. Ophthalmol. **55**:99-109, 1950.

409. Wright, K.A.: *Trichenella spiralis:* an intracellular parasite in the intestinal phase, J. Parasitol. **65**:441-445, 1979.

410. Yii, C.Y.: Clinical observations of eosinophilic meningitis and meningoencephalitis caused by *Angiostrongylus cantonensis* on Taiwan, Am. J. Trop. Med. Hyg. **25**:233-249, 1976.

411. Yii, C.Y., and Cross, J.H.: Human angiostrongyliasis in Taiwan, Southeast Asian J. Trop. Med. Public Health **1**:154-155, 1970.

412. Zimmerman, W.J., Steele, J.H., and Kagan, I.G.: Trichinosis in the U.S. population, 1966-1970: prevalence and epidemiologic factors, Health Serv. Rep. **88**:606-623, 1973.

Diseases caused by filarial nematodes (filariasis)

413. Bartlett, A., Bidwell, D., and Voller, A.: Preliminary studies on the application of enzyme-immunoassay in the detection of antibodies in onchocerciasis, Tropenmed. Parasitol. **26**:370-347, 1975.

414. Bosworth, W., Ewert, A., and Bray, J.: The interaction of *Brugia malayi* and *Streptococcus* in an animal model, Med. Hyg. **22**:714-719, 1973.

415. Choyce, D.P.: Ocular onchocerciasis in Central America, Africa and British Isles (with a note on equine periodic opthalmia), Trans. R. Soc. Trop. Med. Hyg. **58**:11, 1964.

416. Connor, D.H.: Onchocerciasis, N. Engl. J. Med. **298**:379-381, 1978.

417. de Buen, S.: Onchocerciasis. In Marcial-Rojas, R.A., editor: Pathology of protozoal and helminthic diseases, Baltimore, 1971, The Williams & Wilkins Co.

418. Editorial note. Morbid. Mortal. Weekly Rep. **30**:195, 1981.

419. Enfermedad de Robles, Editiorial Universitaria, Universidad de San Carlos, Guatemala, 1963 (extensive monograph).

420. Galindo, L.: Bancroftian filariasis. In Marcial-Rojas, R.A., editor: Pathology of protozoal and helminthic diseases, Baltimore, 1971, The Williams & Wilkins Co.

421. Galindo L., Von Lichtenberg, F., and Baldizon, C.: Bancroftian filariasis in Puerto Rico: infection pattern and tissue lesions, Am. J. Trop. Med. **11**:739-748, 1962.

422. Gentilini, M., et al.: A case of eosinophilic pleurisy due to *Dracunculus medinensis* infection, Trans. R. Soc. Trop. Med. Hyg. **72**:540-541, 1978.

423. Gibson, D.W., and Connor, D.H.: Onchocercal lymphadenitis: clinicopathologic study of 34 patients, Trans. R. Soc. Trop. Med. Hyg. **72**:137-153, 1978.

424. Gibson, D.W., Heggie, C., and Connor, D.H.: Clinical and pathologic aspects of onchocerciasis, Pathol. Annu. **15**:195-240, 1980.

425. Grove, D.I., and Forbes, I.J.: Immunosuppression in bancroftian filariasis, Trans. R. Soc. Trop. Med. Hyg. **73**:23-26, 1979.

426. Guevara-Rojas, A.: Estudio clinico general. In Oncocercosis, Mexico City, 1948, La Prensa Médica Mexicana.

427. Hashiguchi, Y., et al.: The use of an *Onchocerca volvulus* microfilarial antigen skin test in epidemiological survey of onchocerciasis in Guatemala, Trans. R. Soc. Trop. Med. Hyg. **73**:543-548, 1979.

428. Jackowski, L.A., Jr., González-Flores, B., and Lichtenberg, F.: Relationship of tropical hydrocele to filariasis in Puerto Rico, U.S. Naval Med. Res. Inst. Res. Rep. MR 005.09-1033, **1**:25-52, 1960.

429. Kaliraj, P., Ghirnikar, S.N., and Harinath, B.C.: Enzyme-linked immunosorbent assay (ELISA) for bancroftian filariasis, Trans. R. Soc. Trop. Med. Hyg. **75**:119-120, 1981.

430. Lichtenberg, F., and Medina, R.: Bancroftian filariasis in the etiology of funiculo-epididymitis, periorchitis and hydrocele in Puerto Rico, Am. J. Trop. Med. Hyg. **6**:739-751, 1957.

431. Markell, E.K., and Voge, M.: Medical parasitology, Philadelphia, 1981, W.B. Saunders Co.

432. Meyers, W.M., Neafie, R.C., and Connor, D.H.: Onchocerciasis: invasion of deep organs by *Onchocerca volvolus;* autopsy findings, Am. J. Trop. Med. Hyg. **26**:650-657, 1977.

433. Nelson, G.S.: Filariasis, N. Engl. J. Med. **300**:1136-1139, 1979.

434. Neva, F.A., and Ottensen, E.A.: Tropical (filarial) eosinophilia, N. Engl. J. Med. **298**:1129-1131, 1978.

435. O'Connor, F.W.: Etiology of disease syndrome in *Wuchereria bancrofti* infections, Trans. R. Soc. Trop. Med. Hyg. **26**:13-47, 1932.

436. Ottensen, E.A., et al.: Specific allergic sensitization to filarial antigens in tropical eosinophilia syndrome, Lancet **1:** 1158-1161, 1979.

437. Piessens, W.F., et al.: Antigen specific suppressor cells and suppressor factors in human filariasis with *Brugia malayi,* N. Engl. J. Med. **302:**833-837, 1980.

438. Piessens, W.F., et al.: Antigen-specific suppressor T lymphocytes in human lymphatic filariasis, N. Engl. J. Med. **307:**144-148, 1982.

439. Price, D.L., and Child, P.L.: Dracontiasis (dracunculiasis, dracunculosis, medina worm, guinea worm). In Marcial-Rojas, R.A., editor: Pathology of protozoal and helminthic diseases, Baltimore, 1971, The Williams & Wilkins Co.

440. Price, D.L., and Hopps, H.C.: Loiasis (the eyeworm, loa worm). In Marcial-Rojas, R.A., editor: Pathology of protozoal and helminthic diseases, Baltimore, 1971, The Williams & Wilkens Co.

441. Sacks, H.N., Williams, D.N., and Eifrig, D.E.: Loiasis: report of a case and review of the literature, Arch. Intern. Med. **136:**914-915, 1976.

CHAPTER 13

Immunopathology (Hypersensitivity Diseases)

STEWART SELL

Immunity means protection or security from particular diseases or poisons. Immunopathology is the study of diseases caused by immune mechanisms. The word *immunopathology* illustrates the paradox of immune reactions. On one hand, immune reactions provide efficient protection against infectious organisms; on the other hand, they may destroy the host's own tissues and cause disease.

Specific immune protection is mediated by products generated as a result of an immune response, which involves proliferation and differentiation of cells in the lymphoid system. This specific protection depends on previous exposure of the individual to the particular noxious agent or organism (antigen). As a result of this primary exposure to antigen, serum proteins (antibodies) or altered cells (specifically sensitized cells) develop that have the capacity to recognize, react with, and neutralize the noxious agent or infecting organism.

The term *allergy* has different meanings depending on how it is used. Von Pirquet orginally coined the term to mean altered reactivity to a given agent because of a previous exposure to it, without judging whether the altered effect was good or bad. In Britain allergy designates any nonprotective immune reaction; in the United States the term usually refers to atopic reactions (p. 471). *Hypersensitivity* implies destructive effects of any immune reactions.

Many examples of altered reactivity because of a previous exposure are not reactions of allergy or immunity. Some of these phenomena include the Shwartzman reaction (alteration in the state of blood coagulation), adaptive enzyme synthesis (substrate selection of enzyme production), anaphylactoid reactions (pseudoallergic reactions attributable to nonallergic liberation of pharmacologically active agents that may also be liberated by allergic reactions), untoward reactions to drugs attributable to physiologic hyperreactivity (idiosyncrasy), and other types of adaptations to environmental parameters (heat adaptation, cold adaptation, altitude adaptation, emotional adaptation, and so on).

BASIC IMMUNOLOGY
Antigenicity

In all types of immunologic or allergic reactions an individual's immune system acquires specific information from contact with an antigen (Ag). The acquisition and expression of this immunologic knowledge consist of afferent, central, and efferent phases. The afferent phase includes the delivery of antigen to specifically reactive cells. The central phase consists of proliferation and differentiation of cells in the lymphoid system leading to the production of antibody or cells that recognize and react with the antigen. The efferent phase is initiated by the reaction of antibody or sensitized cells with the antigen. The result of this reaction is protective if the antigen is an infecting agent or noxious material; it is destructive if the antigen is associated with normal tissue.

Essential to an immune response is the capacity of the individual's immune system to recognize an antigen. Most natural antigens are other organisms (bacteria, viruses, fungi). Experimental or therapeutic procedures provide contact with other potential antigens, such as exogenous macromolecules (drugs), serum proteins, blood cells, or tissues (grafts) from individuals of the same or other species. An antigen that can induce an immune response is termed an *immunogen*. The capacity of an individual to respond to a given immunogen depends on a number of factors, such as dose, route, form, degree of foreignness, and number of previous exposures to the immunogen.

Lymphoid tissue and immune response

The introduction of an immunogen into a responsive individual leads to changes in the individual's tissues. These changes characteristically occur in organs that contain large numbers of lymphocytes, macrophages, and plasma cells. These cells are known as lymphoid cells, and the organs where they reside are lymphoid organs.

A feature of active immune responses is the enlargement of small lymphocytes into immature *blast cells*. Blast cells are found in lymphoid organs that drain sites of antigen injection and in active inflammatory lesions, particularly those of delayed hypersensitivity reactions. Blast cells may also be induced in cultures of small lymphocytes by certain mitogenic agents in vitro. Blast cells are a manifestation of the proliferative phase of the immune response.

Lymphoid organs include lymph nodes, spleen, thymus, and the gastrointestinal tract in which lymphoid tissue is concentrated as tonsils, Peyer's patches, appendix and isolated submucosal lymphoid aggregates, and bone marrow.

Functions of lymphoid organs

The *bone marrow* contains the progenitor cells for the other lymphoid organs. Progenitor cells produced in the bone marrow circulate to the thymus or gastrointestinal tract where they develop into more mature lymphoid cells. Populations of bone marrow cells that may have recirculated back to the bone marrow can respond to antigens. The *thymus* produces small lymphocytes (thymus-derived lymphocytes, or T cells), necessary for cellular hypersensitivity and cooperative effects in the induction of circulating antibody. The *gastrointestinal lymphoid tissue* or fetal liver is required for the maturation of plasma cell precursors necessary for antibody production (B cells); these plasma cell precursors may be produced by the bone marrow in the adult. The lymph nodes and spleen contain sites where cells from the thymus (T cells) and cells from the bone marrow or gastrointestinal tract (B cells) are organized into a functional unit for the production of circulating antibody or specifically sensitized cells.

Structure of lymphoid tissue

The size and microscopic appearance of lymphoid organs depend on antigenic stimulation. The structure of the lymph node is an example. Lymph nodes are bean-shaped organs with two layers. The outside layer (cortex) is denser in cells than the inside (medulla). Lymphatic vessels enter through the cortex, drain through the medulla, and exit via a single lymphatic vessel at an indentation in the node known as the hilum. In the medulla, cords of lymphocytes alternate with lymphatic sinusoids that connect the afferent and efferent lymphatics. Lymphoid cells in the lymph node cortex are organized into ball-like clusters called follicles. If the follicle has a less dense center with a rim of lightly packed cells, it is called a secondary follicle; if it is composed of tightly packed cells without a dense center, it is a primary folli-

cle. The development of follicles is a manifestation of the induction of antibody formation.

The induction of an immunoglobulin antibody response is associated with the development of germinal centers in the responding lymphoid organs. Antigens as well as nonantigens are taken up by the phagocytic cells (macrophages) in the medullary areas of lymph nodes and spleen. Antigen can also be found in "dendritic" macrophages in the lymph node cortex or splenic white pulp. Dendritic macrophages are elongated, spindle-shaped cells with cytoplasmic extensions that are closely associated with lymphocytes of the cortex or white pulp. Lymphoid follicles form around dendritic macrophages that contain antigen. Cell proliferation leads to development of a spherical mass of cells that pushes the antigen-containing macrophages to the edge of the proliferation (germinal center). Within 5 to 7 days after immunization, plasma cells appear below the germinal center and migrate into the medullary cords where they produce and secrete antibody, which is then released into the medullary sinusoids. Plasma cells may be observed in large numbers in the adjacent medullary cords or splenic red pulp for at least 10 weeks after immunization. In addition to plasma cells, germinal centers produce memory B cells. On reexposure to antigen these enable the "immunized" individual to produce larger amounts of antibody more quickly.

Morphologic changes that occur in a lymph node during the development of specifically sensitized T cells (delayed hypersensitivity) differ from those that occur during the production of circulating antibody (Fig. 13-1). During the development of delayed hypersensitivity, changes occur not in the follicles or germinal centers but in the other areas of the cortex, which contain tightly packed lymphocytes (the paracortical area). Here, a few days after contact with an antigen, large pyroninophilic "immature" blast cells and mitotic figures may be recognized. A temporary increase in the number of small lymphocytes occurs in this area 2 to 5 days after immunization. Probably these are the specifically sensitized cells that are rapidly released into the draining lymph and disseminated throughout the body.

The role of antigenic stimulation in determining the structure of lymph nodes is illustrated by the effect of immunization in germ-free animals that have little antigenic contact. In germ-free animals, lymph nodes contain few primary follicles, essentially no secondary follicles, and sparse paracortical areas (Fig. 13-2). Serum immunoglobulin levels may be only one-tenth to one-hundredth those of conventional animals. The medullary sinusoids are relatively depleted of mononuclear cells. If antigen is introduced, a sharp increase in cortical follicles and paracortical tissue occurs, and the serum immunoglobulin levels may increase to almost normal levels.

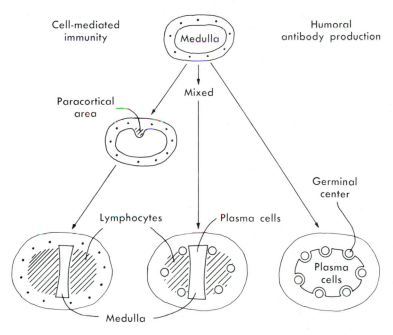

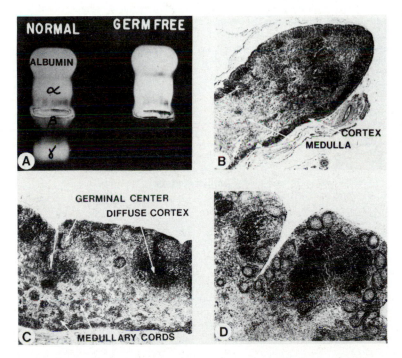

Fig. 13-1. Response of lymphoid tissue to antigenic stimulation. Induction of antibody production is associated with prominent germinal center development in lymph nodes and plasma cell production in medullary cords; delayed hypersensitivity is associated with hyperplasia of paracortical zones. (Modified from Turk, J.L., and Oort, J.: Germinal centers activity in relation to delayed hypersensitivity. In Cottier, H., et al., editors: Germinal centers in immune responses, New York, 1967, Springer-Verlag.)

Fig. 13-2. Serum globulin and lymph nodes of germ-free and normal animals. Serum γ-globulin levels of germ-free animals remain very low, and lymph nodes remain undeveloped owing to lack of antigenic stimulation. Normal animals have well-developed germinal centers and diffuse cortex. These zones become enlarged and more permanent following antigenic stimulation in germ-free animals. **A,** Agar gel electrophoresis of normal and germ-free guinea pig sera. From the top the major protein bands are albumin, α-, β-, and γ-globulin. **B,** Lymph node from germ-free guinea pig. There is narrow rim of cortical tissue with no germinal centers and poorly developed medullary cords. **C,** Normal lymph node (guinea pig). **D,** Lymph node from recently immunized guinea pig.

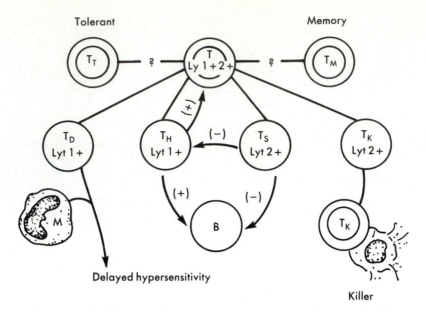

Fig. 13-3. Functional T cell populations: Primitive T cells arise in the thymus and are then distributed to lymph node and spleen where they mature into different functional immune-competent effector populations, including T_D (delayed hypersensitivity), T_H (helper cells for antibody function), T_S (suppressor), and T_K (killer) cells. T_D cells release lymphokines, which act through macrophages to effect delayed hypersensitivity reactions. T_H and T_S cells act to control the extent of immune reactions, with T_H cells providing a positive signal and T_S cells a negative signal. T_K cells specifically kill (lyse) tissue target cells. In addition, T cells may become tolerant (T_T) or memory (T_M) cells. In the mouse different surface markers, such as Lyt 1 or Lyt 2, have been shown to be associated with different functional T cell subpopulations. (From Sell, S.: Immunology, immunopathology and immunity, ed. 3, New York, 1980, Harper & Row, Publishers, Inc.)

Table 13-1. Some properties of T and B lymphocytes

	T cells	B cells
Site of origin	Thymus	Fetal liver, GI tract
Tissue location	Diffuse cortex, germinal centers	Primary follicles, germinal centers
Surface markers		
T antigens	+	−
E rosettes	+	−
EAC rosettes (Creapter)	−	+
Surface Ig	−	+
HLA-A, -B, -C	+	+
HLA-D (Ia)	−	+
FC receptor	−	+
Frequency		
Blood	80%	21%
Lymph node	85%	15%
Spleen	65%	35%
Bone marrow	Rare	Many
Thymus	90%	2%-3%
Mitogen responses		
Soluble con A	+	−
Insoluble con A	+	+
PHA	+	+
Functions	T_H (helper)	Precursor of plasma cell
	T_S (suppressor)	
	T_K (killer)	
	T_D (delayed hypersensitivity)	

+, Present; −, absent.

B and T cells

Functionally the properties of the two major lymphocyte populations are fairly well defined: B cells are the precursors of plasma cells; T cells assist in antibody production and in mediating the various phenomena associated with cell-mediated immunity (delayed hypersensitivity). The regulation of the immune response is a complex phenomenon involving participation of both B and T cells. A number of different functions have been attributed to different subpopulations of T cells (Fig. 13-3).

Distinguishing normal T and B lymphocytes morphologically is impossible. Various techniques have been developed that have been found empirically to correlate with functional indices of T and B cell activity. Table 13-1 presents a list of classically defined T and B cell markers as well as a summary of other features.

B cells have an easily recognized product (cell surface immunoglobulin), making their recognition relatively straightforward. T cells do not have surface immunoglobulin, although they may insert an Ig fragment (V_H) into their cell surface as an antigen receptor. Cell surface immunoglobulin is identified using anti-immunoglobulin reagents. Identification of cytoplasmic or membrane-bound immunoglobulin suffices to classify a cell as a B cell. Primitive B cell precursors may be more difficult to identify, but some investigators claim to have recognized human pre-B cells by detecting cytoplasmic IgM in cells with no surface immunoglobulin. B cells also possess receptors for the Fc fragment of IgG and for complement, as indicated in Table 13-1.

Human T cells are recognized by their ability to form rosettes with sheep erythrocytes (Fig. 13-4). Recently the availability of hybridoma monoclonal antibodies (OK) has enhanced our ability to define and recognize human T cells and T cell subsets. By using labeled antibody preparations containing a single antibody species directed against T cell membrane antigens, we are now able to identify thymus-derived cells as to degree of maturation as well as proposed function. The following are defined T lymphocyte subset phenotypes:

Reagent*	Presumed functional specificity
OK 3 (LEU 4)	Immature T cells
OK 6	Thymocytes
OK 11 (LEU 5)	Mature T cells (pan-T)
OK 4 (LEU 3)	Helper T cells
OK 5, OK 8 (LEU 2)	Cytotoxic-suppressor T cells

A monoclonal antibody to a common monocyte antigen is also available (OKM1). These new reagents together with conventional techniques provide the capacity to distinguish the three lineages important to the definition of benign and malignant immune proliferations: T lymphoid, B lymphoid, and monocytic (macrophage).

The identification of monoclonality and polyclonality is

*OK refers to Ortho reagents, LEU to Becton-Dickinson alternates.

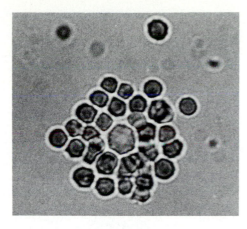

Fig. 13-4. Lymphoid rosette. Central lymphocyte is surrounded by adherent erythrocytes. (Courtesy Antonino Cantanzaro, University of California School of Medicine, San Diego, La Jolla, Calif.)

of great use in dissecting both benign and malignant B lymphocytic lesions. B lymphocytes bear immunoglobulin receptors in their cell membranes. Although these may be of various heavy or light chain types, any given B cell makes only one light chain type. In humans, kappa and lambda light chains are about equally distributed among lymphocytes. A reactive process to a foreign material, since it arises from the stimulation of several clones by foreign material, contains some B cells bearing kappa and some bearing lambda light chains (that is, polyclonal). Malignant B lymphocytic proliferations, on the other hand, contain only the progeny of one malignant clone and thus show only one light chain type (that is, monoclonal). Specific labeled antibodies to kappa and lambda chains on unfixed preparations can be used to determine if a lesion is polyclonal (benign) or monoclonal (malignant).

Subpopulations of T cells have also been identified by their capacity to bind aggregated immunoglobulin of different classes. Tγ cells bind IgG; Tμ bind IgM. There is some evidence that Tγ cells represent a suppressor population and Tμ a helper population.

T and B cell interactions. The interaction of T cells and B cells in the induction phase of humoral antibody formation has been extensively studied. T cells usually recognize large antigenic determinants (carrier molecules), whereas B cells recognize smaller determinants (haptens). A population of T cells may be "carrier primed" by immunization of an animal with uncomplexed carrier. Rabbits primed with the hapten dinitrophenol (DNP) coupled to bovine gamma globulin (BGG) carrier (DNP-BGG) produce a secondary antibody response to DNP only if the boosting agent contained DNP coupled to the same carrier as used for immunization. When carrier-primed T cells are mixed with virgin B cells and exposed to the hapten-carrier complex, the B cells and their progeny produce a much more rapid and increased antibody response to the hapten.

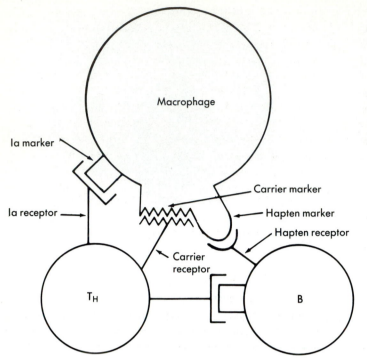

Fig. 13-5. Postulated cellular interactions during induction of antibody formation involving macrophages, T helper cells (T$_H$), and B cells (B). Initiating antigen is processed by macrophages. T$_H$ cell recognizes carrier component of antigen, as well as histocompatibility marker (Ia) on macrophage. T helper cell may also recognize Ia on B cells, but this is not always required. B cells recognize antigen on macrophage and, in presence of T cells that have been stimulated by Ia and carrier reactions, are activated to proliferate and differentiate into plasma cells. B cells also recognize carrier determinants so that antibodies to both hapten and carrier determinants are produced. (From Sell, S.: Immunology, immunopathology and immunity, ed. 3, New York, 1980, Harper & Row, Publishers, Inc.)

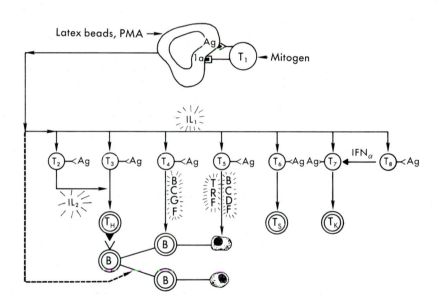

Fig. 13-6. Postulated role of interleukins during induction of immune responses. Interleukin 1 (lymphocyte-activating factor) is produced by macrophages and acts on a number of different subpopulations of precursor T cells, as well as possibly on specific B cells that have also reacted with antigens. Interleukin 1 production by macrophages requires syngenic T cells that recognize MHC marker on macrophage and can be stimulated either by specific antigen or by mitogens. Production of interleukin 1 is therefore MHC restricted, but expression of its activity is not. Interleukin 2 (T cell growth factor) is produced by subpopulation of T cells (T$_2$) that are activated as a result of interleukin 1 or mitogen or both. Interleukin 2 acts on activated T helper cells (T$_3$) to maintain proliferation and differentiation. Interferon (IFN$_\alpha$) is produced by another T cell subset (T$_8$) activated by interleukin 1. It acts on precursors of T$_K$ cells (T$_7$) to expand and differentiate a population of T$_K$ cells. BCGF (B cell growth factor) is produced by a subpopulation of activated T cells (T$_4$) and stimulates proliferation of B cells. BCDF (B cell differentiation factor) stimulates differentiation of B cells. T cell–replacing factor is produced by still another subpopulation of T cells (T$_5$) and acts to maintain further proliferation and differentiation of activated B cells or may act on macrophages to stimulate interleukin 1 production. *Ag*, Immunogenic antigen processed by macrophage; *Ia*, MHC marker on macrophage recognized by T helper cell; *T$_1$*, T helper cell; *B*, B cell; *T$_2$ - T$_8$*, other subpopulations of T cells (precursor cells); *IL$_2$*, interleukin 2; *BCGF*, B cell growth factor; *BCDF*, B cell differentiation factor; *TRF*, T cell–replacing factor; *T$_H$*, memory T helper cell; *T$_S$*, T suppressor cell; *T$_K$*, T killer cell.

The mechanism of cell cooperation during induction of an immune response is not clearly understood. An immunogen is most likely first processed by a macrophage, probably nonspecifically, although the macrophage may have specific receptors transferred from T cells or B cells (cytophilic antibody). The macrophage concentrates antigen and facilitates T and B cell interaction. B cells may be stimulated by a combination of signals, one specific (reaction of B cells with antigen) and one antigenically nonspecific (T cell signal?). Once the B cell is stimulated, it goes through a series of maturation divisions resulting in the appearance of antibody-producing plasma cells. It is likely that continued presence of antigen in some form is required to complete the proliferation-maturation phase.

For macrophages, T cells, and B cells to cooperate during induction of an antibody response, they must be genetically compatible. A simple graphic representation of the nature of the cell surface recognition interactions and the genetically controlled markers involved is given in Fig. 13-5. In the mouse the cell surface markers (Ia markers) are controlled by the Ia region of the major histocompatibility complex (MHC). Similar markers are represented in the HLA-D system of humans. A synopsis of the present understanding of how macrophages, T cells, and B cells cooperate and the postulated role of secreted factors (interleukins) is illustrated in Fig. 13-6.

The ability to fuse B cells from immunized mice with plasma cell tumor lines to produce hybridomas that secrete large amounts of a single "monoclonal" antibody has revolutionized the techniques used to provide specific antibodies for diagnostic, therapeutic, and experimental use. Until a few years ago reagent antibodies had to be produced by immunizing animals. The antibodies produced included a mixture of molecules with different biologic properties and antigen-binding specificities. Hybridoma cell lines produce a homogeneous reactant with antigen-binding specificities that can be clearly defined. The B cells (spleen cells) from the immunized mouse provide the mechanism for production of the antibody (an activated gene). The plasma cell tumor cells provide the mechanism for continued proliferation and immunoglobulin production. Clones are isolated from a population of hybridoma cells by cellular dilution and are grown in vitro. The culture fluids contain large amounts of specific monoclonal antibody that can be harvested and used for a variety of purposes.

Control of the immune response

The extent of proliferation of lymphocytes following antigenic stimulation in vivo must be limited. If the stimulated cells continued to proliferate, the individual would eventually become overwhelmed by lymphocytes. Some postulated mechanisms for control of the immune response include the following: (1) Continued presence of antigen is required to drive reactive cells; degradation of antigenic results in withdrawal of stimulation. (2) Specific circulating antibody provides a feedback signal to block further proliferation of cells. (3) A population of specific T cells (T suppressors) is produced that acts to inhibit both T and B cell proliferation. (4) Antibody to the specific antibody (anti-idiotype) is produced, which acts on similar "idiotypic" antigenic immunoglobulin structures on certain T and B cells. (5) Reactive T and B cell populations may have an inherent refractory period after stimulation. The availability of so many hypotheses is indicative of our poor understanding of this important phenomenon. Loss of control of proliferation of lymphocytes is one of the postulated mechanisms for development of lymphocytic leukemia or lymphoma and production of autoallergic or autoimmune diseases.

Autoallergy and tolerance

If the immune system serves to recognize, react with, and reject organisms or tissues foreign to the host, it would be expected that an individual would not make an immune response to his own tissues. In fact, the possibility that an individual might make an autoallergic reaction was considered such a terrible and irrational event that Ehrlich used the term "horror autotoxicus" for such a possibility. However, it is now clear that many autoallergic reactions do occur. (Diseases caused by autoallergic reactions are discussed in more detail later in this chapter.) Specific mechanisms normally prevent an individual from making an immune response to his own tissue antigens and may also prevent a reaction to foreign antigens. The operation of these mechanisms results in immune tolerance. A break in natural tolerance to self-antigens produces an autoallergic reaction.

Immune tolerance

Immune tolerance is a state of unresponsiveness to a substance that is normally capable of inducing an immune response. It is specific for a given antigen; the immune response to other unrelated antigens remains intact. *Natural tolerance* develops during fetal life so that an individual will not make an immune response to his own tissue antigens but retains the ability to react to tissue antigens from other individuals. *Acquired tolerance* may be induced to foreign antigens if these are contacted when the immune system is compromised, such as early in life or after secondary suppressive events such as irradiation or administration of large doses of immunosuppressive drugs.

The mechanisms responsible for immune tolerance are incompletely understood. Seven major theories have been formulated:

1. *Clonal elimination*. The cells responsible for recognizing and responding to the specific antigen are eliminated from the tolerant animal.

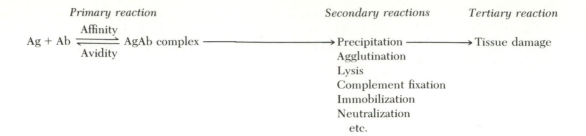

Primary reaction

$$Ag + Ab \underset{\text{Avidity}}{\overset{\text{Affinity}}{\rightleftharpoons}} AgAb \text{ complex} \longrightarrow$$

Secondary reactions

Precipitation
Agglutination
Lysis
Complement fixation
Immobilization
Neutralization
etc.

Tertiary reaction

$\longrightarrow$ Tissue damage

2. *Suppressor cells*. Tolerant animals contain a population of specific suppressor cells, which inhibit the reactive cells present from proliferation or differentiation on reactions with antigen.
3. *Blocking antibody*. Specific circulating antibody or antigen-antibody complexes block the response of potentially responding cells.
4. *Anti-idiotype network control*. Circulating antibodies develop that react with the specific antibody to the antigen because of antigenic determinants on the specific antibody (idiotypes). These idiotypes also are found on the cells responding to the original antigen. Reaction of anti-idiotypes with the cell surface receptors may inhibit the response of these cells.
5. *Antigen processing*. The antigen is not made available to the potentially responding cells because of catabolism in the tolerant animal that bypasses reactive cells.
6. *Tolerant cells*. Tolerance is an active process in which immune reactive cells are able to recognize antigen but do not respond to antigenic stimulation.
7. *Polyclonal B cell activation*. Nonimmune specific events, such as stimulation by endotoxin, may cause activation of B cells that leads to production of autoantibodies.

No single theory can explain all of the natural and experimental phenomena that are included under tolerance or immune unresponsiveness. Different mechanisms may be operative in different situations. Tolerance is most likely an active process involving either the production of tolerant cells or some controlling mechanism that inhibits potentially responding cells.

Tolerance should be clearly differentiated from desensitization. *Desensitization* is a temporary state of immune unresponsiveness induced in an already immunized animal by large doses of antigen administered in a relatively innocuous manner. Desensitization results from consumption of reactive antibodies or cells, thus exhausting the specific immune reactants. Since the antigen is degradable, continued production of antibody or sensitized cells will result in overcoming the desensitized state. Desensitization to IgE reactivity is one of the results of immunotherapy for atopic reactions.

Immune paralysis

An effect similar to tolerance may be induced by injection of moderate amounts of nondegradable antigen (immune paralysis). In such cases, antibody-producing cells may be identified if they are removed from the animal, but secreted antibody is rapidly bound to the circulating antigen. Usually antigens bound to antibody (complexes) are taken up by macrophages (phagocytosis), and both antigen and antibody are degraded. With a nondegradable antigen only the antibody is destroyed, and the antigen is released so that it may again combine with antibody. Thus any antibody formed is removed rapidly by antigen so that circulating antibody is not detectable.

Immunoglobulins and antibodies

Circulating antibodies belong to one or more of several groups of structurally related proteins known collectively as immunoglobulins. The structural features of immunoglobulin molecules are presented in Fig. 13-7. Immunoglobulins may be divided into several major classes (Fig. 13-7; Table 13-2). The manifestation of the reaction of antibody with antigen in vivo depends to a large extent on the class of immunoglobulin or immunoglobulins to which the antibody belongs.

Antibody-antigen reactions

The joining of antibody to antigen to form an antibody-antigen complex depends on the close physical approximation of oppositely charged ionic groups. The unit or part of an antigen molecule with which an antibody reacts is an antigenic determinant. Crystallographic studies of antibody molecules demonstrate a molecular cavity formed by folding of the polypeptide chains of the molecule so that the variable regions of the heavy and light chains line the cavity. This cavity provides a focus for antigen binding (Fig. 13-8).

Primary antibody-antigen reaction. The combination of antigen with antibody to form an antigen-antibody complex is termed the *primary reaction of antibody*. The primary reaction may be considered an equilibrium between free antigen and free antibody on the one hand and bound antigen and antibody (that is, antigen-antibody complex) on the other (see above).

Secondary antibody-antigen reactions. On formation of antibody-antigen complexes, a number of different

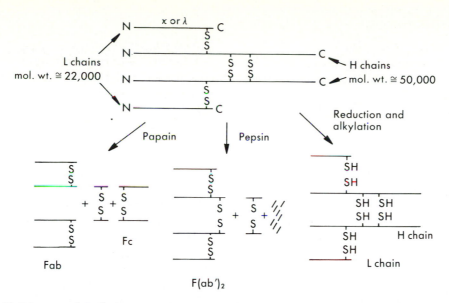

Fig. 13-7. Immunoglobulin fragments. Intact IgG molecule may be fragmented by different reagents into subunits. Digestion with papain results in two major fragments, Fab and Fc, and a minor fragment. Fab fragment consists of L chain and half of H chain joined by a disulfide bond. Fc fragment consists of carboxy terminal segment of H chains joined by a disulfide bond. An additional small peptide containing a disulfide bond is also produced. Fab fragment contains antigen-binding site and reacts with, but does not precipitate, antigen because it is monovalent. Fc portion is responsible for biologic properties such as complement fixation, placental transfer, catabolic rate, and skin fixation. Digestion with pepsin results in two Fab fragments joined by a disulfide bond because of preservation of one of the disulfide bonds joining H chains. This fragment, F(ab')₂, reacts with and precipitates antigen, since it is divalent (contains two antigen-binding sites). Additional peptide fragments, some containing disulfide bonds, are produced by action of pepsin, presumably because of further digestion of Fc fragment. Reduction and alkylation result in liberation of polypeptide chains—two L chains (mol. wt. 22,000) and two H chains (mol. wt. 50,000). Contribution of each polypeptide chain to antigen-binding site is unclear, although separated chains have only a small fraction of antigen-binding capacity of intact Fab fragment. That portion of H chain present in Fab fragment is called Fd piece. Variable domain is located on N terminal half of L chain and N terminal quarter of H chain. Together these make up antibody binding site and are shared among different Ig classes. C terminal portion of H chain consists of three consistent domains for IgG and IgA and four constant domains for IgM and IgE. This part of molecule is virtually the same within each class of Ig but is different from one class to another; class-specific properties of immunoglobulins are determined by H chain. (Modified from Metzger, H.: J.A.M.A. **202:**129, 1967.)

Table 13-2. Some properties of immunoglobulins

Ig class	Structure	Serum concentration (mg/ml)	Size (mol. wt.)	Antigen-binding sites	Complement fixation	Antibody activity	Immune effector function
IgG		12	140,000	2	+	Major class, precipitating	Toxic complex, neutralization, cytotoxic
IgA		2.5	160,000-320,000 (dimer)	4	−	Secretory	Toxic complex (rare)
IgM		1	900,000* (pentamer)	10	++	First formed highly lytic B cell surface	Cytotoxic
IgE	Mast cell	0.0005	180,000	2	−	Binds to mast cells	Anaphylactic
IgD	B cell	0.03	200,000*	2	−	B cell surface	?

−, None; +, some; ++, more.
*μ and α chains contain an *N*-derived polypeptide associated with B cell membrane insertion.

phenomena may be observed, depending on the conditions under which the primary reaction takes place. These phenomena are termed *secondary reactions*. Secondary reactions to the formation of antigen-antibody complexes depend on the nature of the antigen, the nature of the antibody, and other factors such as the presence of complement. A partial list of secondary reactions includes precipitation of the antigen-antibody complex, agglutination of antigen-containing particles by antibody; lysis of antigen-containing cells or organisms; complement fixation; immobilization of motile organisms; and neutralization of organisms or biologically active molecules.

Tertiary antibody-antigen reaction. If antibody-antigen reactions occur in a living animal, tissue damage may occur. This *tertiary effect* of antibody-antigen reactions is considered later in the chapter as an antibody-mediated immunopathologic mechanism.

Immune effector mechanisms

The essence of an immune response is that, as a result of the production of specific antibody or of specifically sensitized cells, the immune individual reacts differently on subsequent exposure to the antigen. This altered reactivity is expressed by the activation of immune effector mechanisms either individually or in combination. Immune effector mechanisms may be divided into six categories: (1) neutralization or inactivation, (2) cytotoxic or cytolytic, (3) atopic or anaphylactic, (4) phenomena (Arthus) related to toxic complexes, (5) cellular (delayed), and (6) granulomatous. The first four types of immunopathologic mechanisms result from circulating antibody combining with a given antigen in vivo. Cellular or delayed reactions are not mediated by humoral antibodies but by specifically sensitized cells. Granulomatous reactions are distinguished from the usual cellular or delayed reactions by morphologic differences in the tissue reaction.

Each immune effector mechanism has a defensive function beneficial for the host (Table 13-3). Antibody-mediated effector mechanisms generally operate against bacteria or bacterial products; cellular effector mechanisms operate against viruses or fungi. The contributions of these mechanisms may vary from one individual to another. Neutralization or inactivation of biologically active toxins by antibody is highly desirable. This is precisely what is accomplished by active immunization with diphtheria toxoid. Cytotoxic or lytic reactions may have direct effects on infecting organisms leading to the death of the offenders. The effect of histamine release (the anaphylactic mechanism) at the usual dose level can result in slight vasodilatation and increased capillary permeability, both effects interpreted in classic pathology as aiding defense. Spasmodic contractions and massive diarrhea produced as a result of gastrointestinal anaphylaxis may serve to eliminate intestinal parasites.

The inflammatory effect of Ag-Ab precipitate in the Arthus mechanism produces stickiness among leukocytes, platelets, and vascular endothelium and results in increased vascular permeability. These effects promote defense by localization, diapedesis of leukocytes, and so on. The delayed types of sensitivity (for example, to tuberculin) at the dose level that occurs in the infection result in local mobilization of phagocytic cells. Granulomatous hypersensitivity may function to isolate or localize insoluble toxic materials or microorganisms. A beneficial effect of granulomatous reactivity occurs in tuberculoid leprosy.

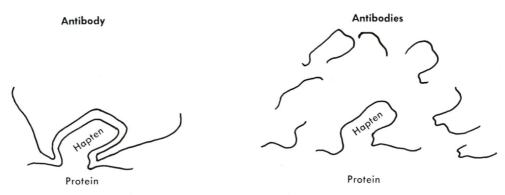

Fig. 13-8. Heterogeneity of antibody binding. Outline labeled "hapten" represents van der Waals outline of *p*-azobenzoate group coupled to protein carrier. *Left drawing,* Idealized antibody that might be formed to such an antigenic structure. The binding site of ideal antibody would present configuration permitting close approximation to the antigenic determinant (in this case, hapten). *Right drawing,* Antibodies actually produced to such a hapten have been found to consist of mixed group of specificities and avidities. Different antibody molecules bind to different parts of hapten and show different affinities. (Modified from Kitagawa, M., Yagi, Y., and Pressman, D.: J. Immunol. **95:**455, l965; copyright 1965, The Williams & Wilkins Co.)

At the abnormal dose levels used in the laboratory or in medical practice, or with the use of nonphysiologic routes of entry (such as intravenous), one may observe disorders that rarely occur naturally, such as anaphylaxis, tuberculin shock, serum sickness, transfusion reaction, and graft rejection. With frequent administration, ingestion, and contact with drugs and other chemicals, other unnatural or iatrogenic diseases occur. There are, however, a large number of naturally occurring immune-mediated diseases: hemolytic anemias, leukopenias, purpura, erythroblastosis fetalis, neonatal thrombocytopenic purpura, atopy, hay fever, polyarteritis nodosa, glomerulonephritis, contact dermatitis, sarcoidosis, and so on. In these naturally occurring diseases, infectious agents do not appear to be primarily involved, and it may properly be said that they occur because the immune apparatus is being used for the wrong purpose.

IMMUNOPATHOLOGIC (ALLERGIC) DISEASES

Tissue alterations that result from the various immune mechanisms may be considered variants of the classic inflammatory reactions. Allergic (immunopathologic) mechanisms are identical to the protective immune effector mechanisms listed previously and may be separated into those mediated by immunoglobulin (neutralization, cytotoxic or cytolytic, Arthus or toxic complex,

Table 13-3. Principal immune defense reactions to infective agents

Type of infection	Immune defense mechanism
Bacterial	Antibody
Viral	Delayed and antibody
Mycobacterial	Granulomatous (delayed)
Protozoal	Delayed and antibody
Worms	Anaphylactic and granulomatous
Fungal	Delayed (granulomatous)

From Sell, S.: Immunology, immunopathology and immunity, ed. 3, New York, 1980, Harper & Row, Publishers, Inc.

Table 13-4. Characteristics of immune effector mechanisms

Mechanism	Immune reactant	Accessory component	Skin reaction	Protective function	Examples of protection	Pathologic mechanism	Disease states
Neutralization	IgG antibody	—	—	Inactivate toxins	Tetanus, diphtheria	Inactivation of biologically active molecules or cell surface receptors	Insulin-resistant diabetes, myasthenia gravis, hyperthyroidism (LATS, LATSP)
Cytotoxic or cytolytic	IgM>IgG antibody	Complement macrophages	—	Kill bacteria	Bacterial infections	Cell lysis or phagocytosis (opsonization)	Hemolytic anemias, vascular purpura, transfusion reactions, erythroblastosis fetalis
Toxic complex	IgG antibody	Complement polymorphonuclear leukocytes	Arthus peaks at 6 hours, fades by 24	Mobilize polys to sites of infection	Bacterial and fungal infections	Polymorphonuclear leukocyte infiltrate, release of lysosomal enzymes	Glomerulonephritis, vasculitis, arthritis, rheumatoid diseases
Anaphylactic	IgE antibody	Mast cells, mediators, end-organ cells	Cutaneous anaphylaxis, peaks at 15-30 minutes, fades in 2 to 3 hours; hives	Open vessels, delivery of blood components to inflammation sites	Parasitic infections	Bronchoconstriction, edema, shock	Anaphylactic shock, hives, asthma, hay fever, insect bites
Delayed hypersensitivity	T_K and T_D cells	Lymphokines, macrophages	Delayed reaction (tuberculin), peaks at 24 to 48 hours	Kill organisms, virus-infected cells	Virus, fungal, and microbacterial infections, cancer (?)	Mononuclear cell infiltrate, target cell killing	Viral skin rashes, graft rejection, autoallergic disease, demyelination
Granulomatous	T_D cells	Macrophages (epithelioid and giant cells)	Granuloma (weeks)	Isolate infectious agents	Leprosy, tuberculosis	Replacement of tissue by granulomas	Sarcoidosis, berylliosis, tuberculosis

T_K, Killer cells; T_D, delayed hypersensitivity cells; LATS, long-acting thyroid stimulator; LATSP, long-acting thyroid stimulator protector.
From Sell, S.: Immunology, immunopathology and immunity, ed. 3, New York, 1980, Harper & Row, Publishers, Inc.

and atopic or anaphylactic) and those mediated by sensitized cells (delayed hypersensitivity and granulomatous reactions). A summary of the features of each type of reaction is presented in Table 13-4.

Antibody-mediated disease

The first four types of allergic reactions result from circulating or humoral antibody combining in vivo with antigen. They share the following properties: (1) The hypersensitive state results from the formation of antibody following exposure to antigen. (2) The first exposure to antigen is followed by a definite induction or latent period (1 to 2 weeks). (3) The allergic reaction occurs only after exposure to the specific antigen or to closely related chemical substances that cross react. (4) The reaction depends not only on the characteristics of the antigen but also on characteristics of the antibody or species of animal (for example, features of anaphylaxis depend on distribution of smooth muscle). (5) The degree of hypersensitivity tends to diminish with time; reexposure to antigen results in the reappearance of hypersensitivity more rapidly and more intensely than does primary exposure (secondary or anamnestic response). (6) The hypersensitive state can be passively transferred with serum or antibody. (7) Administration of antigen with proper precautions can result in temporary desensitization, that is, loss of the ability to react because of saturation of antibody available at the given time.

Cell-mediated disease

Classic delayed hypersensitivity is characterized by the reaction of specifically sensitized cells (lymphocytes) with antigen. As a result of such reactions there may be a release of a number of mediators that increase the intensity of the tissue response by the recruitment of other mononuclear cells. In contrast to reactions characterized in the preceding discussion, delayed hypersensitivity reactions cannot be initiated or transferred by circulating immunoglobulin antibody.

Granulomatous hypersensitivity is characterized by the formation of organized collections of altered mononuclear cells (granulomas). Antigen recognition in granulomatous hypersensitivity is almost certainly by T cells; granulomatous reactivity represents a variation of cellular sensitivity in which macrophages play a predominant role. In tissues the macrophages assume a resemblance to epithelial cells and are termed *epithelioid cells*.

Neutralization or inactivation of biologically active molecules

Neutralization reactions (Fig. 13-9) occur when antibody reacts with an antigen that performs a vital function. Inactivation may occur by reaction of antibody to soluble molecules, such as hormones or enzymes, or by

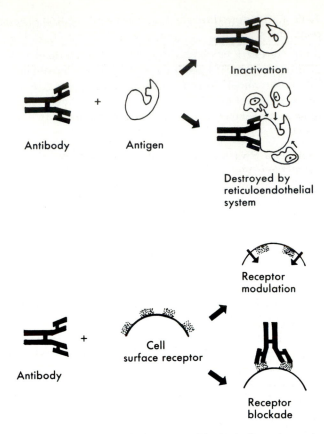

Fig. 13-9. Inactivation and activation of biologically active molecules. (1) Reaction of antibody with antigen results in alteration of tertiary structure of antigen. If antigen is a biologically active molecule such as a hormone or enzyme, this may result in inactivation of active molecule or activation of inactive form. (2) Indirect inactivation occurs as antibody-coated antigen is removed from circulation by reticuloendothelial system. (3) Antibodies may react with cell surface receptors resulting in blockade or (4) modulation of cell surface receptor. Antibodies reacting with some cell surface receptors may also activate cell.

reaction of antibody with cell surface receptors. Reactions with soluble molecules produce changes in the tertiary structure of the biologically active molecule so that it no longer performs its biologic function or is cleared from the circulation by the reticuloendothelial system as an immune complex. Reaction of antibody with cell surface receptors blocks or induces loss of receptor from the cell surface by modulation. Some of the diseases in which neutralization reactions are significant are listed in Table 13-5.

In some of these diseases the patient lacks or has lost the ability to produce a given hormone or factor and is treated by replacement of the missing hormone or factor. Thus the individual is being injected and immunized by *exogenous* molecules. These are recognized as foreign by the immune system, and antibodies are produced that have the capacity to neutralize the hormone or factor used for therapy. In other diseases, antibodies are pro-

Table 13-5. Some diseases associated with neutralization reactions

Disease	Target antigen
Diabetes	Insulin
	Insulin receptors
	Islet cells
Clotting deficiencies	Clotting factors
Pernicious anemia	Parietal cells
	Intrinsic factor
Myasthenia gravis	Acetylcholine receptor
Hyperthyroidism	Thyroid-stimulating hormone receptor (LATS, LATSP)
Hypothyroidism	Thyroid hormone

LATS, Long-acting thyroid stimulator; LATSP, long-acting thyroid stimulator protector.
From Sell, S.: Immunology, immunopathology and immunity, ed. 3, Philadelphia, 1980, Harper & Row, Publishers, Inc.

duced to self-antigen (autoimmune reaction).

Reactions of antibodies with cellular receptors for biologically active molecules have produced both a loss of the ability of the affected cells to respond to stimulatory molecules in some diseases, and the activation of cells by the antibody reaction in other diseases. Antibody to insulin receptors or to acetylcholine receptors blocks the response of the affected cells. On the other hand, antibodies to the thyroid-stimulating hormone receptors (long-acting thyroid stimulator [LATS] and long-acting thyroid stimulator protector [LATSP]) may *stimulate* the thyroid cells and produce hyperthyroidism presumably by mimicking the action of thyroid-stimulating hormone. These are called thyroid-stimulating autoantibodies (TSaab).

Insulin resistance

An example of the variety of antibodies against biologically active materials is antibody-mediated insulin resistance in diabetic patients. Patients receiving heterologous insulin preparations usually produce antibodies with reactivity to the insulin molecule itself. These antibodies are elicited more readily with beef than pork insulin. The functional significance of most of these antibodies is dubious. Large numbers of people demonstrably possess antibodies to insulin without evidence of insulin resistance. Nevertheless, there are a number of people with documented antibodies to insulin in which at least part of the antibody activity is directed to the functional sites on the hormone molecule. Such people develop profound insulin resistance, requiring massive doses of the hormone to activate even a modicum of hypoglycemic activity. It is anticipated that these reactions may be eliminated by the use of recombinant DNA techniques to produce a human insulin for therapy. In another form of diabetes, autoantibodies are directed to the receptor sites for insulin. These antibodies may competitively

bind the end-organ receptor for insulin and prevent effective insulin-receptor binding. In this circumstance massive amounts of insulin are necessary to produce an acceptable blood glucose level.

Myasthenia gravis

A comparison of the naturally occurring disease myasthenia gravis with experimental autoallergic myasthenia and the postulated role of antibodies to acetylcholine receptors (AChR) are illustrated in Fig. 13-10. In this disease, antibodies to AChR result in a loss of receptors at the motor end-plate either because of modulation (endocytosis) or because of an associated lymphocyte inflammation. The loss of receptors is demonstrable by a decreased binding of radiolabeled bungarootoxin, which also binds to AChR.

Idiotype networks, internal images, and hormone receptors

Idiotypes are antigenic determinants that are specific for the VH domains of an antibody and are specific for a given antibody. Immunization of an animal with an antibody (Ab_1) can result in the production of an antiantibody (Ab_2), and in an individual producing a given antibody auto-anti-idiotypic antibodies can be detected, usually transiently and in low amounts. Such anti-idiotypic antibodies may react with the portion of the folded VH region that is the antigen binding site, with adjacent determinants that are not in the antigen binding site, or with portions of both.

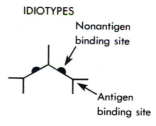

IDIOTYPES
Nonantigen binding site
Antigen binding site

For the present discussion we will explore the anti-idiotype that reacts with the antigen binding site. If Ab_2 does react with the antigen binding site, it may essentially duplicate the structure of the antigenic determinant to which Ab_1 reacts. Thus animals immunized with Ab_2 will be stimulated to produce Ab_1. This implies that Ab_2 (anti-idiotype) contains antigenic determinants (epitopes) conformationally similar to those on the original antigen used to stimulate Ab_1 (idiotype of Ab_2 mimics antigen). It has been shown experimentally that antibodies to viral antigens can be induced by immunization with anti-idiotypic antibody (Ab_2) that was made in response to immunization with antiviral antibody (Ab_1). In this instance Ab_2 acts like the original viral antigen and competes with viral antigen in binding to Ab_1. These

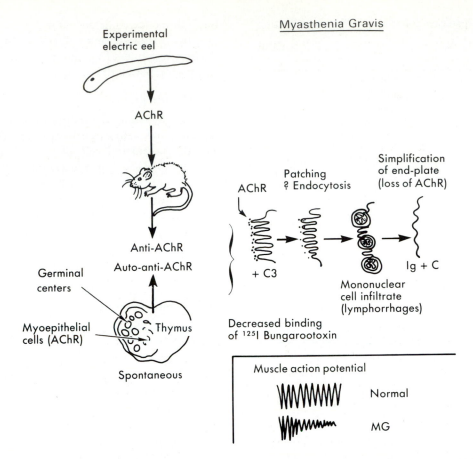

Fig. 13-10. Comparison of experimental allergic and naturally occurring myasthenia gravis. Antibody to acetylcholine receptors (AChR) may be induced in experimental animals by immunization with AChR from electric eel or autologous AChR. Autoantibodies to AChR occur spontaneously in humans with myasthenia gravis. Both experimental animals and affected humans demonstrate progressive muscle weakness, decrease in AChR, associated immunoglobulin and complement deposition, and mononuclear infiltrate at neuromuscular junction. On restimulation, muscle action potential reveals rapid decline. Thymus of affected humans may contain germinal centers not normally found in thymus. Since thymus contains myoepithelial cells with AChR, it is possible that autoantibody production to AChR occurs in thymus. (Modified from Sell, S.: Immunology, immunopathology and immunity, ed. 3, New York, 1980, Harper & Row, Publishers, Inc.)

observations fulfill Jerne's hypothesis of internal images in idiotype networks: Ab_2 contains the internal image of the viral antigen.

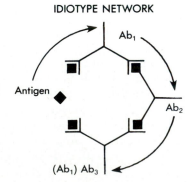

Hormones and neurotransmitter receptors share a number of conceptual analogies with antibodies. Both receptors and antibodies have a recognition domain (for hormone or antigen respectively) and a functional domain that interacts with a unit able to transmit a biologic signal to an effector system. Both receptors and antibodies have the capacity to distinguish fine specificity among ligands (hormones or antigens) with very similar structures. The binding properties of antibodies and receptors for their respective ligands are very similar.

There is convincing evidence that anti-idiotypic antibodies to antihormone or antineurotransmitter antibodies that have antigen binding sites mimicking ligand structure (Ab_{2a}) can actually function biologically as the hormone or neurotransmitter. Other anti-idiotypic antibodies may react to sites on the receptor that are not involved in ligand binding (Ab_{2a}) similar to the anti-idiotypes that react with the nonantigen portion of the VH domain of antibody. These antibodies may block receptors by conformational changes or steric hindrance. Thus anti-idiotypes to antiligand antibodies may either stimulate or block receptors.

LIGANDS, RECEPTORS, AND IDIOTYPES

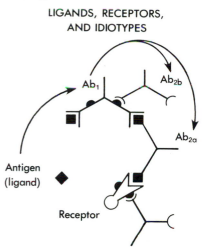

Some examples of molecular mimicry between biologically active ligands and anti-idiotypic antibodies to antiligands follow:

1. Anti-idiotypic antibody to antibodies against insulin receptors interact with the membrane-bound insulin receptor and mimic insulin action.
2. Anti-beta-adrenergic ligand anti-idiotype antibodies bind to the beta-adrenergic receptor and stimulate adenyl cyclase.
3. Antibodies to an agonist of the acetylcholine receptor mimic the binding characteristics of acetylcholine receptor; that is, the antiagonist antibody binding site binds the same ligands as the receptor. Immunization of rabbits with this antibody produces an anti-idiotypic antibody that recognizes acetylcholine receptor, presumably by mimicking the structure of the agonist. Experimental allergic myasthenia gravis is produced in animals making the anti-idiotypic antibody.
4. Rabbits immunized with rat-anti-human thyroid-stimulating hormone (TSH) antibodies produce antibodies that inhibit the binding of TSH to the TSH receptor.

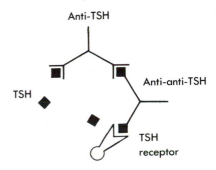

The introduction of hormones and neurotransmitters into the idiotype network opens the door for analyzing a variety of activating and inactivating antibodies, as well as providing a rationale for therapy, since anti-idiotypes can inhibit the production of the antibody to which they are directed (idiotype network).

The protective role of neutralization is obvious. The reaction of antibody to toxic agents, such as diphtheria or tetanus toxins, is beneficial. In fact, this is the goal of immunization against diphtheria or tetanus toxoids. However, when antibody reacts with something vital for normal function, the same mechanism produces disease.

Cytotoxic or cytolytic reactions

In cytotoxic or cytolytic reactions, circulating antibody reacts with either an antigenic component of a cell or an antigen that has become intimately associated with a cell (Fig. 13-11). As a result of this reaction, the complement system is usually activated, with the subsequent death or lysis of the target cell. The ultimate clinical effect depends on the type of cell involved and the severity of the allergic reaction. Cytotoxic or cytolytic reactions caused by humoral antibodies usually affect cells in suspension in the blood (erythrocytes, leukocytes, or platelets) or in the lining of the blood vessels (vascular endothelium). Therefore diseases attributable to this mechanism are often called immunohematologic diseases.

The nature of the clinical disease depends on the type of cell being destroyed and the amount of antibody produced. Destruction of erythrocytes leads to loss of red cells (anemia) and accumulation of released cell contents (hemoglobinemia and hemoglobinuria) and their breakdown products (jaundice and hemosiderosis). The destruction of leukocytes causes increased susceptibility to infection. Platelet loss leads to purpura (purple hemorrhagic lesions caused by the accumulation of red cells in the tissues) and other hemorrhagic manifestations. Similar lesion may be produced by antibodies to vascular endothelium. These diseases are considered in more detail in Chapter 38.

Complement

Complement is made up of at least 11 proteins found in normal serum that interact to produce fragments or complexes with different biologic activities. The first stage of complement activation involves reaction with a receptor site on the Fc portion of an antibody molecule after formation of an antibody-antigen complex. The activation of the entire complement sequence causes alteration of a target cell membrane that permits excess fluid to enter the cell and leads to lysis of the cell. Although the role of complement in inducing cell lysis has been studied for many years, it is now recognized that the activated fragments and complexes of the complement components provide mechanisms for activation or attraction of inflammatory cells. C1 is a macromolecular com-

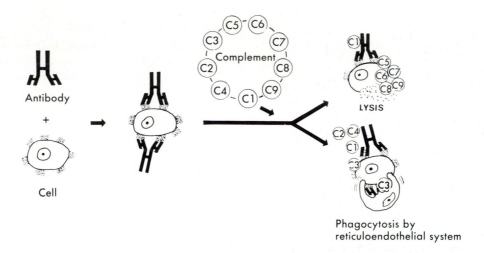

Fig. 13-11. Cytotoxic or cytolytic reactions. Circulating humoral antibody reacts with cell membrane antigens. Through action of complement system, cell membrane integrity is compromised and cell is lysed or altered cell is subject to phagocytosis. These reactions most often affect cells in intimate contact with circulating plasma, such as erythrocytes, leukocytes, platelets, or vascular endothelium.

Table 13-6. Sequence and mechanism of immune hemolysis

Reaction	Biochemical event
$E + A \rightleftharpoons EA$	Erythrocyte reacts with antierythrocyte antibody
$EA + C1 \rightarrow EAC1q^*$	C1 attaches to antibody at a site on C1q and Fc portion of 1g antibody
$C1r \rightarrow \overline{C1r}$	Bound C1q* converts C1r to active form by cleavage of C1r
$C1s \rightarrow \overline{C1s}$	$\overline{C1r}$ activates C1s by cleavage of C1s
$C4 \rightarrow \overline{C4a} + C4b^*$	$\overline{C1s}$ cleaves C4 into $\overline{C4a}$ and C4b* and C2 into $\overline{C2a}$ and C2b*; $\overline{C4a}$
$C2 \rightarrow C2a + \overline{C2b}$	Has anaphylatoxin activity
$C4b^* + C2a^* \rightarrow \overline{C4b2b}$	C4b* and C2b* combine to form C3 convertase
$C3 \rightarrow \overline{C3a} + C3b^*$	$\overline{C4b2b}$ cleaves C3 into $\overline{C3a}$ and C3b; C3a causes degranulation of mast cells (anaphylatoxin)
$C3b^* + C4b2b \rightarrow \overline{C4b2b3b}$	C3b* binds to activated bimolecular complex of C4b2b to form a trimolecular complex that is a specific enzyme for C5, C5 convertase, C3b*; macrophages have receptors for C3b, so that C3b acts as opsonin; C3b on cell surfaces is cleaved by C3b inactivated into C3c and C3d; C3c is released into the fluid phase, whereas C3d remains bound to the cell where it may be detected by antibody to C3d
$C5 \rightarrow \overline{C5a} + C5b^*$	C5 is cleaved into C5a and C5b* by C5 convertase; $\overline{C5a}$ has anaphylactic and chemotactic activity for polymorphonuclear neutrophils
$C5b^* + C6789 \rightarrow \overline{C5b.9}$	C5b* reacts with other complement components to produce a macromolecular complex that has the ability to alter cell membrane permeability; $\overline{C8}$ is most likely the active component with $\overline{C9}$ increasing efficiency of $\overline{C8}$ and producing maximal cell lysis

E, Erythrocyte; A, antibody to erythrocyte; $\overline{C1}$, $\overline{C4}$, etc., line above the C number indicates the active form of the component; C4a, C4b, etc., small letters indicate cleavage products of the parent complement molecule; C4b*, C2b*, asterisk indicates the cleavage product that contains an active binding site for other complement components.
Modified from the lectures of Hans Müller-Eberhard, Scripps Clinic and Research Foundation, La Jolla, Calif. In Sell, S.: Immunology, immunopathology and immunity, ed. 3, New York, 1980, Harper & Row, Publishers, Inc.

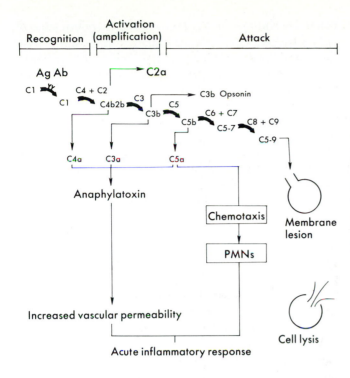

Fig. 13-12. Classical pathway of complement activation. Following reaction of antibody with antigen, cascade reaction of complement components is activated. C1 functions as recognition unit for altered Fc of two IgG or one IgM molecule; C2 and C4 function as activation unit leading to cleavage of C3. C3 fragments have a number of biologic activities: C3a is anaphylatoxin and C3b is recognized by receptors on macrophages (opsonin). C3b also joins with fragments of C4 and C2 to form C3 convertase, which cleaves C5. C5 then reacts with C6 through C9 to form membrane attack unit that produces lesion in cell membranes through which intracellular components may escape (lysis).

Table 13-7. Types of hemolytic drug reactions

Type	Mechanism	Antibody producing direct antiglobulin test positivity	Examples of causative drugs
Hapten	Antibody reacts with drug on cell membrane	Anti-IgG	Penicillin
Immune complex	Antibody-drug complex binds to cells	Anticomplement (C3d)	Quinidine, stibophen
Neoantigen	Antibody reacts to new antigen (frequently Rh)	Anti-IgG	α-Methyldopa
Complement transfer	Complement binds to normal cells after antibody activation	Anticomplement (C3d)	Penicillin
Nonspecific	IgG attaches to altered membrane	Anti-IgG Anticomplement (C3d)	Cephalosporins

plex consisting of three components: C1q, C1r, and C1s. C1 serves as a *recognition unit;* C2, C3, C4, and C5 serve as an enzymatic *activation unit* resulting in a macromolecular assembly of C5, C6, C7, C8, and C9, which serve as an *attack unit* for alteration of the cell membrane. C1 has the ability to bind to the activated Fc receptor of antibody by a reversible ionic reaction through the C1q component. Low serum concentrations of complement may be found in patients with active inflammatory disease attributable to activation of the complement system. The sequence of events involved in the classical pathway of complement activation is shown in Table 13-6 and illustrated in Fig. 13-12.

An alternative pathway for complement activation bypassing the requirement for antibody-antigen complex activation may occur by the C3 shunt mechanism. C3 is cleaved by a serum protein or system of proteins known as properdin. Properdin may be activated by endotoxin

or other microbial products. Therefore the properdin system is a nonimmune-activated alternative mechanism of defense. This system may also play a role in some inflammatory diseases, such as glomerulonephritis and bullous pemphigoid (see "Toxic [immune] complex reactions").

Drug-induced hemolytic reactions

Hemolytic reactions to drugs may be caused by at least five mechanisms (Table 13-7): (1) Drugs may attach to cell membranes and function as haptens. The red cell–hapten complex induces an immune response, and the antibody to the drug reacts with the drug on the cell surface causing lysis of the cell by activation of complement. (2) Immune complexes of antibody and drugs found in the circulation may adhere to cell membranes, cause lysis by complement, and then pass to another cell. In such cases the red cell is an "innocent bystander," since it does not contain the antigen responsible for the hemolytic reaction. (3) Drugs may induce changes in developing cells so that the mature cell expresses a "new" antigen that is autoimmunogenic. The antibody produced reacts with the patient's own cells in the absence of bound drug. (4) Normal erythrocytes may be destroyed by complement components formed by reaction of antibody with another cell if the complement components are not inactivated rapidly or are produced in such large amounts that inactivation of all active components cannot be accomplished quickly. (5) Some drugs appear to alter the cell membrane nonspecifically so that plasma proteins attach to the membrane. If immunoglobulin attaches and forms aggregates, complement activation may occur.

Antiglobulin (Coombs') test

The Coombs' antiglobulin test detects immunoglobulin or complement on the surface of affected cells by agglutination of coated cells by antibodies. There are two tests. In the direct Coombs' test, cells taken from the patient are placed with antibody to IgG or complement in vitro. If the cells in the patient's circulation have been coated with IgG or complement, they will agglutinate in vitro when the antibody is added. In the indirect Coombs' test the patient's serum is added to test cells believed to contain the antigen. These cells are then washed to remove serum proteins, and an antiserum to IgG is added. If the patient's serum contains free antibody that binds to, but does not agglutinate, erythro-

cytes, the addition of anti-IgG will cause agglutination of serum-treated cells. If agglutination occurs, the test demonstrates the presence of antibody in the patient's serum. The results of the direct Coombs' test in the drug-induced hemolytic anemias are listed in Table 13-7. Antibodies to complement are also frequently used to detect the inactivated fragment of C3b on red cells (C3d).

Toxic (immune) complex reactions

A toxic complex reaction is initiated when antibody reacts directly with antigens of basement membranes, when soluble antigen reacts in the tissue spaces with precipitating antibody forming microprecipitates in and around small vessels, or when antigen in excess reacts in the bloodstream with potentially precipitating antibody, forming soluble circulating complexes, which are deposited in the walls of blood vessels. These antigen-antibody complexes fix complement with activation of C3a, C4a, and C5a (anaphylatoxic and chemotactic factors). This results in accumulation of polymorphonuclear leukocytes, which release cathepsins, granulocytic substance, and other permeability factors (Fig. 13-13). These agents cause destruction of the elastic lamina of arteries, alterations in basement membrane (such as glomerulonephritis, p. 469), or dissolution of the basement membranes of vessels (Arthus reaction). Activation of complement chemotactic factors by the C3 shunt may also cause tissue destruction. Anaphylactic mediators released from mast cells after lysis by antibody-antigen complexes and com-

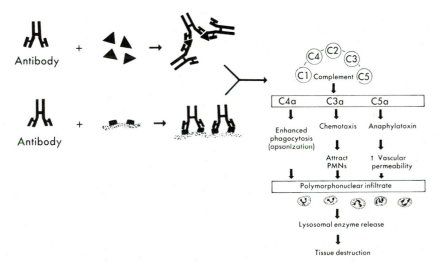

Fig. 13-13. Antibody (usually circulating soluble IgG) reactions with soluble antigens to produce soluble circulating immune complexes or with basement membranes (such as renal glomerular basement membrane). This antibody-antigen complex causes activation of complement with formation of complement fragments. Fragments C3a, C4a, and C5a cause constriction of vascular endothelium (increase vascular permeability), are chemotactic for polymorphonuclear leukocytes, and cause degranulation of polymorphonuclear neutrophils. Released lysosomal polymorphonuclear enzymes digest tissues, producing "fibrinoid" necrosis.

plement (lytic mechanism) may serve to open endothelial cell junctions so that soluble complexes can be deposited in vascular basement membranes.

Arthus reaction

The Arthus reaction is a dermal inflammatory reaction occurring in a properly sensitized individual. The reaction consists of edema, erythema, and hemorrhage, which develop over a few hours, reaching a maximum in 2 to 5 hours or even later if the reaction is severe. Gross necrosis occurs in a reaction of maximal intensity (Fig. 13-14, A). Histologically there are polymorphonuclear leukocyte and platelet thromboses, edema, hemorrhage, vascular fibrinoid necrosis, and massive diapedesis of neutrophils (Fig. 13-14, B). The same lesions may be produced in any vascular organ including the stomach, kidney, liver, brain, and joints. The mechanism of this type of reaction involves formation of intravascular antigen-antibody precipitates leading to accumulation of polymorphonuclear leukocytes and damage to vascular endothelium, followed by blockage of flow in small vessels and ischemic necrosis of the surrounding tissue.

The Arthus reaction differs from the anaphylactic reaction in its time course, gross and histologic features, and physiologic basis. It requires precipitating antibody; nonprecipitating antibody is not effective. Typical lesions may be produced by preformed antigen-antibody complexes and are usually distributed in vessels throughout the body. This type of lesion resembles polyarteritis nodosa and glomerulonephritis in humans.

Serum sickness

The syndrome of serum sickness, first recognized in 1905, includes arthritis, vasculitis (Fig. 13-15), and glomerulonephritis (Fig. 13-16), appearing 10 days to 2 weeks after passive immunization with horse serum (horse tetanus antitoxin). The disease results from the production of circulating, precipitating antibody to horse serum by the treated individual. The disease may be replicated by injection of large amounts of soluble antigen into rabbits. Lesions appear at the time of immune elimination of labeled antigen when soluble complexes are in the serum (Fig. 13-17). By a continuous infusion of antigen, three different immune responses occur in rabbits: (1) Some animals do not respond (immunologic paralysis, a type of tolerance), do not make antibody, and do not

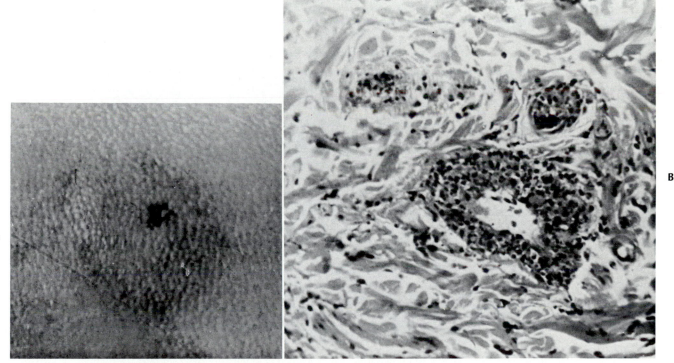

Fig. 13-14. Arthus skin reaction. **A,** Gross appearance of Arthus reaction 6 hours after intradermal injection of antigen into sensitized guinea pig. Dark color in center is caused by escape of red blood cells in places where blood vessels have been severely damaged and may be much larger in more severe reactions. **B,** Microscopic appearance. There is infiltrate of polymorphonuclear leukocytes into wall of small arterioles and fibroid necrosis. Vascular damage permits leakage of blood cells and fluid into dermis, producing edema and erythema. If reaction is severe, thrombosis of affected vessels occurs and may lead to central necrotic area in skin reaction.

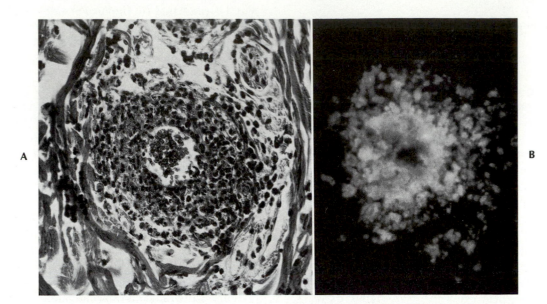

Fig. 13-15. Typical vascular (coronary artery) lesion occurring during course of serum sickness in rabbit after single large intravenous injection of bovine serum albumin (BSA). Photomicrographs of different sections from same block of tissue stained by hematoxylin and eosin, **A,** and fluorescent, anti-BSA, rabbit serum, **B,** with latter demonstrating specific localization of BSA. (Approximately 450×; courtesy Dr. Frank J. Dixon, La Jolla, Calif.)

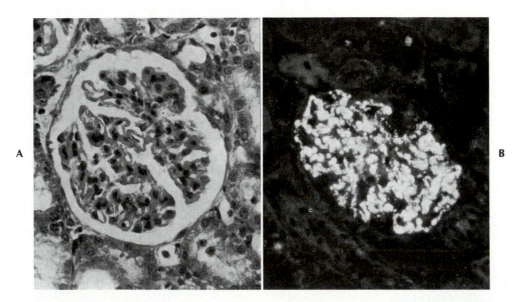

Fig. 13-16. Membranous glomerulonephritis that developed in rabbit after daily small intravenous injections of bovine serum albumin (BSA). Photomicrographs of different sections from same block of tissue stained by hematoxylin and eosin, **A,** and fluorescent, anti-BSA, rabbit serum, **B,** with latter demonstrating specific localization of BSA. (Approximately 450×; courtesy Dr. Frank J. Dixon, La Jolla, Calif.)

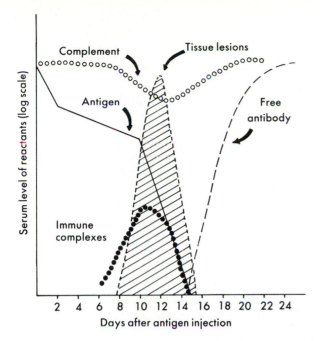

Fig. 13-17. Serum levels of antigen, complement, immune complexes, and antibody during course of experimental acute serum sickness in rabbits. Following intravascular infection of antigen, there are three phases of elimination of antigen from serum: rapid fall owing to equilibration between intravascular and extravascular fluids, a more gradual fall as a result of nonimmune catabolism, and finally rapid immune elimination as antibody is formed. Heart, kidney, or joint lesions are observed shortly after appearance of immune complexes in circulation and are associated with fall in serum complement.

develop serum sickness. (2) Some animals make large amounts of antibody and form complexes in antibody excess, which are rapidly cleared from the bloodstream and do not induce lesions. (3) Most animals produce a moderate amount of antibody, form soluble antigen-antibody complexes in antigen excess, and develop lesions of serum sickness. Complexes formed in vitro and injected into animals can also produce lesions, but only if the complexes are formed in antigen excess.

Antibody excess or complexes in equivalence are cleared by the reticuloendothelial system (RES). The RES recognizes aggregated Ig through Fc receptors. Soluble immune complexes in antigen excess do not have aggregated Ig and are not cleared by the RES. Since Arthus stain reactions occur locally when antigen is injected into the skin, the RES does not play a clearing role and complexes of different composition may induce lesions.

Immune complex disease in humans

Organs of the body that contain capillary basement membrane exposed to the circulating blood (not completely covered by endothelium) are particularly prone to deposition of soluble immune complexes or binding of antibodies to basement membrane. Such organs include the renal glomerulus, lung, joint synovia, choroid plexus of the brain, and uveal tract of the eye.

Glomerulonephritis. The renal glomerular basement membrane is a frequent site for immune complex deposition because of its role as a molecular sieve. Various forms of glomerulonephritis depend on the type of immune complex deposition that occurs. In membranous glomerulonephritis, immune complexes are initially deposited within the basement membrane, resulting in a granular pattern when viewed by immunofluorescence. In the glomerulonephritis following infection with certain serotypes of beta-hemolytic streptococci, subepithelial deposits of complexes that give a "lumpy-bumpy" pattern are seen. Several different patterns are found in systemic lupus erythematosus. One of these, lupus glomerulitis, is characterized by subendothelial deposits. The location of the deposit of immune complexes within the glomerulus appears to depend on the physical and chemical properties of the complexes. Acute inflammation of the glomerulus is caused by complement activation and elaboration of chemotactic fragments that attract and activate polymorphonuclear neutrophils. Glomerular damage is produced by lysosomal enzymes released from these cells. Subacute and chronic inflammation results from a more prolonged deposition of complexes (see the following discussion).

Anti–glomerular basement membrane glomerulonephritis. Experimental allergic glomerulonephritis is induced by immunization of animals with heterologous or homologous glomerular basement membrane, resulting in the production of antibody to glomerular basement membrane. This antibody then localizes on the capillary side of the basement membrane and may be observed by immunofluorescence as a diffuse, thin layer along the endothelial side of the basement membrane (in contrast to the location and form of the toxic complex deposition just described). This linear pattern is seen in about 5% of patients with glomerulonephritis, including those with Goodpasture's disease. The reaction to this antibody with the basement membrane results in the binding of complement, polymorphonuclear leukocyte infiltration, and basement membrane destruction.

Alternate pathway glomerulonephritis. Nonimmune activation of the C3 shunt of the complement system may be the pathogenic mechanism for some cases of glomerulonephritis. Immunofluorescent examination of the glomeruli in these cases may fail to reveal immunoglobulin or antigen, but properdin and complement components above C3 may be detected. It is possible that toxic complexes initiate complement deposition but are undetectable when the examination takes place. Since this type of glomerulonephritis is associated with low serum concentrations of complement, it has been termed *hypocomplementemic glomerulonephritis*.

Relationship of immunopathologic mechanisms to clin-

Table 13-8. Immune findings in some skin diseases

Disease	Lesion	Association	Immune mechanism
Erythema nodosum	Subcutaneous vasculitis	Infection, SLE	Immune complex
Erythema marginatum	Subcutaneous vasculitis	Rheumatic fever	Immune complex (anaphylactic?)
Erythema multiforme	Subcutaneous vasculitis	Drug reaction	Immune complex
Cutaneous vasculitis	Subcutaneous vasculitis	Infection	Immune complex
Dermatitis herpetiformis	Subepidermal bullae	Gluten enteropathy (sprue)	IgA and complement deposition in dermal microfibers and basement membrane (autoantibody or immune complex)
Herpes gestationis	Subepidermal bullae	Pregnancy	Properdin, C3, and IgG in basement membrane (autoantibody, or immune complex)
Pemphigus	Intraepithelial bullae	Autoallergic diseases	Autoantibody to epithelial cells
Pemphigoid	Subepidermal bullae	Neoplasm, autoallergy	Autoantibody to basement membrane
Psoriasis	Corneum parakeratosis, acanthosis	Rheumatoid arthritis	Autoantibody to keratin(?)
Cutaneous lupus	Basement membrane degeneration, subcutaneous vasculitis	Systemic and discoid lupus	Autoantibody to basement membrane or immune complex deposition
Vitiligo	Melanocytes, depigmentation	Autoallergic diseases	Antibody to melanocytes(?)

From Sell, S.: Immunology, immunopathology and immunity, ed. 3, New York, 1980, Harper & Row, Publishers, Inc.

ical findings. Glomerulonephritis is classified as acute, subacute, or chronic according to clinical and pathologic features. Each of the immunopathologic mechanisms—antibody to glomerular basement membrane, deposition of toxic complexes, or alternate pathway deposition of complement—can produce acute, subacute, or chronic glomerulonephritis. The type of lesion depends on the degree of injury produced in a given period of time. Extensive damage from the accumulation of a large number of polymorphonuclear leukocytes in a short period of time results in the pathologic features of focal necrosis and infiltration with leukocytes. Clinical features are caused by extensive destruction of the basement membrane, which permits passage of serum proteins of different sizes (proteinuria) or red cells (hematuria). Subacute glomerulonephritis is associated with proliferation of glomerular cells and smaller lesions in the basement membrane, permitting the passage of only smaller serum proteins (albuminuria) and the clinical picture of nephrosis (hypoproteinemia). Chronic glomerulonephritis may result from pronounced thickening of the glomerular basement membrane caused by the gradual deposition of small amounts of immune complexes over a long period of time (membranous glomerulonephritis). This leads to failure of glomerular filtration, retention of nitrogen (azotemia), and gradual renal failure. The immunopathologic mechanism cannot be identified by routine pathologic examination but requires careful clinical documentation and immunofluorescence or electron microscopic studies.

Skin diseases. A variety of inflammatory cutaneous lesions are believed to be caused by antibody-mediated mechanisms. These include the skin lesions of systemic lupus erythematosus (SLE), pemphigus, pemphigoid, erythema marginatum, erythema nodosum, and erythema multiforme (Table 13-8). Some of these, such as pemphigus, pemphigoid, and the cutaneous lesions of SLE, may be attributable to the direct toxic effect of antibody on epidermal structures, whereas erythema marginatum and erythema nodosum require the action of inflammatory cells.

Collagen diseases. An important group of human diseases variously referred to as "collagen diseases," "connective tissue diseases," or "rheumatoid diseases" has been largely attributed to variations of toxic complex mechanisms. These diseases include polyarteritis nodosa (p. 697), systemic lupus erythematosus (p. 1586), scleroderma (p. 1595), dermatomyositis (p. 1589), rheumatoid arthritis and its variants (p. 1828), and Sjögren's syndrome (p. 1032) (Fig. 13-18).

Other immune complex diseases. Other diseases caused by antibody to basement membrane or deposition of immune complexes include the following: *Goodpasture's disease* is glomerulonephritis associated with pulmonary hemorrhage caused by an antibody that reacts with both pulmonary and renal basement membrane. *Cellular interstitial pneumonia* is an inflammatory disease of the alveolar walls associated with deposition of immunoglobulin and complement in the lung and circulating soluble immune complexes. *Arthritis* is frequently seen transiently during infections. It is believed to be caused by deposition of immune complexes.

Immune complexes have been observed in the choroid plexus in experimental animals injected with immune complexes and in patients with systemic lupus erythematosus. Their role in producing neurologic symptoms remains undefined.

Inflammation of the uveal tract may also be caused by

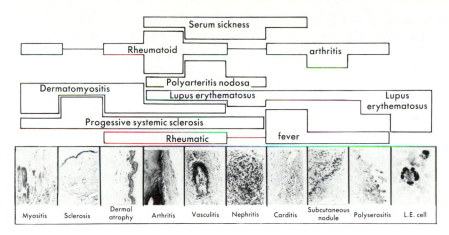

Fig. 13-18. Pathologic features of collagen (rheumatoid) diseases. Lesions assoicated with collagen diseases are shown at bottom of figure. Relative frequency of these lesions within each disease complex is indicated by thickness of overlying bars. Serum sickness is included to illustrate commonality of lesions of known etiology (immune complex–mediated vasculitis, glomerulonephritis, arthritis, and carditis) with lesions of the various naturally occurring collagen diseases. This suggests a role for immune complexes in most collagen disease, but other mechanisms, such as cellular reactions in rheumatoid arthritis, may also be active.

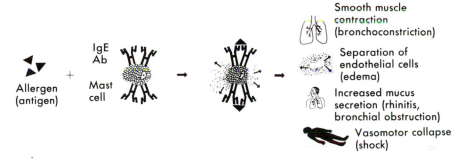

Fig. 13-19. Atopic (immediate-type) reactions. Reaction of allergen (antigen) with IgE antibody fixed to mast cells results in release of pharmacologically active agents. These agents are responsible for an acute reaction consisting of constriction of smooth muscle or endothelial cells. Primary manifestations of this are bronchoconstriction and systemic shock owing to increased vascular permeability. Delayed manifestations of this reaction are caused by other mediators, which induce a cellular inflammatory reaction (see Table 13-9).

immune complex deposition. In humans acute uveitis is associated with circulating immune complexes and immune complexes in the aqueous humor of the anterior chamber of the eye. Other forms of uveitis are caused by cellular reactions.

Atopic and anaphylactic reactions
Atopic (immediate-type) reactions

Atopic reactions are caused by pharmacologically active substances released by the reaction of allergen (antigen) with cells passively sensitized by antibody (Fig. 13-19). The cell type responsible is the mast cell (tissue) or basophil (peripheral blood). After reaction with antigen, a number of pharmacologically active agents may be released or activated (Table 13-9). The exact role of each of the anaphylactic mediators is unclear, although histamine and slow-reacting substance (SRS) appear to be the most important in humans. The effects of these agents

include contraction of smooth muscle, increased vascular permeability, an early increase in vascular resistance (vasoconstriction) followed by collapse (shock), increased gastric secretion, and increased nasal and lacrimal secretions. The lesions observed may be acute because of the sudden release of pharmacologically active agents, or chronic because of the delayed effects of cellular inflammatory infiltrates, primarily polymorphonuclear neutrophils and eosinophils, as in nasal polyps and chronic asthma. Such chronic inflammatory reactions are often associated with repeated contact with small amounts of allergen. Sensitivity may be determined by injection of the antigen into the skin of an affected individual. This results in a central swollen raised area (wheal) surrounded by a red rim (flare) caused by the local release of anaphylactic mediators in the skin (cutaneous anaphylaxis) (Fig. 13-20).

Reaginic antibody (IgE). The antibody responsible for

atopic or anaphylactic sensitivity is called reagin. The term "reagin" was originally applied to the Wassermann reagin, a serum reactant found in patients with syphilis. However, in current terminology reagin is used to designate antibody that has a special ability to bind to mast cells in skin or other tissues, the so-called homocytotropic antibody. This type of activity may be found in any of the major immunoglobulin groups (IgA, IgG, IgM), but in most cases reaginic antibody is found in a separate immunoglobulin class, IgE. In humans atopic or anaphylactic reactions are almost always caused by IgE antibody.

Skin tests are commonly used to detect reaginic antibody activity. Suspected allergens are injected into the skin, and the local reaction is observed within 30 minutes. Skin testing must be done under careful supervision because systemic anaphylactic shock may be induced. Antianaphylactic drugs (epinephrine) must be kept on hand for rapid use if necessary. The local transfer of skin-fixing antibody may be used to demonstrate reaginic activity in serum (passive cutaneous anaphylaxis, Prausnitz-Küstner test).

In vitro tests include the Schultz-Dale test, which uses organs containing smooth muscle (guinea pig intestine or rat uterus) in an organ bath. When the organ is taken from a sensitized animal or incubated with serum from a sensitized individual, contraction will occur when the specific antigen is added. Contraction may also be induced by the addition of mediators (histamine or SRS). The release of histamine from mast cells in vitro may be

Table 13-9. Anaphylactic mediators

Mediator	Physiochemical properties	Biologic activities
Histamine	β-Imidazolylethylamine	Constricts bronchial smooth muscle; increases venular permeability by constricting endothelial cells
Slow-reacting substance	Acidic sulfate ester, mol. wt. <500	Constricts bronchial smooth muscle; increases venular permeability
Eosinophil chemotactic factor	Acidic peptide(s), mol. wt. 500-600	Attracts and deactivates eosinophils
Platelet-activating factor	Phospholipids	Causes aggregation and degranulation of platelets
Basophil kallikrein	Unknown	Causes formation of bradykinin
Neutrophil chemotactic factor	Mol. wt. >10,000	Chemotactic for neutrophils

Modified from Austin, K.F., and Orange, R.P.: Am. Rev. Respir. Dis. **112:**423, 1975.

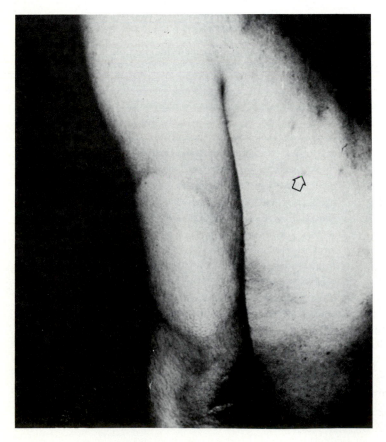

Fig. 13-20. Wheal-and-flare reaction. Massive wheal reaction to bee sting. Central, raised, pale, spongy area (wheal) is surrounded by thin, red flat rim (flare). Wheal is caused by edema, flare by microvascular congestion. Small more typical reactions are present on other areas of stain *(arrow)*. (Courtesy Macy Levine, University of Pittsburgh Medical School, Pittsburgh, Pa.)

induced by contact of sensitized mast cells with antigen. Histamine release may be quantitated spectrophotometrically or by observation of mast cell degranulation. Mast cells may be passively sensitized by incubation with reagin-containing serum. The reactivity of sensitized mast cells to antigen may be inhibited by the addition of blocking serum containing IgG antibody to the same antigen as the IgE antibody. The passive leukocyte-sensitizing (PLS) activity of a given serum is determined by incubation of a reaginic serum with blood leukocytes from nonallergic donors. The cells are then washed and treated with antigen. The extent of histamine release is used as an index of the serum reagin content. The PLS activity of ragweed-sensitive individuals is highest in the early fall (during the pollen season) and lowest in summer just before the pollen season.

The radioallergosorbent test (RAST) depends on the binding of radiolabeled antibody specific for IgE by an antigen–IgE antibody complex. The suspected antigen is first attached to insoluble particles and then added to samples of serum. In sera containing antibodies to the antigen, antibody immunoglobulin binds to the insoluble antigen. Antibody of classes other than IgE may also bind so that excess insoluble antigen is used. The particles are washed and treated with a radiolabeled antibody to IgE. The labeled anti-IgE will bind to the IgE antibody, which is bound to the insoluble antigen. An estimation of the IgE antibody to the specific antigen is made by determination of the amount of labeled anti-IgE bound.

The release of mediators from mast cell granules may occur by one of two mechanisms, nonlytic or lytic. Nonlytic release occurs by fusion of membranes of basophil granules with each other and with the cell membrane, resulting in externalization of granule contents (degranulation) (Fig. 13-21). The mast cell is not destroyed, and the granules reform. Lytic release is caused by antibody-antigen fixation of complement on the mast cell surface, leading to complement-mediated lysis of the cell. IgE-mediated nonlytic release is responsible for the majority of anaphylactic reactions. Lytic release provides a mechanism whereby IgG or IgM antibody may produce anaphylactic symptoms.

The mechanism of nonlytic release after reaction of allergen with reaginic antibody fixed to the mast cell is not known. A secretory process involving microtubules is suspected, since colchicine, which inhibits microtubule function, blocks mediator release. A proteolytic enzyme system that controls the metabolic activity of the mast cell is most likely involved. The activity of this proteolytic system is controlled by cellular concentrations of cyclic nucleotides.

Mast cells do not contain all of the important anaphylactic mediators. IgE-dependent activation of mast cells results in the release of arachidonic acid. Arachidonic acid is metabolized by cells other than mast cells to form prostaglandins and a group of biologically active metab-

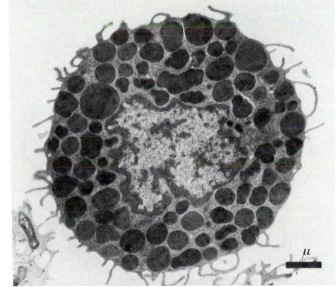

Fig. 13-21. Mast cell degranulation. **A,** Electron micrograph of mast cell. Many homogeneous, electron-dense granules are seen in cytoplasm. **B,** Higher magnification of mast cell granules surrounded by perigranular membranes *(arrows)*. **C,** Degranulation of sensitized mast cell 60 seconds after exposure to antigens *(double arrows)*. Granule membranes oppose *(single arrows)* and fuse with each other and with cell membrane *(double arrows)*. (**A,** 9000×; **B,** 26,000×; **C,** 8000×; from Anderson, P., Slorach, S.A., and Uvnäs, B.: Acta Physiol. Scand. **88:**359, 1973. Courtesy Börje Uvnäs, Karolinska Institutet, Stockholm, Sweden.)

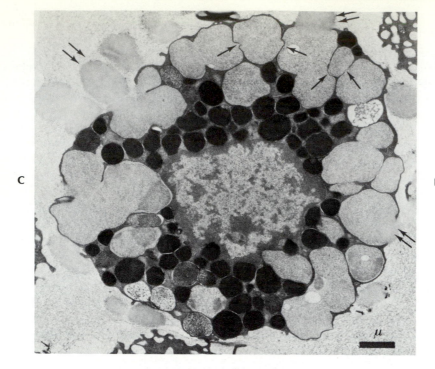

C

Fig. 13-21, cont'd. For legend see page 473.

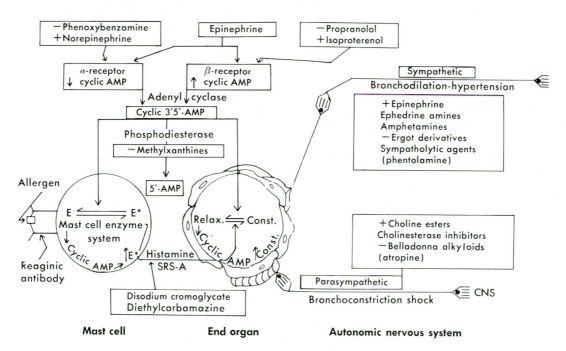

Mast cell **End organ** **Autonomic nervous system**

Fig. 13-22. Pharmacologic control of atopic-anaphylactic reactions. Effects of atopic or anaphylactic reactions are mediated by biologically active mediators released by mast cells and affecting end-organ smooth muscle. Amount of mediators released and reactivity of end organ to mediators are controlled by cellular messenger systems. Mast cell sensitivity depends on amount of reaginic antibody sensitizing the cell and on intracellular level of cyclic AMP. Cyclic AMP levels are controlled by adrenergic receptors. Stimulation of α-receptors causes decrease of cyclic AMP and increased reactivity; stimulation of β-receptors activates adenyl cyclase and produces increased cyclic AMP and decreased reactivity. Similar mechanism is operative for end-organ smooth muscle. Degree of mast cell and end-organ excitability may be modified by pharmacologic agents that operate through adrenergic or autonomic systems. Cyclic AMP is broken down to 5'-AMP by phosphodiesterase, so that inhibition of phosphodiesterase activity by methyxanthines increases cyclic AMP and decreases sensitivity of mast cell and end organs. Epinephrine stimulates both α- and β-receptors but generally has pronounced ability to reverse acute allergic reactions at the usual therapeutic dose. Disodium cromoglycate and diethylcarbamazine inhibit histamine release from mast cells. Excitation of end organs is controlled by a balance of autonomic nervous system. Parasympathetic effects are similar to anaphylactic effects (bronchial constriction, endothelial contraction, increased peristalsis, dilatation of bladder sphincter, and so on, whereas sympathetic effects are the opposite. Certain situations may result in temporary imbalance of these systems and increase severity of reaction, as in patients with chronic asthma. (From Sell, S.: Immunology, immunopathology, and immunity, ed. 3, New York, 1980, Harper & Row, Publishers, Inc.)

olites called leukotrienes. The exact identity of these metabolizing cells is not known. Leukotrienes are believed to be the active agents in slow-reacting substance preparations and are responsible for delayed inflammatory effects.

Anaphylactic reactions

Cutaneous reactions. Cutaneous anaphylaxis (urticaria, wheal and flare, hives) is elicited in a sensitive individual by skin test (scratch or intradermal injection of antigen). Grossly visible manifestations include erythema, formation of a wheal with pseudopods, and a spreading flare that reaches a maximum in 15 to 20 minutes and fades in a few hours (Fig. 13-23). Histologically there is dermal edema with essentially no cellular infiltration. The mechanism is the same as in systemic anaphylaxis, but the reaction is localized because of antibody fixation in the skin. The release of histamine or histamine-like substances into the skin produces local changes in vascular permeability. Cutaneous anaphylaxis should be differentiated from the Arthus reaction in terms of time, appearance, and morphology of the reaction.

Systemic reactions. Anaphylactic shock may occur in an atopic individual following either systemic or local exposure to allergen. Smooth muscle contraction is prominent, with increased permeability of small vessels, leukopenia, fall in temperature, hypotension, incoagulability of blood, bradycardia, and decreased serum complement levels. Circulatory shock with dizziness and faintness may be the only manifestation, but collapse, unconsciousness, and death can occur. Death may result from hypotension or from obstruction and edema of the upper respiratory tract. Acute systemic anaphylaxis in humans is usually iatrogenic, produced by injection of drugs (penicillin), but may occur naturally, for example, after an insect (bee, wasp) sting.

Angioedema. Angioedema is a hereditary condition in which edema and swelling are more extensive than in localized hives. The lesion may involve the eyelids, lips, tongue, or area of the trunk (Fig. 13-24). Involvement of the gastrointestinal tract may produce acute abdominal distress. The symptoms almost always disappear in a few days without surgical intervention. A potentially life-threatening complication is severe pharyngeal involvement that may lead to asphyxia. The pathologic lesion is a firm, nonpitting edema of the dermis and subcutaneous tissue that differs from the wheal-and-flare reaction, which has no erythema. Antihistamines have no effect on angioedema, and the lesions cause a burning or stinging sensation rather than itching. Urticaria may accompany

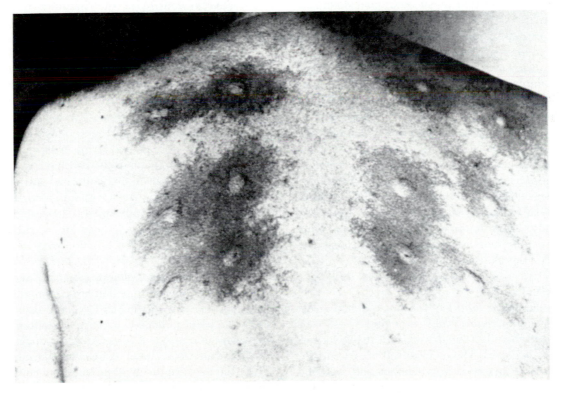

Fig. 13-23. Cutaneous wheal-and-flare reactions following injection of horse dandruff extract into skin sites on back of nonreactive person who has previously been injected with dilutions of sera from person sensitive to horse dandruff (Prausnitz-Küstner test). Central raised edematous area (wheal) is surrounded by flat erythematous zone (flare). (Courtesy Dr. Dennis R. Stanworth, University of Birmingham, Eng.)

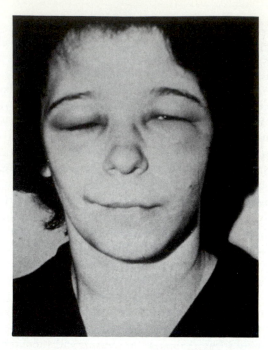

Fig. 13-24. Angioedema. Massive swelling of face occurs with rapid onset and resolves quickly. Swelling shown here was gone 24 hours later. (Courtesy Macy Levine, Pittsburgh, Pa.)

angioedema but is clearly a separate lesion.

Angioedema is inherited as an autosomal dominant trait in which C1 esterase inhibitor is either deficient or inactive. C1 esterase is the active form of the first component of complement. During attacks the C4 and C2 levels in the serum are decreased, indicating that activation of the complement system is important in this phenomenon. The injection of C1 esterase into the skin of normal individuals produces a wheal-and-flare reaction, but the injection of C1 esterase into the skin of patients with angioedema produces a firm, nonpitting induration with no flare (localized angioedema). Therefore production of the lesions of angioedema must involve factors other than lack of C1 esterase inhibitor. The kinin system (p. 27) may be activated by tryptic enzymes. C1 esterase inhibitor is also an inhibitor of the kinin system. Thus interactions of different inflammatory systems may be responsible for the clinical picture observed.

Other allergic reactions

Other human atopic (allergic) reactions include asthma, rhinitis-conjunctivitis, and eczema. These are termed atopic when IgE mediated and anaphylactoid when not IgE mediated. The mechanisms are essentially the same as those involved in cutaneous and systemic cutaneous anaphylaxis. The clinical features of atopic allergy are itching and the production of wheals, sneezing, and respiratory distress. The pathologic features include edema, smooth muscle contraction, and leukopenia. The pharmacologic characteristics are histamine

release and partial protection by antihistamines. The type of reaction seen clinically depends on four factors:

1. *Route of contact with antigen.* If contact occurs with the skin, hives (wheal and flare) predominate. If contact is with respiratory mucous membranes, asthma and rhinitis occur. If contact occurs with the eyes, conjunctivitis will predominate, or if with the ears, serous otitis. If contact occurs in the gastrointestinal tract, food allergy with cramps, nausea, vomiting, and diarrhea results.

2. *Dose of antigen.* In systemic anaphylaxis, large doses of antigen are usually introduced. In other atopic allergies the doses are relatively small and are repeated.

3. *Shock organ.* Individual differences in reactivity depend on individual idiosyncrasy, pharmacologic abnormality of the target tissue (increased histamine content), or increased susceptibility of a given organ because of nonspecific inflammation or adrenergic balance. Many affected individuals have an atopic reaction that involves primarily one organ system (for example, the lungs in asthma) while sparing other organs.

4. *Familial susceptibility.* Members of atopic families have an increased incidence of atopic reactions. It is possible, although not yet established, that genetic control of the immune responses may extend to the IgE immunoglobulin class; certain individuals inherit genes that select an IgE antibody response to a given antigen rather than a response with another immunoglobulin class.

Asthma. Patients with asthma have repeated attacks of respiratory distress because of obstruction of the airway that results from constriction of the smooth muscle in the small bronchi and increased secretion of mucus (Fig. 13-25). There are at least two forms of asthma: one clearly mediated by the anaphylactic mechanism ("allergic" or "extrinsic" asthma) and a nonallergic "intrinsic" form in which the mechanism is not well understood but is probably the result of an imbalance in smooth muscle tone. Specific external antigens cannot be identified and immune mechanisms are not believed to be involved (see also p. 874).

Hay fever (seasonal allergic rhinitis). Seasonal upper respiratory reactions to pollen are commonly referred to as hay fever. The eliciting antigens represent a variety of airborne plant pollens that cause a reaction in the nasal passages and eyes of affected individuals. Symptoms include sneezing, nasal congestion, watery discharge from the eye, conjunctival itching, and cough with mild bronchoconstriction. Usually there is edema of the submucosal tissue with an infiltration of eosinophils, which is entirely reversible. The degree of reaction and severity of symptoms are directly related to the amount of exposure to the allergen responsible.

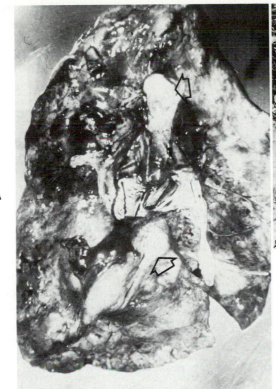

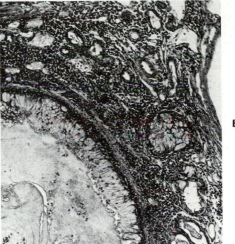

Fig. 13-25. Lung in asthma. **A,** Whole lung. Major bronchi are completely occluded with mucus *(arrows)*. **B,** Microscopic view. Bronchus illustrates characteristic features of asthma: mucus occluding lumen, hyperplastic mucous glands and goblet cells lining bronchus, thickened basement membrane, and infiltration of bronchial wall with inflammatory cells. (**A,** Courtesy William M. Thurlbeck, University of British Columbia, Vancouver.)

Nasal polyps. Nasal polyps may form in the nasal air passages, causing chronic airway obstruction and rendering nasal breathing difficult or impossible. The relationship between nasal polyps and allergic rhinitis (inflammation of the nasal mucous membranes because of atopic reactivity) is uncertain, although some observers believe that sinusitis and polyps may be caused by bacterial allergy. Surgical removal is the most consistently effective therapy.

Food allergy. Ingestion of allergens may lead to gastrointestinal reactions known collectively as food allergy. The relationship of the gastrointestinal reaction to atopic sensitivity is not clear, since many individuals with positive skin reactions to an allergen do not react to ingestion of the allergen, whereas individuals with repeated episodes of vomiting or diarrhea after eating a given food do not produce a skin reaction to the food. Allergy to cow's milk protein is the most frequently suspected gastrointestinal reaction to food. In addition, unsuspected additives to cattle food, such as penicillin, may be present in milk and elicit allergic reactions. Food allergy may lead to hypoproteinemia attributable to loss of protein in the gastrointestinal tract and persistent diarrhea. Other manifestations of food allergy are extensive skin eruptions (urticaria or eczema) and systemic shock.

Aspirin intolerance. Aspirin, one of the world's most widely used drugs, is responsible for a variety of atopic and anaphylactic reactions, including asthma, rhinitis, nasal polyps, and even anaphylactic shock. Aspirin is a chemically active molecule that acetylates serum proteins, including human serum albumin; therefore it is possible that chronic aspirin intolerance may be caused by alteration in the antigenicity of albumin or by aspirin acting as a hapten. An idiosyncratic effect of aspirin in disruption of the physiologic control of smooth muscle and mucus secretion has also been proposed as responsible for aspirin intolerance. Aspirin intolerance may develop in children or appear in adults with no history of atopy.

Insect allergy. Atopic or anaphylactic reactions to contact with insects may be divided into three groups: (1) inhalant or contact reactions to insect body parts or products, (2) skin reactions (wheal and flare) to bites by insects, and (3) systemic reactions to insect stings. Asthmatic or hay fever–like reactions may result from airborne exposure of sensitive individuals to large numbers of insects or their body parts. This occurs outdoors with insects that periodically appear in large numbers, such as cicadas or grasshoppers, and more chronically indoors with beetles, flies, spiders, and so on. Biting insects may produce delayed hypersensitivity or acute wheal-and-flare skin reactions. In a given individual a delayed reaction may convert with age to an anaphylactic one. The common reaction to a mosquito or flea bite is a localized cutaneous anaphylactic reaction; there is a very limited, direct toxic effect of the saliva introduced by the insect bite. Systemic reactions occur frequently from stinging insects, such as bees and wasps; more people die each year as a result of insect stings than from snake bites. Deaths from stinging insects usually occur within 1 hour of the sting. Therefore immediate therapy is required. This may be provided by injection of epinephrine.

Atopic allergens. Atopic reactions may occur to very unusual antigens. Systemic anaphylactic reactions have been unleashed by ingestion of beans, rice, shrimp, fish, milk, cereal mixes, potatoes, Brazil nuts, and tangerines. Men have complained about being allergic to their wives, but usually they are reacting to some component of makeup, hair spray, or other cosmetic agent. There is a documented case of a young wife who developed systemic anaphylactic symptoms shortly after intercourse; appropriate tests demonstrated that she was extremely anaphylactically sensitive to her husband's seminal fluid. Many individuals who work with laboratory animals develop anaphylactic reactions to the dander from these animals. The incidence of such sensitivity increases with the amount of contact with the animals. During the days of cavalry, as many as 20% of cavalrymen had to be discharged or assigned to different tasks because of allergic reactions to horse dander. Documentation of allergic reactions of horses to humans has not been found.

Atopic eczema. This is a chronic skin eruption of varied etiology that usually occurs in young individuals who develop atopic reactions (hay fever) at a later age. The pathologic changes in the skin are consistent with those of a severe contact dermatitis (see p. 481). Erythema, papules, and vesicles are accompanied by intense pruritus. There often follows a more acute wheal-and-flare reaction. There is perivascular accumulation of mononuclear cells, followed by infiltration into the epidermis with epidermal spongiosis. As the affected child becomes older, thickening of the skin of the affected areas occurs (lichenification). Identification of an antigen that elicits the eczema is very difficult, but in some cases there is evidence that the antigens are those that also elicit atopic reactions (pollen, house dust, animal dander). Atopic eczema is morphologically more like a reaction of cellular or delayed hypersensitivity but is discussed here because of its association with atopic conditions. It is believed to occur in individuals with a predisposition to atopic reactivity. An allergic etiology of all eczema must be questioned, since typical eczema may occur in children with severe combined immunologic deficiency and typical atopic eczema may occur in individuals with no personal or family history of atopy.

Anaphylactoid reactions. Any event causing histamine release may cause atopic symptoms that may be confused with a true allergic reaction. Anaphylactoid shock can be produced in normal (nonimmune) animals by injection of a variety of agents capable of releasing histamine, without the mediation of an antigen-antibody reaction. The clinical, physiologic, and pathologic picture that results is virtually indistinguishable from true anaphylaxis but is not produced by an immune reaction. Physical agents (heat, cold), trauma (dermatographia), emotional disturbances, or exercise may evoke pharmacologic mechanisms that mimic allergic reactions. Dermatographia is most likely caused by the release of anaphylactic mediators from mast cells of susceptible individuals by a degree of physical trauma that does not induce a reaction in normal individuals. Such a reaction may confuse the results of skin testing, since a wheal may result simply from insertion of a needle. Cholinergic urticaria is believed to be produced by an abnormal response to acetylcholine released from efferent nerves after exposure to emotional stress, physical activity, or trauma. Cholinesterase levels of the skin may be reduced in cholinergic urticaria leading to prolonged persistence of acetylcholine, which may act to release histamine from tissue mast cells.

The clinical findings in an atopic reaction are often complicated by associated nonimmune factors. Thus asthma is frequently complicated by infection or bronchiectasis, which may overshadow the allergic condition. The severity and duration of asthmatic attacks may be greatly influenced by psychologic conditions, and typical attacks may occur during periods of emotional stress with no known contact with an allergen. These anaphylactoid reactions may be mediated by nonimmunologic mediator release, an imbalance of the sympathetic nervous system, or hyperreactivity of end-organ smooth muscle.

Control of atopic and anaphylactic reactions

The severity of an anaphylactic reaction depends not only on the amount of allergen and reaginic antibody present but also on the reactivity of mast cells, the responsiveness of the end organ (such as smooth muscle), and the influences of the autonomic nervous system (Fig. 13-22). Imbalances among these homeostatic control mechanisms may explain how exposure to various nonimmunologic stimuli, such as heat, cold, physical exercise, light, or psychologic stress, may in some individuals excite reactions that mimic allergic reactions (anaphylactoid reactions). Atopic individuals are more sensitive to histamine than are nonatopic individuals. The lymphocytes of atopic individuals have a decreased ability to respond to certain stimuli by increasing cyclic AMP levels. Thus atopic individuals may not be able to balance the effects of alpha-receptor stimulation or allergen contact (decreased cyclic AMP).

The pharmacologic treatment of atopic reactions may be effective at the level of the mast cell, end organ, or autonomic nervous system. Agents that stimulate beta receptors or sympathetic nerves or agents that block alpha receptors or the parasympathetic system should dampen the effects of atopic reactions.

Cellular or delayed hypersensitivity

Delayed hypersensitivity reactions are mediated by specifically modified lymphocytes capable of responding specifically to allergen at a local site (Fig. 13-26). It is

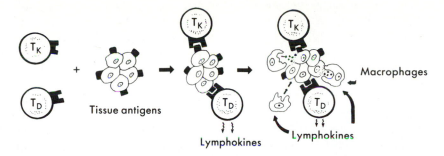

Fig. 13-26. Delayed hypersensitivity (cellular) reactions are mediated by specifically sensitized lymphocytes capable of recognizing antigen. Most likely mechanism is through activation of T_D (delayed hypersensitivity) cells. T_D cells, upon reacting with antigen, release variety of inflammatory mediators (lymphokines), which mainly attract and activate macrophages. Tissue destruction occurs when macrophages phagocytose and digest cells or other tissue components. In some cases antigen is on target cell surface; in others cells are destroyed because macrophages have been activated by lymphokines released from T_D cells reacting with ambient antigen ("innocent bystander effect"). Another T cell, T_K or T killer cell, which has been demonstrated to kill target cells in vitro without macrophages, may also cause tissue damage, but role of T_K cells in vivo is unclear.

manifested by the infiltration of cells, beginning as a perivascular accumulation of lymphocytes and monocytes. The main pathologic feature is the direct destruction of tissue elements (target cells) that contain the antigen. The time course is measured in days or even weeks, in contrast to the cutaneous anaphylactic reaction, which peaks in a few minutes, and to the Arthus type of lesion, which occurs in 4 to 6 hours. The term *tuberculin type of hypersensitivity* is applied because for many years the study of delayed hypersensitivity was the study of the response to tubercle bacilli or products of tubercle bacilli. It is now known that delayed hypersensitivity also contributes to graft rejection and autoallergic diseases and can be induced by purified protein antigens. It differs from the allergic reactions mentioned previously in that (1) humoral antibody is not involved, and reactivity cannot be transferred by serum but only by cells, (2) the time course of the development of the lesion is prolonged, and (3) the gross and microscopic appearances of the lesions differ from those mediated by circulating antibody.

Delayed skin reaction

After injection of antigen into the skin of a sensitive individual, there is little or no reaction for 4 to 6 hours. Induration and swelling usually reach a maximum at 24 to 48 hours (Fig. 13-27). Histologically there is accumulation of mononuclear cells around small veins. Later mononuclear cells may be seen throughout the area of the reaction with massive infiltration in the dermis (Fig. 13-28). Polymorphonuclear cells usually constitute less than one third of the cells at any time, and very few are present at 24 hours or later unless the reaction is severe enough to cause necrosis. The skin reaction is firmer than that in the Arthus reaction. Deposition of fibrin may be seen between collagen fibers in the dermis. Delayed reactions may occur in tissues other than skin.

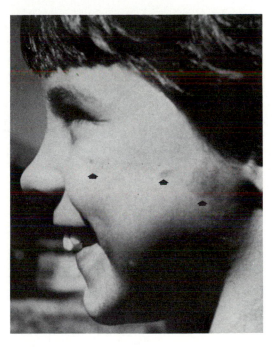

Fig. 13-27. Delayed dermal reactions to mosquito bites. Arrows indicate three reactions at different stages of development or resolution. Just in front of ear is firm, erythematous raised lesion that represents reaction to bite occurring approximately 24 hours previously. Just in front of this is resolving reaction of about 5 to 7 days' duration. Under eye is reaction of 3 to 4 days' duration.

Lymphocyte mediators

The immunologic activity of lymphocytes (T cells) as effector cells in delayed hypersensitivity reactions is amplified and extended by a variety of mediators (lymphokines). These mediators may either be extracted from sensitized cells or released from sensitized cells after reaction with specific antigen; some mediators may also be released from unsensitized lymphocytes activated by mitogens. Extractable factors include transfer factor, a

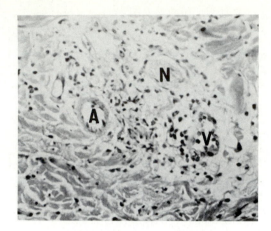

Fig. 13-28. Delayed skin reaction in sensitized guinea pig (microscopic view). There is accumulation of mononuclear cells in and around small venules; later these extend into adjacent dermal tissue. Arterioles (primary site of involvement in Arthus reactions) are not involved. *A,* Arterioles; *N,* nerve; *V,* venule.

low–molecular weight material extractable from sensitized lymphocytes that can confer specific reactivity to a previously unsensitized person; lymphocyte permeability factor, which increases vascular permeability when injected into skin; and interferon, a nonimmune factor that inhibits viral growth. Antigen-stimulated factors released from sensitized cells include migration inhibitory factor (MIF), which suppresses the movement of macrophages in vitro; skin reactive factor, which produces an inflammatory reaction when injected into skin; cytotoxic factor, which kills certain target cells; macrophage chemotactic factor; lymphocyte blastogenic factor; macrophage aggregation factor, which causes clumping of macrophages and lymphocytes; macrophage activation factor, which causes macrophages to adhere to plastic surfaces more avidly; and proliferation inhibitory factor, which inhibits growth of certain target cells.

Lymphokines are identified by their activity. The role that these mediators might play in delayed hypersensitivity reactions remains uncertain, but it is likely that they have a significant function. On contact with antigen,

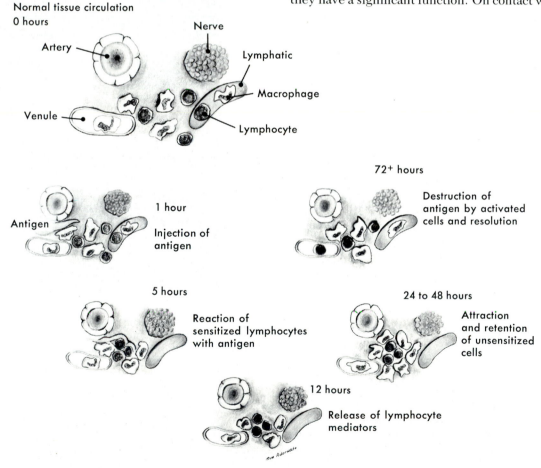

Fig. 13-29. Evolution of delayed hypersensitivity skin reaction. Lymphocytes normally pass through skin from venules to lymphatics, but sensitized lymphocytes in presence of specific antigen become immobilized and activated at site of antigen. These activated lymphocytes release mediators that attract, hold, and activate macrophages. After 24 to 48 hours macrophages destroy antigen and lesion resolves as reacting cells either disintegrate or return to circulation. (From Sell, S.: Immunology, immunopathology and immunity, ed. 2, New York, 1975, Harper & Row, Publishers, Inc.)

sensitized lymphocytes might release factors that attract, hold, and activate macrophages. The number of reacting cells may be increased by transfer factor, cytophilic antibody, or blastogenic factor. Cytotoxic or proliferation inhibitory factors may act on target cells. Each of these may contribute to the protective or destructive effects of delayed hypersensitivity reactions by amassing effector cells or products that serve to kill invading organisms or tissue target cells (Fig. 13-29).

Cutaneous basophil hypersensitivity. A group of lymphocyte-mediated tissue reactions that contain a large number of cells with basophilic granules has been termed *cutaneous basophil hypersensitivity* (CBH). Basophils are infrequent in delayed hypersensitivity but may make up 50% of the cells in CBH reactions. Basophils may also be observed in graft rejections, viral reactions, and contact allergic reactions. The ultrastructural appearance of the granules of basophils in CBH seems to be different from that of mast cells responsible for anaphylactic reactions. The basophils in CBH do not degranulate. Their role in the tissue reaction is not known, but they may serve as a phagocytic cell to supplement the macrophage.

Contact dermatitis. Contact dermatitis (contact eczema, dermatitis venenata) is best represented by the reaction to poison ivy. It also occurs as an allergic response to a wide variety of simple chemicals in ointments, clothing. cosmetics, dyes, adhesive tape, and so on. The allergens are all highly reactive chemical compounds capable of combining with proteins, but they also have lipid solubility, which permits them to penetrate the epidermis. These allergens combine with some constituent of the epidermis to form complete antigens (allergen acting as hapten).

The characteristic skin reaction is elicited in sensitized individuals by exposure of the skin to allergen (natural exposure, patch tests). It is a sharply delineated, superficial skin inflammation with an onset as early as 24 hours after exposure and a maximum at 48 to 72 hours. Its appearance is characterized by redness, induration, and vesiculation. Histologically the dermis shows characteristic perivenous accumulation of lymphocytes and histiocytes and some edema. The epidermis is invaded by these cells and reveals intraepidermal edema (spongiosis), progressing to vesiculation and death of epidermal cells (Fig. 13-30). Hematogenous lymphocytes are the carriers of sensitivity, and epidermal cell death is comparable to the destruction of parenchyma (that is, of the cells bearing the antigen) in graft rejection and the cell-mediated autoallergies.

Graft rejection (see p. 484). The solid tissue from one individual of a species transplanted to a genetically dif-

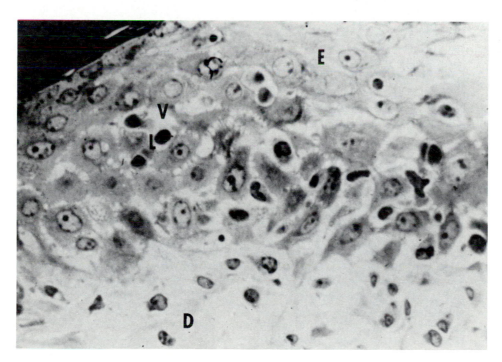

Fig. 13-30. Minimal lesion in contact dermatitis. Mononuclear cells pass from veins in dermis through basement membrane into epidermis where they separate and detach the epidermal cells, producing small spaces (vesicles) that coalesce to form larger vesicles seen grossly. Note separation of epidermal cells as indicated by prominent intracellular bridges. Resolution occurs by regeneration of epidermal cells from basal layer and sloughing of upper epidermis. *D,* Dermis; *E,* epidermis; *L,* lymphocyte; *V,* microscopic vesicle. (Courtesy Martin Flax, Tufts University, Boston, Mass.)

ferent individual of the same species will evoke a characteristic *allograft* (homograft) rejection. If transplantation occurs from one part of the body of an individual to another part of the same individual *(autograft)* or between two genetically identical individuals *(synograft)* such as monozygotic twins, this reaction will not take place. If transplantation is made between individuals of different species *(xenograft)*, rejection is generally similar to that of an allograft but surprisingly is sometimes less intense.

The reaction is perhaps best illustrated by the rejection of two skin grafts from the same donor to the same recipient with the second graft placed about 1 month after the first graft. Revascularization begins during the second or third day after the first grafting procedure and is complete by the sixth or seventh day. A similar response is observed in autografts, synografts, allografts, or xenografts, in that each of these grafts will become vascularized. However, after about a week, the first signs of rejection appear in the deep layers of an allograft or a xenograft. A perivascular (perivenular) accumulation of mononuclear cells occurs similar to that seen in the early stages of a tuberculin skin reaction. The infiltration steadily intensifies, and the graft becomes grossly edematous. The lymphocytic infiltrate extends into the epidermis resulting in an appearance similar to that of contact dermatitis. After 9 to 10 days, thrombosis of the dermal vessels occurs with necrosis and sloughing of the graft. This entire process usually requires 11 to 14 days and is called a *first-set rejection*. (A synograft or autograft does not undergo this process but remains viable with little or no inflammatory reaction.) When a second graft from the same genetically unrelated donor who provided the first graft is transplanted, a more rapid and more vigorous rejection occurs *(second-set rejection)*. During the first 3 days after the second transplant the second graft will be handled in essentially the same way as the first graft. However, vascularization is abruptly halted at 4 to 5 days with the sudden onset of ischemic necrosis. Because the graft never becomes vascularized and the blood supply is

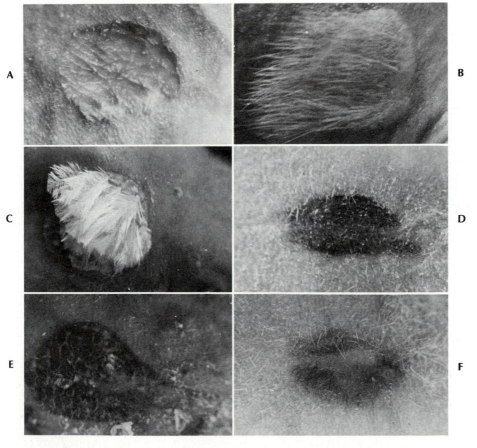

Fig. 13-31. Gross appearance of skin xenografts on nude mice. **A,** Human skin after 60 days. **B,** Cat, 51 days. **C,** Chicken, 32 days. **D,** Chameleon, 41 days. **E,** Fence lizard, 28 days. **F,** Tree frog, 40 days. White stripe in center of frog skin graft represents normal pigmentation of living frog. Nude mice have a characteristic deficiency in delayed hypersensitivity, which permits survival of organ grafts that would be rejected by normal mice. (From Manning, D.D., Reid, H.D., and Shaffer, C.F.: J. Exp. Med. **138**:488, 1973.)

cut off by the second-set rejection, there is little chance for cellular infiltration to occur. The primary target for the second-set rejection appears to be the capillaries taking part in revascularization. Similar events occur after grafting other solid organs such as the kidney or heart.

The experimental evidence strongly indicates that graft rejection is mediated by the cellular allergic reaction: (1) The ability to reject a solid graft by a second-set reaction may be transferred from a sensitized individual to an unsensitized individual with cells, but not with serum except under unusual circumstances (see p. 484). (2) Extracts of donor tissue injected into the skin of a sensitive recipient induce a delayed type of skin reaction. (3) Individuals with depressed cellular reactivity but apparently normal ability to produce antibody, such as persons with Hodgkin's disease, manifest prolonged homograft survival. (4) Antilymphocyte serum or other agents that affect delayed sensitivity more than humoral antibody are effective in prolonging the survival of homografts. (5) Nude mice with greatly suppressed T cell functions will accept grafts even from distant species (Fig. 13-31).

Although graft rejections are more closely linked to delayed or cellular hypersensitivity than to humoral reactions, there is some evidence that circulating antibody plays a role in graft rejection. An acute necrotic rejection of skin allografts occurs when specific antiserum to the graft is injected directly into the site of the skin graft. The failure of any circulation to be established results in complete ischemic necrosis, the "white graft" reaction.

The role that different hypersensitivity mechanisms play in graft rejection can be seen in the morphologic changes observed in rejected renal allografts. The morphology of first-set rejections in untreated recipients is entirely consistent with cellular mechanisms. The main feature is the accumulation of mononuclear cell infiltrate. Within a few hours small lymphocytes collect around small venules. Later many more mononuclear cells appear in the stroma. After a few days these mononuclear cells are much more varied in structure with many small and large lymphocytes, immature blast cells, and more typical mature plasma cells. Invasion of the renal tubular cells occurs with isolation, separation, and death of these cells very similar, if not identical, to that described for tissue-culture monolayers (Fig. 13-32). The interstitial tissue of the rejecting kidney accumulates large quantities of fluid (edema). Finally the afferent arterioles and small arteries become swollen and occluded by fibrin–white cell thrombi. Occasionally these vessels show fibrinoid necrosis and contain immunoglobulins and complement consistent with deposition of antibody-antigen complexes. Therefore the first-set renal allograft rejection by an untreated recipient appears to occur primarily by cellular mechanisms, although there is evidence that humoral antibody may play a role.

A second renal allotransplant from the same donor who provided the first graft may be rejected much more rapidly (within 1 to 3 days). There is little mononuclear cell infiltrate, presumably because adequate circulation

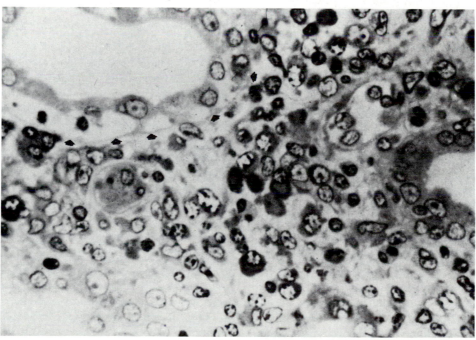

Fig. 13-32. Renal graft rejection. Mononuclear cells have invaded renal stroma and have passed through basement membrane of renal tubule *(arrows)* causing separation, detachment, and death of tubular lining cells. Stroma contains lymphocytes, macrophages, and plasma cells. (Courtesy Martin Flax, Tufts University, Boston, Mass.)

for the accumulation of blood mononuclear cells is never established. There is destruction of peritubular capillaries and fibrinoid necrosis of the walls of the small arteries and arterioles. By 24 hours there is widespread tubular necrosis, and the kidney never assumes any functional activity. Perfusion of a renal homotransplant with plasma from an animal hyperimmunized against the donor of the kidney produces a similar reaction. Therefore the hyperacute second-set rejection of renal allografts appears to be mediated by preformed circulating antibodies. This type of hyperacute rejection of a renal allograft has been observed in humans when grafting was attempted across ABO blood group types. A renal allograft from an A or a B donor to an O recipient resulted in a complete failure of circulation in the graft with distension and thrombosis of afferent arterioles and glomerular capillaries with sludged red cells, presumably because of the action of cytotoxic anti–blood group antibodies on blood group antigens in the vasculature of the grafted kidney.

Immunosuppressive therapy is now widely used to postpone allograft rejection, and the use of immunosuppressive agents has resulted in a prolonged survival of human renal allografts. Such therapy appears to be effective in suppressing the early development of rejection but does not prevent later rejection. Many patients have now survived for several years with renal allografts. However, rejection may still occur. Morphologically the major finding in such late rejected kidneys is a pronounced intimal proliferation and scarring of the walls of medium-sized arteries. The appearance is much like that of a healed or late-stage polyarteritis nodosa. These late rejections are most likely caused by a slowly accumulating antibody-mediated toxic-complex reaction.

An important factor in the survival of a renal transplant is the original disease that caused renal failure. In some recipients whose renal failure was caused by glomerulonephritis, glomerulonephritis develops in the transplanted kidney. This may result from the continued presence of circulating antibody in the recipient's blood that reacts with glomerular antigens. It supports the concept that some stages of poststreptococcal glomerulonephritis are caused by antibodies that react directly with glomerular antigens and not streptococcal antigen deposited on the membranes.

Major histocompatibility complex. The major histocompatibility complex (MHC) is a series of linked genes controlling the extent of the immune response to some antigens (immune response [IR] genes, I region), as well as the expression of cell surface markers that are recognized by the allograft rejection reaction. Because the markers are detected readily on lymphocytes by serologic tests, these genes in humans are called human lymphocyte antigen (HLA) genes. A map of the HLA genes is illustrated in Fig. 13-33. HLA-A, -B, and -C markers are located on essentially all nucleated cells. HLA-D is found primarily on B cells and macrophages.

The inheritance of the HLA markers usually occurs as a block (unless crossing-over has occurred). Thus a given child inherits one MHC complex containing linked HLA-A, -B, -C, and -D from one parent and another set of four HLA markers from the other parent. The linked block of markers is termed a *haplotype*. A given set of parents can produce four different sets of haplotypes in their children as follows:

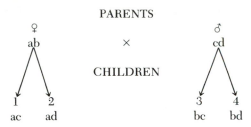

where a, b, c, and d represent a given haplotype of four HLA specificities. Because there are multiple specificities within each HLA gene (HLA-A ≈ 20; HLA-B ≈ 20, HLA-C ≈ 5, HLA-D ≈ 11) there is a minimum of 22,000 different haplotypes ($20 \times 20 \times 5 \times 11$). The number of possible HLA genotypes present in a population may be calculated using the formula

$$\frac{n(n-1)}{2}$$

in which n = the number of haplotypes. The number of possible genotypes is 500 million. Thus the chance of completely matching two unrelated individuals is 1 in 500 million.

Transplantation in humans

The surgical techniques required for solid-tissue grafts are well established, and efforts are being directed mainly toward preventing allograft rejection. The results with kidney grafts are now good enough to indicate that allografting is the treatment of choice for many types of chronic, irreversible renal failure. Clearly the use of sibling or parent donors is far superior for graft survival. Most kidneys, however, come from cadaver donors, since cadaver donors are much easier to obtain. For renal transplants done in 1968, 60% of sibling donor kidneys, 50% of parent kidneys, and 30% of cadaver kidneys remained functional after 5 years.

At transplantation centers the success rate is now much higher. For instance, at the University of California at San Francisco there is a 100% 2-year survival of HLA-matched kidneys from living related donors, 91% for HLA-matched kidneys from living nonrelated donors, and 86% for kidneys from cadaver donors. The cumulative 5-year survival rates are 80%, 75%, and 50% for the respective donor-recipient groups, and better results can be anticipated as postoperative management becomes more sophisticated. New immunosuppressive agents, such as cyclosporin A, which provide more specific suppression of the rejection reaction without a high

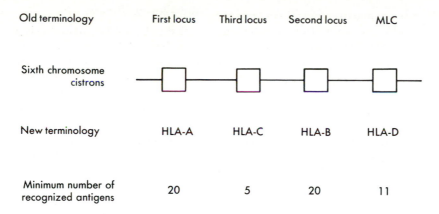

Old terminology	First locus	Third locus	Second locus	MLC
Sixth chromosome cistrons				
New terminology	HLA-A	HLA-C	HLA-B	HLA-D
Minimum number of recognized antigens	20	5	20	11

Fig. 13-33. Proposed genetic map of human major histocompatibility complex. Genes for HLA antigenic specificities are located on sixth human chromosome in order shown. Each genetic locus is believed to contain information for one specificity in each HLA series. There is room in this part of chromosome for many other genes. A given individual expresses a maximum of two specificities in each segregant series. Because each individual inherits a maternal and a paternal chromosome, one person usually expresses eight HLA specificities controlled by the four genetic loci. The centromere is located to the right of HLA-D. (From Sell, S.: Immunology, immunopathology and immunity, ed. 3, New York, 1980, Harper & Row, Publishers, Inc.)

incidence of clinically significant infections, appear to offer the best approach. Postoperative infection is the major complication affecting graft recipients. If infection occurs, immunosuppressive measures must be reduced. In many cases this results in rejection of the graft. The incidence of cancer is also greatly increased in graft recipients compared with age-matched controls. This finding may have important implications for the role of the immune system in resistance to cancer.

Transplantation of other solid organs, such as heart, lung, liver, and pancreas, has received great publicity, but the long-term results have not been encouraging. The number of heart transplants fell from 101 in 1968 to about 30 a year during the 1970s. Transplantation of the heart is not a widely acceptable therapeutic approach at the present time and is restricted to a few experimental centers. The transplantation of solid organs other than the kidney and heart has failed as much from physiologic and surgical difficulties as from immunologic rejection, but with the availability of cyclosporin A, transplantation of liver, pancreas, and other organs is becoming more popular. The kidney is a simple organ to transplant and has considerable reserve; if damaged, a portion of the organ will maintain function. Patients with temporary renal failure or rejection reaction can be maintained on dialysis until measures can be taken to reverse rejection. The transplantation of bone marrow is discussed later in the chapter.

Because of the nature of the data and the presence of multiple uncontrolled variables, many of the results reported for human organ transplantation are uninterpretable. However, one thing appears clear: the survival of the recipient depends less on exact tissue matching, organ source, choice of immunosuppressive treatment, or even surgical skill than on careful pretransplant work-up and conditioning and thorough and painstaking post-transplant follow-up monitoring of the patient by the physicians.

Graft facilitation (tumor enhancement). Humoral antibody to grafted tissue may suppress or block the rejection of a graft by the cellular mechanism (blocking antibody). This paradoxic effect was first noted when transplanted tumor tissue that should have been rejected actually survived longer if the recipient was immunized to produce humoral antibody to the tumor before transplantation (tumor enhancement). Nontumor tissue grafts also survive longer if the recipient has humoral antibody to the graft, either by active or passive immunization (graft facilitation). The enhancement-facilitation effect may interfere with a potential delayed hypersensitivity–mediated rejection reaction (1) by blocking delivery of antigen to the potentially responding cells (afferent effect), (2) by preventing responding cells from recognizing the antigen (central effect), or (3) by protecting the target graft or tumor cells from reaction with any sensitized cells that might be produced (efferent effect). Interference with effector cells is supported by the fact that humoral antibodies may block immune attack of sensitized killer cells in vitro. The exact mechanism of facilitation or enhancement may vary from one situation to another so that no single explanation covers all facilitation-enhancement phenomena.

Graft-versus-host reactions. Graft-versus-host reactions result when immunologically competent cells from allogenic or xenogenic donors are transferred to a recipient whose own immune response is impaired. The transferred lymphoid cells colonize in the recipient. The transferred cells will then recognize and react to the histocompatibility antigens in the recipient. Graft-versus-host reactions become important clinically when grafts of lymphoid tissue, such as bone marrow, which contains immunologically reactive cells, are made. In some situations when the lymphoid tissue of the recipient is not completely destroyed, regeneration of this tissue in the presence of the proliferating donor tissue produces a state of mutual tolerance in which the recipient maintains both its own and the donor lymphoid components.

The reaction of grafted immunoreactive cells produces a wasting syndrome (runting) or a secondary disease in the recipient. This consists of two components: (1) infiltration of tissues, especially the skin, intestine, spleen, and liver, with proliferating lymphocytes resulting in hepatosplenomegaly, diarrhea, and scaly contact dermatitis–like skin lesions, and (2) loss of immune reactivity to other antigens (immune deficiency). The hyperplasia of spleen and other lymphoid tissue is followed by atrophy, presumably because the grafted cells have attacked and destroyed the host's lymphoid tissue. Proliferating host cells make the major contribution to the lymphoid hyperplasia, and it is the recipient's lymphopoietic tissue that bears the brunt of the attack. The success of bone marrow grafting depends on preventing a graft-versus-host reaction.

Bone marrow transplantation. Bone marrow grafts are used to treat patients with aplastic anemia (failure of blood cell production), with immune deficiencies, and with leukemia after radiation treatment. With careful matching and follow-up monitoring, good results are obtained in about half the cases of aplastic anemia or immune deficiency if an HLA-identical sibling donor is used. In treated leukemia, irradiation leads to loss of blood cell production and reduction in immune function.

Unless an identical twin is available, some degree of graft-versus-host reactivity seems inevitable. Efforts in improving bone marrow transplantation have centered on reducing the severity of the graft-versus-host reaction while providing sufficient bone marrow stem cells to reconstitute the recipient. Techniques used have included HLA matching, particularly using HLA-matched siblings; the use of mixtures of cells from a number of related donors with the hope that the most compatible donor cells will survive; the administration of immunosuppressive agents such as cyclophosphamide or antilymphocyte serum; the fractionation of cells in an attempt to eliminate the immunologically reactive cells that would produce the graft-versus-host reaction; and the use of preserved autologous bone marrow obtained during a remission. None of these procedures can be considered satisfactory as yet, although long-term remissions have been obtained in some patients. In most remissions a transient graft-versus-host reaction occurs and the treated individual demonstrates both host and donor cells after the reaction (chimerism).

Autoallergic diseases

The criterion for inclusion of a disease process in the autoallergic category is the demonstration of an endogenous immune response to an endogenous antigen. Acquired hemolytic anemia, idiopathic thrombocytopenic purpura, experimental allergic glomerulonephritis, rheumatoid arthritis, and systemic lupus erythematosus are examples. Many autoallergic diseases are believed to be the result of a delayed type of reaction. Experimentally, lesions are produced by immunizing an animal with constituents of its own tissues. When the hypersensitive state appears, reactions occur where antigen is situated in its tissues and result in lesions. Thus far lesions have been produced by immunization of animals with lens, uvea, central nervous system (CNS) myelin, peripheral nervous system myelin, acetylcholine receptors, thyroid, adrenal, testes, glomerular basement membrane, and salivary gland. The lesions are irregularly distributed in regions of high antigen concentration, for instance, in the white matter of the CNS in experimental allergic encephalomyelitis (Fig. 13-34). Local inflammatory reactions occur around small veins and consist of lymphocytes, histiocytes, epithelioid cells, and giant cells. Necrosis, hemorrhage, and polymorphonuclear infiltration occur in severe acute reactions, and these reactions may be caused by humoral antibody (toxic complex reaction). Parenchymal destruction is coexistent with inflammation (that is, demyelination, destruction of uveal pigment, thyroid colloid, and so on). Within the involved tissue, the degree of destruction is determined to a great extent by blood-tissue barriers. Antibody and sensitized cells may act synergistically or antagonistically in the autoallergic process.

The experimental autoallergic diseases provide good models for the human diseases of unknown etiology (Table 13-10). The acute monocyclic diseases may result from allergic reactions to viruses or bacterial product–tissue combinations.

Autoantibodies. A variety of autoantibodies have been described in different human diseases. The pathogenic significance of most autoantibodies is unknown. A pathogenic importance has been convincingly demonstrated for some of these in vivo, but until more evidence is obtained, it is more likely that most such antibodies are the result of tissue alteration or breakdown rather than the cause of the lesion. It has been postulated that such antibodies actually function to clean up or clear the body fluids of abnormal or damaged tissue components, since it is known that the presence of circulating antibody results in a rapid clearance of antigen from the bloodstream.

Autoallergic mechanism. The reasons why autoallergic reactions develop are many. When an immunotolerant animal becomes responsive to an antigen to which it was previously tolerant, tolerance is said to have been bro-

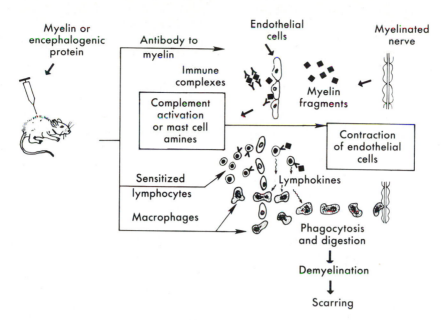

Fig. 13-34. Possible pathogenic events in experimental allergic encephalomyelitis. Immunization of experimental animals with myelin or encephalogenic protein results in production of humoral antibody and specifically sensitized cells, which together lead to demyelination by macrophages. Antibody reacting with myelin released into circulation through endothelial venules in white matter (that is, myelinated area of brain and spinal cord) activates either anaphylatoxin (complement) or mast cell (IgE) degranulation. Contraction of endothelial cells opens up gaps in small venule walls. Sensitized small lymphocytes move into white matter, react with myelin antigen, and release lymphocyte mediators. Macrophages, attracted and activated by these mediators, phagocytose and digest antibody-coated myelin or myelin affected by reaction with sensitized lymphocytes. If zones of demyelination are large, fibrosis will occur and permanent loss of function will result. (From Sell, S.: Immunology, immunopathology, and immunity, ed. 3, New York, 1980, Harper & Row, Publishers, Inc.)

Table 13-10. Relationship of experimental autoallergic diseases to human diseases

Experimental disease	Tissue involved	Histologically similar human diseases	
		Acute monocyclic	Chronic relapsing
Allergic encephalomyelitis	Myelin (CNS)	Postinfectious encephalomyelitis	Multiple sclerosis
Allergic neuritis	Myelin (peripheral nervous system)	Guillain-Barré polyneuritis	
Phakoanaphylactic endophthalmitis	Lens		Phakoanaphylactic endophthalmitis
Allergic uveitis	Uvea	Postinfectious iridocyclitis	Sympathetic ophthalmia
Allergic orchitis	Germinal epithelium	Mumps orchitis	Nonendocrine chronic infertility
Allergic thyroiditis	Thyroglubulin	Mumps thyroiditis	Subacute and chronic thyroiditis
Allergic sialadenitis	Glandular epithelium	Mumps parotiditis	Sjögren's syndrome
Allergic adrenalitis	Cortical cells		Cytotoxic contraction of adrenal
Allergic gastritis	Gastric mucosa		Atrophic gastritis
Experimental allergic nephritis	Glomerular membrane	Acute glomerulonephritis	Chronic glomerulonephritis

Modified from Waksman, B.H.: Medicine **41**:93, 1962.

ken. Autoimmunization is breaking of natural tolerance to self-antigens. Some explanations for autoimmunization are (1) reappearance of previously deleted clones by somatic mutation (clonal selection theory), (2) loss of suppressor cell activity, (3) decline in blocking antibody activity, (4) loss of anti-idiotype network control, (5) release of previously sequestered antigen so that contact with the immune system occurs, (6) alteration of self-antigens by physical damage or infection so that part of self-molecules are recognized as foreign, and (7) polyclonal activation of B cells.

Other mechanisms for overcoming self-tolerance undoubtedly exist as well. The etiology of many autoimmune diseases is still obscure, even if the pathophysiology of the diseases is becoming clearer. As is true for the induction of tolerance, breaking tolerance need not proceed by only one mechanism in a given disease. Only when these mechanisms are sorted out on a disease-by-disease, patient-by-patient basis can progress toward understanding and preventing some of these diseases occur.

The association of a number of diseases believed to be of autoallergic etiology with certain HLA types strongly suggests that the human MHC may control the type and extent of the immune response to certain antigens (Table 13-11). For instance, an inflammatory disease of spinal articulations, termed ankylosing spondylitis, develops in persons who are HLA-B27 positive following infection

with certain gram-negative bacteria, such as *Shigella*, *Salmonella*, and *Yersinia*. Although ankylosing spondylitis also develops in HLA-B27–negative individuals, the incidence is much lower. Thus there may be an immune response gene region in the human MHC that corresponds to the mouse IR region. This immune response region may determine the susceptibility to a variety of autoallergic diseases.

Granulomatous hypersensitivity

Granulomatous hypersensitivity produces space-occupying masses of inflammatory cells in reactions mainly to antigens that cannot be degraded by macrophages (Fig. 13-35). Granulomatous hypersensitivity reactions are identified by the appearance of reticuloendothelial cells, including phagocytes, histiocytes, epithelioid cells, and giant cells. The characteristic epithelioid cell has a prominent eosinophilic amorphous cytoplasm and a large, oval, pale-staining nucleus with a sharp, thin, nuclear membrane and large nucleoli. These cells have been called "epithelioid cells" because of their superficial resemblance to epithelial cells. The epithelioid cells are arranged into tubercles or granulomas, the most characteristic feature of granulomatous hypersensitivity reactions. Granulomatous reactions are considered to be responses to poorly soluble substances and may arise in response to foreign bodies or be ascribed to a peculiar form of hypersensitivity reaction to insoluble antigens. If soluble protein antigen from a tuberculin extract is injected into the skin of a sensitive individual, a typical delayed skin reaction is elicited. However, if a poorly soluble, waxy preparation is used, a granulomatous lesion is produced.

Granulomatous reactions are dependent on T cell recognition of antigen. Because of the nature of the antigen or the immune characteristics of the host, macrophages accumulate in the lesions and produce a lesion that is distinctly different but overlaps with delayed-hypersensitivity reactions. Epithelioid cells are believed to be "activated" macrophages or to represent macrophages that have already performed phagocytosis and digestion of

Table 13-11. HLA disease association

HLA specificity	Disease
B27	Reiter's syndrome, ankylosing spondylarthritis, psoriatic rheumatism
A1	Hodgkin's disease
A2	Acute lymphoblastic leukemia
D3 (A1, B8)	Myasthenia gravis, Graves' disease, Addison's disease, Sjögren's syndrome, systemic lupus erythematosus, chronic active hepatitis, juvenile diabetes
D2	Multiple sclerosis
D4	Chronic polyarthritis
D5	Juvenile rheumatism

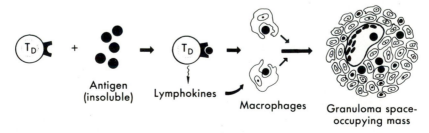

Fig. 13-35. Granulomatous hypersensitivity reactions. Reaction of sensitized cells with poorly degradable antigens results in focal collection of macrophages, lymphocytes, epithelioid cells, and giant cells arranged in oval laminated structure called a granuloma. Granulomas are space-occupying lesions that result in loss of tissue function.

antigen. Experimental animals with depressed T cell activity (thymectomized mice, nude mice, or antilymphocyte-treated mice) also have little or no ability to develop granulomatous reactivity to appropriate challenge. The onset of granulomatous hypersensitivity reactions is much more delayed than that of true delayed hypersensitivity, requiring weeks or even months to develop. Granulomas frequently form around foreign bodies such as suture material. These may or may not be immune mediated. Granulomatous reactions may also occur to antibody-antigen complexes, particularly if the antigen is not readily catabolized.

The diseases in which granulomatous reactions are involved include tuberculosis, histoplasmosis, sarcoidosis, leprosy, many parasitic infections, zirconium granulomas, berylliosis, and granulomatoses associated with vasculitis (Fig. 13-36). The morphologic features of these diseases are discussed in other chapters of this book.

Tuberculosis is a classic example of the role of granulomatous reactivity in producing tissue damage. Infection with tubercle bacilli leads to different types of immune reactivity, including antibody formation, classic delayed hypersensitivity, increased macrophage activity (activated macrophages), and granulomatous reactivity. Granulomatous reactivity is necessary for isolation of infectious organisms. Individuals who have recovered from tuberculosis usually have evidence of old granulomas in tissues that were infected. In some individuals the infection may become disseminated before the immune response is able to localize it, or a previously localized infection may become disseminated if there is a decrease in granulomatous reactivity. That fatal tuberculosis is associated with multiple granulomatous lesions does not

mean that granulomatous reactivity is not protective. Immune reactivity is not always successful in limiting an infection, particularly if the infection is well established before full immune reactivity develops or if other factors such as age or poor condition contribute to a lowered resistance.

Allergic granulomatosis or Churg-Strauss syndrome includes necrotizing vasculitis, extravascular granulomas, and tissue infiltration with eosinophils occurring in association with bronchial asthma. Such a combination of allergic lesions suggests the involvement of different immune effector mechanisms—such as toxic complex, anaphylactic, and granulomatous mechanisms—in a single individual.

The protective function of granulomatous reactivity is best exemplified by leprosy (Table 13-12). It is clear that a favorable response to therapy occurs in patients with granulomatous lesions (tuberculoid leprosy), whereas the prognosis and response to therapy are not good in patients without granulomatous reactivity (lepromatous leprosy). The granulomatous form is associated with a low tissue content of organism and a high resistance, whereas the opposite is true for the lepromatous form. Granulomatous reactivity most likely plays a similar role in tuberculosis and other infections.

Drug allergy

True allergic reactions to drugs fall into one of the preceding categories. Many drug allergies involve in vivo combinations of drugs with body constituents to produce complete antigens. This is apparently almost always true in contact allergies and probably is also the case with atopic disease attributable to aspirin and other chemi-

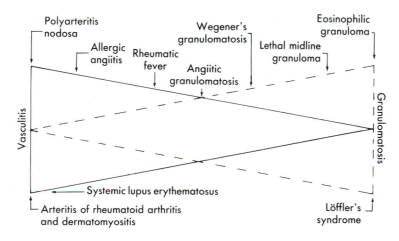

Fig. 13-36. Spectrum of diseases with mixed features of granulomatous lesions and vasculitis. Lesions of Löffler's syndrome and eosinophilic granuloma are essentially pure granulomas with little or no vasculitis. Lesions of polyarteritis nodosa and other rheumatoid diseases are primarily vascular, although some granulomatous lesions (subcutaneous nodules) are associated with these diseases. A number of other diseases demonstrate different mixtures of vasculitis and granulomatous lesions. (Modified from Alarcon-Segovia, D., and Brown, A.L.: Mayo Clin. Proc. **39:**205, 1964.)

Table 13-12. Immunologic characteristics of leprosy

Characteristics	Form of leprosy		
	Tuberculoid	Borderline	Lepromatous
M. leprae in tissues	− or ±	+ or ++	++++
Granuloma formation	++++	+++	−
Lymphocytic infiltration	+++	−	−
Lymph node morphology			
Paracortical lymphocytes	++++	++	−
Paracortical histocytes	−	++	++++
Germinal center formation	+	++	++++
Plasma cells	±	+	+++
Lepromin test	+++	−	−
Delayed hypersensitivity (%)			
To dinitrochlorobenzene	90	75	50
To hemocyanin	100	100	100
Antimycobacterial antibodies (% patients with precipitins in serum)	11-28	82	95
Autoantibodies in serum (%)	3-11		30-50
Immune complex disease (erythema nodosum leprosum)	−	±	+++

− to ++++, Extent of the observation noted.
Modified from Turk, J.L., and Bryceson, A.D.M.: Adv. Immunol. **13**:209, 1971.

cals. Drug reactions may produce asthma and vasomotor rhinitis, urticaria and angioneurotic edema, serum sickness, drug rashes, agranulocytosis, aplastic anemia and thrombocytopenia, contact dermatitis, fixed eruptions, exfoliative dermatitis, photosensitization, and erythema nodosum. Drug-induced hemolytic anemia has already been discussed.

Penicillin reactions are excellent examples of the complexities of drug allergies. Penicillin acts as a hapten (incomplete antigen) that combines with serum or tissue proteins to form a complete antigen. Such combinations may be found in three different chemical forms because of the ability of benzyl penicillin (penicillin G) to attach to proteins by different bonds. The administration of the simple compound benzyl penicillin to experimental animals and to humans may lead to the production of antibodies with at least three different specificities. This opens the possibility of a given individual's producing reaginic type (atopic type) of antibody to one determinant and delayed sensitivity or precipitating antibodies (Arthus type) to another, or even different types of hypersensitivity to the same determinant, thus causing a complex clinical picture because of a combination of different types of allergic reactions.

FINAL COMMENT

Immune mechanisms that serve as defensive reactions to invasion of the body by foreign organisms or to the effects of toxic agents may actually cause disease in certain circumstances. When immune mechanisms are used in a destructive way, the reactions are termed "allergic" or "hypersensitivity" reactions. In most cases of human disease in which immune reactions are believed to play a role, it is difficult to rule out other mechanisms. The characteristics ideally found in experimental immune responses can rarely if ever be established for human diseases. These include (1) a well-defined immunizing event (infection, immunization, or vaccination), (2) a latent period (usually 6 to 14 days), (3) a secondary response (a more rapid and intense reaction on second exposure to the antigen), (4) passive transfer of the disease state with cells or serum from an affected individual, (5) specific depression of the disease by large amounts of antigen (desensitization), and (6) identification and isolation of the antigen.

Presumptive findings consistent with, but not proving, an allergic mechanism in disease states include (1) a morphologic picture consistent with known allergic reactions, (2) the demonstration of antibody or a positive delayed skin reaction, (3) a depression of complement during some stage of the disease, (4) a beneficial effect of agents that are known to inhibit some portion of an allergic reaction (steroids, radiation, nitrogen mustard, aminopterin, and so on), (5) identification of a reasonable experimental model in animals that mimics the human disease, (6) an association with other possible allergic diseases, and (7) an increased familial susceptibility to the same disease or other allergic diseases. An immune etiology for a number of other diseases not included in this chapter, such as inflammatory bowel disease, is suspected but not yet proved. With further understanding of both normal and abnormal immune reactions, many other diseases of unknown etiology may well be shown to be caused by immune mechanisms.

REFERENCES
General

1. Bellanti, J.A.: Immunology, Philadelphia, 1971, W.B. Saunders Co.
2. Boyd, W.C.: Fundamentals of immunology, ed. 4, New York, 1966, Interscience Publishers.
3. Eisen, H.N.: Immunology, ed. 2, Hagerstown, Md., 1980, Harper & Row, Publishers, Inc.
4. Fudenberg, H.H., et al.: Basic and clinical immunology, ed. 3, Los Altos, Calif., 1981, Lange Medical Publishers.
5. Gell, P.G.H., Coombs, R.R.A., and Lachmann, P.J.: Clinical aspects of immunology, ed. 3, Oxford, Eng., 1975, Blackwell Scientific Publications.
6. Golub, E.S.: The cellular basis of the immune response, ed. 2, Sunderland, Mass., 1981, Sinauer Associates, Inc.
7. Hobart, M.J., and McConnell, I.: The immune system, Oxford, Eng., 1975, Blackwell Scientific Publications.
8. Hood, L.E., Weissman, I.L., and Wood, W.B.: Immunology, Menlo Park, Calif., 1978, The Benjamin/Cummings Publishing Co.
9. Miescher, P.A., and Muller-Eberhard, H.J.: Textbook of immunopathology, ed. 2, New York, 1976, Grune & Stratton, Inc.
10. Roitt, I.M.: Essential immunology, Oxford, Eng., 1971, Blackwell Scientific Publications.
11. Sampter, M., editor: Immunological diseases, ed. 2, Boston, 1971, Little, Brown & Co.
12. Sell, S.: Immunology, immunopathology, and immunity, ed. 3, Hagerstown, Md., 1980, Harper & Row, Publishers, Inc.
13. Thaler, M.S., Klausner, R.D., and Cohen, H.J.: Medical immunology, Philadelphia, 1977, J.B. Lippincott Co.

Basic immunology
Antigenicity

14. Kabat, E.A.: The nature of an antigenic determinant, J. Immunol. **97**:1, 1966.
15. Kabat, E.A.: Structural concepts in immunology and immunochemistry, New York, 1968, Holt, Rinehart & Winston.
16. Landsteiner, K.: The specificity of serological reactions, New York, 1962, Dover Publications.
17. Sela, M.: Immunological studies with synthetic polypeptides, Adv. Immunol. **5**:30, 1969.

Lymphoid tissue and immune response

18. Benditt, B.P., and Lagunoff, D.: The mast cell: its structure and function, Prog. Allergy **8**:195, 1964.
19. Bianco, C., Patrick, R., and Nussenzweig, V.: A population of lymphocytes bearing a membrane receptor for antigen-antibody-complement complexes, J. Exp. Med. **132**:702, 1970.
20. Cohen, Z.A.: The structure and functions of monocytes and macrophages, Adv. Immunol. **9**:163, 1968.
21. Fox, R., et al.: Cell surface antigens on human lymphoid organs. In Sell, S., and Wahren, B., editors: Human cancer markers, Clifton, N.J., 1981, Humana Press.
22. Goldschneider, I., and McGregor, D.D.: Anatomical distribution of T and B lymphocytes in the rat, J. Exp. Med. **138**:1443, 1973.
23. Gowans, J.L., and McGregor, D.D.: The immunological activities of lymphocytes, Prog. Allergy **9**:1, 1965.
24. Gutman, G.A., and Weissman, I.L.: Lymphoid tissue architecture: experimental analysis of the origin and distribution of T-cells and B-cells, Immunology **23**:465, 1972.
25. Miller, J.R.A.P., and Osoba, D.: Current concepts of the immunological function of the thymus, Physiol. Rev. **47**:437, 1967.
26. Nossal, G.J.V., Ada, G.L., and Austin, C.M.: Antigens in immunity. IV. Cellular localization of ^{125}I-labeled flagella in lymph nodes, Aust. J. Exp. Biol. Med. Sci. **42**:311, 1964.
27. Robertson, M.: The life of a B lymphocyte, Nature **149**:332, 1980.
28. Sell, S., and Asofsky, R.: Lymphocytes and immunoglobulins, Prog. Allergy **12**:86, 1968.
29. Turk, J.L., and Oort, J.: Germinal center activity in relation to delayed hypersensitivity. In Cottier, H., et al., editors: Germinal centers in immune responses, New York, 1967, Springer-Verlag.

30. Waksman, B.H.: The homing pattern of thymus-derived lymphocytes in calf and neonatal mouse Peyer's patches, J. Immunol. **111**:878, 1973.
31. Yoffey, J.M., and Courtice, F.D.: Lymphatics, lymph and the lymphomyeloid complex, New York, 1970, Academic Press, Inc.

B and T cells

32. Benacerraf, B.: Role of MHC gene products in immune regulation, Science **212**:1229, 1981.
33. Burnet, F.M.: The clonal selection theory of acquired immunity, London, 1959, Cambridge University Press.
34. Claman, H.N., and Mosier, D.E.: Cell-cell interactions in antibody production, Prog. Allergy **16**:40, 1972.
35. Ehrlich, P.: On immunity, with special reference to cell life, Proc. R. Soc. Lond. (Biol.) **66**:424, 1900.
36. Hildemann, W.H., Clark, E.A., and Raison, R.L.: Comprehensive immunogenetics, New York, 1981, Elsevier.
37. Jerne, N.K.: The natural selection theory of antibody formation, Proc. Natl. Acad. Sci. U.S.A. **41**:849, 1955.
38. Katz, D.H., and Benacerraf, B.: The role of products of the histocompatibility gene complex in immune responses, New York, 1976, Academic Press, Inc.
39. Klein, J.: Biology of the major histocompatibility complex, New York, 1975, Springer-Verlag.
40. Marshall, W.H., Valentine, F.T., and Lawrence, H.S.: Cellular immunity in vitro: clonal proliferation of antigen-stimulated lymphocytes, J. Exp. Med. **130**:327, 1969.
41. Miller, J.R.A.P., and Osaba, D.: Current concepts of the immunological function of the thymus, Physiol. Rev. **47**:437, 1967.
42. Mitchison, N.A.: The carrier effect in the secondary response to hapten-protein conjugates. II. Cellular cooperation, Eur. J. Immunol. **1**:18, 1971.
43. Möller, G., editor: Accessory cells in the immune response, Immunol. Rev. **53**:1, 1980.
44. Möller, G. editor: T-cell stimulating growth factors, Immunol. Rev. **51**:1, 1980.
45. Möller, G., editor: Interleukins and lymphocyte activation, Immunol. Rev. **63**:1, 1982.
46. Mosier, D.E., and Coppleson, L.W.: A three-cell interaction required for the induction of the primary response in vitro, Proc. Natl. Acad. Sci. U.S.A. **61**:542, 1968.
47. Nossal, G.J.V., and Ada, G.L.: Antigens, lymphoid cells and the immune response, New York, 1971, Academic Press, Inc.
48. Raschke, W.C.: Plasmacytomas, lymphomas and hybridomas: their contribution to immunology and molecular biology, Biochim. Biophys. Acta **605**:113, 1980.
49. Sell, S.: Development of restrictions in the expression of immunoglobulin specificities by lymphoid cells, Transplant. Rev. **5**:19, 1970.
50. Szilard, L.: The molecular basis of antibody formation, Proc. Natl. Acad. Sci. U.S.A. **46**:293, 1960.
51. Uhr, J.W., and Möller, G.: Regulatory effect of antibody on the immune response, Adv. Immunol. **8**:81, 1968.
52. Unanue, E.R.: The regulatory role of macrophages in antigenic stimulation, Adv. Immunol. **15**:95, 1972.
53. Zinkernagel, R.M.: Thymus and lymphohemopoietic cells: their role in T-cell maturation, in selection of T cells, H_2 restriction-specificity and H_2 linked Ir gene control, Immunol. Rev. **42**:224, 1978.

Autoallergy and tolerance

54. Argyris, B.F.: Adoptive tolerance; transfer of the tolerant state, J. Immunol. **90**:29, 1963.
55. Baker, P.J., et al.: Regulation of the antibody response to type III pneumococcal polysaccharide. II. Mode of action of thymic-derived suppressor cells, J. Immunol. **112**:404, 1974.
56. Basten, A., et al.: Cell-to-cell interaction in the immune response. X. T cell-dependent suppression in tolerant mice, J. Exp. Med. **140**:199, 1974.
57. Burnet, F.M.: The clonal selection theory of acquired immunity, London, 1959, Cambridge University Press.
58. Burnet, F.M.: The integrity of the body: a discussion of modern

immunological ideas, Cambridge, Mass., 1962, Harvard University Press.

59. Chiller, J.M., Habicht, G.S., and Weigle, W.O.: Cellular sites of immunologic unresponsiveness, Proc. Natl. Acad. Sci. U.S.A. **65**:551, 1970.

60. Dresser, D.W., and Mitchison, N.A.: The mechanism of immunological paralysis, Adv. Immunol. **8**:129, 1968.

61. Felton, L.D.: The significance of antigen in animal tissue, J. Immunol. **61**:107, 1949.

62. Gershon, R.K., et al.: Suppressor T cells, J. Immunol. **108**:586, 1972.

63. Halliday, J.J.: Immunological paralysis of mice with pneumococcal polysaccharide antigens, Bacteriol. Rev. **35**:267, 1971.

64. Hašek, M., Langerová, A., and Hraba, T.: Transplantation immunity and tolerance, Adv. Immunol. **1**:1, 1961.

65. Katz, D.H., and Benacerraf, B.: Immunological tolerance: mechanisms and potential therapeutic applications, New York, 1974, Academic Press, Inc.

66. Möller, G., editor: Mechanism of B lymphocyte tolerance, Immunol. Rev. **43**:1, 1979.

67. Möller, G., editor: Models of autoimmune diseases, Immunol. Rev. **55**:1, 1981.

68. Möller G., editor: Suppressor T lymphocytes, Transplant. Rev. **26**:1, 1975.

69. Möller, G., editor: Transplantation tolerance, Immunol. Rev. **46**:1, 1979.

70. Mitchison, N.A.: Induction of immunological paralysis with two zones of dosage, Proc. R. Soc. Lond. (Biol.) **161**:275, 1966.

71. Owen, R.D.: Immunogenetic consequence of vascular anastomoses between bovine twins, Science **102**:400, 1945.

72. Parks, D.E., and Weigle, W.O.: Current perspectives on the cellular mechanisms of immunologic tolerance, Clin. Exp. Immunol. **39**:257, 1980.

73. Weigle, W.O.: Termination of acquired immunological tolerance to protein antigens following immunization with altered protein antigens, J. Exp. Med. **116**:913, 1962.

74. Weigle, W.O.: The induction of autoimmunity in rabbits following injection of heterologous or altered homologous thyroglobulin, J. Exp. Med. **121**:289, 1965.

Immunoglobulins and antibodies

75. Amzel, L.M., and Poljak, R.J.: Three dimensional structure of immunoglobulins, Am. Rev. Biochem. **48**:961, 1979.

76. Bernier, B.M.: Structure of human immunoglobulins: myeloma proteins as analogues of antibody, Prog. Allergy **14**:1, 1970.

77. Binz, H., Lindeman, J., and Wigzell, H.: Cell-bound receptors for alloantigens on normal lymphocytes. II. Antialloantibody serum contains specific factors reacting with relevant immunocompetent T lymphocytes, J. Exp. Med. **140**:731, 1974.

78. Cosenza, H., and Kohler, H.: Specific suppression of the antibody response by antibodies to receptors, Proc. Natl. Acad. Sci. U.S.A. **69**:2710, 1972.

79. Edelman, G.M., et al.: The covalent structure of an entire γG-immunoglobulin molecule, Biochemistry **63**:78, 1969.

80. Fazekas De St. Groth, S., and Scheidegger, D.: Production of nonoclonal antibodies: strategy and tactics, J. Immunol. Methods **35**:1, 1980.

81. Gell, P.G.H., and Kelus, A.S.: Anti-antibodies, Adv. Immunol. **6**:461, 1967.

82. Gottlieb, P.D.: Immunoglobulin genes, Mol. Immunol. **17**:1423, 1980.

83. Green, N.N.: Electron microscopy of the immunoglobulins, Adv. Immunol. **11**:1, 1969.

84. Kabat, E.A.: Origins of antibody complementarity and specificity-hypervariable regions and the multigene hypothesis, J. Immunol. **125**:961, 1980.

85. Kelus, A.S., and Gell, P.G.H.: Immunoglobulin allotypes of experimental animals, Prog. Allergy **11**:141, 1967.

86. Liu, C.-P., et al.: Structure of the genes that rearrange in development, Science **209**:1348, 1980.

87. Marquart, M., et al.: Crystallographic refinement and atomic models of the intact immunoglobulin molecule Kol and its antigen-binding fragment at 3.0 Å and 1.9 Å resolution, J. Mol. Biol. **141**:369, 1980.

88. Melchers, F., Potter, M., and Warner, N., editors: Lymphocyte hybridomas, Curr. Top. Microbiol. Immunol. 81, 1978.

89. Natvig, J.B., and Kunkel, H.G.: Human immunoglobulins: classes, subclasses, genetic variants and idiotypes, Adv. Immunol. **16**:1, 1973.

90. Nisonoff, A., Hopper, J.E., and Spring, S.R.: The antibody molecule, New York, 1975, Academic Press, Inc.

91. Seidman, J.G., and Leder, P.: The arrangement and rearrangement of antibody genes, Nature **276**:790, 1978.

92. Winkelnake, J.L.: Immunoglobulin structure and effector functions, Immunochemistry **15**:695, 1978.

Antigen-antibody reactions

93. Avrameas, S., and Ternynck, T.: The cross-linking of proteins with glutaraldehyde and its use for the preparation of immunoadsorbents, Immunochemistry **6**:53, 1969.

94. Coons, A.H.: Histochemistry with labeled antibody, Int. Rev. Cytol. **5**:1, 1956.

95. Crowle, A.J.: Immunodiffusion, New York, 1961, Academic Press, Inc.

96. Farr, R.S.: A quantitative immunochemical measure of the primary interaction between I*BSA and antibody, J. Infect. Dis. **103**:239, 1958.

97. Heidelberger, M.: Lectures in immunochemistry, New York, 1956, Academic Press, Inc.

98. Kabat, E.A., and Mayer, M.M.: Experimental immunochemistry, ed. 2, Springfield, Ill., 1961, Charles C Thomas, Publisher.

99. Karush, F.: Immunological specificity and molecular structure, Adv. Immunol. **2**:1, 1962.

100. Kitagawa, M., Yagi, Y., and Pressman, D.: The heterogeneity of combining sites of antibodies as determined by specific immunoabsorbents, J. Immunol. **95**:446, 991, 1965.

101. Pressman, D., and Grossburg, A.L.: The structural basis of antibody specificity, New York, 1968, W.A. Benjamin, Inc.

102. Rodbard, D., and Weiss, G.H.: Mathematical theory of immunoradiometric (labeled antibody) assays, Anal. Biochem. **52**:10, 1973.

103. Skelley, D.S., Brown, L.P., and Besch, P.K.: Radioimmunoassay, Clin. Chem. **19**:146, 1973.

104. Weir, D.M., editor: Handbook of experimental immunology, ed. 3, London, 1976, Blackwell Scientific Publications.

Immune effector mechanisms

105. Gell, P.G.H., Coombs, R.R.A., and Lachmann, P.J.: Clinical aspects of immunology, ed. 3, Oxford, Eng., 1975, Blackwell Scientific Publications.

Immunopathologic (allergic) diseases
Neutralization or inactivation of biologically active molecules

106. Goldberg, L.S., et al.: Human autoimmunity, with pernicious anemia as a model, Ann. Intern. Med. **81**:372, 1974.

107. Grob, D., editor: Myasthenia gravis, Ann. N.Y. Acad. Sci. **274**:1, 1976.

108. Harrison, L.C., and Kahn, L.C.: Autoantibodies to the insulin receptor: clinical significance and experimental applications, Clin. Immunol. **4**:107, 1980.

109. Kriss, J.P.: Graves' ophthalmopathy: etiology and treatment, Hosp. Pract. **10**:124, 1975.

110. Lennon, V.A., Lindstrom, J., and Seybold, M.E.: Experimental autoimmune myasthenia: a model of myasthemia gravis in rats and guinea pigs, J. Exp. Med. **141**:1365, 1975.

111. Margolius, A., Jackson, D.P., and Ratnoff, O.D.: Circulating anticoagulants: a study of 40 cases and a review of the literature, Medicine **40**:197, 1961.

112. McKenzie, J.M., and Zakarija, M.: LATS in Graves' disease, Rec. Prog. Horm. Res. **33**:29, 1977.

113. Patrick, J., and Lindstrom, J.: Autoimmune response to acetylcholine receptor, Science **180**:821, 1973.

114. Pope, C.C.: The immunology of insulin, Adv. Immunol. **5**:209, 1966.

115. Rotman, M.B., and Celada, F.: Antibodymediated activation of a defective β-D-galactosidase extracted from an *Escherichia coli* mutant, Proc. Natl. Acad. Sci. U.S.A. **60**:660, 1968.

116. Solomon, D.H., and Beall, G.N.: Thyroid-stimulating activity in the serum of immunized rabbits. II. Nature of the thyroid-stimulating material, J. Clin. Endocrinol. Metab. **28:**1496, 1968.

117. Strickroot, F.L., Schaeffer, R.L., and Bergo, H.L.: Myasthenia gravis occurring in an infant born of a myasthenic mother, J.A.M.A. **120:**1207, 1942.

118. Taylor, K.B., et al.: Autoimmune phenomena in pernicious anemia: gastric antibodies, Br. Med. J. **2:**1347, 1962.

119. Volpe, R.: The role of autoimmunity in hypoendocrine and hyperendocrine function, Ann. Intern. Med. **87:**86, 1977.

Cytotoxic or cytolytic reactions

120. Abramson, N., Eisenberg, P.D., and Aster, R.H.: Post-transfusion purpura: immunologic aspects and therapy, N. Engl. J. Med. **291:**1163, 1974.

121. Ackroyd, J.F.: Sedormid purpura: an immunologic study of a form of drug hypersensitivity, Prog. Allergy **3:**531, 1952.

122. Atkinson, J.P., and Frank, M.M.: Studies on the in vivo effects of antibody: interaction of IgM antibody and complement in the immune clearance and destruction of erythrocytes in man, J. Clin. Invest. **54:**339, 1974.

123. Baldini, M.: Idiopathic thrombocytopenic purpura, N. Engl. J. Med. **274:**1245, 1966.

124. Dacie, J.V., and Wolledge, S.M.: Autoimmune hemolytic anemia, Prog. Hematol. **6:**1, 1969.

125. Freda, V.J., Gorman, J.G., and Pollack, W.: Suppression of the primary Rh immune response with passive Rh IgG immunoglobulin, N. Engl. J. Med. **277:**1022, 1967.

126. Goetz, O., and Muller-Eberhard, H.J.: The alternative pathway of complement activation, Adv. Immunol. **24:**1, 1976.

127. Humphrey, J.H., and Dourmashkin, R.R.: The lesions in cell membranes caused by complement, Adv. Immunol. **11:**75, 1969.

128. Karpatkin, S.: Autoimmune thrombocytopenic purpura, Blood **56:**329, 1980.

129. Kerr, R.-O., et al.: Two mechanisms of erythrocyte destruction in penicillin-induced hemolytic anemia, N. Engl. J. Med. **287:**1322, 1972.

130. Mayer, M.M.: The complement system, Sci. Am. **229:**54, 1968.

131. Muller-Eberhard, H.J.: Chemistry and reaction mechanisms of complement, Adv. Immunol. **8:**1, 1968.

132. Pirofsky, B.: Clinical aspects of autoimmune hemolytic anemia, Semin. Hematol. **13:**251, 1976.

133. Race, R.R., and Sanger, R.: Blood groups in man, Philadelphia, 1962, F.A. Davis Co.

134. Waksman, B.H.: Cell lysis and related phenomena in hypersensitivity reactions, including immunohematologic diseases, Prog. Allergy **5:**340, 1958.

135. Watkins, W.M.: Blood group substances, Science **152:**172, 1966.

136. Zmijewski, C.M.: Immunohematology, New York, 1968, Appleton-Century-Crofts.

Toxic (immune) complex reactions

137. Arthus, M.: Injectons repetees de serum de cheval chez le lapin, C.R. Soc. Biol. (Paris) **55:**817, 1903.

138. Benoit, F.L., et al.: Goodpasture's syndrome: a clinicopathologic entity, Am. J. Med. **37:**424, 1964.

139. Beutner, E.H., Chorzelski, T.P., and Bean, S.F.: Immunopathology of the skin, ed. 2, New York, 1979, John Wiley & Sons, Inc.

140. Couser, W.G., and Salant, D.J.: In situ immune complex formation and glomerular injury, Kidney Int. **17:**1, 1980.

141. Dixon, F.J., et al.: Pathogenesis of serum sickness, Arch. Pathol. **65:**18, 1958.

142. Hargraves, M.M., Richmond, H., and Morton, R.: Presentation of 2 bone marrow elements: the "tart" cell and the "LE" cell, Mayo Clin. Proc. **23:**25, 1948.

143. McCombs, R.P.: Systemic "allergic" vasculitis: clinical and pathological relationships, J.A.M.A. **194:**1059, 1965.

144. Ploth, D.W., et al.: Thyroglobulin–anti-thyroglobulin immune complex glomerulonephritis complicating radioiodine therapy, Clin. Immunol. Immunopathol. **9:**327, 1978.

145. Rich, A.R., and Gregory, J.E.: The experimental demonstration that polyarteritis nodosa is a manifestation of hypersensitivity, Bull. Johns Hopkins Hosp. **72:**63, 1943.

146. Rose, G.A., and Spencer, H.: Polyarteritis nodosa, Q. J. Med. **26:**43, 1957.

147. Theofilopoulos, A.N.: Evaluation and clinical significance of circulating immune complexes, Clin. Immunol. **4:**63, 1980.

148. Vaughn, J.J.: Rheumatologic disorders due to immune complexes, Postgrad. Med. **54:**129, 1973.

149. von Pirquet, C.F., and Schick, B.: Serum sickness, 1905, Baltimore, 1951, The Williams & Wilkins Co. (Translated by B. Schick.)

150. Wilson, C.B., and Dixon, F.J.: Immunopathology and glomerulonephritis, Annu. Rev. Med. **25:**83, 1974.

151. Zabriskie, J.B.: The role of streptococci in human glomerulonephritis, J. Exp. Med. **134:**180, 1971.

152. Zvaifler, N.J.: Rheumatoid arthritis: a dissertation on its pathogenesis and future directions for research, Aust. N.Z. J. Med. **8**(suppl.):44, 1978.

Atopic and anaphylactic reactions

153. Aas, K.: Heterogeneity of bronchial asthma, Allergy **36:**3, 1981.

154. Austen, K.F., and Lichtenstein, L.M., editors: Asthma: physiology, immunopharmacology and treatment, New York, 1973, Academic Press, Inc.

155. Austen, K.F., and Orange, R.P.: Bronchial asthma: the possible role of the chemical mediators of immediate hypersensitivity in the pathogenesis of subacute chronic disease, Am. Rev. Respir. Dis. **112:**423, 1975.

156. Barr, S.E.: Allergy to *Hymenoptera* stings—review of the world literature: 1953-1970, Ann. Allergy **29:**49, 1971.

157. Block, K.S.: The anaphylactic antibodies of mammals including man, Prog. Allergy **10:**84, 1967.

158. Coca, A.F., and Grove, E.F.: Studies on hypersensitiveness. XIII. A study of the atopic reagins, J. Immunol. **10:**445, 1925.

159. Epstein, J.H.: Photoallergy, a review, Arch. Dermatol. **106:**741, 1972.

160. Farr, R.S.: Presidential message, J. Allergy **45:**321, 1970.

161. Fein, B.T.: Aspirin shock associated with asthma and nasal polyps, Ann. Allergy **29:**589, 1971.

162. Frazier, C.A.: Biting insect survey: a statistical report, Ann. Allergy **32:**200, 1974.

163. Golbert, T.M., Patterson, R., and Pruzansky, J.J.: Systemic allergic reactions to ingested antigens, J. Allergy **44:**96, 1969.

164. Grolnick, M.: An investigative and clinical evaluation of dermatographism, Ann. Allergy **28:**395, 1970.

165. Halpern, B.N., Ky, T., and Robert, B.: Clinical and immunological study of an exceptional case of reaginic type sensitization to human seminal fluid, Immunology **12:**247, 1967.

166. Hinson, R.F.W., Moon, A.J., and Plummer, N.S.: Bronchopulmonary aspergillosis, Thorax **7:**317, 1952.

167. Ishizaka, K., Ishizaka, T., and Hornbrook, M.H.: Physico-chemical properties of human reaginic antibody. IV. Presence of a unique immunoglobulin as a carrier of reaginic activity, J. Immunol. **97:**75, 1966.

168. James, L.P., and Austen, K.F.: Fatal systemic anaphylaxis in man, N. Engl. J. Med. **270:**597, 1964.

169. Kay, J.W.: Atopic dermatitis: an immunologic disease complex and its therapy, Ann. Allergy **38:**345, 1977.

170. Killby, V.A., and Silverman, P.H.: Hypersensitive reactions in man to specific mosquito bites, Am. J. Trop. Med. Hyg. **16:**374, 1967.

171. Lewis, R.A., and Austen, K.F.: Mediation of local homeostasis and inflammation by leukotrienes and other mast cell-dependent compounds, Nature **293:**103, 1981.

172. Möller, G., editor: Immunoglobulin E, Immunol. Rev. **41:**1, 1978.

173. Paterson, J.W., and Lulich, K.M.: Pharmacology of asthma: a review of certain aspects, Prog. Respir. Dis. **14:**112, 1980.

174. Prausnitz, C., and Kustner, H.: Studies on sensitivity, Zentralbl. Bakteriol. (Orig. A) **86:**160, 1921. (English translation in Gell, P.G.H., and Coombs, R.R.A.: Clinical aspects of immunology, Philadelphia, 1963, F.A. Davis Co.)

175. Rowe, A.H., and Rowe, A., Jr.: Food allergy, Springfield, Ill., 1972, Charles C Thomas, Publisher.

176. Sheffer, A.L., Austen, K.F., and Gigli, I.: Urticaria and angioedema, Postgrad. Med. **54**:81, 1973.

177. Stebbings, J.H., Jr.: Immediate hypersensitivity: a defense against arthropods, Perspect. Biol. Med. **17**:233, 1974.

178. Steinberg, P., Ishizaka, K., and Norman, P.S.: Possible role of IgE-mediated reaction in immunity, J. Allergy Clin. Immunol. **54**:359, 1974.

179. Szentivanyi, A.: The beta adrenergic theory of the atopic abnormality in bronchial asthma, J. Allergy **42**:203, 1968.

180. Wasserman, S.I., and Center, D.M.: The relevance of neutrophil chemotactic factors to allergic disease, J. Allergy Clin. Immunol. **64**:231, 1979.

Cellular or delayed hypersensitivity

181. Albert, E., and Goetz, D.: The major histocompatibility system in man. In Goetz, D., editor: Histocompatibility antigens, Berlin, 1978, Springer-Verlag.

182. Arnason, B.G., and Waksman, B.H.: Tuberculin sensitivity: immunologic considerations, Adv. Tuberc. Res. **13**:1, 1964.

183. Beer, A.E., and Billingham, R.E.: Immunobiology of mammalian reproduction, Adv. Immunol. **14**:1, 1971.

184. Biberfield, P., Holm, G., and Perlmann, P.: Morphologic observations on lymphocyte peripolesis and cytotoxic action in vitro, Exp. Cell Res. **52**:672, 1968.

185. Bloom, R.R., and Jimenez, L.: Migration inhibitory factor and the cellular basis of delayed hypersensitivity reactions, Am. J. Pathol. **60**:453, 1970.

186. Bodmer, W.F., editor: The HLA system, Br. Med. Bull. **34**:1978.

187. Cerottini, J.-C., and Brunner, K.T.: Cell-mediated cytotoxicity, allograft rejection and tumor immunity, Adv. Immunol. **18**:67, 1974.

188. Cohen, S.: The role of cell mediated immunity in the induction of inflammatory responses, Am. J. Pathol. **88**:502, 1977.

189. Dausset, J.: The major histocompatibility complex in man, Nature **213**:1469, 1981.

190. Doniach, D.: Autoimmune aspects of liver disease, Br. Med. Bull. **28**:145, 1972.

191. Dvorak, H.F., et al.: Morphology of delayed type hypersensitivity reactions in man. I. Quantitative description of the inflammatory response, Lab. Invest. **31**:111, 1974.

192. Eylar, E.H.: Amino acid sequence of the myelin basic protein, Proc. Natl. Acad. Sci. U.S.A. **67**:1425, 1970.

193. Flax, M.H.: Experimental allergic thyroiditis in the guinea pig. II. Morphologic studies on the development of the disease, Lab. Invest. **12**:199, 1963.

194. Flax, M.H., Jankovic, D.B., and Sell, S.: Experimental allergic thyroiditis in the guinea pig. I. Relationship of delayed hypersensitivity and circulating antibody to the development of thyroiditis, Lab. Invest. **12**:119, 1963.

195. Gale, R.P., and Opelz, G.: Second International Symposium on Immunobiology of Bone Marrow Transplantation, Transplant. Proc., vol. 10, no. 1, 1978.

196. Griepp, R.B., et al.: Human heart transplantation: current status, Am. Thorac. Surg. **22**:171, 1976.

197. Hellström, K.E., and Hellström, I.: Lymphocyte-mediated cytotoxicity and blocking serum activity to tumor antigens, Adv. Immunol. **18**:209, 1974.

198. Henney, C.S.: On the mechanism of T-cell mediated cytolysis, Transplant. Rev. **17**:37, 1973.

199. Jones, T.D., and Mote, J.R.: The phases of foreign sensitization in human beings, N. Engl. J. Med. **210**:120, 1934.

200. Kaliss, N.: Immunological enhancement of tumor homografts in mice: a review, Cancer Res. **18**:992, 1958.

201. Kaplan, M.H.: Autoimmunity to heart and its relation to human disease, Prog. Allergy **13**:408, 1969.

202. Lampert, P.W.: Autoimmune and virus-induced demyelinating diseases, Am. J. Pathol. **91**:176, 1978.

203. Lawrence, H.S., and Valentine, F.T.: Transfer factor and other mediators of cellular immunity, Am. J. Pathol. **60**:437, 1970.

204. Levy, G.A., and Chisari, F.V.: The immunopathogenesis of hepatitis B virus induced liver disease, Springer Semin. Immunopathol. **3**:439, 1981.

205. Nakumura, R.M., and Weigle, W.O.: Transfer of experimental thyroiditis by serum from thyroidectomized donors, J. Exp. Med. **130**:263, 1969.

206. Paterson, P.Y.: The demyelinating diseases: clinical and experimental correlates. In Sampter, M., editor: Immunological diseases, ed. 2, Boston, 1971, Little, Brown & Co.

207. Perlmann, P., and Holm, G.: Cytotoxic effects of lymphoid cells in vitro, Adv. Immunol. **11**:117, 1970.

208. Rappaport, F.T., Converse, J.M., and Billingham, R.E.: Recent advances in clinical and experimental transplantation, J.A.M.A. **237**:2835, 1977.

209. Snell, G.D., and Stimpfling, J.H.: Genetics of tissue transplantation. In Green, E.L., editor: Biology of the laboratory mouse, ed. 2, New York, 1966, McGraw-Hill Book Co.

210. Stetson, C.A.: The role of humoral antibody in the homograft rejection, Adv. Immunol. **3**:97, 1963.

211. Storb, R.: Bone marrow transplantation for the treatment of hematologic malignancy and of aplastic anemia, Transplant. Proc. **13**:221, 1981.

212. Szulman, A.E.: The A,B and H blood-group antigens in the human placenta, N. Engl. J. Med. **286**:1028, 1972.

213. Voisin, G.A.: Immunological facilitation, a broadening concept of the enhancement phenomenon, Prog. Allergy **15**:328, 1971.

214. Waksman, B.H.: Experimental allergic encephalomyelitis and the "autoallergic" diseases, Int. Arch. Allergy Appl. Immunol. **14**(suppl.):1, 1959.

215. Waksman, B.H.: Autoimmunization and the lesions of autoimmunity, Medicine **41**:93, 1962.

216. Waksman, B.H., and Namba, Y.: On soluble mediators of immunologic regulation, Cell Immunol. **21**:161, 1976.

217. Zoller, K.M., et al.: Cessation of immunosuppressive therapy after successful transplantation: a national survey, Kidney Int. **18**:110, 1980.

Granulomatous hypersensitivity

218. Adams, D.O.: The granulomatous inflammatory response, Am. J. Pathol. **84**:164, 1976.

219. Albert, D.A., Weisman, M.H., and Kaplan, R.: The rheumatic manifestations of leprosy (Hansen disease), Medicine **59**:442, 1980.

220. Chumbley, L.C., Harrison, E.C., Jr., and Deremee, R.A.: Allergic granulomatosis and angiitis (Churg-Strauss syndrome): report and analysis of 30 cases, Mayo Clin. Proc. **52**:477, 1977.

221. Churg, J.: Allergic granulomatosis and granulomatous vascular syndromes, Ann. Allergy **21**:619, 1963.

222. Daniele, R.P., Dauber, J.H., and Rossman, M.D.: Immunologic abnormalities in sarcoidosis, Ann. Intern. Med. **92**:406, 1980.

223. Dannenburg, A.M.: Cellular hypersensitivity and cellular immunity in the pathogenesis of tuberculosis specificity, systemic and local nature, and associated macrophage enzymes, Bacteriol. Rev. **32**:85, 1968.

224. Deodhar, S.D., Barna, B., and Van Ordstrand, H.S.: A study of the immunologic aspects of chronic berylliosis, Chest **63**:309, 1973.

225. Epstein, W.L.: Granulomatous hypersensitivity, Prog. Allergy **11**:36, 1967.

226. Howell, S.B., and Epstein, W.V.: Circulating immunoglobulin complexes in Wegener's granulomatosis, Am. J. Med. **60**:259, 1976.

227. Mackaness, G.B., and Blanden, R.V.: Cellular immunity, Prog. Allergy **11**:89, 1967.

228. McCombs, R.P.: Diseases due to immunologic reactions in the lungs, N. Engl. J. Med. **286**:1186, 1972.

229. Skinsnes, O.K.: Immunopathology of leprosy: the century in review—pathology, pathogenesis and the development of classification, Int. J. Lepr. **41**:329, 1973.

230. Tepper, L.B., Hardy, H.L., and Chamberlin, R.I.: Toxicity of beryllium compounds, Amsterdam, 1961, Elsevier Publishing Co.

231. Turk, J.L., and Bryceson, A.D.M.: Immunological phenomena in leprosy and related disease, Adv. Immunol. **13**:209, 1971.

232. Warren, K.S.: Modulation of immunopathology and disease in schistosomiasis, Am. J. Trop. Med. Hyg. **26**:113, 1977.

CHAPTER 14

Malnutrition and Deficiency Diseases

HERSCHEL SIDRANSKY

The role of nutrition in the pathogenesis of disease has been of great concern to scientists and physicians for many years. The importance of nutrition to well-being has been understood by civilized societies for centuries. Indeed, the state of nutrition in a society has usually correlated well with its socioeconomic development and advancement. Thus humans have been greatly concerned with the availability of adequate and balanced nutrition. Diseases that are consequences of inadequate diets have long plagued humankind. Unfortunately, they remain with us today and most probably will be with us for years to come.

Historically nutrition gained eminence as a medical science with the discoveries that the absence of essential nutrients, such as single vitamins, induced a variety of important and specific nutritional deficiency diseases. These monumental findings led to a clearer understanding of how essential nutrients play vital roles in the normal functioning of cells, tissues, and organs of animals and humans.

In recent years, as knowledge has rapidly expanded in many areas of biologic and medical science, it has become apparent that the nutritional intake and utilization by any host, animal or human, are important not only in the prevention of deficiency states but also in the host's adaptation and responses to environmental stresses and strains. This chapter is a brief review of how malnutrition and deficiency diseases develop, the manifestations of certain deficiency states, nutritional imbalances, and how nutritional alterations may influence the host's responses to certain environmental manifestations.

As an introduction to malnutrition and deficiency diseases, it is essential to mention briefly the dietary components involved in normal and adequate nutrition. The human body requires some 50 to 60 organic and inorganic compounds in quantities ranging from micrograms to grams.[4,35,53] These are included in six basic groups: proteins, carbohydrates, fats, vitamins, minerals, and water. Proteins are made up of amino acids, eight of which must be supplied by dietary intake because they cannot be synthesized by the body in the amounts needed. These are isoleucine, leucine, lysine, methionine, phenylalanine, threonine, tryptophan, and valine. In addition, an exogenous supply of histidine is needed for early growth and development and therefore may also be considered essential. Carbohydrates in themselves are not essential, but they provide needed dietary calories. Fats or their constituent fatty acids also provide calories. However, three fatty acids, linolenic, arachidonic, and especially linoleic, are currently considered essential. Vitamins, certain minerals, and water are indispensable dietary components. The consequences of the absence or imbalance (altered relationships) of these components, leading to malnutrition or deficiency states, are considered later in the chapter.

In an attempt to characterize the various types of malnutrition or deficiency diseases as they affect individuals, one may consider them as (1) single deficiency states, (2) multiple deficiency states, (3) imbalances, and (4) excesses. The term *single deficiency states* implies that the disease results from the absence of a single essential or indispensable compound. Much of the information regarding such deficiency states has been derived from animal experimentation in which the variables were carefully monitored. Single vitamin deficiencies are the best examples. *Multiple deficiency states* develop when more than one necessary component is lacking in the diet. In humans, multiple deficiencies occur frequently because a diet deficient in one component is usually deficient in others. Thus the pathologic changes may reflect each deficiency to some degree. *Nutritional imbalances* occur when the proportion of one dietary component to another or others is such that pathologic changes occur. Nutritional imbalances can occur under a variety of conditions. One example is the disease kwashiorkor, in which there is a protein deficiency in the presence of adequate or even high caloric intake. In contrast, marasmus occurs when there is a deficiency of total food intake (protein and all other components). Experimentally, amino acid imbalances have been demonstrated to induce a variety of pathologic changes.[30] The concept of nutritional imbalances is relatively new but has been gaining recognition. It stresses that the quantity of intake of each dietary component in relation to other components is of great importance and must be carefully evaluated. *Nutritional excesses*, single or multiple, are becoming increasingly important, especially in affluent societies. Obesity caused by excessive intake, particularly of calories, is a common condition. Hypervitaminosis occurs when specific vitamins are given in excessive amounts and can have serious pathologic manifestations.

PATHOGENESIS OF DEFICIENCY DISEASES

A nutritional deficiency disease develops when the amounts of essential nutrients provided to the cells are inadequate for their normal metabolic functions. The deficiency may be primary or secondary in origin. A primary nutritional inadequacy is induced by a poor diet—one that lacks essential nutrients in either kind or amount or that provides an imbalance of nutrients. A secondary nutritional inadequacy comes about from factors that interfere with the ingestion, absorption, or utilization of nutrients, as well as from metabolic or functional conditions that increase the requirement for nutrients or cause unusual destruction or abnormal excretion of nutrients.

Fig. 14-1 presents a diagrammatic scheme of the pathogenesis of nutritional deficiency diseases. After a nutritional inadequacy (primary or secondary) begins, there is a time lapse before the onset of a nutritional deficiency disease. The time interval may depend on the degree of nutritional inadequacy and the level of nutrient reserves. An important safety factor is the nutrient reserves on which the tissues may draw during temporary lapses in the supply of nutrients. These reserves may be large or small, depending upon the specific nutrient and the overall state of the reserve tissues. Tissue depletion follows the exhaustion of nutrient reserves and may occur rapidly or slowly, depending on the degree of nutritional inadequacy, the amount of nutrient reserves, and the requirement of the body for essential nutrients.

Biochemical lesions develop as a consequence of tissue depletion. Such lesions can best be illustrated by deficiencies of vitamins that are involved with enzyme systems dealing with the release of energy and other metabolic reactions. Biochemical alterations develop and may result in the accumulation of certain metabolites and in the altered metabolism of others. Functional changes in tissues and organs may then occur. Anatomic lesions develop and often are specific for or related to the missing nutritional component or components. Although this sequence has been presented in a stepwise manner, no one step in the chain of events from nutritional inadequacy to anatomic lesions need necessarily be complete before the next begins.

PRIMARY AND SECONDARY NUTRITIONAL INADEQUACY

Primary nutritional inadequacy is caused by a diet that lacks essential nutrients in either kind or amount or that provides an imbalance of nutrients. Such inadequacy has always existed at one time or another in some parts of the world. It has been especially prevalent during and following wars, after crop failures, and in relation to poverty, ignorance, faddism, and cultural taboos. Throughout the world today, protein-calorie malnutrition is the most prominent example of this form of nutritional inadequacy. This will be reviewed in a subsequent section.

Although malnutrition and nutritional deficiency diseases are usually considered to arise solely from an inad-

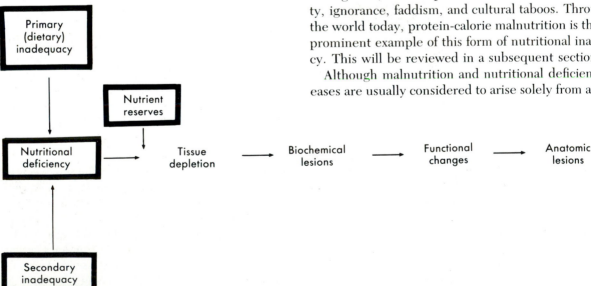

Fig. 14-1. Scheme of pathogenesis of nutritional deficiency diseases.

equate diet, under certain circumstances these may occur in the presence of dietary adequacy. Secondary nutritional inadequacy is caused by a variety of factors other than a poor diet. This type of nutritional inadequacy is of special importance in affluent societies such as in the United States. Factors that may be involved are as follows:

1. Interference with ingestion: gastrointestinal disorders (acute gastroenteritis, gallbladder disease, peptic ulcers, diarrheal diseases, obstructive lesions of the bowel), neuropsychiatric disorders (neurasthenia, psychoneurosis, migraine), anorexia (alcoholism, congestive heart failure, cancer therapy, infectious diseases), food allergy, loss of teeth, pregnancy
2. Increased nutritive requirement: abnormal activity, abnormal environmental factors, fever, hyperthyroidism, pregnancy and lactation
3. Interference with absorption: gastrointestinal diseases (associated with hypermotility or reduction of absorbing surfaces), achlorhydria, biliary diseases
4. Interference with utilization: hepatic dysfunction, hypothyroidism, malignancy
5. Increased excretion: polyuria, lactation, excessive perspiration
6. Increased destruction: achlorhydria

All of the preceding can be influenced by a variety of therapeutic agents that may indirectly induce secondary nutritional inadequacies.

STARVATION

Starvation occurs in individuals of all ages. Much information about this condition was gained from postmortem studies in prison camps during World War II.[37] In general, the overall pathologic changes are minimal; atrophy is the main feature. The changes caused by inanition include great loss of weight, serous atrophy of fat throughout the body, reduced amounts of lymphoid tissue, and marked atrophy of testes or ovaries, cardiac and skeletal muscle, thymus, and liver. Hemosiderosis of the spleen and lipid depletion of adrenal glands are common findings.

PROTEIN-CALORIE MALNUTRITION

The most prevalent form of primary nutritional deficiency disease is protein-calorie malnutrition. According to the World Health Organization (WHO), protein-calorie malnutrition is rampant throughout the world. The two diseases associated with this malnutrition, marasmus and kwashiorkor, affect preschool-aged children in the developing countries of the world. Marasmus is a form of childhood starvation caused by inadequate total food intake. Its manifestations are those of starvation in which pathologic changes are minimal.[36,40] Kwashiorkor, the most important and widespread nutritional deficiency disease in the world today (affecting more than 100 million children) according to WHO, has long been attributed to protein deficiency. In the 1950s it was established that kwashiorkor is caused by a combination of protein deficiency and relatively high carbohydrate intake.[12,18] Such a nutritionally deficient and imbalanced diet leads rapidly to pathologic changes in a number of organs.[81] Many children throughout the world die from this disease. In addition, it has been speculated that children who survive may later develop an enhanced susceptibility to hepatic injury caused by viruses, toxins, or chemical carcinogens, and as adults may have an increased incidence of cirrhosis and primary liver cancer.

Marasmus

Marasmus (Fig. 14-2) is a form of starvation that occurs during childhood. It results from an overall deficit in food intake, including all dietary components (protein, carbohydrate, lipid, vitamins, salts). Therefore it has often been referred to as "balanced starvation."

Marasmus occurs most commonly during the first year

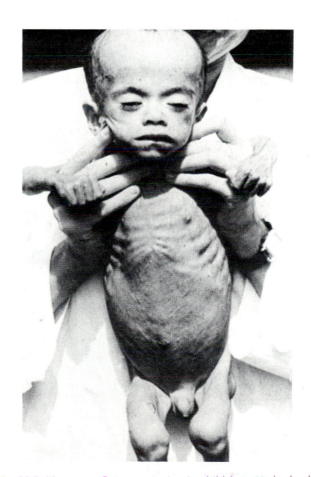

Fig. 14-2. Marasmus. Extreme wasting in child from Netherlands during World War II. (From Latham, M.C., et al.: Scope manual on nutrition, Kalamazoo, Mich., 1972, The Upjohn Co.)

of life and is found in most developing countries. A common cause is early cessation of breast feeding with lack of food intake. The clinical features and findings in marasmus are growth failure (low weight and height, prominent ribs, monkeylike face, protuberant abdomen, thin limbs), muscle wasting and loss of subcutaneous fat, anemia, and diarrhea (common but not a constant feature). Edema is absent, mental changes are uncommon, and appetite is good. Serum protein levels are reduced. Other than the small size or atrophy of organs, no specific gross or microscopic (pathologic) changes are present. The liver is not fatty.

Kwashiorkor[12,18,55,81]

Kwashiorkor (Fig. 14-3) has been recognized for centuries and has been referred to by many names throughout the world. In 1936 Dr. Cicely Williams of the Gold Coast of Africa first described kwashiorkor in detail in the medical literature. Since that time kwashiorkor has gained notoriety as the most widespread and important dietary deficiency disease in the world.

Although kwashiorkor was at first considered to result from protein deficiency alone, the cause is now recognized to be a nutritional imbalance, consisting of protein

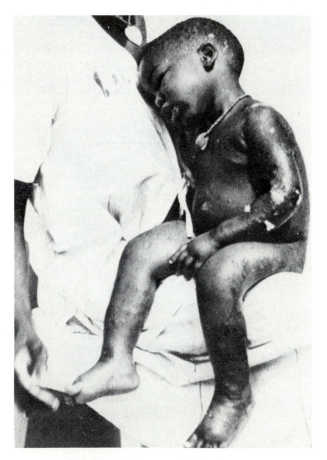

Fig. 14-3. Kwashiorkor. African child showing edema and dermatosis. (From Latham, M.C., et al.: Scope Manual on nutrition, Kalamazoo, Mich., 1972, The Upjohn Co.)

deficiency and adequate or high carbohydrate intake. The disease occurs mainly in children 6 months to 3 years of age. It usually follows weaning when the infant is fed the poor and limited foods of the area (corn, cassava, or other grains and vegetables), which are relatively high in carbohydrate but contain inadequate amounts of proteins that are often of poor quality.

The clinical features and findings in kwashiorkor are growth failure; wasting of muscles of arms and legs but preservation of subcutaneous fat; edema; mental changes, such as apathy, irritability, and lack of interest in surroundings; changes in hair color, texture, and strength; depigmentation of skin; hepatomegaly; diarrhea; and anemia. The main pathologic findings consist of an enlarged, fatty liver with periportal distribution of lipid and atrophy of the pancreas, salivary glands, small intestine glands, and skeletal muscles.

Consequences of kwashiorkor

Although many children die from kwashiorkor, others survive as a consequence of mild involvement or treatment with a well-balanced diet containing adequate and good-quality proteins. Thus in the developing countries there are many adults who have had this nutritional deficiency disease during childhood. In the past, epidemiologists suggested that the fatty liver of kwashiorkor would progress directly to nutritionally induced cirrhosis in adult life. Such adults were thought to have a higher than normal predilection for primary hepatocellular carcinoma. More current views suggest that the liver damage from kwashiorkor makes these individuals more susceptible in later life to injury by hepatotoxic agents (such as viruses or aflatoxin), which then progresses to cirrhosis and in some cases to primary liver cancer.

Much interest has developed in the possibility that stunted mental development may occur as a consequence of kwashiorkor during childhood. In several studies children who had kwashiorkor during early childhood scored lower on IQ tests than did their siblings who did not have kwashiorkor.[10,44]

Although the conclusions from the preceding two examples are still speculative, they deal with important and significant problems that may be consequences of malnutrition during childhood. Absolute proof that these associations are valid is difficult to document. Therefore many investigators have attempted to use experimental kwashiorkor-like models[17,25,58,71,75] in animals to probe the pathogenesis of the induced lesions and the possible consequences of these alterations in later life. Such studies have provided valuable information concerning nutritional deficiencies and imbalances and their effects both on specific organs and on the whole organism.

Experimental kwashiorkor-like models

A number of investigators have developed experimental models of kwashiorkor to attempt to understand the pathogenesis of the lesions in children with this disease. This has been approached by feeding diets deficient in amino acids or protein to experimental animals. The experimental model that probably most closely resembles the pathologic changes reported in infants dying from kwashiorkor[81] is one in which animals are force-fed by stomach tube purified diets devoid of single essential amino acids.[71] Lesions develop within 3 to 10 days in these force-feeding experiments and resemble those described in children with kwashiorkor. The morphologic changes consist of a periportal fatty liver, excess hepatic glycogen, and atrophy of the pancreas, submaxillary gland, stomach, spleen, and thymus. Some of the major conclusions based on these experimental studies are the following:

1. Both total intake and caloric intake of a deficient diet must be adequate to induce pathologic changes. Rats fed a deficient diet ad libitum eat little and develop a marasmus-like rather than a kwashiorkor-like condition. This explains the need for force-feeding the deficient or imbalanced diet to maintain an adequate intake and induce the pathologic changes.
2. Overall, the pathologic changes are similar regardless of which single essential amino acid is eliminated from the diet. This indicates that the results reflect protein deficiency rather than deficiency of a single essential amino acid. Use of poor-quality plant proteins as the sole source of protein with adequate amounts of all other components in force-feeding experiments substantiates this.
3. The pathologic changes are not mediated through adrenal or pituitary hormonal stimulation.
4. Loss of skeletal muscle protein occurs early and is important. Hepatic protein synthesis is maintained at a high level. Marked alterations in hepatic lipid and glycogen metabolism occur.
5. Treatment with a complete, balanced, purified diet rapidly reverses the condition.

VITAMINS

For practical purposes vitamins may be defined as organic catalysts of exogenous origin that are effective in relatively minute amounts and that are essential for the maintenance of the normal structure and function of cells. Vitamins themselves are not utilized to furnish energy but are essential components of the chemical machinery by which the true food substances are metabolized. With certain exceptions they are not synthesized in the body and must be supplied in the diet or from other external sources. Some compounds are vitamins in the above-defined sense for practically all mammals, whereas others are vitamins only for those that are unable to manufacture them. For example, humans, other primates, and guinea pigs are the only mammals that require vitamin C as a dietary component. In these mam-

mals the synthesis of vitamin C from D-glucose proceeds normally except for the final step, the conversion of gluconate to ascorbate. The enzyme necessary for the final step is missing.

Mechanism of action

The biologic action of many vitamins is intimately related to intracellular enzyme systems. Certain vitamins represent components of essential enzyme systems that cannot be synthesized in the body. Moreover, many hormones act through the medium of the intracellular enzyme systems,[24,28] either by regulating their synthesis and breakdown or by stimulating or inhibiting them. An essential difference between hormones and vitamins is that the former are endogenous (synthesized in certain organs for the maintenance of others), whereas the latter are entirely of exogenous origin. The failure of certain enzyme systems also depends on the inheritance of defective genes.[8]

Thus living cells, with normal genic composition and with the aid of hormones and vitamins, may be said to construct and maintain the cytologic machinery that carries out the complex metabolic reactions necessary for their normal life, function, and reproduction. In their efforts to learn the details of these vital processes, investigators have been concerned with morphologic and biochemical events that occur normally and abnormally. With the availability of advanced tools and methods, such as electron microscopy, subcellular fractionation, and biochemical analysis, the intricate picture of the cell as a molecular factory has been developed.

Sources, requirements, and modern uses

Most vitamins are primarily of plant origin and normally enter the body as constituents of ingested plant or animal food. They may be added to the diet or injected parenterally in concentrated or pure form for both prophylactic and therapeutic purposes. The minimum daily requirements of many vitamins for the maintenance of health in normal individuals have been more or less accurately established,[4,35,53] and range from a fraction of a milligram to about 150 mg. The therapeutic dosage necessary to correct certain pathologic states may be many times the prophylactic dose. Although some moderate excess over the minimum requirements is desirable for normal people, there is definite evidence that large doses of vitamins A and D are harmful.

Paths of investigation in humans and animals

Early knowledge of vitamin deficiency was obtained largely by clinical observation of disease entities and empiric discovery that certain foods had preventive or curative value. Based on extensive studies of dietary deficiencies in experimental animals, the complexity of the problem has become evident. The isolation of vitamins in chemically pure form has led to the determination of the structural formulas and in many instances to chemical synthesis. The final step, determination of the mode of action, is under way in many laboratories. Recent developments relating to vitamins A and D have been most revealing.[19-21,27]

The pathologic lesions resulting from vitamin deficiencies are of two types: primary changes caused by metabolic disturbance in the tissues or organs physiologically served by the vitamin involved and secondary effects (notably inanition, organ atrophy, and arrest of growth) on the body as a whole.

Morphologic studies of the primary types of lesions have played an important role in attempts to understand the physiologic action of vitamins. Since vitamins often control the function of specific types of tissue, it has been possible to study not only the retrogressive changes resulting from deficiency but also the mechanisms of repair that occur when the deficiencies are corrected. Studies of this type have made unique contributions to our knowledge of normal cell physiology as well as that of abnormal cell responses. Correlations between morphologic and biochemical alterations are beginning to emerge.

As previously mentioned, vitamins function by entering into complex cytologic mechanisms that also involve enzymes, hormones, and genes. Important vital processes such as detoxication, electron transport, and immune body formation are implemented by these mechanisms. Thus the symptoms of secondary deficiency may appear as a result of disturbances of cellular metabolism from many different causes—from dietary lack to congenital or acquired defects in the intracellular machinery.

Antivitamins

Chemical compounds that are closely related to vitamins will in some cases compete with and replace active vitamins in enzyme systems and thus produce the effects of vitamin deficiencies. Analogs acting in this way have been discovered for ascorbic acid, nicotinic acid, riboflavin, thiamine, pyridoxine, pantothenic acid, vitamin K, and folic acid. Folic acid analogs have been extensively studied because they are beneficial in certain cases of acute leukemia. Different in their mode of action are certain enzymes that destroy vitamins. The best-known example of the latter is thiaminase, which is present in certain types of raw fish and which has been responsible for a rapidly fatal disease in foxes known as Chastek paralysis.

Nomenclature

Chemical names have to some extent replaced letters for the nomenclature of vitamins, but the alphabetic designation is still widely used. All of the well-recognized vitamins are included under the following headings: vitamin A, vitamin B complex (composed of many specific factors), vitamin C (ascorbic acid), vitamin D, vitamin E (alpha-tocopherol and its congeners), and the K vitamins.

Vitamins A, D, E, and K are fat soluble, whereas vitamin C and the members of the B complex are water soluble. Pancreatic disease, hepatobiliary disorders, and prolonged diarrhea are particularly likely to interfere with the absorption of the fat-soluble vitamins. Because vitamins A and D are stored in the liver in large amounts, evidence of deficiencies appears only after malabsorption has existed for many months.

Vitamin A[47,67]
Chemistry and physiology

Vitamin A is a fat-soluble, colorless, primary alcohol that is derived from certain yellow plant pigments known as carotenes. It is available in the diet in two forms, as the vitamin itself or as the provitamin precursors, the carotenes. The carotene molecules are composed of a long chain of carbon and hydrogen atoms, with a ring at each end. In the intestinal mucosa and liver these carotene molecules are split in the center to form, with the addition of two molecules of water, two molecules of vitamin A. Fish-liver oils are important sources of vitamin A itself, whereas the carotenes, primarily of vegetable origin, make up most of the usual dietary intake.

In the small intestine vitamin A esters are hydrolyzed and packaged into micelles with the assistance of bile salts. Carotene is converted into vitamin A and, along with the preformed vitamin A, is esterified preferentially with palmitic acid. Retinyl palmitate is carried in chylomicrons through the lymphatic system to the blood and is stored in the liver. After hydrolysis in the liver, it enters the blood where it is bound to retinol-binding protein and is transported to the tissues where it is needed. Retinoid-binding proteins have also been found to exist in the intracellular compartment in a number of tissues.

The known physiologic activities of vitamin A are as follows:
1. Maintenance of the structure and function of certain of the specialized types of epithelium
2. Formation, by combination with a protein, of expendable photosensitive pigments in the rods and cones of the retina, which transform radiant energy into nerve impulses
3. Maintenance of normal skeletal growth
4. Regulation of cell membrane structure and function

Experimental lesions in animals

The most characteristic effects of experimental vitamin A deficiency are seen in epithelial structures. Many types of epithelium, including that of the salivary glands, respiratory tract, genitourinary tract, pancreatic ducts, skin, conjunctivae, and enamel organs of the teeth, are affected. The epithelial cells involved undergo atrophy, reparative proliferation of the basal layer, and then, regardless of their original structure and function, replacement by stratified keratinizing epithelium. Correction of the deficiency results in autolysis of the keratinized cells and restoration of the original type of epithelium by differentiation of the persisting basal layer.

Vitamin A deficiency in experimental animals causes cessation of endochondral growth, but periosteal bone formation continues normally, so that the long bones become shorter and thicker. Wolbach and Bessey[89] have shown that paralysis and nerve degeneration result not from a direct effect of the deficiency on nerve tissue but from continued growth of the central nervous system after skeletal growth has been arrested. This disproportionate growth rate causes overcrowding of the cranial cavity and spinal cord, with resulting herniation of the brain tissue and nerve roots into the venous sinuses and intervertebral foramina. In this way mechanical damage and degeneration of nerve tissue are brought about.

Recent experimental studies have implicated vitamin A deficiency in enhanced susceptibility to cancer induction by chemical carcinogens. Also, high levels of vitamin A have been found to inhibit the induction of certain cancers in experimental animals. Many studies dealing with vitamin A and its role in chemoprevention of cancer are in progress.[76,77]

Lesions in humans

Vitamin A deficiency leads to retarded growth in children and emaciation in persons of all ages. Atrophy of the skeletal muscles and lymphatic tissue and moderate anemia, probably as a result of bone marrow atrophy, occur.

Xerophthalmia, a dry scaly lesion of the scleral conjunctiva, is the most obvious lesion and often establishes the diagnosis during life. Corneal ulceration may occur, with consequent bacterial infection (keratomalacia). Melanotic pigmentation of the cornea is often seen. Triangular grayish areas in the scleral conjunctiva *(Bitot spots)* represent accumulations of keratinized epithelium. This lesion may be seen in cases of prolonged mild deficiency.

Night blindness, or loss of visual acuity in dim light, is common in vitamin A deficiency. A pigment known as visual purple, or rhodopsin, must be present in the retina for normal vision in partial darkness. This pigment is formed by the combination of vitamin A aldehyde with a protein. The dissociation of this union by light results in an appropriate nerve impulse. Cyclic resynthesis of rhodopsin occurs in the dark, but some of the vitamin A is converted to an inactive compound in the process, and for this reason a continuous source of vitamin A is essential. It has been shown that rhodopsin is the specific stimulator of the retinal rods, which control vision in a weak light, whereas combination of vitamin A aldehyde with a different protein gives rise to idopsin, which stimulates the cones. The cones react to light of high intensity and are necessary for color vision.

A common type of skin lesion is *follicular hyperkeratosis*. Multiple firm papules, 1 to 5 mm in diameter, which may be almost confluent, develop as a result of the formation of keratin plugs in the sebaceous glands, giving the characteristic "toad skin" appearance (Fig. 14-4). Dryness and scaliness of the skin and furunculosis also are commonly present. These skin lesions have been described only in adults, and their specificity for vitamin A deficiency has been debated, since they have been found in scurvy and occasionally in general undernutrition. Histologically degeneration of the sweat glands and hyperkeratinization of the ducts and hair follicles are seen (Fig. 14-5).

Squamous metaplasia is most often seen in the trachea and bronchi and in the pelves of the kidneys, but the uterus, pancreatic ducts, and certain other epithelial structures also may be affected. Death often results from bronchopneumonia. Obstruction of pancreatic ducts by keratotic plugs may lead to cystic dilatation of the ducts

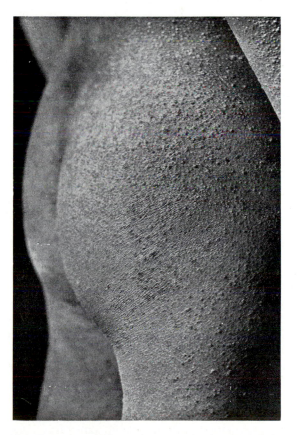

Fig. 14-4. Cutaneous lesions often seen in vitamin A deficiency showing general xeroderma and follicular hyperkeratosis in Chinese patient with xerophthalmia. (Courtesy Dr. Chester N. Frazier; from Sutton, R.L., and Sutton, R.L., Jr.: Diseases of the skin, ed. 10, St. Louis, 1939, The C.V. Mosby Co.)

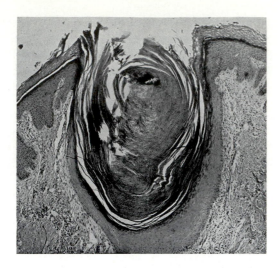

Fig. 14-5. Hyperkeratosis of hair follicle often associated with vitamin A deficiency but found in other nutritional disorders. (Courtesy Dr. Chester N. Frazier; from Sutton, R.L., Jr.: Diseases of the skin, ed. 11, St. Louis, 1956, The C.V. Mosby Co.)

and acini. All of these metaplastic epithelial lesions are far more common in children than in adults. The consequences of long-standing squamous metaplasia with possible progression to anaplasia under certain circumstances have been considered in the pathogenesis of some neoplasms.

Renal calculi are common in vitamin A–deficient animals. In humans, however, there is no evidence that this deficiency is a common cause of nephrolithiasis. The effect of vitamin A deficiency on human teeth is not yet entirely clear. In the continuously growing incisor teeth of rats and guinea pigs, important abnormalities occur as a result of atrophy and squamous metaplasia of the enamel organ. Similar changes in the tooth germs of an infant have been described.

Clinicopathologic correlation

The disease occurs at all ages but has a higher morbidity and mortality in infants. The papular cutaneous lesions, which are seen chiefly in adults, are most numerous on the thighs and forearms but also may involve the shoulders, chest, back, and buttocks. Acnelike lesions may appear on the face, but an etiologic relationship between vitamin A deficiency and acne vulgaris has not been demonstrated.

Bacterial infections, notably conjunctivitis, furunculosis, bronchopneumonia, and pyelonephritis, are common in vitamin A deficiency. There is, however, no proof that such infections are the result of a specific loss of resistance. The development of infection is always explainable on the basis of mechanical effects consequent to the epithelial changes.

The finding of keratinized epithelial cells in the urine, vaginal secretions, and corneal and nasal scrapings is helpful in establishing a diagnosis. Chemical tests for vitamin A concentration in the serum have been applied, but these tests do not have diagnostic value. The most valuable test for vitamin A deficiency is determination of the speed of adaptation to vision in a feeble light. The diagnostic significance of night blindness is increased if there are other reasons for suspecting vitamin A deficiency.

In both naturally occurring and experimentally produced cirrhosis of the liver there is decreased conversion of carotene to vitamin A with decreased storage of vitamin A. The level of vitamin A in the blood falls sharply, and in humans night blindness is often, although not invariably, present. Other types of liver damage may cause similar changes.

Effect of excessive doses

The administration of large amounts of pure vitamin A to experimental animals accelerates the maturation and degeneration of epiphyseal cartilage and the remodeling processes. Because of the excessive loss of cortical bone by increased osteoclastic activity (an exaggeration of the normal sequences), multiple fractures occur. Cutaneous lesions that resemble those seen in deficiency of the B group of vitamins also occur. A clinical picture in children characterized by irritability, anorexia, pruritus, hepatosplenomegaly, bulging fontanels, and painful swelling over the long bones has been ascribed to hypervitaminosis A.

In infants an intake of only 12 times the recommended daily allowance has apparently caused such toxic manifestations.[3,57] In adults toxic symptoms appear only after prolonged ingestion of 20 to 30 times the recommended daily allowance.[53,78] Such huge doses, nearly always self-administered, occasionally result in hospital admission for hyperexcitability, bone pain, and headache. Increased cerebrospinal fluid pressure, together with the history, suggests the correct diagnosis. Symptoms usually disappear shortly after the excessive intake is discontinued.

Vitamin D

Since the pathologic lesions of vitamin D deficiency are manifested almost entirely in the bones, this vitamin is discussed in Chapter 40. It will be noted here that vitamin D is one of the factors involved in the absorption and transportation of calcium and in its normal deposition and maintenance in bone. Deficiency causes rickets in infants and one type of osteomalacia in adults.

Recently, major advances in regard to the biochemistry of vitamin D have been made by DeLuca.[19,20] He demonstrated the existence of biologically active metabolites of vitamin D and that vitamin D must be metabolically altered before it can function. In an attempt to elucidate the mechanism of action of vitamin

D, DeLuca studied physiologic control mechanisms that regulate conversion of vitamin D to its various metabolites and characterized the cellular receptors in the vitamin D target tissues. Transport of vitamin D metabolites from the cytosol to the nucleus in these tissues has been demonstrated. Strong similarities between these metabolites and the steroid hormones have been observed. These findings stress the importance of basic biochemical research, which has now been directed toward clinical applications in attempts to correct metabolic bone diseases of major importance, such as renal osteodystrophy,[73] hypoparathyroidism,[38] glucocorticoid-induced osteoporosis, and vitamin D–resistant rickets.[74]

Hypervitaminosis D

The recommended daily allowance of vitamin D is 400 international units for most age groups. Huge overdosages (1000 to 3000 units/kg body weight/day) lead to hypercalcemia, hypercalciuria, and metastatic calcification.[53] There is some evidence of predisposition to renal calculus formation. Calcium is mobilized from the bones, with resulting osteoporosis. Symptoms include nausea, vomiting, and diarrhea. There is circumstantial evidence that as little as 2000 units per day (only five times the recommended daily allowance) may cause hypercalcemia in infants.[1,2]

Vitamin E (tocopherols)

Alpha-tocopherol is biologically the most active of the naturally occurring tocopherols and is prepared commercially. It is generally accepted that vitamin E acts in metabolism as an antioxidant.[84] Striking effects of vitamin E deficiency are seen in experimental animals of several species. These effects include cessation of growth, complete sterility in both male and female animals, and weakness of the muscles. In male animals degeneration of the seminiferous tubular epithelium occurs, resulting in aspermatogenesis (Fig. 14-6). In female animals the fertilized ova become implanted, but the young embryos become necrotic and are resorbed. The formation of the fetal placenta is retarded, and the maternal-fetal circulation is not properly established. In several species of animals, including guinea pigs and rabbits, degenerative changes occur in skeletal muscle as a result of vitamin E deficiency. Although the pathologic lesions are similar to those seen in the muscular dystrophies of humans, vitamin E has not been found to be of therapeutic value in these diseases.

In vitamin E–deficient animals, particularly if 20% cod-liver oil is present in the diet, an acid-fast lipid material known as *ceroid* is found in fat tissue and also in and about many other types of cells. Apparently this material represents oxidized fat of the unsaturated type, and one function of vitamin E is believed to be its ability to prevent the oxidation of such fats. The greatly increased oxy-

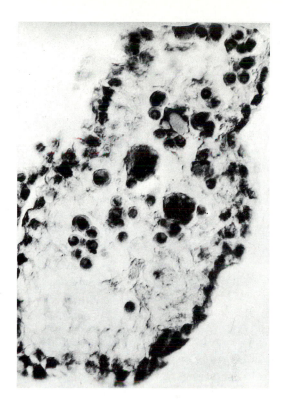

Fig. 14-6. Seminiferous tubule from rat fed diet deficient in vitamin E. Cells have atrophied and desquamated. Crescentic chromatin masses and huge multinucleated cells are typical of advanced vitamin E deficiency. (From Eddy, W.H., and Dalldorf, G.: The avitaminoses, ed. 3; copyrighted 1944 by The Williams & Wilkins Co., Baltimore.)

gen consumption by striated muscle in vitro as a result of experimental vitamin E deficiency suggests that this vitamin has general antioxidant properties.

Infants with cystic fibrosis sometimes show lesions in striated muscle similar to those seen in experimental animals deficient in vitamin E, as well as excessive creatinuria and the presence of ceroid in the intestinal wall. Certain types of megaloblastic anemia in severely undernourished infants have been reported to respond to vitamin E therapy.[7,42,48] The administration of vitamin E to patients with symptoms of porphyria decreases the urinary excretion of aminolevulinic acid, porphobilinogen, coproporphyrins, and uroporphyrins to normal levels.[52] Such observations have suggested that, in humans, vitamin E may have important functions other than the prevention of oxidation of unsaturated fatty acids.[34]

Vitamin K[56,69]

Vitamin K was named from the German word *koagulationvitamin*. It occurs in several closely related forms, its activity apparently being dependent on the component 2-methyl-1,4-naphthoquinone. Although vitamin K is fat soluble, certain active compounds that are water soluble can be prepared. This vitamin was discovered by

Dam in 1935 as a result of careful study of a hemorrhagic disease that he observed in chickens. It was later isolated by Doisy and associates. Physiologically it is necessary for the formation of prothrombin (factor II) and three other coagulation factors, VII, IX, and X; in its absence the mechanism of blood coagulation breaks down. In bacterial and plant cells vitamin K is important in electron transport mechanisms.

Clinically vitamin K is of great importance in preventing hemorrhagic disease of the newborn. In adults simple deficiency is rare because of the abundance of this vitamin in leafy vegetables and other common foods and because of its formation by intestinal bacteria, which are absent for several days in newborn infants. Vitamin K deficiency can occur when there are marked alterations in the intestinal flora or defects in fat absorption. Secondary deficiency occurs frequently in obstructive jaundice, since vitamin K is not absorbed satisfactorily in the absence of bile from the intestine. In the presence of severe liver damage, administration of vitamin K usually is ineffective in preventing hemorrhage. However, it is effective in correcting hemorrhagic lesions resulting from bishydroxycoumarin (Dicumarol) and other anticoagulants that inhibit prothrombin.

Vitamins of B group

The term "vitamin B" was originally applied to the substance capable of curing experimental beriberi, which Funk isolated from rice polishings in 1911. This substance was not chemically pure, and it is now known that thiamine is its most important active component. Concentrates derived from yeast, wheat germ, rice polishings, and other sources contain a number of factors that collectively are known as the vitamin B complex. This complex comprises a group of essential compounds that are chemically unrelated but occur together in certain foods such as liver, milk, and leafy green vegetables. Most compounds in this group are involved in the metabolism of proteins, carbohydrates, and fats. Vitamin B_{12} and folic acid play important roles in blood formation.

Much of our knowledge of the specific effects of deficiency of single members of the B group is derived from studies carried out in experimental animals. To demonstrate the effect of deficiency of a single component, all other components must be supplied in adequate amounts, and the animal must live long enough to become depleted of the component that one desires to study. The effects of riboflavin deficiency, for example, are not seen in animals deprived of the entire B complex. In humans, although deficiency in several of these factors commonly exists simultaneously, several disease entities are associated more or less specifically with the lack of individual factors. No specific disease is recognized as being attributable to lack of the entire B complex, and it is therefore desirable to discuss each factor in the group separately. Thiamine deficiency causes beriberi and is believed to be a factor in Wernicke's disease (see p. 505). Deficiency of niacin (nicotinic acid) is an important factor, although probably not the sole factor, in pellagra. The clinical picture of riboflavin deficiency includes cheilosis, a condition characterized by fissures at the angles of the mouth. Folic acid and vitamin B_{12} are important in hematologic disorders. Pyridoxine, pantothenic acid, biotin, choline, and inositol are also believed to be essential nutrients for humans. Certain effects produced in experimental animals by deprivation of other specific factors will be considered, even though they have not been duplicated in humans.

Thiamine

Chemistry and physiology. Thiamine is found in the thermolabile portion of the B complex, whereas the other members of the B complex that will be considered are thermostabile. Thiamine hydrochloride, which was synthesized in 1937, is composed of a pyrimidine base united to a nitrogen-carbon-sulfur ring containing a pentavalent nitrogen. This compound is phosphorylated to form thiamine pyrophosphate, which acts intracellularly as the coenzyme for carboxylase. The latter enzyme decarboxylates pyruvic acid and participates in the synthesis of fat from carbohydrate. Thus in thiamine deficiency carbohydrate metabolism is interrupted at the pyruvic acid stage, and pyruvic acid accumulates in the tissues and the blood. The lesions of thiamine deficiency are not, however, produced by the simple injection of pyruvic acid, and it is probable that the failure of complete combustion of carbohydrate is the important factor, with the accumulation of pyruvic acid being incidental.

Thiamine is not stored in the body in large amounts. The depletion period before the onset of symptoms is variable, however, depending on the metabolic rate and unknown factors. Recently there have been reports that antithiamine factors in food may play a role in the development of beriberi.

Lesions resulting from deficiency. Human diseases in which thiamine deficiency plays an important role are beriberi, Wernicke's encephalopathy, and Korsakoff's psychosis.

In fatal cases of *beriberi* the findings are somewhat variable. On gross examination the most common lesions are emaciation, muscle atrophy, dilatation (with or without hypertrophy) of the right side of the heart, generalized edema, serous effusions, and chronic passive congestion of the viscera. Death may be caused by high-output cardiac failure, by acute pulmonary edema, or by pneumonia or other complicating infections. The edema is caused in part by cardiac failure, but hypoproteinemia is probably a contributory factor in many cases. This cardiovascular picture is particularly characteristic of the so-called wet type of beriberi, which is usually acute.

Microscopically loss of striation and fatty degeneration of the myocardial fibers are noted. There is diffuse edema, often with slight lymphocytic infiltration of the intestinal tissue of many organs. Skeletal muscles show hyaline and fatty degenerative changes.

Degenerative changes in nerves are more characteristic of the dry or chronic form of the disease, which is seen chiefly in adults. Myelin degeneration and, in severe cases, fragmentation of the axis cylinders are seen in the affected nerves, which may be those of the extremities, the vagi, or the cranial nerves. In thiamine-deficient pigeons, axis cylinder degeneration begins distally and progresses until the neurons are involved. If thiamine is given before neuron death, regeneration of axis cylinders occurs at the usual normal rate. In dogs similar degenerative changes have been described in the central nervous system.

Wernicke's disease, which is associated with chronic alcoholism, is characterized by ganglion cell degeneration and focal demyelinating lesions and hemorrhage in the nuclei surrounding the ventricles and aqueduct, particularly the nuclei of the extrinsic muscles of the eye. There is also some reparative proliferation of neuroglial cells. The picture is often complicated by symptoms of beriberi, scurvy, riboflavin deficiency, and pellagra. An apparently identical lesion may be produced in thiamine-deficient pigeons. In view of the experimental evidence, thiamine deficiency is now believed to be the most important etiologic factor in Wernicke's disease and in the pathologically similar Wernicke-Korsakoff syndrome.[22] Adding thiamine to the diet causes prompt clearing of the neurologic symptoms. *Korsakoff's psychosis*, the result of brain damage after recovery from coma in Wernicke's syndrome, improves more slowly, and underlying psychotic elements often remain.

Clinicopathologic correlation. The mechanism by which thiamine deficiency produces its characteristic lesions is not clear. The degenerative changes in the peripheral nerves and central nervous system are perhaps the result of interrupted carbohydrate metabolism as described previously. This seems logical in view of the fact that the metabolism of nervous tissue is believed to be totally dependent on carbohydrate oxidation. The cardiac manifestations may be related to the experimental observation that the oxygen uptake in vitro of the auricles of thiamine-deficient rats is significantly lower than that of the control animals.

A diet consisting largely of carbohydrate is an important contributing factor in the development of thiamine deficiency, since thiamine requirements are proportional to carbohydrate combustion. Symptoms of peripheral neuritis and mental confusion are explained on the basis of nervous tissue degeneration or anoxia, and cardiorespiratory symptoms such as tachycardia, edema, cyanosis, and pulmonary congestion are at least partially explained

by the cardiac lesions. In the infantile form of beriberi, vomiting, cyanosis, and tachycardia may be followed by death (probably from pulmonary edema) in 24 to 36 hours. The mortality in beriberi varies from 5% to 50%, depending on the severity of symptoms and on the promptness and adequacy of treatment.

Niacin

Chemistry and physiology. Niacin, or nicotinic acid, is prepared by oxidation of the alkaloid nicotine. It is β-pyridine carboxylic acid and is active only in the amide form. Niacin is an essential molecular constituent of diphosphopyridine nucleotide and triphosphopyridine nucleotide, which act as cofactors for several dehydrogenases. Studies have shown that niacin may be synthesized from dietary tryptophan. Pyridoxine aids in this process.

Etiology of pellagra. Although divergent views still exist concerning the etiology of pellagra, there is general agreement that the major factor is deficiency of certain members of the B group of vitamins, particularly niacin. Some investigators believe that niacin deficiency should be regarded as the cause of pellagra, despite the fact that most affected individuals show evidence of multiple dietary deficiencies. The pathologic changes of uncomplicated niacin deficiency have not been described in either humans or experimental animals. Lesions that heal on administration of niacin are assumed to have been caused largely by lack of that compound. Pellagra is apparently a nutritional disease of the "conditioned" type; conditioning factors include exposure to sunlight, alcoholism, organic diseases, and infectious diseases. About 50% of persons with pellagra show achlorhydria. Macrocytic anemia, which is not uncommon, is probably the result of concomitant folic acid deficiency. Qualitative deficiency in the amino acid composition of the protein supply is probably a conditioning factor in pellagra. The relationship of a cornmeal diet to pellagra is probably explainable on the basis of the fact that cornmeal is deficient in tryptophan, which is a precursor of nicotinic acid. There is also some evidence that cornmeal may contain an antagonist of nicotinic acid. Diphosphopyridine nucleotide and triphosphopyridine nucleotide, which have an abnormally low value in the blood and urine of persons with pellagra, rise to normal levels or higher when niacin is administered.

Pellagra occurs frequently in parts of Central America, Yugoslavia, Rumania, and Egypt. In the southern United States, where it was formerly common, it has largely disappeared.[65]

Lesions resulting from deficiency. The pathologic lesions of pellagra involve the skin, mucous membranes, gastrointestinal tract, and nervous system. Emaciation usually is present.

The *cutaneous lesions*, which may be absent in some

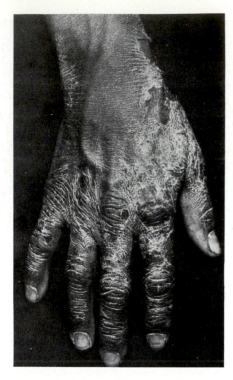

Fig. 14-7. Pellagra. Dermatitis and pigmentation of back of hand. (Courtesy Dr. Grover W. Wende; from Sutton, R.L., Jr.: Diseases of the skin, ed. 11, St. Louis, 1956, The C.V. Mosby Co.)

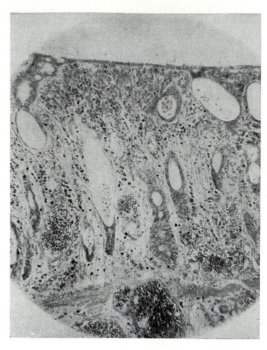

Fig. 14-8. Lesion in colon from patient with pellagra. Photograph of specimen is from collection of Dr. James Denton illustrating cystic glands characteristically found in pellagra, sprue, and possibly other related deficiency diseases. Lesion was formerly known as colitis cystica superficialis and is associated with malnutrition. (From Eddy, W.H., and Dalldorf, G.: The avitaminoses, ed. 3; copyrighted 1944 by The Williams & Wilkins Co., Baltimore.)

cases, are seen particularly in areas exposed to sunlight but may occur in any region exposed to irritation. They show a striking tendency to symmetric distribution, and the affected areas are sharply demarcated from the normal. In the early stages the lesions resemble sunburn, but later the skin becomes roughened, keratotic, scaly, and pigmented (Fig. 14-7). Microscopically congestion of the papillary blood vessels and edema of the papillae are seen. There is moderate lymphocytic infiltration in the corium. The most striking feature is the noticeable thickening of the keratinized layer of the epidermis.

The *tongue*, buccal membranes, gums, and palate become swollen and red, with eventual ulceration. Infection with Vincent's organisms often causes a gray membrane to form. Microscopically the lesions resemble those of the skin.

In the *colon* thickening of the wall with edema and lymphocytic infiltration is seen. Membranous enteritis, with or without ulceration, is often present. Atrophy and cystic dilatation of the crypts of Lieberkühn are said to be characteristic (Fig. 14-8).

Lesions in the nervous system appear late in the course of the disease. Demyelinization of the posterior and lateral columns of the spinal cord and focal demyelinization and ganglion cell degeneration in the cerebrum have been described. Neurologic and even psychotic manifestations are common and clear up rapidly if niacin is administered early. They may be the only manifestations of the deficiency.

The possible occurrence of simultaneous lesions of beriberi or ariboflavinosis has already been mentioned. Nonspecific lesions seen on postmortem examination may include generalized emaciation, visceral atrophy, fatty infiltration and focal necrosis of the liver, and terminal bronchopneumonia.

The key to the production of certain of the lesions in pellagra is undoubtedly the role of niacin in cellular oxidation processes, but this physiologic principle has not been translated into terms that clearly explain the specific lesions found. The occasional appearance of pellagrous dermatitis in the carcinoid syndrome (see p. 573) is of interest. It has been explained on the theory that the formation of serotonin from tryptophan makes less of this amino acid available for niacin synthesis.

The mucous membrane lesions and the gastrointestinal and mental symptoms usually respond promptly to niacin administration. Certain residual signs and symptoms are of the type associated with thiamine, pyridoxine, or riboflavin deficiency, and these often respond to the appropriate treatment.

Riboflavin

Riboflavin (empiric formula $C_{17}H_{20}N_4O_6$) was isolated in 1933 and synthesized in 1935. Historically it was the first vitamin to be identified as a constituent of an enzyme system. It forms the prosthetic group of several

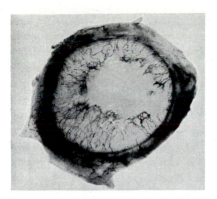

Fig. 14-9. Vascularization of cornea caused by riboflavin deficiency. Photograph of rat eye injected with india ink to demonstrate plexus of newly formed blood vessels. (From Eckardt, R.E., and Johnson, L.V.: Arch. Ophthalmol. **21**:315, 1939.)

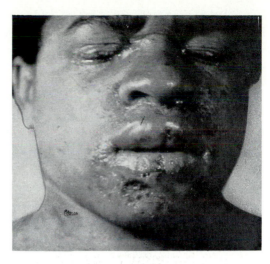

Fig. 14-10. Ariboflavinosis. Cheilosis, nasolabial lesion, and blepharospasm. (From Sydenstricker, V.P., et al.: J.A.M.A. **114**:2437, 1940.)

flavoprotein enzymes, including the "yellow respiratory enzyme" (Warburg), now known as cytochrome oxidase, which, together with the cytochromes, forms an enzyme system of outstanding importance in cellular respiration.

Experimental lesions. The lesions of riboflavin deficiency in young rats are produced only after a period of several weeks during which all other dietary factors are present in adequate amounts. Depletion will not occur if rats are allowed to eat their feces, since the intestinal bacteria synthesize considerable amounts of riboflavin. Failure to gain weight, progressive loss of hair, and swelling and redness of the ears and paws are the outstanding external manifestations. In the late stages extreme weakness and coma develop, with only one or two respirations per minute. From this moribund state, rats recover a considerable amount of vitality and strength almost instantaneously when small doses of crystalline riboflavin are injected. This dramatic result is apparently attributable to the sudden resumption of intracellular respiration.

Lesions in humans. Vascularization of the cornea by capillary sprouts from the limbic plexus (Fig. 14-9) was first noted in riboflavin-deficient rats and later was recognized as an important and early sign of deficiency of the vitamin in humans. In the later stages conjunctivitis develops. The ingrowth of capillaries into the normally avascular cornea probably is an attempt to compensate for the breakdown of oxidation processes in the corneal cells. The ocular lesions in humans and experimental animals progress to the formation of keratitis and ulceration of the cornea.

Ariboflavinosis in humans is characterized also by cheilosis (fissure formation and crusts at the angles of the mouth) and by redness and irritation of the tongue and lips. Of less common occurrence are circumoral pallor and seborrheic dermatitis of the nasolabial folds and ears (Fig. 14-10). Rarely the dermatitis has a more generalized distribution. Riboflavin deficiency may occur in a

pure form or in patients with pellagra or various multiple deficiencies.

Pyridoxine (B₆)[68]

Pyridoxine, a pyridine derivative with the empiric formula $C_8H_{11}NO_3$, was differentiated from other heat-stable members of the B complex by Gyorgyi and associates in 1933. These investigators showed that a characteristic dermatitis in rats is caused specifically by the absence of this vitamin. The paws, snout, and ears become hyperemic and swollen, with eventual desquamation and ulceration. Although the dermatitis has been described as "acrodynia-like," there is no evidence that human acrodynia is caused by pyridoxine deficiency.

Pyridoxine refers to three naturally occurring ring substances: pyridoxine, pyridoxal, and pyridoxamine. All three are converted to the active coenzyme form, pyridoxal 5'-phosphate, whose major function is related to protein or amino acid metabolism. Some metabolic processes in which pyridoxine is involved include transamination, amino acid decarboxylation, transmethylation of methionine, metabolism of tryptophan, and formation of melanin.

In several experimental animals, including pigs, prolonged pyridoxine deficiency causes severe microcytic anemia, which is improved but not entirely alleviated by the administration of pyridoxine. Other lesions found in experimentally induced deficiency in animals are demyelination of peripheral nerves, dorsal root ganglia, and dorsal columns of the spinal cord and fatty infiltration and hemosiderosis of the liver.

The importance of pyridoxine in human nutrition is not clear. Certain residual symptoms in persons with pellagra occasionally respond to pyridoxine administration, apparently because it is a coenzyme for the conversion of tryptophan to niacin. Hyperirritability and convulsions in infants, without other discoverable cause, have been associated rather definitely with pyridoxine deficiency in a commercial formula.

Experimental pyridoxine deficiency has been produced in humans by administration of the antivitamin deoxypyridoxine. The lesions noted include seborrheic dermatitis of the nasolabial folds, cheilosis, and glossitis, as well as a mild normochromic hypoplastic anemia. Thus several of the lesions appear to overlap with those ascribed to riboflavin and niacin deficiency.

The treatment of tuberculosis with isoniazid sometimes results in a conditioned pyridoxine deficiency, with cheilosis and peripheral neuritis. These lesions are resolved by the administration of pyridoxine. Also, pyridoxine deficiency has been reported in patients receiving antihypertensive drugs, patients with Parkinson's disease being treated with L-dopa, and women taking oral contraceptives.[64]

Several B$_6$-dependency syndromes have been described.[26] They respond only to pyridoxine in very large doses, 200 to 600 mg of pyridoxine HC1 per day in contrast to the normal requirement of 1.5 to 2 mg per day. These syndromes are as follows:
1. Convulsions in infants who have become dependent because their mothers were given large doses of the vitamin for hyperemesis gravidarum
2. Hypersideritic anemia with deposition of hemosiderin in the marrow and liver
3. Xanthurenic aciduria
4. Cystothionuria
5. Homocysteinura

The last four conditions usually are related to an inherited enzymatic defect and are examples of "genetically conditioned" deficiencies.

Pantothenic acid

Pantothenic acid is a component of coenzyme A. It prevents or cures a type of dermatitis peculiar to chickens. In rats deficiency of this compound causes a dermatitis, intestinal ulceration, and hemorrhagic necrosis in the adrenal cortex. There is evidence that pantothenic acid may be of importance in preventing the graying of hair that occurs in certain laboratory animals with nutritional deficiencies.

Pantothenic acid is present in most animal tissues and in yeast, and evidence indicates that it may be a growth-promoting substance of almost universal importance. The pantothenate level of the blood is below normal in pellagra, beriberi, and ariboflavinosis. Experimental pantothenic acid deficiency in humans causes malaise, headache, insomnia, and nausea but no significant interference with adrenal function. Despite the physiologic importance of this vitamin, evidence for the spontaneous occurrence of lesions resulting from deficiency remains inconclusive.

Biotin[68]

Biotin (vitamin H or coenzyme R) is a compound essential for the respiration of certain lower organisms and probably of all cells. It combines with avidin, a substance present in uncooked egg white, to form a compound that is not absorbed in the intestines. Our present knowledge of biotin deficiency has been gained largely through observations of animals or humans who have ingested large amounts of raw egg white. In human volunteers fed a diet in which egg white furnished 30% of the total caloric intake, a fine "branny" cutaneous desquamation developed in 3 to 4 weeks. Later, anemia, dryness of the skin, lassitude, mental depression, muscle pains, and other symptoms appeared.[86]

Choline[69]

Choline can be synthesized from dietary methionine. It is an important factor in fat metabolism, and many experimental studies have been concerned with the mechanisms by which it acts.[45] It is an essential component of lecithin, a phospholipid that is a constituent of all cells. Lecithin is probably formed in the liver as a preliminary step in the oxidation of fatty acids. Choline deficiency in experimental animals (dogs, rats, and rabbits), particularly when combined with a high intake of fats with saturated fatty acids, reduces the oxidation of fats in the liver and leads to the accumulation of fat in the liver cord cells (central lobular distribution) and eventually to cirrhosis. Recent experimental studies have suggested that a choline-deficient diet may act as a promoter in liver carcinogenesis induced by chemical carcinogens.[46,70] In young rats, hemorrhagic cortical necrosis of the kidneys, hemorrhages in other organs, and involution of the thymus are found in addition to fatty livers. Cystine-rich diets intensify the liver and kidney lesions, whereas methionine, like choline, reverses the process. Lipocaic, which is obtained by extraction from pancreatic tissue, has a similar effect in removing fat accumulation from the liver (lipotropic action). It is a crude extract, containing choline and inositol, as well as some other lipotropic factor that has not been identified. Choline deficiency has not been shown to occur in humans, and whether choline is an essential dietary factor for humans is not known.

Folic acid and vitamin B$_{12}$[32,68]

Folic acid apparently is identical to the *Lactobacillus casei* factor, a compound essential for the growth of *L. casei*. It is composed of a number of related substances, containing glutamic acid and pteroyl groups, joined together by para-aminobenzoic acid and known collectively as pteroylglutamates. The physiologically active form is a reduction product, tetrahydrofolic acid, formed during absorption.

Folic acid deficiency in monkeys causes a nutritional anemia, with reversal of the lymphocyte-neutrophil ratio. In humans, folic acid is useful in the treatment of sprue and megaloblastic nutritional anemia. It brings about hematologic remission in pernicious anemia but, unlike vitamin B_{12}, does not prevent or improve the degenerative lesions in the spinal cord.

Vitamin B_{12} is the extrinsic factor in pernicious anemia. Its absorption is dependent on the intrinsic factor in gastric mucosa. Like folic acid, vitamin B_{12} consists of a family of compounds. Since a cyano group or cobalt, or both, is present in the molecules, a generic name is the cyanocobalamins. The relation of vitamin B_{12}, liver extract, and folic acid to blood regeneration in various types of anemia is an intricate one (see p. 1329).

Vitamin C (ascorbic acid)
Chemistry and physiology

Ascorbic acid exists in natural sources chiefly in the form of L-ascorbic acid, a six-carbon compound closely related to glucose. In this form, it readily loses two hydrogen atoms to become dehydroascorbic acid, which is reversibly oxidizable in the body. The physiologic action of vitamin C therefore probably depends on its ability to carry out oxidation-reduction reactions, but its role in cellular physiology is incompletely known. There is good evidence that it is essential for the metabolism of phenylalanine and tyrosine and that it maintains certain important sulfhydryl enzymes in the active state.

Ascorbic acid concentration is particularly high in the adrenal glands, but its role in adrenal hormone production is not known. In severe scurvy, it remains in the adrenal glands after it has been depleted in other organs. It is clear that ascorbic acid is necessary for the production and maintenance of several intercellular substances, notably collagen, osseomucin, chondromucin, dentin, and probably the cement substances that hold vascular endothelial cells together in certain animals, including humans and guinea pigs.

Wound repair in scorbutic guinea pigs was studied by Wolbach.[88] The wound fills in normally with blood clot. The clot is then organized by fibroblasts but without blood vessels. No collagen is formed as long as the scorbutic diet is maintained. With the correction of the deficiency, collagen formation begins within 24 hours and proceeds rapidly. The newly formed intercellular material is homogeneous for a time, but argyrophilic fibers and true collagen fibers soon appear. Fibrin is not changed to collagen but is liquefied and removed, and the collagen is laid down independently.

It is apparent that the "homogeneous substance" described in healing wounds by Wolbach is the mucopolysaccharide ground substance of connective tissue from which reticulin and collagen fibrils normally are

formed.[23] In scurvy this formation of fibrils does not occur. There is evidence that ascorbic acid is essential for the formation of hydroxyproline, the most characteristic and essential component of collagen. Radioisotopic studies have shown that the incorporation of labeled sulfur into the chondroitin sulfate of the ground substance is sharply reduced in scurvy, indicating that a basic defect in ground substance formation may exist. Ascorbic acid is vital for collagen formation, serving in the preservation and maturation of fibroblasts and the incorporation of hydroxyproline and hydroxylysine.

Lesions resulting from deficiency

Essentially similar lesions are found in humans and in guinea pigs. The outstanding features are hemorrhages and lesions in the skeleton, including the teeth.

Cutaneous hemorrhage, ranging from petechial to massive extravasation, is almost constantly found at autopsy in adults with vitamin C deficiency. The larger hemorrhages correspond to areas of trauma. Hemorrhage into muscles or along fascial planes is seen particularly at points of mechanical stress. Bleeding occurs from capillaries, presumably because of rupture of the loosened endothelial cells. In infants with vitamin C deficiency, massive subperiosteal hemorrhage is almost always present, especially in the legs. Massive areas of hemorrhage may become infected and suppurate. Ulceration of the gums, loosening of the teeth, and massive hemorrhage from the gums are commonly seen in adults but rarely in infants.

The skeletal lesions, which likewise are the result primarily of the failure to produce intercellular substances, are seen most conspicuously at the ends of growing tubular bones. The changes are described on p. 1742.

Anemia of various types is common in scurvy, particularly in infancy. Although hemorrhage may be a factor, it is rarely the sole cause. Interference with the formation of folic acid compounds has been postulated, and severe megaloblastic anemia in scurvy may respond only to folic acid.

Death most often results from secondary infection, with fatal hemorrhage being a rare cause. Sudden death may follow physical exertion, perhaps from addisonian crisis resulting from stress. Fulminating tuberculosis is particularly common. The failure of the normal localization and repair of tubercles by collagenous scar tissue is a logical explanation for this.

Clinicopathologic correlation

The mortality from scurvy is high in untreated cases but low in recognized cases given adequate therapy.

In infants, pain from subperiosteal hemorrhage is the chief symptom. In general, the symptoms in adults are merely general weakness and depression.

Roentgenographic examination of the bones is an important diagnostic feature in infantile scurvy. Capillary fragility, brought out by means of the tourniquet test or other tests, is of some diagnostic value. Chemical determination of the level of ascorbic acid in the serum and leukocyte layer of centrifuged blood and in the urine is also helpful, but in doubtful cases the response to antiscorbutic treatment often gives the best evidence of deficiency. Experienced clinicians believe that mild cases of anorexia and mental depression that are promptly relieved by vitamin C therapy often are caused by deficiency of that vitamin. In patients with extensive wounds or burns the ascorbic acid level in the blood falls rapidly (perhaps because of mobilization in granulation tissue), and replacement therapy is often indicated.

Vitamins and congenital abnormalities[25,33]

Although definite relationships of dietary deficiencies to congenital abnormalities in humans have not been established, a wide variety of congenital lesions have been produced and studied in lower mammals, notably in rats. The basic principle established by this experimental work is that nutritional factors, particularly vitamins, are more important for fetal differentiation and development than for maternal health. Defects resulting from maternal deficiency in vitamin A, riboflavin, folic acid, vitamin B_{12}, pantothenic acid, and vitamin E and from general undernutrition have been well documented. In general, the similarities between the lesions caused by various dietary deficiencies are more striking than the differences. The lesions involve the eyes and the skeletal, central nervous, cardiovascular, and genitourinary systems. Also included are anophthalmia, cleft palate, exencephaly, hydrocephalus, spina bifida, and ectopia of the abdominal viscera. In the case of vitamin A, defects are caused not only by maternal deficiency but also by excessive maternal intake. Excess intake frequently causes cranial deformities with extrusion of the brain and, sporadically, ocular defects, harelip, and cleft palate. Further study of these phenomena should throw light on the complex and varied (and probably interrelated) mechanisms involved in the production of congenital abnormalities.

SPECIFIC AMINO ACID DEFICIENCIES

In rats and dogs 10 of the amino acids are indispensable for normal growth: tryptophan, lysine, histidine, arginine, phenylalanine, isoleucine, leucine, threonine, methionine, and valine. With the exception of arginine and histidine, these amino acids are essential to produce a positive nitrogen balance in humans. A few specific lesions have been described in animals as a result of deficiency of these elements. However, as mentioned previously in the discussion of experimental kwashiorkor-like models, the pathologic changes with diets deficient in a single essential amino acid are generally similar in rats to those observed with the intake of low-quantity or poor-quality proteins. Thus it may not be worthwhile to review some of the specific single essential amino acid deficiencies as described in the literature.[25,75]

A few specific essential amino acids, particularly tryptophan and the branched-chain amino acids (valine, isoleucine, and leucine) appear to have specific effects other than being mere building blocks for protein synthesis. Tryptophan, in addition to serving as a precursor to serotonin, nicotinic acid, and other metabolites, has been found to have an important regulatory role in hepatic protein synthesis in animals.[72] The branched-chain amino acids, particularly leucine, have been described as having an important role in skeletal muscle protein synthesis.[61]

SPECIFIC FATTY ACID DEFICIENCIES

Linoleic acid deficiency in rats causes scaling of the skin, alopecia, and injury to renal and testicular tubular epithelium. A number of infants fed a formula containing less than 0.1% of calories as linoleic acid failed to grow and showed scaly skin changes.[51] At present there is little evidence for the occurrence of essential fatty acid deficiency in humans under natural conditions. In addition to linoleic acid, linolenic and arachidonic acids are belived necessary for humans.

ESSENTIAL ELEMENTS*

In addition to carbon, hydrogen, oxygen, and nitrogen, 16 elements are considered essential for life: calcium, magnesium, potassium, sodium, sulfur, phosphorus, chlorine, iron, copper, cobalt, manganese, zinc, iodine, selenium, molybdenum, and probably fluorine. Many other elements, however, are present in tissues, and studies of their possible importance are far from complete. In addition to the more obvious functions of calcium, magnesium, phosphorus, sodium, and chlorine—in acting as structural components and in maintaining the electrolyte balance—trace amounts of several metallic elements, such as zinc, copper, manganese, selenium, molybdenum, and magnesium, are of vital importance, since they form essential components of certain enzyme systems. The function of iron as a component of hemoglobin and of intracellular oxidizing enzymes is too well known to require discussion here.

Calcium is important for the contraction of heart muscle and for blood coagulation. Its importance in rickets and osteomalacia and its relation to the parathyroid glands are discussed on p. 1421. Calcium and phosphorus metabolism are discussed in connection with rickets on p. 1723.

Sulfur is extremely important physiologically. However, it would be difficult to produce inorganic sulfur defi-

*References 6, 9, 13, 43, 59, 60, 82, 91.

ciency because, although this element occurs in methionine and cystine, inorganic sulfur cannot be used in the formation of these compounds. Sulfur is most important in the sulfhydryl (—SH) form, in which state it is an active component of many enzymes, vitamins, and hormones. Oxidation of this group to the inactive (S—S) form is believed to be the mechanism of action of many enzyme inhibitors.

Copper is important in hemopoiesis and is an essential constituent of several important enzymes. Experimental deficiency in rats, for example, leads to a microcytic hypochromic anemia, and the rats often die before the anemia becomes severe. Deficiency of this element also causes graying of the hair, which is not prevented by large amounts of pantothenic acid or para-aminobenzoic acid (the other anti–gray hair factors). Certain cases of hyperchromic anemia in children are believed to respond to copper supplementation. The relation of copper metabolism to Wilson's disease is discussed on p. 1164. Copper is also essential for the normal development of bone, the central nervous system, and connective tissue.

Cobalt deficiency in sheep and cattle is the cause of a severe anemia with hemosiderosis of the spleen. Deficiency of this element causes enzootic marasmus in Australian aborigines. Cobalt is a component of vitamin B_{12}.

Manganese deficiency has been largely neglected from the histologic viewpoint. In experimental animals disturbance of growth occurs in the offspring of deficient mothers, with frequent death and osseous defects in surviving animals. Lesions in the humans are unknown.

Zinc is an important component of carbonic anhydrase, uricase, insulin, and phosphatase. Dietary deficiency in rats causes corneal vascularization, alopecia, keratinization of the skin and esophagus, and death in a few weeks. Studies in the Middle East have strongly suggested a relationship of zinc deficiency to dwarfism and hypogonadism, as well as to iron-deficiency anemia and hepatosplenomegaly.[59] These abnormalities are corrected in response to zinc feeding.

Iodine deficiency is related to lesions of the thyroid gland and is discussed in Chapter 33.

Fluorine inactivates phosphatase and several other enzyme systems. Experimental fluorine deficiency in rats has been reported to cause dental caries. For discussion of the effects of fluorine on teeth and bones, see pp. 1005 and 1747.

Selenium apparently substitutes for vitamin E as an antioxidant. *Manganese, chromium, molybdenum,* and *cadmium* have been shown to be active in enzyme systems of plants and lower animals.

MALNUTRITION AND BRAIN FUNCTION

In an earlier section the possibility that stunted mental development occurs secondarily to kwashiorkor was mentioned. Indeed, a number of studies have shown that many types of malnutrition retard the development of the human brain and adversely affect the patterns of learning and behavior in early life.[16,41,62,66] Whether the deficiency is in total calories, total protein, specific amino acids, micronutrients, or combinations of these factors, the result too often is a brain that is far below average size for the age of the child. When the underprivileged are better nourished (and viral and other infections of the central nervous system better controlled), the accepted level of human performance will be raised, and the problems of the social scientist will be considerably simplified.

NUTRITION AND CANCER

Much attention has been given to the possible association between nutrition and cancer (see also Chapter 15). Of the many environmental factors considered to be influential in the induction of cancer, diet and nutrition have gained much notoriety. This association has been derived mainly from diverse epidemiologic data but also from limited experimental studies with animals.*

In relating dietary factors and cancer one must consider the following:

1. Food additives or contaminants, as well as the nutrients themselves, may act as carcinogens, cocarcinogens, promoters, or combinations of these.
2. Nutritional deficiencies or imbalances may lead to biochemical abnormalities that in turn promote neoplastic processes.
3. Excessive intake of certain nutrients may produce metabolic abnormalities that promote neoplasms.

A few of the suspected food contaminants are mycotoxins (specifically aflatoxin) and nitrosamines, which are being investigated as important suspected carcinogens in humans. Studies have revealed that the charred parts of broiled meat and fish contain a series of new heterocyclic amines in the pyrolyzate of amino acids and proteins, which are mutagenic, and that two amines from tryptophan pyrolyzates—3-amino-1,4-dimethyl-5H-pyrido(4,3-b)indole and 3-amino-1-methyl-5H-pyrido(4,3-b)indole—are carcinogenic in animals.[50] Also, the amounts and type of fiber in the diet have been considered to be influential in the induction of bowel cancer in experimental animals.[54,87] Deficiencies of iron, iodine, riboflavin, vitamin A, pyridoxine, and choline have been considered to play a role in the induction of certain types of neoplasms. Based on epidemiologic data and also on animal studies, high dietary fat intake has been reported to increase breast cancer incidence in females.[90] In general, it is believed that the dietary effects occur mainly in relation to promotion, the second stage in the process of carcinogenesis.

*References 15, 54, 63, 79, 80, 87.

A number of experimental studies have revealed that diet or dietary components may act to *prevent* the induction of certain cancers.[85] Certain dietary components have been demonstrated to induce enzyme systems that detoxify chemical carcinogens. Also, some food additives, which are antioxidants, have been demonstrated to act in an inhibitory manner in chemical carcinogenesis. Studies with vitamin A treatment in animals have also suggested an inhibitory effect, particularly in relation to changes in cell differentiation, on the induction of certain types of cancers. A number of experimental studies revealed that selenium supplementation protects against certain neoplasms induced by carcinogens.[54]

Overall, the present knowledge of the association between nutrition and cancer is limited. Further information is needed before their association may be used rationally in the prevention and treatment of cancer in humans.

This chapter has been limited to selected topics dealing with how altered nutrition may induce and influence disease states. It has not covered a number of important areas dealing with nutrition and its interrelationships, such as those with obesity,[83] heart and vessel diseases,[5] infection and the immune system,[14,29,49] aging,[39,92] and drugs.[31,64]

REFERENCES

1. American Academy of Pediatrics, Committee on Nutrition: The prophylactic requirement and the toxicity of vitamin D, Pediatrics **31**:512, 1963.
2. American Academy of Pediatrics, Committee on Nutrition: The relation between infantile hypercalcemia and vitamin D—public health implications in North America, Pediatrics **40**:1050, 1967.
3. American Academy of Pediatrics, Committee on Nutrition: The use and abuse of vitamin A, Pediatrics **48**:455, 1971.
4. American Academy of Pediatrics, Committee on Nutrition: Commentary on breast-feeding and infant formulas, including proposed standards for formulas, Pediatrics **57**:278, 1976.
5. American Heart Association Committee Report: Diet and coronary heart disease, Circulation **58**:762A, 1978.
6. Avioli, L.V.: Major minerals. A. Calcium and phosphorus. In Goodhart, R.S., and Shils, M.E., editors: Modern nutrition in health and disease, ed. 6, Philadelphia, 1980, Lea & Febiger.
7. Baker, S.J., Pereira, S.M., and Begum, A.: Failure of vitamin E therapy in the treatment of anemia of protein calorie malnutrition, Blood **32**:717, 1968.
8. Beadle, G.W.: Genes and the chemistry of the organism, Am. Sci. **34**:31, 1946.
9. Bentler, E.: Iron. In Goodhard, R.S., and Shils, M.E., editors: Modern nutrition in health and disease, ed. 6, Philadelphia, 1980, Lea & Febiger.
10. Birch, H.G., et al.: Relation of kwashiorkor in early childhood and intelligence at school age, Pediatr. Res. **5**:579, 1971.
11. Blix, G., editor: Symposia of the Swedish Nutrition Foundation. I. Mild-moderate forms of protein-calorie malnutrition, Uppsala, 1963, Almqvist & Wiksells.
12. Brock, J.F., and Autret, M.: Kwashiorkor in Africa, WHO Monogr. Ser. **8**:36, 1952.
13. Cavalieri, R.C.: Trace elements. A. Iodine. In Goodhart, R.S., and Shils, M.E., editors: Modern nutrition in health and disease, ed. 6, Philadelphia, 1980, Lea & Febiger.
14. Chandra, P.K.: Interactions of nutrition, infection and immune response: immunocompetence in nutritional deficiency, methodological considerations and intervention strategies, Acta Paediatr. Scand. **68**:137, 1979.
15. Conference on Nutrition and Cancer Therapy, Cancer Res. **37**(7, part 2):2322, 1977.
16. Cravioto, J., and De Licardie, E.R.: Nutrition and behavior and learning, World Rev. Nutr. Diet. **16**:80, 1973.
17. David, H.: Die Leber bei Nahrungsmangel und Mangelernahrung, Berlin, 1961, Akademie-Verlag.
18. Davies, J.N.P.: Nutrition and nutritional diseases, Annu. Rev. Med. **3**:99, 1952.
19. De Luca, H.F.: Recent advances in our understanding of the vitamin D endocrine system, J. Steroid Biochem. **11**:35, 1979.
20. De Luca, H.F.: Vitamin D metabolism and function, Monogr. Endocrinol. **13**:1, 1979.
21. De Luca, L.M., and Shapiro, S.S., editors: Modulation of cellular interactions by vitamin A and derivatives (retinoids), Ann. N.Y. Acad. Sci. **359**:1, 1981.
22. Dreyfus, P.M.: In Beeson, P.B., McDermott, W., and Wyngaarden, J.B., editors: Cecil-Loeb textbook of medicine, ed. 15, Philadelphia, 1979, W.B. Saunders Co.
23. Edwards, L.C., and Dunphy, J.E.: Wound healing. II. Injury and abnormal repair, N. Engl. J. Med. **259**:275, 1958.
24. Einstein, A.B., and Singh, S.P.: Hormonal control of nutrient metabolism. In Goodhart, R.S. and Shils, M.E., editors: Modern nutrition in health and disease, ed. 6, Philadelphia, Lea & Febiger.
25. Follis, R.H., Jr.: Deficiency disease, Springfield, Ill., 1958, Charles C Thomas, Publisher.
26. Frimpter, G.W., Andleman, R.J., and George, W.F.: Vitamin B_6-dependency syndromes: new horizons in nutrition, Am. J. Clin. Nutr. **22**:794, 1969.
27. Ganguly, J., et al.: Systemic mode of action of vitamin-A. In Vitamins and hormones, New York, 1980, Academic Press, Inc.
28. Goodhart, R.S., and Shils, M.E., editors: Modern nutrition in health and disease, ed. 6, Philadelphia, 1980, Lea & Febiger.
29. Gross, R.L., et al.: Role of nutrition in immunologic function, Physiol. Rev. **60**:188, 1980.
30. Harper, A.E., Benevenga, N.J., and Wohlhueter, R.M.: Effects of ingestion of disproportionate amounts of amino acids, Physiol. Rev. **50**:428, 1970.
31. Hathcock, J.N., and Coon, J., editors: Nutrition and drug interrelations, New York, 1978, Academic Press, Inc.
32. Herbert, V., Coleman, N., and Jacob, E.: Folic acid and vitamin B_{12}. In Goodhart, R.S., and Shils, M.E., editors: Modern nutrition in health and disease, ed. 6, Philadelphia, Lea & Febiger.
33. Hillman, R.W., and Goodhart, R.S.: Nutrition in pregnancy. In Goodhart, R.S., and Shils, M.E., editors: Modern nutrition in health and diseases, ed. 5, Philadelphia, 1973, Lea & Febiger.
34. Horwitt, M.K.: Vitamin E. In Goodhart, R.S., and Shils, M.E., editors: Modern nutrition in health and disease, ed. 6, Philadelphia, Lea & Febiger.
35. Irwin, M.I.: Nutritional requirements of man: a conspectus of research, New York, 1980, The Nutrition Foundation, Inc.
36. Jeliffe, D.B., and Welbourn, H.F.: Clinical signs of mild-moderate protein-calorie malnutrition of early childhood. In Blix, G., editor: Mild-moderate forms of protein-calorie malnutrition, Uppsala, Sweden, 1963, Almqvist & Wiksell.
37. Keys, A., et al.: The biology of human starvation, vols. 1 and 2, Minneapolis, 1950, University of Minnesota Press.
38. Kooh, S.W., et al.: Treatment of hypoparathyroidism and pseudohypoparathyroidism with metabolites of vitamin D: evidence for impaired conversion of 25-hydroxyvitamin D to 1α,25-dihydroxyvitamin D, N. Engl. J. Med. **293**:840, 1975.
39. Kritchevsky, D.: Diet, lipid metabolism, and aging, Fed. Proc. **38**:2001, 1979.
40. Lantham, M.: Human nutrition in tropical Africa, Rome, 1965, Food and Agriculture Organization of the United Nations.
41. Latham, M.C.: Protein-calorie malnutrition in children and its relation to psychological development and behavior, Physiol. Rev. **54**:541, 1974.
42. Leonard, P.J., and Losowsky, M.S.: Effect of alpha-tocopherol administration on red cell survival in vitamin E–deficient human subjects, Am. J. Clin. Nutr. **24**:388, 1971.
43. Li, T.K., and Vallee, B.L.: The biochemical and nutritional roles of other trace elements. In Goodhard, R.S., and Shils, M.E., editors:

Modern nutrition in health and disease, ed. 6, Philadelphia, 1980, Lea & Febiger.

44. Lloyd-Still, J.D.: Clinical studies on the effects of malnutrition during infancy and subsequent physical and intellectual development. In Lloyd-Still, J.D., editor: Malnutrition and intellectual development, Littleton, Mass., 1976, Publishing Sciences Group, Inc.

45. Lombardi, B.: Effects of choline deficiency on rat hepatocytes, Fed. Proc. **30:**139, 1971.

46. Lombardi, B., and Shinozuka, H.: Enhancement of 2-acetylaminofluorene liver carcinogenesis in rats fed a choline-devoid diet, Int. J. Cancer **23:**565, 1979.

47. Lui, N.S.T., and Roels, O.A.: The vitamins. A. Vitamin A and carotene. In Goodhart, R.S., and Shils, M.E., editors: Modern nutrition in health and disease, ed. 6, Philadelphia, Lea & Febiger.

48. Majaj, A.S., et al.: Vitamin E responsive megaloblastic anemia in infants with protein-calorie malnutrition, Am. J. Clin. Nutr. **12:**374, 1963.

49. Mata, L.: The malnutrition-infection complex and its environment factors, Proc. Nutr. Soc. **38:**29, 1979.

50. Matsukura, N., et al.: Carcinogenicity in mice of mutagenic compounds from a tryptophan pyrolyzate, Science **213:**346, 1981.

51. McLaren, D.S.: The Vitamins. In Bondy, P.K., editor: Duncan's disease of metabolism: endocrinology and nutrition, ed. 6, Philadelphia, 1969, W.B. Saunders Co.

52. Nair, P.P., et al.: Vitamin E and porphyrin metabolism in man, Arch. Intern. Med. **128:**411, 1971.

53. National Academy of Sciences–National Research Council, Food and Nutrition Board: Recommended dietary allowances, rev. ed. 9, Washington, D.C., 1980, U.S. Government Printing Office.

54. Newell, G.R., and Ellison, N.M., editors: Nutrition and cancer: etiology and treatment, Prog. Cancer Res. Ther. **17:**1, 1981.

55. Olson, R.E.: Protein-calorie malnutrition, New York, 1975, Academic Press, Inc.

56. Olson, R.E.: Vitamin K. In Goodhard, R.S., and Shils, M.E., editors: Modern nutrition in health and disease, ed. 6, Philadelphia, 1980, Lea & Febiger.

57. Persson, B., Tunnell, R., and Ekengren, K.: Chronic vitamin A intoxication during the first half year of life: description of 5 cases, Acta Paediatr. Scand. **54:**49, 1965.

58. Platt, B.S., Heard, C.R.C., and Stewart, R.J.C.: Experimental protein-calorie deficiency. In Munro, H.N., and Allison, J.B., editors: Mammalian protein metabolism, vol. 2, New York, 1964, Academic Press, Inc.

59. Prasad, A.S., editor: Trace elements in human health and disease: zinc and copper, vol. 1, New York, 1976, Academic Press, Inc.

60. Prasad, A.S., editor: Trace elements in human health and disease: essential and toxic elements, vol. 2, New York, 1976, Academic Press, Inc.

61. Rannels, D.E., McKee, E.E., and Morgan, H.E.: Regulation of protein synthesis and degradation in heart and skeletal muscle. In Litwack, G., editor: Biochemical actions of hormones, vol. 4, New York, 1977, Academic Press, Inc.

62. Read, M.S.: Behavioral correlations of malnutrition. In Brazier, M.A.B., editor: Growth and development of the brain, New York, 1975, Raven Press.

63. Reddy, B.S.: Nutrition and its relationship to cancer, Adv. Cancer Res. **32:**238, 1980.

64. Roe, D.A.: Drug-induced nutritional deficiencies, Westport, Conn., 1978, The Avi Publishing Co., Inc.

65. Scrimshaw, N.S.: Pellagra. In Beeson, P.B., McDermott, W., and Wyngaarden, J.B., editors: Cecil-Loeb textbook of medicine, ed. 15, Philadelphia, 1979, W.B. Saunders Co.

66. Scrimshaw, N.S., and Gordon, J.E., editors: Malnutrition, learning and behavior, Cambridge, Mass., 1968, M.I.T. Press.

67. Sebrell, W.H., Jr., and Harris, R.S., editors: The vitamins, ed. 2, vol. 1, New York, 1967, Academic Press, Inc.

68. Sebrell, W.H., Jr., and Harris, R.S., editors: The vitamins, ed. 2, vol. 2, New York, 1968, Academic Press, Inc.

69. Sebrell, W.H., Jr., and Harris, R.S., editors: The vitamins, ed. 2, vol. 3, New York, 1971, Academic Press, Inc.

70. Shinozuka, H., et al.: Enhancement of ethionine liver carcinogenesis in rats fed a choline-deficient diet, J. Natl. Cancer Inst. **61:**813, 1978.

71. Sidransky, H.: Chemical and cellular pathology of experimental acute amino acid deficiency, Methods Achiev. Exp. Pathol. **6:**1, 1972.

72. Sidransky, H.: Nutritional disturbances of protein metabolism in the liver, Am. J. Pathol. **84:**649, 1976.

73. Silverberg, D.S., et al.: Effect of 1,25-dihydroxycholecalciferol in renal osteodystrophy, Can. Med. Assoc. J. **112:**190, 1975.

74. Sockalosky, J.J., et al.: Vitamin D–resistant rickets: end-organ unresponsiveness to $1,25\text{-}(OH)_2D_3$, J. Pediatr. **96:**701, 1980.

75. Sos, J.: Die Pathologie der Eiweissernährung, Budapest, 1964, Verlag der Ungarischen Akademie der Wissenschaften.

76. Sporn, M.B.: Retinoids and cancer prevention, Carcinog. Compr. Surv. **5:**99, 1980.

77. Sporn, M.B., and Newton, D.L.: Chemoprevention of cancer with retinoids, Fed. Proc. **38:**2528, 1979.

78. Stimson, W.H.: Vitamin A intoxication in adults: report of a case with a summary of the literature, N. Engl. J. Med. **265:**369, 1961.

79. Symposium on nutrition and cancer, Fed. Proc. **35:**1307, 1976.

80. Symposium on nutrition in the causation of cancer, Cancer Res. **35**(11, part 2):3231, 1975.

81. Trowell, H.C., Davies, J.N.P., and Dean, R.F.A.: Kwashiorkor, London, 1954, Edward Arnold, Ltd.

82. Underwood, E.J.: Trace elements in human and animal nutrition, ed. 4, New York, 1977, Academic Press, Inc.

83. Van Itallie, T.B.: Obesity: adverse effects on health and longevity, Am. J. Clin. Nutr. **32**(12 suppl.):2723, 1979.

84. Wasserman, R.H., and Taylor, A.N.: Metabolic roles of fat-soluble vitamins D, E and K, Annu. Rev. Biochem. **41:**179, 1972.

85. Wattenberg, L.W.: Inhibitors of chemical carcinogenesis, Adv. Cancer Res. **26:**197, 1978.

86. Williams, R.H.: Clinical biotin deficiency, N. Engl. J. Med. **228:**247, 1943.

87. Winick, M., editor: Nutrition and cancer. In Current concepts in nutrition, vol. 6, New York, 1977, John Wiley & Sons, Inc.

88. Wolbach, S.B.: Controlled formation of collagen and reticulum: study of source of intercellular substance in recovery from experimental scorbutus, Am. J. Pathol. **9**(suppl.):689, 1933.

89. Wolbach, S.B., and Bessey, O.A.: Tissue changes in vitamin deficiencies, Physiol. Rev. **22:**233, 1942.

90. Workshop on fat and cancer, Cancer Res. **41**(9):3677, 1981.

91. World Health Organization: Trace elements in human nutrition: report of a WHO expert committee, Geneva, 1973, WHO Tech. Rep. Ser. no. 532.

92. Young, V.R.: Diet as a modulator of aging and longevity, Fed. Proc. **38:**1994, 1979.

CHAPTER 15   **Neoplasia**

GEORGE Th. DIAMANDOPOULOS
WILLIAM A. MEISSNER

Neoplasms represent a pathologic disturbance of growth characterized by an excessive and unceasing proliferation of cells. Countless varieties arise from essentially all types of human cells. The process of neoplasia is not restricted to humans; neoplasms also develop in most vertebrates and in some insects and plants, and their occurrence in these other forms has been helpful in studying their genesis and behavior. Some neoplasms are called *benign* because they grow slowly and remain so localized that the patient usually experiences little difficulty from them. Others, called *malignant* or *cancerous*, tend to proliferate rapidly and to spread throughout the body so relentlessly that, unless successfully treated, they eventually cause death of the host. Although both types are true neoplasms, it is the malignant ones (cancers) that create such an important problem.

Although tumors must have occurred at all times in humans and animals and in all parts of the world, the earliest evidence available at present is found in the form of tumors in human bones from prehistoric and early historical periods. The *Ramayana*, a manuscript of ancient India (circa 2000 BC), is the first instance in recorded history in which malignant tumors are mentioned. Reference is made in it for the first time to tumor treatment, either with the knife (surgery) or with an arsenical compound (chemotherapy).

Descriptions relating to malignant tumors are also found in the various Egyptian papyri (circa 1500 BC). The Egyptians were the first to realize that tumors arising in various parts of the body differed in their behavior and should be treated differently. Mention is also made of tumors involving the breasts of women in the tablets with cuneiform inscription in the library of Nineveh in Babylonia (circa 800 BC).

In the ancient Greek medical literature, various references to tumors are found. Hippocrates of Cos (460-375 BC), the father of medicine, was the first to divide tumors into two large groups according to their behavior: (1) the innocuous tumors, which included swellings and lumps of various kinds (probably both nonneoplastic and neoplastic) and (2) the dangerous tumors, which killed the patients (probably representing predominantly malignant neoplasms).

Hippocrates coined the terms *karkinos* (for the non-healing [?] neoplastic ulcers) and *karkinōma* (for the solid malignant tumors). Both terms derive from Greek *karkinos*, meaning "crab." The term *cancer* appears much later, deriving from the Latin word *cancrum*, also denoting "crab." The reasons why Hippocrates and his pupils chose the term *crab* to describe malignant tumors are not known. Even as early as the seventh century of our era, there was puzzlement as to the etymologic origins of the word *karkinos*, or *cancer*. Paul of Aegina (AD 625-690), a famous Byzantine physician, writes as follows: "Cancer is particularly frequent in the breasts of women. . . . The veins are filled and stretched around like the feet of an animal called cancer (crab), and hence the disease has gotten its name. But some say that it is so called because it adheres to any part which it seizes upon in an obstinate manner like the crab."

Among the 300 or more books that Galen (AD 131-201) wrote, there is a special monograph on tumors. In it, he divides tumors into three categories: (1) tumors *according* to nature, for example, pregnancy; (2) tumors *exceeding* nature, for example, inflammatory and reparative tumors such as callus around a bone fracture; and (3) tumors *contrary* to nature, for example, true neoplasms. Galen was aware of the phenomenon of tumor metastasis. He was also the first to theorize as to the possible cause of cancer, ascribing it to excess of black bile. It is said that he was the one who coined the term *sarcoma* (Gr. *sarx*, genitive *sarkos*, "flesh") under which he included various tumors with a fleshy gross appearance.

After the fall of the Roman Empire, the hippocratic and galenic traditions were kept viable in Byzantium and Persia and by the Arabs. There was sporadic medical interest in tumors, and from the Middle Ages through the Renaissance medical textbooks contained sections on neoplasia in general and on various tumors in particular, including their effects on the organism. The development of the microscope in the seventeenth century and the founding of histology by Marcello Malpighi (1628-1694) were notable events that led eventually to the introduction of the revolutionary thesis by Rudolf Virchow (1821-1902) that new cells were formed by division of the old: *omnis cellula e cellulā*. From Virchow's concept, modern pathology emerged. It is also the concept on which the classification of tumors is based.

NONNEOPLASTIC GROWTH DISTURBANCES

A neoplasm usually forms a mass. The term *tumor* in older usage referred to any swelling from whatever cause, but currently the term is used almost exclusively as a synonym for neoplasm. Because neoplasms are characterized by a proliferation of cells and the formation of a mass, it is not surprising that other processes, both normal and abnormal, might resemble them in one respect or another. It is appropriate to discuss some of these briefly, partly because they are important in themselves and partly because they need to be compared and contrasted with neoplasms.

Malformations

Defective or abnormal formations of an organ or tissue include complete or partial lack of development, asymmetry, and oversize. Although most malformations bear little resemblance to neoplasms, the lesion called *hamartoma* may be mistaken for a true tumor (Fig. 15-1). It is a focal, often circumscribed overgrowth in improper proportions of tissues normally present in that part of the body. As an example, hamartomas of the lung are well-circumscribed growths of mature cartilage, bronchial epithelium, and mucous glands in abnormal and distorted proportions. Hamartomas arise in many organs and tissues and include many angiomas and benign pigmented nevi. Since they do not have the capacity of continuous growth, they can only be considered to be tumorlike malformations. A *choristoma* is similar to a hamartoma except that the tissues of which it is composed are not normally present in the part of the body in which it is found, for example, adrenal gland tissue in the urinary bladder. Normal-appearing tissue in an abnormal location is called *ectopic* (Fig. 15-2).

Repair

When the organism is damaged from any cause, cell proliferations attempt to repair the injury and restore the tissues to normal structure and function. The process of repair is of great value in terms of preservation of the health of the host. Repair is closely related to the process of inflammation and continues after the inflammation subsides until the injured tissue is restored. Classic examples include the healing of skin wounds and frac-

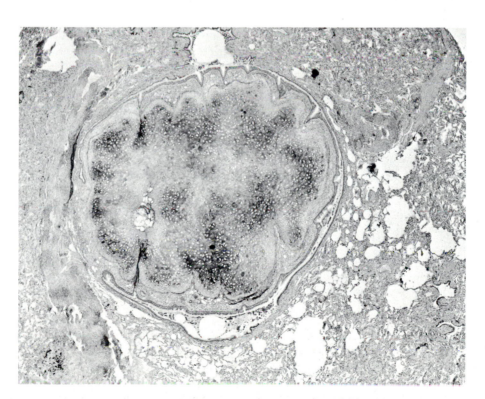

Fig. 15-1. Hamartoma of lung. Although overgrowth contains bronchial epithelium and mucous glands, its chief component is cartilage. (22×.)

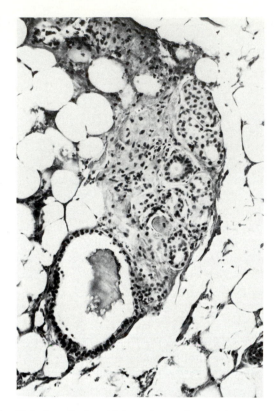

Fig. 15-2. Ectopic thyroid tissue in mediastinal fat. (150×.)

tured bones; in each instance the proliferating cells are appropriate to the region. The cellular proliferation ceases when healing is completed.

Hypertrophy and atrophy

Hypertrophy at the cellular level means an increase in individual cell size. Actually the tissue or organ is usually also increased in total size as a result of the cell change. Hypertrophy occurs with stimulation of the cells to increased work. It may be physiologic, for example, muscle hypertrophy with continued exercise. It may also result from disease conditions such as a deformity of a heart valve causing partial obstruction and an increased workload on the myocardial fibers. Hormonal hypertrophy is brought about by the influence of an excessive hormonal stimulation. The process of hypertrophy regresses when the stimuli are withdrawn, although the organ almost never reverts to its previous (prehypertrophic) state—for example, surgical correction of valvular deformities of the heart does not result in complete alleviation of myocardial hypertrophy.

Atrophy is the diminution in the size of the cells, organ, or tissue after full development has been attained. It occurs whenever the tissue is no longer employed to normal capacity. Such situations include aging, lack of hormonal stimulation, lack of use, and insufficient blood supply.

Hyperplasia

Hyperplasia is an absolute increase in the number of cells per unit of tissue or organ of origin. As a rule, cells that are capable of division, that is, DNA synthesis followed by mitosis, may undergo hyperplasia alone or in combination with hypertrophy when there is a demand for increased work by an organ.

Different cell types vary in their ability to exhibit hyperplasia. For example, surface epithelia, hepatic and renal tubular cells, fibroblasts, endothelium, mesothelium, and reserve hemopoietic bone marrow cells exhibit great capacity to proliferate hyperplastically. Most solid glandular epithelia, bone, cartilage, and smooth muscle of blood vessels and the pregnant uterus show a lesser capacity for hyperplastic proliferation. Neurons, cardiac and skeletal muscle, and smooth muscle of the alimentary tract have little if any capacity for hyperplasia.

Hyperplasia usually affects only a single type of tissue in a given organ. In a few organs, however, hyperplasia is generally of a mixed variety; for example, prostatic hyperplasia includes proliferation of the glandular epithelium, the connective tissue, and even the smooth muscle (Fig. 15-3). In general, cells exhibiting hyperplasia have an increased nucleocytoplasmic ratio, large or multiple nucleoli, and darkly stained nuclei. Some cells are in mitosis. There is also an increase in the number of cytoplasmic organelles (mitochondria, free ribosomes, and a variety of other cytoplasmic alterations). Hyperplastic cells are less specialized, showing partial or complete loss of their normal function and even structure. Once hyperplasia has reached a stage of stability, specialization of cell structure and function returns.

There are several types and causes of hyperplasia. Physiologic hyperplasia results from various types of physiologic (normal) stimuli. For example, cell hyperplasia of breast epithelium is incidental to the onset of puberty or to pregnancy and lactation. Compensatory hyperplasia is the proliferation of cells after a portion of an organ or tissue has been destroyed by disease or surgically excised. For example, surgical removal of part of the liver will induce almost pure hyperplasia of the cells in the remaining liver. Removal of one kidney will result in hypertrophy and hyperplasia of the cells of the remaining kidney. Adaptive hyperplasia is a response to various abnormal stimuli. For example, there is lymphoid tissue hyperplasia occurring after localized inflammation. Pathologic hormonal hyperplasia is brought about by the influence of excessive hormone. An example is endometrial hyperplasia resulting from prolonged estrogen stimulation. The excessive estrogen could come, for example, from a functioning ovarian tumor or from an excessive oral intake.

In terms of histomorphology, hyperplasia may be diffuse or nodular. A diffuse type of hyperplasia such as that seen in Graves' disease of the thyroid consists of the

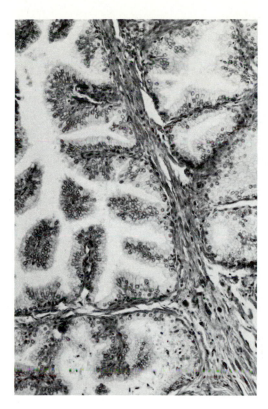

Fig. 15-3. Hyperplasia of prostate. Process mainly involves epithelium, which because of increased number of cells is arranged in fronds with vascular stalk. (200×.)

crowding of the epithelial cells in the form of papillary projections or cell stratification. In nodular hyperplasia (such as prostate, breast, and adrenal), multiple, poorly delineated, highly cellular nodules are formed, compress the surrounding normal tissue, and in places may even destroy it. The factors that determine the development of diffuse rather than nodular hyperplasia, or vice versa, are not well understood. It may be a function of the nature of the target cell participating in the hyperplastic process.

As in hypertrophy, hyperplasia is initiated and controlled by identifiable stimuli. It is nonprogressive in that it is limited in amount and duration. It terminates when the functional need or hormonal stimulus that evoked it has ceased. With the withdrawal of the stimulus the hyperplastic process regresses, but the organ does not always revert to its former state; for example, breast hyperplasia-hypertrophy regresses after pregnancy and lactation, but the breasts do not revert to their original state. Finally, hyperplasia is often useful, at least in compensating for tissue loss or for increase in functional demand.

Metaplasia

Metaplasia denotes the change of one type of adult cell or tissue to another. It usually represents an adaptation

on the part of the organism to abnormal localized environmental changes or to new functional demands. It is often reversible. Although metaplasia may develop in many tissues, it is most prominent in epithelium. An example is change of the bronchial epithelium from the normal columnar, glandular type to squamous epithelium after chronic irritation.

The substitute cells are almost always indigenous to the type of tissue from which the original cells had derived, such as squamous epithelium for columnar epithelium, or bone for connective tissue. Occasionally, however, connective tissue cells or their precursors may exhibit metaplasia possessing epithelial characteristics. This feature can be explained by the fact that during embryogenesis some mesoderm gives rise to epithelium as well as to connective tissue. An example of this type of metaplasia can be seen in organs belonging to the genitourinary system.

The probable mode of genesis of metaplasia is that reserve cells, normally present in the adult organism, may express their latent maturation potential by differentiating into adult cell types. Teleologically, metaplasia represents a protective response by the organism. Thus squamous epithelium, replacing the bronchial ciliated pseudostratified columnar epithelium, is more resistant to injury or inflammation. There is a drawback, however, in that the loss of columnar epithelium along with the goblet cells and glands that secrete mucus deprives the organism of the trapping of bacteria and foreign particles by such protective secretions.

Dysplasia

Dysplasia is a change affecting the size, shape, and orientational relationship of adult types of cells, primarily epithelial cells. Such cells exhibit pleomorphism; that is, they vary in size and shape, possess large, hyperchromatic (darkly stained) nuclei, and exhibit an increase in their nucleus-to-cytoplasm ratio. Mitotic activity is increased, but the mitotic figures are normal. There is disruption of the normal cell layering as seen in stratified squamous epithelium or of the parallel cell arrangement as seen in columnar or glandular epithelium. A synonym for dysplasia is "atypical hyperplasia" (Fig. 15-4).

Dysplastic cell changes are usually brought about by chronic irritation, whatever its cause, or by protracted inflammation. When the inciting stimulus is removed, the dysplastic alterations usually disappear and the participating cells revert to a normal structure and function. The possibility exists that dysplasia precedes neoplasia, as will be discussed later.

Anaplasia

Anaplasia is a term implying a change in a cell or tissue from a more to a less highly differentiated form. A synonym is "undifferentiation," implying that the cells or

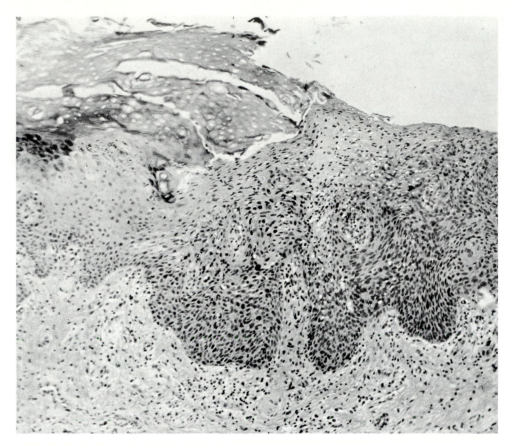

Fig. 15-4. Carcinoma arising in arsenical keratosis showing hyperkeratosis, dysplasia (atypical hyperplasia), and early carcinoma. (125×.)

tissue has become more primitive, even embryonic. The term is used primarily to describe cancers and infrequently for nonneoplastic cellular proliferations.

DEFINITION

Because of the nature and complexity of neoplasia, it is difficult to compose a simple definition that will characterize or be appropriate for all tumors. It is much easier to describe neoplasia than to define it because the differences between tumors and normal tissues or nontumorous proliferations often seem to be a matter of degree rather than type.

Neoplasia is a persistent, abnormal, and relatively autonomous proliferation of cells. It is the result of a permanent cellular defect that is passed on to the cells' progeny. The defect is induced by one factor or a combination of several factors and, once developed, usually becomes independent of them.

Even the preceding definition must be accepted with the following reservations: (1) The abnormal cellular proliferation sometimes produces tissue very similar to normal in appearance. (2) The autonomy of tumors has been overemphasized. Although tumors do consist of perma-

nently altered body cells having the power of continuous growth, their cellular proliferation is only relatively free from the usual restraints. For example, in addition to the tumor's dependence on the host for blood supply and nourishment, its growth may be enhanced or retarded by hormones, drugs, chemicals, and infections, as well as by the systemic condition of the host. (3) On rare occasions the cellular defect is not permanent; spontaneous regression of tumors does occur. (4) Although in many instances the neoplasm becomes completely independent of the causative agent, there is evidence that in some experimental tumors the causative viral genome, or a segment of it, may continue to reside in the genetic apparatus of the tumor cells.

The growth process most like neoplasia is hyperplasia, but differences are readily apparent. Hyperplasia occurs as the result of an identifiable stimulus and ceases when the stimulating agent is removed. It is not an autonomous growth, and there is no permanent cellular defect.

TAXONOMY AND NOMENCLATURE

Many terms used in discussing and describing tumors are seldom applied to other pathologic processes. Furthermore, some tumor terms and their synonyms are not always used properly or consistently. The glossary at the end of the chapter will help clarify their meaning and proper usage.

Many classifications of tumors have been proposed. Although elements of some of them persist, most are of limited or no practical use.

Etiologic classification

Classification based on etiology, a common practice for infectious diseases, is appealing, but impractical for several reasons: (1) The etiology of most tumors is poorly understood. (2) The same agent may produce tumors of several different types. (3) Tumors exactly alike morphologically and clinically may be induced by completely different agents. (4) Once a tumor has arisen, the agent usually is no longer necessary for its continued growth.

Embryogenic classification

At one time it was believed that most neoplasms were derived from embryonic cells or from cells that had reverted to their embryonic state. Because the concept is no longer acceptable, this type of classification is unsatisfactory. The suffix -*blastoma* was used to designate tumors of embryonic cells, and a few such terms persist, mostly for certain tumors in infants. Examples are *nephroblastoma* of the kidney, *neuroblastoma* of the adrenal gland, *retinoblastoma* of the eye, and *hepatoblastoma* of the liver.

Site classification: regional or organ

All organs of the body consist of a variety of tissues, and each of these tissues is capable of giving rise to one or more types of neoplasm. Tumors arising from different tissues of the same organ tend to behave differently, whereas tumors of similar tissues from different organs tend to behave similarly. The tissue of origin rather than the organ of origin determines the behavior of a tumor. The general region of the tumor, such as the arm, the abdominal cavity, or the head, may be descriptive but is not useful in classification.

Functional classification

Many tumors produce various substances, such as mucus, sometimes to great excess. The effects of such function and overfunction are particularly apparent in tumors of endocrine glands, since systemic symptoms may result from increased hormone production. Classifying tumors by substances produced, for example, insulinoma, a tumor that produces insulin, has not been satisfactory because materials such as mucus, or even hormones, may be formed by many different tumors of widely different biologic behavior in a great variety of tissues. Moreover, a tumor may produce multiple sub-

Table 15-1. Some characteristics of typical benign and malignant tumors*

	Benign	Malignant
Growth rate	Slow	Rapid
Mitoses	Few	Many
Nuclear chromatin	Normal	Increased
Differentiation	Good	Poor
Local growth	Expansive	Invasive
Encapsulation	Present	Absent
Destruction of tissue	Little	Much
Vessel invasion	None	Frequent
Metastases	None	Frequent
Effect on host	Often insignificant	Significant

*Many tumors show exception to one or more of these characteristics.

stances; for example, medullary thyroid cancer may secrete calcitonin, histaminase, adrenocorticotropic hormone, and serotonin.

Histogenetic (or cytogenetic) classification

The histogenetic (or cytogenetic) classification is very satisfactory. It is made after microscopic examination of the tumor and recognition of the tissues or cells from which the neoplasm seems to arise or to consist. Such a classification is particularly valuable because the cell type of a tumor is its most important constant element. Because there are tumors corresponding to almost all kinds of normal tissues and cells, the classification of tumors by this method roughly parallels the classification of normal tissues. The method works best for tumors arising from tissues that are distinct; minor difficulties arise because some normal tissues are themselves difficult to classify and do not have distinctive names or because some tumors do not differentiate sufficiently to allow comparison with normal tissues.

Behavioral classification

A second satisfactory method of classifying tumors takes into account their known or anticipated biologic behavior. By this method, tumors are divided (sometimes arbitrarily!) into two groups, one representing relatively innocuous neoplasms designated as benign and the other more rapidly growing, destructive, and dangerous tumors designated as malignant. The synonym for malignant tumor is "cancer." Some of the differences between benign and malignant neoplasms are listed in Table 15-1. The distinction between the two groups is sometimes difficult, since not all tumors are clearly benign or clearly malignant. The most important distinguishing characteristics of cancers are their relative lack of differentiation, their usually rapid growth rate, their

Table 15-2. Some examples of tumor classification*

Tissue	Benign tumor	Malignant tumor
Connective tissue		
Adult fibrous tissue	Fibroma	Fibrosarcoma
Embryonic fibrous tissue	Myxoma	Myxosarcoma
Cartilage	Chondroma	Chondrosarcoma
Bone	Osteoma	Osteosarcoma
Fat	Lipoma	Liposarcoma
Muscle		
Smooth muscle	Leiomyoma	Leiomyosarcoma
Striated muscle	Rhabdomyoma	Rhabdomyosarcoma
Endothelium		
Lymph vessels	Lymphangioma	Lymphangiosarcoma
Blood vessels	Hemangioma	Hemangiosarcoma
Lymphoid tissue	Nonrecognized	Lymphosarcoma
Bone marrow	Nonrecognized	Leukemia
Neural tissue		
Nerve sheath	Neurilemoma	Neurogenic sarcoma
Nerve cells	Ganglioneuroma	Neuroblastoma
Epithelium		
Squamous epithelium	Papilloma	Squamous cell carcinoma (epidermoid carcinoma)
Transitional epithelium	Papilloma	Transitional cell carcinoma
Glandular epithelium	Adenoma	Adenocarcinoma
Liver cells	Benign hepatoma	Malignant hepatoma
Sweat glands	Hidradenoma	Hidradenoid carcinoma
Islets of Langerhans	Islet cell adenoma	Islet cell carcinoma
Miscellaneous		
Trophoblasts	Hydatid mole	Choriocarcinoma
Totipotential cells	Benign teratoma	Malignant teratoma

*Since there are almost limitless varieties of tumors, a complete table of classification would require many pages. Any shortened version is not only necessarily incomplete but also likely to be confusing. This table is meant only to show some examples and to be a general guide to nomenclature. Extensive classifications of tumors of respective organs and tissues, including synonyms and related terms, are presented particularly well in the various fascicles of the *Atlas of Tumor Pathology,* published by the Armed Forces Institute of Pathology, and in the *International Histologic Classification of Tumors,* published by the World Health Organization.

invasion of local tissues, and their spread to other parts of the body to establish discontinuous colonies (metastases).

Currently used classification

The currently used classification is a combination of two approaches, one based on the histogenetic or the presumed tissue of origin and the other on the anticipated behavior. Usually the two methods are combined in the final nomenclature.

To complete the nomenclature of tumors, various suffixes are useful. The suffix *-oma* implies tumor. Benign tumors are usually named by adding the suffix to the name of a cell type of tissue; for example, a benign tumor of fibrous tissue is called a *fibroma* and a benign tumor of glandular epithelium, an *adenoma*. Malignant tumors of epithelium are called *carcinomas*, whereas malignant tumors of mesenchymal tissues are designated *sarcomas*, both terms being used either independently (such as renal cell carcinoma) or as suffixes (such as fibrosarcoma).

Tumors are named and classified, therefore, on a his-

togenetic or cytogenetic basis, together with an interpretation of the biologic behavior and with addition of appropriate suffixes. Examples of classification of tumors are given in Table 15-2.

CHARACTERISTICS OF TUMOR TISSUES AND CELLS

The great diversity of tumor types results in a wide spectrum of characteristics of tumor tissues and cells. Some tumors resemble normal tissues and cells so closely—not only histologically but also biochemically, functionally, and immunologically—that they are nearly indistinguishable from the normal tissues and cells. Such a close resemblance is especially true in benign tumors, but it also holds in some better-differentiated cancers. The more malignant the tumor, the more deviation from normal, the ultimate being changes so extreme as to bear little or no resemblance to normal tissues and cells. It should be emphasized in any discussion of tumor tissue and cell characteristics that the degrees of deviation from normal vary widely and that there are no specific or constant features present in all neoplasms.

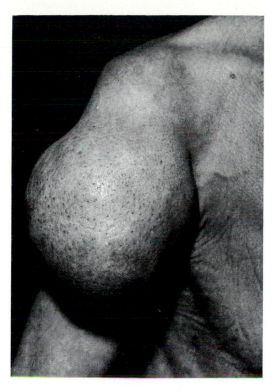

Fig. 15-5. Subcutaneous lipoma that had gradually increased in size over period of 6 to 8 years in 70-year-old man. Note stretching of skin as evidenced by widely separated pores.

Gross pathologic condition

The gross appearance of tumors is so variable and inconsistent, even with tumors of the same type, that one can only generalize on the most typical features. Since it is often impossible on the basis of gross examination alone to distinguish a neoplasm from swellings produced by inflammation, hyperplasia, and other growth disturbances, true identification requires microscopic examination. Tumors tend to have a different color, texture, and consistency from the tissue of origin. Benign tumors usually are spherical or ovoid and, if not encapsulated, at least well circumscribed (Fig. 15-5). They are freely movable and often firm and uniform in gross appearance unless retrogressive changes such as hemorrhage, infarction, and fibrosis occur (Figs. 15-6 and 15-7). In contrast, malignant tumors are more likely to be irregularly shaped and poorly circumscribed, with projections of the main growth extending into the adjacent structures so as to make the entire mass fixed (Fig. 15-8). Sarcomas, as their name implies, typically have a fleshy consistency, whereas many carcinomas are very firm. The retrogressive changes seen in benign tumors are even more frequent in malignant tumors, with ulceration and infarction being particularly common (Fig. 15-9). Such secondary changes alter the appearance of the primary tumor so extensively that the gross appearance is not of much

assistance in classification. Nevertheless, gross descriptive terms continue to be used, often denoting tumor characteristics of little significance. Terms such as papillary (Fig. 15-10), hemorrhagic, stenosing, infiltrating, fungating, diffuse, ulcerative, solid, and cystic are interesting descriptively but not always of much practical importance.

Architecture

The microscopic arrangements and growth patterns of tumor cells are of considerable importance in their recognition and classification. For example, tumors of glandular origin may be recognized on the basis of gland formation; tumors of the islets of Langerhans tend to recapitulate the arrangement of the cells in the normal islet (Fig. 15-11). Some benign tumors and tumors of low-grade malignancy may duplicate the structural pattern of the normal tissue prototype so well that they are unrecognizable as tumors. The more usual finding in cancers is that the microscopic arrangement of the cells is quite different from that in normal tissues. The relationship of the cells to each other or to a basement membrane (polarity) is disrupted, and the orderly maturation of cells is lost. In addition to the altered orientation and alignment of the tumor cells to each other, their relationship to the stroma also is changed. Invasion of the stroma by tumor cells is one of the most important diagnostic criteria of cancer.

There are some tumors that have a mixed pattern of cell types and architectural arrangement. One of these is the teratoma (Figs. 15-7 and 15-12), which is a true neoplasm arising from totipotential cells. Teratomas often are composed of numerous types of tissue representing all classic germ layers. Teratomas may be benign or malignant. Although they most commonly arise in the ovary or testis, they may occasionally be seen in other locations, such as the neck and mediastinum. The rather common dermoid or hair-filled cyst of the ovary is a variant of a teratoma in which the tumor forms well-differentiated skin and skin appendages as a prominent feature. The differentiation of some parts of a teratoma is at times quite impressive, some of the structures being histologically indistinguishable from the normal and even capable of function, for example, struma ovarii (goiter of the ovary), an ovarian teratoma containing thyroid tissue. When teratomas become malignant, it may be only one element that does so, although some malignant teratomas metastasize with multiple elements. Many forms of teratomas, frequently quite complex, have been encountered. The term *teratology* often has been applied to include the study of imperfectly developed embryos in which loss of key embryonic cell blocks has led to malformations. These malformations, however, are not neoplasms and therefore are not teratomas.

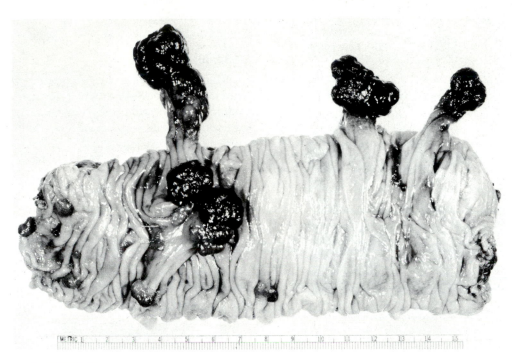

Fig. 15-6. Multiple polyps of segment of colon. Larger polyps are pedunculated and hemorrhagic.

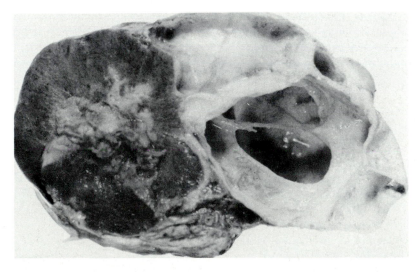

Fig. 15-7. Cystic teratoma of ovary. This benign neoplasm shows both solid and cystic foci. Microscopically various types of tissue composed tumor.

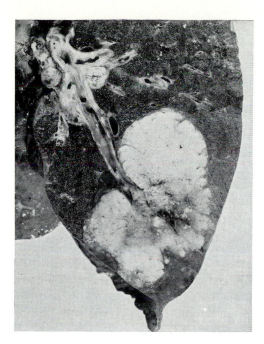

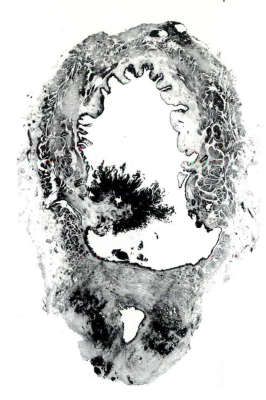

Fig. 15-8. Adenocarcinoma of bronchus of lower right lobe showing origin from bronchus and extension into surrounding pulmonary tissue, together with metastatic involvement of peribronchial lymph nodes.

Fig. 15-10. Section through bladder, prostate, and urethra showing papillary tumor arising from lateral bladder wall. (From Austen, G., Jr., and Friedell, G.H.: J. Urol. **93:**224, 1965.)

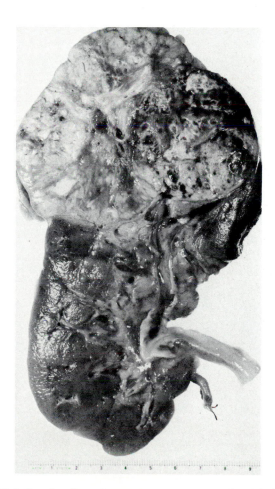

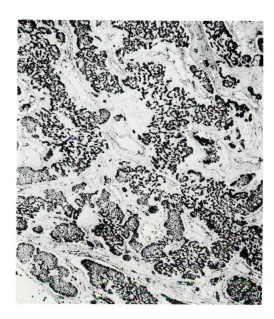

Fig. 15-9. Renal cell carcinoma occupying one pole of kidney. Tumor is partly hemorrhagic and necrotic.

Fig. 15-11. Islet cell tumor. Solid clusters and ribbonlike growth are reminiscent of normal islet of Langerhans. (30×.)

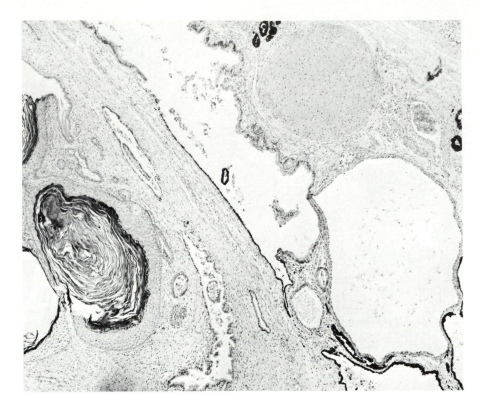

Fig. 15-12. Teratoma of testis. In addition to several types of glandular epithelium centrally, nodule of cartilage is present in upper right and masses of keratinizing squamous epithelium at left. (50×.)

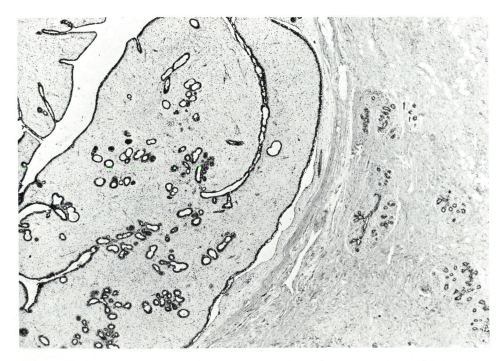

Fig. 15-13. Portion of adenofibroma of breast. Breast tissue at right is normal except for compression by tumor. (26×.)

Tumors may be composed of two or more elements without necessarily being teratomas. Sometimes the elements are related and of the same general type of tissue. At other times they are unrelated. The adenofibroma of the breast is a benign neoplasm consisting of glandular epithelium and fibrous tissue of the breast lobule; each of the types of tissue is a part of the neoplasm (Fig. 15-13). The carcinosarcoma of the uterus is a malignant neoplasm in which carcinoma of the endometrium and sarcoma of the endometrial stroma (supporting matrix) grow together as joint cancer. Tumors containing several closely related elements are rather common; for example, adenoacanthoma is the term for formation of some

squamous epithelium by a glandular carcinoma. A tumor containing several types of sarcoma growing as one unit is called a malignant mesenchymoma. In addition to tumors' being composed of several types of tissues, multiple independent tumors of similar or different types may arise from the same region, perhaps in response to a common stimulus. These are not synonymous with the tumors just described.

Although tumors of mixed elements might well be designated mixed tumors, this term, unfortunately, has been used almost exclusively for a specific type of neoplasm arising in the salivary glands and occasionally in other, comparable structures. Actually, the term "mixed tumor of salivary gland" is a misnomer, since it was used originally under the assumption that the cartilaginous or myxomatous stroma so common in such tumors was a true part of the neoplasm. It is now believed that the tumor is an epithelial neoplasm with a metaplastic stromal response.

Cytology

Cytologic changes of tumor cells may involve only the cytoplasm, with or without the nucleus, or the cell as a whole. Cells of benign tumors differ little from their normal counterparts. Cells of malignant tumors tend to be larger than normal, to have irregular outlines with bizarre forms, and to show a pleomorphism or variation in size and shape (Fig. 15-14). Giant cells, often with multiple nuclei and unusual shapes, are common in high-

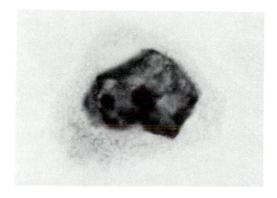

Fig. 15-14. Cancer cell showing irregular outline of cell and nucleus, hyperchromatism of nucleus, and prominent nucleoli. (1200×.)

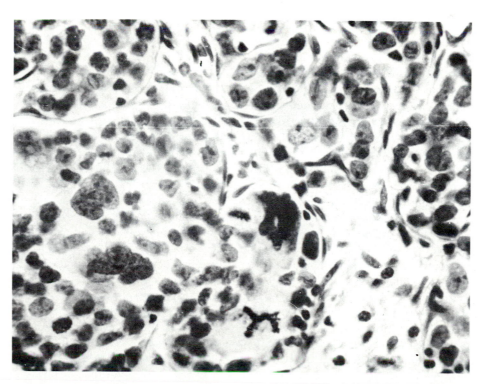

Fig. 15-15. Extremely anaplastic cancer showing abnormal mitoses, multinucleated tumor giant cells, and extensive pleomorphism. (800×.)

ly malignant cancers (Fig. 15-15). Degenerative changes, such as vacuolization, are common in both cytoplasm and nucleus.

In well-differentiated tumor cells, the *cytoplasm* contains the characteristic constituents, secretions, and products (such as cross striations, mucus, keratin) present in the normal cell prototypes. Even enzymes formed by the normal cell may be found in better-differentiated cancers, and their presence may assist in the proper classification of the neoplasm. With increasing anaplasia, the tumor cells lose such refinements. For example, it is unusual for a cancer cell arising from bronchial epithelium to show cilia. Some cytoplasmic changes are seen better by the electron microscope, such as variation in size and decrease in number of mitochondria and degenerative changes of the mitochondria, the endoplasmic reticulum, and the microfilaments. None of the electron microscopic alterations is constant or diagnostic, and the chief value of the electron microscope in tumor study is in assisting in the classification of the individual tumor by identifying specific cytoplasmic substances such as myofibrils. Although there are frequent plasma membrane defects in cancer cells, there is none that is constant in all neoplastic cells. In fact, the opposite is the case because variability of plasma membrane composition is a common aspect of neoplasia.

The *nuclei* of the tumor cells show the most obvious deviations from normal, but again it must be emphasized that the nucleus of a tumor cell may look microscopically identical to the nucleus of a normal cell. Usually the nuclei of cancer cells are enlarged, often disproportionate to the cell size (Figs. 15-14 and 15-15). The chromatin is increased or condensed, and nucleoli become more prominent. The amount of nucleoprotein is increased. Nuclei are frequently lobed or otherwise irregular in shape and may show the same tendency to pleomorphism as the cell itself. Mitoses are usually more frequent than in normal tissues, and atypical mitoses, often resulting in multinucleated cells, occur (Fig. 15-16). The nuclear membrane generally is thickened.

Although there may be no obvious change from the normal, cells of many neoplasms, particularly malignant neoplasms, may show a slight to an extreme deviation in both morphology and number of *chromosomes* (Fig. 15-17). For example, in 80% to 90% of patients with chronic granulocytic leukemia, a marker chromosome, the Philadelphia (Ph[1]) chromosome, is present in granulocyte, monocyte, erythrocyte, and megakaryocyte precursors. It results from the translocation of part of the long arm of chromosome 22 to the long arm of chromosome 9 (t9;22) and perhaps also from the reciprocal translocation of a smaller part of the long arm of chromosome 9 to the long arm of chromosome 22. Moreover, leukemic cells from patients with acute myeloblastic leukemia may exhibit translocation of the long arm of chromosome 8 to the long arm of chromosome 21 (t8;21), whereas leukemic cells

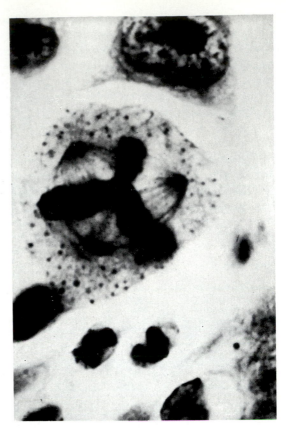

Fig. 15-16. Abnormal tripolar mitosis occurring in malignant melanoma. (Phosphotungstic acid–hematoxylin; 2350×.)

from patients with acute promyelocytic leukemia may show a translocation from the long arm of chromosome 17 to the long arm of chromosome 15 (t17;15). Finally, in the majority of patients with Burkitt's lymphoma, the neoplastic cells exhibit reciprocal translocation between chromosomes 8 and 14 (t8;14) and, less often, between chromosomes 8 and 2 (t8;2) or 8 and 22 (t8;22). Chromosomal aberrations seen in solid tumors usually involve deletions. For example, a deletion in chromosome 11 may be present in Wilms' tumor cells, a deletion in chromosome 13 may be found in a proportion of retinoblastoma cells, and chromosome 22 may be lost in human meningioma cells. In summary, cytogenetic studies indicate that cells in the majority of human neoplasms exhibit some chromosomal defect and that in as many as half of the cases such defect is recurrent; that is, it is characterized by the presence of a marker chromosome. There has been no conclusive evidence that any of the aforementioned chromosomal defects are causally related to the initiation or the persistence of the neoplastic state. Nevertheless, the recurrent presence of marker chromosomes strongly suggests that there might be some cause-effect relationship between the two.

It has been found that various types of neoplasms are more likely to develop in persons who exhibit inherited or acquired chromosomal defects in their somatic cells.

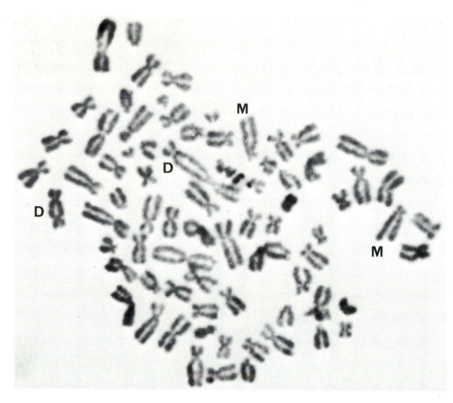

Fig. 15-17. Chromosome preparation of tumor cell from patient with breast cancer. Cell is hyperdiploid showing 74 chromosomes, including two markers, *M,* and two dicentrics, *D.*

For example, chromosome 21 is present in triplicate in patients with Down's syndrome; it is noteworthy that acute lymphoblastic or myeloblastic leukemia is 20 times as common in patients with this syndrome as in the general population. Patients with Fanconi's anemia whose cells are characterized by chromosomal aberrations have a higher risk of monocytic or myelomonocytic leukemia. Finally, chromosomal defects that result in somatic cells from exposure to x-ray irradiation may predispose an individual to cancer development.

Although any one of the foregoing cytoplasmic, nuclear, or chromosomal changes may at times be seen in nonneoplastic and benign neoplastic tissues, the multiple and severe changes described previously are found predominantly in cells of malignant tumors. The appreciation that some cancer cells are so atypical that they can be recognized individually as such, without any knowledge of their relationship to each other and to the surrounding normal tissues, has allowed the development of a diagnostic technique known as exfoliative cytology. This technique, which was developed by Dr. George Papanicolaou and is usually called the Pap smear, is based on two principles: (1) individual cancer cells often can be diagnosed as such microscopically by their large size, their pleomorphism, their increased nucleus-to-cytoplasm ratio, their hyperchromasia of nuclei, their prominent nucleoli, and their abnormal mitoses (see Fig. 15-25), and (2) cancer cells exfoliate more readily than

normal cells, most likely because their cohesiveness is lowered as a result of either a decrease in the number of tight junctions or a lowered calcium content.

The study of exfoliated cells permits the diagnosis of cancer at its earliest possible stages, even when still in situ, that is, while it is noninvasive and has not produced signs or symptoms recognizable clinically. This is of great importance in terms of prognosis because early diagnosis usually means high curability. Although exfoliative cytology has limitations, its great value is that it can be employed as a screening procedure for large numbers of people at low cost. We emphasize, however, that a positive Pap smear should be verified by a biopsy of the tissue in question. As a test, it is of the greatest value in the early diagnosis of cancer of the uterine cervix. It is of lesser value for diagnosis of cancer of the lung, endometrium, stomach, kidney, and urinary bladder.

Some tumors do not exfoliate, but cells still may be aspirated with a needle and syringe and recognized as cancerous by means of similar criteria. This technique, fine needle aspiration, is particularly useful for solid tumors such as those of the thyroid, breast, and pancreas.

Tumor cells, benign or malignant, growing in vitro usually do not show any structural features that are pathognomonic of neoplasia. However, some of these cells growing in culture may show altered morphology characterized by pleomorphism and an increase in growth rate, and cytogenetic studies often reveal chromosomal abnormalities. Such morphologic alterations are most likely epiphenomena of the neoplastic process because in vitro, established lines of nonmalignant normal cells may exhibit similar morphologic and cultural characteristics, but to a lesser extent.

Tumor stroma

In addition to the tumor cells proper (parenchyma), a tumor has a stroma, that is, a supporting framework of connective tissue and vascular supply. The stroma is derived from the normal tissues of the host and is a part of the tumor only in a passive sense. The amount and vascularity of the stroma vary greatly. In general, rapidly growing tumors, particularly sarcomas, have a highly vascular stroma with little connective tissue. More slowly growing tumors are less well vascularized. In some cases most of the tumor consists of dense connective tissue stroma. The formation of excessive connective tissue stroma in a tumor is called *desmoplasia* (Fig. 15-18), and cancers showing such a change are called *scirrhous*. Some tumors stimulate the formation of cartilage or bone in the stroma. Tumors with little stroma and composed mostly of tumor cells are called *medullary*.

New blood vessels and vascular channels in a tumor arise from older, preexisting vessels (angiogenesis). It has been known for a long time that tumor cells in vivo elicit an early and sustained ingrowth of new capillaries from the host's vessels. Only recently, however, has a substance been isolated from various human and animal neoplasms that has a mitogenic effect on capillary endothelium. This *tumor-angiogenesis factor* (TAF) appears to be secreted by the tumor parenchymal cells themselves. Of practical interest is the fact that no solid tumor can grow to more than 2 to 3 mm in diameter without neovascularization; if the activity of TAF could be blocked by a specific antibody or a chemical, angiogenesis would not occur, and the tumor would not continue to grow.

Lymphocytes, histiocytes, and plasma cells at times infiltrate the stroma of various benign and malignant tumors. This mononuclear cell reaction may represent response to local irritation by the tumor, but it also may be a host immunologic defense mechanism to the neoplastic process.

Although nerves may be present in tumors as a result of survival during infiltration of preexisting normal structures, and although nerve filaments may be found, chiefly in relation to stromal vessels, tumors are not under nervous control. Some tumors actually have neurons as components, but they appear to be nonfunctioning. Until tumors are large enough to impinge on preexisting nerves, pain does not result.

Biochemistry

Numerous attempts to delineate basic biochemical differences between tumor cells and normal cells have thus far been inconclusive. Of particular concern in studying

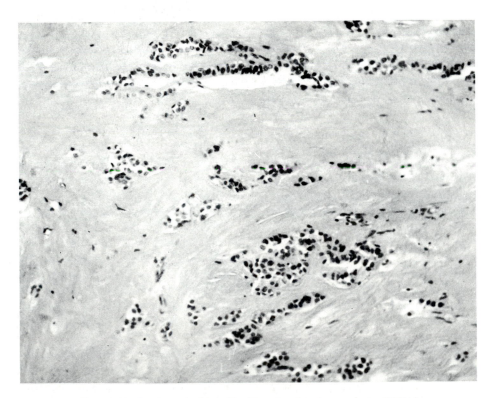

Fig. 15-18. Carcinoma of breast with extensive desmoplasia. (125×.)

the biochemistry of tumor cells is the composition of the enzymes that distinguishes normal cells from cancer cells. Also of concern is the determination of the particular pathways of biosynthesis that might be drug sensitive and thus amenable to chemotherapeutic measures. The vast diversity of detail in basic biochemical reactions on which both normal and tumorous cell growth and division depend makes the problem extremely difficult. One of the early theories was that of Warburg, who discovered anaerobic glycolysis in cancer tissue and hypothesized that it characterized all cancer tissue, but not normal tissue; he postulated a fundamental problem of intermediary metabolism and its regulation. The theory of Greenstein emphasizes the convergence in tumors toward common and more primitive enzymes and a general loss of enzymes not necessary for the basic existence of the cell. Another theory suggests that cancer may be the result of a loss or an alteration of proteins that, although essential for control of growth, are not essential for survival. More recently, altered feedback mechanisms and cell interactions have been emphasized.

Tumor cells do not have specific enzymes, proteins, or metabolic changes that are common to all tumors, nor are such changes consistently different from normal cells. There is a great diversity of biochemical characteristics of both normal and neoplastic tissue, and as yet no differences are constant or specific enough to be of diagnostic value. Tumor enzyme patterns, however, do tend to resemble each other more than those of normal tissue. It has been suggested that there may be a minimal enzyme pattern common to all tumors; other enzyme patterns added to the minimal pattern perhaps influence the nature and characteristics of the tumor.

Functional characteristics

Although in most instances neoplastic cells expend their energy on proliferation rather than on production, often they make various substances, in varied amounts, either intracellularly or extracellularly.

Neoplastic epithelial cells may produce substances; for example, keratin may be produced by squamous cell carcinoma of the epidermis, mucus by adenocarcinoma of the colon, or bile by hepatoma. Mesenchymal tumor cells may produce large amounts of extracellular substances such as cartilage matrix, for example, produced by chondroma or chondrosarcoma, or osteoid produced by osteoma or osteosarcoma. Neoplastic melanocytes usually produce melanin (Fig. 15-19). Lymphosarcoma cells may produce macroglobulins, whereas plasma cells of multiple myeloma usually secrete Bence Jones or other abnormal proteins.

Benign or malignant tumors of endocrine organs, especially if well differentiated, are of special interest because they may produce hormones that cause host

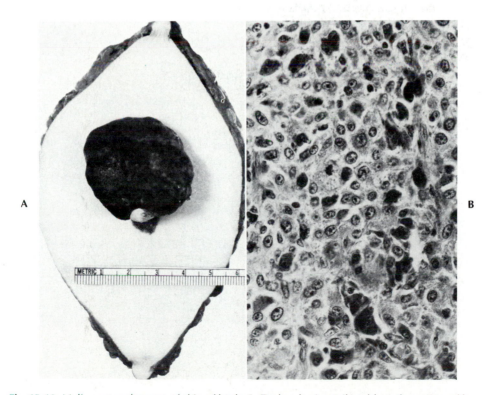

Fig. 15-19. Malignant melanoma of skin of back. **A,** Dark color is attributable to formation of large amounts of melanin by tumor cells. **B,** Photomicrograph of same tumor as **A.** Dark tumor cells contain much melanin pigment. (400×.)

effects disproportionate to their size and location. At times the presence of a tumor of an endocrine organ may be suggested by symptoms of excessive hormone production. Various clinical syndromes produced by hyperfunction of endocrine tumors, such as hyperinsulinism, acromegaly, and hyperparathyroidism, are discussed in other chapters. The following generalizations may be made regarding tumors arising in endocrine organs:

1. Endocrine tumors may or may not produce effective hormone.
2. If the tumor produces hormone, the production tends to be unregulated and may or may not be excessive.
3. Benign tumors are more likely to function than are malignant tumors.
4. The size of the tumor is not necessarily related to the degree of functional activity.
5. Metastases from endocrine cancers may function or hyperfunction.

With increasingly sensitive determinations of respective hormone levels in the blood, it is becoming possible to determine that a patient has a specific endocrine tumor not otherwise detectable by physical examination or usual diagnostic procedures. For example, radioimmunoassays of thyrocalcitonin might show an elevated blood level and indicate the presence of a medullary carcinoma of the thyroid that otherwise would be occult, that is, undetectable by the usual clinical examinations.

In addition to hormone production by tumors of endocrine glands, hormones or hormonelike substances may be produced by tumors seemingly unrelated in structure to the appropriate endocrine gland. Such ectopic or inappropriate hormone production may be found in tumors of endocrine, as well as nonendocrine, organs and tissues. The phenomenon is not entirely random, since some tumors are more likely to produce ectopic hormone than are others. For example, adrenocorticotropic hormone may be secreted by small-cell undifferentiated carcinomas of the lung (Fig. 15-20), islet cell tumors of the pancreas, thymomas, medullary carcinomas of the thyroid, and other tumors of both endocrine and nonendocrine tissues. Moreover, small-cell carcinomas of the lung may secrete antidiuretic hormone. Some adenocarcinomas of the colon and of the breast have parathyroid hormonelike activity. Hepatocellular carcinomas may secrete hormones similar to gonadotropic hormone, resulting in sexual precocity. This type of tumor function has been termed *ectopic hormone syndrome*. It may signify gene derepression leading to the expression of new gene func-

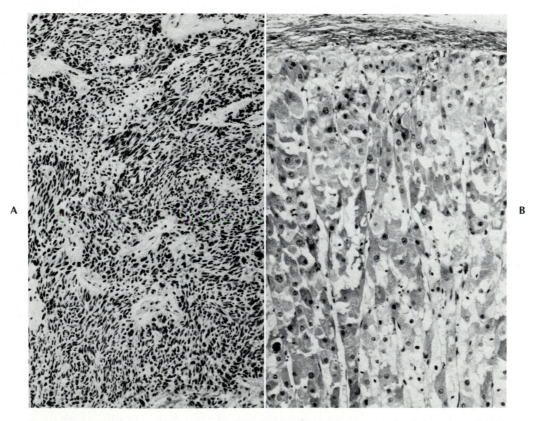

Fig. 15-20. A, Carcinoma of bronchus, small-cell type. Since tumor cells are often spindle shaped, cancer is sometimes called "oat cell." This tumor secreted excessive ACTH resulting in adrenocortical hyperplasia, **B,** and Cushing's syndrome. (**A,** 125×; **B,** 300×.)

tions. Frequently tumors with seemingly inappropriate secretions arise from cells originating in the neural crest and have common cytochemical properties of amine precursor uptake and decarboxylation (APUD). Such APUD cells include, for example, the C cells of the thyroid, the argentaffin cells of the lung and gastrointestinal tract, the islet cells of the pancreas, and cells of the adrenal medulla.

Neoplastic cells may produce excessive amounts of enzymes. For example, the level of acid phosphatase of prostatic origin is elevated in 75% of patients with disseminated carcinoma of the prostate, but in only 20% of patients in whom the carcinoma is confined within the prostatic capsule. Serum amylase levels are elevated in 25% of patients with pancreatic carcinoma. Many cancers produce a plasminogen-activating enzyme, which by lysing fibrin may contribute to the invasive or metastatic properties of the tumor. On the other hand, neoplastic cells may lose a marker enzyme. For example, granulocytes of chronic granulocytic leukemia have a decreased or absent alkaline phosphatase content, whereas cells of endocrine tumors may lack specific enzymes, which usually results in the production of unfinished hormonal products, for example, the manufacturing of proinsulin by a pancreatic islet cell adenoma.

Neoplastic cells may produce a number of systemic pathologic states by introducing into the host abnormal amounts of chemical substances. For example, carcinoma of the stomach or pancreas may induce increased coagulability of blood that could result in thrombotic and thromboembolic episodes (see "Interrelationships of tumor and host").

Tumor-specific and tumor-associated antigens

The demonstration that inbred animals immunized against tumors from syngeneic (isologous) hosts reject tumors but not skin grafts from the same hosts has established the fact that tumor cells possess specific antigens differing from those of normal cells and capable of eliciting an immune response in the competent host. The antigens induced experimentally by chemicals differ from those induced by viruses; those found in spontaneous human tumors also differ.

Experimental tumors induced by chemical carcinogens

Two main features characterize the cellular antigens of tumors induced by chemical carcinogens. First, there is antigenic individuality: tumors induced by the same chemical carcinogen, either at different sites in the same animal or in different animals of the same inbred strain, do not cross-immunize against each other. Subpopulations of a single tumor may also possess antigenic individuality. Second, the degree of antigenicity among tumors induced by chemical carcinogens differs: tumors

induced at multiple sites in the same animal, or in different animals of the same strain, vary in their antigenic strength. For example, whereas appropriately immunized animals will reject as many as 10^6 to 10^7 cells of a given tumor, similarly immunized animals may be incapable of rejecting more than 10^3 to 10^4 cells of another tumor induced by the same chemical carcinogen.

Antigens that are found in cells of tumors induced by chemical carcinogens are located on the plasma membrane of the cells. In most cases these antigens are either weak or present in very small amounts so that they are incapable of eliciting a humoral response. In a few cases, however, the antigens are strong enough to stimulate antibody formation. This antibody can be used in immunofluorescence tests to localize tumor-specific antigens for visual inspection. It is likely that the carcinogenic agent plays a direct and decisive role in determining both antigenic individuality and differences in antigenic strength of chemically induced tumors. Possibly the chemical carcinogen, either directly or indirectly, induces random mutations at the level of the histocompatibility genes. As a result, the histocompatibility antigens are altered and become the tumor-specific transplantation antigens characteristic of the carcinogenic event.

Experimental tumors induced by oncogenic viruses

In contrast to the antigenic individuality exhibited by chemically induced tumors, neoplasms induced by a given oncogenic virus, at different sites in the same animal or in different animals belonging to the same or to different species, consist of neoplastic cells that share common antigens. In addition, the same antigens are present in various types of cells that are transformed in vitro by the same oncogenic virus. These antigens differ, however, from those found in cells rendered neoplastic in vivo or in vitro by another oncogenic virus. The main features of the antigenic components of tumors arising under the influence of DNA or RNA viruses follow.

Cells rendered neoplastic by oncogenic DNA viruses, such as simian virus 40 (SV40) or polyoma virus, contain new protein-antigens that are coded for by the viral genome. For example, cells transformed neoplastically by SV40 contain a nuclear protein—the large tumor (T) antigen (Fig. 15-21) of mol. wt. 90,000 daltons—and a cytoplasmic protein—the small T antigen of mol. wt. 17,000 daltons. Cells transformed neoplastically by polyoma virus always express two proteins, the middle T antigen of mol. wt. 56,000 daltons and the small T antigen of mol. wt. 22,000 daltons. The polyoma large T antigen of mol. wt. 100,000 daltons is not essential for neoplastic cell transformation, and its expression varies with different types of cells. In addition to these virus-coded proteins, which are identified in cells by immunologic or biochemical means, there are other types of virus-coded

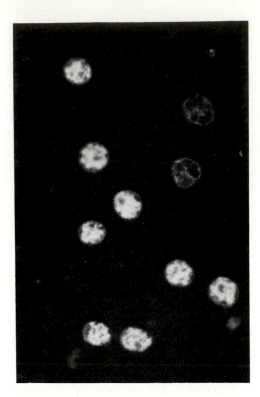

Fig. 15-21. Peripheral blood smear of hamster bearing lymphocytic leukemia induced by oncogenic DNA simian virus 40 (SV40). White (reacting) nuclei of leukemic lymphocytes have been stained by indirect immunofluorescence for SV40-mediated tumor (T) antigen. Two normal polymorphonuclear neutrophilic leukocytes are shown with nonreacting nuclei. Erythrocytes are faintly visible. (800×.)

cellular proteins, the tumor-specific transplantation (TST) antigens, which are identified on the plasma membrane of virus-transformed cells by in vivo transplantation rejection or oncogenesis prevention tests.

Cells rendered neoplastic by oncogenic RNA viruses release infectious virus continuously and as a result contain antigens specific for viral core proteins and viral envelope glycoproteins. It is also likely, although difficult to demonstrate because of the virus shedding, that they possess new virus-coded cell surface antigens that may be important in tumor regression or rejection. The killing by cytolytic T cells of murine hematopoietic cells rendered leukemic by the murine leukemia virus (an oncogenic RNA virus) seems to be determined by the ability of the killer cells to identify tumor-specific antigens in association with normal histocompatibility (H-2) antigens. This histocompatibility restriction of cell killing, known as the Zinkernagel-Doherty phenomenon, may explain how the immune system of a tumor-bearing host can identify and destroy tumor cells without harming normal cells. By understanding how the immune recognition of tumor cells takes place, we may be able to enhance the means by which the organism rejects tumors and thus be in a position to improve prognosis.

Human tumors developing spontaneously

Regression of malignant neoplasms in humans has been observed only rarely. Although in some of these instances regression was most likely caused by nonimmunologic factors such as hormone dependency and nutritional requirements, there are some malignant neoplasms, most notably choriocarcinoma and Burkitt's lymphoma, in which tumor regression may have had an immunologic basis. Humoral immune response to human tumors has been demonstrated recently by the immunofluorescence technique for cells of Burkitt's lymphoma, malignant melanoma, and osteosarcoma. In addition, cellular immunity, namely the presence of lymphocytes sensitized against tumor cells, has been shown to exist in patients with neuroblastoma and in those with other malignant tumors. Neoplastic cells may dedifferentiate morphologically and functionally and manifest an ability to produce substances usually found only in embryonic cells. For example, cells of many adenocarcinomas of the colon contain and secrete a glycoprotein identical to a component present in cells of embryonic colonic mucosa, whereas cells of most hepatocellular carcinomas contain and secrete an alpha$_1$ globulin that is normally produced by fetal hepatic parenchymal cells. Because the presence of these carcinoembryonic or oncofetal substances has been demonstrated in heterologous hosts, they have been called tumor-associated antigens. They do not behave, however, as antigens in the autologous host. From a practical point of view the identification of these substances in the serum of patients bearing such tumors can be of diagnostic and prognostic significance.

TUMOR BEHAVIOR
Growth rate

As a general rule, benign tumors grow slowly and malignant tumors rapidly. Many malignant tumors increase remarkably in size in weeks or months, whereas benign tumors often require years to attain a large size. Actually, however, there is a broad range of growth rates in tumors, even in tumors of the same histologic type.

An intriguing concept of tumor growth is based on doubling time of the tumor cells: after a tumor cell undergoes mitosis to become two, each daughter cell then divides to become four, eight, 16, and so on, with each successive division resulting in a doubling of the tumor mass (Fig. 15-22). If the growth rate were constant, the time for each doubling would be constant. A 10 μm diameter cancer cell would require 20 doublings to reach a tumor diameter of 1 mm, 30 doublings for 1 cm diameter, and 40 doublings to reach a weight of 1 kg. Thus, if all the cells of a tumor had a short interval between mitoses, the tumor size would increase rapidly unless there were other factors to prevent it. The doubling time of Burkitt's lymphoma has been estimated at 5

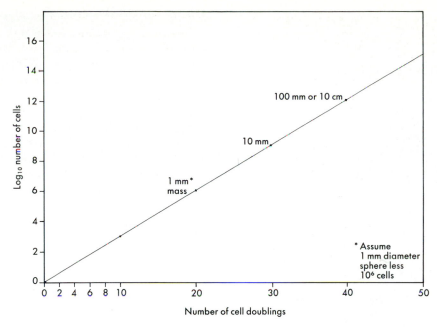

Fig. 15-22. Theoretical growth curve relating number of tumor doublings to number of tumor cells present and size of tumor.

days; other tumors have an estimated doubling time up to 200 days or more. As the tumor becomes larger, each doubling becomes more dramatic, even though the time for doubling remains constant. Although this concept may be true for some tumors, doubling times are inconstant often even in the same tumor, and there are many biologic and treatment influences that increase or decrease growth rates. For example, increase in bulk may be largely a result of necrosis, hemorrhage, and edema, any of which may occur suddenly and rapidly.

Microscopically, increased growth rate is demonstrated by the presence of mitoses and of young cells, which are frequent in cancer but relatively rare in benign tumors and most normal tissues. As many as 20 or more mitoses per thousand cells is a common proportion in a malignant tumor, whereas less than one mitosis per thousand cells is usual in benign tumors or normal tissues. It must be emphasized that neither rapidity of growth nor the presence of numerous mitoses is in itself necessarily an indication of tumor. Even abnormal mitoses are not pathognomonic of cancer, although they occur much more frequently in malignant tumors than in other tissues. Some tissues normally have a rapid turnover of cells. For example, the mitotic activity of the intestinal epithelium and the bone marrow may even be in excess of that found in adenocarcinoma of the colon and chronic granulocytic leukemia, respectively. Even at its maximum, the growth rate of a malignant tumor rarely exceeds that of embryonic tissues. The excessive mitotic rate in many cancers would lead one to expect even more rapid growth than actually occurs. The discrepancy is attributable to such factors as production of some nonvi-

able cells, desquamation of superficial cells when ulceration occurs, necrosis resulting from inadequate stromal blood supply with or without secondary bacterial infection, and loss of proliferative activity through cell differentiation.

There are indications that growth-controlling or regulatory mechanisms influence mitotic activity of neoplastic cells, but they are not well understood. Occasionally a tumor, either benign or malignant, becomes inactive (dormant) for a period of time and then resumes its active growth. Some experimental tumors have been found to produce lesser amounts of specific mitotic inhibitors, called *chalones*. Most likely control of neoplastic cell proliferation is the end product of the interplay of a variety of factors whose identity and relative importance await further investigation. The ability of cells and their daughter cells to proliferate excessively is of course a major concern in the study and treatment of tumors. Because a tumor cell that does not proliferate is of little importance to the patient, a great deal of cancer therapy, both by ionizing radiation and by chemotherapy, is directed at bringing about a cessation or suppression of mitosis in tumor cells.

Local growth and invasion

All tumors grow by expansion with a progressive increase in bulk and a resultant compression of the surrounding tissues. Most benign tumors merely push aside the surrounding normal tissues, and the compressed adjacent stroma often forms a capsule delineating the tumor. The growth of benign tumors becomes significant when expansion compresses important adjacent struc-

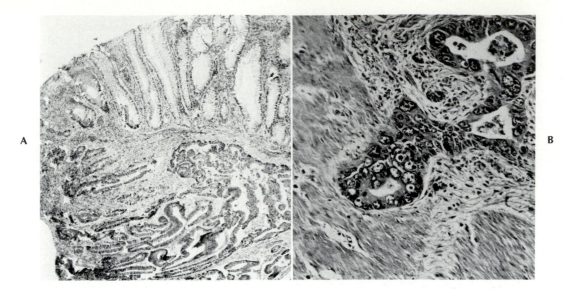

Fig. 15-23. A, Invasion of submucosa and muscularis by well-differentiated adenocarcinoma of colon. Some normal mucosa remains. **B,** Colonic adenocarcinoma invading muscularis. Same case as **A.** (**A,** 125×; **B,** 300×.)

tures or when the tumor is large enough to be unsightly. In addition, various retrogressive changes such as hemorrhage, infarction, and infection may cause a rapid increase in size of the benign neoplasm.

Malignant tumors also grow by expansion, and some low-grade cancers may develop partial encapsulation by the same mechanism as in benign neoplasms. Usually, however, malignant tumors invade, infiltrate, and destroy the adjacent normal tissues, and as a consequence their outlines usually are irregular and vague, rather than rounded and encapsulated as in benign tumors.

A primary characteristic of malignant tumors is their invasive ability, resulting in a continuous spread of the disease (Fig. 15-23). Locally, the invasion extends into the interstices of the surrounding normal tissues. The extent of such infiltration is of very practical importance in terms of therapy because if surgical removal of the tumor does not include adequate excision of the surrounding tissues, recurrence of the neoplasm is inevitable. The mechanisms responsible for the ability of malignant neoplastic cells to invade and destroy neighboring tissues are not well understood. It cannot be explained by the rapidity of growth of cancer cells and increased tissue pressures, since there are highly invasive tumors that grow rather slowly. Although many neoplastic cells are motile and possess phagocytic properties, these features are also found in normal cells, which lack the ability to invade. It is likely that cancer cells elaborate products that directly or indirectly are responsible for the phenomenon of invasion. For example, proteolytic enzymes or lytic factors formed by the tumor could modify the stroma at the growing margin, making the tissues more vulnerable to invasion. Collagenolytic substances have

been identified in cells of squamous cell carcinoma of the skin and in various sarcomas. Many tissues are resistant to invasion because they are resistant to the action of various products being elaborated by cancer cells. For example, structures such as cartilage, tendon, ligament, dense fibrous tissue, and the elastica of arteries are almost completely impervious to tumor invasion. As a result, they act like natural barriers to the invading cancer cells. Soft tissues and muscle, on the other hand, are easily invaded.

Carcinoma in situ is a growth disturbance in which there is sufficient atypicality of the epithelial cells and their arrangement to warrant the diagnosis of cancer in the absence of invasion (Fig. 15-24). The exact line of demarcation between carcinoma in situ and severe atypical hyperplasia cannot be defined consistently. Although there is still some controversy regarding the nature of carcinoma in situ, with some investigators believing that it represents a reversible change, most pathologists consider it a true intraepithelial neoplasm that frequently progresses to invasive carcinoma. It may be seen in many tissues of the body, but particularly in the epidermis, the mucosa of the cervix, the endometrium, and the bronchial epithelium. Cells desquamating from carcinoma in situ often are recognizable cytologically as cancer cells (Fig. 15-25).

Metastasis

The invasive property of cancer not only accounts for continuous local extension of the disease but also initiates and promotes the development of another important method of tumor spread. Metastasis is a process in which malignant tumor cells invade vessels or local tissue spaces in such a manner that they may detach and

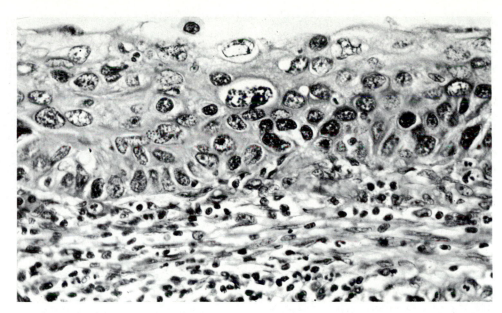

Fig. 15-24. Carcinoma in situ of cervix. Note extreme atypicality of cells near surface and that one cell has desquamated. From such desquamated cells, cytologic diagnosis of cancer can be made. (500×.)

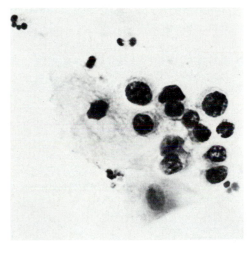

Fig. 15-25. Exfoliated cancer cells in Papanicolaou smear from uterine cervix. (500×.)

migrate or be transported to a distant site, where they finally lodge and grow in the new location to form a secondary tumor mass. The term *metastasis* is used not only for the process itself but also for the new discontinuous secondary growth. The ability to metastasize is a property of many malignant tumors but not of any benign tumors. The usual routes of dissemination of detached tumor cells are through lymphatic vessels or blood vessels as emboli, through serous cavities, occasionally by transport in the spinal fluid, through hollow structures such as bronchi or ureters, and rarely by contact with an apposing structure.

The most common route for the metastatic spread of cancer is through the lymphatic vessels. In general, car-

cinomas tend to metastasize this way, whereas sarcomas favor the venous route. Once tumor cells have invaded lymphatic vessels, they may detach to become emboli or they may form a continuous growth within the vessel itself. The latter type of growth is known as lymphatic permeation and usually accounts only for local spread of the disease; extension by growth along nerves, often by what appears to be permeation of lymphatic spaces, is an important method of local extension in many cancers (Fig. 15-26). The more common process is for detached tumor cells to be carried as emboli to the peripheral sinus of a regional lymph node where the tumor cells multiply and eventually invade the lymphoid pulp and develop supporting stroma (Fig. 15-27). The entire lymph node gradually becomes replaced and considerably enlarged by the metastatic tumor. Sooner or later the capsule will be invaded, but it often remains intact for a long time.

The role of the lymph node as a filter or barrier to the spread of cancer cells is not well understood. Lymph nodes are often believed to damage tumor cells but, conversely, they also seem to provide a fertile soil for their growth. Perhaps an initial barrier, filter, or destructive function is eventually overcome because of intensity or duration of cancer cell embolization.

With a knowledge of the primary site, the most likely distribution of lymph node metastasis can be surmised. For example, a carcinoma of the breast commonly metastasizes to the axillary lymph nodes, carcinoma of the scrotum to inguinal lymph nodes, and carcinoma of the stomach to the lymph nodes along the greater and lesser curvatures. Sometimes, however, because of vagaries of lymphatic flow or obstruction of lymphatics, metastasis in a distant or unusual site may be the first to appear. For example, carcinoma of the left side of the lip occasionally may metastasize to one of the posterior cervical lymph nodes on the right side or a carcinoma of the prostate may metastasize to the supraclavicular lymph nodes.

Metastasis through blood vessels is the common route for sarcomas, but frequently carcinomas also metastasize this way. Certain carcinomas such as those of the lung, breast, kidney, prostate, and thyroid are particularly likely to show blood-borne metastases. Once cancer cells of the main tumor mass have invaded blood vessels, they may detach as tumor emboli, either as single cells or, especially if a thrombus forms around them, as cellular aggregates of various sizes (Fig. 15-28). Although occasionally a large mass of tumor (for example, of sufficient size to cause fatal pulmonary embolism) becomes detached, the most frequent size is a few hundred micrometers or less. The mechanism of embolization of tumor cells is simple: they are transported like all emboli through their respective vascular system. Thus cancers of an organ that drains normally into the portal vein system tend to metastasize to the liver (Fig. 15-29); most other cancers metastasize through the caval veins to the lungs. Since it is easier for tumor cells to invade venules and veins than to invade arteries, metastasis by the arterial route is of less significance except in the case of tumors of the lung. As with lymphatic metastases, blood-borne metastases may at times appear at unusual sites

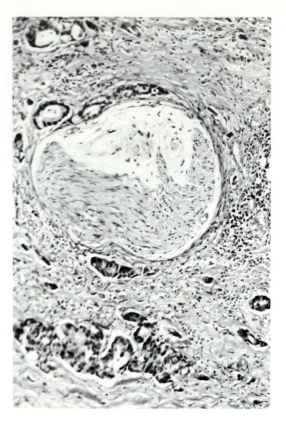

Fig. 15-26. Adenocarcinoma of lung with perineural invasion. Part of nerve shows degeneration. (125×.)

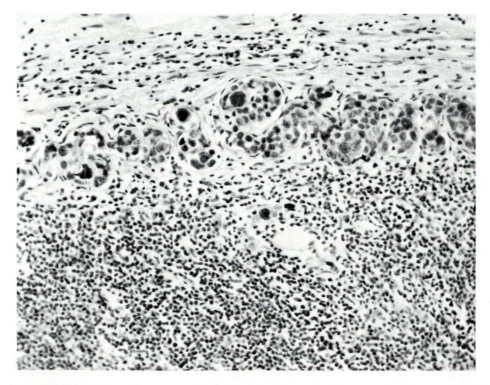

Fig. 15-27. Metastatic carcinoma in peripheral sinus of inguinal lymph node. Tumor lies just beneath capsule and is beginning to invade pulp. (250×.)

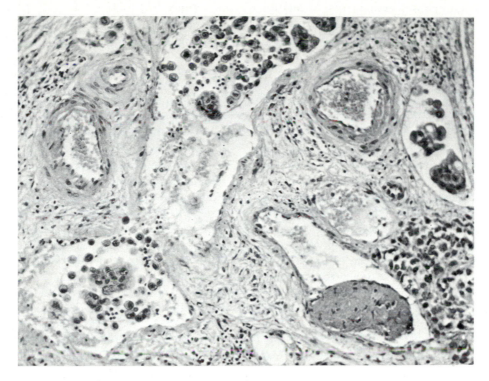

Fig. 15-28. Extensive blood vessel invasion by carcinoma of pancreas. Note thrombus in one small vein. (250×.)

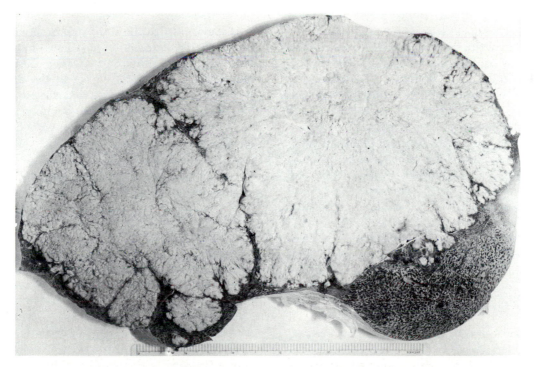

Fig. 15-29. Section of liver showing almost complete replacement of parenchyma by metastatic carcinoma. Primary tumor was in colon.

because of retrograde metastasis occurring after venous obstruction or aberrant vascular anastomoses. An anastomotic paravertebral plexus of veins (Batson's plexus) may allow tumor emboli to be diverted from the regular systemic venous circulation into the vertebral veins, particularly when there is increased intra-abdominal pressure; this mechanism may partially account for the high incidence of metastasis to the vertebrae from posterior midline cancers such as carcinoma of the prostate.

For cancers in the appropriate locations, a spread through serous cavities, such as peritoneum, is common once the tumor has invaded the serosa of its organ so that it may become detached and mechanically disseminated. Metastases developing through the transcoelomic route in the peritoneum tend to gravitate to the pelvis into the rectovaginal or rectovesicle pouches. Other possible routes of metastatic spread, such as through the spinal fluid, through ureters, through bronchi, or to apposing tissues (as from the lower lip to the upper lip) are infrequent. For some reason, tumor cells implanted on the intact surface of normal tissue do not seem to grow well. Cancers may, however, be mechanically transported and implanted by a surgeon's scalpel, needle, or sutures; care must be taken during surgery not to contaminate the wound with cancer cells.

Since a metastasis represents a colony of the primary tumor, it is not surprising that it usually resembles the primary mass in color, consistency, and microscopic appearance. As a general rule, however, the metastasis is less invasive than the primary tumor, tends to be more regular in outline, and sometimes is even encapsulated (for example, a metastatic carcinoma to the brain is better demarcated than a primary glioma of the brain). Although the metastasis may be either more or less differentiated than the parent tumor, the histologic resemblance is usually such that it is possible to make a shrewd estimate as to the nature and site of the primary tumor from a study of the metastasis. At times there is a problem of distinguishing a primary tumor from its metastasis, since a primary neoplasm may be large with small metastases or small with large metastases. Even occult cancers (those not detectable by clinical methods alone) may give rise to metastases, and the secondary growth may be the first indication of cancer. If there are multiple cancerous nodules in an organ, they are probably metastatic. Some tumors metastatic in bone stimulate excessive new bone formation. Such osteoplastic metastases are particularly frequent in cancers arising from the prostate or breast.

Because the local growth of many cancers can be eradicated or controlled effectively, the presence or absence of metastases is one of the most important criteria in determining the prognosis of an individual cancer case. It is obvious that if multiple metastases are present, local therapy will not cure the disease. It is not surprising that

the mechanisms of metastasis continue to be studied intensively.

Three steps, as previously noted, are necessary for production of metastasis: (1) invasion of cancer cells into lymphatics or blood vessels or into appropriate tissue spaces, (2) detachment of the cells with embolization or other mechanical transport, and (3) lodgment and progressive growth of the cells in a new location. Every cancer has its own particular growth characteristics, including the ability to invade and metastasize, the time required for metastasis, and the place to which metastases occur. Metastatic ability of a tumor is, of course, influenced by its location, since the nature of the vascular supply of the primary site is important. Many cancers seem to be capable of entering the first step in the development of metastasis without necessarily continuing the process to the point of completion. For example, blood vessel invasion is relatively common in many cancers, but it does not necessarily mean that metastasis has already taken place, or that it will. Transport, the second step in the development of metastasis, is more or less mechanical. It is assisted by natural movements of the part, such as peristalsis, and by excessive manipulation of the tumor by the patient or physician. Again, however, even the presence of tumor cells in the bloodstream does not necessarily mean that metastasis will take place. There is considerable evidence that tumor cells are often embolic in blood or lymphatic vessels without production of metastasis. Many tumor cells must be lost along the course.

It is evident that the third step in the development of metastasis is of much importance—tumor cells must lodge and grow in their new location. Not all organs and tissues are equally susceptible to the development of metastases. For example, metastases are relatively uncommon in the spleen or in skeletal muscle, although both must receive many tumor emboli. Conversely, metastases grow well in the liver. Such differences in the "soil" are not well understood and may be related to such factors as variation in vascular size and permeability, local nourishment, and local resistance.

GRADING AND STAGING OF CANCERS

At times an estimate of the degree or grade of malignancy of a cancer may be useful for prognosis and for determination of type of treatment. Such grading is applied only to malignant tumors. Cancers in some locations may be graded roughly by their gross appearance because often those that show an exophytic or fungating type of growth are less malignant than those that are diffusely infiltrating. More frequently, tumors are graded microscopically, with two factors being considered: (1) the degree of anaplasia or undifferentiation of the tumor and (2) an estimate of the rate of growth. Customarily tumors are graded numerically into three or four grades,

Table 15-3. Grading of epidermoid carcinoma of the oral mucosa

	Grade		
	I	II	III
Evidence of differentiation			
Intercellular bridges	+	±	−
Keratinization	+	+	±
Epithelial pearls	+	±	−
Evidence of rapid, abnormal proliferation			
Mitoses per high-power field	<2	2-4	>4
Atypical mitoses	−	±	+
Nuclear and cellular pleomorphism	±	+	+
Multinucleated and tumor giant cells	−	−	+

+, Present; ±, may or may not be present; −, absent.

with the low numbers implying a lesser degree of malignancy. Evidence of differentiation is based on the resemblance of the tumor to the normal tissue prototype. For example, a well-differentiated tumor arising from squamous epithelium would be expected to form considerable amounts of keratin and intercellular bridges. The estimate of rapidity of growth is based on the number of mitoses per unit of tissue (for example, per high-power field) and the increase of nuclear chromatin. Table 15-3 shows as an example the histologic grading of epidermoid carcinoma of the oral mucosa.

Sometimes tumors that were once low grade become increasingly malignant with passage of time so that a cancer that was once growing very slowly becomes high grade and invades and metastasizes widely and rapidly. For example, papillary carcinoma of the thyroid, one of the lowest grade and slowest growing of all cancers, may transform into a giant cell carcinoma, which is one of the most highly malignant of all tumors; chronic granulocytic leukemia may progress into myeloblastic leukemia ("blast crisis"), which is much more malignant. Rarely, tumors become more differentiated and of a lower grade; an example is the malignant neuroblastoma, which at times differentiates into a benign ganglioneuroma.

Although grading of tumors is a fairly common practice, it has limited clinical usefulness because of several difficulties. Although, in general, tumors are uniform throughout in histologic appearance, some vary considerably from portion to portion; hence, a biopsy from one region may give a false impression of the degree of malignancy present in another area. The estimation of degree of malignancy must also take into consideration the primary site of the tumor, since normal tissues vary in their degree of differentiation. In any event, the prognosis achieved by gross or histologic grading obviously does not take into account such factors as the duration of the tumor, the presence or absence of metastasis, and the age of the patient, all of which are of great clinical importance in determining prognosis. Consequently, the chief value of grading is in the field of group prognosis and in evaluation of therapy of groups rather than individual cases.

The stage of a cancer is the evaluation of its extent, based usually on gross and clinical findings. It is not judged by the grade of the tumor. Consideration is given to the size and extent of the primary tumor (T), the presence and extent of lymph node (N) metastases, and the presence of distant metastases (M). By combining these three evaluations a staging system (TNM) has been developed as a useful method of describing the extent of spread of an individual tumor at a given time. As an example, p. 1474 shows a suggested method of staging of carcinoma of the cervix, and on p. 1554 is a reference to the TNM system of staging as applied to breast cancer.

INTERRELATIONSHIPS OF TUMOR AND HOST

Benign tumors affect the host primarily because of their size or location. A large benign tumor is a nuisance and a cosmetic problem, and it may compress important structures. Because benign tumors, especially the larger ones, often undergo retrogressive changes, such as infarction and hemorrhage, they may show a sudden increase in size, giving the false impression of rapid cellular growth. Even a small benign tumor, however, may at times be of importance to the host because of location; for example, a tumor in the region of the ampulla of Vater may be less than 1 cm in diameter and still cause severe biliary obstruction. Similarly, some benign endocrine tumors, even when small, may produce excessive amounts of hormone and in this way be harmful to the host.

Malignant neoplasms have the same potential effects on the host as the benign tumors, but the effects are accentuated by the more rapid, invasive growth. Cancers have a greater tendency than do benign tumors to necrosis, infarction, ulceration, and hemorrhage. Symptoms of anemia produced by hemorrhage or by the presence of tumor products, symptoms of obstruction attributable to involvement of hollow viscera, and symptoms of pressure attributable to both compression and destruction of tissue are all common findings in cancer (Figs. 15-30 and 15-31). Most patients with cancer eventually become so weakened and often immunodeficient from the disseminated disease that they become highly susceptible to infection, especially bronchopneumonia, which is the most common immediate cause of death in cancer patients. Many patients who die from cancer, particularly if the tumor is widely disseminated, show an extreme wasting or malnutrition called *cachexia*. It has a number of causes, including the ulceration, hemorrhage, and infection, the necrosis of tissues with release of toxins,

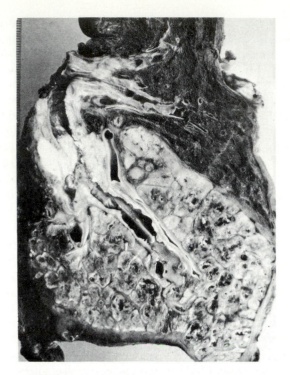

Fig. 15-30. Carcinoma of bronchus with secondary infection. Relatively small tumor surrounds and occludes lobar bronchus near hilum. Distal to tumor, bronchi are dilated and suppuration is extensive.

the immunodeficiency, and the sleeplessness and anxiety that many terminal cancer patients experience. The cachexia of cancer is not caused primarily by the extravagant nutritional demands of widespread tumor, nor is it caused by any specific toxin that the cancer produces; similar cachexia is seen in patients dying of other wasting diseases, such as disseminated tuberculosis.

There are innumerable other but inconstant systemic effects produced by tumors. Since the mechanisms of their development are rarely understood, only a few are mentioned as examples: dermatomyositis may develop in patients with various types of cancer; unexplained peripheral neuritis and degenerative brain changes may occur in cancer patients; and acanthosis nigricans (a hyperpigmented, keratotic skin lesion) suggests the likelihood of carcinoma, usually of the stomach. Many tumor effects are biochemical. For example, there may be a disturbed salt metabolism in some patients who have carcinoma of the stomach; there may be a diminution or elevation of various serum enzymes, such as the acid phosphatase that often is elevated in patients with prostatic cancer. Many changes in the blood, especially in serum proteins, have been reported in cancer patients, such as a deficiency in specific proteins or the presence of abnormal proteins. Since increased coagulability of the blood may complicate cancers, particularly those of the pancreas and stomach, the development of sudden unexplained thrombotic episodes indicates the possibility of cancer of the upper abdomen. Unfortunately none of

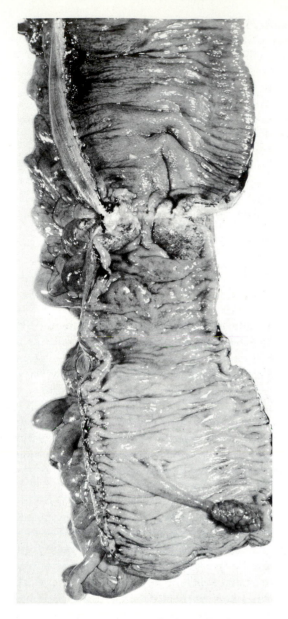

Fig. 15-31. Constricting carcinoma of colon with dilatation of bowel proximal to tumor. Pedunculated polyp is an incidental finding.

these changes is constant enough to be reliable as a diagnostic test for cancer. The following are some further examples of inconstant effects produced by tumors:

Hematologic
    Anemia, erythrocytosis, thrombocytopenia, thrombocytosis, leukemoid reaction, abnormal serum proteins
Dermatologic
    Pruritus, urticaria, erythema, hyperpigmentation, dermatomyositis
Neurologic
    Neuropathy, myelopathy, encephalopathy
Skeletal
    Osteoporosis, osteomalacia
The nature of the mechanisms of host resistance

against the development and growth of tumors is still incompletely understood. There is a wide range of virulence with cancers of the same histologic and clinical types in different individuals. Most malignant neoplasms exhibit more aggressive behavior in the young; a few, however, such as carcinoma of the thyroid, seem more malignant in older persons. Many tumors are either hormonally dependent or can be influenced by hormone therapy. The presence or absence of adequate blood supply also may alter tumor growth. Finally, in both human and experimental tumors host-mediated immunity seems to play either a synergistic or an antagonistic role in the pathogenesis of neoplasia.

COURSE AND TREATMENT

The biologic behavior of a tumor depends on multiple factors, some of which are inherent in the tumor itself and others in the host. Certainly there is an interplay of tumor-host relationships so that multiple factors combine to determine the ultimate biologic behavior of the neoplasm. Benign tumors not only grow slowly but also at times reach a point where they seem to become dormant or even to regress. This is true, for example, with leiomyomas of the uterus, which often cease growing after menopause. Occasionally even malignant tumors enter a stage of dormancy, and in rare, but well-documented, instances they may regress spontaneously. Spontaneous regression is defined as the complete or partial disappearance of cancer that cannot be attributed to treatment. The explanations for the phenomenon are inconclusive. Cancers of many different sites and types have shown such regression, the more common being renal cell carcinoma, neuroblastoma, choriocarcinoma, and malignant melanoma.

The more typical and usual course of untreated cancer is continuous local and metastatic extension with progressive systemic effects, all of which combine to weaken the host in diverse ways until cachexia and death from bronchopneumonia ensue. About half of the deaths in cancer patients result from infections, the most common being bronchopneumonia, septicemia, and peritonitis. The majority of infections are caused by gram-negative bacilli. Other causes of death in these patients include organ failure, tumor infarction and hemorrhage, and carcinomatosis (widespread dissemination of the tumor).

With treatment, many tumors, though not cured, may persist for years before ultimately causing death. Some patients live many years with cancer even without treatment. Daland[9] studied 100 cases of untreated cancer of the breast and found that 22% of the patients were alive at the end of 5 years and 5% at the end of 10 years; the last surviving patients died 13 years after their first symptoms. Usually, the course of a cancer nowadays is influenced by therapy, but it is often difficult to distinguish between therapeutic response and biologic predeterminism of the tumor.

Since many lesions may be confused with tumor clinically, treatment should not be started until there is microscopic confirmation of neoplasm. Treatment is based on the gross and microscopic evaluation and classification of the tumor by the pathologist and on the extent and location of the tumor. During an operation the microscopic diagnosis and classification of a tumor may be carried out with a high degree of accuracy by the pathologist's use of a rapid frozen-section technique. Surgery, irradiation, anticancer drugs, immunotherapy, or any combination of these may be selected to treat a particular tumor. The goal of therapy is complete eradication or destruction of all the cancer and thus a cure. Unfortunately this is not always possible, and palliative therapy is then directed at slowing the rate of growth and eradicating portions of the tumor to prolong the patient's life and alleviate pain and suffering. In general, surgical removal, when feasible, continues to be the most common and practical approach to the treatment of cancer.

In recent years, there has been great progress in the use of drugs as specific therapeutic agents against cancer. Since some tumors are hormone dependent, effective palliation may result from a change in the accustomed hormonal environment on which the tumor depends. For example, carcinoma of the prostate may be controlled for a time by the lowering of androgen levels (orchiectomy) or by administering estrogen in large amounts. Cancer of the breast in premenopausal women may respond favorably to removal of estrogen (oophorectomy, adrenalectomy, hypophysectomy) or to testosterone administration. Anticancer drugs now in use, in addition to hormones and other steroid compounds, include alkylating agents, antimetabolites, and miscellaneous drugs, such as urethan and actinomycin D. In some instances chemotherapeutic drugs produce a favorable and even a prolonged response. Since such agents interfere with the synthesis of nucleic acids and proteins, not only tumor cells but normal cells as well may be destroyed. New drugs are continually being developed that have more selective anticancer effects. Some tumors that are highly responsive to chemotherapy include Hodgkin's disease, Wilms' tumor, choriocarcinoma, and acute lymphatic leukemia.

Although the effects of radiation on tissues in general have been described in Chapter 6, certain aspects deserve mention here. The therapeutic effects of radiation on a tumor depend on (1) the direct effect on the tumor cells, (2) the impairment of blood supply, and (3) fibrosis and hyalinization of the stroma, both of which impair nutritional exchange and hinder the spread of tumor cells. Much more irradiation is required to kill tumor cells in tissue culture than is necessary to kill them in the organism. Tumors, both benign and malignant, vary in their response to radiation according to their cell type, vascularity, and stromal support.

Radiosensitivity means the responsiveness of a given

tumor to ionizing radiation therapy, as evidenced by shrinkage with partial or complete regression of the tumor. This is brought about through attenuation or disruption of the reproductive ability of the neoplasm. In general, the so-called law of Bergonié and Tribondeau holds: poorly differentiated tumors respond to radiation well and better-differentiated tumors respond poorly. There are, however, major exceptions to this. It is important to remember that radiosensitivity and radiocurability are not synonymous. In fact, some of the most radiosensitive tumors seldom are cured by this treatment. Thus less than an erythema dose of roentgen radiation will induce considerable regression of a lymphosarcoma, but cures of lymphosarcoma by radiation therapy are uncommon.

Much of our information regarding radiosensitivity rests on empiric grounds. For convenience, tumors may be grouped into three general classes from the standpoint of their response to radiation: radiosensitive, radioresponsive, and radioresistant. Radiosensitive tumors such as lymphosarcoma will regress with treatment that does no, or merely transient, damage to adjacent normal tissues. Such amounts range up to 2500 rad when administered in the conventional manner. Radioresponsive tumors such as carcinoma of the breast are those that will regress when subjected to a course of radiation that does only minor damage to the adjacent normal tissues. The amounts effective in this group range from 2500 to 5000 rad. Tumors such as osteosarcoma that are no more sensitive than their surrounding tissues are considered radioresistant. They require 5000 rad or more to bring about regression. Sometimes the radiation response of tumors is more effective when chemotherapeutic agents are administered simultaneously. Similarly, increased

oxygen tension enhances the effectiveness of the radiation. The periphery of a tumor, being better oxygenated, is more radiosensitive than the core. For some cancers, radioisotopes have proved to be useful in concentrating the radiation effects in the tumor, for example, radioiodine in thyroid carcinoma.

Normal tissues vary in sensitivity to radiation, with lymphocytes being most sensitive and adult neurons most resistant. In general, the tumors derived from a given cell type tend to follow the relative sensitivity of that type. Vascularity of stroma increases the sensitivity of a tumor, as does rapidity of growth.

Unfortunately, tumors that are initially radiosensitive may become radioresistant if they recur after treatment. This change in response to radiation is not accompanied by recognizable gross or histologic alterations.

RECURRENCE

Recurrence is a clinical term used to describe the reappearance of a tumor, after its apparent removal or destruction (Fig. 15-32). Recurrence indicates that some of the original tumor cells have survived and have eventually multiplied to such an extent that the tumor is again clinically obvious. Usually recurrence appears within the length of time required for a few tumor cells left behind by the attempted extirpation of the tumor to multiply to a recognizable mass. There are instances, however, that cannot be explained by the time required for multiplication of cells alone. Carcinoma of the breast has recurred in the scar 28 years after removal of the primary tumor. Liver metastases from malignant melanoma of the eye may be latent for many years before becoming clinically detectable or significant. The factors that keep the cells viable yet dormant over the years and then permit recur-

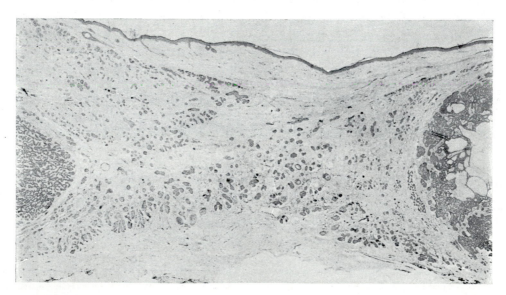

Fig. 15-32. Two masses of basal cell carcinoma recurring on both sides of scar, also diffusely infiltrated by basal cell carcinoma. This was caused by incomplete removal of primary tumor. (16×.)

rent growth are difficult to understand. Sometimes, as in the buccal mucosa or urinary bladder, new tumors develop in the same general region and may simulate recurrence.

ETIOLOGY AND PATHOGENESIS

There is no one cause for the development of tumors. Although some factors in their production are established, in both animals and humans, many are still unknown. The statement that cancer is a disease of civilization has had to be corrected as our knowledge of more primitive peoples has increased. The causes of tumors are those initiating factors that produce irreversible intracellular changes resulting in the abnormal growth that we recognize as tumor. Some of the factors seem to be inherent in the host or dependent on the host. These are called the intrinsic, endogenous, or host factors and include (1) heredity, (2) race, (3) age, (4) sex and hormones, and (5) immunologic status. Other apparent causes of tumor are listed as extrinsic or exogenous and include physical, chemical, and biologic agents. A study of the epidemiologic and geographic distribution of cancer has been most interesting in evaluating the relative significance of the various factors in the production of cancer. It is apparent that tumors often are the result of multiple causes, and it is usually difficult to separate various possible causative factors in the individual instance.

Tumors are not limited to humans but arise in all species of animals and in plants. They have been studied extensively, not only in primates but also in other mammals, domestic and captive, birds, reptiles, amphibians, fishes, and invertebrates. As in humans, tumors in animals show a great diversity of structure and behavior. Some are surprisingly similar to the human counterpart in gross and microscopic structure, but the biologic behavior is not necessarily the same. Nevertheless, the knowledge that spontaneous tumors do arise in animals

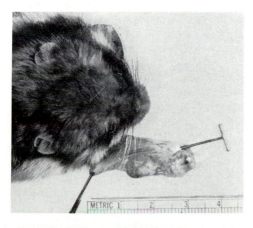

Fig. 15-33. Everted cheek pouch of hamster bearing human malignant melanoma. Implant is 35 days old.

has allowed the investigation of the biologic characteristics of tumors in general. Furthermore, the fact that tumors can be induced experimentally in animals by a variety of techniques has aided considerably in investigation of mechanisms of cancer induction in humans and of the agents responsible.

Transplantation of tumors is a good example of a technique that has been successful in many animals, and tumors often may be transmitted in this fashion from animal to animal for many generations. A wide variety of carcinomas and sarcomas and even benign tumors have been transplanted in this way. Heterologous transplantation may be made from a number of malignant tumors, including those of humans. The anterior chamber of the eye in rats, guinea pigs, and rabbits; the mouse brain; the hamster cheek pouch (Fig. 15-33); and the chorioallantoic membrane of chick embryos are particularly serviceable foci for tumor transplantation. Such tumors may ultimately adapt themselves to the host and give rise to metastases.

Intrinsic factors
Heredity

There is considerable proof that heredity plays a role in the development of tumors. For example, cancer of the same organ in monozygous twins is more common than chance would dictate. Multiple cancers in the same individual are more common than the expected incidence. An increased incidence of certain types of tumor in a family is often difficult to prove conclusively in humans because one type might well be concentrated in a family by chance alone. There are a few neoplasms, however, that are found more commonly in members of the same family, appearing earlier in life and usually arising multifocally within the affected organ. For example, retinoblastoma of the eye, which occurs in 1 in 20,000 live births, exhibits a familial occurrence in 5% to 10% of cases; when familial it is often found bilaterally. This familial predisposition has been interpreted to represent an inherited susceptibility that is the result of a defective gene.

A tendency toward development of tumors in multiple endocrine organs also is familial. Tumors of the multiple endocrine adenoma (MEA I) syndrome usually include adenomas of the pancreas, pituitary gland, and parathyroid gland. Another familial (MEA II) syndrome has an association of medullary thyroid carcinoma, tumor of the adrenal medulla (pheochromocytoma), and tumor or hyperplasia of the parathyroid glands. For example, in one family, a father had carcinoma of the thyroid gland, pheochromocytoma, and parathyroid adenoma; thyroid cancer and pheochromocytoma developed in his son; and his son's daughter already had thyroid carcinoma. It is difficult to explain such a familial incidence except by inheritance of defective genes.

In addition to an inherited tendency for the development of specific cancers, a state or condition that predisposes to the development of cancer also may be inherited. An example of such a state is multiple polyposis of the large intestine, a familial condition in which hundreds of polypoid adenomas arise in the mucosa of the large intestine; usually cancer of the colon also develops in early adult life. Another comparable familial condition that predisposes to cancer is neurofibromatosis, in which neurofibrosarcomas and other tumors may arise. There are a few metabolic disturbances found in members of the same family that predispose to neoplasia. For example, xeroderma pigmentosum, a familial disease that is transmitted as a mendelian recessive disorder, is characterized by extreme sensitivity to ultraviolet radiation. It manifests itself early in childhood and with advancing age is associated with the development of various types of skin cancer, such as basal cell carcinoma, squamous cell carcinoma, and malignant melanoma. The defect in xeroderma pigmentosum results from the inability of epidermal cells to repair ultraviolet radiation damage to their DNA bases.

The genetic background or determination in human cancers is usually difficult to separate from the various environmental influences. In experimental animals, however, there is strong evidence that genetic factors play an important role in influencing the incidence of both spontaneous and experimentally induced tumors. Animal experiments have given the best evidence for the hereditary aspects of tumors because animals can be better observed and controlled than humans, both in breeding and in environment. By selective breeding it has been possible to develop and observe groups of genetically identical animals; the incidence of types of spontaneous tumors within a strain may be concentrated or bred out. For example, C3H mice have a high incidence of mammary and liver tumors, whereas C57 black mice show a low incidence of development and even a resistance to the development of many tumors. Although the genetic makeup of the animal host may not by itself be a sufficient condition for cancer production, it nevertheless may be an important predisposing or contributing factor.

Racial and geographic factors

The different racial incidences of specific types of tumor in humans may be in part genetic, but many of the differences are more likely the result of environmental conditions that are distributed throughout the whole population in a given area. Factors such as climate, soil and water, diet, habits, and customs may act alone or in combination. Study of the reasons for racial and geographic differences is important in evaluating definitive causes of cancers. One cancer that has been the subject of much speculation is liver cancer, which is relatively rare in Americans and Europeans as compared with Orientals. Cancer of the breast is uncommon in Japanese women but is a very common neoplasm in American women. Cancer of the uterine cervix is rare in Jewish women. In Europe and America, cancer of the penis is rare, but in Uganda it is the most common type of cancer in humans, accounting for 10% of all male cancers. Epidermoid and basal cell carcinomas of the skin are very common in whites but rare in blacks.

Age

Although tumors appear in any age group, malignant tumors tend to occur in older individuals. Whether this is caused by an alteration of the cells of the host with increasing age, by a decreased ability to mount an immune response, by a longer chance for the cells to express a latent malignant potential, or by a longer exposure to environmental factors is unknown. For some tumors, however, there are two peaks of incidence. For example, for leukemia there is an incidence peak in childhood, suggesting that inherent host factors may be of great significance; a second peak occurs in the older age groups, suggesting that environmental factors may be at work.

Tumors in adults occur mostly in epithelia lining the various internal and external body surfaces and in organs that undergo changes during life—for example, the prostate in men and the breast, uterus, and ovaries in women—or in organs exposed to carcinogens. In children, tumors rarely arise from epithelial tissues. Instead, childhood neoplasms arise most frequently in tissues and organs that exhibit rapid absolute and differential growth, for example, bone marrow (leukemia), bone (osteosarcoma), immature neural elements (neuroblastoma or retinoblastoma), and mesenchymal elements (various sarcomas).

There is less correlation between the histologic characteristics of tumors in children and their biologic behavior than is the case with tumors of adults. For example, morphologically "benign" tumors of children may exhibit a malignant course, whereas morphologically "malignant" tumors may have a benign course. The reasons for these differences in clinical behavior between childhood and adult tumor histologic conditions are not known.

Sex and hormones

The difference in incidence of specific types of tumors, particularly cancers, in males and females is often striking. Although the difference may be partially explained by genetics, habits, occupation, environment, and immunologic factors, it is quite possible that the presence of specific sex hormones also may have a direct relationship to the high and low incidence of certain tumors. Some cancers of both endocrine and nonendocrine tissues can be alleviated and partially controlled by alteration of the accustomed hormonal environment. Even though beneficial effects usually are only temporary, there is no doubt that some cancers are hormone dependent to a degree. There is considerable experimental evidence that hormone imbalances, deficiencies, and excesses may in themselves be causes of tumors or at least contribute in some way to their development. Furth and co-workers[14] have shown that derangement of physiologic feedback mechanisms can lead to neoplasm. For example, ablation of the thyroid gland in the mouse causes sustained suppression of the thyroid hormone levels, leading to sustained stimulation of the pituitary thyrotropes and consequent tumorigenesis of the pituitary gland.

Immunologic factors

Host-mediated immunity plays an important role in both spontaneously appearing human tumors and experimentally induced animal tumors. In an immunocompetent host, cancers perhaps arise anew rather frequently but are recognized by the cellular immune surveillance as foreign and are destroyed. This is primarily true for experimental neoplasms that are induced by oncogenic viruses and consist of neoplastic cells bearing moderately strong tumor-specific transplantation antigens. It is less so for tumors that are induced by chemical carcinogens or develop spontaneously and consist of cells with very weak antigens. As a result, the host cannot mount an immune reaction severe enough to render them ineffective.

There are instances also in which there is an apparent association between an increased cancer incidence and a decreased or altered effectiveness of the host's immune mechanism. For example, the weakened immune response of advancing age may be a reason for a higher tumor incidence. Moreover, immunodeficiency states either genetically inherited or the result of suppression of the cell-mediated immune mechanism (such as after administration of immunosuppressant drugs) are associated with an increased cancer incidence and with cancers that grow more rapidly than in the general population. The types of malignant neoplasms developing in immunodeficient persons are not characteristic of those found in the general population, tending to a predominance of tumors of the lymphoreticular systems. Patients with lymphoproliferative diseases may also exhibit immunodeficiency states; for example, patients with malignant lymphoma or Hodgkin's disease may display a deficiency of T cell function, whereas patients with multiple myeloma may manifest deficient B cell immunity. Finally, patients with chronic lymphocytic leukemia may be deficient in both T cell and B cell immunity. Immunologic deficiencies often become worse as the cancer progresses, which may account in part for the more rapid tumor growth with time.

The presence of circulating blocking factors (tumor antigens or antigen-antibody complexes) may prevent sensitized lymphocytes from attacking tumor cells effectively, whereas a weak immune response, such as that present during the initial stages of tumor development, may have a stimulatory rather than an inhibitory effect on tumor growth. Of course, enhancement of the host's immune mechanism by nonspecific stimulants, such as BCG vaccine and *Corynebacterium parvum*, or the development of unblocking antibodies by the host, may assist in restraining tumor growth and, at times, in tumor rejection at both primary and metastatic sites.

Although the prospects of developing and using various techniques for active and passive immunization against cancer are exciting, one should understand that at present the strong intrinsic oncogenic potential characteristics of the majority of cancers will circumvent the various immunoprotective mechanisms of the host and cause its death.

Extrinsic factors
Physical agents

It is doubtful that a single trauma (meant here as the result of physical violence) can lead to the production of a cancer. The incidence of carcinoma in scars is somewhat higher than in adjacent normal skin, but in such cases the development of the tumor can be ascribed to the abnormal environment of the cells in the scar rather than to the trauma from which the scar arose. Medicolegal claims for compensation for development of a tumor ascribed to a single trauma are frequent but rarely have a basis in fact. The criteria essential before a positive relationship between a tumor and a given trauma can be considered are as follows:
1. The part in which the tumor arose must be proved to have been normal before the injury.
2. The tumor must develop within a reasonable time after the trauma.
3. The tumor must be of a type that could originate from the cells traumatized.
4. Trauma must have been adequate to produce tissue disruption and ecchymosis.

Even when these criteria are fulfilled, coincidence may still explain the appearance of a cancer.

A number of inert materials such as plastic films and glass spheres and fibers, when implanted into various body sites of experimental animals, cause the production of malignant neoplasms, mostly sarcomas. It appears that the size and shape rather than the chemical nature of the foreign body are responsible for tumor development. Moreover, the genetic background of the host animal and its age and sex are factors that influence the expression of the oncogenic state.

Tumorigenesis caused by artificial implants into humans must be a rare event considering the large number of patients who have received a variety of prostheses. The low tumor incidence may be attributable to a long tumor-latency period, which exceeds the life expectancy of the person receiving an implant late in life. Since implantation of prostheses into humans will increase in future years, physicians dealing with these problems should be aware of the possibility of tumor induction as the result of therapeutic implantation of inert substances.

Ionizing radiation (see also Chapter 6) is not a common cause of cancer, but there is no doubt that it is a factor in the production of some tumors both in humans and in experimental animals. Many of the early workers using x rays at the beginning of this century received excessive radiation on their hands that led to radiation dermatitis with later development of cancer (Fig. 15-34). Although the majority of these skin tumors were epidermoid or basal cell carcinomas, some fibrosarcomas also developed. Postradiation skin cancer of the hands among radiologists has now virtually disappeared with adoption of appropriate safety standards and the use of technologically advanced x-ray equipment.

All types of ionizing radiation have been found to be associated with an increased incidence of leukemia in humans. For example, radiation workers exhibit an increased incidence of acute and chronic granulocytic

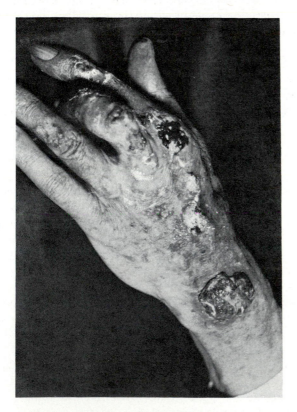

Fig. 15-34. X-ray dermatitis and multiple carcinomas of 5 years' duration in 83-year-old male physician after 15 years of repeated small exposure to x-ray irradiation.

leukemia. Acute leukemia develops more frequently in children exposed to x rays either in utero or postnatally than in children in the general population. A high proportion of patients with ankylosing spondylitis, treated with x rays over the spine for long periods, showed an increased incidence of leukemia. Japanese atomic bomb survivors exhibited a profound increase in the incidence of chronic granulocytic leukemia that reached a peak 4 to 8 years after radiation exposure.

Although skin and hemopoietic tumors are the ones most often caused by ionizing radiation, other tissues may also be stimulated to produce cancers. For example, osteosarcomas developed among New Jersey watch workers who inadvertently ingested radioactive materials while applying luminous radium- and mesothorium-containing paints to dials of watches. Carcinoma of the lung has been noted among workers in the uranium mines of Central Europe and the United States, probably caused by minute amounts of radon present in the inspired air. Finally, carcinoma of the thyroid is much more common in individuals who received x rays to the neck region as infants.

The factors responsible for the induction of cancer after exposure to radiation are not clearly defined. It is possible that radiation alters cellular DNA or interferes with the regulation of gene function. It is also possible that radiation may activate latent oncogenic viruses, which may ultimately be responsible for cancer induction. Probably the induction of cancer by radiation involves a variety of modes. The cancers, once produced, tend to be similar clinically and histologically to those that arise from other causes; their treatment, including response to therapeutic radiation, is also similar. The latent period between the radiation exposure and the development of a neoplasm may vary from a few years to several decades.

There is both experimental and clinical proof that overexposure to ultraviolet rays increases the incidence of skin cancer. Much more carcinoma of the skin develops among white farmers of the southwestern United States where there is considerably more exposure to the sun than among city dwellers in the north. The skin cancers are mostly epidermoid and basal cell carcinomas. As mentioned previously, patients with xeroderma pigmentosum exhibit a high incidence of skin cancer because of the extreme sensitivity of their skin to ultraviolet rays.

Chemical agents

The first hint that there might be specific causes for cancer was found by Pott in 1775. He noted that a far greater number of carcinomas of the scrotum occurred in chimney sweeps in London than in the general population. This was the first report of occupational cancer. As a result of his observations, there was continued interest in soot and coal tar as a possible stimulus for the development of tumors, as well as in the possibility of other occupational cancers. The latter have included cancer of the urinary bladder in aniline dye workers and cancer of the skin in workers using arsenic or coal tar. In 1914, two Japanese investigators, Yamagiwa and Ichikawa, successfully produced experimental cancer of rabbits' skin by repeatedly painting the ears of rabbits with coal tar, thus proving conclusively that cancer could be induced chemically. Since that time a wide variety of compounds of diverse chemical structure have been found to exhibit carcinogenic potential in experimental animals and in humans (Fig. 15-35). Some of the more important examples are as follows:

1. Alkylating agents, for example, beta-propiolactone, epoxides, mustard gas, nitrogen mustard
2. Polycyclic aromatic hydrocarbons, for example, benzo[a]pyrene, dibenz[a,h]anthracene, methylcholanthrene, soot, tar, cigarette smoke
3. Aromatic amines, for example, acetylaminofluorene, aminobiphenyl, benzidine, naphthylamine
4. Nitrosamines and other nitroso compounds
5. Naturally occurring products, for example, aflatoxin B_1, actinomycin D, mitomycin C, safrole
6. Drugs, for example, chlorambucil, cyclophosphamide, diethylstilbestrol
7. Metals, for example, arsenic compounds, cadmium compounds, chromium compounds, asbestos
8. Industrial products, for example, chloromethyl ether, vinyl chloride
9. Food additives, for example, azo dyes ("butter yellow")
10. Miscellaneous products, for example, carbon tetrachloride, ethionine, thiourea, urethane

Chemicals that are responsible for carcinogenesis can be grouped on the basis of their mode of action into three major classes. (1) Direct-acting carcinogens possess a chemical structure that empowers them to react irreversibly, usually by means of an electrophilic region, that is, an electron-deficient segment, with the electron-rich regions of the various cell constituents, resulting in molecular alterations that can lead to neoplastic transformation. (2) Procarcinogens are not carcinogenic in themselves. They become active only after metabolic conversion, usually by a microsomal mixed-function oxidase mechanism, in the living host organism. That some chemical compounds exhibit carcinogenicity for certain target organs may imply that these organs possess the specific activation enzymes necessary for their conversion. In rare instances procarcinogens may be activated by microorganisms such as those comprising the intestinal flora. (3) Promotors of carcinogenesis, compounds such as croton oil and phenols, lack an intrinsic carcinogenic potential and cannot be converted into true carcinogens by the host. They are capable, however, of enhancing the effect of either direct-acting carcinogens or procarcinogens.

There are several possible mechanisms by which a chemical carcinogen may trigger the oncogenic event at the cellular level. Direct-acting carcinogenic compounds such as the alkylating agents, which are strong mutagens, may, because of their electrophilic properties, bind covalently to preferred regions of the cell DNA. Similarly, procarcinogens, such as the polycyclic aromatic hydrocarbons, aromatic amines, nitrosamines, and even naturally occurring products such as aflatoxin B_1, which are not by themselves mutagenic, are converted into strong electrophilic metabolites by the host and become capable of binding covalently to the cell DNA. This binding to DNA may lead either to base substitution or to frame shift mutations that may result eventually in neoplastic transformation in daughter cells after division. A chemical carcinogen may, on the other hand, bind to cell RNA and modify it. The altered RNA could be transcribed into cell DNA, through the reverse transcriptase system, leading to the establishment of permanent misinformation. Finally, a chemical carcinogen may modify mRNA or tRNA, resulting in the formation of aberrant proteins, or it may bind to a preexisting protein, modifying it directly. If the altered protein is an enzyme such as DNA polymerase, it could lead to faulty DNA replication. If,

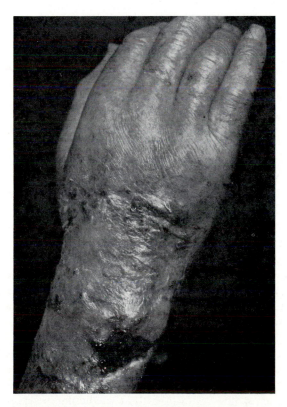

Fig. 15-35. Multiple epidermoid carcinomas and keratoses that developed as result of repeated exposure to oil and tar over 30 years in 68-year-old man. Carcinoma had previously been excised from same area.

on the other hand, it is a repressor protein controlling host regulatory genes, its modification could lead to stable epigenetic changes.

It is not possible at present to determine if the oncogenic event mediated by a chemical carcinogenic compound results from the direct alteration of cell DNA or indirectly from interference with the regulation of gene function. Most likely, different chemical carcinogens transform cells neoplastically by different mechanisms. Moreover, it is probable that the initiating oncogenic event may not be as important a factor in the development of clinical cancer as are the subsequent changes brought about by proliferation and selection. For example, the expression of the oncogenic state may be related to epiphenomenal alterations that take place long after exposure to the carcinogen. These may consist of (1) plasma membrane changes involving mechanisms of growth control, (2) the ability to secrete collagenolytic and fibrinolytic enzymes, and (3) the capacity to initiate angiogenesis, to invade locally, and to metastasize to distant sites. In addition, the genetic background, age, and sex of the host, as well as the immunologic, hormonal, and nutritional (particularly riboflavin and vitamin A) state, may determine the nature of the expression and progression of the oncogenic state. Finally, the chemical carcinogen may influence the clinical expression of cancer by inducing immunosuppression in the host organism.

Tests with *Salmonella* bacteria and mammalian microsomal enzymes have shown that up to 90% of the known chemical carcinogens are also mutagens. Consequently, it appears highly probable that chemicals found to be mutagenic may turn out to be carcinogenic as well. Therefore the *Salmonella* and microsomal enzyme mutagenicity test has been suggested as a screening procedure to identify chemicals with a carcinogenic potential. The mutagenic substances thus detected could be evaluated further for oncogenicity by the expensive and time-consuming but more reliable technique of animal testing. It should be emphasized, however, that the hypothesis that the carcinogenic event is a mutagenic event, that is, caused by somatic cell mutation, has not been confirmed. There is evidence that not all carcinogenic transformation has a genetic basis. For example, transplantation of frog carcinoma cell nuclei into frog eggs results in normal tadpoles, and mouse teratocarcinoma cells implanted into early embryos lose their oncogenic potential.

The histologic types of tumors that develop after exposure to a chemical carcinogen depend to a great extent on the route of its administration. If the agent is painted on the skin, a neoplasm of the squamous epithelium is induced. If the same agent is injected into deeper tissues, a sarcoma may result. Some chemical carcinogens after injection or oral administration produce tumors of specific organs; for example, the aromatic amine 2-naph-

1. POLYCYCLIC HYDROCARBONS—experimental skin tumors and sarcomas

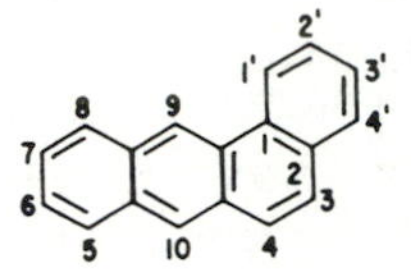

Benzanthracene

(weak carcinogen)

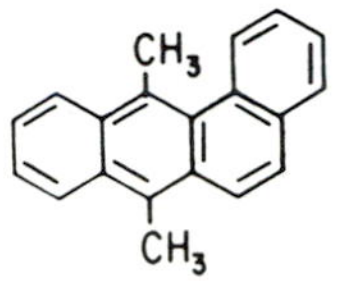

9,10-Dimethyl-1,2-benzanthracene

(potent carcinogen)

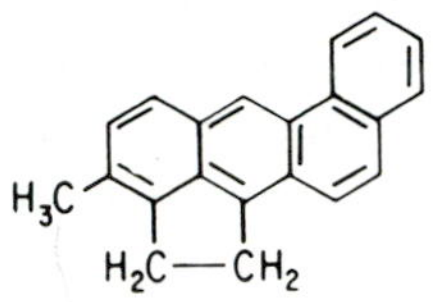

Methylcholanthrene

(potent carcinogen)

Has been prepared from desoxycholic and cholic acid

2. AZO DYES—experimental liver tumors

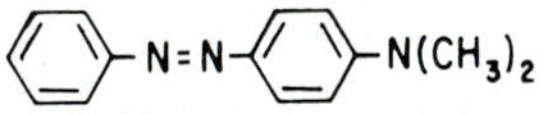

p-Dimethylaminoazobenzene "butter yellow"

3. AROMATIC AMINES—bladder cancer in man

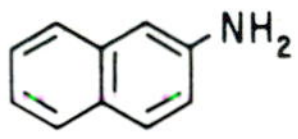

2-Naphthylamine

4. URETHAN—lung adenomas in mice

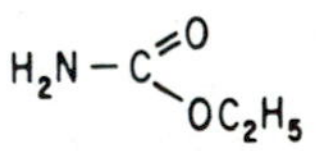

Ethyl carbamate "urethan"

5. ARSENIC—skin cancer in man

Fig. 15-36. Structural formulas for some carcinogenic chemicals.

thylamine produces cancer of the urinary bladder in humans and dogs, and the azo dye butter yellow causes cancer of the liver in rodents.

Although a wide variety of chemical compounds have been shown to manifest carcinogenic properties in experimental animals, this effect can be demonstrated only when the dose of the chemical is high and the exposure to it is prolonged. Many carcinogens present in the environment in minute amounts are not known to produce cancer in humans. There are some carcinogenic substances, however, such as the aflatoxins, that are present in relatively small amounts as contaminants in food or water and to which a given population is exposed over prolonged periods. This situation appears to be responsible for the high incidence of hepatocellular carcinoma among people living in certain parts of Africa and the Orient. Finally, although many of the known carcinogenic compounds are not found as such in nature, they are nevertheless rather similar to substances that are produced normally by the human organism. For example, the steroid hormones and the bile salts have structural formulas not very different from those of many of the carcinogenic chemicals (Fig. 15-36). This feature suggests that some of these naturally occurring substances may possess carcinogenic properties that manifest themselves only in special situations conducive to cancer development in the human host.

Biologic agents

There is little to suggest that bacteria, higher organisms, or parasites directly cause human cancer. The only implications are indirect ones through the provision of a source of chronic irritation that ultimately may become cancerous, such as schistosomiasis and carcinoma of the urinary bladder, or through the production of substances such as fungal aflatoxins that may be carcinogenic in minute amounts.

The role of viruses in the causation of cancer is more significant. The contagious nature of the human wart was established in 1907 when the disease was transmitted to volunteers with cell-free filtrates. In 1908, Ellerman and Bang succeeded in transmitting avian leukemia to chickens with cell-free filtrates, and in 1911 Rous demonstrated that an avian sarcoma was caused by a filterable agent. Bittner in 1936 showed that a viral agent, acting in concert with genetic and hormonal factors, could cause mammary adenocarcinoma in mice, and Gross in 1951 demonstrated that murine lymphatic leukemia could be caused by a virus. These important pioneer discoveries have been followed more recently by additional data demonstrating beyond doubt that many types of benign and malignant animal tumors can be caused by viruses.

As of now there is only suggestive evidence that viruses can cause malignant neoplasms in humans. The clear demonstration that viruses can induce cancer in experimental animals, however, makes it probable that similar induction may occur in humans. A summary of the experimental work on the viral etiology of cancer is therefore of interest.

There are two broad classes of oncogenic or tumor-producing viruses based on their nucleic acid content: those that contain deoxyribonucleic acid (DNA) as their genetic material and those that contain ribonucleic acid (RNA).

Oncogenic DNA viruses belong to four distinct subgroups: the papovaviruses, the adenoviruses, the herpesviruses, and the poxviruses. Each of these viruses can cause one or more histologic types of neoplasms (Fig. 15-37) in the appropriate host (Table 15-4).

Cells that are exposed in vitro to oncogenic DNA viruses may either lyse after virus replication or transform. Cells that transform develop morphologic, biochemical, antigenic, and behavioral alterations that are heritable. Most important, transformed cells can establish permanent cell lines that quite often exhibit oncogenic properties as shown by their ability to form progressively growing tumors in the appropriate animal host. As mentioned previously, cells transformed by oncogenic DNA viruses develop both nuclear (T) and plasma membrane (TST) antigens that are virus related but are not virion antigens.

The viral specificity of the T and TST cellular antigens provides indirect evidence that the information for their synthesis is derived from the viral genome. Direct evidence that viral genes persist indefinitely in cells rendered neoplastic in vivo or transformed in vitro by one of the oncogenic DNA viruses can be derived by nucleic acid hybridization techniques when virus-specific DNA sequences are found within the cell DNA and virus-specific messenger RNA is localized within the cell cytoplasm. Moreover, infectious virus can be rescued from the neoplastic cells that are not shedding virus, by fusing them with indicator cells that permit viral replication. Recent evidence indicates that the viral DNA is covalently linked to the cell DNA. It is not known at present whether integration of the viral genome within the cell genetic apparatus is necessary for the maintenance and expression of the oncogenic state. From a teleologic point of view, integration seems to protect the viral DNA from the host's immune mechanisms.

Oncogenic RNA viruses have basic similarities in physical characteristics, chemical composition, and antigenic properties. They are naturally transmitted from parent to offspring through the germinal cells or by a congenital infection and, less often, by direct contact. They can be transmitted also experimentally by inoculating the virus into susceptible animals. Usually when transmitted congenitally, and occasionally when transmitted by direct contact, they cause neoplasms in their

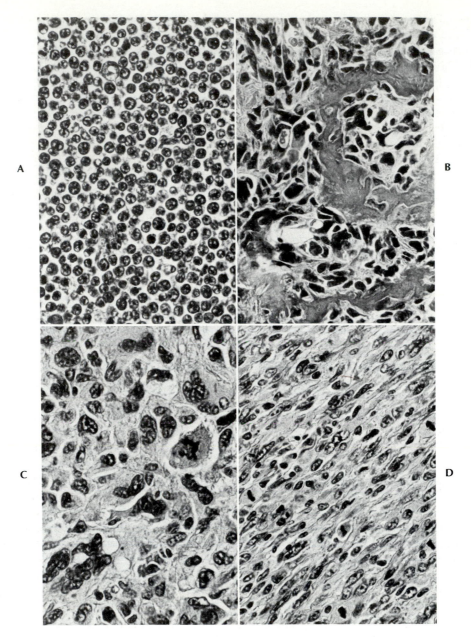

Fig. 15-37. Four types of malignant neoplasms induced in hamsters by the oncogenic DNA, simian virus 40 (SV40). **A,** Lymphosarcoma. **B,** Osteogenic sarcoma. **C,** Pleomorphic sarcoma. **D,** Spindle cell sarcoma. (500×.)

host of origin and in experimental hosts. Morphologically similar neoplasms can be induced by different types of oncogenic RNA viruses, and the same virus can cause different types of neoplastic and nonneoplastic lesions (Table 15-5).

In contrast to cells that are infected by oncogenic DNA viruses in vitro, which may either lyse after virus replication or transform, cells infected by oncogenic RNA viruses do not lyse. Instead they shed virus continuously. In addition, although oncogenic DNA viruses can induce cellular DNA synthesis, which is usually followed by cell transformation, oncogenic RNA viruses lack this

capacity. As a result, freshly prepared cell cultures that are actively proliferating are the cells best suited for transformation. Once transformation has occurred under the influence of an oncogenic RNA virus, the cells develop morphologic, biochemical, antigenic, and behavioral alterations that are heritable. They may also establish permanent cell lines that at times exhibit oncogenic properties. Transformed cells usually contain biochemical markers that establish the persistence of viral genes within the genetic apparatus of the cell. It is not known definitely whether the persistence of the viral genome within the transformed cells is a prerequisite for the

Table 15-4. Oncogenic DNA viruses

Virus	Host in which oncogenic	Types of neoplasms induced
Papovaviruses		
Papilloma	Human, cow, dog, rabbit	Squamous cell papilloma
Polyoma	Mouse, hamster	Sarcoma, carcinoma
Vacuolating agent (SV40)	Hamster	Sarcoma, osteosarcoma, leukemia, lymphoma
SV40-like agents (human)	Hamster	Sarcoma
Adenoviruses	Hamster	Small-cell sarcoma
Herpesviruses		
Lucké's virus	Frog	Renal adenocarcinoma
Marek's disease	Chicken	Neurolymphomatosis
Sylvilagus	Rabbit	Lymphoma
Saimiri	Monkey	Lymphoma
Ateles	Monkey	Lymphoma
Epstein-Barr virus	Human	Burkitt's lymphoma (?), nasopharyngeal carcinoma (?)
Simplex, type 2	Human	Carcinoma of uterine cervix (?)
Poxviruses		
Fibroma-myxoma	Rabbit, squirrel, deer	Fibroma, myxoma
Yaba	Monkey	Fibroma
Molluscum contagiosum	Human	Squamous cell papilloma
Other viruses		
Hepatitis B virus	Human	Hepatocellular carcinoma (?)
Unidentified	Human	Kaposi's sarcoma (?)

Table 15-5. Oncogenic RNA viruses

Virus	Host in which oncogenic	Types of neoplasms induced
Myeloblastosis	Chicken	Myeloblastic leukemia
Lymphomatosis	Chicken	Lymphoblastic leukemia
Erythroblastosis	Chicken	Erythroblastic leukemia
Rous sarcoma	Chicken	Sarcoma
Gross	Mouse	T cell leukemia, lymphoma
Abelson	Mouse	B cell leukemia, lymphoma
Graffi	Mouse	Myeloid leukemia
Friend, Rauscher	Mouse	Erythroid leukemia
Kaplan, Rich	Mouse	Reticulum cell sarcoma
Harvey, Moloney	Mouse	Sarcoma
Bittner	Mouse	Mammary adenocarcinoma
Leukemia, lymphoma	Other mammals	Leukemia, lymphoma
Sarcoma	Other mammals	Sarcoma
Leukemia, lymphoma	Human	T cell leukemia (?), lymphoma (?)

maintenance and expression of the oncogenic state.

The events of the interaction between the susceptible cell and the oncogenic RNA virus at the molecular level (Fig. 15-38) have been elucidated. After adsorption of the virus onto the cell plasma membrane and its penetration into the cytoplasm, an RNA-dependent DNA polymerase that has been termed reverse transcriptase, which is brought into the cell by the virus, transcribes the single-stranded viral RNA into a single-stranded DNA. A DNA-dependent DNA polymerase then transcribes the single-stranded DNA into a double-stranded DNA, the provirus. An endonuclease, an exonuclease, and a ligase presumably cleave the cellular DNA, insert the provirus into it, and then mend the DNA break, with the result that the viral double-stranded DNA is integrated into the host cell DNA after one cell division. The integrated provirus replicates by the enzyme systems intrinsic to the cell, which are also responsible for the replication and repair of the cell DNA. It serves also as template for the transcription of progeny viral RNA. From a teleologic viewpoint, viral integration results in the ability of an oncogenic RNA virus, through its DNA intermediate, to replicate while being protected from the host's immune mechanisms, a phenomenon previously encountered with oncogenic DNA viruses.

Possible mechanisms of viral oncogenesis. Oncogenic RNA viruses are classified into three subgroups on the basis of their oncogenic properties: (1) the acute sarcoma viruses, (2) the acute leukemia viruses, and (3) the chronic lymphoid leukosis viruses. Whereas the acute sarcoma and acute leukemia viruses induce sarcomas or leukemias in vivo within 2 to 3 weeks and transform neoplastically fibroblasts and/or hemopoietic cells in vitro, the chronic lymphoid leukosis viruses induce predominantly lymphoid lymphomas of B cell type in 4 to 12 months and are incapable of transforming cells in culture in detectable frequencies over prolonged periods. The molecular differences in the genomes of the oncogenic RNA viruses, which may be responsible for the differences in their functional capacity, can be summarized as follows.

The acute sarcoma viruses contain three viral genes that direct virus replication: group-specific antigens (gag), coding for viral core proteins; polymerase (pol), coding for viral reverse transcriptase; and envelope (env), coding for viral envelope glycoproteins. In addition, they contain genes that are responsible for the oncogenic or sarcomagenic transformation event affecting the virus-infected cells. Evidence indicates that these genes, designated as onc or src genes, were originally derived from progenitor genes of normal vertebrate cells, which may function during the organism's growth and development. The viral onc or src genes direct the synthesis of phosphoproteins that are similar to the proteins encoded by the homologous cellular genes. Both the viral-coded and cellular-coded proteins have an associated protein kinase activity that catalyzes the covalent

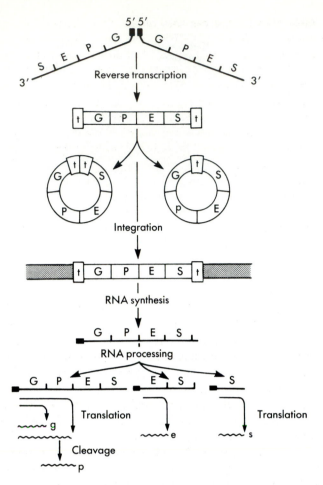

Fig. 15-38. Replication of retroviruses. (The term retrovirus is synonymous with oncogenic RNA virus.) Current knowledge of the molecular events that mediate the replication of retroviruses is summarized in this model; avian sarcoma virus is used as a prototype. *G,* Gene gag; *P,* pol; *E,* env; *S,* src; *g, p, e, s,* proteins encoded by gag, pol, env., and src, respectively; *t,* terminal redundancy in nucleotide sequence of viral DNA; *heavy single lines,* RNA; *wavy single lines,* proteins; *open bars,* viral DNA; *stippled bars,* cellular DNA; *solid bar* (at left end of RNA molecules), nucleotide sequence that is transposed (spliced) during genesis of viral messenger RNAs. (From Bishop, J.M.: N. Engl. J. Med. **303:**675, 1980.)

addition of phosphate to a specific amino acid in protein molecules. Neoplastic transformation in this case may therefore result from the action of virus-coded proteins that function as substitute enhancers or inhibitors of normal cellular regulatory mechanisms.

The acute leukemia viruses are variants of the chronic lymphoid leukosis viruses (see the following paragraph). They possess specific transforming or onc genes, which were acquired from homologous cellular genes. Because these oncogenic sequences interrupt the viral gag, pol, or env genes, they render the viral particles incapable of independent replication. These newly acquired sequences, however, provide the virus with the capacity

for abnormal expression of cellular gene products that cause transformation of infected cells.

The chronic lymphoid leukosis viruses contain only three viral genes: gag, pol, and env. These viruses lack genes similar to the onc or src genes found to be responsible for oncogenesis in the acute leukemia viruses. They seem to induce neoplastic disease by a mechanism different from that of the aforementioned two types of viruses; genetic elements present in their proviral DNA act as transcriptional promoters. By integrating adjacent to cellular genes that control cell proliferation, they activate them and cause their enhanced expression. This in turn leads to uncontrolled cell proliferation—oncogenesis. Thus viral DNA sequences acting as transcriptional promoters activate normal cellular growth regulatory genes resulting in neoplastic cell proliferation.

Oncogenic DNA viruses cause neoplastic cell transformation by mechanisms different from those mentioned for oncogenic RNA viruses. Because simian virus 40 (SV40) and polyoma virus are of relatively small size, having been sequenced recently, their transforming properties have been studied extensively. SV40 and polyoma virus induce a cytologic and histologic variety of malignant neoplasms in vivo and transform neoplastically different types of cells in vitro. They both specify a group of related proteins, called T (tumor) antigens, which are involved in cell transformation and viral replication. The genomic portion of SV40 essential for neoplastic cell transformation codes for two proteins: the large T antigen (mol. wt. 90,000 daltons) and the small T antigen (mol. wt. 17,000 daltons). SV40 mutant viruses defective in production of small T but not of large T antigen are still capable of oncogenesis in vivo and of neoplastic cell transformation in vitro, although the presence of small T antigen enhances the ability of SV40 to transform efficiently. In contrast, polyoma virus codes for three T (tumor) protein-antigens: the large T (mol. wt. 100,000 daltons), the middle T (mol. wt. 56,000 daltons), and the small T (mol. wt. 22,000 daltons). It appears that the middle T is by itself sufficient for neoplastic cell transformation, whereas the large T is involved in viral DNA replication and the control of transcription. Like the onc or src gene products of some of the oncogenic RNA viruses, polyoma middle T antigen has an associated protein kinase activity, which may also be present in the large SV40 T antigens.

The transforming proteins of oncogenic RNA and DNA viruses are often found in association with various proteins of neoplastic cells (similar proteins are found in normal cells), some of which are bound to the cell-membrane fractions. It is possible that the various cell-transforming proteins affect cellular protein kinases, which participate in an elaborate metabolic cascade that controls normal cell division.

Viruses and human cancer. Evidence that viruses can

cause cancer in animals both naturally and experimentally has been accumulating steadily since the early part of this century, yet scientists have been reluctant to accept the possibility that viruses could cause cancer in humans. There are two main reasons for this attitude. First, scientists were fearful of the idea that cancer, which is a disease usually associated with death, could conceivably have a viral etiology and therefore be transmissible. Second, it is obvious that cancer in humans does not behave in ways similar to those characteristic of diseases of known viral origin, since it does not appear to be contagious, that is, transmitted by contact. The view has gradually been advanced that, although the induction of cancer by viruses in animals is no proof that the same phenomenon takes place in humans, there is a distinct possibility that some viruses could be responsible for a number of human neoplasms. Of course, both endogenous (genetic, immunologic, humoral) and exogenous (physical, chemical) factors may play a synergistic or antagonistic role in the clinical expression of cancer in the immunocompetent human host.

As of now there is no conclusive evidence that a virus or viruses cause any of the malignant neoplasms in humans. The only positive proof for a viral origin of human neoplasms derives from the finding that a papillomavirus causes benign papillomatous growths or warts of the epidermis and a poxvirus causes molluscum contagiosum, another benign skin neoplasm. There are only six instances in which some circumstantial epidemiologic relationship has been established between viruses and the development of malignant neoplasms in humans (Tables 15-4 and 15-5). These are (1) an RNA retrovirus and certain forms of adult T cell leukemia and lymphoma; (2) the Epstein-Barr virus and Burkitt's lymphoma; (3) the Epstein-Barr virus and nasopharyngeal carcinoma; (4) herpes simplex virus type 2 and carcinoma of the uterine cervix; (5) hepatitis B virus infection and primary hepatocellular carcinoma; and (6) an as yet unidentified virus and Kaposi's sarcoma. It should be mentioned parenthetically that the Epstein-Barr virus is known to cause infectious mononucleosis in young adults in America and Europe.

Although it has been proved conclusively that viruses cause cancer in animals, the evidence, as mentioned previously, that viruses can cause cancer in humans is weak or absent. This ambiguity is due chiefly to the fact that Koch's postulates, which are applicable primarily to bacterial rather than viral diseases, cannot be fulfilled with oncogenic viruses, particularly since the oncogenic potential of a virus cannot be evaluated in the human host. On the other hand, the demonstration that a human virus, whether in its intact form or partially inactivated, can induce tumors in experimental animals or can transform animal cells neoplastically in vitro is no proof that it is also oncogenic in humans. This point has been amply

illustrated by the case of human adenoviruses that are oncogenic in various experimental animals but are known to be cytopathogenic in humans, causing upper respiratory infections. Finally, the demonstration that a virus, whether of animal or human origin, can transform human cells morphologically in vitro cannot be used as evidence that the transformation event is of neoplastic nature. This has been demonstrated by the inability of Epstein-Barr virus–transformed human lymphocytes and SV40-transformed human cells to cause tumors in adult isogeneic or allogeneic patients (bearing cancer). Of course, these negative findings may be explained on the basis of the fact that, since virus-transformed cells develop new virus-related cellular antigens, they are foreign even to the isogeneic human host. Finally, that a given virus transforms human cells in vitro does not mean that the same virus will be oncogenic in the human host in vivo.

In view of these major difficulties regarding the establishment of unequivocal proof for a cause-effect relationship between viruses and human cancer, one may only hope to demonstrate a regular association between a particular viral agent and a particular type of cancer. In that case, elimination of the virus from large populations through vaccination might curtail or completely suppress the appearance of at least some of the human cancers. Of course, for vaccination to succeed, the virus must be transmitted horizontally. Otherwise, alternative means will have to be found that will prevent the expression of the oncogenic potential of vertically transmitted viruses. Even if successful vaccination were possible, the number of people that must be included in the study, the time that it would take for the results of preventive field trials to become known, and the possible complications that could arise might not justify the advantages that could result from such an effort.

A discussion of viral oncogenesis is not complete without mention of recent observations that cellular genes derived from the DNA of various animal and human cancers are capable, under appropriate experimental conditions, of neoplastically transforming mouse embryo cells grown as cell lines in culture. This type of neoplastic cell transformation could indicate that oncogenesis may result from the alteration of cellular proto-oncogenes that are homologous to the viral oncogenes.

Mode of origin

The exact mechanisms by which the multiple and complex factors produce the changes in cellular metabolism that result in tumor are not understood. Because cancer is a cellular disease, it is appropriate to postulate that one or more somatic cell mutations are induced, resulting in irreversible molecular changes in cell constituents, especially DNA. Many types of molecular abnormalities have been suggested, and perhaps several may be involved in varying combinations in respective tumors. The development of tumors is the result of the interplay of many causative factors. Some of these may act as the initiating agent and then disappear. Others (or perhaps the same agent) may serve as a secondary promoting factor at a later date. The factors may not always even act directly on the cells but may bring about their effect by acting on other tissues of the host. Although little is known as to the mode of origin of any one neoplasm, several models have been proposed on theoretical grounds suggesting different possibilities and necessities for the action of multiple agents in the final production of cancer (Fig. 15-39).

There are several theories that attempt to explain the origin of a tumor in terms of site. One theory states that a tumor may have a unicentric origin, arising from a single cell, for example, monoclonal gammopathy. This does not necessarily imply that the oncogenic agent affected a single cell only. It means, however, that if many cells were originally transformed neoplastically, one clone had a striking proliferative advantage so that it outgrew all other cells and gave rise to the whole neoplasm. A second theory suggests that a tumor may arise from single cells, but multicentrically. This is supported by the finding that multiple biopsies have demonstrated in situ carcinoma over discontinuous areas. Moreover, some neoplasms, such as retinoblastoma of the eye, are often bilateral, implying again a multifocal origin. A third theory asserts that a tumor may arise either unicentrically or multicentrically from a community of cells to be found in a given area or field, for example, cancer of the oral cavity. Still another theory indicates the possibility that,

although a tumor may arise from single or multiple points, it may enlarge not only by cellular proliferation of the original tumor foci but also by neoplastic conversion of the normal tissues in the vicinity of the neoplastic growth. It is currently believed that, as far as site is concerned, different tumors may have different modes of origin depending on a variety of predisposing or contributing factors. A point of practical importance, however, is that tumors that have an actual or potential multicentric origin may be associated with a high rate of recurrence. The multicentric mode of tumor origin would exclude the possibility that cancer arises only by spontaneous mutation of a single somatic cell.

Precancerous lesions

There are certain states or conditions that predispose to the subsequent development of tumors, particularly of cancers. Such precancerous states are important from the clinical viewpoint because by recognition and treatment of them it may be possible to prevent a subsequent cancer from arising, even though one does not understand the exact cause of the cancer.

Chronic irritation has long been blamed as a source of tumors, both benign and malignant. Although often difficult to prove, there is considerable clinical evidence to support this theory. The appearance of cancer on buccal mucosa in relation to a jagged tooth or in the gum in the region of the irritation of an ill-fitting denture plate is too frequent to be attributable to chance alone. Carcinoma of the bronchus in cigarette smokers has been shown to be preceded by metaplasia and atypical hyperplasia, presumably brought about by repeated repair after chronic

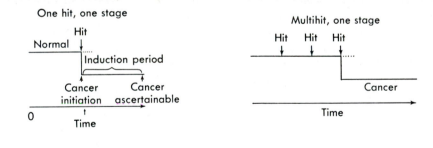

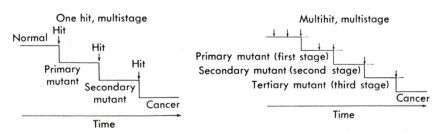

Fig. 15-39. Possible models of cancer induction. (From Barron, B.A., and Richart, R.M.: J. Natl. Cancer Inst. **41:**1343, 1968.)

irritation. On the other hand, there are regions of the body, such as the palm of the hand, that are subject to much irritation and yet the development of tumor in those locations is exceedingly rare.

Many of the precancerous conditions represent hyperplasias, often long standing and somewhat atypical as compared with the usual hyperplasias. One example is the hyperplastic change that arises in skin that has been exposed to excessive irradiation: a hyperplasia that becomes progressively atypical develops, and often multiple foci of cancer appear 5, 10, or even more years later. Many chemical carcinogens experimentally seem to work in a similar manner with hyperplasia of a progressively atypical nature usually preceding the development of at least the recognition of true cancer. Some chemical carcinogens do not act as chronic irritants and still are carcinogenic, and many chemicals are irritants but do not produce cancer.

In the course of the growth of the embryos, groups of cells may fail to develop properly and may become segregated in the tissues, and evidence suggests that such rests are more likely to become tumorous than normal tissues. Either benign or malignant tumors may arise from embryonic rests, but these are not a common source of tumor.

The question of whether a benign tumor may become malignant is difficult to answer with any degree of accuracy. The available evidence indicates that benign tumors do not commonly become malignant. Although such a possibility does exist, most malignant tumors probably are malignant from their inception rather than passing through a benign neoplastic phase.

There are numerous other conditions or states that have been suggested to be precancerous. Some of these, such as hormone imbalances and neurofibromatosis, have been mentioned previously. The list is almost limitless and includes some items with dubious and unproved relationships. The few mentioned here will give an idea as to the scope of changes that have been suggested:

1. Achlorhydria often precedes the development of cancer of the stomach.
2. Lack of circumcision predisposes to cancer of the penis.
3. Gallstones usually precede cancer of the gallbladder.
4. Cirrhosis precedes most liver cancer.
5. Women who were pregnant at an early age have a lower risk of breast cancer than do those older with their first pregnancy.
6. Adenocarcinoma of the vagina is more common in women whose mothers had been administered stilbestrol for threatened abortion.
7. Cancer is far more likely to develop in an undescended testis than in a normally descended testis.
8. Fair-skinned individuals are particularly predisposed to cancer of the lip and skin.

CANCER AS A PUBLIC HEALTH PROBLEM

As previously noted, cancer is a worldwide disease. Although it has often been considered a disease of civilization, humankind must have been exposed to various carcinogens for millions of years, even though new ones may well have been added in recent times. Reports of cancer in the developing countries are numerous, and cancer is a leading cause of death in most parts of the world today.

Much interesting and useful information regarding tumors has been obtained from the study of data compiled from geographic and demographic studies and from statistics from large series of well-documented cancer cases. Opportunities for human experiments in the etiology of cancer are limited, but by collection and study of epidemiologic data it has been possible, for example, to suggest specific agents that might be involved. Such data often have implicated a carcinogenic agent present in occupational or other exposures, and such data led to the conclusion that excessive cigarette smoking is in some way related to the development of cancer of the bronchus.

The varying incidence of types of cancer in different parts of the world suggests endless possibilities for etiologic investigation (Table 15-6). For example, the high incidence of liver cancer in Africa and Asia may represent a two-stage process consisting of liver damage in childhood, possibly from malnutrition, which predisposes the

Table 15-6. Estimated age-adjusted death rates per 100,000 population in various countries

	All sites		Lung		Stomach		Breast	Prostate
Country	**Male**	**Female**	**Male**	**Female**	**Male**	**Female**	**Female**	**Male**
Austria	189	123	52	7	31	16	19	15
Chile	147	121	18	5	50	26	11	12
England and Wales	190	123	74	15	20	9	28	12
Japan	141	88	19	6	57	29	5	2
United States	159	106	51	12	7	4	22	15
Venezuela	101	100	16	7	28	17	9	10

From 1981 Cancer facts and figures, New York, 1980, American Cancer Society.

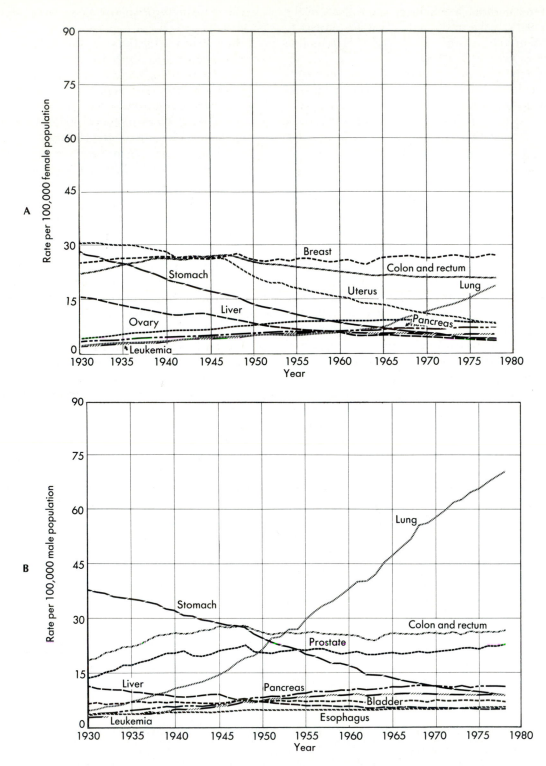

Fig. 15-40. Trend of female, **A,** and male, **B,** cancer death rates by site, United States, 1930-1978. Rate is standardized for age on the 1970 U.S. population. Data from National Vital Statistics Division, Bureau of the Census. (From 1981 Cancer facts and figures, New York, 1980, American Cancer Society.)

Table 15-7. Estimated cancer deaths by sex
for all sites, 1981

Site	Estimated deaths		
	Total	Male	Female
All sites	420,000	227,500	192,500
Buccal cavity and pharynx (oral)	9,150	6,300	2,850
Lip	175	150	25
Tongue	2,000	1,400	600
Salivary gland	700	450	250
Floor of mouth	525	400	125
Other and unspecified mouth	1,550	1,000	550
Pharynx	4,200	2,900	1,300
Digestive organs	110,500	57,600	52,900
Esophagus	8,100	5,800	2,300
Stomach	13,900	8,400	5,500
Small intestine	700	350	350
Large intestine (colon-	46,200	21,500	24,700
Rectum rectum)	8,700	4,700	4,000
Liver and biliary passages	9,400	4,600	4,800
Pancreas	22,000	11,500	10,500
Other and unspecified digestive	1,500	750	750
Respiratory system	110,100	81,000	29,100
Larynx	3,700	3,100	600
Lung	105,000	77,000	28,000
Other and unspecified respiratory	1,400	900	500
Bone, tissue and skin	10,050	5,800	4,250
Bone	1,750	1,000	750
Connective tissue	1,600	800	800
Skin	6,700	4,000	2,700
Breast	37,100	300	36,800
Genital organs	46,400	23,700	22,700
Cervix, invasive uterus	7,200	—	7,200
Corpus, endometrium	3,100	—	3,100
Ovary	11,400	—	11,400
Prostate	22,700	22,700	—
Testis, other male genital	1,000	1,000	—
Other and unspecified genital, female	1,000	—	1,000
Urinary organs	18,700	12,200	6,500
Bladder	10,600	7,300	3,300
Kidney and other urinary	8,100	4,900	3,200
Eye	400	200	200
Brain and central nervous system	10,200	5,600	4,600
Endocrine glands	1,500	600	900
Thyroid	1,050	350	700
Other endocrine	450	250	200
Leukemia	15,900	8,900	7,000
Other blood and lymph tissues	21,600	11,200	10,400
Hodgkin's disease	1,700	1,000	700
Multiple myeloma	6,700	3,400	3,300
Other lymphomas	13,200	6,800	6,400
All other and unspecified sites	28,400	14,100	14,300

From 1981 Cancer facts and figures, New York, 1980, American Cancer Society.

*Carcinoma in situ of the uterine cervix and superficial skin cancers not included in totals.

organ to a carcinogenic stimulus (such as viral hepatitis or a chemical carcinogen) in later life.

There is evidence that a single brief exposure to a carcinogen may cause a rapid rise followed by a slow decline in the incidence of certain cancers, whereas prolonged exposure gives a continuous rise in incidence, such as occurs with cigarette smoke and lung cancer.

Statistical data are, of course, also necessary in emphasizing the relative importance of certain cancers and in pointing out trends for specific cancers to increase or decrease (Fig. 15-40). The death rates of some of the common cancers are shown in Table 15-7.

During the past 25 years the overall incidence of cancer in the United States has decreased slightly. Cancers of the stomach, esophagus, rectum, and uterus have declined, whereas cancers of the lung, pancreas, and colon have increased. In 1981 in the United States there were an estimated 815,000 new cancer cases, of which 412,000 were in females and 403,000 in males. Cancer at present ranks as the second most common cause of death in the United States (Table 15-8).

Obviously, malignant tumors represent a great public health problem. The best approach to the problem would be prevention, but this is difficult because the cause of most cancers is still unknown. Since most cancers are at present unexplained by genetic factors, they must be caused by exogenous factors; theoretically, therefore, if the exogenous factors were better understood, most cancers should be preventable. Early detection also warrants much attention because it allows better chances for cure or palliation. An example of a pathologic technique for early detection is cytologic diagnosis,

Table 15-8. Mortality for leading causes of death in the United States, 1977

Rank	Cause of death	Number of deaths	Death rate per 100,000 population	Percent of total deaths
	All causes	1,899,597	816.3	100.0
1	Diseases of heart	718,850	303.4	37.8
2	Cancer	386,686	168.4	20.4
3	Stroke	181,934	75.3	9.6
4	Accidents	103,202	45.4	5.4
5	Influenza and pneumonia	51,193	21.4	2.7
	Others	248,101	107.3	13.1

From 1981 Cancer facts and figures, New York, 1980, American Cancer Society.

especially in patients believed to be at high risk, for example, sputum examination in uranium workers for early detection of lung cancer. Treatments for cure or palliation have improved both in type and in effectiveness with continually better understanding of the biochemistry and pathology of the disease.

The goals for the control of cancer are prevention, earlier recognition, and better treatment. However, individual cancers have such diverse causes and biologic behaviors that they cannot be attacked as a single disease; this one frustrating fact is the major obstacle to cancer control.

GLOSSARY

adenocarcinoma malignant tumor of glandular epithelium.

adenoma benign tumor of glandular epithelium.

agenesis complete congenital absence of an organ or tissue.

anaplasia backward growth; a change in tumor cells to less differentiated cells with loss of some structural or functional characteristics; often used as a synonym for undifferentiation.

aplasia lack of development of an organ or tissue.

atrophy diminution in size of cells, organ, or tissue after full development has been attained.

benign innocuous; in tumor terms, refers to a neoplasm that grows slowly, remains localized, and usually does little harm; rarely used synonym, benignant.

cachexia severe wasting of body tissues because of a chronic disease such as cancer.

cancer malignant neoplasm.

cancerogen agent that produces cancer; term rarely used, carcinogen being applied, often incorrectly, in its place.

carcinogen strictly, an agent that produces carcinoma; in common although incorrect usage, an agent that produces any type of tumor.

carcinoma malignant tumor of epithelium.

carcinoma in situ malignant epithelial tumor showing no invasion.

carcinoma simplex poorly differentiated adenocarcinoma.

carcinosarcoma a cancer containing a mixture of carcinomatous and sarcomatous elements.

colloid mucinous; excessive production of mucus.

cystadenoma benign tumor of glandular epithelium forming cysts.

cytology literally, study of cells; in current usage, study of exfoliated cells (Papanicolaou technique) for purpose of diagnosing cancer; cytotechnology.

desmoplasia excessive fibrous tissue formation in tumor stroma.

differentiated possessing cellular maturity and organization similar to normal.

dormant resting; a tumor in an inactive state but capable of resuming activity

dysplasia abnormal, atypical cellular proliferation; not tumor.

epidermoid carcinoma cancer of squamous epithelium; synonym, squamous cell carcinoma.

grade estimate of the degree of malignancy of a tumor.

hamartoma malformation of tissues indigenous to area resembling and having some features of tumor.

hyperplasia increase in number of cells per unit of tissue.

hypertrophy increase in size of cells, organ, or tissue.

hypoplasia arrested development of an organ or tissue below normal mature size.

latent not clearly apparent but capable of emerging and developing into clinical significance.

lymphoma broad term used for any cancer arising from lymphoid tissue.

malignancy state or quality of being malignant; not a synonym for cancer.

malignant malicious, of high virulence; in tumor terms, a neoplasm with ability to invade, metastasize, and cause death; synonym rarely used, malign.

medullary marrowlike; gross description term for soft and presumably highly cellular tumor.

mesenchymoma a tumor, benign or malignant, consisting of two or more mesenchymal elements in addition to fibrous stroma.

metaplasia change of a type of adult cell to one not normally present in that tissue.

metastasis secondary discontinuous cancerous growth; term also used for process of formation of such growths.

mixed tumor literally, tumor with mixed elements; in common usage, term often applied to specific type of tumor arising mostly in salivary glands.

neoplasm new growth, tumor (see text).

occult hidden; term used to describe cancers not detectable by the usual clinical examinations.

oncogenic tumor producing; term applied mostly to tumor-producing viruses.

oncology the study of tumors.

papilloma benign epithelial tumor in which neoplastic cells cover fingerlike processes of stroma; also, any benign epithelial tumor growing outward from surface.

pearls collections of keratin formed in well-differentiated epidermoid carcinomas.

pleomorphism variability in morphology, especially in size and shape.

polyp tumor or tumorlike mass projecting from mucosal surface.

prognosis a forecast as to the probable course and outcome of a disease.

sarcoma nonepithelial malignant tumor; includes most cancers of mesodermal tissues, such as connective tissue, muscle, and lymphoid tissue.

scirrhous (pronounced skir'us or sir'us) gross descriptive term for tumor that is firm because of extensive desmoplasia.

squamous cell carcinoma synonym for epidermoid carcinoma.

stage estimate of extent of spread of cancer.

teratology study of abnormal embryonic development and congenital malformations.

teratoma true neoplasm arising from totipotential cells and composed therefore of numerous types of tissues.

tumor in older usage, any swelling; current usage, synonym for neoplasm (see text).

REFERENCES

1. Arrighi, F.E., et al., editors: Genes, chromosomes, and neoplasia, New York, 1980, Raven Press.
2. Atkin, N.B.: Cytogenetic aspects of malignant transformation, New York, 1976, S. Karger.
3. Baserga, R., editor: The cell cycle and cancer, New York, 1971, Dekker.
4. Becker, F.F., editor: Cancer: a comprehensive treatise, 6 vols., New York, 1975-1977, Plenum Press.
5. Bodansky, O.: Biochemistry of human cancer, New York, 1975, Academic Press, Inc.
6. Cairns, J.: Cancer: science and society, San Francisco, 1978, W.F. Freeman & Co.
7. Castro, J.E., editor: Immunological aspects of cancer, Baltimore, 1978, University Park Press.
8. Clark, R.L., et al., editors: The year book of cancer, Chicago, annual, Year Book Medical Publishers.
9. Daland, E.M.: Untreated cancer of breast, Surg. Gynecol. Obstet. **44:**264, 1927.
10. Day, S.B., et al., editors: Cancer invasion and metastasis: biologic mechanisms and therapy, New York, 1977, Raven Press.
11. del Regato, J.A., and Spjut, H.J., editors: Cancer: diagnosis, treatment and prognosis, ed. 5, St. Louis, 1977, The C.V. Mosby Co.
12. Doll, R., et al.: The causes of cancer: quantitative estimates of avoidable risks of cancer in the United States today—special report, J. Natl. Cancer Inst. **66:**1191, 1981.
13. Essex, M., et al., editors: Viruses in naturally occurring cancers, Cold Spring Harbor, N.Y., 1980, Cold Spring Harbor Laboratory.
14. Furth, J., Kim, U., and Clifton, K.H.: Cancer progression from dependence to autonomy, Natl. Cancer Inst. Monogr. 2:149, 1960.
15. Gross, L.: Oncogenic viruses, ed. 3, New York, 1981, Pergamon Press, Inc.
16. Grundman, N.E., editor: Recent results in cancer research, New York, annual, Springer-Verlag.
17. Harris, J.E., et al.: The immunology of malignant disease, St. Louis, 1976, The C.V. Mosby Co.
18. Hartmann, W.H., et al., editors: Atlas of tumor pathology, Washington, D.C., Armed Forces Institute of Pathology.
19. Hiatt, H.H., et al., editors: Origins of human cancer, Cold Spring Harbor, N.Y., 1977, Cold Spring Harbor Laboratory.
20. Holland, J.F., et al., editors: Cancer medicine, Philadelphia, 1973, Lea & Febiger.
21. Homburger, F., editor: Progress in experimental tumor research, Basel, annual, S. Karger.
22. Hynes, R.O., editor: Surface of normal and malignant cells, New York, 1979, John Wiley & Sons, Inc.
23. Kaiser, H.E., editor: Neoplasms—comparative pathology of growth in animals, plants, and man, Baltimore, 1981, The Williams & Wilkins Co.
24. Klein, G., et al., editors: Advances in cancer research, New York, annual, Academic Press, Inc.
25. Lynch, H.T., editor: Cancer genetics, Springfield, Ill., 1976, Charles C Thomas, Publisher.
26. Manual for staging of cancer, Chicago, 1980, American Joint Committee for Cancer Staging and End Results Reporting.
27. Papanicolaou, G.N.: Atlas of exfoliative cytology, Cambridge, Mass., 1954, Harvard University Press.
28. Park, W.W.: The histology of borderline cancer—with notes on prognosis, Berlin, 1980, Springer-Verlag.
29. Pierce, G.B., et al.: Cancer, a problem of developmental biology, Englewood Cliffs, N.J., 1978, Prentice-Hall, Inc.
30. Prescott, D.M.: Reproduction of eukaryotic cells, New York, 1976, Academic Press, Inc.
31. Rosenberg, S.A., editor: Serologic analysis of human cancer antigens, New York, 1980, Academic Press, Inc.
32. Schottenfeld, D., editor: Cancer epidemiology and prevention: current concepts, Springfield, Ill., 1975, Charles C Thomas, Publisher.
33. Sherman, M.I., et al., editors: Teratomas and differentiation, New York, 1975, Academic Press, Inc.
34. Slaga, T.J., editor: Modifiers of chemical carcinogenesis: an approach to the biochemical mechanism and cancer prevention, New York, 1980, Raven Press.
35. Slaga, T.J., et al., editors: Mechanisms of tumor promotion and cocarcinogenesis, New York, 1978, Raven Press.
36. Sobin, L.H., et al., editors: A coded compendium of the international histological classification of tumors, Geneva, 1978, World Health Organization.
37. Tooze, J., editor: DNA tumor viruses, ed. 2, Cold Spring Harbor, N.Y., 1981, Cold Spring Harbor Laboratory.
38. Waters, H., editor: The handbook of cancer immunology, New York, 1978, Garland STPM Press.
39. Weiss, L., editor: Fundamental aspects of metastasis, Amsterdam, 1976, North Holland Publishing Co.
40. Weiss, R.A., editor: RNA tumor viruses, ed. 2, Cold Spring Harbor, N.Y., 1981, Cold Spring Harbor Laboratory.
41. Woodruff, M.F.A.: The interaction of cancer and host—its therapeutic significance, New York, 1980, Grune & Stratton, Inc.
42. Yuhas, J.M., et al., editors: Biology of radiation carcinogenesis, New York, 1976, Raven Press.

CHAPTER 16 **Heart**

THOMAS M. SCOTTI
DONALD B. HACKEL

The cardiovascular system consists of the heart, blood vessels, and lymphatics. Although the heart and blood vessels are considered separately as a matter of convenience, it is evident that functionally the system is a unit. The heart is essentially a pump, provided with valves and powered by muscular walls. It is enclosed within the pericardium, a fibroserous sac containing a small amount of fluid, which basically is a lubricated compartment in which it can move. The visceral pericardium (the epicardium) forms the outer layer of the heart.

Heart disease is a major cause of illness and disability and is the leading cause of death in the United States[1]; in 1978 heart disease was responsible for almost two fifths (37.8%) of all deaths. In that year there were 1,927,788 deaths from all causes, of which 729,510 were attributed to cardiac disease, a total death rate of 334.3 per 100,000 population.[1] This is a marked increase compared with the mortality from heart disease of about 60 years earlier. For example, in 1920 cardiac deaths (124,143) represented only 10.9% of all deaths (1,142,558), a rate of 141.9 per 100,000 population.[2] However, in the 1960s yearly mortality for heart disease generally exceeded that of 1978, reaching a peak in 1963 when the rate was 375.2 per 100,000 population.[3] Thus it appears that there has been a downward trend in mortality from heart disorders in recent years.[3,5,6]

The four major cardiac disorders are (1) ischemic heart disease, particularly the atherosclerotic type, (2) hypertensive heart disease (hypertensive cardiopathy), (3) rheumatic heart disease, and (4) congenital heart disease.

Ischemic heart disease and hypertensive heart disease are the most important health problems in the United States among middle-aged and elderly persons.[4] By far the leading type of fatal cardiac disease is ischemic heart disease,[3,5] and considerable attention will be given to this subject.

Syphilitic heart disease and bacterial endocarditis are still important diseases, but they do not occur as frequently as in previous years. Morbidity and mortality for other types of infectious heart disease also are low. Likewise, nutritional cardiovascular diseases, such as cardiac beriberi, are of little significance in the United States.[4]

The order of presentation of the material will be first a consideration of the noninflammatory conditions other than growth disturbances (for example, degenerative diseases, metabolic disturbances, nutritional disturbances, traumatic diseases, radiation injury, endocrine disturbances, fluid and electrolyte disturbances, and disturbances of circulation of blood, including particularly ischemic heart disease), followed by the various inflammatory diseases, and then the disturbances of growth, such as atrophy, hypertrophy and dilatation, cysts, and tumors. The final items to be discussed briefly will be disturbances of the conduction system, biopsy of the pericardium and myocardium, and rejection of cardiac transplants. Congenital heart disease is dealt with in Chapter 17.

Before discussing the various heart diseases, it is fitting to review briefly some pertinent aspects of cardiac failure, since frequent references will be made to this condition.

CARDIAC FAILURE

Cardiac failure is a clinical state in which the heart is unable to maintain an adequate circulation for bodily needs. The basic factors that cause or contribute to heart failure may be summarized as follows:

1. The heart muscle may be weakened by disease processes that cause sufficient loss of muscle tissue or impairment of contractility so that the heart is unable to function as an efficient pump. Among the lesions producing myocardial weakness are myocardial infarction, myocardial fibrosis, coronary insufficiency, myocarditis, and metabolic disorders.

2. There may be a mechanical overload of the heart that in time may lead to myocardial failure. Such an

increased demand on the myocardium results from (a) an increased resistance to ejection of blood, as in valvular stenosis or hypertension, or (b) an excessive demand for increased cardiac output, as in valvular insufficiency, arteriovenous shunts, and increased tissue needs (such as thyrotoxicosis).

3. Impaired filling of the heart chambers, as may result from cardiac tamponade or constrictive pericarditis, may be responsible for a decreased cardiac output.

In some instances heart failure may result from a combination of these basic factors.

Cardiac failure is either acute or chronic. Acute failure is caused by such conditions as coronary occlusion, obstruction to cardiac outflow as in massive pulmonary embolism, or cardiac tamponade resulting from sudden hemopericardium incident to rupture of the heart. In acute heart failure there is a sudden reduction or cessation of cardiac output. Dyspnea, orthopnea, and pulmonary edema may be present, and in some instances the symptoms of shock develop. Chronic heart failure is most commonly seen in association with coronary atherosclerosis, hypertensive cardiopathy, and valvular deformities. However, it may occur as a result of any disease that weakens the heart directly or causes an increased demand on the myocardium. Whenever the cardiovascular system makes sufficient adjustments to maintain adequate output, a state of compensation is reached. The principal compensatory phenomena are tachycardia, cardiac dilatation, and cardiac hypertrophy. When the adjustments are inadequate, a state of cardiac decompensation is said to exist.

Heart failure may involve one side of the heart more than the other. In left-sided heart failure the major manifestations are those associated with passive congestion and edema of the lungs. In more severe cases, pulmonary hypertension results, leading to failure of the right side of the heart. Although failure of the right side of the heart is usually combined with that of the left, there are instances of isolated right-sided failure. The manifestations of right-sided heart failure include subcutaneous edema (particularly in the dependent parts of the body), hydrothorax, ascites, passive congestion of the liver and spleen, generalized venous congestion, cyanosis, and, usually, increased blood volume. The clinical syndrome with the foregoing features is termed congestive heart failure. The cardiac output in typical congestive heart failure usually is reduced, although in some patients at rest it may be normal. Cardiac failure associated with certain diseases (such as hyperthyroidism, severe anemias, and arteriovenous shunts, including arteriovenous fistulas and the shunts in the bones in osteitis deformans) may be accompanied by an elevated cardiac output; thus it is given the designation *high-output heart failure*.

The terms *backward failure* and *forward failure* have been applied to the manifestations of congestive heart failure. In backward failure there is an increase in diastolic pressure within the failing ventricle or ventricles, followed by a rise in atrial pressure that is transmitted backward, producing an elevated pressure in the veins. In forward failure the manifestations result from failure of the heart to pump a sufficient output, causing a diminished flow of blood to the tissues, particularly to the kidneys. Actually, these two mechanisms do not function independently of each other, since in a continuous circulation one does not occur without the other.

The pathogenesis of edema in cardiac failure is an intriguing problem that has held the interest of investigators for a long time but is still not completely solved. For many years the edema has been explained as a consequence of increased venous pressure, leading to a rise in capillary blood pressure, increased filtration, and edema. Although increased venous pressure plays a part in the development of edema, the emphasis today is on the importance of retention of sodium and water in the body. The role of intrinsic renal mechanisms and hormonal or neural factors (for example, reduction in glomerular filtration rate, enhanced renal tubular reabsorption of sodium, hypersecretion of aldosterone, and an increased release of antidiuretic hormone) has been discussed in Chapter 3 (p. 73).

NONINFLAMMATORY DISEASES OTHER THAN GROWTH DISTURBANCES
Degenerative diseases and disturbances in metabolism

The degenerative processes affecting the heart, particularly the myocardium, include atrophy and the disturbances in protein, fat, carbohydrate, and mineral metabolism.

Atrophy

Since atrophy is brought about by some disturbance of intracellular metabolism (p. 95), it deserves mention in this section. However, the details are considered later under disturbances of growth (p. 638).

Disturbances in protein metabolism
Parenchymatous and hydropic degeneration

If the heart is affected by either parenchymatous or hydropic degenerative changes, the myocardium is usually soft and flabby and there is likely to be some degree of dilatation of the ventricles. On the cut surface the muscle of the left ventricle is gray or grayish brown and characteristically has a swollen, opaque, frosted-glass appearance (the reason for the term *cloudy swelling*). In parenchymatous degeneration the microscopic picture is that of swollen, indistinct muscle cells with increased granularity of the cytoplasm from the presence of innumerable, small protein particles. In hydropic degeneration, an extension of the process of cloudy swelling, there is vacuolization of the cytoplasm resulting from the accumulation of small droplets of water. These degenerative processes are the result of cellular injury occurring in a variety of conditions, including infectious diseases, especially those associated with high fevers, intoxications from chemical and metallic poisons, extensive burns, and anoxemia from many causes.

Basophilic or mucoid degeneration of myocardium

Basophilic or mucoid degeneration of the myocardium is a common but often overlooked alteration of the muscle fibers (Fig. 16-1). The term *basophilic degeneration* is applicable because in sections stained with hematoxylin and eosin there is an accumulation of a basophilic material within the cytoplasm of the muscle cells. The lesion occurs in the muscle of all chambers, but the left ventricle is most frequently affected. Characteristically the distribution is focal or patchy, with involvement of occasional or many fibers throughout the myocardium. The change also has been observed in Purkinje fibers. The basophilic material usually accumulates at first in the perinuclear portion of the fiber. In the early lesion it is very pale, separating the myofibrils and causing little if any fragmentation of them. The affected fiber often is swollen. Later the cytoplasmic substance extends throughout the fiber, replacing the myofibrils. It may be light blue and granular, sometimes producing a slightly vacuolated appearance of the affected area, or there may be small, irregular, homogeneous masses of deeper blue material in the degenerated foci. The nucleus generally is not disturbed, although occasionally in more extensively involved fibers it appears to be undergoing partial dissolution. The degenerated fibers frequently contain abundant lipofuscin pigment.

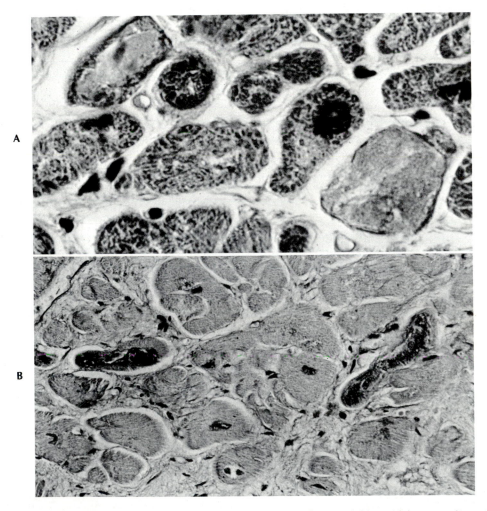

Fig. 16-1. Basophilic degeneration of myocardium. **A,** Mucoid material (blue with hematoxylin stain) within two muscle fibers. Only thin rim of sarcoplasm remains. In greatly swollen fiber *(lower right)* intracytoplasmic substance is finely vacuolated. In other fiber *(upper left)* few darker homogeneous clumps are present with paler substance. **B,** Two fibers containing mucoid material stained by periodic acid–Schiff method.

Significant histochemical findings include a positive periodic acid–Schiff reaction, even after digestion with diastase; metachromasia with toluidine blue; bright blue-green stain with Alcian blue; light red stain with Mayer's mucicarmine; negative Feulgen reaction; and negative reactions with ribonuclease and hyaluronidase.[38,39] The basophilic intracytoplasmic substance, sometimes referred to as mucinous degeneration[38] or cardiac colloid,[19] has been considered to be a mucoprotein or acid mucopolysaccharide. Since it does not stain for lipids, it probably is not a glycolipid.[19] The results of certain histochemical and electron microscopic studies have led some investigators to suggest that the basophilic material is a product of a disorder of carbohydrate (mainly glycogen) metabolism, being composed essentially of a glycoprotein[35] or a glucan (polyglucosan).[27,33]

Basophilic degeneration occurs most frequently in persons over 40 years of age, although it is observed occasionally in younger individuals. The cause is unknown, but it may be related to ischemia of the myocardium.[38] A possible relationship to myxedema has been considered.[9,16] However, it is apparent that basophilic degeneration of the myocardium is not specific for this disease (see "Hypothyroidism [myxedema heart]", p. 572). Instances of this myocardial lesion have been observed in progressive familial myoclonic epilepsy, possibly the result of actual or relative ischemia that may be associated with the muscle spasm and epileptic attacks occurring in this disease.[30] As a rule this degenerative change does not produce functional cardiac disturbances, but the possibility that severe degrees of the process may be clinically significant should be considered.

Hyaline degeneration

In certain acute infectious diseases, individual muscle fibers may become swollen, and their sarcoplasm may be deeply eosinophilic and homogeneous while the nuclei are pyknotic or disappear. This change resembles Zenker's (waxy) degeneration or necrosis of striated voluntary muscle. Hyaline degeneration often is present in the muscle fibers remaining in an old healed myocardial infarct. It also is observed in the myocardium in nutritional disturbances such as beriberi. The hyaline change in these conditions, however, is not apparent grossly. A more prominent hyalinization, seen grossly as well as microscopically, occurs in areas of connective tissue proliferation—for example, old myocardial infarcts replaced by scar tissue; areas of fibrosis of the myocardium resulting from the healing of an inflammatory lesion; and fibrous thickening of the mural endocardium such as that adjacent to an old myocardial infarct, that resulting from abnormal currents of the bloodstream as in valvular insufficiency, or that associated with endocardial fibroelastosis (p. 646).

Amyloidosis*

In secondary amyloidosis deposits of amyloid occur most abundantly in the spleen, kidneys, liver, and adrenal glands. The heart also may be involved in this variant of the disease, but the deposits of amyloid usually are small. Amyloid infiltration of the heart is observed most frequently in primary systemic amyloidosis. The latter occurs without apparent preexisting disease and is characterized by widespread deposits of amyloid in the tongue, gastrointestinal tract, lungs, skeletal muscles, skin, and other mesodermal tissues and organs, in addition to deposits in the heart. Amyloidosis associated with multiple myeloma, in which the distribution of amyloid is much like that seen in the primary systemic form, is sometimes accompanied by cardiac involvement.

A distinctive type of amyloidosis has been described in which amyloid is restricted largely to the heart. Deposits either do not appear in other organs or are present in insignificant amounts. This is in contrast to the systemic forms of amyloidosis in which involvement of other organs is extensive. It is of considerable interest that the average age of persons with amyloid confined to the heart is higher than that of those with primary systemic amyloidosis or amyloid disease complicating multiple myeloma. The disease affects elderly persons, usually in the seventh to ninth decades, and thus seems to be a manifestation of senescence. It is sometimes referred to as senile cardiac amyloidosis.

In addition to the foregoing forms of amyloidosis, certain hereditary types have been reported in which the heart may become involved, and in one type it is the organ predominantly affected.[11]

The deposits of amyloid in the heart may be so slight that they produce no significant gross morphologic alterations, but generally they are widely distributed throughout the organ in a nodular or diffuse fashion, causing characteristic macroscopic changes. In severe involvement the heart is usually enlarged. The walls of the various chambers, particularly the atria, are thick and rigid, so that they do not collapse when the blood escapes. The cut surface of the myocardium is tan and glistening, and sometimes translucent streaks, bands, or nodular masses of amyloid may be seen. In the endocardium of the atria there are minute, translucent gray or pink-gray, slightly elevated nodules arranged diffusely or in localized collections, often causing a mottled or speckled appearance of the endocardium. Similar nodules may appear in the epicardium, or there may be diffuse, indurated, grayish, thickened areas of both layers of the pericardium. Nodular or diffuse thickening of the valvular endocardium occurs in some instances.

Microscopically, amyloid appears interstitially as scat-

*References 10-12, 23, 24, 26, 31, 41.

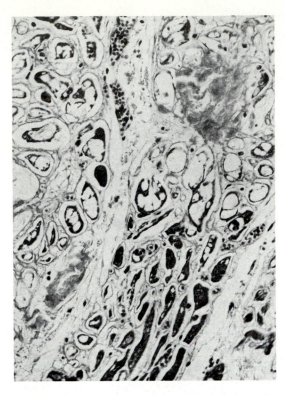

Fig. 16-2. Amyloidosis of myocardium. Microscopic section discloses clumps of hyaline material interstitially and also surrounding myocardial fibers. Cytoplasm of many fibers has disappeared. Other fibers are atrophic.

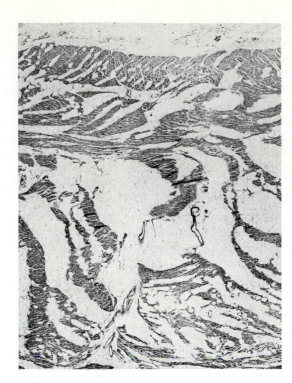

Fig. 16-3. Extensive stromal fatty infiltration of myocardium with replacement of muscle.

tered foci with little effect on adjacent muscle fibers or as nodular or diffuse deposits that compress the muscle cells and sometimes form ringlike structures around the fibers (Fig. 16-2). The more extensive infiltrations cause atrophy, vacuolization, and even disappearance of muscle fibers. Deposits of amyloid may be seen in the walls of small and medium-sized arteries and veins. Discrete masses of amyloid are seen in the connective tissue of the endocardium. In the epicardium the hyaline material may surround the fat cells, producing characteristic amyloid rings. Special stains are used to identify amyloid in the heart, but often the reactions are variable or atypical. (see also p. 90).

Clinically, there may be evidence of cardiomegaly and congestive heart failure and electrocardiographic changes. Cardiac amyloidosis may be suspected if a patient, especially an elderly one, develops congestive heart failure in the absence of any recognizable cause of failure.

Disturbances in fat metabolism
Fatty infiltration

Fatty infiltration of the heart consists of an abnormal accumulation of adipose tissue interstitially in the myocardium, usually associated with an excessive amount of adipose tissue in the stromal layer of the epicardium. It is not to be confused with fatty degeneration, in which lipid

is present within the cytoplasm of the myocardial fibers (see the following discussion). Fatty infiltration occurs most commonly in the ventral wall of the right ventricle. It also affects the wall of the right atrium, where it may involve the sinoatrial and the atrioventricular nodes. Sometimes it occurs in the left ventricle, particularly in the subendocardial myocardium.

Grossly, on the cut surface of the myocardium there is loss of the normally sharp demarcation of the muscle from the overlying epicardial fat. From the latter site, yellow streaks and bands extend into the myocardium. If the involvement is extensive, slightly elevated yellow areas may be seen beneath the endocardium.

Microscopically, the excessive adipose tissue in the myocardium is continuous with the epicardial fat, except when fatty infiltration is localized in the subendocardial myocardium of the left ventricle. The fatty tissue separates muscle bundles and individual fibers, causing compression and atrophy of the fibers. Sometimes the adipose tissue may replace all or almost all of the muscle of a particular area (Fig. 16-3).

Fatty infiltration of the heart occurs most often in patients with generalized obesity. As a rule, the lesion does not cause significant clinical manifestations even when it is severe. Impairment of cardiac function is said to be present occasionally, but only in instances of very extensive involvement of the myocardium. Fatty infiltration of the myocardium is rarely the primary cause of death, but in some patients it may be contributory. When other diseases place an extra load on a right ventricle that is already affected by fatty infiltration, this chamber may be unable to compensate. Only rarely has cardiac rupture occurred at the site of fatty infiltration.

Fatty degeneration

Fatty degeneration of the myocardium is characterized by the presence of lipid droplets or globules within the cytoplasm of the muscle fibers as a result of injury sustained by the cells. Causes of this lesion include anoxic, toxinic, and toxic injury. Anoxia may be associated with severe anemias, particularly pernicious and aplastic anemias. Sometimes leukemia is responsible. Severe loss of blood or coronary insufficiency may have a similar result. Bacterial toxins (as in diphtheria), septicemias with high fever, and intoxications from chemicals, such as phosphorus, chloroform, arsenic, ether, and alcohol, also may cause fatty degeneration of the myocardium. The lesion has been attributed to uremic intoxication, but it is possible that the concomitant anemia, rather than uremia itself, is responsible.[28] Fatty degeneration is observed in the myocardium of newborns who die soon after delivery or within the first few days of life and in whom there is clinical and postmortem evidence of cardiac failure. The causes of death in the newborn fall into three categories: (1) pulmonary atelectasis, hyaline membrane disease, or hypoplasia, (2) unavoidable loss of fetal blood in utero, hemolytic disease of the newborn, or placental insufficiency, and (3) congenital heart disease.[37]

Grossly, two forms of fatty degeneration are observed: patchy and diffuse.[14] In the patchy form the subendocardial portion of the myocardium and the papillary muscles are affected, particularly in the left ventricle. This type is especially characteristic of the anemias. Beneath the surface a yellowish mottling can be seen, that is, irregular yellowish streaks or lines of involved muscle alternating with lines of unaffected muscle, producing a "tigroid," "tabby cat," or "thrush-breast" appearance. Foci of fatty degeneration may be seen in other layers of the myocardium, but these are usually of minor degree. In the diffuse form, which appears most often in severe infections and toxic states, there is a pale yellowish discoloration throughout the entire myocardium of both ventricles. The heart is soft and flabby. If there is only a slight degree of involvement, the fatty change may not be apparent in the gross specimen and can be recognized only by microscopic examination. In newborns the lesion tends to occur in the right side of the heart, but in older babies both ventricles are equally involved. The amount of fat appears to be related to the duration of cardiac stress and is especially noticeable in those whose death is caused by hyaline membrane disease.[37]

Microscopically, the cytoplasm of the degenerated muscle fibers appears finely vacuolated in sections stained with hematoxylin and eosin (Fig. 16-4, A). The fat droplets are clearly seen in the cells of tissue treated with special stains such as Sudan IV and osmic acid (Fig. 16-4,

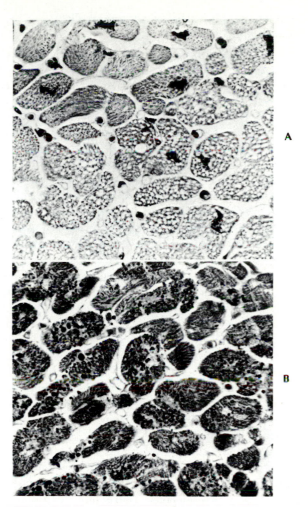

Fig. 16-4. Fatty degeneration of myocardium. **A,** Rather uniform, fine vacuolization in myocardial fibers. **B,** Degeneration in phosphorus poisoning. Black droplets in myocardial fibers are globules of fat (osmic acid stain). Occasional fat globules in interstitial tissue appear to have been expelled from fibers.

B). Many investigators believe that cardiac disturbances are not caused by this lesion. However, in one report, no explanation for a patient's cardiac failure and death was found except severe fatty degeneration of the myocardium that occurred without any apparent cause.[17] In view of such an instance as this, one must consider the possibility that fatty degeneration, especially if severe, may affect myocardial efficiency in some cases.

Lipid-storage diseases

Focal collections of histiocytes, with or without lipid in the cytoplasm, may be found in the endocardium, the myocardium, or the walls of the coronary arteries in any of the lipidoses.[8] A low-grade inflammatory reaction may be associated with the nodular accumulations of cells. The type of lipid depends on the nature of the disease process. Although the cardiac involvement is usually part of a generalized disorder, a rare instance of lipidosis limited to the heart has been reported.[34]

Disturbances in carbohydrate metabolism
Mucopolysaccharidosis

A rare entity in infancy and childhood, whose exact place in the category of storage diseases was not well defined until recently, is gargoylism or Hurler's disease. It was formerly classified as lipochondrodystrophy because the storage material was believed to be a lipid. Now the disease is regarded as one of the genetic mucopolysaccharidoses, in which the cellular storage substance is an acid mucopolysaccharide.[32]

Aggregations of vacuolated mononuclear cells may be present in the mural or valvular endocardium, the myocardium, the pericardium, and the walls of coronary arteries.[13,40] Varying degrees of fibrosis are associated with the lesions. Grossly, there is usually enlargement of the heart. Minute nodules on the valvular surfaces and thickening of the valve leaflets occur. Cardiac failure has been reported as a cause of death in patients with gargoylism.

Glycogen infiltration

In diabetes mellitus, there may be an increase of glycogen within the myocardial fibers associated with the high concentration of glucose in the blood (p. 1467). Glycogen infiltration also can be seen in muscle cells surrounding a healed myocardial infarct, especially in fibers near the endocardium.

Among the disorders associated with a disturbance of carbohydrate metabolism are the glycogen-storage diseases, in which the liver, kidneys, heart, and skeletal muscles may be affected. These familial diseases are caused by an inherited genetic defect. At least eight different types of glycogen-storage diseases have been described, each characterized by a deficiency of a different enzyme (p. 103). The most common is the hepatic type (the classic von Gierke's disease) with involvement primarily of the liver and the kidneys, causing enlargement of these organs. In 1929, von Gierke named the entity *hepato-nephromegalia glycogenica*. The enzymatic defect is a reduction or absence of glucose-6-phosphatase, so that glycogen is not converted to glucose in the liver. The result is an abnormal accumulation of glycogen that has a normal chemical structure.

A less common form of glycogen-storage disease is the cardiac type. This is actually a generalized glycogenosis in which the major manifestation is involvement of the heart. An intracellular enzyme believed to be localized in the lysosomes, α-1,4-glucosidase, which hydrolyzes maltose and glycogen into glucose, has been found to be absent from the tissues of children affected by this type of glycogen-storage disease.[15,21,22] The chemical structure of the glycogen is normal. In 1932, Pompe named the disorder *cardiomegalia glycogenica*. Although the disease is sometimes referred to as Pompe's disease because of his description of the lesion, it should be pointed out

that two other investigators (Bischoff and Putschar) at the same time independently described patients dying in infancy with pronounced enlargement of the heart caused by diffuse deposition of glycogen in this organ.[36]

The main features of the cardiac form of glycogen-storage disease are as follows:

1. Occurrence in infancy, usually at 4 months to 1 year of age
2. Diffuse glycogen infiltration of the heart, with distortion, rounding, and great enlargement of the organ
3. Death attributable to cardiac failure, usually in the first year of life
4. A characteristic microscopic appearance in which there are enlargement and pronounced vacuolization of almost all myocardial fibers because of the deposition of abundant glycogen, so that the fibers appear as clear or hollow cylinders surrounded by a thin rim of cytoplasm (Fig. 16-5)—often described as a "lacework" appearance of the myocardium

Best's carmine and periodic acid–Schiff stains are useful in demonstrating the glycogen. This substance may be demonstrated even in tissue fixed in formalin for a long time. An occasional associated feature is a thickened opaque endocardium, especially of the left ventricle—a form of secondary endocardial fibroelastosis. It has been suggested that the degree of this change is related to length of survival.[43]

In addition to the diffuse form of glycogen-storage dis-

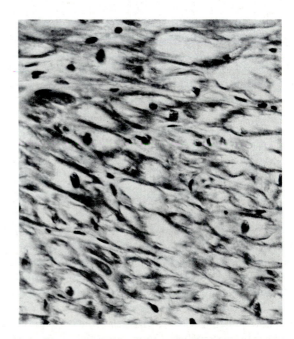

Fig. 16-5. Glycogen-storage disease of myocardium. In formalin-fixed, hematoxylin and eosin–stained preparations, muscle fibers appear as clear spaces surrounded by thin rim of sarcoplasm.

ease, there is a type characterized by a spotty or localized distribution of glycogen referred to as circumscribed glycogen disease of the heart (cardiomegalia glycogenica circumscripta). In some instances of the localized type, single or multiple large circumscribed but not encapsulated masses appear in the myocardium (nodular form of glycogen-storage disease).[20] The nodules, which previously were regarded as neoplastic (so-called rhabdomyomas), often are associated with tuberous sclerosis of the brain. Rhabdomyomas are discussed later in the chapter under tumors of the heart (p. 649).

Disturbances in mineral metabolism
Calcification

The more common form of pathologic calcification in the heart is the dystrophic type. It occurs most frequently in valves, usually the aortic and mitral, especially those affected by old rheumatic disease. A striking example of valvular calcification is that seen in calcific aortic stenosis, in which the cusps become distorted and rigid and often are the site of massive calcified nodules (p. 622). Calcification also may occur in vegetations of bacterial endocarditis. Various forms of inflammation, particularly tuberculosis, may predispose to the deposition of calcium in the pericardium. In an occasional instance, almost the entire pericardium may be involved, so that the heart becomes encased in a rigid, calcified shell that sometimes interferes with cardiac function. Dystrophic calcification occurs also in the myocardium, especially in hyalinized scars of healed myocardial infarcts. Calcification may be so extensive that it can be demonstrated in roentgenograms. Foci of necrosis of the myocardium attributable to a variety of causes, such as ischemia and infections, may be the sites of calcification.[18] In these foci the calcium is deposited within necrotic muscle fibers (Fig. 16-6). Calcification of the myocardium also may result from damage sustained during open-heart surgery.[7] Sometimes this postoperative calcification develops rapidly and prominently within a few days after surgery.

Whereas dystrophic calcification may appear in the absence of an elevated calcium level in the blood, metastatic calcification is associated with an increased serum calcium that may be the result of hyperparathyroidism, destructive bone lesions, hypervitaminosis D, or renal insufficiency. There is a tendency for localization of the mineral in the kidneys, lungs, gastric mucosa, and walls of blood vessels (pp. 88 and 1421). In the heart, calcium is deposited chiefly in the elastica of the coronary arteries and the endocardium of the right atrium. If degenerated and necrotic foci are present in the myocardium, there will be an acceleration of dystrophic calcification because of the increased availability of calcium.[18]

Pathologic ossification

Osseous metaplasia in the heart is not common, but it may be present in areas of calcification, especially in the valves or pericardium and rarely in the myocardium. In the latter site the underlying lesion usually is a scar of an old, healed myocardial infarct (see p. 594).

Hemochromatosis

The heart is almost always affected in hemochromatosis. The degree of involvement may be slight and without evidence of gross changes, but often it is sufficient to produce a brownish discoloration of the myocardium. Microscopically, hemosiderin granules are identified within myocardial fibers and occasionally in the connective tissue cells (Fig. 16-7). Varying degrees of degeneration, edema, and fibrosis of the myocardium can be seen.[25] The fibrosis may be related to concomitant disease, such as coronary artery sclerosis, and not to the presence of the pigment itself.[25] Electrocardiographic changes and even cardiac failure may ensue.[29] Arrhythmias may occur as a result of iron deposits in the fibers of the conduction system.[42]

Nutritional disturbances
Malnutrition

In severe inanition or starvation, the heart is decreased in size and often is brown as a result of accumulation of granules of yellow-brown pigment in the

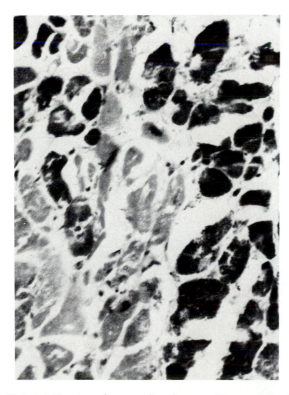

Fig. 16-6. Calcification of myocardium in area of degeneration and necrosis (in uremia). Dark, calcium-impregnated fibers stand out sharply in contrast to pale necrotic fibers without calcification.

muscle fibers. In other words, brown atrophy occurs (p. 86). Interstitial edema and degeneration of muscle cells are associated with the atrophic fibers. Atrophy of the epicardial fat also may be evident.

A form of heart disease that is considered to be caused by chronic malnutrition associated particularly with a lack of animal protein in the diet has been described in South African Bantus.[53] Cardiac failure is likely to occur in these patients. At autopsy the heart is usually dilated, subendocardial fibrosis may be prominent, and mural

thrombi may be seen in the cardiac chambers. Microscopically, alterations are noted in the myocardium—hydropic vacuolization of muscle fibers, interstitial edema, and fibrosis. Although certain of the changes are suggestive of those seen in beriberi, there is no evidence that vitamin B_1 deficiency is responsible. A similarity has been observed between this form of cardiomyopathy in adult Africans and that seen in kwashiorkor in infants.[58] Kwashiorkor is a nutritional disease caused by ingestion of a diet deficient in proteins but usually rich in carbohydrates. Coexistent vitamin deficiencies often are present.

Vitamin deficiencies
Beriberi

Among the vitamin deficiencies, the most important cause of cardiac disease is lack of vitamin B_1 (thiamine). This deficiency causes beriberi, a disease long known among peoples of the Orient but also seen in the United States, particularly in chronic alcoholics. Heart failure with edema develops in patients with the cardiac form of beriberi. Hypoproteinemia may contribute to the edema (see p. 630). An important clinical feature is widespread peripheral vasodilatation leading to an elevated cardiac output. The resulting increased work required of the heart undoubtedly contributes to the cardiac failure.

Grossly, the heart usually is enlarged, frequently increased in weight, and often globose. The enlargement is caused chiefly by dilatation of the chambers, particularly the right ventricle, but hypertrophy also may be present (Fig. 16-8). Mural thrombi are evident in some instances.

The microscopic features are not specific. The most characteristic change is interstitial edema. This is often pronounced and may be accompanied by hydropic

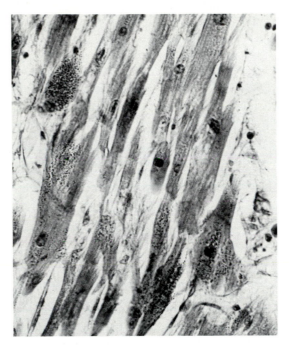

Fig. 16-7. Hemochromatosis of myocardium. Fine, granular, hemosiderin pigment is present in many muscle fibers. (Hematoxylin and eosin.)

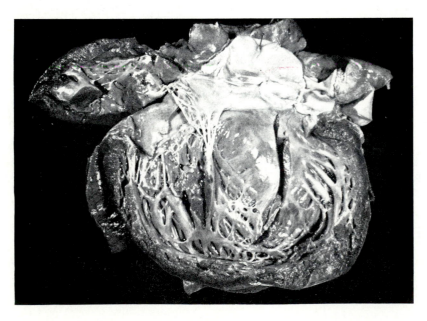

Fig. 16-8. Heart of 46-year-old chronic alcoholic with beriberi. Note globular form with hypertrophy and dilatation of left ventricle.

degeneration of myocardial fibers.[45,47] Slight fibrosis, especially in the subendocardial muscle and the conduction bundle, has been described.[8] Although retrograde changes of the muscle cells in hearts of patients affected with beriberi are not striking, they are seen more regularly and more prominently in experimental, thiamine-deficient animals.[51] They include loss of striations, vacuolization, hyalinization, and focal necrosis of myocardial fibers. Infiltration by polymorphonuclear and mononuclear leukocytes occurs but is not prominent. Lesions identical to those caused by thiamine deficiency have been observed in animals with lack of potassium.[51]

The myocardial changes seen in chronic alcoholism (ethyl alcohol), including various forms of degeneration, are generally believed to be attributable to the accompanying nutritional disturbance. Some investigators, however, believe that excessive alcohol may produce injurious effects directly on the myocardium in the absence of the beriberi syndrome—so-called alcoholic cardiomyopathy (see below).

Scurvy (vitamin C deficiency)

Children who exhibit severe manifestations of vitamin C deficiency in the skeleton may die suddenly.[50] These deaths have been attributed to cardiac hypertrophy, particularly of the right ventricle. Microscopic findings in the heart, however, are not significant. Myocardial degeneration has been reported in vitamin C deficiency in humans and experimentally in guinea pigs.[60]

Vitamin E deficiency

Vitamin E deficiency is not an important cause of heart disease in humans, but it produces changes in the cardiac muscle in animals.[51] In animals on a vitamin E–deficient diet, necrosis of myocardial fibers followed by fibrosis has been described. Ceroid pigment is present in muscle fibers and in macrophages. In one experiment the foci of necrosis were accompanied by acute myocarditis, and calcification of cardiac muscle was sometimes seen.[48]

Alcoholic cardiomyopathy

As noted previously, the heart may be affected in chronic alcoholism because of the accompanying nutritional disturbance (beriberi). Direct damage to the myocardium by excessive, habitual intake of ethyl alcohol is said to occur also (alcoholic myocardiopathy or cardiomyopathy).[49] In the latter condition the pathologic features include fibrosis (either sparse or larger and more confluent areas) and cardiac enlargement, particularly of the left ventricle, caused by compensatory hypertrophy of the myocardial fibers.[49] In an occasional instance, the characteristics of both cardiac beriberi and alcoholic cardiomyopathy may be present. In an electron microscopic study of myocardium obtained by needle biopsy from patients with alcoholic cardiomyopathy, the following ultramicroscopic alterations have been described: (1) degeneration or absence of contractile elements, (2) increase in number of mitochondria, (3) swollen mitochondria with reduction in number or absence of their cristae ("mitochondrial ghosts"), and sometimes (4) distension of sarcoplasmic reticulum to cystic proportion and increase in fat deposits.[44]

The adverse effects produced by alcohol ingestion include loss of cardiac contractility and disturbances in mitochondrial respiration, in calcium uptake by the mitochondria and sarcoplasmic reticulum, and in myocardial lipid metabolism.[46] It has been suggested that alcohol may exert its effect on the heart by means of its circulating metabolite, acetaldehyde.[56]

A form of cardiomyopathy has been observed in patients who ingested large quantities of beer, so-called beer-drinkers' myocardosis.[52,54,55,57,59] In some of these patients, pericardial effusion (sometimes massive) occurred in addition to the myocardial involvement, and the term *perimyocardiopathy* has been used to describe the entity.[54] Some investigators consider beer-drinkers' myocardosis to be a more advanced stage or a special type of alcoholic cardiomyopathy.[59] Others express the opinion that cobalt (added to the beer to stabilize and improve the appearance of its foam or "head") causes direct toxic injury to the heart, although other factors probably increase the susceptibility of these patients to the cobalt.[54,55] According to another view, the disease is an acute fulminating form of beriberi, resulting from a thiamine deficiency associated with the high alcoholic intake and exaggerated by cobalt, the effect of the latter being either a direct block of thiamine utilization or an interference with intracellular enzymatic functions necessary for thiamine utilization.[52] By light microscopy, the beer-drinker's heart shows interstitial edema, hydropic and lipid vacuolization and hypertrophy of myocardial fibers, and a decrease in myofibrils. Electron microscopically, there may be loss of myofibrils and fragmentation of the remaining ones, damaged sarcoplasmic reticulum, and swollen, distorted, vacuolated, or ruptured mitochondria.

Traumatic disease[61-63]

Included in the category of traumatic heart disease are injuries to the heart and the pericardium resulting from physical force. The injuries are classified as penetrating and nonpenetrating.

Penetrating injuries

Penetrating injuries of the heart may be caused by flying missiles (bullets, shell fragments), stab wounds from slender rigid objects (knife, ice pick, long pin or needle, splinter of glass, sharp end of broken rib, various metal or wood objects), or foreign bodies migrating from elsewhere in the body. Swallowed or aspirated foreign bodies may erode through the wall of the esophagus or bronchus and penetrate the pericardium and the myocardium. Occasionally an object such as a needle or a bullet enters the body at a distant site and migrates to the heart by way of the circulation.

A serious effect of penetrating wounds of the heart, one that is responsible for most of the early deaths, is hemopericardium with cardiac tamponade (cardiac compression). As a result of the tamponade, there is an impediment to the filling of the cardiac chambers, as well as compression of the great veins, interfering with return of blood to the heart. Severe hemorrhage without tamponade, as external hemorrhage or as a hemothorax, may occur when the laceration of the pericardium is sufficiently large to allow escape of blood from the pericardial sac. Infection may complicate penetrating wounds and may be followed by the development of pericarditis and abscesses of the pericardium or myocardium, or both. Valvular defects caused by direct injury or by a severing of papillary muscles are not common. Laceration of a coronary artery, with or without myocardial infarction, may be produced. Coronary thrombosis occasionally occurs as a result of contusive injury of the artery by the penetrating object. Sometimes the penetrating object is lodged within the wall of the heart and is retained as a foreign body for years without causing symptoms, but there is always the danger that it may be mobilized as an embolus in the pulmonary or systemic circulation. Embolic complications of penetrating wounds are also seen in association with a mural thrombus that results from endocardial injury or in association with a superimposed bacterial endocarditis. The development of an aneurysm at the site of myocardial injury has been reported. Arrhythmias may be slight or severe, and in some instances they may be the cause of death immediately after the cardiac trauma—for example, if ventricular fibrillation occurs. It has been estimated that one out of every four persons with a penetrating heart wound will survive the immediate effects of the injury and will live long enough to receive adequate medical care.[63]

Nonpenetrating injuries

Nonpenetrating injuries of the heart are frequently caused by direct forces applied to the thorax, such as a direct blow to the precordium or a sudden compression of the heart between the sternum and the vertebrae as in the common steering wheel accidents. Cardiac injury also may be caused by indirect forces—for example, sudden compression or crushing of the abdomen and extremities during a cave-in accident, unaccompanied by injury to the thoracic cage. The damage produced by these indirect forces is the result of a sudden increase in hydrostatic pressure and a forcing of blood into the heart and great vessels, which already are filled with blood. Blast forces, particularly when transmitted through water, and decelerative forces as in elevator accidents are other factors that may cause nonpenetrating injuries of the heart.

Nonpenetrating cardiac trauma may produce a variety of lesions, including rupture of the heart, myocardial contusion and laceration, pericardial laceration, pericarditis, hemopericardium, and lacerations of valves, chordae tendineae, papillary muscles, and coronary arteries. The relationship of nonpenetrating trauma to the production of coronary thrombosis is controversial. In a study of 546 cases of nonpenetrating cardiac trauma in the files of the Armed Forces Institute of Pathology, not one instance of coronary thrombosis of the major vessels was found.[62] The authors of this survey favor the impression that coronary thrombosis rarely occurs, especially in a previously normal vessel. It is possible that sufficient localized injury caused by a blunt impact in an already diseased artery may precipitate thrombosis.[61]

Myocardial contusion or hemorrhage, which is one of the most common traumatic heart lesions encountered clinically, may lead to serious complications or sequelae such as cardiac rupture, formation of a myocardial aneurysm, calcification of the injured area, and cardiac failure. In some cases a prominent leukocytic infiltration may be associated with severe myocardial hemorrhage, consisting mainly of neutrophils but also with a few eosinophils and mononuclear cells. Focal necrosis of muscle fibers may be seen in the midst of the inflammatory cells.[62] At autopsy it is sometimes difficult to distinguish between contusions and certain nontraumatic interstitial extravasations of blood such as those caused by anoxia and poisons, and in some instances contusions may simulate early infarcts.[61] The most common traumatic cardiac lesion found at autopsy in cases of nonpenetrating injuries is rupture of the heart.[62] A fibrinous pericarditis occasionally is observed in association with nonpenetrating trauma, but purulent pericarditis is rare and usually is the result of contamination from concomitant injuries to the esophagus or respiratory tract.[62]

Functional disturbances of the heart, particularly arrhythmias, are significant consequences of nonpenetrating cardiac injury. There is no definite correlation between the extent of myocardial damage and the production of arrhythmias. Occasionally, fatal ventricular arrhythmias or cardiac standstill may follow an apparently minor trauma. Such an occurrence may be encountered in the so-called concussive type of nonpenetrating wound, which is characterized by jarring of the heart without the production of significant lesions.[62] For example, a person hit in the chest by a stick and another struck in the precordium by a pitched ball died a few minutes after the injuries. No evidence of cardiac damage was found at autopsy other than a few petechiae seen especially in the pericardium; no other anatomic cause of death was discovered.[62]

Radiation injury

Cardiac muscle is one of the tissues most resistant to the effects of ionizing radiation. Fairly heavy doses of radiation may be absorbed by the heart without any perceptible effects. However, there are a number of reports in the literature that attribute various nonspecific changes in the heart and pericardium to the effects of radiation. In 1942, Warren[71] noted certain myocardial lesions that were considered to be the result of radiation therapy—for example, slight interstitial fibrosis, hyaline and fatty degeneration and necrosis, and lymphocytic infiltration in some cases.

In a more recent study of cardiac lesions in patients receiving radiation therapy to the mediastinum, Fajardo, Stewart, and Cohen[65] regarded the following as late radiation effects: (1) pericardial fibrosis, adhesions, and effusions (sometimes with clinical manifestations of tamponade or chronic constrictive pericarditis), (2) diffuse myocardial fibrosis, and, less frequently, (3) focal endocardial fibroelastosis and (4) pronounced thickening of the intima by fibroblasts, collagen, endothelial cells, and histiocytes, some with large foamy cytoplasm. These authors noted the similarity of the myocardial lesion to that produced experimentally in rabbits with single doses of radiation varying from 3150 to 8250 rad. The pericardium was less affected in the rabbits than in the patients. The occurrence of occlusive coronary artery disease following mediastinal radiation in several young adults who did not have any major risk factors for coronary atherosclerosis has been cited as evidence that ionizing radiation might induce severe coronary atherosclerosis.[64]

Among the early radiation effects on the heart observed in victims of the atomic bomb explosions at Hiroshima and Nagasaki,[68] the most prominent were hemorrhages in the different layers, particularly in the epicardium. Also present in some instances were perivascular edema of the myocardium and infiltration of the endocardium and myocardium by leukocytes—plasma cells and sometimes small and large mononuclear cells. Only rarely were lesions observed in the cardiac muscle itself, such as fatty change and focal necrosis. Evidence of myocardial injury was rarely seen in swine subjected to total body irradiation during the 1946 atomic bomb explosion at Bikini or in swine with total body exposure to million-volt x radiation.[70]

Apparently, massive doses of radiation are necessary to induce histologic changes in the myocardium. In an experiment in which adult rats received doses of 750 to 20,000 rad through a precordial portal, at least 10,000 rad delivered in a single dose was required to produce myocardial damage (degeneration of muscle fibers, interstitial edema, capillary hemorrhages, and lymphocytic infiltration).[67] The microscopic changes were evident as early as 7 days after irradiation. The pericardium and endocardium were intact in those receiving 10,000 rad. In animals observed over 1 year in whom single doses up to 7500 rad were given, no late changes such as muscular atrophy or myocardial fibrosis were observed. In the previously mentioned experiment in rabbits, however, in which single radiation doses ranging from 3150 to 8250 rad were employed, myocardial fibrosis was produced.[65] The electrocardiographic disturbances reported in animals exposed to total body irradiation may be attributed, at least in part, to associated changes in the potassium concentration of the serum.[66]

In one study, dogs that had received cardiac irradiation exhibited an increased survival rate after the production of myocardial infarction by coronary artery ligation.[69] The lesions produced did not involve the entire thickness of the ventricular wall as did the myocardial infarcts in the nonirradiated dogs. The beneficial effects of irradiation in these animals have been attributed to the dilatation of existing myocardial capillaries and precapillary arterioles, resulting in improvement of the collateral circulation and augmentation of the coronary blood flow. Apart from the vascular changes in this experiment, there was no lesion in the heart and pericardium that could be attributed to the radiation itself.

Endocrine disturbances
Hyperthyroidism (see also p. 1401)

The association between heart disease and thyrotoxicosis is well known, but the exact relationship of hyperthyroidism to the development of the cardiac abnormalities is a subject of controversy.[93] Cardiac disability in thyrotoxicosis often is the result of aggravation of an underlying primary disturbance of the heart (such as coronary artery disease, hypertensive cardiopathy, congenital defect, or rheumatic heart disease) that may or may not have been clinically evident before hyperactivity of the thyroid gland. Some investigators believe that thyrotoxicosis by itself can be a cause of heart disease and cardiac failure. This view is based principally on clinical studies of thyrotoxic patients with congestive heart failure in whom no evidence of associated primary cardiac disease could be recognized. Although relatively few postmortem examinations of such patients have been made, some support for this contention has been derived from autopsies that did not reveal any other cause for the cardiac disorder.[93]

The clinical features of a thyrotoxic heart, with or without a preexisting cardiac disorder, include tachycardia, increased cardiac output, atrial fibrillation, angina pectoris, cardiac enlargement, and cardiac failure. No constant microscopic lesions are attributable to the effects of thyrotoxicosis per se, but foci of fatty degeneration, fibrosis, and lymphocytic infiltration of the myocardium have been described in a few cases.[83] The structural alterations characteristic of other forms of heart disease may be present. There is a lack of uniformity in the results reported in experimentally produced hyperthyroidism in animals. However, in some investigations, definite changes have been described—hypertrophy and dilatation of the heart, foci of degeneration and necrosis of myocardial fibers, myocardial fibrosis, and an infiltration by lymphocytes and a few neutrophils and eosinophils.[92]

The cardiac effects of hyperthyroidism have been attributed to increased work of the heart, deficient nutrition of the myocardium, and an increased vulnerability of the heart to even mild intoxications and infections.[92] There is some evidence that the cardiac damage is caused by direct hormonal action on the heart muscles.[88] It has been suggested that thyroid hormone potentiates the stimulating and hypoxia-inducing effects of the adrenergic catecholamines, especially epinephrine, on the heart.[88]

Hypothyroidism (myxedema heart)
(see also p. 1399)

In long-standing myxedema, cardiovascular disturbances are likely to occur. These may result solely from the myxedematous state or from preexisting lesions that are aggravated by the metabolic changes present in myxedema.[86] Among the disturbances of the heart and circulation that have been noted are the following: bradycardia, decreased cardiac output, lowered cardiac tonus, prolonged circulation time, reduced blood volume, increased capillary permeability, pericardial effusion, angina pectoris, and characteristic electrocardiographic changes. Congestive heart failure has been described,[75,86] but there is some question as to whether this is a constituent of the syndrome of uncomplicated myxedema.[88] Associated disease such as coronary atherosclerosis or hypertension may be responsible. Cardiac enlargement is observed in the majority of patients with severe myxedema. Although hypertrophy has been reported in the relatively few detailed pathologic studies of the heart in myxedema, true cardiac hypertrophy usually is ascribed to other accompanying cardiovascular diseases.[72]

Grossly, the myxedema heart is pale, flabby, and dilated. Microscopically, interstitial edema may be present[79] and is a possible factor causing enlargement of the heart. An increase in fluid content has been demonstrated by actual measurement in the heart of rabbits in which myxedema was experimentally induced.[100] Other features described are hydropic vacuoles, loss of striations, small pyknotic nuclei in muscle cells,[82] and basophilic degeneration of the myocardium.[9,16] The latter change is not specific for myxedema, since it is observed in association with other diseases.[16,19,31,38] However, certain investigators believe it is more pronounced in patients with thyroid disease,[16] and others report morphologic differences between the intracellular basophilic substance in myxedema and that encountered in nonmyxedematous conditions.[19] Myocardial fibrosis may be present, which usually can be explained by coexisting coronary sclerosis.

The frequent association of coronary atherosclerosis with myxedema has been noted,[75] and its development has been attributed, at least in part, to hypercholesterolemia, which is characteristic of the myxedematous state. Coronary sclerosis has been described also in young myxedematous patients.[101] Experimental evidence suggesting a relationship between myxedema and coronary atherosclerosis is provided by the production of atherosclerosis of large arteries after the postnatal surgical removal of the thyroid gland of sheep and goats.[77] In more recent experiments in dogs (which have a high resistance to formation of atherosclerotic lesions by cholesterol feeding alone), atherosclerosis generally is produced by the combination of procedures leading to hypothyroidism, including surgical thyroidectomy, and the administration of cholesterol or other dietary factors.[94] Despite these clinical and experimental observations, some investigators are not convinced that myxedema itself augments or enhances the development of atherosclerosis.[72-74]

Pituitary disease

In hypopituitarism, as in Simmonds' disease, atrophy of the heart occurs in association with atrophy of other organs such as the liver, kidneys, spleen, and adrenal cortex (p. 1382). A more severe form of heart disease resulting in death may be associated with pituitary adenomas causing acromegaly (p. 1384).

Acromegaly

A common cardiovascular feature in patients with acromegaly is hypertrophy of the heart, affecting all chambers but especially the left ventricle. Cardiac failure commonly occurs in these patients. The heart may be enormous, with weights as much as 1300 g being recorded.[84] The hypertrophy may not be accounted for by any intracardiac lesion, such as valvular or coronary artery disease. Hypertension is present in some patients with acromegaly and may be partly responsible for the hypertrophy, but it is not a regular feature. Cardiac hypertrophy occurs even in the absence of hypertension.[87] In the case of acromegalic patients whose cardiomegaly cannot be explained by coexisting cardiac abnormalities or hypertension, the possibility that growth hormone from the pituitary adenoma is the stimulus for the hypertrophy has been considered.[87,88] The possibility that humoral substances other than growth hormone may be responsible cannot be excluded.[84]

Since the histologic picture is not characteristic, it is not possible to distinguish the enlarged heart of an acromegalic patient from enlarged heart of other causes. In addition to hypertrophy of muscle fibers, there may be moderate to severe interstitial fibrosis of the myocardium.[87] The sizes of muscle fibers in individual cases vary. Pronounced enlargement of fibers does not occur in every instance. Other features sometimes seen are small vessel disease, interstitial foci of lymphocytes and histiocytes, and myocarditis resembling that induced by catecholamines.[84]

Changes induced by catecholamines

Adrenosympathogenic hormones, which enhance myocardial oxygen consumption, are believed by some investigators to induce hypoxic injury when they are excessive.[88,89] It is postulated that, as a result of an increased amount of catechalomines, oxygen consumption by the heart muscle may be so excessive as to cause exhaustion of the available oxygen brought to the heart by the coronary arteries (even if the blood flow is augmented by their dilatation), leading to myocardial hypoxia.[88] It also has been suggested that even a moderate or slight increase in oxygen-consuming cardiac sympathoadrenomedullary activity may produce manifestations of severe local hypoxia if compensatory dilatation of the coronary arteries is impaired by vascular disease.[89] The possibility exists that changes in serum potassium brought about by catecholamines (initial elevation and subsequent depression[88]) may be deleterious to the myocardium.[89]

Myocardial alterations have been observed in experimental animals and in patients treated with epinephrine and *l*-norepinephrine.[97,98] The microscopic lesions are basically focal, consisting of edema, hemorrhages, and degeneration and necrosis of muscle fibers, followed by leukocytic infiltration and subsequent fibrosis. The term *norepinephrine myocarditis* has been applied to the lesions produced in dogs and patients who received *l*-norepinephrine.[97] Investigators have produced infarctlike cardiac necrosis in animals by administration of isoproterenol.[80,91] There was a close correlation between the dose injected and the degree of severity of necrosis, thus allowing production of standardized myocardial lesions. Furthermore, they found that, unlike the natural catecholamines (epinephrine and norepinephrine), isoproterenol, even in high doses, was associated with a low mortality, making it valuable for production and study of myocardial infarction of uniform severity. The necrosis was attributed to relative ischemia resulting from the effect of isoproterenol on the myocardium (that is, greatly increasing the oxygen requirement of myocardial fibers) and on the peripheral circulation (that is, vasodilatation with reduction of blood pressure). In an experiment by other investigators, in which lesions were caused by overdoses of isoproterenol, norepinephrine, and epinephrine, those produced by isoproterenol were most severe, consisting of infarctlike areas of myocardial

necrosis with hyalinization or vacuolization of the muscle fibers, interstitial and cellular edema, and extensive inflammation.[76] Histochemical and electron microscopic studies made on the hearts of the animals revealed that some of the changes were similar to those produced by ischemia, although other changes were attributed to the metabolic effects of the drugs on the muscle fibers or to the action of the agents on cellular growth and proliferation.

Lesions similar to norepinephrine myocarditis are seen in some patients with pheochromocytomas.[81,97] They do not affect large areas but are focal, consisting of swollen and granular degenerated fibers, foci of eosinophilic fibers, leukocyte infiltration, and sometimes interstitial fibrosis. The cells are lymphocytes, histiocytes, Anitschkow cells, and a few neutrophils. The myocarditis is not of infectious origin, nor is it considered to be a hypersensitivity reaction. It is attributed to a secretory product of pheochromocytomas (norepinephrine).[81] Hypertrophy of the heart is a feature in many patients with pheochromocytomas. This is probably caused by the coexistent chronic hypertension, but a possible contributory factor may be the tendency of the heart to absorb readily the circulating catecholamines.[88]

A special form of necrosis has been described in patients with pheochromocytomas, as well as in animals in shock or that have been injected with norepinephrine. The terms *myofibrillar degeneration* and *contraction band necrosis* have been applied to this lesion, which is characterized by dense irregular banding of the myocyte and other signs of cell necrosis (mitochondrial densities, nuclear pyknosis, and so on; see p. 630 and Fig. 16-55).

Carcinoid syndrome (carcinoid heart disease)

The syndrome associated with metastasizing carcinoid tumors is characterized by distinctive episodic flushing of the skin, mottled cyanosis, telangiectases, asthmalike attacks, intestinal hyperperistalsis with diarrhea, an increased level of serotonin (5-hydroxytryptamine) in the blood, and an excess of 5-hydroxyindoleacetic acid in the urine. Cardiac manifestations that develop in some patients with this syndrome are principally a result of tricuspid and pulmonary valve involvement (see p. 624). The lesions in carcinoid heart disease are characteristic and can be differentiated from those found in the heart in congenital, degenerative, infectious, and collagen diseases.[85] They consist of focal or diffuse plaques of a peculiar type of fibrous tissue (often referred to as cartilagelike), which is free of elastic fibers and is superimposed upon the endocardium of the valvular cusps, upon the mural endocardium of the cardiac chambers, and upon the intima of the great veins, the coronary sinus, and occasionally the great arteries.[90] These carcinoid fibrous plaques are sharply demarcated from the otherwise normal underlying endocardium of the valves and heart chambers by the elastic lamina. Likewise, the carcinoid plaques in the vessels rest upon an intact inner elastic lamina. Cellular infiltration in the lesions is not pronounced, but some lymphocytes, plasma cells, and mast cells may be present, along with newly formed blood vessels.

In the majority of cases the distinctive lesions are limited to the right side of the heart. The fibrous lesions have been noted on both sides of the valve cusps,[85] although when the pulmonary valve is affected, frequently the fibrous tissue is deposited almost entirely on the arterial aspect of the pulmonic valve cusps.[90] The fibrous thickening and contraction of the cusps usually cause pulmonary stenosis and tricuspid regurgitation, but some degree of pulmonary regurgitation and tricuspid stenosis also may be present. The process on the tricuspid valve may extend onto the chordae tendinae and the papillary muscles. The chordae tendineae may become thickened, shortened, and fused. Similar carcinoid lesions are known to occur in the left side of the heart but much less commonly than in the right side.[90] Occasionally, both sides of the heart may be affected in the same patient.[90] Myocardial hypertrophy and dilatation may be present, in most cases as the result of the valvular lesions.[99]

The pathogenesis of the carcinoid heart lesions is not clearly established. Serotonin has been implicated as the substance most likely responsible for the development of the fibrous plaques, but the evidence for this assumption is not conclusive. It is not clear why cardiac disease develops in some patients with hyperserotonemia and the carcinoid syndrome but not in others. It is often presumed that serotonin is inactivated during its passage through the lungs and that left-sided lesions do not occur unless a right-to-left cardiovascular shunt exists or unless the syndrome is caused by a bronchial adenoma of the carcinoid type. However, instances of left-sided cardiac lesions have been found in patients without such a shunt or pulmonary tumor,[90] which suggests that the probable causative principle, serotonin, is not totally inactivated in the lungs. In view of the demonstrations of elevated levels of bradykinin, in addition to serotonin, in the serum of patients with the carcinoid syndrome, bradykinin may play a contributory role in carcinoid heart disease.[96] Practically all attempts to produce the lesion experimentally in animals have been unsuccessful; however, in one investigation,[95] intimal and endocardial proliferative lesions resembling, yet not identical to, the carcinoid heart disease in humans have been produced in animals when a combination of three factors was present:

1. Hyperserotonemia (following injection of 5-hydroxytryptamine)
2. Periodic tryptophan deficiency
3. Altered liver function induced by a hepatotoxic agent

Other endocrine disturbances

In Addison's disease, or chronic adrenal insufficiency, the heart is sometimes atrophic and contains an abundance of brown pigment (brown atrophy) (p. 86). Cardiac hypertrophy may result from the hypertension associated with Cushing's disease (p. 1384). Glycogen infiltration of the myocardium in diabetes mellitus has been referred to previously (p. 566). The association of coronary atherosclerosis with diabetes mellitus is discussed on p. 583. Also, alterations in the small coronary vessels with myocardial dysfunction may occur in diabetics without large coronary artery involvement (diabetic cardiomyopathy).[78]

Fluid and electrolyte disturbances
Hydropericardium

Normally, the pericardial cavity contains about 5 to 50 ml of clear, straw-colored fluid that includes a small amount of protein and is of low specific gravity (that is, a transudate). An excessive quantity, usually more than 100 ml, of this transudate in the pericardial sac is referred to as hydropericardium. This term is not applied to the effusion associated with serous or serofibrinous pericarditis, which includes the elements of an inflammatory exudate—increased protein content, higher specific gravity, and leukocytes. The color of the fluid in hydropericardium may be altered under certain conditions. It may be bile stained if jaundice is present, deep red or brown if there is hemorrhage, or red as a result of postmortem hemolysis.

The causes of hydropericardium are those conditions associated with a noninflammatory type of edema. It is seen most frequently as a part of the picture of congestive heart failure. It also occurs in the nephrotic syndrome, the hypoproteinemic state associated with malnutrition or chronic wasting diseases, myxedema, and beriberi, and as a result of interference with the venous return from the pericardial circulation such as that caused by neoplastic or inflammatory lesions of the mediastinum.

The clinical significance of hydropericardium depends more on the rapidity of accumulation than on the total quantity of fluid. Large effusions up to 1000 ml or more that collect slowly in the pericardial cavity may cause no embarrassment of the heart provided that the pericardium is not thickened by disease and is permitted to stretch. On the other hand, a smaller amount (for example, 150 to 250 ml) of fluid accumulating quickly will usually cause serious disturbances by producing cardiac tamponade.

Edema of myocardium

Interstitial edema of the myocardium may be present in a wide variety of disorders, among which are severe inanition or starvation, beriberi, cardiac trauma, radiation injury, endocrine disturbances (especially myxedema), intoxication by drugs and chemical poisons, electrolyte imbalances (for example, hypopotassemia), uremia, infectious and other forms of myocarditis, and conditions associated with stasis of blood or ischemia of the myocardium. In some instances, hydropic change of the myocardial fibers may accompany the interstitial edema. When edema is severe, as in myxedema, cardiac enlargement may occur even in the absence of true myocardial hypertrophy. It is not certain if long-standing myocardial edema stimulates connective tissue overgrowth leading to myocardial fibrosis.

When there is a pronounced interstitial edema, often with prominence and perhaps proliferation of connective tissue cells, some pathologists make a diagnosis of so-called serous myocarditis.[411,412] However, such histologic alterations should not be regarded as evidence of a true myocarditis. As will be seen later, the common feature of the different forms of myocarditis is the presence of an exudate containing leukocytes of various kinds. A diagnosis of myocardosis, a seldom-used term, is sometimes made to denote noninflammatory diseases of the myocardium and retrograde changes not related to coronary artery disease, which may include pronounced interstitial edema.[384]

Effects of potassium disturbances
Hypopotassemia

The pathologic effects of hypopotassemia have been observed in animals fed a diet deficient in potassium.[51,102] Microscopically, the essential feature of the myocardial lesion is a degeneration of muscle fibers, with swelling, loss of striations, and hyaline change followed by necrosis and disintegration of the fibers. Resulting from the degeneration are changes in the interstitial tissue consisting of edema, proliferation of vascular endothelium and fibroblasts, and infiltration by histiocytes. The muscle debris is removed by phagocytes, and healing is accomplished by hypertrophy of the surviving muscle and condensation of connective tissue.[102] On the basis of electron microscopic studies of the focal lesion of experimentally produced potassium depletion, there is evidence that an important change is the alteration of membrane permeability of muscle cells induced by electrolyte imbalance.[105] Cytoplasmic alterations with little nuclear loss are prominent throughout the process and suggest the degenerative nature of the lesion. This is in contrast to the disruption of vital cellular components seen in the early lesion of ischemic necrosis of the myocardium.[105]

Myocardial lesions similar to those produced experimentally in animals have been observed in potassium deficiency in humans—a neutrophilic, lymphocytic, and macrophagic infiltration associated with necrosis of muscle fibers.[103] In some patients with severe and prolonged potassium deficiency, myocardial fibrosis as well as myocardial necrosis have been reported.[104] Clinically, cardiac disturbances may occur in hypopotassemia, including atrial and ventricular arrhythmias, potentiation of digitalis effects, and characteristic electrocardiographic changes.

Hyperpotassemia

Hyperpotassemia may have a profound effect on the heart, producing bradycardia and a distinctive electrocardiographic pattern. If the serum potassium level is high, ventricular fibrillation and cardiac standstill may occur. The morphologic changes in the heart caused by hyperpotassemia have not been defined. However, certain of the myocardial alterations in uremia, such as cloudy swelling and interstitial edema, may be the result of hyperpotassemia.[28]

Disturbances of circulation of blood
Hemopericardium

The presence of blood in the pericardial cavity is known as hemopericardium, or hematopericardium. Among the common causes of hemorrhage in the pericardial sac are ruptured aneurysms of the aorta, trauma of the heart and great vessels, and rupture of a recent myocardial infarct. Sometimes hemopericardium accompanies myocardial infarction in the absence of cardiac rupture as a result of bleeding from the newly formed vessels in the associated organizing fibrinous pericarditis. Although this complication has been observed in connection with anticoagulant therapy,[108,109] it can occur spontaneously in patients not treated with anticoagulants.[106,107] Leukemia, scurvy, and other diseases characterized by a hemorrhagic diathesis may cause hemopericardium. Neoplasms involving the pericardium may produce bloody effusions, particularly secondary cancers. Inflammations of the pericardium, such as tuberculosis, can cause a hemorrhagic exudate. Rare instances of hemopericardium occur after rupture of the heart in an area of the myocardium involved by an abscess or by extensive fatty infiltration.

The essential morphologic feature of hemopericardium in fatal cases is distension of the pericardial sac by the blood that fills the space. The blood may be fluid or clotted (Fig. 16-9). If a small amount of fluid blood is present, it may be largely resorbed. Blood not resorbed will clot and become organized. Instances of constrictive pericarditis have been reported as a sequel to hemopericardium.[110,111]

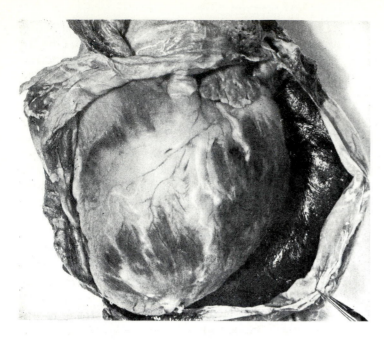

Fig. 16-9. Hemopericardium caused by rupture of aneurysm into pericardial sac. (From Anderson, W.A.D., and Scotti, T.M.: Synopsis of pathology, ed. 10, St. Louis, 1980, The C.V. Mosby Co.)

The clinical effects of hemopericardium depend on the amount and rapidity of bleeding. As little as 150 to 250 ml of blood, rapidly filling the pericardial cavity, can cause cardiac tamponade and death. Pericardiocentesis for relief of acute tamponade may be a lifesaving procedure in some cases.

Intracardiac hemorrhages

Cardiac hemorrhages occur in a variety of conditions, including the following:

1. Traumatic injuries of the heart—for example, nonpenetrating forces causing contusions of the myocardium or minute penetrating wounds such as those caused by needle punctures
2. Diseases associated with a hemorrhagic diathesis, such as leukemia, scurvy, and the thrombocytopenias
3. Anoxia resulting from suffocation, shock, and other causes
4. Fulminating septicemias—for example, meningococcemia
5. Poisoning by chemicals or carbon monoxide
6. Administration of anticoagulants
7. Exposure to ionizing radiation

Sometimes, hemorrhage of the myocardium is associated with other diseases of the heart, as in myocardial infarction (Fig. 16-22).

Morphologically, hemorrhages in the heart are frequently in the form of petechiae or ecchymoses. They occur in any layer of the heart but are particularly prominent on the epicardial and mural endocardial surfaces and are seldom seen on the heart valves. Occasionally a more massive hemorrhage may be seen, as in leukemia.

Shock

The heart may be involved in the shock syndrome in two ways. In cardiogenic shock, sudden impairment of cardiac function, resulting in a decreased cardiac output, is the primary factor that initiates the shock. A common cause of this type of shock is acute myocardial infarction, usually with involvement of 40% or more of the left ventricle.[118] On the other hand, the heart can be secondarily damaged as a result of the compensatory mechanisms that are activated in response to shock,[112] whether of the cardiogenic type[118] or caused by noncardiogenic factors, such as hemorrhage, trauma, or burns. In various studies of experimental hemorrhagic shock, it has been shown that the heart may develop anatomic lesions,[113,114,117] as well as signs of cardiac failure[119] and of metabolic abnormalities.[113]

Anatomic changes have been described in the hearts of human subjects in shock,[119] as well as in the hearts of various animals after experimental induction of hemorrhagic shock.[113,114,117] Fatty degeneration of the myocardium occurs in humans who die of traumatic shock[115] and also in dogs after a hemorrhagic shock episode.[116] In addition, there are three other kinds of lesions that involve the myocardium in shock: (1) subendocardial hemorrhage, (2) necrosis, including myofibrillar degeneration (p. 630 and Fig. 16-55), and (3) zonal lesions.[116,117] The zonal lesions are areas of intense contraction of a myocyte adjacent to the intercalated disc, associated with disruption of sarcomeres and displacement of mitochondria.

The etiologic basis for the myocardial lesions lies in the abnormal physiologic and metabolic situation in which the heart is operating. There is a low head of arterial pressure so that coronary blood flow tends to be low and inadequate, even though coronary vascular resistance is decreased and the percentage of the cardiac output that goes to the heart is increased. In addition, the heart rate is greatly increased, the left ventricular blood volume is decreased, the blood pH is decreased (metabolic acidosis), and there is a marked increase in the concentration of circulating catecholamines. Experimental studies have suggested that the subendocardial hemorrhage and the necrotic lesions of the myocardium are caused by oxygen lack, since they can be prevented by treating dogs in shock with oxygen.

Anemia

In the presence of advanced and chronic forms of anemia, fatty degeneration of the myocardium is evident, usually in a patchy, streaking, "tigroid" or "tabby cat" pattern. The myocardium is flabby, and frequently cardiac hypertrophy[122] and dilatation occur. The associated myocardial anoxemia is responsible for the degeneration and may be a stimulus leading to cardiac hypertrophy. It is probable, however, that overwork of the heart, evidenced by an increased cardiac output to compensate for the oxygen lack in the tissues, is a significant factor causing the cardiac enlargement. The clinical manifestations include palpitations, shortness of breath on exertion, tachycardia, murmurs, cardiac enlargement, and electrocardiographic changes. Angina pectoris and congestive heart failure may occur in some patients, especially those with preexisting heart disease.

In sickle cell anemia, profound alterations may be produced in the heart in addition to the lesions just mentioned. Interstitial edema of the myocardium, disappearance of striations and hyaline change of muscle fibers, and polymorphonuclear leukocytic infiltration have been described.[123] Some of the changes in this disease may not be caused by the anemia itself but may be the result of circulatory stasis and thrombosis. The latter occasionally occurs in the small arteries of the heart. In some instances, pulmonary arteriolar thrombosis may lead to pulmonary heart disease (cor pulmonale).[120]

Cardiac lesions have been reported in newborns dying of hemolytic disease attributable to Rh incompatibility.[121] Heart failure is considered to be an important factor in the death of these patients. The heart is flabby, dilated, and increased in weight. The nuclei of the myocardial fibers are enlarged. Other findings include epicardial hemopoietic foci and petechiae, nucleated red cell precursors in the blood vessels, and microscopic evidence of a mild degree of fibroelastosis in all chambers in the more severe cases. Sometimes minute myocardial infarcts (1 to 2 mm in size) are seen that are confined to the inner part of the myocardium, most frequently in the tips of the papillary muscles in both ventricles. Fatty degeneration also is observed in the myocardium in hemolytic disease of the newborn.[37]

Coronary artery and ischemic heart disease

Of the variety of diseases that affect the coronary arteries, the most important and most common is atherosclerosis. In the restricted sense, the term *coronary artery disease* does not indicate heart disease. The vascular disorder may exist with or without clinical or pathologic evidence of myocardial damage. The terms *coronary heart disease* and *ischemic heart disease* are preferred when myocardial lesions or clinical manifestations occur as a result of disturbances of the coronary circulation. The World Health Organization's Study Group on Atherosclerosis and Ischemic Heart Disease defined ischemic heart disease as the "cardiac disability, acute and chronic, arising from reduction or arrest of blood supply to the myocardium in association with disease processes in the coronary arterial system."[126] Subsequently, the Expert Committee on Cardiovascular Diseases and Hypertension accepted the term coronary heart disease as synonymous with ischemic heart disease.[124] It should be emphasized that coronary heart disease includes cardiac disturbances from other lesions of the coronary arteries in addition to atherosclerosis.

Cardiac disease resulting from coronary atherosclerosis and its complications, referred to as atherosclerotic coronary heart disease, includes such features as angina pectoris, myocardial infarction, myocardial atrophy and fibrosis, congestive heart failure, cardiac hypertrophy and dilatation, and sudden death caused by cardiac standstill or ventricular fibrillation with or without anatomic evidence of myocardial disease. Actually, these are the same manifestations that may occur in any other type of coronary heart disease. Valvular atherosclerosis with or without calcification is not included in this discussion of atherosclerotic coronary heart disease, although atherosclerosis may affect the valves, as in some instances of calcific aortic disease (p. 622).

Some authors use the term *arteriosclerotic heart disease* for that type of myocardial derangement associated with coronary atherosclerosis that is characterized by a slowly progressive diminution of blood supply to the heart, leading to atrophy and fibrosis of the myocardium, and they often include atherosclerosis of the aortic valve with calcification (that is, calcific aortic stenosis of nonrheumatic origin). Also, in earlier statistics reference is made to the item *arteriosclerotic heart disease including coronary disease*, which is considered to be synonymous with coronary (or ischemic) heart disease. Only recently has the item *ischemic heart disease* been included in the International Classification of Diseases.[128]

Incidence

Just as heart disease is the leading cause of death in the United States, coronary heart disease, especially the atherosclerotic type, is the chief form of fatal cardiac disease. In 1978, there were 1,927,788 deaths from all causes in the United States. Among these, 729,510 resulted from cardiac disease of all types and 642,270 from ischemic heart disease (a total death rate of 294.3 per 100,000 population).[1] Thus ischemic (coronary) heart disease accounts for 88% of the mortality from all forms of heart disease. Most of the deaths from ischemic heart disease occur at ages 35 to 74 years.[5] Generally, death rates for the various age groups are higher for males than for females. The difference decreases progressively with advance in age. The sex differentials in mortality are lower among nonwhites than among whites.[5]

The recent data from the National Center for Health Statistics, which are tabulated as age-adjusted death rates, indicate a downward trend in mortality from ischemic heart disease.[3,5,125] The death rate for ischemic heart disease in 1978 decreased 2.2% from the rate in 1977 and was 25.1% below the rate in 1968.[1]

Anatomic features

Two coronary arteries normally arise from the aorta: the left and the right (Fig. 16-10). In anatomic studies a variability in the pattern of distribution of the coronary arteries has been demonstrated.[132,137,138] The anatomic patterns are classified as right coronary artery preponderant or left coronary artery preponderant, depending on which artery crosses the posterior crux of the heart, or balanced circulation if both arteries extend to the crux and neither crosses it. The crux is that region of the pos-

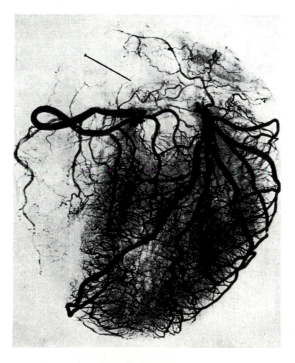

Fig. 16-10. Roentgenogram of injected coronary circulation in normal adult heart. (From Gross, L.: The blood supply to the heart, New York, 1921, Paul B. Hoeber, Inc.)

terior surface of the heart where all four chambers and the interatrial and interventricular septa meet. In right artery preponderance (or predominance), the most common pattern in human hearts in both sexes, the right coronary artery supplies the entire right ventricle, the posterior half of the interventricular septum, and a part of the posterior wall of the left ventricle and gives rise to the atrioventricular nodal and posterior descending arteries. In the heart with a balanced circulation, which is the next most frequent pattern, each ventricle receives its blood supply from the correspondingly named coronary artery, and the posterior branch of the right coronary artery supplies practically all of the posterior part of the interventricular septum, while the anterior part of the septum receives its blood supply from the left coronary artery. In left artery preponderance, the least frequent pattern, there are variable degrees of preponderance, but in the most exaggerated form, the left coronary artery supplies all of the left ventricle, the entire interventricular septum, and a part of the posterior wall of the right ventricle, and it gives rise to the atrioventricular nodal and posterior descending arteries. In any of these patterns, variable branches from both coronary arteries supply blood to the two atria.

Schlesinger[137] produced evidence that the anatomic patterns varied in incidence according to sex and that they were associated with different reactions of the heart to coronary artery disease. In his study the balanced circulation was more prevalent in women, and hearts with this pattern suffered least from the effects of coronary artery disease. Left artery preponderance was seen more often in men and increased the vulnerability of the heart to the effects of coronary artery disease. Whereas Schlesinger found that hearts with left artery preponderance had the greatest incidence of myocardial infarction and the worst prognosis after infarction, Pitt and associates[167] were unable to correlate the pattern of the coronary arteries with the incidence of coronary occlusions or with the prognosis after myocardial infarction. Despite the convenient classification of the topography of the coronary circulation, one anatomic fact of great importance must not be overlooked. The left ventricle and the interventricular septum make up the predominant mass and weight of the heart, and the major portion of these structures (even in hearts with right artery preponderance) receives blood from the left coronary artery. Because this artery provides the greatest number of arterial radicles and supplies the major myocardial mass, it is anatomically and functionally the predominant artery.[132,138]

The presence of anastomoses between coronary arteries in the normal heart is an established fact,[135] but the size of these communications is not agreed on by all. It is commonly believed that they are not more than 40 μm in diameter unless there is an associated disease of the coronary arteries or myocardium.[131] A number of investigators, however, have demonstrated anastomoses up to several hundred micrometers in diameter in some normal hearts. Sizes up to 180,[134] 200,[130] 300,[132] and even 350 μm[129] have been reported. It has been observed that the anastomoses are comparatively small and thin walled under normal circumstances when they probably do not participate much in the coronary flow and that they elongate and become thick walled and tortuous under stress of a major amount of pulsatile flow.[132] Collateral circulation is developed as a result of an increase in size of the anastomotic channels, which occurs in response to the need of the heart and not because of advancing age—that is, in relation to considerable narrowing or old complete occlusions of the coronary arteries or their main branches or in response to a myocardial need even in the absence of significant coronary artery disease.[131] The collateral circulation may be a factor limiting the size of a myocardial infarct after coronary occlusion. Also, in some instances it may prevent significant clinical manifestations or morphologic changes in the myocardium in the presence of long-standing obstructive arterial lesions.[131]

In addition to these coronary anastomoses, there are luminal channels that pass from the arterioles, the capillary beds, the sinusoids, and the coronary veins within the myocardium directly into the cavity of the heart.[136] These are sometimes referred to as thebesian vessels, an all-inclusive term that includes the following:

1. Arterioluminal vessels, which connect branches of the coronary arteries with the lumen of the heart
2. Capillary-luminal vessels, the capillary network connecting the lumen of the heart with either the coronary arteries or veins
3. Sinusoid-luminal channels, which are connections between the cavities of the heart and the myocardial sinusoids in which some small coronary arteries terminate
4. Venoluminal channels, the openings between the cavities of the heart and the coronary veins (the type originally described by Thebesius in 1708)[136]

Some of the blood within the vessels of the myocardium drains directly into the lumen of the heart by way of these channels. However, the channels may function as routes of collateral circulation. For example, in instances of right coronary artery occlusion, the rarity of infarction of the right ventricle may be explained, at least in part, by the fact that the thin wall of this ventricle is sufficiently nourished by blood derived directly from the lumen of the heart as a result of reversal of blood flow through these luminal vessels.

Types of coronary artery disease

A variety of diseases affect the coronary arteries, the most prevalent being atherosclerosis, which accounts for

more than 90%, with the other lesions being responsible for less than 10%. These diseases may be limited to the vessels themselves without any associated cardiac disease. By means of lead-agar injections of the coronary arteries, many complete occlusions have been demonstrated in the absence of significant anatomic or clinical evidence of myocardial damage. The apparent inconsistency of such a finding is explained by the presence of large anastomoses that bypass the obstructed area.[131] On the other hand, coronary atherosclerosis can produce varying degrees of narrowing and complete occlusion of the arteries (Fig. 16-11), resulting in ischemic heart disease. It should be noted that there are examples of myocardial damage (such as infarction) and even sudden death in patients in whom significant disease of the coronary arteries is not demonstrated at autopsy. Perhaps these patients have an acute coronary insufficiency brought on by an increased demand by the myocardium for more oxygen, as in exercise or the increased cardiac output associated with emotion.[144] It is also possible that a spasm of a coronary artery may be the basis for the acute coronary insufficiency.[133] The following is a list of the lesions of the coronary arteries that are potential causes of coronary occlusion:

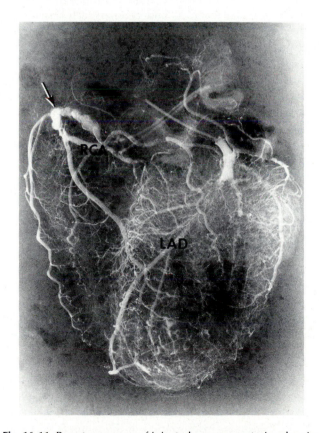

Fig. 16-11. Roentgenogram of injected coronary arteries showing complete occlusion of left anterior descending coronary artery (*LAD*) and aneurysm of right coronary artery (*RCA*). Aneurysm (*arrow*) is a rare complication of coronary atherosclerosis.

1. Atherosclerosis
   a. With progressive luminal narrowing
   b. With thrombosis
   c. With hemorrhage in atheromatous plaque
   d. With rupture of atheromatous plaque
2. Stenosis of coronary ostia
   a. Caused by syphilitic aortitis
   b. Caused by aortic atherosclerotic plaque
3. Inflammations
   a. Rheumatic arteritis
   b. Polyarteritis nodosa
   c. Thromboangiitis obliterans
   d. Tuberculosis
   e. Other bacterial infections
4. Embolism
5. Thrombotic diseases
6. Neoplasms
7. Trauma
8. Aneurysms
9. Congenital anomalies
10. Medial calcification in infancy
11. Other diseases (such as scleroderma, xanthomatosis, and amyloidosis)

Coronary atherosclerosis. Coronary atherosclerosis is the major cause of ischemic heart disease. Other terms such as coronary sclerosis and coronary arteriosclerosis sometimes are used synonymously but, more correctly, arteriosclerosis is a generic term that includes several variants, one of which is atherosclerosis.

Morphologic aspects. The basic lesion in atherosclerosis is in the intima, being characterized by focal thickenings (plaques) of fibrous and lipid nature that tend to narrow the lumen and reduce the blood flow. In addition, the plaques tend to undergo various changes, such as calcification (Fig. 16-12), hemorrhage, ulceration, and superimposed thrombosis (complicated lesions).

There is some disagreement as to what constitutes the initial changes in atherosclerosis. A common opinion is that the earliest lesions are fatty flecks or streaks resulting from deposition of plasma lipid in the intima.[177] In contrast to this view, other theories maintain that certain changes on or within the intima, which precede lipid deposition, are the initial lesions (see also discussion of early events in atherogenesis, p. 582).

Although the primary event in the development of atherosclerotic lesions is debated, many investigators are in agreement that the presence of lipid in the vessel wall stimulates certain mesenchymal changes that eventually lead to fibrous tissue proliferation. Thus the early lesions develop into elevated lipid-laden fibrous lesions that protrude into the lumen (fibrofatty or fibrous plaques). In advanced lesions, hyalinization of the connective tissue occurs, and the lipid appears as large globules, as cholesterol crystals, and within large macrophages. Calcification is prominent and is present mainly at the junction of the intima and media, but it also extends into the hyalin-

ized plaques. The elastic tissue is greatly degenerated and in some areas may be absent. Lymphocytic infiltration of the adventitia may be noted. As a result of the plaque formation, narrowing of the lumen ensues. When necrosis occurs in the plaque, the necrotic tissue, together with the lipid material, produces a noticeable softening of the lesion; thus the designation *atheroma* (porridgelike mass) is appropriate. Encroachment of the intimal lesions on the media may cause a thinning of this layer.

Most investigators agree that atherosclerotic lesions occur more frequently in the left coronary artery than in the right, although a few authors state that in their experience the right coronary artery is involved as commonly as or more commonly than the left. The incidence is highest in the anterior descending branch of the left coronary artery, less in the right coronary artery, and still less in the circumflex branch of the left coronary artery. The area of severest involvement is about 3 to 4 cm from the coronary ostia. In a study of the coronary arteries in American soldiers killed in the Korean conflict,[145] the disease was found most commonly at or just beyond the bifurcation of the arteries, giving the impression that hemodynamic forces about the bifurcations (for example, eddying of the bloodstream during the diastolic recoil of

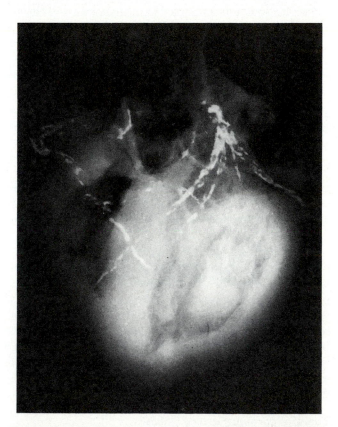

Fig. 16-12. Roentgenogram of heart, not injected, illustrating extensive and severe calcification of coronary arteries. This is a feature of atherosclerosis and is more severe in this instance than usual.

the dilated coronary arteries) are a factor in the mechanism of plaque formation. The fact that atherosclerosis is greater in the coronary arteries (which come off a part of the aorta that is usually not severely affected by atherosclerosis) than in the renal arteries (which come off a part of the aorta that is usually considerably involved by the disease) favors the concept that hemodynamic factors are related to a selective involvement of the coronary arteries.[146]

The atherosclerotic plaques are usually patchy and situated eccentrically along one side of the lumen, although occasionally there may be concentric thickening of the

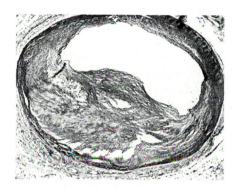

Fig. 16-13. Atherosclerosis of small branch of anterior descending coronary artery (main branch occluded by thrombus). Note thick fibrous and atheromatous plaque on one side, considerably reduced lumen, and greatly thinned media. Patient, 47-year-old white woman, died of myocardial infarction.

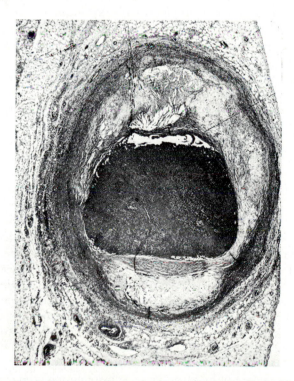

Fig. 16-14. Coronary atherosclerosis and thrombosis. Intima is irregularly thickened and media is thinned because of advanced atheromatosis.

wall of the vessel (Fig. 16-13). One of the complications of coronary atherosclerosis is gradual encroachment of the lesion on the lumen of the artery, leading to luminal narrowing that sometimes is extreme, even to the point of complete occlusion. Other complications are coronary thrombosis, intramural hemorrhage, rupture of an atheromatous plaque, and, rarely, aneurysm formation (Fig. 16-11).

In association with atherosclerosis, coronary thrombosis is a major cause of coronary occlusion (Fig. 16-14). Thrombi usually are found at sites of narrowing in the sclerotic arteries. They occur, in order of descending frequency, in the left anterior descending coronary artery, the right coronary artery, and the left circumflex artery.[153] Occasionally, thrombi are present in more than one artery. The initiation of thrombi is attributed to several possible factors.:

1. Roughening of the endothelium over the degenerated area, producing a suitable site for platelet deposition
2. Softening, breakdown, rupture, and ulceration of a plaque
3. Narrowing of the lumen by a plaque, resulting in local disturbance of blood flow
4. Hemorrhage in an atheromatous lesion, with disruption of tissue and release of thromboplastic substances
5. Increased coagulability of the blood associated with lipids in the blood

If the patient survives for several weeks, organization of a thrombus ensues, followed usually by canalization (Fig. 16-15). Some investigators have stressed that thrombosis is not merely a terminal event but rather a recurring process. According to this idea, a thrombus

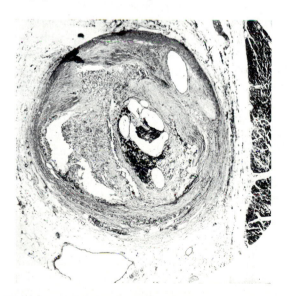

Fig. 16-15. Organization and canalization of thrombosed coronary artery in 43-year-old man. Note extreme atheromatous degeneration. Dark central masses consist of old fibrin. This is left circumflex branch.

forms on the surface of an atherosclerotic plaque, organizes, and becomes incorporated into the intima.[143] The process is repeated, and thus a gradual narrowing of the lumen occurs.

The formation of new capillaries can be demonstrated in atherosclerotic plaques[165,180] that are said to be derived from the intimal endothelium of the artery or from the vasa vasorum in the media and adventitia. Hemorrhage into the plaque may result from increased pressure within the capillaries as in hypertension, increased fragility of the capillary walls, or lack of support from the surrounding degenerated tissue in the lesion. An intramural hemorrhage is sometimes large enough to cause expansion of the plaque without rupture of the intimal lining and thereby to produce coronary occlusion. Or, as the hemorrhage disrupts the tissue, the latter probably liberates thromboplastic substances that can initiate thrombosis.[165] It is difficult to determine if occlusion of the coronary artery is produced by a spasm of the vessel wall induced by the hemorrhage in an atherosclerotic lesion. This possibility has been suggested.[144]

Rupture of the atheromatous plaque does not occur as frequently as sclerotic narrowing, thrombosis, or intramural hemorrhage. When the soft, atheromatous plaque ruptures, it may cause occlusion of the lumen at the site, form an embolus, or initiate the formation of a thrombus.

Early events in atherogenesis. The development of the atherosclerotic process is a controversial subject, particularly in regard to the nature of the early lesions. As already pointed out, it is commonly believed that infiltration of lipid from the blood into the intima is the primary event, leading to the formation of fatty streaks.[176,177] In some studies the first change noted after lipid infiltration is damage to the internal elastic lamina resulting from accumulation of extracellular lipid.[164] However, many investigators contend that the lipid first accumulates within mesenchymal cells, which are believed to be multipotential smooth muscle (myointimal) cells capable of producing collagen, elastic, and muscle fibers. It has been proposed that these cells are derived from cells normally present in the media, which proliferate and then migrate to the intima in response to lipid deposition.[181] Some of the lipid-containing cells may be macrophages. It has been suggested that not only are the smooth muscle cells a site for accumulation of lipids but they also may be involved in synthesizing them or in modifying the lipids that enter the intima from the blood.[150] Later, the lipids appear extracellularly after release from the cells that have undergone necrosis.[150]

Another view is that local alterations in the vascular wall, resulting from some form of injury (hemodynamic, endocrine, metabolic, immunologic, hypoxic, and so on), precede lipid deposition. Some investigators describe the early changes as fragmentation and degeneration of the inner elastic lamina, along with an increase in acid mucopolysaccharide and subendothelial fibroblastic proliferation[163]; others, as proliferative fibromuscular intimal thickening[149]; and still others, as increased vascular permeability and an increased production of sulfated glycosaminoglycans.[179] It is believed that these alterations facilitate the infiltration of plasma lipids and lead to their entrapment within the intima.

One theory emphasizes encrustation of fibrin as the significant factor in the early development of atherosclerotic lesions; that is, mural thrombi form on the intimal surface, organize, and become incorporated in the intima. When fatty deposits are superadded, the picture of atherosclerosis is completed.[143] Another hypothesis maintains that platelet-mediated endothelial permeability is the first step in atherogenesis[148]; that is, the platelets adhere to the endothelium, agglutinate, and then disintegrate, releasing vasoactive amines, which increase vascular permeability to lipids and protein.

It is generally agreed that the intimal smooth muscle cells are an important component of atherosclerotic lesions. Many investigators believe that the proliferation of these cells is related to lipid deposition. However, it has been suggested recently that a focal increase in the number of intimal smooth muscle cells precedes lipid deposition. According to some investigators, the stimulus for cell proliferation is a growth-promoting factor in the blood, probably of protein nature, which is able to pass through the endothelial barrier into the intima because of local injury to the endothelium.[172] Other investigators have proposed that the intimal cells are altered initially by mutagenic agents (such as chemicals or viruses), and then they proliferate under the influence of certain promoting factors. The implication is that the proliferative lesions have properties resembling those of benign neoplasms.[142]

Etiology. The cause or causes of atherosclerosis are not known, but there are a number of predisposing or risk factors.[140] Among these are the hemodynamic forces of the bloodstream that have already been mentioned. In recent years the importance of diet and blood lipids has been stressed. Other influential factors are heredity, sex, age, race, body build, hypertension, infections, smoking, emotional stress, physical inactivity, other diseases (for example, diabetes mellitus or obesity), and hormones (see also discussion of atherosclerosis on p. 689).

It is generally believed that a disturbance of lipid metabolism is an important predisposing cause of coronary atherosclerosis. Diet is closely associated with such a derangement. Practically all of the blood lipids are conjugated to proteins to form particles of varying size and composition known as the lipoproteins. There are four major classes of lipoproteins: (1) chylomicrons, the form in which ingested lipids are transported to the circulation and the tissues, (2) very low–density lipoproteins (VLDL) or pre-beta lipoproteins, which are heavily laden with triglycerides, (3) low-density lipoproteins (LDL) or beta lipoproteins, which contain a greater proportion of cholesterol, and (4) high-density lipoproteins (HDL) or alpha lipoproteins.

Considerable evidence in the literature suggests that abnormalities such as an increase in the serum LDL fraction, hypercholesterolemia, and an increased cholesterol phospholipid ratio in the blood are associated with the development of atherosclerosis. Many surveys have indicated that patients with coronary heart disease tend to have higher serum cholesterol values than do normal subjects.[157] Furthermore, in a number of follow-up studies of healthy men in whom predisease serum levels were analyzed, it was noted that the incidence of new coronary heart disease in later years was three times greater in men who had higher predisease cholesterol levels than in men with low levels.[157] In follow-up studies of middle-aged men in the United States, the frequency of subsequent myocardial infarction was about three times greater in men with predisease cholesterol values greater than 230 mg/100 ml of blood than in men with lower values.[157]

In contrast to the LDL fraction, which shows a positive relationship to the incidence of coronary heart disease, the HDL fraction appears to be inversely related.[140] Low concentrations of HDL in the blood are apparently associated with an increased risk of coronary heart disease.[140,162] It has been suggested that HDL may be important for normal clearance of cholesterol from tissues, including the arterial wall, so that an increase in the plasma HDL concentration may have a protective effect against the development of atherosclerosis and ischemic heart disease.[162]

There are reports that emphasize the importance of triglycerides in relation to atherosclerosis. It has been claimed that the triglyceride-rich, very low–density type of lipoprotein is more commonly involved in coronary heart disease than is the low-density type in which cholesterol predominates.[139] Some studies of the role of serum lipids in the clotting process point to a possible link between thrombosis and the triglyceride abnormality.[139] Serum triglyceride levels were elevated in South African European males, particularly those over 40 years of age, among whom the incidence of ischemic heart disease is high, and the values were low in African Bantu subjects, who have a low incidence of ischemic heart disease.[141]

Certain diseases such as diabetes mellitus, usually associated with hyperlipemia, have a definite relationship to coronary atherosclerosis, although the disturbance of lipid metabolism may not be the only factor. Coronary atherosclerosis occurs more frequently in diabetics than in the general population, and the disease occurs at an earlier age and is usually more severe. Obesity predisposes to coronary atherosclerosis, but its role is not clear. Some investigators suggest that it is associated with an abnormality of lipid metabolism but, because hypertension is often present in obese patients, it may be that the abnormal blood pressure is contributory. Also to be considered is the possibility that excess weight adds an extra load to a heart already burdened.

Differences in the incidence of heart disease in various countries of the world have been noted. The low incidence in certain countries has been attributed to low fat in the diet, but other factors cannot be excluded. As an example, in a comparative autopsy study in a Japanese city and in a city of the United States, coronary atherosclerosis was found to be less severe in Japan, and myocardial infarction was seven times more frequent in the United States.[147] The Japanese diet has a low fat content as compared with the American diet.

Evidence derived from various studies suggests a familial or hereditary predisposition to coronary atherosclerosis,[160] but whether this is related to inheritance of anatomic differences of the coronary arteries or to familial patterns of lipid metabolism has not been ascertained. The disease is more prevalent with advancing age but is not limited to old age. In a post–World War II study, data on 866 cases of coronary heart disease in soldiers between 18 and 39 years of age were accumulated. Of these cases, 450 were examined at autopsy, and advanced coronary atherosclerosis with its various complications was demonstrated.[183] In a group of U.S. soldiers killed in action in Korea, averaging 22 years of age, evidence of coronary atherosclerosis was observed in 77.3%.[145] The disease process varied from fibrous thickening to large atheromatous plaques causing complete occlusion of one or more of the major vessels. In comparison to the Korean investigation, a postmortem study of American soldiers killed in action in the Vietnam conflict, also averaging 22 years of age, showed that the percentage of those affected by some degree of coronary atherosclerosis was less but still significant (45%) and that severe narrowing of the coronary arteries was less striking.[161]

The influence of sex and race was mentioned previously. In brief, women are less prone to atherosclerotic coronary heart disease than are men, and it tends to develop at a later age in women; there is a lower incidence of the disease in nonwhites than in whites. Some reports indicate that the disease is more common in women with obesity, diabetes mellitus, hypertension, or surgical extirpation of the ovaries,[170,182] and that it develops at an earlier age; others state that the incidence and severity of atherosclerosis are less in men treated with estrogens for carcinoma of the prostate than in nontreated men.[169] Partly because of such reports, it has been suggested that female sex hormones, especially estrogens, protect against coronary heart disease. However, some investigators have reported that they found no difference in the incidence of this disease in castrated women compared to noncastrated women,[169] thus differing from the previously mentioned reports. Of interest is the evidence that intimal proliferation of vessels (arteries and veins), with and without thrombosis, is associated with oral contraceptives as well as with female steroid hormones related to pregnancy and the postpartum state.[155] Also, the results of recent studies in the United Kingdom strongly suggest that women who use oral contraceptives are at a greater risk of myocardial infarction than are nonusers.[158,159]

Clinically, hypertension is present in many patients with coronary heart disease. Also, in autopsy studies, there is evidence of more extensive atherosclerosis and coronary heart disease among hypertensive patients than among nonhypertensive patients. The increased blood pressure probably is not a primary cause of atherosclerosis but rather an aggravating one; perhaps it accentuates the local hemodynamic factors in the vessels or, when hypercholesterolemia is also present, the high intravascular pressure probably accelerates infiltration of lipid through the arterial wall. Hypertension is more common in individuals with diabetes mellitus, gout, kidney disease, or obesity and in women who are taking oral contraceptives.[140]

Certain studies indicate that emotional stress and physical inactivity play roles in the development of atherosclerosis. In a survey of physicians, it was assumed that general practitioners and anesthesiologists were subject to greater stress than dermatologists and pathologists, and coronary disease appeared to be three times more prevalent in the general practitioners and two times more prevalent in the anesthesiologists than in dermatologists and pathologists.[174]

Epidemiologic, autopsy, and experimental data suggest a causal relationship between cigarette smoking and cardiovascular morbidity and mortality.[151] Recent epidemiologic studies on different populations have shown a strong relationship between cigarette smoking and an increased death rate from coronary heart disease in men,[151,175] with approximately a twofold higher risk of death from this disease for all male cigarette smokers compared with nonsmokers.[151] Also, these smokers have a greater probability of dying of coronary heart disease at an earlier age than do nonsmokers. Furthermore, the evidence seems to suggest that women who smoke cigarettes have a greater risk of sudden death from this disease than do nonsmoking women.[151] Autopsy studies have shown a greater frequency and severity of coronary and aortic atherosclerosis, as well as greater myocardial arteriolar wall thickening, among cigarette smokers than among nonsmokers.[151] Experimental studies suggest that certain pathophysiologic, biochemical, and anatomic changes associated with coronary heart disease may be induced by elevated carboxyhemoglobin levels, which have been demonstrated in smokers, and by cigarette smoke and nicotine.[151]

A recent prospective epidemiologic investigation that confirmed the relationship between coronary heart disease and the usually accepted risk factors (such as hypertension, diabetes mellitus, cigarette smoking, elevated serum levels of cholesterol, triglyceride, and beta lipoproteins, and a history of parental ischemic heart disease) also indicated a significant association with type A behavior pattern.[171] This behavior pattern is characterized by enhanced aggressiveness, ambitiousness, competitive drive, and a chronic sense of time urgency. The more relaxed type B subject, on the other hand, was found to have a lower incidence of coronary heart disease. However, not all cardiologists accept this finding, and more rigorous testing is necessary to show that type A behavior plays a significant role in coronary heart disease.[152]

Some investigators have reported a lower incidence of myocardial infarction among necropsy subjects with hepatic cirrhosis,[154] suggesting that the latter protects against myocardial infarction by interfering in some way with the development and progression of coronary atherosclerosis. However, such a relationship based solely on necropsy data has been questioned. It is considered likely that a high mortality of hepatic cirrhosis, rather than a lower frequency of myocardial infarction among patients with cirrhosis, is the factor responsible for the rarity of myocardial infarction at necropsy.[173]

Among other factors believed to be associated with coronary heart disease is the quality of drinking water. A number of studies have shown a higher death rate from ischemic heart disease in communities with soft water than in areas with hard water. It is not known why hard water seems to have a protective effect, but some investigators suggest that the high content of mineral, chiefly calcium, is responsible for this action. Many studies have reported the association of coronary heart disease with a lack or increase of various elements in the water supply,[166,168] but the results are not conclusive.

Effects and complications. The effects of coronary atherosclerosis include angina pectoris, myocardial fibrosis, myocardial infarction, congestive heart failure, cardiac hypertrophy and dilatation, and sudden death. The details will be discussed after a consideration of other types of coronary artery disease that may produce the same effects.

Stenosis of coronary ostia. Narrowing of the openings of the coronary arteries can occur as the result of syphilitic aortitis and is an important cause of coronary insufficiency. One or both ostia may be involved. The incidence of this complication in patients with syphilitic aortitis is said to be between 8% and 35%[184] but has been reported to be as high as 51%.[192] The ostia are narrowed as a result of encroachment of intimal plaques upon the openings or by extension of the inflammatory process into that part of the coronary arteries passing through the aortic wall. Ostial involvement is more likely to occur if the coronary arteries originate above the upper level of the sinuses of Valsalva where the aortitis tends to be prominent. The lesion seldom extends beyond the coronary orifices into the vessels, but if it does, it usually involves less than 15 mm of the proximal part of the arteries. Syphilitic coronary arteritis of the distal branches is uncommon. Coronary arterial thrombosis and aneurysm formation are rare complications. However, varying degrees of concomitant coronary atherosclerosis may be present. The manifestations of coronary ostial stenosis usually are seen in patients under 40 years of age and include angina pectoris and dyspnea on exertion or paroxysmal nocturnal dyspnea. A relatively prolonged terminal illness with cardiac failure is the rule, but sudden death may occur.[184] Myocardial infarction is not a common complication, probably because of the extensive collateral circulation that develops as a result of the gradual occlusion of the coronary ostia. Myocardial fibrosis is the chief evidence of cardiac damage attributable to diminished blood supply.

Occlusion of the ostium of a coronary artery in a non-syphilitic patient occasionally may be caused by an aortic atherosclerotic plaque encroaching on the orifice, especially if the artery originates high in the aorta.

Inflammations

Rheumatic arteritis.[189] In active rheumatic fever, lesions occur mainly in the small intramyocardial branches of the coronary arteries and less frequently in the main coronary arteries. Probably these vascular lesions contribute to myocardial damage, but in the presence of an active rheumatic myocarditis it is difficult to determine how much of the damage is caused by them. One type of lesion is an exudative and necrotizing panarteritis characterized by edema and a mild or pronounced leukocytic infiltration by lymphocytes, plasma cells, neutrophils, and sometimes basophilic cells like those found in the Aschoff bodies. Fibrinoid swelling of the collagen may be present. The more extensive lesions with prominent necrosis of the vessel wall resemble polyarteritis nodosa. Frequently, Aschoff bodies are noted in proximity to the blood vessels. Thrombi may form within the lumina of the intramyocardial vessels in association with the inflammation, followed by organization and canalization (see Fig. 16-33). Rare instances of thrombotic occlusion of a main coronary artery with or without myocardial infarction have been reported.

Polyarteritis nodosa. The coronary arteries are affected in the majority of patients (approximately 70%) with polyarteritis nodosa as part of a widespread involvement of the smaller and medium-sized arteries. Rarely is the disease limited to the coronary arteries. This relatively uncommon disease of unknown cause is a form of necrotizing arteritis accompanied by aneurysm formation and thrombosis in the coronary arteries. Myocardial infarction may occur.

Thromboangiitis obliterans. Thromboangiitis obliterans (Buerger's disease) is an inflammatory disease affecting chiefly the vessels of the extremities, but occasionally it involves the visceral vessels, including the coronary arteries. The lesion may lead to coronary thrombosis and myocardial infarction.

Other forms. Other forms of coronary arteritis such as those caused by tuberculosis or other bacterial infections are sometimes observed.

Embolism.[191] An infrequent cause of coronary occlusion is embolism, which most commonly involves the left coronary artery and its branches. The usual forms of emboli are those derived from bland thrombi and those associated with bacterial endocarditis. Bland emboli usually arise from thrombi on atherosclerotic plaques in the root of the aorta but also may originate from a thrombus in a main coronary artery or from mural thrombi in the left ventricle, left atrium, or left atrial appendage. Thrombi in the pulmonary veins caused by suppurative disease of the lungs, or as a result of invasion by tumor, may give rise to emboli. Rarely does a coronary embolus originate from thrombi in peripheral veins (paradoxical embolism). The vegetations of bacterial endocarditis are important sources of emboli, particularly those growing in the sinuses of Valsalva in proximity to the coronary ostia. Sometimes it is difficult to determine morphologically if a coronary occlusion is the result of thrombosis or embolism. Sudden death and myocardial infarction are possible effects of these emboli. Multiple minute emboli may be the cause of myocardial failure. Atheromatous plaques in a coronary artery may rupture and give rise to emboli. Fat embolism and air embolism may occur in the coronary circulation. The former usually produces no significant clinical manifestations, but the latter may be a cause of death.

Thrombotic diseases. Coronary thrombosis occasionally occurs in disorders other than atherosclerosis, as in diseases associated with stasis and sludging of blood or with hypercoagulability of the blood, such as sickle cell anemia, polycythemia vera, and shock. Hyaline thrombi in the small intramyocardial vessels may be demonstrated in thrombotic thrombocytopenic purpura (Fig. 16-16).

Neoplasms. Primary or metastatic tumors of the heart may cause compression of a vessel and, in rare instances, result in coronary occlusion.

Trauma. Penetrating injuries may cause laceration of a coronary artery, with or without myocardial infarction. Occasionally, the penetrating object produces coronary thrombosis by causing contusion of an artery. It is believed that if nonpenetrating cardiac trauma induces

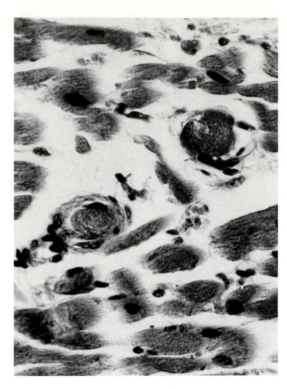

Fig. 16-16. Hyaline thrombi in small vessels of myocardium in thrombotic thrombocytopenic purpura.

coronary thrombosis in a previously normal vessel, it does so rarely.[62] It is possible that sufficient localized blunt injury in an already diseased artery may precipitate thrombosis (p. 570).[61]

Aneurysms.[185-187] Aneurysms are not common in the coronary arteries. The types of aneurysms include congenital, mycotic, atherosclerotic, syphilitic, dissecting, rheumatic, and those caused by polyarteritis nodosa. Dissecting aneurysm of a coronary artery usually results from extension of the process from the aorta, but dissection of the coronary arteries without involvement of the aorta may occur.[186] It causes coronary occlusion by pressure of the blood within the wall of the vessel. Among the complications of the other forms of aneurysms are thrombotic coronary occlusion and rupture with hemopericardium and cardiac tamponade.

Congenital anomalies. One of the most significant abnormalities of the coronary arteries is an anomalous origin of one or both arteries from the pulmonary artery. The coronary artery most frequently involved is the left. Myocardial hypoxia caused by venous blood supplying the left ventricle may lead to severe myocardial damage and cardiac failure. Other congenital lesions of the coronary arteries include aneurysms and arteriovenous fistulas.

Medial calcification in infancy.[188,190] Coronary atherosclerosis as it is seen in adults rarely affects infants and children. The usual type of occlusive coronary artery dis-

ease occurring in infancy and occasionally in childhood is a distinct pathologic entity known by several names: medial calcification, medial coronary sclerosis, medial calcification with fibroblastic proliferation of the intima, coronary sclerosis of infancy, or idiopathic arterial calcification in infancy. This lesion is characterized by a fibroblastic proliferation of the intima associated with calcification that starts close to the internal elastic lamina and extends into the media and into the thickened intima, with involvement being more prominent in the media. Coronary occlusion may result, followed by infarction and calcification of the myocardium or sudden death. The occlusion is attributable chiefly to the intimal proliferation rather than to the medial calcification. Occasionally, thrombosis occurs.

This is usually a generalized disease that affects many vessels throughout the body, although involvement of the coronary arteries frequently is the most prominent feature. In some instances the arterial lesions are associated with advanced renal disease, hypervitaminosis D, or congenital anomalies of the heart or great vessels. There is one interesting group, however, in which no primary cause is demonstrated, namely, the idiopathic type of arterial calcification.

Effects of myocardial ischemia

As mentioned previously, lesions of the coronary arteries in themselves are not necessarily accompanied by clinical or pathologic evidence of heart disease. Manifestations occur when a sufficient degree of myocardial ischemia is produced to disturb the metabolism and performance of the heart. The nature of the cardiac disease depends on the suddenness of onset, duration, and degree of myocardial ischemia, as well as the location and extent of the area affected by the insufficient blood supply. Myocardial ischemia may be brought about by one or a combination of the following:

1. Diminution of coronary blood flow (as in coronary artery disease, aortic stenosis, or shock)
2. Demand of the myocardium for more oxygen in certain situations such as during or after exercise, increased cardiac output associated with emotions,[144] or rapid cardiac arrhythmias
3. Hypertrophy of the heart and increased cardiac work without concurrent increase of coronary blood flow (as in hypertensive or valvular heart disease)

A significant factor that may prevent the development of myocardial ischemia is an adequate collateral circulation through anastomotic channels. The effect of a sudden myocardial ischemia, such as that which follows an acute and complete occlusion of a coronary artery, may be sudden death or myocardial infarction. A temporary myocardial ischemia is responsible for the symptom angina pectoris. Progressive narrowing of the coronary arteries, as in coronary atherosclerosis, may be associated with a more chronic ischemia that leads to atrophy and fibrosis of the myocardium.

Myocardial infarction. A consequence of coronary occlusion is myocardial infarction, although the relationship is not an invariable one. The collateral circulation may be adequate, so that muscle necrosis is prevented, or the patient may die before any visible changes of an infarct develop. Conversely, infarction of the myocardium can occur in the absence of sudden occlusion. In such instances, old atherosclerotic lesions with narrowing of the vessel lumen or old organized atherosclerotic thrombi frequently are found at autopsy. In these cases myocardial ischemia apparently is the result of coronary insufficiency brought on by factors that increase the demand of the myocardium for more oxygen.[144] A suggestion has been made that myocardial infarction unassociated with acute coronary thrombosis may be the clinical equivalent of Selye's experimentally produced electrolyte-steroid cardiopathy with necrosis (ESCN).[225] The latter is characterized by large infarctoid necroses caused by the combined action of certain steroids and sodium salts in the absence of coronary occlusion.[225]

The role that undue exertion plays in precipitating an attack of myocardial infarction is difficult to determine. A history of severe activity at the time of onset of symptoms of infarction seldom is obtained. For example, in one study of acute myocardial infarction in a large industrial population, the activity at the time of an attack was listed as follows: heavy activity or severe exertion, 4.5%; moderate activity, 42%; at rest, 39.2%; and asleep, 14.3%[220]

Cause of infarct. In the majority of instances of acute myocardial ischemia, the causative lesion is atherosclerosis of the coronary arteries, with or without intramural hemorrhage or thrombosis.[153] In a study of 141 cases of myocardial infarct in human hearts, severe narrowing (that is, 70% or greater compromise of the lumen) was observed in two or three of the major arterial trunks in 81% of the hearts.[153] Most of the remainder had severe narrowing in one major artery or a moderate degree of atherosclerosis in one or more arteries. In 29% of the hearts, coronary atherosclerosis alone was the cause of the infarct. Coronary thrombosis was demonstrated in nearly half (45%) and intramural hemorrhage in 39%, both almost always associated with severe atherosclerosis. Hemorrhage and thrombosis occurred together in some arteries, and it is possible that the thromboses were precipitated by the hemorrhage. Although numerous intramural hemorrhages were encountered in this series, they were generally of moderate or slight degree and did not appear extensive enough to compromise the arterial lumen in themselves[153] but at times may have accentuated the luminal narrowing already existing in a diseased vessel.

Of the major arteries, the most frequently occluded is the left coronary artery, and particularly its left anterior descending branch. In a survey of 1495 cases of occlusion obtained from several sources in the literature, the distribution of the occlusion was as follows: left main artery, 71; left anterior descending branch, 834; left circumflex artery, 211; and right coronary artery, 379.[221]

Although coronary atherosclerosis is the most common lesion leading to myocardial infarction, any of the other less common diseases affecting the coronary arteries (pp. 579-586) may be causative. Also, there have been several reports in which infarction has occurred in the presence of normal coronary arteries. In some of these patients a pathophysiologic cause of ischemia of the myocardium (for example, aortic stenosis or insufficiency, carbon monoxide poisoning, or prolonged hypotension as in shock) may have been responsible.[199] In others, however, no known cause was found, and in these instances other mechanisms have been considered (for example, spasm of coronary artery, platelet aggregation or thrombosis followed by resolution, or disease of small coronary vessels).[213]

Recently a controversy has arisen as to the relationship of coronary thrombosis to myocardial infarction.[197] The classic view that coronary thrombi cause myocardial infarcts has been reexamined by some investigators.[222,229] There appears to be general agreement that coronary arterial thrombi occur infrequently in patients who die suddenly and in those with infarcts limited to the subendocardial region of the myocardium, although coronary atherosclerosis with luminal narrowing is usually present. On the other hand, more extensive infarcts involving one half or more (sometimes the entire thickness) of the septal or ventricular wall are commonly associated with coronary thrombosis.[197,222] According to one view, coronary thrombosis in these instances is the result rather than the cause of infarction and is particularly likely to occur in association with cardiac failure or cardiogenic shock.[222,229] The thrombus is believed to form secondarily in an already narrowed atherosclerotic artery as a result of diminished cardiac output and consequent slowing of the coronary blood flow. However, other investigators point out that the consistent location of thrombi in a proximal position in the artery or arteries supplying the infarcted area of the myocardium, commonly at sites of rupture or ulceration of atherosclerotic plaques, favors the classical concept that thrombi play a causal role.

Location and types of infarcts. Almost all infarcts occur in the left ventricle. The most frequent site is the anterior region of the left ventricle near the apex, usually including the anterior two thirds of the interventricular septum, because of disease of the descending branch of the left coronary artery. The next most common site is the posterior part of the left ventricle, together with the posterior third of the interventricular septum, which generally is related to disease of the right coronary artery. Less commonly, infarcts are confined to the lateral wall of the left ventricle, usually as a result of disease of the left circumflex artery.

Myocardial infarcts are classified as anterior, posterior, lateral, septal, and circumferential, depending on the general region of the left ventricle involved,[144] or according to combinations of these terms, such as anterolateral, posterolateral, and anteroseptal. Although the septum often is involved in infarcts of the anterior or posterior types, only rarely are infarcts limited to the ventricular septum. The unusual circumferential infarct may result from disease of the anterior descending coronary artery when the posterior descending coronary artery is small, or it may represent the result of several independent infarcts in the three major vascular regions of the left ventricle.[144] An infarct that is designated *posterior* by this classification may be referred to as either *diaphragmatic* or *inferior* in electrocardiographic terminology. The right ventricle is infrequently involved, and when it is, the lesion usually is an extension of an infarct of the left ventricle. Rarely is the lesion limited to the right ventricle. Some writers have suggested that the relatively thin wall of this ventricle is sufficiently nourished by blood directly from the lumen of the heart through the luminal vessels, thus preventing infarction. Others reason that the right ventricle is less susceptible to infarction because its metabolic requirements are not as great as those in the left ventricle or because there is less interference with coronary blood flow in the thin muscle of the right ventricle as a result of constriction of intramyocardial vessels during systole than in the thick left ventricular wall.

Infarcts of the atria frequently are unrecognized during life and even at autopsy. Statistics vary greatly as to the incidence of atrial infarcts, depending a great deal on the thoroughness with which one searches for them. In a study of 182 consecutive cases of myocardial infarct, 31 (17%) of the hearts examined were found to have atrial infarcts.[200] Most of the infarcts occur in the right atrium (especially in the right atrial appendage). They often are accompanied by mural thrombi and seldom occur alone. They usually are associated with infarcts of the left ventricle. It is believed that the oxygenated blood of the left atrium tends to protect this chamber from infarction. In many atrial infarcts, obstructive disease of the nutrient blood vessels is not identified.

Sometimes, one may see what is referred to as infarction at a distance. When there is a gradual occlusion of one coronary artery, the myocardium that is ischemic derives its blood supply chiefly from anastomotic channels of the other coronary artery. Then if the latter becomes suddenly occluded, an acute infarct develops in the area originally supplied by the first artery.

Myocardial infarcts may be classified on the basis of the degree of thickness of the ventricular wall they occupy[230]:

1. Full-thickness or transmural infarcts, with involvement of the entire thickness of the ventricular wall
2. Large or massive infarcts but not involving the full thickness
3. Laminar infarcts, involving less than half of the thickness of the wall, most frequently the inner or subendocardial half—thus sometimes called "subendocardial infarcts"

The pattern of infarcts has been found to correspond to portions of one or more of the four chief muscle bundles of the heart, with the laminar type involving usually one and never more than two bundles, and the others involving two or more bundles.[230] The thickness of the infarct may be important in determining the complications and sequelae that may develop. For example, in one study,[230] rupture of the heart occurred only in the full-thickness infarcts. Aneurysms of the ventricular wall and mural thrombosis were associated most frequently with such infarcts, less commonly with massive but not full-thickness lesions, and rarely with laminar infarcts.

Infarcts also are classified according to the age of the lesions. *Acute*, *fresh*, and *recent* are terms for newly formed infarcts, whereas *old*, *healing*, *organizing*, *healed*, and *organized* are terms applied to the more advanced lesions.

Morphologic features. The following microscopic and gross features are based on an investigation of the hearts of 72 patients with myocardial infarcts. In these patients there was definite clinical evidence of the time of onset of myocardial ischemia, so that the ages of the lesions could be determined.[215]

FIRST WEEK. Usually no definite histologic changes are detected by routine light microscopy for the first 5 or 6 hours after the onset of myocardial ischemia (see p. 590 for studies of early infarcts). After that, coagulative necrosis of the myocardium becomes evident, characterized by hyaline change in the fibers, with loss of striations and a more deeply eosinophilic appearance. Karyolysis of muscle nuclei is prominent, and pyknosis and karyorrhexis also can be seen. The connective tissue and to a lesser extent the small blood vessels also undergo necrosis. Neutrophils are attracted to the necrotic area, beginning peripherally and then spreading centrally. During the first 24 hours the leukocytic infiltration is slight, and from the second to the fourth day it increases progressively. By the fourth day the infiltration is pronounced, with degenerative changes and necrosis occurring in many of the infiltrating cells (Fig. 16-17). By the fifth or sixth day, many of the neutrophils are necrotic and gradually disappear. Edema and focal hemorrhages may be present. On the fourth or fifth day the first signs of removal of muscle fibers appear. Blood capillaries and fibroblasts penetrate the infarct from the periphery.

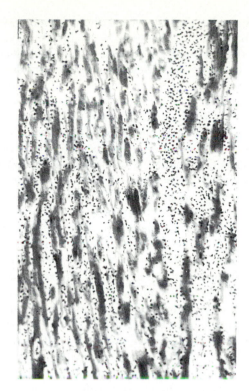

Fig. 16-17. Acute myocardial infarction. Necrotic muscle fibers are separated by heavy neutrophilic infiltration.

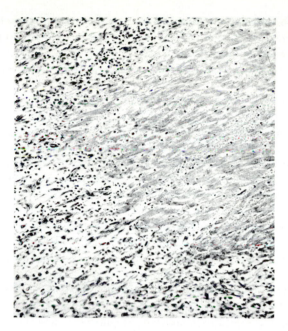

Fig. 16-18. Organizing myocardial infarct. Necrotic muscle is surrounded by granulation tissue, lymphocytes, and macrophages.

Simultaneously, macrophages penetrate the necrotic area. Single muscle fibers or small clumps of fibers may undergo phagocytosis and removal by the seventh day.

SECOND WEEK. During the second week the removal of peripheral muscle fibers is a prominent feature. By the tenth day there is a peripheral zone from which the necrotic muscle fibers are almost completely removed. Numerous pigmented macrophages are present, with most of the pigment being the yellow-brown lipofuscin formerly present in muscle cells but some of it representing hemosiderin granules resulting from the breakdown of erythrocytes in hemorrhagic areas. The ingrowth of blood vessels and connective tissue is more prominent, and a moderate number of eosinophils, lymphocytes, and plasma cells may be seen (Fig. 16-18). Active phagocytosis and removal of muscle fibers occur along the edge of the remaining necrotic muscle. By the end of the second week, practically all the necrotic muscle is removed in very small infarcts (3 to 4 mm in diameter). Neutrophils are almost gone. Fine, newly formed collagen fibers usually are found in the periphery at about the twelfth day.

THIRD WEEK. Removal of muscle fibers continues in larger infarcts, and there is progressive ingrowth of the vascularized connective tissue. Pigmented macrophages are numerous, eosinophils are decreasing, and lymphocytes and plasma cells are still prominent. Collagen fibers produced by the fibroblasts particularly in the periphery are moderately prominent at the end of 3 weeks.

FOURTH TO SIXTH WEEKS. There is a gradual increase of collagenous connective tissue with progressive removal of the necrotic muscle. By the end of this period, collagen is a prominent feature. There is a decrease in the vascularity and in the infiltrating pigmented macrophages and lymphocytes, and the scar becomes contracted. Some of the pigmented macrophages may persist for as long as 1 to 2 years after absorption of the infarct.[215] Isolated intact muscle fibers that were spared may be present throughout the scar.

AFTER 6 WEEKS. Some of the sequelae of myocardial infarction include left ventricular aneurysm formation (p. 594), mural thrombosis, and cardiac hypertrophy. An old aneurysm may be markedly thinned, but its scarred wall is strong and rarely ruptures. Mural thrombi frequently form in the aneurysm and may be the source of thromboemboli to the brain, spleen, kidneys, intestines, and lower extremities.

PERICARDIUM. In many infarcts, particularly those in which the subepicardial muscle is affected, a fibrinous pericarditis appears after 24 hours and begins to organize about the eighth or ninth day. Unless the exudate is unusually thick, it is completely organized about 4 weeks after the onset of the infarct.

MURAL THROMBOSIS. Endocardial thrombi may occur as early as the fifth day after the onset of the infarct, their organization beginning on the ninth day and becoming complete about the sixteenth day. Fresh thrombi and partially organized ones may be found in relation to comparatively old infarcts.

ANOTHER VIEW OF HEALING. In the usual description of an infarct, as noted in the foregoing paragraphs, it is stated that the connective tissue and small blood vessels also undergo necrosis and that, as the necrotic muscle is removed, the area is replaced by newly formed granulation tissue. According to some investigators,[193] however, there is a certain critical size of an infarct under which the stroma does not share in the necrosis. This is the so-called miliary infarct. Neutrophilic infiltration is not a prominent feature in this type of infarct, but macrophages gain access to all parts of the lesion and phagocytose all the dead muscle rapidly and evenly. It is believed that the original stroma becomes condensed without new connective tissue formation. These same investigators claim that an exactly similar sequence of events occurs at the border of all larger infarcts. Furthermore, their explanation differs from the usual interpretation of the fate of the central portions of the infarct where muscle, connective tissue, and blood vessels are necrotic. Their concept is that the necrotic muscle is absorbed slowly by macrophages, leaving the reticular framework of the endomysium intact. Instead of replacement by granulation tissue, there is said to be recolonization of the endomysial sheaths by fibroblasts and endothelial cells, and in time the reticular fibers become thicker and hyalinized.

The gross appearance of an infarct is not striking during the first few hours of myocardial ischemia. The earliest change is that the myocardium appears paler and drier than normal. Sometimes, focal, blotchy, red-purple areas of hemorrhage are present. These changes are seen during the first 48 to 72 hours and are slight at first but become progressively more distinct. With the infiltration of neutrophils, the area becomes yellowish. At about the fourth day a definite yellow border appears in the periphery, which gradually becomes broader until about the sixth to eighth days, when the entire infarct is yellow or yellow-green. At about 8 to 10 days a reddish purple zone is noticed at the periphery of the infarct as a result of the granulation tissue, and the infarcted area shrinks somewhat because of the resorption of necrotic muscle (Fig. 16-19). The peripheral reddish zone of granulation tissue is depressed below the surface. As healing progresses, the infarct becomes pale gray, and ultimately, a gray-white or white fibrous shrunken scar replaces the resorbed dead muscle in about 2 to 3 months. The speed with which an infarct heals depends on the size of the lesion and the adequacy of the collateral circulation.

Special studies of early infarcts. As already pointed out, definite myocardial changes usually are not detected by routine light microscopy within 5 or 6 hours after onset of ischemia. Some investigators, however, believe that "waviness" as well as elongation of myocardial fibers

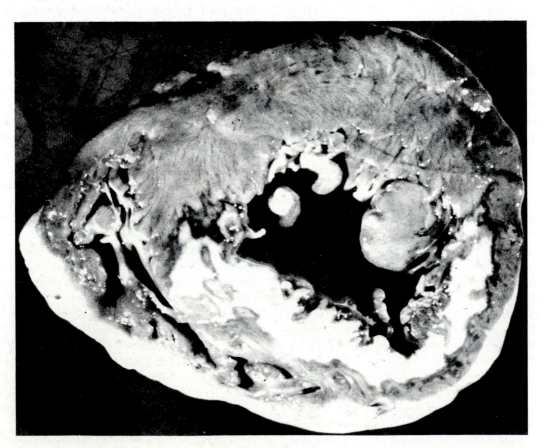

Fig. 16-19. Recent infarct of myocardium of left ventricle, anteroseptal.

(as a result of passive stretching of damaged fibers at each systole) can be observed before that time as the earliest histopathologic change.[208,214] This feature has been demonstrated in rats within 5 to 10 minutes after ligation of coronary arteries.[214]

By means of chemical, histochemical, and electron microscopic studies, changes can be demonstrated in early myocardial infarcts, often before the onset of the histologic alterations observed in routine light microscopy. By chemical analysis, it can be determined that a loss of glycogen and an increase in lactic acid occur in the ischemic myocardium within a few minutes after coronary occlusion. Glycogen depletion has been demonstrated histochemically in experimentally induced myocardial infarcts in dogs within 30 to 60 minutes after coronary occlusion, followed in a few hours by a degenerative change characterized by the appearance of nonglycogenic, periodic acid–Schiff–positive material.[212,232] Investigations by electron microscopy[196] have shown that as early as 5 minutes after coronary occlusion in rabbits there is a disappearance of perinuclear glycogen granules, as well as nuclear alterations such as clumping of the nucleoplasm. Swelling of mitochondria appeared in 20 to 30 minutes, followed by their rupture in 3½ to 4 hours. At the same time there was a disruption of sarcolemma. After 4 to 5 hours, transverse tearing of myofilaments was evident. In experimental studies in dogs it was shown that microscopic changes occurring after ligation of a vessel such as the left circumflex coronary artery were reversible for about 20 minutes, after which they tended to become irreversible.[156]

A decrease in succinic dehydrogenase activity has been described in a patient who died 2 hours after the onset of myocardial ischemia.[228] Decreased activity of this enzyme has been demonstrated in the ischemic myocardium in dogs 15 hours after ligation of the coronary artery.[212] Enzymes other than succinic dehydrogenase (SDH), such as glutamic-oxaloacetic transaminase (GOT) and lactic dehydrogenase (LDH), are known to be released from the myocardium after ischemia.[210] Appreciable amounts of GOT and LDH can be demonstrated in the serum after myocardial infarction.[231] Other serum enzymes, which together with GOT and LDH are most frequently assayed for the confirmation of the clinical diagnosis of acute myocardial infarct, are the isoenzymes of LDH, α-hydroxybutyric dehydrogenase (HBD), and creatinine phosphokinase (CPK).[194] The use of histochemical techniques has been investigated for the purpose of detecting decreased enzymatic activity in early myocardial infarcts in human hearts in which no gross microscopic ischemic changes were observed by conventional means.[217]

By chemical analysis of tissues and by histochemical techniques, it can be shown that potassium is lost from ischemic myocardial fibers. Chemical analysis of the infarct discloses about 10% loss of potassium during the first 60 to 90 minutes, but after this time it rapidly disappears, and at about 12 hours the intracellular potassium is nearly equal to the concentration of this ion in the extracellular fluid. By histochemical methods, no change is observed until after 6 hours, at which time a decrease in the potassium in the cells is observed, and by 12 to 15 hours there is a complete loss of potassium.[209] Electrolyte changes in ischemic myocardium, including loss of potassium and increase of sodium, are noted to be more severe in dogs with transient occlusions of the coronary arteries than in those with permanently occluded arteries.[211] The reduced blood flow through the infarct is the factor that slows the development of electrolyte changes in muscle made ischemic by permanent occlusion of a coronary artery.[211]

Complications and causes of death. Frequently the onset of myocardial infarction is characterized by agonizing, intense pain after weeks or months of prodromal precordial distress or pain of varying degree and intensity with or without other cardiac symptoms. However, the onset may be ushered in by sudden pain without prodromal symptoms, and sometimes myocardial infarction comes on without pain of any type—so-called silent myocardial infarction. The incidence of old, healed silent infarcts was reported to be as high as 3.5% of all autopsies in one investigation.[204] Only a minority of patients who enter the hospital with myocardial infarction die from the particular attack.[144]

The immediate mortality from acute myocardial infarction in several large series has been shown to vary between 14% and 30%, with the average in 3721 cases being 24%.[201] With more precise methods of clinical diagnosis, as well as newer methods of cardiac monitoring, resuscitation, and therapy, the incidence of immediate mortality is found to be generally lower (15%).[201] The immediate mortality, however, is increased (48%) when serious arrhythmias develop in myocardial infarction, and the mortality is progressively greater with increasing degrees of atrioventricular heart block.[201] In a study of hospitalized patients during the years 1946, 1954, and 1961, the American Medical Association's Commission on the Cost of Medical Care found a 50% reduction in mortality among patients suffering acute coronary occlusion, with the rate falling from 48.9% in 1946 to 24.4% in 1961. According to the Commission,[227] the reasons for the reduction are as follows:

1. Earlier recognition of coronary occlusion
2. Newer forms of cardiac resuscitation
3. More extensive use of oxygen
4. Availability of effective means of maintaining blood pressure during shock
5. Greater use of electrocardiograms

The most common cause of death in myocardial infarction is congestive heart failure, including right ventricular failure, left ventricular failure, or both. This represents about 30%[226] to 43%[216] of the deaths from infarction. Many of the other deaths are attributed to acute coronary failure (23%),[216,226] which refers to the type of death in patients who, while convalescing from acute myocardial infarction, have recurrent attacks of chest pain as a result of acute coronary insufficiency. With few exceptions these patients do not have another fresh infarct in addition to the original one when examined at autopsy. Sudden death occurs in these patients with acute coronary failure, during or after an attack of pain, apparently resulting from ventricular asystole or fibrillation.[226] Other causes of sudden death include two complications, massive pulmonary embolism and rupture of the heart. Cardiogenic shock may be the cause of death in about 9% of patients with myocardial infarction[216]; this develops shortly after the onset of the lesion. The shock results from a loss of the pumping ability of the heart, with power failure and a decreased cardiac output occurring when infarction has affected 40% or more of the ventricular muscle.[118]

The foregoing serious cardiac manifestations (excluding pulmonary embolism and cardiac rupture) are regarded by some investigators not as complications but as inherent features of myocardial infarction. Thromboembolism and rupture of the heart are complications that in themselves may be significant causes of death in patients with acute myocardial infarcts. Other complications of myocardial infarcts include ventricular aneurysms, myocardial calcification, and postmyocardial infarction syndrome.

MURAL THROMBOSIS AND THROMBOEMBOLISM. In large myocardial infarcts the endocardium is commonly involved, thus favoring formation of a thrombus. The size of the thrombus depends on the area of subendocardial damage. In small infarcts the overlying endocardium may escape, since the blood supply to the subendocardial area may not be interrupted. Slowing of the heart rate and bed rest no doubt aid the formation of mural thrombi. The bed rest also predisposes the patient to the development of venous thrombi in the lower extremities and in the pelvis, thus adding another possible source of emboli. As the myocardial infarct undergoes organization, the overlying mural thrombus tends to soften as a result of proteolytic enzyme action. Such thrombi are a constant menace, since portions are likely to break away from time to time. These thrombi or the ones in the veins of the legs or pelvis commonly give rise to thromboemboli that may obstruct the pulmonary, renal, mesenteric, splenic, pancreatic, or cerebral arteries. In one autopsy series the incidence of thromboembolism was 45%, and this complication was the main cause of death in 12% of cases of myocardial infarction and a contributing cause in an additional 15%.[207] In other studies, emboli were responsible for 6%[216] and 14%[226] of deaths.

There is disagreement among different observers concerning the value of anticoagulant therapy in lowering the incidence of thromboembolic complications in acute myocardial infarction, although a significant reduction in such complications is frequently reported.

RUPTURE OF HEART. The heart may rupture as a complication of acute myocardial infarction.[202,219,226] The

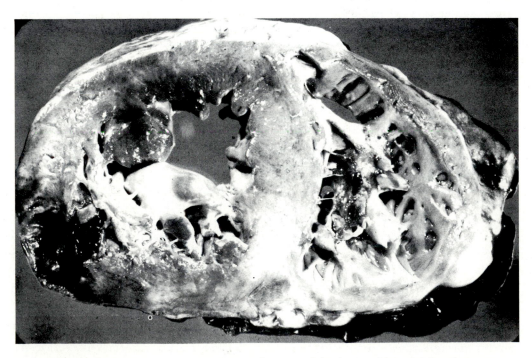

Fig. 16-20. Ruptured left ventricle through myocardial infarct and hemopericardium.

rupture may be either through the free wall with resulting hemopericardium and tamponade (70%), or through the ventricular septum (20%), or may be a combination of both (10%). Furthermore, a papillary muscle may rupture as a result of infarction. The incidence of myocardial rupture in patients with an acute infarct varies in different reports from 5.5%[219] to 24%.[226] The rupture usually occurs within the first week of the infarction while the necrotic region is soft (Figs. 16-20 to 16-22), and rarely occurs after the third week, by which time significant healing has usually occurred. The incidence of rupture is increased in patients with hypertension.[219] It has been noted that the acutely infarcted myocardium may be stretched and thinned.[224] This expansion may be demonstrated during life by two-dimensional echocardiography and may be used as a predictor of infarct rupture.

Rupture of a papillary muscle is a rare lesion resulting from infarction of the left ventricle. This leads to mitral valvular insufficiency because of the failure of the ruptured papillary muscle to anchor the valve and to keep it closed during ventricular systole. In some cases there is a spiral twisting of the chordae tendineae attached to the necrotic avulsed papillary tip (Fig. 16-23). Death occurs in a matter of hours whether or not twisting is present.[205] A lesser degree of papillary muscle involvement in a left ventricular infarct may result in papillary muscle dysfunction rather than in rupture.[195] In this case the infarcted papillary muscle will be unable to contract and to anchor the mitral valve during systole, so that mitral regurgitation will develop.

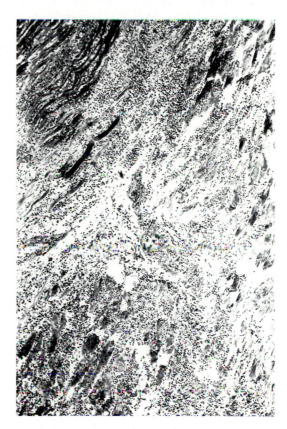

Fig. 16-22. Ruptured myocardial infarct. Hemorrhage is present among darker muscle fibers.

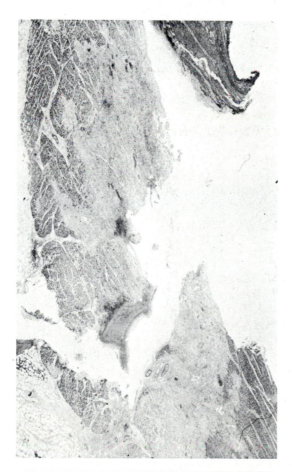

Fig. 16-21. Ruptured myocardial infarct (low power).

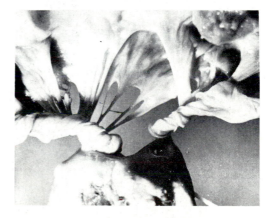

Fig. 16-23. Torsion pattern of chordae tendineae in rupture of papillary muscle. Inferior surface of mitral valve shows double spiral twisting of chordae tendineae, avulsed papillary tip, and anterior commissure. (From Harder, H.I., and Brown, A.F.: Calif. Med. 83:452, 1955.)

Less common causes of cardiac rupture include various lesions of the myocardium: fatty infiltration, abscess, gumma, tuberculosis, and malignant tumor. Traumatic rupture has already been discussed (p. 570).

ANEURYSM OF HEART. A ventricular aneurysm may appear during the acute phase of a myocardial infarct, but most often it is evident in the healed stage. Healed infarcts of the heart are composed of fibrous tissue and constitute relatively thin places in the wall, since they are rarely more than one third to one half as thick as the normal ventricle. Such scarred areas, especially if they are large, tend to bulge or stretch under the force of the systolic pressure. Since the scar tissue is not elastic, it fails to recoil, and in time an old infarct may exhibit a rounded, saclike bulge in the wall of the ventricle. An aneurysm of the heart usually is located in the left ventricle near the apex, the most common site of infarction. Mural thrombi often are present, partly filling the sac (Fig. 16-24). Calcification of the wall of the aneurysm

may occur. Cardiac aneurysms are reported in 10% to 38% of patients with myocardial infarction.[198] Congestive heart failure commonly occurs in association with aneurysms of the ventricle. Spontaneous rupture of an aneurysm is not common and, when it occurs, usually does so during the acute stage of a myocardial infarct. Infrequent causes of cardiac aneurysms include trauma, myocardial abscesses, erosive bacterial endocarditis, and congenital defects.

CALCIFICATION OF MYOCARDIUM. An uncommon effect of myocardial infarction, calcification of the myocardium tends to occur in old myocardial infarcts with or without ventricular aneurysms (Fig. 16-25). Plaquelike areas of calcification may be demonstrated in the lesions, particularly in a roentgenogram of the chest, and sometimes the calcification is extensive. Rarely, osseous meta-

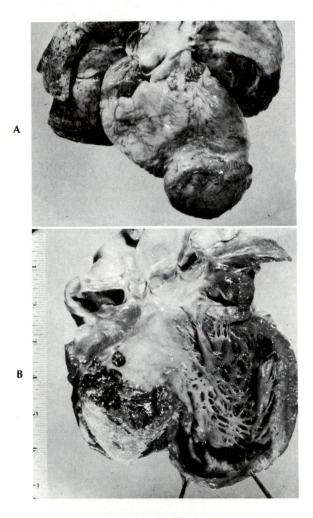

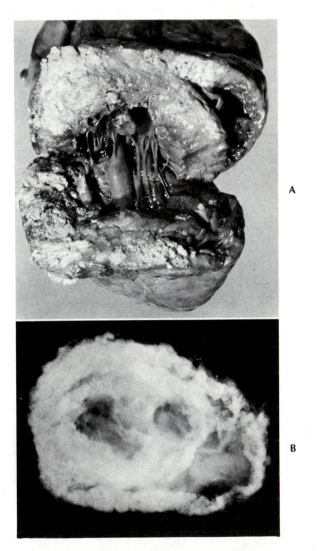

Fig. 16-24. Aneurysm of left ventricle, a sequela of myocardial infarct. **A,** External view. **B,** Interior view, bisected. On right, between forceps, is thin fibrotic wall. On left, sac is filled with organizing thrombus. Note prominent secondary endocardial fibrosis in left ventricle.

Fig. 16-25. **A,** Extensive calcification of myocardium occurring as sequela of massive myocardial infarct. **B,** Extensive calcification of myocardium and coronary arteries; portion of heart shown in **A.** Roentgenogram was made at time of autopsy. (**A,** From Rezek, P.R., and Millard, M.: Autopsy pathology, Springfield, Ill., 1963, Charles C Thomas, Publisher.)

plasia is present. Occasionally, calcium deposits may occur in acute myocardial infarcts.

POSTMYOCARDIAL INFARCTION SYNDROME. An infrequent complication of a myocardial infarct is the postmyocardial infarction syndrome (Dressler's syndrome) characterized by fever, chest pain, pericarditis, pleuritis, and pneumonitis. It tends to occur within the second to the sixth week after the onset of the infarct but can occur during the first week and as late as 3 months after the acute attack. The mechanism of production of this syndrome is not known, but an autoimmune reaction has been implicated. Circulating antiheart antibodies have been demonstrated in patients with postmyocardial infarction syndrome, as well as in those with acute myocardial infarcts without this syndrome.[206]

Noninfarct effects of myocardial ischemia. Effects of myocardial ischemia other than infarct include angina pectoris, sudden death, and myocardial fibrosis.

Angina pectoris. The usual concept of angina pectoris is that paroxysmal pain in the chest is provoked by an increase in the demands of the heart and relieved by a decrease of the work of the heart. The physiologic mechanism in the production of this syndrome is a relative oxygen deficiency of the myocardium. The underlying cause of ischemia of the heart muscle is usually coronary atherosclerosis, with narrowing or occlusion of one or more branches of the coronary arteries. Other causes are narrowing of the coronary ostia attributable to syphilitic aortitis, aortic stenosis or insufficiency (which reduces the coronary blood flow and at the same time increases the work of the heart, producing a relative oxygen deficiency of the myocardium), and severe anemias. Other conditions that increase the oxygen needs of the heart are cardiac hypertrophy, cardiac failure, and violent exercise. The factors that tend to precipitate an attack of angina pectoris are exertion, eating, emotion, and cold, since the oxygen requirement is increased by each of these.

A variant form of angina pectoris occurs in some patients who have recurrent attacks of chest pain at rest (variant angina or Prinzmetal's angina). This syndrome has been attributed to episodes of acute myocardial ischemia brought about by spasm of a coronary artery.[133]

Sudden death. Sudden death may occur during an attack of myocardial infarction, as mentioned previously. Sudden death without myocardial infarction may be the termination of coronary artery disease in patients who have had typical anginal attacks, although it commonly occurs also in persons who appear healthy and have had no previous telltale symptoms. It is generally agreed that, excluding trauma and poisoning, heart disease is the most common cause of sudden or instantaneous death, and in these instances, coronary atherosclerosis is the predominant lesion. Usually, severe coronary atherosclerosis with or without old organized thrombi is found at autopsy in persons who die suddenly either at

work or at home.[144] Recent coronary thrombosis is responsible for the sudden death in some persons. Coronary vasospasm[133] and systolic compression of the left anterior descending coronary artery by an overbridging left ventricular muscle during strenuous exercise[218] have been considered as possible causes of sudden death in certain patients. Other cardiac diseases such as hypertensive cardiac hypertrophy, calcific aortic stenosis, and various forms of myocarditis are factors that favor syncope and lead to instantaneous death. The mechanism by which myocardial ischemia causes sudden death is believed to be ventricular asystole or fibrillation.[226]

Myocardial fibrosis. Focal or diffuse fibrosis of the myocardium is the lesion characteristically found in patients with a chronic, progressive type of myocardial ischemia, as in severe coronary atherosclerosis and stenosis of the coronary ostia. The myocardial lesion is commonly observed in the heart of patients who have had a history of attacks of angina pectoris or who died suddenly as a result of coronary insufficiency without myocardial infarction. It is conceivable that with each episode of angina pectoris, which signifies a relative oxygen deficiency of the myocardium, there is sufficient damage to the heart muscle to account for the development of myocardial fibrosis (see Fig. 16-48).

Many observers contend that the lesions represent fibrous replacement of atrophic muscle fibers. However, others attribute them to healing of minute infarcts involving scattered groups of muscle fibers.[144] An interesting concept is that focal myocytolysis is responsible for the genesis of myocardial fibrosis.[223] In this process the muscle fibers disintegrate within small and discrete areas. The myofibrils disappear, but the muscle nuclei are intact and remain visible for some time. The stroma is unaffected. Eventually, all that remain are small areas of empty but intact endomysial sheaths in the meshes of which are macrophages that may be filled with brown pigment. Healing of these foci is largely the result of collapse and condensation of the preserved stroma rather than of fibroblastic proliferation and collagen formation. There is a resemblance of focal myocytolysis to miliary infarcts, which were described previously. In fact, some investigators believe focal myocytolysis is not a lesion in a class by itself but is in reality a miliary infarct.[193] Aside from its relationship to coronary atherosclerosis, myocytolysis can occur also in association with noncoronary diseases, such as cardiomegaly and congestive heart failure of unknown origin, myocarditis of various types, and other diseases.[223]

The heart affected by myocardial fibrosis may be normal in size or hypertrophic. There is some question as to whether cardiac hypertrophy can result from coronary insufficiency alone. Since many patients with coronary artery disease have coexistent hypertension, the latter may be the significant factor causing hypertrophy of the heart in these instances. However, it has been suggested that myocardial anoxia from coronary atherosclerosis in itself may result in muscle strain or dilatation and subsequent hypertrophy.[433] The degree of hypertrophy is proportional to the extent of coronary artery disease, and it is greater in the presence of congestive heart failure.[433]

INFLAMMATORY DISEASES

A variety of inflammations may affect any or all layers of the heart. The individual lesions are known as endocarditis, myocarditis, and pericarditis. Involvement of all layers of the heart is termed pancarditis. The classic example of a pancarditis is that associated with rheumatic fever, which will be discussed first.

Rheumatic fever and rheumatic heart disease

Rheumatic fever is a systemic, poststreptococcal nonsuppurative inflammatory disease of protean manifestations and of varying severity and duration affecting many structures in the body.[239] The connective tissues and the smaller blood vessels of various organs are the principal sites of lesions, with the greatest damage usually occurring in the heart. Also involved are the joints, tendons, fasciae, muscles, subcutaneous tissue, arteries, serous membranes, lungs, and brain. Because of the protean manifestations of rheumatic fever and the lack of a specific laboratory diagnostic test, it is sometimes difficult to differentiate this disease clinically from others. For guidance in the diagnosis, the revised Jones criteria[253] have been generally accepted. The criteria are divided into major and minor categories, dependent on their relative occurrence in rheumatic fever and in other disease syndromes from which the disease must be differentiated. In addition, it is necessary that these criteria be supported by evidence of a preceding streptococcal infection. The major criteria are as follows:

1. Carditis
2. Polyarthritis
3. Chorea
4. Subcutaneous nodules
5. Erythema marginatum

The minor diagnostic criteria include the following:

1. Fever
2. Arthralgia
3. Prolonged P-R interval in the electrocardiogram
4. Increased erythrocyte sedimentation rate, presence of C-reactive protein, or leukocytosis
5. History of rheumatic fever or the presence of inactive rheumatic heart disease

Rheumatic fever is not only a disease of protean manifestations but also one of great variability in degree of severity. In many rheumatic patients the symptoms at onset are so vague that the disease is not recognized. On the other hand, rheumatic fever may be a fulminating disease with severe carditis. The heart enlarges rapidly, severe valvulitis of the mitral and aortic valves often develops, and congestive failure sets in, followed by death within weeks or months. This occurs most frequently in patients between 10 and 15 years of age. In other instances the disease is relatively severe at the onset in childhood but goes on to a subacute phase in the second decade, with recurrent acute attacks from time to time.

Incidence

On the basis of several studies in the United States and elsewhere, it appears that the incidence and severity of rheumatic fever and rheumatic heart disease have been on the decline during the twentieth century. In the United States a continuous decrease in the mortality from these diseases has been observed since the turn of the century.[4] During the 1950s the fall was approximately 74% in children 5 to 14 years of age. A decreased mortality from rheumatic heart disease in the middle-aged group was also recorded (26% to 46% for persons 45 to 49 years of age, and 8% to 38% for persons 50 to 54 years of age).[4] Within the 20-year period 1944 to 1964, the number of deaths from rheumatic fever and rheumatic heart disease in the United States decreased from 27,930 per year (20.6 per 100,000) to 17,315 per year (8.7 per 100,000).[280] In 1978 the death rate was 6.1 per 100,000.[1] In a study of 139 cases of acute rheumatic fever in adolescent and adult patients in Britain from 1954 to 1961, there were no fatalities and only two patients had a severe form of the illness.[233] Before the advent of penicillin and the other antibiotics, it is probable that improvement in socioeconomic conditions was an influential factor in the decline,[255,294] and perhaps a natural mutation of the disease played some part.[294] The introduction of chemotherapy and antibiotics did not initiate the decline but undoubtedly accelerated it.[4,294]

It is generally stated that there is no significant sex or racial predilection. Some authors note a slight prevalence among females, but the difference is not striking. The racial factor is more difficult to evaluate because of the presence of important coexistent factors, such as socioeconomic and environmental.[127] In 1920 the mortality for rheumatic fever was lower for nonwhite persons (essentially blacks) than for whites. After that time all groups experienced decreased death rates, but the decline for nonwhites was less than for whites, so that by 1940 the rates for whites were lower than those for nonwhites.[4] The relatively higher mortality among nonwhites was not attributed to racial predisposition but to sociologic factors that resulted from the migration of these people to urban centers where substandard living conditions and inadequate medical care prevailed.[4]

Since 1940 the reduction in mortality from rheumatic fever and rheumatic heart disease has continued among whites and nonwhites, but, interestingly, in the period 1962-1964 whites registered lower death rates up to the age of 45 years but higher rates beyond this age than did nonwhites.[280] The changed situation is not adequately explained, although a conjecture that may partially account for it is that the greater improvement in mortality among the younger whites (perhaps because of better medical care) resulted in a larger portion of them surviving to manifest the disease and its effects beyond the age of 45 years.[280] It has been noted that a black who has acquired the disease tends to have a more severe course, to have greater residual heart damage, and to die at an earlier age.[127] Severe, fulminating, often fatal first attacks of rheumatic fever frequently occur in young adult blacks and Puerto Ricans who are recent migrants to northern U.S. cities. This has been ascribed to the sudden change in mode of living.[4]

Despite the decline in incidence and the decreased severity in the United States, rheumatic fever is still a threat among children and young adults. It continues to leave its crippling mark on the heart. The disease strikes most frequently in childhood between 5 and 15 years of age, with the onset occurring with greatest frequency between the ages of 6 and 10 years.

Etiology and pathogenesis

The cause and pathogenesis of rheumatic fever have been the subject of controversy for a long time. Many of the theories in the past have considered a number of organisms as etiologic agents, such as viruses, diplococci, and nonhemolytic streptococci. But today it is generally agreed that acute rheumatic fever occurs after an infection with beta-hemolytic streptococci of group A. The various manifestations of the disease in the heart and other regions of the body, excluding the initial infection (tonsillitis, nasopharyngitis), are not the result of a direct infection of the tissues. The organisms characteristically are not cultured from the lesions in the heart, joints, and blood during the active phase of the disease. According to the current concept, induction of hypersensitivity or autoimmunity by products of beta-hemolytic streptococci of group A is responsible for the changes in rheumatic fever.

Some clinical and experimental observations that give support to the view that these organisms are the cause of rheumatic fever and that an immunologic mechanism is involved are the following:

1. An increase in incidence of rheumatic fever has been observed after epidemics caused by beta-hemolytic streptococci of group A.[235]
2. The first attack usually occurs after a latent period of about 2 to 3 weeks after infection by this micro-

organism in the nasopharynx, suggesting a period of sensitization to the bacteria.
3. Exacerbations of the disease frequently follow subsequent streptococcal infections.
4. Use of antibiotics has contributed to the reduction of the incidence and severity of rheumatic fever and has lowered the rate of recurrences.
5. In patients with rheumatic fever, elevated titers of antibodies to antigens of the beta-hemolytic group A streptococci have been demonstrated, such as antistreptolysin, antistreptokinase, and antistreptohyaluronidase.
6. Experimentally, lesions similar (but not identical) to those of rheumatic carditis have been produced by sensitization of animals to foreign protein.[245]
7. Cardiac lesions, including those resembling Aschoff bodies, have been produced in rabbits after the induction of repeated infections with group A hemolytic streptococci.[241]

It is not clear which of the streptococcal products is responsible for the pathogenesis of rheumatic fever. According to one theory, streptococcal materials have the ability to render autogenous tissue substances antigenic, so that autoantibodies are formed that react specifically with respective tissue components to cause the lesions of rheumatic fever.[236] This concept is based on experiments in which rats, immunized with mixtures of killed streptococci and emulsions of rat heart or connective tissues, were observed to form autoantibodies to the respective tissues. In these animals, changes in the valves and connective tissue of the heart that resembled those seen in rheumatic carditis in humans were identified.[236] Such antibodies were not produced in these animals by injections of the homologous tissue emulsions alone (without streptococci).[236] Evidence for the induction of autoantibody to heart tissue by antecedent group A streptococcal infection in humans has been provided by investigations demonstrating that the sera of patients with uncomplicated streptococcal infections, rheumatic fever, rheumatic heart disease, or glomerulonephritis often contain streptococcal antibody that is cross-reactive with heart tissue.[240]

Rheumatic fever develops in only a small number of patients with streptococcal infection. The attack rate varies from less than 1%[252] to about 3%.[244] It is difficult to account for the relatively low incidence of rheumatic fever despite the large number of streptococcal infections. However, undoubtedly the interrelationship between infection with beta-hemolytic streptococci of group A and subsequent development of rheumatic fever is dependent on other factors in addition to the presence of the organism.[249] The suggestion that a concomitant virus can enhance the effects of streptococci (or vice versa)[237,243] is of interest in this regard.

Predisposing factors

Among the predisposing factors that influence the incidence of rheumatic fever are age, sex, race, climate, socioeconomic conditions, nutrition, and heredity. The factors of age, sex, and race have been referred to in the discussion of the incidence of the disease.

According to many reports, the incidence of rheumatic fever is dependent on the climate. It is sometimes believed that the disease is especially common in the temperate zones and less frequent in the subtropical and tropical regions and that a higher incidence occurs in cold, damp regions, particularly in proximity to low-lying areas near rivers and waterways, as in certain northern cities of the United States. For example, earlier studies have shown that rheumatic fever in southern states occurred much less frequently than in northern states and that the death rate, recurrence rate, and frequency of heart damage were less in rheumatic patients in Miami, Florida, than in similar groups in some of the northern cities.[246-249] However, other investigators have reported evidence that there are no significant differences in the occurrence and severity of rheumatic fever and rheumatic heart disease related to geographic and climatic variations.[238,250,251,254] Their impression is that socioeconomic factors are important in the development of the disease anywhere in the world regardless of geography and climate. A recent study from Miami, Florida,[254] presents data that differ from the earlier investigations,[246-249] indicating that rheumatic fever in Miami is not unlike the pattern of illness in other endemic areas of the United States.

The significance of socioeconomic factors is reflected in the observation that rheumatic fever occurs more frequently among the poor than among the well-to-do classes. The disease appears to coincide closely with density of population, overcrowding of living quarters (especially for sleeping), and poor nutrition. These factors tend to favor the spread of upper respiratory infections. The rise in the number of these infections and the lack of proper medical attention may contribute to the increased incidence of rheumatic fever. The observation that rheumatic fever "runs in families" has led to genetic analyses of families with this disease. As a result of such investigations, it has been suggested that susceptibility to rheumatic fever is hereditary (as a simple recessive trait), although the nature of the inherent defect is not yet clear.[255] Although the importance of heredity cannot be denied, it is probably not the only reason for a high incidence of rheumatic fever in some families. Susceptibility may be attributable to poor nutrition, group crowding, or the presence of a streptococci carrier in the home.

Basic pathologic processes

A widely accepted concept of the nature of rheumatic fever is that it is one of the so-called immune disorders of connective tissue, the principal lesions being in the connective tissues throughout the body, especially in the heart. In the early phase of development of the lesions, edema of the connective tissues is associated with an increase in acid mucopolysaccharide. The collagen fibers are pushed apart by the accumulating basophilic ground substance, and subsequently they undergo swelling, fraying, fragmentation, and disintegration. The affected areas, including the collagen fibers and the ground substance, are altered considerably and take on a deeply eosinophilic appearance resembling fibrin; thus, the change is referred to as fibrinoid degeneration or necrosis (Fig. 16-26). This fibrinoid change is a characteristic feature of many hypersensitivity reactions, but it is not a pathognomonic manifestation of hypersensitivity, since the alteration can be seen in lesions from other causes.

The early exudative and degenerative features are followed by proliferation, that is, an infiltration by lymphocytes, plasma cells, histiocytes, and fibroblasts. The most distinctive proliferative lesion is the granulomatous phase of the Aschoff body (described in the following discussion). The granulomatous lesions in the extracardiac tissues, such as the lesions in the synovial membranes of the joints, may bear a resemblance to the Aschoff bodies. As the rheumatic lesions advance in age, they undergo fibrosis and scar formation.

Aschoff bodies or nodules

The Aschoff bodies occur in the interstitial tissue of the heart, especially in the myocardium and the endocardium, often in the vicinity of small blood vessels (Figs. 16-27 and 16-28). Occasionally, they are present in the pericardium.[262] Aschoff bodies have been described in the adventitia of the aorta,[273] but they are uncommon and usually are present in the proximal part of the aorta. Lesions elsewhere in the body may be suggestive of, but should not be confused with, Aschoff bodies.[277] Aschoff nodules are globular, elliptic, or fusiform microscopic structures. They are seldom large enough to be detected by the unassisted eye. Three phases or stages in the development of the Aschoff body are recognized:

1. Early (exudative, degenerative, or alterative) phase
2. Intermediate (proliferative or granulomatous) phase
3. Late (senescent, fibrous, healing, or healed) phase

It is in the granulomatous stage that the lesion is identifiable as an Aschoff body and is regarded as pathognomonic for rheumatic carditis. This lesion, according to our present knowledge, does not occur in any other disease. Attempts have been made to correlate the various stages of the lesion with the clinical course of the disease.[263] It should be emphasized, however, that it is possible to find different stages in the same heart, since

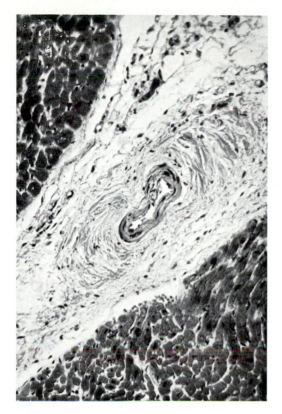

Fig. 16-26. Fibrinoid change around coronary arteriole.

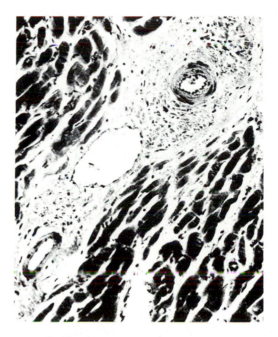

Fig. 16-27. Aschoff bodies in myocardium. Low-power view shows interstitial perivascular location.

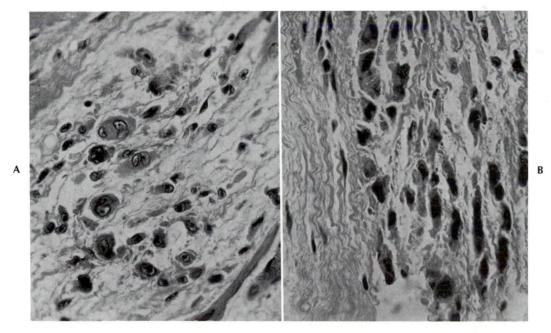

Fig. 16-28. Aschoff bodies in myocardium in 15-year-old white boy. **A,** Intermediate phase with distinct Aschoff cells. **B,** More advanced lesion with elongation of cells, pyknosis, and smudging of nuclei.

some patients have recurrences of rheumatic fever.

The early phase of the life cycle of the Aschoff body, said to occur up to the fourth week of the illness, is represented by exudative, degenerative, and fibrinoid changes in the collagenous tissue, as described in the foregoing paragraphs. There is usually a varying number of lymphocytes and plasma cells in the affected area.

In the intermediate phase, which is evident during the fourth to the thirteenth weeks of the disease, swelling and fragmentation of collagen fibers and fibrinoid change are present in the nodule, but proliferation is the dominant feature. There is an accumulation of cardiac histiocytes, the so-called Anitschkow cells. These large mononuclear cells are found in normal hearts but are increased in number in the Aschoff bodies. In themselves, they do not represent a specific response to rheumatic fever.[258] These cells have a moderate amount of faintly stained cytoplasm with vaguely defined borders. Their nuclei are large and vesicular and contain a prominent central chromatin mass that in longitudinal section is serrated (caterpillar-like). In cross section a halo is observed about the chromatin bar so that the nucleus has an owl-eye appearance. Also present in the nodule are large cells with abundant basophilic cytoplasm, ragged cell borders, and one to four nuclei of the type seen in the Anitschkow cells. These characteristic mononuclear or multinucleated giant cells, known as Aschoff cells, are modified Anitschkow histiocytes. Other cells usually seen are lymphocytes, plasma cells, and occasional neutrophils. As this phase progresses, the exudative and fibrinoid alterations gradually disappear.

In 3 to 4 months, the healing phase is reached, characterized by regression and fibrosis of the nodule. The Aschoff body is elongated or fusiform, the cytoplasm of the component cells is diminished in amount, the cells become elongated and spindle shaped, and their nuclei stain solidly. Frequently, fibrillar material appears between the cells, crowding them into rows. It has been suggested that the mononuclear as well as the multinucleated giant cells are transformed into connective tissue cells.[263] The collagenous fibers fuse to form dense collagenous bundles, resulting in small scars between the muscle bundles, frequently perivascularly.

The nature of the Aschoff body, particularly in regard to the origin of the Aschoff cells, is a controversial subject. The generally accepted view, as suggested in the foregoing discussion, is that changes in the ground substance and the collagen fibers are primary and precede the formation of Aschoff cells, which are exponents of a mesenchymal reaction.[282] The Anitschkow cell, from which the Aschoff cell is derived, was originally considered to be a cardiac myocyte but now is widely held to be a cardiac histiocyte.[258] Some investigators call the cell a myocardial reticulocyte.[260]

In contrast to this view is the concept, which is receiving considerable attention, that Aschoff bodies originate and evolve from primary injury to muscle cells in the heart.[272] The proponents of this view claim that the so-called interstitial Aschoff bodies in the myocardium are lesions of the striated heart muscle fibers in aggregates or bundles among or between other aggregates or bundles of heart muscle fibers, that the Anitschkow or Aschoff cells are myogenic elements and are misinterpreted as being connective tissue cells, and that nonnucleated sarcoplasmic fragments are erroneously interpreted as altered collagen fibers and fibrinoid change. The endocardial Aschoff bodies are considered to be lesions of nonstriated or smooth muscle cells, which normally occur in the zone between endothelium and myocardium. Evidence obtained from a recent study using immunofluorescence microscopy has given support to this concept.[256] In this investigation, actomyosin antigenically similar to that of normal cardiac striated muscle cells was demonstrated in the cells and cell fragments of myocardial Aschoff bodies, and actomyosin antigenically similar to that of smooth muscle cells was observed in the cells of endocardial Aschoff bodies.

According to other investigators, the Aschoff bodies are derived from diseased lymphatic vessels.[283] They are of the opinion that proliferation of the endothelial cells of the lymphatics is the primary response in the pathogenesis of the rheumatic lesions and that these cells give rise to the characteristic Aschoff cells. The lymphedema resulting from blockage of the vessels by the proliferating endothelial cells is believed to be responsible for secondary damage to connective tissue and cardiac muscle. Among the secondary myocardial alterations observed in the vicinity of some of the Aschoff bodies were clumps of degenerating muscle cells that closely resembled Aschoff cells.

Aschoff bodies in resected atrial appendages

The development of surgical valvulotomy for mitral stenosis has made it possible to examine the left atrial appendage microscopically and to observe the rheumatic process in a part of the heart during life. The incidence of rheumatic lesions in resected atrial appendages has been reported as 16%[268] to 74%.[276] The patients who were subjected to mitral commissurotomy were said to have no clinical or laboratory evidence of rheumatic activity, even those with Aschoff bodies in the surgical specimens. The rather high incidence of Aschoff nodules in some of the reports may be caused by a lack of adherence to strict criteria of what constitutes an Aschoff body.[277] Nevertheless, true Aschoff nodules have been found in a significant proportion of appendages.

There is a difference of opinion regarding the significance of the lesions identified in the appendages. Some investigators believe that these lesions resemble, but are not typical of, Aschoff bodies.[261] However, others, using rigid criteria, are able to recognize true Aschoff bodies, which they regard as histologic evidence of rheumatic activity, despite the inability to correlate the lesions with clinical activity of the disease.[270] In such instances the disease has been referred to as being in a subclinical phase.[269] According to one report, the rheumatic process is considered to be active only in the presence of exudative changes, alterations in collagen, and fibrinoid appearance in the Aschoff bodies.[281]

Some observers have demonstrated a significant relationship between the preoperative clinical course and the presence of Aschoff bodies in the resected atrial appendages.[259] Patients who had progressive worsening of cardiac symptoms for 18 months or less before operation had a much higher rate of occurrence of Aschoff bodies than those whose severe cardiac symptoms had remained stationary for at least 2 years before operation.[259] The authors suggest that this correlation strongly indicates that Aschoff bodies in themselves are diagnostic of rheumatic heart disease, believing that such activity may be responsible for the progressive deterioration of the cardiac status. On the basis of follow-up studies, it appears that the presence of Aschoff bodies is of little prognostic importance. The postoperative mortality and morbidity, as well as clinical improvement, are generally the same for the group of patients in whom biopsy results are positive for Aschoff bodies and the group in whom they are negative.[270] An interesting observation has been reported recently concerning a difference in the incidence of myocardial Aschoff bodies in necropsy and surgical specimens. Aschoff bodies were found in the left atrium at necropsy in only 4% of 206 patients with chronic mitral stenosis, whereas they were identified in surgically resected left atrial appendages in 21% of 192 patients.[275] The reason for this difference is not known.

Pathologic anatomy of rheumatic heart disease

The cardiac lesions in rheumatic fever are those of a pancarditis, that is, endocarditis, myocarditis, and pericarditis. Rheumatic lesions of the coronary arteries were reviewed earlier in this chapter with the diseases of these vessels. After discussion of rhuematic carditis, a brief consideration will be given to various extracardiac changes associated with rheumatic fever.

Endocarditis

Endocarditis associated with rheumatic fever may be valvular or mural (parietal). Among the most serious effects of rheumatic heart disease is the valvular lesion, which is best referred to as valvulitis, since the entire substance of the valve is involved, not merely the endocardium. In the active stage of the disease there are thickening and loss of transparency of the valve leaflets or cusps, followed by the formation of characteristic tiny, wartlike nodules (verrucae or wartlike vegetations) ranging from 1 to 3 mm in diameter, mainly along the closure line or contact edges of the cusps. Thus the lesion is given the designation *verrucous endocarditis*. The mitral valve is the most common site of vegetations, followed in descending order of frequency by the mitral and aortic valves combined, the aortic valve, and, less commonly, the tricuspid and pulmonic valves. The vegetations are located on the atrial surfaces of the atrioventricular valves and on the ventricular surfaces of the semilunar valves. Sometimes verrucae extend onto the mural endocardium of the left atrium. The lesions may be present also on the chordae tendineae, particularly on their attachments to the leaflets and rarely on the papillary muscles of the left ventricle. In descriptions of this disease, usually no mention is made of the presence of verrucae in the valve pockets, but in a detailed study of rheumatic valvulitis some years ago,[265] valve pocket verrucae were described. However, these lesions are rather inconspicuous or are observed only on microscopic examination, in contrast to the prominent verrucae that sometimes occur in the atrioventricular valve pockets in Libman-Sacks endocarditis.[323]

The verrucae in the earlier stage are slightly translucent, later becoming more opaque and gray or tawny. They may appear in rows, in small groups or clusters, or as isolated lesions. Since they are usually firmly attached, they are not readily dislodged to produce embolic phenomena (Fig. 16-29).

Microscopically, the earliest lesion is said to occur in the valve rings (the attachments of the cusps to the fibrous anulus).[265] It then extends throughout the substance of the entire leaflet. Edema with swelling of the leaflet, an increased number of capillaries, and an infiltration by lymphocytes and occasionally neutrophils are seen. Plasma cells and fibroblasts may be present. In some instances this nonspecific inflammatory reaction may be all that occurs. Usually, however, there is also an increase in acid mucopolysaccharide, with alteration of collagen and fibrinoid change near the surface of the valve. The inflammatory cells are increased in number, and sometimes Aschoff cells are present. The proliferating cells at the base of the fibrinoid area may be lined up in a palisading fashion with their long axes at right angles to the surface. Aschoff bodies may occur, but not commonly. In the uncomplicated case, bacteria are not present in the vegetations.

The mechanism of development of the verrucae is a matter about which there is some dispute. It is probable that the degenerated fibrinoid foci are extruded beyond the surface of the valve, followed by the superimposition of platelet thrombi from elements in the bloodstream (Fig. 16-30). The incidence of vegetations is high in the left side of the heart, where the pressure is greatest, and their formation is along the line of closure of the valve

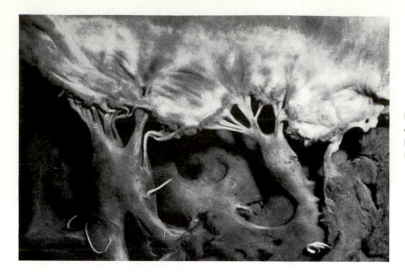

Fig. 16-29. Acute recurrent rheumatic endocarditis. Verrucae are present along closing edges of tricuspid leaflets. Note thickened chordae tendineae. (Courtesy Dr. Orlyn B. Pratt, Los Angeles, Calif.)

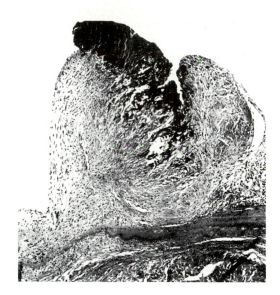

Fig. 16-30. Verrucous nodule. Dark cap consists of fibrin that is being organized by connective tissue cells from valve.

cusps. These features suggest that a role in the pathogenesis of the vegetations is played by mechanical trauma related to intracardiac tension and to the impact and mutual compression of the surfaces of the valve leaflets. It is suggested that a healthy endothelium can sustain the trauma without any injury, but when there is an inflammatory lesion of the valve immediately beneath it, the endothelium may be disrupted by the trauma.[266]

Lesions of the mural endocardium also may occur in rheumatic fever. They are seen most commonly in the posterior wall of the left atrium just above the posterior leaflet of the mitral valve. The lesion at this site is known as MacCallum's patch, and it consists of a thickening of the endocardium with a tawny-gray, ridged, and furrowed surface that, on healing, is converted to a thick-

ened, gray-white, wrinkled plaque. The microscopic picture of the acute lesion is similar to that of the valvulitis.

Healing of rheumatic valvulitis. Sometimes valvulitis is mild, and little if any fibrous thickening of the valve and chordae tendineae results. Usually, however, there is moderate to severe fibrosis with varying degrees of distortion of the valve leaflets. The changes that take place are as follows:

1. Fibroblastic proliferation and collagen formation throughout the valve, with scarring, thickening, and rigidity of the leaflets
2. Organization of the vegetations, with greater thickening of the leaflets along the line of closure
3. Adhesions between the lateral portions of the cusps, particularly in the region of the commissures
4. Thickening, shortening, and fusion of the chordae tendineae
5. Frequently, calcification, which contributes to the rigidity of the valve

The final result is deformity of one or more valves, especially the mitral and aortic (Figs. 16-31, 16-32, 16-42 to 16-44, and 16-46). The incidence of deformity of the various valves, singly or in combination, is as follows in descending order of frequency[257]:

1. Mitral
2. Mitral and aortic
3. Aortic
4. Mitral, aortic, and tricuspid
5. Mitral and tricuspid
6. Mitral, aortic, tricuspid, and pulmonary

The pulmonary and tricuspid valves rarely are involved by themselves. The most characteristic type of deformity is mitral stenosis. Another common lesion is aortic stenosis, which may develop into greatly deformed, calcific cusps (calcific aortic stenosis). Valvular

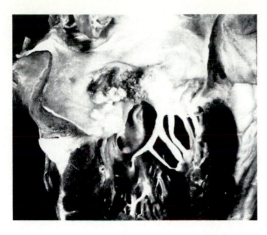

Fig. 16-31. Mitral stenosis. Mitral leaflets are thickened, fused, and ulcerated. Note greatly thickened chordae tendineae.

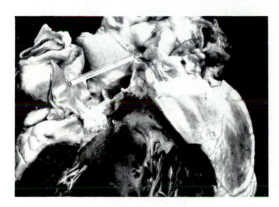

Fig. 16-32. Aortic stenosis. Note fusion of cusps along commissures. Patient had history of rheumatic disease. (From Hall, E.M., and Ichioka, T.: Am. J. Pathol. 16:761, 1940.)

insufficiency may result because of retraction of the scarred leaflets in the vertical diameter, leading to shortening of the cusps. Mitral insufficiency and stenosis are commonly combined.

It must be emphasized that, since recurrences occur in rheumatic fever, there may be fresh verrucae superimposed on the healed lesions. Thrombi may be found in the chambers of the heart, particularly in the left atrium or its appendage, in association with mitral stenosis (see Fig. 16-42). At times, secondary nonspecific vegetations of the nonbacterial thrombotic type, which are not associated with active rheumatic inflammation, may be superimposed on the healed valves. These may reach considerable size.[265]

Microscopically, the healed valves are thickened as a result of an increase in fibrous tissue with hyalinization. The inflammatory cells usually have disappeared. Vascularization may be evident, consisting of capillaries that often are distorted by scar tissue and of thick-walled vessels with narrowed lumina. Calcification of varying degree is frequently present. Metaplasia, with bone and

bone marrow formation, may occur occasionally. In the atrial lesion, healing results in fibrous thickening of the endocardium associated with an increase in distorted elastic fibers and newly formed vessels.

Myocarditis

In the acute stages, rheumatic myocarditis is characterized by the presence of (1) specific Aschoff bodies, (2) nonspecific interstitial myocarditis, and (3) parenchymal damage. The most distinctive lesions are the Aschoff bodies or nodules described previously. The nodules are scattered throughout the interstitial tissue of the myocardium and also may be seen in the subendocardial connective tissue. They are most prevalent in the interventricular septum and in the upper part of the posterior wall of the left ventricle,[263] but they also may be found in the other areas of the ventricles and in the atria and their appendages. Rheumatic myocarditis is most readily differentiated from other forms of myocarditis in the intermediate phase of the disease, when the Aschoff nodules are most typical because of the presence of mononuclear or multinucleated Aschoff cells. Associated with these granulomatous lesions is the nonspecific feature, that is, an infiltration of lymphocytes, plasma cells, histiocytes, occasionally many neutrophils, and sometimes a few eosinophils throughout the edematous interstitial connective tissue. The nonspecific inflammatory reaction is present not only in the vicinity of Aschoff bodies but also in areas where there are none of these specific structures. Furthermore, there is evidence of parenchymal damage varying from degenerative changes to foci of necrosis of the muscle tissue. The areas of necrosis are surrounded by various cells, including cardiac histiocytes and multinucleated giant cells. The giant cells are believed to be syncytial myogenic masses that represent an attempt at regeneration. These muscle lesions resemble but are not true Aschoff bodies.[277] As mentioned previously, however, certain investigators are of the opinion that myocardial Aschoff bodies originate from primary injury to heart muscle cells.[272]

Any of the three types of lesions just discussed may affect the conduction system and be responsible for various electrocardiographic changes; but it has been suggested that the nonspecific inflammation with the associated foci of muscle necrosis, rather than the isolated interstitial Aschoff bodies, is more significant in this regard.[278]

In the later stages of the disease there is gradual subsidence of the inflammatory reaction, and the Aschoff bodies become converted to small scars. After exacerbations, recent lesions may be found side by side with the older, healed ones. Myocardial fibrosis is common and more extensive in hearts with severe chronic valvular deformities, which may in part be attributable to myocardial anoxia, as in aortic stenosis.

Pericarditis

Rheumatic heart disease is almost invariably associated with inflammatory changes in the pericardium. The tendency to affect serous membranes is one of the distinctive features of rheumatic fever. The typical lesion is a fibrinous pericarditis resembling that associated with other causes. The exudate varies from a thin film of fibrin to a heavy shaggy coat with adhesions between the layers of the pericardium, thus the designation *shaggy heart*, or cor villosum (Latin *villus*, "shaggy hair"). The fibrinous exudate is sometimes likened to bread and butter (because of the resemblance to the buttered surfaces of slices of bread after a bread-and-butter sandwich has been pulled apart), an expression retained in the litera-

ture since its use by Hope in 1832.[262] Serofibrinous exudate with a variable amount of fluid in the pericardial sac may be encountered, but the fibrinopurulent type is rare. The thick, shaggy, fibrinous exudate with adhesions is more likely to be seen in those instances of recurrent attacks.

Microscopically, in addition to fibrin, an infiltrate of lymphocytes, plasma cells, histiocytes, and occasionally neutrophils is present. Also, the characteristic foci of fibrinoid change and Aschoff bodies may be seen. Fibroblasts and Aschoff cells often are arranged in a palisading fashion adjacent to fibrinoid areas. Subsequently, organization of the fibrin by vascularized connective tissue may be observed. If much fluid is present, recovery may

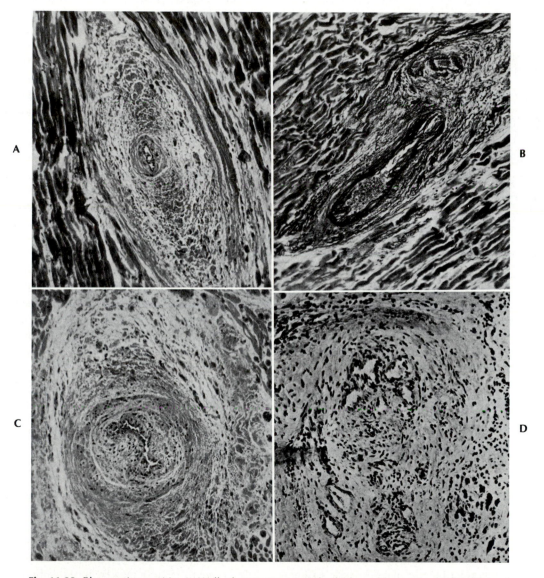

Fig. 16-33. Rheumatic arteritis. **A,** Wall of coronary arteriole thickened because of infiltration of fibrinoid. Edema and masses of fibrinoid are seen in perivascular tissue. Patient, 15-year-old white boy, died of rheumatic pancarditis. **B,** Swelling and proliferation of elastic tissue. **C,** Verrucous nodules (fibrin and platelets) almost fill lumen of this coronary arteriole. Same case as shown in **A.** **D,** Late stage in canalization of artery. Arterial wall almost obliterated by scar tissue. (**D,** Courtesy Dr. R.W. Huntington, Jr.)

occur without pericardial fibrous adhesions. On the other hand, when fibrin is abundant, organization of the exudate leads to fibrous thickening of the pericardial layers, fibrous adhesions between their surfaces, adhesions to neighboring extracardiac structures, and partial or complete obliteration of the pericardial cavity. The result is chronic adhesive pericarditis.

Coronary arteries

The lesions of the coronary arteries in rheumatic fever (Fig. 16-33) are considered in the discussion of coronary artery disease (p. 585). It is not possible to determine the degree of myocardial damage produced by the vascular disease in the presence of active carditis. Whether rheumatic arteritis does or does not predispose the coronary vessels to atherosclerosis is a debatable point.

Stigmas

It is customary for many pathologists to make a diagnosis of "old rheumatic" endocarditis or valvulitis on the basis of certain morphologic features, even in the absence of Aschoff bodies. In these instances the diagnosis may be partly influenced by a known history of rheumatic fever, but sometimes such a clear-cut history is not obtained. The usual morphologic criteria (rheumatic stigmas[267,279]), both gross and microscopic, that are accepted as evidence of antecedent rheumatic fever include changes in the valves, mural endocardium, myocardium, and pericardium. They are as follows:

1. Fibrous thickening of the valve leaflets, particularly at the line of closure
2. Valvular deformities, especially mitral or aortic stenosis and, more significantly, the two lesions occurring at the same time
3. Thickening and shortening of the chordae tendineae
4. Thickening and rugose elevations of the posterior wall of the left atrium just above the posterior leaflet of the mitral valve (MacCallum's patch or plaque)
5. Pericardial adhesions, especially circumscribed obliteration of the pericardial sac near the apex
6. Certain microscopic changes such as endocardial reduplication and vascularization in the valves, especially by thick-walled musculoelastic arteries and arterioles, distortion and interruption of elastic fibers in the left atrial wall, and interstitial scars in the myocardium chiefly adjacent to vessels
7. Aschoff bodies

The Aschoff bodies may be found in a significant number of hearts with mitral stenosis in patients who exhibited no evidence of active rheumatic heart disease before death.[271] As was pointed out before, Aschoff bodies also are observed frequently in surgically resected atrial appendages despite the absence of any clinical or laboratory evidence of rheumatic activity in the patients preoperatively.

Several investigators have cautioned that the evidence must be weighed carefully before a diagnosis of rheumatic heart disease is made, especially when specific Aschoff bodies are not demonstrated. They call attention to the fact that other diseases, particularly various forms of bacterial endocarditis, may produce valvular distortions indistinguishable from those caused by rheumatic fever.[274,279,379]

Extracardiac lesions
Subcutaneous nodules

Lesions in the subcutaneous tissues tend to occur more often in children than in adults. They vary from 0.5 to 2 cm in diameter and are spherical or ovoid. They may be attached to deeper structures such as tendons or tendon sheaths, periarticular ligaments, fasciae, or periosteum. The nodules are usually somewhat mobile except when attached to the periosteum.[289] They are frequently multiple (average, three or four), are painless, and last 4 to 6 days, occasionally longer. In contrast, the nodules of rheumatoid arthritis, which are similar histologically, tend to be larger, are characterized by pain and tenderness, and persist for months or even years.

Microscopically, the nodules are nonencapsulated and consist of three distinct zones: a central necrotic area with some fibrinoid change; bordering this, a zone of histiocytes and fibroblasts in a radial and palisade arrange-

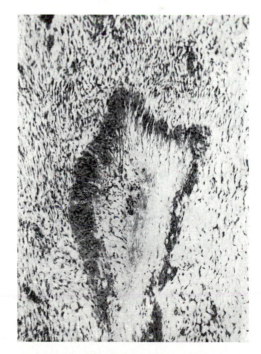

Fig. 16-34. Subcutaneous nodule. Note area of fibrinoid necrosis surrounded by pale edematous tissue supporting many fusiform mesenchymal cells. (75×; AFIP.)

ment; and a surrounding zone of edematous connective tissue in which some degree of nonspecific, chronic inflammation may be seen (Fig. 16-34). Within the outer zone, there may be proliferation of blood vessels, but this is not a conspicuous feature.[291] Foci similar to Aschoff bodies sometimes are noted. The subcutaneous nodules usually occur in association with evidence of rheumatic carditis.[289] A lesion has been described in apparently nonrheumatic children that simulates the rheumatic nodule but is believed to represent an unusual reaction to trauma.[285]

Arterial lesions

Rheumatic arteritis is present in many instances of rheumatic fever. The lesions are not confined to the coronary arteries but may be seen in arteries in various organs of the body. They are described in the discussion of coronary artery diseases earlier in this chapter (Fig. 16-33). When the aorta is involved, the lesions are found predominantly in the proximal part of the vessel.

Polyarthritis

The rheumatic changes in the joints are not as well known as those in the heart. The synovial membrane and the periarticular connective tissues are the sites of hyperemia, edema, neutrophilic infiltration, fibrinoid change, and foci of necrosis of connective tissue, followed by proliferative changes of a granulomatous character. Focal lesions similar to Aschoff bodies are observed. Serous or serosanguineous fluid may be present in the joint cavity. This usually subsides, without leaving a residuum.[284]

Pleural and pulmonary lesions

Pleuritis may develop in association with polyarthritis or carditis. Pleural effusion usually is present, and the pleural surfaces appear slightly opaque as a result of a fine film of fibrin. No definite Aschoff bodies are described in the pleura. Rheumatic pneumonia has been described, but there is a question about its specificity. There is no pathognomonic picture. Grossly, the lungs are large, bluish or purplish, firm, and rubbery. Microscopic changes include edema, capillary hemorrhages, and a patchy fibrinous exudate in the alveoli. The fibrin is in the form of globular masses or hyaline-like membranes and often is associated with monocytes.[290] Organization of the fibrinous masses occurs with formation of so-called Masson bodies. Fibrinoid changes and angiitis may be seen, but Aschoff bodies are not evident.

Lesions of central nervous system

One of the major manifestations of rheumatic fever is chorea minor (Sydenham's chorea, St. Vitus' dance), although this entity has been reported in association with other clinical states. The word chorea (Greek *choreia*, "dance") refers to the disordered and involuntary movements of the trunk and extremities that are characteristic

of the disease. Chorea minor, often associated with or preceded by acute rheumatic fever, is seen in childhood and early adolescence, more commonly in girls. It has been shown to be associated most frequently with a benign form of rheumatic fever.[295]

Chorea minor must be differentiated from Huntington's chorea, a chronic hereditary disorder occurring usually in adults. The cerebral lesions in chorea minor consist of a diffuse meningoencephalitis of mild degree that is not pathognomonic. Grossly, changes are not striking, but there may be evidence of edema, hyperemia, and petechiae. Microscopically, lesions have been described in the cerebral hemispheres, the brainstem, and, most frequently, the basal ganglia. Small hemorrhages, edema, and perivascular exudation of lymphocytes are commonly seen. The ganglion cells may show some changes, but these are not specific.

Late sequelae of rheumatic heart disease in the brain include chronic obliterating endarteritis and embolism. Rheumatic obliterating endarteritis and other vascular changes, including thrombosis, involve particularly the meningeal and cortical vessels, with subsequent gross or microsopic softenings in the brain.[286,287] Cerebral embolism results especially from thrombi in the left atrium or its appendage, most frequently in patients with mitral stenosis and atrial fibrillation. Other sources of emboli may be the vegetations of nonspecific, nonbacterial thrombotic endocarditis and bacterial endocarditis, either of which may be superimposed on the deformed valves.

Prognosis and causes of death

The outlook today for patients with acute rheumatic fever is much better than it was several decades ago. In one study of children admitted to the hospital with presumably initial attacks, exclusive of chorea, a comparison was made of the number of fatalities among the first 100 consecutive patients seen during the first year of each of four decades. The percentages of deaths were as follows: 1920-1921, 24%; 1930-1931, 20%; 1940-1941, 8%; 1950-1951, 3%.[294] The 3% mortality represents an eightfold decrease since the beginning of the study. Other observations in this investigation were a modest decline in the incidence of cardiac involvement and a twofold improvement in the severity of carditis.

The decline in incidence and severity of rheumatic fever was noted even before the advent of antibiotics in the 1940s. Among the factors that contributed to the favorable state was improvement in standards of living for the poorer classes of urban areas after the extreme privation and crowded quarters of the depression years. There also was an awareness of the role of streptococcal infections in the first and succeeding attacks of the disease, so that the medical profession instituted measures to protect the patient and to isolate carriers. Natural mutation of the disease as a result of a new generation of more resistant hosts and less vigorous organisms also may have been a factor.[294] With the development of antimicrobial prophylactic programs and the use of potent antirheumatic agents, there was acceleration of the decline in mortality and lessening severity of the disease.[294]

Certain factors, such as the nature of the attack of rheumatic fever and the cardiac status at the time the patient is first seen by the physician, have been shown to influence the subsequent course of the disease. Many patients who initially had arthritis or chorea but no significant murmurs remain free of rheumatic heart disease.[296] The frequency, duration, and severity of recurrences (the last being most significant) affect the prognosis.[295] The more frequent and more severe the recurrences, the greater are the disability and mortality. In patients who have evidence of rheumatic heart disease when first observed, there is a greater likelihood that the cardiac damage will disappear during subsequent years (1) in those who had no previous attacks of rheumatic heart disease than in those who had previous attacks, (2) in those without diastolic murmurs, and (3) in those with no cardiomegaly.[296] Patients who have considerable cardiomegaly or congestive heart failure at the onset of rheumatic fever do poorly, and it is unusual for the ones who survive adolescence to reach 30 years of age.[295] Patients with little or no cardiac enlargement early in the disease are relatively free from serious recurrences and have a longer life.[295]

The chief causes of death in patients with rheumatic heart disease[295,298,299] are cardiac failure with or without associated rheumatic activity, bacterial endocarditis, and embolism. Death also may be attributed to other complications, such as bronchopneumonia.

Cardiac failure is the most frequent cause of death from rheumatic heart disease, and it often coexists with and is caused by active rheumatic fever, particularly in early life. In young or middle-aged adults, heart failure is likely to be caused by various valvular deformities. In older patients, other types of lesions, such as coronary heart disease, often are superimposed on old rheumatic heart disease and may be the cause of death. Patients with heart failure are more susceptible to the development of other lesions (pulmonary infarcts).

Bacterial endocarditis, usually of the subacute type, shows a downward trend as a cause of death in rheumatic heart disease, probably because of the use of antibiotics and chemotherapeutic agents in the treatment of the disease and their use in prophylactic programs in the management of patients with rheumatic heart disease. The peak incidence of bacterial endocarditis in rheumatic patients occurs at about 20 to 39 years of age.[298] Older patients are more likely to have the acute type of bacterial endocarditis.[298]

Embolism as a cause of death in rheumatic heart disease shows a substantial increase, in contrast to the downward trend of deaths caused by bacterial endocarditis.[298] The organ most frequently affected is the brain, followed by the kidneys, spleen, and lungs. The majority of emboli are bland, but occasionally they may be septic, the latter arising from superimposed bacterial endocarditis. Most of the emboli originate in mural thrombi within the left atrium or its appendage, particularly in association with mitral stenosis and atrial fibrillation. Another possible source of emboli is a concomitant, nonspecific nonbacterial thrombotic endocarditis on a valve.[298] In contrast to emboli from the atrium or its appendage, emboli from nonbacterial thrombotic endocarditis are not dependent on atrial fibrillation, for they may occur whether the rhythm is regular or not.[298,299] At times the source of the emboli cannot be identified in the heart at autopsy. In such instances it has been suggested that mural thrombi or vegetations of nonbacterial thrombotic endocarditis were washed away completely. If roughened surfaces from which they were dislodged cannot be found, one may assume that the areas healed. Because of the high frequency of occurrence of thrombosis of the left atrial appendage, there is a danger of causing an arterial embolism during the course of mitral commissurotomy for mitral stenosis by inadvertently dislodging a fragment of a thrombus.[293] Occasional cases have been reported in which death was caused by emboli arising from calcific fragments of a greatly calcified mitral valve during valvulotomy.[292] Calcific emboli also have been reported to occur spontaneously, as well as in association with surgical procedures on the aortic valve, in patients with calcific aortic stenosis.[297] Another source of embolism, particularly pulmonary, is a thrombus in the veins of the lower extremities.

Sudden death may occur as a result of obstruction of a stenotic mitral orifice by a ball thrombus in the left atrium or as a result of coronary insufficiency associated with aortic stenosis.

Heart in rheumatoid arthritis

The possible relationship of rheumatic fever to rheumatoid arthritis has long been a subject of discussion in the literature. Many pathologic investigations have shown that rheumatic heart disease and rheumatoid arthritis frequently coexist. The reported proportion of patients with rheumatoid arthritis who have postmortem evidence of associated rheumatic heart disease varies from 7% to 65.7%.[309] There is, of course, the possibility that use of less rigid criteria of what constitutes rheumatic heart disease may account for the high incidence of this disease in some of the investigations. In a comparative study, one investigator observed that the incidence of rheumatic heart disease was somewhat higher (12.2%) in the group with rheumatoid arthritis than in the general population, in whom the incidence was 6.1%.[309] These data, together with those in the other published cases, suggest that coexistence of the two diseases is not merely fortuitous. Despite the autopsy evidence suggesting a predisposition to rheumatic heart disease in patients with rheumatoid arthritis, most of the clinical studies have failed to bring out a high incidence of rheumatic heart disease in such patients.[309] The apparent discrepancy between the pathologic and clinical investigations is not satisfactorily explained. The possibility that healed lesions of a specific rheumatoid heart disease can produce deformities indistinguishable from those of rheumatic heart disease may be considered, but proof of such a hypothesis is lacking at present.[309]

In recent years, characteristic types of cardiovascular heart disease that are distinct from rheumatic heart lesions have been described in association with (1) peripheral rheumatoid arthritis and (2) ankylosing spondylitis. In the first instance, any or all of the three layers of the heart are involved, and the disease often is referred to as rheumatoid heart disease. In ankylosing spondylitis, the characteristic changes are principally in the aorta and aortic valve. Although once considered a variant of rheumatoid arthritis, ankylosing spondylitis is now generally regarded as a separate entity (see discussion later in the chapter).

Rheumatoid heart disease[300,302,305,309]

In some patients with rheumatoid arthritis (about 1% to 5%), characteristic granulomatous lesions resembling the rheumatoid subcutaneous nodule may be found in the pericardium, myocardium, and valves, together with a nonspecific chronic inflammatory response. The center of the granulomatous lesions is necrotic, with some fibrinoid change, and this is surrounded by a zone of large palisaded histiocytes and fibroblasts, along with lymphocytes and plasma cells. The rheumatoid granulomas differ from true Aschoff bodies in that they are larger, there is more necrosis in the center, and typical Aschoff cells are not present. Segmental or focal vasculitis—acute, chronic, granulomatous, or healed—may be encountered in the myocardium or epicardium.[304,305]

Ankylosing spondylitis[301,303,308,310]

Ankylosing spondylitis (Marie-Strümpell disease) was formerly referred to as rheumatoid spondylitis, but there are certain features of this disease that have influenced investigators to consider it an entity separate from peripheral rheumatoid arthritis:

1. There is a high incidence in men, whereas peripheral rheumatoid arthritis occurs mainly in women.
2. It frequently exists without peripheral arthritic manifestations.
3. The serologic reaction for the rheumatoid factor is usually negative in the absence of peripheral joint involvement, and even when the latter is also present, the incidence of positive tests is low.

The type of cardiovascular disease associated with ankylosing spondylitis is distinct from the rheumatoid heart disease described previously. The clinical manifestations are aortic insufficiency, persistent atrioventricular conduction defects, cardiac enlargement, and, less commonly, pericarditis. The morphologic picture is that of an aortitis with aortic valvulitis that mimics syphilitic heart disease. The major changes are as follows:

1. Dilatation of the aortic valve ring
2. Thickening and shortening of the aortic valve leaflets
3. Thickened, rolled, free margins of the aortic valve cusps
4. Adhesions and partial fusion of the aortic valve commissures in some instances and nonadherent or even widened commissures in others
5. Pericardial adhesions
6. Foci of necrosis of the aortic media, with chronic inflammation and vascularization in the vicinity of the valve ring

Occasionally, foci of chronic inflammation with vascularized fibrous tissue are demonstrated in the region of the atrioventricular node; this accounts for conduction disturbances.[308] The other cardiac valves generally are unaffected unless they show evidence of other types of disease. Aschoff bodies and rheumatoid granulomas are not present. Gross hypertrophy and dilatation of the left ventricle may develop as a result of the aortic insufficiency. This form of cardioaortic disease is said to occur only rarely, if at all, in patients with peripheral rheumatoid arthritis without spinal involvement.[303] Spondylitic heart disease, as this cardioaortic disease is sometimes called, has been reported to occur occasionally in patients with Reiter's syndrome[307] and in those with psoriatic arthritis with spondylitis.[306]

Syphilitic heart disease

In syphilitic cardiovascular disease the main lesion is aortitis (p. 316). Lesions of the heart itself are caused mainly by syphilitic aortic valvulitis or pathologic changes in the aortic valve ring, with dilatation of the latter. The result is aortic insufficiency, which, in turn, produces gross hypertrophy and dilatation of the left ventricle. Narrowing or closure of the coronary ostia in syphilis also is dependent on aortitis. Angina pectoris and other manifestations of coronary insufficiency may ensue. Primary myocarditis, which is usually gummatous, occurs rarely.

In a compilation of statistics from several articles in the literature, it was found that in the preantibiotic era in the United States, syphilitic heart disease, a manifestation of tertiary syphilis, ranked as the third most frequent type of heart disease,[127] but in the antibiotic era a sharp decrease in incidence of syphilitic heart disease has occurred.

Despite the decline of syphilitic cardiovascular disease, syphilis remains a public health problem of major importance. According to a recent report from the Centers for Disease Control,[311] syphilis was the third most frequently reported communicable disease in the United States in 1980. Reported primary and secondary syphilis cases totaled 27,204 for 1980, an increase of 9.4% from the number reported for 1979.

Syphilitic aortic valvulitis

The term valvulitis is more accurate than endocarditis, which is sometimes used to describe this form of syphilitic heart disease (Fig. 16-35). The primary lesion in the aorta spreads to the aortic ring and valve and, according to current belief, produces aortic insufficiency by separation of the valvular commissures, thickening and retraction of the cusps, and stretching of the aortic ring. Vegetations are not seen on the valves unless there is a superimposed bacterial endocarditis, which occurs infrequently.[315]

As for the pathogenesis of these changes, it can be seen microscopically that the lesion of the aorta in the vicinity of the valve ring is an obliterative endarteritis of the vasa vasorum, with perivascular lymphocytic infiltration followed by medial degeneration, necrosis, loss of elastic fibers, and fibrosis.[321] As a result of the pressure of the blood, the weakened aortic ring dilates. In some instances of syphilitic aortitis there may be sufficient dilatation of the aortic ring to produce aortic insufficiency, even without separation of the valve cusps at the commissures. Usually, however, there is extension of the regressive and inflammatory changes into the base of the valve and the most lateral parts of the leaflets, followed by the appearance of granulation tissue, which leads to fibrosis with hyalinization and widening of the commissures. The most widely held view is that adhesions between the lateral portions of the leaflets and the adjacent aortic wall of the sinus of Valsalva are mainly responsible for the separation of the commissures.[321] Thickening, eversion, and rolling of the free margins of the valve cusps frequently are seen, but these changes are probably the result of continuous mechanical pressure of the regurgitating blood, associated with insufficiency of the aortic valve.[321] Microscopically, the midportions of the valves and free margins of the cusps exhibit only fibrosis and hyalinization and no chronic inflammation or granulation tissue.

Other views have been expressed, in addition to that noted in the preceding paragraph, which attempt to explain the reason for the separation of the cusps at the commissures. The valvular defect has been attributed to a wedge-shaped inflammatory and sclerotic lesion in the aortic wall that separates the cusps,[317] although this is probably not a frequent cause. Another concept that has not received much attention but is worthy of consider-

ation is that the primary factor in the genesis of the deformity of the commissures is not the reparative fibrosis but a destructive process associated with syphilitic inflammation; first the inflammation of the aortic wall results in destruction and dislodgment of the cusp attachments at the commissures and then reparative fibrosis occurs.[314] The loss of valve substance at the commissures is believed to be responsible for certain valvular distortions, such as folding back of a cusp into the ventricle and an inequality of attachment of the two cusps at the same commissure. Whatever may be the basic cause of the valve cusps at the commissures, dilatation of the aortic ring probably contributes to this defect.

From the foregoing, it can be seen that the characteristic functional disturbance in syphilitic valvulitis is aortic insufficiency, not stenosis. It is conceivable that aortic stenosis may occur occasionally, but only when there is an associated lesion such as rheumatic valvulitis or calcification of the valve. A few instances of combined syphilitic and rheumatic valvulitis have been reported.[315,316,319] Calcium rarely infiltrates the ring or cusps in syphilitic valvulitis, but such infiltration has been known to happen.[192,319] Extension of syphilitic aortitis to the mitral valve is a rare event. Because of the aortic insufficiency, hypertrophy and dilatation of the left ventricle occur. The trauma of the regurgitating blood causes characteristic endocardial changes, such as fibrous thickening of the endocardium of the left ventricle and the formation of endocardial pockets or "birds' nests" with their opening toward the aortic orifices.[317]

Coronary ostial stenosis

Extension of syphilitic aortitis to the coronary ostia and possibly to the proximal parts of the coronary arteries is an important component of syphilitic heart disease leading to coronary insufficiency. This complication of aortitis and its effects on the heart, such as myocardial fibrosis, have been discussed previously.

Syphilitic myocarditis[320]

Essentially two types of myocardial lesions have been described in syphilis: (1) a granulomatous inflammation characterized by the presence of gummatous lesions that have the characteristics of gummas elsewhere in the body (diffuse and localized gummatous myocarditis[322]) and (2) a primary nonspecific myocarditis,[313] which is a subject of dispute. The termination of the latter lesion is believed to be fibrosis, thus the designation *fibrous myocarditis*.

Gummas are seen rarely and may involve any part of the myocardium but usually are located near the base in the interventricular septum. These granulomatous lesions are single or multiple, localized or diffuse, and often recognizable grossly. In congenital syphilis a diffuse microscopic gummatous myocarditis, in the absence

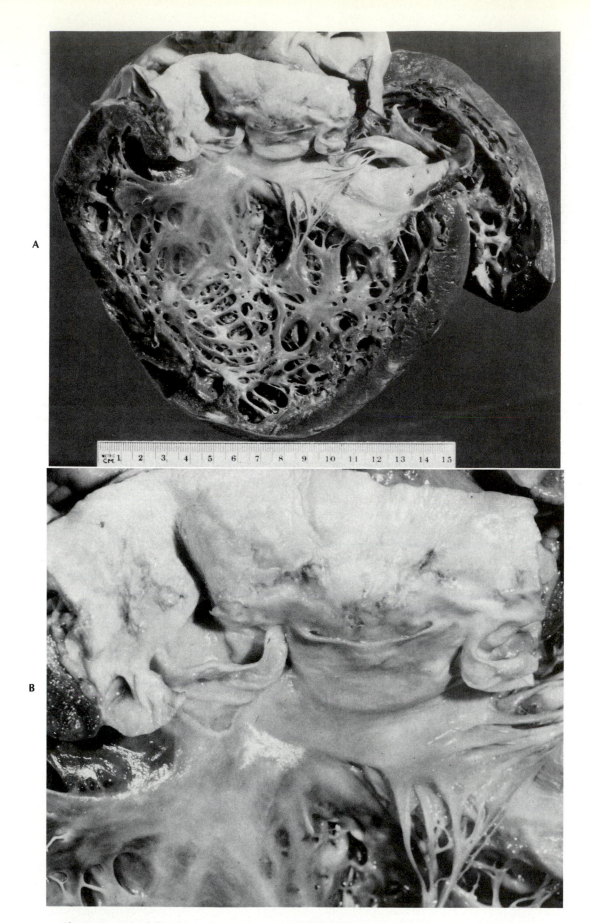

Fig. 16-35. A, Syphilitic heart disease. Left ventricular hypertrophy and dilatation and endocardial fibrosis are associated with insufficiency of aortic valve. **B,** Involvement of aortic valve (close-up view of **A**) in syphilitic aortitis. Note separation of commissures of aortic valve, deformity of cusps, and intimal changes of aorta.

of macroscopic gummas, has been reported in which spirochetes may be demonstrated.[318] Whether an entity exists known as diffuse syphilitic myocarditis, consisting of chronic inflammation (lymphocytes, plasma cells, histiocytes, and fibroblasts) comparable to other fibrosing lesions in acquired syphilis and with demonstration of spirochetes, is highly controversial. If such an entity exists, it is exceedingly rare. Except for gummas, the myocardial changes in cardiovascular syphilis can almost always be attributed to vascular changes such as narrowing of the coronary ostia or associated coronary atherosclerosis.[312] The conduction system may be affected by lesions of the myocardium such as the gumma, or by extension of lesions from the aortic valve or the sinuses of Valsalva, resulting in electrocardiographic changes.[501]

Syphilitic pericarditis

Rarely, gummas may involve the epicardium, usually as an extension from lesions in the myocardium. Except for this granulomatous inflammation of the pericardium, which may lead to fibrous adhesions, it is questionable whether any other form of syphilitic pericarditis occurs.

Endocarditis

Depending on the site of endocarditis, this lesion can be classified as valvular, mural or parietal, chordal, trabecular, or papillary when it involves the valvular endocardium, the inner lining of the heart cavities, the endocardium of the chordae tendineae, the trabeculae carneae, or the papillary muscles, respectively. It is the practice of many to use the word "endocarditis," without a qualifying adjective, to indicate inflammation of the valvular endocardium, which is the area most frequently involved. In some instances, as in rheumatic fever, the entire valve substance usually is affected, so that the term "valvulitis" is more appropriate. With few exceptions the various types of endocarditis are characterized by the presence of vegetations, which are excrescences projecting from the endocardial surface at a point of damage or inflammation. These may be small and wartlike (verrucae) as in rheumatic endocarditis or large, sometimes massive, as in bacterial endocarditis.

The inflammatory lesions of the endocardium may be grouped as to whether they are noninfective or infective. Those in the latter category are characterized by direct invasion of the endocardium by microorganisms, although in certain instances the organisms are usually not demonstrable (for example, syphilitic endocarditis). Rheumatic endocarditis, one of the noninfective group, is related to an infection elsewhere but is the result of hypersensitivity or autoimmunity, not of a direct microbial attack on the endocardium. The types of endocarditis include the following:

1. Noninfective
   a. Rheumatic
   b. Atypical verrucous (Libman-Sacks)
   c. Nonbacterial thrombotic
2. Infective
   a. Bacterial
   b. Tuberculous
   c. Spirochetal (for example, syphilitic)
   d. Fungal
   e. Viral
   f. Rickettsial

Rheumatic endocarditis

For a detailed discussion of rheumatic endocarditis, see p. 601.

Atypical verrucous (Libman-Sacks) endocarditis

A peculiar type of endocarditis first recognized by Libman in 1911[325] and later described by Libman and Sacks[326] is a cardiac manifestation of a grave connective tissue disease, acute disseminated lupus erythematosus (p. 1587). Endocardial lesions of Libman-Sacks endocarditis, which occur in probably less than 50% of patients with this disease, consist of vegetations that sometimes resemble the verrucae of acute rheumatic endocarditis or the vegetations of bacterial endocarditis in size and distribution but usually are larger than the former and smaller than the latter (Fig. 16-36).

The characteristic lesions of atypical verrucous endocarditis are the flat spreading type, appearing as flat, granular, tawny vegetations on the valve, which are not confined to the line of closure but have a tendency to spread over both valve surfaces, often occurring at the base of the valves (in the region of the ring and commissures), in the valve pockets, and even on the ventricular and atrial endocardium.[323] In some instances, verrucae in the pockets of the mitral or tricuspid valves are very conspicuous and are the predominant or sole lesions. This is a diagnostic feature of the disease and is in contrast to the valve pocket lesions sometimes found in rheumatic endocarditis, which are either inconspicuous or observed only on microscopic examination.[323] Verrucae often are present in the pockets formed by the attachments of the chordae tendineae to the valve leaflets, along the chordae themselves, and on the chordal attachments to the papillary muscles.[323] Gross ulceration or perforation of the valves is not a feature of Libman-Sacks endocarditis, and bacteria are not present in the lesions unless there is a superimposed bacterial endocarditis. Although these lesions may heal and cause fibrous thickening of the valves, they do not tend to produce valvular deformities. If deformities are present, a careful search should be made for previous rheumatic disease.[323] Verrucae commonly and characteristically affect multiple valves at the same time, especially the mitral and tricuspid. It is common to see these lesions on the tricuspid valve alone or in combination with mitral and pulmonic valve verrucae. The aortic valve is not involved as frequently as in rheumatic fever. Embolic phenomena are not characteristic of Libman-Sacks endocarditis.

Microscopically, distinctive lesions may be seen in the endocardium even in the absence of macroscopic vegetations. There are areas of edema, fibrinoid change, and an accumulation of histiocytes, plasma cells, occasionally lymphocytes and neutrophils, and later fibroblasts. Included in the lesions are "hematoxylin bodies" of Gross,[323] the specific feature of the disease, which represents clumps of nuclear material that appear to be analogous to the bodies in the L.E. cells of the bone marrow. The verrucae consist of fibrinoid, necrotic portions of the valve substance admixed with fibrin and platelet thrombi. Hematoxylin bodies may be present within the granular thrombotic material. Associated with the vegetations is a variable degree of valvulitis, characterized by the presence of young capillaries with swelling and proliferation of endothelial cells, between which is an infiltrate of inflammatory cells of the types just mentioned.

Frequently associated with the endocarditis are alterations in the pericardium. Early there may be typical fibrinoid changes, followed by a fibrinous or serofibrinous pericarditis. Usually, the fibrinous exudate is not very abundant,[323] but there may as much as 600 to 950 ml of fluid in the pericardial sac.[324] Organization of the exudate leads to fibrous adhesions of the pericardium, with partial or complete obliteration of the cavity (chronic adhesive pericarditis).

In the myocardium, focal myocarditis with lymphocytes, plasma cells, and histiocytes may be present. Often there are foci of edema and fibrinoid change interstitially. Sometimes, fibrinoid necrosis and acute inflammation of the myocardial vessels can be demonstrated. Aschoff bodies are not present in the myocardium, endocardium, or pericardium.

Nonbacterial thrombotic endocarditis

Various terms refer to the nonbacterial thrombotic form of endocarditis: *terminal endocarditis, cachectic* or *marantic endocarditis, endocarditis simplex,* and *degenerative verrucal endocardiosis.* The verrucae exhibit various gross forms.[327,330] In some instances they are small,

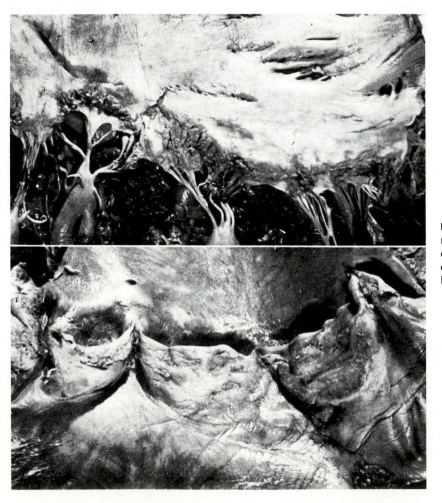

Fig. 16-36. Atypical verrucous endocarditis of mitral and aortic valves (Libman-Sacks) in 38-year-old woman. Diagnosis was lupus erythematosus disseminatus. (Courtesy Dr. Reuben Straus, Portland, Oreg.)

single or multiple, brownish nodules measuring less than 3 mm in diameter, usually arranged along the line of closure. Sometimes they are seen on the nodules of Arantius of the aortic valve. These small lesions often resemble the verrucae of rheumatic valvulitis but usually are larger and more friable than the rheumatic type. Other vegetations are larger. They may be single, tawny, and usually granular but sometimes are smooth and polypoid or occasionally shaggy, or they are multiple, at times conglomerate, soft friable lesions that can be mistaken for vegetations of bacterial endocarditis. These larger lesions are located along the line of closure and have a tendency to involve the commissures of the mitral and aortic valves.[330] A healed verruca may be observed, consisting of a fibrous nodule or tag or a slightly bulbous thickening of the edge of a valve. Lamblian excrescences on the nodules of Arantius may be examples of this variant.[327]

The vegetations are confined to the cardiac valves, chiefly the mitral and, next in descending frequency, the aortic and tricuspid. The pulmonic valve is not commonly affected. The lesions are on the surfaces of the valves exposed to the impact of the bloodstream. Unlike the verrucae of atypical verrucous endocarditis, they do not involve both surfaces of the valves, the mural endocardium, or valve pockets.[330] There is a tendency for this lesion to occur on scarred, thickened, and deformed valves such as those of healed rheumatic valvulitis.[327,330]

Microscopically, there are areas of swollen collagen, with fibrinoid change beneath the surface of the valve. Tufts of capillaries may be seen in the midst of the degenerated collagen, but only a few inflammatory cells are present in and about the lesions. The verrucae consist of small mounds of degenerated collagen admixed with serum, fibrin, and platelets. Some investigators are of the opinion that these blood elements are derived from permeable or eroded vessels of the valves,[327] whereas others are convinced that the vegetations are made up of bland thrombi originating from the blood within the cardiac chambers and superimposed on the degenerated valvular substance.[329,331] Bacteria are not present in the verrucae.

The pathogenesis of these lesions is not clear. Some of the factors, alone or in combination, that have been considered to play a role in the development of the valvular degeneration that precedes verrucal formation are allergy, vitamin C deficiency, hemodynamic trauma to valves, and existence of sclerotic, deformed valves.[327] In addition to the underlying valvular degeneration, another factor that may contribute to the production of vegetations in this disease is increased coagulability of the circulating blood with intravascular deposits of fibrin clots.[332] This is suggested by the fact that nonbacterial thrombotic endocarditis, often with associated venous thrombi, appears commonly in patients who have under-

lying diseases (such as cancer) in which disseminated intravascular coagulation is a relatively frequent manifestation.

In the past, it was held that nonbacterial thrombotic endocarditis was an incidental occurrence in the course of any fatal disease and of no appreciable clinical significance.[330] This is not the opinion among most investigators today. The lesion is known to occur in other than terminal wasting diseases. It is observed during acute and chronic illnesses, in the young and in the aged, and in the well-nourished as well as in the cachectic or marantic patient.[327] Thus the terms "terminal," "cachectic," and "marantic" are not appropriate. According to the findings in several studies, these lesions are clinically significant in that they are a common source of emboli.[329,331] Infarcts in the brain, lungs, and elsewhere ensue. Apparently, these lesions serve as a nidus for the development of bacterial endocarditis.[327,328,334] Since the advent of the antibiotic era, the incidence of nonbacterial thrombotic endocarditis has increased, while there has been a corresponding decrease in incidence of bacterial endocarditis. According to some observers, this implies a control of factors formerly leading to infection of the thrombotic lesions and favors the concept that bacterial endocarditis often arises as a result of infection of nonbacterial thrombotic endocarditis.[328]

Bacterial endocarditis

Included in the category of bacterial endocarditis are infections of the valvular or mural endocardium caused by bacteria other than the tubercle bacilli and spirochetes. Endocarditis caused by these organisms and the endocardial lesions caused by fungi and other nonbacterial organisms are considered under their respective headings. A characteristic of bacterial endocarditis is the presence of vegetations, usually on the valves, which contain microorganisms. Although the vegetations may be small, they often are massive and thus interfere to some degree with the proper functioning of the valves. The clinical picture of bacterial endocarditis is that of a generalized infection associated with cardiac manifestations and evidences of embolism resulting from fragments of vegetations that have been set free into the circulation.

For years it has been customary to classify bacterial endocarditis into acute and subacute forms. The former referred to the fulminant acute infection that, without treatment, almost invariably terminated fatally in a period of 2 weeks to 2 months. In the earlier literature, the term *subacute* was coined to designate infections ranging from 6 weeks to 3 months in duration and the term *chronic* was applied to the disease that lasted for more than 3 months, sometimes years. Subsequently, all chronic cases were grouped with the subacute ones.[350] Sometimes the designation *endocarditis lenta* (Latin *len-*

ta, "slow," "lingering," "lasting") was used for the so-called subacute cases because of the milder course and longer duration compared with acute bacterial endocarditis. It is apparent that current effective treatment has changed the course of the two varieties of endocarditis, so that there is now an overlapping in their clinical, bacteriologic, and pathologic features. Accordingly, a view is expressed that a distinction between acute and subacute bacterial endocarditis is no longer necessary, that it is an academic one, and that nomenclature should be based on the etiologic agent, for example, *Streptococcus viridans* endocarditis and staphylococcal endocarditis. There is no question that identification of the causative microorganisms is all important in ensuring that adequate therapy be instituted as early as possible. Nevertheless, various writers still recognize at least a clinical distinction between acute and subacute bacterial endocarditis,[339,346,347,366] although it is difficult to distinguish the two varieties at autopsy on the basis of the morphologic features.

The major distinction between acute and subacute endocarditis exists in the invasive and destructive capabilities of the infecting microorganisms. Acute bacterial endocarditis is caused by virulent and destructive organisms (such as the staphylococci) that have a tendency to produce extensive necrosis of the heart valves as well as abscesses in the heart and elsewhere in the body, resulting in an acute fulminant clinical course. On the other hand, subacute bacterial endocarditis is the result of less virulent organisms (such as *Streptococcus viridans*) that cause relatively little necrosis or suppuration in the host's tissues. Consequently, the disease usually is prolonged. However, it is not always possible to determine what the severity of the disease will be on the basis of the etiologic agent. In some instances, organisms that are generally of low virulence may produce a clinically acute disease, whereas certain highly virulent pathogens may induce a more indolent form of the disease. Furthermore, serious complications, such as valvular ulceration and rupture, may develop suddenly in patients with subacute illness, resulting in a rapid downhill course, although it is not possible to predict which patient will have complications.

Bacterial endocarditis is not as common as it was in the preantibiotic era, but it is still an important disease. As a matter of fact, in a study by one group of investigators, the incidence of the disease again increased in recent years.[335] Since the introduction of antimicrobial agents in clinical medicine, changes have occurred in the incidence of the various causative organisms and in the pathologic picture.[339,347,351,366-368] *S. viridans* is still the most frequent cause of bacterial endocarditis, although it has decreased somewhat in importance during the antibiotic era. On the other hand, infections from other forms of streptococci (including enterococci), staphylococci, certain gram-negative bacteria, and various unusual organisms have increased in incidence. There has been a striking decrease in the number of cases of bacterial endocarditis caused by pneumococci and gonococci.

Age and sex

Although bacterial endocarditis may occur in any period from childhood to old age, most cases including subacute bacterial endocarditis[347,351] and acute bacterial endocarditis[357] occur over 50 years of age. The change in age distribution of infective endocarditis has been rather striking during the past 30 years, as noted in the following data[366]: In the period 1913 to 1948, 10% to 25% of patients with this infection were over 50 years of age and 2% to 10% were more than 60 years of age. Since 1948, 50% to 60% have been more than 50 years of age and 20% to 30% have been over 60 years of age. There is a preponderance of the disease among males, but the ratio of males to females differs in the various reported series.

Causative organisms

About 90% of cases of bacterial endocarditis are caused by streptococci (such as *S. viridans*, enterococci, and microaerophilic strains) and staphylococci.[339,351] *S. viridans* is still the most common cause of subacute disease, although it has diminished in frequency during the antibiotic era. It had been reported as the causative organism in 70% to 90% of cases of subacute bacterial endocarditis,[338,350,355,356] but more recently it appeared to be responsible for about 50% of cases.[366] Virulent staphylococci, predominantly *Staphylococcus aureus*, cause more than 50% of cases of acute bacterial endocarditis. In some reports, they are the etiologic agent in from 60%[355] to 82%[357] of cases. Pneumococci and gonococci, which were once prominently associated with bacterial endocarditis, particularly acute, have been demonstrated infrequently as causes since the advent of antibiotics. Other less common organisms that may produce either type of endocarditis include other strains of streptococci and staphylococci, gram-negative enteric bacilli (such as *Escherichia coli*, *Klebsiella*, *Pseudomonas*, *Salmonella*, *Serratia*), *Listeria*, and *Haemophilus influenzae*. An occasional instance of acute bacterial endocarditis attributed to organisms of the tribe Mimeae, particularly the genus *Herellea*, has been reported.[348,364]

The increase in frequency of unusual microorganisms, including fungi as well as bacteria, as causes of infective endocarditis may be related to the use of antimicrobial and immunosuppressive agents, unsterile techniques of self-inoculation of narcotics by drug addicts, and various types of cardiovascular surgery, including placement of prosthetic valves.[366]

Predisposing conditions

The two groups of factors that predispose to the development of the subacute form of the disease are (1) factors initiating bacteremia that is usually transient and (2) the presence of underlying heart disease, mainly acquired or congenital valvular lesions. Transient bacteremia has been demonstrated in association with everyday procedures, such as brushing of teeth or gum chewing; minor dental procedures, particularly extraction; manipulation of the genitourinary tract, as in catheterization or cystoscopy; and even normal deliveries.[344] In a group of patients with subacute bacterial endocarditis, the most common initiating factors were believed to be upper respiratory infections, dental manipulations, and operative genitourinary procedures.[356] Endocarditis was found occasionally in obstetric patients after normal delivery or abortion, in patients with genitourinary infections, and occasionally after cardiac catheterization.[356] In many patients the source of the organisms responsible for subacute disease is not known.

The highly pathogenic organisms that tend to produce clinically acute endocarditis commonly arise from infections elsewhere in the body (for example, pneumonia, skin infections, and renal infections) or may be introduced intravenously by narcotic addicts who administer the drug to themselves without using aseptic techniques. These organisms may also appear as a result of bacteremia initiated by certain procedures performed in patients of the older age group, such as extensive surgery for cancer, skin incisions for intravenous infusions (cutdowns), cystoscopy, and urethral catheterization.[357] Organisms may be introduced into the heart inadvertently during cardiac surgery for rheumatic or congenital heart disease[336,341] or for implantation of prosthetic valves,[352] which may result in either acute or subacute valvular infection.[366]

The presence of underlying heart disease predisposes to bacterial endocarditis, particularly that caused by less virulent organisms resulting in the more protracted (subacute) form of the disease. The bacteria implant most frequently on valves that are thickened and fibrotic as a result of rheumatic fever (Fig. 16-37, A), although the frequency of this association has decreased during the antibiotic era.[366] According to one report, the underlying heart disease in more than 50% of the patients was rheumatic and in about 20% there was congenital heart disease.[356] Bicuspid aortic valves are commonly associated with bacterial endocarditis, but it is not always possible to be certain whether the valvular defect is of congenital or rheumatic origin. Congenital lesions predisposing to the infection are interventricular septal defects, subaortic stenosis, and pulmonary stenosis. Similar lesions occur at sites of coarctation of the aorta and patent ductus arteriosus, but these are properly termed bacterial end-

arteritis. Interatrial septal defects are not common sites of bacterial endocarditis. Only occasional instances of bacterial endocarditis are superimposed upon valves damaged by syphilis. When the infection is associated with syphilitic valve disease, a combined rheumatic valvulitis is likely to be present, casting some doubt upon syphilis as a predisposing cause.[315] In recent years, atherosclerotic valvular disease has been observed as a fairly common underlying lesion.[365,366] Myxomatous transformation of cardiac valves may also predispose to bacterial endocarditis.[376,377] Although acute bacterial endocarditis may be superimposed on previously diseased valves, it commonly affects previously normal valves much more than does subacute bacterial endocarditis. Reports have indicated that 40% to 60% of patients with the acute infection have no underlying cardiac disorder.[366]

Pathogenesis

The microorganisms enter the bloodstream by one of the portals of entry mentioned previously. It is generally believed that the bacteria are implanted on the valves or mural endocardium directly from the bloodstream rather than by means of bacterial embolism through blood vessels supplying the area. The infection seems to occur at sites that are under a strain, for example, the valvular surfaces affected by mechanical trauma associated with intracardiac tension and force of contact, or an area exposed to a jetlike stream of blood such as that forced through an interventricular septal defect or a patent ductus arteriosus. According to one theory, infection of a valve does not occur primarily as a result of localization of bacteria on the endothelium but as a consequence of contamination of a nonbacterial thrombotic vegetation. It is postulated that prolonged stress leads to changes in the valve resulting in a nonbacterial thrombotic endocarditis; this lesion then becomes the focus for localization of bacteria.[334] Although healthy valves show such valvular alterations after stressful conditions, these changes are found more frequently on previously damaged valves.[334]

Endocardial lesions

The characteristic pathologic feature of bacterial endocarditis is the presence of vegetations on the valve cusps or leaflets. Infective endocarditis limited to the mural endocardium is uncommon. The valve most frequently affected is the mitral. The aortic valve is the next most commonly involved. The occurrence of vegetations on the mitral and aortic valves simultaneously is fairly common, but the valves on the right side of the heart seldom are affected. In most instances of clinically subacute endocarditis, the valve is the seat of a preexisting disease (Fig. 16-37, A), but occasionally it may have been previously normal. The vegetations of the acute disease

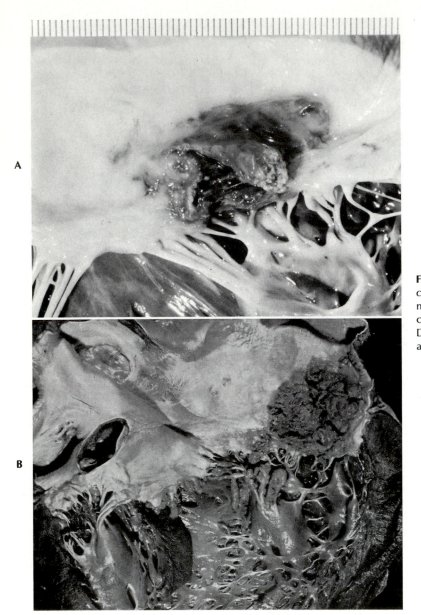

Fig. 16-37. Bacterial endocarditis of mitral valve *(Streptococcus viridans)*. **A,** Lesion in combination with old rheumatic valvulitis. Note thickening, shortening, and fusion of chordae tendineae characteristic of rheumatic lesion. **B,** Different lesion. Note large vegetation on wall of left atrium and involvement of chordae tendineae.

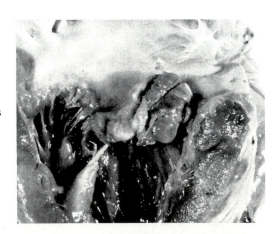

Fig. 16-38. Bacterial endocarditis of mitral valve (clinically subacute) with bulbous type of vegetation.

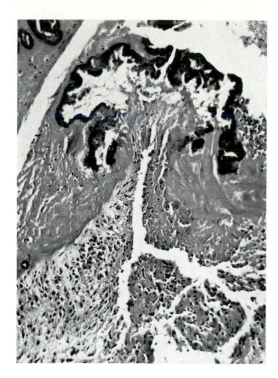

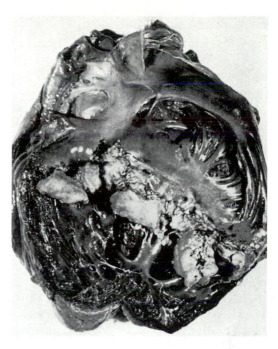

Fig. 16-39. Vegetation of mitral valve in bacterial endocarditis (same heart as that shown in Fig. 16-37, *B*). Note dark masses of bacteria at top, partly embedded in fibrin. Thickened valve leaflet *(below)* is diffusely infiltrated with large mononuclear cells and fibroblasts. Note necrotic core *(right center)* that appears to involve part of valve leaflet. Few neutrophils are seen in fibrin.

Fig. 16-40. Bacterial endocarditis of tricuspid valve *(Staphylococcus aureus)* in 56-year-old black patient with abscess of testicle and scrotal fistula.

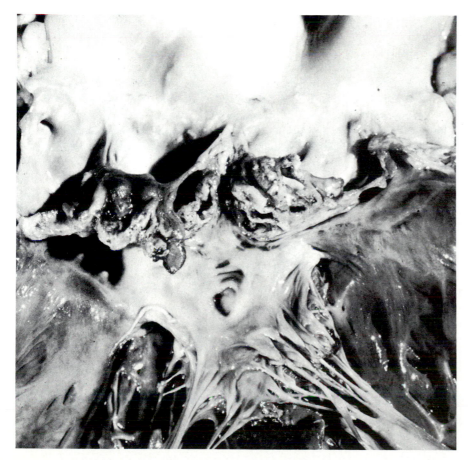

Fig. 16-41. Bacterial endocarditis (clinically acute). Prominent vegetations appear on aortic valve cusps, which are perforated. Smaller vegetations on mitral valve are not seen so well in this view.

caused by highly pathogenic organisms are often found on otherwise normal valves.

The vegetations vary in size from a few millimeters to a centimeter or more and are gray, tawny, reddish, or brown, fairly firm but friable, single or multiple, and flat, filiform, fungating, or polypoid (Figs. 16-37, 16-38, 16-40, and 16-41). It has been said that vegetations caused by very virulent organisms tend to be larger, more globose, and smoother than in subacute endocarditis (Fig. 16-40); however, it is not possible to distinguish the acute from the subacute form of the disease on the basis of these or other gross features of the lesions. Because the vegetations are friable, they give rise to emboli, in contrast to rheumatic lesions, which do not. The vegetations tend to localize on the atrial surfaces of the atrioventricular valves and on the ventricular surfaces of the semilunar valves. They arise from the contact areas of the cusps or leaflets but tend to spread along the valve surfaces onto the adjacent mural endocardium (Fig. 16-37, *B*). The chordae tendineae may be involved. Ulceration and perforation of the valve leaflets or cusps may develop (Fig. 16-41). Sometimes in the acute disease there are ulcerations that are not covered but are surrounded by vegetations.[360]

Microscopically, the vegetations consist of fibrin, platelets, leukocytes, and bacteria, and in the underlying valve a nonspecific inflammatory reaction with varying degrees of necrosis is present. In the acute, fulminant cases, neutrophils are prominent and there may be extensive necrosis with abscess formation. The abscess may extend to the valve rings. In the prolonged cases, varying degrees of granulation tissue and fibroblastic proliferation with mononuclear inflammatory cells are seen (Fig. 16-39). Sometimes, foreign body giant cells are encountered in the necrotic area.[360] Histologic evidence of preexisting rheumatic valvulitis and even Aschoff bodies in the myocardium may be found in association with vegetations of subacute bacterial endocarditis. As a rule, bacterial masses are present in the periphery of the fibrin, in a position to seed the bloodstream with organisms (Fig. 16-39). Occasionally the bacteria are deeply embedded in the vegetation. In such instances, organisms may not be present in the embolic fragments.

Healing of a vegetation may take place, particularly after antibiotic therapy.[343,354] There is invasion of the fibrinous layer by granulation tissue, resulting in fibrosis. The bacteria are phagocytosed and destroyed. Hyalinization and calcification of the vegetation subsequently occur, and endothelialization may be evident. If calcification is extensive, a severely deformed nodular valve may develop.

Bacteria-free cultures

In some patients with proved bacterial endocarditis, premortem blood cultures are sterile despite ideal laboratory procedures.[349] This is particularly so in subacute bacterial endocarditis. In an analysis of patients with bacterial endocarditis, no organisms were cultured in 17% of 182 cases of subacute bacterial endocarditis,[356] whereas in only one (2%) of 50 cases of acute bacterial endocarditis was the blood culture negative.[357] In some patients whose premortem blood cultures are sterile, organisms can be demonstrated in vegetations at autopsy by smear or by culture.[338]

The reasons for negative blood culture are not always apparent unless the patient had received recent antibiotic therapy. The most likely factor responsible for sterile cultures, particularly in subacute bacterial endocarditis, is the presence in the blood of immune bodies that are capable of destroying the infecting organisms. If relatively few organisms enter the bloodstream from the vegetations, the blood may be rapidly sterilized, so that repeated cultures will be negative. Organisms can be demonstrated in the blood only if they enter the circulation faster than immune bodies can destroy them.[360]

Complications and sequelae

Complications and sequelae of bacterial endocarditis may be divided into two categories: cardiac changes and extracardiac complications.

Cardiac changes. Various degenerative changes, petechial hemorrhages, and focal necrosis of the myocardium may occur as a result of the associated infection, and sometimes a focal or diffuse nonspecific myocarditis is present. Myocardial abscesses occur more often in the acute than in the subacute form. Abscesses of the valve rings may be encountered in patients with acute bacterial endocarditis, perhaps more frequently since the advent of antibiotic therapy.[361] Apparently the antimicrobial agents control the infection on the valves and elsewhere but do not penetrate the lesions in the valve rings.[361] Embolism of the larger coronary arteries is rare, but minute embolic fragments of vegetations may be found frequently in the intramyocardial branches of the coronary arteries. Cardiac failure may result not only from the myocardial changes, but also from progressive valvular impairment. Complications produced by the destructive effects of the endocardial lesions include perforation of valve leaflets, aneurysm of valve leaflets, which may subsequently rupture, perforation of the sinuses of Valsalva, rupture of the chordae tendineae, and rupture of the interventricular septum. Despite successful therapy, a variety of serious sequelae may occur in subsequent years.[355] In particular, there may be valvular changes associated with the healing of bacterial endocarditis—aortic insufficiency, valvular perforation, and aneurysm.

Extracardiac complications. A very common and serious complication of bacterial endocarditis is embolism resulting from the breaking off of fragments of vegetations into the bloodstream. Since, in the majority of instances, vegetations are located on the mitral and aortic valves, emboli most frequently enter the systemic circulation and affect particularly the spleen, kidneys, and brain, causing infarcts, abscesses, or mycotic aneurysms. Abscesses are more likely to occur in acute than in subacute bacterial endocarditis because of the greater virulence of the causative organisms. Pulmonary abscesses may be seen in association with bacterial endocarditis of the right side of the heart.

Petechiae in the skin, conjunctivae, and eye grounds are common. It is not certain whether they are attributable to emboli or to toxic damage of the capillaries. Small, raised, red, tender areas on the hands and feet and especially on the fingertips are characteristic lesions known as Osler's nodes. They are thought to be the result of toxic or allergic inflammation of the vascular walls and are more characteristic of subacute bacterial endocarditis.[360] Janeway lesions, which are more likely to occur in acute bacterial endocarditis, are painless, hemorrhagic, slightly raised areas occurring usually in the palms and soles.

Focal necrotizing glomerulonephritis is more common in subacute bacterial endocarditis than in the acute disease. This lesion is no longer believed to be caused by emboli (whence the old term "embolic"). Rather, it probably represents an immunoallergic vascular response to antigenic products of the bacteria (p. 736).[333] Occasionally a diffuse glomerulonephritis occurs. The usual effects of septicemia involving many organs and tissues of the body are evident in bacterial endocarditis. These are similar to septicemia of other causes.

Prognosis and causes of death

The prognosis in bacterial endocarditis has changed decidedly in recent years. Before the advent of antimicrobial therapy, the prognosis was almost hopeless. Now with the availability of effective treatment the outlook is much better. The overall recovery rate from the active phase of bacterial endocarditis (sometimes referred to as bacteriologic cure) is reported in several series to be about 65% to 80%,[342] although in some reports the rate is less.[356,357] There is a considerable difference, however, in the rates between the two forms of the disease. For example, in one study the overall cure rate of the active infection among patients with both forms of bacterial endocarditis was 83%; for subacute bacterial endocarditis, 89%; and for the acute disease, 25%.[342] In other reports, only eight of 53 patients (15%)[355] and two of 54 patients[357] with acute bacterial endocarditis survived the active phase of the infection. It is apparent that acute bacterial endocarditis is still a more ominous disease than subacute bacterial endocarditis.

Unfortunately, the optimistic picture in regard to cure of the active phase of bacterial endocarditis is marred by the occurrence of serious sequelae in patients with healed endocardial lesions after successful therapy. The defects that are associated with healing of the endocardi-

al lesions include aortic insufficiency, perforation of valve leaflets, and valvular aneurysms.[355]

Since the institution of antibiotic therapy, there has been a change in the causes of death in bacterial endocarditis.[358] In the preantibiotic era, infection was the primary cause of death. Today the most common cause is usually reported to be congestive heart failure, which may occur during or after treatment. Cardiac failure may be caused by valvular alterations or by an accompanying myocarditis and only rarely by coronary embolism. Other causes of death include persistent infection, embolism to major organs, rupture of mycotic aneurysms of cerebral arteries, and renal insufficiency. However, in a fairly recent autopsy study of 47 patients with infective endocarditis, infection and not congestive heart failure was found to be the major cause of death.[359] The authors of this study suggest that the increased number of deaths resulting from infection may be in part related to the fact that infective endocarditis was not recognized clinically in many of the patients, who therefore were not treated for the disease. Also, the disease in the majority of patients who did not have prosthetic valves was less than 6 weeks in duration, so that death occurred before intractable cardiac failure resulting from valve destruction had a chance to develop.

Tuberculous endocarditis

Tuberculous endocarditis is a rare form of cardiac disease. It may consist of tubercles throughout the endocardium as part of a miliary tuberculosis, polypoid tubercles and tuberculous nodules on the valves, or tuberculous thrombi. Tuberculous thrombi contain entrapped tubercle bacilli and undergo transformation into granulomatous masses.[360]

Spirochetal endocarditis

Syphilitic valvulitis is discussed in the section of this chapter dealing with syphilitic heart disease. Endocarditis with vegetations caused by *Spirillum minus* has been reported.

Fungal endocarditis

Endocardial involvement by higher bacteria, yeasts, and fungi is uncommon. Actinomyocosis occasionally attacks the heart but infrequently produces valvular endocarditis.[340] Fungal endocarditis from *Candida albicans*, *Histoplasma capsulatum*, *Coccidioides immitis*, *Aspergillus*, *Cryptococcus neoformans*, *Blastomyces dermatitidis*, and *Mucor* has been reported.[353] Two forms are recognized clinically. In one group of patients, fungal endocarditis is not clinically evident and occurs as an apparently minor manifestation of an overwhelming generalized mycotic infection. The other clinical type resembles the picture of bacterial endocarditis. At autopsy, vegetations similar to those of bacterial endocarditis are encountered chiefly on the valves.

Microscopically, many organisms are usually present in the vegetations. The inflammation in the underlying endocardium is consistent with the nature of the infecting organism and includes granulomatous or acute and chronic nonspecific inflammation with or without suppuration. Recently, endocarditis from *Candida albicans* has increased as a result of widespread use of antibiotics and adrenal corticosteroids and the advent of cardiac surgery.[363] It has been noted in narcotic addicts who use unsterile procedures in injecting the narcotic intravenously and occasionally has been seen in a patient who has received prolonged intravenous penicillin therapy.[353,363]

Aspergillus, as well as *Candida*, has been observed as a cause of endocarditis after the insertion of artificial valves (allografts and prostheses) in the heart.[336]

Viral and rickettsial endocarditis

As yet, viral endocarditis has not been firmly established as a clinical entity in man, but it has been demonstrated that viruses may produce endocarditis in experimental animals.[243,337,362] An occasional instance of endocarditis in patients with Q fever has been reported.[345]

Valvular deformities

Among the diseases producing valvular deformities, rheumatic fever is the most common. The effects produced are the same, regardless of the cause. Valvular deformities commonly result in cardiac failure. At times it may be difficult to distinguish clinically between insufficiency caused by disease of the valve leaflets and that caused by dilatation of the ring.

The mitral valve is most often affected by chronic deforming processes, followed next in frequency by the aortic valve. The valves on the right side of the heart are seldom involved. Combinations of valvular deformities, especially mitral and aortic, are common (Figs. 16-42 and 16-43).

Mitral stenosis

Mitral stenosis is the result of rheumatic endocarditis in most instances. Occasional cases are caused by bacterial endocarditis, particularly if the latter is healed. Only rarely is mitral stenosis attributable to other forms of endocardial disease such as Libman-Sacks endocarditis, endocardial fibroelastosis, or a congenital anomaly of the valve. Severe calcification of the mitral anulus fibrosus unassociated with mitral valvulitis has been reported as a cause of mitral stenosis, but this lesion more often is associated with mitral insufficiency.[375] The cause of massive noninflammatory calcification of the mitral anulus is not known, but it has been suggested that it is a degenerative change associated with aging.[375] Occasionally the calcific mass may extend into the ventricular septum, with invasion of the conduction system leading to conduction disturbances.

The gross appearance of the stenotic valve varies greatly according to the degree of involvement. Fibrous adhesions at the commissures may be slight or extensive. The leaflets are fibrotic and thickened, especially toward the closing edges. Contraction of scar tissue takes place, the valve leaflets become more rigid, and calcification of the mitral cusps and ring frequently is present to a greater or lesser degree (Fig. 16-43). Ulceration of the thickest part of the deformed valve is a common occurrence. The orifice becomes considerably narrowed. When the valves are less extensively involved and the bases of the leaflets are still somewhat pliable, the narrowed opening is surrounded by puckered, thickened tissue—so-called purse-string puckering. As the entire valve becomes more rigid and nonpliable, it takes on the appearance of a fixed diaphragm with a narrow oval or curved opening—"buttonhole" or "fishmouth" orifice (Fig. 16-44). Thickening, shortening, and fusion of the chordae tendineae and broadening of their attachments to the valve leaflets are evident. There also may be fibrosis of the tips of the

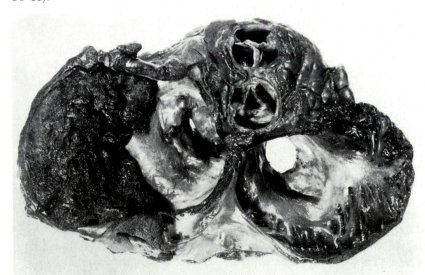

Fig. 16-42. Stenosis of mitral, tricuspid, and aortic valves caused by chronic rheumatic endocarditis. Mitral orifice is mere slit. Note large thrombus in dilated left atrium.

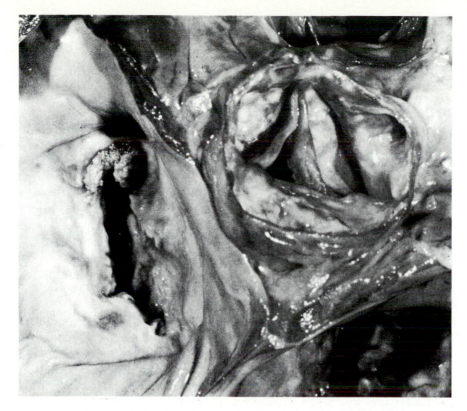

Fig. 16-43. Mitral and aortic stenosis with calcification of both valves.

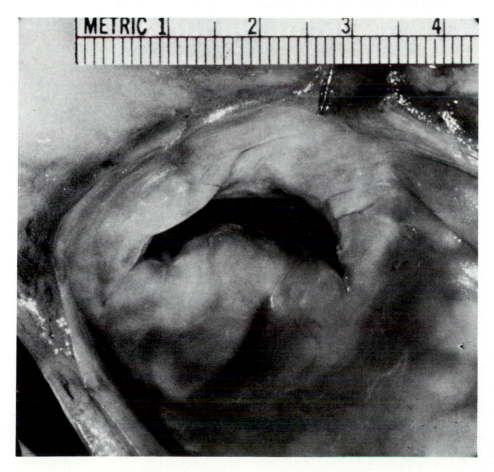

Fig. 16-44. Mitral stenosis with "fishmouth" orifice.

papillary muscles. In some instances the changes in the chordae tendineae and the fusion of the valve leaflets may progress to such an extent that the valve becomes transformed into a funnel-shaped structure, with further narrowing of the orifice.

The effects of mitral stenosis develop as a consequence of obstruction to the outflow of blood from the left atrium and include the following:

1. Dilatation and hypertrophy of the left atrium, which occasionally appears as a huge saclike structure (so-called giant left atrium)
2. Endocardial fibrous thickening of the left atrium
3. Pronounced chronic passive congestion of the lungs
4. Hypertrophy and dilatation of the right ventricle as a result of pulmonary hypertension
5. Dilatation of the right atrium as right-sided heart failure develops
6. A normal-sized left ventricle or, in prolonged mitral stenosis, atrophic left ventricle caused by reduced inflow of blood, with possible hypertrophy of this ventricle if mitral insufficiency also is present

Some of the complications that may occur in mitral stenosis are atrial fibrillation, thrombosis in the left atrial appendage and left atrium—sometimes in the form of a ball thrombosis, and embolism after thrombosis (Figs. 16-42 and 16-45).

Mitral insufficiency

Mitral insufficiency caused by organic disease frequently is associated with mitral stenosis to some degree, but occasionally it occurs as a pure lesion without stenosis. Organic diseases producing insufficiency are the same as those causing mitral stenosis. In addition, myxomatous transformation of the mitral valve or rupture of a leaflet or of the chordae tendineae caused by trauma or bacterial endocarditis or rupture of a papillary muscle as a result of myocardial infarction or bacterial endocarditis may cause insufficiency. Functional or relative mitral insufficiency may be caused by dilatation of the mitral ring associated with myocarditis, myocardial infarction, left ventricular failure in hypertension, myocardial failure from anemia, mediastinopericarditis, or dilated left ventricle in aortic regurgitation.

When mitral insufficiency is the main alteration, the effects are as follows:

1. Dilatation and hypertrophy of the left ventricle
2. Dilatation of the left atrium, often greater than in mitral stenosis
3. Chronic passive congestion of the lungs
4. Effects on the right side of the heart as in mitral stenosis after left-sided failure

Aortic stenosis

Aortic stenosis may be of the noncalcific or calcific type, the latter being the most frequent. Noncalcific stenosis frequently is associated with aortic insufficiency, and its cause is usually rheumatic fever. Congenital valvular and subaortic stenosis may occur. The valvular form is sometimes associated with a bicuspid aortic valve. Aortic stenosis is commonly combined with mitral valve disease.

The usual form of aortic stenosis is the calcific nodular

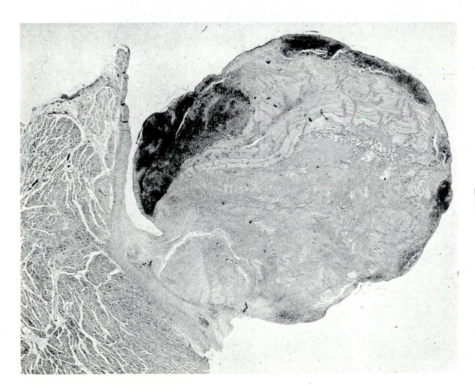

Fig. 16-45. Pedunculated mural thrombus in left atrium associated with mitral stenosis.

type (that is, calcific aortic stenosis), which tends to occur in older patients more frequently than does the noncalcific type. Although there is a wide range in age, most cases are seen in persons in the sixth and seventh decades. The disease occurs predominantly in men. In most clinical and pathologic studies the majority of cases of calcific aortic stenosis are considered to be of rheumatic origin.[372,374] Mönckeberg[378] classified many of the solitary aortic lesions as atherosclerotic in origin. The condition came to be well recognized by the designation *Mönckeberg's aortic sclerosis*. In some instances isolated calcific aortic stenosis has been considered to be a consequence of a congenital malformation.[381] Rarely, severe calcific aortic stenosis is reported in familial hypercholesteremic xanthomatosis.[369]

Healed bacterial endocarditis is another cause of aortic stenosis. In a study of brucellosis and its relationship to heart disease, the theory that rheumatic fever is responsible for the majority of cases of calcific aortic stenosis has been questioned.[379] On the basis of pathologic, clinical, and immunologic studies, the author of this study considered most of the cases to be the result of healed *Brucella* endocarditis. In a review of fatal brucellosis, endocarditis was found to be the most important cardiac lesion, since it was found in 35 (80%) of 44 cases, with the aortic valve being involved in 29 (83%) of the 35 cases.[380] Many investigators agree that infection with *Brucella* is probably responsible for some instances of calcific aortic stenosis, but they believe that rheumatic fever continues to be the main etiologic factor.

The gross appearance of calcific aortic stenosis is characteristic. Because of fibrous thickening and calcification, the closing edges of the cusps stand out rigidly. The commissures are fused and calcified. Occasionally, the fusion of the cusps may be so great that a bicuspid valve resembling the congenital form results. On the ventricular side, buttresses of calcific material usually reinforce the cusps at their bases. Calcified nodules often are found in the sinuses of Valsalva. The orifice of the valve is reduced by the foregoing changes to a mere slitlike opening (Figs. 16-46 and 16-47).

The primary effect of aortic stenosis is hypertrophy of the left ventricle as a result of increase in work of that chamber. When cardiac failure occurs, there is dilatation of the left ventricle as well, and there may be dilatation and hypertrophy of the other chambers later. The aorta is small as a rule, and the intima is smooth because of low intra-aortic pressure and reduced blood volume. Angina pectoris is noted frequently in aortic stenosis. The cause of the pain is myocardial anoxia attributable to functional coronary insufficiency resulting from the reduced coronary blood flow. Associated coronary atherosclerosis with narrowing of the lumina of the vessels may be a factor in some instances. Multiple small scars in the myocardium are believed to result from the anoxia (Fig. 16-48). Clinical manifestations of left ventricular failure may appear

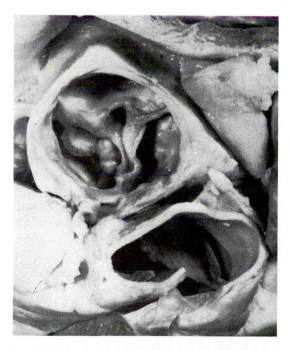

Fig. 16-46. Nodular calcific aortic stenosis. Note perpendicular slitlike opening. Patient, 60-year-old white man, had history of rheumatic fever at age of 12 years. Heart weight was 715 g. (From Hall, E.M., and Ichioka, T.: Am. J. Pathol. **16**:761, 1940.)

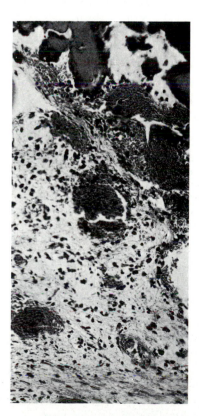

Fig. 16-47. Root of nodular calcific aortic valve. Dark masses at top are calcified areas. Many dilated capillaries and many large mononuclear cells are seen throughout. (From Hall, E.M., and Ichioka, T.: Am. J. Pathol. **16**:761, 1940.)

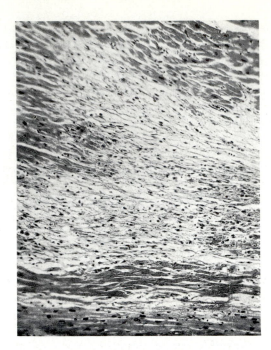

Fig. 16-48. Scarring in myocardium caused by anoxia. Patient was 20-year-old girl who died of left ventricular failure because of aortic stenosis. Heart weight was 550 g. (From Hall, E.M., and Ichioka, T.: Am. J. Pathol. **16:**761, 1940.)

later and may become severe enough to cause pulmonary congestion and right-sided heart failure. Sudden death may occur in aortic stenosis.

Aortic insufficiency

Aortic insufficiency occurs most frequently in syphilitic heart disease and in rheumatic endocarditis involving the aortic valve. A variety of less common causes also may produce aortic insufficiency[370]: bacterial endocarditis with or without rupture of the valve cusps, traumatic rupture of the valve, dissecting aneurysm and Marfan's syndrome, ankylosing spondylitis, fenestrations of the aortic valve, high interventricular septal defect and other congenital abnormalities involving the aortic valve, functional insufficiency caused by dilatation of the aortic valve ring in hypertensive heart disease, and atherosclerosis and myxomatous transformation of the aortic valve cusps.

The major effect of aortic insufficiency is cardiac enlargement as a result of hypertrophy and dilatation of the left ventricle, which is frequently very pronounced. Some of the largest hearts are associated with aortic insufficiency. Fibrosis of the endocardium and endocardial pockets of Zahn ("birds' nests") with their openings toward the aortic orifice commonly occur. Endocardial valvuloids (valvelike structures) may also be associated with aortic insufficiency.[373] They are observed at the inferior margin of the subaortic bulge of the myocardium. It has been suggested that they result from prolifer-

ation of the endothelium induced by the regurgitant stream. Valvuloids differ from endocardial pockets in that their openings are directed away from the aortic valves. When left ventricular failure occurs, right-sided failure may be superimposed. Angina pectoris may result from functional coronary insufficiency attributable to diminished coronary flow (resulting from the low diastolic blood pressure) and an increased demand of the hypertrophied heart for more oxygen. However, associated coronary artery disease also may be responsible. In syphilis, the narrowing of the coronary orifices and concomitant coronary atherosclerosis are the usual causes of cardiac pain. Other characteristic clinical manifestations are the low diastolic and high pulse pressures, Corrigan's pulse with the typical waterhammer or collapsing quality, capillary pulsations, the pistol-shot sound heard over the femoral artery, and the systolic and diastolic murmurs detected over the femoral artery when it is compressed (Durozier's sign).

Tricuspid stenosis

Tricuspid stenosis is almost always attributable to rheumatic fever or congenital disease. It also may be caused by bacterial endocarditis. There are a number of other but infrequent causes, including the carcinoid syndrome.

Tricuspid insufficiency

Tricuspid insufficiency is more common than stenosis and is most often functional, resulting from failure and dilatation of the right ventricle. Insufficiency may be the result of rheumatic valvulitis, rupture of the leaflets or chordae tendineae, or the unusual carcinoid syndrome.

Pulmonary stenosis

Pulmonary stenosis is, as a rule, a congenital lesion. Rheumatic endocarditis may involve the pulmonary valve but infrequently produces a deformity. Bacterial endocarditis as a cause of stenosis of the pulmonary valve is rare. Involvement of the valve is reported in the carcinoid syndrome, usually resulting in stenosis, although sometimes insufficiency occurs.

Pulmonary insufficiency

Pulmonary insufficiency may result from congenitally defective or absent pulmonic cusps and rarely from rheumatic valvulitis. More often, it is of the functional type, being associated with a general dilatation of the right side of the heart with failure.

Myxomatous transformation of valves[371,376,377]

A peculiar deformity of cardiac valves, which is characterized by myxomatous change in the valvular connective tissue with resultant thickening, stretching, and redundancy of the leaflets or cusps, is known as myxomatous transformation or mucoid degeneration of heart valves or as blue valve or floppy valve syndrome. This alteration occurs without inflammation, intense fibrosis, or calcification. The cause of the lesion is not known, but some investigators consider it to be an incomplete expression (*forme fruste*) of Marfan's syndrome. It has been described in some instances of congenital or rheumatic heart disease, but frequently it is not associated with any other cardiovascular disease. The myxomatous valvular change seen in elderly patients may be unrelated to this entity. Any valve may be the site of involvement, but the mitral and aortic valves are affected most often. Patients with this abnormality may have no symptoms. However, serious complications may occur, such as valvular insufficiency, rupture of a valve or chordae tendineae, and predisposition to infective endocarditis. Valvular insufficiency may be related to loss of valve substance caused by the myxomatous transformation, defective coaptation of valve cusps or leaflets, mucinous change in chordae tendineae, or superimposed infective endocarditis.

In the mitral valve the posterior leaflet is severely affected as a rule. Occasionally the posterior leaflet only may be involved. A striking feature is ballooning or aneurysmal protrusion of the leaflets, particularly the posterior leaflet, into the ventricular chamber. A ballooning posterior leaflet syndrome has been described, in which the deformity of the mitral valve is associated with a mid-systolic click or late systolic murmur, or both. Patients with this syndrome may be asymptomatic, but mitral insufficiency and cardiac failure may occur. In an occasional patient, syncope or sudden death has been observed.[377]

Myocarditis

Inflammation of the muscular layer of the heart is termed *myocarditis*. The statistical incidence of this disease has undergone a profound change over the past three to four decades. Formerly, clinicians designated almost every disease of the heart muscle as myocarditis.[386] It was common to attribute death to chronic myocarditis, particularly in elderly persons, when focal or diffuse fibrosis of the myocardium was found at autopsy. Since it has been recognized that myocardial fibrosis is commonly the result of coronary artery disease, the diagnosis of chronic or fibrous myocarditis has been made less frequently.

In a survey of 5626 consecutive autopsies at Michael Reese Hospital in Chicago in 1941,[411,412] 240 cases of myocarditis (4.3%) were encountered, of which 186 (approximately 78%) were nonrheumatic. In a study of the autopsies accessioned at Armed Forces Institute of Pathology (1947),[393] 1402 cases of myocarditis were collected, with the estimated incidence being 3.5%.[384] More than 90% of the 1402 cases were nonrheumatic.

These incidence figures are in agreement with the statistics obtained in later investigations, for example, 3.3% at Bellevue Hospital in New York (1954)[386] and 3.4% at Cincinnati General Hospital (1956).[384]

There are various classifications of myocarditis, none of which is entirely satisfactory to both the pathologist and the clinician. An older division into interstitial and parenchymatous types is not used much today. This classification is based on whether the inflammation is limited to the interstitial connective tissue or causes prominent parenchymal change. Actually, both the stroma and the parenchyma are affected in many forms of myocarditis. The terms *specific* and *nonspecific* are sometimes applied to the morphologic pattern of an inflammatory reaction in the various forms of myocarditis. A specific inflammation is one characterized by a well-recognized histologic picture that is highly suggestive or diagnostic of a disease or group of diseases, for example, the granulomatous lesions of tuberculosis and syphilis or the pathognomonic Aschoff body of rheumatic carditis. A nonspecific reaction does not conform to any distinctive pattern, as may be seen in many forms of myocarditis associated with infectious agents in which focal or diffuse collections of a variety of inflammatory cells are evident. In some forms of myocarditis, both specific and nonspecific inflammations are represented; for example, in rheumatic myocarditis the specific lesion is the Aschoff body, and commonly associated with it is a nonspecific inflammation consisting of the presence of lymphocytes, plasma cells, histiocytes, and occasionally neutrophils throughout the edematous interstitial tissue.[278] A separation of myocarditis into acute, subacute, and chronic forms is sometimes made.

Most commonly, the disease is classified according to etiologic factors. The following classification is based on that proposed by Manion[400] at the Armed Forces Institute of Pathology:

1. Myocarditis caused by infectious agents
   a. Bacterial
   b. Rickettsial
   c. Viral
   d. Protozoal and parasitic
   e. Fungal
   f. Spirochetal
2. Idiopathic myocarditis
   a. Diffuse, interstitial
   b. Granulomatous
3. Myocarditis in connective tissue diseases
   a. Rheumatic fever
   b. Rheumatoid arthritis
   c. Lupus erythematosus
   d. Polyarteritis nodosa
   e. Dermatomyositis
4. Myocarditis caused by physical agents, chemical poisons, drugs, and metabolic disorders

a. Trauma
b. Irradiation
c. Chemical poisons
d. Drugs
e. Uremia
f. Hypokalemia
g. Others

Myocarditis caused by infectious agents

In the myocardial lesions associated with infectious diseases, the inflammation may be attributable to an actual invasion of the myocardium by the organisms or to the action of their toxins, although it is possible that an allergic mechanism is responsible in some instances.

The microscopic picture of acute myocarditis varies. The inflammation may be patchy (focal) or diffuse. In certain bacterial infections, degenerative changes and necrosis of the muscle are likely to be prominent, whereas interstitial inflammation is slight. In other instances a nonsuppurative inflammation of the supporting connective tissue is the predominant change, with a cellular infiltrate consisting of lymphocytes, plasma cells, eosinophils, and Anitschkow cells. Neutrophils usually are not present in great numbers and frequently are absent. The stroma may be edematous. Not uncommonly, both the parenchymal and interstitial features are prominent. Abscesses may be caused by pyogenic organisms (especially staphylococci and beta-hemolytic streptococci) either as a complication of a pyemia from a suppurative inflammation elsewhere in the body or as a consequence of bacterial endocarditis (Figs. 16-49 and 16-50). Rarely, abscesses develop in the myocardium as the result of certain fungal infections, for example, actinomycosis and blastomycosis. Pyogenic organisms sometimes may produce a more diffuse suppurative myocarditis. Fibrosis is seen in the later phase of certain myocardial lesions, particularly if there has been a significant degree of parenchymal destruction (as in diphtheria).[391] In regard to the effects of diphtheria on the heart, some authors are reluctant to accept the myocardial changes as evidence of a true myocarditis because the primary lesions are degenerative and necrotic. But since a secondary inflammatory cell infiltrate occurs in response to the primary toxic injury of muscle, it seems proper to designate this as diphtheritic myocarditis.[391]

The gross appearance of the heart in acute myocarditis is not distinctive, but usually the myocardium is pale and flabby and the chambers are dilated. Some degree of hypertrophy may be seen, especially in those instances associated with cardiac failure. Abscesses appear as small, yellow, round or streaky foci that sometimes become confluent. Some of the abscesses may be surrounded by a hemorrhagic zone.

Granulomatous inflammation of the myocardium is produced by certain bacterial infections, such as tuberculosis, tularemia, and brucellosis. Tuberculous myocarditis is rare and occurs as nodular, miliary, and diffuse infiltrative types.[411,412] The nodular lesions also are referred to as tuberculomas. Involvement of the myocardium is mainly the result of hematogenous spread from infection elsewhere in the body but also can be caused by extension from a tuberculous pericarditis. Foci of granulomatous inflammation and fibrosis are reported in brucellosis, although in this disease there may also be myocardial abscesses, particularly associated with *Brucella* endocarditis.[380]

Sarcoidosis is not proved to be an infectious disease, but it is mentioned at this point because of the close

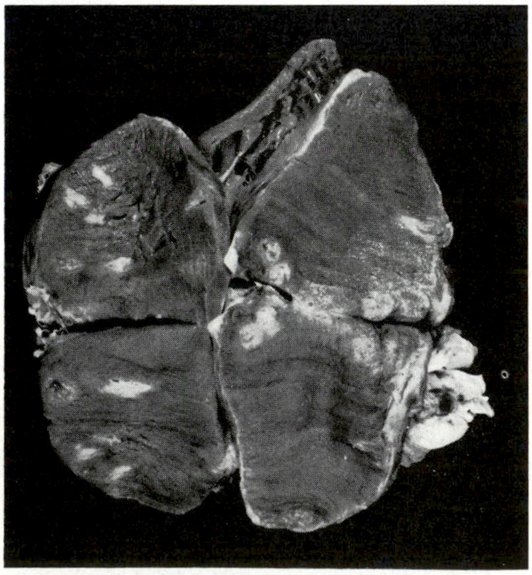

Fig. 16-49. Pyemic abscesses in myocardium *(Staphylococcus aureus).*

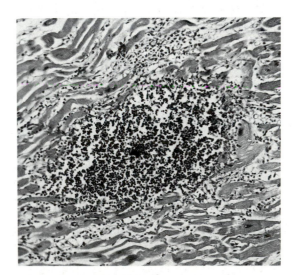

Fig. 16-50. Abscess of myocardium in patient with acute bacterial endocarditis (staphylococcal). Small dark mass in center of abscess is clump of organisms.

microscopic resemblance of its lesions to the noncaseating forms of tuberculosis. Within the past few decades, sarcoidosis has been recognized with increasing frequency as a cause of heart disease unrelated to cor pulmonale.[406] The granulomatous inflammation may be accompanied by a considerable degree of fibrosis, and myocardial damage may result from both active and fibrotic lesions.[414] Electrocardiographic changes, cardiac failure, and even sudden death[403,405,414] may ensue. Sarcoid lesions also occur in the endocardium and epicardium. More common than direct sarcoid involvement in the heart is cor pulmonale, resulting from extensive pulmonary sarcoidosis.

A form of myocarditis that is often overlooked occurs in association with acute nasopharyngitis and acute tonsillitis (Fig. 16-51).[392] The inflammation in these cases may be focal or diffuse, sometimes with extensive parenchymal and interstitial changes within the myocardium. The usual cells of the inflammatory reaction are lymphocytes, mononuclear cells larger than lymphocytes, Anitschkow cells, and polymorphonuclear leukocytes. Abscesses are not present. Lesions simulating Aschoff bodies occasionally are seen. It is suspected that one of the streptococci is the etiologic agent in these instances, but apparently septicemia is not the cause of the myocarditis.[392] The possibility that a bacterial toxin is responsible must be considered. The role of hypersensitivity has not been determined.

Myocarditis frequently is seen in rickettsial diseases. It is uniformly present in scrub typhus and occurs in about 50% of the cases of epidemic typhus and Rocky Mountain spotted fever (Fig. 16-52).[393] Microscopic fea-

tures include interstitial edema and focal or patchy infiltration by inflammatory cells—mainly lymphocytes, plasma cells, macrophages, Anitschkow cells, mast cells, and eosinophils, usually in close association with a small vessel. Neutrophils are scanty unless necrosis is present, but a significant degree of degeneration and necrosis usually is not evident. A more diffuse myocarditis occurs in some instances (p. 337). Occasionally, vascular changes such as capillary and arteriolar endothelial swelling and phlebitis with thrombosis may be noted in the heart.[382] Necrotizing arteritis of the myocardium is sometimes present in epidemic typhus.[382]

Myocarditis has been reported in a variety of viral diseases, including some of the common infections: poliomyelitis, varicella, influenza, viral pneumonia, infectious hepatitis, mumps, infectious mononucleosis, psittacosis, lymphocytic choriomeningitis, and infections caused by group B coxsackievirus. Generally, the microscopic picture of the myocardial lesions in many of the viral infections is similar. At first, the interstitial tissue is infiltrated by lymphocytes and neutrophils and there is necrosis of individual muscle fibers. Later, lymphocytes and histiocytes predominate and some degree of connective tissue proliferation occurs. The mechanism by which the organism produces cardiac changes is not known, but it has been suggested that the virus induces damage in the heart by affecting essential energy systems in the cells or by participating in an antigen-antibody complex that gives rise to an autoimmune disease.[410]

Two of the protozoal diseases in which myocarditis

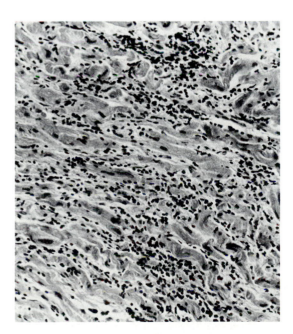

Fig. 16-51. Diffuse, nonspecific myocarditis in child with upper respiratory infection.

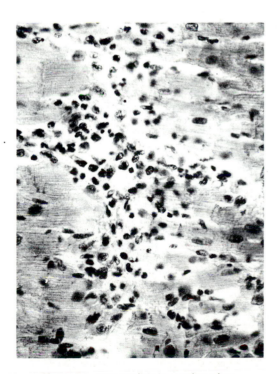

Fig. 16-52. Myocarditis in scrub typhus.

occurs are infection with *Trypanosoma cruzi* (Chagas' disease) and toxoplasmosis. In Chagas' disease, many organs and tissues are invaded by the organism, but the myocardium, skeletal muscle, and central nervous system are most frequently attacked (p. 467). The inflammation in the myocardium usually is intense, with a cellular infiltration consisting of histiocytes, plasma cells, lymphocytes, and some polymorphonuclear leukocytes. Degeneration and necrosis of muscle fibers may be prominent. *Leishmania* organisms are found within muscle fibers (Figs. 12-9 and 16-53). Toxoplasmosis caused by an intracellular protozoan, *Toxoplasma gondii*, is said to be widespread in humans and animals (p. 415). There are congenital and acquired forms. Microscopic changes in the myocardium include focal necrosis, edema, and accumulation of inflammatory cells (plasma cells, macrophages, and lymphocytes). Occasional pseudocysts containing organisms are seen in the myocardium within or outside muscle fibers, often separate from the foci of inflammation (Fig. 12-14, *A*).[395]

Among the intestinal helminthic parasites that affect the heart are *Trichinella spiralis* and *Echinococcus granulosus*. Myocarditis is a serious complication in trichino-

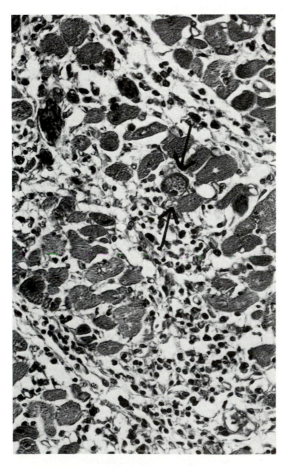

Fig. 16-53. Diffuse myocarditis in Chagas' disease. *Arrows,* Muscle fiber containing organisms.

sis and may lead to cardiac failure. The inflammatory reaction is a response to the larvae, but the latter are rarely identified in the lesions. The parasites either are destroyed or pass on into the circulation and do not encyst within the myocardium (p. 427). Microscopically, both muscle and intersitial tissue are involved. There is focal necrosis of the muscle fibers, along with an accumulation of lymphocytes and eosinophils predominantly. Sometimes there is an increased amount of fluid in the pericardial sac, in which few larvae may be found. *Echinococcus* disease is uncommon in the United States. However, in sheep-grazing countries such as Uruguay, Argentina, Australia, and New Zealand and in the Mediterranean area the disease is frequent.[387] Hydatid cysts occasionally occur in the myocardium. The primary hydatid cyst of the heart tends to rupture into the lumen of a cardiac chamber or into the pericardial sac.[387] Rupture into an adjacent cardiac chamber, with release of hydatid fluid and daughter cysts into the circulation, may result in anaphylactic reactions or peripheral emboli.[394]

Since the advent of antibiotic therapy, the incidence of cardiac involvement by fungal infections has increased. Instances of blastomycosis, actinomycosis, cryptococcosis, coccidioidomycosis, histoplasmosis, and aspergillosis affecting the myocardium have been reported. The lesions are similar to those seen in other organs (Chapter 11). Syphilitic myocarditis was discussed earlier in this chapter under syphilitic heart disease.

Idiopathic (Fiedler's) myocarditis

Idiopathic myocarditis occurs without the usual apparent causes. As more is learned about the etiologic factors of heart disease, it is to be expected that various conditions will be separated from this category, as has occurred in the past. Idiopathic myocarditis sometimes is termed *isolated* because typically the inflammation is limited to the myocardium and is not accompanied by endocarditis, pericarditis, or any other disease in the body that is known to cause myocarditis. There is often rapidly progressive myocardial failure or sudden death. The gross appearance of the heart is not unlike that seen in myocarditis associated with known infectious agents, the essential features being dilatation and sometimes hypertrophy. When the lesions are extensive, they appear as yellow-gray or gray foci throughout the myocardium. Mural thrombi are commonly present. Microscopically, two forms usually are described: the diffuse type without the formation of granulomas and the granulomatous type.[411-413]

Diffuse myocarditis is encountered more frequently than is the granulomatous type. It is characterized by a nonspecific inflammation consisting of lymphocytes, plasma cells, macrophages, eosinophils, and a few neutrophils throughout the interstitial tissue. Involvement of the parenchyma with destruction of muscle fibers may be noted. Variability of the lesion is emphasized. Some are very cellular, and others culminate in fibrosis.

In the granulomatous variety, throughout the myocardium are small or large granulomas without caseation, consisting of macrophages, giant cells, other forms of leukocytes, and areas of muscle necrosis. The giant cells are of the foreign body and Langhans' types, but some giant cells of myogenic origin also may be present (Fig. 16-54).[413] Acid-fast bacilli and spirochetes cannot be demonstrated. The possible relationship of granulomatous myocarditis to sarcoidosis has been suggested, and the problem has been posed as to whether it represents a rare form of the latter disease.[399] However, at the present time, granulomatous myocarditis is not regarded as sarcoidosis. Sarcoid lesions are known to occur in the heart, but they are secondary to the generalized disease.

Several reports have appeared in the literature describing a lesion known as giant cell myocarditis,[385,388,398,416] the cause and nature of which are not known. This lesion is regarded by some authors as a third variant of idiopathic myocarditis. However, on the basis of the descriptions in the literature, it appears that some of the cases should be classified with the granulomatous form of idiopathic myocarditis, since granulomas of the tuberculoid type are described in them. Others are characterized by the formation of myogenic giant cells without typical granulomas and perhaps should be designated simply as idiopathic diffuse myocarditis with myogenic giant cells. In this connection, Saphir,[411,412] in his early review of isolated myocarditis, made reference to the occasional presence of myogenic giant cells in the diffuse form of the disease.

Myocarditis in connective tissue diseases

Myocarditis in rheumatic fever, rheumatoid arthritis, and lupus erythematosus is described elsewhere in the text. The lesion in the myocardium in polyarteritis nodosa is a necrotizing vasculitis with extension of the inflammatory reaction to the adjacent perivascular tissue. With formation of thrombi in the vessels, secondary ischemic changes, including infarction, may occur in the myocardium.

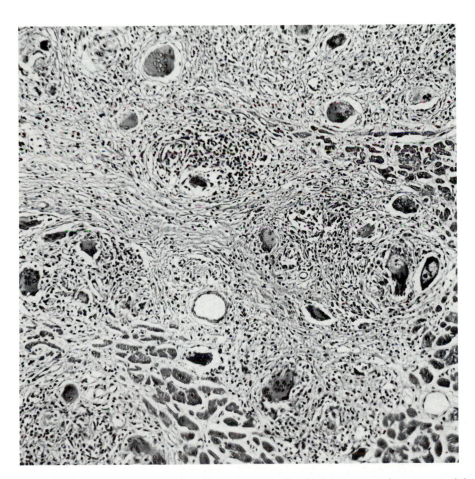

Fig. 16-54. Granulomatous myocarditis with many giant cells. Coalescent granulomatous nodules with fibrous replacement of muscle. Giant cells are of foreign body and Langhans' types, with asteroid bodies in some cells. No lesions are in rest of body.

Microscopic changes in the heart muscle reported in dermatomyositis are similar to those found in the skeletal muscle but are less severe.[417] Degeneration, loss of striations, vacuolization, and necrosis of muscle fibers may be seen. Sometimes there is interstitial edema, and in some instances an inflammatory cell infiltration (mainly lymphocytes and some histiocytes) is present interstitially or perivascularly.[417] Hyalinized thickening of the intramyocardial arterioles with narrowing of the lumina may be evident. Scleroderma is said to bear a relationship to dermatomyositis. However, the lesions in the heart consist of irregular areas of fibrous tissue replacement of the myocardium without any significant inflammatory component. Only an occasional lymphocyte and histiocyte may be present. The connective tissue appears cellular because of prominence of connective tissue cells and not because of an inflammatory cell infiltration.[418] Slight intimal or medial thickening of the arterioles may be noted.

Myocarditis caused by physical agents, chemical poisons, drugs, and metabolic disorders

In cardiac trauma a nonspecific myocarditis may be seen in association with contusions of the myocardium, with the lesion consisting of an infiltrate of neutrophils and a few eosinophils and mononuclear cells, together with focal necrosis of muscle fibers and hemorrhage (p. 569).[62] Myofibrillar degeneration, differing from ordinary coagulation necrosis and characterized by a segmented or banded appearance of the myocardial cytoplasm, is said to be a common form of cardiac muscle injury (Fig. 16-55).[407] It has been produced experimentally by shock, as well as by several chemical and metabolic means (pp. 573 and 576), and has been observed in the human myocardium after cardiac surgery. Associated with the cell injury may be an interstitial cellular reaction, chiefly of the mononuclear type.

The changes in the myocardium caused by certain chemical poisons or drugs consist primarily of degeneration (parenchymatous, hydropic, or fatty) and focal necrosis of myocardial fibers. Edema and small hemorrhages also may be present. Some of the toxic agents are carbon monoxide, phosphorus, cadmium, and arsenic. In some instances, a nonspecific inflammatory reaction, consisting chiefly of lymphocytes and histiocytes, occurs in response to the necrotic tissue. Myocarditis characterized by an interstitial exudate with many eosinophils has been observed in association with sulfonamide therapy.[389,390] This is generally interpreted as a manifestation of hypersensitivity. In some instances, necrotizing arteritis accompanies the myocarditis. Myocardial changes induced by catecholamines with the production of so-called norepinephrine myocarditis are described on p. 573.

Myocardial lesions have been reported in patients dying suddenly and unexpectedly, who had been receiving tranquilizers (phenothiazine compounds). The lesions consisted of foci of myocardial degeneration, associated with hyperplastic changes in arterioles and increased acid mucopolysaccharide in and about these vessels.[408]

A nonspecific myocarditis has been reported in ure-

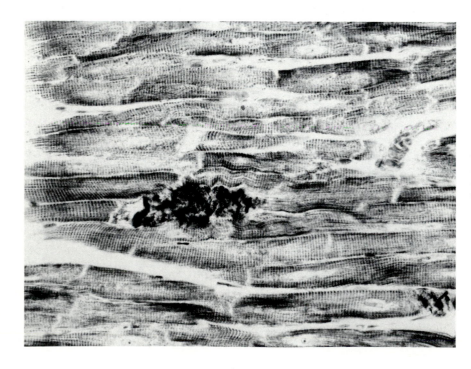

Fig. 16-55. Myofibrillar degeneration (or contraction band necrosis). Dark area near the center contains thick, irregular, distorted cross bands in involved myocytes, which contrast with regular, fine cross striations in other myocytes. (Phosphotungstic acid–hematoxylin stain; 400×.)

mia,[411,412] but some investigators do not accept such an entity, although they recognize the presence of fatty degeneration and edema of the myocardium attributable to uremic intoxication.[28] Hypopotassemia (hypokalemia) leads to degeneration and necrosis of myocardial fibers, edema of the interstitial tissue, and a leukocytic infiltration.

In Friedreich's ataxia, myocardial fibrosis, focal degeneration of myocardial fibers, and a scanty cellular infiltration (chiefly lymphocytes) have been described. The lesion has been referred to as a chronic, progressive myocarditis,[409] but in some instances alterations in the small intramyocardial coronary arteries have been observed (that is, medial degeneration followed by intimal proliferation and narrowing of the lumen) that have been considered to be the cause of the myocardial changes.[397] The possibility has been raised that a state of autoimmunization may exist as a result of antigens liberated by degenerating myocardium.[397] It has been postulated that there is a close relationship between the cardiac manifestations of Friedreich's ataxia and familial cardiomegaly.[401]

Myocardial degeneration and necrosis with secondary inflammatory reaction have been reported in the hearts of patients with myasthenia gravis.[402] The microscopic picture varies. There may be slight focal atrophy and vacuolization of muscle fibers with accompanying mild lymphocytic infiltration of the interstitial tissue (resembling the lymphorrhages found in the skeletal muscles), or there may be extensive myocardial necrosis associated with abundant inflammatory cell response—neutrophils, lymphocytes, histiocytes, and occasionally multinucleated giant cells. In some instances the presence of multinucleated cells is the striking feature ("giant cell myocarditis").[385] Autoantibodies to skeletal and cardiac muscle have been demonstrated in patients with myasthenia gravis.[383]

In progressive muscular dystrophy,[404,415] the microscopic picture is not that of a distinct inflammatory reaction, but there are significant myocardial alterations, that is, areas of muscle replacement by fibrous and adipose tissues in which only a few lymphocytes and histiocytes are present. The myocardial fibers in and about these areas are atrophied or hypertrophied and exhibit degenerative changes. Cardiac arrhythmias and sudden death, which sometimes occur in this disease, have been attributed to alterations in fibers of the sinus node and coronary arteries supplying both the sinus node and the atrioventricular node.[396]

Pericarditis

Pericarditis is an inflammation of the epicardium or the parietal layer of the pericardium. It may be classified as acute, subacute, or chronic. Quite frequently, it is designated according to anatomic features, such as (1) fibrinous, (2) serous, (3) serofibrinous, (4) fibrinopurulent or purulent, (5) hemorrhagic, (6) cholesterol, (7) granulomatous, (8) chronic adhesive (or obliterative), and (9) chronic constrictive. The various forms of pericarditis may be classified on the basis of etiologic factors as follows:

1. Acute nonspecific (idiopathic)
2. Infectious
   a. Bacterial (acute)
   b. Tuberculous
   c. Viral
   d. Other infectious forms
3. Immunologic
   a. Rheumatic fever
   b. Other connective tissue disorders
4. Neoplastic
5. Metabolic
   a. Uremic
   b. Myxedema
   c. Gout
6. Traumatic (including postcardiac surgery)
7. Associated with myocardial infarction

In the following discussion, the anatomic types of pericarditis will be considered first, followed by examples of the etiologic forms.

Anatomic types
Fibrinous, serous, and serofibrinous pericarditis

The most common response of the pericardium to various injurious agents, infectious and noninfectious, is an inflammation characterized by a fibrinous exudate with or without a serous effusion (Fig. 16-56). The usual known causes are uremia, acute bacterial infections, rheumatic fever, myocardial infarction, and tuberculosis. Acute nonspecific pericarditis, usually of unknown origin but occasionally caused by a virus, is commonly associated with a fibrinous or serofibrinous exudate. When the pericarditis is caused by infections, the organisms gain entrance to the pericardium by way of the bloodstream or by direct extension from a nearby infection such as pleural empyema or, in the case of tuberculosis, a caseous lymph node.

Occasionally, acute pericarditis is of the serous type, which is characterized by an effusion of fluid that is richer in protein and of a higher specific gravity than the transudate of hydropericardium. More often, however, the reaction is a fibrinous pericarditis that may be accompanied or followed by an effusion, hence the term serofibrinous pericarditis. The character and extent of the reaction vary in individual cases. The exudate may be dry or moist, thin or thick, finely granular or shaggy (like bread and butter). In the early stages the fibrin may be barely perceptible, but the pericardial surfaces lose their

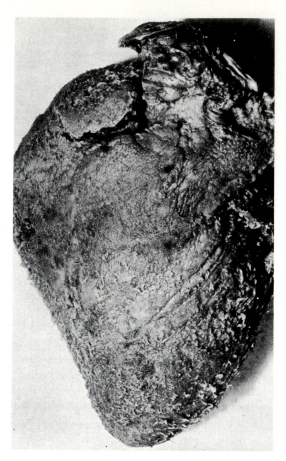

Fig. 16-56. Acute fibrinous pericarditis. Note shaggy coat of fibrin covering surface of heart. (From Anderson, W.A.D., and Scotti, T.M.: Synopsis of pathology, ed. 10, St. Louis, 1980, The C.V. Mosby Co.)

glistening sheen and assume a dull, opaque appearance, or the fibrin may consist of a thin film that, at times, covers only part of the pericardial surfaces. The amount of fluid accompanying the laying down of fibrin is variable.

Fibrinous pericarditis is clinically manifested by the presence of a friction rub. As fluid accumulates in the pericardial sac, the friction rub disappears. In some instances, particularly in serous pericarditis or in the less extensive forms of acute fibrinous pericarditis, the exudate is completely resorbed and the serosal surfaces return to normal. When fibrin is more abundant, the pericarditis is likely to heal by organization after the penetration of the exudate by newly formed granulation tissue, terminating in localized or diffuse thickening of the pericardium with adhesions. In rheumatic and tuberculous pericarditis, the distinctive lesions of these diseases are present in the serosal tissue in addition to the fibrinous or serofibrinous exudate.

Purulent or fibrinopurulent pericarditis

Purulent or fibrinopurulent pericarditis is caused by pyogenic organisms such as the staphylococci, strepto-

cocci, and pneumococci, which reach the pericardium by way of the bloodstream from a focus of infection elsewhere, by direct extension from nearby tissues, or by direct implantation in wounds. Certain nonbacterial organisms (such as fungi and, rarely, viruses) also may cause a suppurative inflammation of the pericardium. Purulent or suppurative pericarditis occurs less frequently than in previous years because of the present-day antimicrobial therapy. A serofibrinous pericarditis commonly precedes the development of fibrinopurulent or purulent inflammation. On inspection, the pericardial surfaces are seen to be covered with a yellowish or slimy gray layer of exudate. If much fibrin is present, the layer is thick, shaggy, and gelatinous. There are varying amounts of fluid, which at first is serous and then gradually becomes cloudy and purulent. Many organisms usually are found in the fluid. Cardiac tamponade may occur even if there is a relatively small amount of exudate present, apparently because the inflammation and thickening of the pericardial walls interfere with the usual degree of stretching. Microscopically, in addition to the fibropurulent or purulent exudate on the surface, there are many neutrophils throughout the serosal walls. Extension into the myocardium, pleura, or mediastinum may be noted.

Purulent pericarditis occurs less commonly than the fibrinous (or serofibrinous) type but is much more severe. Patients are acutely ill, with constitutional signs and symptoms of infection along with the manifestations of pericardial disease. As in fibrinous pericarditis, there is a friction rub. It is not likely that the purulent exudate will resorb completely. Healing by organization takes place, and the result is fibrosis, adhesions, and even calcification. The termination is adhesive pericarditis or, in some instances, chronic constrictive pericarditis.

Hemorrhagic pericarditis

A hemorrhagic pericarditis is one in which blood is present in addition to the features of one of the other inflammatory exudates (serous, serofibrinous, or purulent). The causes include tuberculosis, uremia, severe acute infections, and neoplastic involvement of the pericardium. Patients with hemorrhagic diseases in whom pericarditis of any type develops are likely to have an associated hemorrhagic effusion.

Cholesterol pericarditis

A rare occurrence is pericardial effusion containing cholesterol (commonly referred to as cholesterol pericarditis). It usually is associated with myxedema.[420] Another cause of this type of effusion is tuberculosis. In the latter instance, cholesterol results probably from the breakdown of blood that sometimes accompanies tuberculous pericarditis. Any form of hemorrhagic pericarditis or hemopericardium may be responsible for the presence of cholesterol in the pericardial fluid. In some patients, the

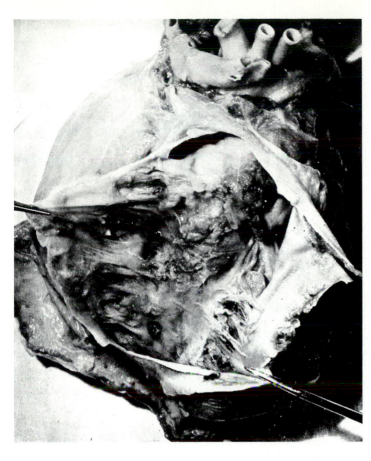

Fig. 16-57. Chronic adhesive pericarditis. Pericardial sac has been opened, displaying fibrous bands joining visceral and parietal pericardium. (From Anderson, W.A.D., and Scotti, T.M.: Synopsis of pathology, ed. 10, St. Louis, 1980, The C.V. Mosby Co.)

origin of the lipid-laden effusion is unknown. In one instance, cholesterol pericarditis of unknown cause progressed to constrictive pericarditis.[420] Microscopic examination of the pericardium removed surgically disclosed hyalinized connective tissue infiltrated by lymphocytes, plasma cells, lipid-containing foamy macrophages, foreign body giant cells, and cholesterol crystals.

Granulomatous pericarditis

The most frequent form of granulomatous inflammation involving the pericardium is tuberculosis (described later). Gummatous (syphilitic) pericarditis is rare and usually represents an extension from myocardial gummas. Frankly granulomatous pericarditis sometimes occurs in rheumatoid arthritis.

Chronic adhesive (or obliterative) pericarditis

Fibrinous exudates exhibit a tendency to undergo organization. In the early phase of healing, vascularized granulation tissue can be seen between islands of the denser fibrinous deposits that still remain. In places where the surface layer has not been destroyed, the mesothelial cells may become cuboid and appear as proliferating masses of epithelial-like cells that sometimes form structures resembling ducts or glands. As organization progresses, fibrous adhesions develop between the pericardial surfaces. The cavity may become completely

obliterated, or pockets of varying sizes may remain. At first, the fibrous adhesions are thin and easily separated, but later they become firmer and more difficult to tear apart (Fig. 16-57). Some authors prefer the term "adherent pericardium" to "adhesive pericarditis" because there often is no evidence of chronic inflammation. Chronic adhesive pericarditis usually causes no embarrassment of the heart, thus differing from chronic constrictive pericarditis.

Sometimes, chronic adhesive pericarditis is accompanied by fibrous adhesions between the parietal pericardium and adjacent structures—mediastinum, pleura, diaphragm, and thoracic cage. This condition is referred to as mediastinopericarditis. Some observers regard the lesion as an added burden to the heart and a possible factor in the development of cardiac hypertrophy and failure in patients who have some underlying disturbance such as valvular disease.[360]

Chronic constrictive pericarditis

A most significant sequel of some types of pericarditis is chronic constrictive pericarditis, the result of healing of the inflammatory exudate. It is characterized by a pronounced fibrous thickening of the pericardium, which becomes so rigid that it mechanically interferes with the heart action and the circulation (Fig. 16-58). The pericardial cavity may be completely or partially obliterated, and sometimes small collections of fluid are entrapped

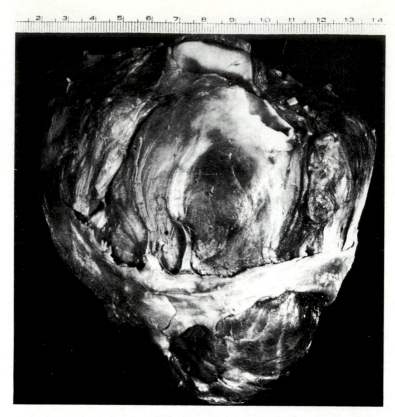

Fig. 16-58. Constrictive pericarditis. Note band of calcified tissue (6 to 1.5 cm in width), which definitely constricts heart. Thickened fibrous pericardium, which covered rest of heart, has been removed. Patient, 38-year-old white woman, had severe recurring ascites.

between adhesions. Calcification of the thickened, hyalinized pericardium may occur. Constrictive pericarditis may or may not be associated with mediastinopericarditis. When the latter is present, it usually accentuates the functional disturbances.

The main effect of the rigid pericardium is interference with diastole of the heart. The dense fibrous tissue could cause narrowing of the orifices of the venae cavae, but this has been demonstrated in only an occasional case.[425] The heart is usually normal or smaller than normal in size but may be enlarged.[421,424]

Pick's disease is a syndrome consisting of chronic constrictive pericarditis with severe venous congestion of the liver that may lead to fibrosis (cardiac cirrhosis) and ascites. Perihepatic and perisplenic fibrosis with hyalinization also may be associated. Polyserositis (Concato's disease) is characterized by large effusions into the various serous cavities: pericardial, pleural, and peritoneal. This syndrome may terminate in constrictive pericarditis and perihepatic and perisplenic fibrosis. The cause of Concato's disease is not known.

Regarding the etiologic basis for constrictive pericarditis, no definite cause can be determined in most patients. However, among the cases in which a cause has been established, tuberculosis is commonly considered to be the most frequent,[421] although recently the incidence of tuberculous pericarditis has been diminishing. Purulent pericarditis and hemopericardium (traumatic and nontraumatic types)[110,111,421] also are regarded as possible etiologic factors. Rheumatic fever is not a significant cause of constrictive pericarditis, although it has been reported to be responsible for an occasional case.[421] In one report the coexistence of rheumatic heart disease and constrictive pericarditis was observed in five cases, but the author remarked that there was no evidence that the two conditions were causally related.[424] There is some evidence that occasionally acute nonspecific (idiopathic) or viral pericarditis may progress to constrictive pericarditis. Isolated instances of constrictive pericarditis have been reported in rheumatoid arthritis, disseminated lupus erythematosus, infectious mononucleosis, neoplastic diseases, and other disorders.[419]

Pericardial plaques

Sometimes referred to as milk spots, pericardial plaques are white, smooth, glistening, opaque, well-circumscribed areas of fibrosis of the pericardium occurring principally on the epicardial surface of the anterior wall of the right ventricle. They are observed frequently as incidental findings at autopsy. They may be single or multiple and measure about 1 to 3 cm in diameter. The cause is not known, but they are generally believed to be the result of healed circumscribed pericarditis.[360] In the earlier literature the term "soldier's spots" or "plaques" was used, originating in the old idea that the straps of knapsacks carried by soldiers in World War I produced pressure against the chest wall, causing chronic irritation of the visceral pericardium.[360]

Etiologic types

Acute nonspecific pericarditis

Also known as acute idiopathic pericarditis and acute benign pericarditis, nonspecific pericarditis is today one of the most frequently encountered forms of pericarditis in clinical practice. According to some writers, it is probably the most frequent.[427,428] A lowering of the incidence of the former leading causes of acute pericarditis—acute bacterial infections and rheumatic fever—has been brought about apparently as a result of extensive use of antibiotics.[427] The prognosis of acute nonspecific pericarditis is usually good, although a few instances of fatal cardiac compression have been reported.[428] In most of the patients there is a history of antecedent respiratory infection followed in 1 to 20 days by an onset of acute pericarditis, which is ushered in by severe precordial and substernal pain, pericardial friction rub, fever, chills, anorexia, and malaise. The duration of the acute illness averages 2 weeks, but there may be recurrences within 2 weeks to several months.[428]

Pericardial fibrinous inflammation and effusion are common.[422,428] Sometimes the effusion is hemorrhagic. Associated pleuritis with or without evidence of pneumonitis is common.[428] Apparently this disease may lead to a constrictive pericarditis, as judged from the occasional case histories that suggest such a relationship.[419,428] The possibility that acute nonspecific (benign) pericarditis is of viral origin has been proposed. In a study of 34 cases of this disease, five instances were observed in which there was evidence for a viral infection (a group B coxsackievirus, echovirus type 8, adenovirus type 3, mumps, and infectious mononucleosis), but in 29 (85%) of the 34 cases, no cause was demonstrated.[423]

Bacterial (acute) pericarditis

See previous discussion of fibrinous, serous, serofibrinous, purulent, and hemorrhagic pericarditis.

Tuberculous pericarditis

In some cases tuberculous pericardial lesions are trivial and transient. In others they are serious and progressive.[426] In regard to its pathogenesis, tuberculous pericarditis arises either by extension from adjacent mediastinal, pulmonary, or osseous lesions or by metastatic dissemination from concurrent active tuberculosis in more distant areas.[426] Extension from adjacent structures is the most important mode of infection, and usually it is by means of retrograde lymphatic spread from lesions in the tracheobronchial lymph nodes. Occasionally a caseous lymph node adhering to the parietal pericardium ulcerates into the pericardial sac.

Anatomically, there may be scattered subserosal granulomas, which arise from hematogenous spread and may be associated with small effusions. These may be difficult to identify by biopsy or at autopsy. However, the more usual form of tuberculous pericarditis is characterized by a fibrinous exudate with effusion that progresses from an acute to a chronic phase (Figs. 16-59 and 16-60). The epicardium is covered by thick, shaggy, blood-stained fibrin that often is arranged in ridges caused by contractions of the heart. The entire pericardium becomes thickened and leathery as a result of progressive disease and gradual fibrosis. Gray tubercles may be seen throughout the parietal and visceral pericardium, and sometimes caseous areas coalesce to form a yellowish white interrupted layer. Organization of the fibrinous exudate contributes to the fibrosis. Effusions of fluid may occur soon after fibrin formation. The amount varies from a few hundred milliliters to several liters, so that cardiac tamponade may occur occasionally. The fluid often contains fibrin and blood and sometimes liquefied caseous debris. In some instances the effusion persists for a prolonged period. In others there is abundant fibrin with little fluid. The surfaces of both pericardial layers adhere to each other, but localized pockets of fluid or liquefied debris may be seen. The typical tuberculous granulomatous lesions can be demonstrated microscopically within the pericardial walls (Fig. 16-61). Calcification may occur in the late stages. The end result may be chronic constrictive pericarditis.

Viral pericarditis

See previous discussion of acute nonspecific pericarditis.

Other infectious forms of pericarditis

Rare instances of pericardial involvement have been described in association with actinomycosis and fungal infections of the heart. Pericarditis may be caused by *Entamoeba histolytica*, usually as a result of extension of an amebic abscess of the liver into the pericardial sac. Organisms sometimes are demonstrated in the pericardial exudate.

Rheumatic pericarditis

The features of pericarditis associated with rheumatic fever have been reviewed previously (p. 604).

Pericarditis associated with other connective tissue diseases

Pericarditis sometimes occurs in association with connective tissue diseases other than rheumatic fever. Evidences of pericarditis commonly are found in patients with rheumatoid arthritis.[309] In a certain proportion of these patients the pericarditis is caused by an intercur-

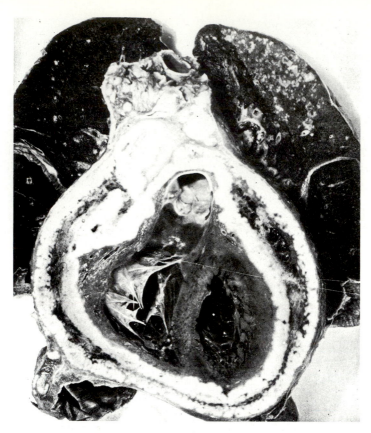

Fig. 16-59. Tuberculous pericarditis. Note pronounced caseous thickening of visceral and parietal pericardium, massive caseation of mediastinal lymph nodes, and tuberculous areas in lung tissue. (From Anderson, W.A.D., and Scotti, T.M.: Synopsis of pathology, ed. 10, St. Louis, 1980, The C.V. Mosby Co.)

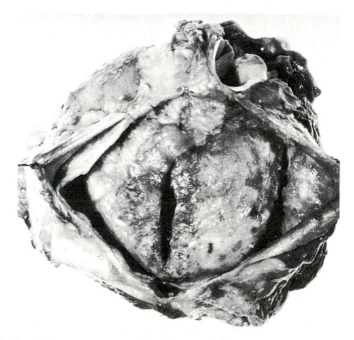

Fig. 16-60. Healing tuberculous pericarditis in 51-year-old white man. Roughened epicardium is covered with organizing fibrin. Parietal pericardium is thickened. Heart and pericardium weighed 930 g.

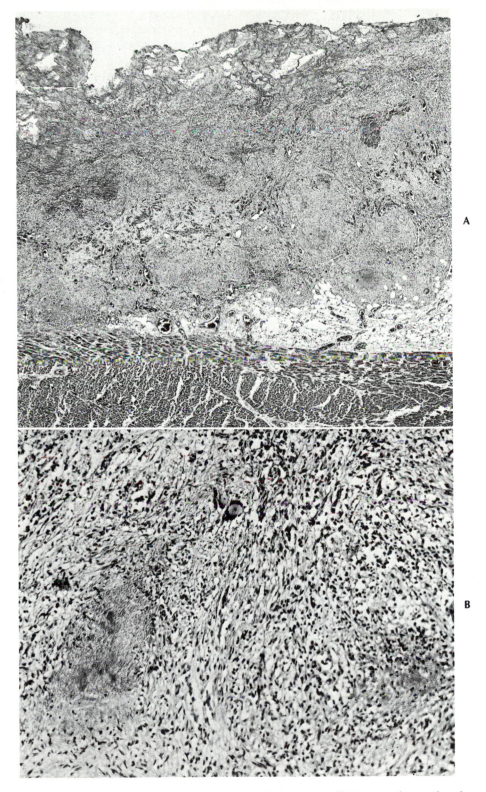

Fig. 16-61. Tuberculous pericarditis with fibrinous exudate. **A,** Note fibrin on surface and coalescent granulomatous nodules in epicardium. Caseation in nodule in lower right part of inflammatory mass. **B,** High-power magnification of area in **A.** Note coalescent tubercles with foci of caseation necrosis.

rent disease that is not related to the arthritis. In most of the patients, evidences of healed obliterative or adhesive pericarditis of unknown cause are present. The possibility that these represent instances of previous rheumatoid granulomatous pericarditis that has completely healed has been considered.[309] Frankly granulomatous pericarditis occurs occasionally in rheumatoid arthritis. Acute fibrinous pericarditis may occur in association with the cardioaortic disease found in patients with ankylosing spondylitis and may result in fibrous adhesions of the pericardium. In systemic lupus erythematosus, a fibrinous or serofibrinous pericarditis may accompany the underlying fibrinoid changes in the pericardial wall that are characteristic of this disease. Organization of the exudate leads to chronic adhesive pericarditis. Acute pericarditis occasionally is reported in other collagen disease, including polyarteritis nodosa and thrombotic thrombocytopenic purpura.

Neoplastic pericarditis

The details of involvement of the pericardium by primary or secondary neoplasms are discussed later in this chapter. Associated with the neoplastic infiltration, there may be a pericarditis characterized by a fibrinous or hemorrhagic exudate. Pericardial effusion is common and may be serous or bloody. The pericarditis usually is sterile, but a purulent pericarditis may occur as a result of contamination from an esophageal carcinoma extending directly into the pericardium.

Uremic pericarditis

In patients dying of uremia the pericardial surfaces frequently are covered by a thin film of fibrin. Occasionally the exudate consists of a fairly thick layer. Characteristically the fibrinous pericarditis is dry. If an effusion is present, it is usually not abundant and, at times, is hemorrhagic. This is a sterile form of pericarditis unless secondary infection supervenes. The responsible factor is not known, but it is believed to be a metabolic chemical disturbance associated with uremia. Microscopically, in addition to the fibrinous exudate, lymphocytes are present, but few if any polymorphonuclear leukocytes are seen. There is evidence of organization of the exudate in patients who survive for several days or weeks after the onset of pericarditis (Fig. 16-62).

Traumatic pericarditis

Fibrinous, serofibrinous, and hemorrhagic pericarditis occur as a result of penetrating injuries. A purulent pericarditis may ensue because of contamination of a wound by bacteria. Less commonly, a fibrinous pericarditis is caused by nonpenetrating cardiac trauma, but purulent pericarditis rarely occurs with this type of injury and usually is caused by contamination from associated injuries to the esophagus or the respiratory tract.[62]

After cardiac surgery a brief and usually insignificant episode of traumatic pericarditis with a transient friction rub occurs.[428] In addition, there is another type of acute pericarditis that develops in some patients subjected to any type of cardiac surgery. This is known as the postpericardiotomy, postcardiotomy, or postcommissurotomy syndrome.[428] The onset is from the first week to the sixth month after surgery, and it is characterized by pericardial pain, friction rub, and low-grade fever. A sterile pericardial effusion may be present. The cause of the pericarditis is unknown, although an autoimmune reaction has been implicated.[206] Recovery is the rule. A similar syndrome may occur after myocardial infarction (Dressler's syndrome).

Pericarditis in myocardial infarction

Pericarditis associated with an infarct of the heart is characterized by a sterile fibrinous exudate. Effusions of serous or serosanguineous type occasionally occur but rarely are large enough to cause cardiac compression. In most patients the pericardial lesion is limited to the area overlying the infarct, but in some instances the entire pericardium is affected.[428] Organization of the exudate occurs, with complete healing taking place in about 4 weeks. Pericarditis with effusion, sometimes hemorrhagic, occurs in the postmyocardial infarction syndrome, which may have an immunologic basis and is known as Dressler's syndrome (p. 595).

DISTURBANCES OF GROWTH
Atrophy

The term *atrophy* indicates a reduction in the size of a heart that had previously reached full development. This is an acquired disease, in contrast to hypoplasia, which is a congenitally small, underdeveloped heart. The

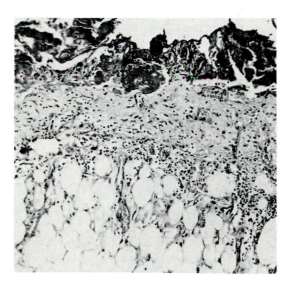

Fig. 16-62. Fibrinous pericarditis with partial organization in uremic patient. Note scanty cellular (lymphocytic) infiltration.

reduced size of the heart in atrophy is caused chiefly by a decrease in size of the individual muscle fibers, but there is also a reduction in the number of fibers, since some of them actually disappear. The number of nuclei is greatly increased in proportion to the number of fibers. This may be evidence of an attempted regeneration, but mitotic figures are not seen.[436] Associated changes may be evident in the myocardium of an atrophic heart, such as cloudy swelling, fatty degeneration, and pigmentation. A conspicuous accumulation of a granular, yellow-brown pigment (lipofuscin) occurs in the sarcoplasm of the muscle fibers, usually near the poles of the nuclei, in so-called brown atrophy of the heart. This term refers to the brownish discoloration imparted to the heart by the pigment that is observed in the gross specimen. In instances of very extensive pigmentation, some of the pigment may appear between muscle fibers, probably that which formerly existed in fibers that disappeared. Brown atrophy is seen particularly in elderly persons, but it may occur in young adults as well. Atrophy of the heart is seen in severe inanition or starvation, in endocrine disturbances (such as Addison's disease and Simmonds' disease), and in chronic wasting diseases such as pulmonary tuberculosis and cancer.

Atrophy of the epicardial fat also may be seen in long-standing malnutrition, together with atrophy of adipose tissue in other sites of the body. Edema, which is associated with this change, produces a gelatinous appearance of the fat (gelatinous or serous atrophy of fat). Microscopically, the fat cells are small and show increased density of the cytoplasm, which often contains water droplets. Pale fluid (edema) is present between the cells.

Hypertrophy and dilatation

An important objective sign of cardiac disease is enlargement of the heart. This may be attributed to hypertrophy or dilatation or both.

Hypertrophy

Hypertrophy is characterized by an increase in mass of the myocardium, resulting in an increased weight of the heart and a thickening of the muscle of the affected chambers. When dilatation of the heart also is present (that is, an increased volume capacity of the cardiac chambers because of elongation or stretching of the muscle fibers), the increase in thickness of the musculature may not be obvious. Hypertrophy sometimes is referred to as concentric when the myocardium is thickened in the absence of dilatation and as eccentric when dilatation also is evident. An increase in heart weight because of excessive epicardial fat or myocardial edema is not indicative of true hypertrophy.

The normal thickness of the wall of the left ventricle is about 10 to 12 mm and that of the right ventricle 3 to 4 mm, not including the papillary muscles and the trabeculae carneae of these chambers. A left ventricular wall 15 mm in thickness represents significant hypertrophy, provided that the chamber is well dilated. In concentric hypertrophy of the left ventricle, the wall may be 20 mm or more in thickness, and the lumen of the chamber appears smaller than usual (Fig. 16-63). Grossly, in addi-

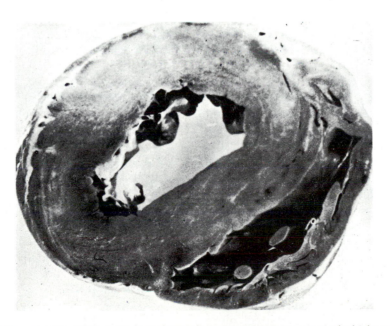

Fig. 16-63. Hypertrophy of left ventricle in chronic hypertension. Note excessively thickened wall of left ventricle as compared with wall of right ventricle. Heart has been cut transversely through ventricles. (From Anderson, W.A.D., and Scotti, T.M.: Synopsis of pathology, ed. 10, St. Louis, 1980, The C.V. Mosby Co.)

tion to thickening of the walls of the chambers, the cardiac muscle is firm. When the ventricles are involved, the papillary muscles and the trabeculae carneae are rounded and enlarged, and in atrial hypertrophy the muscle fasciculi are prominent, especially the musculi pectinati of the right atrium. However, if there is also a significant degree of cardiac dilatation, the papillary muscles and the other muscular prominences of the affected chambers tend to become flattened. The weight of the heart is increased. The normal heart weighs between 300 and 350 g in men and between 250 and 300 g in women. Variability of heart weight occurs in accordance with certain factors such as body weight[444] and body length.[447] Techniques have been devised to study the weight and various structural features of individual heart chambers.[434,435] As part of these procedures, excess tissue such as epicardial fat is removed, so that a more accurate weight of the myocardium of each chamber is obtained.

Microscopically, myocardial hypertrophy is characterized by an increase in size of individual muscle fibers, which is evidenced chiefly by their increased width or diameter. The nuclei often are enlarged and variable in shape. In a comparison of a normal heart (300 g) with an enlarged heart (500 g) and an atrophic heart (165 g), the ratio of fiber size was found to be about 5:9:4 respectively.[436] A proliferation of muscle fibers (hyperplasia) is not the cause of enlargement of the heart—at least not in adults. Certain investigators, however, contend that hyperplasia of the myocardium may play a role in causing an increase of myocardial mass in some infants.[431,439] An interesting hypothesis concerning enlargement of the heart in adults is that there is no increase in the number of fibers but only an increase in fiber diameter in hypertrophied hearts up to 500 g (critical heart weight), but beyond this weight the thickened fibers split longitudinally, causing an increase in the number of muscle fibers.[438]

Electron microscopy has been used to study the fundamental changes taking place in cardiac hypertrophy. The contractile material of the myocardial fibers consists of myofibrils, which in turn are composed of hundreds of myofilaments, the basic structural units of the muscle fibers. In electron microscopic studies of hypertrophied human hearts, evidence has been obtained indicating that enlargement of heart muscle cells is attributable principally to an increase in the number of myofilaments of the normal variety, through formation of new myofibrils and possibly by addition of filaments to preexisting myofibrils.[442] The increased number of myofilaments was confirmed in a study of experimentally induced cardiac hypertrophy in animals.[432] It appears that ultrastructural investigations have not settled the question as to whether new myofibrils are formed by longitudinal splitting of existing myofibrils, although this has been suggested.[430] Mitochondrial changes also have been described in hypertrophied hearts,[430] particularly as to size and number, but the findings differ in the various studies. Multiple intercalated discs have been frequently observed in muscle cells of hypertrophied hearts in experimental animals[437] and in human patients.[440] These structures are characterized by two, three, or four transverse segments of discs lying along the same myofibrils, each two of which are separated by one to 10 sarcomeres.[437] It has been suggested that the multiple intercalated discs may be metabolically active and the site for formation of new sarcomeres.

Support for the view that increased myocardial mass is predominantly the result of an increase in size of cells rather than in their number is gained from nucleic acid determinations of heart tissue in experimental cardiomegaly.[445] Among the significant findings in the enlarged hearts of experimental animals that suggested an increase in the amount of cytoplasm per cell were (1) increased ratio of ribonucleic acid (largely a cytoplasmic constituent) to deoxyribonucleic acid (a component of the nucleus) and (2) an increase in total ribonucleic acid content of the heart (as well as an increased total protein content) without concomitant increase in deoxyribonucleic acid content.

Certain degenerative changes within muscle fibers (among them basophilic degeneration) and multiple minute foci of myocardial necrosis followed by connective tissue replacement have been described in cardiac hypertrophy.[438] In the absence of other causes, such as coronary artery disease, these changes are attributed to a state of relative hypoxia of the muscle as a result of the vascular supply's becoming less adequate as the fiber size increases. It has been shown that, as the muscle fibers enlarge in the hypertrophied heart, the capillaries do not multiply, so that the concentration of capillaries decreases with increase in the diameter of the myocardial fibers and heart weight.[443] The ischemia is at the capillary level and is in direct proportion to the degree of hypertrophy.[136] Exception is taken to the foregoing concept by certain investigators who believe that in advanced hypertrophy there is an increase in capillaries as well as in myocardial fibers, although a ratio of one capillary per fiber is maintained. The myocardial hypoxia in these hearts is not considered to be attributable to failure of capillary blood supply but rather to restriction of coronary perfusion resulting from insufficient widening of the coronary ostia and inadequate growth of the coronary arteries and their branches as hypertrophy becomes greater.[438]

Causes of hypertrophy

In general, the causes of hypertrophy of the heart are the same as those responsible for dilatation (see the following discussion). However, the basic factors that stimulate the myocardial fibers to hypertrophy are not known. Stretching of the muscle fibers in response to stresses imposed on the heart is believed to be the essential factor that induces the cells to enlarge. With elongation of the muscle fibers, the surface area of the cells is increased, allowing for better nutrition and growth of the fibers. Other factors that may influence the muscle cells to increase in size are anoxia and hormonal stimulation, but the mechanism by which hypertrophy occurs as a result of these factors is not clearly understood. Chronic anemia is regarded as a stimulus for cardiac hypertrophy[122,441]; however, it is likely that the hypertrophy is induced not only by anoxic injury to the myocardium but also by overwork of the heart brought about by an increased cardiac output to compensate for the oxygen lack in the tissues. It has been suggested that coronary atherosclerosis without hypertension results in cardiac hypertrophy by causing anoxic myocardial damage and subsequent muscle strain or dilatation.[433] The role of hormones, such as the catecholamines and the pituitary growth hormone, in stimulating cardiac hypertrophy has been referred to previously.[88] Further investigations are necessary to determine if specific biochemical lesions in the myocardium are responsible for the development of hypertrophy. The possibility has been considered that an increase in ribonucleic acid and protein may be involved in the initial growth stimulus, but the mechanisms by which ribonucleic acid and protein synthesis is stimulated are not known. It has been suggested that a transient adenosine triphosphate depletion may trigger the synthetic process.[453]

Hypertrophy with or without dilatation may involve predominantly the left side of the heart or the right side or both. The degree and location of hypertrophy and dilatation are related to the character of the stress or burden imposed on the heart.

Some of the causes of left ventricular hypertrophy are systemic hypertension, aortic valvular disease (either stenosis or, more particularly, insufficiency), mitral insufficiency, occlusive coronary artery disease, coarctation of the aorta, septal defects, patent ductus arteriosus, and increased output attributable to hypermetabolic states (such as hyperthyroidism) or arteriovenous fistulas. The increased vascularity of the bones in osteitis deformans (Paget's disease of bone) is similar, in effect, to an arteriovenous fistula. When the heart is greatly enlarged chiefly as a result of left ventricular hypertrophy (usually weighing 800 g or more), the descriptive term *cor bovinum* ("ox heart") is sometimes used.

Hypertrophy of the right ventricle results from pulmonary stenosis (isolated or in tetralogy of Fallot), pulmonary insufficiency, tricuspid insufficiency, and especially from the various conditions producing an increased resistance to the pulmonary blood flow (pulmonary arterial hypertension), which include mitral stenosis, wide patent ductus arteriosus, lung diseases (for example, chronic emphysema, long-standing bronchiectasis, and pulmonary fibrosis as in pneumoconiosis), pulmonary vascular disorders (for example, multiple organizing pulmonary arterial thrombi[429] and pulmonary arteriolosclerosis, which may be secondary or primary), and severe kyphoscoliosis. The existence of primary pulmonary vascular disease, formerly a dubious entity, is now accepted, although its incidence is very low. The disease is described in the literature as idiopathic pulmonary hypertension.[446]

In patients with left ventricular hypertrophy, failure of the left ventricle may ensue, leading to pulmonary hypertension and right ventricular hypertrophy. Thus there is hypertrophy of both ventricles. Both ventricles also may be hypertrophied in instances of valvular disease involving both sides of the heart, in diffuse myocardial disease as in certain forms of myocarditis, or in idiopathic hypertrophy of the heart.

Dilatation

Hypertrophy of the heart is commonly associated with cardiac dilatation and may be preceded by it. One form of dilatation occurs when there is a significant degree of damage to the myocardium (so-called *myogenic dilatation*), as in degenerative myocardiopathies, various types of myocarditis, and coronary heart disease. The features are prominent cardiac enlargement, increased diameter of the heart, flabbiness of the muscle, inefficiency of the myocardium of the involved chambers, and cardiac failure. Another form of dilatation results from the excessive demands imposed on the heart as a result of structural defects (such as valvular disease) or increased peripheral resistance (hypertension) and is said to precede the cardiac hypertrophy associated with these cardiovascular alterations. Elongation of the cardiac chambers is a characteristic feature that early writers attributed to an increased muscle tonus, thus the designation *tonogenic dilatation*. In some instances, cardiac dilatation results from a combination of a weakened diseased myocardium and an increased load on the heart.

Cor pulmonale

The term *cor pulmonale* (pulmonary heart disease) in the restricted sense refers to disease of the right side of the heart (right ventricular dilatation or hypertrophy, or both, with or without failure) that results from disorders originating in the lungs and involving the parenchyma or the pulmonary circulation. However, the term is used by some authors in a broad sense to include also the effects on the right side of the heart of intrinsic cardiac diseases such as mitral stenosis or congenital septal defects that secondarily cause pulmonary hypertension. Cor pulmonale may be acute or chronic. Acute cor pulmonale is especially noticeable after massive pulmonary embolism and is characterized by rapid dilatation of the pulmonary trunk, conus, and right ventricle. Chronic cor pulmonale, which is more common than the acute type, is associated with diseases causing chronic pulmonary hypertension, and as a result there is sufficient time for development of hypertrophy of the right ventricle. Among the various pulmonary disorders causing chronic pulmonary hypertension are diffuse pulmonary emphysema, bronchiectasis, tuberculosis, pneumoconiosis, sarcoidosis, scleroderma, fibrosis of undetermined cause, pulmonary effects of kyphoscoliosis, multiple organized small pulmonary emboli, and hypoventilation associated with extreme obesity (pickwickian syndrome).

Cardiac hypertrophy in hypertension
Systemic hypertension

In a study by the National Center for Health Statistics,[448] adults between 18 and 79 years of age in the United States were classified in one of three groups in accordance with the following levels of blood pressure:

1. Nonhypertensive—systolic pressure below 140 mm Hg and diastolic pressure below 90 mm Hg
2. Definite hypertension—systolic pressure 160 mm Hg or above or diastolic pressure 95 mm Hg or above
3. Borderline hypertension—systolic and diastolic pressures between those specified in 1 and 2

The frequency of hypertension increases steadily with age. About 20% of men between 20 and 29 years of age have a mild degree of hypertension, but only about 5% have a more severe degree. Hypertension of at least mild degree is common in middle-aged and elderly people, occurring in about 40% of both men and women between 45 and 49 years of age and in 60% of those between 60 and 64 years.[450] It is frequently stated that the disease is more common in women than in men (in a ratio of 2:1).[452] However, in one study of a representative group of the average working population, hypertension was found to occur more commonly in men up to 45 years of age and more frequently in women thereafter.[450] In the United States, more blacks than whites are found to have hypertension.[127]

Systemic hypertension is classified into two main groups according to the cause:

1. That caused by known disease of renal or extrarenal nature, referred to as secondary hypertension
2. That in which the cause is obscure, designated as idiopathic, primary, or essential hypertension

The majority of cases of hypertension (about 90%) are of the latter type, which is further subdivided into the more frequent benign and the less common malignant varieties. The principal causes of systemic hypertension may be classified as follows[451]:

1. Renal
   a. Vascular diseases (arteriosclerosis, arteritis, polyarteritis nodosa, mechanical obstruction attributable to thrombosis, embolism, tumors, and so on)
   b. Parenchymal diseases (glomerulonephritis, pyelonephritis, hydronephrosis, polycystic disease, amyloidosis, tumors, and so on)
   c. Perinephric diseases (perinephritis, tumors, hematoma, and so on)
   d. Obstructive uropathies (prostatic hyperplasia, stones, tumors, and so on)
2. Cerebral
   a. Increased intracranial pressure (trauma, inflammation, tumors)
   b. Anxiety states
   c. Lesions of brainstem (poliomyelitis and so on)
3. Cardiovascular
   a. Heart failure
   b. Arteriovenous fistula
   c. Heart block
   d. Coarctation of aorta
4. Endocrine
   a. Pheochromocytoma
   b. Adrenocortical tumors
   c. Pituitary adenomas
   d. Hyperthyroidism
   e. Arrhenoblastoma
5. Preeclampsia and eclampsia
6. Unknown causes (essential hypertension)

The pathogenesis of hypertension is discussed in Chapter 19 (p. 750). The prognosis is variable. Some patients remain asymptomatic for many years, whereas others have disabling and even fatal complications.[455] There is a definite relationship between the mean age at death and the severity of hypertension. In the mildest form of the disease, the mean age is 61.7 years, and in the most severe group it is 47 years.[454] Women tolerate the disease much better than do men.[450,456] One factor that may be responsible for the more serious prognosis in men is the development of a complication, coronary atherosclerosis, that is more likely to occur in men.[450,452] In the United States the death rate is higher among blacks than among whites.[127]

The morphologic effects of systemic hypertension are manifested as lesions in the heart, peripheral vessels, kidneys, and brain. The cardiac manifestations will be considered here. The other lesions are described elsewhere.

Hypertensive heart disease

Hypertensive heart disease (hypertensive cardiopathy) is an important and common form of heart disease in the United States. The causes of death among hypertensive patients are the following[454]: (1) congestive heart failure, 26.1%; (2) coronary artery disease, 9.8%; (3) cerebrovascular accidents, 14.9%; (4) uremia, 20.2%; and (5) causes unrelated to hypertension, 29%. The cardiac complications therefore account for 35.9% of the deaths. It should be pointed out that in other series in the literature, the proportion of deaths from cardiac complications is somewhat higher.

Among the pathologic features of hypertensive cardiopathy, the most striking is hypertrophy of the heart involving chiefly the left ventricle. The average weight of the heart is 500 to 600 g, but it may be as much as 1100 g.[454] There is a correlation between the weight of the heart and the severity of hypertension, but there is no correlation between the weight of the heart and the duration of the disease.[454,456] The left ventricular wall is thickened (up to 20 mm or more), the papillary muscles and trabeculae corneae are rounded and prominent, and the cardiac chamber is small (concentric hypertrophy) (Fig. 16-63). When cardiac failure ensues, dilatation of the chamber also may be prominent. Endocardial fibrous thickening may be present in the left ventricle in instances of long-standing hypertension. After the onset of left ventricular failure, there may be dilatation and hypertrophy of the right side of the heart. In a significant number of patients there is associated coronary atherosclerosis, which is probably enhanced by the hypertension. Complications of coronary artery disease (such as myocardial infarction) can occur. Fibrinous pericarditis may be evident in patients who die as a result of uremia. Microscopically, the features include enlargement and degenerative changes of individual muscle fibers and focal myocardial fibrosis, although the latter is frequently the result of coexisting coronary atherosclerosis. Myocardial edema and foci of necrosis characterized either by intense eosinophilia or by complete dissolution of the muscle fibers occur in malignant hypertension.[449]

Cardiac hypertrophy in heart diseases of obscure origin

In most instances of hypertrophy or dilatation of the heart, an obvious preexisting disorder can be demonstrated. In some patients, however, cardiomegaly occurs in the absence of any known cause of heart disease and is referred to as idiopathic. The examples of this type of disorder that will be discussed are idiopathic congestive and hypertrophic cardiomyopathies, endocardial fibroelastosis, and endomyocardial fibrosis. These diseases are sometimes classified among the group of conditions termed *primary cardiomyopathies.*

Regarding the cardiomyopathies, different viewpoints and some confusion concerning terminology and classification have appeared in the literature,[461,465] although it is generally agreed that the term *cardiomyopathy* literally means a disorder of heart muscle, as does the term *myocardiopathy.* As used by many investigators, the term *cardiomyopathy* excludes disorders of cardiac muscle caused by coronary artery disease, hypertension (systemic or pulmonary), valvular defects, or congenital cardiovascular lesions. Some writers prefer to use the term *cardiopathy* instead of *cardiomyopathy,*[465] since certain

conditions commonly classified as the latter exhibit changes in areas of the heart other than the myocardium. For example, in endocardial fibroelastosis, which some investigators include among the primary cardiomyopathies,[468] there is a prominent endocardial lesion that results in impairment of myocardial contractile function.

The cardiomyopathies are usually divided into primary and secondary types. In primary cardiomyopathy the disease process is limited to the heart and usually its cause is obscure or unknown. In secondary cardiomyopathy the heart is involved as part of a generalized disorder. Examples of secondary cardiomyopathy are infectious myocarditis, endocrine and nutritional disorders, alcoholic cardiomyopathy, hemochromatosis, sarcoidosis, amyloidosis, glycogen-storage disease, immunologic connective tissue disorders, and Friedreich's ataxia. These diseases are discussed elsewhere in this chapter. In common use today is a clinical or pathophysiologic classification of the cardiomyopathies.[463] Thus the cardiomyopathies may be classified as congestive, hypertrophic, constrictive (restrictive), and obliterative types. The first two types, the most common and most important, are considered in the following. The constrictive or restrictive form is uncommon, its most frequent cause being amyloid infiltration of the heart. Endomyocardial fibrosis, also discussed in the following, is an example of obliterative cardiomyopathy.

Idiopathic congestive and hypertrophic cardiomyopathies

Congestive (dilated) cardiomyopathy occurs more frequently in adults than in children or infants and more often in men than in women. Clinically, it is characterized by cardiomegaly, progressive and recurrent or intractable heart failure, and often signs of systemic or pulmonary embolism. Anatomically, a major feature is prominent dilatation of the ventricles. The heart is usually heavier than normal, although in some patients the weight is within the normal range. Mural thrombi frequently are present in one or both ventricles. The ventricular walls may be thicker than normal but often do not appear thickened. It is likely that a slight or moderate degree of cardiac hypertrophy may be masked by the marked dilatation of the ventricles. Microscopically, there may be no alteration of the myocardium other than an increase in size of many muscle fibers. Sometimes degenerative changes and small areas of fibrosis are seen in the myocardium. When a significant degree of myocardial fibrosis is present, without concomitant coronary artery disease, it is difficult to exclude healed myocarditis as the underlying disease.[462,472] A familial form of cardiomyopathy occurs that, except for the familial occurrence, is clinically and anatomically similar to idiopathic congestive cardiomyopathy. In addition to the microscopic features already described, basophilic (mucoid) degeneration of the myocardium has been observed in some cases.[457-459]

In idiopathic hypertrophic cardiomyopathy the ventricular cavities are normal in size or smaller than normal, in contrast to the dilated cavities of idiopathic congestive cardiomyopathy. The heart weight is usually increased, the ventricular walls are thicker than normal, and often there is a disproportionate or asymmetric hypertrophy of the ventricular septum (that is, it is thicker than the free wall of the left ventricle).[470] Although the asymmetric septal hypertrophy is characteristic of this form of cardiomyopathy, it occasionally occurs in other acquired or congenital heart diseases.[466] Idiopathic hypertrophic cardiomyopathy may be divided into nonobstructive and obstructive types. In the latter type, obstruction to the left ventricular outflow is particularly evident, causing manifestations of subaortic stenosis,[460,469] so-called idiopathic hypertrophic subaortic stenosis. Sometimes an associated obstruction is found in the right ventricle. In an occasional instance the disturbance is restricted to the right ventricle, causing subpulmonic obstruction to right ventricular ejection.[471]

Another characteristic feature of idiopathic hypertrophic cardiomyopathy is myocardial cell disorganization in the ventricular septum.[467,470] Microscopically, this is characterized by disorderly myofiber orientation in which bundles of muscle cells are irregularly arranged and course in various directions. This feature occasionally occurs in hearts of normal infants or of infants with congenital cardiac diseases; however, the areas of septal disorganization tend to be smaller than in idiopathic hypertrophic cardiomyopathy.[466,467] It has been suggest-

ed that idiopathic hypertrophic cardiomyopathy may represent an inherited disorder of ventricular muscle growth, leading to irregular contraction and abnormal excessive hypertrophy.[463]

Endocardial fibroelastosis

The primary type of endocardial fibroelastosis[473-477] is a disease of obscure origin that occurs predominantly in infants and children but is also observed in adults.

Grossly, there is usually a diffuse (but occasionally a patchy) thickening of the mural endocardium caused by overgrowth of collagenous and elastic tissues. The left ventricle is the chamber most frequently affected, and in some instances it is the only one. The endocardium of the other chambers, particularly the left atrium, also may be involved, but usually in conjunction with that of the left ventricle. The altered endocardium is several times thicker than normal, smooth, opaque, and white or gray-white (Fig. 16-64). The valves may be affected, usually the aortic and mitral. In some series, valvular involvement is said to occur in almost 50% of the cases. The cusps are thickened and sometimes nodular, or there may be rolling of the edges. Stenosis or insufficiency of the valve orifices may result. Mural thrombi are common in the adult form of the disease, and frequently these give rise to emboli. Thrombi are not usually seen in the infantile and childhood cases. Cardiac enlargement is present and is attributable mainly to left ventricular hypertrophy. Dilatation with flattening of the papillary muscles and trabeculae carneae may also occur.

Microscopically, the most striking feature is the thickened endocardium as a result of a proliferation of colla-

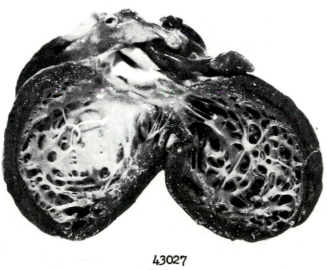

43027

Fig. 16-64. Endocardial fibroelastosis in 7-month-old black female infant. Heart weight was 77 g. Note left ventricle hypertrophy and dilatation.

gen and elastic fibers, which tend to run parallel to the surface (Fig. 16-65). The endocardial thickening usually is more severe in the infantile form of the disease. The fibroelastic tissue often extends into the sinusoids. There is usually a clear line of demarcation between the altered endocardium and the adjacent myocardium. Fibrosis of the myocardium is not a prominent feature. There may be only occasional small patches of myocardial fibrosis, particularly near the endocardium. Sometimes, especially in infants, the myocardial thin-walled vascular channels are prominently dilated and filled with blood. Inflammation is not a feature of the lesion.

Clinically, in infants there may be a sudden onset of cardiac failure in the first few weeks of life, characterized by shortness of breath, cyanosis, and death within minutes or hours, or the signs of heart failure may develop later, between 6 weeks and 6 months of age, followed by death in days or weeks. Occasionally, death occurs in the latter part of the first year or during the second year, preceded by symptoms for several months. The symptoms of the disease in childhood are similar to those in infancy, but there is usually a latent period between

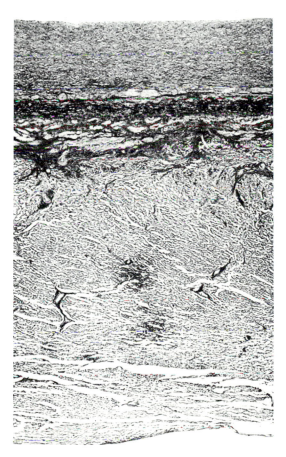

Fig. 16-65. Endocardial fibroelastosis. Section has been treated with elastic tissue stain to emphasize thickened endocardium with abundant elastic fibers running parallel to surface. There is slight degree of fibrosis in subendocardial myocardium.

birth and the onset of the symptoms. In the adult form of the disease the duration of symptoms is generally longer, chronic congestive heart failure is more prominent, and the embolic phenomena are a notable feature of the clinical picture.

The cause of the primary type of endocardial fibroelastosis is not known. The lesion that occurs in infancy and childhood is believed to be congenital. A popular theory implicates anoxia as the causative factor. It has been suggested that the fibroelastosis results from intrauterine endocardial anoxia from premature closing of the foramen ovale at a crucial stage in the development of the heart. In support of this theory is the observation that secondary endocardial fibroelastosis occurs in association with known congenital anoxia-inducing lesions such as an anomalous origin of the left coronary artery from the pulmonary artery or one of its branches. According to other theories, the endocardial proliferation is the result of an abnormality of development, a congenital metabolic disorder, organization of fibrin deposits, lymph stasis, or certain mechanical stresses.

The disease in adults is even more difficult to explain. Some writers contend that the adult form arises from the congenital infantile or childhood disease, despite the long interval between birth and the onset of symptoms. However, the majority believe that the adult lesion is etiologically different. Among the suggested theories are the following:

1. The endocardial disease is caused by an underlying myocardial injury such as that resulting from thiamine deficiency (beriberi heart disease) or from a preceding idiopathic myocarditis.
2. It represents a form of connective tissue disorder.
3. It bears a relationship to the entity endomyocardial fibrosis (the nature of this lesion and how it differs from endocardial fibroelastosis are considered later in the discussion of endomyocardial fibrosis).
4. Chronic impairment of cardiac lymph flow is important in the pathogenesis of the lesion.

The development of cardiac hypertrophy and subsequent heart failure may be explained by two mechanisms. First, there is increased work of the heart as the thickened endocardium interferes with proper contraction and relaxation, mimicking the decreased diastolic filling of chronic constrictive pericarditis (thus the designation *constrictive endocardial sclerosis*). Second, the thickened endocardium, by its blockage of the openings of the luminal channels connecting the myocardial vessels with the lumen of the heart, interferes with the blood supply to the adjacent muscle, causing myocardial injury.

The primary or idiopathic form of endocardial sclerosis must be differentiated from the secondary type of endocardial fibroelastosis, which is related to known cardiac disorders. The secondary form is probably brought about by intracardiac hypoxia, by abnormalities of the blood current within the chambers, or by lymphatic obstruction. This form is associated with congenital cardiac defects, anomalous coronary arteries, and metabolic disorders influencing myocardial function in infants and children and with hypertensive cardiopathy, healed myocardial infarction, and valvular deformities in adults.

Endomyocardial fibrosis

Endomyocardial fibrosis is an unusual form of heart disease of uncertain cause that is particularly prevalent among East Africans.[478-481] In Uganda the important cardiac diseases are hypertensive, syphilitic, and rheumatic heart disease, in addition to endomyocardial fibrosis. The endomyocardial disease accounts for 15% of all cases of heart failure in autopsies at Mulage Hospital in Uganda. In contrast to what is seen in the United States, atherosclerosis, coronary artery disease, cor pulmonale, and thyrotoxicosis are insignificant cardiac problems in Africa.[480]

Grossly, endomyocardial fibrosis is characterized by a massive, destructive, scarring process involving one or both ventricles. The lesion is in the apices and inflow tracts, extending to behind the posterior atrioventricular valve leaflets. The papillary muscles and the chordae tendineae are affected and fused, and the posterior leaflet of the atrioventricular valve is sealed to the mural endocardium. Mural thrombosis may be evident, and in some instances the ventricular apex (particularly the right) may be obliterated by the fibrous tissue and the thrombus. The outflow tracts are not affected except for a nonspecific jet effect resulting in slight endocardial fibroelastosis. The semilunar valves are not involved unless there is a coexisting disease such as rheumatic valvulitis. Typical lesions also may be present in the atria. Cardiac hypertrophy is not as constant and frequently not as striking as in idiopathic endocardial fibroelastosis. In fact, in some instances the heart size may be normal. Dilatation of the cardiac chambers may be evident.

Microscopically, in the scarred areas there is destruction of the original endocardium and of the adjacent myocardium, with replacement by granulation tissue. The superficial layer of the scar is composed of hyalinized connective tissue. A few inflammatory cells of the mononuclear type are present in the lesion. Elastosis is minimal or absent in the fibrous area, and the elastic fibers of the original endocardium remain as broken irregular masses. This is in contrast to the lesion of endocardial fibroelastosis. Calcification of the scarred area may occur. The destructive feature is responsible for the use of the term *endomyocardial necrosis* for this lesion. The inner one third to one half of the myocardium may be invaded irregularly by fibrous tissue, although in some cases myocardial involvement is not extensive. The pathologic changes of endomyocardial fibrosis in the Ugandan patients apparently differ from those observed in cryptogenic heart disease in the South African Bantu. The latter disease resembles the idiopathic cardiac hypertrophy described in the American and European literature.[464]

The clinical manifestations of endomyocardial fibrosis are somewhat similar to those of the adult form of endocardial fibroelastosis insofar as the patients present a picture of congestive heart failure of obscure origin. There may be signs of mitral or tricuspid insufficiency, rarely stenosis, and the features of constrictive pericarditis may be simulated. Embolic phenomena are uncommon.

Several theories have been proposed regarding the cause of this disease. One is that the heart lesion may be of infectious, possibly viral, origin. Another is that it represents an autoimmune alteration that leads to formation of autoantibodies, followed by an inflammatory reaction and diffuse fibrosis. A third theory implicates malnutrition as the cause of the disease. Also under consideration is the possible relationship of the disease to increased consumption of African plantain, which is rich in serotonin.[481]

Cysts

Cysts of various types occur in the pericardium, in the heart itself, and in the heart valves.

Pericardial cysts[486] are congenital malformations characterized by a thin fibrous wall lined by flattened mesothelial cells that are sometimes difficult to distinguish from vascular endothelial cells. These cysts occur in the anterior mediastinum and are in contact with the thoracic wall, the parietal pericardium, and sometimes the diaphragm and one of the lungs.[483] It has been suggested that the lesions result from failure of fusion of the primitive coelomic lacunae, which normally coalesce to form the pericardial cavity. The cysts must be differentiated from those caused by *Echinococcus granulosus* and from other types of mediastinal cysts. Pericardial cysts frequently cause no symptoms and are identified by roentgenogram in the course of a routine examination or are found incidentally at autopsy. At times they produce symptoms such as thoracic pain.

Epithelial cysts of the heart itself are extremely rare malformations.[484,485] There are two types: those lined by ciliated epithelium and those lined by nonciliated epithelium. The ciliated cysts arise in the left ventricle and are usually solitary. The nonciliated cysts occur in the atria and often are multiple. Stratified squamous epithelium has been identified in some of the cysts. Several theories have been proposed to explain the origin of the cysts, among which is the theory that the cysts represent forms of heterotopia—inclusions of the more cranial endoderm (thyroglossal, pharyngeal, respiratory, and esophageal primordia)[487] or inclusions of pericardial origin.[488] A rare tumor in the region of the atrioventricular node composed of multiple, closely grouped, nonciliated cystic structures has been described as a mesothelioma or lymphangioendothelioma. Conduction disturbances, including complete heart block, may result from the presence of intramyocardial epithelial cysts.

Blood cysts of the cardiac valves are small, dark red nodules, usually less than 1 or 2 mm in diameter, that are present most frequently on the atrial side of the atrioventricular leaflets and rarely on the ventricular surface of the semilunar cusps. These lesions, sometimes referred to as telangiectases, consist of unilocular spaces lined by endothelial cells and filled with blood. The origin of the cysts is not definitely known. They have been regarded variously as hematomas, angiomas, hamartomas, or dilatation of blood vessels assumed to exist in the cusps. Another explanation of their origin is that blood is pressed into crevices on the surface of the cusps, and subsequently the blood cysts are formed by fusion of the mouth of the crevices.[482] Usually, blood cysts produce no significant clinical manifestations.

Tumors

Tumors of the heart may be classified as primary or secondary, as benign or malignant, and as pericardial or intracardiac (myocardial or endocardial).

Primary tumors

Neoplasms are known to originate in any part of the heart, including the pericardium, but such tumors are rare. In some reports no tumors have been recorded in as many as 30,000 autopsies, whereas in other studies as many as three cases of primary heart tumors in 1200 autopsies were reported (0.25%). According to the American Medical Association statistics, 480,331 autopsies were performed in the United States from 1938 to 1942. During this period, reports of eight cases of primary heart tumors were published—an incidence of 0.0017% if all cases were reported.[499] In another survey of autopsy material the incidence was 0.05%.[498]

Primary pericardial tumors

Primary pericardial tumors are rarer than those of intracardiac origin and include fibromas, lipomas, angiomas, leiomyomas, teratomas, mesotheliomas, and sarcomas. Of this group, the most common are mesotheliomas and sarcomas, the latter being mainly fibrosarcomas. The mesothelioma consists of tumor nodules or masses, often confluent, on the visceral and parietal pericardium, or it may be a diffuse, firm, gray-white mass obliterating the pericardial cavity and encasing the heart. In the nonobliterating form the pericardial cavity may be distended by fluid that is frequently hemorrhagic. Mesotheliomas exhibit malignant tendencies, as evidenced by invasion of the underlying cardiac muscle and occasionally by metastases to the hilar lymph nodes and elsewhere.

Microscopically, these neoplasms are made up of masses of epithelium-like mesothelial cells, at times forming tubulelike, glandlike, or papillary structures. In some tumors the epithelium-like elements may be admixed with bundles of spindle cells. If the latter are the prominent feature, the appearance may be that of a fibrosarcoma. When the epithelium-like component is conspicuous, there is a striking resemblance to carcinoma. Sometimes a misdiagnosis of mesothelioma is made in instances of secondary carcinoma of the pericardium in which the primary growths elsewhere are unrecognized. The existence of benign mesothelioma of the pericardium has been questioned by some investigators who regard such a lesion as reactive mesothelial hyperplasia.[493]

Primary intracardiac tumors

Primary intracardiac tumors[497] are benign or malignant. The benign tumors include myxomas, rhabdomyomas, fibromas, lipomas, angiomas, and so-called mesotheliomas. The most common of this group are the myxomas. The next most frequently reported are the rhabdomyomas, although they are much less common than the myxomas. The malignant tumors are sarcomas, which closely follow myxomas in the number reported.[497] Most of the sarcomas are spindle cell tumors—fibrosarcomas, myxosarcomas, and leiomyosarcomas. Others are rhabdomyosarcomas, angiosarcomas, reticulum cell sarcomas, and lymphosarcomas. The exact nature of myxomas and rhabdomyomas is not agreed on by all. The following discussion will deal with these two lesions.

Myxoma. The most common primary tumor of the heart is the myxoma arising from the mural endocardium (Fig. 16-66). Myxomas are found almost exclusively in the atria, with about three fourths occurring in the left atrium in the region of the fossa ovalis. This location is in contrast to that of cardiac sarcomas, which arise most frequently in the right atrium. Only occasionally do myxomas occur in the ventricles. Cardiac myxomas are usually single tumors, but they may be multiple in some patients, appearing in the same chamber or in different chambers.[500] Myxomas occur at any age, but the majority are observed in persons between 30 and 60 years of age. The sex distribution usually is reported as being equal. The tumors are generally polypoid, frequently pedunculated, externally glistening and smooth or slightly lobular, and occasionally villous. They may be soft or firm. On section, their cut surfaces are yellow-white or red-brown, with evidence of hemorrhage, and they are often gelatinous in appearance.

Microscopically, myxomas consist of a loose, sparsely cellular stroma with stellate, spindle, polyhedral, and multinucleated cells scattered throughout. Vessels of capillary size lined by plump endothelial cells, foci of

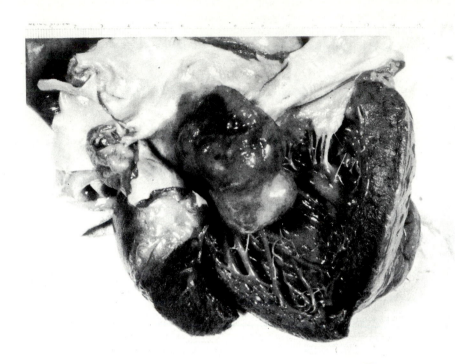

Fig. 16-66. Myxoma of heart. Note smooth glistening tumor attached to septal wall of left atrium and partly blocking mitral orifice.

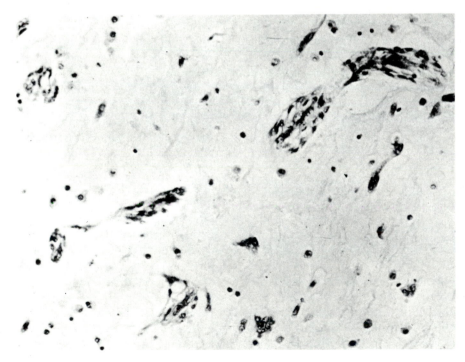

Fig. 16-67. Myxoma of heart. Note myxomatous stroma, few lymphocytes and plasma cells, and capillaries lined by prominent endothelial cells.

lymphocytes, and varying amounts of collagen are present (Fig. 16-67). Hemorrhage and granules of hemosiderin pigment commonly are seen in the stroma. Stains for mucin are usually positive. The lesions are covered by normal endothelial cells, and thrombi sometimes overlie the tumors. In one reported instance of a primary myxomatous tumor of the right atrium, epithelium-like cells forming glandlike and cystic spaces were incorporated in the mass. It was believed that these cells resulted from inclusions of pericardial elements during cardiac development.[488]

There has been some controversy concerning the nature of cardiac myxomas, but the prevalent opinion appears to be that they are true neoplasms. A number of investigators have considered them to be organizing mural thrombi. However, ultrastructural characteristics of thrombi have not been demonstrated in these lesions.[491] Although most authors maintain that myxomas are neoplastic, there is no general agreement as to their origin. One opinion is that the tumors arise from remnants of the myxoid tissue that composes the embryonic endocardium. Another view is that they are simple connective tissue tumors in which a myxoid change occurs as a result of stresses to which they are subjected within the cardiac chamber.[497] On the basis of recent electron microscopic studies, various investigators have described the cell of origin as smooth muscle cells derived from the subendocardium,[494] multipotential mesenchymal cells capable of producing various cell types,[490] or endocardial lining cells.[495]

A less frequent type of myxoma affects the cardiac valves. This is a papillary lesion. Its nature is also controversial, being sometimes reported as a true neoplasm and in other instances as an organized thrombus[496] or as peristent embryologic myxomatous tissue.[489]

Rhabdomyomas. Rhabdomyomas of the myocardium appear as single or multiple, circumscribed but not encapsulated, gray or gray-white nodules in any part of the heart. The masses often bulge into the cardiac lumen and rarely are pedunculated.

Microscopically, the nodules consist of large, swollen myocardial fibers filled with glycogen. In routine histologic preparations the cells appear as empty spaces surrounded by a rim of cytoplasm, but the characteristic feature is the presence of spider cells. These are cells with a central nucleus that appears suspended by threads of cytoplasm separated by large, glycogen-filled vacuoles. In some cells the vacuoles are not large and the cytoplasm is abundant and granular.

Rhabdomyomas usually occur in children and infants, often in association with tuberous sclerosis of the brain, but survival into adulthood is possible. Although the lesion is regarded as the most common primary tumor of the heart in infants and children, its neoplastic nature has been questioned. The belief that rhabdomyomas are developmental anomalies or hamartomas is a strong one.[496,497]

Secondary tumors

Any part of the heart, and particularly the pericardium, may be involved by malignant tumors originating in another organ or tissue. Most of these are metastatic growths resulting from hematogenous or lymphatic dissemination. Direct extension of an intrathoracic malignant tumor may also occur into the pericardium, from which invasion of the heart itself may ensue. Secondary neoplasms of the heart occur much more frequently then primary tumors. In an analysis of several autopsy studies, the incidence of secondary cancer in the heart was 0.03% to 5.3% of all autopsies and 1.5% to 18.3% in patients dying of cancer.[492] Primary cancers in almost any organ may involve the heart secondarily, but the most frequent are carcinoma of the lung and breast, malignant lymphoma, leukemia, and malignant melanoma (Figs. 16-68 to 16-70).[492]

Morphologically, the secondary tumors appear as small or large nodules involving the pericardium more often than the myocardium or endocardium. The resemblance to the primary lesions may be apparent both grossly and microscopically. Metastatic melanomas may be pigmented or nonpigmented. Leukemic involvement may not be recognized in the gross specimen but microscopically appears as diffuse or focal infiltrations. With neoplastic involvement of the pericardium, a fibrinous or hemorrhagic exudate frequently occurs. Occasionally, there may be an extensive infiltration of the pericardium by a firm, nodular tumor that encases the heart.

Effects of cardiac tumors

The clinical features of tumors of the heart are variable. In some instances there may be no significant symptoms or signs. Pericardial effusion is a sign commonly associated with neoplastic involvement of the pericardium. The effusion may be serous or bloody, the latter particularly with secondary cancers. Neoplastic cells may be found in the aspirated pericardial fluid. Rarely, signs of constrictive pericarditis occur. Complete heart block and bundle-branch block may result from involvement of the conduction system. Manifestations of obstruction of the superior or inferior vena cava may be produced by secondary growths or primary sarcomas involving the right atrium.

Much attention is being focused on intracardiac myxomas because of the increasing number of correct diagnoses being made during life, followed by the successful surgical removal of these tumors.[489] Intermittent positional symptoms from occlusion of the mitral valve orifice such as dyspnea, weakness, palpitation, faintness, and substernal discomfort or pain suggest the diagnosis. Electrocardiographic features, cardiac catheterization,

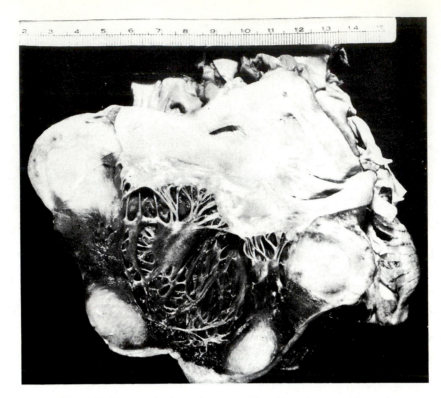

Fig. 16-68. Metastatic tumor in myocardium (from hypernephroma).

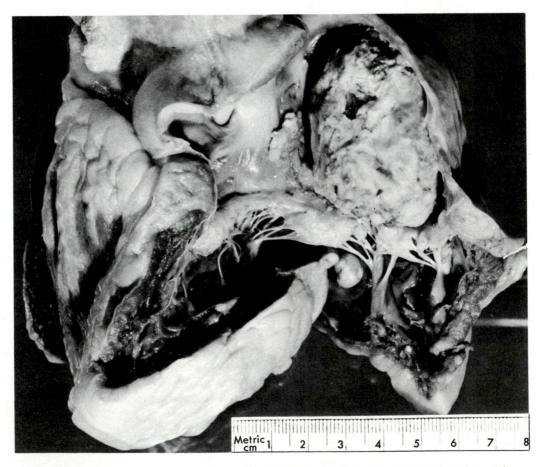

Fig. 16-69. Metastatic carcinoma of heart (from thyroid gland). Tumor mass projects into right atrium from appendage. Smaller tumor nodules are evident in right ventricle.

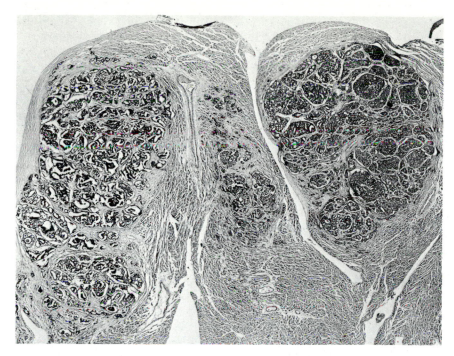

Fig. 16-70. Metastatic carcinoma involving myocardium (from thyroid gland).

and roentgenographic findings are aids in making a diagnosis, but angiocardiography and echocardiography are particularly useful in demonstrating a space-occupying lesion in the heart. Occasionally, tumor fragments cause embolic phenomena, and a tissue diagnosis of myxoma sometimes can be made by microscopic examination of the intravascular mass removed at embolectomy.[489] Recurrences of cardiac myxomas after surgical excision have been reported. Inadequate resection, tumor implantation, and unrecognized multicentric myxomas are considered possible causes of recurrence.[500]

DISTURBANCES OF CONDUCTION SYSTEM

The Wolff-Parkinson-White (WPW) syndrome, characterized by a short P-R interval and a prolonged QRS complex[505] is an entity whose etiology and mechanism of production are controversial. The explanations of the mechanism involved in this syndrome are many, among which are two commonly held theories. One theory postulates the presence of an accessory pathway, presumably a congenital anomaly, which may be either the bundle of Kent or some other connection between the atrium and ventricle. The atrial impulse passes over the aberrant anatomic bundle and reaches one ventricle early, setting off a premature ventricular response and accounting for the short P-R interval. Shortly after this occurs, the ventricles are activated in the normal manner through the atrioventricular pathway. This slightly asynchronous ventricular excitation is said to be responsible for the QRS aberration. According to the other theory, the transmission of atrial impulses to the ventricles is by

way of the normal atrioventricular node and is not dependent on the presence of anomalous anatomic atrioventricular connections. The impulses are transmitted in an abnormal manner via the normal conducting system, the basic disorder being a failure of part of the atrioventricular node to delay the atrial impulse for the normal period of time before allowing its passage to the ventricle while the rest of the node delays its share of the impulse in a normal manner.[504] The term *accelerated conduction syndrome* has been suggested for the WPW syndrome.[504]

Actually, it is possible that a different mechanism is responsible in different cases. From histopathologic studies it appears that some cases of WPW syndrome are associated with accessory communications and others are not, and accessory communications may be present without this syndrome.[503] In the majority of patients with WPW syndrome the heart is anatomically normal. However, in some patients, associated cardiac abnormalities may be present.

The conduction system is involved in many of the diseases affecting the heart.[501,502] In congenital heart disease the atrioventricular node, the bundle, and the bundle branches may be abnormally positioned or may show areas of disruption or fibrous tissue replacement. In addition, accessory bundles may be present, either replacing or accompanying the normal structures. Complete or incomplete atrioventricular block and bundle branch block may occur. Acute inflammatory diseases may produce lesions at various locations in the conduction system. Their effects frequently are transient. This group includes diphtheria, staphylococcal abscesses in the myocardium, scarlet fever, bacterial endocarditis, viral infections, Fiedler's myocarditis, and Chagas' disease. Rheumatic heart disease, sarcoidosis, and *Echinococcus* cysts are subacute to chronic in their effects.

Atherosclerotic coronary heart disease, especially with myocardial infarction or myocardial fibrosis, angiitis from such diseases as polyarteritis nodosa, and purpuras may cause damage by interference with the blood supply to the conduction system. Hypertensive cardiopathy causes physiologic changes by elongation and stretching of the pathways. Also, associated coronary atherosclerosis may contribute to conduction disturbances in hypertensive heart disease. Drugs such as the sulfonamides may produce an actual myocarditis. Neoplasms, primary and secondary, may be responsible for disturbances in conduction. The sinoatrial and atrioventricular nodes and the beginning of the bundle branches may be involved by fatty infiltration, and in rare instances atrioventricular block may occur. Fatty degeneration of the myocardium in anemia, diabetes mellitus, or toxic states may affect the conduction system, especially the bundle branches. In pericarditis the sinoatrial node may be involved.

BIOPSY OF PERICARDIUM AND MYOCARDIUM

For many years the pathologist was not accustomed to receiving specimens obtained from the living human heart, with the exception of pericardial fluids or occasionally pericardial tissue removed at operation for constrictive pericarditis. With the further development of cardiac surgery, other tissue specimens are now being submitted to the laboratory for study. The portion of atrial appendage amputated at the time of mitral valvulotomy, essentially for technical reasons, provides the pathologist an excellent opportunity to study the myocardium of a living patient. The common finding of Aschoff bodies in resected atrial appendages has been discussed previously in connection with rheumatic carditis. Additional investigations (such as pharmacodynamic, electron microscopic, immunochemical, and histochemical) of the surgically removed appendages serve to further our understanding of the human myocardium.[509,511]

More recently, interest has grown in regard to biopsy of the heart as a help in establishing the diagnosis of cardiac disease.[506,508,512-514] Among the indications for biopsy of the pericardium and ventricular myocardium are the following[513]:

1. Chronic or recurrent pericarditis of uncertain cause
2. Unexplained hemopericardium
3. Possible constrictive or adhesive pericarditis
4. Significant myocardial disease without sufficient evidence of the usual causes of heart disease to explain the myocardial failure

In addition, endomyocardial biopsy has been used to study the pathological changes of cardiac allograft rejection after cardiac transplantation.[507,516,522]

One may obtain the tissue by means of special needles, using a cardiac catheterization technique[506] or percutaneous puncture, or by means of a catheter introduced intravenously (for example, through the internal jugular vein).[507] Some investigators suggest that for more adequate diagnostic study it may be advisable to obtain several separate specimens of pericardium, pericardial fluid, and myocardium by an open surgical procedure.[513] Although the primary purpose of these procedures is to establish as definite a diagnosis as possible by histologic and bacteriologic means, other studies (biochemical, electron microscopic, and so on) may assist in augmenting our knowledge of the metabolism of the myocardium and the myocardial behavior in various forms of heart disease. As with biopsies of other organs and tissues, the pericardial or myocardial specimens in some instances may be insufficient or inadequate for diagnosis or may not be representative of the disease.

REJECTION OF CARDIAC TRANSPLANTS

In a histopathologic study of orthotopic canine cardiac allografts, the vascular injuries of acute and chronic cardiac rejection were said to be similar to those in renal and probably other rejected visceral allografts.[517] Acute rejection of these transplants resulted in death of the average untreated host by the seventh day. Histologically, the chief features in the myocardium were capillary and venular damage manifested by endothelial swelling and necrosis, vascular engorgement often associated with exudation of fibrin and red blood cells, microthrombi, and infiltration by monocytes and lymphocytes. By 96 hours, groups of myocardial fibers were affected by ischemic degeneration followed later by myocytolysis and myocyte necrosis that persisted as small scars when the rejection episode was arrested by immunosuppressive therapy. The major changes in hearts rejected after 1 to 15 months (chronic rejection) consisted of widespread destructive arteritis and intimal fibrosis, both causing luminal narrowing and myocardial ischemia.

In another investigation a study was made of the pathologic events of rejection of heterotopic canine cardiac allografts placed in the neck of untreated recipient dogs. The technique that was used made it possible to obtain sequential biopsies.[521] The initial histologic change was observed within 2 days, at first primarily in subepicardial and subendocardial areas but very shortly throughout the entire myocardium. The early lesion consisted of a perivascular exudate made up almost exclusively of small lymphocytes. By 4 to 6 days the infiltrating cells were medium lymphocytes and plasma cells, frequently in close association with myocardial fibers, some of which were necrotic. Between 6 to 8 days, the cellular infiltration and myocardial necrosis were more widespread, and vascular changes were seen in the myocardium. At 9 to 14 days the inflammation continued to be widespread, and only a few viable myocardial fibers were seen. The vessels were more severely altered, with hypertrophied endothelium, subendothelial deposits, and thickened walls. Much of the damaged myocardium was replaced by fibroblasts and small capillaries. Morphologic evidence of graft rejection was not evident during immunosuppressive therapy, but when therapy was stopped, the pathologic events of rejection occurred as in untreated animals.

The first human recipient of a cardiac transplant died 18 days postoperatively of bilateral pneumonia.[523] The pathologic findings in the heart, in addition to changes apparently unrelated to rejection such as fibrinous pericarditis and infarctlike areas in the atria, included edema and cellular infiltrate. The latter was more prominent in the donor's left atrium and ventricles and consisted chiefly of lymphocytes, with some plasma cells and Anitschkow cells. The infiltrate was not as impressive as that seen in transplanted dog hearts but was difficult to explain without evoking rejection as its basis. Foci of necrotizing arteritis were observed in both ventricles, but it was not certain whether the vascular lesions resulted from rejection. The patient was receiving steroid therapy after transplantation.

Since this study there have been a number of reports dealing with the pathology of cardiac allograft rejection in humans. The following is a summary of the various changes in the acute and chronic (late) allograft rejection reactions.[515,516,518,520,522] In acute rejection the heart at autopsy appears dark red, swollen, firm, and edematous. Fibrinous pericarditis is a constant feature, and subendocardial and myocardial hemorrhage is usually present. The microscopic findings include swelling and disruption of the endothelium of vessels with platelet and fibrin deposition on the intimal surface, interstitial infiltration of the myocardium (especially around vessels) by mononuclear (lymphoid) cells, a similar infiltration in the thickened intima of the coronary arteries, arterial medial necrosis, edema and hemorrhages in the myocardium, and foci of myocardial degeneration and necrosis.

In chronic or late allograft rejection, the principal morphologic features are an infiltrate of mononuclear cells (lymphocytes, plasma cells, histiocytes) in the intima of coronary arteries and in the myocardium (mainly in perivascular areas), intimal proliferation and fibrosis of coronary arteries, and foci of myocytolysis and fibrosis of the myocardium. In long-term survivors the intimal lesion may progress and become atherosclerotic. It has been suggested that the initiating factor in cardiac allograft atherosclerosis may be immunologic injury to the intima, but that intimal platelet and fibrin microthrombi and elevated serum lipids may contribute to its development.[520]

The use of human heart valves as allografts to replace defective valves had been in effect several years before the first human cardiac transplant. In a morphologic study of 34 orthotopically transplanted human allograft aortic valves, which had been in place from 1 day to 2½ years, there was no evidence of rejection, although they were found to be subject to mechanical failure from rupture of the cusps or from other causes.[519] The initial change, microscopically, at the junction of the graft with the host's tissue was an infiltration by a few neutrophils along with deposition of fibrin. Later, there was evidence of organization associated with a mild lymphocytic and plasma cell infiltrate. The myocardial portion of the graft was gradually removed by macrophages, and vascularization of its tissue became evident. Along the superior and inferior margins of the graft, fibrin became organized and formed a fibrous intimal sheath that extended over the edges of the allograft to the base of its cusps. In one instance, endothelium extended over the fibrous intimal sheath onto the cusps. The allograft was secured in place by the fibrous intimal sheath and by healing at its junction with the tissues of the host.

REFERENCES

1. Monthly vital statistics report: Final mortality statistics, 1978, vol. 29, no. 6, suppl. 2, September 17, 1980, U.S. Department of Health and Human Services.
2. Mortality statistics, 1920, U.S. Bureau of the Census, Department of Commerce, Washington, D.C., 1922, U.S. Government Printing Office.
3. Mortality trends for leading causes of death: United States, 1950-69, National Center for Health Statistics. Data from National Vital Statistic, series 20, no. 16, Department of Health, Education, and Welfare Pub. No. (HRA) 74-1853, March 1974.
4. Stamler, J.: Cardiovascular diseases in the United States, Am. J. Cardiol. **10**:319, 1962.
5. Statistical bulletin, Metropolitan Life Insurance Co. **61**:8-12, Oct.-Dec., 1980 (Cardiovascular diseases, United States, Canada, and Western Europe).
6. Why the American decline in coronary heart disease? (editorial), Lancet **1**:183, 1980.

Noninflammatory diseases other than growth disturbances
Degenerative diseases and disturbances in metabolism

7. Bajusz, E.: Myocardial calcification and cardiac surgery, Lancet **1**:174, 1964.
8. Batsakis, J.G.: Degenerative lesions of the heart. In Gould, S.E., editor: Pathology of the heart and blood vessels, ed. 3, Springfield, Ill., 1968, Charles C Thomas, Publisher.
9. Brewer, D.B.: Myxoedema: autopsy report with histochemical observations on nature of mucoid infiltrations, J. Pathol. Bacteriol. **63**:503, 1951.
10. Briggs, G.W.: Amyloidosis, Ann. Intern. Med. **55**:943, 1961.
11. Cohen, A.S.: Amyloidosis, N. Engl. J. Med. **277**:522, 1967.
12. Dahlin, D.C., and Edwards, J.E.: Cardiac clinics: amyloid localized in heart, Proc. Staff Meet. Mayo Clin. **24**:89, 1949.
13. Dawson, I.M.P.: Histology and histochemistry of gargoylism, J. Pathol. Bacteriol. **67**:587, 1954.
14. Dible, J.H.: Is fatty degeneration of heart muscle a phanerosis? J. Pathol. Bacteriol. **39**:197, 1934.
15. Field, R.A.: The glycogenoses: Von Gierke's disease, acid maltase deficiency, and liver glycogen phosphorylase deficiency, Am. J. Clin. Pathol. **50**:20, 1968.
16. Fisher, C.E., and Mulligan, R.M.: Quantitative study of correla-

tion between basophilic degeneration of myocardium and atrophy of thyroid gland, Arch. Pathol. **36**:206, 1943.

17. Garvin, C.F.: Fatty degeneration of heart causing myocardial insufficiency: report of case, Arch. Intern. Med. **66**:603, 1940.
18. Gore, I., and Aarons, W.: Calcification of myocardium: pathologic study of 13 cases, Arch. Pathol. **48**:1, 1949.
19. Haust, M.D., et al.: Histochemical studies on cardiac "colloid," Am. J. Pathol. **40**:185, 1962.
20. Haymond, J.L., and Giordano, A.S.: Glycogen storage disease of heart, Am. J. Clin. Pathol. **16**:651, 1946.
21. Hers, H.G.: α-Glucosidase deficiency in generalized glycogen storage disease (Pompe's disease), Biochem. J. **86**:11, 1963.
22. Hsia, D.Y.Y.: The diagnosis and management of the glycogen storage diseases, Am. J. Clin. Pathol. **50**:44, 1968.
23. Jones, R.S., and Frazier, D.B.: Primary cardiovascular amyloidosis, its clinical manifestations, pathology and histogenesis, Arch. Pathol. **50**:366, 1950.
24. Josselson, A.J., Pruitt, R.D., and Edwards, J.E.: Amyloid localized to heart: analysis of 29 cases, Arch. Pathol. **54**:359, 1952.
25. Keschner, H.W.: Heart in hemochromatosis, South. Med. J. **44**:927, 1951.
26. King, L.S.: Atypical amyloid disease, with observations on new silver stain for amyloid, Am. J. Pathol. **24**:1095, 1948.
27. Kosek, J.C., and Angell, W.: Fine structure of basophilic myocardial degeneration, Arch. Pathol. **89**:491, 1970.
28. Langendorf, R., and Pirani, C.L.: Heart in uremia: electrocardiographic and pathologic study, Am. Heart J. **33**:282, 1947.
29. Levin, E.B., and Golum, A.: Heart in hemochromatosis, Am. Heart J. **45**:277, 1953.
30. Manion, W.C.: Basophilic mucoid degeneration of the heart, Med. Ann. D.C. **34**:60, 1965.
31. Mathews, W.H.: Primary systemic amyloidosis, Am. J. Med. Sci. **228**:317, 1954.
32. McKusick, V.A., et al.: The genetic mucopolysaccharidoses, Medicine **44**:445, 1965.
33. Rosai, J., and Lascano, E.F.: Basophilic (mucoid) degeneration of myocardium, Am. J. Pathol. **61**:99, 1970.
34. Ross, C.F., and Belton, E.M.: A case of isolated cardiac lipidosis, Br. Heart J. **30**:726, 1968.
35. Roy, P.E.: Basophilic degeneration of myocardium, Lab. Invest. **32**:729, 1975.
36. di Sant' Agnese, P.A.: Diseases of glycogen storage with special reference to the cardiac type of generalized glycogenosis, Ann. N.Y. Acad. Sci. **72**:439, 1959.
37. Scott, J.M.: Fatty change in the myocardium of newborn infants, Am. Heart J. **64**:283, 1962.
38. Scotti, T.M.: Basophilic (mucinous) degeneration of myocardium, Am. J. Clin. Pathol. **25**:994, 1955.
39. Scotti, T.M.: Basophilic degeneration of the myocardium in a whale and a horse, Am. J. Clin. Pathol. **38**:530, 1962.
40. Strauss, L.: The pathology of gargoylism; report of case and review of the literature, Am. J. Pathol. **24**:855, 1948.
41. Thomashow, A.I., Angle, W.D., and Morrione, T.G.: Primary cardiac amyloidosis, Am. Heart J. **45**:895, 1953.
42. Vigorito, V.J., and Hutchins, G.M.: Cardiac conduction system in hemochromatosis, Am. J. Cardiol. **44**:418, 1979.
43. Wilson, R.A., and Clark, N.: Endocardial fibroelastosis associated with generalized glycogenesis: occurrence in siblings, Pediatrics **26**:86, 1960.

Nutritional disturbances

44. Alexander, C.S.: Electron microscopic observations in alcoholic heart disease, Br. Heart J. **29**:200, 1967.
45. Benchimol, A.B., and Schlesinger, P.: Beriberi heart disease, Am. Heart J. **46**:245, 1953.
46. Bing, R.J.: Cardiac metabolism: its contribution to alcoholic heart disease and myocardial failure, Circulation **58**:965, 1978.
47. Blankenhorn, M.A., et al.: Occidental beriberi heart disease, J.A.M.A. **131**:717, 1946.
48. Bragdon, J.H., and Levine, H.D.: Myocarditis in vitamin E–deficient rabbits, Am. J. Pathol. **25**:265, 1949.
49. Evans, W.: Acoholic cardiomyopathy, Am. Heart J. **61**:556, 1961.
50. Follis, R.H., Jr.: Sudden death in infants with scurvy, J. Pediatr. **20**:347, 1942.
51. Follis, R.H., Jr.: Deficiency disease, Springfield, Ill. 1958, Charles C Thomas, Publisher.
52. Grinvalsky, H.T., and Fitch, D.M.: A distinctive myocardiopathy occurring in Omaha, Nebraska: pathologic aspects, Ann. N.Y. Acad. Sci. **156**:544, 1969.
53. Higginson, J., Gillanders, A.D., and Murray, J.F.: Heart in chronic malnutrition, Br. Heart J. **14**:213, 1952.
54. Kesteloot, H., et al.: An enquiry into the role of cobalt in the heart disease of chronic beer drinkers, Circulation **37**:854, 1968.
55. Morin, Y., Tetu, A., and Mercier, G.: Québec beer-drinkers' cardiomyopathy: clinical and hemodynamic aspects, Ann. N.Y. Acad. Sci. **156**:566, 1969.
56. Rubin, E.: Alcoholic myopathy in heart and skeletal muscle, N. Engl. J. Med. **301**:28, 1979.
57. Sullivan, J.F., Egan, J.P., and George, R.P.: A distinctive myocardiopathy occuring in Omaha, Nebraska: clinical aspects, Ann. N.Y. Acad. Sci. **156**:526, 1969.
58. Swanepoel, A., Smythe, P.M., and Campbell, J.A.H.: The heart in kwashiorkor, Am. Heart J. **67**:1, 1964.
59. Wellmann, K.F.: Beer drinkers myocardosis: report of a case with electron microscopic observations, Am. J. Clin. Pathol. **50**:444, 1968.
60. Wolbach, S.B.: Pathologic changes resulting from vitamin deficiency, J.A.M.A. **108**:7, 1937.

Traumatic disease

61. Moritz, A.R.: Injuries of heart and pericardium by physical violence. In Gould, S.E., editor: Pathology of the heart, ed. 3, Springfield, Ill., 1968, Charles C Thomas, Publisher.
62. Parmley, L.F., Manion, W.C., and Mattingly, T.W.: Nonpenetrating wounds of the heart and aorta, Circulation **18**:371, 1958.
63. Parmley, L.F., Mattingly, T.W., and Manion, W.C.: Penetrating wounds of the heart and aorta, Circulation **17**:953, 1958.

Radiation injury

64. Fajardo, L.F., and Stewart, J.R.: Coronary artery disease after radiation, N. Engl. J. Med. **286**:1265, 1972.
65. Fajardo, L.F., Stewart, J.R., and Cohen, K.E.: Morphology of radiation induced heart disease, Arch. Pathol. **86**:512, 1968.
66. Fulton, G.P., and Sudak, F.N.: Effect of total body x-irradiation on serum electrolyte levels and electrocardiograms of golden hamster, Am. J. Physiol. **179**:135, 1954.
67. Leach, J.E.: Some of the effects of roentgen irradiation on cardiovascular system, Am. J. Roentgenol. **50**:616, 1943.
68. Liebow, A.A., Warren, S., and DeCoursey, E.: Pathology of atomic bomb casualties, Am. J. Pathol. **25**:853, 1949.
69. Senderoff, E., et al.: The effects of cardiac irradiation upon the normal canine heart, Am. J. Roentgenol. **86**:740, 1961.
70. Tullis, J.L.: Response of tissue to total body irradiation, Am. J. Pathol. **25**:829, 1949.
71. Warren, S.: Effects of radiation on normal tissues, Arch. Pathol. **34**:1070, 1942.

Endocrine disturbances

72. Andrus, E.C.: Thyroid and circulation, Circulation **7**:437, 1953.
73. Baker, S.M., and Hamilton, J.D.: Capillary changes in myxedema, Lab. Invest. **6**:218, 1957.
74. Blumgart, H.L., Freedberg, A.S., and Kurland, G.S.: Hypercholesterolemia, myxedema and atherosclerosis, Trans. Assoc. Am. Physicians **65**:114, 1952.
75. Fahr, G.: Myxedema heart, report based upon study of 17 cases of myxedema, Am. Heart J. **8**:91, 1932.
76. Ferrans, V.J., et al.: Histochemical and electron microscopical studies on the cardiac necroses produced by sympathomimetic agents, Ann. N.Y. Acad. Sci. **156**:309, 1969.
77. Goldberg, S.A.: Changes in organs of thyroidectomised sheep and goats, Q.J. Exp. Physiol. **17**:15, 1927.
78. Hamby, R.I., Zoneraich, S., and Sherman, L.: Diabetic cardiomyopathy, J.A.M.A. **229**:1749, 1974.
79. Higgins, W.H.: Heart in myxedema: correlation of physical and postmortem findings, Am. J. Med. Sci. **191**:80, 1936.

80. Kahn, D.S., Rona, G., and Chappel, C.I.: Isoproterenol-induced cardiac necrosis, Ann. N.Y. Acad. Sci. **156**:285, 1969.

81. Kline, I.K.: Myocardial alterations associated with pheochromocytomas, Am. J. Pathol. **38**:539, 1961.

82. LaDue, J.S.: Myxedema heart: pathologic and therapeutic study, Ann. Intern. Med. **18**:332, 1943.

83. Lewis, W.: Question of specific myocardial lesion in hyperthyroidism (Basedow's disease), Am. J. Pathol. **8**:255, 1932.

84. Lie, J.T., and Grossman, S.J.: Pathology of the heart in acromegaly, Am. Heart J. **100**:41, 1980.

85. MacDonald, R.A., and Robbins, S.L.: Pathology of the heart in the carcinoid syndrome: a comparative study, Arch. Pathol. **63**:103, 1957.

86. McGavack, T.H., and Schwimmer, D.: Problems in treatment of cardiac failure in myxedema, J. Clin. Endocrinol. **4**:427, 1944.

87. Piggott, J.A.: Pathologic changes in rheumatic heart disease, Bull. Pathol. **10**:15, 1969.

88. Raab, W.: Hormonal and neurogenic cardiovascular disorders, Baltimore, 1953, The Williams & Wilkins Co.

89. Raab, W.: Pathophysiologic fundamentals of the origin and prevention of degenerative heart disease, Ann. N.Y. Acad. Sci. **156**:281, 1969.

90. Roberts, W.C., and Sjoerdsma, A.: The cardiac disease associated with the carcinoid syndrome, Am. J. Med. **36**:5, 1964.

91. Rona, G., et al.: An infarct-like myocardial lesion and other toxic manifestations produced by isoproterenol in the rat, Arch. Pathol. **67**:443, 1959.

92. Rosen, S.H.: Goiter heart, U.S. Armed Forces Med. J. **2**:1593, 1951.

93. Sandler, G., and Wilson, G.M.: The nature and prognosis of heart disease in thyrotoxicosis: a review of 150 patients treated with ^{131}I, Q.J. Med. **28**:347, 1959.

94. Schenk, E.A., Penn, I., and Schwartz, S.: Experimental atherosclerosis in the dog: a morphologic evaluation, Arch. Pathol. **89**:102, 1965.

95. Spatz, M.: Pathogenic studies of experimentally induced heart lesions and their relation to the carcinoid syndrome, Lab. Invest. **13**:288, 1964.

96. Spatz, M.: Ann. N.Y. Acad. Sci. **156**:142, 1969.

97. Szakacs, J.E., and Cannon, A.: *l*-Norepinephrine myocarditis, Am. J. Clin. Pathol. **30**:425, 1958.

98. Szakacs, J.E., and Mehlman, B.: Pathologic changes induced by *l*-norepinephrine: quantitative aspects, Am. J. Cardiol. **5**:619, 1960.

99. Thorson, A.H.: Studies on carcinoid disease, Acta Med. Scand. **161**(suppl. 334):1, 1958.

100. Webster, B., and Cooke, C.: Morphologic changes in heart in experimental myxedema, Arch. Intern. Med. **58**:269, 1936.

101. Willius, F.A.: Cardiac clinics: clinic on advanced coronary sclerosis with congestive heart failure in young adults; juvenile myxedema, Proc. Staff Meet. Mayo Clin. **11**:551, 1936.

Fluid and electrolyte disturbances
Effects of potassium disturbances

102. French, J.E.: Histologic study of heart lesions in potassium-deficient rats, Arch. Pathol. **53**:485, 1952.

103. Reye, J.D., Jr.: Death in potassium deficiency: report of case including morphologic findings, Circulation **5**:766, 1952.

104. McAllen, P.M.: Myocardial changes occurring in potassium deficiency, Br. Heart J. **17**:5, 1955.

105. Molnar, Z., Larsen, K., and Spargo, B.: Cardiac changes in the potassium depleted rat, Arch. Pathol. **74**:339, 1962.

Disturbances of circulation of blood
Hemopericardium

106. Anderson, M.W., Christensen, N.A., and Edwards, J.E.: Hemopericardium complicating myocardial infarction in absence of cardiac rupture: report of 3 cases, Arch. Intern. Med. **90**:634, 1952.

107. Dressler, H., Yurkofsky, J., and Starr, M.C.: Hemorrhagic pericarditis, pleurisy, and pneumonia complicating recent myocardial infarction, Am. Heart J. **54**:42, 1957.

108. Goldstein, R., and Wolf, L.: Hemorrhagic pericarditis in acute myocardial infarction treated with bishydroxycoumarin, J.A.M.A. **146**:616, 1951.

109. Izzo, P.A., et al.: Hemopericardium associated with anticoagulant therapy, Arch. Intern. Med. **92**:350, 1953.

110. Laslo, M.H.: Constrictive pericarditis as sequel to hemopericardium: report of a case following anticoagulant therapy, Ann. Intern. Med. **46**:403, 1957.

111. McKusick, V.A., Kay, J.H., and Isaacs, J.P.: Constrictive pericarditis following traumatic hemopericardium, Ann. Surg. **142**:97, 1955.

Shock

112. Bing, R.J., and Ramos, H.: The role of the heart in shock, J.A.M.A. **181**:871, 1962.

113. Hackel, D.B., and Goodale, W.T.: Effects of hemorrhagic shock on the heart and circulation of intact dogs, Circulation **11**:628, 1955.

114. Hackel, D.B., Ratliff, N.B., and Mikat, E.M.: The heart in shock, Circ. Res. **25**:895, 1974.

115. Mallory, T.B.: Systemic pathology consequent to traumatic shock, J. Mt. Sinai Hosp. **16**:137, 1949.

116. Martin, A.M., Jr. and Hackel, D.B.: The myocardium of the dog in shock: a histochemical study, Lab. Invest. **12**:77, 1963.

117. Melcher, G.W., and Walcott, W.W.: Myocardial changes following shock, Am. J. Physiol. **164**:832, 1951.

118. Page, D.L., et al.: Myocardial changes associated with cardiogenic shock, N. Engl. J. Med. **285**:133, 1971.

119. Siegel, H.W., and Downing, S.E.: Reduction of left ventricular contractility during acute hemorrhagic shock, Am. J. Physiol. **218**:772, 1970.

Anemia

120. Akenhead, W.R., and Jaques, W.E.: Pulmonary edema, cardiomegaly, and anemia, Am. J. Clin. Pathol. **26**:926, 1956.

121. Hogg, G.R.: Cardiac lesions in hemolytic disease of the newborn, J. Pediar. **60**:352, 1962.

122. Paplanus, S.H., Zbar, M.J., and Hays, J.W.: Cardiac hypertrophy as a manifestation of chronic anemia, Am. J. Pathol. **34**:149, 1958.

123. Winsor, T., and Burch, G.E.: Electrocardiogram and cardiac state in active sickle-cell anemia, Am. Heart J. **29**:685, 1945.

Coronary artery and ischemic heart disease
Incidence

124. Coronary heart disease, WHO Tech. Rep. Ser. No. 168, 1959.

125. Coronary heart disease death rates (medical news), J.A.M.A. **231**:691, 1975.

126. Ischemic heart disease, WHO Tech. Rep. Ser. No. 117, 1957.

127. Phillips, J.H., Jr., and Burch, G.E.: A review of cardiovascular diseases in the white and black races, Medicine **39**:241, 1960.

128. Vital health statistics, National Center for Health Statistics, ser. 4, no. 6, Washington, D.C., Sept. 1966, U.S. Department of Health, Education, and Welfare (eighth revision of international classification of diseases).

Anatomic features

129. Baroldi, G., Mantero, O., and Scomazzoni, G.: Collaterals of coronary arteries in normal and pathologic hearts, Circ. Res. **4**:223, 1956.

130. Bellman, S., and Frank, H.A.: Intercoronary collaterals in normal hearts, J. Thorac. Surg. **36**:584, 1958.

131. Blumgart, H.L., Schlesinger, M.J., and Davis, D.: Studies on relation of clinical manifestations of angina pectoris, coronary thrombosis, and myocardial infarction to pathologic findings with significance of collateral circulation, Am. Heart J. **19**:1, 1940.

132. James, T.N.: Anatomy of the coronary arteries, New York, 1961, Paul B. Hoeber, Inc.

133. Maseri, A., Chierchia, S., and L'Abbate, A.: Pathogenetic mechanisms underlying the clinical events associated with atherosclerotic heart disease, Circulation **62**(suppl. V): 3, 1980.

134. Prinzmetal, M., et al.: Studies on coronary circulation: collateral circulation of normal human heart by coronary perfusion with radioactive erythrocytes and glass spheres, Am. Heart J. **33**:420, 1947.

135. Rees, J.R.: The myocardial collateral circulation, Br. Heart J. **31**:1, 1969.

136. Roberts, J.T.: Vessels of heart. In Luisada, A.A., editor: Development and structure of the cardiovascular system, New York, 1961, McGraw-Hill Book Co.
137. Schlesinger, M.J.: Relation of anatomic pattern to pathologic conditions of coronary arteries, Arch. Pathol. 30:403, 1940.
138. Truex, R.C.: Distribution of coronary arteries. In Likoff, W., and Moyer, J.H., editors: The distribution of the human coronary arteries, Coronary heart disease, New York, 1963, Grune & Stratton, Inc.

Coronary atherosclerosis

139. Albrinck, M.J.: Triglycerides, lipoproteins, and coronary artery disease, Arch. Intern. Med. 109:345, 1962.
140. American Association Committee Report: Risk factors and coronary disease, Circulation 62:449A, 1980.
141. Antonis, A., and Bersohn, I: Serum-triglyceride levels in South African Europeans and Bantu and in ischaemic heart-disease, Lancet 1:998, 1960.
142. Benditt, E.P.: Evidence for a monoclonal origin of human atherosclerotic plaques and some implications, Circulation 50:650, 1974.
143. Duguid, J.B.: Role of connective tissue in arterial disease. In Page, I.H., editor: Connective tissue, thrombosis, and atherosclerosis, New York, 1959, Academic Press, Inc.
144. Edwards, J.E.: Pathologic spectrum of occlusive coronary arterial disease, Lab Invest. 5:475, 1956.
145. Enos, W.F., Holmes, R.H., and Beyer, J.: Coronary disease among United States soldiers killed in action in Korea: preliminary report, J.A.M.A. 152:1090, 1953.
146. Glagov, S., Rowley, D.A., and Kohut, R.I.: Atherosclerosis of human aorta and its coronary and renal arteries: a consideration of some hemodynamic factors which may be related to the marked differences in atherosclerotic involvement of the coronary and renal arteries, Arch. Pathol. 72:558, 1961.
147. Gore, I., et al.: Coronary atherosclerosis and myocardial infarction in Kyushu, Japan and Boston, Massachusetts, Am. J. Cardiol. 10:400, 1962.
148. Gresham, G.A.: Early events in atherogenesis, Lancet 1:614, 1975.
149. Hardin, N.J., Minick, R., and Murphy, G.E.: Experimental induction of atheroarteriosclerosis by the synergy of allergic injury to arteries and lipid-rich diet. III. The thickening in the pathogenesis of later developing atherosclerosis, Am. J. Pathol. 73:301, 1973.
150. Haust, M.D.: The morphogenesis and fate of potential and early atherosclerotic lesions in man, Hum. Pathol. 2:1, 1971.
151. The health consequences of smoking, Jan. 1974, U.S. Department of Health, Education, and Welfare, Public Health Service. DHEW Publ. No. (CDC) 74-8704.
152. The heart in type A behavior, Medical World News, pp. 103-104, Feb 24, 1975.
153. Horn, R.C., Jr., and Fine, G.: Types of coronary obstruction and their morphologic characteristics. In James, T.N., and Keyes, J.W., editors: The etiology of myocardial infarction, Boston, 1963, Little, Brown & Co.
154. Howell, W.L., and Manion, W.C.: The low incidence of myocardial infarction in patients with portal cirrhosis of the liver: a review of 639 cases of cirrhosis of the liver from 17,731 autopsies, Am. Heart J. 60:341, 1960.
155. Irey, N.S., and Norris, H.J.: Intimal vascular lesions associated with female reproductive steroids, Arch. Pathol. 96:227, 1973.
156. Jennings, R.B., et al.: Myocardial necrosis induced by temporary occlusion of a coronary artery in the dog, Arch. Pathol. 70:68, 1960.
157. Keys, A., and Blackburn, H.: Background of the patient with coronary heart disease, Prog. Cardiovasc. Dis. 6:14, 1963.
158. Mann, J.I., Inman, W.H.W., and Thorogood, M.: Oral contraceptive use in older women and fatal myocardial infarction, Br. Med. J. 2:445, 1976.
159. Mann, J.I., et al.: Myocardial infarction in young women with special reference to oral contraceptive practice, Br. Med. J. 2:241, 1975.
160. McKusick, V.A.: Genetic factors in arteriosclerosis, with particular reference to atherosclerosis of the coronary arteries. In Blumenthal, H.T., editor: Cowdry's arteriosclerosis, ed. 2, Springfield, Ill., 1967, Charles C Thomas, Publisher.
161. McNamara, J.J., et al.: Coronary artery disease in combat casualties in Vietnam, J.A.M.A. 216:1185; 1971.
162. Miller, G.J., and Miller, N.E.: Plasma-high-density-lipoprotein concentration and development of ischemic heart-disease, Lancet 1:16, 1975.
163. Moon, H.D., and Rinehart, J.F.: Histogenesis of coronary arteriosclerosis, Circulation 6:481, 1952.
164. Parker, F.: An electron microscopic study of experimental atherosclerosis, Am. J. Pathol. 36:19, 1960.
165. Paterson, J.C.: The reaction of the arterial wall to intramural hemorrhage. In Symposium on atherosclerosis, Washington, D.C., 1954, National Academy of Sciences–National Research Council.
166. Peacock, P.B.: Atherosclerotic heart disease and the environment, Trans. N.Y. Acad. Sci. 35:631, 1973.
167. Pitt, B., et al.: Location of coronary arterial occlusions and their relation to the arterial pattern, Circulation 28:35, 1963.
168. Punsar, S., et al.: Coronary heart disease and drinking water: a search in two Finnish male cohorts for epidemiologic evidence of a water factor, J. Chronic Dis. 28:259, 1975.
169. Ritterband, A.B., et al.: Gonadal function and the development of coronary heart disease, Circulation 27:237, 1963.
170. Rivin, A.U., and Dimitroff, S.P.: The incidence and severity of atherosclerosis in estrogen-treated males, and in females with a hypoestrogenic or a hyperestrogenic state, Circulation 9:533, 1954.
171. Rosenman, R.H., et al.: Coronary heart disease in Western Collaborative Group Study: final follow-up experience of 8½ years, J.A.M.A. 233:872, 1975.
172. Ross, R., and Glomset, J.A.: Atherosclerosis and the arterial smooth muscle cell: proliferation of smooth muscle is a key event in the genesis of the lesions of atherosclerosis, Science 180:1332, 1973.
173. Ruebner, B.H., Miyai, K., and Abbey, H.: The low incidence of myocardial infarction in hepatic cirrhosis: a statistical artifact? Lancet 2:1435, 1961.
174. Russek, H.I.: Emotional stress and coronary heart disease in American physicians, dentists and lawyers, Am. J. Med. Sci. 243:616, 1962.
175. Smoking and health: report of the Advisory Committee to the Surgeon General of Public Health Service, Public Health Service Pub. No. 1103, 1964.
176. Spain, D.M.: Atherosclerosis, Sci. Am. 215:48, 1966.
177. Strong, J.P., and McGill, H.C.: The natural history of coronary atherosclerosis, Am. J. Pathol. 40:37, 1962.
178. Thomas, W.A., Hartcroft, W.S., and O'Neal, R.M.: Myocardial infarction in man and experimental animals, Arch. Pathol. 69:104, 1960.
179. Walton, K.W.: Pathogenic mechanisms in atherosclerosis, Am. J. Cardiol. 35:542, 1975.
180. Wartman, W.B.: Occlusion of coronary arteries by hemorrhage into their walls, Am. Heart J. 15:459, 1938.
181. Wissler, R.W.: Development of the artherosclerotic plaque. In Braunwald, E., editor: The myocardium: failure and infarction, New York, 1974, HP Publishing Co., Inc.
182. Wuest, J.H., Jr., Dry, T.J., and Edwards, J.E.: Degree of coronary atherosclerosis in bilaterally oophorectomized women, Circulation 7:801, 1953.
183. Yater, W.M., et al.: Cornoary artery disease in men 18 to 39 years of age: report of 866 cases, 450 with necroscopy examinations, Am. Heart J. 36:334, 1948.

Other lesions of coronary arteries

184. Burch, G.E., and Winsor, T.: Syphilitic coronary stenosis with myocardial infarction, Am. Heart J. 24:740, 1942.
185. Crocker, D.W., Sobin, S., and Thomas, W.C.: Aneurysms of the coronary arteries: report of three cases in infants and review of the literature, Am. J. Pathol. 33:819, 1957.
186. Foord, A.G., and Lewis, R.D.: Primary dissecting aneurysms of peripheral and pulmonary arteries: dissecting hemorrhage of media, Arch. Pathol. 68:553, 1959.
187. Gore, I., Smith, J., and Clancy, R.: Congenital aneurysms of the coronary arteries with a report of a case, Circulation 19:221, 1959.

188. Gower, N.D., and Pinkerton, J.R.H.: Idiopathic arterial calcification in infancy, Arch. Dis. Child. **38**:408, 1963.
189. Gross, L., Dugel, M.A., and Epstein, E.Z.: Lesions of coronary arteries and their branches in rheumatic fever, Am. J. Pathol. **11**:253, 1935.
190. Moran, J.J.: Idiopathic arterial calcification of infancy: a clinicopathologic study. In Sommers, S.C., editor: Pathology annual, New York, 1975, Appleton-Century-Crofts.
191. Shrader, E.L., Bawell, M.B., and Moragues, V.: Coronary embolism, Circulation **14**:1159, 1956.
192. Woodruff, I.O.: Cardiovascular syphilis, Am. J. Med. **4**:248, 1948.

Myocardial infarction

193. Barrie, H.J., and Urbach, P.G.: The cellular changes in myocardial infarction, Can. Med. Assoc. J. **77**:100, 1957.
194. Batsakis, J.G.: Serum enzymes in cardiovascular diseases, Laboratory Scope **1**:2, 1969.
195. Burch, G.E., DePasquale, N.P., and Phillips, J.H.: Clinical manifestations of papillary muscle dysfunction, Arch. Intern. Med. **112**:158, 1963.
196. Caulfield, J., and Klionski, B.: Myocardial ischemia and early infarction: an electron microscopic study, Am. J. Pathol. **35**:489, 1959.
197. Chandler, A.B.: Relationship of coronary thrombosis to myocardial infarction, Mod. Concepts Cardiovasc. Dis. **44**:1, 1975.
198. Chapman, D.W., Amad, K., and Cooley, D.A.: Ventricular aneurysm: fourteen cases subjected to cardiac bypass repair using the pump oxygenator, Am. J. Cardiol. **8**:633, 1961.
199. Cheitlin, M.D., McAllister, H.A., and de Castro, C.M.: Myocardial infarction without atherosclerosis, J.A.M.A. **231**:951, 1975.
200. Cushing, E.H., et al.: Infarction of cardiac auricles (atria): clinical, pathological, and experimental studies, Br. Heart J. **4**:17, 1942.
201. Dreifus, L.S., Oslick, T., and Likoff, W.: Cardiac arrhythmias in acute myocardial infarction. In Likoff, W., and Moyer, J.H., editors: Coronary heart disease, New York, 1963, Grune & Stratton, Inc.
202. Edmondson, H.A., and Hoxie, H.J.: Hypertension and cardiac rupture, Am. Heart J. **24**:719, 1942.
203. Friedberg, C.K.: Controversial problems regarding coronary heart disease. In Lidoff, W., and Moyer, J.H., editors: Coronary heart disease, New York, 1963, Grune & Stratton, Inc.
204. Gould, S.E., and Cawley, L.P.: Incidence of unsuspected healed myocardial infarction in a general hospital. In Rosenbaum, F.F., and Belknap, E.L. editors: Work and the heart, New York, 1959, Harper & Row, Publishers.
205. Harder, H.I., and Brown, A.F.: Torsion patterns of papillary muscle: review of literature; report of case, Calif. Med. **83**:452, 1955.
206. Heine, W.I., et al.: Antibodies to cardiac tissue in acute ischemic heart disease, Am. J. Cardiol. **17**:798, 1966.
207. Hellerstein, H.K., and Martin, J.W.: Incidence of thromboembolic lesions accompanying myocardial infarction, Am. Heart J. **33**:443, 1947.
208. Hoch-Ligeti, C., and Lan, C.W.: Morphology and frequency of early myocardial damage in various diseases, Am. J. Clin. Pathol. **62**:455, 1974.
209. Jennings, R.B., Crout, R., and Smetters, G.W.: Studies on distribution and localization of potassium in early myocardial ischemic injury, Arch. Pathol. **63**:586, 1957.
210. Jennings, R.B., Kaltenbach, J.P., and Smetters, G.W.: Enzymatic changes in acute myocardine ischemic injury, Arch. Pathol. **64**:10, 1957.
211. Jennings, R.B., et al.: Electrolyte alterations in acute myocardial ischemic injury, Circ. Res. **14**:260, 1964.
212. Kent, S.P., and Diseker, M.: Early myocardial ischemia: study of histochemical changes in dogs, Lab. Invest. **4**:398, 1955.
213. Khan, A.H., and Haywood, L.J.: Myocardial infarction in nine patients with radiologically patent coronary arteries, N. Engl. J. Med. **291**:427, 1974.
214. Majno, G., Bouchardy, B., and Joliat, G.: Histopathology of myocardial infarcts: the earliest cellular lesion, Am. J. Pathol. **70**:82a, 1973.
215. Mallory, G.K., White, P.D., and Salcedo-Salgar, J.: Speed of healing of myocardial infarction: study of pathologic anatomy in 72 cases, Am. Heart J. **18**:647, 1939.
216. McQuay, N.W., Edwards. J.E., and Burchell, H.B.: Types of death in acute myocardial infarction, Arch. Intern. Med. **96**:1, 1955.
217. Morales, A.R., and Fine, C.: Early human myocardial infarction: a histochemical study, Arch. Pathol. **82**:9, 1966.
218. Morales, A.R., Romanelli, R., and Boucek, R.J.: The mural left anterior descending coronary artery, strenuous exercise, and sudden death, Circulation **62**:230, 1980.
219. Naeim, F., de la Maza, L.M., and Robbins, S.L.: Cardiac rupture, myocardial infarction, Circulation **45**:1231, 1972.
220. Pell, S., and D'Alonzo, C.A.: Acute myocardial infarction in a large industrial population: report of a 6-year study of 1356 cases, J.A.M.A. **185**:831, 1963.
221. Plotz, M.: Coronary heart disease, New York, 1957, Paul B. Hoeber, Inc.
222. Roberts, W.C., and Buja, L.M.: The frequency and significance of coronary arterial thrombi and other observations in fatal acute myocardial infarction: a study of 107 necropsy patients, Am. J. Med. **52**:425, 1972.
223. Schlesinger, M.J., and Reiner, L.: Focal myocytolysis of heart, Am. J. Pathol. **31**:443, 1955.
224. Schuster, E.H., and Buckley, B.H.: Expansion of transmural myocardial infarction: a pathophysiologic factor in myocardial rupture, Circulation **60**:1532, 1979.
225. Selye, H.: The pluricausal cardiopathies, Springfield, Ill. 1961, Charles C Thomas, Publisher.
226. Spiekerman, R.E., et al.: The spectrum of coronary heart disease in a community of 30,000: a clinicopathologic study, Circulation **25**:57, 1962.
227. Survey of coronary occlusion, A.M.A. News, July 6, 1965.
228. Wachstein, M., and Meisel, E.: Succinic dehydrogenase activity in myocardial infarction and in induced myocardial necrosis, Am. J. Pathol. **31**:353, 1955.
229. Walson, A., Hackel, D.B., and Estes, E.A.: Acute coronary occlusion and the "power failure" syndrome, Am. Heart J. **79**:613, 1970.
230. Wartman, W.B., and Souders, J.C.: Localization of myocardial infarcts with respect to muscle bundles of heart, Am. Heart J. **79**:613, 1970.
231. White, L.P.: Serum enzymes: serum lactic dehydrogenase in myocardial infarction, N. Engl. J. Med. **255**:984, 1956.
232. Yokoyama, H.O., et al.: Histochemical studies of early experimental myocardial infarction: periodic acid–Schiff method, Arch. Pathol. **59**:347, 1955.

Inflammatory diseases
Rheumatic fever and rheumatic heart disease
Incidence and etiology

233. Begg, T.B., Kerr, J.W., and Knowles, B.R.: Rheumatic fever in adolescents and adults, Br. Med. J. **2**:223, 1962.
234. Cardiovascular diseases in the United States—facts and figures: The American Heart Association in cooperation with the National Heart Institute and the Heart Disease Control Program, Public Health Service, New York, 1965, U.S. Department of Health, Education, and Welfare.
235. Catanzaro, F.J., et al.: Symposium on rheumatic fever and rheumatic heart disease: role of streptococcus in pathogenesis of rheumatic fever, Am. J. Med. **17**:749, 1954.
236. Cavelti, P.A.: Studies on pathogenesis of rheumatic fever: experimental production of autoantibodies to heart, skeletal muscle, and connective tissue, Arch. Pathol. **44**:1, 13-27, 1947.
237. Coburn, A.F., and Pauli, R.H.: Interaction of host and bacterium in development of communicability by *Streptococcus haemolyticus*, J. Exp. Med. **73**:551, 1941.
238. Garcia-Palmieri, M.R.: Rheumatic fever and rheumatic heart disease as seen in the tropics, Am. Heart J. **64**:577, 1962.
239. Griffith, G.C.: Rheumatic fever: its recognition and treatment, J.A.M.A. **133**:974, 1947.
240. Kaplan, M.H., and Svec, K.H.: Immunologic relation of streptococcal and tissue antigens. III. Presence in human sera of strep-

tococcal antibody cross-reactive with heart tissue: association with streptococcal infection, rheumatic fever, and glomerulonephritis, J. Exp. Med. **119**:651, 1964.

241. Murphy, G.E., and Swift, H.F.: Induction of rheumatic-like cardiac lesions, closely resembling those of rheumatic fever, in rabbits following repeated skin infections with group A streptococci, J. Exp. Med. **89**:687, 1949.

242. Murphy, G.E., and Swift, H.F.: Induction of rheumatic-like cardiac lesions in rabbits by repeated focal infections with group A streptococci: comparison with cardiac lesions of serum disease, J. Exp. Med. **91**:485, 1950.

243. Pearce, J.M.: Heart disease and filterable viruses, Circulation **21**:448, 1960.

244. Rammelkamp, C.H., Jr., Wannamaker, L.W., and Denny, F.W.: Epidemiology and prevention of rheumatic fever, Bull. N.Y. Acad. Med. **28**:321, 1952.

245. Rich, A.R., and Gregory, J.E.: Experimental evidence that lesions with basic characteristics of rheumatic carditis can result from anaphylactic hypersensitivity, Bull. Johns Hopkins, Hosp. **73**:239, 1943.

246. Saslaw, M.S.: Rheumatic fever in subtropical climate: clinical behavior and management, J. Florida Med. Assoc. **41**:357, 1954.

247. Saslaw M.S., and Johnson, L.C.: Frequency of rheumatic heart disease in Miami, Florida: autopsy findings, Am. Heart J. **53**:814, 1957.

248. Saslaw, M.S., Hernandez, F.A., and Randolph, H.E.: Five and ten year follow-up study of rheumatic patients: role of climate and environment, Am. J. Cardiol. **3**:754, 1959.

249. Saslaw, M.S., and Streitfeld, M.M.: Group A beta hemolytic streptococci in relation to rheumatic fever: study of school children in Miami, Florida, Am. J. Dis. Child. **92**:550, 1956.

250. Shaper, A.G.: Cardiovascular disease in the tropics. I. Rheumatic heart, Br. Med. J. **3**:683, 1972.

251. Shefferman, M.M., et al.: Acute rheumatic fever in Puerto Rico, Am. J. Dis. Child. **110**:239, 1965.

252. Siegel, A.C., Johnson, E.E., and Stollerman, G.H.: Controlled studies of streptococcal pharyngitis in a pediatric population. I. Factors related to the attack rate of rheumatic fever, N. Engl. J. Med. **265**:559, 1961.

253. Special Committee Report of the American Heart Association: Jones criteria (revised) for guidance in the diagnosis of rheumatic fever, Circulation **32**:664, 1965.

254. Tamer, D.M.: Acute rheumatic fever in a south Florida county hospital, Circulation **50**:765, 1974.

255. Wilson, M.G.: Advances in rheumatic fever, New York, 1962, Harper & Row, Publishers, Inc.

Pathologic anatomy

256. Becker, C.G., and Murphy, G.E.: Demonstration of contractile protein in endothelium and cells of the heart valves, endocardium, intima, arteriosclerotic plaques, and Aschoff bodies of rheumatic heart disease, Am. J. Pathol. **55**:1, 1969.

257. Clawson, B.J.: Rheumatic heart disease: analysis of 796 cases, Am. Heart J. **20**:454, 1940.

258. Clawson, B.J.: Relation of "Anitschkow myocyte" to rheumatic inflammation, Arch. Pathol. **32**:760, 1941.

259. Dalldorf, F.G., and Murphy, G.E.: Relationship of Aschoff bodies in cardiac arterial appendages to the natural history of rheumatic heart, Am. J. Pathol. **37**:507, 1960.

260. Ehrlich, J.C., and Lapan, B.: Anitschkow "myocyte," Arch. Pathol. **28**:361, 1938.

261. Enticknap, J.B.: Biopsy of left auricle in mitral stenosis, Br. Heart J. **15**:37, 1953.

262. Friedberg, C.K., and Gross, L.: Pericardial lesions in rheumatic fever, Am. J. Pathol. **12**:183, 1936.

263. Gross, L., and Ehrlich, J.C.: Studies on myocardial Aschoff body: descriptive classification of lesions, Am. J. Pathol. **10**:467, 1934.

264. Gross, L., and Friedberg, C.K.: Lesions of cardiac valve rings in rheumatic fever, Am. J. Pathol. **12**:469, 1936.

265. Gross, L., and Friedberg, C.K.: Lesions of cardiac valves in rheumatic fever, Am. J. Pathol. **12**:855, 1936.

266. Hadfield, G., and Garrod, R.P.: Recent advances in pathology, ed. 5, Philadelphia, 1947, McGraw-Hill Book Co.

267. Hall, E.M., and Anderson, L.R.: Incidence of rheumatic stigmas in hearts which are usually considered nonrheumatic, Am. Heart J. **25**:64, 1943.

268. Janton, O.H., et al.: Results of surgical treatment for mitral stenosis: analysis of 100 consecutive cases, Circulation **6**:321, 1952.

269. Lannigan, R.: The rheumatic process in the left auricular appendage, J. Pathol. Bacteriol. **77**:49, 1959.

270. Manchester, B., et al.: Aschoff bodies in left auricular appendages of patients with mitral stenosis: clinicopathologic study, including postoperative follow-up, Arch. Intern. Med. **95**:231, 1955.

271. McKeown, F.: Left auricular appendage in mitral stenosis, Br. Heart J. **15**:433, 1953.

272. Murphy, G.E.: The characteristic rheumatic lesions of striated and of non-striated or smooth muscle cells known as Aschoff bodies and those myogenic components known as Aschoff cells or as Anitschkow cells or myocytes, Medicine **42**:73, 1963.

273. Pappenheimer, A.W., and von Glahn, W.C.: Lesions of aorta associated with acute rheumatic fever, and with chronic cardiac disease of rheumatic origin, J. Med. Res. **44**:489, 1924.

274. Peery, T.M.: Brucellosis and heart disease: shaky foundations of "rheumatic" heart disease, Postgrad. Med. **19**:323, 1956.

275. Roberts, W.C., and Virmani, R.: Aschoff bodies at necropsy in valvular heart disease, Circulation **57**:803, 1978.

276. Sabiston, D.C., Jr., and Follis, R.H., Jr.: Lesions in auricular appendages removed at operations for mitral stenosis of presumed rheumatic origin, Bull. Johns Hopkins Hosp. **91**:178, 1952.

277. Saphir, O.: The Oschoff nodule, Am. J. Clin. Pathol. **31**:534, 1959.

278. Saphir, O., and Langendorf, R.: Nonspecific myocarditis in acute rheumatic fever, Am. Heart J. **46**:432, 1953.

279. Saphir, O., and Lowenthal, M.: Changes in endocardium of pigs simulating rheumatic stigmata of man, Am. J. Pathol. **27**:211, 1951.

280. Statistical bulletin, Metropolitan Life Insurance Co. **47**:8, 1966.

281. Tedeschi, C.G., Wagner, B.M., and Pani, K.C.: Studies in rheumatic fever: clinical significance of Aschoff body based on morphologic observations, Arch. Pathol. **60**:408, 1955.

282. Wagner, B.M., and Tedeschi, C.G.: Studies in rheumatic fever: origin of cardiac giant cells, Arch. Pathol. **60**:423, 1955.

283. Wedum, B.G., and McGuire, J.W.: Origin of the Aschoff body, Ann. Rheum. Dis. **22**:127, 1963.

Extracardiac lesions

284. Angevine, D.M.: Pathology of rheumatic disease, Radiology **49**:1, 1947.

285. Beatty, E.C., Jr.: Rheumatic-like nodules occurring in nonrheumatic children, Arch. Pathol. **68**:154, 1959.

286. Bruetsch. W.L.: Late cerebral sequelae of rheumatic fever Arch. Intern. Med. **73**:472, 1944.

287. Bruetsch, W.L.: Rheumatic brain disease: late sequel of rheumatic fever, J.A.M.A. **134**:450, 1947.

288. Denst, J., and Neuberger, K.T.: Intracranial vascular lesions in late rheumatic heart disease, Arch. Pathol. **46**:191, 1948.

289. Keil, H.: Rheumatic subcutaneous nodules and simulating lesions, Medicine **17**:261, 1938.

290. Scott, R.F., Thomas, W.A., and Kissane, J.M.: Rheumatic pneumonitis: pathologic features, J. Pediatr. **54**:60, 1959.

291. Sokoloff, L., McCluskey, R.T., and Bunim, J.J.: Vascularity of early subcutaneous nodule of rheumatoid arthritis, Arch. Pathol. **55**:475, 1953.

Prognosis and causes of death

292. Adams, M.J.T.: Multiple calcific embolism following mitral valvotomy, Br. Heart J. **23**:333, 1961.

293. Bailey, C.P., and Morse, D.P.: Mitral commissurotomy performed from the right side, J. Thorac. Surg. **33**:427, 1957.

294. Bland, E.F.: Declining severity of rheumatic fever: a comparative study of the past four decades, N. Engl. J. Med. **262**:597, 1960.

295. Bland, E.F., and Jones, T.D.: Rheumatic fever and rheumatic heart disease: 20 year report on 1000 patients followed since childhood, Circulation 4:836, 1951.

296. Feinstein, A.R., et al.: Rheumatic fever in children and adolescents: a long term epidemiologic study of subsequent prophylaxis, streptococcal infections, and clinical sequelae: VII. Cardiac changes and sequelae, Ann. Intern. Med. 60:87, 1964.

297. Holley, K.E., et al.: Calcific embolization associated with valvotomy for calcific aortic stenosis, Circulation 28:175, 1963.

298. Wallach, J.B., Borgatta, E.F., and Angrist, A.A.: Rheumatic heart disease, Springfield, 1962, Charles C Thomas, Publisher.

299. Wallach, J.B., Lukash, L., and Angrist, A.A.: Mechanism of death in rheumatic heart disease in different age periods, Am. J. Clin. Pathol. 26:360, 1956.

Heart in rheumatoid arthritis

300. Baggenstoss, A.H., and Rosenberg, E.F.: Unusual cardiac lesions associated with chronic multiple rheumatoid arthritis, Arch. Pathol. 37:54, 1944.

301. Clark, W.S., Kulka, J.P., and Bauer, W.: Rheumatoid aortitis with aortic regurgitation: an unusual manifestation of rheumatoid arthritis (including spondylitis), Am. J. Med. 22:580, 1957.

302. Cruickshank, B.: Heart lesions in rheumatoid disease J. Pathol. Bacteriol. 76:223, 1958.

303. Graham, D.C., and Smythe, H.A.: Bull. Rheum. Dis. 9:171, 1958.

304. Kulka, J.P.: The vascular lesions associated with rheumatoids arthritis, Bull. Rheum. Dis. 10:201, 1959.

305. Lebowitz, W.B.: The heart in rheumatoid arthritis (rheumatoid disease): a clinical and pathological study of sixty-two cases, Ann. Intern. Med. 58:102, 1963.

306. Reed, W.B.: Psoriatic arthritis: a complete clinical study of 86 patients, Acta Derm. Venereol. 41:396, 1961.

307. Rodnan, G.P., et al.: Reiter's syndrome and aortic insufficiency, J.A.M.A. 189:889, 1964.

308. Sobin, L.H., and Hagstrom, J.W.C.: Lesions of cardiac conduction tissue in rheumatoid aortitis, J.A.M.A. 180:1, 1962.

309. Sokoloff, L.: Heart in rheumatoid arthritis, Am. Heart J. 45:635, 1953.

310. Toone, E.C., Pierce, E.L., and Hennigar, G.R.: Aortitis and aortic regurgitation associated with rheumatoid spondylitis, Am. J. Med. 26:255, 1959.

Syphilitic heart disease

311. Centers for Disease Control annual summary 1980: reported morbidity and mortality in the United States, Morbid. Mortal. Weekly Rep. 29:78, 1981.

312. Gore, I.: Myocarditis in infectious diseases, Am. Pract. 1:292, 1947.

313. Hamman, L., and Rich, A.R.: Clinical pathological conference: case of syphilitic myocarditis, Int. Clin. 4:221, 1934.

314. Jason, R.S.: Insufficiency of aortic valve due to syphilis: study of its genesis, Arch. Pathol. 32:409, 1941.

315. Koletsky, S.: Syphilitic cardiovascular disease and bacterial endocarditis, Am. Heart J. 23:208, 1942.

316. Lisa, J.R., Solomon, C., and Eckstein, D.: Heart in combined syphilitic aortic valvulitis and rheumatic heart disease, Arch. Pathol. 33:37, 1942.

317. Martland, H.S.: Syphilis of aorta and heart, Am. Heart J. 6:1, 1930.

318. Pratt-Thomas, H.R.: Diffuse gummatous myocarditis, Arch. Pathol. 36:80, 1943.

319. Sager, R.V., and Sohval, A.R.: Combined syphilitic and rheumatic disease of aortic valve: report of 3 cases, Arch. Pathol. 17:729, 1934.

320. Saphir, O.: Syphilitic myocarditis, Arch. Pathol. 13:266, 1932.

321. Saphir, O., and Scott, R.W.: Involvement of aortic valve in syphilitic aortitis, Am. J. Pathol. 3:527, 1927.

322. Spain, D.M., and Johannsen, M.W.: Three cases of localized gummatous myocarditis, Am. Heart J. 24:689, 1942.

Endocarditis

Atypical verrucous (Libman-Sacks) endocarditis

323. Gross, L.: Cardiac lesions in Libman-Sacks disease, with consideration of its relationship to acute diffuse erythematosus, Am. J. Pathol. 16:375, 1940.

324. Humphreys, E.M.: Cardiac lesions of acute disseminated lupus erythematosus, Ann. Intern. Med. 28:12, 1948.

325. Libman, E.: Characterization of various forms of endocarditis, J.A.M.A. 80:813, 1923.

326. Libman, E., and Sacks, B.: A hitherto undescribed form of valvular and mural endocarditis, Arch. Intern. Med. 33:701, 1924.

Nonbacterial thrombotic endocarditis

327. Allen, A.C., and Sirota, J.H.: Morphogenesis and significance of degenerative verrucal endocardiosis (terminal endocarditis, endocarditis simplex, nonbacterial thrombotic endocarditis), Am. J. Pathol. 20:1025, 1944.

328. Angrist, A.A., and Marquiss, J.: Changing morphologic picture of endocarditis since advent of chemotherapy and antibiotic agents, Am. J. Pathol. 30:39, 1954.

329. Barry, W.E., and Scarpelli, D.: Nonbacterial thrombotic endocarditis: a clinicopathologic study, Arch. Intern. Med. 109:151, 1962.

330. Gross, L., and Friedberg, C.R.: Nonbacterial thrombotic endocarditis: classification and general description, Arch. Intern. Med. 58:620, 1936.

331. MacDonald, R.A., and Robbins, S.L.: The significance of nonbacterial thrombotic endocarditis: an autopsy and clinical study of 78 cases, Ann. Intern. Med. 46:255, 1957.

332. McKay, D.G.: Disseminated intravascular coagulation, New York, 1965, Harper & Row, Publishers, Inc.

Infective endocarditis

333. Allen, A.C.: The kidney, ed. 2, New York, 1962, Grune & Stratton, Inc.

334. Angrist, A.A., and Oka, M.: Pathogenesis of bacterial endocarditis, J.A.M.A. 183:249, 1963.

335. Angrist, A.A., Oka, M., and Nakao, K.: Prevention and control of bacterial endocarditis, N.Y.J. Med. 68:1824, 1968.

336. Braimbridge, M.V.: Cardiac surgery and bacterial endocarditis, Lancet 1:1307, 1969.

337. Burch, G.E., and De Pasquale, N.P.: Viral endocarditis, Am. Heart J. 67:721, 1964.

338. Cates, J.E., and Christie, R.V.: Subacute bacterial endocarditis: review of 442 patients treated in 14 centres appointed by Penicillin Trials Committee of Medical Research Council, Q. J. Med. 20:93, 1951.

339. Chase, R.M., Jr.: Infective endocarditis today, Med. Clin. North Am. 57:1383, 1973.

340. Cornell, A., and Shookhoff, H.B.: Actinomycosis of heart simulating rheumatic fever: report of 3 cases of cardiac actinomycosos with review of literature, Arch. Intern. Med. 74:11, 1944.

341. Denton, C., et al.: Bacterial endocarditis following cardiac surgery, Circulation 15:525, 1957.

342. Friedberg, C.K., Goldman, H.M., and Field, L.E.: Study of bacterial endocarditis, Arch. Intern. Med. 107:6, 1961.

343. Geiger, A.J., and Durlacher, S.H.: Fate of endocardial vegetations following penicillin treatment, Am. J. Pathol. 23:1023, 1947.

344. Glaser, R.J., and Rifkind, D.: The diagnosis and treatment of bacterial endocarditis, Med. Clin. North Am. 47:1285, 1963.

345. Grist, N.R.: Rickettsial endocarditis, Br. Med. J. 53:8, 1963.

346. Hamburger, M.: Acute and subacute bacterial endocarditis, Arch. Intern. Med. 112:1, 1963.

347. Hayward, G.W.: Infective endocarditis: a changing disease, Br. Med. J. 2:706, 1973.

348. Hirsch, S.R., and Koch, M.L.: *Herellea (Bacterium anitratum)* endocarditis, J.A.M.A. 187:148, 1964.

349. Keefer, C.S.: Subacute bacterial endocarditis: active cases without bacteremia, Ann. Intern. Med. 11:714, 1937.

350. Kerr, A., Jr.: Subacute bacterial endocarditis, Springfield, Ill., 1955, Charles C Thomas, Publisher.

351. Lerner, P.I., and Weinstein, L.: Infective endocarditis in the antibiotic era, N. Engl. J. Med. 274:199, 1966.

352. Madison, J., et al.: Prosthetic aortic valvular endocarditis, Circulation 51:940, 1975.

353. Merchant, R.K., et al.: Fungal endocarditis: review of the literature and report of three cases, Ann. Intern. Med. 48:242, 1958.

354. Moore, R.A.: Cellular mechanism of recovery after treatment with penicillin: subacute bacterial endocarditis, J. Lab. Clin. Med. **31**:1279, 1946.

355. Morgan, W.L., and Bland, E.F.: Bacterial endocarditis in the antibiotic era: with special reference to the later complications, Circulation **19**:753, 1959.

356. Pankey, G.A.: Subacute bacterial endocarditis at the University of Minnesota Hospital, 1939 through 1959, Ann. Intern. Med. **55**:550, 1961.

357. Pankey, G.A.: Acute bacterial endocarditis at the University of Minnesota Hospitals, Am. Heart J. **64**:583, 1962.

358. Robinson, M.J., and Ruedy, J.: Sequelae of bacterial endocarditis, Am. J. Med. **32**:922, 1962.

359. Robinson, M.J., et al.: Infective endocarditis at autopsy, Am. J. Med. **52**:492, 1972.

360. Saphir, O.: Nonrheumatic inflammatory diseases of the heart. In Gould, S.E., editor: Pathology of the heart, ed. 2, Springfield, Ill., 1960, Charles C Thomas, Publisher.

361. Sheldon, W.H., and Golden, A.: Abscesses of valve rings of heart, frequent but not well recognized complication of acute bacterial endocarditis, Circulation **4**:1, 1951.

362. Sohal, R.S., and Burch, G.E.: Electron microscopy study of the endocardium in coxsackie virus B4 infected mice, Am. J. Pathol. **55**:133, 1969.

363. Soler-Bechara, J., et al.: *Candida* endocarditis, Am. J. Cardiol. **13**:820, 1964.

364. Sorrell, W.B., and White, L.V.: Acute bacterial endocarditis caused by variant of genus *Herellea*: report of case, Am. J. Clin. Pathol. **23**:134, 1953.

365. Uwaydah, M.M., and Weinberg, A.N.: Bacterial endocarditis—a changing pattern, N. Engl. J. Med. **273**:1231, 1965.

366. Weinstein, L.: "Modern" infective endocarditis, J.A.M.A. **233**:260, 1975.

367. Wilson, L.M.: Etiology of bacterial endocarditis before and since the introduction of antibiotics, Ann. Intern. Med. **58**:946, 1963.

368. Wilson, L.M.: Pathology of fatal bacterial endocarditis before and since the introduction of antibiotics, Ann. Intern. Med. **58**:84, 1963.

Valvular deformities

369. Barr, D.P., Rothbard, S., and Eder, H.A.: Atherosclerosis and aortic stenosis in hypercholesteremic xanthomatosis, J.A.M.A. **156**:943, 1954.

370. Darvill, F.T.: Aortic insufficiency of unusual etiology, J.A.M.A. **184**:753, 1963.

371. Frable, W.J.: Mucinous degeneration of the cardiac valves: the "floppy valve" syndrome, J. Thorac. Cardiovasc. Surg. **58**:62, 1969.

372. Hall, E.M., and Ichioka, T.: Etiology of calcified nodular aortic stenosis, Am. J. Pathol. **16**:761, 1940.

373. Hutchins, G.M., and Maron, B.J.: Development of endocardial valvuloids with valvular insufficiency, Arch. Pathol. **93**:401, 1972.

374. Karsner, H.T., and Koletsky, S.: Calcific disease of the aortic valve, Philadelphia, 1947, J.B. Lippincott Co.

375. Korn, D., De Sanctis, R.W., and Sell, S.: Massive calcification of the mitral annulus: a clinicopathological study of fourteen cases, N. Engl. J. Med. **267**:900, 1962.

376. McCarthy, L.J., and Wolf, P.L.: Mucoid degeneration of heart valves; "blue valve syndrome," Am. J. Clin. Pathol. **54**:852, 1970.

377. Marshall, C.E., and Shappell, S.D.: Sudden death and the ballooning posterior leaflet syndrome: detailed anatomic and histochemical investigation, Arch. Pathol. **98**:134, 1974.

378. Monckeberg, J.G.: Der normale histologische Bau und die Sclerose der Aortenklappen, Virchows Arch. (Pathol. Anat.) **176**:472, 1904.

379. Peery, T.M.: Brucellosis and heart diseases. IV. Etiology of calcific aortic stenosis, J.A.M.A. **166**:1123, 1958.

380. Peery, T.M., and Belter, L.F.: Brucellosis and heart disease. II. Fatal brucellosis: a review of the literature and report of new cases, Am. J. Pathol. **36**:673, 1960.

381. Roberts, W.C.: Anatomically isolated valvular disease, Am. J. Med. **49**:151, 1970.

Myocarditis

382. Allen, A.C., and Spitz, S.: Comparative study of pathology of scrub typhus (tsutsugamushi disease) and other rickettsial diseases, Am. J. Pathol. **21**:603, 1945.

383. Beutner, E.H., et al.: Studies on autoantibodies in myasthenia gravis, J.A.M.A. **182**:46, 1962.

384. Blankenhorn, M.A., and Gall, E.A.: Myocarditis and myocardosis: clinocopathologic appraisal, Circulation **13**:217, 1956.

385. Burke, J.S., Medline, N.M., and Katz, A.: A giant cell myocarditis and myasthenia gravis, Arch. Pathol. **88**:359, 1969.

386. de la Chapelle, C.E., and Dossmann, C.E.: Myocarditis, Circulation **10**:747, 1954.

387. Dighiera, J., et al.: Echinococcus disease of the heart, Circulation **17**:127, 1958.

388. Dilling, N.V.: Giant-cell myocarditis, J. Pathol. Bacteriol. **71**:295, 1956.

389. French, A.J.: Hypersensitivity in pathogenesis of histopathological changes associated with sulfonamide chemotherapy, Am. J. Pathol. **22**:679, 1946.

390. French, A.J., and Weller, C.V.: Interstitial myocarditis following clinical and experimental use of sulfonamide drugs, Am. J. Pathol. **18**:109, 1942.

391. Gore, I.: Myocardial changes in fatal diphtheria: summary of observations in 221 cases, Am. J. Sci. **215**:257, 1948.

392. Gore, I., and Saphir, O.: Myocarditis associated with acute nasophryngitis and acute tonsillitis, Am. Heart J. **34**:831, 1947.

393. Gore, I., and Saphir, O.: Myocarditis: classification of 1402 cases, Am. Heart J. **34**:827, 1947.

394. Heilbrunn, A., Kittle, C.F., and Dunn, M.: Surgical management of echinococcal cysts of the heart and pericardium, Circulation **27**:219, 1963.

395. Hooper, A.D.: Acquired toxoplasmosis: report of a case with autopsy findings, including a review of previously reported cases, Arch. Pathol. **64**:1, 1957.

396. James, T.N.: Observations on the cardiovascular involvement, including the cardiac conduction system, in progressive muscular dystrophy, Am. Heart J. **63**:48, 1962.

397. James, T.N., and Fisch, C.: Observations on the cardiovascular involvement in Friedreich's ataxia, Am. Heart J. **66**:164, 1963.

398. Kean, B.H., and Hoekenga, M.T.: Giant cell myocarditis, Am. J. Pathol. **28**:1095, 1952.

399. Long, W.H.: Granulomatous (Fiedler's) myocarditis with extracardiac involvement: a case report with sudden death, J.A.M.A. **177**:184, 1961.

400. Manion, W.C.: Scientific exhibits: myocarditis; frequent complication of systemic diseases, Arch. Pathol. **61**:329, 1956.

401. Manning, G.W.: Cardiac manifestations in Friedreich's ataxia, Am. Heart J. **39**:799, 1950.

402. Mendelow, H., and Genkins, G.: Studies in myasthenia gravis: cardiac and associated pathology, J. Mt. Sinai Hosp. **21**:218, 1954.

403. Morales, A.R., et al.: Sarcoidosis of the heart. In Sommers, S.C., editor: Pathology annual, New York, 1975, Appleton-Century-Crofts.

404. Nothacker, W.G., and Netsky, M.G.: Myocardial lesions in progressive muscular dystrophy, Arch. Pathol. **50**:578, 1950.

405. Pascoe, H.R.: Myocardial sarcoidosis: report of a case with unexpected death, Arch. Pathol. **77**:299, 1964.

406. Porter, G.H.: Sarcoid heart disease, N. Engl. J. Med. **263**:1350, 1960.

407. Reichenbach, D., and Benditt, E.P.: Myofibrillar degeneration: a common form of cardiac muscle injury, Ann. N.Y. Acad. Sci. **156**:164, 1969.

408. Richardson, H.L., Graupner, K.I., and Richardson, M.E.: Intramyocardial lesions in patients dying suddenly and unexpectedly, J.A.M.A. **195**:254, 1966.

409. Russell, D.S.: Myocarditis in Friedreich's ataxia, J. Pathol. Bacteriol. **58**:739, 1946.

410. Sanders, V.: Viral myocarditis, Am. Heart J. **66**:707, 1963.

411. Saphir, O.: Myocarditis: general review, with analysis of 240 cases, Arch. Pathol. **32**:1000, 1941.

412. Saphir, O.: Myocarditis: general review, with analysis of 240 cases, Arch. Pathol. **33**:88, 1942.

413. Saphir, O.: Isolated myocarditis, Am. Heart J. **24**:167, 1942.

414. Scotti, T.M., and Mckeown, C.E.: Sarcoidosis involving heart: report of case with sudden death, Arch. Pathol. **46**:289, 1948.

415. Storstein, O., and Austarheim, K.: Progressive muscular dystrophy of heart, Acta Med. Scand. **150**:431, 1955.

416. Tesluk, H.: Giant cell versus granulomatous myocarditis, Am. J. Clin. Pathol. **26**:1326, 1956.

417. Wainger, C.K., and Lever, W.F.: Dermatomyositis: report of 3 cases with postmortem observations, Arch. Dermatol. Syph. **59**:196, 1949.

418. Weiss, S., et al.: Scleroderma heart disease, with consideration of certain other visceral manifestations of scleroderma, Arch. Intern. Med. **71**:749, 1943.

Pericarditis

419. Cortes, F.M., editor: The pericardium and its disorders, Springfield, Ill., 1971, Charles C Thomas, Publisher.

420. Creech, O., et al.: Cholesterol pericarditis: successful treatment by pericardiectomy, Circulation **12**:193, 1955.

421. Deterling, R.A., Jr., and Humphreys, G.H., II: Factors in etiology of constrictive pericarditis, Circulation **12**:30, 1955.

422. Herrmann, G.R., et al.: Pericarditis: clinical and laboratory data of Am. Heart J. **43**:641, 1952.

423. Johnson, R.T., et al.: Acute benign pericarditis: virologic study of 34 patients, Arch. Intern. Med. **108**:823, 1961.

424. Kaltman, A.J., Schwedel, J.B., and Strauss, B.: Chronic constrictive pericarditis and rheumatic heart disease, Am. Heart J. **45**:201, 1953.

425. McPhail, J.L., et al.: Surgical management of constrictive pericarditis, J. Thorac. Cardiovasc. Surg. **53**:360, 1961.

426. Schepers, G.W.H.: Tuberculous pericarditis, Am. J. Cardiol. **9**:248, 1962.

427. Sodeman, W.A., and Smith, R.H.: Re-evaluation of the diagnostic criteria for acute pericarditis, Am. J. Med. Sci. **235**:672, 1958.

428. Spodick, D.H.: Acute pericarditis, New York, 1959, Grune & Stratton, Inc.

Disturbances of growth
Atrophy: hypertrophy and dilatation

429. Barnard, P.J.: The pathology of corpulmonale, pulmonary arteriosclerosis, and pulmonary hypertension secondary to thromboembolism, Prog. Cardiovasc. Dis. **1**:371, 1959.

430. Bishop, S.P., and Cole, C.R.: Ultrastructural changes in the canine myocardium with right ventricular hypertrophy and congestive heart failure, Lab. Invest. **20**:219, 1969.

431. Black-Schaffer, B., and Turner, M.E.: Hyperplastic infantile cardiomegaly: a form of "idiopathic hypertrophy" with or without endocardial fibroelastosis; and a comment on cardiac "atrophy," Am. J. Pathol. **34**:745, 1958.

432. Carney, J.A., and Brown, A.L., Jr.: Myofilament diameter in the normal and hypertrophic rat myocardium, Am. J. Pathol. **44**:521, 1964.

433. Connolly, E.P., and Littman, D.: Coronary arteriosclerosis and myocardial hypertrophy, N. Engl. J. Med. **245**:753, 1951.

434. Grant, R.P.: Architectonics of heart, Am. Heart J. **46**:405, 1953.

435. Jones, R.S.: Weight of heart and its chambers in hypertensive cardiovascular disease with and without failure, Circulation **7**:357, 1953.

436. Karsner, H.T., Saphir, O., and Todd, T.W.: Cardiac muscle in hypertrophy and atrophy, Am. J. Pathol. **1**:351, 1925

437. Laks, M.M., et al.: Presence of widened and multiple intercalated discs in the hypertrophied canine heart, Circ. Res. **27**:391, 1970.

438. Linzbach, A.J.: Heart failure from the point of view of qualitative anatomy, Am. J. Cardiol. **5**:370, 1960.

439. MacMahon, H.E.: Hyperplasia and regeneration of myocardium in infants and in children, Am. J. Pathol. **13**:845, 1937.

440. Maron, B.J., and Ferrans, V.J.: Significance of multiple intercalated discs in hypertrophied human myocardium, Am. J. Pathol. **73**:81, 1973.

441. Norman, T.D., and McBroom, R.D.: Cardiac hypertrophy in rats with phenylhydrazine anemia, Circ. Res. **6**:765, 1958.

442. Richter, G.W., and Kellner, A.: Hypertrophy of the human heart at the level of fine structure: an analysis and two postulates, J. Cell Biol. **18**:195, 1963.

443. Roberts, J.T., and Wearn, J.T.: Quantitative changes in capillary-muscle relationship in human hearts during normal growth and hypertrophy, Am. Heart J. **21**:617, 1941.

444. Rosahn, P.D.: Weight of normal heart in adult males, Yale J. Biol. Med. **14**:209, 1941.

445. Summer, R.G., and McIntosh, H.D.: Nucleic acid studies in experimental cardiomegaly, Circ. Res. **12**:170, 1963.

446. Whitaker, W., and Heath, D.: Idiopathic pulmonary hypertension: etiology, pathogenesis, diagnosis, and treatment, Prog. Cardiovasc. Dis. **1**:380, 1959.

447. Zeek, P.M.: Heart weight: weight of normal human heart, Arch. Pathol. **34**:820, 1942.

Cardiac hypertrophy in hypertension

448. Gordon, T., and Waterhouse, A.M.: Hypertension and hypertensive heart disease, J. Chronic Dis. **19**:1089, 1966.

449. Koepsell, J.E., Kuzma, J.F., and Murphy, F.D.: Hypertensive cardiovascular disease (acute) (malignant hypertension): clinical and pathologic study of 39 cases, Arch. Intern. Med. **85**:432, 1950.

450. Master, A.M., Garfield, C.I., and Walters, M.B.: Normal blood pressure and hypertension, Philadelphia, 1952, Lea & Febiger.

451. Page, I.H., and Corcoran, A.C.: Arterial hypertension: its diagnosis and treatment, Chicago, 1945, Year Book Medical Publishers.

452. Perera, G.A.: Hypertensive vascular disease: description and natural history, J. Chronic Dis. **1**:33, 1955.

453. Rabinowitz, M.: Overview on pathogenesis of cardiac hypertrophy, Circ. Res. **35**:3, 1974.

454. Smith, D.E., Odel, H.M., and Kernohan, J.W.: Causes of death in hypertension, Am. J. Med. **9**:516, 1950.

455. Sokolow, M., and Perloff, D.: The prognosis of essential hypertension treated conservatively, Circulation **23**:697, 1961.

456. Stein, B.R., and Barnes, A.R.: Severity and duration of hypertension in relation to amount of cardiac hypertrophy, Am. J. Med. Sci. **216**:661, 1948.

Cardiac hypertrophy in heart disease of obscure origin
Idiopathic cardiac hypertrophy

457. Barry, M., and Hall, M.: Familial cardiomyopathy, Br. Heart J. **24**:613, 1962.

458. Battersby, E.J., and Glenner, G.G.: Familial cardiomyopathy, Am. J. Med. **30**:382, 1961.

459. Bishop, J.M., Campbell, M., and Jones, E.W.: Cardiomyopathy in four members of a family, Br. Heart J. **24**:715, 1962.

460. Brent, L.B., et al.: Familial muscular subaortic stenosis: an unrecognized form of "idiopathic heart disease" with clinical and autopsy observations, Circulation **21**:167, 1960.

461. Burch, G.E., and Giles, T.: Cardiomyopathy: diagnostic criteria and classification. In Chung, E.K., editor: Controversy in cardiology, New York, 1976, Springer-Verlag.

462. Dammin, G.J., Glaser, R.J., and Roberts, J.C.: Isolated myocarditis, myocardial fibrosis, and intractable myocardial failure, Am. J. Pathol. **27**:695, 1951.

463. Goodwin, J.F.: Congestive and hypertrophic cardiomyopathy, Lancet **1**:731, 1970.

464. Higginson, I., Isaacson, C., and Simson, I.: The pathology of cryptogenic heart disease: a study of the pathological pattern in eighty cases of obscure heart failure in the South African Bantu black, Arch. Pathol. **70**:497, 1960.

465. Korb, G.: Heart diseases of unknown etiology: problems of terminology and classification. In Bajusz, E., and Rona, G., editors: Cardiomyopathies, Baltimore, 1973, University Park Press.

466. Maron, B.J., and Epstein, S.E.: Hypertrophic cardiomyopathy, Am. J. Cardiology **45**:141, 1980.

467. Maron, B.J., et al.: Quantitative analysis of cardiac muscle cell disorganization in the ventricular septum, Circulation **60**:685, 1979.

468. McKinney, B.: Pathology of the cardiomyopathies, London, 1974, Butterworth & Co. (Publishers) Ltd.

469. Pare, J.A., et al.: Hereditary cardiovascular dysplasia: a form of familial cardiomopathy, Am. J. Med. **31**:37, 1961.

470. Roberts, W.C., and Ferrans, V.J.: Pathologic anatomy of the cardiomyopathies, Hum. Pathol. **6**:287, 1975.

471. Taylor, R.R., Bernstein, L., and Jose, A.D.: Obstructive phenomena in ventricular hypertrophy, Br. Heart J. **26**:193, 1964.

472. Ware, E.R., and Chapman, B.M.: Chronic fibroplastic myocarditis, Am. Heart J. **33**:530, 1947.

Endocardial fibroelastosis

473. Black-Schaffer, B.: Infantile endocardial fibroelastosis: a suggested etiology, Arch. Pathol. **63**:281, 1957.

474. Johnson, F.R.: Anoxia as cause of endocardial fibroelastosis in infancy, Arch. Pathol. **54**:237, 1951.

475. Kline, K., et al.: The relationship between human endocardial fibroelastosis and obstruction of the cardiac lymphatics, Circulation **30**:728, 1964.

476. McCormick, W.F.: Endocardial fibrolaslosis: a summary of the literature and a review of 24 new cases, South. Med. J. **51**:1232, 1958.

477. Thomas, W.A., et al.: Endocardial fibroelastosis: factor in heart disease of obscure etiology: study of 20 autopsied cases in children and adults, N. Engl. J. Med. **251**:327, 1954.

Endomyocardial fibrosis

478. Ball, J.D., Williams, A.W., and Davies, J.N.P.: Endomyocardial fibrosis, Lancet **1**:1049, 1954.

479. Coelho, E., and Pimentel, J.C.: Diffuse endomyocardial fibrosis, Am. J. Med. **35**:569, 1963.

480. Davies, J.N.P.: The heart of Africa: cardiac pathology in the population of Uganda, Lab. Invest. **10**:205, 1961.

481. Shaper, A.G.: Plantain diets, serotonin, and endomyocardial fibrosis, Am. Heart J. **73**:432, 1967.

Cysts

482. Boyd, T.A.B.: Blood cysts on heart valves of infants, Am. J. Pathol. **25**:757, 1949.

483. Laipply, T.C.: Cysts and cystic tumors of mediastinum, Arch. Pathol. **39**:153, 1945.

484. Marshall, F.C.: Epithelial cyst of the heart, Arch. Pathol. **64**:107, 1957.

485. Morris, A.W., and Johnson, I.M.: Epithelial inclusion cysts of the heart: a case report and review of literature, Arch. Pathol. **77**:36, 1964.

486. Schlumberger, H.G.: Tumors of the mediastinum. In Atlas of tumor pathology, Sect. V, Fasc. 18, Washington, D.C., 1951, Armed Forces Institute of Pathology.

487. Willis, R.A.: The borderland of embryology and pathology, ed. 2, London, 1962, Butterworth & Co. (Publishers) Ltd.

Tumors

488. Anderson, W.A.D., and Dymtrk, E.T.: Primary tumor of heart containing epithelium-like elements, Am. J. Pathol. **22**:337, 1946.

489. Diferding, J.T., Gardner, R.E., and Roe, B.B.: Intracardiac myxomas with report of two unusual cases and successful removal, Circulation **23**:929, 1961.

490. Ferrans, V.J., and Roberts, W.C.: Structural features of cardiac myxomas, Hum. Pathol. **4**:111, 1973.

491. Fine, G.: Neoplasms of the pericardium and heart. In Gould, S.E., editor: Pathology of the heart and blood vessels, ed. 3, Springfield, Ill., 1968, Charles C Thomas, Publisher.

492. Hanfling, S.M.: Metastatic cancer to the heart: review of the literature and report of 127 cases, Circulation **22**:474, 1960.

493. McAllister, H.A., and Fenoglio, J.J.: Tumors of the cardiovascular system. In atlas of tumor pathology, second series, Fasc. 15, Washington, D.C., 1978, Armed Forces Institute of Pathology.

494. Merkow, L.P., et al.: Ultrastructure of a cardiac myxoma, Arch. Pathol. **88**:390, 1969.

495. Morales, A.R., et al.: The ultrastructure of smooth muscle tumors with a consideration of the possible relationship of glomangiomas, hemangiopericytomas, and cardiac myxomas. In Sommers, S.C., editor: Pathology annual, New York, 1975, Appleton-Century-Crofts.

496. Pomerance, A.: Papillary "tumours" of the heart valves, J. Pathol. Bacteriol. **81**:135, 1961.

497. Prichard, R.W.: Tumors of heart: review of subject and report of 150 cases, Arch. Pathol. **51**:98, 1951.

498. Ravid, J.M., and Sachs, J.: Tumors of heart, with report of primary fibromyxosarcoma with multiple tumors of mesentery and alimentary tract, Am. Heart J. **26**:385, 1943.

499. Straus, R., and Merliss, R.: Primary tumor of heart, Arch. Pathol. **39**:74, 1945.

500. Wold, L.E., and Lie, J.T.: Cardiac myxomas: a clinicopathologic profile, Am. J. Pathol. **101**:217, 1980.

Disturbances of conduction system

501. Lev, M.: The conduction system. In Gould, S.E., editor: Pathology of the heart, ed. 3, Springfield, Ill., 1968, Charles C Thomas, Publisher.

502. Lev, M., and Bharati, S.: Atrioventricular and intraventricular conduction disease, Arch. Intern. Med. **135**:405, 1975.

503. Lev, M., et al.: A histopathologic study of the atrioventricular communications in two hearts with the Wolff-Parkinson-White syndrome, Circulation **24**:41, 1961.

504. Prinzmetal, M., et al.: Accelerated conduction: the Wolff-Parkinson-White syndrome and related conditions, New York, 1952, Grune & Stratton, Inc.

505. Wolff, L., Parkinson, J., and White, P.D.: Bundle-branch block with short P-R interval in healthy young people prone to paroxysmal tachycardia, Am. Heart J. **5**:685, 1930.

Biopsy of pericardium and myocardium

506. Bulloch, R.T., Murphy, M.L., and Pearce, M.B.: Intracardiac needle biopsy of the ventricular septum, Am. J. Cardiol. **16**:227, 1965.

507. Caves, P.K., et al.: Percutaneous transvenous endomyocardial biopsy, J.A.M.A. **225**:288, 1973.

508. Proudfit, W.L., and Effler, D.B.: Diagnosis and treatment of chronic pericarditis by percardial biopsy, J.A.M.A. **161**:188, 1956.

509. Rosenblum, I., Stein, A.A., and Kausel, H.: Pharmacodynamic studies on isolated human auricular myocardium, J.A.M.A. **182**:532, 1962.

510. Stein, A.A., Change, K.S., and Alley, R.: Histochemical observations on enzyme distribution in surgically resected human myocardium, J.A.M.A. **182**:534, 1962.

511. Stein, A.A., Thibodeau, F., and Stranahan, A.: Electron microscopic observations in alcoholic heart disease, J.A.M.A. **182**:537, 1962.

512. Sutton, D.C., and Sutton, G.C.: Needle biopsy of the human ventricular myocardium: review of 54 consecutive cases, Am. Heart J. **60**:364, 1960.

513. Sutton, G.C., et al.: Study of the pericardium and ventricular myocardium: exploratory mediastinotomy and biopsy in unexplained heart disease, J.A.M.A. **185**:786, 1963.

514. Weinberg, M., Fell, E.H., and Lynfield, J.: Diagnostic biopsy of the pericardium and myocardium, Arch. Surg. **76**: 825, 1958.

Rejection of cardiac transplants

515. Bieber, C.P., et al.: Cardiac transplantation in man. VII. Cardiac allograft pathology, Circulation **41**:753, 1970.

516. Hastillo, A., Hess, M.L., and Lower, R.R.: Cardiac transplantation: expectations and limitations, Mod. Concepts Cardiovasc. Dis. **50**:13, 1981.

517. Kosek, J.C., Hurley, E.J., and Lower, R.R.: Histopathology of orthotopic canine cardiac homografts, Lab. Invest. **19**:97, 1968.

518. Milam, J.D., et al.: Morphologic findings in human cardiac allografts, Circulation **41**:519, 1970.

519. Reichenbach, D.: Pathologic changes in homografts of human aortic valves, Bull. Pathol. **10**:93, 1969.

520. Rider, A.K., et al.: The status of cardiac transplantation, 1975, Circulation **52**:531, 1975.

521. Rowlands, D.T., Jr., et al.: Rejection of canine cardiac allografts, Am. J. Pathol. **53**:617, 1968.

522. Sagar, K.B., et al.: Left ventricular mass by M-mode echocardiography in cardiac transplant patients with acute rejection, Circulation **64**:215, 1981.

523. Thomson, J.G.: Heart transplantation in man—necropsy findings, Br. Med. J. **2**:511, 1968.

CHAPTER 17 Congenital Heart Disease

MAURICE LEV
SAROJA BHARATI

Knowledge concerning congenital heart disease has increased rapidly in the past 40 years because of advances in physiology, clinical medicine, and surgery. It is more important for students of pathology to understand mechanisms and hemodynamics than to remember detail. Intended primarily for students, the consideration herein of congenital heart disease is not exhaustive, and for more comprehensive reading the publications of Edwards,[1] Lev,[2] Lev and Bharati,[3] and Netter,[4] and their bibliographies may be consulted.

The pathology of congenital heart disease may be considered from the standpoint of the individual abnormality or from the standpoint of the complex. A *complex*, as the term is used here, is a single abnormality or a group of abnormalities that have a tendency to be associated and the effects of that individual abnormality or group of abnormalities on the economy of the heart. Effects on economy include those on the myocardium, endocardium, valves, and conduction system.

Complexes will be dealt with exclusively in this chapter. They may conveniently be divided into those associated with (1) isolated shunts, (2) isolated obstructions, and (3) obstructions combined with shunts. A few complexes that do not fit into these categories also will be discussed.

A shunt is a transfer of blood from one side of the circulation to the other through an abnormal pathway. It is self-evident that life is normally maintained only with adequate transfer of blood from the systemic to the pulmonary circulation and back again. Such transfer through an abnormal pathway may produce pathologic change. Likewise, it is clear that the entire circulation is characterized by passage of blood through narrower and wider regions. The narrower regions are not necessarily obstructions. An obstruction is one that goes beyond the limits of physiologic narrowing.

Because of the tremendous advances made in the field of congenital heart disease by physiologists, clinicians, and surgeons in the last 40 years, it is necessary to introduce certain terms not ordinarily used in discussing the pathology of heart disease. In this chapter the term *hypertrophy* of a chamber means an increase in muscle mass of that chamber. When this increase is obtained by contraction of the chamber on an increased volume, the term *volume hypertrophy* is used, but when the increase is obtained by contraction of the chamber against increased resistance, the term *pressure hypertrophy* is used. The term *atrophy* of a chamber means a decrease in the muscle mass of that chamber, which again is related to a decrease in volume or pressure. The term *enlargement* of a chamber implies an increased volume in that chamber unrelated to failure of the myocardium. When such enlargement is attributable to failure, the term *dilatation* is used. It is self-evident that volume hypertrophy is accompanied by enlargement. In pressure hypertrophy, the chamber is normal or smaller than normal. The term *endocardial hypertrophy* implies a diffuse or focal increase in thickness of the endocardium because of altered hemodynamics. When diffuse, it is considered to be related to an increase in tension. When focal, it is related to turbulent flow. Increase in tension or turbulence may be obtained either by an increase in pressure or flow or by abnormally directed flow. The histologic counterpart of endocardial hypertrophy is proliferation of the elastic tissue, collagen, and in some cases the smooth muscle components of the endocardium and sometimes also of the subendocardium. When degenerative changes have set in, the term *endocardial sclerosis* is used. The term *hemodynamic changes of valves* implies focal or diffuse thickenings at the edge, the line of closure, the ring, the anulus, or the body of the valve related to altered hemodynamics, whether of pressure or flow. Pressure produces mostly a thickening of the line of closure and edge, whereas flow produces a generalized thickening of the valve.

Aided by Grant HL 30558-01 from the Heart, Lung and Blood Center of the National Institute of Health, Bethesda, Md.

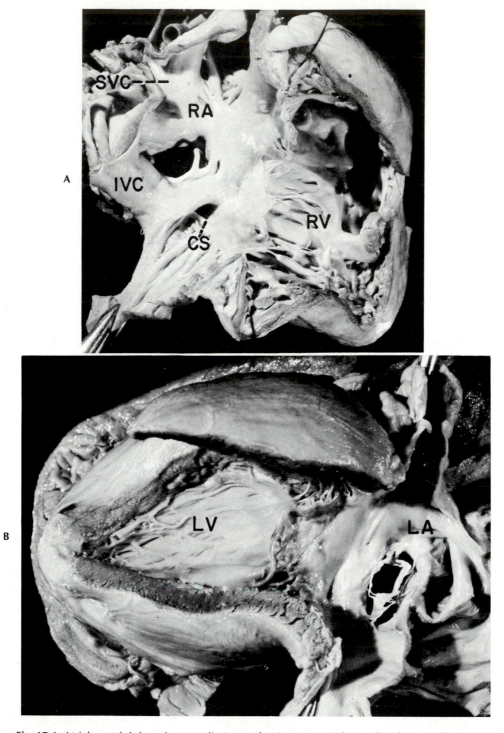

Fig. 17-1. Atrial septal defect, fossa ovalis (secundum) type. **A,** Right atrial and ventricular view of one heart. **B,** Left atrial and ventricular view of another heart. *CS,* Coronary sinus; *IVC,* inferior vena cava; *LA,* left atrium; *LV,* left ventricle; *RA,* right atrium; *RV,* right ventricle; *SVC,* superior vena cava.

In the description of complexes it will be understood that changes in the endocardium and valves occur with increased pressure or flow or with turbulent flow as in jet lesions. To simplify matters, these will not always be mentioned.

PATHOLOGY OF ISOLATED SHUNTS

A shunt may occur from the left to the right side or from the right to the left side of the circulation. In instances of isolated shunts (those unaccompanied by obstructive phenomena), if there is no increase in pulmonary resistance, the shunt should be left to right because pulmonary resistance is normally less than peripheral systemic resistance. Such isolated shunts, without pulmonary hypertension, will be discussed first, followed by such shunts with pulmonary hypertension and then other shunts that are frequently or invariably associated with pulmonary hypertension.

Left-to-right shunt at atrial level—isolated atrial septal defect complexes

Anomaly. A defect in the atrial septum may occur in the region of the fossa ovalis—called *atrial septal defect, fossa ovalis type* (or *secundum type*) (Fig. 17-1). It may occur distally, in the region adjacent to the mitral and tricuspid valves—called *atrial septal defect, primum type (persistent ostium primum)* (Fig. 17-2). The latter is always associated with a cleft aortic leaflet of the mitral valve. Or a defect may occur in the proximal portion of the atrial septum— called *proximal septum (sinus venosus) type* (Fig. 17-3). This type of defect is always associated with entry of some or all of the right pulmonary veins into the right atrium, a straddling superior vena cava, a straddling inferior vena cava, or any combination of these. The fourth type of defect is the coronary sinus

type. This is a defect in the atrial septum above or in the region of the coronary sinus. Thus the coronary sinus may enter both atria (straddling coronary sinus).

Complex. In the fossa ovalis type of atrial septal defect (Fig. 17-4), there is volume hypertrophy of the right atrium and right ventricle, enlargement of the tricuspid and pulmonic orifices, hemodynamic changes of the tricuspid and pulmonic valves, focal or diffuse endocardial hypertrophy of the right atrium and right ventricle, and enlargement of the pulmonary trunk. The left atrium and left ventricle show volume atrophy, with the mitral and aortic orifices smaller than normal. There may be considerable hemodynamic change of the mitral valve. The mitral valve may be redundant and floppy.

These findings are related to left-to-right shunt at the atrial level with increased pulmonary flow. The shunt is in this direction because the right ventricle fills more easily than the left and the pressure in the left atrium is higher than that in the right.

In the primum type of atrial septal defect, the pathologic changes in the right side are the same as in the secundum type. However, because of the presence of the cleft in the aortic leaflet of the mitral valve and the manner of attachment of the aortic leaflet of the mitral valve to the septum, the left side of the heart may be different. The cleft aortic leaflet of the mitral valve may result in mitral insufficiency. When this condition is present, the left ventricle will show volume hypertrophy, whereas the left atrium may be normal in size or even show volume hypertrophy. The more anterior attachment of the aortic leaflet of the mitral valve uncommonly limits the outflow tract, producing subaortic stenosis, which may lead to pressure hypertrophy of the left ventricle.

The complexes formed in the sinus venosus type of

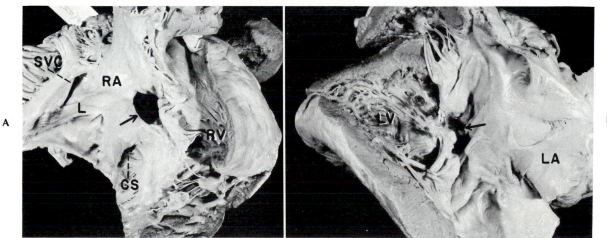

Fig. 17-2. Atrial septal defect, primum type (persistent ostium primum). **A,** Right atrial and ventricular view. **B,** Left atrial and ventricular view. Arrows point to persistent ostium primum. *CS,* Coronary sinus; *L,* limbus; *LA,* left atrium; *LV,* left ventricle; *RA,* right atrium; *RV,* right ventricle; *SVC,* mouth of superior vena cava.

atrial septal defect are variable, depending on the place of entry of the superior and inferior venae cavae. In general, there is volume hypertrophy of the right atrium and right ventricle, with the left atrium and ventricle ranging from hypertrophy to atrophy.

The coronary sinus defect is usually associated with other complexes, but occasionally it is isolated, producing a secundum type of complex.

Left-to-right shunt at ventricular level—isolated ventricular septal defect

Anomaly (Fig. 17-5). Ventricular septal defects may be present anywhere in the ventricular septum, but they have a predilection for the subaortic area. When present in the subaortic area, they may be anterior to but not involving the pars membranacea, anterior to and involving the pars membranacea, within and limited to the pars membranacea, or within the pars membranacea and involving the muscular septum both anterior and posterior to it. When more apical, they may be present along the line of junction of the anterior and posterior septa, within the posterior septum at the base close to the mitral valve anulus, or in any area in the muscular ventricular septum. Depending on their position, they enter the right ventricle beneath the pulmonic orifice, adjacent to the tricuspid valve, within the lower part of the infundibulum, or in the sinus away from the tricuspid valve.

Complex (Fig. 17-6). The ventricular septal defect complex is characterized by volume hypertrophy of the right ventricle, enlargement of the pulmonic orifice, hemodynamic changes of the tricuspid and pulmonic valves, endocardial hypertrophy of the right ventricle, pressure hypertrophy of the right atrium, volume hypertrophy of the left atrium and left ventricle, enlargement of the mitral orifice, hemodynamic changes of the mitral and aortic valves, and in some cases endocardial hypertrophy of the left atrium and left ventricle.

These findings are related to left-to-right shunt at the ventricular level, increased pulmonary flow, and increased volume in the left side of the heart. If left alone, many small or medium-sized ventricular septal defects may close spontaneously.

Left-to-right shunt at ductus level—isolated patent ductus arteriosus

Anomaly (Fig. 17-7). A ductus arteriosus is a muscular connection between the aorta, distal to the left subclavian artery and the left pulmonary artery at its junction with the main pulmonary trunk. A ductus arteriosus that is patent after 3 months of age is considered abnormal. A ductus may be considered abnormally large before 3 months of age, but an exact criterion of judgment is lacking today. A patent ductus may be as long as 2 cm or so brief as to constitute a windowlike structure between the aorta and the left pulmonary artery in the usual position of the ductus. Its diameter may range from 2 mm up to as much as 1 cm, and it may be a straight tube or slightly cirsoid.

Complex (Fig. 17-8). In the patent ductus arteriosus

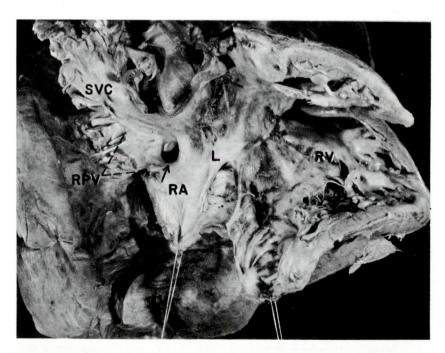

Fig. 17-3. Atrial septal defect, proximal septum (sinus venosus) type. Right atrial and right ventricular view. Arrow points to defect. *L,* Limbus; *RA,* right atrium; *RPV,* right pulmonary veins; *RV,* right ventricle; *SVC,* superior vena cava.

complex there are volume hypertrophy of the left atrium and left ventricle with or without endocardial hypertrophy, enlargement of the mitral and pulmonic orifices with hemodynamic changes of the valves, enlargement of the pulmonary trunk and the two pulmonary arteries with or without atherosclerotic changes, and enlargement of the ascending aorta.

These are the effects of left-to-right shunt at the ductus level, with increased pulmonary flow and increased volume in the left side of the heart.

Pulmonary hypertension associated with shunts

In the consideration of the shunts discussed so far, it was assumed that no pulmonary hypertension was present. Such may be the case; despite the increased pulmonary flow, the greatly distensible pulmonary vascular tree is able to accommodate it without increasing the pressure in the pulmonary circuit. However, pulmonary hypertension may develop for one or all of the following reasons:

1. A flow beyond the distensibility of the lung vasculature
2. A vasoconstriction of the pulmonary bed
3. Secondary pathologic changes in the intima or

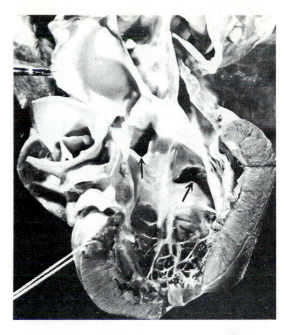

Fig. 17-5. Ventricular septal defects. Left ventricular view. Arrows point to two defects, one beneath aortic valve and one beneath mitral valve.

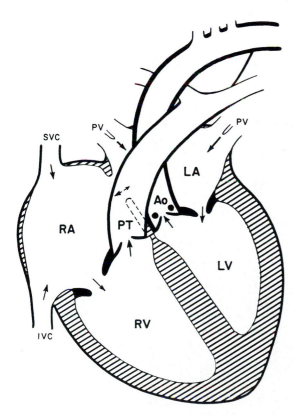

Fig. 17-4. Schematic diagram of heart in atrial septal defect, fossa ovalis type, complex. Arrows indicate direction of flow. *Ao,* Aorta; *IVC,* inferior vena cava; *LA,* left atrium; *LV,* left ventricle; *PT,* pulmonary trunk; *PV,* pulmonary veins; *RA,* right atrium; *RV,* right ventricle; *SVC,* superior vena cava.

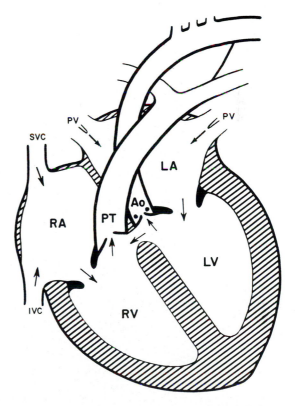

Fig. 17-6. Schematic diagram of ventricular septal defect complex. *Ao,* Aorta; *IVC,* inferior vena cava; *LA,* left atrium; *LV,* left ventricle; *PT,* pulmonary trunk; *PV,* pulmonary veins; *RA,* right atrium; *RV,* right ventricle; *SVC,* superior vena cava.

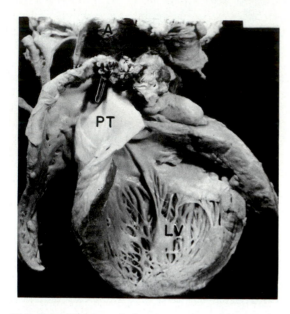

Fig. 17-7. Patent ductus arteriosus complex, without pulmonary hypertension. Probe passes through ductus. *A,* Aorta; *LV,* left ventricle; *PT,* pulmonary trunk; *RV,* right ventricle. (From Lev, M.: Autopsy diagnosis of congenitally malformed hearts, Springfield, Ill., 1953, Charles C Thomas, Publisher.)

media of the muscular arteries and arterioles of the lungs, restricting the pulmonary bed

Thus pulmonary hypertension may occur most commonly in ventricular septal defect, less commonly in patent ductus arteriosus, and least commonly in atrial septal defect.

The pathologic effects of pulmonary hypertension on the heart, developing in left-to-right shunts, are related to an increase in pressure on the right side, with or without a decrease in flow to the left side (Fig. 17-9). The former leads to pressure hypertrophy on the right side and the latter to a decrease in the previously present volume hypertrophy of the left side. This decrease may reach the point of less than normal flow, with volume atrophy on the left side. When this occurs, there is usually a reversal of shunt from left-to-right to right-to-left.

Common atrioventricular orifice

Anomaly (Fig. 17-10). In common atrioventricular (AV) orifice, there is one undivided common orifice for the mitral and tricuspid orifices, and this is guarded by a

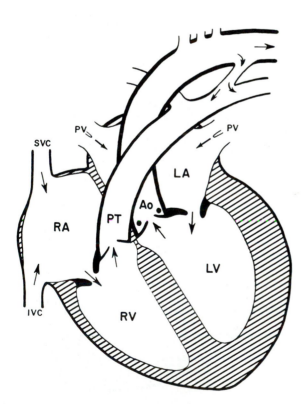

Fig. 17-8. Schematic diagram of patent ductus arteriosus complex. *Ao,* Aorta; *IVC,* inferior vena cava; *LA,* left atrium; *LV,* left ventricle; *PT,* pulmonary trunk; *PV,* pulmonary veins; *RA,* right atrium; *RV,* right ventricle; *SVC,* superior vena cava.

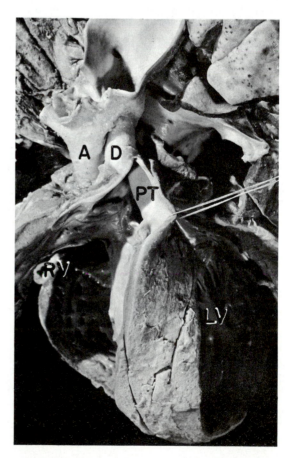

Fig. 17-9. Patent ductus arteriosus complex with left-to-right shunt, pulmonary hypertension, and hypoplasia of ascending aorta. *A,* Aorta; *D,* ductus arteriosus; *LV,* left ventricle; *PT,* pulmonary trunk; *RV,* right ventricle.

valve consisting either of four leaflets (anterior and posterior and right and left lateral) or of five leaflets (there may be a fifth leaflet on the right side). This anomaly is always associated with a septal defect at the base of the heart, which consists of a persistent ostium primum combined with a basal ventricular septal defect. Also, there is often an associated secundum defect, with displacement of the atrial septum to the left. The common atrioventricular orifice may be divided into tricuspid and mitral portions of relatively normal size (balanced type), or either the tricuspid (right ventricular type) or mitral (left ventricular type) side may dominate.

Complex (Fig. 17-11). Thus in the balanced form both ventricles are hypertrophied and enlarged. In the dominant right form the right ventricle is hypertrophied and enlarged, whereas the left ventricle is smaller and usually thinner than normal. In the dominant left form the left ventricle is hypertrophied and enlarged, whereas the right ventricle is smaller but thicker than normal.

The pathologic changes in the balanced form are related to left-to-right shunt at the atrial and ventricular levels with pulmonary hypertension and to varying mitral or tricuspid insufficiency. The reasons for the dominant right and dominant left forms are not yet understood.

Isolated aorticopulmonary septal defect

Anomaly (Fig. 17-12). In the aorticopulmonary septal defect an opening is present between the ascending aorta and the pulmonary trunk, usually situated above the aor-

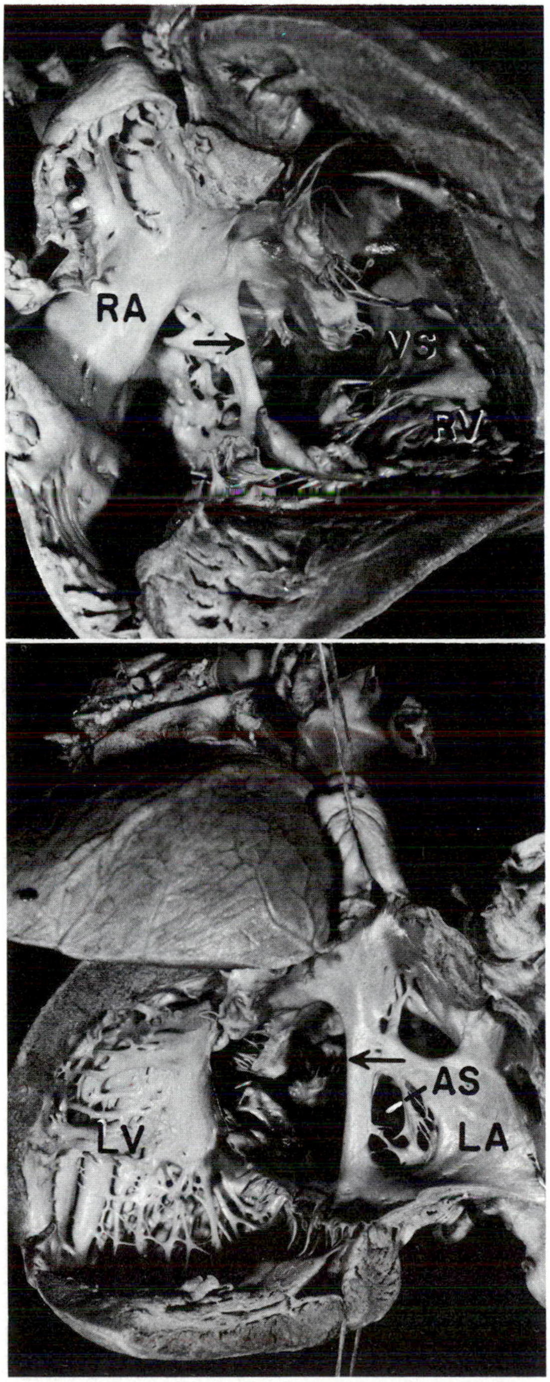

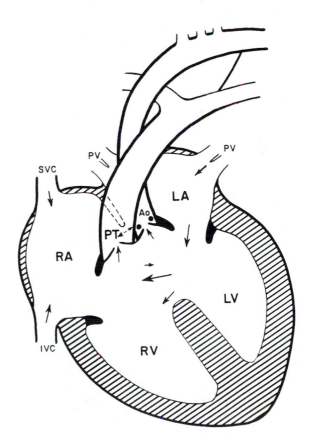

Fig. 17-10. Common atrioventricular (AV) orifice. **A,** Right atrial and right ventricular view. **B,** Left atrial and ventricular view. Arrows point to distal edge of septum primum. *AS,* Atrial septal defect, secundum type; *LA,* left atrium; *LV,* left ventricle; *RA,* right atrium; *RV,* right ventricle; *VS,* ventricular septum.

Fig. 17-11. Schematic diagram of common atrioventricular (AV) orifice complex. *Ao,* Aorta; *IVC,* inferior vena cava; *LA,* left atrium; *LV,* left ventricle; *PT,* pulmonary trunk; *PV,* pulmonary veins; *RA,* right atrium; *RV,* right ventricle; *SVC,* superior vena cava.

tic and pulmonic valves. This opening may be only a few millimeters in diameter or may be massive.

Complex. In the aorticopulmonary septal defect complex, there are pressure hypertrophy of the right atrium and right ventricle, enlargement of the pulmonary trunk and orifice, volume hypertrophy of the left atrium and left ventricle, and enlargement of the mitral and aortic orifices.

These are the effects of left-to-right shunt at the ascending aorta–pulmonary trunk level usually associated with pulmonary hypertension, with increased pulmonary flow and increased volume on the left side.

Total anomalous pulmonary venous drainage

Anomaly (Fig. 17-13). In total anomalous pulmonary venous drainage, all of the pulmonary veins enter the right atrium, directly or indirectly. When they do so directly, they enter a pouchlike formation that fuses with the right atrium. When they enter indirectly, they usually form a common pulmonary vein that empties into a partial left superior vena cava, the innominate vein, the right superior vena cava, the azygos vein, the portal vein, the inferior vena cava, the coronary sinus, the left gastric

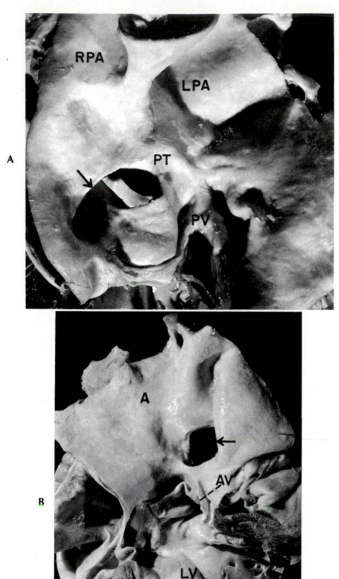

Fig. 17-12. Aorticopulmonary septal defect. **A,** Pulmonary trunk view. **B,** Aortic view. Arrows point to defect. *A,* Aorta; *AV,* aortic valve; *LPA,* left pulmonary artery; *LV,* part of left ventricle; *PT,* pulmonary trunk; *RPA,* right pulmonary artery.

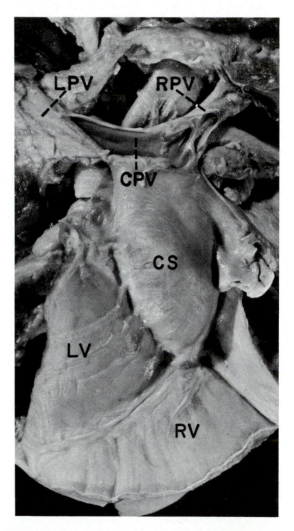

Fig. 17-13. Total anomalous pulmonary venous drainage into coronary sinus. Left posterior view. *CPV,* Common pulmonary vein; *CS,* coronary sinus; *LPV,* left pulmonary veins; *LV,* left ventricle; *RPV,* right pulmonary veins; *RV,* right ventricle. (From Lev, M.: The pathology of congenital heart disease. In Banyai, A.L., and Gordon, B.L., editors: Advances in cardiopulmonary disease; copyrighted 1964 by Year Book Medical Publishers, Inc, Chicago; used by permission.)

vein, or the ductus venosus. There is always an atrial septal defect of the fossa ovalis type.

Complex (Fig. 17-14). In total anomalous pulmonary venous drainage there are in general two types of complexes: those without pulmonary venous obstruction and those with pulmonary venous obstruction.

Complexes without pulmonary venous obstruction. In complexes without pulmonary venous obstruction, the heart is greatly enlarged. There are volume and pressure hypertrophy of the right atrium and right ventricle, enlargement of the tricuspid and pulmonic orifices, enlargement of the pulmonary trunk, a structurally small left atrium, a normal left ventricle, or volume atrophy of the left ventricle, and a small aortic orifice, with hypoplasia of the aorta.

These changes are related to left-to-right shunt at the pulmonary venous level, increased pulmonary flow, right-to-left shunt at the atrial level, and usually pulmonary hypertension.

Complexes with pulmonary venous obstruction. When the pulmonary veins make connection with veins in the abdomen, and sometimes with those in the chest, there is an obstruction of the venous return either along the course of the common pulmonary vein or along its junction with the other vein. Under these circumstances,

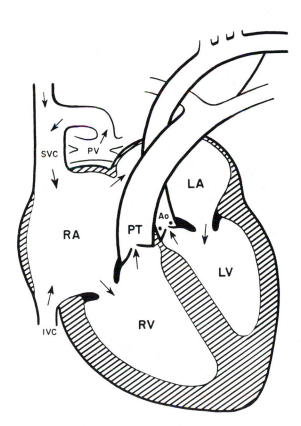

Fig. 17-14. Schematic diagram of total anomalous pulmonary venous drainage into superior vena cava complex. *Ao*, Aorta; *IVC*, inferior vena cava; *LA*, left atrium; *LV*, left ventricle; *PT*, pulmonary trunk; *PV*, pulmonary vein; *RA*, right atrium; *RV*, right ventricle; *SVC*, superior vena cava.

although the heart shows the same essential characteristics as in this complex without pulmonary obstruction, the heart is smaller, being either normal in size or slightly enlarged. The size difference in this complex with pulmonary venous obstruction is considered to be attributable to a lesser volume and greater pressure hypertrophy of the right side.

PATHOLOGY OF ISOLATED OBSTRUCTIONS

In this chapter only three types of obstructions will be discussed: (1) obstruction to outflow from the right ventricle, (2) obstruction to outflow from the left ventricle, and (3) obstruction in the transverse aorta.

Isolated pulmonary stenosis (pulmonary stenosis with normal aortic root)

Anomaly (Fig. 17-15). The pulmonic valve usually consists of a diaphragm-like structure with only an incipient formation of cusps. This diaphragm may have a minute or larger opening. Uncommonly, the valve is fairly well formed but its cusps are agglutinated at the commissures. Thus the obstruction is usually valvular. However, in a few cases the valve is not obstructed, but the obstruction is at the mouth of the infundibulum of the right ventricle. Here, the septal and parietal bands are greatly thickened and together form a ring of obstruction into the conus.

Complex (Fig. 17-16). In the isolated pulmonary stenosis complex there are pressure hypertrophy of the right ventricle, often poststenotic dilatation of the pulmonary trunk, hemodynamic changes in the tricuspid valve with or without mild stenosis, and endocardial hypertrophy of the right ventricle.

We are dealing here with the effects of obstruction to the outflow of the right ventricle with, however, sufficient left-sided flow to sustain life.

Isolated aortic stenosis

Anomaly (Fig. 17-17). There are three types of aortic stenosis: valvular, subvalvular (subaortic), and supravalvular.

In valvular stenosis the aortic valve consists of one, two, or three cusps that are greatly irregularly thickened, often consisting of just nubbins of tissue. In the younger age groups, the anulus also is smaller than normal. Thus the stenosis is both anular and valvular in younger age groups, but chiefly valvular in older age groups.

There are several varieties of subvalvular (subaortic) stenosis. In one variety a sheet of fibroelastic tissue extends over the ventricular septum to the aortic leaflet of the mitral valve, a varying distance from the aortic valve. In a second variety a fibrous diaphragm-like structure is situated in this region. In a third variety a muscular bulge on the septum beneath the aorta narrows the subaortic area. This muscular bulge is part of a disease

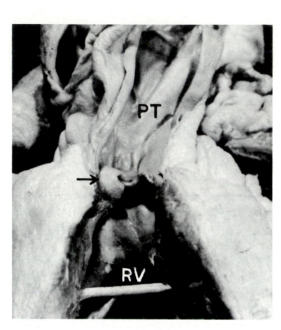

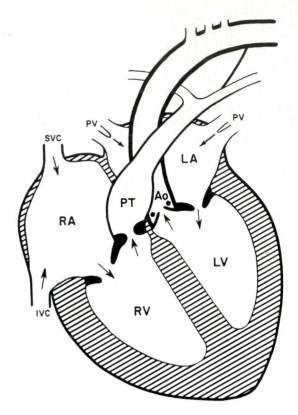

Fig. 17-15. Isolated pulmonary stenosis. Arrow points to diaphragm-like pulmonary valve. *PT,* Pulmonary trunk; *RV,* right ventricle. (From Lev, M.: Autopsy diagnosis of congenitally malformed hearts, Springfield, Ill., 1953, Charles C Thomas, Publisher.)

Fig. 17-16. Schematic diagram of isolated pulmonary stenosis complex. *Ao,* Aorta; *IVC,* inferior vena cava; *LA,* left atrium; *LV,* left ventricle; *PT,* pulmonary trunk; *PV,* pulmonary veins; *RA,* right atrium; *RV,* right ventricle; *SVC,* superior vena cava.

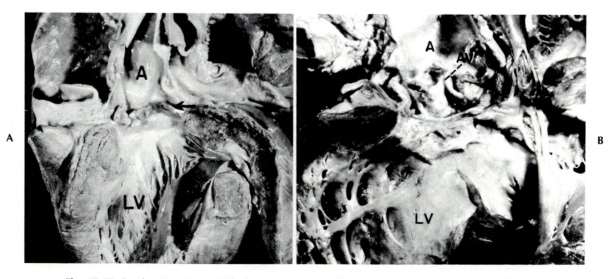

Fig. 17-17. Aortic stenosis. **A,** Valvular type. Arrow points to abnormal aortic valve with aortic stenosis. **B,** Subvalvular (subaortic) type. Note large fibroelastic plaque producing subaortic stenosis. (**A** and **B,** From Lev, M.: Autopsy diagnosis of congenitally malformed hearts, Springfield, Ill., 1953, Charles C Thomas, Publisher.)

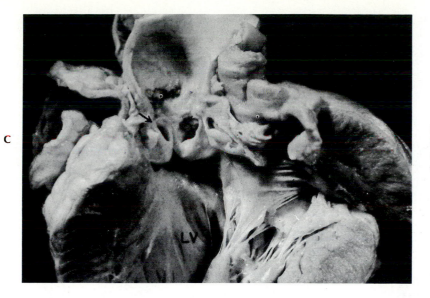

C

Fig. 17-17, cont'd. C, Supravalvular type with subacute bacterial aortitis. Arrow points to narrowing at upper margins of sinuses of Valsalva. *A,* Aorta; *AV,* Aortic valve; *LV,* left ventricle.

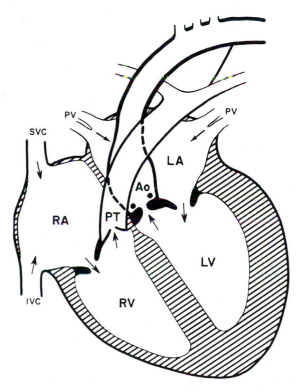

Fig. 17-18. Schematic diagram of aortic stenosis complex. *Ao,* Aorta; *IVC,* inferior vena cava; *LA,* left atrium; *LV,* left ventricle; *PT,* pulmonary trunk; *PV,* pulmonary veins; *RA,* right atrium, *RV,* right ventricle; *SVC,* superior vena cava.

entity called idiopathic hypertrophic subaortic stenosis (IHSS). In this disease there is more hypertrophy of the ventricular septum than of the parietal wall of the left ventricle. The architecture of the left ventricle shows a chaotic arrangement of muscle, which is congenital and often familial.

There are two varieties of the supravalvular type. One consists of a thickening and accentuation of the normal supravalvular aortic rim at the upper margins of the sinuses of Valsalva. The other consists of a ridge of thickening about 1 cm above the sinuses of Valsalva.

Complex (Fig. 17-18). The aortic stenosis complex is characterized by pressure hypertrophy of the left ventricle and often of the left atrium and hemodynamic changes at the mitral valve, in some cases with insufficiency of the valve. In the subvalvular and supravalvular types the aortic valve is always thickened. This may be either a hemodynamic change or a structural part of the malformation. Supravalvular aortic stenosis may be associated with supravalvular or peripheral pulmonary stenoses, abnormal facies in children, and abnormalities in calcium metabolism.

Coarctation of aorta

Coarctation of the aorta means a narrowing of the aorta. As used in this chapter, the term does not necessarily imply a constrictive region. Such narrowings may occur in any part of the aorta. The only one that concerns us here is the one in the region of the isthmus.

The isthmus of the aorta is the segment between the origins of the left subclavian artery and the ductus or ligamentum arteriosum. In a number of newborns this region is smaller than the regions of the aorta proximal and distal to it because in fetal life the left ventricular flow passes into the brachiocephalic region, whereas the right ventricular flow passes through the ductus into the descending aorta. Thus the isthmus is a site of lessened flow and at birth may be smaller than normal. The isthmus usually attains normal size after birth.

There are three types of coarctation: fetal (nonconstrictive, preductal), transitional, and adult (paraductal). These terms pertain chiefly to the complexes produced

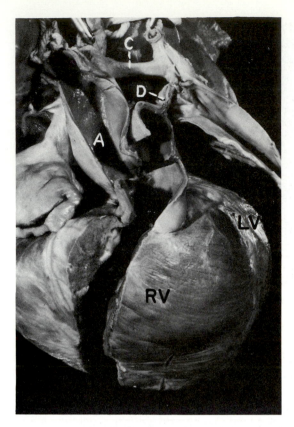

Fig. 17-19. Fetal coarctation complex. *A,* Ascending aorta; *C,* coarctation; *D,* ductus arteriosus; *LV,* left ventricle; *RV,* right ventricle.

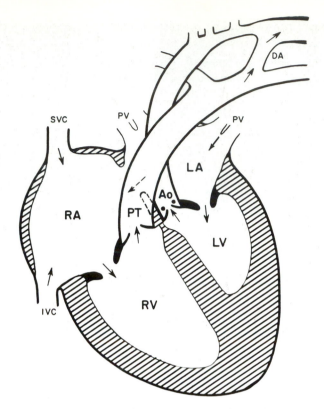

Fig. 17-20. Schematic diagram of fetal coarctation complex. *Ao,* Aorta; *DA,* ductus arteriosus; *IVC,* inferior vena cava; *LA,* left atrium; *LV,* left ventricle; *PT,* pulmonary trunk; *PV,* pulmonary veins; *RA,* right atrium; *RV,* right ventricle; *SVC,* superior vena cava.

rather than to the topography of the narrowing of the aorta.

Fetal coarctation

Anomaly (Fig. 17-19). In fetal coarctation there is a narrowing of the transverse aorta that involves the entire isthmus or, more commonly, extends from the innominate or left common carotid artery. The left subclavian artery is given off a considerable distance from the origin of the left common carotid artery. The ascending aorta is smaller than normal.

Complex (Fig. 17-20). In the fetal coarctation complex there is always an atrial septal defect of the fossa ovalis type and a widely patent ductus arteriosus. Volume and pressure hypertrophy of the right ventricle is present, accompanied by enlargement of the tricuspid and pulmonic orifices, enlargement of the pulmonary trunk, and volume atrophy of the left atrium and left ventricle with smallness of the mitral orifice.

It is assumed that the pathogenesis of this complex is as follows. Since the complex just described is found in the newborn heart, the smallness of the left side and largeness of the right side are caused by insufficient blood reaching the left side of the heart and more blood reaching the right side. The small amount of blood entering the ascending aorta results in the small ascending

aorta and, of course, even smaller isthmus. Thus the coarctation and the hypoplasia of the ascending aorta may be considered to be caused by insufficient flow. After birth there may be a left-to-right shunt at the atrial level and a right-to-left shunt at the ductus level.

Transitional coarctation

There is evidence that some cases of fetal coarctation pass through a transitional phase (transitional coarctation) and that, if the infant survives this stage, the anomaly develops to become converted adult coarctation. This is theorized to take place in the following manner.

After birth, if the child with fetal coarctation survives, the pulmonary pressure falls sufficiently to invite more blood into the left atrium and ventricle, at the same time causing the progressive closure of the ductus arteriosus and the foramen ovale. These chambers comply with this added volume and throw more blood into the aorta. The added volume in the aorta converts the narrow isthmus into a constrictive lesion. Thus the right ventricle becomes more normal in thickness, while the left ventricle takes on size and weight. When seen in the transitional phase, both chambers may be hypertrophied. If the child survives this stage, pulmonary hypertension becomes minimal and the complex takes on the physiologic features of typical adult coarctation.

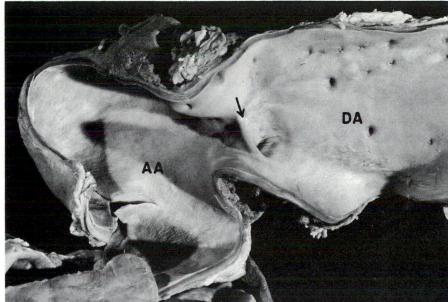

Fig. 17-21. Adult coarctation. Arrow points to coarctation. *AA,* Ascending aorta; *DA,* descending aorta. (From DeBoer, A., et al.: Arch. Surg. **82:**801, 1961.)

Paraductal (juxtaductal, adult) coarctation

Anomaly (Fig. 17-21). In adult coarctation there is a maximum point of narrowing just proximal to, at, or just distal to the ductus arteriosus. A patent ductus may be present proximal or distal to the obstruction.

Complex (Fig. 17-22). In the adult coarctation complex, pressure hypertrophy of the left ventricle and in some cases of the left atrium is present, the mitral and aortic orifices are enlarged, and the ascending aorta is dilated.

This is a constrictive lesion in the aorta, with hypertension proximal and hypotension distal to the constriction and with pressure hypertrophy of the left atrium and ventricle. Collateral anastomoses occur between the proximal and distal portions of the aorta by way of the subclavian, dorsal scapular, internal mammary, and intercostal arteries.

PATHOLOGY OF OBSTRUCTIONS COMBINED WITH SHUNTS

When an obstruction is combined with a shunt, the total effect depends on the extent of the obstruction and the direction and extent of the shunt. These principles will become evident in the discussion of the following entities: tetralogy of Fallot, double-outlet right ventricle, transposition, tricuspid atresia, and hypoplasia of the aortic tract complex.

Tetralogy of Fallot

Anomaly (Fig. 17-23). In tetralogy of Fallot the aorta overrides (straddles) the interventricular septum over a defect in this septum and emerges from both ventricles. The pulmonary trunk emerges from the right ventricle.

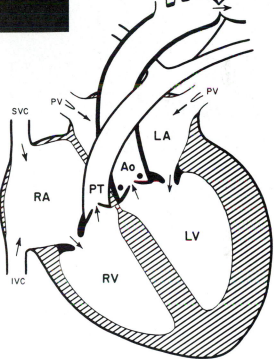

Fig. 17-22. Schematic diagram of adult coarctation complex. *Ao,* Aorta; *IVC,* inferior vena cava; *LA,* left atrium; *LV,* left ventricle; *PT,* pulmonary trunk; *PV,* pulmonary veins; *RA,* right atrium; *RV,* right ventricle; *SVC,* superior vena cava.

There is stenosis of the infundibulum somewhere along its course, and this may be associated with stenosis of the pulmonic orifice itself.

Depending on the extent of the stenosis and the size of the defect, there are two types of complexes—cyanotic and acyanotic. In the cyanotic type the stenosis predominates, whereas in the acyanotic type the stenosis is relatively mild and the ventricular septal defect predominates.

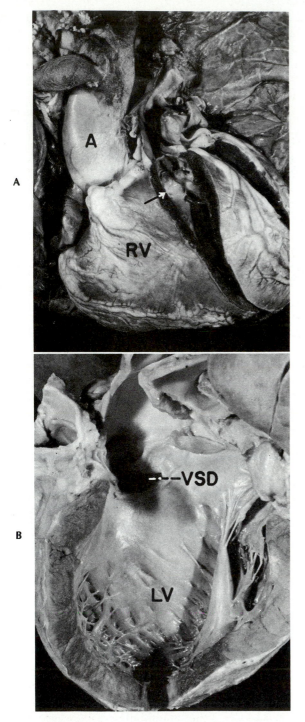

Fig. 17-23. Tetralogy of Fallot. **A,** Anterior view of one heart. **B,** Left ventricular view of another heart. *A,* Aorta; *LV,* left ventricle; *RV,* right ventricle (arrow points to infundibular stenosis); *VSD,* ventricular septal defect. (From Lev, M.: The pathology of congenital heart disease. In Banyai, A.L., and Gordon, B.L., editors: Advances in cardiopulmonary disease; copyrighted 1964 by Year Book Medical Publishers, Inc., Chicago; used by permission.)

Complexes (Fig. 17-24). In *cyanotic tetralogy* there is pressure hypertrophy of the right atrium and right ventricle. The tricuspid orifice has a tendency to be smaller than normal, with abnormalities in structure of the valve. There often is pronounced endocardial hypertrophy (fibroelastosis) in the infundibular region. The left atrium and left ventricle have a tendency to be smaller than normal, with corresponding smallness of the mitral orifice, whereas the aortic orifice is enlarged.

We are dealing with the effects on the right side of the heart, which are related to systemic and infundibular resistance, decreased pulmonary flow, and the predominant right-to-left shunt at the ventricular level.

In *acyanotic tetralogy* there are pressure and volume hypertrophy of the right ventricle, pressure hypertrophy of the right atrium, volume hypertrophy of the left atrium and left ventricle, and enlargement of the mitral and aortic orifices.

We are dealing with predominant left-to-right shunt at the ventricular level, increased pulmonary flow, and increased volume on the left side of the heart.

Double-outlet right ventricle

In double-outlet right ventricle, both arterial trunks emerge completely or almost completely from the right ventricle, and there may or may not be aortic-mitral or

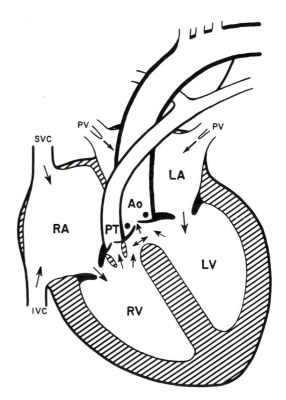

Fig. 17-24. Schematic diagram of cyanotic tetralogy of Fallot complex. *Ao,* Aorta; *IVC,* inferior vena cava; *LA,* left atrium; *LV,* left ventricle; *PT,* pulmonary trunk; *PV,* pulmonary veins; *RA,* right atrium; *RV,* right ventricle; *SVC,* superior vena cava.

pulmonic-mitral continuity. There are simple and complicated types. The simple types may be classified according to the position of the ventricular septal defect (VSD) in relation to the great vessels as follows: (1) with subaortic VSD (VSD related to the aorta), (2) with subpulmonic VSD (VSD related to the pulmonary trunk), (3) with doubly committed VSD (VSD related to both vessels), and (4) with noncommitted VSD (VSD related to neither vessel). Any of these types may be associated with pulmonary stenosis. The complicated types are associated with (1) mitral atresia, (2) common atrioventricular orifice, or (3) total anomalous pulmonary venous drainage. Only the simple types with subaortic and subpulmonic VSD are discussed in this chapter.

Double-outlet right ventricle with subaortic VSD and pulmonary stenosis

Anomaly (Fig. 17-25). In this anomaly both the aorta and the pulmonary trunk emerge almost completely from the right ventricle. The aorta lies adjacent to the defect. The infundibular stenosis resembles that in tetralogy.

Complex (Fig. 17-26). In this complex there is pressure hypertrophy of the right side atrium and ventricle and volume atrophy of the left atrium, whereas the left

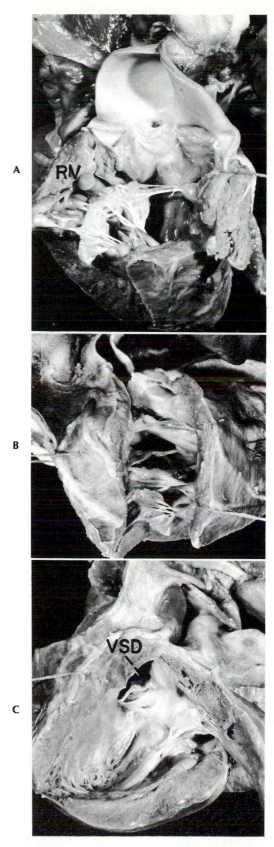

Fig. 17-25. Double-outlet right ventricle with subaortic ventricular septal defect. **A,** Base of aorta. **B,** Base of pulmonary trunk. **C,** Left ventricle. *RV,* Right ventricle; *VSD,* with pulmonary stenosis.

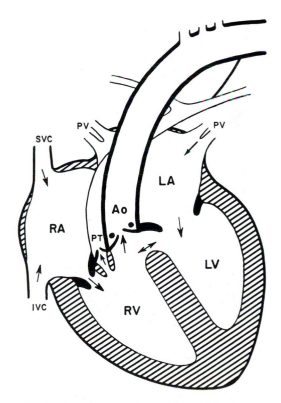

Fig. 17-26. Schematic diagram of double-outlet right ventricle with subaortic ventricular septal defect with pulmonary stenosis. *Ao,* Aorta; *IVC,* inferior vena cava; *LA,* left atrium; *LV,* left ventricle; *PT,* pulmonary trunk; *PV,* pulmonary veins; *RA,* right atrium; *RV,* right ventricle; *SVC,* superior vena cava.

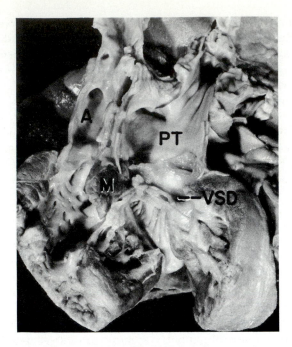

Fig. 17-27. Double-outlet right ventricle with subpulmonic VSD (Taussig-Bing heart). Right ventricular view. *A*, Aorta; *M*, muscular separation between aorta and pulmonary trunk; *PT*, pulmonary trunk; *VSD*, ventricular septal defect.

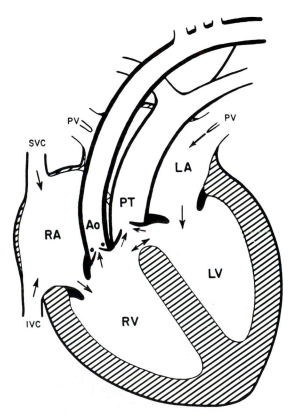

Fig. 17-28. Schematic diagram of double-outlet right ventricle with subpulmonic VSD (Taussig-Bing heart). *Ao*, Aorta; *IVC*, inferior vena cava; *LA*, left atrium; *LV*, left ventricle; *PT*, pulmonary trunk; *PV*, pulmonary veins; *RA*, right atrium; *RV*, right ventricle; *SVC*, superior vena cava.

ventricle varies from atrophy to hypertrophy.

We are dealing with the right side related to peripheral and infundibular resistance, right-to-left shunt at the ventricular level, decreased pulmonary flow, and decreased volume in the left side of the heart. When the left ventricle is hypertrophied, this may be caused by obstruction of this chamber by an inadequately sized ventricular septal defect.

Double-outlet right ventricle with subpulmonic VSD (Taussig-Bing heart)

Anomaly (Fig. 17-27). In this anomaly the aorta emerges completely from the right ventricle removed from the defect of the ventricular septum. The pulmonary trunk is related to the defect and either comes off completely from the right side or straddles the interventricular septum.

Complex (Fig. 17-28). In this complex there are pressure and volume hypertrophy of the right ventricle, pressure hypertrophy of the right atrium, enlargement of the pulmonary orifice and trunk, smallness of the aortic orifice, volume hypertrophy of the left atrium and ventricle, and enlargement of the mitral orifice.

We are dealing with the right side being related to systemic and pulmonary resistance, the left side related to pulmonary resistance, left-to-right shunt at the ventricular level, increased pulmonary flow, pulmonary hypertension, and increased volume on the left side.

Transposition of the arterial trunks

Transposition is a controversial term with varying interpretations. It may be considered as that abnormality in which the aorta or its remnant is abnormally placed vis-à-vis the pulmonary trunk or its remnant, or one or both of these vessels emerge from the wrong chambers, or the vessels are abnormally placed vis-à-vis the atrioventricular orifices. Normally the aorta is situated to the right and posterior with the pulmonary trunk to the left and anterior. In *regular* (d-) transposition the aorta is displaced anteriorly but remains to the right. It may emerge from both ventricles or from the right ventricle. In that sense, tetralogy of Fallot and double-outlet right ventricle are mild or partial forms of transposition. When the aorta emerges from the right ventricle and the pulmonary trunk from the left ventricle, there is *regular complete* transposition. The aorta may emerge anterior but distinctly to the left of the pulmonary trunk. This is inverted (l-) transposition. In that situation the ventricles are also inverted, with the left ventricle situated to the right and anterior, giving rise to the pulmonary trunk, while the right ventricle is situated to the left and posterior, giving rise to the aorta. This is called *corrected transposition* because the circulation is physiologically corrected, with systemic venous blood going to the pulmonary trunk, and pulmonary venous blood going to the aorta.

There are many complexes associated with transposition of the arterial trunks. In this chapter we deal only with simple regular (d-) complete transposition.

Simple regular (d-) complete transposition

Anomaly (Fig. 17-29). In this entity the aorta emerges from the right ventricle, while the pulmonary trunk comes off the left ventricle. The aorta is in most cases anterior and to the right, whereas the pulmonary trunk is posterior and to the left.

Complex (Fig. 17-30). In simple complete transposition complex, there may or may not be a ventricular septal defect, an atrial septal defect, or a patent ductus.

There is pressure hypertrophy of the right atrium and ventricle and, in many cases, volume hypertrophy of the left side. In still other cases, where pulmonary hypertension develops, pressure hypertrophy of the left side ensues.

We are dealing with two separate circulations, systemic and pulmonic, which communicate only by shunts at the atrial, ventricular, or ductus level. The direction of shunting at the atrial level is usually left to right, at the ventricular level right to left, and at the ductus level variable.

Tricuspid stenosis or atresia complexes

There is a group of complexes that have tricuspid stenosis or atresia as their base. These may or may not be associated with transposition. In this chapter, only some of those without transposition will be discussed.

Tricuspid atresia without transposition

Anomaly (Fig. 17-31). In tricuspid atresia the tricuspid orifice is absent. In its stead there may be a slight dimple in the distal portion of the atrium where the orifice should be.

Complex (Fig. 17-32). In tricuspid atresia without transposition there is always an associated atrial septal

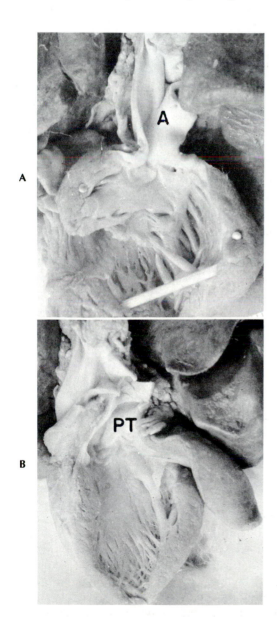

Fig. 17-29. Simple, regular complete transposition. **A,** Right ventricular view. **B,** Left ventricular view. *A,* Aorta; *PT,* pulmonary trunk. (From Lev, M.: Autopsy diagnosis of congenitally malformed hearts, Springfield, Ill., 1953, Charles C Thomas, Publisher.)

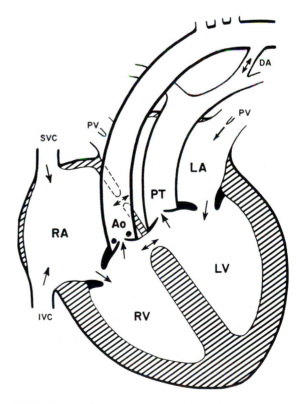

Fig. 17-30. Schematic diagram of simple, regular complete transposition complex. *Ao,* Aorta; *DA,* ductus arteriosus; *IVC,* inferior vena cava; *LA,* left atrium; *LV,* left ventricle; *PT,* pulmonary trunk; *PV,* pulmonary veins; *RA,* right atrium; *RV,* right ventricle; *SVC,* superior vena cava.

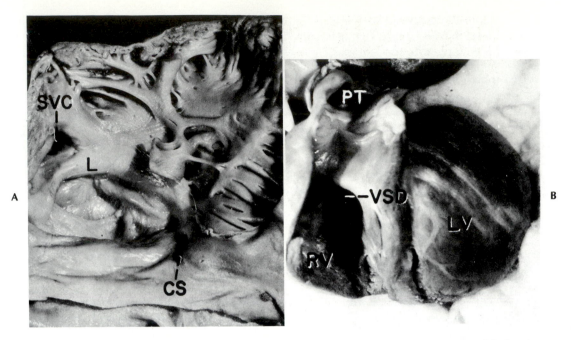

Fig. 17-31. Tricuspid atresia without transposition. **A,** Right atrial view. **B,** Anterior view. *CS,* Coronary sinus; *L,* limbus; *LV,* left ventricle; *PT,* pulmonary trunk; *RV,* right ventricle; *SVC,* superior vena cava; *VSD,* ventricular septal defect. (From Lev, M.: Autopsy diagnosis of congenitally malformed hearts, Springfield, Ill., 1953, Charles C Thomas, Publisher.)

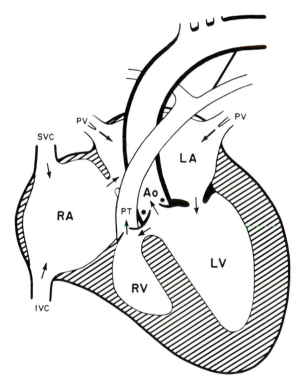

Fig. 17-32. Schematic diagram of tricuspid atresia without transposition complex. *Ao,* Aorta; *IVC,* inferior vena cava; *LA,* left atrium; *LV,* left ventricle; *PT,* pulmonary trunk; *PV,* pulmonary veins, *RA,* right atrium; *RV,* right ventricle; *SVC,* superior vena cava.

defect of the fossa ovalis type and in most cases a small ventricular septal defect. Pressure hypertrophy of the right atrium and volume hypertrophy of the left atrium and ventricle are present. The right ventricle shows volume atrophy, with infundibular stenosis, and small pulmonary orifice with or without a bicuspid pulmonic valve.

We are dealing with right-to-left shunt at the atrial level, left-to-right shunt at the ventricular level, decreased pulmonary flow, increased volume on the left side, and decreased volume on the right side.

Tricuspid stenosis with severe pulmonary stenosis or atresia (pulmonary atresia with intact ventricular septum)

Anomaly (Fig. 17-33). In tricuspid stenosis with pulmonary stenosis or atresia, the tricuspid anulus is small and the tricuspid valve consists of three poorly differentiated thickened leaflets, some of which may be displaced downward into the right ventricle. The right ventricle is a small chamber with a thick wall and frequently diffuse endocardial hypertrophy. The infundibular musculature is greatly thickened, and there is infundibular stenosis. The pulmonic orifice may be minute or obliterated. The pulmonic valve, when present, may show a diaphragm-like arrangement. The pulmonary trunk is minute. There is always an atrial septal defect of the fossa ovalis type. The left atrium and left ventricle are hyper-

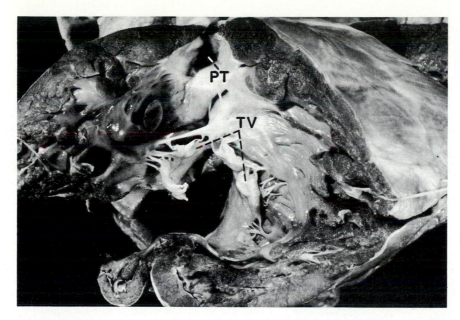

Fig. 17-33. Tricuspid stenosis with pulmonary stenosis. Right ventricular view. *PT*, Exit of pulmonary trunk; *TV*, tricuspid valve.

trophied and enlarged, with enlargement of the aortic and mitral orifices.

Complex (Fig. 17-34). In tricuspid stenosis with pulmonary stenosis or atresia, there are pressure hypertrophy of the right atrium and volume hypertrophy of the left atrium and ventricle, with enlargement of the aortic orifice.

We are dealing with the effects of right-to-left shunt at the atrial level, increase in volume on the left side, decreased volume but increased pressure on the right side, and decreased pulmonary flow.

Hypoplasia of aortic tract (hypoplastic left heart) complexes

Anomaly (Fig. 17-35). Hypoplasia of the aortic tract complexes are a group of complexes associated with severe aortic stenosis or atresia and with smallness of the left side of the heart. There are two types of such complexes: one with open mitral orifice and the other with mitral atresia. When the orifice is open, there is a small left ventricle with a relatively thick wall and diffuse endocardial hypertrophy (fibroelastosis). When it is closed, the left ventricle may be grossly absent or may be a small endocardium-lined slit.

Complexes (Fig. 17-36). Hypoplasia of aortic tract complexes are typified by volume and perhaps pressure hypertrophy of the right atrium and right ventricle, an atrial septal defect of any type, and a widely patent ductus arteriosus. We are dealing with volume atrophy of the left side and volume hypertrophy of the right side before birth. After birth there is left-to-right shunt at the atrial level and right-to-left shunt at the ductus level. The

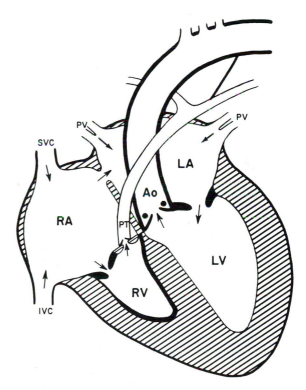

Fig. 17-34. Schematic diagram of tricuspid stenosis with pulmonary stenosis complex. *Ao*, Aorta; *IVC*, inferior vena cava; *LA*, left atrium; *LV*, left ventricle; *PT*, pulmonary trunk; *PV*, pulmonary veins, *RA*, right atrium; *RV*, right ventricle; *SVC*, superior vena cava.

ascending aorta and the coronary arteries are fed retrograde from the ductus arteriosus. Thus there is a ductus-dependent circulation. The reason for the peculiar left ventricle when the mitral orifice is open is not understood.

CAUSE OF DEATH

Increased pulmonary flow may lead to pneumonitis that may kill or contribute to the death of the patient. When there is decreased pulmonary flow, the patient may die from the effects of anoxia. Right or left ventricular failure, acute or chronic, may follow volume or pressure hypertrophy of either side. Subacute bacterial endocarditis may be engrafted on a bicuspid aortic valve, patent ductus arteriosus, or pulmonary stenosis and may be superimposed on persistent ostium primum and small ventricular septal defects. There is a tendency for this disease also to attack regions just distal to obstructions, as in coarctation and supravalvular aortic stenosis. Depending on the severity of the lesion, there is a wide range of longevity in some of the complexes without surgery (isolated pulmonary stenosis, tetralogy of Fallot, isolated patent ductus arteriosus, isolated aortic stenosis, and adult coarctation of the aorta), whereas other com-

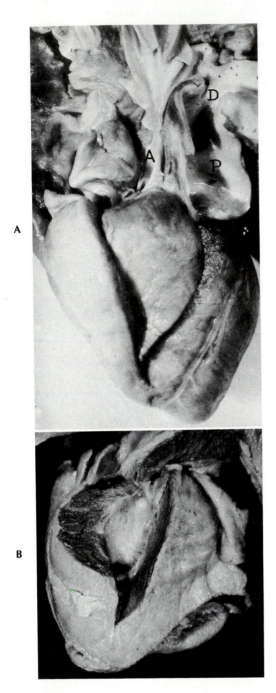

Fig. 17-35. Hypoplasia of aortic tract, with aortic and mitral stenosis. **A,** Anterior view of one heart. **B,** Left ventricular view of another heart. *A,* Aorta; *D,* ductus orteriosus; *P,* pulmonary trunk. In **B,** note small left ventricle, thick wall, and fibroelastosis. (**A,** From Lev, M.: Autopsy diagnosis of congenitally malformed hearts, Springfield, Ill., 1953, Charles C Thomas, Publisher.)

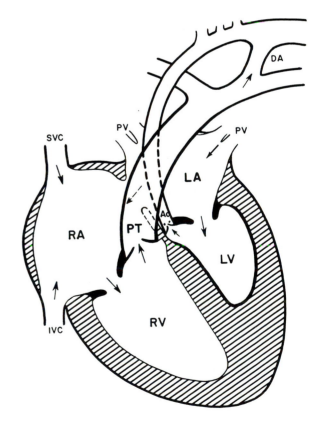

Fig. 17-36. Schematic diagram of hypoplasia of aortic tract complex. *Ao,* Aorta; *DA,* ductus arteriosus; *IVC,* inferior vena cava; *LA,* left atrium; *LV,* left ventricle, *PT,* pulmonary trunk; *PV,* pulmonary veins; *RA,* right atrium; *RV,* right ventricle; *SVC,* superior vena cava.

plexes do not permit long survival (tricuspid atresia, fetal coarctation, hypoplasia of the aortic tract complex, and complete transposition).

RECENT ADVANCES IN THE TREATMENT OF CONGENITAL HEART DISEASE

The last 40 years have seen tremendous advances in the treatment of congenital heart disease. Patent ductus arteriosus, coarctation of the aorta, isolated pulmonary stenosis, tetralogy of Fallot, total anomalous pulmonary venous drainage, and many other lesions are treated definitively with success. Treatment of other diseases produces considerable palliation. New surgical procedures are being created almost daily. It therefore behooves the pathologist to be well grounded in the details of this disease entity.

REFERENCES

1. Edwards, J.E.: Congenital malformations of heart and great vessels. In Gould, S.E., editor: Pathology of the heart, ed. 3, Springfield, Ill., 1968, Charles C Thomas, Publisher.
2. Lev, M.: Congenital heart disease. In Saphir, O., editor: A text on systemic pathology, vol. 1, New York, 1958, Grune & Stratton, Inc.
3. Lev, M., and Bharati, S.: Embryology of the heart and pathogenesis of congenital malformations of the heart. In Ravitch, M.M., et al., editors: Pediatric surgery, ed. 3, Chicago, 1979, Year Book Medical Publishers, Inc.
4. Netter, F.H., Alley, R.D., and van Mierop, L.H.S.: Diseases; congenital anomalies. In Netter, F.H.: The CIBA collection of medical illustrations, vol. 5—Heart, Summit, N.J., 1969, CIBA Pharmaceutical Co.

CHAPTER 18

Blood Vessels and Lymphatics

JACK L. TITUS

HAN-SEOB KIM

ARTERIES
Normal structure and age changes

Arteries conventionally are divided into three types depending on their size and certain histologic features: (1) large, elastic arteries; (2) medium-sized, distributing, muscular arteries; and (3) arterioles, which connect to capillaries. The three types are not sharply divided; elastic arteries gradually merge with muscular arteries and muscular arteries with arterioles. Histologically all arteries have three layers: the tunica intima on the luminal side of the vessel, the tunica media as a middle layer, and the tunica adventitia as the outermost layer (Fig. 18-1, A). These three layers become less definite as the arteries diminish in size and usually are not clearly identifiable in arterioles. Arteries and veins of all sizes and types are lined by an endothelium, which is a single layer of cells. The endothelial cells, basement membranes, and different amounts of connective tissues in different vessels form the tunica intima. Endothelial cells are not well demonstrated in routine histologic preparations; special techniques and electron microscopic study show them to be flattened cells with specialized junctions, intracellular organelles for transport of substances, and, in some cases, secretory organelles.

The elastic arteries include the aorta and its major branches and the major pulmonary arteries. In the first decade of life the tunica intima of these vessels is composed of endothelial cells with their basement membranes, a scanty amount of ground substance, collagen and elastic fibers, and the internal elastic lamina. The intima is bounded by the internal elastic lamina, a fenestrated sheet of elastic fibers that may be regarded both as part of the intima and as the beginning of the tunica media. The tunica media of elastic arteries constitutes the bulk of the arterial wall and consists chiefly of concentrically arranged, fenestrated laminae of elastic tissue with intervening smooth muscle cells and histologically amorphous ground substance, which biochemically is proteoglycans. The elastic laminae become thicker and increase in number in adulthood compared to childhood. The outermost elastic lamina of the media is the external elastic lamina. The large number of elastic laminae in the media of large elastic arteries have the capacity to absorb and transmit the pulsatile stroke of left ventricular systole and maintain intra-arterial pressure during diastole, effecting relatively constant pressure and flow of blood. The tunica adventitia consists of irregularly arranged collagen and elastic fibers. Small nutrient vessels of the arteries themselves, the vasa vasorum, are present in the adventitia together with lymphatics and nerves. In humans the outer portion of the media of the thoracic aorta also has vasa vasorum.

Muscular arteries (Fig. 18-1) generally are branches of elastic arteries, with internal diameters ranging from 0.3 to 3 mm. The definition of a muscular artery is mainly a histologic one related to near absence of well-defined elastic laminae in the media. The intima of a muscular artery is similar to that of an elastic artery, but thinner. The internal elastic lamina in muscular arteries in usual light microscopic preparations appears to be a single, continuous, wavy line; it is not continuous, however, but fenestrated, and is not wavy in life, the waviness being a postdeath artifact. The media of the muscular arteries is thick compared with the other two layers and consists of primarily circularly disposed, spindle-shaped smooth muscle cells, fine collagen and elastic fibers, and ground substance. The external elastic lamina is less prominent than that of elastic arteries and is not present in cerebral arteries. The tunica adventitia is thinner than the media and consists of collagen fibers, coarse and irregular elastic fibers, vasa vasorum, lymphatics, and nerves.

In both elastic and large muscular arteries the intima and the inner part of the media derive nutrition from the vascular lumen by permeation, whereas the nourishment of the outer media is derived from the vasa vasorum. There is therefore a nutritional boundary zone (watershed area) within the media that is especially susceptible to damage resulting from changes such as increased thickness of the intima, mural thrombosis within the arterial lumen, impaired oxygenation or oxygen release by the circulating blood, and obstruction of the vasa vasorum.

Arterioles are the smallest arteries, with an internal diameter of 0.3 mm or less. The larger arterioles have the usual three tissue layers including a poorly defined internal elastic lamina. In the smaller arterioles the media is one or two smooth muscle cells in thickness. The adventitia, consisting chiefly of collagen and elastic fibers, is relatively thick in larger arterioles and less prominent in smaller ones.

Changes that are roughly proportional to age occur in arteries as a result of the constant hemodynamic stresses of intraluminal blood pressure and flow. With time the walls of all arteries become more rigid, thus the term *senile arteriosclerosis*. These age changes are reflected in dilatation (ectasia) of some large elastic arteries and in tortuosity of some large muscular arteries. The structural basis of arterial aging, which can be regarded as an inevitable physiologic process, is most conspicuous in the intima but also involves the media.

Intimal thickening. In the fetus and neonate the intima is composed almost exclusively of endothelial cells with basement membranes (Fig. 18-1, *A* and *B*). In older infants (Fig. 18-1, *C* and *D*) some splitting of the internal elastic lamina and accumulation of fine elastic fibrils between the internal elastic lamina and the basement

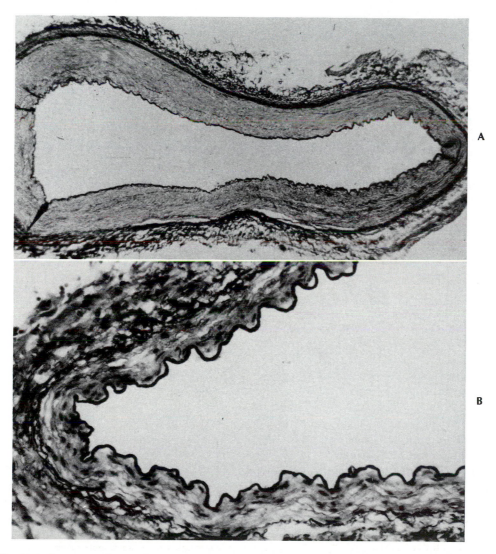

A

B

Fig. 18-1. Structure of normal muscular arteries at different ages in cross sections of coronary arteries, each stained to demonstrate elastic tissue. **A,** From a neonate. Wavy black line lining lumen is internal elastic lamina; endothelial cells and intima cannot be seen. Prominent muscular media is surrounded by black line of external elastic lamina. Adventitia is composed of loosely disposed connective tissue fibers. **B,** From a neonate. Higher-power view of a coronary artery emphasizes apparent absence of intima at this age.

Continued.

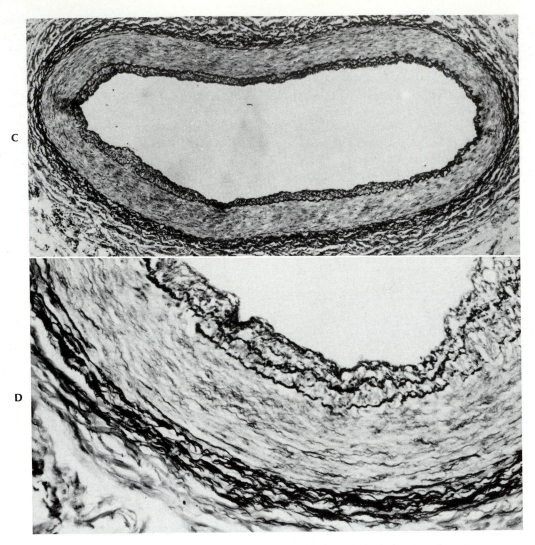

Fig. 18-1, cont'd. C, From 2-year-old child. True intima is evident. **D,** From 4-year-old. Higher-power view demonstrates fibromuscular intimal layer and reduplication of internal elastic lamina.

membrane of the endothelium are found. These changes are the beginning of intimal thickening that is a part of normal growth and remodeling processes. By 6 to 12 months of age, smooth muscle cells are found in the intima adjacent to the internal elastic lamina, creating a musculoelastic intimal layer. These smooth muscle cells synthesize basement membrane material, collagen, elastin, and proteoglycan (ground substance) of extracellular material.[7] Throughout life, intimal thickening progresses with the addition of more elastic and collagen fibers and eventual loss of cellular elements. These changes are seen most commonly in coronary arteries, the abdominal aorta (more on the dorsal than the ventral aspect), and the larger arteries of the lower extremities, all of which tend to manifest severe atherosclerotic lesions.[3]

Medial fibrosis. Progressive increase in the amount of collagen and ground substance of the media of arteries creates medial fibrosis, which begins at an early age. Medial fibrosis is associated with loss of smooth muscle cells, so that the media is hyalinized in advanced age. In small arteries and arterioles these changes occur more commonly in the viscera and lower extremities and are similar to those of chronic hypertension. When fibrosis is severe, luminal narrowing leading to tissue ischemia may ensue, but in general, medial fibrosis has little functional effect.

Changes in chemical composition Chemical analyses demonstrate a gradual increase in calcium salts in the arterial wall with increasing age. In addition, elastin content of the aorta increases along with changes in its amino acid composition. Aging arteries accumulate lipoproteins and glycosaminoglycans.

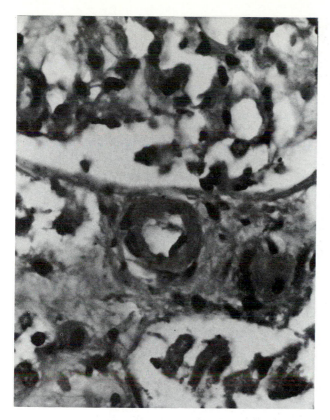

Fig. 18-2. Hyaline arteriolosclerosis of renal arteriole *(center)*. Portion of glomerulus is above arteriole, and round dark mass to right of arteriole is another hyalinized arteriole cut obliquely.

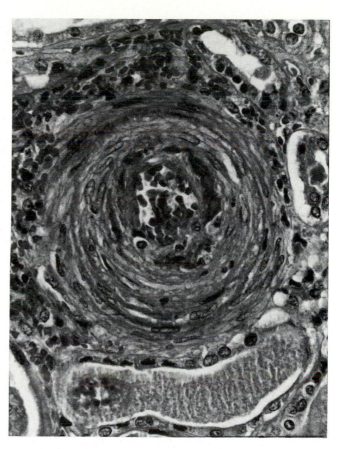

Fig. 18-3. Hyperplastic (proliferative) arteriolosclerosis of renal arteriole from patient with malignant hypertension. Concentrically arranged layers of intimal modified smooth muscle cells narrow lumen ("onion-skin" lesion). Dark amorphous material near lumen is fibrinoid necrosis.

Arteriosclerosis

Arteriosclerosis is a generic, inclusive term that describes thickening and hardening of the arterial wall. Included in this term are four pathologic entities: arteriolosclerosis, hypertensive arteriosclerosis, Mönckeberg's medial calcific sclerosis, and atherosclerosis. Some confusion results from the use of the term *arteriosclerosis* for the more specific disease entity of *atherosclerosis*, and the use of the unqualified term to indicate the arterial changes associated with aging (senile arteriosclerosis), hypertension (hypertensive arteriosclerosis), and reparative response of the artery to injuries (reparative arteriosclerosis). The term *hyaline arteriosclerosis* usually means hyaline arteriolosclerosis.

Arteriolosclerosis

Two morphologic abnormalities of arterioles, hyaline arteriolosclerosis (arteriolar hyalinosis) and hyperplastic (proliferative) arteriolosclerosis, constitute arteriolosclerosis.

Hyaline arteriolosclerosis. Hyaline arteriolar thickening (sclerosis) is a common pathologic lesion. Arteriolar hyalinosis (Fig. 18-2) pathologically is manifested by a subendothelial, homogeneous, glassy pink material in

hematoxylin and eosin–stained sections. It may accompany hypertensive disease, be a physiologic phenomenon of aging, or occur in patients with diabetes mellitus. The usual hyalinosis of visceral arterioles begins as a focal, segmental process that spreads to involve the entire circumference of the vessel. Some of the hyaline material, which is not homogeneous chemically, appears to be derived from precipitated plasma proteins,[1] and it also contains some lipid material. Moderate reduplication and thickening of endothelial basement membranes are usually present. The hyaline arteriolosclerosis of aging cerebral arterioles differs from that of visceral arterioles in that it appears to result from progressive fibrotic thickening of the adventitia and fibrosis of the media leading to the hyalinized vessel.

Hyperplastic (proliferative) arteriolosclerosis. Intimal thickening with consequent luminal reduction of hyperplastic arteriolosclerosis is a characteristic lesion of malignant hypertension, but identical changes may be found in patients with the hemolytic-uremic syndrome, progressive systemic sclerosis (scleroderma), and possibly toxemia of pregnancy. The process has been studied most extensively in accelerated hypertension, especially in renal interlobular arterioles and small arteries. Three main intimal morphologic patterns that can be distinguished are the "onion-skin lesion," mucinous intimal thickening, and fibrous intimal thickening.[8] The onion-skin intimal lesion consists of loosely disposed layers of modified smooth muscle cells (Fig. 18-3). The mucinous intimal thickening consists mainly of lucent amorphous material, probably proteoglycans, with few cells. Fibrous intimal thickening, which is less common, has hyaline deposits, reduplicated elastic fibers, and coarse bundles of collagen. The fine structural features of the cells of the thickened intima are those of modified smooth muscle cells, including a basement membrane, pinocytic vesicles, cytoplasmic myofilaments, and, most characteristically and constantly, spindle-shaped dense bodies or attachment devices associated with myofilaments. The pathogenesis of these intimal changes is unclear, but plasma proteins probably gain entry into the intima following endothelial injury such as increased pressure (hypertension), hypoxia, or immune damage. The common pathway is endothelial injury with increased permeability and a healing reaction of the vessel wall that involves smooth muscle cell migration from the media and proliferation of these cells with fibrosis.

Hypertensive arteriosclerosis

Regardless of its etiology, hypertension may be divided, clinically and to some degree pathologically, into chronic ("benign") and accelerated ("malignant") types. Accelerated hypertension may occur de novo, or it may supervene in patients who are chronically hypertensive. Sustained elevation of the arterial blood pressure is associated with apparently adaptive structural changes in arteries of all sizes. The changes in the larger arteries are similar in all types of hypertension, but different processes occur in the smaller arteries and arterioles in chronic and accelerated hypertension. The possibility that the structural changes of arteriolosclerosis initiate the hypertensive state is unlikely, for such changes are sometimes absent, particularly in early cases[2]; moreover, structural changes do not develop in arterioles that are protected from hypertension by occlusive changes in the larger arteries supplying them.

The classic hypertensive arterial change of large and medium-sized arteries as found in young individuals is medial hypertrophy resulting from increased numbers of smooth muscle cells and elastic fibers. The intima of these vessels may have increased numbers of longitudinally oriented smooth muscle fibers. With time, these hyperplastic and hypertrophic changes are replaced by collagenization with the thickened arterial wall becoming less resilient and the lumen dilated and tortuous.

In benign hypertension smaller arteries may show medial thickening as in the larger arteries, but the intimal thickening is more pronounced and results in luminal narrowing. The major change is hyaline arteriolosclerosis (Fig. 18-2). In both benign and malignant forms of hypertension, reduplication of basement membranes, elastosis, fibrosis, and hyaline deposits commonly are present.

In malignant hypertension the intima of smaller arteries and arterioles is thickened by hyperplastic (proliferative) lesions described previously. In addition to the hyperplastic and hyaline changes, arterioles, especially in the kidney, may undergo fibrinoid necrosis manifested by pyknotic nuclei, polymorphonuclear leukocytes, and intramural extravasation of red blood cells (Fig. 18-3). Fibrin thrombi within the narrowed lumina may be present and an additional cause of ischemia.

Mönckeberg's medial calcific sclerosis

Mönckeberg's medial calcification is an age-related degenerative process of calcification of the media of large and medium-sized muscular arteries (Fig. 18-4) that is fundamentally a different process from occlusive atherosclerosis and has little or no clinical significance.[4] The vessels most commonly affected are the femoral, tibial, radial, ulnar, and uterine arteries. This calcific arteriosclerotic lesion may occur with atherosclerosis in the same vessels of an individual. Affected vessels, which are hard when palpated and are demonstrable on roentgenograms, generally are dilated and show transverse ridges of medial calcification under the intima. Sometimes medial calcification shows osseous metaplasia containing marrow elements (Fig. 18-4). The etiology is unknown, but it is probably a misconception to consider Mönckeberg's medial calcification as a disease process. Similar medial calcific lesions have been produced in experimental animals by repeated infusions of vasoactive pharmacologic agents such as epinephrine or nicotine.

Medial calcification also occurs in pseudoxanthoma elasticum and in idiopathic arterial calcification of infancy. In pseudoxanthoma elasticum, a recessively inherited disease, changes occur in the elastic fibers of the skin, eyes, and vessels. The earliest detectable histologic vascular lesion is accumulation of calcium in elastic fibers, followed by fragmentation of the fibers.[6] Calcification is often found in the internal elastic lamina of the gastric arteries and in all medial elastic tissue of the coronary and large peripheral arteries. Coronary arterial occlusion may occur. Idiopathic arterial calcification of infancy is a rare but serious disease often involving coronary and systemic arteries[5] in babies less than 6 months old. The calcification is found in the internal elastic lamina and in the media, often associated with fibrous intimal thickening. When the coronary arteries are involved, the heart is enlarged and myocardial infarction

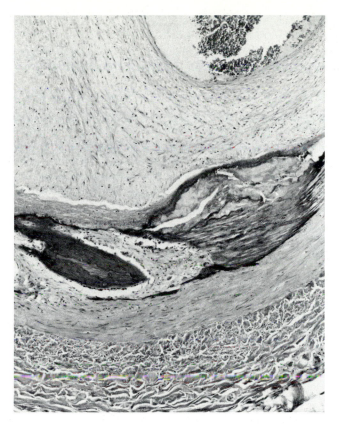

Fig. 18-4. Medial calcification (Mönckeberg's medial calcific sclerosis) of femoral artery of elderly man. Dark, irregular mass in center of photograph is calcification of inner media with osseous metaplasia; below calcific mass are normal medial muscle and adventitia. Vascular lumen containing red blood cells is in upper right of photograph. Intima is thickened by fibromuscular tissue.

may cause death. No pathogenic mechanism is known; results of studies of calcium and other mineral metabolism, lipid metabolism, and endocrine functions have all been normal.

Atherosclerosis

Atherosclerosis (AS), a specific form of arteriosclerosis, is primarily an intimal disease characterized by fibrous (fibrolipid, atheromatous) plaques. The most distinctive feature of AS is the localized accumulation of lipids, forming an atheroma (fibrofatty plaque) in the intima of large elastic arteries and medium-sized muscular arteries. The atheromatous plaque is a raised, localized lesion within the intima that has a central core of lipid, which is mostly cholesteryl esters complexed with proteins, and an overlying tissue plate. In addition to lipids, various cells, connective tissue fibers, and blood products accumulate in the lesions. Complications including thrombosis, calcification, hemorrhage into the plaque, and ulceration can occur. The term *atherosclerosis* derives from the combination of *athero-* (porridge), referring to the soft, lipid-rich material in the center of a typical intimal plaque, and *sclerosis* (scarring), referring to the connective tissue components.

The major clinical syndromes related to AS result from ischemia produced by narrowing of the vascular lumen (coronary heart disease, peripheral vascular disease, cerebral infarction), or from weakening of the arterial wall leading to an aneurysm. Although AS in humans begins early in life and develops progressively over years, it is rarely symptomatic in the first three decades, but thereafter the frequency of clinical atherosclerotic events increases logarithmically with age.[29]

Epidemiology. Because of its prevalence, AS can be considered epidemic in industrialized nations. In 1967, in about 50 countries on all continents, the most common causes of death (37% overall) were cardiovascular diseases, most of which were related to atherosclerosis.[41] Every year approximately 1 million persons in the United States experience either a myocardial infarct or sudden cardiac death. Nearly all of these are the result of atherosclerotic coronary artery disease (CAD). An encouraging fact is that, beginning in the mid-1960s, there has been more than a 20% decline overall in coronary heart disease mortality in the United States[24] and a decline in the prevalence of CAD.[46] Similar or greater decreases in mortality are recorded for cerebrovascular diseases, most of which also are atherosclerotic in origin.[45]

According to the International Atherosclerosis Project,[27] the geographic distribution of AS showed both geographic and ethnic differences in average extent of involvement of arterial intimal surfaces at all ages, with significantly higher numbers from industrialized populations, which also had higher mortalities from CAD. The study suggested that geographic factors probably are more important than racial factors, supporting the belief that AS is in part an environmental disease. It has been observed repeatedly that populations that move from an area with a low incidence of atherosclerotic diseases to one with a high incidence tend gradually to acquire the higher rates of the country of adoption.

Epidemiologic investigations of living populations have disclosed risk factors that are associated with an increased likelihood of developing clinical atherosclerotic disease.[44] These risk factors, which are best defined for CAD and cerebrovascular diseases, include age, sex, genetic background, hyperlipoproteinemia, hypertension, cigarette smoking, diabetes mellitus, and obesity. These factors are not mutually exclusive, and some are irreversible, whereas others are reversible or potentially reversible.

Age. Although the natural history of AS is most often an age-related phenomenon,[11,47] AS is not simply the result of unmodified, intrinsic, biologic aging processes. Some populations age without showing clinical evidence of AS, and most mammalian species age without spontaneously developing AS. Although aging appears to play a role, particularly in relation to the changes in cells of the arterial wall, AS can best be considered an age-related disease that can be influenced by both environmental and genetic factors.

Sex. There is a striking difference in the incidence and severity of atherosclerosis between the two sexes. Atherosclerotic coronary heart disease is predominantly a disease of men, especially at younger ages; the prevalence in men in the fourth decade is three times that in women.[13] This difference decreases with age but remains higher at all ages in men. Possible explanations for the sex differences include levels of estrogenic hormones[30] and higher levels of high-density lipoprotein, which is known to be antiatherogenic,[18] in premenopausal women than in men.

Genetic factors. The significance of racial differences in atherogenesis may reflect the genetic background of different populations. Although such differences vary with the location of the lesions,[33] coronary atherosclerosis is generally less severe in blacks than in whites. Apparent genetic roles in familial predisposition to AS may be related to genetic effects on other risk factors, especially hyperlipoproteinemia, hypertension, and diabetes mellitus.

Hyperlipoproteinemia and diet. Atherosclerotic lesions are more severe in patients with hyperlipoproteinemia, including those with diabetes mellitus, myxedema, nephrosis, xanthomatosis, and familial hypercholesterolemia. A directly proportional relationship between the level of serum cholesterol and the risk of atherosclerotic coronary heart disease has been repeatedly established in epidemiologic, clinical, and pathologic studies.[3,34] In most animal models, elevation of the plasma cholesterol level by increased dietary cholesterol and saturated fat leads to atherosclerotic lesions similar to those in humans. The precise mechanisms by which the plasma lipoproteins contribute to the pathogenesis of AS are not known, but the lipids found in atherosclerotic lesions are thought to originate primarily from the plasma lipoproteins. Controversy exists as to the significance of elevations of serum triglyceride levels.[18] Many studies have demonstrated the specific effects of diet on lipid and lipoprotein levels, including the amount of dietary cholesterol ingested, the ratio of polyunsaturated to saturated fat, the total number of calories from carbohydrates, protein, and fat, and the intake of alcohol and concentrated sweets.[19]

Hypertension. Hypertension has been shown to be a major risk factor for atherosclerotic CAD, cerebrovascular disease, and peripheral vascular disease.[13] Experimentally, hypertension augments the induction of atherosclerosis. The atherogenic mechanism of hypertension may be related to increased workload on arterial smooth muscle, mechanical injury to the arterial wall, or increased filtration pressure and increased permeability of the endothelium. Abnormalities of the humoral mediators of blood pressure control, including catecholamines, renin, angiotensin, kallikrein, kinin, and prostaglandins, may play a role in atherogenesis.

Cigarette smoking. The relationship between cigarette smoking and a higher risk of atherosclerotic CAD, especially sudden cardiac death, is unequivocal. Autopsy studies have shown a greater extent of coronary and aortic AS in smokers than in nonsmokers.[48] The component of cigarette smoking responsible for the acceleration of atherosclerotic events is not known. It may be related to effects of the cigarette smoking on thrombosis or to increased concentration of carboxyhemoglobin in the blood of smokers.

Diabetes mellitus. Diabetes mellitus contributes importantly to all manifestations of atherosclerotic diseases, including CAD, peripheral arterial disease, and cerebrovascular disease. Although other risk factors, particularly elevated blood cholesterol levels, high blood pressure, obesity, and low plasma levels of high-density lipoprotein, are significantly related to diabetes mellitus, these factors do not totally explain the added risk of diabetes mellitus.

Other risk factors. Other risk factors suggested to be associated with AS include obesity, physical activity, hyperglycemia, water hardness, personality type, stress, hemoglobin values, alcohol intake, coffee consumption, and nonatherosclerotic cardiac abnormalities. The role of obesity may be by virtue of its association with other risk factors for AS such as hyperlipoproteinemia, hypertension, diabetes mellitus, and hyperglycemia, but individuals 20% or more above the ideal weight have an increased risk of CAD or cerebrovascular disease. Sedentary men have approximately three times the rate of coronary heart disease of physically active men, but whether exercise has a direct effect on atherogenesis is not certain, although increased serum levels of high-density lipoprotein have been reported in the physically active. Although epidemiologic studies have identified personality attributes associated with increased risk of CAD, it has not been established that such attributes are related to the development of AS per se. The role of the other proposed risk factors listed is controversial.

Morphology. Although the fibrous and complicated plaques are the atherosclerotic lesions associated with disturbances in blood flow that cause clinical disease states, the morphologic changes of diffuse intimal thickening, fatty dots and streaks, and gelatinous lesions may be either precursors of the basic atherosclerotic lesion or stages in its development.

Diffuse intimal thickening. Diffuse fibromuscular intimal thickening of arteries that develops with age has been viewed as an integral part of the atherosclerotic process or at least a requisite change for the development of atherosclerosis.[3] The process is most rapid during the first two decades of life, occurs in all humans, and is found in most arteries, but it is not clearly related to advanced atherosclerotic lesions.

Fatty dots and streaks. Fatty dots and streaks are well-circumscribed, yellow (lipid-laden), flat or minimally raised foci that vary in size from barely visible dots to elongated, beaded streaks (Fig. 18-5). They begin to appear in the aorta in the first year of life just above the aortic valve and at the site of the closed ductus arteriosus. In the first decade of life, fatty streaks (juvenile fatty streaks) are found near the ostia of intercostal arteries, in the aortic arch, and in the posterior wall of the thoracic and abdominal aorta. Most individuals have at least some intimal fatty dots and streaks by 3 years of age, and their extent increases in the second decade of life. These lesions are found at puberty in the proximal segments of the coronary arteries. Fatty dots and streaks begin to develop in carotid and intracranial arteries during the third and fourth decades of life. Blacks have more extensive lesions than whites or other racial groups, and females of all racial groups have more extensive lesions than do males of the same populations.[26] Fatty dots and streaks are not consistently associated with diet, serum lipids, geographic residence, or other risk factors for AS.

The histologic features of fatty dots and streaks vary. All have lipids in the intima, either intracellularly or extracellularly. Most often the lipids are present in closely packed foam cells immediately beneath the endothelium or in elongated fat-containing cells scattered within the intima (Fig. 18-6). In both human and experimental models the foam cells have been shown to be derived from either smooth muscle cells[15] or macrophages.[16]

The origin and significance of fatty dots and streaks and their relationship to atherosclerotic disease are uncertain. The location of these lesions mainly in the thoracic aorta contrasts with the more frequent location of recognized AS in the abdominal aorta. Although fatty streaks are present in the coronary arteries of most juveniles, great variations exist in the incidence of atherosclerotic CAD in different adult populations. The cholesteryl esters in foam cells of fatty dots and streaks differ chemically from those in the lipid core of atheromatous fibrous plaque.[42] These dissimilarities might be explained on the basis of two types of fatty streaks, which differ in morphology, cellular genotype, and lipid content, with one type related to the fibrous plaque and the other type not related.[35] Fatty streaks are uncommon in older persons, suggesting that they may be absorbed.

Gelatinous lesions. Gray gelatinous elevations, which sometimes have been regarded as precursors of the fibrous plaque,[3] are difficult to detect on inspection of the arterial intimal surface. They may be circumscribed, round, or oval, occasionally reaching a diameter of 1 cm, or they may extend along the long axis of the artery. They can be observed in the abdominal aorta of children, even in the absence of fatty dots and streaks. Microscopically the lesions are foci of intimal edema representing an insudate of plasma that separates the formed extracellular elements.[43] Little information is available as to age of appearance and frequency distributions. The concept that gelatinous lesions are precursors of atherosclerosis remains in question.

Fibrous plaques. The term *fibrous plaque*[23,51] refers to the gross morphologic appearance of the lesion that is the hallmark of AS. Other names include atherosclerotic plaque, atheromatous plaque, fibrolipid plaque, and fibrofatty plaque. The lesions are raised, pearly white to gray, smooth-surfaced, plaquelike structures in the intima that vary in diameter from a few millimeters to over a centimeter. They usually are elongated in the direction of the long axis of the artery, and lesions may become confluent. The plaques, which are in the intima but may extend into the media, may encroach considerably on the vascular lumen, especially in muscular arteries such as the coronary arteries. On cross section (Fig. 18-7) a typical lesion has a soft, yellow central zone with gruel-like material (atheroma) covered on the luminal aspect by a

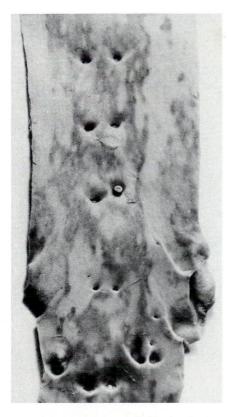

Fig. 18-5. Opened aorta of 11-year-old boy has been stained with Oil Red O to demonstrate fatty streaks, which are dark vertical streaks on wall of aorta and about orifices of branches. In the natural state these streaks are pale yellow.

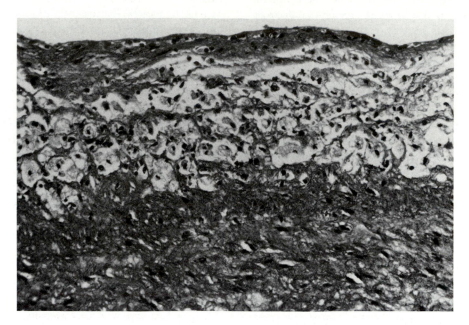

Fig. 18-6. Foam cells in intima of aorta. Lumen and endothelium are above. Media is lower third of photograph.

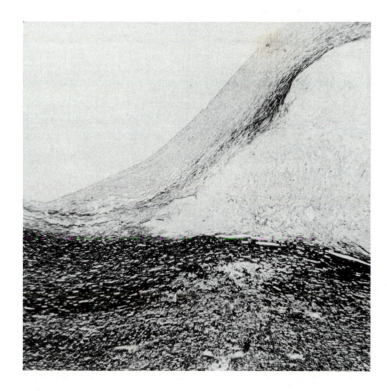

Fig. 18-7. Portion of typical fibrous (atheromatous) plaque of aorta demonstrates fibrous cap adjacent to lumen *(above left)* and central atheromatous material *(pale, amorphous tissue to right of center)* with darkly stained media in lower third of photomicrograph.

layer of dense fibromuscular tissue (fibrous cap). Intact plaques do not stain with fat stains because the lipids in the center are covered by the fibrous cap. Not all grossly typical fibrous plaques contain central atheromatous material; some are made up entirely of fibrous or fibromuscular tissue.

The distribution, frequency, time of appearance, and extent of surface involvement of fibrous plaques vary in different arteries and in different segments of the same artery. In general, plaques are found most often in the abdominal aorta, large arteries of the lower limbs, carotid arteries, proximal portions of the coronary arteries, and circle of Willis. The prevalence, extent, and location of fibrous plaques parallel the frequency of clinical diseases attributable to AS.

Microscopically the central atheroma of an uncomplicated fibrous plaque consists of acellular, granular or amorphous, electron-dense material that contains lipids, especially crystals of cholesteryl esters, cellular debris, proteoglycans, fibrin, and other plasma proteins. Extra-

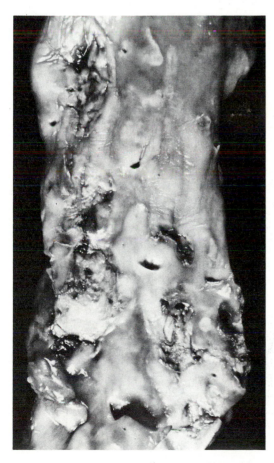

Fig. 18-8. Opened abdominal aorta shows variety of lesions of advanced atherosclerosis. White raised areas are fibrous plaques. Irregular areas along both cut edges are complicated plaques, some of which are ulcerated with superimposed thrombi *(black material)*. Orifices of some branches are narrowed by atherosclerotic process.

cellular lipid in the lipid core originates mainly from necrosis of fat-laden cells. The fibrous cap is composed of avascular connective tissues and elongated smooth muscle cells covered by endothelium.[22] The connective tissue contains glycosaminoglycans (acidic mucopolysaccharide), elastic and collagen fibers synthesized by the smooth muscle cells,[37,38] and reticulin fibrils. Inflammatory cells, including macrophages, may be present. The histologic appearance of lesions varies considerably depending on the relative amounts of the different components. In apparently older or more advanced lesions the collagen of the fibrous cap is dense and hyalinized, and the smooth muscle cells are atrophic, although occasional fat-laden foam cells of uncertain origin may be present near the lipid core. The smooth muscle cells in the fibrous cap[15] differ ultrastructurally in shape and cytoplasmic organelles from typical medial smooth muscle cells. In the cap they are slender, oriented in the long axis of the artery, have few cytoplasmic projections, and have few myofilaments, which are near the plasma membrane.

Complicated plaques. Complicated plaques develop from preexisting fibrous plaques as a result of one or a combination of several pathologic changes that include calcification, ulceration, thrombosis, and hemorrhage. The complicated lesion (Fig. 18-8) is the most common type of atherosclerotic lesion that produces significant circulatory change and clinical disease in adults.

CALCIFICATION. In advanced fibrous plaques, calcification is common. The intima is brittle and cracks like an eggshell when the vessel is opened. Microscopically the dystrophic calcific process involves both the fibrous cap and the atheromatous portion of the plaque. This form of atherosclerotic intimal calcification is to be differentiated from Mönckeberg's medial calcific arteriosclerosis, which affects only the tunica media. In experimental atherosclerosis the size of calcific complicated lesions has been shown to decrease on removal of the atherosclerotic stimulus.[12]

ULCERATION AND THROMBOSIS. Advanced fibrous plaques with soft pultaceous atheromas, especially those with calcification, may ulcerate as a result of mechanical or hemodynamic forces. With ulceration, cholesterol or lipid debris from the atheroma may be discharged and embolize. Mural thrombi may form on the ulcer or at sites of endothelial damage or mural hemorrhage. Such thrombi also may embolize, or they may become organized and incorporated within the intimal plaque. Mural thrombi in medium-sized arteries may progress to occlusive thrombi that may recanalize.

HEMORRHAGE. Hemorrhage into atherosclerotic plaques is a common finding in advanced lesions, especially in the coronary arteries. The blood may reach the lesion from the vascular lumen through surface ulcerations or from rupture of capillaries that vascularized the atheroma from adventitial vasa vasorum.[40] Hemosiderin pigment as evidence of prior hemorrhage is common.

Changes in the media and adventitia. Although AS is a disease of the intima, the more advanced lesions are associated with secondary changes in the media (Fig. 18-9). With encroachment of the expanding atherosclerotic lesion into the media, the internal elastic lamina is attenuated and fragmented, and smooth muscle cells and elastic lamina atrophy with thinning of the media. Aneurysmal dilatation may follow, especially in elastic arteries. Fibrosis of the adventitia and foci of lymphocytes in the adventitia are common accompaniments of complicated atherosclerotic lesions.

Pathogenesis. AS is a multifaceted and multifactoral disease whose exact pathogenesis is unknown. Theories proposed in the past have been based on aging, mechanical injury, intraintimal hemorrhage, anoxia, insudation of blood products following endothelial injury, and encrustation (thrombosis). The insudation, imbibition, inflammation, and perfusion theory proposed that organization of proteins in the insudate contributed the fibrous component and the plasma lipids contributed the lipid component of advanced lesions. The encrustation (thrombogenic) theory suggested that breakdown and organization of a fibrin-platelet thrombus led to the atherosclerotic plaque. Elements of both these theories, especially the role of coagulation factors, are incorporated into current concepts of atherogenesis, which involve specific roles of arterial smooth muscle cells, endothelial cells, platelets, and lipoproteins.

Arterial smooth muscle cells. Arterial smooth muscle cells can synthesize each of the three characteristic connective tissue matrix proteins—collagen, elastic fiber proteins, and proteoglycans—and are the principal source of connective tissue in the intima. Smooth muscle cells can take up and degrade some lipids, including low-density lipoprotein and can synthesize cholesterol.[10]

Smooth muscle cell migration and proliferation can be stimulated by platelet-derived growth factor, a macrophage factor, a possible endothelial cell factor, hyperlipidemic serum, lipoproteins, cholesterol, cholesteryl esters, some lipids, and insulin.[38] Smooth muscle cells in areas of increased glycosaminoglycan content are more responsive to proliferative stimuli. The proliferation or function of these cells is inhibited by prostaglandins, fatty acids, oxidative derivatives of cholesterol, high-density lipoprotein, heparin, thrombocytopenia in some models, estrogens, antirheumatic drugs, and age.[50]

For some agents one concentration may stimulate proliferation whereas another concentration causes cellular injury that may provoke the usual inflammatory-reparative processes and thus contribute to the formation of a lesion. Knowledge of the quantitative aspects of stimuli for smooth muscle cell proliferation is minimal. Although considerable information about the pathobiology of arterial smooth muscle cells is available, the combined effects of multiple factors on the behavior of these cells is less well known, particularly in intact animals and in the complex environment of a developed or developing plaque.

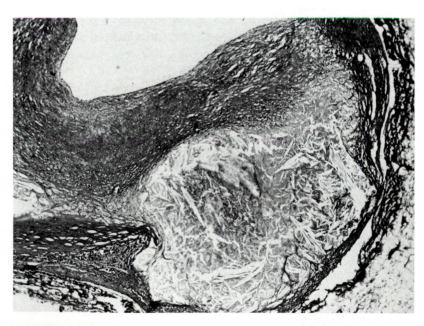

Fig. 18-9. Lumen *(above, left of center)* of coronary artery is narrowed, and media *(darkly stained tissue in lower part and right side of photograph)* are thinned by atherosclerotic process, which consists of central atheroma with cholesterol clefts, fibrin, and cellular debris covered on luminal aspect by thick fibromuscular tissue.

Endothelial cells. Structural and functional integrity of the endothelial cell layer is fundamental for maintenance of normal structure and function of the vascular system. Glycosaminoglycans of the endothelial cell plasma membrane prevent activation of blood coagulation, platelets, and leukocytes. The endothelial cell can synthesize the powerful anti-platelet-aggregatory vasodilator substance prostacyclin (PGI_2); factor VIII (antihemophilic factor); plasminogen activator; a heparin-like anticoagulant substance; and basement membrane materials including collagen, elastin, and glycosaminoglycans.[21,25]

That endothelial injury is important in atherogenesis has been known for many years. Experimentally, endothelial injury can be induced mechanically, chemically, immunologically, and by diet-induced chronic hyperlipidemia, bacterial endotoxin, viruses, hypoxia, carbon monoxide, tobacco proteins, and hemodynamic forces. The responses of the vessel to endothelial injury may be modified by insulin, vasoactive peptides, platelet and white blood cell products, and plasma lipoproteins.[32]

Among this staggering array of factors, many of which are interrelated, that can affect the endothelium, some stand out as probably primary in atherogenesis. Endothelial denudation or injury permits platelet adherence, aggregation, and release of products at the site of exposed subendothelial connective tissue. Plasma constituents, such as lipoproteins, have access to the underlying arterial wall, since the permeability barrier has been altered. The interaction of the platelet products and plasma constituents leads to smooth muscle cell migration into and proliferation within the intima.

Platelets. Platelets adhere to sites of endothelial injury, aggregate to form platelet masses, release granules rich in a variety of secretory products including platelet-derived growth factor (PDGF), which is mitogenic for smooth muscle cells, and synthesize products including some prostaglandins. The most important stimulus to platelet adherence is the exposure of collagen fibrils to the circulating blood.

Thrombin, which stimulates adherence of platelets to each other, activates the formation of the cyclic prostaglandin endoperoxides from arachidonic acid. The cyclic endoperoxides are converted into potent prostacyclin (PGI_2) in the endothelium and thromboxane A_2 in the platelets. Thromboxane A_2 is a proaggregatory, vasoconstrictive substance; prostacyclin is an antiaggregatory, vasodilatory substance.[31] Platelet aggregation also is promoted by antigen-antibody complexes, fatty acids, smoking, and hypercholesterolemia.

Lipoproteins. The plasma lipoproteins—chylomicrons, very low–density lipoprotein (VLDL), low-density lipoprotein (LDL), and high-density lipoprotein (HDL)—have a role in atherogenesis. Triglycerides of dietary and endogenous origin are transported, respec-

tively, by the chylomicrons and VLDL. Chylomicrons are catabolized to a triglyceride-poor, cholesterol-enriched lipoprotein particle (remnant), which has been postulated to be atherogenic.[53] LDL, which is derived from VLDL, is bound by fibroblasts, smooth muscle cells, lymphocytes, and endothelial cells and is degraded to the amino acids of the protein moiety and to the cholesterol and fatty acids of the cholesteryl ester. Intracellular accumulation of cholesterol shuts off synthesis of LDL receptors, inhibits cholesterol synthesis by enzyme inhibition, and stimulates enzymatic esterification of cholesterol.[17] Accumulation of cholesteryl esters, cholesterol, and lipoproteins is characteristic in atherosclerotic plaques, but the specific mechanisms by which hypercholesterolemia, hyperlipoproteinemia, and hyperlipemia cause AS are not known.[28,52] The antiatherogenic effect of HDL may be related to its role in the transport of cholesterol to the liver for breakdown and to competition of HDL with LDL for cellular binding.[18,49]

Current theories of pathogenesis. The current major theories of the pathogenesis of atherosclerosis postulate that it is myogenic in nature, involving proliferation of smooth muscle cells.

RESPONSE TO INJURY HYPOTHESIS. This hypothesis, proposed by Ross,[38] incorporates aspects of the older insudation and encrustation theories. Endothelial injury permits adherence and aggregation of platelets with release of PDGF, which, together with plasma constituents, causes intimal proliferation of smooth muscle cells. Prostacyclin deficiency, related to hyperlipidemia,[20] increases platelet aggregability and endothelial permeability. Intimal proliferation of smooth muscle cells is accompanied by the synthesis of connective tissue matrix proteins and often by the deposition of intracellular and extracellular lipids. Although restoration of the endothelial barrier may allow the lesion to regress if both the injury to the endothelium and the response to it are limited, repeated or chronic cycles of injury over a period of years result in lesions. According to this theory, platelets play a key role in the stimulation of intimal smooth muscle cells, leading to the development of the atherosclerotic lesion; experimental support for this key issue exists.[14]

MONOCLONAL (MUTAGENIC) HYPOTHESIS. Benditt[9] suggested that each fibrous plaque begins with proliferation of a single, genetically transformed smooth muscle cell. The hypothesis is based on the finding that fibrous plaques from black females who were heterozygotes for glucose 6-phosphate dehydrogenase (G-6-PD) frequently contained only one of the two G-6-PD isoenzymes. In these women normal arterial and other tissues should be heterozygous for G-6-PD isoenzymes (mosaicism) because of random inactivation of one X chromosome in embryonic life. The finding of monotypism of the smooth muscle cells of the plaques suggested their origin from a single cell, similar to the known monoclonal nature of uterine leiomyomas, which presumably arise by mutation. Known mutagenic agents include endogenous or environmental chemical agents, radiation and some viruses, some chemicals in cigarette smoke, and some cholesterol metabolic products that are carried by the lipoproteins. Whether the monoclonal nature of the lesion is by selection processes of a certain cell line or by mutation is controversial.[36] Animal models with similar cellular markers to test the monoclonal hypothesis experimentally have not been found.

Animal models. Identification of etiologic and pathogenic factors in AS is a problem because of the difficulty in obtaining tissues at appropriate times and intervals from living persons, the limitations of materials derived from autopsy, and the long time course of the disease, which apparently begins in childhood. Accordingly, a variety of experimental animal models including pigs, nonhuman primates, rabbits, rats, mice, birds (chickens, pigeons, and turkeys), and dogs have been used for the study of AS. Since in most of these clinical atherosclerotic disease does not develop in the natural state, abnormal diets, with or without other measures, are needed to produce AS. Some common laboratory animals such as dogs and rats are relatively resistant to atherosclerotic disease induced by dietary measures alone. Certain swine and some nonhuman primates appear to be most suitable, although specific questions may be answered by use of other experimental models. Animal models are particularly suitable for regression studies, studies of the metabolism of the arterial wall, and studies of the cellular pathobiology of AS.

Arteritis

Arteritis means any type of inflammatory process of an artery or arteriole. The terms *vasculitis* and *angiitis* are essentially synonyms. Veins and capillaries also may be involved synchronously or metachronously in many types of arteritis. The inflammatory process may result from invasion of the vessel by microbiologic agents or from immunologic, chemical, mechanical, or radiant energy injuries. Pathologic classification of the apparently primary, noninfective vasculidites is not entirely satisfactory because there is considerable overlap of size, type, location, and histopathologic features of involved vessels and organs among reasonably well-delineated clinical syndromes and diseases.[66,70]

Endarteritis obliterans

Endarteritis obliterans is intimal cellular proliferation and thickening that narrows the lumen of small arteries and arterioles. The suffix "-itis" is misleading because there is minimal if any inflammatory cell infiltrate, although inflammatory processes may have been involved in the development of the lesion. The term is a descriptive pathologic designation, not a specific disease. Endarteritis obliterans is common in chronic cutaneous or gastrointestinal ulcers, tuberculous foci, chronic pulmonary abscesses, chronic meningitis, end-stage kidney disease, and functionally atrophic vessels or organs such as the ductus arteriosus, umbilical arteries, postpartum and postmenopausal uterine arteries, and arteries supplying surgically removed organs. Microscopically the lumen of the vessel is reduced or obliterated by orderly arranged, proliferated intimal fibrous tissue, which is

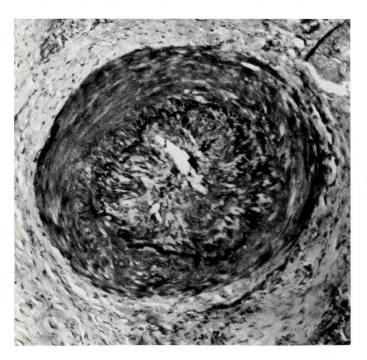

Fig. 18-10. This small artery exhibits endarteritis obliterans with vascular lumen markedly narrowed by cellular intimal proliferation. Black wavy line is internal elastic lamina.

often in a concentric pattern (Fig. 18-10). This lesion is to be distinguished from organized, recanalized thrombi.

Infective arteritis

Nonsyphilitic arteritis. Direct invasion of the artery by bacteria, fungi, parasites, rickettsiae, or viruses from adjacent infected foci, by hematogenous spread including infected thrombi from distant foci, or from septicemia may result in segmental inflammation (mycotic arteritis). Infective endocarditis is the most frequent condition causing infective arteritis. Weakening of the arterial wall may lead to a mycotic aneurysm or to rupture of the vessel. Vasa vasorum are the route of entry of organisms into large vessels such as the aorta,[81] whereas direct invasion from the lumen occurs mainly in vessels small enough to entrap the infectious particles. Microscopically an inflammatory infiltrate permeates the vessel wall and causes destruction of tissues. Thrombosis with stenosis or occlusion of the vascular lumen may occur. The organ or tissue affected may suffer ischemic necrosis (infarction).

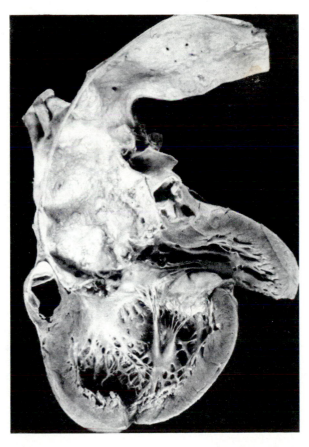

Fig. 18-11. Left ventricle, aortic valve, and thoracic aorta have been opened to demonstrate late changes of syphilitic aortitis. Intimal surface of aorta is irregularly wrinkled and thickened ("tree bark" appearance), and ascending aorta is aneurysmally dilated.

Syphilitic arteritis. Syphilitic (luetic) vascular involvement occurs late in the course of luetic disease as a type of tertiary syphilis. It is relatively rare today owing to improved control and treatment of syphilis, but the increase of primary syphilis in the last decade may result in an increase of syphilitic vascular disease in the future. Cardiovascular complications occur in approximately 10% of syphilitic patients.[78] Clinical vascular disease results mainly from aortitis, leading to an aneurysm; small arteries are infrequently involved.

Syphilitic aortitis, which affects primarily the ascending aorta and aortic arch, is the most common manifestation of cardiovascular syphilis. The predilection for the proximal aorta may result from the rich vascular and lymphatic circulation in this segment and the frequent infection of mediastinal lymph nodes in the early secondary stage of syphilis. Grossly the intima of the involved aorta has pearly-white, thickened plaques separated by normal intima that is wrinkled and has small depressions so that the overall appearance vaguely resembles tree bark (Fig. 18-11). Superimposed atherosclerotic lesions may obscure the syphilitic lesions. The aortic lesions may extend to the branches of the aortic arch. Histologically the characteristic findings are adventitial thickening with endarteritis of the vasa vasorum and perivascular accumulation of plasma cells and lymphocytes, and destruction of the elastic tissue and smooth muscle cells of the media in a patchy ("moth-eaten") fashion (Fig. 18-12). Stellate medial scars result from tissue destruction and cause the wrinkling of the intima. The intimal plaques are foci of subendothelial, avascular, dense fibrosis in which hyaline degeneration and calcification are common. The multiple foci of inflammatory destruction and scarring of the media weaken the aortic wall, leading to dilatation of the aorta and aneurysm formation. Often the process extends into the aortic valve anulus and aortic cusps, with dilatation of the anulus and fibrosis of the cusps creating aortic valvular insufficiency and narrowing of the ostia of the coronary arteries resulting in myocardial ischemia.

Syphilitic involvement of small arteries is most prominent in larger arterioles and arteries of the brain and meninges (Heubner's arteritis) characterized by striking endothelial cellular proliferation, which, however, is not specific since similar changes are seen in tuberculous disease.[85] Cerebral ischemia results, and involved vessels may thrombose, leading to cerebral infarction. Similar changes occur rarely in other arteries, including the coronary arteries.[74]

Noninfective vasculitides

Polyarteritis nodosa. Initially described by Kussmaul and Maier[80] in 1886 as periarteritis nodosa because grossly visible nodules were seen under the skin, polyarteritis nodosa (PAN) is a necrotizing vasculitis of small

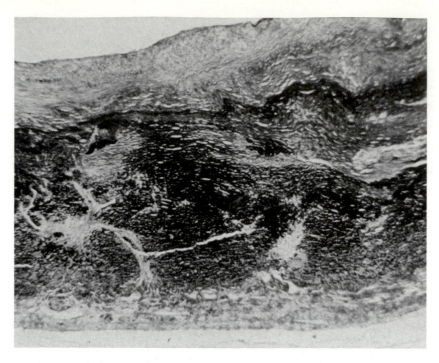

Fig. 18-12. Healing of syphilitic aortitis leads to scarring of media *(light, irregular areas)* with loss of medial elastic tissue (elastica is black in this stain) and secondary intimal fibrous thickening. Lumen of aorta is at top and adventitia at bottom of photograph.

and medium-sized muscular arteries. Polyarteritis is the appropriate term because the inflammatory process involves all layers of the arterial wall. Vessels in any part of the body may be affected, and multiple organs and tissues are involved. Males are more commonly affected than females by a ratio of 2.5:1. The mean age at onset of the disease is 45 years.[66]

PAN appears to be related to deposition of immune complexes, although such complexes may not be demonstrable in all cases. When immune complexes, such as hepatitis B surface antigen-antibody,[86] are present, the necrotizing vasculitis also may be regarded as a hypersensitivity vasculitis (see discussion later in the chapter). PAN may occur in association with, or as part of, connective tissue diseases that have a high incidence of circulating immune complexes, especially systemic lupus erythematosus[90] and rheumatoid arthritis. Tumor-related antigens may be involved in the development of some cases of PAN.[68]

The anatomic sites most commonly involved in PAN are the kidneys (85%), heart (75%), liver (60%), gastrointestinal tract (50%), muscle (40%), pancreas (35%), testes (33%), peripheral nerves (30%), central nervous system (25%), and skin (20%). The pulmonary, but not the bronchial, arteries are spared in classic PAN. Involvement of the vessel is characteristically segmental and often at branching points. Nodular, beaded indurations may be seen in larger muscular arteries.

Classically the histopathologic changes are divided

into four stages, which are considered to be sequential.[55] These are the alternative-degenerative stage, acute inflammatory stage, granulation tissue stage, and healed or scar tissue stage. All stages may be seen simultaneously in the same vessel and in the same organ or tissue, suggesting persistence of the inciting factors. In the acute inflammatory stage, panarteritic inflammation with neutrophilic leukocytes, eosinophils, and mononuclear cells and fibrinoid necrosis of the vessel are found (Fig. 18-13, *A*). Thrombosis with luminal obstruction occurs frequently, and aneurysms may form and possibly rupture. Repair of destruction of the degenerative and acute stages characterizes the granulation tissue stage, which leads to a scar. The healed phase of PAN (Fig. 18-13, *B*) is a vascular fibrous scar that distorts the normal architecture and often contains hemosiderin pigment and scattered round cells; an organized and recanalized thrombus may be present.

The clinical manifestations of PAN are protean, are generally nonspecific, and reflect dysfunction of multiple organ systems. Although there are no specific diagnostic laboratory findings, the erythrocyte sedimentation rate invariably is increased during the active phase of the disease, and results of serum immunologic tests are frequently abnormal.[94]

Hypersensitivity vasculitis. Hypersensitivity vasculitis includes a heterogeneous group of clinical syndromes in which inflammation of venules, capillaries, and arterioles is found. Synonyms are allergic vasculitis, microscopic

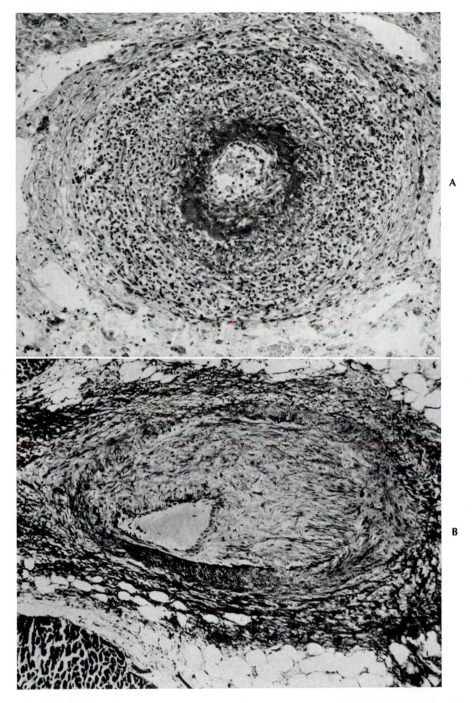

Fig. 18-13. Polyarteritis nodosa (PAN). **A,** Acute inflammatory stage of PAN is characterized by panarteritic and periarteritic inflammation with polymorphonuclear leukocytes, eosinophils, and round cells, destruction of vascular tissues, and fibrinoid necrosis *(dark, amorphous material about lumen)*. **B,** In healing and healed stages of PAN, reparative fibrosis distorts vascular wall with loss of most of internal elastic lamina *(black wavy line)* and marked narrowing of original lumen by organized thrombus and reparative fibrosis.

polyarteritis, and leukocytoclastic vasculitis. The anatomic sites of involvement are skin, mucous membrane, lung, brain, heart, gastrointestinal tract, kidney, and muscle; skin involvement dominates the clinical picture. Hypersensitivity vasculitis is an immunologic response to antigenic material. Various agents postulated as etiologic factors are infectious agents (*Streptococcus*, *Staphylococcus*, hepatitis B virus, influenza virus, cytomegalovirus, malaria, mycobacterial organisms), foreign proteins (animal serum, hyposensitization antigens), chemicals (insecticides, herbicides, petroleum products), and drugs (aspirin, phenacetin, phenothiazines, penicillin, sulfonamides, tetracycline, propylthiouracil, quinidine). The disease usually occurs 7 to 10 days after exposure to the stimulus. It is usually self-limited but can recur or become chronic.

The most common histopathologic pattern is a polymorphonuclear leukocytic infiltrate in which the cells often are fragmented (leukocytoclastic reaction), fibrinoid necrosis, endothelial cellular swelling, and extravasation of erythrocytes (Fig. 18-14). A second histopathologic pattern is a predominantly lymphocytic infiltrate of the involved vessel. The first pattern is associated with hypocomplementemia thought to be caused by deposition of immune complexes. The second pattern is believed to result from delayed hypersensitivity or cellular immune mechanisms, and the serum complement level is normal. In a given patient usually all lesions appear to be of similar duration.

Within the general group of hypersensitivity vasculitis

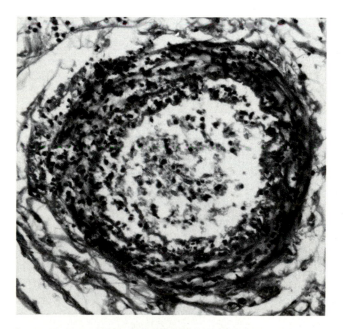

Fig. 18-14. Hypersensitivity vasculitis of small artery is characterized by diffuse inflammatory infiltrate of polymorphonuclear leukocytes, many of which are fragmented, and small round cells and extravasation of red blood cells.

are subgroups that have distinctive clinicopathologic characteristics but identical histopathologic features. These include serum sickness, Henoch-Schönlein purpura, mixed cryoglobulinemia, vasculitis associated with some collagen-vascular disease[95] such as rheumatoid arthritis or systemic lupus erythematosus, and vasculitis associated with certain malignancies.[66]

Wegener's granulomatosis. Wegener's granulomatosis is a clinicopathologic complex of acute necrotizing granulomas of the upper and lower respiratory tracts, glomerulonephritis, and widespread small-vessel vasculitis of both arteries and veins, particularly of the lungs and upper airways. "Limited" Wegener's granulomatosis is the same entity without renal involvement.[62] Classic instances of the generalized form lead to death in months, although the use of immunosuppressive agents in recent years has given substantial remissions. Males are more frequently affected than females (3:2), and the peak occurrence is in the fourth and fifth decades of life. The etiology of the disease is unknown; the findings of subepithelial immunoglobulin deposits on the glomerular basement membrane and the presence of circulating immune complexes[76] in some patients suggest that immune-complex deposition in tissues has a pathogenic role. The approximate frequencies of organ system involvement pathologically are lungs (100%), paranasal sinuses (95%), nasopharynx (90%), kidneys (80%), joints (60%), skin (50%), eyes (40%), ears (40%), heart (30%), and nervous system (25%).[97]

Necrotizing granulomatous inflammation of the tissues and necrotizing vasculitis with or without granulomas are the histopathologic hallmarks of Wegener's granulomatosis (Fig. 18-15). The granulomas consist of necrotic tissue, sometimes fibrinoid necrosis, a dense infiltrate of polymorphonuclear and mononuclear cells, multinucleated giant cells, epithelioid cells, and fibroblastic proliferation. The vascular involvement may be segmental or circumferential; when it is segmental, the involved area is adjacent to a granuloma. The acute lesions heal by fibroblastic repair and scarring. Lesions in all stages may be present at the same time. The renal lesions are usually those of focal necrotizing glomerulonephritis; sometimes diffuse proliferative glomerulonephritis with crescent formation may be found, especially with rapidly progressive renal dysfunction.

Wegener's granulomatosis should be differentiated from the systemic necrotizing vasculitides PAN and the Churg-Strauss syndrome, the neoplastic diseases lymphoma and midline malignant reticulosis, and granulomatous diseases such as tuberculosis, sarcoidosis, and syphilis.[92] Lymphomatoid granulomatosis may be differentiated from Wegener's granulomatosis by the absence of glomerulonephritis and the presence of atypical lymphoid cells. The relationship of the disseminated form of Wegener's granulomatosis to the limited form and of both to idiopathic (lethal) midline granuloma is controversial. Idiopathic lethal midline granuloma, a highly destructive, progressive, necrotic disease of the upper airway, may be part of a pathogenic spectrum that encompasses generalized and limited forms of Wegener's granulomatosis, or it may be a separate disease that needs to be distinguished from Wegener's granulomatosis.[67]

Allergic angiitis and granulomatosis (Churg-Strauss syndrome). Churg and Strauss[64] in 1951 reported a form of disseminated necrotizing vasculitis occurring exclusively among asthmatics and characterized by tissue and blood eosinophilia and intravascular and extravascular granulomas. Characteristic findings are vasculitis of small and medium-sized arteries, veins, arterioles, and venules of the lungs and eosinophilic pneumonia-like areas. Levels of serum IgE are elevated in some cases. The pathogenesis of the disease involves an immunologic mechanism.[63,65]

Tissues and organs found at autopsy to be involved by the Churg-Strauss syndrome are, in order of decreasing frequency, the spleen, kidney, heart, liver, lung, gastrointestinal tract, musculoskeletal system, and central nervous system.[66] Histologically eosinophils and granulomas are seen in and around small vessels. Fibrinoid necrosis, thrombosis, infarction, and aneurysm formation may occur but are less frequent than in PAN.

Although there are similarities in clinical symptomatology between PAN and Churg-Strauss syndrome, the latter differs in the high frequency of pulmonary findings, which usually are the initial ones, and less frequent renal and central nervous system involvement. Diseases to be distinguished from the Churg-Strauss syndrome that also have pulmonary eosinophilia, granulomas, or vasculitis with or without asthma, and blood eosinophilia include eosinophilic pneumonia, allergic bronchopulmonary aspergillosis, bronchocentric granulomatosis, eosinophilic granuloma, Wegener's granulomatosis, necrotizing sarcoid-granulomatosis, and drug vasculitis.[79]

Giant cell arteritis (temporal arteritis, cranial arteritis, granulomatous arteritis). Giant cell arteritis is a systemic vascular disease with granulomatous inflammation of medium-sized and large arteries. The inflammation often appears clinically to be limited to the cranial arteries, particularly the temporal. Most patients have granulomatous inflammation, but giant cells are not always found. It is a disease of protean manifestations, with fever, headache, visual symptoms, scalp tenderness, malaise, jaw claudication, anemia, and elevated erythrocyte sedimentation rate. Epidemiologic features include an average age of onset of symptoms of about 70 years (onset rarely occurs before 50 years of age),[73,75] increased prevalence with age, a female preponderance by a ratio of 2 or 3 to 1, greater frequency in northern areas and among individuals of Scandinavian descent, unusual occurrence in black people, seasonal peaks in the spring and summer, and familial clusterings. An association has been observed between giant cell arteritis and polymyalgia rheumatica[69]; the two conditions may be manifestations of the same systemic disorder.

Although the cause of this arteritis is unknown, it has been suggested that damaged vascular elastic tissue,

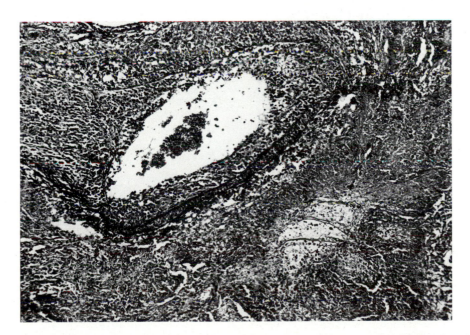

Fig. 18-15. Wegener's granulomatosis with necrotizing and granulomatous inflammation of medium-sized pulmonary artery *(center and left of photograph)* and necrotizing granulomatous inflammation of the pulmonary parenchyma *(right of pulmonary artery)*.

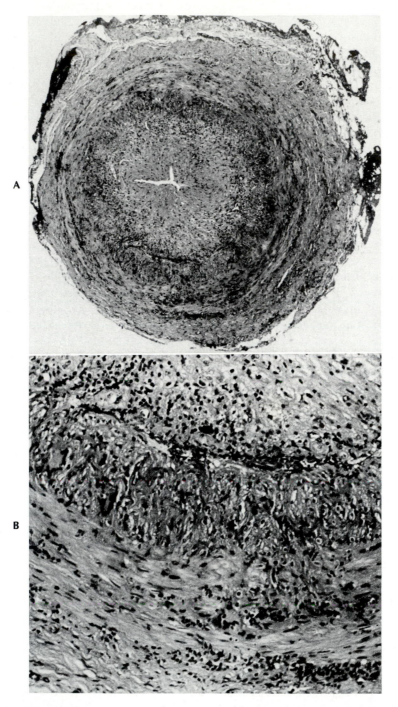

Fig. 18-16. Giant cell (temporal, cranial) arteritis. **A,** Low-power photomicrograph of biopsy of temporal artery shows near occlusion of lumen (reduced to central cross-shaped slit) by granulation tissue and granulomatous inflammation of all layers of vessel. **B,** Higher-power view of portion of vessel in **A** demonstrates intimal granulation tissue *(upper one third of photograph)*, giant cells in and about internal elastic lamina *(central area of photograph)*, and inflammatory cells in outer media and adventitia *(lower one third of photograph)*.

especially of the internal elastic lamina, acts as an antigen that incites vascular inflammation. Immunoglobulin deposits have been found in affected arteries.[58]

Preferential sites of involvement include the ophthalmic and posterior ciliary branches of the internal carotid artery and the temporal, occipital, facial, and maxillary branches of the external carotid system. Autopsy studies have shown active arteritis in many vessels including the aorta and the common carotid, axillary, brachial, femoral, and mesenteric arteries, but clinical symptoms related to these sites of involvement are uncommon or subtle.

The histologic features vary in different patients and even in the same vessel of one individual. Granulomatous arterial inflammation with or without giant cells, nonspecific inflammatory infiltrates throughout the wall with both polymorphonuclear and mononuclear cells, and intimal thickening by granulation tissue are the usual findings (Fig. 18-16). The granulomatous reaction is usually around the internal elastic lamina and typically involves the whole circumference of the vessel. Giant cells, either foreign body type or Langhans' type, are found in about half to two thirds of cases [84] and are usually close to the internal elastic lamina, which is often fragmented or focally absent. Occasionally only panarteritic inflammation or eccentric or concentric intimal cellular proliferation with marked narrowing of the lumen is present, without disruption of the internal elastic lamina. Thrombosis of the narrowed lumen may occur. The segmental distribution of the process creates "skip-lesions."

Clinically this form of granulomatous arteritis appears to be a self-limited disease, but blindness may develop rapidly as a result of involvement of the ophthalmic artery. Rarely death results, usually from systemic, especially aortic, involvement. Histopathologic diagnosis from examination of a biopsy specimen of a cranial artery, frequently the temporal, requires complete sampling because of skip-lesions, as well as clinical correlations.

Takayasu's arteritis. Takayasu's arteritis is an inflammatory disease of large arteries, especially the aorta and its larger branches, that causes luminal stenosis and aneurysms. Synonyms include pulseless disease, primary arteritis of the aorta and its branches, idiopathic medial aortopathy and arteriopathy, obliterative brachiocephalic arteritis, panaortitis, aortic arch syndrome, aortitis syndrome, giant cell arteritis of the aorta, reverse coarctation, nonspecific aortoarteritis, and occlusive thrombo-aortopathy. The disease most frequently affects the young with 80% being 11 to 30 years of age; women account for 90% of cases.[83] The disease is worldwide in distribution and affects all races. The most common causes of death associated with Takayasu's disease are congestive heart failure, myocardial infarction, and sudden unexplained death.

Four types of Takayasu's disease have been defined. Type I is characterized by active or chronic inflammation of the ascending aorta, the arch, and the great vessels, usually associated with the pulseless syndrome. Type II, also called atypical coarctation of the aorta, involves the descending thoracic aorta and the abdominal aorta without involving the aortic arch. Type III, which is the most common (occurring in about two thirds of reported cases[93]), is a combination of involvement of the aortic arch, its branches, and the abdominal aorta. Type IV is a combination of one of the other three types with involvement of the pulmonary artery.

The etiology of Takayasu's arteritis has not been elucidated. It is not entirely certain whether the condition is a specific disease or a symptom complex that can result from a variety of pathologic processes. Although tuberculous infection has been suggested as a possible cause, such a relationship is doubtful in most cases of Takayasu's arteritis. An autoimmune reaction to aortic tissues[72,88] may be causative.

The aorta in Takayasu's arteritis is diffusely thickened, and the intima has a gray, pebbly appearance with localized, plaquelike elevations. Skip areas of involvement are common with focal stenoses or aneurysms of different sizes alternating with nearly normal segments. Occasionally organization of superimposed thrombi contributes to the plaque formation. Aneurysms are common in the distal thoracic and abdominal aorta, especially in older patients.[91] The histologic findings in affected vessels vary according to the stage of the disease (Fig. 18-17). Inflammation with polymorphonuclear and mononuclear cells and occasional Langhans' giant cells may be present in all layers but usually is more marked in the adventitia than in the media or the intima. Perivascular inflammation about vasa vasorum mimics syphilitic aortitis. Foci of medial destruction with reparative fibrosis are prone to the formation of aneurysms. In apparently late stages of the process, adventitial fibrosis and extensive intimal proliferation and fibrosis result in marked luminal narrowing, producing the pulseless syndrome when the subclavian arteries are involved. Segments of large arteries damaged by the inflammatory process often manifest secondary atherosclerotic changes, which may mask the basic condition. Although Takayasu's arteritis characteristically involves large arteries, medium-sized arteries, especially the coronary arteries, may be involved.

Differentiation from syphilitic aortitis may be aided by serologic tests for syphilis, by involvement of the abdominal aorta (which is uncommon in lues), and by the young age of most patients with Takayasu's arteritis. Giant cell (cranial) arteritis involving aortic segments may be indistinguishable histologically from Takayasu's arteritis,[61] but usually medial inflammation and repair are more prominent in the former, which occurs mainly at older ages and always affects medium-sized muscular arteries.

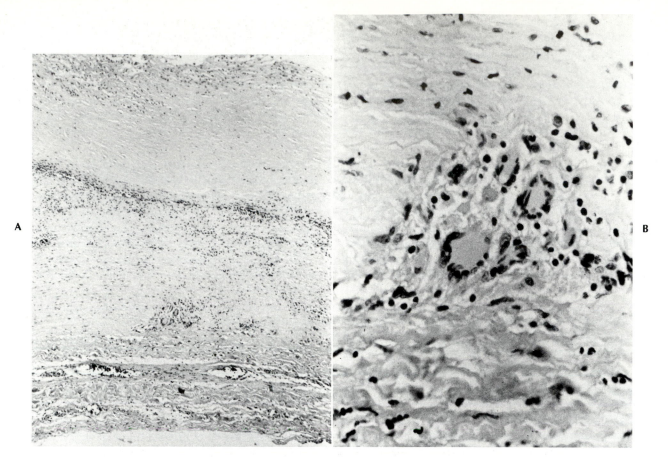

Fig. 18-17. Takayasu's arteritis involving aortic arch. **A,** Intima *(upper one third of photograph)* is thickened by fibrosis; media *(center portion of photograph)* has scattered foci of inflammatory cells, giant cells, and scarring; adventitia *(lower one fifth of photograph)* is fibrotically thickened with scattered plasma cells and lymphocytes, especially near vasa vasorum. **B,** Higher-power view of giant cells and inflammatory cells shown in **A.**

Tissue obtained for pathologic study during surgery on an affected vessel may not be diagnostic, since surgical treatment most often occurs late in the disease to treat stenotic or aneurysmal complications; nonspecific fibrotic scarring may be the main histopathologic finding.

Mucocutaneous lymph node syndrome (Kawasaki disease). Mucocutaneous lymph node syndrome (MCLS, Kawasaki disease) is an acute or subacute febrile systemic illness of unknown cause, occurring mainly in young children.[57,98] It is worldwide in distribution with a mortality of 1% to 2%. Possible causes considered are infectious, toxic, genetic, and allergic-immunologic agents.[87,89]

The most striking pathologic finding at autopsy is necrotizing panarteritis of the coronary arteries with multiple aneurysms (Fig. 18-18).[54] The inflammation may be acute or chronic depending on the duration of the illness. Fibrous arterial scars with luminal stenosis are seen in later stages. Necrotizing panarteritis often is found in iliac, renal, mesenteric, hepatic, and pancreatic arteries, occasionally with aneurysms. Similar vascular lesions

may be present in veins. Parenchymal, nonpurulent, nondestructive, inflammatory lesions may be seen in many tissues; these lesions heal without structural sequelae. Death from MCLS usually is the result of coronary arterial complications.

Retrospective analysis of instances of infantile polyarteritis nodosa (IPAN)[82] leads to the conclusion that IPAN and MCLS are essentially identical. Both differ clinically and pathologically from adult PAN.

Rheumatic vasculitis. At autopsy, fatal cases of acute rheumatic fever may have vasculitis involving the aorta, carotid and coronary arteries, and medium-sized arteries and veins of the viscera. Early aortic lesions are perivascular foci of inflammation and fibrinoid change in the adventitia and medial fibrinoid change in linear zones.[56,71] Although these lesions may have large basophilic histiocytes, typical Aschoff nodules in their granulomatous phase are rare. Healed lesions are perivascular fibrotic areas that, unlike those resulting from syphilis, do not involve the entire thickness of the media of the

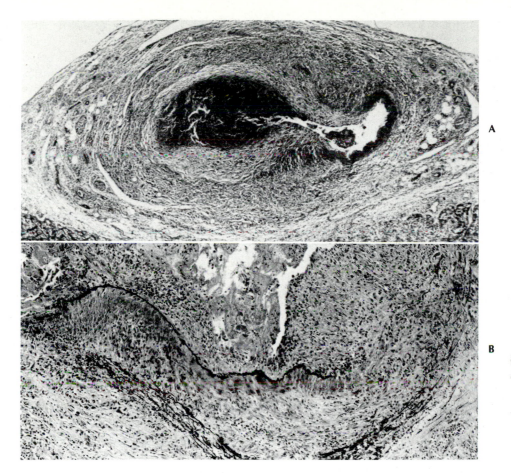

Fig. 18-18. Kawasaki disease (mucocutaneous lymph node syndrome) with panarteritis of coronary arteries. **A,** Necrotizing panarteritis of epicardial coronary artery with aneurysm that is filled with thrombus *(center of photograph).* **B,** Higher-power view of wall of coronary artery shows granulation tissue and organizing thrombus *(upper),* inflammation and necrosis of media *(lower)* with interruption of internal elastic lamina, and adventitial inflammatory tissue *(lower left and right).*

aorta. Active and healed intimal lesions analogous to those of the atrial endocardium have been reported. Involved muscular arteries, such as the coronary arteries, usually have rheumatic inflammation of all mural layers with prominent intimal lesions whose healing sometimes leads to luminal stenosis. Rheumatic vasculitis and aortitis are uncommon and generally not significant functionally. Rarely hypersensitivity vasculitis may be found in fatal acute rheumatic fever.

Rheumatoid aortitis. In the diseases rheumatoid arthritis and ankylosing spondylitis, aortitis or its sequelae may occur in the ascending thoracic aorta and may lead to aortic valvular insufficiency.[56] The pathologic lesions are nonspecific and primarily medial with loss of normal elements, focal scars, and scattered foci of lymphocytes and plasma cells. Mild to moderate intimal and adventitial fibrosis is present. In rheumatoid arthritis with aortitis, specific rheumatoid granulomas similar to the subcutaneous nodules of rheumatoid arthritis may be found rarely.

Thromboangiitis obliterans. Thromboangiitis obliterans (TAO, Buerger's disease) is an uncommon inflammatory occlusive disease involving small and medium-sized arteries and veins of the extremities in a segmental fashion. The disease affects mainly males under 35 years of age who are cigarette smokers.[59] Although the specificity of TAO has been questioned, it is generally accepted to be a distinct clinical symptom complex[77] with reasonably characteristic pathologic features. The symptom complex consists of intermittent claudication followed by ischemic necrosis of the toes or fingers with gangrene that progresses toward the trunk. The etiology of TAO is unknown, but toxic effects of cigarette smoking are important. Among other possible pathogenic mechanisms are altered immune mechanisms, hypercoagulability, and genetic factors because of the slightly greater prevalence in Orientals and Ashkenazi Jews.

Vessels of the lower extremities are affected more commonly than those of the upper extremities. TAO rarely has been observed in vessels of the heart, lung, brain, gastrointestinal tract, and male genitalia, almost exclusively only when the disease is severe and progressive in the extremities.

The lesions are characteristically focal or segmental, and involved segments are occluded. Microscopically, early lesions have inflammatory infiltrate of all layers of the vessel by polymorphonuclear leukocytes and always are thrombosed (Fig. 18-19). The thrombi are quite cellular and frequently have microabscesses. The intima is diffusely thickened by cellular proliferation; no lipid aggregates or calcium deposits are present. The internal elastic lamina characteristically is intact. In later or more advanced stages, mononuclear cells predominate in the inflammatory infiltrates and occasional epithelioid cell granulomas with Langhans' giant cells are present in the thrombus. The architecture of the medial muscle layer is preserved. As the disease becomes more chronic, more fibrosis and fewer inflammatory cells are found and the thrombus is recanalized. Neither arterial wall necrosis nor aneurysm occurs. TAO can be distinguished from atherosclerosis and bland thrombi or emboli on the basis of the cellular thrombus, the well-preserved media, the inflammatory reaction in the intima, media, and adventitia, the size of vessels involved, and the synchronous involvement of veins as well as arteries.

Raynaud's phenomenon and disease. Raynaud's phenomenon is episodic symmetric ischemia of the fingers and rarely the hands provoked primarily by cold but also by other stimuli such as emotion, trauma, hormones, and drugs. The affected digits show pallor followed by cyanosis and then redness, reflecting underlying arterial ischemia, venostasis, and reactive hyperemia, respectively. Uncommonly, ulceration and necrosis of digits occur. Raynaud's phenomenon may be associated with many conditions, including occlusive arterial disease, trauma, neurogenic lesions, and many of the connective tissue syndromes.[96] When Raynaud's phenomenon occurs without an associated condition in an otherwise normal individual, the condition may be termed Raynaud's disease or primary Raynaud's phenomenon. Although the digital arteries of patients with Raynaud's disease may not have structural abnormalities, a study of biopsies of the fingertips of a few patients showed segmental inflammatory and fibrinoid changes of the capillaries and regressive changes of glomus bodies.[60]

Aneurysms

An aneurysm is a permanent, abnormal dilatation of a blood vessel caused by weakening or destruction of the wall of the vessel. Aneurysms may be congenital or acquired. Most commonly elastic arteries and their major branches are involved. Larger muscular arteries are less frequently involved. Aneurysms of all types tend to enlarge with time; the enlargement and the production of clinical problems may be a slow or rapid process. Deleterious effects of aneurysms include alterations in blood flow distally, thrombosis with the potential for thromboembolism, rupture, and compression of adjacent structures.

Aneurysms can be classified by the composition of the

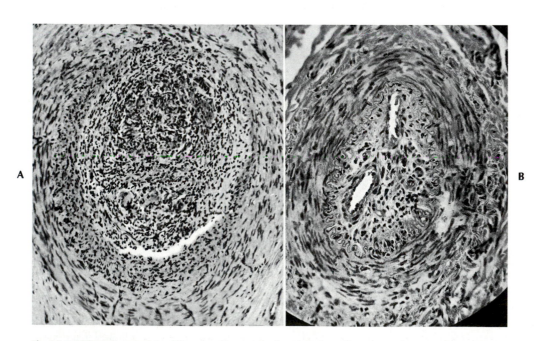

Fig. 18-19. Thromboangiitis obliterans (Buerger's disease) of small arteries of extremities. **A,** Panarteritic inflammation without mural necrosis, and beginning organization of cellular thrombus that has microabscesses and scattered giant cells. **B,** Recanalization of an organized thrombus has occurred. Internal elastic membrane *(wavy line)* is intact.

wall of the dilatation (true, false), shape (saccular, fusiform, cylindroid, serpentine, racemose), or pathogenic mechanisms (arteriovenous, mycotic, dissecting, traumatic, artherosclerotic, syphilitic, congenital). A *true* aneurysm is composed of all layers, or parts of them, of the normal vessel. A *false* aneurysm has a fibrous wall and is the result of rupture of the vessel with the formation of a cavity contained by adventitial and perivascular tissues. *Saccular* aneurysms are more or less spherical outpouchings with reasonably well-defined origins or necks. *Fusiform* aneurysms are spindle shaped and involve more or less uniformly the entire circumference of the vascular segment. *Cylindroid* aneurysms are variants of the fusiform type. A *serpentine* aneurysm is a tortuous, dilated vessel whose enlargement usually is the result of senile ectasia. An *arteriovenous* aneurysm refers to the dilated vessels associated with an arteriovenous fistula; *racemose (cirsoid)* aneurysms are forms of arteriovenous aneurysms in which there are masses of intercommunicating small arteries and veins. *Mycotic* aneurysms result from weakening of the arterial wall by infection with a microbiologic agent. *Dissecting* aneurysm, more appropriately termed dissecting hematoma, is the separation of the layers of the vascular wall by a column of blood from the lumen.

Aortic aneurysms

Most aneurysms of the aorta and its major elastic or musculoelastic branches are true aneuryms; false aneurysms principally result from traumatic rupture of the vessel. Medial weakness is the immediate factor leading to the development of the aneurysm. The common types are atherosclerotic, syphilitic, and dissecting aneurysm.

Atherosclerotic aneurysm. Atherosclerosis is the most common cause of aortic aneurysms in the Western world. The abdominal aorta is the most common location. Atherosclerotic aneurysms of the abdominal aorta are more common in males and after the age of 60 with frequency increasing with age. The cause is advanced atherosclerosis, that is, complicated lesions that encroach on the media and cause thinning and destruction of medial elastic tissue with atrophy of the media resulting from pressure phenomena and from impaired nutrition of the media. In the thoracic aorta, especially the ascending and arch portions, atherosclerosis may be the basic problem, but in many cases primary medial degeneration is the underlying condition, and the atherosclerosis is a secondary, and contributory, factor.

Most atherosclerotic aortic aneurysms are fusiform (Fig. 18-20, *A*). In the abdominal aorta most are infrarenal, beginning 1 to 3 cm distal to the renal arteries. Many extend into one or both common iliac arteries and their external and internal branches; often separate iliac arterial aneurysms also are present. The aneurysm may involve the origins of the superior mesenteric artery and the celiac axis. The suprarenal and infrarenal portions of the abdominal aorta and the descending thoracic aorta may form one large aneurysmal structure constituting a thoracoabdominal aneurysm. Abdominal aortic aneurysms may be any size; clinically significant ones usually are greater than 5 or 6 cm in diameter.

Usually the aneurysm contains mural thrombus, composed primarily of laminated fibrin that develops on the ulcerated, roughened atherosclerotic intimal surface (Fig. 18-20, *B*). Abnormal local hemodynamic effects contribute to the thrombosis. Branches of the aorta may be obliterated by the thrombus with resultant localized ischemic effects in the region supplied by the branch. Fragments of the thrombus may embolize distally into peripheral arteries. The thrombus may build up to large size and cause aortic luminal narrowing. Large aneurysms may compress adjacent vessels and, rarely, nerves.

Abdominal aortic aneurysms may rupture into either the peritoneum or, more commonly, the retroperitoneum, and thoracic aneurysms can rupture into the mediastinum with or without intrapleural extension. Rupture may be sudden and massive with death in minutes. Generally, the likelihood of rupture increases with size. Ruptures may be small and slowly progressive amounting to a "leaking" aneurysm. Infection of an atherosclerotic aneurysm is uncommon and occurs more often when there is rupture.[126] Occasionally the aneurysm may impinge on vertebral bodies, in which event the posterior wall of the aneurysm is formed by the anterior spinal ligament or cancellous bone.

Microscopic examination of the wall of an atherosclerotic true aneurysm shows marked loss of normal arterial structure, so that the wall consists of fibrous tissue with only portions of normal medial components (Fig. 18-21). The adventitia is fibrotically thickened and has mild to moderate chronic inflammatory infiltration, mainly foci of lymphocytes. Remnants of medial smooth muscle and elastic tissue are present, and atheromatous materials, fibrin, and thrombus replace the normal intima and part of the media.

Inflammatory aneurysms are a special type of atherosclerotic aneurysms. The wall of the aneurysm is composed of dense fibrotic tissue with abundant inflammatory cell infiltrates that involves adjacent structures, making operative dissection difficult. Although some workers have suggested that an autoimmune reaction to transudation of blood constituents through the thinned wall of the aneurysm contributes to the formation of an inflammatory aneurysm, at this time they are best regarded as a type of atherosclerotic aneurysm.[121]

The natural course of most atherosclerotic aneurysms is gradual enlargement and eventual rupture or thrombosis. Although acute rupture has a grave prognosis, the

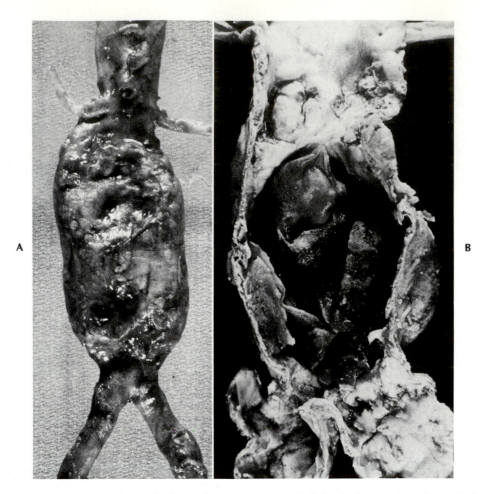

Fig. 18-20. A, Intact infrarenal atherosclerotic aneurysm of abdominal aorta viewed anteriorly. Origins of celiac axis and superior mesenteric artery, as well as the right and left renal arteries, are above aneurysm. Aortic bifurcation and common iliac arteries are below. **B,** Opened atherosclerotic aneurysm of distal abdominal aorta demonstrates laminated fibrin thrombus *(dark material)* in aneurysm. Renal arteries are at top of photograph, and aortic bifurcation with severely atherosclerotic and aneurysmal common iliac arteries is at bottom.

outlook with elective surgical treatment today is good.[101-103]

Syphilitic aneurysm. Syphilitic (luetic) aneurysms are complications of syphilitic aortitis that develop in the tertiary stage of syphilis. They occur predominantly in the thoracic aorta, especially in the ascending and arch portions. In the past syphilis was a common cause of aneurysms of the thoracic aorta, but today atherosclerotic[105] and medial degenerative causes are far more common.[115]

Syphilitic aneurysms usually become manifest after the age of 50. They are usually saccular but can be cylindroid or fusiform (see Fig. 18-11), and more often attain larger size (15 to 20 cm in diameter) than do atherosclerotic aneurysms. These aneurysms often displace, compress, or erode adjacent structures, leading to respiratory, esophageal, or skeletal complications. Rupture may occur into the mediastinum, pericardial space, pleural

cavities, trachea, bronchi, or esophagus or externally through the chest wall. Although the syphilitic aneurysm per se does not necessarily cause cardiac dysfunction, commonly the aortic root and valve also have syphilitic aortitis leading to aortic valvular incompetence and cardiac failure.

The histologic features of syphilitic aneurysms, which are true aneurysms, are those of healed luetic aortitis (see Fig. 18-12). The adventitia is moderately thickened by fibrosis, and vasa vasorum manifest endarteritis obliterans with narrowing or occlusion of their lumina. The scars may extend from the adventitia through the media and into the intima. Fibrosis of the intima is common and often is continuous with that of the media. Typical atherosclerotic lesions frequently are superimposed on and may mask the underlying luetic process, especially on gross morphologic examination. Spirochetes are rarely if ever demonstrated in typical luetic aneurysms.

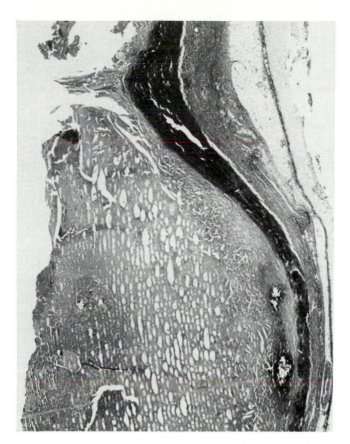

Fig. 18-21. Portion of wall of atherosclerotic aneurysm of aorta. Black tissue is medial elastica. At top is nondilated aorta with complicated atherosclerosis and fibrin thrombus. Bulge to right is wall of aneurysm, which contains fibrin thrombus on luminal side *(toward left)*, and complicated atherosclerosis with focal calcification *(irregular black masses near media)*.

Dissecting aneurysm. A dissecting aneurysm (DA) is a dissecting hematoma in which blood is present within the wall of the vessel and spreads (dissects) longitudinally, creating a cavity by separation of the tissues. In nearly all instances the dissection is in the media. The aorta is the most common site, but the lesion can occur in any artery. Generally the onset of the event is acute and is a dramatic clinical emergency. Modern treatment has improved the outlook for patients with acute aortic dissections with a decrease in mortality from some 90% within 3 months in untreated persons in the past to 20% to 35% with modern medical and surgical treatment.[108,130] The estimated frequency is 5 to 10 per 1 million population, which is two to three times the frequency of ruptured abdominal atherosclerotic aneurysms. DA occurs more often in men by a ratio of 2 or 3 to 1, mainly in the age range of 50 to 70 years. Before the age of 40 there is nearly equal male to female distribution.[116] Half of the dissections in women occur during pregnancy.[117] In persons under the age of 40 years DA occurs mainly in those with a familial predisposition,[113]

Marfan's syndrome,[125] or congenital heart disease such as coarctation of the aorta[129] and bicuspid aortic valve.[109] DA is more common in blacks,[131] perhaps because of their greater incidence of hypertension.

Morphologic and pathogenic features. The dissecting column of blood is located primarily between the outer and middle thirds of the aortic media (Figs. 18-22 and 18-23). In more than 95% of cases an intimal tear (Fig. 18-24) that continues into the media is present and presumed to be the origin of the dissecting hematoma (Fig. 18-25), but rare instances of DA without an intimal tear have been reported. Generally the intimal tear is 4 to 6 cm in length and perpendicular to the long axis of the aorta; rarely it may be nearly circumferential in the aortic root. Most intimal tears in the ascending aorta are in its proximal portion, less than 4 cm from the aortic valve cusps—that is, at the junction of the sinus and tubular portions of the aorta[118,120]—and are most often on the right lateral aspect of the aorta with the dissection following the greater curvature of the thoracic aorta. The dissection commonly extends proximally and distally from the tear. The dissecting column of blood may simply end in the media and adventitia, may rupture into adjacent tissues or body cavities, or may reenter the lumen of the aorta or one of its branches. True reentry sites occur in 10% to 20% of cases with about half communicating with the aorta, most often the abdominal aorta, and the other half with a major artery, most often an iliac. Often the dissecting process involves the major branches of the aortic arch, the right coronary artery, the left intercostal arteries, the left renal artery, or the left iliac artery. Muscular branches of the aorta may be completely severed from their aortic origin and originate from the dissected cavity (false lumen).

DeBakey and co-workers[107,108] classified DA into three types according to the apparent origin and extent of the condition. Type I (75% of cases) begins in the ascending thoracic aorta and extends distally for a variable distance; type II (5% of cases) is confined to the ascending aorta and often is found in patients with Marfan's disease; and type III (20% of cases) begins in the descending thoracic aorta, just distal to the origin of the left subclavian artery in the aortic isthmus. A modification of this classification also is used; type A dissections involve the ascending aorta and include DeBakey types I and II; type B does not involve the ascending aorta.[104] Dissection that begins in the abdominal aorta is rare, can progress proximally (retrograde in regard to blood flow), and usually is traumatic in origin, including iatrogenically produced lesions. When the dissection is localized to just a few centimeters from the intimal tear and does not reenter, the process is termed "incomplete" DA. Sometimes DA may heal resulting in a "double-barreled" or even a "triple-barreled" aorta, referring to second or third aortic false channels. These channels are endothelialized and

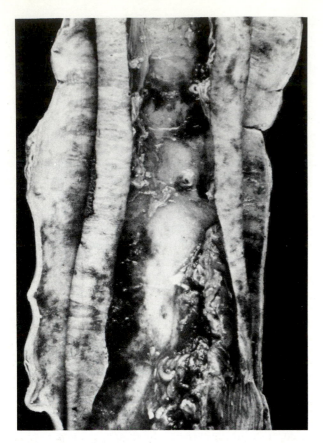

Fig. 18-22. Acute dissecting aneurysm (hematoma) of aorta. Adventitial surface of aorta is in center (note orifices of aortic branches), and dissected channel (false lumen) that partly surrounded true aorta has been opened. Column of blood that separated medial layers to form false lumen has been removed.

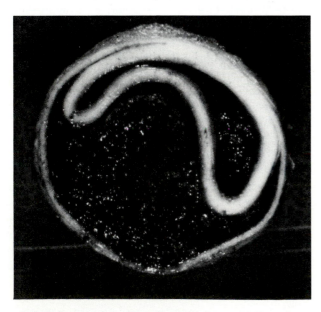

Fig. 18-23. Cross section of aorta that has acute dissecting aneurysm shows true aortic lumen *(above and right)* compressed by dissecting column of blood that separates media and creates false lumen.

may develop atherosclerotic and thrombotic changes as does the native aorta.

Death from DA most often results from rupture. Rupture sites frequently associated with rapid demise include the pericardial sac leading to acute hemopericardium, the mediastinum, the left pleural space, and the retroperitoneum. Extension of the medial dissection into the arch branches may lead to cerebral ischemia. Extension into a major coronary artery, usually the right, may cause fatal myocardial infarction. Extension to a cardiac chamber rarely may occur. DA involving the renal arteries may lead to renal failure, and involvement of intercostal arteries may cause infarction of the spinal cord. Aortic valvular insufficiency may result from loss of commissural support of the valve. Patients who survive the acute episode ("healed" or chronic DA) may develop a saccular aneurysm of the false channel.

About 70% of patients with DA clinically have systemic hypertension, and in autopsy studies about 90% of patients have left ventricular hypertrophy, suggesting that hypertension had been present. The frequency of DA appears greater in patients with malignant (accelerated) hypertension than in those with benign hypertension.[99] Although hypertension is the most common clinical finding associated with DA, its exact role in the pro-

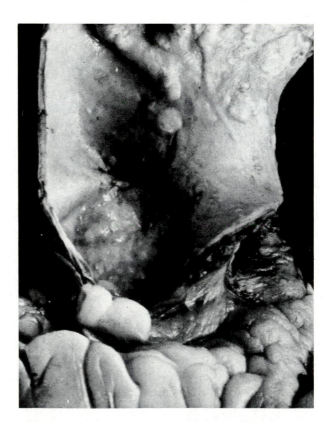

Fig. 18-24. Opened proximal ascending thoracic aorta has intimal tear *(dark hockey stick–shaped structure)* that leads to disseecting hematoma. Unopened left ventricle is below.

duction of the condition has not been defined. Other clinical or pathologic states associated with DA include pregnancy, Marfan's syndrome, atherosclerosis, trauma, aortic valvular stenosis (especially of the congenitally bicuspid valve), and coarctation of the aorta; in all of these conditions except Marfan's syndrome, DA is rare.[109,111,132]

The focus of study of the pathogenesis of DA is the tunica media. Histologic and electron microscopic examinations show a variety of abnormalities that may or may not be pathogenically significant, but some morphologic alteration usually is present. Cystic medial necrosis (CMN) is one such process.[110] It is characterized by focal accumulations of mucoid (myxoid) material in the aortic media in areas with loss of normal smooth muscle cells and elastic fibers, but rarely with true necrosis or inflammation (Fig. 18-26). True cysts with a limiting membrane or lining are not present; the accumulations are gel-like ground substance. Fibrosis of slight to moderate degree may exist. CMN occurs mainly in persons over 40 years of age[100,111] except in Marfan's syndrome with aortic dilatation when it is found at any age. The exact relationship of CMN to DA is uncertain. In Marfan's syndrome, congenital bicuspid aortic valve, and coarctation of the aorta, the occurrence of CMN may be coincidental rather than causal for DA. Although DA is associated with hypertension, no certain correlation of hypertension and CMN exists, and a specific medial defect to explain the susceptibility of patients with hypertension to DA has not been established.[123,124]

The media of the aorta in the majority of instances of DA does not show typical cystic medial degeneration ("necrosis") but rather manifests loss and fragmentation of elastic fibers and slight fibrosis, usually with some increase in ground substance. In many cases these nonspecific changes do not appear to be greater in frequency or extent in DA than in nondissected aortic media of age- and sex-matched controls. These medial changes are likely the result of the processes of injury and repair initiated by hemodynamic events as part of aging.

At this time it can be concluded that while the typical lesion of cystic medial "necrosis" and the medial degenerative changes are commonly found in DA, their pathogenesis and their precise role in DA are not yet certain. Identification of a specific biochemical abnormality, especially in Marfan's syndrome, would clarify the situation. The higher incidence of intimal-medial tears in the ascending aorta than in other aortic segments may be related to hemodynamic factors,[115] and the location of the dissection in the media might be related to the nutritional watershed zone of the media.

Atherosclerosis (AS) does not appear to be a significant factor in most instances of DA, although it may play a role by disrupting normal medial and intimal architecture. AS often is found coincidentally. The medial scarring of syphilitic aortitis seems virtually to preclude DA; at least the finding of the two conditions in the same aorta is an extreme rarity.

Aortic sinus aneurysms. Aneurysms of the aortic sinuses of Valsalva are uncommon.[106] Such aneurysms may be congenital or acquired and are to be distinguished from simple dilatation of the sinuses that occurs with aging and hypertension, and from annuloectasia associated with DA or fusiform aneurysm of the ascend-

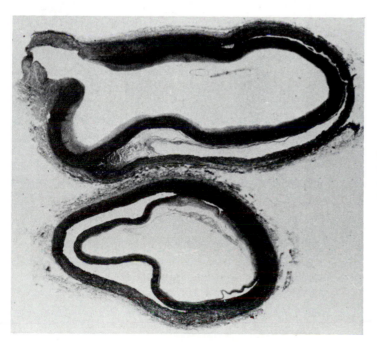

Fig. 18-25. Cross section of dissecting aneurysm of aorta. Native lumen in center is partly surrounded by false lumen that resulted from separation of media (*black tissue*) by dissecting hematoma.

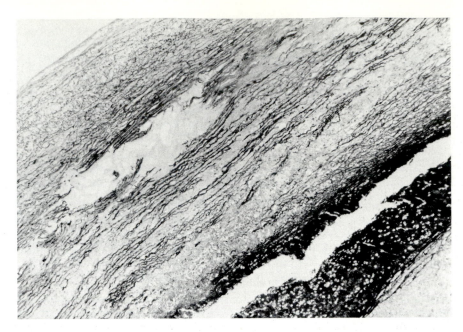

Fig. 18-26. Severe cystic medial degeneration (necrosis) of aorta with dissecting aneurysm. Lumen is in upper left corner of photograph. Bulk of photograph is markedly abnormal media, which has marked loss of elastic fibers *(black wavy lines)* and large areas of mucoid material *(pale areas)*. Empty space and dark material obliquely crossing right lower quadrant of photograph are dissected channel partly filled with blood.

ing aorta. Recognized causes include congenital absence or hypoplasia of medial elements, Marfan's syndrome, syphilis, ankylosing spondylitis, and infective endocarditis. In contrast to congenital forms, acquired aortic sinus aneurysms commonly involve more than one sinus of Valsalva and also the ascending aorta.

The major clinical problems relating to aneurysms of the aortic sinuses are caused by rupture into a cardiac chamber, the pericardial cavity, or an extracardiac site. Death most commonly is the result of congestive heart failure related to arteriovenous shunting, or acute pericardial tamponade from rupture into the pericardial cavity. Surgical correction often is possible.[106]

Coronary artery aneurysms

Coronary artery aneurysms may be congenital, atherosclerotic, inflammatory, or traumatic in nature. They may be single or multiple and saccular or fusiform in shape.[119] The congenital forms have hypoplasia of the media, but secondary histopathologic changes in the wall of the aneurysm often make the distinction between congenital and atherosclerotic forms difficult. Most of the apparent congenital aneurysms occur before age 40, but atherosclerotic coronary arterial aneurysms occur at older ages. Inflammatory coronary aneurysms may be associated with syphilis, infective endocarditis, possibly rheumatic carditis or other connective tissue disorders, and Kawasaki disease and may not become apparent until after resolution of the causative disease. Traumatic

coronary aneurysms often are associated with fistulous communications to one of the right-sided cardiac chambers. Dissecting aneurysms of the coronary artery most often are the result of aortic DA or trauma. Death caused by coronary artery aneurysm is usually related to occlusion or embolism with myocardial ischemia, and less frequently to rupture.

Pulmonary artery aneurysms

Aneurysms of the pulmonary arterial trunk[127] or of its major branches are rare. Most involve the main trunk of the pulmonary artery, with or without involvement of its branches. Frequently aneurysms of the pulmonary artery are associated with, or result from, congenital cardiovascular defects. Causes of acquired pulmonary arterial aneurysms include trauma, atherosclerosis, syphilitic and tuberculous inflammation, mycotic foci from infective endocarditis, and medial degenerative changes. The clinical manifestations depend on the etiology and the location and size of the aneurysm. The right ventricle frequently is enlarged. Congestive heart failure and rupture of the aneurysm are the common causes of death.

Aneurysms of other arteries

Aneurysms of systemic arteries are uncommon.[127] Aneurysms of the splenic artery may be atherosclerotic or congenital in origin, and their rupture in late stages of pregnancy is a well-recognized but rare event. Renal artery aneurysms, apart from those associated with fibro-

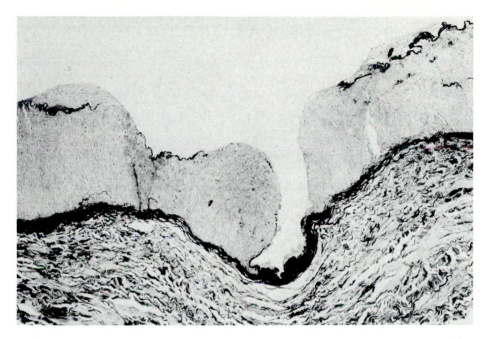

Fig. 18-27. Medial fibroplasia type of fibromuscular dysplasia of renal artery caused renovascular hypertension. In this longitudinal section of renal artery *(lumen at top),* focal marked thickenings of media *(left and right halves of photograph)* caused focal stenoses. Between areas of medial thickening, media is nearly absent, permitting small aneurysmal outpouching *(center of photograph).* Thin, wavy black line near lumen is internal elastic lamina that is absent in some areas. Heavy black lines, constituting external elastica, and adventitial tissues occupy lower part of photomicrograph. Intima is essentially normal; it can be identified in foci of slight, nonspecific thickening.

muscular dysplasia, are most commonly atherosclerotic, although congenital and traumatic types occur; renal hypertension and infarction are the most frequent complications. The most common peripheral arterial aneurysms are atherosclerotic types in the lower extremities, especially of the popliteal and femoral arteries. In the upper extremities, traumatic, mycotic, and arteritic aneurysms are more common than atherosclerotic ones.

Arteriopathy
Fibromuscular dysplasia

Fibromuscular dysplasia (FMD) is a disease of unknown etiology characterized by nonatherosclerotic, segmental stenosing lesions with or without focal aneurysmal outpouchings of the affected artery. Clinically significant lesions are most frequent and best defined in the renal arteries, but the condition also has been found in the coronary, superior mesenteric, celiac, common hepatic, axillary, internal carotid, and intracerebral arteries, often in association with FMD of other vessels, especially the renal artery. The major clinical conditions resulting from FMD are hypertension, cerebral ischemia, and intestinal ischemia. Renal arterial involvement is bilateral in approximately half of patients; unilateral lesions are more often on the right than on the left by a ratio of 3:1 in adults. The mean age at diagnosis is in the fourth decade, and females predominate. Pathogenic factors considered to be important include a developmental error, hormonal effects, mechanical stress, and anatomic variations in vasa vasorum leading to mural ischemia. Pathologic lesions are found more frequently in all vessels with age, but apparently they are clinically unimportant.

The general term *fibromuscular dysplasia* includes the pathologic processes of medial fibroplasia, perimedial dysplasia, medial hyperplasia, and intimal fibroplasia.[114,128] Medial fibroplasia (Fig. 18-27) is the most common type. Grossly the involved vessel has luminal ridges that narrow the lumen. Between the stenosed areas the wall is thinned and may have, or appear to have, aneurysms of the thin areas. The lesions are best demonstrated pathologically in the longitudinally opened vessel and in longitudinally oriented histologic sections. The stenosing ridges are areas of medial thickening by fibromuscular tissue in which the smooth muscle cells may show architectural disarray with loss of the normal, orderly, parallel arrangement of cells. The intervening thin areas are composed of histologically normal medial smooth muscle, which may be greatly decreased in quantity from normal. The alternating stenosed areas and thinned or aneurysmal areas give the appearance of a string of beads

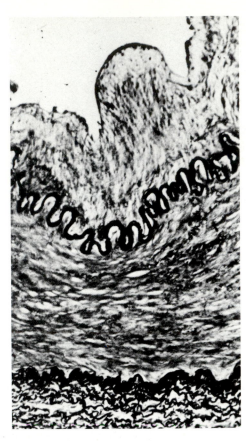

Fig. 18-28. Intimal fibroplasia form of fibromuscular dysplasia of renal artery. Focal intimal thickenings *(top)* produced focal stenoses. Upper wavy black line is internal elastic lamina; below it are normal media, external elastic lamina, and adventitia.

in arteriograms. Mild to moderate intimal fibrosis may be present; true atherosclerosis is uncommon and when present is a coincidental or complicating lesion. Perimedial dysplasia probably is the second most common form of fibromuscular dysplasia and is characterized by the accumulation of circumferential aggregations of elastic-like tissue between the media and the adventitia, creating the narrowed regions. Medial hyperplasia is an uncommon form of FMD characterized by foci of apparent hyperplasia of normal medial smooth muscle with minimal architectural disorganization. Intimal fibroplasia (Fig. 18-28), a rare form of fibromuscular dysplasia, is characterized by focal eccentric or circumferential subendothelial mesenchymal cell proliferations that are somewhat similar to the histopathologic change of endarteritis obliterans, with essentially normal medial and adventitial structures.

Cystic adventitial disease of the popliteal artery

Cystic adventitial disease of the popliteal artery is a rare condition characterized by an adventitial ganglion-like cyst containing mucoid fluid that compresses the

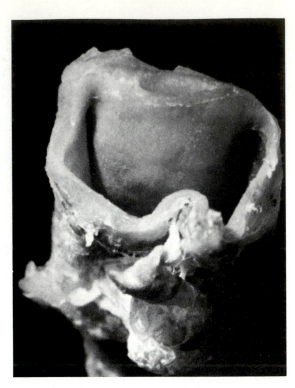

Fig. 18-29. Cystic adventitial disease of popliteal artery compressing arterial lumen (seen in oblique view of cross section at top of photograph). Large cystic structure is thick-walled intra-adventitial cyst.

popliteal artery and causes intermittent claudication.[112] The male-to-female ratio is 8:1, and the average ages at diagnosis are 36 years in men and 49 years in women. The grossly fusiform-shaped cyst is present within the adventitia (Fig. 18-29) and may or may not be lined by mucus-containing cells. Cystic adventitial disease also has been reported in the radial, ulnar, femoral, and external iliac arteries and in the saphenous and femoral veins.[122] Theories of pathogenesis include repetitive trauma and inclusion of mucin-secreting cells within the adventitia during development.

VEINS
Normal structure and age changes

Normal veins (Fig. 18-30) differ from arteries of the same size in that the wall of a vein is thinner, the three tunicae are less well demarcated, elastic tissue is scanty and not clearly organized into distinct internal and external elastic laminae, and medial smooth muscle cells are relatively fewer in number, widely separated by collagen fibers, and arranged in both circular and longitudinal fashions. All veins, except the vena cavae and common iliac veins, have valves. The valves, which are best developed in the leg veins, are paired folds of intimal tissue with collagen and elastin but little smooth muscle. Valves occur every 1 to 6 cm, often just distal to the point

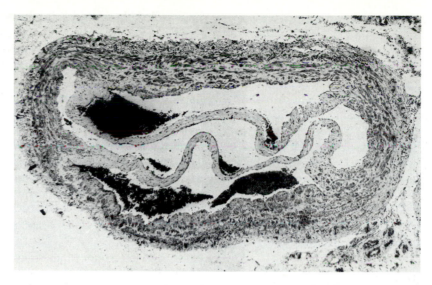

Fig. 18-30. Transverse section of normal saphenous vein shows pair of valves crossing lumen. Intima, media, and adventitia are not as well demarcated in veins as in arteries, well-defined elastic laminae are not present, and medial smooth muscle bundles are separated by collagen.

of entry of a tributary vein, and prevent retrograde venous blood flow. The venous system is a reservoir or capacitance unit for the cardiovascular system, containing 60% to 75% of the blood volume.[135]

The principal age change in veins is the development of a definite fibromuscular intimal layer, which often is eccentric in thickness at a given site. This intimal fibromuscular layer hyalinizes with age and may calcify focally. Although this change rarely produces luminal narrowing, the advanced forms create phlebosclerosis.

Varicosities
Varicose veins

Varicose veins are abnormally dilated and tortuous veins.[139] Although this pathologic condition of veins may occur in any part of the body, including the lower esophagus, anal region, and spermatic cord, the most common sites are the superficial veins of the lower extremities, particularly the long saphenous vein and its tributaries. More than 20 million people in the United States are affected by varicose veins of the legs, with the peak occurrence being in the fourth and fifth decades. Women are affected three to six times more often than men. The condition appears to be more prevalent in Western countries. The etiology and pathogenesis of varicosities are multifactorial. Major considerations include hereditary (familial) weakness of the venous wall and valves, increased intraluminal pressure in leg veins from the upright posture with incompetence of the valves resulting from dilatation of the vessel, pregnancy because of compression of iliac veins and increased blood volume, and hormonal effects on smooth muscle. Less common etiologic and pathogenic factors are obesity and aging

with atrophy of perivenous soft tissues. Scarring changes and thrombotic or neoplastic obstructions may be associated with varicosities distal to the involved venous segment.

Varicose veins of the legs are dilated, tortuous, elongated, and nodular. Histologic changes are similar to those of age but more marked. Calcific foci related to degeneration of medial elastic fibers may be present. Thrombosis is common, and organization of the thrombi may lead to intimal fibrous and hyaline plaques. All of these changes are considered to be secondary, not causal. Prolonged venous stasis leads to skin changes of edema, stasis dermatitis, cellulitis, erosion, and ulceration and is a major factor in the development of thrombophlebitis in varicose veins. Pulmonary thromboembolism from varicose veins is uncommon.

Esophageal varices

Esophageal varices are tortuous and distended coronary veins of the distal esophagus and cardia of the stomach. They are almost always the result of obstruction of portal venous flow, most often caused by cirrhosis of the liver, since the coronary veins serve as collateral channels. In addition to hepatic cirrhosis, esophageal varices result from superior vena caval obstruction, portal vein thrombosis, hepatic vein thrombosis (Budd-Chiari syndrome), pylephlebitis, and tumor compression of the major portal trunk. Rupture and bleeding are the problems related to esophageal varices.

Hemorrhoids

Hemorrhoids are varicosities of the hemorrhoidal venous plexuses.[133] External hemorrhoids are varicosities of the inferior hemorrhoidal plexus, which is located below the dentate line of the anal canal, is covered by squamous epithelium, and drains to the internal iliac veins of the systemic venous system. Internal hemorrhoids are varicose veins of the submucosal internal hemorrhoidal plexus, which is located above the dentate line, is covered by transitional and columnar epithelium, and drains to the portal venous system. Factors implicated in hemorrhoidal disease are heredity, erect posture, obstruction of venous return caused by increased intra-abdominal pressure as with pregnancy, straining during bowel movement and diarrhea, and portal hypertension by virtue of the hemorrhoidal plexus serving as a collateral channel. Thrombosis, ulceration, hemorrhage, and perianal infection are frequent complications of hemorrhoids.

Varicoceles

A varicocele is a mass of varicose veins of the pampiniform plexus of the spermatic cord. This plexus is formed by the veins draining the testes and epididymis and drains by a single channel into the renal vein on the left and into the inferior vena cava on the right side of the body. Primary (idiopathic) varicocele is common on the left side but rare on the right. Secondary (symptomatic) varicocele may occur on either side and results from increased pressure on or in the spermatic veins as with hepatosplenomegaly, marked hydronephrosis, and abdominal tumors.

Phlebothrombosis and thrombophlebitis

In the past, two types of venous thrombosis were recognized: thrombophlebitis resulting from inflammation of the vein owing to injury or to neighboring inflammation, and phlebothrombosis as a primary condition related to hemodynamic and coagulation alterations. Today this distinction is recognized to be more theoretical than practical, since in most cases the initial problem is phlebothrombosis and the thrombus itself causes inflammatory reaction in the wall of the affected vein manifested by local and systemic signs and symptoms of an inflammatory state. The terms commonly are used synonymously.

The pathogenesis of venous thrombosis is summarized in Virchow's triad, which emphasizes the importance of changes in the vessel, particularly endothelial damage; changes in the composition of the blood; and disturbance of blood flow, especially stasis. One or more of these pathogenic factors are likely to be present in certain clinical situations,[135] including use of estrogen-containing compounds, malignancy, cardiac disease with congestive heart failure or arrhythmia, postoperative states, and inactivity or immobilization for any reason.

Phlebographic, pathologic, and radioactive tracer studies in the legs have shown that venous thrombosis develops initially in calf veins, mainly in the soleal sinuses and the related valves (Fig. 18-31). Most of these spontaneously lyse or organize. Only some enlarge to form a thrombus of sufficient size to cause luminal obstruction or embolize. Thrombosis of larger veins,

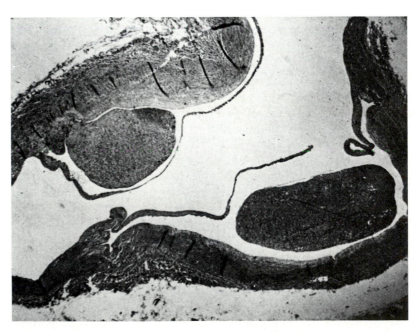

Fig. 18-31. Histologic section of leg vein with phlebothrombosis shows thrombi originating in sinuses of venous valves. Point of attachment of one thrombus *(upper left)* is shown; plane of section did not pass through attachment of other thrombus *(lower right)*.

such as those of the iliofemoral system, which may be an extension of thrombi originating in calf veins,[143] has a higher risk of pulmonary thromboembolism. Pulmonary thromboemboli originate from veins of the legs in approximately 95% of cases. Approximately half of patients with acute venous thrombosis will have pulmonary thromboembolic episodes, but the majority of these are clinically inapparent.[136]

The affected vein may appear normal or may be distended and firm to palpation. Internally a mural or an occlusive thrombus is present. The attachment of the thrombus to the wall may be delicate and easily separated. If the initial site of attachment of the thrombus can be determined, most often it is in the sinus of a valve. At the point of attachment an inflammatory-reparative process is present in thrombi that have been present for more than several hours (Fig. 18-32). This reaction initially consists of an ingrowth of fibroblasts into the thrombus from the venous intima, along with the deposition of scattered lymphocytes, macrophages, and a few polymorphonuclear leukocytes. Later, granulation tissue organizes the thrombus, and complete resolution may lead to a focus of fibrous intimal thickening or to an organized, recanalized thrombus.

Special types of venous thrombosis

Superficial thrombophlebitis. Superficial venous thrombosis of the legs usually results from varicose veins, while that of the arms usually is caused by the administration of intravenous fluids. The local inflammatory response generally is aseptic. Pulmonary thromboembolism is rare, and when it occurs it is most often the result of extension of the thrombotic process into the common femoral vein or of the coexistence of deep vein thrombosis.

Thrombophlebitis migrans. Thrombophlebitis migrans is a clinical, but not morphologic, condition characterized by recurrent episodes of venous thrombosis of the extremities and viscera. It is most commonly associated with malignant tumors, Buerger's disease, connective tissue disorders, and blood disorders such as polycythemia rubra vera and sickle cell disease. Malignant neoplasms particularly associated with migratory thrombophlebitis are carcinomas of the lung, female reproductive tract, pancreas, gastrointestinal tract, prostate, and breast. Frequently this syndrome is accompanied by nonbacterial thrombotic endocarditis of the cardiac valves.

Phlegmasia alba dolens. The clinical finding of "white, painful leg" refers to massive swelling of the leg that is associated with some, but not all, cases of iliofemoral venous thrombosis. The massive swelling is postulated to result from blockage of veins and perivenous lymphatics by an inflammatory process. The condition is much more common in the left than the right leg, probably because the left iliac vein is compressed by the right common iliac artery or by the aortic bifurcation. It occurs most often in women in the third trimester of pregnancy or after childbirth or in patients who have had extensive pelvic surgery. The frequent absence of valves within the iliac

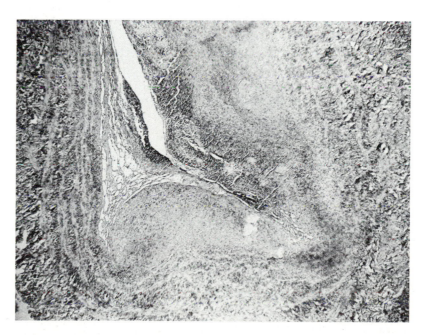

Fig. 18-32. Thrombophlebitis of leg vein shows thrombus narrowing lumen *(upper left of center)* and inflammatory cells in venous wall and thrombus.

veins and the proximity of the iliofemoral system to the inferior vena cava may account for the development of pulmonary embolism in this condition.

Phlegmasia cerulea dolens. In some patients with massive iliofemoral venous thrombosis, the extremity is markedly swollen, the skin is blue, and bullae or superficial gangrene develops. The basis for this complication of venous thrombosis is thrombosis of collateral channels and decreased arterial blood flow. It is a serious condition with a mortality that ranges from 27% to 42%, depending on the presence or absence of venous gangrene.[134]

Superior vena caval syndrome. Obstruction of the superior vena cava (SVC) most often results from external compression.[140] Thrombosis is present in less than half of patients and most often results from the process that compresses or invades the wall of the SVC. Although in the past the SVC syndrome was caused by syphilitic aortic aneurysm or tuberculous mediastinitis in 40% of patients, today most instances result from malignant disease.[141] Bronchogenic carcinoma accounts for 75% of patients with the SVC syndrome, and about half of these have small-cell undifferentiated carcinoma, 15% have lymphoma, and 7% have metastatic neoplasms from various sites. Rare causes of the SVC syndrome include primary SVC thrombosis, pericardial constriction, idiopathic sclerosing mediastinitis, and goiter. The clinical syndrome of obstruction of the SVC consists of dilatation of veins of the upper part of the thorax and neck, edema and plethora of the face, neck, and upper part of the torso including the breasts, edema of the conjunctiva, and central nervous system symptoms of headache, visual distortion, and disturbed state of consciousness.

Inferior vena caval syndrome. The most common cause of obstruction of the inferior vena cava (IVC) is thrombosis, usually by extension from thrombosed iliac and femoral veins. Neoplastic involvement by external compression, invasion, or direct intraluminal extension is the other major cause of IVC obstruction. Renal cell carcinoma is the tumor that most commonly causes IVC obstruction (Fig. 18-33). Less frequent causes are external pressure from abdominal aortic aneurysm, ascites, pregnancy, retroperitoneal fibrosis, paravertebral lymphadenopathy, pelvic lipomatosis, pelvic inflammatory disease, and extension of hepatic and renal vein thrombi into the IVC. In childhood, IVC obstruction may result from right-sided Wilms' tumor, neuroblastoma, or multicystic kidneys. Symptoms and signs of IVC obstruction are swelling and edema of the lower extremities, distension of the superficial veins of the lower limbs, and the appearance of collateral venous channels in the lower abdomen.

Thrombosis of hepatic veins (Budd-Chiari syndrome). The Budd-Chiari syndrome is thrombotic obstruction of the major hepatic veins resulting in hepatic congestion

and portal hypertension.[137] The IVC may be involved by direct extension. Secondary slowing of blood flow in the portal vein may lead to thrombosis of the portal system. The cause can be identified in about two thirds of cases. In decreasing order of frequency the identified factors are hepatic tumors, use of birth control pills, polycythemia rubra vera, amebic abscess, pregnancy, paroxysmal nocturnal hemoglobinuria, and trauma. Intense hepatic congestion with a "nutmeg" appearance, centrilobular or panlobular necrosis and hemorrhage, and replacement fibrosis are the major pathologic features in the liver. Acute forms, characterized by abdominal pain, ascites, and acute hepatic failure, are associated with complete sudden obstruction. Subacute to chronic forms, characterized by abdominal pain, ascites, and hepatosplenomegaly, are associated with incomplete occlusion of the veins.

Portal vein obstruction. Extrahepatic obstruction of the portal vein may be caused by thrombosis (pylethrombosis), compression by intra-abdominal tumors or cysts, congenital venous atresia with cavernous malformation

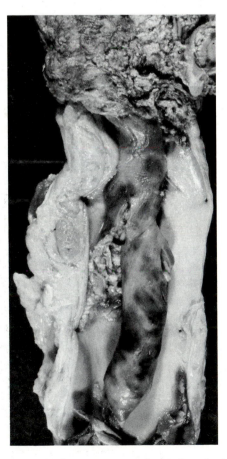

Fig. 18-33. Opened inferior vena cava shows thrombotic obstruction *(lower three fourths of photograph)* resulting from intraluminal extension *(upper one fourth of photograph)* of renal cell carcinoma.

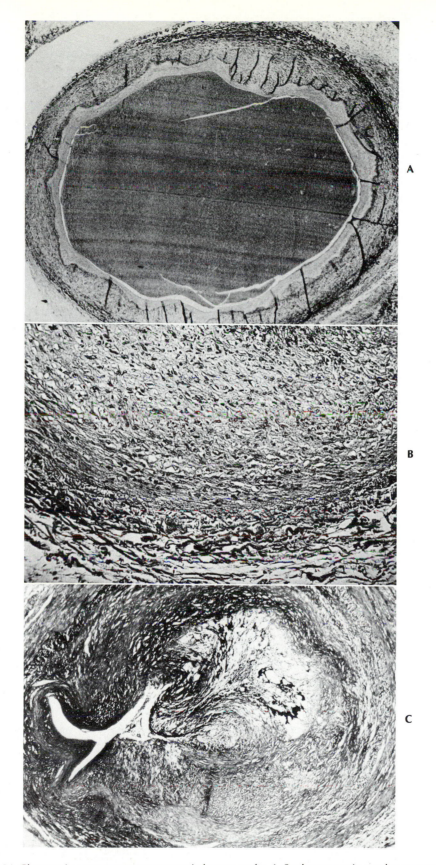

Fig. 18-34. Changes in aortocoronary artery vein bypass grafts. **A,** Saphenous vein used as coronary arterial bypass graft has slight intimal thickening 1 month after operation. Vascular lumen is filled by barium-gelatin mixture used for postmortem arteriogram. Light region surrounding lumen is thickened intima. Media and adventitia are slightly fibrotic. **B,** Proliferating smooth muscle cells and fibroblasts *(upper two thirds of photograph)* and their extracellular products produce intimal thickening. Fibrotic media and adventitia are in lower part of photograph. **C,** Fibromuscular intimal thickening and true atherosclerosis reduced lumen of this vein graft to cruciate slit *(left of center)* 8 years after operation.

in childhood, and inflammation (pylephlebitis) that usually results from an intra-abdominal infection.[145] Thrombosis of the portal vein may be a complication of liver cirrhosis, visceral carcinoma, or polycythemia rubra vera. The thrombus may undergo organization and become a fibrous cord or undergo cavernous transformation to form a spongy, trabeculated venous lake involving the area of the portal vein and extending into the gastroduodenal ligament. Acute complete thrombosis of the portal vein in the absence of formed collaterals is catastrophic, leading to hemorrhagic infarction of the small bowel. Chronic forms have signs of portal hypertension with abdominal pain, ascites, splenomegaly, hematemesis, and melena.

Aortocoronary vein bypass grafts

Segments of veins, usually autologous saphenous veins, are used to bypass obstructed coronary arteries, as well as peripheral arteries, with generally good results for long periods. Changes in these venous grafts influence their long-term function. The major morphologic alteration is fibromuscular intimal proliferation (Fig. 18-34, A and B) that begins a few days after operation but is not necessarily steadily progressive with time, although it may cause severe luminal narrowing or total occlusion of the bypass graft.[142,144] Occlusion of these grafts in the early postoperative period is thrombotic and is mainly related to arterial disease distal to the coronary anastomosis or to technical surgical factors. The proliferating intimal cells are longitudinally oriented smooth muscle cells similar to those found in atherosclerotic lesions. They are capable of synthesizing collagen, elastin, and glycosaminoglycans. With time, the intimal lesion becomes less cellular and has more collagen fibers and ground substances. Factors implicated in the ubiquitous intimal proliferation in coronary artery bypass vein grafts are arterial intravascular pressure and flow, angle of anastomosis, tension on the graft, ischemic insult caused by severance of vasa vasorum of the graft, and mural deposits of fibrin that accumulate as a result of endothelial damage. True atherosclerotic changes in saphenous vein bypass grafts (Fig. 18-34, C) are uncommon until years after operation, although they are more common and appear earlier in patients with hyperlipidemic states.[138]

LYMPHATICS
Normal structure

The lymphatic system consists of lymphatic capillaries, lymphatic vessels (collecting vessels), and lymph nodes. Lymphatic capillaries are similar but not identical to blood capillaries. They consist of a single layer of endothelium with an interrupted basal lamina and scattered single smooth muscle cells. Lymphatic vessels resemble veins, and those larger than 200 to 500 μm in external diameter have poorly defined intimal, medial, and adventitial layers whose structure quantitatively shows great variations. Virtually all lymphatic vessels have valves, which may be either bicuspid or tricuspid. The vessels often are dilated in the segments between valves. Lymphatic capillaries and vessels unite to form superficial and deep plexuses in and about many tissues and organs. The larger lymphatic vessels, such as the thoracic duct, have nerves and small blood vessels in their adventitia.

Lymphangitis

Acute lymphangitis results from the introduction of microorganisms, especially pyogenic bacteria, into the subcutaneous tissue. The superficial lymphatics are affected. Common organisms are beta-hemolytic streptococci and staphylococci. The affected lymphatics are visible as cutaneous erythematous streaks that spread up the arm or leg to the axillary or inguinal lymph nodes. Microscopically the lymphatics are dilated and contain leukocytes, cell debris, and coagulated lymph. The perilymphatic tissues are hyperemic and edematous with an inflammatory exudate. Recovery from acute lymphangitis with or without treatment usually is complete and without sequelae, but recurrent acute lymphangitis or incomplete resolution may lead to chronic lymphangitis. Chronic lymphangitis may cause permanent lymphatic obstruction by fibrosis resulting in chronic lymphedema.

Lymphedema

Lymphedema is swelling of soft tissue, especially the limbs, caused by a localized increase in the quantity of lymph.

Primary (idiopathic) lymphedema

Congenital lymphedema.[149] A familial-hereditary form (Milroy's disease) and a nonfamilial (simple) form of congenital lymphedema are recognized. In both forms, from birth, part or all of one extremity is diffusely swollen but is not painful or ulcerated. Milroy's disease, which also may be associated with other congenital anomalies, appears to be transmitted as an autosomal dominant trait with high penetrance, variable expression, and a predilection for males. The simple form, whose etiology is unknown, may be associated with Turner's syndrome.[146] Histologic study of the involved region in either form shows dilatation of the subcutaneous lymphatics, increased interstitial fluid, and some fibrosis in longstanding cases.

Lymphedema praecox.[148] In this condition, which primarily affects females in the second or third decade of life, lymphedema begins in the foot or ankle and progresses slowly up the leg to involve the entire extremity in months or years. The skin of the extremity becomes roughened, and the edema becomes nonpitting. Other abnormalities have been observed in patients with lymphedema praecox, including yellow nails, pleural effusion, primary pulmonary hypertension, bronchiectasis, cerebrovascular malformations, small pelvis, hypospadias, abnormal bone length, osteosclerosis, pes cavus, fused lumbar vertebrae, fixed flexion of the finger, distichiasis, hemangiomas of the feet and hands, and micrognathism.[147] The etiology is unknown, but a relationship to the reproductive system is suspected because of age of onset, female preponderance, and increased swelling during menses.

Secondary (obstructive) lymphedema

The most common cause of obstructive lymphedema is a malignant tumor that occludes the lymphatic vessels or the lymph nodes. Surgical removal of lymphatics or lymph nodes and destruction of lymphatics by irradiation also are frequent causes. Less common causes include sclerosing retroperitoneal fibrosis, granulomatous processes such as sarcoidosis and tuberculosis of retroperitoneal or inguinal lymph nodes, and nematodal parasitic infestation (filariasis) of lymphatics producing elephantiasis. Because of the numerous anastomotic connections among lymphatic vessels, obstruction must be widespread or involve a critical site for draining lymph nodes, such as the axilla or the groin, for secondary lymphedema to develop. Lymphatics distal to the point of obstruction are markedly dilated and the interstitial vessels are edematous and become fibrotic with time. Rupture of distended large lymphatics may occur, permitting the escape of milky lymphatic fluid that may create, depending on site of drainage, chylous ascites (chyloperitoneum), chylothorax, chylopericardium, or chyluria.

TUMORS AND TUMORLIKE CONDITIONS

The distinction between true vascular neoplasms that have the potential for autonomous growth and a variety of other vasoproliferative lesions including vascular hamartomas often is not clear, leading to imprecise terminology and classification.

Arteriovenous fistula (aneurysm)

An arteriovenous (AV) fistula or aneurysm is a communication between an artery and vein without an intervening capillary bed.[162] It may be either a congenital malformation or an acquired condition. In acquired forms, morphologic changes are found mostly in the veins, which are distended and have a thickened wall. Congenital AV fistulas have vessels that are thickened and hyalinized and a fibrotic stroma that may be calcified focally. The functional consequences of an AV communication

depend on its size and include cardiomegaly and congestive heart failure, varicose veins, ulceration or gangrene of the skin, bluish red birthmarks, and increased length of an involved limb.

Hemangiomatous and telangiectatic conditions
Hemangiomas

Hemangiomas are typically of capillary origin, but they may also arise from venules and arterioles. Any organ can be affected, but the skin, especially of the face, is by far the most common site. Many are congenital; one third of all babies have a hemangioma of some type.[178] The gross appearances of hemangiomas vary depending on the size and density of the tangled vessels forming the lesion, the degree of arteriovenous shunting present, the degree of thrombosis or fibrosis, the degree of endothelial cell proliferation, and the organ involved.

Capillary hemangioma. The most common hemangiomas are of the capillary type.[163,167] In the skin they are small or large, single or multiple, flat to slightly elevated, strawberry marks that are bright red to purple, well-circumscribed, warm, soft, often lobulated lesions. The lesions are present at birth or first appear between the third and fifth weeks of life, increase in size for several months, regress spontaneously by thrombosis and fibrosis, and most often involute completely within a few years. Histopathologically, capillary hemangiomas are composed of small thin-walled vessels (Fig. 18-35) of capillary size that are lined by a single layer of flattened or plump endothelial cells that usually are surrounded by a discontinuous layer of pericytes and reticulin fibers. Nevus flammeus is a cutaneous telangiectatic capillary hemangioma that is a nonelevated, port wine–colored macule appearing at about 10 years of age and gradually increasing with age.

Cavernous hemangioma. Hemangiomas of the cavernous type are most common in or beneath the skin of the face, neck, and extremities, sometimes forming a subcutaneous mass with normal overlying skin. They also may be found in the oral mucosa, stomach, small intestine, liver, and bones. Lesions may be single or multiple, discrete or diffuse, red to blue, soft masses that are spongy on sectioning. Histopathologically lesions are composed of tangles of thin-walled, cavernous blood vessels and spaces separated by scanty connective tissue stroma that resembles erectile tissue. Cavernous hemangiomas rarely involute spontaneously. The Kasabach-Merritt syndrome[176] is an extensive cavernous hemangioma, usually of the liver, and thrombocytopenic purpura with consumption coagulopathy resulting from coagulation in the hemangioma.

Combined capillary and cavernous hemangioma. Some hemangiomas histologically show a spectrum from pure capillary hemangioma through mixed capillary and

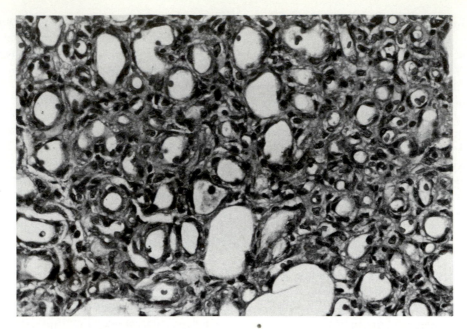

Fig. 18-35. High-power photomicrograph of capillary hemangioma of skin. Small, endothelial-lined vascular channels vary in size.

cavernous types to pure cavernous structure. Clinically lesions with these histopathologic features usually resemble cavernous hemangiomas and are frequently found on the head and face in children.[160] Such hemangiomas, especially those of skeletal muscles, may recur after incomplete resection and the histopathologic picture may cause concern because of nuclear pleomorphism, but the lesions never metastasize.[151]

Hereditary hemorrhagic telangiectasia (Osler-Weber-Rendu disease)

Hereditary hemorrhagic telangiectasia (HHT, Osler-Weber-Rendu disease, Osler's disease)[153] is a genetic disorder transmitted as an autosomal dominant trait of high penetrance that is characterized by multiple telangiectases of the skin, mucous membranes, and viscera. The usual clinical presentation is recurrent bleeding from the involved site that tends to increase in frequency and severity with age. The lesions are superficial, punctate, purplish spots from 1 to 4 mm in diameter that blanch with pressure. Microscopically collections of dilated small blood vessels, lined by a single layer of endothelium and based on delicate connective tissue, are found. A pulmonary arteriovenous fistula develops in an estimated 15% of patients with HHT, and 40% to 60% of patients with pulmonary arteriovenous fistula have HHT.[164]

Angiomatosis

Angiomatosis refers to the presence of multiple, diffuse hemangiomatous lesions in association with other congenital malformations. Specific syndromes, which are probably inborn dysplastic states, are recognized. All are quite rare.

The Klippel-Trenaunay syndrome[168] is a rare developmental entity consisting of nevus flammeus, congenital varices, arteriovenous fistula, and hypertrophy of the soft tissue and bones. The lesions may involve only a digit, a portion of a hand or a foot, or an entire extremity and may extend to the upper or lower trunk. The lesions usually continue to enlarge as the patient matures but do not progress after adulthood.

The Sturge-Weber syndrome[150] is a rare congenital disorder with a nevus flammeus on one side of the face in the area of the distribution of the trigeminal nerve, as well as ipsilateral retinal and leptomeningeal angiomatosis leading to ipsilateral buphthalmos and to contralateral hemiparesis or epilepsy with mental deficiency. Calcium and iron deposits outlining the contour of cerebral gyri and sulci in a railroad track pattern are seen on plain roentgenograms of the skull.

The Maffucci syndrome[152] is a congenital condition of dyschondroplasia with abnormal ossification of bone, skeletal deformities, and hemangiomas that may be capillary, cavernous, or combined types. Malignant neoplasms, especially of bones and blood vessels, occur frequently.

In the blue rubber-bleb nevi syndrome[153,171] bluish, rubbery, nipplelike vascular lesions of the skin and angiomas of the gastrointestinal tract are found. As a rule the skin lesions are cavernous hemangiomas, but a capillary hemangiomatous pattern with endothelial cell proliferation also may be seen.

The von Hippel-Lindau syndrome is a rare autosomal

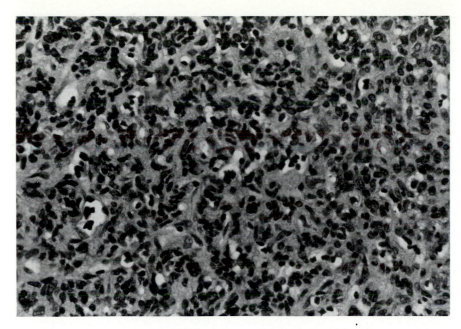

Fig. 18-36. High-power photomicrograph of benign hemangioendothelioma from skin of child. Proliferation of endothelial cells obscures scattered small vascular lumina.

dominant disorder[165] in which hemangioblastomas are present in the cerebellum (Lindau's tumor) and retina (von Hippel's tumor) in association with cysts of the pancreas, kidneys, or liver. Other benign or malignant tumors of many organs may occur, including renal cell carcinoma in about 25% of patients.

Hemangioendothelioma

Most hemangioendotheliomas are true neoplasms of vascular origin with autonomous growth characteristics, in contrast to most hemangiomas, which are hamartomas.

Benign hemangioendothelioma[167] is a cellular, hyperplastic (juvenile) hemangioma found in any organ but especially the skin, subcutaneous tissue, and liver of children. Grossly the lesion is a well-demarcated, gray-red mass. Microscopically proliferation of uniform, endothelial cells in layers makes identification of vascular lumina difficult (Fig. 18-36). The tumor is not malignant. Juvenile hepatic hemangioendothelioma is associated with a high mortality as a result of hepatic failure or congestive heart failure.[158]

Hemangioendothelioma also has been used to designate the entity first described as vegetant intravascular hemangioendothelioma which resembles a vascular malignancy. This entity is the same as intravascular papillary endothelial hyperplasia.[157] These lesions may be unusual organizing thrombi with florid cellular proliferation. Perhaps the most common use of the term *hemangioendothelioma* is in reference to the malignant endothelial tumor, malignant hemangioendothelioma, which will be discussed with hemangiosarcoma.

Glomus tumor (glomangioma)

A glomus tumor is an uncommon, benign neoplasm usually found in the dermis, submucosal tissue, or superficial soft tissues. It arises from a neuromyoarterial body (Sucquet-Hoxer anastomosis) containing contractile glomus cells. Most glomus tumors are found in the subungual region[156] and are typically painful, a feature that is absent in other sites.[166,173] These tumors are usually a few millimeters in maximum diameter and in the skin appear as rounded, red-blue, painful nodules. Histologically the tumors are composed of blood vessels lined by normal endothelial cells and surrounded by sheets of uniform, round to oval glomus cells with many nonmyelinated nerve fibers (Fig. 18-37). Although tissue culture studies identified glomus cells as pericytes, ultrastructural studies show them to resemble modified smooth muscle cells.[177]

Hemangiopericytoma

Pericytes are perivascular cells that are found in place of smooth muscle cells in the wall of the terminal arteriole as it becomes the precapillary (metarteriole), and around capillaries, external to the basement membrane. Electron microscopic studies indicate that the tumor, hemangiopericytoma, originates from pericytes.[179]

Hemangiopericytomas[161,163] are rare tumors that can occur at any age and in any site. They vary in size from less than 1 cm up to large masses that are circumscribed or thinly encapsulated. Histologically the tumors are composed of small vessels whose lumina are surrounded by spindle-shaped pericytes in a radial arrangement out-

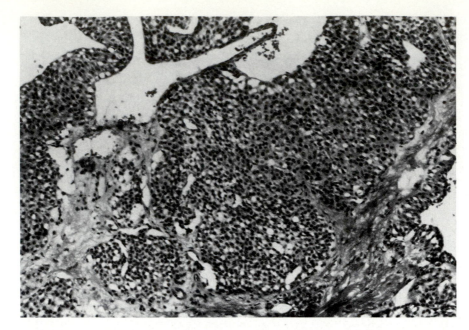

Fig. 18-37. Glomus tumor is composed of sheets of small, round to oval glomus cells surrounding vascular spaces. Nonmyelinated nerve fibers are present.

side the capillary basement membrane. Most are benign tumors, but local recurrence or distant spread eventuates in about 20% of patients.

Hemangiosarcoma (angiosarcoma)

Hemangiosarcoma (angiosarcoma, malignant hemangioendothelioma) is a malignant tumor of vascular tissue occurring at all ages, most frequently in skin and subcutaneous tissue, liver, spleen, bone,[155] lung, and soft tissue.[163,167] They are usually bulky, firm masses that histologically may be relatively well-differentiated tumors with multilayering of endothelial cells in well-formed vascular channels, or poorly differentiated lesions composed of solid clusters of cells with poorly formed vascular channels. Hepatic hemangiosarcomas have been associated with prior remote exposure to arsenic, thorium dioxide (Thorotrast), and gaseous vinyl chloride.[172]

Histiocytoid hemangioma[174] is a recently described entity characterized by the indolent behavior of a group of lesions, including hemangioendothelioma of bone, in which the main proliferating cell is a histiocytoid endothelial cell. These entities need to be distinguished from true angiosarcomas, which they resemble microscopically.

Kaposi's sarcoma

Kaposi's sarcoma is a multicentric, malignant neoplastic process[175] usually classified as an angiosarcomatous lesion occurring mainly in older men. The usual clinical finding is a dark blue to reddish purple macule or nodule on the extremities, although mucous membranes, lymph nodes, and internal organs also may be involved. On histologic examination, interweaving bands of malignant spindle cells and vascular structures forming clefts between the cells are found (Fig. 18-38). The nature and origin of the sarcomatous cells have not been established. Altered immunologic status has been implicated in the pathogenesis of Kaposi's sarcoma because of a higher incidence in patients receiving immunosuppressive therapy and because of an association of Kaposi's sarcoma, cytomegalovirus infection, and *Pneumocystis carinii* pneumonia in homosexual men,[159] drug abusers, and other epidemiologic groups (acquired immune deficiency syndrome, AIDS).

Primary tumors of large veins and arteries

Primary, true tumors arising in the major blood vessels are quite rare.[169] About two thirds are in large veins in which smooth muscle tumors, especially leiomyosarcoma, are the most frequent. Virtually all primary tumors of the aorta and pulmonary artery and their large branches are sarcomatous neoplasms including intimal (endothelial) sarcoma, fibrosarcoma (fibromyxoid sarcoma), leiomyosarcoma, and undifferentiated sarcoma.

Lymphangioma

Lymphangiomas are benign overgrowths of lymphatic vessels; whether these are congenital malformations, hamartomas, or true neoplasms is not certain. Lymphangiomas are classified as capillary, cavernous, or cystic (hygroma) types, and combinations are frequent.

Capillary lymphangioma (lymphangioma simplex) is an

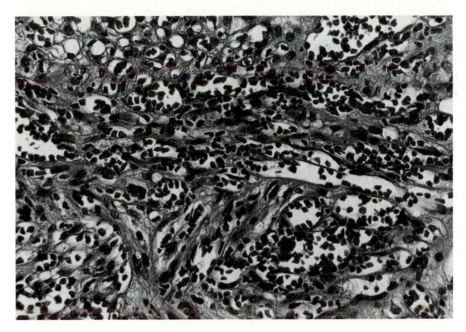

Fig. 18-38. Kaposi's sarcoma. Interweaving bands of malignant spindle-shaped stromal cells separate proliferating endothelial cells that form slitlike vascular spaces.

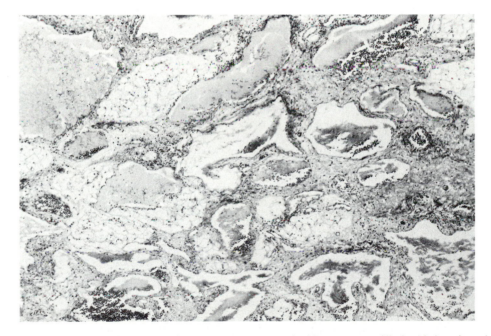

Fig. 18-39. Cystic hygroma (lymphangioma) is composed of large spaces filled with lymph and scattered collections of lymphocytes. This lesion is from neck of child.

apparently congenital lesion of the skin or mucous membranes of the head and neck that grows slowly if at all. The small, circumscribed, pale white to pink tumors are composed of a network of endothelium-lined, thin-walled lymphatic spaces often separated by lymphoid aggregates.

Lymphangiomyoma, which can be regarded as a variant of capillary lymphangioma, has proliferating smooth muscle cells and branching, slitlike lymphatic channels.[180] It is a rare, acquired or congenital lesion most commonly involving abdominal and thoracic lymphatics of females[170] and may be associated with chylothorax.

Cavernous lymphangioma[154] is more common than the capillary variety. It also is an apparently congenital lesion that grows slowly and is composed of numerous dilated lymphatic spaces filled with lymph (chylangioma), which may be coagulated and hyalinized or calcified. The distinction from capillary lymphangioma on the basis of size of channels is somewhat arbitrary. Mixed lesions of cavernous lymphangioma and hemangioma are more common.

Cystic lymphangioma (hygroma)[154] occurs principally in the neck (hygroma colli cysticum) as a disfiguring congenital lesion. The cystic mass usually is multilocular and contains serous fluid or lymph. The histologic structure is similar to that of cavernous lymphangioma except for the large size of the spaces (Fig. 18-39). Large collections of lymphocytes may be present in the stroma. Total excision of large lesions may be difficult, and incomplete excision leads to recurrence. Infection of cystic hygroma is a serious problem.

Lymphangiosarcoma

Lymphangiosarcoma occurs chiefly in areas of chronic lymphedema, most often in edematous arms after radical mastectomy and radiotherapy for carcinoma of the breast.[181] This usually fatal tumor is manifested by multiple, purple or blue, macular skin lesions that may form a hemorrhagic mass composed of proliferating vascular channels lined by anaplastic endothelial cells. The histopathologic features may be quite similar to those of hemangiosarcoma or Kaposi's sarcoma.

REFERENCES
Normal structure and age changes; arteriosclerosis
1. Biava, C.G., et al.: Renal hyaline arteriosclerosis: an electron microscopic study, Am. J. Pathol. 44:349, 1964.
2. Castleman, B., and Smithwick, R.H.: The relation of vascular disease to the hypertensive state: adequacy of renal biopsy as determined from a study of 500 patients, N. Engl. J. Med. 239:729, 1948.
3. Haust, M.D.: Atherosclerosis in childhood. In Rosenberg, H.S., and Bolande, R.P., editors: Perspectives in pediatric pathology, vol. 4, Chicago, 1978, Year Book Medical Publishers.
4. Mönckeberg, J.G.: Über die reine Mediaverkalkung der Extremitatenarterien und ihr Verhalten zur Arteriosklerose, Virchows Arch. (Pathol. Anat.) 171:141, 1903.
5. Moran, J.J.: Idiopathic arterial calcification of infancy: a clinicopathologic study, Pathol. Annu. 10:393, 1975.
6. Neufeld, H.N., and Blieden, L.C.: Pediatric atherosclerosis: genetic aspects. In Strong, W.B., editor: Atherosclerosis: its pediatric aspects, New York, 1978, Grune & Stratton, Inc.
7. Ross, R., et al.: Cells of the artery wall and atherosclerosis. In Brinkley, B., and Porter, K., editors: International cell biology, New York, 1977, Rockefeller University Press.
8. Sinclair, R.A., Antonovych, T.T., and Mostofi, F.K.: Renal proliferative arteriopathies and associated glomerular changes: a light and electron microscopic study, Hum. Pathol. 7:565, 1976.

Atherosclerosis
9. Benditt, E.P.: The monoclonal theory of atherogenesis. In Paoletti, R., and Gotto, A.M., Jr., editors: Atherosclerosis reviews, vol. 3, New York, 1978, Raven Press.
10. Bierman, E.L., and Albers, J.J.: Lipoprotein uptake by cultured human arterial smooth muscle cells, Biochim. Biophys. Acta 388:198, 1975.
11. Bierman, E.L., and Ross, R.: Aging and atherosclerosis. In Paoletti, R., and Gotto, A.M., Jr., editors: Atherosclerosis reviews, vol. 2, New York, 1977, Raven Press.
12. Daoud, A.S., et al.: Regression of advanced atherosclerosis in swine, Arch. Pathol. Lab. Med. 100:372, 1976.
13. Dawber, T.R.: The Framingham study: the epidemiology of atherosclerotic disease, Cambridge, Mass., 1980, Harvard University Press.
14. Fuster, V., Fass, D.N. and Bowie, E.J.W.: Resistance to atherosclerosis in pigs with genetic and therapeutic inhibition of platelet function, Thromb. Haemost. 42:270, 1979.
15. Geer, J.C., and Haust, M.D.: Smooth muscle cells in atherosclerosis: monograph on atherosclerosis, vol. 2, Basel, 1972, S. Karger.
16. Gerrity, R.G.: The role of monocyte in atherogenesis. I. Transition of blood-borne monocytes into foam cells in fatty lesions, Am. J. Pathol. 103:181, 1981.
17. Goldstein, J.L., and Brown, M.S.: The low density lipoprotein pathway and its relationship to atherosclerosis, Annu. Rev. Biochem. 56:259, 1977.
18. Gotto, A.M., Jr.: Status report: plasma lipids, lipoproteins, and coronary artery disease. In Paoletti, R., and Gotto, A.M., Jr., editors: Atherosclerosis reviews, vol. 4, New York, 1979, Raven Press.
19. Gotto, A.M., Jr., Foreyt, J.P., and Scott, L.W.: Hyperlipidemia and nutrition: ongoing work. In Hegyeli, R., editor: Atherosclerosis reviews, vol. 7, New York, 1980, Raven Press.
20. Gryglewski, R.J.: Prostacyclin and atherosclerosis—a hypothesis. In Gotto, A.M., Jr., Smith, L.C., and Allen, B., editors: Atherosclerosis, vol. 5, New York, 1980, Springer-Verlag.
21. Harker, L.A., and Ross, R.: Pathogenesis of arterial vascular disease, Semin. Thromb. Haemostas. 5:274, 1979.
22. Haust, M.D., More, R.H., and Movat, H.Z.: The role of smooth muscle cells in the fibrogenesis of arteriosclerosis, Am. J. Pathol. 37:377, 1960.
23. Haust, M.D.: Light and electron microscopy of human atherosclerotic lesions, Adv. Exp. Med. Biol. 104:33, 1978.
24. Havlik, R.J., and Feinleib, M.: Proceedings on the conference on the decline in coronary heart disease mortality, NIH Publication No. 79-1610, Washington, D.C., 1979, U.S. DHEW, Public Health Service.
25. Hoak, J.C., et al.: Interaction of thrombin and platelets with vascular endothelium, Fed. Proc. 39:2606, 1980.
26. McGill, H.C., Jr.: Fatty streaks in the coronary arteries and aorta, Lab. Invest. 18:100, 1968.
27. McGill, H.C., Jr., editor: The geographic pathology of atherosclerosis, Lab. Invest. 18:463, 1968.
28. McGill, H.C., Jr.: problems in pathogenesis. In Paoletti, R., and Gotto, A.M., Jr., editors: Atherosclerosis reviews, vol. 2, New York, 1977, Raven Press.
29. McGill, H.C., Jr., Geer, J.C., and Strong, J.P.: Natural history of human atherosclerotic lesions. In Sandler, M., and Bourne, G.H., editors: Atherosclerosis and its origin, New York, 1963, Academic Press, Inc.
30. McGill, H.C., Jr., and Stern, M.P.: Sex and atherosclerosis. In Paoletti, R., and Gotto, A.M., Jr., editors: Atherosclerosis reviews, vol. 2, New York, 1977, Raven Press.

31. Mitchell, J.R.A.: Prostaglandins in vascular disease: a seminal approach, Br. Med. J. **282**:590, 1981.
32. Mustard, J.F., Packham, M.A., and Kinlough-Rathbone, R.: Platelets, thrombosis and atherogenesis, Adv. Exp. Med. Biol. **104**:127, 1978.
33. National Heart and Lung Institute: Task force on genetic factors in atherosclerotic disease, DHEW Publication No. (NHH) 76-922, Washington, D.C., 1976, U.S. DHEW, Public Health Service.
34. Oalmann, M.C., et al.: Community pathology of atherosclerosis and coronary heart disease: post-mortem serum cholesterol and extent of coronary atherosclerosis, Am. J. Epidemiol. **113**:396, 1981.
35. Pearson, T.A., et al.: Evidence for two populations of fatty streaks with different roles in the atherogenic process, Lancet **2**:496, 1980.
36. Pearson, T.A., et al.: Clonal characteristics of cutaneous scars and implications for atherogenesis, Am. J. Pathol. **102**:49, 1981.
37. Ross, R.: The smooth muscle cell. II. Growth of smooth muscle cell in culture and formation of elastic fibers, J. Cell. Biol. **50**:172, 1971.
38. Ross, R.: Atherosclerosis: a problem of the biology of arterial wall cells and their interactions with blood components, Arteriosclerosis **1**:293, 1981.
39. Ross, R., and Klebanoff, S.I.: The smooth muscle cell. I. In vivo synthesis of connective tissue proteins, J. Cell. Biol. **50**:159, 1971.
40. Sakurai, I.: Coronary arterial changes in childhood and young adults with respect to progression of coronary sclerosis and a brief comment on thrombosis as a complication. In Schettler, G., et al., editors: Atherosclerosis, vol. 4, New York, 1976, Springer-Verlag.
41. Schettler, G., Nüssel, E., and Buchholz, L.: Epidemiological research in Western Europe. In Paoletti, R., and Gotto, A.M., Jr., editors: Atherosclerosis reviews, vol. 3, New York, 1978, Raven Press.
42. Smith, E.B.: The relationship between plasma and tissue lipids in human atherosclerosis, Adv. Lipid Res. **12**:1, 1974.
43. Smith, E.B.: Molecular interactions in human atherosclerotic plaques, Am. J. Pathol. **86**:665, 1977.
44. Stamler, J.: Lifestyles, major risk factors, proof and public policy, Circulation **58**:3, 1978.
45. Stamler, J.: Data base on the major cardiovascular diseases in the United States. In Hegyeli, R., editor: Atherosclerosis reviews, vol. 7, New York, 1980, Raven Press.
46. Strong, J.P., and Guzman, M.A.: Decrease in coronary atherosclerosis in New Orleans, Lab. Invest. **43**:297, 1980.
47. Strong, J.P., Restrepo, C., and Guzman, M.: Coronary and aortic atherosclerosis in New Orleans. II. Comparison of lesions by age, sex, and race, Lab. Invest. **39**:364, 1978.
48. Strong, J.P., and Richards, M.L.: Cigarette smoking and atherosclerosis in autopsied men, Atherosclerosis **23**:451, 1976.
49. Tall, A.R., and Small, D.M.: Current concepts: plasma high-density lipoproteins, N. Engl. J. Med. **299**:1232, 1978.
50. Titus, J.L., and Weilbaecher, D.G.: Smooth muscle cells in atherosclerosis. In Gotto, A.M., Jr., Smith, L.C., and Allen, B., editors: Atherosclerosis, vol. 5, New York, 1979, Springer-Verlag.
51. Wissler, R.W.: Development of the atherosclerotic plaque. In Braunwald, E., editor: The myocardium: failure and infarction, New York, 1974, H.P. Publishing.
52. Wissler, R.W.: Principles of the pathogenesis of atherosclerosis. In Braunwald, E., editor: Heart disease: a textbook of cardiovascular medicine, Philadelphia, 1980, W.B. Saunders Co.
53. Zilversmit, D.B.: Atherogenesis: a postprandial phenomenon, Circulation **60**:473, 1979.

Arteritis

54. Amano, S., et al.: General pathology of Kawasaki disease: on the morphological alterations corresponding to the clinical manifestations, Acta Pathol. Jpn. **30**:681, 1980.
55. Arkin, A.: A clinical and pathological study of periarteritis nodosa: a report of five cases, one histologically healed, Am. J. Pathol. **6**:401, 1930.
56. Baggenstoss, A.H., and Titus, J.L.: Rheumatic and collagen disorders of the heart. In Gould, S.E., editor: Pathology of the heart and blood vessels, ed. 3, Springfield, Ill., 1968, Charles C Thomas, Publisher.
57. Bell, D.M., et al.: Kawasaki syndrome: description of two outbreaks in the United States, N. Engl. J. Med. **304**:1568, 1981.
58. Bonnetblanc, J.M., et al.: Immunofluorescence in temporal arteritis, N. Engl. J. Med. **298**:458, 1978.
59. Buerger, L.: Thromboangiitis obliterans: a study of the vascular lesions leading to presenile spontaneous gangrene, Am. J. Med. Sci. **136**:567, 1908.
60. Burch, G.E., Harb, J.M., and Sun, C.S.: Fine structure of digital vascular lesions in Raynaud's phenomenon and disease, Angiology **30**:361, 1979.
61. Cairns, S.A., and Oleesky, S.: Takayasu's disease and giant cell arteritis—a single disease? Br. Med. J. **2**:127, 1977.
62. Carrington, C.B., and Liebow, A.A.: Limited forms of angiitis and granulomatosis of Wegener's type, Am. J. Med. **41**:497, 1966.
63. Chumbley, L.C., Harrison, E.G., and DeRemee, R.A.: Allergic granulomatosis and angiitis (Churg-Strauss syndrome): report and analysis of 30 cases, Mayo Clin. Proc. **52**:477, 1977.
64. Churg, J., and Strauss, L.: Allergic granulomatosis, allergic angiitis and periarteritis nodosa, Am. J. Pathol. **27**:277, 1951.
65. Conn, D.L., et al.: Immunologic mechanism in systemic vasculitis, Mayo Clin. Proc. **51**:511, 1976.
66. Cupps, T.R., and Fauci, A.S.: The vasculitides, Philadelphia, 1981, W.B. Saunders Co.
67. DeRemee, R.A., et al.: Wegener's granulomatosis: anatomic correlates, a proposed classification, Mayo Clin. Proc. **51**:777, 1976.
68. Elkon, K.B., et al.: Hairy-cell leukemia with polyarteritis nodosa, Lancet **2**:280, 1979.
69. Ettlinger, R.E., Hunder, G.G., and Ward, L.E.: Polymyalgia rheumatica and giant cell arteritis, Annu. Rev. Med. **29**:15, 1978.
70. Fan, P.T., et al.: A clinical approach to systemic vasculitis, Semin. Arthritis Rheum. **9**:248, 1980.
71. Fassbender, H.G.: Pathology of rheumatic diseases, Berlin, 1975, Springer-Verlag.
72. Fehér, J., et al.: Changes induced by vascular antigens in the aorta of guinea-pigs: immunological and morphological studies, Br. J. Exp. Pathol. **59**:237, 1978.
73. Goodman, B.W., Jr.: Temporal arteritis, Am. J. Med. **67**:839, 1979.
74. Herskowitz, A., Cho, S., and Factor, S.M.: Syphilitic arteritis involving proximal coronary arteries, N.Y. State J. Med. **80**:971, 1980.
75. Huston, K.A., et al.: Temporal arteritis: a 25-year epidemiologic, clinical and pathologic study, Ann. Intern. Med. **88**:162, 1978.
76. Israel, H.L., Patchefsky, A.S., and Saldana, M.J.: Wegener's granulomatosis, lymphomatoid granulomatosis, and benign lymphocytic angiitis and granulomatosis of lung: recognition and treatment, Ann. Intern. Med. **87**:691, 1977.
77. Juergens, J.L.: Thromboangiitis obliterans (Buerger's disease, TAO). In Juergens, J.L., Spittell, J.A., Jr., and Fairbairn, J.F., II, editors: Allen-Barker-Hines peripheral vascular diseases, ed. 5, Philadelphia, 1980, W.B. Saunders Co.
78. Kampmejer, R.H.: Manifestations of late syphilis, South. Med. Bull. **53**:17, 1965.
79. Koss, M.N., Antonovych, T., and Hochholzer, L.: Allergic granulomatosis (Churg-Strauss syndrome): pulmonary and renal morphologic findings, Am. J. Surg. Pathol. **5**:21, 1981.
80. Kussmaul, A., and Maier, R.: Über eine bisher nicht beschriebene eigentümliche Arterienerkrankung (periarteritis nodosa), die mit Morbus Brighti und rapid fortschreitender allgemeiner Muskellähmung einhergeht, Dtsch. Arch. Klin. Med. **1**:484, 1866.
81. Lande, A., and Berkmen, Y.M.: Aortitis: pathologic, clinical and arteriographic review, Radiol. Clin. North Am. **14**:219, 1976.

82. Landing, B.H., and Larson, E.J.: Are infantile periarteritis nodosa with coronary involvement and fatal mucocutaneous lymph node syndrome the same? Comparison of 20 patients from North America with patients from Hawaii and Japan, Pediatrics **59**:651, 1977.

83. Lupi, H.E., et al.: Takayasu's arteritis: clinical study of 107 cases, Am. Heart J. **93**:94, 1977.

84. Mambo, N.C.: Temporal (granulomatous) arteritis: a histopathological study of 32 cases, Histopathology **3**:209, 1979.

85. McCormick, W.F., and Schochet, S.S., Jr.: Atlas of cerebrovascular disease, Philadelphia, 1976, W.B. Saunders Co.

86. Michelak, G.: Immune complexes of hepatitis B surface antigen in the pathogenesis of periarteritis nodosa, Am. J. Pathol. **90**:619, 1978.

87. Morens, D.M.: Thoughts on Kawasaki disease etiology (editorial), J.A.M.A. **241**:399, 1979.

88. Nakao, K., et al.: Takayasu's arteritis: clinical report of eighty-four cases and immunological studies of seven cases, Circulation **35**:1411, 1967.

89. Newton-John, H.F.: Kawasaki disease in Melbourne: a report of eleven cases, Aust. Paediatr. J. **16**:57, 1980.

90. Paronetto, F., Deppisch, L., and Tuchman, L.R.: Lupus erythematosus with fatal hemorrhage into the liver and lesions resembling those of periarteritis nodosa and malignant hypertension: immunocytochemical observations, Am. J. Med. **36**:948, 1964.

91. Rose, A.G., and Sinclair-Smith, C.C.: Takayasu's arteritis: a study of 16 autopsy cases, Arch. Pathol. Lab. Med. **104**:231, 1980.

92. Scully, R.E., Galdabini, J.J., and McNeely, B.U.: Case records of the Massachusetts General Hospital (Case 19-1976), N. Engl. J. Med. **294**:1052, 1976.

93. Scully, R.E., Galdabini, J.J., and McNeely, B.U.: Case records of the Massachusetts General Hospital (Case 43-1978), N. Engl. J. Med. **299**:1002, 1978.

94. Sheps, S.G., and McDuffie, F.C.: Vasculitis. In Juergens, J.L., Spittell, J.A., Jr., and Fairbairn, J.F., II, editors: Allen-Barker-Hines peripheral vascular disease, ed. 5, Philadelphia, 1980, W.B. Saunders Co.

95. Soter, N.A., Austen, K.F., and Gigli, I.: The complement system in necrotizing angiitis of the skin: analysis of complement component activities in serum of patients with concomitant collagen-vascular disease, Invest. Dermatol. **63**:219, 1974.

96. Spittell, J.A., Jr.: Raynaud's phenomenon and allied vasospastic diseases. In Juergens, J.L., Spittell, J.A., Jr., and Fairbairn, J.F., II, editors: Allen-Barker-Hines peripheral vascular disease, ed. 5, Philadelphia, 1980, W.B. Saunders Co.

97. Wolff, S.M., et al.: Wegener's granulomatosis, Ann. Intern. Med. **81**:513, 1974.

98. Yanagihara, R., and Todd, J.K.: Acute febrile mucocutaneous lymph node syndrome, Am J. Dis. Child. **134**:603, 1980.

Aneurysms; arteriopathy

99. Burchell, H.B.: Aortic dissection (dissecting hematoma: dissecting aneurysm of the aorta), Circulation **12**:1068, 1955.

100. Carlson, R.G., Lillehei, C.W., and Edwards, J.E.: Cystic medial necrosis of the ascending aorta in relation to age and hypertension, Am. J. Cardiol. **25**:411, 1970.

101. Crawford, E.S., and Schuessler, J.S.: Thoracoabdominal and abdominal aortic aneurysms involving celiac, superior mesenteric, and renal arteries, World J. Surg. **4**:643, 1980.

102. Crawford, E.S., et al.: Graft replacement of aneurysm in descending thoracic aorta: results without bypass or shunting, Surgery **89**:73, 1981.

103. Crawford, E.S., et al.: Infrarenal abdominal aortic aneurysm: factors influencing survival after operation performed over a 25-year period, Ann. Surg. **193**:699, 1981.

104. Daily, P.O., et al.: Management of acute aortic dissections, Ann. Thorac. Surg. **10**:237, 1970.

105. DeBakey, M.E., and Noon, G.P.: Aneurysms of the thoracic aorta, Mod. Concepts Cardiovasc. Dis. **44**:53, 1975.

106. DeBakey, M.E., and Noon, G.P.: Aneurysms of the sinuses of Valsalva. In Sabiston, D.C., and Spencer, F.C., editors: Gibbon's surgery of the chest, Philadelphia, 1976, W.B. Saunders Co.

107. DeBakey, M.E., et al.: Surgical management of dissecting aneurysms of the aorta, J. Thorac. Cardiovasc. Surg. **4**:130, 1965.

108. DeBakey, M.E., et al.: Dissecting aneurysms of the aorta. In Bergan, J.J., and Yao, J.S.T., editors: Aneurysms, diagnosis and treatment, New York, 1981, Grune & Stratton, Inc.

109. Edwards, W.D., Leaf, D.S., and Edwards, J.E.: Dissecting aortic aneurysm associated with congenital bicuspid aortic valve, Circulation **57**:1022, 1978.

110. Erdheim, J.: Medionecrosis aortae idiopathica cystica, Virchows Arch. (Pathol. Anat.) **276**:187, 1930.

111. Gore, I.: Dissecting aneurysms of the aorta in persons under forty years of age, Arch. Pathol. **55**:1, 1953.

112. Haid, S.P., Conn, J., Jr., and Bergan, J.J.: Cystic adventitial disease of the popliteal artery, Arch. Surg. **101**:765, 1970.

113. Hanley, W.B., and Bennett, J.N.: Familial dissecting aortic aneurysm: a report of three cases within two generations, Br. Heart J. **29**:852, 1967.

114. Harrison, E.G., and McCormack, L.J.: Pathologic classification of renal arterial disease in renovascular hypertension, Mayo Clin. Proc. **46**:161, 1971.

115. Klima, T., et al.: Morphology of ascending aortic aneurysms. Hum. Pathol. **14**:810, 1983.

116. Kolata, J.B., and Marx, J.: Epidemiology of heart disease: search for causes, Science **194**:509, 1976.

117. Mandel, W., Evans, E.W., and Walsford, R.L.: Dissecting aortic aneurysm during pregnancy, N. Engl. J. Med. **251**:1059, 1954.

118. Murray, C.A., and Edwards, J.E.: Spontaneous laceration of ascending aorta, Circulation **48**:848, 1973.

119. Norwood, W.I., and Aretz, T.H.: Case records of the Massachusetts General Hospital (Case 35-1980), N. Engl. J. Med. **303**:571, 1980.

120. Roberts, W.C.: Aortic dissection: anatomy, consequences, and causes, Am. Heart J. **101**:195, 1981.

121. Rose, A.G., and Dent, D.M.: Inflammatory variant of abdominal atherosclerotic aneurysm, Arch. Pathol. Lab. Med. **105**:409, 1981.

122. Roth, J.A., Kearney, P., and Wittmann, C.J.: Cystic adventitial degeneration of the common femoral artery, Arch. Surg. **112**:210, 1977.

123. Schlatmann, T.J.M., and Becker, A.E.: Histologic changes in the normal aging aorta: implication for dissection aortic aneurysm, Am. J. Cardiol. **39**:13, 1977.

124. Schlatmann, T.J.M., and Becker, A.E.: Pathogenesis of dissecting aneurysm of aorta, Am. J. Cardiol. **39**:21, 1977.

125. Sinclair, R.J., Kitchen, A.H., and Turner, R.W.: Marfan's syndrome, Q. J. Med. **29**:19, 1960.

126. Sommerville, R.L., Allen, E.V., and Edwards, J.E.: Bland and infected arteriosclerotic abdominal aortic aneurysms, Medicine **38**:207, 1959.

127. Spittell, J.A., Jr., and Wallace, R.B.: Aneurysms. In Juergens, J.L., Spittell, J.A., Jr., and Fairbairn, J.F., II, editors: Allen-Barker-Hines peripheral vascular disease, Philadelphia, 1980, W.B. Saunders Co.

128. Stanley, J.C., et al.: Arterial fibrodysplasia: histopathologic character and current etiologic concepts, Arch. Surg. **110**:561, 1975.

129. Strauss, R.G., and McAdams, A.J.: Dissecting aneurysm in childhood, J. Pediatr. **76**:578, 1970.

130. Wheat, M.W.: Acute dissecting aneurysms of the aorta: diagnosis and treatment—1979, Am. Heart J. **99**:373, 1980.

131. Wheat, M.W., Jr., et al.: Acute dissecting aneurysms of the aorta, J. Thorac. Cardiovasc. Surg. **58**:344, 1969.

132. Wilson, S.K., and Hutchins, G.M.: Aortic dissecting aneurysms, Arch. Pathol. Lab. Med. **106**:175, 1982.

Veins

133. Goldberg, S.M., Gordon, P.H., and Nivatvongs, S.: Essentials of anorectal surgery, Philadelphia, 1980, J.B. Lippincott Co.

134. Haimovici, H.: Ischemic forms of venous thrombosis: phlegmasia cerulea dolens and venous gangrene, Heart Bull. **16**:101, 1967.

135. Kazmier, F.J., and Juergens, J.L.: Venous thrombosis and obstructive diseases of the veins. In Juergens, J.L., Spittell, J.A., Jr., and Fairbairn, J.F., II, editors: Allen-Barker-Hines periph-

eral vascular disease, ed. 5, Philadelphia, 1980, W.B. Saunders Co.

136. Kistner, R.L.: Incidence of pulmonary embolism in the course of thrombophlebitis of the lower extremities, Am. J. Surg. **124:**169, 1972.

137. Langer, B., Rotstein, L.E., and Campbell, V.M.: The Budd-Chiari syndrome. In Orloff, M.J., Stipa, S., and Ziparo, V., editors: Medical and surgical problems of portal hypertension, Proceedings of the Serono Symposia, vol. 34, New York, 1980, Academic Press, Inc.

138. Lie, J.T., Lawrie, G.M., and Morris, G.C., Jr.: Aortocoronary bypass saphenous vein graft atherosclerosis: anatomic study of 99 vein grafts from normal and hyperlipoproteinemic patients up to 75 months postoperatively, Am. J. Cardiol. **40:**906, 1977.

139. Lofgren, K.A.: Varicose veins. In Juergen, J.L., Spittell, J.A., Jr., and Fairbairn, J.F., II, editors: Allen-Barker-Hines peripheral vascular diseases, Philadelphia, 1980, W.B. Saunders Co.

140. Lokich, J.J., and Goodman, R.: Superior vena cava syndrome: clinical management, J.A.M.A. **236:**58, 1975.

141. Parish, J.M., et al.: Etiologic considerations in superior vena cava syndrome, Mayo Clin. Proc. **56:**407, 1981.

142. Spray, T.L., and Roberts, W.C.: Changes in saphenous veins used as aortocoronary bypass, Am. Heart J. **94:**500, 1977.

143. Strandness, D.E., Jr., and Thiele, B.L.: Selected topics in venous disorders: pathology, diagnosis and treatment, New York, 1981, Futura Publishing.

144. Unni, K.K., et. al.: Pathologic changes in aortocoronary saphenous vein grafts, Am. J. Cardiol. **34:**526, 1974.

145. Webb, L.J., and Sherlock, S.: The aetiology, presentation and natural history of extrahepatic portal venous obstruction, Q. J. Med. **48:**627, 1979.

Lymphatics

146. Alvin, A., et al.: Lymph vessel hypoplasia and chromosome aberrations in six patients with Turner's syndrome, Acta Derm. Venereol. (Stock.) **47:**25, 1967.

147. Kinmonth, J.B.: The lymphatics: diseases, lymphography and surgery, Baltimore, 1972, The Williams & Wilkins Co.

148. Schirger, A., Harrison, E.G., Jr. and Janes, J.M.: Idiopathic lymphedema: review of 131 cases, J.A.M.A. **182:**14, 1962.

149. Schirger, A., and Peterson, L.F.: Lymphedema. In Juergens, J.L., Spittell, J.A., Jr., and Fairbairn, J.F., II, editors: Allen-Barker-Hines peripheral vascular diseases, Philadelphia, 1980, W.B. Saunders Co.

Tumors and tumorlike conditions

150. Alexander, G.L., and Norman, R.W.: The Sturge-Weber syndrome, Baltimore, 1960, The Williams & Wilkins Co.

151. Allen, P.W., and Enzinger, F.M.: Hemangioma of skeletal muscle, Cancer **29:**8, 1972.

152. Bean, W.B.: Dyschondroplasia and hemangiomata (Maffucci's syndrome). II., Arch. Intern. Med. **102:**544, 1958.

153. Bean, W.B.: Vascular spiders and related lesions of the skin, Springfield, Ill., 1958, Charles C Thomas, Publishers.

154. Burbank, M.K., and Spittell, J.A., Jr.: Tumors of blood and lymph vessels. In Juergens, J.L., Spittell, J.A., Jr., and Fairbairn, J.F., II, editors: Allen-Barker-Hines peripheral vascular diseases, Philadelphia, 1980, W.B. Saunders Co.

155. Campanacci, M., Boriani, S., and Giunti, A.: Hemangioendothelioma of bone: a study of 29 cases, Cancer **46:**804, 1980.

156. Carroll, R.E., and Berman, A.T.: Glomus tumor of the hand: review of the literature and report of 28 cases, J. Bone Joint Surg. **54:**691, 1972.

157. Clearkin, K.P., and Enzinger, F.M.: Intravascular papillary endothelial hyperplasia, Arch. Pathol. Lab. Med. **100:**441, 1976.

158. Dehner, L.P., and Ishak, K.G.: Vascular tumors of the liver in infants and children: a study of 30 cases and review of the literature, Arch. Pathol. **92:**101, 1971.

159. Durack, D.T.: Opportunistic infections and Kaposi's sarcoma in homosexual men (editorial), N. Engl. J. Med. **305:**1465, 1981.

160. Edgerton, M.T.: The treatment of hemangiomas: with special reference to the role of steroid therapy, Ann. Surg. **183:**517, 1976.

161. Enzinger, F.M., and Smith, B.H.: Hemangiopericytoma: an analysis of 106 cases, Hum. Pathol. **7:**61, 1976.

162. Fairbairn, J.F., II, and Bernatz, P.E.: Arteriovenous fistulas. In Juergens, J.L., Spittell, J.A. Jr., and Fairbairn, J.F., II, editors: Allen-Barker-Hines peripheral vascular diseases, ed. 5, Philadelphia, 1980, W.B. Saunders Co.

163. Hajdu, S.I.: Pathology of soft tissue tumors, Philadelphia, 1979, Lea & Febiger.

164. Hodgson, C.H., and Kaye, R.L.: Pulmonary arteriovenous fistula and hereditary hemorrhagic telangiectasia: a review and report of 35 cases of fistula, Dis. Chest **43:**449, 1963.

165. Horton, W.A.: Von Hippel-Lindau disease: clinical and pathological manifestations in nine families with 50 affected members, Arch. Intern. Med. **136:**769, 1976.

166. Kohout, E., and Stout, A.P.: The glomus tumor in children, Cancer **14:**555, 1961.

167. Landing, B.H., and Farber, S.: Tumors of the cardiovascular system: atlas of tumor pathology, fascicle 7, Washington, D.C., 1956, Armed Forces Institute of Pathology.

168. Lindenauer, S.M.: The Klippel-Trenaunay syndrome: varicosities, hypertrophy and hemangioma with no arteriovenous fistula, Ann. Surg. **162:**303, 1965.

169. McAlister, H.J., Jr., and Fenoglio, J.J.: Tumors of the cardiovascular system: atlas of tumor pathology, second series, fascicle 15, Washington, D.C., 1978, Armed Forces Institute of Pathology.

170. McCarty, K.S., et al.: Pulmonary lymphagiomyomatosis responsive to progesterone, N. Engl. J. Med. **303:**1461, 1980.

171. Morris, S.J., et al.: Blue rubber-bleb nevus syndrome, J.A.M.A. **239:**1887, 1978.

172. Popper, H., et al.: Development of hepatic angiosarcoma in man induced by vinyl chloride, Thorotrast, and arsenic: comparison with cases of unknown etiology, Am. J. Pathol. **92:**349, 1978.

173. Rosai, J.: Ackerman's surgical pathology, ed. 6, St. Louis, 1981, The C.V. Mosby Co.

174. Rosai, J., Gold, J., and Landy, R.: The histiocytoid hemangiomas, Hum. Pathol. **10:**707, 1979.

175. Safai, B., and Good, R.A.: Kaposi's sarcoma: a review and recent developments, CA **31:**2, 1981.

176. Straub, P.W., et al.: Chronic intravascular coagulation in Kasabach-Merritt syndrome, Arch. Intern. Med. **129:**475, 1972.

177. Venkatachalam, M.A., and Greally, J.G.: Fine structure of glomus tumor: similarity of glomus cells to smooth muscle, Cancer **23:**1176, 1969.

178. Waisman, M.: Common hemangiomas: to treat or not to treat, Postgrad. Med. **43:**183, 1968.

179. Waldo, E.D., Vuletin, J.C., and Kaye, G.I.: The ultrastructure of vascular tumors: additional observations and review of the literature, Pathol. Annu. **12**(2):279, 1977.

180. Wolff, M.: Lymphangiomyoma: clinocopathologic study and ultrastructural confirmation of its histogenesis, Cancer **31:**988, 1973.

181. Woodward, A.H., Ivins, J.C., and Soule, E.H.: Lymphangiosarcoma arising in chronic lymphedematous extremities, Cancer **30:**562, 1972.

CHAPTER 19 **Kidneys**

DAVID B. JONES

STRUCTURE AND FUNCTION[83]

The kidneys of normal humans each contain about 1¼ million nephrons. The rich vascular network of these nephrons is perfused by roughly one fourth of the cardiac output under basal conditions. The renal arteries branch into interlobar, arcuate, and interlobular arteries. The interlobular arteries course perpendicularly from the medulla to the renal cortex, giving off a succession of afferent arterioles. After perfusing the high-pressure glomerular capillaries, the blood recollects into the smaller efferent arterioles. The efferent arterioles in the juxtamedullary region branch into the vasa recta, which course straight down into the papilla and loop back to collect into veins. The veins of the kidney have thin walls and course with the arteries.

The afferent arteriole enters the glomerular tuft and breaks into about eight branches, which, in turn, branch into the anastomosing capillary network of each of eight glomerular lobules. These capillaries are lined by a unique endothelium with specialized holes or fenestrations of about 1000 Å in diameter that permit free access of the plasma to the glomerular basement membrane. The connective tissue support of the glomerular capillaries is almost entirely basement membrane substance; only a rare collagen fibril is seen in healthy or diseased glomeruli. This basement membrane is composed of a special amorphous form of collagen, type IV, with prominent carbohydrate components.[45] It has been suggested that the amount of carbohydrate packed between cross-linked protein may partly determine porosity of the basement membrane to macromolecules. The visceral glomerular epithelial cell, or podoctye, appears to be the major source for basement membrane synthesis. Where the basement membrane covers the outer perimeter of the capillary endothelium, it measures about 0.3 μm in thickness. The central dense part of the basement membrane (lamina densa) is covered by less dense inner and outer layers (lamina rara interna and lamina rara externa). The laminae rarae interna and externa contain sialic acid and heparan sulfate, which may act as a charge barrier to proteins with a net negative charge.[42]

The podocytes cover the external surface of each glomerular capillary basement membrane with octopus-like processes that branch and interdigitate with one another (foot processes) (Fig. 19-1). These foot processes are separated by a filtration slit of 200 to 500 Å in width, but a thin film of plasma membrane connects the foot processes (the filtration slit membrane) (Fig. 19-2).[43,83] The barrier to leakage of macromolecules apparently depends on maintenance of the charge barrier of the lamina rara, a normal lamina densa, and a healthy covering of glomerular epithelial cells.

Where the capillaries adjoin in the central portion of the lobule, the basement membrane thickens and encloses the mesangium (Fig. 19-3). The mesangium is composed of a spongelike meshwork of basement membrane (mesangial matrix) that encloses mesangial cells.[39] It extends from the hilum of the glomerulus up the center of each lobule like a contorted Eiffel Tower. The mesangial cells, which are analogous to pericytes, have been shown to be phagocytic and may be responsible for laying down mesangial matrix in scarring.[59]

The glomerular tuft is enclosed by Bowman's capsule, which opens into the proximal tubule and is lined by flattened capsular epithelial cells.

The juxtaglomerular apparatus consists of a collar of granulated and ungranulated cells that replace the smooth muscle cells of the afferent arteriole at the hilum of the glomerulus. Nonmyelinated nerve fibers are found amid these cells. Where the distal tubule of each nephron passes adjacent to these arteriolar cells, the tubular cells form a compact plaque of highly specialized cells (macula densa), which are in intimate contact with the juxtaglomerular apparatus cells. There is much evidence that this apparatus monitors pulse pressure and sodium content of the distal tubule and is concerned with their control.

The proximal and distal tubules with their complex

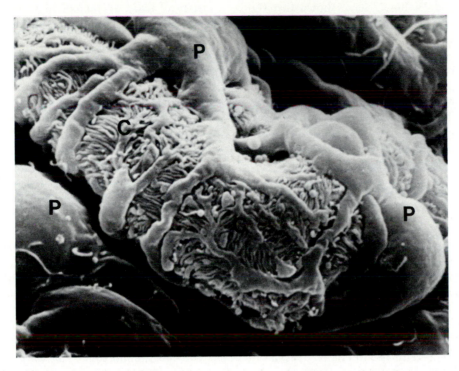

Fig. 19-1. Scanning electron micrograph of normal glomerular capillary, *C*, enclosed by podocytes, *P*, with primary processes and interdigitating foot processes. (5200×.)

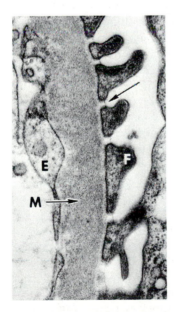

Fig. 19-2. Glomerular capillary wall showing foot processes of podocytes, *F*; filtration slit membrane *(arrow)*; basement membrane, *M*; and fenestrated endothelium, *E*. (40,000×.)

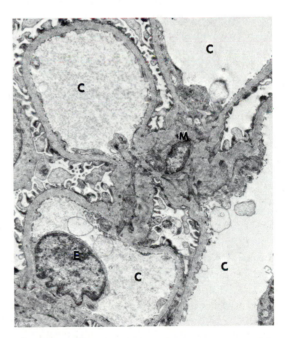

Fig. 19-3. Portion of human glomerulus showing endothelial cell, *E*; mesangial cell, *M*; and capillaries, *C*. Basement membrane is somewhat thickened by hypertension. (3600×.)

cytologic specialization are highly adapted to the resorption of nutrients (amino acids, glucose) and electrolyte pumping. Welling and Welling[89] have shown that the brush border microvilli of the proximal tubules increase the luminal surface area 30 fold, and the complex interdigitations of the basal antiluminal surface increase that area 20 fold. Such a large surface is critical for the resorptive and electrolyte pumping functions. In the medullary portion of the kidney, the loops of Henle and the loops of the vasa recta form the anatomic basis for the countercurrent multiplier system whereby a high osmotic gradient is produced in the renal papilla, permitting the water resorption characteristic of mammals.

PRINCIPLES OF RENAL PATHOPHYSIOLOGY
Glomerular disease

Acute injury. When glomeruli are involved with acute inflammation, as in other capillary beds, there is increased capillary permeability and sometimes actual discontinuity of capillary basement membranes. This increased permeability permits plasma proteins (proteinuria), red cells (hematuria), and white blood cells to leak into the urine. Tamm-Horsfall glycoprotein may precipitate and entrap these components, forming casts. The identification of casts, protein, and red blood cells in the urine is important in diagnosing glomerular inflammation.

With acute inflammation the glomeruli become swollen and hypercellular because of infiltration with neutrophils and monocytes and because of proliferation and hydropic swelling of mesangial and endothelial cells. This may result in blockage of blood flow through most of the glomerular capillary loops, so that only a few capillaries shunt blood to the efferent arteriole. The sharp fall in filtration fraction results in the paradox of a low glomerular filtration rate with relative preservation of tubular function. This may lead to oliguria (little urine formation) or anuria (no urine formation).

As inflammation subsides, hydropic swelling decreases, and inflammatory cells leave, a resolution to near-normal function can occur.

Chronic injury. Glomeruli undergo progressive scarring as a result of chronic injury. Scar tissue in the glomerular tuft is composed of new deposits of basement membrane. The continued glomerular injury may be manifest by some increased capillary permeability with proteinuria and perhaps microscopic hematuria. Continued glomerular scarring results in destruction of whole glomeruli or obliteration of capillary channels in glomeruli that are injured to a lesser degree. This scarring causes a progressive decrease in glomerular filtration rate, and renal plasma flow decreases because of the obstruction of the arterial bed by the scarred glomeruli. The sharp fall in glomerular filtration rate eventually results in renal failure and death.

Tubular disease

Acute injury. Ischemia, immunologic injury, and a variety of toxic substances may result in acute tubular injury or necrosis, which may produce oliguria or anuria if most or all nephrons are involved. The failure of urine formation in the presence of morphologically normal arteries and glomeruli may be explained by the following[81]:

1. Arterial vasoconstriction
2. Mechanical plugging of tubules by necrotic tubular debris and precipitated protein (casts)
3. Back-diffusion of glomerular filtrate into the interstitium through gaps in the walls of necrotic tubules and ruptured peritubular basement membranes
4. A rise in tissue turgor pressure from this back-diffusion, resulting in decreased glomerular filtration

In the great variety of acute tubular injuries, part or all of these factors may play a role.

If oliguria persists, azotemia (sharp rise in nitrogenous waste products in the blood) and acute renal failure may result. If the patient survives for 14 to 21 days, the remarkable regenerative capacity of the tubules permits a return to normal or near-normal function.

Chronic tubular loss or atrophy. In chronic renal disease, whether caused by chronic glomerular disease, chronic arteriosclerotic renal disease, or chronic interstitial inflammatory disease, the tubules may be destroyed or may develop irregular atrophy with interstitial fibrosis and thickened peritubular basement membranes. Such chronic tubular changes are associated with decreased ability to pump sodium, synthesize ammonium ions, exchange hydrogen ions, and form a concentrated urine. The large reserve of proximal tubular function in resorbing many substances such as amino acids and glucose usually prevents their appearance in the urine even in advanced tubular atrophy. The formation of urine of fixed, nearly isotonic osmolality is attributable in part to the structural and functional alteration of the countercurrent multiplier system and in part to the solute load of accumulated waste products (urea) that force an osmotic diuresis in the few remaining functioning nephrons.

Vascular disease

Acute arterial obstruction. Renal vasoconstriction may result in a decrease or even a cessation of glomerular filtration and urine formation. Such vasoconstriction may occur in shock and hypovolemia. Persistent poor renal perfusion because of hypovolemia, arterial vasoconstriction, and perhaps low cardiac output may result in oliguria and azotemia. Such azotemia caused by extrarenal factors is termed prerenal azotemia.

More severe degrees of arterial obstruction may result from extreme arterial vasoconstriction, embolism, or thrombosis and may cause renal infarction.

Chronic arterial obstruction. With progressive narrowing and perhaps obliteration of the arterial and arteriolar lumina by hyperplastic or hyaline intimal arteriosclerotic changes, there is a progressive ischemia of the part of the kidney supplied by those vessels. This results in ischemic collapsed glomeruli, tubular atrophy, and interstitial fibrosis. When a sufficiently large proportion of nephrons is involved by this process, the glomerular filtration rate falls to critical levels, and renal function fails. This arteriosclerotic disease of the kidney (nephrosclerosis) may be the primary process, but obliteration of the renal vascular bed because of glomerular, chronic tubular, or chronic interstitial disease also may result in noticeable arteriosclerotic changes.

Chronic venous obstruction. High intrarenal venous pressure, whether attributable to renal vein thrombosis or high systemic venous pressure from such causes as congestive heart failure, may result in renal congestion and proteinuria. It is presumed that such congestion causes increased capillary permeability.

Edema of renal disease

The edema of renal disease is of three types: water and salt overload, hypoproteinemic (nephrotic) edema, and congestive heart failure. Water and salt overload develops in patients with damaged kidneys when water and salt intake exceeds excretory capacity. This edema may characteristically accumulate in the face and eyelids, since such patients may comfortably lie flat unlike patients with congestive heart failure. When water and salt overload is extreme, pulmonary edema and death may result.

Hypoproteinemic (nephrotic) edema may occur in a number of glomerular diseases that result in pronounced proteinuria and hypoproteinemia. The low serum albumin level results in a fall in plasma osmotic pressure, loss of blood volume into the interstitial tissues, and a contracted blood volume. The low effective blood volume results in reflex sodium saving and thus water saving through the juxtaglomerular apparatus–renin–aldosterone mechanism.

Many patients with acute or chronic renal disease have severe arterial hypertension. This increased load on the heart may result in congestive heart failure and contribute to the formation of edema.

Uremia

Uremia is a systemic toxic state resulting from acute or chronic failure to eliminate urine. It may be caused by urinary tract obstruction, as well as by parenchymal renal disease. Although the problems seen in uremia may differ to a degree depending on whether the renal failure is acute or chronic, many of the manifestations are seen in both—central nervous system toxicity, pericarditis, pulmonary edema and pneumonitis, immunologic depression, pancreatitis, gastroenteritis, anemia, bleeding tendency, acidosis, electrolyte imbalance, azotemia, and uremic frost. When severe and progressive, uremia results in death.

Central nervous system toxicity. Manifestations of central nervous system toxicity include tremor, twitching, lethargy, convulsions, and coma. These may be the result of accumulating waste products, acidosis, hyponatremia, and hypocalcemia. Cerebral edema is common, particularly with hypertension, when vascular lesions of the central nervous system may trigger convulsive episodes.

Pericarditis. When the accumulating waste products reach a high level, a fibrinous pericarditis and perhaps pleuritis may develop. The mechanism of production is not understood.

Pulmonary edema and pneumonitis. With renal failure, hypervolemia and heart failure are common, and varying degrees of pulmonary congestion and edema occur. Radiologists recognize a characteristic central butterfly pattern of edema and congestion in roentgenograms of the chest that has been termed uremic pneumonitis. At autopsy, such lungs contain a fibrin-rich edema fluid.

Immunologic depression. In severe renal failure patients are very susceptible to infection, which may be the coup de grace. In addition to this poorly understood susceptibility to bacterial infection, there are depression of the cellular immunity mechanism and impaired ability to reject homografts. Although these are beneficial if renal transplantation is carried out, the dangers of infection are ever present.

Gastroenteritis. A nonspecific gastroenteritis may occur in uremia. It may be manifested as vomiting with gastritis, intestinal obstruction resulting from paralytic ileus, or bloody diarrhea caused by uremic colitis. Bleeding from small acute ulcers may occur anywhere along the gastrointestinal tract.

Pancreatitis. The uremic state often results in the plugging of pancreatic ducts by inspissated secretions. This may result in asymptomatic focal pancreatitis and sometimes in painful clinical pancreatitis.

Anemia. The anemia of renal failure is often striking and may be the feature bringing the patient to the physician. It appears to result from both decreased production of red cells and shortened red cell life. Depression of red cell production may be the consequence of decreased renal erythropoietin production. Increased red cell destruction may be the result of the uremic toxic state alone, but, in addition, the acute arteriolar and glomerular lesions of a variety of renal diseases cause traumatic damage to red cells known as microangiopathic hemolytic anemia.

Bleeding tendency. Contributing to the anemia of renal failure is the bleeding tendency so commonly seen.

The cause of this bleeding may be capillary fragility or interference with platelet aggregation by accumulation of metabolites such as guanidinosuccinic acid.

Uremic frost. The skin of the anemic uremic individual is pale, and with the accumulation of carotene-like pigments, the skin assumes a sallow yellow color. The urea content rises in the perspiration as well as in the plasma, and as facial perspiration evaporates, the urea remains as a powdery "uremic frost."

Renal failure

Acute renal failure. In acute renal failure certain problems are related to sudden development of oliguria. Water intake often is maintained before the patient or physician is aware of the renal problem. The resulting water overload may cause pulmonary edema or cardiac failure. Another problem of oliguria is hyperkalemia resulting from lack of excretion of dietary potassium and endogenous potassium from the breakdown of blood, necrotic tissue, and the catabolism of negative nitrogen balance. Hyperkalemia may result in cardiac arrhythmias and sudden death.

Chronic renal failure. In chronic renal failure acidosis is a big problem, since the kidney fails to excrete hydrogen ions as ammonia and fails to reabsorb adequately all the filtered bicarbonate. Phosphates, sulfates, and other anions accumulate, and acidosis results.

Because the chronically damaged kidney fails to convert 25-vitamin D to the active principle 1,25-vitamin D, defective absorption of calcium from the intestinal tract results in hypocalcemia. Hypocalcemia leads to secondary parathyroid hyperplasia with concomitant demineralization and resorption of bone osteomalacia. Bone pain and bony deformities (renal rickets) may develop in children with long-standing chronic renal disease and acidosis.

In long-standing chronic renal failure, peripheral nerve degeneration may develop and cause disturbing sensory and motor problems.

RENAL DISEASES
Classification

No single method of classification of renal disease is easily applicable. The basic method used herein is based in part on the portion of the kidney primarily involved in the disease process and in part on the biologic nature of the disease process. A general attempt is made to have this classification correlate with the clinical behavior of the diseases. In the past the classification of renal disease was based on the gross and microscopic appearance at autopsy. These objective findings seen only at the end of a disease process were sometimes misinterpreted and failed to correlate with the clinical findings in life. The use of the percutaneous renal biopsy at various stages in renal disease has been of great value.[66] In the biopsy a core of tissue is obtained by a special needle that is thrust into the kidney through the back. This tissue may be studied by light, electron, and fluorescence microscopy. Serial biopsies are possible. As a result of following patients who have had careful clinical, laboratory, and biopsy workups, we are able to understand better the nature of certain human kidney diseases and to assess the effects of various forms of therapy on these diseases. Following is the classification of renal diseases:

1. Glomerulonephritis
   a. Diffuse
      (1) Acute poststreptococcal
      (2) Acute nonstreptococcal
      (3) Rapidly progressive
      (4) Chronic progressive
      (5) End-stage chronic
   b. Focal
      (1) With systemic bacterial infection
      (2) Of probable immunologic origin—IgA focal glomerulonephritis
      (3) Hereditary
2. Nephrotic syndrome
   a. Minimal change disease, lipoid nephrosis, or nil disease
   b. Focal segmental glomerular sclerosis
   c. Congenital nephrotic syndrome
   d. Membranoproliferative glomerulonephritis
   e. Idiopathic membranous nephropathy (membranous glomerulonephritis)
   f. Systemic lupus erythematosus
   g. Systemic infection or hypersensitivity reactions
   h. Circulatory disturbances and renal vein thrombosis
   i. Amyloidosis
   j. Toxemia of pregnancy
3. Disease of vascular origin
   a. Hypertensive vascular disease
   b. Benign nephrosclerosis
   c. Malignant nephrosclerosis
   d. Diabetic nephropathy
   e. Renal infarction
   f. Polyarteritis nodosa and Wegener's granulomatosis
   g. Thrombotic renal disease
      (1) Disseminated intravascular coagulation
      (2) Bilateral renal cortical necrosis
      (3) Hemolytic uremic syndrome
      (4) Thrombotic thrombocytopenic purpura
   h. Scleroderma
   i. Radiation nephritis
4. Tubular disease
   a. Acute tubular necrosis
      (1) Toxic nephropathy
      (2) Ischemic tubular necrosis
   b. Osmotic nephrosis
   c. Hypokalemic nephropathy

5. Chronic interstitial and tubular disease
   a. Interstitial nephritis
   b. Pyelonephritis
   c. Tuberculous pyelonephritis
   d. Urinary tract obstructive disease
   e. Renal papillary necrosis
   f. Analgesic abuse nephropathy
   g. Multiple myeloma nephropathy
   h. Gout nephropathy
   i. Hypercalcemic nephropathy and renal calcinosis
   j. Renal lithiasis
6. Congenital malformations and anomalies
   a. Agenesis and hypoplasia
   b. Fusion, ectopia, and reduplication
   c. Dysplasia and polycystic dysplasia
   d. Congenital obstructive microcystic disease
   e. Simple cysts
   f. Infantile polycystic disease
   g. Adult polycystic disease
   h. Medullary cystic disease
7. Renal neoplasms
   a. Benign tumors
      (1) Adrenocortical nodules
      (2) Hamartomas
      (3) Mesenchymal tumors
      (4) Cortical tubular adenomas
   b. Malignant tumors
      (1) Adenocarcinoma
      (2) Wilms' tumor
      (3) Leukemic infiltration
      (4) Transitional cell carcinoma

Glomerular disease
Pathogenesis of glomerular injury

Glomeruli may be injured by immunologic, metabolic, vascular, thrombotic, hereditary, toxic, and as yet unknown mechanisms. Immunologic mechanisms are of particular importance in both experimental and human glomerular disease. Immunoglobulins IgG, IgM, and IgA can be demonstrated in both human and experimental glomerulonephritis.[91] In addition, components of the classical and alternative pathways of complement may be demonstrated in such lesions and at times appear to be the principal deposit with little immunoglobulin. Three important mechanisms of glomerular immunologic injury are anti–glomerular basement membrane disease, immune complex disease, and alternative pathway injury.

Anti–glomerular basement membrane disease

Lindeman[51] first demonstrated that antibodies develop when a kidney of one species is injected into another species and that when such antibodies (nephrotoxic serum) are reinjected into the original species, acute glomerular inflammation results. Subsequent research has shown that the critical antigens involved are in the glomerular basement membrane. It was then shown that the injection of the foreign-species glomerular basement membrane along with adjuvants results in antibodies that cross-react with the animal's own glomerular basement membrane and induce inflammation.[80] In some cases of human glomerular inflammation (glomerulonephritis) it has been possible to isolate anti–glomerular basement membrane antibody from the serum and to elute or split off combined antibody from the glomeruli of such patients and identify it as anti–glomerular basement membrane antibody.[18]

One can couple fluorescein dye to antibodies against gamma globulin or complement components (fluorescent antibodies) and react these reagents with frozen sections of either experimental or human anti–glomerular basement membrane diseased glomeruli. Fluorescence microscopy reveals a linear deposition of anti–glomerular basement membrane antibody and complement along the glomerular basement membrane (Fig. 19-4). Electron microscopy may show a thin, fluffy, linear layer of material between the capillary endothelium and basement membrane in such cases.[18]

Studies indicate that anti–glomerular basement membrane disease is the basis for all cases of Goodpasture's syndrome and about half the cases of rapidly progressive glomerulonephritis. The mechanism by which one develops antibodies against one's own glomerular basement membrane is not known, but it is possible that one

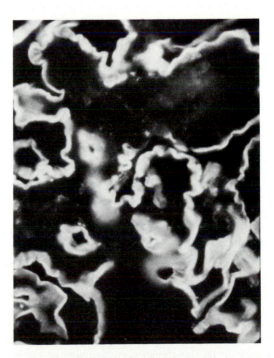

Fig. 19-4. Rapidly progressive glomerulonephritis of antiglomerular basement membrane type showing linear staining of glomerular basement membrane with fluorescent antihuman IgG. (Courtesy Dr. Claude Cornwall, Syracuse, N.Y.)

develops antibodies either against one's own basement membrane or against other endogenous or exogenous antigens that cross-react with glomerular basement membrane.

Immune complex disease

The experimental injection of certain foreign non-glomerular antigens into animals stimulates antibody formation. The antibody then combines with still circulating antigen, and the complex is deposited in glomeruli along with complement. This complex of antigen, antibody, and complement plus neutrophils and monocytes causes glomerular injury.[66] Fluorescent antibody reagents show that the immune complexes are deposited as lumpy deposits just outside the basement membrane and in the mesangium. Electron microscopy confirms the presence of deposits between the podocytes and the glomerular basement membrane and in the mesangium. This type of glomerular deposit occurs when there is moderate antigen excess to antibody because such small aggregates are trapped in the glomerular filter. With antibody equivalence or excess, large aggregates are formed that are taken up by the reticuloendothelial system. With great antigen excess, only small, soluble aggregates form and remain in the circulation or are filtered.

Naturally occurring immune complex disease has been demonstrated in mice infected with lymphochoriomeningitis virus at birth.[19] These mice have continued viremia (moderate antigen excess) and deposit virus antigen-antibody complexes in their glomeruli. New Zealand black mice are chronically infected with one or more viruses and develop antinuclear antibodies. Complexes of antibodies, complement, and nuclear antigens are deposited in glomeruli and cause glomerular damage. This antinuclear antibody disease resembles human systemic lupus erythematosus (SLE). Antinuclear antibody, nuclear antigen, and complement have been demonstrated in the lumpy deposits characteristically seen in SLE. Other human diseases that appear to be of this immune complex type are acute glomerulonephritis, membranous glomerulonephritis (see Fig. 19-25), and some cases of rapidly progressive and chronic glomerulonephritis.

Alternate pathway disease

Certain patients with membranoproliferative glomerulonephritis have greatly depressed serum complement component C3 levels but normal levels of C1, C2, and C4.[23,30] The glomeruli of such patients show little immunoglobulin deposition by immunofluorescence studies but heavy deposits of complement C3 and also deposits of properdin of the alternative pathway of the complement system.[62] A circulating nephritic anticomplementary factor, C3NeF, has been found in such patients.

Nephritic factor (NeF) has been found to be an immunoglobulin that acts to stabilize C3 convertase and enhance alternative pathway activity. With electron microscopy these sites of complement and properdin deposition are shown to be very electron dense (see Fig. 19-23). Such glomerular lesions have been called dense deposit disease.[30] Alternative pathway disease also occurs in some patients with rapidly progressive glomerulonephritis. Acute poststreptococcal glomerulonephritis usually shows striking activation of the alternative pathway of complement, and to a lesser extent SLE shows activation of this pathway as a supplement to the classical complement pathway activation by immune complex deposition.[91] Focal glomerulonephritis induced by IgA deposits appears also to implicate the alternative pathway.

Role of fibrin deposits in glomerular disease

Fibrin deposition in glomerular capillaries and Bowman's space is seen in severe glomerular injury, particularly rapidly progressive glomerulonephritis (see Fig. 19-10). Experimental and clinical evidence suggests that minimization of the deposition of fibrin by anticoagulation decreases the amount of irreversible scarring.[87,90]

Diffuse glomerulonephritis

Acute diffuse glomerulonephritis is characterized by an acute inflammatory process involving all the glomeruli of both kidneys. This inflammation results in blockage of many of the glomerular capillaries with cellular exudate and hydropic swelling, thus decreasing glomerular filtration. The inflammation also results in increased capillary permeability so that plasma proteins, red blood cells, and white blood cells appear in the urine.

Acute poststreptococcal glomerulonephritis.[26] Careful epidemiologic, bacteriologic, and serologic studies indicate that at least two thirds of the cases of acute diffuse glomerulonephritis follow hemolytic streptococcal infections after about a 10-day latent period. Only certain strains of hemolytic streptococci (types 12, 4, 1, and Red Lake) seem to be nephritogenic. Although most of these infections are of the upper respiratory tract, skin and wound infections may be responsible. The streptococcal infection may be identified by culture, or it may be inferred later by a rising titer of antibodies against streptococcal antigens, that is, antistreptolysin O (ASO) titer. The inflammation is clearly not attributable to the local presence of streptococci in the glomeruli, since cure of the infection with antibiotics does not prevent the development of nephritis. Immunologic, fluorescence, and electron microscopic studies indicate that poststreptococcal diffuse glomerulonephritis is an immune complex disease because streptococcal antigen and human antibody are trapped in the glomerulus.

Clinical features. Acute poststreptococcal glomerulonephritis is seen mostly in children, particularly from 3 to 7 years of age, and in young adults. The disease affects males with about twice the frequency of females. It is common and occurs throughout the world.

Characteristically the patient notices a smoky, rusty, reddish brown urine (gross hematuria) that is passed in smaller than usual volume (oliguria). In very severe cases there may be anuria. Edema is present in about two thirds of the patients and most often involves the face and eyelids.

Hypertension occurs in about half of patients sufficiently ill to enter the hospital. In 5% to 10% the hypertension may be sufficiently severe to cause cerebrovascular damage and cerebral edema (hypertensive encephalopathy). This may result in headache, vomiting, convulsions, and coma. The cause of the hypertension is unknown but has been attributed to hypervolemia or to neurogenic or humoral influences.

After a few days the hematuria, proteinuria, and hypertension diminish, and in the favorable cases all findings have returned to normal in 6 months. About 80% to 90% of children have a good outcome, whereas only 50% to 70% of adults do as well. About 2% to 5% of patients die in the acute phase as a result of uremia, infection, or cardiovascular problems.[20] Some patients surviving the acute phase may have persistent, active, progressive disease, which heals with a large loss of nephrons, or they may have a slow, smoldering, downhill course.[7]

Pathologic anatomy. The kidney in acute diffuse glomerulonephritis is moderately swollen and may be either pale or congested. Microscopically the changes are mainly in the glomeruli. The glomeruli are swollen and distend Bowman's capsule. There is a sharp increase in the number of cells within the glomerular tuft, and because of this stuffing of capillary channels with swollen cells and inflammatory cells, few red blood cells are seen. The individual glomerular tuft lobules often are club shaped because of the ballooning of the tuft (Figs. 19-5 and 19-6). Electron microscopy and immunofluorescence microscopy show "humps" of immune complex deposit between the basement membrane and podocytes (Figs. 19-7 and 19-8).

The increased cellularity is caused by proliferation of mesangial and endothelial cells and the infiltration of the tuft by neutrophils and monocytes. When there are many neutrophils in most of the glomeruli, the disease is called *acute exudative glomerulonephritis*, whereas when the cellularity is predominantly caused by mesangial cells, endothelial cells, and monocytes,[14] the term *acute proliferative glomerulonephritis* is used. When damage is more serious, rupture and thrombosis of capillaries may occur with pronounced red cell leakage and fibrin clot formation in Bowman's space. A proliferation of Bowman's capsular cells in this exudate may result in a loose epithelial crescent partially or completely filling

Bowman's space. Such a condition is called acute necrotizing glomerulonephritis. The severity of the clinical picture and the eventual outcome correlate well with the degree of glomerular inflammation and destruction as seen in renal biopsy. Whereas acute exudative or proliferative lesions may resolve with only a minor increase in mesangial thickening and cellularity, acute necrotizing lesions may be irreversible.

Acute nonstreptococcal glomerulonephritis. About one third of the cases of acute diffuse glomerulonephritis are apparently not of hemolytic streptococcal origin. Pneumococcal infections, viral infections, bacterial endocarditis, and similar infections have been associated with acute diffuse glomerulonephritis in some cases, whereas other cases have no evidence of a preceding infection. It appears that the outlook of nonstreptococcal glomerulonephritis may not be as good as in the poststreptococcal variety.

Rapidly progressive glomerulonephritis.[73] A few patients have acute nephritis that manifests continuous active progression, with death from renal failure occurring within 3 to 12 months. Other patients may have the same progressive lesions without a clinically manifest acute stage. Evidence of streptococcal origin usually is absent. At autopsy the kidneys are characteristically enlarged, pale, and soft; this was referred to in older literature as large white kidney. There may be some irregularity of the surface of the kidney and some adherence of the capsule. The cut surface of the thick cortex is pale.

Microscopically fairly uniform involvement of all glomeruli is seen. Capsular epithelial proliferation admixed with monocytes results in the formation of capsular crescents (Fig. 19-9) and deposition of fibrin (Fig. 19-10). The fibrin may cause the capsular epithelial proliferation.[86] Adhesions of glomerular tufts to the capsule and obliteration of Bowman's space are common. Scarring of the glomerular tufts is striking, with few patent capillaries remaining. Tubular atrophy is diffuse and of a moderate to severe degree. Interstitial edema and fibrosis often are striking. Many tubules contain casts. Arteries show little evidence of change.

Because glomerular lesions resembling crescentic glomerulonephritis may be seen with systemic arteritis, membranoproliferative glomerulonephritis, and Goodpasture's syndrome, the correct diagnosis is reached only when all factors are considered.[79] In Goodpasture's syndrome, acute necrotizing or rapidly progressive glomerulonephritis is associated with pulmonary hemorrhage and pulmonary hemosiderosis. In some cases in young adults, men particularly, hemoptysis is the initial symptom with the glomerulonephritic symptoms appearing later. The disease progresses rapidly, with death occurring from renal failure in weeks to a few months. At death the kidneys grossly and microscopically usually resemble those of rapidly progressive glomerulonephritis. The lungs show alveolar hemorrhage, hemosiderin-filled macrophages, and thickening of the alveolar walls. Immunologic studies indicate that the glomerular lesion is caused by anti–glomerular basement membrane antibodies. It is probable that cross-reaction of these antibodies with lung basement membrane causes the pulmonary hemorrhages.

Chronic progressive glomerulonephritis. Chronic progressive glomerulonephritis is characterized by smoldering activity over a period of years. Proteinuria and microscopic hematuria may be the only signs for a long time. Some cases occur after a clinical attack of acute glomerulonephritis, but most appear insidiously with no preceding history of renal problems. In some patients, early or late in the disease, such severe proteinuria occurs that hypoproteinemia and a nephrotic syndrome develop. As the scarring progresses in the kidneys, hypertension is often seen. Renal failure slowly develops as the number of functioning nephrons is depleted.

Renal biopsy during the smoldering active phase of the disease shows two types of reaction, a chronic proliferative pattern in which most glomeruli show at least some degree of scarring or the focal pattern in which normal glomeruli are associated with scattered glomeruli in various stages of scarring (Fig. 19-11). Tubular atrophy, interstitial fibrosis, and arteriosclerosis increase with the degree of glomerular involvement and loss. Two special variations of chronic progressive glomerulonephritis— nephrotic syndrome with focal segmental glomerular

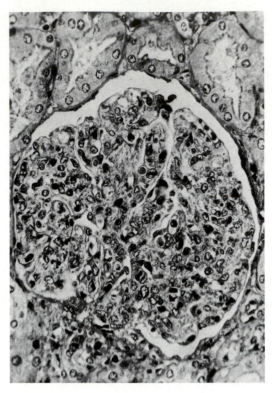

Fig. 19-5. Acute poststreptococcal glomerulonephritis. Swollen, hypercellular glomerular lobules with few open capillaries. (250×.)

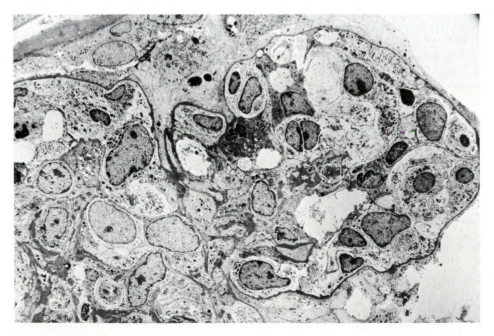

Fig. 19-6. Acute poststreptococcal glomerulonephritis. Electron micrograph showing swollen, hypercellular glomerular lobules. (1600×.)

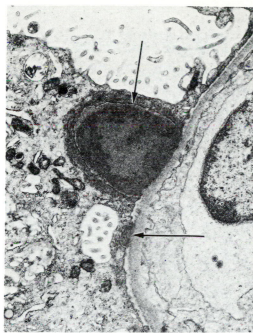

Fig. 19-7. Acute poststreptococcal glomerulonephritis. "Humps" of immune complex outside basement membrane are indicated by arrows. (6000×.)

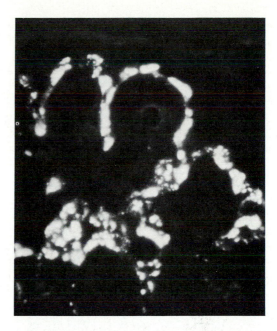

Fig. 19-8. Acute poststreptococcal glomerulonephritis. "Humps" of immune complex stained with fluorescent antihuman complement (C3). (1000×; courtesy Dr. Claude Cornwall, Syracuse, N.Y.)

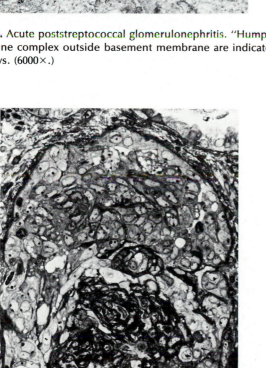

Fig. 19-9. Rapidly progressive glomerulonephritis, antiglomerular basement membrane type. Note crescent of epithelial cells encircling compressed glomerular tuft.

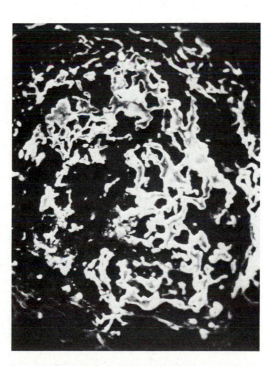

Fig. 19-10. Rapidly progressive glomerulonephritis stained with fluorescent antihuman fibrin. Both tuft and crescent contain fibrin. (Courtesy Dr. Claude Cornwall, Syracuse, N.Y.)

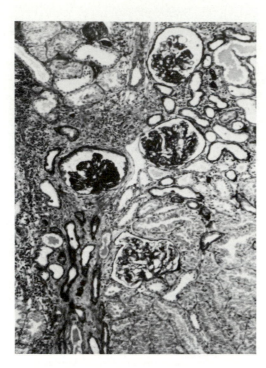

Fig. 19-11. Chronic progressive glomerulonephritis. Note glomeruli in various stages of scarring and patchy tubular atrophy.

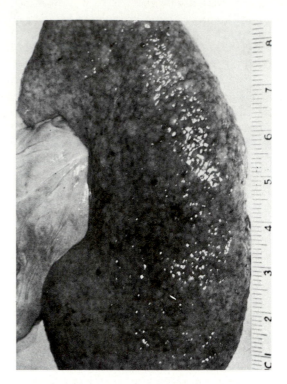

Fig. 19-12. End-stage chronic glomerulonephritis. Pebbly surface corresponds to surviving hypertrophied nephrons amid atrophy.

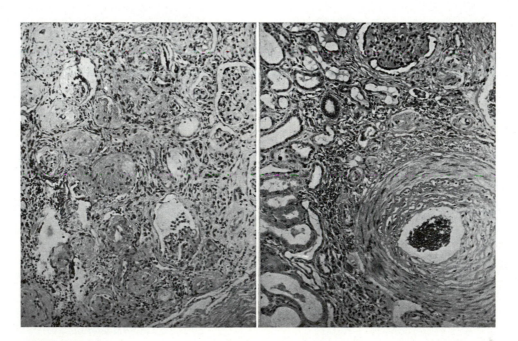

Fig. 19-13. Chronic glomerulonephritis. Note glomerular capsular adhesions and hyalinization and thickening of blood vessels.

sclerosis and membranoproliferative glomerulonephritis—are discussed with the nephrotic syndrome.

End-stage chronic glomerulonephritis.[32] A small, contracted, scarred kidney appears to be the final common pathway of a group of glomerular diseases. It is difficult in this late stage to recognize the nature of the preceding process because of the extensive scarring. Such a kidney may be formed from the progression of acute glomerulonephritis, poststreptococcal or nonstreptococcal rapidly progressive glomerulonephritis, hereditary nephritis, lipoid nephrosis, membranous glomerulonephritis, and focal glomerulonephritis. A large group is first recognized in terminal renal failure with no antecedent history. Clinically, end-stage chronic glomerulonephritis is characterized by hypertension and all the features of chronic renal failure.

Pathologic anatomy. At the end stage the kidneys are small and firm with a granular, pebbly surface to which the renal capsule is adherent (Fig. 19-12). The renal cortices are irregularly thinned and scarred with loss of normal architectural markings. Microscopically the majority of the glomeruli are the site of intense scarring and hyalinization (Fig. 19-13). Many old glomerular scars have been resorbed so that the number of glomeruli is decreased. Tubular atrophy is pronounced, with irregular dilated tubules interspersed with small shrunken tubules. There is a high degree of interstitial fibrosis, and a mild infiltrate of lymphocytes and histiocytes often is

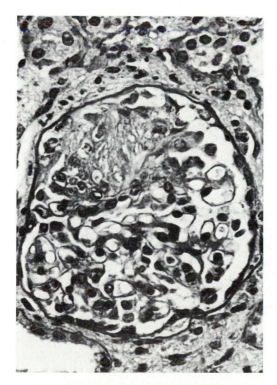

Fig. 19-14. Focal glomerulonephritis with focal crescent and scarring.

seen in the stroma. A few less severely damaged nephrons remain with enlarged, partially scarred glomeruli and hypertrophied tubules. Medium-sized and small arteries commonly show pronounced intimal and medial proliferation. This hyperplastic arteriosclerosis is partly a reaction to the obliterated renal vascular bed and partly from the hypertension that is usually present. In some cases in which the hypertension has become severe there may be evidence of fibrinoid necrosis and hemorrhage in the vessel walls.

Focal glomerulonephritis

Focal glomerulonephritis is the pathologic name applied to a process that involves some glomeruli and spares others. If the diseased glomeruli are totally involved, the process is called global; if only parts of the glomeruli are involved, it is called segmental. The pattern of partial involvement of glomeruli may be an expression of systemic diseases as well as diseases affecting only the kidney.

Focal glomerulonephritis with systemic bacterial infection. For many years physicians have recognized that patients may have hematuria and proteinuria during the height of bacterial infections. When death occurs at this time, some glomeruli show hypercellularity, focal necrosis, thrombosis of glomerular lobules, or even focal capsular epithelial proliferation, producing epithelial crescents or adhesions (Fig. 19-14). Since this involves only a small proportion of glomeruli, it is not surprising that survivors generally show no abnormalities of renal function. The term *glomerulitis* has been used by some for such changes.

A striking lesion of this type known as focal embolic glomerulonephritis is seen in patients with subacute bacterial endocarditis. Of patients having endocarditis for at least 6 weeks, approximately two thirds develop thrombonecrosis of individual glomerular lobules with leakage of red cells from ruptured capillaries into Bowman's space and down the tubules, producing hematuria. A small epithelial crescent often develops at the site of this necrotic lobule. Red blood cells in the proximal and the distal convoluted tubules, leaking from a damaged glomerulus, produce small reddish spots on the capsular or cut surface. This produces the so-called flea-bitten kidney of subacute bacterial endocarditis. In patients whose endocarditis is of longer duration, scarring of the glomerular lobule and adjacent crescent is seen, the so-called fibrous lesion.

The term *focal embolic glomerulonephritis* implies that the necroses are the result of small emboli from the valvular vegetations. Although microemboli might produce such a lesion, bacteria rarely are seen in the lesions, and the disease may occur with valvular lesions of the right side of the heart.

Immunofluorescence and electron microscopy study

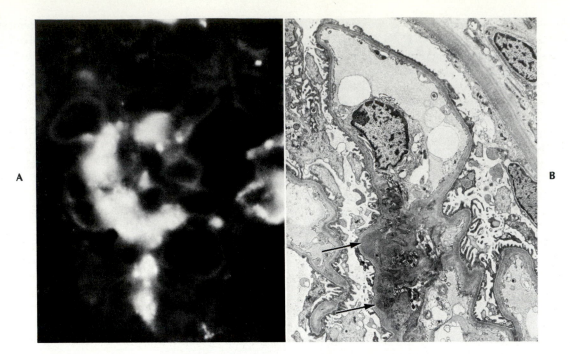

Fig. 19-15. Berger's IgA focal glomerulonephritis. **A,** Stained fluorescent with antihuman IgA. IgA is limited to mesangium. **B,** Deposits in mesangium *(arrows)*. (**A,** Courtesy Dr. Claude Cornwall, Syracuse, N.Y.; **B,** 3000×.)

of renal specimens from patients with bacterial endocarditis has revealed immune complex deposits in the glomerular lesions, indicating that bacterial antigenemia is the cause of the disease.[27]

Focal glomerulonephritis of probable immunologic origin other than systemic infection. Immunologic glomerular injury may be focal as well as diffuse. Such injuries may be divided clinically into recurrent hematuria (IgA focal glomerulonephritis) and glomerular injury as part of systemic immune complex diseases, discussed under systemic lupus erythematosus, polyarteritis nodosa, and Schönlein-Henoch purpura (anaphylactoid purpura).[16]

IgA focal glomerulonephritis. Certain patients with recurrent hematuria or proteinuria on renal biopsy have a few glomeruli with focal hypercellularity, thrombonecrosis, or scarring of glomerular lobules.

Immunofluorescence and electron microscopy demonstrate prominent immunoglobulin deposits of IgA and traces of IgG in the mesangium of these glomeruli (Fig. 19-15).[12] The majority of such patients recover with no clinical residua. In a few patients the nephrons are progressively destroyed until chronic renal failure develops, and they become part of the large group of end-stage chronic glomerulonephritis cases.

Hereditary nephritis (Alport's syndrome). A hereditary form of chronic renal disease has been studied in many families. Often associated with nerve deafness, it affects males more seriously, and few live beyond 30 years of age. Recurrent hematuria is the usual initial symptom. The renal changes seen are those of a progressive focal chronic glomerulonephritis. A prominent microscopic feature is the occurrence of foam cells in the renal cortex, sometimes in large collections. The glomerular basement membranes under electron microscopy show peculiar laminations or splitting and many small dense granules. Immunoglobulin deposits are absent.

Nephrotic syndrome

A group of diseases involving the kidney, although dissimilar in pathogenesis and many clinical features, has in common the clinical findings of massive proteinuria, hypoproteinemia, edema or anasarca, hyperlipemia, and lipiduria.

The basic underlying process appears to be excessive glomerular tuft permeability resulting in the massive proteinuria, with other changes occurring after the severe depletion of the plasma protein pool. Although the exact mechanism of hyperlipidemia is not known, most investigators believe that the liver stressed by the need for massive synthesis of plasma protein in response to urinary loss also overproduces these lipids. The low plasma albumin level results in a fall in plasma volume because of the loss of its osmotic effect. This leads to increased aldosterone release with conservation of sodium and water, resulting in edema formation. Facial edema is common, and ascites and hydrothorax often are present. The urinary sediment contains many hyaline and granular casts and casts containing highly refractile birefringent lipid droplets. The prognosis of a patient with the nephrotic syndrome is determined by the nature of the underlying disease.

A few of the important causes of the nephrotic syndrome are as follows:

1. Immune complex, autoantibody, or hypersensitivity disease
    a. Chronic progressive glomerulonephritis
    b. Lipoid nephrosis, minimal change disease
    c. Focal segmental glomerular sclerosis
    d. Idiopathic membranous glomerulonephritis (membranous nephropathy)
    e. Membranoproliferative glomerulonephritis
    f. Systemic immune complex disease (systemic lupus erythematosus)
    g. Immune complex disease from systemic infection (syphilis, malaria)
    h. Hypersensitivity reaction (bee sting, snake bite, heavy metal compounds such as mercury or gold, drugs such as trimethadione)
2. Circulatory diseases (bilateral renal vein thrombosis, constrictive pericarditis)
3. Metabolic diseases (diabetic glomerulosclerosis, amyloidosis)
4. Pregnancy (toxemia of pregnancy)
5. Hereditary (congenital nephrotic syndrome)

Lipoid nephrosis

In the past the term *lipoid nephrosis* included two entities: minimal change disease (nil disease, or foot-process disease) and focal glomerular sclerosis. Minimal change disease is a major cause of the nephrotic syndrome. It is a disease primarily of small children (1 to 3 years of age) but may occur in older children and occasionally in adults. Clinically it is characterized by the insidious onset of a gross nephrotic syndrome without significant hypertension, hematuria, or azotemia, except late in the course in patients with unremitting disease. Remissions and exacerbations of the nephrotic syndrome are common in this disease with or without treatment. Renal biopsy specimens studied with the light microscope characteristically reveal normal or near-normal glomeruli. Many studies have failed to show deposits of immunoglobulins or complement in these glomeruli, and the etiology remains obscure. Electron microscopy shows no abnormality of glomerular basement membranes of mesangium and no immune deposits. The foot processes of the glomerular epithelial cells or podocytes show flattening, loss of filtration slit pores, and development of tight junctions between adjacent epithelial cell processes (Fig. 19-16).[29]

Scanning electron microscopic studies of human minimal change disease and experimental nephrotic syndrome induced by aminonucleoside have shown that the

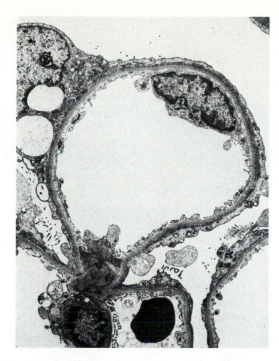

Fig. 19-16. Lipoid nephrosis (minimal change disease). Note foot-process flattening. (4000×.)

flattening of foot processes results from rounding up of the injured epithelial cells and thus diminished interdigitation with the processes of adjacent podocytes (Fig. 19-17).[6,35] This interpretation of the apparent loss of foot processes rather than so-called fusion explains the reversibility to normal foot processes with clinical remission. With incomplete remission, in which mild proteinuria persists, areas of foot-process flattening may persist. The tubular epithelium may show hyaline droplets as evidence of proteinuria and fatty droplets as evidence of hyperlipemia and lipiduria. This lipid probably produces the pale yellow renal cortex seen at autopsy. The kidneys usually are enlarged or of normal size.

In the preantibiotic era, death from intercurrent bacterial infection was common, so that about 60% of the patients died within 5 years. With antibiotic therapy the mortality at 5 years fell to about 25%. With modern steroid therapy perhaps combined with immunosuppressive drugs, complete remission or control occurs in most cases, and the mortality is less than 10%.

Focal segmental glomerular sclerosis (focal sclerosis)[28]

Until recently nephrotic syndrome with focal segmental glomerular sclerosis was included with minimal change disease in studies of lipoid nephrosis. Focal segmental glomerular sclerosis differs in that, in addition to the diffuse foot-process changes in all the glomeruli, focal sclerosis of glomerular lobules with thick basement membranes, adhesions, and fibrinoid nodules develop

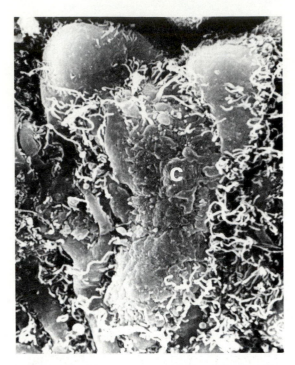

Fig. 19-17. Scanning electron micrograph of glomerular capillary, C, in minimal change disease. Note loss of foot processes and many microvilli. Similar appearance is seen in membranous nephropathy. (1800×.)

first in the juxtamedullary glomeruli and then in others (Fig. 19-18). Early in the course of the disease such lesions may be missed by biopsy, and the erroneous diagnosis of minimal change disease is made. As in minimal change disease, immunofluorescence studies show no immunoglobulin or complement deposits in focal glomerulosclerosis except for nonspecific traces of IgM in old scars.

Focal segmental glomerular sclerosis tends to be resistant to steroid therapy and to progress to renal failure in many cases. The incidence is greater in adults than in children.

Congenital nephrotic syndrome[33]

Congenital nephrotic syndrome is a clinical variant of lipoid nephrosis that is sometimes familial and is characterized by onset of severe nephrotic syndrome within the first few days or weeks of life. Death usually occurs within the first year. Some patients have minimal change disease, whereas others have a peculiar variant that at autopsy shows a characteristic microcystic dilatation of proximal tubules and glomerular scarring.

Membranoproliferative glomerulonephritis (mesangiocapillary glomerulonephritis)[30,36,82]

Membranoproliferative glomerulonephritis is the variant in 10% to 15% of patients with nephrotic syndrome and is most common in the second decade. The glomeruli by light microscopy are large and hypercellular and show distinctive club-shaped glomerular lobules (Fig. 19-19). There is a striking increase in mesangial cells and

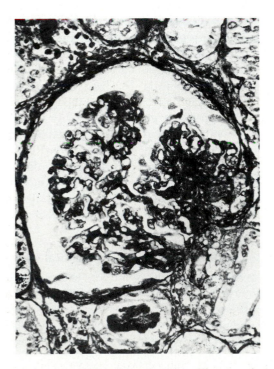

Fig. 19-18. Focal glomerular sclerosis. (Silver methenamine stain.)

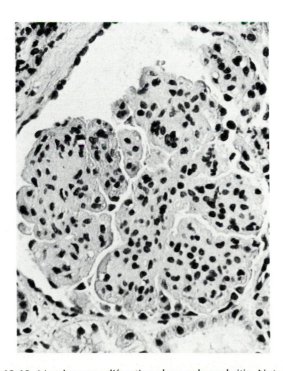

Fig. 19-19. Membranoproliferative glomerulonephritis. Note cellular, swollen lobules.

mesangial basement membrane substance. The glomerular capillary walls are often double contoured from splitting of the basement membrane (Fig. 19-20). Neutrophils are often seen in these tufts during peaks of clinical activity. Electron microscopy and immunofluorescence have revealed that there are two types of this disease. Type I is an immune complex disease with lumpy immunoglobulin deposits in the mesangium and in the capillary walls of the tuft (Figs. 19-21 and 19-22). The splitting of the capillary basement membrane results from the enlarged mesangium extending out to encircle the capillary.[36]

Type II (hypocomplementemic glomerulonephritis) is an alternative pathway disease. Although immunoglobulin deposits are slight or absent, there is a striking deposit of complement in the capillary walls. This complement deposit is associated with peculiar "dense deposits" in the capillary walls (Fig. 19-23).[30] It has been suggested that these dense deposits are remnants of components of the alternative pathway of complement activation (Fig. 19-24). Such patients have very low serum complement levels and often have a circulating anticomplementary gamma globulin, C3NeF (nephritic factor).[62,75]

These two types of membranoproliferative glomerulonephritis may be indistinguishable clinically except for serum complement levels. In acute exacerbations of disease the clinical picture of membranoproliferative glomerulonephritis may resemble acute diffuse glomerulonephritis. The nephrotic syndrome is resistant to steroid therapy, and the disease tends to progress to renal failure in a few months or years.

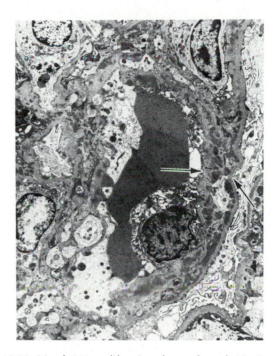

Fig. 19-21. Membranoproliferative glomerulonephritis, immune complex type. Note double layer of basement membrane *(arrows)* and immune complex deposits. (3000×.)

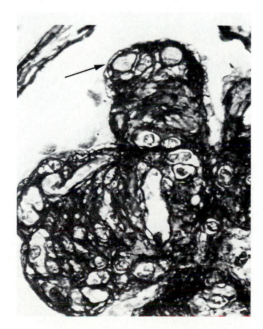

Fig. 19-20. Membranoproliferative glomerulonephritis. Note duplication of capillary basement membrane *(arrow).* (Silver methenamine stain.)

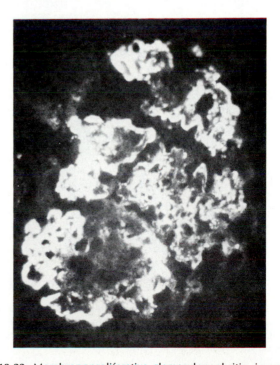

Fig. 19-22. Membranoproliferative glomerulonephritis, immune complex type, stained with fluorescent antihuman complement (C3). (Courtesy Dr. Claude Cornwall, Syracuse, N.Y.)

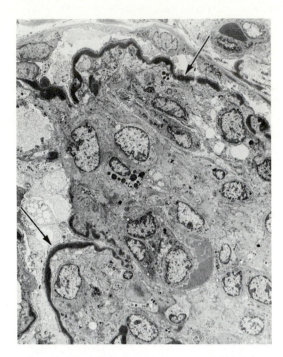

Fig. 19-23. Membranoproliferative glomerulonephritis, dense deposit type. Note dense linear deposits about periphery of lobules *(arrows).* (3000×.)

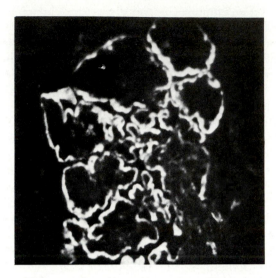

Fig. 19-24. Membranoproliferative glomerulonephritis, dense deposit type, stained with fluorescent antihuman complement (C3). (Courtesy Dr. Claude Cornwall, Syracuse, N.Y.)

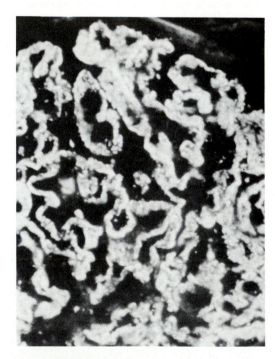

Fig. 19-25. Idiopathic membranous nephropathy, an immune complex disease, showing lumpy staining of glomerular immune complex deposits with fluorescent antihuman IgG. (Courtesy Dr. Claude Cornwall, Syracuse, N.Y.)

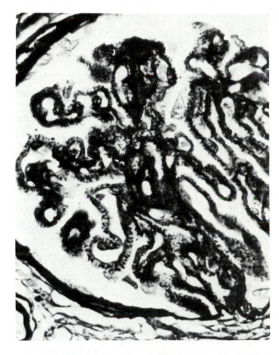

Fig. 19-26. Membranous nephropathy. Note spikes of basement membrane between deposits. (Silver methenamine stain.)

Stife and co-workers[82] have described a variant of this lesion in which there are massive deposits disrupting the glomerular basement membranes, so-called type III membranoproliferative glomerulonephritis.

Idiopathic membranous glomerulonephritis[72]

Idiopathic membranous glomerulonephritis (membranous nephropathy) is the most important cause of nephrotic syndrome in adults, although occasional cases occur in children. The disease is characterized by insidious onset of proteinuria and the nephrotic syndrome. This lesion has a common association with cancer.[21] The process tends to have a long course not greatly modified by steroid therapy. Even with clinical improvement there may be little morphologic change in the glomerular lesions. This disease may progress to pronounced glomerular scarring, tubular atrophy, and uremia after a period of years. Immunologic and structural evidence indicates that this is an immune complex disease (Fig. 19-25).[66,72]

Grossly the kidneys may be of normal size or slightly enlarged early in the disease but somewhat shrunken and granular in the late stages. The yellowish cast of the cut surface is attributed to lipid in the tubules. Light microscopy reveals normal glomeruli in early lesions, but later a uniform thickening of the capillary basement membrane is seen. With the periodic acid–silver methenamine stain, thin clublike projections of the basement membrane may be seen extending out between minute, beadlike, hyaline droplets (Fig. 19-26). These droplets

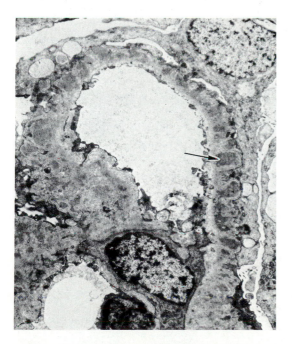

Fig. 19-27. Membranous nephropathy. *Arrow,* Nodular deposits in outer part of thickened basement membrane. (6000×.)

are shown to be immunoglobulin deposits by immunofluorescence. Electron microscopy even in early lesions reveals nodular protein deposits outside the basement membrane under the flattened podocytic foot processes (see Fig. 19-17). As the disease progresses, the basement membrane thickens, and clublike processes of new basement membrane form between the protein deposits (Fig. 19-27). In advanced stages of the disease, basement membranes, including the deposits, may become five to 10 times the usual thickness. The mesangium shows very little involvement in this disease.

Systemic lupus erythematosus

The immunologic disorder systemic lupus erythematosus (SLE) involves the kidney mildly to severely in 60% to 70% of cases. The renal glomeruli are the prime sites of injury from this disease, apparently as the result of the deposition of immune complexes, particularly between the endothelium and the glomerular basement membrane and in the mesangium. Examination of the urine reveals proteinuria, hematuria, oval fat bodies, and casts. The nephrotic syndrome develops in 20% to 30% of the patients, and the prognosis in this group is unusually poor. Renal biopsy may reveal normal kidney, moderate mesangial lesions (mesangitis), focal glomerulitis, diffuse lupus glomerulonephritis, or a membranous lesion similar to idiopathic membranous nephropathy.[5,53]

The characteristic glomerular lesions of SLE include irregular hypercellularity of glomerular lobules associated with "fibrinoid" necrosis and nuclear karyorrhexis. The fibrinoid immune complex material is deposited as a thick coat in the mesangium and inside the glomerular basement membranes. This produces thick-walled capillary loops, the so-called wire loop lesion (Figs. 19-28 and 19-29).

Electron microscopy in the characteristic case shows clearly the deposits of electron-dense protein between the endothelium and the lamina densa of the basement membrane. The deposits also accumulate in the mesangium adjacent to the basement membrane (Fig. 19-30). In reaction to this inflammation, epithelial crescents, adhesions to Bowman's capsule, and glomerular scarring occur. Occasional hyaline thrombi are seen in glomerular capillary lumina. Fuzzy basophilic aggregates of nuclear material (hematoxylin bodies) occasionally may be seen in zones of necrosis. In severe cases a lymphoid and plasma cell intertubular infiltrate is present.

Those cases having a membranous pattern by light microscopy (uniform, thick basement membranes) appear to be similar to idiopathic membranous nephropathy by electron microscopy.

The prognosis is the poorest in diffuse lupus glomerulonephritis, but aggressive steroid therapy may be lifesaving. The uncommon membranous pattern of lupus nephritis runs a protracted course similar to that of membranous nephropathy. Focal lupus glomerulitis seldom results in progressive destruction of renal function.

Systemic infection or hypersensitivity reactions

In general, the outlook of patients with nephrosis resulting from infection or hypersensitivity reactions is better than that of patients with the nephrotic syndrome

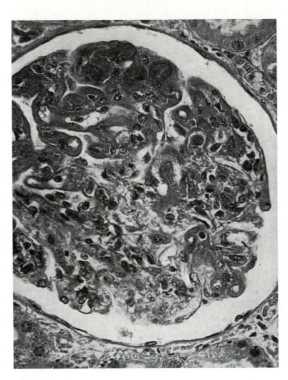

Fig. 19-28. Diffuse lupus glomerulonephritis with "wire loop" lesions and immune deposits.

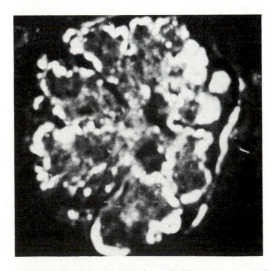

Fig. 19-29. Diffuse lupus glomerulonephritis stained with fluorescent antihuman IgG. Note coarse loops and lumps of deposits. (Courtesy Dr. Claude Cornwall, Syracuse, N.Y.)

of other causes if the underlying cause is properly treated (treatment of syphilis, cessation of offending drug therapy, and so on). Electron microscopy may reveal immune complex deposits of a membranous type as in syphilis or even foot-process changes as in lipoid nephrosis.

Circulatory disturbances

Proteinuria of a mild degree is common in congestive heart failure. In certain severe forms of heart failure, such as occur in constrictive pericarditis, a frank nephrotic syndrome may result. Bilateral renal vein thrombosis in adults may be associated with the nephrotic syndrome. Renal biopsy usually reveals membranous nephropathy but may demonstrate amyloidosis. Studies suggest that the thrombosis is the result rather than the cause of the renal disease.[85]

In infants, acute renal vein thrombosis may occur as a complication of severe gastroenteritis and may result in hemorrhagic renal infarction.[56]

Amyloidosis[25]

The kidney is the site of amyloid deposit in most cases of secondary amyloidosis and about a third of the cases of primary amyloidosis. The glomeruli are the most important deposit site, but amyloid may be found in arterial walls and surrounding the tubules and the vasa recta of the medulla. Glomerular amyloidosis results in proteinuria and, in some cases, nephrotic syndrome. Chronic renal failure develops in advanced cases. The kidneys usually are enlarged, pale, and firm. Microscopically the

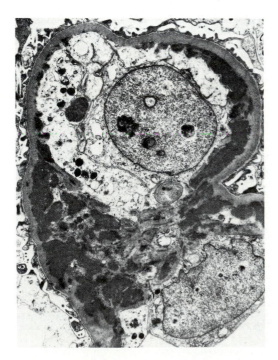

Fig. 19-30. Systemic lupus erythematosus with subendothelial and mesangial deposits. (6000×.)

glomeruli show irregular capillary wall thickening and distension of the mesangium with an eosinophilic homogeneous deposit. Capillary lumina are narrowed. In advanced lesions the entire capillary bed of the tuft is obliterated by massive deposits. The diagnosis of amyloidosis may be confirmed by special stains (crystal violet, Congo red, and polarized light or thioflavin T and ultraviolet microscopy) or by electron microscopy. The electron microscope reveals the amyloid deposits to be composed of masses of fibrils 80 to 100 Å wide. Such fibrillary deposits are seen inside and outside the capillary basement membrane and in the mesangium (Figs. 19-31 and 19-32).

Toxemia of pregnancy (preeclampsia and eclampsia)

In the third trimester of pregnancy, often the first pregnancy, proteinuria, edema, and hypertension may develop. This is called preeclampsia. If the condition becomes more severe with decreased renal function, convulsions, and perhaps death, it is called eclampsia. Women whose mothers had toxemia have a high risk of the condition. This syndrome may be simulated by essential hypertension or chronic glomerulonephritis or other chronic renal disease.

In true toxemia of pregnancy the glomeruli are the main site of involvement. By light microscopy the glomeruli are revealed to be swollen without increased cellularity but are relatively bloodless because of narrowed or collapsed capillary channels. The mesangium is swollen, and the capillary walls often appear thickened as a result of deposition of a thin layer of pink fibrinoid material and also as a result of endothelial cell swelling. Elec-

tron microscopy reveals hydropic swellings of endothelial and mesangial cell cytoplasm and also electron-dense protein deposits between the endothelium and glomerular basement membrane and in the mesangium (Fig. 19-33).[67] Fluorescent antibody studies have shown that the glomerular protein deposits are predominantly fibrin.[87] It appears that circulating partially polymerized fibrinogen is present as a result of activation of the clotting

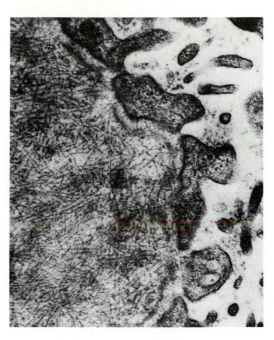

Fig. 19-32. Amyloid filaments with foot processes covering them. (40,000×.)

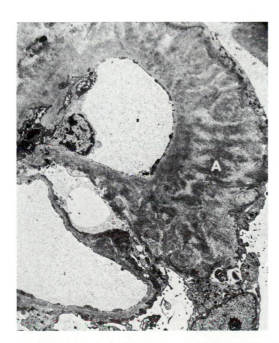

Fig. 19-31. Amyloidosis. Capillary wall thickened by amyloid filaments, A. (3400×.)

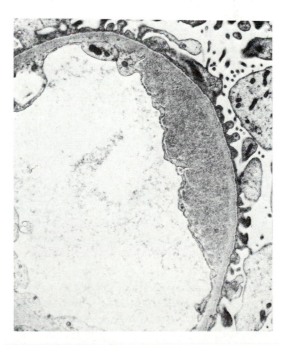

Fig. 19-33. Toxemia of pregnancy. Fibrin between endothelium and basement membrane of glomerular capillary. (7000×.)

mechanism and is trapped in the glomerulus. This apparently leads to the increased glomerular permeability and proteinuria. The tubular changes seen in toxemia of pregnancy (hyaline droplets, fatty droplets, and cloudy swelling) are believed to be the result of glomerular disease.

After delivery of the baby, a remarkable resolution of glomerular morphology to normal may be expected, and urinary findings return to normal.[67] Hypertension occurs after toxemia of pregnancy in 40% to 50% of patients. It is not clear whether toxemia causes this hypertension or merely hastens its onset.

Vascular renal disease

The enormous renal blood flow and the contribution of the kidney to the homeostasis and pathophysiology of the circulation of the blood make renal vascular disease of utmost importance. This renal blood flow is modulated by systemic and local hydrodynamic and hormonal factors and incompletely understood intrinsic intrarenal control. In disease these flow control mechanisms are modified and may contribute to renal dysfunction and damage, such as arterial hypertension, shock, and vascular obstruction.

Hypertensive vascular disease

Hypertension is the most common serious chronic disease, affecting about half the population over 60 years of age. Arterial hypertension is defined clinically as borderline when it reaches 140/90 mm Hg and hypertensive when 165/95 mm Hg. Elevation of systolic pressure alone (systolic hypertension) or elevation of both systolic and diastolic pressure (diastolic hypertension) both have an increased risk of serious complications, but diastolic hypertension is more dangerous.[40,41] The arterial changes and vascular complications increase with the severity and duration of the hypertension but are modified by genetic factors, environmental factors, sex (females tolerate hypertension better), and associated diseases (diabetes mellitus).

The increased peripheral resistance resulting in sustained hypertension may arise from (1) increased sympathetic tone, (2) increased release of renin and generation of angiotensin II, (3) the presence of vasoconstrictive substances in the circulation, (4) increased sodium load and extracellular fluid load, and finally (5) a postulated excessive responsiveness to the other factors. In a given individual hypertension may be attributable to a combination of these factors.

Role of renin.[64] It is now generally believed that the juxtaglomerular cells at the hilum of the glomerulus synthesize renin. These cells release renin when stimulated by baroreceptors in the afferent arteriole, by sympathetic nervous system stimulation, or on detection of changes of sodium or other electrolyte levels in the distal tubule.

Released renin hydrolyzes plasma renin substrate into angiotensin I. Convertase in the lung causes conversion of angiotensin I to the potent octapeptide, angiotensin II, which both causes arteriolar smooth muscle contraction and triggers the release of aldosterone, in turn facilitating renal sodium conservation. This physiologic homeostatic mechanism may be disrupted in pathologic states. The juxtaglomerular apparatus may misinterpret chronic renal cortical ischemia as inadequate blood volume. This results in increased renin release and increased sodium load. In severe cases hyperplasia of juxtaglomerular cells (see Fig. 19-37) and an excessive release of renin occur, and hyperrenin hypertension results.

Essential hypertension—nature and pathogenesis. Essential hypertension comprises about 90% of hypertensive individuals. Although the cause of essential hypertension is unknown, a number of factors are related to its development. Genetic factors are indicated by a strong family history of essential hypertension and the inordinately high incidence in the black population, about double that of the white population. The absence of any sharp separation between normal, mild hypertension and severe hypertension suggests that a mosaic of factors causes hypertension, including electrolyte control, nervous system reactivity, arterial reactivity, vasoactive chemical substances, and other environmental factors. The inability of patients with essential hypertension to handle sodium properly is believed to be an important factor, since populations with a high salt dietary intake have more hypertension. Tobian and Binion[84] have shown that chemical analyses of the arterial wall of patients with essential hypertension show an increased sodium content. Also, control of sodium intake and output is one of the most effective ways of treating essential hypertension. It appears that cerebrocortical and sympathetic excessive stimulation contributes to the peripheral resistance, and modern treatment of hypertension combines sedation and autonomic blockade. Direct attack on the hyperreactivity of vascular smooth muscle is an aim of pharmacologic therapy. Unlike secondary hypertension there is usually no elevation of renin or angiotensin in essential hypertension. It is only when malignant hypertension supervenes that renin and angiotensin levels rise.

Secondary hypertension. Following is the classification of secondary hypertension with examples:
1. Central nervous system disease (increased intracranial pressure, neoplasms)
2. Cardiovascular disease (coarctation of the aorta, severe atherosclerosis)
3. Endocrine disease (adrenocortical hyperplasia or neoplasms, pheochromocytoma)
4. Toxemia of pregnancy
5. Drugs (oral contraceptives, methamphetamine abuse)

6. Renal arterial stenosis (atherosclerosis, renal artery fibromuscular dysplasias, thromboembolism or thrombosis, atheromatous embolism, dissecting aneurysm)

7. Parenchymatous renal disease (bilateral—chronic glomerulonephritis, polycystic kidneys, chronic pyelonephritis; unilateral—chronic pyelonephritis, renal tumors, hydronephrosis)

Hypertension is generally induced in central nervous system disease by a rise in sympathetic tone or endocrine stress stimulation. Both coarctation of the aorta and severe atherosclerosis generate hypertension by sympathetic vasoconstriction and the stimulation of the renin system. Endocrine hypertension results either from the release of vasoconstrictive catecholamines of a pheochromocytoma or from the sodium load expansion induced by adrenal corticosteroids.

Toxemia of pregnancy hypertension is believed to be induced by placental production of a vasoactive substance. In addition, there is often an increased sodium load. Oral contraceptives in susceptible women result in increased levels of renin substrate and hypertension, which are reversed on cessation of the medication.

Renal arterial obstruction when exceeding 50% results in decreased renal blood flow. When obstruction is severe, there is striking activation of the renin-angiotensin system, and juxtaglomerular hyperplasia and hypertension from excessive renin may result. Important causes of renal artery stenosis producing hypertension are atheroma near the renal artery ostia and thromboemboli of the renal artery or main branches. Atheromatous emboli produce ischemia and hypertension, but the obstructions are in small intrarenal arteries.[38] Fibromuscular dysplasia causing stenosis of renal arteries may lead to severe hypertension in children or young women. Surgery repairing these congenital dysplasias or acquired arterial stenosis may be curative.[31]

Many chronic parenchymatous renal diseases may result in hypertension—chronic glomerulonephritis, chronic pyelonephritis, polycystic kidneys, radiation nephritis, diabetic nephropathy, or hydronephrosis. When unilateral disease is present, as in hydronephrosis, nephrectomy may be curative. The mechanisms of hypertension induction by parenchymal disease are sodium and water load increase attributable to chronic renal failure and in some cases to renin and aldosterone. In many cases of chronic renal disease there is an endarterial intimal proliferation caused by so-called endarteritis obliterans induced by a shrunken vascular bed in the scarred kidney and intimal hyperplasia induced by hypertension. This may exaggerate the hypertension and even induce malignant hypertension.

Malignant hypertension is severe diastolic hypertension (for example, 230/150), which results in vascular injury, necrotizing arteriolitis, papilledema, hypertensive encephalopathy, cardiac decompensation, and rapidly progressive renal failure.

Complications of hypertension. Even though the kidney is adversely affected in hypertension, developing arteriolar nephrosclerosis, it is uncommon for a patient to die of chronic renal failure (less than 5%) except with malignant hypertension. The most common complications are cardiac. Hypertension is accompanied by concentric left ventricular hypertrophy. When the cardiac hypertrophy is extreme, it may progress to failure with dilatation, known as hypertensive myocardiopathy. Hypertension appears to accelerate the progression of atherosclerosis, and coronary atherosclerosis is the major mechanism of death in the hypertensive patient. These deaths include sudden cardiac death syndrome, myocardial infarction, and arteriosclerotic myocardiopathy with failure. Although such deaths occur in nonhypertensive patients, hypertensive patients have an increasing risk of such problems as the level of hypertension rises. Men have about twice the incidence of coronary artery disease of women, but women are still at great risk compared with the normotensive population.[40] Central nervous system vascular disease is a major risk for hypertensive patients, particularly women, with cerebral thrombosis and infarction or cerebral hemorrhage. Hemorrhage arises from rupture of either Charcot-Bouchard microaneurysms of the cerebral arteries (cerebral hemorrhage) or berry aneurysms of the circle of Willis (subarachnoid hemorrhage).[41]

Other complications of hypertension are dissecting aneurysm of the aorta and all the complications of severe atherosclerosis.

Benign nephrosclerosis (arterionephrosclerosis)

Benign nephrosclerosis is the most common form of renal disease and is seen in most persons over 60 years of age. Long-standing moderate arterial hypertension induces arteriosclerotic proliferative and hyaline changes in small muscular branches of the renal arteries and renal arterioles. This results in focal atrophy of tubules and sclerosis of glomeruli. The intervening kidney is relatively uninvolved; thus renal function is usually fairly well maintained. Even when it is severe, benign nephrosclerosis causes chronic renal failure in less than 5% of patients. Mild arteriosclerotic intimal thickening may occur in the elderly without hypertension, but extensive nephrosclerosis is consistently associated with hypertension. Clinical problems of the patient are usually related to hypertensive complications in other organs. The vessels of the human retina mirror the visceral arteriolar changes, and an ophthalmoscopic estimation of the severity of vascular involvement is of great clinical value.

With increasing severity of the nephrosclerosis, mild shrinking of the kidneys results because of a loss of tubular mass. The renal cortex is thinned, and the surface of the kidney develops a punctate scarring resembling grained leather. The fibrosis in the minute foci of ischemic atrophy makes the kidney firmer and slightly paler than normal. Muscular arteries with thickened walls may be seen.

Microscopically the small muscular arteries show intimal thickening because of proliferation of intimal smooth muscle cells, which deposit new elastic fibers, the lamina of basement membrane, and collagen fibrils. Under the light microscope this material has a pink hyaline appearance. Although some intimal thickening occurs with age, it is most striking when associated with hypertension.

Hyaline arteriolar sclerosis is a characteristic lesion of benign nephrosclerosis. A pink, homogeneous protein is deposited in the intima narrowing the lumen. The electron microscope shows this vascular hyaline as a finely granular protein deposit often containing minute lipid inclusions. It is believed to be the result of insudation of plasma proteins into the arteriolar wall where the proteins are denatured into insoluble residues. With more severe hypertension, hypertrophy of the smooth muscle cells and some intimal proliferation of smooth muscle cells occur (Fig. 19-34).[34]

The glomeruli in benign nephrosclerosis may appear normal by light microscopy except for old sclerosed scars in foci of ischemic atrophy. With more severe hypertension, mild thickening of the basement membranes may be seen in most glomeruli, but some show various stages of ischemic wrinkling of capillaries and collagenous scarring (glomerular ischemic obsolescence).

Malignant nephrosclerosis

A vicious complication called malignant or accelerated hypertension develops in about 5% of patients with hypertension of whatever cause. This is characterized by very high systolic and diastolic blood pressure, papilledema, hypertensive encephalopathy, and rapidly developing renal failure (malignant nephrosclerosis). High renin and angiotensin blood levels are present. Life expectancy without adequate treatment is less than 2 years. Only rarely does malignant nephrosclerosis develop anew in a normal kidney. Most commonly malignant hypertension arises in a patient with benign hypertension whose kidneys would show the changes of benign nephrosclerosis. Thus the acute renal changes of malignant nephrosclerosis are superimposed on benign nephrosclerosis. The acute changes in arteries and arterioles[34] are (1) striking intimal proliferation of smooth muscle cells with loose laminae of collagen and basement membrane (onion-skin proliferation) and (2) so-called arteriolar necrosis. The necrotic arterioles show extravasation of red blood cells and proteins through incompetent endothelium into the vessel wall (so-called fibrinoid deposits) and often show thrombosis of the lumen. This

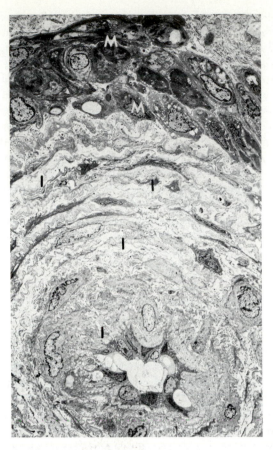

Fig. 19-34. Hyperplastic changes in small artery with hypertension. Hypertrophied medial cells, *M*, "onion-skin" layers of intimal cells and basement membrane, *I*. (1200×.)

process is distinguished from arteritis by the presence of few or no inflammatory cells. Immunofluorescence studies of these lesions show fibrinogen, gamma globulins, complement, and albumin in the fibrinoid (Figs. 19-35 and 19-36). Even though gamma globulin and complement may be seen in these lesions, many believe that this is a passive trapping of these plasma proteins rather than an immunologic process. Glomerular changes in malignant nephrosclerosis combine an exaggeration of the glomerular basement membrane thickening and ischemic wrinkling seen in benign nephrosclerosis. In addition, thrombonecrotic and hemorrhagic lesions develop in some glomeruli, analogous to the arteriolar necrosis. These acute glomerulitic lesions heal with scarring. Hypertrophy of the juxtaglomerular apparatus and hypergranularity of these cells correlate well with the hyperreninism of these patients (Fig. 19-37). With the progression of the obstruction of the vascular bed by arterial and glomerular lesions, tubular atrophy and interstitial fibrosis develop.

The gross appearance of the kidney in malignant nephrosclerosis reflects the processes just described (Fig. 19-38). The kidney is usually somewhat reduced

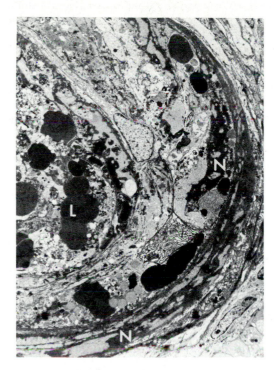

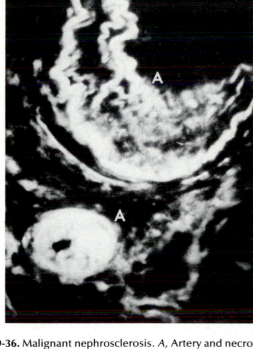

Fig. 19-35. Malignant nephrosclerosis with necrotic arteriole showing laminar insudation of plasma proteins and red cells into necrotic wall, *N*, and cell debris and red cells in lumen, *L*. (2500×.)

Fig. 19-36. Malignant nephrosclerosis. *A*, Artery and necrotic arteriole stained with fluorescent antihuman fibrin. (Courtesy Dr. Claude Cornwall, Syracuse, N.Y.)

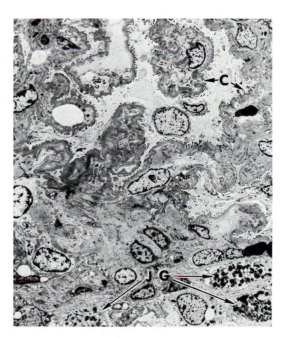

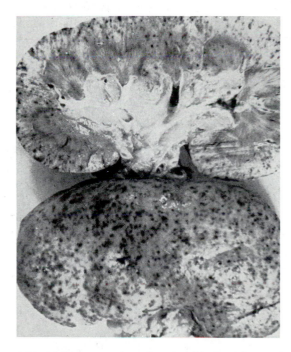

Fig. 19-37. Malignant nephrosclerosis. Thick, wrinkled capillary basement membranes, *C*, and heavily granulated juxtaglomerular cells, *JG*. (1000×.)

Fig. 19-38. Malignant nephrosclerosis with focal hemorrhages caused by thrombonecrosis of arterioles and glomeruli.

in size, has a finely granular cortex with tiny hemorrhages (flea-bitten kidney), and may show tiny cortical infarcts.

When malignant hypertension is superimposed on other diseases such as chronic glomerulonephritis, a composite of the acute hyperplastic and thrombonecrotic lesions is added to the primary disease changes.

Diabetic nephropathy

Nephropathy, a common complication of diabetes, is composed of three entities: severe arteriolar nephrosclerosis, glomerulosclerosis (Kimmelstiel-Wilson disease),[46] and often some acute or chronic pyelonephritis. The most severe form of hyaline arteriolar sclerosis occurs in diabetes mellitus, and a unique hyaline involvement of both afferent and efferent arterioles is often seen. Hypertension accompanies this severe vascular change. In about 25% of diabetics, in addition to nephrosclerosis, a peculiar massive deposition of basement membrane matrix occurs in the mesangium of some or many glomeruli (nodular intercapillary glomerulosclerosis or Kimmelstiel-Wilson disease).[17] This produces a typical globular hyaline ball in the center of a glomerular lobule with the capillaries displaced to the periphery (Fig. 19-39). Mesangial cells are increased but are peripherally displaced by the hyaline matrix. The basement membranes of the glomerular capillaries may be normal or thickened. Bright red deposits of fibrinoid material may block some of these capillaries. More commonly the glomeruli show a diffuse moderate thickening of capillary basement membranes and increased mesangial cells and coarse mesangial matrix (diffuse diabetic glomerulosclerosis).[17] This diffuse process may or may not accompany the nodular form of Kimmelstiel-Wilson disease. The diffuse glomerular change mirrors the vascular basement membrane thickening of many small vessels in the body (diabetic angiopathy). Although the microscopic lesions of diffuse glomerulosclerosis are difficult to differentiate from benign nephrosclerosis when they are well developed with associated severe hyaline arteriolar sclerosis, accurate diagnosis can usually be made. Electron microscopy of renal biopsy specimens reveals diffuse basement membrane thickening of capillaries and mesangium even in diabetes of relatively short duration, although this may not be discernible by light microscopy (Fig. 19-40).[17] Chemical analysis of diabetic glomeruli indicates increased carbohydrate content in the basement membrane. This may explain the increased permeability and proteinuria noted in these patients. Hyaline nodular deposits in Bowman's capsule when present are said to be quite specific for diabetes.[46]

Foci of acute or chronic inflammation from pyelonephritis are common in the diabetic kidney and reflect the continuing problem diabetics have with bacterial infections. Tubular atrophy and interstitial fibrosis parallel

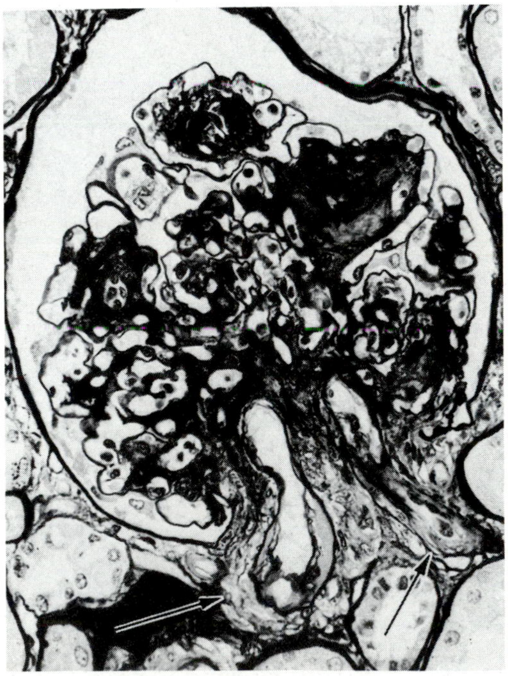

Fig. 19-39. Diabetic glomerulosclerosis. Note nodules in glomerular lobules, basement membrane thickening, and hyaline arteriolar sclerosis involving both afferent and efferent arterioles *(arrows)*. (Silver methenamine stain.)

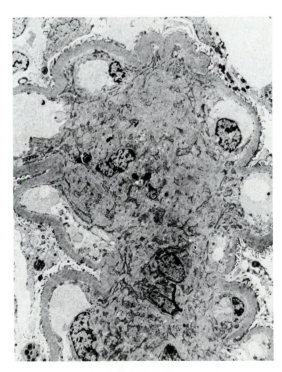

Fig. 19-40. Diabetic glomerulosclerosis. Capillaries with thick basement membranes surrounding mesangium enlarged by thick strands of mesangial matrix. (1300×.)

vascular, glomerular, and pyelonephritic involvement. Necrotizing papillitis in diabetics is discussed on p. 762.

Clinically, proteinuria and hypertension reflect the development of diabetic nephropathy, which may progress slowly resulting in renal or heart failure. In about 5% of diabetics proteinuria is heavy enough to produce a nephrotic syndrome. Renal biopsy typically shows diffuse diabetic glomerulosclerosis in these nephrotic diabetics, correlating with a more diffuse capillary alteration than is seen in the nodular form.

In lethal untreated diabetic coma, extensive glycogen deposits in the loops of Henle (Armani-Ebstein vacuoles) may be the only pathologic clue to the mechanism of death.

Renal infarction

Renal infarctions are common, are often multiple, and usually result from emboli arising from cardiac vegetations or mural thrombi. Less commonly atheromatous emboli from the aorta, usually associated with atheromatous aortic aneurysm, may cause renal infarction, hypertension, and renal failure.[38] Intrinsic renal artery occlusion from dissecting aneurysm, arteritis, or thrombosis also causes infarction. Although the infarcts may cause back pain and hematuria, acute renal failure is seen only with extensive bilateral occlusion and with dissecting aneurysm of the aorta. Ischemic renal tissue adjacent to infarcts may be a source of excessive renin production and hypertension.

Polyarteritis nodosa and Wegener's granulomatosis[22]

The kidneys are affected in 70% to 80% of patients with polyarteritis nodosa, an acute inflammatory disease of arteries, and renal failure is common.

This disorder is divided into a classic form with predominant involvement of larger muscular arteries often producing aneurysms and infarcts and the microscopic form with predominantly small artery and glomerular involvement. Immunofluorescence studies fail to show evidence of immunologic origin in most cases; however, some cases do show immunoglobulin deposits in both arteries and glomeruli. The prognosis of these cases with allergic vasculitis is much better than that with the other types. Hypertension is common with polyarteritis, and renal failure is often the mode of death, particularly in the microscopic form. The effects on the rest of the kidney are similar to malignant nephrosclerosis. The characteristic leukocytic and often eosinophilic infiltrate in the arterial wall distinguishes polyarteritis. The glomeruli may show ischemic wrinkling, focal glomerulitis with necrosis and epithelial crescents, or acute glomerulonephritis with the allergic variety of polyarteritis. Wegener's granulomatosis is closely related to polyarteritis nodosa, with similar arteritis and renal disease, but in addition has necrotizing granulomatous lesions of the nasal passages, nasal sinuses, and lungs.

Thrombotic renal disease

A group of diseases is characterized by fibrin and platelet thrombus formation in arterioles and glomeruli of the kidney causing acute renal failure. These cases may result from initiation of disseminated intravascular coagulation triggered by such things as bacteremia (gram-negative endotoxic shock, gram-positive bacterial sepsis) and accidents of childbirth (abruptio placentae, amniotic fluid embolism, toxemia of pregnancy).[57] Often the renal involvement in these states is overshadowed by other systemic symptomatology. When arterial and capillary fibrinous thrombosis is massive and associated with shock, as in abruptio placentae or endotoxic shock, bilateral renocortical necrosis may develop.[76] Even if the patient survives the primary disease, the renal lesion is usually lethal. Bilateral renocortical necrosis exhibits symmetric infarction of the renal cortex and columns of Bertin and thrombotic occlusion of small arteries adjacent to the infarction.

If vascular obstruction is less extreme, even though there is acute impairment of renal function, permanent loss of renal function is not to be expected. Apparently, most of the thrombi are rapidly lysed and only focal scars result.

Hemolytic uremic syndrome is closely related to the aforementioned diseases. It usually occurs in children but is seen in adults.[24,88] An acute episode of arteriolar and glomerular thrombotic process associated with thrombocytopenia is present, with damage limited to the kidney (Figs. 19-41 and 19-42). Viral infections have been clinically associated with onset of the disease. The thrombi cause acute renal failure; in addition, extensive fragmentation of red blood cells results from blood perfusing the damaged vessels. The fragmented cells hemolyze, and anemia results. Most patients recover, but with severe involvement there may be fatal bilateral cortical necrosis or residual severe damage to arterioles and glomeruli.

Thrombotic thrombocytopenic purpura closely resembles the hemolytic uremic syndrome, but it involves various organs such as the central nervous system and has prolonged or recurrent activity usually ending in death.[58]

Scleroderma renal disease (progressive systemic sclerosis)

About 40% of patients dying of scleroderma show severe renal involvement and renal failure.[11] The striking changes are intimal proliferation of arcuate arteries and afferent arterioles. Severe hypertension may develop with severe renal involvement, contributing to the changes. Acute thrombonecrotic changes in arterioles

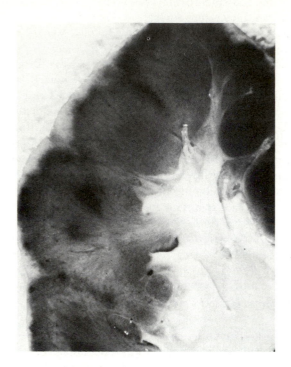

Fig. 19-41. Hemolytic uremic syndrome with cortical necrosis. Note white infarcted outer cortex.

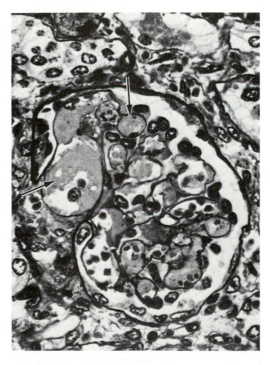

Fig. 19-42. Hemolytic uremic syndrome. Note thrombi in entering arteriole and glomerular capillaries *(arrows).* (Silver methenamine stain.)

and glomeruli closely resemble those in malignant nephrosclerosis but may develop before severe hypertension. Severe interstitial fibrosis and tubular atrophy accompany the vascular involvement.

Radiation nephritis

Treatment of the abdomen with high doses of ionizing radiation may result in renal damage, hypertension, and renal failure after a latent period of 6 to 12 months.[52] Thrombonecrotic (fibrinoid) changes develop in the particularly susceptible glomeruli and in arterioles.[52,60] Tubular atrophy is moderate early in the disease but may become severe. Changes resulting from severe or malignant hypertension may be superimposed.

Tubular disease

The term *nephrosis* is an ambiguous word that, for historical reasons, came to be applied to a variety of pathogenetically unrelated degenerative lesions. For instance, lipoid nephrosis or its clinical contraction, "nephrosis," is a primary glomerular disease with secondary changes as previously discussed, whereas mercury nephrosis, osmotic nephrosis, and so on refer to primary tubular diseases. The general term *nephropathy* is now commonly used (for example, mercury nephropathy).

Acute tubular necrosis

Acute tubular necrosis resulting from a variety of mechanisms is the most important and common cause of acute renal failure. Because of the reparative and regenerative capability of renal tubules, if the patient can survive the initial period of renal failure and concurrent disease, excellent recovery of renal function can be expected.

Clinical picture. The onset of the acute renal failure may be abrupt when associated with severe injury or may be gradual if the injury develops slowly. Pronounced oliguria develops, with a progressive rise in nitrogenous waste products in the blood. Complete anuria is rarely seen. This oliguric phase may last from 4 days to a month but usually is about 10 to 12 days. Continuous injury as seen in uncontrolled infection prolongs the oliguric phase. It is during this stage that water and salt overload and hyperkalemia are dangerous problems. The small amount of urine formed is of low osmolality and may contain tubular cell casts, red blood cells, and some protein. When hemolysis has been a feature of the disease, hemoglobin also is present in the urine.

After 10 to 12 days the urinary volume in such a patient will typically be increased to over 1 liter per 24 hours. In this early diuretic phase the urine is still of low osmolality, and considerable sodium, potassium, and chloride may be lost in the urine. Up to 25% of deaths occur during this critical period. There may be little lowering of blood urea and creatinine levels despite the diuresis. As tubular regeneration is completed, about the seventeenth day, renal concentrating ability improves, and there is a rapid fall in blood urea levels.

Prognosis of acute tubular necrosis depends, to a considerable extent, on the causative agents. In patients with associated severe lesions, such as peritonitis, extensive burns, or severe surgical trauma, which are life threatening in themselves, there is a high mortality. Patients with acute tubular necrosis uncomplicated by severe systemic disease, as is seen in a hemolytic transfusion reaction or a toxic injury, have an excellent prognosis with modern therapy, which includes water and electrolyte control and peritoneal dialysis or hemodialysis.

Acute tubular necrosis may be associated with a large variety of diseases, but the immediate causes may be divided into (1) those of toxic origin (toxic nephropathy) and (2) those related to pronounced hypovolemia, shock, and renal vasoconstriction (ischemic acute tubular necrosis). Often, toxic and ischemic factors complement each other in producing the tubular injury.

Toxic nephropathy. Toxic nephropathy may result from general poisons damaging tubular epithelium such as mercuric chloride, carbon tetrachloride, ethylene glycol (antifreeze), phosphorus, and insecticides or may result from an idiosyncratic reaction in an individual susceptible to drugs such as sulfonamides, antibiotics such as polymyxin and amphotericin B, barbiturates, salicy-lates, and iodinated organic compounds used for contrast materials in roentgenographic studies.[74]

Acute mercury nephropathy is a characteristic example of this type of injury. Mercuric chloride is sometimes taken in a suicide attempt. Those patients who do not die of shock within the first day develop acute renal failure with pronounced oliguria. If the kidneys are examined between the fifth and tenth days, they are found to be swollen and pale. Microscopically the epithelium of the proximal convoluted tubules is necrotic and desquamated into the lumen and may undergo striking dystrophic calcification (Fig. 19-43). The regenerating epithelium is seen lining the tubular basement membrane and is flat and thin and contains occasional mitoses (Fig. 19-43).

Oliver, MacDowell, and Tracey[63] have demonstrated by dissection of damaged nephrons that although mercuric chloride causes selective proximal tubular necrosis, the vasomotor collapse seen in human poisoning results in ischemia of the kidneys and also irregular distal tubular injury.

Other poisons may produce relatively characteristic appearances. Ethylene glycol (antifreeze) has been consumed by alcoholics and produces not only brain damage but also tubular necrosis with innumerable calcium oxalate crystals in the tubular lumina. A few round, slightly greenish concretions of calcium oxalate may be seen in a variety of cases of acute tubular necrosis, particularly those associated with liver damage. Dioxane and diethy-

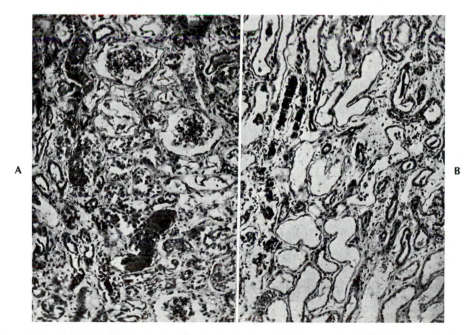

Fig. 19-43. Mercury bichloride poisoning in kidney. **A,** Kidney on seventh day after ingestion of mercury. Note desquamation and destruction of tubular epithelium. **B,** Kidney on eleventh day. Note loss of tubular epithelium, flattened tubular lining, and dark calcium masses in tubular lumina.

lene glycol produce a distinctive ballooning hydropic degeneration of proximal convoluted tubules, progressing to focal hemorrhagic cortical necrosis. The tubular necrosis of carbon tetrachloride poisoning is characterized by large amounts of neutral fat in the basal portions of proximal convoluted tubules.

Ischemic acute tubular necrosis. Although many names have been used for this common cause of acute renal failure (lower nephron nephrosis, hemoglobinuric nephrosis, vasomotor nephropathy), the common underlying feature appears to be renal vasoconstriction of uncertain cause.

The factors that provide the background for development of ischemic acute tubular injury are dehydration, hypovolemia, shock, renal arterial vasoconstriction, and often the presence of hemoglobinuria, myoglobinuria, jaundice, or perhaps toxins from bacterial infections. Typical clinical situations in which such tubular injury occurs are as follows:

1. Mismatched blood transfusion with massive hemolysis
2. Massive crushing injury in which myoglobin is released from damaged muscle in the presence of surgical shock (this "crush syndrome" was a prominent clinical entity in bombing raids of World War II)
3. Massive cutaneous burns with hemolysis of red cells and inadequate fluid replacement
4. Severe bacterial infection, such as generalized peritonitis
5. Massive hemorrhage with inadequate replacement, particularly in pregnancy

Oliver and associates[63] have studied such kidneys by dissecting out individual nephrons. They have shown in both proximal and distal tubules irregular patches of cast formation, tubular degeneration, and basement membrane disruption (tubulorrhexis). They believe that the tubulorrhexic lesions are of ischemic origin. Others are of the opinion that toxic breakdown products of hemoglobin, myoglobin, and other toxic substances are important in causing the tubular necrosis. Following are five hypotheses for the pathogenesis of the oliguria of acute tubular necrosis:[81]

1. Continued poor renal perfusion resulting from vasoconstriction
2. Tubular obstruction resulting from casts and necrotic tubular debris
3. Strong rise in intrarenal tissue turgor pressure from leaking tubules and depression of glomerular filtration
4. Back-leakage of glomerular filtrate through damaged tubules into the interstitial tissues and the renal capillaries
5. Glomerular lesions

Experimental and clinical data indicate that renocorti-

cal ischemia occurs in either toxic or ischemic tubular necrosis. The importance of the other factors is less clear.

The kidneys of patients dying after about 10 days of renal failure are grossly swollen and show a pale cortex and a darker medulla with accentuated striations. Microscopically the kidney of ischemic tubular necrosis frequently shows somewhat dilated proximal convoluted tubules lined by a low epithelium (Fig. 19-44). The distal tubules characteristically are dilated with flattened cells having basophilic cytoplasm. Granular reddish or brownish casts (heme casts) may be seen in the distal tubules or collecting ducts, particularly at the juxtamedullary zone. The tubular epithelium adjacent to the cast is often degenerating, and the basement membrane may be disrupted (tubulorrhexis). The casts that rupture into the interstitial tissues may result in small granulomas and in thrombosis of adjacent venules. Solez, Morel-Maroger, and Sraer[78] have demonstrated that severe deficiency of the brush borders of proximal tubules is particularly characteristic of acute tubular necrosis. Jones[37] confirmed this brush border deficiency with scanning and transmission electron microscopy and also demonstrated severe decrease in the basal interdigitations of the tubular cells. The tremendous normal luminal and antiluminal surface areas necessary for pumping electrolytes are

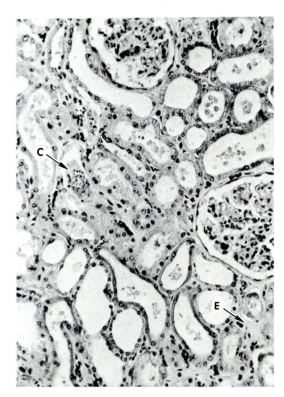

Fig. 19-44. Ischemic acute tubular necrosis with low regenerating tubular epithelium, dilated lumina, casts, *C*, and intertubular edema, *E*. (120×.)

severely decreased.[8] This may result in a sodium- and chloride-rich fluid reaching the juxtaglomerular complex, which may produce vasoconstriction (tubuloglomerular feedback) and sustained oliguria.[63] The glomeruli characteristically show no lesions. A prominent interstitial edema separating the tubules often is seen.

Reversible tubular lesions

Osmotic (sucrose) nephrosis. When hypertonic solutions of sucrose or mannitol or similar substances are given intravenously, as in the treatment of cerebral edema, a hydropic swelling of the proximal tubules of the kidney results (Fig. 19-45). This change is caused by the filling of the cytoplasm of these cells with innumerable, small, pinocytic vesicles. This is generally an asymptomatic and promptly reversible lesion.

Hypokalemic (vacuolar) nephropathy. In severe chronic potassium depletion such as that seen in chronic diarrhea, impairment of the renal concentrating mechanism may result, with the development of large vacuoles at the basal portion of the cytoplasm of mainly the proximal convoluted tubules (Fig. 19-46). Electron microscopy shows these vacuoles to be the result of pronounced distension of the basal infoldings of these cells. These distended infoldings are believed to be caused by disturbance of electrolyte pumping. With potassium therapy the functional and structural changes revert to normal.

Chronic tubular disease

Chronic atrophy of tubules is most commonly a secondary effect of chronic glomerulonephritis, chronic interstitial nephritis, and the long-standing ischemia of nephrosclerosis. It also may result from a variety of lesions, to be discussed subsequently, that obstruct outflow of urine in the tubules or from the kidney. This secondary atrophy may result from direct injury as part of the primary disease, from ischemia developing from vascular changes, or from a poorly understood trophic atrophy after injury to any of the interdependent parts of the nephron. Whatever the cause, this atrophy results in defective tubular function.

Interstitial nephritis[15]

The term *interstitial nephritis* is used for the variety of acute and chronic inflammatory processes that predominantly involve the renal interstitial tissue. This diagnosis is made difficult clinically and pathologically in that glomerular, vascular, tubular, and obstructive disease may result in secondary interstitial inflammation. Primary interstitial nephritis may be divided into acute and chronic nonbacterial interstitial nephritis and acute and chronic pyelonephritis.

Acute diffuse nonbacterial interstitial nephritis in many cases appears to be attributable to drug sensitivity (for example, sulfonamides, phenytoin, and methicillin).

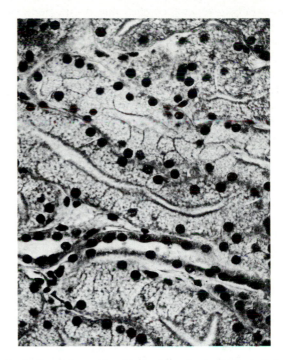

Fig. 19-45. Osmotic nephrosis. Note proximal tubular cells laden with pinocytic vesicles.

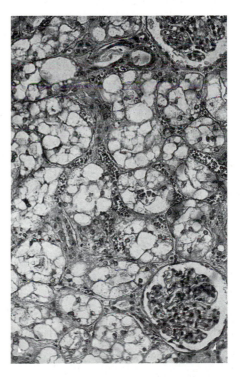

Fig. 19-46. Hypokalemic (vacuolar) nephropathy of potassium deficiency from case of regional enteritis. (Courtesy Dr. Joseph F. Kuzma; from Anderson, W. A. D.: Synopsis of pathology, ed. 10, St. Louis, 1980, The C.V. Mosby Co.)

Fever, skin rash, eosinophilia, and azotemia develop. On withdrawal of the drug recovery may occur. Renal biopsy shows lymphocytes, plasma cells, eosinophils, histiocytes, and some neutrophils in an edematous interstitial stroma. Tubular necrosis, degeneration, or atrophy is seen depending on the duration of the process. In methicillin-associated interstitial nephritis, antibodies have been demonstrated that bind to a benzylpenicilloyl hapten–tubular basement membrane antigen present in the renal tubular basement membranes.[8] The occurrence of a similar acute interstitial nephritis in certain infectious diseases such as diphtheria and scarlet fever suggests that hypersensitivity may also play a role in pathogenesis. An interstitial nephritis occurs in leptospirosis (Weil's disease), but the organisms may be seen in the lesion.

Chronic, diffuse, nonbacterial, interstitial nephritis is usually caused by other processes such as the papillary necrosis of analgesic abuse, sarcoidosis, and ischemia. After chronic pyelonephritis and other causes are excluded, the cause of some cases of diffuse chronic interstitial nephritis remains unknown.

Balkan nephritis is a remarkable chronic interstitial nephritis that occurs commonly in certain areas of Yugoslavia and Bulgaria. It progresses to uremia and is characterized by chronic interstitial inflammation, intense fibrosis, and tubular atrophy. A nephrotoxin is suspected but has not been identified.

Pyelonephritis

The etiology and pathogenesis of lower as well as upper urinary tract infection are discussed, since they are interrelated and most acute pyelonephritis follows infection of the lower tract.

Escherichia coli is the cause of 85% of urinary tract infections. Other common pathogens are *Proteus*, *Enterococcus*, *Pseudomonas*, *Klebsiella*, and *Staphylococcus*. With acute recurrent attacks these latter organisms are more common and may be more resistant to antibiotics. All of the organisms excluding *Staphylococcus* are inhabitants of the colon and normally contaminate urethral orifices, awaiting an opportunity for invasion.

The pathogenesis of lower urinary tract infection depends on introduction of the organism and depression of normal antibacterial mechanisms. Organisms may more readily gain access to the female bladder because of the shorter urethra and a urethrovesical reflux in which straining forces bladder urine into the contaminated upper urethra. This urine may then undergo reflux into the bladder. These features help explain the higher incidence in females. Catheterization of the bladder is of profound significance in urinary infection. The combination of carrying in organisms plus mechanical damage is important. Indwelling catheters routinely cause cystitis. Normal antibacterial mechanisms in the lower urinary tract may be depressed by mechanical obstruction and stasis of urine. Infection of the urinary tract is common therefore in congenital urinary tract anomalies, prostatic hyperplasia, spinal cord injury with cord bladder, and pregnancy. Diabetes mellitus also causes depression of antibacterial factors and infection is common. By contrast, voluminous hypotonic urine and frequent micturition aid local antibacterial factors.

Once acute cystitis is established, the pathogenesis of infection of the kidney is not so clear. Although lymphogenous spread to the kidney is generally discounted, hematogenous and direct transureteral ascending spread may occur. Animal experiments indicate both mechanisms may induce bacterial infection of the kidney and renal pelvis, although at least transient obstruction is needed to lower resistance in a normal kidney to permit infection except with the *Staphylococcus*. In humans there is little evidence that bacteremia precedes nonstaphylococcal acute pyelonephritis. Yet in acute pyelonephritis, characteristically, with absence of obstruction one sees a wedge-shaped zone of inflammation involving papilla and cortex with the remaining kidney free of disease, a condition suggesting vascular inoculation. Ureterovesical reflux is demonstrable in some patients and so indicates a direct manner of carrying organisms to the kidney.[15] The problem of hematogenous versus the ascending route of infection remains unsettled. Once the kidney is infected, the papilla in particular is susceptible because its high stromal osmolality interferes with white blood cell and complement function. Intrarenal scarring in the healing process causes intrarenal obstruction, which also lowers resistance and aids intrarenal spread of infection.

Clinically, lower tract infection is characterized by dysuria, frequency, and bacteriuria. A bacterial colony count on cultured urine over 100,000 colonies per milliliter indicates an established infection, not just urethral contamination. Patients with acute pyelonephritis clinically exhibit fever, chills, flank pain, and costovertebral angle tenderness. Urinalysis will show mild proteinuria, red blood cells, many white blood cells (pyuria), and white cell inclusion casts. In absence of bilateral obstruction the blood urea nitrogen is not elevated. Acute pyelonephritis in the absence of obstruction is characterized grossly by a swollen wedge-shaped area involving papilla and adjacent cortex infiltrated by gray-white foci of inflammatory reaction. Microscopically there may be neutrophils in the tubules and in the edematous stroma. Microabscesses may be present. The glomeruli are relatively spared. The adjacent, uninvolved kidney is without lesions.

With acute obstruction the process may spread to extensively involve the kidney and even to produce necrosis of the renal papillae.

Hematogenous pyelonephritis from *Staphylococcus*

differs in that multiple cortical abscesses may be seen occurring after bacteremia. Sometimes these produce a large, localized, tumorlike, multilocular abscess—carbuncle of the kidney—which may be confounding clinically. A serious complication of staphylococcal acute pyelonephritis is extrarenal rupture of a cortical abscess and development of a huge perinephric abscess.

If obstruction is absent or corrected, acute pyelonephritis responds well to treatment, leaving one or more depressed wedge-shaped zones of fibrosis, tubular atrophy, and collapsed atrophic glomeruli.

Recurrent and chronic pyelonephritis. Unfortunately the very features that resulted in the first attack of acute pyelonephritis are inclined to result in a recurrent attack often by a new and more resistant organism. Thus ensues the problem of recurrent and chronic pyelonephritis in which multiple foci of bacterial infection gradually destroy renal function until the reserve of normal kidney is consumed and chronic renal failure supervenes, if the disease is bilateral. When the process is unilateral, extreme destruction, scarring, and contraction may occur, so the end-stage scar may be difficult to distinguish from a dysplastic maldevelopment.

Pathologically the kidney in chronic pyelonephritis may be recognized by multiple wedge-shaped scars involving cortex and papillae. The surface of the kidney exhibits a U-shaped depression over these scars in contrast to the sharply depressed V-shaped scars of vascular disease. The corresponding minor calyx is dilated. Intervening zones of relatively normal kidney lie between the scars. Microscopically one sees in the kidney chronic interstitial inflammatory reaction with lymphocytes and plasma cells, often with foci of acute neutrophilic reaction. The tubules show varying degrees of dilated or atrophic tubules, often containing many colloidlike casts. There is pronounced interstitial fibrosis. The glomeruli, although relatively spared, may exhibit varying degrees of periglomerular fibrosis and may collapse, and some have converted to atrophic scars. Secondary intimal hyperplasia of small muscular arteries is present, but severe vascular changes are usually associated with concomitant hypertension (Fig. 19-47).

In the literature there is a great discrepancy in the supposed incidence of chronic pyelonephritis seen at autopsy, varying from 1.4% to 33%. Using rigid criteria to eliminate other causes of chronic interstitial inflammation, most authors believe that the incidence is only about 1.5% to 3%.[47] It appears that cases of chronic renal failure that may have been loosely called chronic pyelonephritis in the past were actually nonbacterial chronic interstitial nephritis or of other origin such as nephrosclerosis.[47]

Tuberculous pyelonephritis. Hematogenous spread to the kidneys occurs from pulmonary or other foci of infection. Progressive renal tuberculosis results from hema-

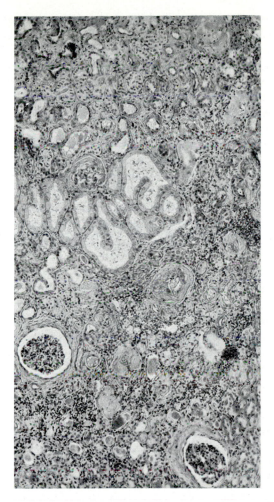

Fig. 19-47. Chronic pyelonephritis. Capsular thickening of glomeruli, interstitial fibrosis and cellular infiltrate, hyaline casts in some tubules, and enlargement of other tubules. (AFIP 76640.)

togenous seeding of the renal cortex to form small caseous foci that spread to the medulla where a progressive caseous ulcerative lesion develops. Involvement of the pelvis and other renal papillae follows, with caseous ulceration of the papillae and extensive intrarenal spread of tuberculous inflammation eventually causing loss of function, hydronephrosis, and spread to the lower urinary tract. The opposite kidney is often involved to some degree. In miliary tuberculosis (tuberculous sepsis) the kidney may be as involved as other organs with many miliary tubercles, but renal dysfunction is not significant.

Obstruction of urinary tract

Mechanical obstruction to urinary outflow causes a rise in luminal pressure and proximal dilatation of the ureter (hydroureter) and renal pelvis (hydronephrosis). The etiology of obstruction may be congenital anomalies (particularly in children), neuromuscular defects such as cord bladder, benign and malignant tumors, renal and bladder calculi, infection and subsequent fibrosis, pregnancy, anomalous arteries at the ureteropelvic junction, and numerous other causes.

Pathogenesis of the progressive dilatation of the ureter and renal pelvis depends on the pressure of continued glomerular filtration to replace urine that is resorbed by the lymphatics, vasa recta of the papilla, capillaries of the pelvic mucosa, or a hypothesized direct pyelovenous outflow.

The progression of the process is determined by the degree and location of obstruction. Unilateral, rapidly developing, complete ureteral obstruction without infection results in moderate proximal dilatation of ureter and renal pelvis. Renal blood flow rapidly falls, and intimal vascular hyperplasia and intense atrophy of tubules and glomeruli follow. Partial obstruction by maintenance of more renal function results in a slow but progressive dilatation of the renal pelvis to often extreme degrees when unilateral. With advanced hydronephrosis the renal parenchyma is stretched over the dilated calyceal system and undergoes intense fibrous atrophy of all components. When hydronephrosis is bilateral and early, the kidney may show only moderate tubular dilatation and flattening and mild chronic interstitial inflammatory infiltrate. When renal biopsy is performed on such a patient with unexplained renal failure as a result of unrecognized bilateral ureteral obstruction from pelvic cancer, the pathologic diagnosis can be difficult.

Clinical manifestations of obstruction are pain, renal enlargement, polyuria, or anuria. Recurrent pyelonephritis or refractory urinary tract infections may be an important problem. When a hydronephrotic kidney becomes infected, it may become a sac filled with purulent exudate (pyonephrosis) usually requiring surgery. With relief of the cause of mechanical obstruction the recovery of renal function depends on the duration of the obstruction and the degree of vascular change and tubular atrophy. After relief of the obstruction, renal concentrating power is reduced but usually improves with time. Occasionally relief of severe obstruction is followed by massive polyuria with electrolyte loss, which may be life threatening.

Renal papillary necrosis (necrotizing renal papillitis)

Acute or chronic necrosis of the renal papilla of one or both kidneys results in extreme impairment of renal function. Although it was first recognized chiefly in diabetics with pyelonephritis, investigators now recognize that acute pyelonephritis with acute obstruction, analgesic abuse, and sickle cell disease may induce human papillary necrosis. The incidence has increased greatly in the last few years, and this is attributed mainly to analgesic abuse and better recognition.

Diabetic patients with pyelonephritis even in the absence of obstruction may exhibit fever, back pain, pyuria or hematuria, and perhaps ureteral colic from sloughed necrotic papillae passing down the ureter. Oliguria and renal failure follow. It is believed that the diabetic vascular disease results in ischemic papillae that are sensitized to further injury by pyelonephritis.

Papillary necrosis also occurs in nondiabetic patients with acute pyelonephritis and acute obstruction of the drainage of one or both kidneys (Fig. 19-48). This often occurs in older men and is often clinically overshadowed by the problems of the accompanying obstruction and infection. Papillary ischemia induced by the acute obstruction is believed to be an important pathogenic mechanism.

Pathologic examination of the kidney of acute necrotizing papillitis reveals yellow or opaque grayish papillae, some of which may have sloughed away. The necrosis generally involves the distal two thirds and is sharply defined from the often congested surviving medulla. The renal cortex may show whitish streaks and mottled areas of inflammatory reaction and small abscesses. Microscopically the papilla usually shows an acellular necrotic remnant of stroma with some acute inflammation at the junction with the medulla. Bacterial colonies may sometimes be seen in the necrotic zone with obstructive necrosis.

Sickle cell disease may show spotty, partial sclerosis

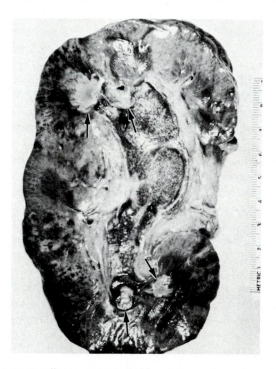

Fig. 19-48. Papillary necrosis resulting from acute pyelonephritis and obstruction. Note necrotic papillae *(arrows)*, mottled patchy cortical infiltrate of acute pyelonephritis, and congested, dilated renal pelvis.

and necrosis of the renal papilla. These probably contribute to the parenchymal changes of sickle cell nephropathy.

Analgesic abuse nephropathy

Analgesic abuse (phenacetin nephropathy) is a major cause of papillary necrosis and chronic renal failure. These patients tend to be middle-aged women who have consumed several kilograms of phenacetin-aspirin mixtures over a number of years. Recurrent pyelonephritis, hypertension, and renal colic from passing necrotic papillae are common clinical manifestations.

Experimental data are confusing but suggest that aspirin as well as phenacetin may contribute to the process. The prognosis of analgesic abuse nephropathy is better than the other papillary necrosis processes, and about two thirds remain stable or improve after stopping drug abuse.[48]

Pathologically the appearance of the kidney of analgesic abuse is variable in that the process often extends over a long time period.[10] At first only yellow necrotic tips of papillae are seen. Later the papillae become dark, shrunken, sloughed, or even calcified. The surface of the renal cortex overlying these necrotic papillae is depressed while the intervening cortex between papillae is raised so that nodules or ridges are produced. Microscopically the necrotic papillae are structureless and sclerotic. The renal cortex shows tubular atrophy, interstitial fibrosis, and varying amounts of chronic inflammatory reaction.

It has been reported that analgesic abuse patients appear to have an increased incidence of renal transitional cell carcinomas.

Myeloma nephropathy

Renal insufficiency develops in multiple myeloma in 30% to 50% of cases.[54] Amyloidosis, renal calcinosis, and pyelonephritis contribute to this failure, but the basic lesion is a chronic interstitial nephritis with tubular atrophy and laminar "hard" casts showing a multinucleated giant cell reaction. Bence Jones proteinuria (light-chain excretion) appears to result in this tubular injury by overloading of proximal tubules with light chain, which may form intracytoplasmic crystalloids or may be converted into insoluble amyloid in innumerable giant lysosomes (Fig. 19-49). Exocytosis of the amyloid into the tubular lumen results in amyloid-containing casts, which are commonly seen in myeloma (Fig. 19-50). The often massive formation of casts may result in obstruction and contribute to the tubular atrophy and renal failure.

Gout nephropathy

Renal problems in gout result from hypertension, renal stones, and formation of gouty tophi in the renal

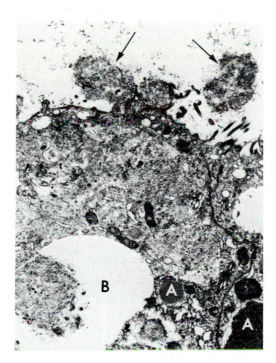

Fig. 19-49. Multiple myeloma nephropathy. Light-chain protein is absorbed in proximal tubular cells, *A*, polymerizes in lysosomes, *B*, and is extruded in lumen as amyloid fibrils *(arrows)*.

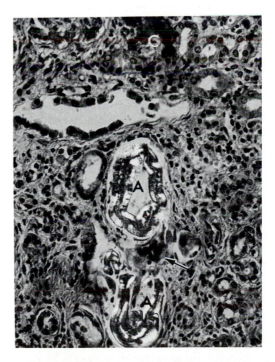

Fig. 19-50. Multiple myeloma nephropathy. Congo red stain under polarized light. Note laminar casts showing bright green dichroism characteristic of amyloid, *A*, foreign body giant cell *(arrow)*, tubular atrophy, and renal calcinosis, *C*.

medulla. These tophi show the usually histiocytic inflammatory reaction to the crystalline urates. When renal insufficiency develops in about 20% to 25% of gouty patients, interstitial inflammation, fibrosis, tubular atrophy, arterionephrosclerotic changes, and gouty tophi are characteristically seen.

Amorphous urates within tubules may be seen in neonatal kidneys as yellow streaks in the medulla, the so-called uric acid infarcts. These arise from the normal striking breakdown of blood cells in the neonatal period and are of no clinical significance.

Hypercalcemia and renal calcinosis

Hypercalcemia and hypercalciuria may cause calcium deposition in the kidney (renal calcinosis), renal injury, dysfunction, or failure and commonly result in formation of renal calculi. Hypercalcemia results from excessive bone resorption attributable to hyperparathyroidism, vitamin D intoxication, extensive bone destruction by cancer, hyperthyroidism, excessive calcium intake as in milk-alkali syndrome, sarcoidosis, and the rare idiopathic infantile hypercalcemia (see p. 1421).

Clinically hypercalcemia may result in renal stones and renal colic, band keratopathy (calcium deposits of the cornea), calcified conjunctival deposits, polyuria from loss of concentrating ability, and renal failure. Pronounced hypercalcemia (over 15 mg/dl) may produce a crisis with polyuria changing to oliguria and severe central nervous system symptoms. Massive visceral metastatic calcification may occur, with a poor prognosis.

Renal calcinosis results either from dystrophic calcification of necrotic tissue, as may be seen in calcified necrotic tubular cells in acute mercury chloride poisoning, or from hypercalcemia. In calcinosis attributable to hypercalcemia the major site is in the basement membranes of Henle's loop and collecting ducts, particularly in the medulla near the cortex, but in severe disease, extensive cortical deposition is also seen. The calcium tends to be deposited in concretions on the inner aspect of the tubular basement membrane. These concretions enlarge, damage cells, and obstruct the lumen. When renal calcinosis is very severe, there may be linear deposition along many tubular basement membranes. Secondary tubular atrophy, interstitial fibrosis, and nonspecific chronic inflammation then occur.

Renal lithiasis

Renal stones have been recognized since antiquity, and renal colic resulting from ureteral passage of a stone is legend because of the characteristic pain produced.

Pathogenesis. Renal stone formation is believed to be the result of both excessive concentration of the stone constituents and conducive physicochemical situations. Important factors are excess concentration of urinary excretory products because of highly concentrated urine

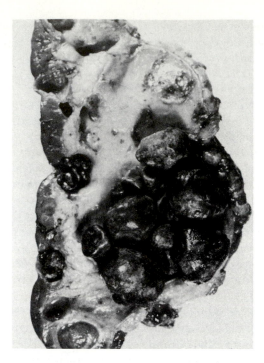

Fig. 19-51. Hydronephrosis with renal stones in renal pelvis and calyces.

resulting from environmental or habitual chronic dehydration. Hypercalciuria from various causes, excessive oxalate, or uric acid production on an acquired or genetic basis and hereditary cystinuria are important causes. Of equal if not greater importance are those factors conducive to precipitation of the crystalloid. An alkaline pH favors calcium phosphate stone formation, whereas an acid pH encourages stone formation in a child with cystinuria.

Stabilization of the solution supersaturated with phosphates and other constituents in the urine is of great importance.[13] Failure of stabilization mechanisms results in deposition onto a nidus of an endogenous or exogenous foreign body (such as necrotic tissue, fibrin, a true foreign body in the bladder, or a Randall's plaque). A Randall's plaque is a minute focus of stromal calcification at the tip of the papilla.[70] When the epithelium is eroded, it acts as a nidus for stone formation of considerable size before the stone tears free from its attachment and becomes free in the pelvis. Stasis of urine induced by partial obstruction tends to facilitate stone formation.

Types of stones.[69] Calcium stones are the most common (50% to 70%) and may be pure or mixtures of oxalate, phosphate, and hydroxyapatite. Massive phosphate stones called staghorn calculi may form a cast of the entire renal pelvis and calyces.

Magnesium ammonium phosphate pure or mixed stones are common in infection with urea-splitting bacteria such as *Proteus*. Uric acid stones comprise from 5% to 10% and cystine stones from 2% to 3%.

Phosphate stones are white, smooth, and soft, whereas oxalate stones are hard, crystalline with sharp edges, and dark brownish. Uric acid stones are dark brown when pure. On fracture most stones show a concentric laminar structure.

Effects of stones are obstruction of the outflow of urine and production of hydronephrosis, the promotion of infection, and the production of renal colic by the passage of small stones down the ureter. Stones and infection often combine to destroy renal function in the involved kidney (Fig. 19-51).

Congenital malformations and anomalies
Agenesis and hypoplasia

Fortunately bilateral renal agenesis is uncommon (about 2 per 1000 autopsies on fetuses and newborns). It is associated with pulmonary hypoplasia and the peculiar facies described by Potter[68] of wide-set eyes, parrot-beak nose, receding chin, and low-set ears.

Unilateral renal agenesis is at least twice as common and is more commonly seen in males. When an isolated anomaly, it is compatible with full life, but frequent association of unilateral agenesis with anomalies such as esophageal atresia or congenital heart disease causes unilateral agenesis to be often encountered in stillborn or infant autopsies.

True renal hypoplasia is relatively uncommon, and most tiny kidneys are the result of acquired disease. True hypoplasia is usually bilateral, and the kidneys have decreased numbers of calyces and papillae and a decreased nephron population. A variant of such hypoplasia is oligomeganephronia in which the nephrons are not only greatly reduced in number but are very hypertrophied with huge glomeruli.

Anomalies of renal ectopia, fusion, and reduplication[49]

Kidneys may be displaced downward, even into the pelvis, and acquire their blood vessels from the large vessels nearby. Crossed ectopia describes the rare occurrence of both kidneys lying on the same side with the ureter of one crossing the midline. The kidneys may be fused, usually at the lower pole (horseshoe kidney), and are usually displaced somewhat caudally. The renal pelvis of one or both kidneys may be reduplicated along with ureteral reduplication. Obstruction and infection often complicate such anomalies of renal position and formation.

Defective renal differentiation, renal dysplasia, and polycystic dysplastic kidney

Defective renal differentiation consists of disturbed nephrogenesis in which one sees abnormal ducts surrounded by concentric collars of undifferentiated mesenchyme often containing smooth muscle or even cartilage

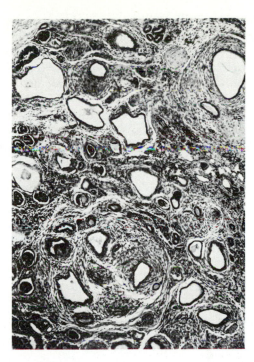

Fig. 19-52. Dysplasia of kidney. Note disorganized renal structure with embryonic type of peritubular stromal proliferation.

(Fig. 19-52). The kidney may be small, or such dysplastic collecting ducts may become cystic, producing the large polycystic dysplastic kidney (Potter type II). Such dysplasia may partially or completely involve one or rarely both kidneys. Unilateral cystic dysplasia is without familial tendency and occurs equally in both sexes. It is often associated with other malformations. Bilateral total polycystic dysplastic kidneys result in death in infancy. Lesser degrees of involvement have a variable life expectancy.

Congenital obstructive microcystic dysplasia (Potter type IV)[50,65]

Intrauterine obstruction to urinary outflow interferes with the genesis of new waves of nephrons. Depending on the location of the obstruction, it may involve part of one kidney or more commonly both kidneys. In addition to other dysplastic changes, the conspicuous feature is cystic dilatation, particularly of subcapsular Bowman's capsule about glomeruli, producing a microcystic kidney. The prognosis depends on the severity of the obstruction (Figs. 19-53 and 19-54).

Simple cystic disease of the kidney

Simple cysts, solitary or multiple, of the kidney are very common. Their common association with nephrosclerosis and chronic pyelonephritis suggests tubular obstruction resulting from scarring. Their greatest significance is confusion with solid tumors of the kidney.

Bilateral polycystic kidney

Infantile polycystic kidney (Potter type I).[50,60] Infantile polycystic kidney is a rare defect in renal differentiation that is lethal at birth and apparently is attributable to a homozygous phenotype of an autosomal recessive trait. The kidneys are large and smooth in external contour, but on section the kidneys are uniformly replaced by radially oriented cysts that produce a remarkable spongelike appearance (Fig. 19-55). Dissection of the nephrons of such kidneys indicates that the primary defect is excessive proliferation, and cystic dilatation of the collecting ducts with other changes is secondary. Multiple cysts of the liver or bile ductule proliferations uniformly accompany this disease.

Adult polycystic kidney (Potter type III).[50,65] Adult polycystic kidney characteristically involves only a portion of the collecting ducts and nephrons so that much of the renal structure and function is retained. Patients usu-

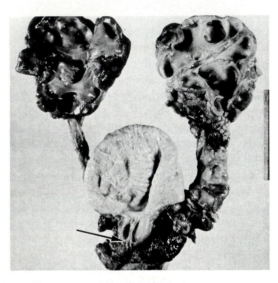

Fig. 19-53. Congenital bilateral hydronephrosis from posterior urethral obstruction *(arrow).*

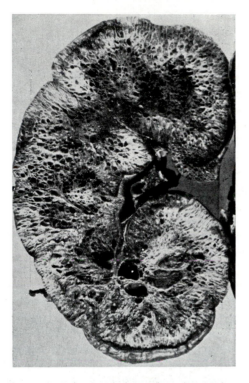

Fig. 19-55. Polycystic kidney of newborn infant.

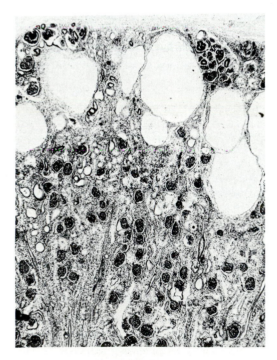

Fig. 19-54. Congenital bilateral hydronephrosis with microcystic dysplasia of renal cortex.

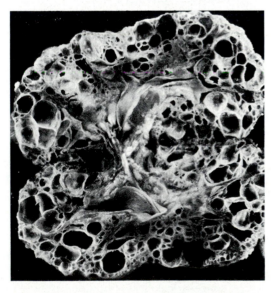

Fig. 19-56. Polycystic kidney of adult.

ally survive to the fifth or sixth decade although a few die in childhood. This disease is always bilateral and in most cases is attributable to an autosomal dominant trait. Grossly the kidneys are often huge, weighing more than 1500 g apiece. The innumerable cysts, varying from barely visible to 5 cm in size, produce a cobblestone-like external surface (Fig. 19-56). On cross section the cysts contain straw-yellow, hemorrhagic, or even gelatinous fluid. The renal pelvis and calyces are stretched, compressed, and distorted by the cysts, and this results in a characteristic roentgenographic appearance. The intervening islands of renal parenchyma may be normal in appearance or may show secondary compression, atrophy, and fibrous arterionephrosclerosis, or pyelonephritis, resulting in eventual renal failure. Dissections of the nephrons and collecting ducts in such cases[65] have shown that the cystic dilatations and proliferations occur in any part of the nephron but have a special predilection for the angle of Henle's loop and Bowman's capsule.

Associated with adult polycystic disease are multiple liver cysts in about one third of cases and, much less commonly, cysts of the pancreas and spleen. About 15% of cases are associated with berry aneurysms of cerebral arteries.

Medullary cystic diseases[50]

Closely related to polycystic disease are medullary sponge kidney and uremic medullary cystic disease. The pathogenesis of these lesions is not known but is assumed to be from abnormal development. Medullary sponge kidney is generally a benign, asymptomatic cystic dilatation of collecting ducts of the renal medulla, which is seen as an incidental finding in adults by x-ray examination of the upper urinary tract with radiocontrast materials. There is some tendency for urinary calculus formation and secondary pyelonephritis, but generally the abnormality causes no problem.

Medullary cystic disease is a lethal disease of older children and young adults. This entity also is called familial nephrophthisis (Fanconi's familial nephronophthisis). There is a familial tendency in these cases, and an autosomal recessive trait has been suggested.

Clinically the patients usually have anemia, salt-losing syndrome, concentration defect, and azotemia. Pathologically such kidneys are shrunken, have granular surfaces, and show many small cysts in the medulla, particularly at the corticomedullary junction (Fig. 19-57). These cysts of the medulla are lined by flattened tubular epithelium. In the cortex there are intense tubular atrophy, interstitial fibrosis, and some lymphoid interstitial infiltrate. The arteries show little change. The number of glomeruli is greatly reduced. The remaining glomeruli show old scars, active scarring, and some large, hypertrophic glomeruli. Renal biopsy may not be diagnostic, for the medullary cysts may be missed, and the other changes may suggest chronic glomerulonephritis or chronic pyelonephritis. The prognosis of the patient is poor.

Renal neoplasms
Benign tumors

Benign renal tumors are usually small and are seen incidentally at nephrectomy or autopsy. They include ectopic adrenocortical nodules, hamartomas, benign mesenchymal neoplasms, and cortical tubular adenomas.

Adrenocortical nodules are small and resemble adrenal cortex morphologically. Ectopic adrenocortical nodules may be found in other locations along the embryologic urogenital ridge.

Hamartomas. Angiomyolipomas are one common form seen in the kidney. They are composed of single or multiple nodules of vessels, smooth muscle, and fat cells. When these tumors are large and show bizarre large nuclei, an erroneous diagnosis of cancer may be made. Hamartomatous nodules are frequently associated with the hereditary disease tuberous sclerosis, which is also manifested by hamartomas and neoplasms in the skin, brain, heart, and other viscera.

Mesenchymal neoplasms. Medullary fibromas are common small white nodules seen incidentally at autopsy in the renal medulla. They are composed of swirls of interstitial connective tissue cells and collagen enclosing renal tubules. These cells contain lipid droplets and apparently arise from medullary interstitial cells, which

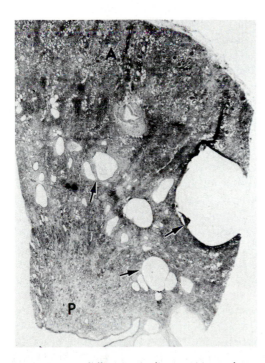

Fig. 19-57. Uremic medullary cystic disease. Macrophotograph of tissue section. Renal cortex with atrophy, *A,* papilla, *P,* and medullary cysts *(arrows).*

they appear to resemble electron microscopically. Opinion is divided as to whether these represent hamartomas or hyperplasia of medullary interstitial cells. Small cortical fibromas, lipomas, and leiomyomas are seen occasionally. Hemangiomas are rare but can cause hematuria. Large benign stromal neoplasms are very rare.

Cortical tubular adenomas. Cortical tubular adenomas vary from 0.1 to 3 cm in diameter, are white or yellow, and are four times more common in males. They are frequently seen in the kidney with benign nephrosclerosis or chronic pyelonephritis. Microscopically they are relatively encapsulated, are composed of tubular cords or papillary structures, and may be cystic. Since many of these nodules closely approach or match adenocarcinomas of the kidney in histologic appearance, Bennington[9] and others believe that such nodules are either precancerous or small carcinomas. If these nodules are less than 3 cm in diameter, metastases are rare. Large adenomas, even though histologically innocent in appearance, are considered at least potentially malignant. Electron microscopy of renal "adenomas" and adenocarcinomas indicates that both show ultrastructural features of proximal tubules of the kidney.[9]

Malignant tumors[6]

Adenocarcinoma of kidney (hypernephroma). Hypernephroma is an old misnomer indicating adrenal rest origin. Histologic, ultrastructural, and immunologic studies indicate renal proximal tubular origin, but like many old names hypernephroma stays with us. This cancer comprises 70% to 80% of renal cancer and occurs most commonly at 50 to 70 years of age. The prevalence is twice as great in men as in women. The most common clinical presentation of the tumor is with hematuria, usually painless. Less commonly it is manifested by flank pain, unexplained fever, and abdominal mass, or metastatic lesions in lungs or bones. Anemia is often present, and polycythemia, presumably resulting from release of erythropoietin by the tumor, may occur. Cancer cells can occasionally be recognized in cytologic smears. Diagnosis usually depends on roentgenographic studies such as intravenous pyelogram, angiogram, and radioisotopic renal scans.

Adenocarcinoma of the kidney is generally fairly slow in growth, and metastases may appear fairly late. Prognosis depends on the extent of spread and vascular invasion. McDonald and Priestly[55] found a 54% incidence of venous invasion by the tumor (Fig. 19-58). Kaufman and Mims[44] found that if the cancer was confined to the kidney, a 60% 5-year and a 50% 10-year survival were seen. When venous invasion or perirenal extension had occurred, the survival was halved. The presence of metastases meant little or no long-term survival. Overall cure rate at 10 years is from 17% to 28%.

Gross pathologic studies show that these tumors may arise from any part of the cortex of either kidney. They are usually large and golden yellow, with central cystic areas containing fresh or old blood. White zones of fibrosis and coagulative necrosis are common in the central zone. When lipid content of the tumor cells is low, a cream or tan color is seen.

Dissection of the renal veins may reveal a thrombus composed partly or completely of tumor (Fig. 19-58). This thrombus may extend into the vena cava.

At autopsy this carcinoma most commonly has metastasized to the lungs, but lymph node, liver, and bone metastases are common. Pathologic fracture of an osseous metastasis may be the initial picture with this disease.

Histologically this cancer shows a wide variety of growth patterns often in the same tumor. Most characteristically the tumor is composed of clear cells with prominent cell borders and relatively regular nuclei growing in sheets, nests, cords, or tubules or in a papillary manner (Fig. 19-59). Such cells are rich in glycogen and lipid. Granular cells with pink granular cytoplasm are seen. Most carcinomas show mixtures of cell types, but when the tumor is predominantly a granular cell, the prognosis is somewhat poorer. Rarely there is a spindling sarcomatoid component of the tumor (carcinosarcoma) associated with foci of clear cell carcinoma. There is disagreement whether these represent true sarcomas or are sarcomatoid metaplasia. The prognosis of this type is poor.

Nephroblastoma (Wilms' tumor).[61] This cancer of embryonic renal cells is the most common of the malignant abdominal tumors of young children, although it accounts for only 6% of renal cancers in all ages. It occurs equally in males and females. The cancer may be present at birth, 28% occur in the first year, and 96.5% occur before 6 years of age. Clinically it appears most commonly as a palpable abdominal mass. Fever and hypertension are present half the time. Pain is sometimes present, but hematuria is uncommon.

Grossly the tumor is usually large, rounded, and dwarfing but not invading the kidney until late. The cut surface reveals a soft, gray-white to cream-colored tumor. Extension into adjacent tissues is common. Microscopically the tumor is composed of small anaplastic tumor cells that make poorly formed tubules and also grow in a diffuse sarcomatoid pattern. Sometimes cross-striated rhabdomyoblasts can be seen (Fig. 19-60).

Early metastases to lungs, liver, and lymph nodes and rapid local invasion are seen. Prognosis in this tumor has improved greatly in recent years with modern surgery, radiotherapy, and chemotherapy. Survival of 80% with the addition of chemotherapy is an improvement over the 50% survival with surgery and radiotherapy. This

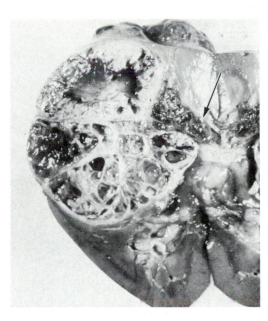

Fig. 19-58. Adenocarcinoma of kidney. *Arrow,* Tumor thrombus in renal vein branch.

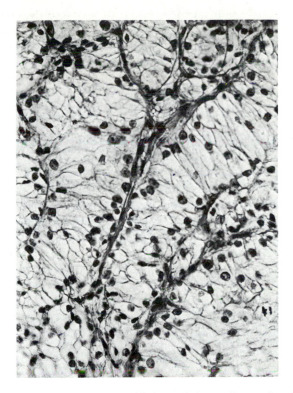

Fig. 19-59. Adenocarcinoma of kidney of clear cell type showing papillary structure. (350×; courtesy Dr. S.E. Gould.)

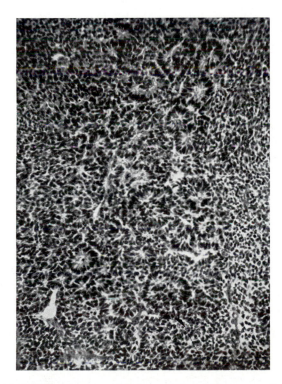

Fig. 19-60. Wilms' tumor of kidney. Note tubular or rosettelike structures amid tissue of sarcomatous appearance.

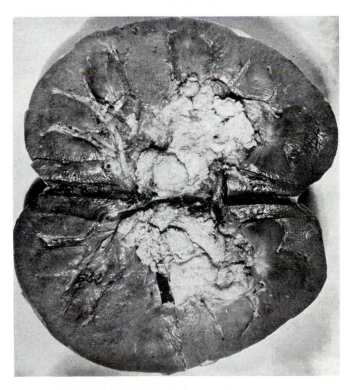

Fig. 19-61. Papillary carcinoma of renal pelvis.

cancer is one of the few that may be cured even after visceral metastasis has occurred.

Leukemic infiltration. Leukemic infiltration of the kidneys is a common finding, particularly in chronic lymphatic leukemia. The infiltrate may be bilateral, nodular, or diffuse and may cause renal enlargement and even renal failure. Histologically, monotonously uniform leukemic cells distend the stroma between tubules and glomeruli. Hemorrhages in the pelvic tissues are common.

Tumors of renal pelvis. These cancers arise from the urothelium, the transitional epithelium (Fig. 19-61). These tumors are twice as common in males as in females and comprise about 8% of renal cancers. The presenting clinical picture is usually of hematuria, either painless or painful if blood clots are passed. The tumor cells may be shed in the urine and recognized in cytologic smears, affording an opportunity for early diagnosis. Roentgenographic demonstration of the tumor in the renal pelvis is the usual diagnostic tool. The cancers vary from very low-grade transitional carcinoma or "papilloma" composed of cells resembling transitional epithelium all the way to solid, infiltrating, anaplastic carcinoma. Multicentric new foci of in situ or invasive transitional cell carcinoma may be present in the ureter in 70% of cases at the time of surgery or later. Of renal pelvic cancers, 15% are keratinizing squamous cell carcinomas arising from metaplasia of the urothelium, and they have a poor prognosis. Riches[71] found that all patients with so-called papillomas survived; 57% of patients with low-grade papillomas survived 5 years, 38% of those with high-grade papillary tumors survived 5 years, and none of those with various solid, infiltrating cancers survived after 5 years.

REFERENCES
General

1. Brenner, B.M., and Rector, F.C., editors: The kidney, ed. 2, Philadelphia, 1981, W.B. Saunders Co.
2. Hamburger, J., Crosnier, J., and Grünfeld, J.P.: Nephrology, New York, 1979, John Wiley & Sons, Inc.
3. Heptinstall, R.H.: Pathology of the kidney, ed. 2, Boston, 1974, Little, Brown & Co.
4. Spargo, B.H., Seymour, A.E., and Ordóñez, N.G.: Renal biopsy: pathology with diagnostic and therapeutic implications, New York, 1980, John Wiley & Sons, Inc.

Specific

5. Appel, G.B., et al.: Renal involvement in systemic lupus erythematosus, Medicine **57**:371, 1978.
6. Arakawa, M.: A scanning electron microscopy of the glomerulus of normal and nephrotic rats, Lab. Invest. **23**:489, 1970.
7. Baldwin, D.S.: Poststreptococcal glomerulonephritis: a progressive disease? Am. J. Med. **62**:1, 1977.
8. Baldwin, D.W., et al.: Renal failure and interstitial nephritis due to penicillin and methicillin, N. Engl. J. Med. **279**:1245, 1968.
9. Bennington, J.L.: Cancer of the kidney: etiology, epidemiology, and pathology, Cancer **32**:1017, 1973.
10. Burry, A.: Pathology of analgesic nephropathy: Australian experience, Kidney Int. **13**:34, 1978.
11. Cannon, P.J., et al.: The relationship of hypertension and renal failure in scleroderma (progressive systemic sclerosis) to structural and functional abnormalities of the renal cortical circulation, Medicine **53**:1, 1974.
12. Clarkson, A.R., et al.: IgA nephropathy: a syndrome of uniform morphology, diverse clinical features and uncertain prognosis, Clin. Nephrol. **8**:459, 1977.
13. Coe, F.L., and Favus, M.J.: Disorders of stone formation. In Brenner, B.M., and Rector, F.C., editors: The kidney, ed. 2, Philadelphia, 1981, W.B. Saunders Co.
14. Cotran, R.S.: Monocytes, proliferation and glomerulonephritis, J. Lab. Clin. Med. **92**:837, 1978.
15. Cotran, R.S.: Interstitial nephritis. In Churg, J., et al., editors: Kidney disease: present status, Baltimore, 1979, The Williams & Wilkins Co.
16. Counahan, R., and Cameron, J.S.: Henoch-Schönlein nephritis. In Massy, S.G., editor: Kidney in systemic disease, vol. 7, Basel, 1977, S. Karger.
17. Dachs, S., et al.: Diabetic nephropathy, Am. J. Pathol. **44**:155, 1964.
18. Dixon, F.J.: The pathogenesis of glomerulonephritis, Am. J. Med. **44**:493, 1968.
19. Dixon, F.J., Oldstone, M.B.A., and Fonietti, G.: Pathogenesis of immune complex glomerulonephritis of New Zealand mice, J. Exp. Med. **134**(suppl.):65s, 1971.
20. Dodge, W.F., et al.: Poststreptococcal glomerulonephritis: a prospective study in children, N. Engl. J. Med. **286**:273, 1972.
21. Eagen, J.W., and Lewis, E.J.: Glomerulopathies of neoplasia, Kidney Int. **11**:297, 1977.
22. Fauci, A.S., Haynes, B.F., and Katz, P.: The spectrum of vasculitis: clinical, pathologic, immunologic, and therapeutic considerations, Ann. Intern. Med. **89**:660, 1978.
23. Gerwurz, H., et al.: The complement profile in acute glomerulonephritis, systemic lupus erythematosus and hypocomplementemic chronic glomerulonephritis: contrast and experimental correlations, Int. Arch. Allergy Appl. Immunol. **34**:556, 1968.
24. Gianantonio, C., et al.: The hemolytic uremic syndrome, J. Pediatr. **61**:478, 1964.
25. Glassock, F.J., and Cohen, A.H.: Secondary glomerular diseases. In Brenner, B.M., and Rector, F.C., editors: The kidney, ed. 2, Philadelphia, 1981, W.B. Saunders Co.
26. Glassock, R.J., et al: Primary glomerular diseases. In Brenner, B.M., and Rector, F.C., editors: The kidney, ed. 2, Philadelphia, 1981, W.B. Saunders Co.
27. Gutman, R.A., et al.: The immune complex glomerulonephritis of bacterial endocarditis, Medicine **51**:1, 1977.
28. Habib, R.: Focal glomerulosclerosis, Kidney Int. **4**:355, 1973.
29. Habib, R., and Kleinkneckt, C.: The primary nephrotic syndrome of childhood: classification and clinicopathologic study of 406 cases. In Sommers, S.C., editor: Pathology Annual, New York, 1971, Appleton-Century-Crofts.
30. Habib, R., et al.: Dense deposit disease: a variant of membranoproliferative glomerulonephritis, Kidney Int. **7**:204, 1975.
31. Harrison, E.G., and McCormack, L.J.: Pathologic classification of renal arterial disease in renovascular hypertension, Mayo Clin. Proc. **46**:161, 1971.
32. Heptinstall, R.H.: Pathology of end stage renal disease, Am. J. Med. **44**:656, 1968.
33. Huttenen, N.P.: Congenital nephrotic syndrome: a study of 75 patients, Arch. Dis. Child. **51**:344, 1973.
34. Jones, D.B.: Arterial and glomerular lesions associated with severe hypertension: light and electron microscopic studies, Lab. Invest. **31**:303, 1974.
35. Jones, D.B.: Correlative scanning and transmission electron microscopy of glomeruli, Lab. Invest. **37**:569, 1977.
36. Jones, D.B.: Membranoproliferative glomerulonephritis: one or many diseases? Arch. Pathol. Lab. Med. **101**:457, 1977.
37. Jones, D.B.: Ultrastructure of human acute renal failure, Lab. Invest. **46**:254, 1982.
38. Jones, D.B., and Iannaccone, P.M.: Atheromatous emboli in renal biopsies: an ultrastructural study, Am. J. Pathol. **78**:261, 1975.
39. Jones, D.B., Mueller, C.B., and Menefee, M.: The cellular and

extracellular morphology of the glomerular stalk, Am. J. Pathol. **41**:373, 1962.

40. Kannel, W.B., Schwartz, M.J., and McNamara, P.M.: Blood pressure and risk of coronary heart disease: the Framingham study, Dis. Chest **56**:43, 1969.

41. Kannel, W.B., et al.: Epidemiologic assessment of the role of blood pressure in stroke: the Framingham study, J.A.M.A. **214**:301, 1970.

42. Kanwar, Y.S., and Farquhar, M.G.: Anionic sites in the glomerular basement membrane: in vivo and in vitro localization to the laminae rarae by cationic probes, J. Cell. Biol. **81**:137, 1979.

43. Karnovsky, M.J.: The structural bases for glomerular filtration. In Churg, J., et al., editors: Kidney disease—present status, Baltimore, 1979, The Williams & Wilkins Co.

44. Kaufman, J.J., and Mims, M.M.: Tumors of the kidney, Curr. Probl. Surg. **1**:1, 1966.

45. Kefalides, N.A.: Current status of chemistry and structure of basement membranes. In Kefalides, N.A., editor: Biology and chemistry of basement membranes, New York, 1978, Academic Press, Inc.

46. Kimmelstiel, P., and Wilson, C.: Intercapillary lesions in glomeruli of kidney, Am. J. Pathol. **12**:83, 1936.

47. Kimmelstiel, P., et al.: Chronic pyelonephritis, Am. J. Med. **30**:589, 1961.

48. Kincaid-Smith, P.: Analgesic nephropathy, Ann. Intern. Med. **68**:949, 1968.

49. Kissane, J.M.: Congenital malformations. In Heptinstall, R.H., editor: Pathology of the kidney, ed. 2, Boston, 1974, Little Brown & Co.

50. Kissane, J.M.: The morphology of renal cystic disease. In Gardner, K.D., Jr., editor: Cystic diseases of the kidney, New York, 1976, John Wiley & Sons, Inc.

51. Lindeman, W.: Sur la mode d'action de certain poison renaux, Ann. Inst. Pasteur **14**::49, 1900.

52. Luxton, R.W.: Radiation nephritis: a long-term study of fifty-four patients, Lancet **2**:1221, 1961.

53. Mahajan, S.K., et al.: Changing histopathology patterns in lupus nephropathy, Clin. Nephrol. **10**:1, 1978.

54. Martinez-Maldonado, M., et al.: Renal complications in multiple myeloma: pathophysiology and some aspects of clinical management, J. Chronic Dis. **24**:221, 1971.

55. McDonald, J.R., and Priestly, J.T.: Malignant tumors of kidney: surgical and prognostic significance of tumor thrombosis of renal vein, Surg. Gynecol. Obstet. **77**:295, 1943.

56. McFarland, J.B.: Renal vein thrombosis in children, Am. J. Med. **34**:269, 1965.

57. McKay, D.G.: Disseminated intravascular coagulation: an intermediary mechanism of disease, New York, 1965, Harper & Row, Publishers, Inc.

58. McWhinney, J.B., et al.: Thrombotic thrombocytopenic purpura in childhood, Blood **19**:181, 1962.

59. Michael, A.F., et al.: The glomerular mesangium, Kidney Int. **17**:14, 1979.

60. Mostofi, F.K.: Radiation effects on the kidney. In Mostofi, F.K., and Smith, D.E., editors: The kidney, Baltimore, 1966, The Williams & Wilkins Co.

61. Mostofi, F.K.: Tumors of the renal parenchyma. In Churg, J., et al., editors: Kidney disease: present status, Baltimore, 1979, The Williams & Wilkins Co.

62. Mueller-Eberhardt, H.J.: Complement abnormalities in human disease, Hosp. Pract. **13**:65, 1978.

63. Oliver, J., MacDowell, M., and Tracey, A.: The pathogenesis of acute renal failure associated with traumatic and toxic injury: renal ischemia, nephrotoxic damage and the ischemuric episode, J. Clin. Invest. **30**:1307, 1951.

64. Oparil, S., and Haber, E.: The renin-angiotensin system, N. Engl. J. Med. **291**:389, 1974.

65. Osathanondli, V., and Potter, E.L.: Pathogenesis of polycystic kidneys, Arch. Pathol. **77**:459, 1964.

66. Pirani, C.L., and Salinas-Madrigal, L.: Evaluation of percutaneous renal biopsy, Pathol. Annu. **3**:249, 1968.

67. Pirani, C.L., et al.: The renal glomerular lesions of pre-eclampsia: electron microscopic studies, Am. J. Obstet. Gynecol. **87**:1047, 1963.

68. Potter, E.L.: Bilateral renal agenesis, J. Pediatr. **29**:68, 1946.

69. Prien, E.L., and Frondel, C.: Studies in urothiasis: composition of urinary calculi, J. Urol. **57**:949, 1947.

70. Randall, A.: Etiology of primary renal calculus, Surg. Gynecol. Obstet. **71**:209, 1940.

71. Riches, E.: Tumors of the kidney and ureter, Edinburgh, 1964, E.&S. Livingstone, Ltd.

72. Rosen, S.: Membranous glomerulonephritis: current status, Hum. Pathol. **2**:209, 1971.

73. Rosen, S.: Crescentic glomerulonephritis: occurrence, mechanisms, and prognosis, Pathol. Annu. **10**:37, 1975.

74. Schreiner, G.E., and Maher, J.F.: Toxic nephropathy, Am. J. Med. **38**:409, 1965.

75. Scott, D.M., et al.: The immunoglobulin nature of nephrotic factor (NeF), Clin. Exp. Immunol. **32**:12, 1978.

76. Sheehan, H.L., and Moore, H.C.: Renal cortical necrosis and the kidney of concealed accidental hemorrhage, Springfield, Ill., 1954, Charles C Thomas, Publisher.

77. Sherman, R.L., Churg, J., and Yudis, M.: Hereditary nephritis with a characteristic renal lesion, Am. J. Med. **56**:44, 1974.

78. Solez, K., Morel-Maroger, L., and Sraer, J.D.: The morphology of "acute tubular necrosis" in man: analysis of 57 renal biopsies and a comparison with the glycerol model, Medicine **58**:362, 1979.

79. Spargo, B., et al.: The differential diagnosis of crescentic glomerulonephritis, Hum. Pathol. **8**:187, 1977.

80. Steblay, F.W.: Glomerulonephritis induced in sheep by injection of heterologous glomerular basement membrane and Freund's complete adjuvant, J. Exp. Med. **116**:253, 1962.

81. Stein, J.H., Lifschitz, M.D., and Barnes, L.D.: Current concepts on the pathophysiology of acute renal failure, Am. J. Phys. **234**:F171, 1978.

82. Stife, C.F., et al.: Membranoproliferative glomerulonephritis with disruption of the glomerular basement membrane, Clin. Nephrol. **7**:65, 1977.

83. Tisher, C.C.: Anatomy of the kidney. In Brenner, B.M., and Rector, F.C., editors: The kidney, ed. 2, Philadelphia, 1981, W.B. Saunders Co.

84. Tobian, L., and Binion, J.: Tissue cations and water in arterial hypertension, Circulation **5**:754, 1952.

85. Trew, P.A., et al.: Renal vein thrombosis in membranous glomerulonephritis: incidence and association, Medicine **57**:69, 1978.

86. Vassalli, P., and McCluskey, R.T.: The pathogenic role of the coagulation process in rabbit masugi nephritis, Am. J. Pathol. **45**:653, 1964.

87. Vassalli, P., Morris, R.H., and McCluskey, R.T.: The pathogenic role of fibrin deposition in the glomerular lesions of toxemia of pregnancy, J. Exp. Med. **118**:467, 1963.

88. Vitsky, B.H., et al.: The hemolytic uremic syndrome: a study of renal pathologic alterations, Am. J. Pathol. **57**:627, 1969.

89. Welling, L.W., and Welling, D.J.: Surface areas of brush border and lateral cell walls in the rabbit proximal nephron, Kidney Int. **8**:343, 1975.

90. Whitaker, A.N., et al.: Disseminated intravascular coagulation and intravascular hemolysis in glomerular disease: the response to heparin therapy. In Kincaid-Smith, P., Mathew, T.H., and Becker, E.L., editors: Glomerulonephritis: morphology, natural history and treatment, New York, 1973, John Wiley & Sons, Inc.

91. Wilson, C.B., and Dixon, F.J.: The renal response to immunological injury. In Brenner, B.M., and Rector, F.C., editors: The kidney, ed. 2, Philadelphia, 1981, W.B. Saunders Co.

CHAPTER 20

Lower Urinary Tract

R.C.B. PUGH

THE URETER
Congenital anomalies

Congenital anomalies of the ureter are not uncommon and, although often asymptomatic, are often associated with urinary tract infection, which they sometimes initiate and frequently perpetuate. Most result from maldevelopment of the ureteric bud and comprise anomalies of number, position, and termination, and some affect the structure of the ureter itself.

In the most extreme and rarest form there is complete failure of development of the ureteral bud with renal aplasia; usually the bladder on the affected side is hypoplastic. Much more commonly the anomaly is less severe, the bladder and ureteral orifice are normally formed, and the ureter can be traced from the bladder into the true pelvis or loin and is surmounted by a dysplastic kidney. Part of such a ureter may be apparently normal, but frequently it is reduced to a fibrous string in the upper part of its course.

The most common ureteral anomaly is duplication (duplex ureter), which is complete when there are two separate ureteral orifices and incomplete when the two ureters join before they enter the bladder (Fig. 20-1). There are usually as many renal pelves as there are ureters, and the kidney related to the upper ureter and pelvis is often small and dysplastic. In about half the cases of incomplete duplication the two ureters join in the lower third. In the complete form they pass down side by side and just before reaching the bladder the ureter from the lower pelvis crosses the one from the upper, which frequently has an ectopic opening (in the male within the external sphincter and into the posterior urethra, vas deferens, epididymis, or seminal vesicle, and in the female either into the urethra or adjacent to the external meatus). An extremely rare form of duplication is the so-called inverted Y in which there are two ureteral orifices and two ureters that fuse into a single tube that passes up to a single kidney. Triplication is also recorded.

Pelviureteral obstruction is frequently seen in children and young adults and is the most common form of congenital ureteral constriction. Depending on its degree, there is a varying amount of back pressure with dilatation of the pelvicalicine system and renal functional impairment. Some patients with less severe lesions first show symptoms in middle age. The etiology is not known, but aberrant vessels, adhesions between the upper ureter and pelvis, altered disposition of the muscle bundles in the upper ureter, excess of collagen in the muscle coat, and a mucosal valve have at various times been believed to be responsible.

Primary obstructive megaureter, a condition analogous to pelviureteral obstruction, is more common in males than in females and is sometimes bilateral. The greater part of the ureter is dilated and hypertrophied, but there is a short terminal segment of normal caliber that does not permit reflux. The pathology of the condition is not known, but the abnormality is believed to be within the narrow segment. In the megaureter-megacystis syndrome there is a large-capacity bladder, capable of emptying without residue, with reflux into grossly dilated ureters.

A ureterocele is a ballooning of the lower end of the ureter, forming an intravesical cyst that is lined externally by vesical mucosa and internally by ureteral mucosa. The ureteral meatus may be small and like a pinpoint, and the upper ureter is often distended. The condition occurs more often in girls than in boys and is frequently associated with duplex and ectopic ureters and congenital ureteral strictures.

Other, less common anomalies include postcaval ureter (a right-sided anomaly in which the ureter passes behind the inferior vena cava), herniation (in which the ureter enters a hernial sac), diverticulum (usually juxtavesical), kinks, torsions, and valves. Long atretic segments are sometimes seen in association with multicystic disease of the kidney, and, very rarely, aberrant vessels obstruct the lower ureter in children. In the "prune bel-

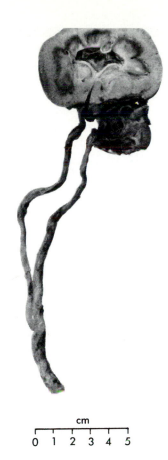

cm

0 1 2 3 4 5

Fig. 20-1. Incomplete duplication of ureter. Kidney has been rotated, and small upper (dysplastic) part lies to right and inferiorly.

ly" syndrome there is anomalous development of the entire genitourinary system and the ureters are usually dilated, elongated, and tortuous.

Trauma

Ureteral damage caused by external violence is rare, usually results from road traffic accidents, and is more common in children than in adults. Rupture or avulsion may occur at or just below the pelviureteral junction, and clinically the condition is often masked by the severity of other injuries. Penetrating wounds of the abdomen do not usually involve the ureters, but on rare occasions they may be damaged during gynecologic operations, by the passage of a stone, by the use of a Dormia basket, or by overvigorous attempts at retrograde pyelography. Pelvic irradiation sometimes leads to ureteral fibrosis and obstruction.

Obstruction and dilatation

The ureter may be obstructed by pressure from without (as in retroperitoneal fibrosis, retroperitoneal tumors, and pelvic lipomatosis), by changes in its wall (caused by amyloidosis, endometriosis, bilharzial fibrosis, and neoplasms), by intraluminal lesions (such as pol-

yps), or by the impaction of calculi, tumor fragments, blood clots, or fungus balls. There may be actual stricturing, or the obstruction can be caused by kinking of the ureter and, depending on the completeness of the obstruction and the length of time that obstruction of whatever cause has been present, there will be a variable amount of proximal myohypertrophy and luminal dilatation. Temporary obstruction often occurs when the ureteral orifice becomes edematous during an episode of acute cystitis. Dilatation is also seen when there is bladder outflow obstruction, as with the enlarged prostate, and in pregnancy when there is loss of tone, possibly caused by hormonal influences, or actual pressure on the ureter at the pelvic brim.

Vesicoureteral reflux

The urine secreted by the kidney passes down the ureter by peristaltic action. When the peristaltic wave reaches the lower end, the ureterovesical opening relaxes to allow the urine to enter the bladder and then closes again and remains closed until the next wave arrives. Peristalsis is essentially myogenic, and musculomuscular junctions allow transmission of the contractions. There is also adrenergic and cholinergic innervation of the ureter with scanty neuromuscular junctions, and ganglion cells are found only in its terminal parts.

The prevention of reflux depends on the integrity of the ureterovesical junction, which in turn depends on compression of the submucosal portion of the ureter against the underlying detrusor muscles and the active contraction of the trigonal muscles. Any interference with either of these components will result in reflux, allowing bladder pressures, which always rise during micturition and may be abnormally high at other times, to be transmitted to the kidney. Any rise in intracaliceal pressure above the filtration pressure will inevitably alter intrarenal hemodynamics. Reflux itself is not necessarily harmful, but when it is accompanied by intrarenal reflux, parenchymal scarring (reflux nephropathy) is likely to develop, especially if the urine is infected. The mechanism of scarring is not yet known, but experimental evidence suggests that the configuration of the renal papillae determines whether intrarenal reflux is likely. There may also be alterations in concentrations of antibody against Tamm-Horsfall protein.

Reflux may be primary, when the intramural portion of the ureter is unduly short or there is lack of the firm muscular backing at the ureteral hiatus in the bladder, or secondary as a result of, for example, urethral valves, neuropathic bladder, or a diverticulum. There is evidence of racial differences in incidence and possibly of a familial predisposition to the condition. Reflux in children may be reversible.

Local lesions of acquired type that cause damage to and dilatation of the ureter are not infrequently accompanied by reflux. Cystitis, if localized to the region of the ureteral orifice, is liable to cause rigidity of the periureteral tissues, which allows reflux to occur.

Calculous disease

Ureteral stones are rarely primary and have usually migrated from the renal pelvis. They are of several types—endemic uric acid, oxalate, or ammonium acid urate stones occurring in certain specific localities throughout the world and usually associated with a high proportion of cereal in the diet; infective stones composed of magnesium ammonium phosphate or calcium phosphate, occurring in association with urinary tract infection (most commonly with *Proteus* organisms), and, in about a fourth of the cases, complicating a local urologic abnormality; and metabolic stones associated with disorders of calcium, oxalate, purine, or amino acid metabolism. In the presence of infection, endemic or metabolic stones may acquire a coating of phosphates. The majority of ureteral stones occur in men between the ages of 20 and 50. The stones may impact anywhere in the lumen of the ureter, the sites of predilection being the pelviureteral junction, the pelvic brim, the point where the ureter enters the bladder, and the ureteral orifice itself. Stone impaction usually leads to proximal dilatation of the ureter or of the renal pelvis and calices with pyelonephritis or pyonephrosis if infection is present. At the site of impaction there may be local inflammation, sometimes leading to ulceration and periureteritis. Very occasionally the ureteral orifice prolapses into the bladder, producing an intravesical mass that has to be distinguished from a ureterocele.

Inflammation

Nonspecific inflammation of the ureter is usually part of a more generalized inflammatory process, also affecting the renal pelvis or the bladder, and frequently is associated with and results from vesicoureteral reflux. Trauma to the mucosal surface by the passage of a calculus or by instrumentation may be an aggravating factor. The gross and microscopic features do not call for particular comment. Sometimes the mucosal surface has a granular appearance because of subepithelial collections of lymphoid cells (ureteritis follicularis). Malakoplakia sometimes affects the ureter.

Tuberculosis is the most common specific inflammation. The ureter is almost always involved by downward spread of the disease from the kidney, occurring either by continuity of tissue or by lymphatics. When healing occurs, there is often dense fibrosis that may completely obliterate the lumen or occlude its lower end and cause obstructive hydronephrosis and hydroureter.

Proliferative mucosal lesions

In response to inflammation, and often adjacent to urothelial tumors, the lesions of ureteritis cystica and von Brunn's nests are sometimes seen. Essentially similar lesions are seen in both the renal pelvis and bladder, and the mode of their production and significance are considered in more detail later. The lesions of ureteritis cystica may be so large as to produce a curious cobblestone appearance on the intravenous urogram. The condition occurs especially in elderly patients and is most often seen in the upper third of the ureter.

Tumors

The benign tumors most often seen in the ureter are the fibroepithelial polyps, which have a central core of loose connective tissue and a covering of transitional epithelium (Fig. 20-2). The lesions are usually single, but occasionally multiple, and are commonly found in the upper ureter but are sometimes seen lower down and may protrude through the ureteral orifice. On rare occasions fibromas, myomas, and angiomas involve the ureter.

The most common primary malignant tumors arise from the transitional epithelium, usually as a part of generalized urothelial neoplasia. About 5% of all urothelial tumors are primary within the ureter and occur with about equal frequency on the right and left sides. Males are more commonly affected than females, and patients are usually in their sixth or seventh decade although no age is exempt. Macroscopically the lesions are papillary (or, less often, sessile) and may be single or multiple. The

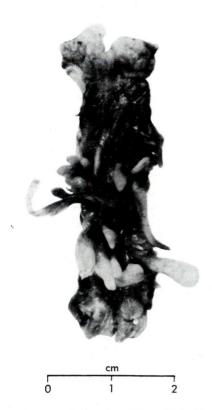

Fig. 20-2. Excised segment of ureter with multiple fibroepithelial polyps.

majority are situated in the lower ureter. Invasion of the ureteral wall is not often seen. The etiology and general characteristics of ureteral tumors are similar to those of the urothelial tumors of the bladder and will be considered later. Uncommon forms are the so-called stump tumors arising in the residual ureter months or years after simple nephrectomy, often for benign disease. Tumors occasionally arise at the site of a ureterocolic anastomosis.

The ureter is sometimes involved in metastatic disease with deposits in the ureteral wall itself or in adjacent retroperitoneal nodes from primary tumors in the testis, prostate, breast, colon, lung, or lymphoid system.

THE BLADDER
Congenital anomalies

Congenital anomalies of the bladder are of many types and of varying severity and complexity, the rarest being agenesis, duplication, and hourglass deformity. Failure of closure of the urachus may result in complete patency or the formation of cysts or fistulas, as described later. Diverticula occur either at the ureteral hiatus in the bladder wall or in the region of the urachus, but often become evident only if there is also lower urinary tract obstruction. Vesicovaginal or vesicorectal fistulas are found if the urorectal septum fails to develop.

By far the most important anomaly is vesical exstrophy from incomplete fusion of the mesodermal elements that normally form the genital tubercle, the anterior bladder wall, and the infraumbilical part of the anterior abdominal wall (Fig. 20-3). It is generally stated to be present in about 1 of every 50,000 births. Males are more often affected than females, the proportions being variously estimated to be between 7 to 1 and 2 to 1. In the complete forms in males the bladder is very small and is everted on the anterior abdominal wall, forming a reddened, extremely tender mass on which the ureteral orifices and trigone are seen. The penis is rudimentary and stumpy with epispadias, the scrotum is often bifid, and the testes are commonly undescended. The pubic bones fail to unite in the midline, resulting in a waddling gait, and there is a high incidence of congenital anomalies affecting the skeleton and gastrointestinal tract. The appearances are very similar in females, in whom the clitoris is cleft. As a result of infection, areas of squamous and glandular metaplasia of the epithelium develop and there is often a mucoid exudate on the surface. The prognosis in untreated cases is poor because of upper urinary tract infection. Tumors are sometimes seen and are usually adenocarcinomas.

Trauma

The bladder may be damaged by gunshot wounds and in other penetrating injuries, and occasionally it is inadvertently opened during surgical operations (such as those on large sliding hernias), or in the course of transurethral procedures, or is damaged by attempts to procure abortion. Rupture of the bladder may result from direct violence to the lower abdomen, as with a kick, and is commonly seen in those who have been in road traffic accidents, especially when there is a fractured pelvis. When the bladder is full at the time of the accident, the rupture may be intraperitoneal, but much more commonly it is extraperitoneal, with the wall being either torn open or penetrated by a spicule of bone. The mucosal surface is sometimes damaged by an indwelling catheter or a foreign body, producing an area of ulceration or polypoid cystitis, often with a heavy local eosinophil infiltration.

Dilatation

The bladder dilates to a varying degree in the presence of organic outflow obstruction caused by congenital lesions, such as urethral valves, or by acquired conditions, such as prostatic enlargement or urethral stricture, or when there are neurologic disorders. These conditions may be congenital (such as spina bifida) or may occur after trauma, inflammation, other disease (tabes dorsalis or disseminated sclerosis), or neoplasms—all of which can interfere with the normally smooth interaction of the sphincters, which are under cerebral control through the somatic nerves, and the detrusors controlled by the autonomic system. The effects produced depend on the level of the lesion and the extent to which local conditions within the bladder are modified by urinary infection. In cauda equina and conus lesions there is partial or complete interruption of the sacral reflex arc, which affects detrusor action. Initially the bladder distends painlessly, but later irregular detrusor activity returns and the blad-

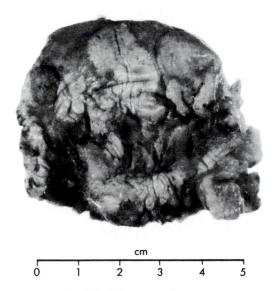

cm

| 0 | 1 | 2 | 3 | 4 | 5 |

Fig. 20-3. Exstrophied bladder excised from middle-aged man (in whom transitional cell carcinoma subsequently developed at site of ureterocolic anastomosis). Note pale smooth areas of squamous metaplasia.

der hypertrophies and becomes coarsely trabeculated (hypertonic or autonomic bladder). Reflux and ascending infection are common. When the cord lesion is above the sacral level, the initial stage of spinal shock and retention with overflow is followed by reflex micturition mediated through the spinal reflex arc (reflex or automatic bladder). If there is urinary infection, the bladder capacity may become greatly reduced. The uninhibited neurogenic bladder occurs when there is loss of higher cortical control, as with a cerebral tumor, and the large atonic neurogenic bladder, with a thin wall and atrophied muscle, develops when there is overdistension from lack of sensation because of interruption of the sensory limb of the reflex arc.

Simple obstruction of short duration will result in dilatation that is usually recoverable when the cause is removed, but when it is of long standing, the bladder wall gradually hypertrophies because of the rise in intravesical pressure and becomes trabeculated, and diverticula may appear. Eventually decompensation occurs and the bladder wall then thins and dilates, usually with reflux and hydroureter. Evidence suggests that the abnormality in bladder neck obstruction without prostatic enlargement (Marion's disease) is a disorder of function rather than a mechanical obstruction attributable to local fibrosis.

Diverticula of the bladder are occasionally congenital but are much more commonly seen in patients with acquired outflow obstruction, being especially frequent in elderly patients with an enlarged prostate and a trabeculated bladder. They are particularly common in the posterolateral wall and are often large and multiple. They usually fail to empty completely on micturition, leading to urinary stasis within their lumina. Their walls consist of fibrous tissue and a variable amount of smooth muscle with an inner lining of transitional epithelium, which often undergoes squamous metaplasia. Complications include ulceration, stone formation, and neoplastic change in the lining mucosa.

Herniation and displacement

The bladder may occasionally herniate through the inguinal or femoral rings, usually in elderly patients. A cystocele is a protrusion of the bladder into the vagina in multiparous women. In pelvic lipomatosis the bladder has a characteristic inverted pear shape and its base is pushed up out of the pelvis by the mass of perivesical fat.

Calculous disease

Many of the calculi seen in the bladder are secondary, since they originate in the upper urinary tract or form on a nucleus of dead tissue or a foreign body, especially when the urine is infected with urea-splitting organisms. Urinary stasis is often an added factor and predisposes to the "recumbency" calculi occurring in bedridden patients. Endemic calculi—once frequently seen, but now rare, in parts of England—are rare in blacks but are common in certain nonindustrialized Mediterranean and Far Eastern countries where there is a high cereal content in the diet. In children these endemic stones are more common in boys than in girls, occur more frequently in the bladder and urethra than in the upper urinary tract, and usually consist of ammonium acid urate and calcium oxalate. Endemic stones in adults in these countries usually consist of uric acid, calcium oxalate, and ammonium acid urate. In westernized areas of the world, bladder stones in children are infection stones, whereas in adults they are composed of pure calcium oxalate or a mixture of calcium oxalate and phosphate or are infection stones. Metabolic stones, similar to those seen in the ureter, also occur in the bladder and in the presence of infection may become coated with phosphates.

Calculi composed of phosphates are gray or gray-white and may be hard, or soft and friable. Oxalate stones are usually hard and either are smooth, rounded or nodular, resembling mulberries, or are irregularly spiculated; if there has been much local bleeding, they are frequently black or a very dark brown. Uric acid and urate stones are smooth, yellow or brown, and round or oval. Cystine stones are hard, smooth, and yellow and have a somewhat waxy appearance.

Fistulas

A vesicovaginal fistula between the posterior wall of the bladder and the upper anterior wall of the vagina may occur after obstetric injuries or irradiation damage or is attributable to direct extension of tumor from one viscus to another. A vesicointestinal fistula between the bladder and either the rectum, or sigmoid or small intestine occurs most commonly in diverticulitis or malignant disease of the large bowel and is seen only infrequently in regional ileitis (Fig. 20-4).

Inflammation

A variety of bacterial and fungal infections can cause inflammatory changes in the bladder, which may also occur with parasitic infestation or direct exposure to chemical irritants, with foreign bodies, or after local trauma. Any congenital or acquired lesion causing obstruction and stasis is liable to exacerbate an inflammatory process.

Since the normal bladder epithelium is very resistant to bacterial infection, primary cystitis is rare. Most cases are caused by spread of infection from the upper urinary tract, as occurs with tuberculosis, or from the urethra as when cystitis follows instrumentation. Cystitis occurs much more commonly in females than in males because of the short urethra, which is liable to fecal contamination and to mechanical trauma during intercourse. Pros-

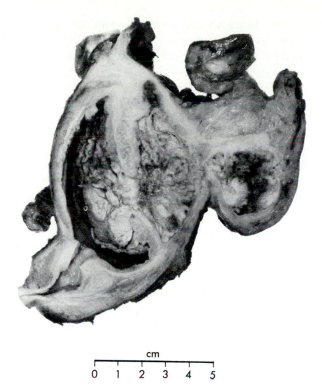

Fig. 20-4. Vesicointestinal fistula. Adenocarcinoma of colon invading posterior wall of bladder.

tatic obstruction is a very frequent cause in males.

It is often difficult to correlate symptoms with the presence or absence of bacteria in the urine, and patients with clinical cystitis may at various times be asymptomatic with or without bacteriuria or symptomatic either way. Asymptomatic bacteriuria is a common disorder in childhood, occurring, according to different estimates, between 5 and 30 times more frequently in girls than in boys. It is also seen in both nonpregnant and pregnant women, and in a significant number of the latter asymptomatic bacteriuria in early pregnancy may be followed by symptomatic urinary tract infection—and in particular by acute pyelonephritis—the nearer it is to term. The particular danger of infection is the frequency with which it is complicated by vesicoureteral reflux and residual urine, which may lead to chronic renal disease, hypertension, and renal failure. In children with urinary infection there is probably little if any permanent structural damage to the urinary tract in the absence of reflux.

For treatment to be effective, it is important to localize the infection and, in particular, to distinguish between upper and lower tract infection. This is often difficult. In addition to microbiologic examinations of midstream and clean-catch specimens of urine, many techniques, including ureteral catheterization, suprapubic bladder aspiration, bladder washouts, detection of antibody-coated bacteria, and determinations of nonspecific C-reactive

protein concentrations and serum antibodies to O antigens of *Escherichia coli* may have to be employed.

The most common causative organisms are *E. coli*, *Staphylococcus aureus*, and *Streptococcus faecalis*. In hospital practice, infection with *Proteus* and *Pseudomonas aeruginosa* occurs quite commonly. Specific cystitis caused by tuberculosis is not uncommon, and a number of viruses, including herpesvirus and adenovirus, and fungi such as *Actinomyces* and *Candida* are sometimes responsible. Urinary tract infection is usually accompanied by an immune response with a rise in antibody titer to the somatic antigens of the infecting organisms, but it is generally believed that specific antibodies play little or no part in protecting against or eradicating urinary infection. During the course of an infection there may be rises in IgA, IgG, and IgM levels in the urine, and secretory IgA (half of which is derived from urethral secretions) is also found in increased amounts, which may be partly responsible for protecting the urethra against infection and may also explain the relative infrequency of cystitis as a complication of urethritis.

The variable severity of urinary tract infection from patient to patient may be related to the virulence of the responsible organism, owing to the presence of bacterial capsules or the ability to produce an endotoxin. The tendency for certain organisms to colonize different parts of the tract preferentially is thought to be due to their "adhesiveness" (capacity to attach to a particular type of epithelium and not to others).

Acute cystitis, or an acute exacerbation of chronic cystitis, may be of variable severity. In mild cases there is mucosal congestion with some local edema and polymorphonuclear leukocyte infiltration. With severe infection the congestion and edema are pronounced and the epithelium is either hyperplastic or ulcerated; there is widespread inflammatory cell infiltration, principally by polymorphonuclear leukocytes, which affects the lamina propria and may spread into the muscle coat. The vessels are thick walled, and their lining endothelium is often prominent. Abscesses may occur. Chronic nonspecific cystitis occurs after persistent or repeated attacks of acute cystitis. The epithelium may be deficient, irregularly hyperplastic, or sometimes polypoid, and in long-standing cases there is often squamous metaplasia. The lamina propria is usually broadened, contains more fibrous tissue than is usual, and is congested and diffusely or focally infiltrated with inflammatory cells. These are mainly lymphocytes and plasma cells, with a few eosinophils here and there, and the lymphoid cells may be collected into follicles. The process spreads into the muscle coat to a varying depth, and the blood vessels throughout the bladder wall are usually thickened. In the later stages of the disease the fibrous tissue contracts and the bladder capacity is greatly reduced.

Descriptive adjectives are sometimes used to indicate

the predominant change (for example, hemorrhagic cystitis or ulcerative cystitis), and the term follicular cystitis describes the accumulation of lymphoid cells that is often seen deep to the mucosa in many types of chronic cystitis and that can be recognized as pale granular lesions when viewed through the cystoscope or in the fixed specimen. Bullous cystitis is a rare form in which there is localized edema of the lamina propria resulting in a folded or polypoid mucosa that appears cystic. There may be local hemorrhages, and macroscopically the lesion may simulate the grapelike masses of embryonal sarcoma. Emphysematous cystitis, seen in diabetics or in association with infection with gas-forming organisms, is a very rare condition in which the bladder wall is studded with gas-filled cysts lying in the lamina propria.

Special forms of cystitis

In abacterial cystitis inflammatory changes are often severe and accompanied by mucosal ulceration, although the urine is persistently sterile. The cause is not known, but some of the patients have Reiter's disease characterized by conjunctivitis, arthritis, and nonspecific urethritis, cystitis, or prostatitis, and attributable possibly to *Mycoplasma hominis* or *Chlamydia*. In Britain and North America Reiter's disease frequently complicates nongonococcal genital infections, whereas in Scandinavia and on the European continent it is more likely to occur after a dysenteric type of illness.

Gangrenous cystitis (also described as croupous, diphtheritic, membranous, or pseudomembranous cystitis) has a wide variety of causes, such as chemical irritants, physical damage by excess heat or irradiation, infections, overdistension, extravesical pressure from an impacted gravid uterus, damage to blood vessels, and thrombosis or embolism, which either interfere with the blood supply of the bladder or produce severe inflammation. Very rarely gangrene occurs after transurethral resection of the prostate. Cystoscopically, gray sloughing areas are seen and the mucosa and parts of the lamina propria may be passed as a cast of the bladder. The mucosa is often covered with a layer of fibrin, pus, degenerated epithelium, and organisms.

In encrusted cystitis, when the urine is infected with urea-splitting organisms, and especially when the bladder wall has been damaged (for example, by local irradiation or repeated diathermy), deposits of calcium phosphate or calcium magnesium phosphate occur on the damaged area. Macroscopically there are grayish white gritty plaques or crusts on the mucosal surface, and microscopically there is irregular ulceration or hyperplasia of the epithelium with adherent calculous material, which sometimes elicits a local foreign-body giant cell reaction.

In irradiation cystitis the bladder is damaged by local or external irradiation of the bladder wall itself or of adjacent organs. The first changes to be noted are mucosal congestion and a variable amount of local edema, sometimes progressing to the formation of bullae. More prolonged exposure results in mucosal ulceration, edema of the lamina propria with acute necrotizing arteriolitis, and some inflammatory cell infiltration. In the later stages mucosal ulceration persists, but there are often epithelial proliferation and hyperplasia, with or without squamous metaplasia, as well as considerable fibrosis of the lamina propria and muscle coat, leading to contraction of the bladder. There are varying degrees of endarteritis, and if tissue damage is severe, fistulas are liable to form.

Interstitial cystitis characteristically occurs in middle-aged or elderly women, who complain of distressing and disabling frequency, dysuria, and suprapubic pain and are found on cystoscopy to have a hyperemic, usually contracted, bladder that bleeds easily when distended. Most of the changes are seen on the posterior wall or at the vault. Microscopically the mucosa may or may not be ulcerated, but the most stiking changes are seen in the lamina propria, which is broadened and more fibrous than normal and is diffusely infiltrated with lymphocytes, plasma cells, and some eosinophils and polymorphonuclear leukocytes. The fibrous septa in the muscle coat are also widened and infiltrated with inflammatory cells, and there may be fibrous tissue replacement of muscle fibers and spread of the inflammatory process through the full thickness of the bladder wall. The capillaries in the lamina propria are usually very prominent, and the arterioles are frequently thick walled. The cause is not known. Although hormonal changes, infection, and lymphatic obstruction have been believed to play a part, recent work has suggested that the disease has an autoimmune basis. Interstitial cystitis is essentially a disease of women; any male patient with symptoms that in a female would immediately suggest the diagnosis is much more likely to have malignant disease in his bladder. He should be thoroughly investigated and kept under regular surveillance with cytologic examinations of the urine and, if necessary, repeated bladder biopsies.

Cyclophosphamide, when administered as a cytotoxic agent, may produce a hemorrhagic cystitis that can eventually lead to bladder contracture. The changes are caused by the breakdown products of cyclophosphamide rather than by the drug itself and are not dose dependent. Tumor formation is a very rare complication.

The local infiltration of the bladder wall with eosinophils commonly seen in the base of ulcers caused by indwelling catheters and during the reparative stages after bladder biopsy, and as a constant feature of the acute stages of bilharzial infestation, needs to be distinguished from eosinophilic cystitis. This is a rare condition believed to be attributable to infection or to food or drug allergy occurring in young patients (sometimes children) and often accompanied by blood eosinophilia. Cystoscopically the bladder mucosa is usually polypoid and the appearances may resemble a tumor, but microscopically the bladder wall, especially the lamina propria, is diffusely and heavily infiltrated with eosinophils and there is no suggestion of neoplasia. Granulomatous cystitis has been reported in the rare syndrome of chronic granulomatous disease of childhood in which the bactericidal activity of the leukocytes is depressed, probably because of a genetically determined enzyme deficiency.

Malakoplakia is a rare condition that was first described in the urinary tract and has subsequently been found in the testes, epididymides, prostate, and, very occasionally, the gut. In the bladder yellowish, round or oval, plaquelike or occasionally polypoid lesions are scattered over the mucosal surface, and the lamina propria contains dense collections of large histiocytes with granular cytoplasm (von Hansemann cells). These contain small, rounded, sometimes apparently laminated bodies (Michaelis-Gutmann bodies, Fig. 20-5) that stain for iron and with the von Kossa and periodic acid–Schiff tech-

niques and are believed to be altered bacteria or breakdown products of bacteria that have become mineralized. There is often a clinical history of urinary tract infection, and the condition is considered to be an atypical form of granulomatous response to coliform infection. The lesions should not be mistaken for neoplasms.

The bladder is involved in most cases of renal tuberculosis, and in tuberculous cystitis the changes are usually first seen near the ureteral orifices. The early lesions are hyperemic and granular but soon progress to ulceration, whereas fibrosis occurs in the later stages of the disease and may result in very gross contracture of the bladder. The histologic appearance is in no way different from that seen in tuberculous lesions elsewhere in the body.

The bladder is very occasionally affected in fungal infections, especially actinomycosis and candidiasis, sometimes by direct spread from adjacent organs or more commonly through the bloodstream in generalized systemic disease, which may complicate the prolonged use of antibiotics, steroids, or immunosuppressive drugs.

The bladder is frequently involved in bilharzial disease and is occasionally affected in infestation with *Echinococcus* and *Strongyloides stercoralis*.

Proliferative and metaplastic mucosal lesions

Von Brunn's nests, cystitis cystica, and cystitis glandularis are three related conditions commonly seen in the inflamed bladder or around the stalk of papillary tumors and the margins of sessile or invasive tumors, both in experimental animals and in humans. To consider the cystic and glandular lesions as types of cystitis is both unfortunate and inaccurate, since (in common with von Brunn's nests) they are really reactive in nature and would be better designated as examples of cystic or glandular metaplasia. For the present, however, they will continue to be referred to as "cystitis." It is sometimes stated that these lesions are precancerous, but, although undoubtedly they sometimes have a malignant potential, the association with neoplasia is by no means invariable and all three are better regarded as being indicative of mucosal instability, which is often capable of complete resolution.

Von Brunn's nests are formed by buds or sprouts of transitional epithelium that grow down from the surface into the underlying lamina propria and later become surrounded by a condensed layer of connective tissue that eventually separates them from the overlying cells (Fig. 20-6). Central cavitation of the cysts or infolding of the surface epithelium, with the formation of crypts that become obstructed, will lead to the formation of cystitis cystica (Fig. 20-7). In the fully formed cysts there is a

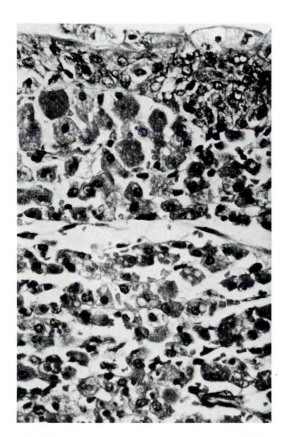

Fig. 20-5. Malakoplakia. Lamina propria contains many large macrophages with granular cytoplasm. Note round, targetlike, Michaelis-Gutmann bodies. (Hematoxylin and eosin; 600×.)

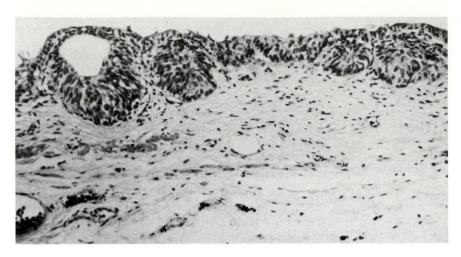

Fig. 20-6. Von Brunn's nests dipping down into lamina propria; one on left shows commencing cavitation. (Hematoxylin and eosin; 240×.)

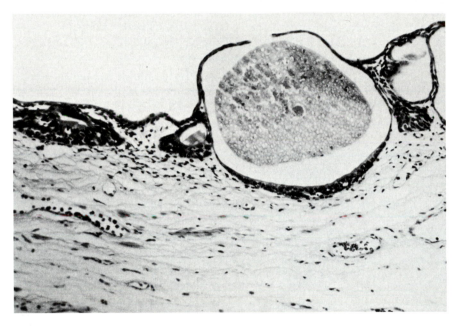

Fig. 20-7. Cystitis cystica. (Hematoxylin and eosin; 240×.)

lining of flattened or low cuboid cells, and if the cysts are of sufficient size, the mucosal surface becomes irregular and has a granular appearance. Cystitis glandularis is produced when the cells lining the cysts differentiate into columnar epithelium.

Squamous metaplasia of the transitional epithelium of the bladder is commonly seen in inflammatory disease and is not necessarily precancerous. The same cannot be said with certainty when the change occurs in cells lining a diverticulum, where there is a much higher incidence of both squamous metaplasia and squamous carcinoma than in the bladder. The type of squamous change in which, because of estrogen stimulation, the cell cyto-

plasm becomes vacuolated (and is therefore often referred to as vaginal metaplasia), is frequently seen as a white patch with clear-cut edges on the trigone of young women with the urethral syndrome. It has no association with neoplastic disease. Leukoplakia, a rare condition more common in men than in women, is distinguished from squamous metaplasia by surface keratinization with or without parakeratosis and the presence of a stratum granulosum and intercellular bridges. It is frequently associated with chronic or recurrent urinary tract infection, and malignancy (commonly squamous carcinoma) occurs in about one fourth of cases.

Polypoid cystitis commonly occurs with incipient or

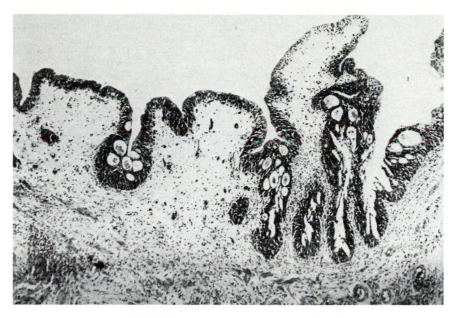

Fig. 20-8. Polypoid cystitis. Note broad-based mucosal projections. (Hematoxylin and eosin; 96×.)

established vesicointestinal fistula or when the bladder is stimulated locally, for example, by the tip of an indwelling catheter. It is distinguished from a papillary tumor by the shape of the papillae, which taper from a broad base to a narrow tip (Fig. 20-8).

Epithelial (urothelial) tumors

More than 90% of all bladder tumors arise from the transitional epithelium, which is continuous with a similar epithelium that lines the renal pelves, the ureters, and the greater part of the urethra. Many workers object to the term "urothelium" to describe this common cell lining, but its use has the distinct advantage of emphasizing the basic fact that the various parts of the urinary tract form a coherent whole and that tumor formation in any one area, such as the bladder, must be considered and treated in the light of the changes elsewhere in the urinary system. Urothelial neoplasia is therefore a single, potentially multifocal disease that may affect any part of the urothelium. That several areas may be involved simultaneously suggests a single common cause, but in many cases the disease pattern becomes evident only over a period of years. For example, a renal pelvic tumor on one side may be followed by a bladder tumor, with a urethral tumor developing later (Fig. 20-9). Common causes may again be operative, but other factors, such as implantation of cells in the lower tract from a lesion higher up, lymphatic spread, or direct surface spread of tumor by continuity along an epithelial surface, may be responsible for the multicentricity of the tumors. Local conditions may be important in determining where neoplastic change will occur.

Etiology

The association between bladder cancer and industrial occupation was first recognized in aniline dye workers in Germany at the turn of the century, and the list of occupations in which there is risk now includes the chemical, rubber, and cable industries, gas retort house workers, rat catchers, sewage workers, and laboratory technicians. The toxic substances responsible for neoplasia are the metabolic products of α- and β-naphthylamine, benzidine, and 4-aminodiphenyl, some of which are carcinogenic in experimental animals. Occupational tumors occur at an earlier age than do spontaneous ones, after an induction period, sometimes as long as 20 or more years, between contact with the chemical and the clinical appearance of tumor. Histologically, industrial bladder tumors are similar to spontaneous lesions. It has been estimated that in heavily industrialized areas of the United States and United Kingdom between 20% and 30% of bladder tumors in men are associated with occupation. Cigarette smoke, phenacetin-containing analgesics, and antineoplastic drugs such as cycloplosphamide and chlornaphazin can act as carcinogens, but coffee and the artificial sweeteners saccharine and cyclamate are no longer considered to be harmful.

Local lesions in the urinary tract itself may also be important. Within a short time of birth, areas of squamous and glandular metaplasia develop in the mucosa of the exstrophied bladder as a result of repeated infection and trauma, and in very rare cases malignancy supervenes. The tumors occur at a younger age than those in patients with normally developed bladders, and adenocarcinomas are particularly common, although they rare-

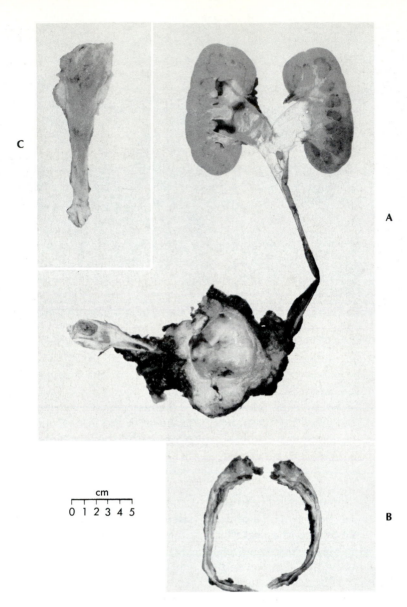

Fig. 20-9. Multiple urothelial tumors in middle-aged man. **A,** Nephroureterocystoprostatectomy (in 1969) for tumors in left renal pelvis, lower end of left ureter, region of internal meatus, and right ureter. **B,** Urethrectomy (early 1972) for tumor. *Inset,* Right ureterectomy (late 1972) for multiple urothelial tumors.

ly metastasize. The proliferative changes in the mucosa may persist after the exstrophy is corrected surgically, with a continued risk of tumor formation. The same considerations apply in the defunctionalized bladder after urinary diversion, since pyocystis is not uncommon and tumors occasionally develop. A vesical diverticulum also predisposes to tumor formation; squamous metaplasia frequently occurs in the epithelial lining and there is a higher incidence of squamous carcinoma within a diverticulum than in the bladder itself. The significance of leukoplakia and the mucosal proliferative lesions has already been discussed. The association between bladder cancer and schistosomiasis is frequently reported, and

there is a high incidence of squamous carcinoma in some parts of the world where infestation is common. The belief that there is a direct causal relationship between the two is yielding place to the concept that neoplasia might be initiated by urine-borne carcinogens, possibly nitrosamines formed during attacks of urinary tract infection, and accelerated by irritation from the presence of ova.

Incidence and frequency

In the United States, bladder cancer accounts for about 4% of all cancers in males and about 2% of cancers in females, the comparable figures for England and

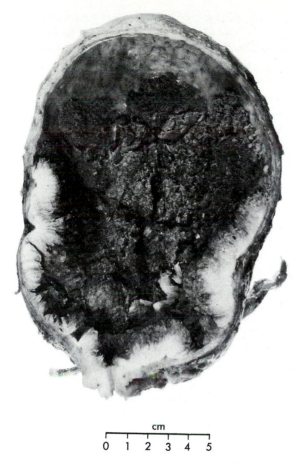

cm
0 1 2 3 4 5

Fig. 20-10. Cystectomy specimen. Multiple papillary tumors cover greater part of bladder wall. There was no histologic evidence of invasion of lamina propria or muscle.

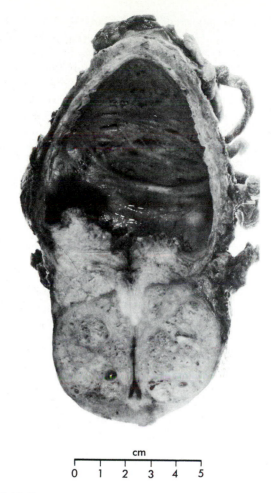

cm
0 1 2 3 4 5

Fig. 20-11. Cystoprostatectomy specimen. There is sessile invasive tumor at bladder base and in prostatic urethra. Note enlarged prostate and vesical trabeculation.

Wales being 7% for males and 2.5% for females. In both countries tumors occur more commonly in males than in females, in ratios of between 2 and 4 males to 1 female. Although tumors may occur at any age, neoplasia is rare in the first five decades but thereafter shows a sharp rise in incidence.

Gross appearance

Urothelial tumors may be single or multiple (Fig. 20-10), finely or coarsely fronded, papillary, sessile (Fig. 20-11), nodular, or ulcerated or, in the in situ disease, recognizable only as areas of mucosal reddening or granularity. When a tumor extends into the bladder wall, there is a variable amount of thickening in and around its base. Tumors may occur anywhere in the bladder but have a predilection for the trigone, the region of the ureteral orifices, and the posterolateral walls.

Microscopic appearance

The recognition of neoplastic change in urothelium using only the light microscope is often difficult, subjective, and dependent in no small measure on the experi-

ence of the observer. Recent work correlating transmission and scanning electron microscope studies with light microscopic findings is beginning to introduce some degree of objectivity and helping to establish more firmly the diagnostic characteristics of normal, premalignant, and malignant epithelium. Pleomorphic microvilli, seen with the scanning electron microscope, are reported in premalignant and malignant epithelia but are not specific features, since they sometimes occur in inflammatory lesions. The luminal membrane of normal urothelium seen with transmission electron microscopy has a unique appearance, and the superficial cells are seen to be joined by tight junctions and desmosomes. The deeper cells similarly are joined by desmosomes whose numbers may be increased in noninvasive tumors and decreased when invasion has occurred. The electron microscope can also reveal discontinuities in the basal lamina that are not seen with the light microscope.

To fully assess a bladder tumor, one needs to determine four specific features: the pattern of its growth, the cell type, the degree of tumor differentiation (or grade), and the depth of invasion of the bladder wall (pathologic stage).

The pattern is determined by examination of histologic sections with a hand lens or the low power of the microscope and can be described as papillary, solid (infiltrating), papillary and solid, or noninvasive (in situ). In the first, tumor growth is into the lumen of the bladder and the tumor can be seen to have a finely fronded pattern with delicate papillary processes. In the solid tumors, growth occurs mostly into the bladder wall, and in a papillary and solid tumor, both types of growth pattern are seen. In the noninvasive tumor there may be very little to see other than, possibly, some localized thickening of the epithelium.

The cell type may be transitional, squamous, or glandular, and it is important to distinguish between squamous metaplasia and squamous carcinoma and between glandular metaplasia and adenocarcinoma. The most practical distinction is that if the squamous or glandular areas are focal within a tumor that is otherwise transitional in type, the correct designation is metaplasia, whereas an overall change indicates a squamous or glandular carcinoma. Another feature of the pure squamous carcinoma is that the infiltrating processes of tumor cells sometimes have a somewhat spiky or angular outline and are surrounded by a fibroblastic or fibrous stroma (Fig. 20-12). The incidence of squamous carcinoma is difficult to assess. Figures of 1% to 7% of all bladder tumors are quoted, with the differences being attributable to failure to distinguish between tumor and metaplasia. Pure adenocarcinoma of the bladder is another rare type of primary tumor and, indeed, most of the grandular tumors

seen in the bladder are extravesical tumors arising, for example, in the bowel and growing into the contiguous bladder wall. Glandular tumors arising at the apex of the bladder may originate in the urachus, and the extremely rare examples occurring at the bladder base are believed to arise either from endodermal remnants or from areas of cystitis glandularis arising by a process of metaplasia in the trigonal epithelium. Pure adenocarcinomas comprise less than 1% of all bladder tumors.

Before describing the grades of transitional cell carcinoma, it is first necessary to define the papilloma and establish the means of distinguishing it from a carcinoma. The papilloma is a papillary lesion with a central core of loose, rather delicate, connective tissue and a covering of transitional epithelium up to four or five layers in thickness. The individual cells vary little, if at all, from normal bladder epithelial cells and are of regular size and shape; they lie at right angles to the basement membrane except for the most superficial layer, which often lies parallel to it. Mitoses are absent. Characteristically the papilloma is a cylindrical structure and, when seen in longitudinal section, has parallel sides, which distinguishes it from polypoid cystitis in which there are tapering fingerlike processes broader at their bases than at their tips. With these criteria the papilloma will be diagnosed only rarely. All other papillary lesions should be considered as carcinomas, provided that polypoid cystitis has been excluded. In many carcinomas there is evidence of penetration of the basement membrane and invasion of the bladder wall, but the diagnosis of carcinoma can and should be made in their absence if the changes in the epithelium justify it.

Transitional cell carcinomas can be divided into three

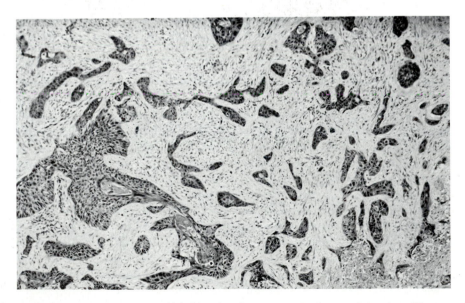

Fig. 20-12. Squamous carcinoma of bladder showing pronounced stromal reaction. (Hematoxylin and eosin; 96×.)

grades depending on their degree of dedifferentiation. In the differentiated (grade I) tumor the cells are clearly of transitional type, but the criteria of papilloma are not fulfilled (Fig. 20-13). The most noticeable difference is a significant increase in the number of layers of cells, usually accompanied by some loss of polarity and minor degrees of hyperchromicity. Occasional mitoses are often seen. The intermediate (grade II) tumor is still recognizable as being of transitional origin (Fig. 20-14). There are more cell layers than in the normal epithelium or papilloma, and this is associated with a greater loss of polarity and more pronounced nuclear hyperchromicity and

mitotic activity than is seen in the differentiated tumor. There may also be some irregularity of the luminal aspect of the epithelium. The anaplastic or undifferentiated (grade III) tumor (Fig. 20-15) is no longer clearly recognizable as having originated in transitional epithelium. All the features noted in the previous grades are much more pronounced, and the superficial layers of cells have often become loosened and been shed into the lumen of the bladder. Squamous and glandular metaplasia may occur in any type of transitional cell tumor, but both are much more common in the less well-differentiated ones.

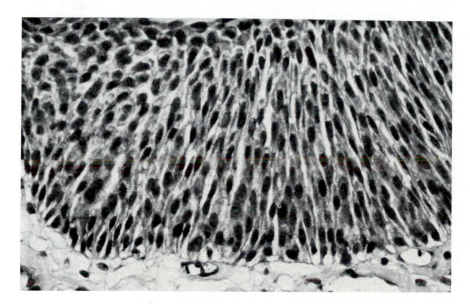

Fig. 20-13. Differentiated (grade I) transitional cell carcinoma. (Hematoxylin and eosin; 600×.)

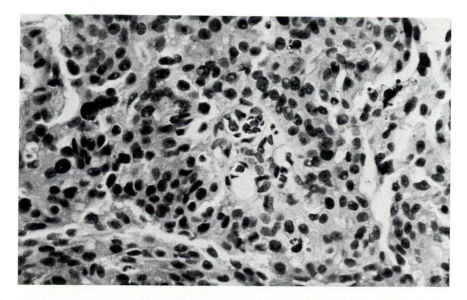

Fig. 20-14. Intermediate grade (grade II) transitional cell carcinoma. (Hematoxylin and eosin; 600×.)

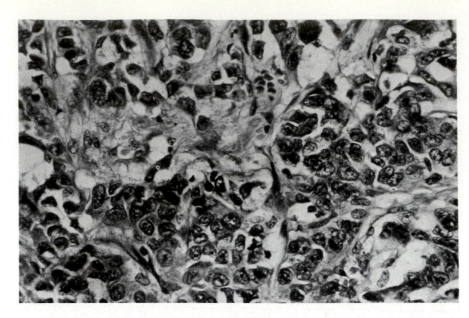

Fig. 20-15. Anaplastic (grade III) carcinoma. (Hematoxylin and eosin; 600×.)

The squamous carcinomas and adenocarcinomas can each be graded similarly according to their degree of differentiation.

From the prognostic point of view it is important to assess the depth to which the bladder wall is invaded by a tumor, that is, to determine the pathologic stage. The greater the amount of tissue available to the pathologist, the more comprehensive and accurate the staging is likely to be, but even in very small specimens the amount of infiltration should always be assessed. The following pathologic stages are recognized in the 1978 edition of the International Union against Cancer (UICC) booklet:

pTis   Preinvasive (in situ) carcinoma
pTa   Papillary noninvasive carcinoma
pT1   Tumor not extending beyond lamina propria
pT2   Invasion of superficial muscle
pT3   Invasion of deep muscle or perivesical tissue
pT4   Invasion of prostate or other extravesical structures
pTO   No tumor found
pTX   Extent of invasion cannot be assessed

It is important to stage a tumor according to the greatest depth reached by its advancing edge. Lymphatic or vascular invasion ahead of the main tumor mass should not increase the stage, although it should be noted.

Proliferative changes, consisting of epithelial hyperplasia, von Brunn's nests, cystitis cystica, and sometimes polypoid cystitis, are commonly seen in the bladder mucosa around the base of the tumor and between multiple tumors even when there is little or no obvious abnormality on unassisted-eye or cystoscopic examination. The specific red cell adherence test, which needs to be further refined before it can be recommended unre-servedly, has been used to assess the invasive potential of bladder tumors.

Carcinoma in situ

Carcinoma in situ, or noninvasive bladder cancer, is an important type of tumor whose natural history is not yet fully known. In some patients it progresses within a relatively short time to papillary or invasive tumor, but in others it remains latent for several years and constitutes an extremely difficult therapeutic problem. It can be defined simply as diffuse or localized histologic change in the epithelium resembling carcinoma, but without evidence of invasion, and characterized by some or all of the following features: an increase in the number of cell layers, crowding of the nuclei, loss of the regular arrangement and polarity of the cells, hyperchromatic nuclei, increased mitotic activity, presence of mitoses above the basal layer of cells, and, frequently, lack of cohesion of the superficial layers of cells, which desquamate into the lumen of the bladder. In fully developed examples one should have no problem in making the diagnosis but may sometimes have difficulty in distinguishing carcinoma in situ from reactive hyperplasia. In some patients monitored with serial biopsies it is possible to see the in situ disease evolve through the stages of hyperplasia and hyperplasia with atypia, but the precise point at which the diagnosis of carcinoma will be made is likely to vary from observer to observer. Regularly repeated cytologic examinations of the urine are essential for diagnosis and for monitoring therapy.

Differential diagnosis

Care should be taken to distinguish between polypoid cystitis and papilloma or papillary carcinoma and not to

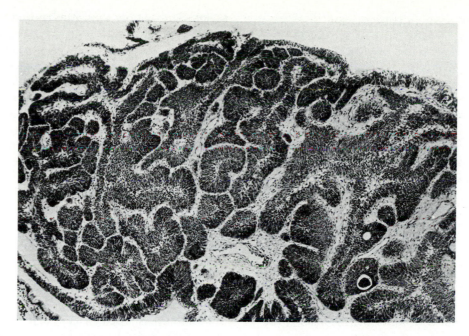

Fig. 20-16. Inverted papilloma of bladder. There is thin surface layer of epithelium, continuous with solid, and occasionally cystic, transitional epithelial masses in lamina propria. (Hematoxylin and eosin; 96×.)

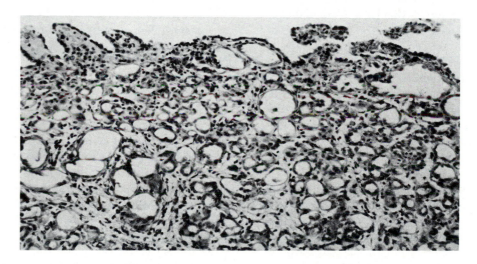

Fig. 20-17. Nephrogenic adenoma. Surface epithelium is cuboid and lamina propria contains many acini and tubules lined by flattened cells. (Hematoxylin and eosin; 96×.)

confuse von Brunn's nests with invasive tumor. There should be no difficulty when the nests are in continuity with the surface, but one should remember that in a late stage of their development they may become separated from the overlying epithelium by a layer of connective tissue. The inverted papilloma (Fig. 20-16), in which there is a localized subepithelial proliferation of epithelium producing a rounded or oval nodule that histologically combines the features of von Brunn's nests and cystitis cystica, is sometimes seen at the bladder base and may be mistaken for a tumor. In the nephrogenic adenoma

(Fig. 20-17), which is almost certainly a reparative lesion occurring after previous mucosal damage, the transitional epithelium is usually replaced by a single layer of cuboid cells from which small acini and tubular structures extend into the underlying lamina propria. This lesion may be mistaken for an adenocarcinoma.

Inflammatory lesions such as eosinophilic cystitis and malakoplakia may simulate a tumor on gross examination, although there should be no difficulty when they are examined microscopically. Problems may also arise with certain types of chronic cystitis, and the practical difficulties that may occur in patients with the clinical picture of interstitial cystitis have already been mentioned. Primary amyloidosis of the bladder may cause profuse hematuria. Histologic examination will reveal deposits of amyloid in the lamina propria, bladder muscle, or blood vessels. The overlying epithelium is frequently thickened and hyperplastic, and if it is unduly polypoid, there may be some resemblance to an epithelial tumor. Endometriosis occasionally involves the bladder and causes hematuria.

Specimens of epithelial tumors at the bladder base obtained by transurethral biopsy are often a problem in histologic diagnosis, and one should remember that a bladder tumor may invade the superficial prostate, that a prostatic carcinoma occasionally spreads upward into the lamina propria of the bladder and masquerades as a bladder tumor, and that very occasionally carcinoma of the bladder and prostate may coexist. The bladder is commonly invaded by gastrointestinal adenocarcinomas, with incipient or actual vesicointestinal fistula and preceding or accompanying polypoid cystitis, and cervical tumors may spread into the bladder base. Other forms of metastasis are uncommon and include transcoelomic spread from upper abdominal malignancies, hematogenous spread in malignant melanoma, and implantation of renal parenchymal carcinomas that have invaded the pelvicalicine system and spread down the ureter.

Spread of urothelial tumors

The most important method of spread is by direct extension into and eventually through the bladder wall and the subsequent invasion of adjacent organs and tethering of the bladder to the pelvic wall. Involvement of one or another ureteral orifice or intramural ureter sometimes occurs relatively early and has an importnat bearing on prognosis.

The tendency for vesical tumors to be associated with tumors elsewhere in the urothelium has already been emphasized. A tumor may recur at its original site after local treatment, but it is difficult, if not impossible, for the urologist always to make a clear distinction between a true recurrence and new multicentric tumor formation. Spread by lymphatics occurs commonly; when the superficial lymphatics in the bladder wall are invaded, there may be centrifugal spread deep to the surface mucosa producing a subepithelial plaque-like mass of tumor, whereas spread by the deeper lymphatics, which is particularly liable to occur with the anaplastic types of tumor, leads to involvement of the regional lymph nodes in the pelvis and abdomen. Blood-borne metastases often occur in the later stages of the disease with deposits in the liver, lungs, bone, and adrenals. Other sites include the heart, brain, and kidney.

Cytologic diagnosis of urothelial tumors

Exfoliative cytology is playing an increasingly important part in the diagnosis of urothelial tumors and is of special value in screening asymptomatic individuals who are at industrial risk. It is also useful as an additional diagnostic aid in patients with hematuria, but the technique has serious limitations if it is used as a method of routine follow-up examination of patients who have already been treated for a bladder tumor. The accuracy of the technique varies from observer to observer, and false-positive results may occur with urinary tract infections and in patients with urinary calculi, and false negatives with low-grade tumors, which in general tend to exfoliate less readily than do high-grade ones. To obtain reproducible results and improve accuracy, it is essential that the techniques of collection and preparation of the specimens be standardized.

Immunologic aspects

Genitourinary malignancy may be associated with changes in both cell-mediated and humoral immunity. Although there is a high incidence of neoplasia in the elderly, and it is known that tumors sometimes occur in patients receiving immunosuppressive therapy, there is as yet no proof that depression of the immune system always precedes or is associated with the early stages of malignancy. The evidence indicates that only in disseminated neoplastic disease is there serious immunodeficiency.

Other tumors

Connective tissue tumors of all types, some benign and some malignant, and taking origin from fibrous tissue, smooth muscle, nerves, and blood vessels, account for only about 5% of all bladder tumors. A number are symptomless and are incidental findings at autopsy or operation, whereas others cause hematuria or, much less commonly, produce hormonal effects such as occur with pheochromocytomas. Some neurofibromatous tumors develop in patients with von Recklinghausen's disease. Lymphomas of the bladder are rare tumors, occurring particularly in middle-aged and elderly patients, producing rounded masses in the lamina propria that have a characteristic appearance when seen with the cystoscope.

The most common bladder tumor in infants and young children is the embryonal sarcoma (Fig. 20-18), which produces pale, fleshy, polypoid, grapelike masses that typically arise over a large area at the base of the bladder. Microscopically the bladder epithelium is usually thinned but is otherwise normal, and the lamina propria is occupied by embryonic mesenchyme consisting of masses of pleomorphic, darkly stained, often stellate cells in a loose, almost myxomatous background. In

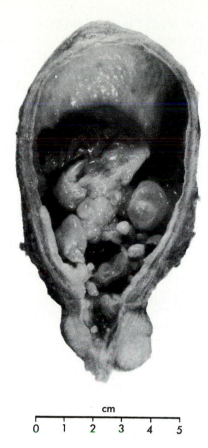

cm

0 1 2 3 4 5

Fig. 20-18. Embryonal sarcoma ("grapelike sarcoma") of bladder base and prostate in young boy.

about half the cases the tumor cells have eosinophilic cytoplasm in which cross-striations can be identified (rhabdomyoblasts). The tumor may also involve the lower ends of the ureters, the prostate, and the seminal vesicles, and in females polypoid masses may be present at the introitus.

THE URACHUS

The urachus is the remains of the narrow allantoic canal, which in fetal life runs between the apex of the bladder and the umbilicus and in adults is not infrequently found incidentally in histologic sections taken from the fundus of the bladder. The central lumen is usually small, and the wall consists of a layer of cuboid, low columnar, or transitional epithelium, a small amount of connective tissue, and a smooth muscle sheath, which is distinct from the surrounding bladder muscle. Part or all of the urachus may remain patent after birth. If the entire canal is open (urachal fistula), urine is discharged at the umbilicus. Patency at the vesical end only leads to the formation of a urachal diverticulum, and if the other end is patent at the umbilicus, there is a urachal sinus. A urachal cyst forms if the two ends are closed off and the

central portion becomes distended. The tumors arising in the urachus are derived from its epithelial lining or, less commonly, from the surrounding fibrous tissue and muscle. The most frequent type is an adenocarcinoma, which only rarely involves the mucosal surface of the bladder and grows either in the deeper part of the bladder wall or outside it in the supravesical area, where it may form a mass of considerable size. The prognosis is not good, and the tumors must be excised widely to prevent local recurrence.

REFERENCES

1. Alroy, J., Pauli, D.U., and Weinstein, R.S.: Correlation between numbers of desmosomes and the aggressiveness of transitional cell carcinoma in human urinary bladder, Cancer **47:**104, 1981.
2. Andersen, D.A.: Historical and geographical differences in the pattern of incidence of urinary stones considered in relation to possible aetiological factors. In Hodgkinson, A., and Nordin, B.E.C., editors: Renal Stone Research Symposium, London, 1969, J. & A. Churchill, Ltd.
3. Andersen, J.A., and Hansen, B.F.: The incidence of cell nests, cystitis cystica and cystitis glandularis in the lower urinary tract revealed by autopsies, J. Urol. **108:**421, 1972.
4. Aquilina, J.N., and Bugeja, T.J.: Primary malignant lymphoma of the bladder: case report and review of the literature, J. Urol. **112:**64, 1974.
5. Babaian, R.J., et al.: Metastases from carcinoma of the urinary bladder, Urology **16:**142, 1980.
6. Barlebo, H., Sorensen, B.L., and Ohlsen, A.S.: Carcinoma in situ of urinary bladder—flat intraepithelial neoplasia, Scand. J. Urol. Nephrol. **6:**213, 1972.
7. Barrett, J.C.: Gangrenous cystitis, Br. J. Urol. **34:**312, 1962.
8. Booth, C.M., Cameron, K.M., and Pugh, R.C.B.: Urothelial carcinoma of the kidney and ureter, Br. J. Urol. **52:**430, 1980.
9. Brannan, W., Lucas, T.A., and Mitchell, W.T., Jr.: Accuracy of cytologic examination of urinary sediment in the detection of urothelial tumors, J. Urol. **109:**483, 1973.
10. Brumfitt, W., and Asscher, A.W.: Urinary tract infection: proceedings of the Second National Symposium held in London, 1972, London, 1973, Oxford University Press.
11. Carpenter, A.A.: Pelvic lipomatosis: successful surgical treatment, J. Urol. **110:**397, 1973.
12. Carswell, J.W.: Intraperitoneal rupture of the bladder, Br. J. Urol. **46:**425, 1974.
13. Catalona, W.J.: Practical utility of specific red cell adherence test in bladder cancer, Urology **18:**113, 1981.
14. Clayson, D.B.: Recent research into occupational bladder cancer. In Connolly, J.G., editor: Carcinoma of the bladder, New York, 1981, Raven Press.
15. Cohen, G.H.: Obstructive uropathy caused by ureteral candidiasis, J. Urol. **110:**285, 1973.
16. Cole, P.: Coffee drinking and cancer of the lower urinary tract, Lancet **1:**1335, 1971.
17. Cole, P., et al.: Smoking and cancer of the lower urinary tract, N. Engl. J. Med. **284:**129, 1971.
18. Cullen, T.H., Popham, R.R., and Voss, H.J.: An evaluation of routine cytological examination of the urine, Br. J. Urol. **39:**615, 1967.
19. Cyr, W.L., Johnson, H., and Balfour, J.: Granulomatous cystitis as a manifestation of chronic granulomatous disease of childhood, J. Urol. **110:**357, 1973.
20. Dale, G.A., and Smith, R.B.: Transitional cell carcinoma of the bladder associated with cyclophosphamide, J. Urol. **112:**603, 1974.
21. Davies, R., and Hunt, A.C.: Surface topography of the female bladder trigone, J. Clin. Pathol. **34:**308, 1981.
22. de Klotz, R.J., and Young, B.W.: Conservative surgery in the management of benign ureteral polyps, Br. J. Urol. **36:**375, 1964.

23. Doctor, V.M., Phadke, A.G., and Sirsat, M.V.: Pheochromocytoma of the urinary bladder, Br. J. Urol. **44:**351, 1972.
24. Finlay-Jones, L.R., Blackwell, J.B., and Papadimitriou, J.M.: Malakoplakia of the colon, Am. J. Clin. Pathol. **50:**320, 1968.
25. Friedman, N.B., and Ash, J.E.: Tumors of the urinary bladder, AFIP atlas of tumor pathology, sect. VIII—sect. 31a, Washington, D.C., 1959, Armed Forces Institute of Pathology.
26. Friedman, N.B., and Kuhlenbeck, H.: Adenomatoid tumors of the bladder reproducing renal structures (nephrogenic adenomas), J. Urol. **64:**657, 1950.
27. Gettel, R.R., Lee, F., and Ratliff, R.K.: Ureteral diverticula, J. Urol. **108:**392, 1972.
28. Gordon, H.L., et al.: Immunologic aspects of interstitial cystitis, J. Urol. **109:**228, 1973.
29. Halawani, A., Al-Waidh, M., and Said, S.M.: Serology in the study of the relationship between S. haematobium infestation and cancer of the urinary bladder, Br. J. Urol. **42:**580, 1970.
30. Hanna, M.K.: Bilateral retroiliac-artery ureters, Br. J. Urol. **44:**339, 1972.
31. Hanson, L., et al.: Biology and pathology of urinary tract infections, J. Clin. Pathol. **34:**695, 1981.
32. Harmer, M.H., editor: TNM classification of malignant tumours, ed. 3, Geneva, 1979, International Union against Cancer.
33. Hicks, R.M.: Carcinogenesis in the urinary bladder: a multistage process. In Connolly, J.G., editor: Carcinoma of the bladder, New York, 1981, Raven Press.
34. Hicks, R.M., et al.: Demonstration of n-nitrosamines in human urine: preliminary observations on a possible aetiology for bladder cancer in association with chronic urinary tract infections, Proc. R. Soc. Med. **70:**413, 1977.
35. Highman, W., and Wilson, E.: Urine cytology in patients with calculi, J. Clin. Pathol. **35:**350, 1982.
36. Hodge, J.: Avulsion of a long segment of ureter with Dormia basket, Br. J. Urol. **45:**328, 1973.
37. Jacobs, J.B., et al.: Scanning electron microscopic features of human urinary bladder cancer, Cancer **48:**1399, 1981.
38. Javadpour, N., Solomon, T., and Bush, I.M.: Obstruction of the lower ureter by aberrant vessels in children, J. Urol. **108:**340, 1972.
39. Johansson, S., et al.: Uroepithelial tumors of the renal pelvis associated with abuse of phenacetin-containing analgesics, Cancer **33:**743, 1974.
40. Johnson, F.R.: Some proliferative and metaplastic changes in transitional epithelium, Br. J. Urol. **29:**112, 1957.
41. Lambird, P.A., and Yardley, J.H.: Malakoplakia: report of a fatal case with ultrastructural observations on Michaelis-Gutmann bodies, Johns Hopkins Med. J. **126:**1, 1970.
42. Malek, R.S., Greene, L.F., and Farrow, G.M.: Amyloidosis of the urinary bladder, Br. J. Urol. **43:**189, 1971.
43. Marshall, F.F., and Middleton, A.W., Jr.: Eosinophilic cystitis, J. Urol. **112:**335, 1974.
44. Morgan, R.J., and Cameron, K.M.: Vesical leukoplakia, Br. J. Urol. **52:**96, 1980.
45. Marshall, V.F., and Keuhnelian, J.G.: Crossed ureteral ectopia with solitary kidney, J. Urol. **110:**176, 1973.
46. Mostofi, F.K., Sobin, L.H., and Torloni, H.: W.H.O. international histological classification of tumours, no. 10—Histological typing of urinary bladder tumours, Geneva, 1973, World Health Organization.
47. Newman, J., and Hicks, R.M.: Detection of neoplastic and pre-neoplastic urothelia by combined scanning and transmission electron microscopy of urinary surface of human bladders, Histopathology **1:**125, 1977.
48. O'Flynn, J.D., and Mullaney, J.: Vesical leukoplakia progressing to carcinoma, Br. J. Urol. **46:**31, 1974.
49. O'Grady, F., and Brumfitt, W.: Urinary tract infection. Proceedings of the First National Symposium held in London, 1968, London, 1968, Oxford University Press.
50. O'Kane, H.O.J., and Megaw, J. McI.: Carcinoma of the exstrophic bladder, Br. J. Surg. **55:**631, 1968.
51. Ormond, J.K.: Idiopathic retroperitoneal fibrosis: an established clinical entity, J.A.M.A. **174:**1561, 1960.
52. Packham, D.A.: The epithelial lining of the female trigone and urethra, Br. J. Urol. **43:**201, 1971.
53. Peterson, L.J., Paulson, D.F., and Bonar, R.A.: Response of human urothelium to chemical carcinogens in vitro, J. Urol. **111:**154, 1974.
54. Peterson, L.J., Paulson, D.F., and Glenn, J.F.: The histopathology of vesical diverticula, J. Urol. **110:**62, 1973.
55. Potts, I.F., and Hirst, E.: Inverted papilloma of the bladder, J. Urol. **90:**175, 1963.
56. Prall, R.H., Wernett, C., and Mims, M.M.: Diagnostic cytology in urinary tract malignancy, Cancer **29:**1084, 1972.
57. Price, D.A., Morley, A.R., and Hall, R.R.: Scanning electron microscopy in the study of normal inflamed and neoplastic human urothelium, Br. J. Urol. **52:**370, 1980.
58. Ransley, P.G.: Vesico-ureteric reflux. In Hendry, W.F., editor: Recent advances in urology/andrology, ed. 3, New York, 1981, Churchill Livingstone.
59. Reiter's disease, Br. Med. J. **4:**576, 1969.
60. Rose, G.A., and Wallace, D.M.: Observations on urinary chemiluminescence of normal smokers and non-smokers and of patients with bladder cancer, Br. J. Urol. **45:**520, 1973.
61. Rubin, L., and Pincus, M.B.: Eosinophilic cystitis: the relationship of allergy in the urinary tract to eosinophilic cystitis and the pathophysiology of eosinophilia, J. Urol. **112:**457, 1974.
62. Schulman, C.C.: Electron microscopy of the human ureteric innervation, Br. J. Urol. **46:**609, 1974.
63. Slater, R.B., and Kirkpatrick, J.R.: A case of closed injury of the upper ureter, Br. J. Urol. **43:**591, 1971.
64. Smith, A.F.: An ultrastructural and morphometric study of bladder cancer, Virchows Arch. (Pathol. Anat.) **390:**11, 1981.
65. Stamey, T.A.: Pathogenesis and treatment of urinary tract infections, Baltimore, 1980, The Williams & Williams Co.
66. Stanton, M.J., and Maxted, W.: Malacoplakia: a study of the literature and current concepts of pathogenesis, diagnosis and treatment, J. Urol. **125:**139, 1981.
67. Sutor, D.J., Wooley, S.E., and Illingworth, J.J.: A geographical and historical survey of the composition of urinary stones, Br. J. Urol. **46:**393, 1974.
68. Tannenbaum, M., Tannenbaum, S., and Romas, N.A.: Conformational membrane changes in early bladder cancer. In Connolly, J.G., editor: Carcinoma of the bladder, New York, 1981, Raven Press.
69. Turner-Warwick, R., et al.: A urodynamic view of the clinical problems associated with bladder neck dysfunction and its treatment by endoscopic incision and transtrigonal posterior prostatectomy, Br. J. Urol. **45:**44, 1973.
70. Union Internationale contre le Cancer: Cancer incidence in five continents, vol. 2, Geneva, 1970, Springer-Verlag.
71. Utz, D.C., Hanash, K.A., and Farrow, G.M.: The plight of the patient with carcinoma in situ of the bladder, Trans. Am. Assoc. Genitourin. Surg. **61:**90, 1969.
72. Utz, D.C., et al.: Carcinoma in situ of the bladder, Cancer **45:**1842, 1980.
73. Wallace, D.M.: Urothelial neoplasia: causes, assessment and treatment, Ann. R. Coll. Surg. Eng. **51:**91, 1972.
74. Wallace, D.M., Chisholm, G.D., and Hendry, W.F.: T.N.M. classification of urological tumours (U.I.C.C.), 1974, Br. J. Urol. **47:**1, 1975.
75. Watson, N.A., and Notley, R.G.: Urological complications of cyclophosphamide, Br. J. Urol. **45:**606, 1973.
76. Wesolowski, S.: Bilateral ureteral injuries in gynaecology, Br. J. Urol. **41:**666, 1969.
77. Whitaker, R.H., Pugh, R.C.B., and Dow, D.: Colonic tumours following uretero-sigmoidostomy, Br. J. Urol. **43:**562, 1971.
78. Whitehead, E.D., and Tessler, A.N.: Carcinoma of the urachus, Br. J. Urol. **43:**468, 1971.
79. Williams, D.I.: Urology in childhood. Handbuch der Urologie [Encyclopedia of urology], vol. XV, supplement, New York, 1974, Springer-Verlag.
80. Wisheart, J.D.: Primary tumours of the ureteric stump following nephrectomy, Br. J. Urol. **40:**344, 1968.
81. Zincke, H., Furlow, W.L., and Farrow, G.M.: Candida albicans cystitis: report of a case with special emphasis on diagnosis and treatment, J. Urol. **109:**612, 1973.

CHAPTER 21 Male Reproductive System and Prostate

F. KASH MOSTOFI
CHARLES J. DAVIS, Jr.

TESTES

Normally the adult testicle is located in the scrotum. Its main components are the seminiferous tubules. Germ cells in various stages of maturation comprise the major population of adult normal seminiferous tubules, and their sole function is to produce spermatozoa. In addition to these cells, the seminiferous tubules also contain the sustentacular cells of Sertoli, which have three functions: (1) they support the germ cells; (2) they produce estrogens and some androgens; and (3) they form the basement membrane of the seminiferous tubules. The seminiferous tubules drain into collecting ducts, which join to form the rete testis, thence vasa efferentia, and finally the epididymis; these serve to transmit the spermatozoa out of the gonad. The seminiferous tubules are surrounded by a delicate basement membrane (tunica propria) and are supported by a delicate fibrovascular stroma in which varying numbers of interstitial cells of Leydig are seen. The main functions of Leydig cells are to constitute part of the supporting stroma of the gonad and to produce hormones; they are the main source of testosterone and other androgenic hormones in men, and they produce estrogens and possibly progesterone and corticosteroids. Sertoli and Leydig cells are thus the hormone-producing cells of the male gonad and, along with their homologues in the ovary (theca-granulosa cell), are designated the specialized stromal cells of the gonad to differentiate them from the usual fibrovascular stroma that the gonads have in common with all other organs. The entire structure is covered by tunica, which contains the smooth muscle layer of Dartos. The outer layer is covered by mesothelium. Thus, in addition to the testicle, the scrotum contains the testicular adnexa.

Anomalies

Excluding malposition of the testicle, anomalies are very rare. Anorchidism (congenital absence) and monorchidism (one testicle) have been reported. Synorchidism (fusion of testicles) occurs intra-abdominally. Polyorchidism has been found at operation and necropsy.

Ectopic testis

Ectopic testis is a congenital malposition of the testicle outside the normal channel of descent. This ectopia, according to its location, is classified as interstitial, pubopenile, femoral, crural, transverse, or perineal.

Cryptorchidism

When the congenital malposition results in retention of the testicle anywhere along the route of descent, it is known as cryptorchidism. The cause of cryptorchidism is not always evident. The various apparent causes are short spermatic vessels of vas deferens, adhesions to the peritoneum, poorly developed inguinal canal or superficial abdominal ring, maldevelopment of the scrotum or cremaster muscles, and hormonal influences. Incomplete descent is found quite frequently during the first few months of infancy. The incidence is about 4% in boys under 15 years of age and about 0.2% in adults. Histologically the cryptorchid testis before puberty does not differ from the normally descended organ (Fig. 21-1). After puberty, however, it is always smaller than normal. The capsule is somewhat thickened and wrinkled. The epididymis is separated from the mesorchium. There is progressive loss of germ cell elements. The tubules may be lined only with spermatogonia and spermatids, but occasionally there is spermatogenesis. In fact, foci of spermatogenesis are found in 10% of undescended testes. This condition has also been reported in abdominal testis. It is estimated that 10% of men with untreated cryptorchidism remain fertile. The basement membrane of the tubules thickens and hyalinizes. In later stages spermatogenesis is rare or absent and the tubules are lined only with Sertoli cells. Tubules with completely occluded lumina are not uncommon. The collecting tubules and rete may be quite prominent, a condition

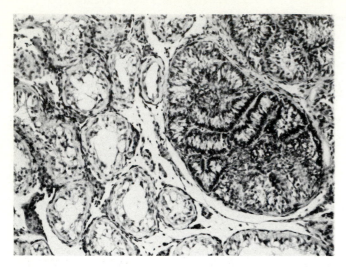

Fig. 21-1. Cryptorchid testis. Note the two islands of immature tubules. (100×.)

that suggests hyperplasia and even adenoma. The intertubular tissue is sparsely cellular and becomes more dense with age. The interstitial cells of Leydig are conspicuous and vary in number. In some cases the Leydig cells are decreased in number, and in other cases they are increased both in size and in number. They are found singly, in small groups, and occasionally in large masses. In some cryptorchid testicles most of the atrophied organ is composed of large groups of polyhedral Leydig cells, between which may be found scanty fibrous tissue and a few fibrosed tubules. In rare instances very few cellular elements are encountered and the entire testes become completely fibrosed.

The cause of atrophy of undescended and ectopic testes is not known. There is convincing evidence that an optimum temperature is necessary for spermatogenesis and that temperatures higher than that within the scrotum suppress spermatogenesis. When aspermia or hypospermia exists, the testicle atrophies. The chief function of the scrotum is to regulate the temperature for the testes. Ischemia caused by pressure, stressed by some authors, is definitely a minor factor in causing suppression of spermatogenesis in cryptorchidism. There is a high incidence of tumors of the testes in cryptorchidism.

Intersexuality

A true hermaphrodite or ambisexual is one who possesses an ovary and a testicle or true ovotestes with or without external genitalia of both sexes. A pseudohermaphrodite possesses gonads of one sex and genitalia of either both sexes or the opposite sex. In the male pseudohermaphrodite the testes are present but the internal genitalia are of both sexes, and the penis and scrotum are poorly developed. In the female pseudohermaphrodite the ovaries are present, usually in their normal position,

the vagina is rudimentary and opens into the urethra, and the clitoris is hypertrophied.

Testis in male infertility

About 15 of every 100 marriages in the United States are barren, and male infertility accounts for about half of the cases. In all such patients quantitative determination of urinary 17-ketosteroids, estrogens, and gonadotropins, karyotyping, and testicular biopsy are essential to determine the specific cause of the male infertility and whether it is curable. Wong, Straus, and Warner[64-66] have proposed a simple classification of male infertility: pretesticular, testicular, and posttesticular.

Pretesticular causes of infertility are mainly hypopituitarism, endogenous or exogenous estrogen or androgen excess, hypothyroidism, diabetes mellitus, and glucocorticoid excess.

Hypopituitarism may be prepubertal or postpubertal. Prepubertal causes include lesions in or adjacent to the pituitary, for example, craniopharyngiomas, trauma, and cysts. Such patients eventually manifest sexual infantilism, failure of somatic growth, and varying degrees of adrenal and thyroid hypofunction. Testicular biopsy shows small immature seminiferous tubules and immature Leydig cells similar to those in prepubertal testis.

Postpubertal hypopituitarism results from tumors, trauma, or infarction. Testicular biopsy shows maturation arrest, loss of germ cells, reduced diameter of tubules, and progressive thickening and hyalinization of tunica propria. The Leydig cells are small and shriveled.

Hypopituitarism may be the result of genetic defects in gonadotropin secretion. There are no demonstrable lesions of the pituitary or deficiencies of adrenal and thyroid function or growth. The patients may show deficiency of both follicle-stimulating hormone (FSH) and luteinizing hormone (LH), or the FSH may be normal but the LH deficient. Testicular biopsy in the former shows small and immature seminiferous tubules resembling prepubertal testis. In the latter the seminiferous tubules show a greater degree of development than do the Leydig cells. In both cases the patients are generally tall and eunuchoid.

Estrogen excess may be endogenous (hepatic cirrhosis, adrenal tumor, Sertoli or Leydig cell tumor) or exogenous (administered to patients with cancer of prostate). Initially the biopsy shows failure of maturation, progressive decrease of germinal elements, diminished diameter of seminiferous tubules, and thickening and hyalinization of tunica propria. Eventually there are complete sclerosis of tubules and atrophy of Leydig cells. The findings are identical to those in postpubertal hypopituitarism.

Androgen excess may be endogenous (adrenogenital syndrome or androgen-producing adrenocortical or testicular tumors) or exogenous (oral administration). Pathologic findings depend on whether the condition developed before or after puberty. If prepubertal, the result is virilism and failure of the testis to mature. If postpubertal, there are progressive loss of germ cells and, unless recognized and remedied, tubular sclerosis.

Glucocorticoid excess, whether endogenous (Cushing's syndrome) or exogenous (administered for treatment of ulcerative colitis, rheumatoid arthritis, or bronchial asthma) can result in oligospermia and maturation arrest or hypospermatogenesis.

Hypothyroidism and diabetes mellitus may result in decreased fertility. Hypospermatogenesis is followed by thickening of tunica propria. In uncontrolled diabetes autonomic neuropathy may result in impotence.

Testicular causes of infertility are agonadism, cryptorchidism, maturation arrest, hypospermatogenesis, absence of germ cells (Sertoli cell–only syndrome), Klinefelter's syndrome, mumps orchitis, and irradiation damage.

Agonadism

Congenital agonadism is extremely rare and consists of total absence of the testes. If this occurs in early embryonic life, the infant will be female. Occasionally in cryptorchid boys the epididymis ends blindly, but careful search fails to show any gonadal tissue (vanishing testis syndrome). The chromosomal pattern is XY. Because testes must have been present in fetal life to initiate development, they must have been resorbed after that period.

Bilateral anorchia may be associated with incomplete differentiation of male genitalia. The gonads and the internal genital structures may be absent or rudimentary. These findings suggest that the testes must have been present to initiate male sex development but vanished before maturity.

Jost[62] showed that fetal testis plays an important role in the early development of the wolffian structures and regression of müllerian elements. The development of wolffian structures is related to the local androgen production, whereas regression of müllerian elements seems to be influenced by additional nonandrogenic factors. Federman's[57] excellent discussion of the situation may be summarized as follows: If the male fetus begins life with dysgenetic testis, varying degrees of pseudohermaphroditism may ensue; if gonadal failure occurs before organization of the genital tract, female external genitalia will result; if gonadal failure occurs during the period of male sexual differentiation, ambiguous genitalia may result; if, however, testicular failure occurs after the sixteenth week of gestation, the male structures are established and the fetus will develop as a male but without testes.

Cryptorchidism

The histology of cryptorchidism is described on p. 791.

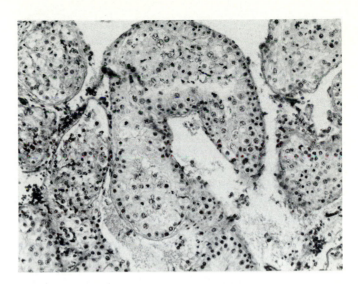

Fig. 21-2. Maturation arrest. (160×.)

Maturation arrest

Maturation arrest is manifested in a testicular biopsy by the failure of normal spermatogenesis at some stage. Complete maturation arrest consists of failure of spermatogenesis beyond one of the immature phases of the process (Fig. 21-2). No secondary spermatocytes, spermatids, or spermatozoa are present. Incomplete maturation arrest is similar except that in some areas maturation has progressed to the spermatid stage and in some areas even to spermatozoa. The Sertoli cells, tunica propria, and Leydig cells are normal, as is the diameter of the seminiferous tubules. Oligospermia or azoospermia is present. Levels of urinary FSH, LH, and 17-ketosteroids are normal.

Hypospermatogenesis

Hypospermatogenesis is more difficult to detect (Fig. 21-3). All cells of spermatogenic series are present in the same proportions as normal, but the number of each variety is decreased. The seminiferous tubules are of normal size. Sertoli and Leydig cells and the tunica of the tubules are normal. Patients have oligospermia with normal urinary FSH, LH, and 17-ketosteroid levels.

Absence of germ cells (Sertoli cell–only syndrome)

Two categories of germ cell absence are recognized: congenital (Del Castillo syndrome) and acquired. In the former there is usually complete absence of germ cells (Fig. 21-4); in the latter some seminiferous tubules may show persistent germ cell elements. The diameter of seminiferous tubules is decreased, the tunica propria of the tubule is not thickened, and the Leydig cells are normal. The secondary sex characteristics are well developed; the patients are potent but infertile. The urinary 17-ketosteroid levels are normal, but urinary FSH and LH levels are invariably high.

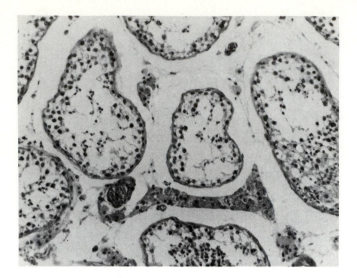

Fig. 21-3. Hypospermatogenesis. (160×.)

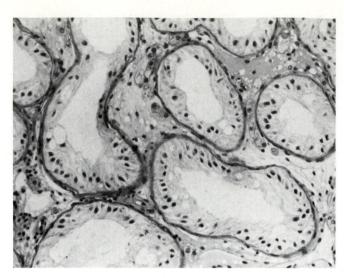

Fig. 21-4. Sertoli cell–only syndrome. (100×.)

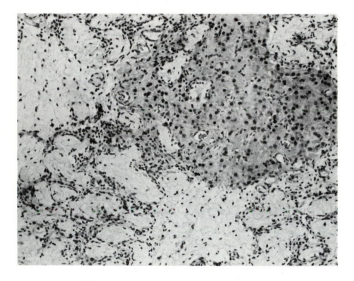

Fig. 21-5. Klinefelter's syndrome. (70×.)

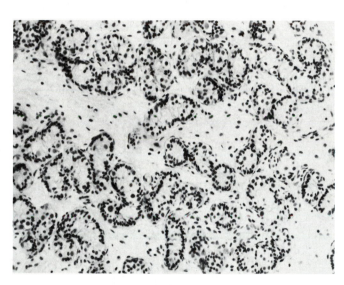

Fig. 21-6. Kallman's syndrome. (100×.)

Klinefelter's syndrome

About 3% of male sterility is attributable to primary hypogonadism. This syndrome is characterized by testicular hypoplasia, azoospermia, gynecomastia, eunuchoid build, increase in urinary gonadotropin, and, not infrequently, subnormal intelligence (Fig. 21-5). The diagnosis is seldom made before puberty. Chromosome studies reveal an XXY intersexuality caused by fertilization of an ovum in which the divided X chromosome failed to separate. Such individuals have a sex-chromatin pattern similar to genetic females. However, other individuals with a similar or nearly similar syndrome are genetically males. There is increased urinary excretion of pituitary gonadotropic hormones.

The testes are usually small (1.5 × 0.5 cm). The histologic findings vary widely. The tubules are sclerosed and

hyalinized, and there is an apparent increase in the number of interstitial cells. Tubular fibrosis is progressive and is associated with retardation of spermatogenesis. Spermatogenic activity varies greatly. Careful examination of a biopsy specimen may fail to show any activity whatsoever, but it may be found on examination of the entire testis. Maturation as far as primary spermatogenesis, even to the stage of secondary spermatogenesis and spermatids and, in rare instances, spermatozoa, has been reported. The release of sperm from the testis to the ejaculate is uncommon, but a few have been observed.

Kallman's syndrome

Kallman's syndrome is a form of hypogonadotropic hypogonadism also referred to as olfactory-genital syndrome. It is characterized by anosmia, occasional color

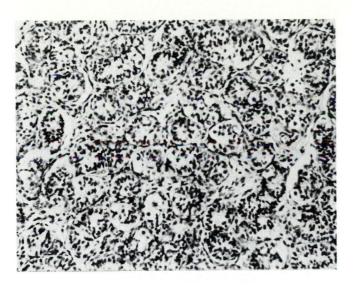

Fig. 21-7. Immature testes. (100×.)

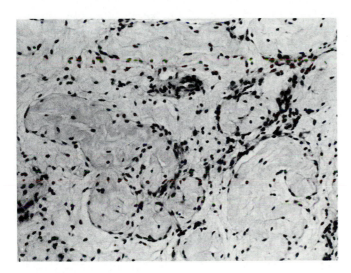

Fig. 21-8. Tubular interstitial sclerosis. (100×.)

blindness, and congenital absence of Leydig cells, resulting in eunuchoidism and infantile testes, scrotum, and penis (Fig. 21-6).

Immature testes

As the name indicates, the testes are morphologically identical to those of prepubertal individuals (Fig. 21-7). The condition is seen in prepubertal gonadotropin deficiency (isolated gonadotropin deficiency and Kallman's syndrome).

Tubular and interstitial sclerosis

Tubular and interstitial fibrosis is an end stage in which all the seminiferous tubules are sclerotic and the interstitium is fibrotic (Fig. 21-8). The testes are small, and there is total absence of spermatogenesis.

Excurrent duct obstruction

Obstruction at any point from the epididymis to the ejaculatory ducts results in zero sperm count (azoospermia), but the testes are of normal size and testicular biopsy shows active but not necessarily normal spermatogenesis.

Mumps orchitis

The histologic findings in mumps orchitis are described on p. 791. Ten to 20 years after the initial infection, depending on the extent of testicular involvement, there may be oligospermia or azoospermia. The 17-ketosteroid and LH levels are normal, but the level of FSH is elevated.

Irradiation damage

Permanent germ cell destruction results from exposure to radiation so that in time the tubules are lined by Sertoli cells only. The diameter of seminiferous tubules is progressively smaller, and the tunica is thicker, terminating in sclerosis. Leydig cells are preserved. The patient is azoospermic or oligospermic. The urinary FSH level is elevated, but the 17-ketosteroid and LH levels are normal.

Posttesticular causes of infertility

Posttesticular causes of infertility consist mainly of block, which may be congenital (absence or atresia of vas deferens or epididymis) or acquired. Acquired is more frequent and may result from infection (such as gonorrhea) or surgical intervention (voluntary or iatrogenic). The clinical manifestation is azoospermia. The testicular biopsy specimen in such patients shows active spermatogenesis. The seminiferous tubules may be dilated, and there may be hypospermatogenesis or cellular sloughing or both.

Another cause of posttesticular infertility is impaired sperm mobility. Wong and associates[64-66] reserve this term specifically for those patients in whom sperm counts are adequate and testicular biopsy specimens are normal, yet the mobility of spermatozoa in the semen is either greatly impaired or absent.

In all men with infertility, testicular biopsy is necessary for proper categorization and prognosis.

Acquired atrophy

Excluding undescended testicles, acquired atrophy occurs in senility, prolonged hyperpyrexia, debility, avitaminosis, cirrhosis of the liver, hypothyroidism, schizophrenia, estrogen medication for carcinoma of the prostate, and diseases of the pituitary gland and hypothalamus. Faulty or suppressed spermatogenesis without other changes may questionably be considered mild atrophy. The early findings in atrophy are degenerative changes of the spermatogonia cells. As atrophy progresses, the germinal epithelial cells disappear, leaving

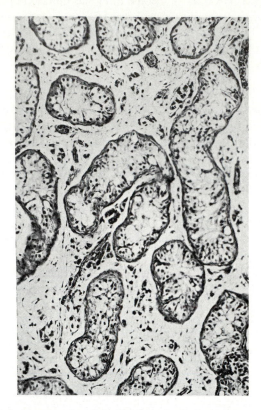

Fig. 21-9. Atrophy of testicle. Thickened tubular basement membranes are lined with degenerated spermatogonia and Sertoli cells. Leydig cells are prominent in interstitial tissue. (100×.)

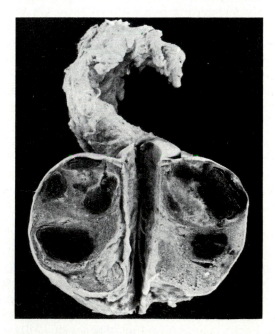

Fig. 21-10. Multiple infarcts of testicle in polyarteritis nodosa.

only Sertoli cells resting on a thickened basement membrane. The seminiferous tubules become small and farther apart, and the interstitial cells of Leydig appear prominent (Fig. 21-9).

Thrombosis and infarction

Hemorrhage, thrombosis, and infarction of the testicle occur in trauma, torsion, leukemias, bacterial endocarditis, and polyarteritis nodosa (Fig. 21-10). Birth trauma may cause hemorrhage of the testicle. Many such hemorrhages are small hematomas that resorb rapidly.

Torsion

A sudden twisting of the spermatic cord results in strangulation of the blood vessels serving the testicle and epididymis. The predisposing causes of torsion are free mobility and high attachment of the testicle. These anatomic features are found in such conditions as failure of the tunica vaginalis to close, large tunica vaginalis, absence of scrotal ligaments, gubernaculum testis or posterior mesorchium, or elongation of the globus minor. Abnormal attachment of the common mesentery and vessels to the globus minor and lower pole of the testicle provides attachment of the testicle by a narrow stalk instead of a wide band. The exciting cause may be violent exercise or straining. The majority of the cases of torsion involve undescended testicles. Torsion may occur at any age; cases have been reported in newborn infants and in very elderly persons. The twist is commonly located in the free intravaginal portion of the cord. It may be a half turn to two full turns in either direction. The gross and microscopic findings depend on the degree of strangulation. Usually the picture is that of congestion and hemorrhage followed by necrosis of the testicle. The interstitial tissue may or may not be infiltrated with leukocytes. The tubules suffer varying degrees of degeneration and necrosis. At times the entire testicle is found to be necrotic and acellular, and "ghost" tubules remain as conspicuous components in the histologic picture.

Inflammation orchitis

Acute orchitis. Acute orchitis is (1) an infection via the vas deferens and epididymis, (2) a combination epididymo-orchitis, or (3) a metastatic lymphogenous or hematogenous infection. Epididymo-orchitis is predominantly caused by urethritis, cystitis, and seminal vesiculitis. Acute orchitis may be a complication of mumps, smallpox, scarlet fever, diphtheria, typhoid fever, glanders, dengue fever, influenza, typhus fever, pneumonia, malaria, filariasis, and Mediterranean fever. Acute orchitis also has been encountered as a complication in focal infections such as sinusitis, osteomyelitis, cholecystitis, and appendicitis.

In acute orchitis the testicle becomes firm, tense, and swollen. In gonorrheal orchitis, which is usually an extension from the epididymis, single or multiple abscesses develop or the testicle may be diffusely infiltrated with neutrophilic leukocytes, lymphocytes, and plasma cells.

Mumps orchitis. The incidence of orchitis as a complication of parotitis is between 20% and 30%. This complication occurs mostly in adults. Grossly the testicle is enlarged, and the tunica albuginea contains punctate hemorrhages. In the early stages the parenchyma appears edematous. Microscopically the acute inflammatory process is characterized by diffuse interstitial infiltration with polymorphonuclear neutrophils, lymphocytes, and histiocytes. Similar cellular elements fill the lumina and distend the tubules. Very few tubules suffer necrosis, but in severe cases the germinal epithelial cells and spermatogonia undergo degeneration with subsequent loss of spermatogenesis. In subacute and chronic phases of mumps orchitis, the interstitial tissue is infiltrated with lymphocytes. When degeneration has been extensive, the testicle becomes smaller and the thickened tubules are lined with a few Sertoli cells. The incidence of testicular atrophy and consequent sterility in this type of orchitis is not known.

Chronic orchitis. Acute inflammation of the testicle may completely resolve, or the inflammation may continue in a chronic form. The inflammation may be focal or diffuse, unilateral or bilateral. In some cases fibrosis may be seen grossly. There is a varying degree of degeneration and disappearance of the tubular cells, and the basement membranes of the tubules become thickened and hyalinized. Many patients with testicular tumors give a history of some form of orchitis.

Granulomatous orchitis. The etiology and pathogenesis of a rather characteristic type of nonspecific granulomatous orchitis that may be misinterpreted as tuberculosis have not been entirely clarified despite excellent research and studies of the lesion. It occurs predominantly among middle-aged men and frequently is associated with trauma. Grossly the testis is enlarged, and the tunica albuginea may be normal or thickened. The tissue is usually grayish, white, tan, or brownish. Histologically there is a striking tuberculoid pattern. The relatively circumscribed microscopic tubercles originate from and within the tubules. They are composed of epithelioid cells, lymphocytes, plasma cells, some polymorphonuclear neutrophils, and multinucleated giant cells. The walls of the tubules are thickened by fibrous proliferation and, with the inflammatory cellular infiltrate, blend with the contiguous interstitial tissue. The interstitial tissue shows fibrosis and is predominantly infiltrated with lymphocytes and plasma cells. The origin of the epithelioid cells is Sertoli cells lining the tubules. The transformation of the Sertoli cells to epithelioid or histiocytic cells is the result of the effect of a lipid fraction of spermatozoa. Berg[2] has produced granulomas in hamsters with an acid-fast staining lipid fraction of human spermatozoa.

Malakoplakia. One type of granulomatous orchitis, often with abscess formation, is characterized by infiltration with large histiocytes with small round or oval nuclei and "ground-glass" granular cytoplasm containing Michaelis-Gutmann bodies. The lesion is described on p. 777.

Tuberculosis of testicle and epididymis

Tuberculosis of the testicle without involvement of the epididymis is rare. Discrete tubercles in the testicle may be encountered in generalized miliary tuberculosis. Tuberculosis of the epididymis is usually unilateral, may occur at any age, and frequently is associated with tuberculosis of the lungs and genitourinary tract. The location of the primary focus of genital tuberculosis has stimulated considerable controversy among many investigators. Young's extensive surgical experience[36] has convinced him that, in most of the cases of genital tuberculosis, the primary site is in the seminal vesicles. Walker[33] lends support to advocates of the theory that the prostate gland or seminal vesicles harbor the primary focus.

The earliest lesions are seen as discrete or conglomerated, yellowish, necrotic areas in the globus minor. Microscopically these reveal either characteristic tubercles or disorganized inflammatory cellular reaction consisting of polymorphonuclear leukocytes, plasma cells, desquamated epithelial cells, some large monocytes, occasional multinucleated giant cells, and many acid-fast bacilli. The early lesion may regress and become calcified. Usually, however, there is progressive invasion until the entire epididymis becomes involved. When the tunica vaginalis is invaded, a considerable amount of serofibrinous or purulent exudate develops. Usually the tunica vaginalis serves as a barrier against extension into the testicle, and it is often surprising to find complete destruction of the epididymis with no invasion of the testicle.

Syphilis

The testicles are involved in almost every syphilitic patient. Syphilitic orchitis occurs either as a diffuse interstitial inflammation with fibrosis or as single or multiple gummas. Either of these types of lesion may be found in the acquired or congenital forms of syphilis. In contrast to tuberculosis, acquired syphilitic orchitis affects the testicle before the epididymis.

Grossly in the diffuse interstitial type the testis is enlarged, the cut surface is bulging grayish to yellowish white, and there is loss of normal architecture. The gummatous testicle is enlarged, firm, globular, smooth, and, rarely, nodular. When sectioned, the yellowish white or grayish white gummas bulge from the surrounding parenchyma. Extension of the gumma into the tunica vaginalis causes adhesion to the scrotum, and secondary infection induces ulceration of the scrotum with herniation of the testicle. In fibrous syphilitic orchitis the testicle is small and hard. When fibrosis is not pronounced, however, the testicle is of normal size and somewhat indurated.

Microscopically in secondary syphilis both the interstitial tissue and the seminiferous tubules are involved. The inflammatory reaction is similar to that seen in other organs. There is heavy infiltration with plasma cells, lymphocytes, and monocytes. The inflammatory reaction often surrounds small and large blood vessels that show hyperplasia of their walls. Angiitis of small arteries is characteristic. The involved seminiferous tubules resemble those of granulomatous orchitis with replacement of normal cell population with histiocytes, lipophages, and proliferating Sertoli cells. Spirochetes are readily demonstrable with Levaditi or Warthin-Starry stains.

Microscopically the gummas of the testicle are similar to those found elsewhere. The gumma is composed of a central area of necrosis surrounded by a zone of edematous fibrous tissue infiltrated with plasma cells, lymphocytes, and occasional multinucleated giant cells. There are decreased spermatogenesis and thickening of the basement membrane of the tubules. Spirochetes are readily demonstrable in this stage. In later stages there are diffuse fibrosis, peritubular and basal hyalinization with necrosis of the tubular cells, and shrinking of the tubules. The interstitial cells usually are well preserved and often are hypertrophied. Spirochetes are rarely found in the fibrotic state.

Chronic vaginalitis (chronic proliferative periorchitis, pseudofibromatous periorchitis)

Chronic proliferative periorchitis frequently has been designated as multiple fibromas of the tunica vaginalis. The etiology of this peculiar inflammatory lesion is unknown. Some cases are definitely associated with trauma. The age incidence is between 20 and 40 years.

Grossly the tunica vaginalis is found to be greatly thickened and nodular (Fig. 21-11). The surface is smooth and glistening. The nodules are multiple, scattered irregularly throughout the tunica vaginalis, and more numerous along the epididymis. They range from 1 mm to 2 cm in diameter. On sectioning, some of the nodules are found to be circumscribed and resemble uterine fibroids, whereas others are ill defined or confluent. Occasionally some nodules become calcified.

Microscopically the sections reveal a scanty cellular collagenous fibrous tissue, often interlacing or having a whorling architecture, infiltrated with lymphocytes and plasma cells. In other cases there is very little inflammatory cellular reaction.

Spermatic granuloma

Invasion of spermatozoa into the stroma of the epididymis provokes an inflammatory reaction designated as

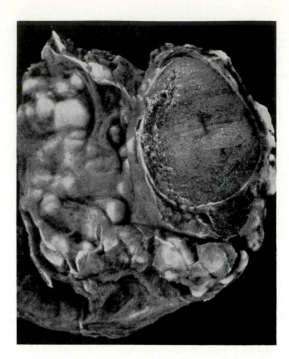

Fig. 21-11. Nodular vaginalitis (pseudofibromatous periorchitis). (Courtesy Dr. Robert S. Haukohl, Tampa, Fla.)

spermatic granuloma. The lesions are not uncommon, and similar lesions occur within the testes. Trauma or inflammation injures the wall of the tubule, and spermatozoa are spilled into the stroma. In some patients who have had vasectomies, loss of ligature from the proximal (testicular) end of the vas allows extravasation of spermatozoa resulting in sperm granuloma. Such loss of ligature may also result in reestablishing communication between severed ends of the vas. The lesions range from 3 mm to 3 cm in diameter. They are firm and white and may contain soft yellow or yellowish brown areas. They may be located in any part of the epididymis, but the majority occur in the upper pole.

Histologically the early reaction is infiltration with neutrophilic leukocytes and phagocytes, followed by various mononuclear cells, among which are histiocytes and epithelioid cells. At this stage the lesion is tuberculoid in character, with a center containing spermatozoa and debris. Lymphocytes appear among the epithelioid cells, and a mild fibroblastic proliferation replaces the epithelioid cells. The late lesions consist of hyalinized fibrous tissue, spermatozoa, granules of calcium, and very few inflammatory cells. Lipochrome pigment may be present in some lesions.

Tumors

Intrascrotal tumors may be divided into six categories (Fig. 21-12). The most common of these are germ cell tumors, and the least common are various benign and malignant tumors of fibrovascular stroma and the adnexa. Unless otherwise designated, "testicular tu-

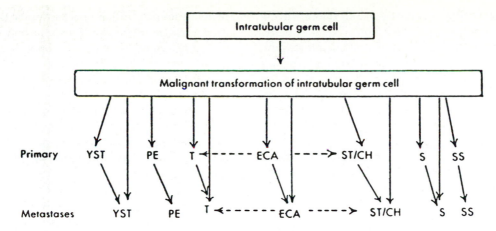

Fig. 21-12. Schematic relationship of testicular germ cell tumors. Neoplastic germ cell may remain intratubular and undifferentiated, or it may invade testicular parenchyma, vascular spaces, and rete testis. In adults embryonal carcinoma may progress to teratoma or choriocarcinoma, or both, either in primary tumor or in metastases, as indicated by broken lines. *CH*, choriocarinoma; *ECA*, embryonal carcinoma; *PE*, polyembryoma; *S*, seminoma; *SS*, spermatocytic seminoma; *ST*, syncytiotrophoblast; *T*, teratoma; *YST*, yolk sac tumors, infantile embryonal carcinoma, endodermal sinus tumor.

mors" refers to those of germ cell origin.

One of the products of World War II was the realization that germ cell tumors of the testis, although rare among the general population, are common in young men. The work of U.S. Army clinicians and pathologists who studied these tumors initiated an unusual interest in the biology and pathology of these neoplasms and the management of the patients. In the last decade tremendous advances have been made, justifying the claim that progress in treating testicular germ cell tumors is among the greatest developments in cancer research in this century.

It has been learned that a malignant germ cell tumor is capable of producing markers that can be used to diagnose a tumor accurately and monitor its progression reliably, that the neoplastic germ cell is capable of responding to the influence of organizers, and that some malignant germ cell tumors can undergo transformation into a benign phenotype. More important, the introduction of multimodal treatment, using various chemotherapeutic agents with or without radiotherapy, has brought about a miraculous improvement in the prognosis of these tumors. Complete elimination of malignancy in these tumors is still a great challenge to the imagination of the biologic scientist.

Incidence and prevalence

The incidence of germ cell tumors is 2 to 3 per 100,000 white male population. They are rare among blacks in the United States and among Africans and Asians.

In the 20- to 39-year age group the incidence of germ cell testis tumors is 5.8 to 7.2 per 100,000. In this group they are the most common solid tumors and the most common cause of death from malignancy. In the white male population in the United States about 90% of germ cell tumors occur before the age of 45, but the tumors have a trimodal age distribution with peaks during infancy, in late adolescence and early adulthood, and after 60 years of age. The histologic findings and behavior of the tumors vary with age. A doubling of mortality from these testicular tumors was reported between the mid-1940s (1943-1947) and the late 1950s and early 1960s (1958-1962).

Etiology

The cause of testicular germ cell tumors is unknown, but several factors are suspect. Genetic factors apparently play a role in the high incidence of testicular tumors in brothers, identical twins, monozygous twins, and members of the same family. Muller[22a] has reported a history of malignant disease of the testis in the next of kin in 16% of cases. Patients with one testis tumor have a high incidence of another tumor in the opposite testis. Tumors commonly develop in dysgenetic gonads. There is a high incidence of testicular tumor in certain strains of mice, and this can be genetically manipulated.

Maldescent of the testis is associated with a high incidence of testicular tumors. Of 2200 testis tumors we have seen, 72 were in undescended testes. Because cryptorchidism after 21 years of age affects only 1 in 250 men, this would indicate an incidence of 2.6% of maldescent in this group. The high incidence is attributed to the higher temperature to which undescended testis is subjected in the groin or abdomen. Other possible factors are abnormal structure of the undescended testis and interference with blood supply. In humans there is a slightly higher incidence of tumors on the right side (52% versus 48% on the left).

Many patients with testicular germ cell tumors give a history of mumps or other form of orchitis. Many patients give a history of trauma, but whether trauma initiates the process or simply brings to focus an abnormal testis has not been settled. In connection with trauma it may be mentioned that induction of teratomas in fowl by intratesticular injection of zinc salts, alone or with pituitary gonadotropic hormones, is attributed to the necrotizing effects of the injection.

In recent years testicular germ cell tumors have been reported in two men after the use of lysergic acid diethylamide (LSD), in patients who have received certain drugs for long periods, and in those exposed to microwave radiation.

Endocrine abnormalities may play a role in development of testicular tumors. As mentioned previously, there is a high incidence of testicular germ cell tumors in young adulthood, when sexual activity is at its highest. Levels of pituitary gonadotropins, chorionic gonadotropins, and estrogens may be elevated in some patients with testicular tumors, and this may play a role in the genesis of testicular tumors. A seminoma was reported in a man who had received hormone therapy for sterility. Experimentally germ cell tumors have been induced in fowl by injection of zinc or copper; zinc-induced fowl teratomas occur only during the period of maximal pituitary gonadotropin secretion. In strain 129 mice, which have a high incidence of spontaneous testicular germ cell tumors, transplantation of genital ridge of 12½- to 13½-day embryos to the testes of adult mice of the same strain induces large numbers of testicular teratomas and embryonal carcinomas.

In summary, maldescent, mumps orchitis, and trauma to the testes are the three most important factors in the genesis of testicular germ cell tumors in humans, but most testicular tumors occur in individuals who appear to be otherwise normal.

Symptoms

There are no early symptoms of testicular tumor other than gradual enlargement of the testis, pain, and a heavy or dragging sensation. Presence of a nodule or hardness with or without pain may be detected incidentally by a patient, his physician, or sexual partner. Gynecomastia is seen in 2% to 10% of patients, indicating the desirability of examining the testes in all patients with gynecomastia. In about 10% the symptoms are acute, simulating epididymitis, torsion, or infarction of the testis. About 25% of patients are found to have generalized metastases. Rarely the initial symptom may be infertility.

Diagnosis

A complete physical examination should be done. The testis may be enlarged and have a rubbery consistency. There may be one or more nodules. The shape of the testis is often maintained. The tumor is usually distinct from the epididymis and not attached to the overlying scrotal tunica or the skin. The epididymis and the spermatic cord are usually uninvolved. In boys a painful, tender intrascrotal mass may be caused by torsion. With an associated abdominal mass, care should be taken in the examination to avoid rupture of the mass.

Discussion of specific diagnostic procedures used in suspected cases of testicular tumors is beyond the scope of this presentation, but mention should be made that these are directed toward the determination of (1) whether the tumor is confined to the testis, has extended beyond but is still confined to the scrotum, or has already metastasized and how extensively and (2) whether the tumor is producing any hormones or markers and the serum level of such markers.

For many years it has been known that patients with testicular tumor may show positive pregnancy test results. The crude bioassays of Ascheim-Zondek and Friedman's tests have now been superseded by more specific and more sensitive tests.

At present two tumor markers are widely used in diagnosis, staging, and follow-up monitoring of patients with testicular tumors: beta fraction of human chorionic gonadotropin (HCG) and alpha fetoprotein (AFP). After some initial confusion the cell of origin of these markers has now been established. In testicular tumors HCG is synthesized by syncytiotrophoblasts either alone or as choriocarcinoma. Any preorchiectomy elevation of HCG or its persistence after orchiectomy indicates the presence of one of these elements in the primary tumor or in the metastasis. Ectopic production of HCG has been demonstrated in about 8% of patients with a variety of nontesticular, non–germ cell tumors; thus the presence of elevated HCG level or its demonstration in a nongerminal tumor cell does not per se indicate choriocarcinoma or syncytiotrophoblasts.

The situation is a little more complex with AFP. This fetoprotein was initially demonstrated in human fetal serum and in mice with hepatomas. In the human embryo it is produced first by the yolk sac and later by the liver. Thus in adults pregnancy is the only normal state in which AFP is elevated. In testicular tumors AFP is most often associated with yolk sac elements, whose epithelium usually demonstrates this fetal albumin. Rarely, embryonal carcinoma cells and some columnar mucus-containing epithelial cells of mature and immature teratomas also contain AFP. One or both of these markers are present in about 70% of testicular germ cell tumors. The half-life of HCG is 24 hours; that of AFP is 5 days. Persistence of one or both of these markers 1 week after the removal of the tumor-bearing testis indicates the presence of metastasis.

Follicle-stimulating hormone (FSH) levels are also frequently elevated, but this has no clinical significance. In addition to these three markers, carcinoembryonic antigen (CEA), human placental lactogen (HPL), pregnancy-specific antigen 1 (SP1), testosterone, estrogens, luteinizing hormone, placental alkaline phosphatase (PLAP), and human chorionic somatomammotropin are also being evaluated.

There is no satisfactory clinical classification of testicular germ cell tumors beyond distinguishing those that are confined to the parenchyma of the testis from those that have extended to the adnexa, metastasized below the diaphragm, or spread above the diaphragm.

Testicular biopsy is contraindicated in patients with suspected testicular tumor because biopsy has been associated with a high incidence of local recurrence, which is otherwise rare. Orchiectomy is done in all such patients. Wide sampling of the tumor and the nontumorous testicular tissue is indicated because sometimes a small focus of more malignant cell types is found in a tumor that is predominantly of a different histology. The application of stains for tumor markers is the only reliable means to find their specific site of origin.

Because most testicular germ cell tumors have the potentiality of metastasis, many patients are given some type of postorchiectomy treatment—radiation, surgery, or chemotherapy. The decision to give further treatment and the choice of specific type of therapy are based on three factors: (1) the clinical evidence of metastasis, (2) the histology of the primary tumor, and (3) the persistence of tumor markers after orchiectomy. Most patients who are destined to die of germ cell tumors of the testis do so within 2 years after orchiectomy.

The rarity of testicular germ cell tumors, the heterogeneity of their structure, ranging from simple to complex neoplasms, and the absence of readily available experimental models have resulted in considerable confusion about the histogenesis, pathology, natural history, and behavior of these tumors. The classic work of Friedman and Moore[12] and Dixon and Moore,[9] who reported their observations on 1000 cases of testicular tumors collected at the Army Institute of Pathology (now the Armed Forces Institute of Pathology) in Washington during World War II, followed by Mostofi's studies[19] of an additional 10,000 testicular tumor cases collected in the American Testicular Tumor Registry, housed at the Institute, and Sesterhenn's work[29a] with tumor markers have clarified many of the problems. The discussion of pathology of these neoplasms is based on these studies, the work of the World Health Organization Scientific Advisory Group on Testicular Tumors, and the experimental research of Stevens[31] and Pierce and Beals.[23]

Histogenesis

Willis[35] advocated two distinct sites of origin of testicular tumors: seminomas arise from cells in the seminiferous tubules, and all other tumors arise from foci of plu-

ripotential embryonic tissue that escaped the influence of the primary organizer during embryonic development. Based on this, he proposed a classification of these tumors into seminoma and teratoma. Because the latter category included tumors of different structure and behavior, the classification has not been accepted, although it has been somewhat modified in recent years by some English investigators. The American writers, on the other hand, have maintained that all of these tumors originate from the germ or sex cell (Fig. 21-12). This position has now been conclusively confirmed. Stevens[31] demonstrated experimentally the origin of murine embryonal carcinoma and teratoma from the germ cells. Pierce and Beals[23] showed that, ultrastructurally, embryonal carcinoma cells resemble the primitive germ cells. Mostofi[17a,19] has conclusively demonstrated that all human testicular germ cell tumors, except teratomas, originate directly from malignant transformation of intratubular germ cells.

To understand the pathology and the modern pathologic classification of germ cell tumors of the testis, one must remember the potentialities of the fertilized germ cell. Almost immediately this cell divides into two groups: the precursors of embryonic (somatic) elements and of extraembryonic (trophoblastic) elements. The progression of these precursors is in an orderly, organized, controlled manner to result in the embryo and the placenta, respectively. Very early in embryogenesis one cell is destined to become the germ cell and eventually develop into the gonads.

The malignant germ cell has the same potentialities except that the growth is disorganized, haphazard, and uncontrolled. Stevens has demonstrated that teratomas in mice originate from malignant transformation of germ cells. Mostofi has demonstrated that malignant transformation of intratubular germ cell may progress while the cells are still intratubular to form one or more of the following basic histologic types: seminoma, spermatic seminoma, embryonal carcinoma, yolk sac tumor, syncytiotrophoblast, and by implication, choriocarcinoma. He also demonstrated that the malignant germ cell can invade the stroma and the lymphatics and metastasize. The undifferentiated intratubular malignant germ cells or any of the basic cell types may be seen in the seminiferous tubules adjoining the main tumor. The undifferentiated intratubular malignant germ cells have sometimes been called carcinoma in situ.

Histopathologic classification

Modern histopathologic classification of testicular germ cell tumors initially separates them into two main categories: tumors of one histologic pattern, which constitute about 38% of testicular germ cell tumors, and tumors of more than one histologic pattern, which are seen in 62% of cases:

A. Tumors of one histologic pattern
  1. Seminoma
  2. Spermatocytic seminoma
  3. Embryonal carcinoma
  4. Yolk sac tumors, infantile embryonal carcinoma, endodermal sinus tumor
  5. Polyembryoma
  6. Choriocarcinoma syncytiotrophoblasts
  7. Teratoma
B. Tumors of more than one histologic pattern

Any combination of the seven basic patterns may occur. The specific types and the relative proportions of each should be mentioned.

Tumors of one histologic type

Seminoma. Compared with the incidence of other germ cell tumors, seminoma occurs in the older age group and is relatively less malignant. Undescended testes harbor this tumor more frequently than other forms of teratoid tumors. Seminoma constitutes 31% of all germ cell tumors and 72% of germ cell tumors of one histologic type. Clinically in pure seminoma no elevation of AFP or beta fraction of HCG is seen; if either of these is detected in the serum, the tumor contains other elements.

The involved testis may be only slightly enlarged or may be 10 times larger than normal, yet it usually maintains almost its normal contour. This gross feature is attributable to the fact that the tunical covering is rarely invaded. The neoplasm is opaque grayish white or yellowish white and sometimes contains yellowish and yellowish brown areas of necrosis (Fig. 21-13). Some tumors are homogeneous, whereas others are distinctly lobulated. The large tumors replace the entire testis, whereas small tumors are circumscribed but not encapsulated. Hemorrhagic necrosis is rare, and cysts are never found in pure seminomas.

Microscopically seminomas are readily recognized because of their monocellularity. The cells are moderately large, round, cuboid, or polyhedral and quite uniform in size, and most reveal distinct cell borders. The cytoplasm usually is quite clear, containing glycogen, but occasionally it is slightly stained. The relatively large, round, centrally located nucleus may occupy one third to one half of the cell. The nucleolus is prominent and slightly eosinophilic, and some nuclei have two nucleoli (Fig. 21-14).

The cells are quite regular, and mitotic figures are infrequent. In about 10%, however, there is increased mitotic activity (high mitotic seminoma), indicating a more aggressive tumor. The seminoma cells occur in cords, columns, or sheets; they may be infiltrating or intratubular. The stroma is usually delicate but almost invariably shows varying degrees of lymphocytic infiltration that may sometimes be quite prominent. In some the stroma may be granulomatous and in a few, very fibrous. The stroma divides the tumor into lobules. The reaction of the stroma is interpreted as an immunologic response of the body to the tumor. The tumors are very radiosensitive, and the 5-year mortality is less than 5% in tumors confined to the testis, and 20% to 60% in those that have already metastasized at the time of orchiecto-

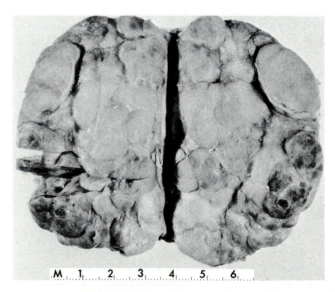

Fig. 21-13. Seminoma of testis.

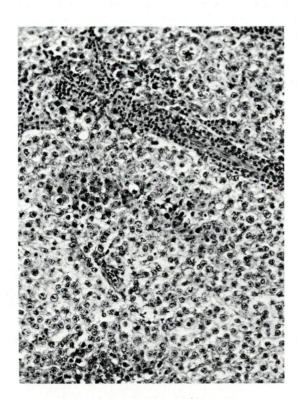

Fig. 21-14. Seminoma of testis. (145×.)

my. Most deaths from germ cell tumors occur in 2 years, and almost all in 5 years, of discovery.

Spermatocytic seminoma. Spermatocytic seminoma (Fig. 21-15) usually occurs in older patients. Grossly it is softer and more yellowish and mucoid than is seminoma and has small or large spaces containing pinkish fluid. Microscopically, although the major cell population is of intermediate size as in seminoma, there are a number of cells resembling secondary spermatocytes and huge mononucleate or multinucleate giant cells. The cytoplasm has no glycogen. The nuclei of the intermediate and large cells have a distinct chromatin distribution, which resembles the meiotic phase of normal primary spermatocytes and is described as filamentous or spireme.

Lymphocytic and granulomatous reactions are absent.

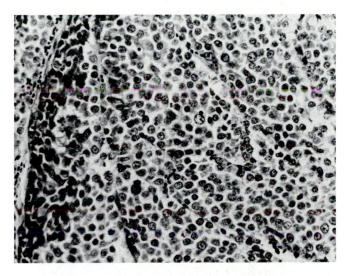

Fig. 21-15. Spermatocytic seminoma. (250×.)

The tumors are believed to be radiosensitive, and the prognosis is very good. To date, spermatocytic seminomas have not been reported in any site other than the testis.

Embryonal carcinoma. Pure embryonal carcinoma constitutes 3% of germ cell tumors, but areas of embryonal carcinoma are found in 47% of all tumors. HCG levels are not elevated in pure embryonal carcinoma, but some elevation of AFP may be found. Grossly the tumors are among the smallest. They distort the contour of the testicle more than the seminoma because of their invasion of the capsule and epididymis. The cut surfaces reveal a soft gray or grayish red tissue with areas of hemorrhage and necrosis (Fig. 21-16). The tumors are rarely cystic.

Microscopically the characteristic feature of these tumors is that they are made up of definitely carcinomatous cells—large, highly anaplastic with amphophilic cytoplasm, often with indistinct cell borders (Fig. 21-17). The nuclei are prominent and eosinophilic and may be quite large. Mitotic figures are always present and often numerous. The cells usually form glandular, tubular, papillary, or pseudocystic structures or rarely solid sheets. Hemorrhage and necrosis are not uncommon. The stroma does not have the distinct pattern of the seminoma. It may be imperceptible or abundant, fibrous, primitive, or even sarcomatous. The tumors are less sensitive to radiation than are seminomas. Chemotherapy has miraculously reduced the mortality.

A few tumor cells contain AFP, but none of the cells of pure embryonal carcinoma contains HCG. Ultrastructural studies have shown that embryonal carcinoma consists of primitive cells intermingled with more mature cells. Some investigators believe that the primitive cells have the capability of differentiating into embryonic or trophoblastic tissue.

For many years retroperitoneal lymph node dissection

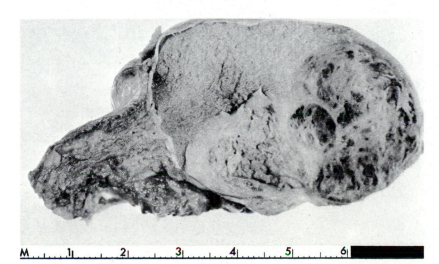

Fig. 21-16. Embryonal carcinoma of testis.

(RPLND) was carried out in all patients with embryonal carcinoma. If results were positive, the patients were further treated by radiation or chemotherapy or both. This regimen is under scrutiny, and it is possible that RPLND will be eliminated.

One of the most dramatic results of current treatment of cancer has occurred in testicular embryonal carcinoma. In the 1970s, 75% of patients with embryonal carcinoma died within 5 years; today, through chemotherapy, over 80% of those whose tumor is confined to the testis survive after orchiectomy. If metastases have occurred, 70% may survive.

Yolk sac tumors (infantile embryonal carcinoma). These tumors have also been designated as endodermal sinus tumors because they resemble a yolk sac or an endodermal sinus. They are the most common testicular tumor in infants and children. AFP levels are usually high. Grossly the testis is usually enlarged, and the cut surface is yellowish gray, mucinous, and greasy. Microscopically the tumor has a reticular pattern with epithelial cells that range from flattened to cuboid and even low columnar cells forming anastomosing tubular structure (Fig. 21-18).

AFP is demonstrable in many tumor cells. The survival in infants and children is over 80%. Pure yolk sac tumors are rarely seen in adults and have poor prognoses, but yolk sac tumor areas are found in over 40% of adult testicular tumors of more than one cell type.

Polyembryoma. This very rare tumor is composed predominantly of embryoid bodies. These are structures containing a disc and cavities surrounded by loose mesenchyme simulating an embryo of about 2 weeks' gestation. Tubular structures resembling endoderm and syncytiotrophoblastic elements may be present. Polyembryoma as defined is very rare, but embryoid bodies are found frequently with embryonal carcinoma and teratoma.

Choriocarcinoma. Pure choriocarcinomas are the most malignant of germ cell tumors, but fortunately they are extremely rare (18 in 6000). They are usually small and always hemorrhagic and necrotic with a small rim of viable tissue at the periphery. Frequently the patients, who are usually in their early twenties, initially have symptoms of metastasis. Sometimes, because of its small size, the primary lesion is completely missed until autopsy. The level of chorionic gonadotropins is markedly elevated and there is gynecomastia.

To diagnose choriocarcinoma, one must recognize two types of cells, the cytotrophoblast and the syncytiotrophoblast (Fig. 21-19). The cytotrophoblasts are polyhedral cells having a clear or pinkish cytoplasm with relatively large hyperchromatic nuclei. They lie in sheets or make up the major portion of the villuslike structures, which are usually bordered by syncytiotrophoblasts. The syncytiotrophoblasts are large, often huge, irregular, bizarre cells with pseudopodia extending between other cells. Their cell wall is indistinct. They possess a large

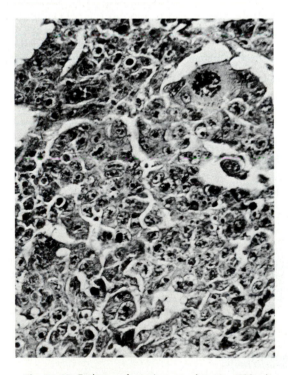

Fig. 21-17. Embryonal carcinoma of testis. (230×.)

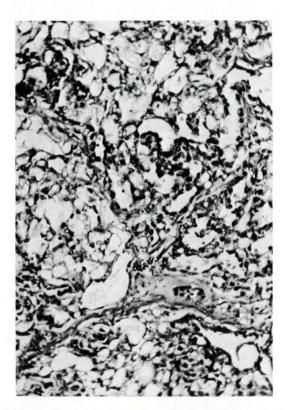

Fig. 21-18. Yolk sac tumor (infantile embryonal carcinoma) of testis. (130×.)

amount of azurophilic cytoplasm, which frequently is vacuolated. Their deeply staining nuclei are large, irregular, and pyknotic. Some of the cells are multinucleated.

The syncytiotrophoblasts are usually located (as in choriocarcinoma of the uterus) in the advancing edge of the tumor, but distinct villus formation is very rare. None of the current markers is demonstrable in cytotrophoblasts. Syncytiotrophoblasts contain HCG, human placental lactogen (HPL), and pregnancy-specific antigen 1 (SP1). All of our patients with pure choriocarcinoma of the testes were dead within 35 weeks of the diagnosis.

In contrast to the rarity of pure choriocarcinoma, syncytiotrophoblasts or areas of choriocarcinoma are not infrequently seen in association with other testicular tumors. This will be discussed under tumors of more than one histologic pattern. In a number of cases in which the primary tumor has no demonstrable chorionic elements, the metastasis may show choriocarcinoma.

Teratoma. Teratoma in the testis is defined as a complex tumor with recognizable elements of more than one germ layer. It constitutes about 3% of all germ cell tumors, 7% of tumors of one histologic type in adults, and about 40% of infantile testicular tumors. Teratomatous areas are found in 47% of tumors of more than one histologic type. The AFP level may be slightly elevated. Grossly the tumors are of moderate size, grayish white, cystic, and honeycombed with areas of cartilage and bone (Fig. 21-20). The cysts mostly contain keratohyaline matter but may contain mucin. In contrast to the ovaries, dermoid tumors are rare in the testes.

Microscopically the testicular teratoma is a complex tumor revealing a disorderly arrangement of a great variety of fetal and adult structures originating from the three germ layers: ectoderm, mesoderm, and entoderm. The most common well-differentiated structures are squamous cysts filled with keratohyaline substance, cartilage, smooth muscle, mucous glands, respiratory and gastrointestinal structures, and, in infants and children, nerve tissue. Such tumors are designated mature teratoma (Fig. 21-21). Occasionally the tumors are quite immature, showing primitive cartilage, mesenchyme, neuroectodermal canals, and abortive intestinal and respiratory tubules. Such tumors are designated as immature teratoma.

AFP is demonstrable in columnar mucus-containing epithelial cells of mature and immature teratomas. Rarely a teratoma shows malignant transformation, for example, squamous carcinoma, mucinous adenocarcinoma,

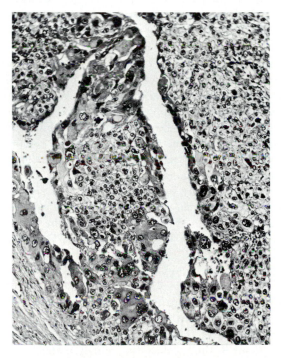

Fig. 21-19. Choriocarcinoma of testis. (100×.)

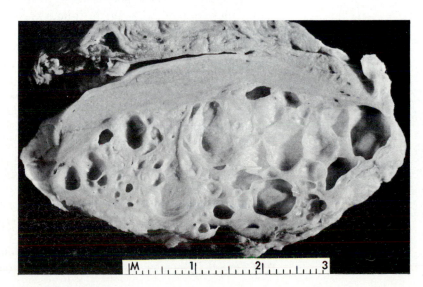

Fig. 21-20. Teratoma of testis.

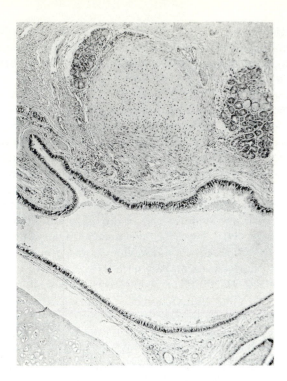

Fig. 21-21. Teratoma of testis. (48×.)

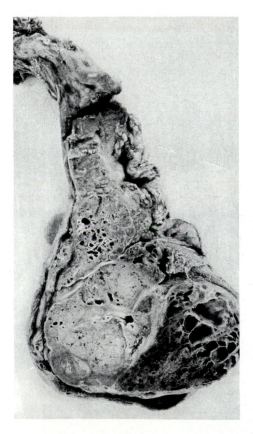

Fig. 21-22. Teratoma and embryonal carcinoma (teratocarcinoma) of testicle infiltrating spermatic cord.

carcinoid, or rhabdomyosarcoma. Although no malignant areas may be encountered, mature and immature teratomas should not be regarded as benign, since about 29% show metastases and terminate fatally in 5 years. In infants and children the prognosis is much better.

Tumors of more than one histologic type. In 62% of patients with testicular germ cell neoplasms the tumor consists of more than one histologic type. Except for spermatocytic seminoma, which tends to occur in pure form, all other cell types may occur in combination. The detection of the various types that may be present and the designation of the mixtures have been the source of considerable confusion. The application of tumor markers to the tissue has clarified the presence of various elements and provided the proper explanation for the bizarre clinical behavior of this group of tumors and the divergence between the histologic findings in primary tumor and the metastasis. For a long time the prevalent concept was that the most frequent combination was embryonal carcinoma and teratoma, to which the term *teratocarcinoma* was applied; it has now been demonstrated that, in fact, the most frequent combination is embryonal carcinoma, teratoma, yolk sac tumor, and syncytiotrophoblasts. Thus both HCG and AFP may be present in the serum.

Grossly these tumors are usually quite large and solid with cystic areas. They may have areas of hemorrhage and necrosis (Fig. 21-22). Histologically the embryonal carcinoma segment is readily identifiable. The teratomatous component may consist of mature or immature teratoma. The yolk sac elements and the syncytiotrophoblasts are often overlooked and are likely to be missed unless the sections are stained for tumor markers. The second most frequent combination is seminoma and syncytiotrophoblasts. Any one or more of the elements that are present in the primary tumor may metastasize.

In these tumors of more than one histologic type, one clinical finding causes considerable consternation—serum elevation of HCG in the range of below 2000 units, particularly in patients with seminoma. Such a finding raises the suspicion of choriocarcinoma. Sometimes a focus of choriocarcinoma is readily detected and the problem is resolved. More often, either some syncytiotrophoblasts are seen, or nothing is found that can explain the elevated HCG. In such cases staining for tumor markers and thorough examination of the tumor and the testis will reveal the presence of syncytiotrophoblasts in the tumor, in the supporting stroma, or in the adjacent seminiferous tubules. Syncytiotrophoblasts may recapitulate any of the forms that they show in various stages of placenta. Where no explanation can be found in the testis for the elevated HCG levels, the existence of HCG-producing cells in metastasis should be ruled out; this can be done by postorchiectomy determination of HCG levels. Elevation 1 week after orchiectomy indicates the existence of metastasis. A normal tumor marker level, however, does not exclude metastasis of components that do not produce markers.

One of the fascinating features of testicular germ cell tumors is that, although the histology of the metastases reflects the histology of the primary tumor in over 90%, occasionally the metastases are entirely different histologically from the primary tumor, or metastatic foci may have different histologic patterns. A primary tumor that may consist of embryonal carcinoma, teratoma, or a mixture of these may metastasize as such or as choriocarcinoma, or the metastases in the lymph nodes may be different histologically from those in the liver, lung, or kidney. A primary lesion may consist of a small mature teratoma or seminoma, either alone or in association with an area of scarring and calcific and hemosiderin deposition, but the widespread metastases may consist of choriocarcinoma, embryonal carcinoma, or teratocarcinoma. In many testicular tumors of all types it is not unusual to find intratubular undifferentiated malignant germ cells, intratubular seminoma, embryonal carcinoma, yolk sac tumor, or syncytiotrophoblasts. Any of these may invade the parenchyma.

The observed histologic discrepancies between the primary lesion and the metastases may be explainable on one of several bases: a small focus of the cell type present in the metastasis may have been missed in the primary; the totipotential malignant germ cell or the primitive embryonal carcinoma cell may have been carried away to develop into another cell type in the metastasis; or the location may have influenced the histology of the metastasis. In recent years it has also been demonstrated that, after treatment with radiation or chemotherapeutic agents, a histologically proven metastatic embryonal carcinoma or embryonal carcinoma and teratoma may reveal only mature teratoma cells. Whether this is a result of the therapeutic agent acting as an organizer or its cytotoxic action on embryonal carcinoma, thus permitting the growth of the histologically resistant mature teratoma, has not been resolved. These observations, however, challenge the oncologist to find means of converting a rapidly growing malignant tumor destined to destroy the host if left untreated into a slowly growing, nonlethal, histologically benign tumor that may then be surgically removed.

Metastasis

Extratesticular spread of germ cell tumors constitutes the ominous progression of these neoplasms. It can be lymphogenous or directly or indirectly hematogenous. Lymphogenous metastasis occurs much more frequently than hematogenous except in choriocarcinoma. The lymph nodes predominantly involved are the iliac, periaortic, mediastinal, and supraclavicular groups. Eventually hematogenous spread occurs either directly through testicular vascular channels or indirectly through lymphatic drainage into superior vena cava. The organs most frequently harboring metastases are the lungs, liver, and kidneys, but no organ is immune.

Burned-out testicular tumors

Discovery of an apparent extragonadal germ cell tumor—choriocarcinoma, embryonal carcinoma, seminoma, or teratocarcinoma—should lead to careful and thorough examination of the testis before the tumor is accepted as extragonadal. Not infrequently one of the testes of patients with such tumors shows a well-defined, acellular, rather dense scar with or without hemosiderin deposition and with or without dark blue staining masses (hematoxyphilic bodies). A small focus of mature teratoma, seminoma, or embryonal carcinoma may be seen, or there may be intratubular malignant germ cells.

Tumors derived from specialized gonadal stroma

To understand the hormonal and morphologic features of tumors derived from specialized gonadal stroma, one should remember that the primitive mesenchyme of the genital ridge forms the whole gonad of each sex except for the germ cells that migrate from their site of origin in the yolk sac entoderm. These primitive mesenchymal cells constitute the supporting stromal elements for the germ cells. In the female they give rise to theca, granulosa, and lutein cells and in the male, to the sustentacular cells of Sertoli and the interstitial cells of Leydig. The cells of origin of the testis and ovary are identical, and in neoplastic proliferation one might suppose that the strict control that directs the differentiation of these two dissimilar structures might be deranged so that structures reminiscent of either ovary or testis may develop. Thus Sertoli and Leydig cell tumors may be found in the ovary (in addition to granulosa cell, theca cell, and lutein cell tumors), and the latter three tumors may be seen in the testis (in addition to Sertoli cell and Leydig cell tumors).

Nodules consisting of Sertoli cell–lined or immature tubules are not infrequent in the undescended testis, and although sometimes erroneously designated as adenomas, they are persistent or hyperplastic nodules. Unless there is a distinct grossly visible tumor, the lesion should not be so designated. Sertoli, granulosa, or theca cell tumors or those showing admixtures occur in all ages but more commonly in infants and children. They correspond to arrhenoblastoma and androblastomas of the ovary. About one third of adult patients show gynecomastia. Grossly the tumors are usually fairly large, well circumscribed, round or oval, firm, and yellowish or yellowish gray. The cut surfaces are bulging and somewhat greasy.

Microscopically three basic patterns may be recognized: tubular, stromal, or mixed. In the tubular type, tubules are lined by high or low columnar Sertoli-like cells (Fig. 21-23) or cuboid cells resembling granulosa cells. The stromal type shows closely packed rounded or spindle-shaped cells with dark-staining nuclei and a small amount of cytoplasm, which resemble theca cells. The mixed type contains all cell types and even Leydig cells. The cells contain estrogens. These tumors have been designated as "androblastoma" by Teilum,[32] who reported three cases with gynecomastia. Mostofi, Theiss, and Ashley[22] have reported a series of 23 cases and suggested the designation "tumors of specialized gonadal stroma." These tumors are mostly benign—only about 10% are malignant and those that metastasize do so within 1 year.

The manifestations of Leydig cell tumors are extremely interesting. Normally Leydig cells produce mostly testosterone but some estrogens and other hormones as well. They undergo morphologic and endocrine involutional changes beginning in fetal and newborn life, when they are stimulated by gonadotropins to appear as large epithelium-like cells; in infancy and childhood they resemble fibroblastic cells; in adulthood they are large and granular; and in old age they are small and vacuolated, have a dark-staining nucleus, and are often again spindly.

Clinically all children with Leydig cell tumors manifest macrogenitosomia, with voice changes, enlargement of the penis, pubic and axillary hair, and precocious body development. If the condition is not recognized and the tumor-bearing testis is not removed, premature closure of the epiphysis may occur, resulting in dwarfism. In others, gynecomastia develops as the child approaches adolescence. In adult patients no supermasculinizing features are observed, but about half show gynecomastia and other feminizing features. Gynecomastia may be attributable to estrogen production or to metabolism of increased or altered androgens. The tumors produce testosterone, estrogens, progesterone, and even corticosteroids.

Grossly the testis usually is enlarged, although this may not be detected. About half of the patients consult a physician because of gynecomastia, with the breasts about two times larger than normal. The testicular tumors are lobulated, well circumscribed, and homogeneously yellowish to mahogany brown. Areas of necrosis and hemorrhage are extremely rare, but calcification may be encountered.

Microscopically the most common cell type is large polyhedral cells with vacuolated or eosinophilic cytoplasm, a round or oval vesicular nucleus, and a single or double nucleolus (Fig. 21-24). Binuclear and trinuclear cells are not uncommon. In addition to lipids, testosterone and other hormones, and brown pigment, the cytoplasm may contain Reinke's crystals, which are characteristic of interstitial cells but seem to have no function. The tumors may recapitulate the various types of interstitial cells encountered in the normal testis in its involution. The cells are arranged in columns and cords sep-

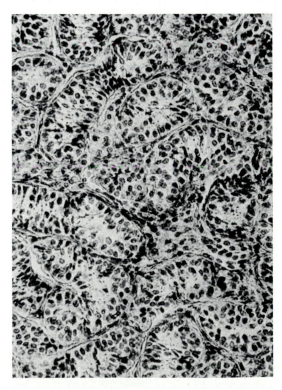

Fig. 21-23. Sertoli cell tumor of testis. (205×.)

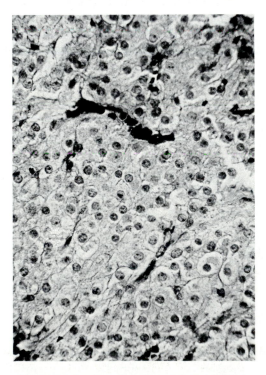

Fig. 21-24. Leydig cell tumor of testis. (250×.)

arated by well-vascularized fibrous tissue, frequently giving the tumors an endocrine pattern.

Differentiation between hyperplasia and tumor (adenoma or carcinoma) is sometimes difficult, especially in children and in patients with adrenogenital syndrome. In tumors there is a distinct mass, and there usually are no entrapped seminiferous tubules. Differentiation between a benign and a malignant interstitial cell tumor is difficult on a histologic basis, but cellular anaplasia, increased mitoses, and vascular invasion are disturbing features. Fortunately, 90% of the tumors are benign. The only criterion for malignancy is metastasis, and this usually is late in development. It is important to do hormone assays in such patients because a rise in or a persistently elevated androgen level after orchiectomy may indicate the development of metastasis. Differentiation from a tumor derived from an adrenal rest is sometimes difficult, but adrenal rests occur almost entirely outside the tunica of the testis and tumors in the substances of the testis must be regarded as interstitial cell tumors. Histologically and endocrinologically the two tumors frequently are indistinguishable.

Tumors and tumorlike conditions containing both germ cell and gonadal stromal elements

These are usually seen in dysgenetic gonads but rarely also in undescended testis and, more rarely, in normally located testis. The tumors, designated as gonadoblastoma, show large cells resembling seminoma and rarely embryonal carcinoma and small cells resembling immature Sertoli-granulosa cells and occasionally Leydig cells. The tumors are usually benign, but the germ cell element may metastasize.

Lymphoid tumors initially manifested as testicular tumors

These tumors, which may occur at any age, are more frequent in older patients and are often the initial manifestation of the systemic disease. In recent years, with the control of generalized lymphoma by chemotherapeutic agents, a number of patients have shown involvement of the testis, which is usually enlarged. The cut surface is grayish or yellowish, and areas of necrosis are frequent.

Microscopically there is massive infiltration of the testicular parenchyma with one or more types of reticuloendothelial cells and compression and atrophy of seminiferous tubules. Generalized lymphoma develops in many patients within 2 years.

Secondary tumors

The testis may be a site of metastases from the lungs, prostate, stomach, kidney, colon, pancreas, bladder, and rectum. Although in most cases these are autopsy findings, occasionally they may simulate a primary tumor.

Characteristically the infiltrate does not resemble a germ cell or stromal tumor, and it is interstitial with extensive location in vascular and lymphatic channels.

EPIDIDYMIS

Anomalies. Absence of the epididymis is rare. The testis in such instances may or may not be present. Duplication of the epididymis is usually associated with polyorchidism. Abnormal descent is associated with abnormal descent of the testis. On occasion the epididymis may be located anterior to the testis, which further complicates the often difficult problem of distinguishing between lesions in the epididymis and those in the testis. Anomalies of fusion are rare. In this situation there is a lack of fusion between the ducts and the seminiferous tubules.

Inflammation. Epididymitis is the most common intrascrotal inflammatory process and usually results from the spread of organisms from the prostatic urethra, prostate, or seminal vesicle. Less often the process is hematogenous. The usual causative agents are the common pyogenic organisms, although in patients under 35 years of age, gonococci and chlamydiae are more common. Histologically epididymitis may be acute or chronic, with or without abscesses and ductal destruction. Not infrequently the epididymal epithelium undergoes squamous metaplasia to produce a picture that has been confused with squamous carcinoma. The so-called traumatic epididymitis has been a subject of controversy for many years. The question is whether straining or heavy lifting can cause retrograde passage of sterile urine down the vas to produce irritation and inflammation. Tuberculous epididymitis generally occurs in patients with renal tuberculosis, and frequently the disease also exists in the prostate and seminal vesicle. Tuberculous epididymitis is more likely to be bilateral than other types of inflammation; in the well-developed disease nodules may be found along the spermatic cord. Inflammation of the epididymis frequently extends into the adjacent parenchyma of the testis, and a diagnosis of epididymo-orchitis is applicable.

Tumors. With the exception of the adenomatoid tumor, tumors of the epididymis are uncommon. Longo and associates[43] collected 134 cases of primary tumors of the epididymis from the world literature. The adenomatoid tumor (Fig. 21-25) has been reported under a variety of names such as mesothelioma, lymphangioma, and adenomyoma. Similar tumors are encountered in the tunica vaginalis, spermatic cord, posterior aspect of the uterus, fallopian tube, and ovary; thus such tumors develop along the course of the mesonephric duct.

Adenomatoid tumors are believed to originate from mesothelial cells. Most of the tumors occur in persons between 20 and 40 years of age. About 80% are attached to the epididymis, usually the globus minor, and the remainder are located on the tunica of the testes and in the cord. They are painless, single, firm, round or ovoid nodules ranging from less than 1 cm to 5 cm in greatest diameter. The cut surfaces are homogeneous, grayish white, and fibrous, having a whorled appearance; they occasionally reveal yellow areas. Histologically they have glandlike structures and irregular spaces, and some contain cords of epithelium-like cells (Fig. 21-26). The stroma varies in amount and is composed of a loose or dense

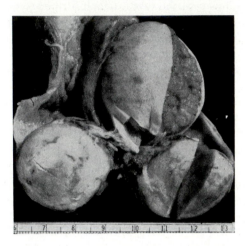

Fig. 21-25. Large adenomatoid tumor of lower pole of epididymis. Tumor is bisected and almost as large as testis above. (Courtesy Dr. Paul C. Dietz, La Crosse, Wis.)

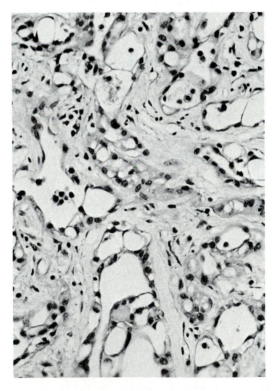

Fig. 21-26. Adenomatoid tumor of epididymis. (225×.)

fibrous connective tissue in which broad smooth muscle fibers are recognized. The glandlike structures may be lined with flat, cuboid, or low columnar cells. Many of the cells, particularly those arranged in cords, are vacuolated.

Leiomyoma, the second most common tumor of the epididymis, may be associated with a hydrocele. Other benign tumors that have been reported are angiomas, fibromas, and lipomas. Adrenocortical rests are rather common but are seldom large enough to be detected clinically. Splenic rests may also descend with the testis (gonadal-splenic fusion). Papillary cystadenoma of the epididymis occurs as a small nodule in the head of the organ. The size range is from 1 to 5 cm (mean, 2.3 cm). They may have a solid, cystic, or multicystic appearance and are well circumscribed. Histologically the ducts are dilated and lined by clear or vacuolated cells that protrude into the lumen as papillations. The appearance is similar to a low-grade, clear cell carcinoma of the kidney, but they are apparently benign. Price[49] found that these lesions represent the epididymal component of Lindau's disease. Patients with bilateral lesions showed manifestations of the syndrome in other organs, whereas unilateral cystadenomas were interpreted as a forme fruste of the disease. Carcinomas of epididymis and adjacent structures (appendix testis, appendix epididymis, and rete testis) occur but are rare, and it is often difficult to be certain one is not dealing with metastatic carcinoma or mesothelioma of tunica vaginalis. To date, epididymal carcinoma has not been established as a distinct clinicopathologic entity.

SPERMATIC CORD

Anomalies. Anomalies of the spermatic cord consist of congenital absence or congenital atresia of the vas deferens. Sterility is present when either of these conditions is bilateral. Complete or incomplete duplication of the vas deferens has been reported.

Inflammation. Inflammation of the vas deferens is known as vasitis or deferentitis, whereas inflammation of the entire spermatic cord is termed funiculitis. Lymphangitis, phlebitis, and thromboangiitis may be attributed to a variety of causes. Vasitis may be caused by extension of epididymitis or lymphogenous transportation from urethritis and cystitis. The etiology of some cases of both vasitis and funiculitis is not definitely known, but trauma and focal and general infections are suspected. Tuberculosis of the spermatic cord results from tuberculous epididymitis and seminal vesiculitis. Filarial funiculitis is associated with elephantiasis of the penis and scrotum. There are lymphangiectasia and fibrosis of the interstitial tissue. The walls of the lymph vessels become thickened and frequently reveal obliterative lymphangitis, with calcific and crystalline deposits. Calcified filariae may be found in whorls of hyalinized fibrous tissue. The various inflammatory cells encountered in filarial funiculitis are lymphocytes, plasma cells, eosinophils, and, in some cases, multinucleated giant cells.

Cysts. Cysts of the epididymis (spermatocele) or the testicular appendix (hydatid of Morgagni) or epididymal appendices are quite common. The most important are spermatoceles, which may be unilateral or bilateral, unilocular or multilocular. The epithelium is flattened or cuboid or may be ciliated and surrounded by various amounts of hyalinized fibrovascular tissue and occasionally cholesterol crystals. The lumen is filled with fluid that is either neutral or slightly alkaline. The sediment contains lymphocytes, cellular debris, fat globules, and sometimes cholesterol. The presence of spermatozoa distinguishes these cysts from hydrocele.

Varicocele. Varicocele is a common condition in which the veins of the pampiniform plexus are dilated and elongated and their tortuosity is increased. The cause of primary or idiopathic varicocele is not definitely known. Secondary or symptomatic varicocele is the result of pressure on the spermatic veins or its tributaries by an enlarged liver and spleen, pronounced hydronephrosis, muscle strain, and abdominal tumors. Primary varicocele usually involves the left spermatic cord and occurs predominantly in young boys.

Tumors. Lipoma is the most common tumor of the spermatic cord. Leiomyomas and neurofibromas occur less frequently. Vasitis nodosa is a benign tumorlike lesion of the vas that is more frequently seen as more men resort to vasectomy as a means of contraception. Several years after vasectomy a nodule may appear near the surgical site. Histologically it is composed of numerous tubular structures lined by cuboidal or columnar epithelium. The tubules usually contain spermatozoa. These structures occur in and adjacent to the wall of the vas and are usually associated with sperm granulomas. Olson[47] attributed this lesion to obstruction. Less frequently the lesion occurs in the epididymis (Fig. 21-27) in the absence of a history of ligation, but obstruction is the most likely causative factor. Malignant tumors of the spermatic cord are chiefly sarcomas. In the first three decades of life this is almost invariably embryonal rhabdomyosarcoma. The bulk of such lesions are generally found in the spermatic cord, but there may be extension into the epididymis and even into adjacent areas of the testis. The parietal tunica vaginalis may also be invaded. Other sarcomas occur chiefly between the ages of 50 and 80 as liposarcoma, malignant fibrous histiocytoma, fibrosarcoma, and leiomyosarcoma (Fig. 21-28). Liposarcomas are usually the well-differentiated sclerosing variety. These and most of the histiocytomas tend to be of low-grade malignancy; they are prone to local recurrence, but metastases are uncommon.

SCROTUM

Anomalies. Arrest of development may result in the formation of a separate pouch for each testicle. Half of the scrotum corresponding to undescended testicle may be rudimentary. A cleft scrotum resembling labia majora is encountered in pseudohermaphroditism. Partial cleft scrotum may accompany other congenital defects of the genitourinary system.

Dermatologic lesions. The common skin diseases of the scrotum are scabies (*Sarcoptes scabiei*), pediculosis, prurigo, eczema, erysipelas, psoriasis, and, not infrequently, syphilitic lesions. Sebaceous and epidermal

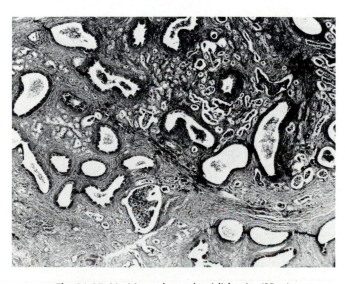

Fig. 21-27. Vasitis nodosa of epididymis. (25×.)

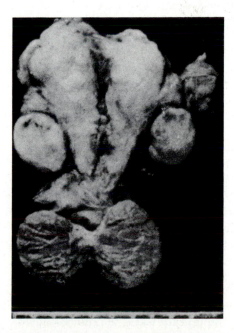

Fig. 21-28. Testis and spermatic cord. Fibrosarcoma of spermatic cord. (Courtesy Dr. Joseph L. Teresi, Brookfield, Wis.)

cysts are common and are frequently multiple and calcified.

Gangrene. Gangrene of the scrotum may be caused by trauma or may be a complication of infectious diseases, phimosis, chancroid, balanitis, or periurethritis. Idiopathic or spontaneous gangrene is unassociated with trauma or infection. There is often associated gangrene of the penis.

Hematoma. Hematoma of the scrotum is an effusion of blood within the tissue of the scrotal wall. The blood may collect beneath the tunica dartos, between the tunica vaginalis and the fibrous coat (paravaginal hematoma), or in the scrotal septum. Hematomas are usually of traumatic origin.

Elephantiasis. Elephantiasis of the scrotum is characterized by diffuse increase and fibrosis of the subcutaneous tissue and obvious thickening of the skin resembling elephant's hide and resulting in enlargement of the scrotum. The disease is the result of lymph stasis either from blocking of the lymphatics by microfilaria (*Wuchereria bancrofti*) or from cicatricial closure of the lymph channels caused by chronic inflammation after trauma, excision of lymph nodes, or chronic lymphadenitis. In filariasis the adult worm obstructs the lymph channels. Secondary infection, according to some investigators, is necessary to produce elephantiasis. The live worm apparently provokes little or no inflammation. The dead and disintegrating forms stimulate proliferation of the intima, followed by thrombosis and organization.

Tumors. The most common tumor of the scrotum, squamous cell carcinoma, has been declining in frequency, probably because of its recognized association many years ago with environmental carcinogens. The well-known and almost legendary "chimney-sweep's cancer" has been replaced by that arising among workers with tar, paraffin, and mineral oil, as well as in mule spinners in cotton mills. Squamous cell carcinomas of the scrotum do not differ appreciably from similar lesions of the penis, including the age of prevalence. They appear initially as a nodular, ulcerative, or exophytic lesion and may be multiple. Most are well or moderately differentiated and grow slowly. Metastases involve the inguinal nodes, and distant spread is uncommon. Death usually results from extensive local disease. According to Dean,[69] there is an increased incidence of multiple primary malignancies in patients with scrotal carcinoma. A variety of soft tissue tumors, benign and malignant, occur in the scrotal wall, but none is particularly common.

TUNICA VAGINALIS

Hydrocele. A hydrocele is an abnormal accumulation of serous fluid in the sac of the tunica vaginalis (Fig. 21-29). Normally there are a few drops of serous fluid between the visceral and parietal layers.

In the congenital type of hydrocele, there is a direct communication with the abdominal cavity as a result of failure of closure of the funicular process. In infantile hydrocele there is an accumulation of fluid in the partly closed funicular process and the sac of the tunica vaginalis, but there is no communication with the abdominal cavity. Acute hydrocele may be a complication of gonorrhea, tuberculosis, syphilis, erysipelas, rheumatism, typhoid, or neoplasms. Between 25% and 50% of acute hydroceles are the result of trauma.

The fluid of the hydrocele is odorless, viscid, and straw to amber colored. The usual amount varies from 10 to 300 ml and in one case was 4.5 liters. It has a neutral reaction, and its specific gravity varies from 1.020 to 1.026. It contains about 6% protein (serum albumin, cholesterol, serum globulin, and fibrinogen), alkaline carbonates, and sodium chloride. Occasionally fibrous bodies coated with fibrin are found floating in the fluid. The bodies originate from detached villous projections of the tunica vaginalis. If the hydrocele is infected, the fluid may be cloudy, or it may be brownish red if slight hemorrhage has occurred. Microscopic examination of comparatively clear hydrocele fluid reveals a few mesothelial cells, lymphocytes, cholesterin crystals, and lecithin bodies.

The sac of the hydrocele may be a single- or multiple-chambered structure. The inner surface of the tunica vaginalis is usually smooth, but there may be adhesions and fibrous projections. The wall is variously thickened, composed of scanty cellular fibrous tissue infiltrated with lymphocytes and some plasma cells. Calcific deposits occasionally are encountered. Following meconium peritonitis, extensive deposits of calcification and mucin may be found over the tunica.

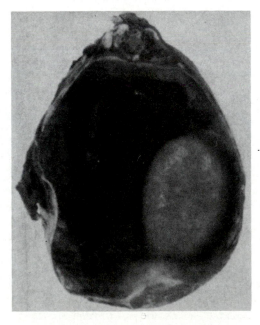

Fig. 21-29. Hydrocele. Normal testicle.

Hematocele. Hemorrhage in the sac of the tunica vaginalis is known as hematocele. Spontaneous hematocele is slow and insidious in its development, whereas a rapidly developing hematocele is invariably the result of trauma. The blood coagulates, fibrin settles out and organizes, and the wall becomes thick and rough. In long-standing hematocele the tunica vaginalis becomes enormously thickened with dense fibrous tissue, which occasionally becomes partly calcified. Trauma may result in the formation of both hematoma and hematocele.

Tumors. Fibrous pseudotumor (nodular periorchitis) is a tumorlike lesion that typically occurs as well-circumscribed, round, ovoid, or localized plaquelike nodules over the tunica. It is very firm in consistency and is white. It consists almost entirely of mature collagen, although it may contain foci of calcific deposits, scattered inflammatory cells, and mesothelial cell inclusions. The cause is unknown. About one third of the patients have a history of trauma or epididymo-orchitis. Many such tumors are associated with hydrocele; they appear as asymptomatic nodules from the third through the sixth decades and are benign.[46]

Mesothelial lesions of the tunica. Hyperplasia of the mesothelial cells lining the tunica vaginalis and tunica albuginea is common and may be found in association with any inflammatory process that involves the tunica. Histologically, small acinar, tubular, or papillary structures lined by small mesothelial cells are found within the zone of inflammation. This process typically rather sharply outlines the deep margin of this zone. The presence of solid sheets of such cells or their extension into normal tissue such as epididymis or normal adipose tissue of the cord should raise the question of malignancy. A second form of benign mesothelial proliferation has been referred to as nodular mesothelial hyperplasia.[48] This occurs as small nodules of tissue within the fluid of hydroceles or hernia sacs, particularly in infants and children. Microscopically the nodules are composed of viable sheets of mesothelial cells enmeshed in fibrin. Malignant mesothelioma of tunica is a tumor usually associated with hydrocele. Multiple, friable excrescences are found studding the visceral and parietal tunica vaginalis and the tunica albuginea. The tumor grows into the structures of the cord and testicular adnexa and invades the periphery of the testis. It should be noted that invasion of rete testis by mesothelioma is frequently confused with a primary tumor of rete testis. Spread is to regional lymph nodes. Not infrequently these tumors represent the early manifestation of generalized mesothelioma of peritoneum or pleura; the latent period may be as long as 4 years.

PENIS

Anomalies

Phimosis. Phimosis is a condition in which the preputial orifice is too small to permit retraction of the prepuce behind the glans. It is independent of inflammation of the foreskin. An acquired phimosis may result from inflammation, trauma, or edema that narrows the preputial opening so that the prepuce cannot be retracted. Congenital phimosis predisposes to development of preputial calculi and squamous cell carcinoma. Paraphimosis is a condition in which the retracted prepuce cannot be reduced, with swelling of the prepuce and ulceration of the constricting tissue. It is usually a complication of gonorrhea, chancre, chancroid, balanitis, or trauma.

Hypospadias. Hypospadias is a developmental arrest in which the urethral meatus is present on the undersurface of the penis. It is probably a result of disturbance of sex differentiation, causing imperfect closure of the urethral groove. The arrest may take place anywhere along the urethral groove, thus resulting in hypospadias with location from the glans penis to the perineum. Hypospadias is associated with a rather high incidence of genital anomalies such as cryptorchidism, enlarged prostatic utricle, and bifid scrotum. In about 25% of the cases hypospadias is inherited as a recessive trait.

Epispadias is a rare form of congenital defect in which the urethral meatus is located at the upper surface of the penis. Its incidence in newborn infants is 1 in 50,000, and it frequently is associated with cryptorchidism, exstrophy of the urinary bladder, or absence of the prostate gland. In fact, it is a mild form of exstrophy.

Inflammation

Syphilis. The common site of a hard chancre is on the glans near the frenum or on the inner surface of the prepuce. It also may occur within or at the site of the urethral meatus, or rarely, on the shaft (see p. 316).

Chancroid. An acute venereal disease caused by *Haemophilus ducreyi* and usually transmitted by sexual intercourse, chancroid produces a painful ulcer on the corona, prepuce, or shaft of the penis. This ulcer is necrotic and suppurative and bleeds readily. It is not as indurated as the syphilitic chancre and is therefore termed soft chancre (see p. 300).

Herpes progenitalis. Herpes progenitalis is characterized by development of a group of vesicles on the glans or prepuce. The surrounding tissue is inflamed. The vesicles rupture, and small discrete or confluent ulcers develop that heal with a short time.

Granuloma inguinale. Granuloma inguinale usually begins in the inguinal region and spreads to the perineum, scrotum, and penis. Nodules and serpiginous ulcers develop on the prepuce, and these spread to the glans and the shaft (see p. 313).

Lymphopathia venereum. Lymphopathia venereum is often confused with granuloma inguinale, but it is a specific venereal disease caused by a filterable agent (see p. 342).

Fusospirochetosis. Erosive and gangrenous balanitis is a disease comparable to Vincent's angina and is caused by a fusiform bacillus (*Vibrio*) and a spirochete (see p. 319).

Plastic induration. Plastic induration (Peyronie's disease) is a fibrositis of the penis involving Buck's fascia and the sheath of one or both corpora cavernosa. The cause is unknown. It resembles Dupuytren's contracture and keloids, and 25% of patients do show Dupuytren's contracture. The disease is more common than reports in the literature indicate. About 5% to 10% of cases reveal mild lesions. Two types are described: (1) thickening and contracture of the median septum and (2) localized nodules or indurated thickened areas involving the sides and underportion of the sheath of the corpus cavernosum. There are curvature of the penis and pain on erection and difficult or impossible intromission. Microscopically there is a scanty cellular fibrous tissue in which there are few blood vessels and mild evidence of inflammation. The lesion often resembles scar tissue. Occasionally the fibrous tissue undergoes ossification.

Sclerosing lipogranuloma (paraffinoma). Sclerosing lipogranuloma is a subcutaneous granulomatous reaction seen most often in the penis and scrotum. It appears as painful or painless nodules, plaques, or fistulas and can be demonstrated by infrared absorption spectrophotometry to result from the presence of exogenous lipid (paraffin hydrocarbons). Microscopically the involved area exhibits diffuse hyalinized tissue with variable numbers of inflammatory cells and numerous vacuoles. The latter vary in size from several micrometers to those that are grossly visible. Some vacuoles have no lining, whereas others may be partially outlined by flattened multinucleated, foreign body–type giant cells. A history of lipid injection is rarely volunteered, but the lesion is believed to result from an effort to facilitate erection or increase potency.

Tumors

Benign tumors. Squamous cell papillomas occur on the glans and shaft under various names, the most common being the condyloma. Hemangioma is the most common mesodermal lesion of the glans. Neurofibromas and leiomyomas occur rarely as small nodules of the glans, frenulum, prepuce, or shaft.

CONDYLOMA ACUMINATUM. Incorrectly termed venereal wart, condyloma acuminatum is a raspberry- or cauliflower-shaped tumor usually located on the sulcus. The tumor may be a single papilloma, or there may be multiple or conglomerated papillomas. These tumors frequently are associated with or occur after various inflammatory diseases of the penis. A viral etiology cannot be excluded. Microscopically these are essentially squamous papillomas characterized by pronounced acanthosis and hyperplasia of the prickle cell layer. Parakeratosis is present. The rete ridges are elongated and may be branching, but they all extend to about the same level. The growth is characteristically upward toward the surface and not downward into the tissue. Sometimes the tumor is quite extensive. A histologically similar lesion

has received attention. It has been designated giant condyloma, Buschke-Lowenstein tumor, or verrucous carcinoma. It forms grotesque cauliflower-like warty masses of large size with a strong tendency to extend, perforate the prepuce, destroy the underlying tissue, ulcerate, become infected, and produce many fistulas. Clinically the masses behave as cancer, and recurrence is the rule, but histologically they are benign. In contrast to the usual condylomas, the stratum corneum is thicker, parakeratosis is present, and there is pronounced acanthosis and papillation, as well as pronounced hyperplasia of the prickle cell layer. The papillae extend much deeper. Mitoses are limited to the basal layers, and stratification is normal. The tumors rarely metastasize.

VERRUCA. Verruca is an ordinary squamous cell papilloma revealing hyperkeratosis and thus differing from a single condyloma, in which the epithelium is piled up in the middle layer (acanthosis).

BOWENOID PAPULOSIS. The benign lesions of bowenoid papulosis occur chiefly on the penile shaft and adjacent perigenital skin of men between the ages of 20 and 45 years. Mucosal lesions may also occur but seldom without involvement of adjacent skin. The lesions may be solitary but usually are multiple and typically vary from 1 to 10 mm in size. The appearance is that of a shiny, flesh-colored, pink to red-brown, black, or violaceous papular or verrucoid lesion. Histologically there may be hyperkeratosis, frequently parakeratosis, focal hypergranulosis, vacuolated keratinocytes, irregular acanthosis, and occasional papillomatosis. There is orderly maturation with scattered hyperchromatic nuclei, dysplastic cells, and mitoses. Many of the last are in the same stage of development, chiefly metaphase. The most important feature that distinguishes bowenoid papulosis from erythroplasia and Bowen's disease is the absence of full-thickness involvement by atypical keratinocytes. Recent evidence points to the human papilloma virus and herpes simplex virus (type 2) as the etiologic agents. Treatment should be conservative.

Premalignant lesions

ERYTHROPLASIA OF QUEYRAT. Erythroplasia of Queyrat is a pinkish pagetoid lesion that usually involves the glans but occasionally may occur on the coronal sulcus or prepuce. It is shiny, pinkish red, flat, faintly elevated, and sharply marginated. The surface is smooth, slightly eroded, "velvety," more firm than the surrounding normal tissue, quite pliable, and with definite evidence of fixation to the underlying tissue. Histologically erythroplasia of Queyrat shows an area of irregular acanthosis in which the keratin layer is decreased and there is parakeratosis. The epidermis is thickened and composed of atypical cells with loss of normal polarity and of normal maturation. Many of the cells are vacuolated, and numerous mitotic figures are seen at all levels. The rete ridges are elongated and extend into the underlying stroma and sometimes are attached to each other. The subepithelial layer of dermis is edematous and shows infiltration that is predominately plasmacytic. It is important to distinguish between erythroplasia, which occurs on the penile mucosa, and Bowen's disease, which occurs on penile skin. Unlike erythroplasia, Bowen's disease is associated with a high incidence of primary malignant tumors of skin and viscera.

Malignant tumors

SQUAMOUS CELL CARCINOMA. In the United States less than 2% of all cancers in men arise in the penis. The incidence on other parts of the world is as follows: China, 18.3%; continental Europe, 4.9%; Great Britain, 1.27%. In the United States, penile cancer occurs about three or four times more frequently in blacks than in whites. The greatest incidence is between the ages of 45 and 60 years. Rare cases in childhood and early adult life have been reported.

It would not be an exaggeration to state that the presence of a foreskin is a predisposing cause for squamous cell carcinoma of the penis, since without this structure the incidence is insignificant. In India carcinoma of the penis rarely develops in Muhammedans, who practice circumcision in infancy as a religious rite, whereas Hindus, who do not circumcise, have about a 10% incidence. Among Jews, who are also regularly circumcised in infancy, the disease is almost unknown. The exciting causes of this neoplasm are irritation by retained smegma, phimosis, and trauma. Smegma has been shown to be possibly carcinogenic. Many patients give a history of previous venereal disease.

The location of the neoplasm, in order of frequency, is the (1) frenum and prepuce, (2) glans, and (3) coronal sulcus. The tumors may be papillary or flat and ulcerating. They grow slowly. Histologically they are of low malignancy. Metastasis to the inguinal lymph nodes occurs in about 50% of the cases. Visceral metastasis is extremely rare.

SARCOMA. Fibrosarcoma, leiomyosarcoma, Kaposi's sarcoma, endothelioma, and malignant melanoma are seen rarely. Metastatic carcinoma to the penis usually is a terminal event in the course of carcinomatosis. The tumor characteristically fills the vascular spaces of erectile tissue to produce a rather generalized induration of the organ. The primary lesions are most commonly in the prostate, bladder, kidney, or gastrointestinal tract.

URETHRA

Mechanical disturbances

Diverticula. Urethral diverticula are fairly common in females but rare in males. They may be congenital or acquired. Congenital true diverticula, arising from the periurethral glands, always occur on the ventral wall of the anterior portion of the urethra, whereas acquired diverticula develop in the posterior portion. The acquired

diverticula are caused by inflammation, trauma, or, in the male, obstruction of the urethra.

Prolapse. Prolapse of the urethra occurs almost exclusively in females. It usually involves the entire circumference, and the lumen is located in the center. Unless reduced promptly, pressure and infection produce vascular engorgement and acute inflammation.

Obstruction. Strictures of the urethra may be congenital or acquired. The former occurs usually in male infants at either the corona or the membranous urethra. Infant girls also may manifest congenital stricture of the distal portion of the urethra. Acquired strictures are the most common, and at one time most of them were complications of gonorrheal urethritis. This will probably be the case again with the recent increase in the incidence of venereal disease. About 10% are the result of trauma, but tuberculosis, other venereal diseases, periurethral abscesses, and caruncles also may cause urethral strictures. In women, obstetric trauma is the chief cause. Whatever the cause, the urethra heals by proliferation of fibroblasts and scarring, resulting in contraction. If left untreated, eventually there are back pressure, dilatation of the urethra, hypertrophy of the vesical musculature, and finally hydroureter and hydronephrosis.

Inflammation

Gonococcal urethritis. Acute urethritis may be attributed to a variety of bacteria. Gonococcal urethritis in the male, as a rule, involves the portion of urethra anterior to the triangular ligament (p. 298).

Nonspecific urethritis. Trauma, injection of chemical irritants, masturbation, coitus (in which the female partner may suffer a nonspecific vaginitis), redundant foreskin, and pinhole meatus are causes of nonspecific urethritis. The same conditions that predispose to cystitis act similarly in the urethra. Various bacteria have been isolated, among which staphylococci, streptococci, and colon bacilli predominate. In recent years nongonococcal urethritis has been recognized with increasing frequency; it is most commonly caused by *Chlamydia trachomatis*. Gonococci and chlamydiae produce similar symptoms and often coexist. Thus treatment of gonococcal urethritis with penicillin is often followed by recurrent symptoms (postgonococcal urethritis) because of the resistant *Chlamydia* organisms. Because laboratory procedures have now progressed to the point that both organisms can be readily identified, tetracycline has been advocated when both are present.

Abscesses. Abscesses within and continuous with the urethra are infrequent. They are usually complications of gonorrhea, but they may be complications of nonspecific infections. These abscesses develop when the urethral glands are infected and their ducts occluded.

Reiter's disease. Urethritis, conjunctivitis, and arthritis form a clinical triad known as Reiter's disease. The cause of this disease is not known, and tissue changes have not been investigated. Several workers have recovered viruslike agents by inoculating embryonated eggs with filtered urethral and conjunctival exudates. Spontaneous recovery is the rule, but relapses occur in about 25%, sometimes after a considerable silent period.

Urethrolithiasis. Calculi are rarely formed in the urethra. They either are dislodged bladder calculi or, when primary, originate in a urethral diverticulum.

Tumors

Benign tumors. The most common benign tumors and tumorlike lesions of the urethra are caruncles, cysts, leiomyomas, and condylomas. The last is the most common lesion in young adult males, in whom it is frequently multifocal and recurrent. A lesion that has been designated ectopic prostate occurs in the prostatic urethra. The latter, including the verumontanum, are normally lined in part by prostatic acinar epithelium. When this tissue projects into the urethral lumen as a result of either hyperplasia or mucosal redundancy, it is said to be ectopic. Such a lesion can cause hematuria or hematospermia if in proximity to the orifices of the ejaculatory ducts.

CARUNCLES. Urethral caruncles are confined almost entirely to the female urethra. Their cause is unknown. There are several theories: regional or circumscribed prolapse of urethral mucosa caused primarily by postmenopausal shrinkage of vaginal tissue with secondary trauma and infection, infection and chronic irritation resulting from lack of proper hygiene, and trauma consequent to coitus or childbirth.

Histologically there are three somewhat arbitrary types. The papillomatous type is frequently grossly lobulated as a result of clefts or crypts. The surface is covered by transitional and stratified squamous epithelium in various places. The epithelium continues along the crypts, from which sprouts extend deep into the stroma. Some of the epithelium-lined crypts on cross section appear as deep-seated nests of epithelial cells. Such areas may be confused with carcinoma. The stroma is usually infiltrated with inflammatory cellular elements.

The telangiectatic caruncle is highly vascular. The vessels are so numerous that the lesion has an appearance similar to the papillomatous type.

The granulomatous type lacks epithelial hyperplasia and is almost entirely composed of granulation tissue.

CYSTS. Cysts of the urethra may be congenital or acquired. Acquired cysts are more common and result from inflammatory occlusion of the urethal glands. The cysts of the posterior urethra arise from occlusion of the periurethral and subcervical ducts. Polyps are usually encountered in the folds of the urethra. Some of the polyps are difficult to differentiate from fibromas and papillomas. Papillomas occur in any part of the urethra, but the majority are encountered about the vesical neck at or near the meatus.

Malignant tumors. Malignant tumors of the urethra include squamous cell carcinoma, transitional cell carcinoma, adenocarcinoma, mesonephric carcinoma, and, rarely, melanoma. Squamous cell carcinoma of either male or female urethra is uncommon, but vulvourethral carcinoma is not infrequent. Transitional cell carcinomas occur chiefly in the posterior urethra and most often are associated with similar lesions in the bladder. Some of the urethral adenocarcinomas probably originate from periurethral glands, but others clearly arise via glandular metaplasia of the transitional cell epithelial lining of the mucosa. Some urethral carcinomas have a tubular pattern composed of cells with clear or granular cytoplasm, reminiscent of renal cell carcinoma. These are designated as mesonephric carcinomas, although their origin is uncertain. Urethral melanomas are usually seen in older women. Malignant tumors of Cowper's gland are rare. They occur as ulcerative, nodular, or fungating lesions in the perineum and histologically show a mucinous or adenoid cystic appearance.

PROSTATE GLAND

The prostate gland, the largest accessory sex organ in males, is situated immediately below the internal urethral orifice. In embryonic life the prostate is formed by a number of evaginations from the posterior and lateral walls of the posterior urethra. At about the twelfth week of embryonic development, the prostate reveals five lobes—anterior, middle, posterior, and two lateral lobes. These lobes fuse during the last half of fetal life so that at birth the divisions are imperceptible. During the third trimester of fetal life, the prostate enlarges as a result of gonadal and gonadotropic hormones of the mother. The hyperplasia persists for a few days after birth, and then the organ atrophies and does not fully develop until puberty.

From 15 to 30 branching tubular glands embedded in fibromuscular tissue make up the adult prostate. The glandular epithelium consists of two layers: tall columnar luminal cells and flattened cuboidal basal cells. The epithelium rests on a thin basement membrane. The supporting stroma consists of equal amounts of smooth muscle and fibrous tissue.

Functionally, three different types of glands are recognized (Fig. 21-30):

1. The smallest, the mucosal glands, lie in the periurethral tissue and open at various points around the urethra.
2. The submucosal glands are situated in the tissue around the periurethral area. Their ducts are longer and open into the urethral sinuses. The mucosal and submucosal glands together form the inner gland group, which is of mixed embryologic origin and develops from the dorsal wall of the urethra above the mesonephric ducts. They are par-

tially separated from the main mass of prostatic glands by an indefinite capsule.

3. The external or main glands are derived entirely from the endodermal epithelium of the urogenital sinus and form the outer and largest portion of the prostate. Their ducts also open into the urethral sinuses. The inner group of glands, commonly referred to as the female prostate, give rise to benign nodular hyperplasia. For this reason benign

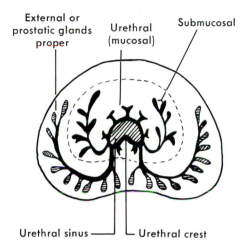

External or prostatic glands proper   Urethral (mucosal)   Submucosal

Urethral sinus   Urethral crest

Fig. 21-30. Distribution of normal prostatic glands slightly modified. Urethral (mucosal) and submucosal glands together form inner group, which is separated from outer gland group by an inconstant capsule. (From Grant, J.C.B.: A method of anatomy, ed. 5, Baltimore, 1952, The Williams & Wilkins Co.)

enlargement mainly produces urinary symptoms. Prostatic cancer almost invariably begins in the outer groups of glands, commonly referred to as the male prostate.

Although it has been customary to divide the adult prostate gland into five lobes (two lateral lobes, a median lobe, a posterior lobe, and an anterior lobe), there are no sharp lines of demarcation between the lobes (Fig. 21-31). Based on embryologic, ultrastructural, and arterial injection studies, the prostate is now regarded as essentially two separate organs: (1) the periurethral, female portion, which is sensitive to estrogens and androgens, and (2) the subcapsular true male prostate, which is sensitive to androgens; the latter forms a horseshoelike sheath around the former.

The normal development and maintenance of the prostate depend on testicular androgens. The prostate undergoes certain involutional changes with age. It atrophies after orchiectomy or administration of estrogens.

Nontumorous conditions

Acute prostatitis. Acute inflammation usually results from ascent of bacteria from the urethra or descent from the upper urinary tract or bladder. It may be spontaneous, but it is a fairly frequent complication of urethral manipulation by catheterization, urethral dilatation, and cystoscopy, especially if the patient has had a quiescent (chronic) prostatitis. Infection also may occur via hematogenous and lymphogenous spread. The most common bacteria are gonococci, staphylococci, streptococci, and the coliform bacilli. Not infrequently, smears and cultures are negative, but both must always be examined.

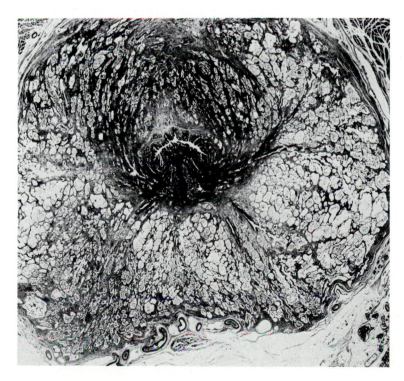

Fig. 21-31. Transverse section of prostate showing main mass of outer glands, submucosal glands, and urethral (mucosal) glands. There is no sharp line of separation between submucosal and outer glands in this section. Age unknown. (Approximately 3×.)

Grossly the prostate gland is enlarged, boggy, and edematous and contains multiple abscesses and foci of necrosis. Microscopic sections reveal multiple circumscribed collections of polymorphonuclear leukocytes, the glands being distended with a purulent exudate, or the inflammatory process may be diffuse. Edema, hyperemia, and foci of necrosis are frequent concomitant histologic findings.

Chronic prostatitis. Chronic inflammation of the prostate gland is common, and as with teeth and tonsils, the prostate has been considered to harbor foci of infection, causing arthritis, myositis, neuritis, and iritis. Allergic manifestations also have attributed to chronic prostatitis. Asthma, dermatitis, and pseudoangina pectoris have been reported to be relieved by adequate treatment of prostatitis. At necropsy the prostate gland of about 70% of men past 50 years of age reveals inflammatory changes.

The etiologic agents of chronic prostatitis are the same as those causing acute prostatitis, although in some types of chronic prostatitis the cause is unknown. Corpora amylacea or prostatic calculi may cause obstruction and stasis of secretion, leading to secondary inflammatory changes. A great number of cocci and bacilli are isolated from the chronically inflamed prostate. Frequently, however, the cultures are entirely negative.

Several forms of chronic prostatitis may be seen. The most common reveals diffuse, patchy, or very discrete foci of lymphocytic and plasma cell infiltration with or without changes in the acini and ducts. Some of these may be intact with the lumina empty and others with the lumina filled with debris and desquamated epithelial cells. Still others may show transformation to squamous epithelium. Some acini may become dilated as a result of intraluminal occlusion of ducts by various cellular elements and corpora amylacea, with loss of the epithelial lining and abscess formation.

Granulomatous prostatitis. An interesting chronic inflammatory lesion is nonspecific granulomatous prostatitis, the cause of which is unknown but is believed to be related to prostatic secretions. It is postulated that, as a result of inflammation, the integrity of ductal epithelial lining is lost and the secretions escape into the adjacent prostatic tissue. The resulting inflammatory reaction consists of many macrophages and lipophages as well as lymphocytes, plasma cells, and monocytes. Occasionally eosinophils, epithelioid cells, and Langhans'-type giant cells also are seen. Sometimes fragments of corpora amylacea are present amid the inflammatory reaction.

The significance of this type of reaction is twofold: (1) it may be confused with tuberculosis, and (2) it may be mistaken clinically and pathologically for carcinoma. In such patients rectal examination may reveal stony hardness of the prostate gland and lead to a clinical diagnosis of carcinoma. The biopsy specimen may be misinter-preted as clear cell carcinoma of the prostate.

Specific granulomas. Primary tuberculosis of the prostate gland is rare, and tuberculous involvement is almost always the result of either direct spread from the urethra, vas deferens, or bladder or spread via hematogenous or lymphatic routes. It occurs in younger people. Granulomatous and fibrocaseous forms are the most common types. Syphilitic, blastomycotic, and coccidiomycotic granulomas are rare.

Parasitic infection. Echinococcal cyst of the prostate gland is quite rare, and its occurrence is limited to the regions in which the parasite is endemic. Bilharzial involvement of the prostate is common among men in endemic regions and is considered a possible contributing factor to the obstruction of the bladder neck that occurs in these patients. *Trichomonas vaginalis* also may infect the prostate gland.

Cavitary or diverticular prostatitis. Diverticula or cavities may develop in any type of prostatitis in which there is stagnation of exudate in ducts and acini. Prolonged stagnation causes reactive fibrous tissue proliferation, which constricts the ducts. Acini dilate, and intra-acinar septa become thin and break down, resulting in formation of cavities. Prostatic diverticula may develop in cases of urethral stricture owing to dilatation of prostatic ducts opening into the posterior urethra as a result of back pressure. Urine may enter the cavities, and salts may precipitate to form calculi. The end stage of various types of chronic prostatitis is fibrosis and scarring.

Corpora amylacea and calculi. Corpora amylacea are found in increasing numbers with age. They are formed from desquamated epithelial cells producing concentric lamellae around inspissated prostatic secretions that accumulate because of partial ductal obstruction. They are composed largely of protein and nucleic acid. Cyclic growth of corpora amylacea results from addition of concentric layers. Corpora amylacea may block the ducts with dilatation and further inspissation of secretions. Inflammatory reaction of the ducts may result in deposition of calcium salts (phosphate and carbonate) to form calculi.

Prostatic calculi are quite common, occurring in 20% to 30% of all men over the age of 50 years, but they are rarely of clinical importance. Two types are identified: true (endogenous) and false (exogenous). Endogenous calculi are formed around the nuclei of corpora amylacea as already described. Other calculi may form from a nucleus of compact cellular debris, blood clots, or necrotic tissue. The number may vary from a few to hundreds and the size from 1 mm to 5 cm or larger. There may be one in a dilated acinus or duct or several packed in a cavity. They may be round, ovoid, or triangular and, when grouped together, may have faceted surfaces. Their color varies from white or grayish white to various shades of brown. Some are very firm and brittle, whereas others are somewhat plastic. Exogenous calculi occur less frequently. They arise from urine and are always brittle and rough.

The type of calculus may be determined by chemical examination of the nucleus. The nucleus of an exogenous calculus contains urates and phosphates, whereas the nucleus of an endogenous calculus is composed of organic material. Prostatic calculi may lead to the erroneous diagnosis of carcinoma of the prostate gland on rectal examination of the prostate because of its hardness. They are easily identified by roentgenographic examination unless they are radiolucent.

Thrombosis and infarction. A common necropsy finding, especially in bedridden patients, is thrombosis of the periprostatic venous plexus. Some investigators doubt that thrombi of these veins are an important source of pulmonary embolism. The thrombosed areas usually organize and form phleboliths, which often are seen on roentgenograms. Infarcts may be caused by vascular changes associated with arteriosclerosis, hypertension, or polyarteritis and occasionally may be of embolic origin, as in bacterial endocarditis. Local changes resulting from trauma caused by the passage of sounds, catheters, and cystoscopes, by massage of the prostate gland, and by transurethral prostatic resection have initiated infarction. The glands around the infarcts frequently undergo squamous cell metaplasia.

Recent investigations indicate the possible role of estrogens of testicular or adrenal origin in stimulating squamous cell metaplasia. Squamous cell nests may persist in the zone of a healed infarct and occasionally be misinterpreted as carcinoma.

Tumorlike lesions

Cysts. Cysts of the prostate gland may be congenital or acquired. Congenital cysts are symmetric and are associated with other abnormalities, such as patent urachus and spina bifida. The müllerian duct cyst is usually retroprostatic. The müllerian duct, if it were patent, would extend from the appendix testis in a groove between the testicle and epididymis and up the spermatic cord and lie between the vas deferens and bladder, where it would join the duct from the opposite side. It would then become incorporated in the musculature of the bladder wall, pass through the prostate gland, and end in the utricle. Thus it is understandable that such cysts, forming from abnormal remnants of the müllerian duct, may form anywhere along its course. Müllerian duct cysts vary in size from a small dilatation of the utricle to huge masses containing several liters of clear, straw- to chocolate-colored fluid. The wall of the cyst is composed of a laminated collagenous fibrous tissue lined by flat or low cuboidal epithelial cells. Acquired forms are retention, echinococcal, and bilharzial cysts.

Amyloid deposits. Amyloid deposits may form in the prostate. They may be part of primary amyloidosis or may be confined to the prostate. They occur around the blood vessels and in periglandular areas. Amyloidosis of the prostate is asymptomatic but may be responsible for postprostatectomy bleeding.

Hyperplasia. Nonneoplastic nodular enlargement of the prostate—nodular hyperplasia, benign prostatic hypertrophy—is the most common symptomatic tumorlike condition in humans. It seldom occurs before the age of 50, but the incidence increases with age, and it can be found at autopsy in 75% to 80% of men over age 80. It is rare in Orientals.

Prostatic hyperplasia appears a decade earlier in American blacks than in whites, and it is rare among Koreans, Indians, Japanese, and Bantus. It is common in the dog and the mastomys. Prostatic hyperplasia occurs more frequently in men of the digestive, pyknic, or endomorphic type. The normal prostate in an adult weighs about 20 g. The enlarged prostate can be two to four times larger but seldom weighs more than 200 g, although one weighing 820 g has been reported.

Despite extensive clinical and laboratory research, the cause of hyperplasia has not been fully established. Clinical research at various times has pointed to inflammation, arteriosclerosis, and sexual indulgence or perversion as etiologic factors or has suggested that the nodules in hyperplastic prostate glands are akin to adenomas and leiomyomas of the uterus. Laboratory investigations, both anatomic and endocrinologic, have presented considerable evidence to suggest an endocrine basis for hyperplasia.

Prostatic hyperplasia occurs in the inner zone of the prostate, whereas carcinoma is usually found in the outer portion (Fig. 21-32). It occurs at a time in a man's life

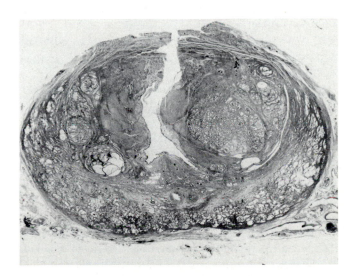

Fig. 21-32. Transverse section of prostate showing distinct nodules of stromal hyperplasia in periurethral zone. Large nodules consist of glandular and cystic structures. Tissues of outer prostate are compressed around edges. (3×.)

when there are disturbances of sex hormones. Although males possess a high level of androgens and females a high level of estrogens, both sexes harbor both sex hormones. In the female the ovaries are the major source of estrogens and some androgens, and the adrenal glands are the major source of androgens and probably some estrogens. In the male the testes produce most of the androgens, but some also are produced in the adrenal glands, and both organs contribute to the estrogen pool in the male. With advancing age there is a distinct fall in the level of androgens in the male and of estrogens in the female and a corresponding increase in the other sex hormones—estrogens in the male and androgens in the female. Whether this is a relative or absolute increase has not been settled. Both hormones have a tropic, stimulating effect on the reproductive organs that possess homologous tissues. The periurethral inner prostate and certain other sex organs and the breasts are responsive to the estrogens, whereas the outer prostate and the secondary sex organs of men are responsive to the androgens. Several possibilities may be considered in the endocrine relationship of prostatic hyperplasia:

1. A relative increase in the production of androgens by the active interstitial cells of Leydig associated with decreased function of tubules and decreased estrogen production
2. A relative increase in the production of estrogens by the increased Sertoli cells seen in old age and associated with decreased androgenic production by the interstitial cells of Leydig
3. A simultaneous stimulation of the prostate by both hormones, the action being, however, on different cells—the androgens acting on the epithelium and the estrogens on the fibromuscular stroma
4. A change in the structure of androgens or estrogens or both or some other hormone
5. A synergistic stimulation of the prostate by both the hormones and one or more endogenous or exogenous compounds
6. A change in the response of the endocrine-sensitive target organ, the prostate, brought about by environmental, circulatory, or genetic disturbances
7. A nonhormonal stimulation of the prostate, endogenous or exogenous, acting independent of the endocrine system

Any one or a combination of these factors could result in hyperplasia of the prostate gland.

Evidence based on histologic examination suggests that the etiologic agent of this disease begins to produce changes in the prostate after the age of 40 years, reaches its maximum intensity at about 60 years of age, and continues to be present in sufficient amounts to cause changes during the remainder of life. The majority of investigators in the field believe that in the senile or presenile age groups a shift in the androgen/estrogen ratio results in the dominance of estrogen, and this, act-

ing on the ambisexual estrogen-sensitive tissue of the prostatic area, produces nodular hyperplasia.

The anatomic location of the prostate readily explains the symptoms of hyperplasia. There is interference with and obstruction to the flow of urine. Rectal examination shows a soft, boggy, nodular prostate.

Grossly the enlarged prostate gland is smooth or nodular, firm, and somewhat elastic or rubbery. The appearance of the surfaces made by sectioning depends on whether the greatest amount of hyperplasia involves the glands or the fibromuscular tissue. If the hyperplasia is more glandular, the cut surface reveals many various-sized nodules, some of which are well circumscribed and surrounded by pearl white fibromuscular tissue. Some of the nodules have a honeycombed architecture. The cut surface of an enlarged prostate is yellowish and moist with a milky fluid. Cysts are common, and some of these may contain white or amber-colored corpora amylacea or calculi. If the hyperplasia is predominantly of fibromuscular tissue, the cut surfaces are pallid, glossy, and homogeneous, and very little milky fluid can be expressed. In contrast to the lobular architecture of the normal prostate gland, the rather spongy hyperplastic nodules form a mass that compresses the surrounding tissues into a false capsule, enabling the nodular masses to be shelled out with ease.

The initial lesion has been demonstrated to be a multicentric aglandular fibromuscular nodule (Figs. 21-33 and 21-34) originating in the submucous portion of the prostatic urethra. This stimulates the proliferation of nearby glands, with early invasion of the nodules by the epithelial elements to produce the usual stromal-glandular mixture. The acini are increased in number and size. Many undergo dilatation and invagination, forming villous projections (Fig. 21-35).

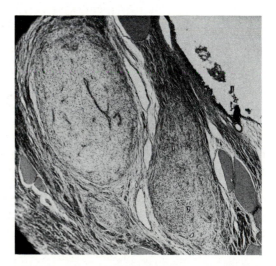

Fig. 21-33. Two small stromal nodules near urethra. Lower nodule has ill-defined margin and merges with surrounding tissues above and below. Well-formed blood vessels can be seen in nodules. (40×.)

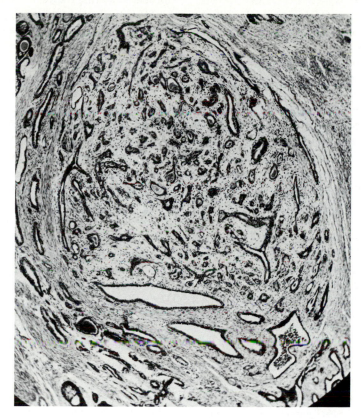

Fig. 21-34. Fibroadenomatous nodule. Epithelium lining the glands is low, cuboidal, and inactive. (65×.)

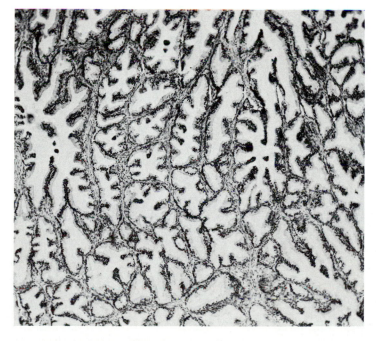

Fig. 21-35. Area of intra-acinar papillary hyperplasia. (65×.)

Some of the acini are lined by active cells and others by inactive cells (Fig. 21-36). The active cells are tall columnar cells with poorly defined borders, abundant finely granular or homogeneous cytoplasm, and basal nuclei often forming a double layer. The papillary infoldings are numerous and elongated, and the intralobular trabeculae are thin and delicate. The inactive cells that line many of the cystic acini are cuboidal or low columnar with well-defined cell walls, scanty vesiculated cytoplasm, and single-layered basal nuclei. The papillae are few and relatively small and the intralobular septa thick and coarse. The lumina contain desquamated epithelial cells, granular secretory material, and occasional corpora amylacea. Lymphocytic infiltration is a frequent accompaniment, but this is probably not an indication of chronic inflammation.

Depending on the relative amounts of stromal and glandular elements, Franks[127a] has recognized the following types of hyperplasia: stromal (fibrous or fibrovascular) nodule, fibromuscular nodule, muscular nodule, fibroadenomatous nodule, and fibromyoadenomatous nodule. To these may be added the purely glandular adenomatous nodule. The true stromal nodules are found only in subepithelial tissues around the urethra above the verumontanum. The smaller nodules are made up of a meshwork of fine fibrils with groups of elongated spindle cells or flat stellate cells arranged around small vascular spaces. No elastic tissues are present in the nodules. The fibromuscular and muscular nodules are similar except that there is more fibrous tissue in the former. Fibroadenomatous and fibromyoadenomatous nodules are also similar except for the presence of smooth muscle elements in the latter.

The purely glandular adenomatous nodule is rare in humans, but it is seen in dogs. It may be so pronounced as to suggest an adenoma.

Secondary changes in the nodule. Areas of chronic and occasionally acute inflammation are seen in almost all nodules. Areas of chronic inflammation often surround distended ducts filled with inspissated secretion.

The mechanical effect of the expanding hyperplastic nodules within the relatively confined prostate is manifested in another important change—prostatic infarction—which occurs in 25% of hyperplastic glands.

The genesis of these infarcts is readily explained by the fact that all the blood supply of the hyperplastic nodules comes from the periphery, and sometimes it is stretched over the nodule. As the nodules expand, they sometimes compress the blood vessels at the periphery, with resultant ischemia in the center of the nodule and a hemorrhagic infarction.

Clinically this may be manifested as hematuria or complete urinary shutdown. The prostate may feel hard, and there may be elevation of prostatic acid phosphatase levels. The infarcted area consists of a lobule with a central hemorrhagic area and necrosis of the tissue. Prostatic infarction is invariably associated with squamous metaplasia of tubuloacinar structures. With healing there are fibrosis of the stroma and development of compact transitional or squamous cell nests. Scattered hemosiderin deposits are seen.

The chief complicaton of the enlarged prostate is ure-

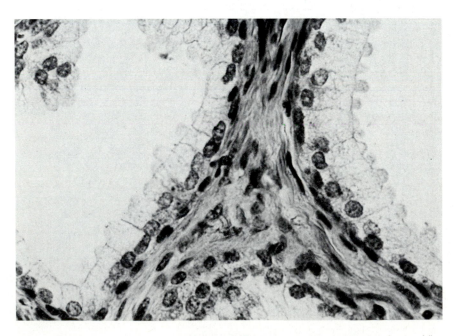

Fig. 21-36. Epithelium in intra-acinar papillary hyperplasia showing inconspicuous layer of flattened basal cells beneath surface epithelium. (870×.)

thral obstruction with secondary effects on the bladder, ureters, and kidneys (Fig. 21-37). The enlarging prostate causes elongation, tortuosity, and compression of the posterior portion of the urethra, and the urinary outlet is elevated above the floor of the bladder. These changes result in retention of urine, and with retention there is usually secondary infection. The enlarged median lobe stretches the sphincter vesicae muscles, resulting in incompetence of the sphincter and constant dribbling. In its efforts to overcome the obstruction, the crisscrossing vesical musculature undergoes compensatory hypertrophy, which produces the characteristic ribbed appearance of the muscle (trabeculation). The bladder wall may be twice its normal thickness. Contractions of the vesical musculature to increase the intravesical pressure in order to overcome bladder neck obstruction lead to outpocketings of the mucosa through the thinner portions of the wall to form diverticula. If not treated, decompensation results in dilatation of the bladder and thinning of the wall.

Normally the ureters enter the bladder at an angle and traverse intramurally before opening into the bladder lumen. This arrangement tends to provide an effective

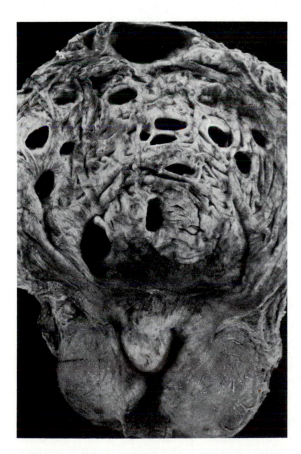

Fig. 21-37. Hyperplasia of prostate gland. Obstruction of urethra by large middle lobe and hypertrophied bladder with cellules and diverticula.

valve action so that as the bladder becomes temporarily filled normally, the elevated intravesical pressure closes off the ureteral orifices to prevent reflux of the urine up the ureters. As soon as the bladder is emptied, pressure on the wall is released and the ureteral orifices open. When dilatation and thinning of the bladder occur following obstruction at the bladder neck, the normal sphincter action of the vesical musculature at the ureteral orifices is removed. The increased intravesical pressure is thus transmitted to the ureters and the renal pelvis, and they also undergo compensatory hypertrophy and dilatation (hydroureter and hydronephrosis). There are usually infection and pyelonephritis. The increased intrapelvic pressure leads to hydronephrotic atrophy of the renal parenchyma as a result of ischemia. If this is bilateral, hypertension may develop. The renal lesions are the most important sequelae of prostatic enlargement.

Benign tumors. If the nodules of nodular hyperplasia of the prostate gland are considered tumors (as some believe they should be), adenomas, fibroadenomas, fibromas, or leiomyomas are very common. Differentiation of stromal hyperplasia from neoplasia is sometimes difficult. Although some of the circumscribed nodules of the enlarged prostate gland are similar to tumors, they should not be designated as neoplasms. Some of the reported adenomas are actually circumscribed areas of glandular hyperplasia. Likewise, many of the recorded leiomyomas are instances of fibromuscular hyperplasia.

Excluding prostatic hyperplasia, benign tumors of the prostate are rare. Kaufman and Berneike[136a] recorded 38 cases of leiomyomas. The average age of the patients was about 60 years. The tumors weighed from about 15 to 1450 g. They were firm, rubbery, yellowish white, and homogeneous. Microscopically the tumors revealed interlacing whorls of smooth muscle with little intervening fibrous tissue. Neurofibromas occasionally involve the prostate gland.

Other benign epithelial abnormalities. Several types of atypical hyperplasia have been described. Lobular hyperplasia is characterized by proliferation of small acini around a central acinus. In postatrophic hyperplasia, groups of irregular small acini are seen distributed aound a central atrophic acinus. This type of hyperplasia is often associated with small acinar carcinoma and is believed to be precancerous. Both of these hyperplasias occur in the outer zone of the prostate. Secondary hyperplasia is the term applied to instances in which large acini are lined partly by a single layer of cuboidal cells and partly by papillary projections covered by similar epithelium. Focal intra-acinar hyperplasia consists of glands within glands. This is distinguished from intra-acinar carcinoma by the presence of a delicate fibrovascular stroma between glands, a distinct basal cell layer, and uniform benign-appearing nuclei. Basal cell hyperplasia—fetalization of the prostate—is characterized by intra-acinar proliferation of small basophilic cells with ovoid nuclei and scant cytoplasm. The lesion may be focal, lobular, or diffuse. All these hyperplasias are associated with varying degrees of stromal hyperplasia and may occur anywhere.

In atrophy the glands are small. They are lined by low cuboidal epithelium with small, densely staining nuclei. There is a central, partly collapsed duct also lined by atrophic epithelium. The stroma is hyalinized. The term "atrophy" would seem to be a misnomer because the cells have been observed to become hyperplastic or even neoplastic. Squamous metaplasia of prostatic epithelium may occur following infection or the use of an indwelling catheter, but it is most often associated with infarction of the prostate or estrogen therapy for carcinoma of the prostate.

Malignant tumors

Carcinoma. Although the large majority of prostatic cancers are glandular and usually referred to as adenocarcinoma, the term *carcinoma* is generally preferred. Carcinoma of the prostate gland is the second most frequent cause of death from cancer in the male population in the United States. The incidence of carcinoma of the prostate is highest among the black population in the United States (blacks, 23 per 100,000; whites, 14.3 per 100,000), whereas the incidence in Israel is 7.3 and in Japan 1.1. In the United States the incidence of prostatic carcinoma is lowest among Jews, intermediate among Catholics, and highest among Protestants. It is high among married men and those with children and among persons living in metropolitan and urban areas; it has a familial incidence. Four categories of carcinoma of the prostate are recognized.

LATENT CARCINOMA. In autopsies of men dying of other causes, carcinoma of the prostate is found unexpectedly in 26% to 37% of prostates. In a worldwide study conducted by the International Agency for Cancer Research,[124] the frequency of such carcinomas was determined from autopsies performed in Hong Kong, Singapore, Israel, Uganda, Germany, Sweden, and Jamaica. It was found that the incidence of small carcinomas was the same; however, the incidence of larger latent carcinomas varied. It was lowest in Hong Kong and Singapore, intermediate in Israel and Uganda, and high in Germany, Sweden, and Jamaica. These figures corresponded to deaths from carcinoma of the prostate, suggesting that environmental factors play a role in incidence and prevalence of carcinoma of prostate; they suggest that, while many of these carcinomas remain dormant during the lifetime of the host, environmental factors must play a role in inciting latent carcinomas into clinical carcinoma in some men.

INCIDENTAL CARCINOMA. In 6% to 20% of tissues removed surgically for clinically benign prostatic hyperplasia, histologic examination shows carcinoma of the prostate. The discovery of incidental carcinoma in a patient who has no symptoms referable to his carcinoma raises many questions. Are these accidental discoveries of carcinomas that would have remained dormant? Should these carcinomas be left alone, or are they the group in which surgical extirpation may be lifesaving?

OCCULT CARCINOMA. A number of patients who have no symptoms of prostatic carcinoma show evidence of metastases on clinical examination, such as roentgenographic changes in the site of a fracture or an enlarged lymph node. Biopsy of the metastatic lesion may reveal carcinoma, the prostatic origin of which is demonstrated by stains for prostatic acid phosphatase and prostatic-specific antigens and is then confirmed by biopsy examination of the prostate. It would seem that at least some, if not most, occult carcinomas originate from latent carcinomas.

CLINICAL CARCINOMA. The category of clinical carcinoma includes all cases in which rectal examination has aroused suspicion of carcinoma of the prostate and the diagnosis is confirmed by pathologic examination of the tissue removed from the prostate.

ETIOLOGY. Although the cause of carcinoma of the prostate is unknown, androgens have been suspect. Androgens are essential for the development and maintenance of the prostate. Carcinoma of the prostate is extremely rare in eunuchs and in patients with Klinefelter's syndrome. Testosterone accelerates the activity of carcinoma cells, whereas orchiectomy or estrogen therapy causes regression of tumor. Ultrastructurally cancer cells resemble testosterone-treated rabbit prostate cells. These observations have led to the theory that androgens are in some way responsible for carcinoma of the prostate. But prolonged administration of androgens has not produced any tumors, and cancer of the prostate occurs at the time of life when the level of androgens is normally low. The most prevalent hypothesis is that carcinoma of the prostate, which is a slow-growing tumor, may begin at the stage of life when androgen levels are high and may remain quiescent in most men whose androgen levels decline with advancing age. In a number of cases, some disturbance of the hypothalamic pituitary adrenal testes prostate axis may stimulate the dormant malignant cells to develop clinical cancer.

Viral inclusions have been observed in carcinoma of the prostate; Paulson, Rabson, and Fraley[144] reported that cultures of hamster prostate tissue infected with simian virus 40 underwent transformation 5 to 8 days after injection. These transformed cells developed into carcinoma when they were injected into the homologous hosts. Histologically the tumor resembled carcinoma of the prostate and gave the chemical and histochemical properties of carcinoma.

Exposure to cadmium has also been suspected.

SYMPTOMS. There are no distinct symptoms of early carcinoma of the prostate, and the symptoms, when present, are indistinguishable from those of benign hyperplasia of the prostate. Late cancers usually manifest themselves through back pain and anemia, which indicate bone metastases. Rectal examination is the only way carcinoma of prostate can be detected and is indicated in every patient over 50 years of age. A hard nodule or an area of induration in the prostate gland should be considered cancerous unless proved otherwise.

DIAGNOSIS. Cytologic, biochemical, roentgenographic, and pathologic methods are employed in the diagnosis of cancer of the prostate. The neoplastic cells in the smears are pleomorphic and hyperchromatic. The nuclear/cytoplasmic and the nucleolar/nuclear ratios are disturbed. The cells occur in clusters, and cell borders are indistinct, but nuclear borders are definite. Prostatic massage is contraindicated because neoplastic cells have been found in the bloodstream of 15% of patients with carcinoma of the prostate who had prostatic massage. Recently fine-needle aspiration has been employed with good results.

Acid phosphatase is present normally in the prostate, blood, urine, and saliva. The demonstration of elevated total serum acid phosphatase and prostatic acid phosphatase levels is a useful test for diagnosis and detection of metastasis, even before x-ray films show the tumor, and for determining response to therapy. The serum acid phosphatase level is elevated in 60% of patients with carcinoma of the prostate and in 80% of those with bony metastases. Further rises in an initially elevated level are indicative of metastases. In patients who respond to treatment, there is a drop in acid phosphatase levels about 1 week after surgical castration and 2 to 3 weeks after estrogen therapy. Because elevation of the total serum acid phosphatase level is found in Paget's disease and other bone diseases, multiple myeloma, Gaucher's disease, and hyperparathyroidism, it is essential to measure the prostatic fraction, prostatic acid phosphatase, and prostatic-specific antigen, which are more reliable indicators than total serum acid phosphatase. However, digital or operative manipulation of the prostate, catheterization, and infarction of the prostate may cause temporary elevation of the prostatic acid phosphatase level. It should be noted that urine acid phosphatase evaluation is of no value, since it is of renal origin.

Roentgenographic examination, including pyelography, chest x-ray examination, CT scan, and bone scan, is essential for diagnosis and staging of carcinoma of prostate. Most often the metastatic lesions of bone are osteoblastic, but osteolytic and mixed osteoblastic and osteolytic lesions also may be seen. A biopsy of bone lesions is necessary for diagnosis of metastatic carcinoma.

CLINICAL CLASSIFICATION. Clinical classification takes into consideration whether the lesion is incidentally found in clinically benign but pathologically cancer-containing prostate or discovered on rectal examination. If the latter, classification depends on whether it is a single nodule or multiple nodules in the prostate, whether the tumor is confined to the prostate or has extended beyond the confines of the prostate to the seminal vesicles, periprostatic tissue, or adjacent structures, and whether there is evidence of metastasis. Such categorization, combined with pathologic findings, determines the specific mode of therapy.

PATHOLOGIC FINDINGS. Grossly the malignant prostate may be large, of normal size, or smaller than normal. Approximately 15% to 20% of nodular hyperplastic prostates harbor carcinoma. Carcinoma may originate in any part of the gland; however, in about 75% it is located mainly in the posterior lobe. About 95% begin in the subcapsular zone (Fig. 21-38). As a rule, the malignant prostate is very firm in consistency, but occasionally it may be soft. The cut surface is dry, fibrous, and homogeneously pallid and often contains irregular yellowish areas.

Microscopically about 96% of malignant neoplasms of the prostate are adenocarcinomas, but they are generally referred to as carcinoma (Fig. 21-39). The tumor may consist of tiny, small, or simple large glands, fused glands, glands within glands, papillary structures, columns and cords, or solid sheets with little or no gland formation (Figs. 21-40 to 21-42). Often a combination of two or more of these is seen. Usually the glands are closely packed with little or no stroma between them, but in some cases the glands may be haphazardly distributed in the stroma. The cells may vary from cuboidal to columnar; they may form a single layer or be piled up. The cytoplasm varies a great deal. It may be pale or dark staining, vacuolated, amphophilic, granular, or eosino-

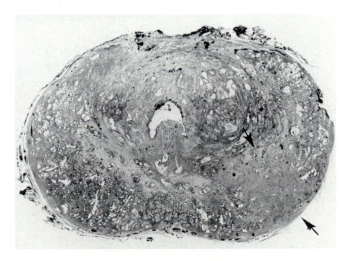

Fig. 21-38. Transverse section of prostate showing large area of carcinoma involving subcapsular zone *(arrows).* (15×.)

philic. It contains varying amounts of prostatic acid phosphatase, prostatic-specific antigen, and other tumor markers.

In many cases the individual cells lack the usual distinct morphologic criteria for malignancy. Cellular anaplasia is slight, and giant cells and mitotic figures are often absent (Fig. 21-43). The nuclei may be small, fairly uniform, and pale or dark staining, membranes may be delicate, and the chromatin distribution may be fairly homogeneous. Other carcinomas may show moderate or marked anaplasia (Figs. 21-44 and 21-45). The characteristic features of nuclei of carcinoma of prostate are coarse chromatin distribution, vacuolization, and a large but ill-defined nucleolus.

In contrast to normal or benign prostatic hyperplasia, in which the distribution of prostatic acid phosphatase and prostatic-specific antigen is fairly uniform and luminal in location, considerable variation is seen in the distribution of these markers in carcinoma of the prostate. Individual cells or clones of cells may contain one marker, both markers, or neither; this is seen in both tumors that form glands and those that do not. Thus carcinomas of the prostate tend to be heterogeneous in regard to pattern of growth, cell population, functional state of the cell, and degree of anaplasia.

Tumors forming regular small or large glands populated by cells that show little or no anaplasia are often diag-

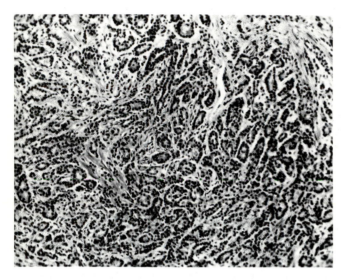

Fig. 21-39. Carcinoma of prostate, small acinar type. (145×.)

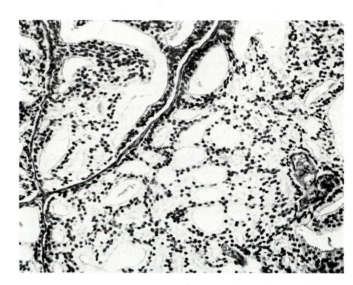

Fig. 21-40. Carcinoma of prostate, cribriform pattern. (63×.)

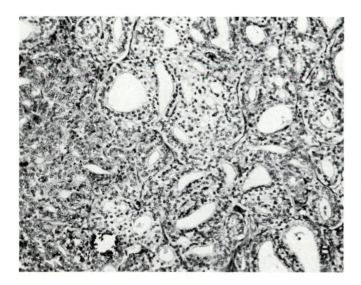

Fig. 21-41. Carcinoma of prostate. Mixed pattern of small and large acini and cribriform patterns. Note that some cells have pale cytoplasm whereas others have darker cytoplasm. (150×.)

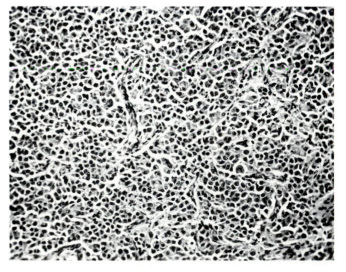

Fig. 21-42. Carcinoma of prostate, undifferentiated pattern. (160×.)

nostic problems. In examining such tumors attention must be focused on disturbances of architecture, evidence of invasion, arrangement and structure of nuclei, and distribution of enzymes. Tiny and small glands, glands back to back, glands inside glands, large glands without convolutions, and haphazard distribution of glands are diagnostic of carcinoma of prostate. Acini lined by a single layer of nuclei that are homogeneously pale or dark staining or vacuolated and contain an irregularly outlined nucleolus are carcinoma. Uneven distribution of prostatic acid phosphatase or prostatic-specific antigen in cell cytoplasm is indicative of carcinoma. Distortion and disruption of the delicate periacinar base-

ment membrane and invasion of the stroma are other helpful criteria. Invasion of the stroma is best detected by finding acini situated directly on muscle bundles or infiltrating them. The most reliable pathologic criterion for diagnosis of carcinoma of the prostate is perineural invasion. We have found this in over 85% of patients with prostate carcinoma (Fig. 21-46). The spaces are not lymphatics, and the finding has no prognostic significance.

It can be assumed that all carcinomas of prostate start as clinically inapparent carcinomas that are eventually detected either during a physical examination or because of symptoms of metastases. Carcinoma of the prostate is usually a slowly growing tumor. In its earliest stages the

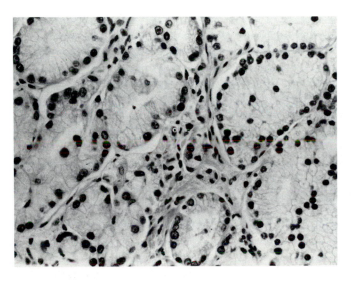

Fig. 21-43. Carcinoma of prostate showing slight anaplasia with fairly uniform nuclei. (160×.)

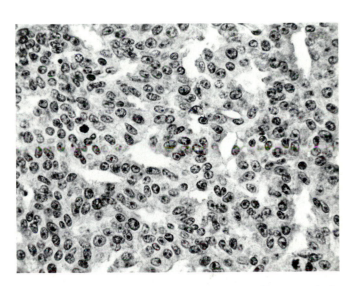

Fig. 21-44. Carcinoma of prostate showing moderate anaplasia, intermediate degree of variation in shape, and staining of nuclei. (160×.)

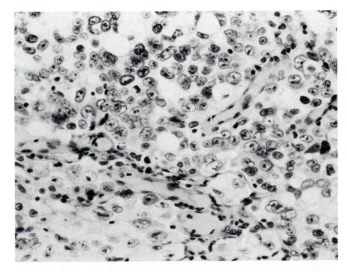

Fig. 21-45. Carcinoma of prostate showing marked anaplasia. Many nuclei are vacuolated and contain large irregular nucleoli. (160×.)

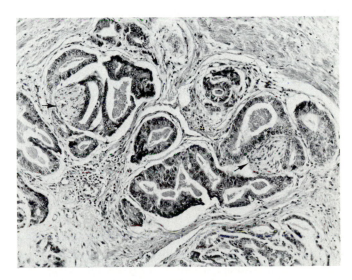

Fig. 21-46. Carcinoma of prostate showing perineural invasion *(arrows).*

neoplastic transformation may be unifocal, but Byar and Mostofi[125] have shown that prostatic carcinoma is multifocal. Whether pathologic examination of the removed tissue shows a unifocal or multifocal lesion is of clinical significance, as is whether the tumor is confined to the prostate, has extended locally, or has metastasized via lymphatics or the bloodstream.

LOCAL EXTENSION. The subcapsular location of the prostate predisposes to early invasion and penetration of the capsule and extension beyond the capsule with resultant anchoring of the prostate. In later stages the tumor may extend to the bladder neck, the seminal vesicles, the trigone, and, not infrequently, one or both ureteral orifices.

METASTASES. Lymphatic metastases have been reported in 7% to 25% of prostatic carcinomas that are confined to the prostate; the incidence increases with local extension. The pelvic, inguinal, periaortic, mediastinal, and supraclavicular lymph nodes are often involved, the earliest and most frequent involvement being in the pelvic nodes.

Hematogenous spread is manifested most frequently by osseous metastases, which occur in 70% of cases. The pelvis and the lumbar spine are the most frequent sites, but the ribs, femur, clavicle, or any other bone may be involved. The route of metastases to the spine has been extensively studied, and considerable disagreement prevails. According to some investigators, the route of metastasis to the spine is by way of lymphatics. However, it has been demonstrated that metastasis also occurs along the vertebral venous plexus. Willis[145] maintained that carcinoma of the prostate invades the systemic circulation in the same manner as other tumors do. By careful necropsy studies, he was able to demonstrate pulmonary metastasis in the majority of his cases.

EFFECTS OF THERAPY. The mode of therapy for carcinoma of prostate is controversial, especially for low-grade "incidental carcinomas" and carcinomas that are confined to the prostate. In such patients, if it is assumed that the tumor constitutes the early and presumably curable stages of the malignancy, complete surgical removal would seem to be the treatment of choice. Some such tumors (5% to 15%), however, have already metastasized at first examination; radical surgery is currently associated with a 90% incidence of impotence and about a 10% incidence of incontinence. There is also evidence that even without treatment some of these patients may live a long time and die of other causes. In recent years there has been a revival of radiation therapy for these patients.

Less controversial is the treatment of patients in whom the carcinoma has extended beyond the prostate or has metastasized. Such patients are given one of several types of internal and/or external irradiation and antiandrogen therapy.

Because androgens are essential for the development and maintenance of the prostate gland, which undergoes atrophy after castration, and because androgens are known to stimulate the growth of carcinoma of the prostate, Huggins and Hodges[135a] demonstrated that removal of the main source of androgen (testes) and treatment with estrogens are beneficial in the control of carcinoma of the prostate. In 80% of cases the tumors respond. The cells show vacuolization of cytoplasm and "ballooning." In such a cell the nucleus is pushed to the periphery (Fig. 21-47). The chromatin of the nucleus becomes condensed, the nucleolus disappears, and the nucleus becomes pyknotic. The swollen cells ultimately rupture and fuse with the stroma, which becomes vacuolated, pale staining, and fibrillar. This stromal change is followed by fibrosis. In some cases estrogen therapy causes inactivity of the neoplastic cells and disappearance of acid phosphatase from the cytoplasm. Squamous cell metaplasia following estrogenic effect may occur in the prostate and in the metastatic areas of the bones. The process may progress to squamous cell carcinoma. Orchiectomy and estrogen do not cure carcinoma of the prostate; the only successful method is early and complete removal of the tumor. The neoplasm may be and usually is controlled by antiandrogen therapy, but eventually the tumor cells fail to respond to such therapy. Massive increase in estrogen levels, adrenalectomy, and hypophysectomy have been tried with temporary beneficial results. Evidence has been presented that the incidence of cardiovascular deaths is increased in the first 9 months after initiation of estrogen therapy in patients with nonmetastatic carcinoma of the prostate, and there is general agreement to limit antiandrogen therapy to patients with biochemical or x-ray evidence of metastasis. The role of other chemotherapeutic agents is being actively explored.

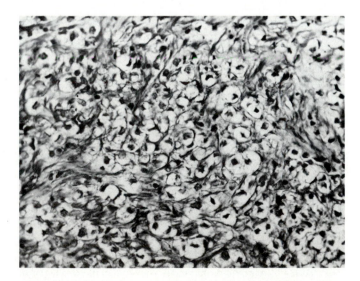

Fig. 21-47. Carcinoma of prostate showing estrogen effect (300×.)

Other carcinomas. A papillary adenocarcinoma, initially believed to be confined to the utricle and to be of müllerian origin, has been designated endometrioid carcinoma. However, it has been demonstrated that the tumor is of prostatic acinar origin, that it may occur in other locations (in the substance of the prostate rather than in the utricle), that the tumor in the utricle is usually associated with a typical carcinoma in the prostate, and that the cells contain both prostatic acid phosphatase (PAP) and prostatic-specific antigen (PSA).

TRANSITIONAL CELL CARCINOMA. Prostatic ducts are lined for the most part with transitional epithelium and partly with acinar epithelium. Thus it is conceivable that the transitional epithelium of the ducts may become malignant. However, in such cases before the diagnosis of primary transitional cell carcinoma of prostatic ductal origin is made, it is essential to rule out a carcinoma of the bladder or posterior urethra because carcinomas in these locations frequently grow into the prostate and replace prostatic ductal epithelium. Occasionally a transitional cell carcinoma is discovered in the bladder, but there is no apparent connection with the prostatic transitional cell carcinoma. In such cases it is probable that the carcinogenic agents that have induced malignant transformation of vesical or urethral epithelium have also acted on the prostatic ductal epithelium to induce neoplasia.

SQUAMOUS CELL CARCINOMA. Squamous cell carcinoma of prostate is also extremely rare; the comments made in reference to transitional cell carcinoma are equally applicable for this tumor. We have seen a number of cases of adenocarcinoma of prostate that, following prolonged administration of estrogens, have been transformed into squamous cell carcinoma.

MUCINOUS ADENOCARCINOMA. Many carcinomas of the prostate have mucin-containing cells, but rarely the tumor is predominantly or entirely mucinous adenocarcinoma. In all such cases PAP and PSA will reveal whether the tumor is prostatic acinar or extraprostatic in origin.

UNDIFFERENTIATED CARCINOMAS. Undifferentiated carcinoma of the prostate is another rarity, but it is more common than transitional or squamous cell carcinoma. In such cases it is essential to stain the tissue for PAP and PSA. This reveals one of several patterns: sheets of positive cells side by side with negative cells or more often scattered PAP/PSA–positive clones among cells that are negative.

Sarcoma. Sarcoma of the prostate gland is rare. It occurs at any age but is much more frequent in the young. We have seen rhabdomyosarcomas, leiomyosarcomas, fibrosarcomas, lymphosarcomas, angiosarcomas, malignant fibrous histiocytoma, and carcinosarcomas of the prostate. In recent years dramatic results have been reported in treatment of rhabdomyosarcoma in children.

SEMINAL VESICLES

The seminal vesicles are bilateral saclike outpouchings from the vas deferens at its termination in the ejaculatory duct. They have irregular, branching lumina with numerous outpocketings lined by pseudostratified epithelium, which often contains yellow pigment and secretory granules. The walls are composed of smooth muscle similar to but thinner than that of the vas.

Congenital anomalies of seminal vesicles are rare. Entrance of ectopic ureter to seminal vesicle may form cysts. Two types have been recognized: congenital and acquired. The former are regarded as malformations of either müllerian or wolffian ducts; the latter result from secondary inflammation, causing stenosis of the terminal portion of the duct and cystic dilatation in the proximal portion.

Grossly the cut surface shows a thin-walled structure filled with gray mucoid material. Histologically the inner surface is covered with a single layer of flattened and attenuated cuboidal epithelial cells. The cytoplasm is scant and contains occasional brownish granules and relatively large, irregularly shaped hyperchromatic nuclei. The lamina propria is usually thick and fibrotic.

Inflammation. Inflammation may be categorized as nonspecific seminal vesiculitis (acute or chronic), abscess, or specific vesiculitis such as tuberculosis, trichomoniasis, and schistosomiasis. Inflammatory reaction of the seminal vesicles usually results from urethral or prostatic infection.

Tumors and tumorlike lesions. Two tumorlike lesions merit mention: amyloid deposition and calcification.

Amyloidosis of seminal vesicle is similar to amyloid deposition elsewhere. It consists of deposits of a pale, pinkish, homogeneous substance in the connective tissue, in muscle, and in blood vessels. Some lymphocytic or granulomatous reaction may be seen.

Calcification of seminal vesicles is rare. It may follow chronic infection, such as tuberculosis in older patients, especially those with diabetes. It may be unilateral or bilateral. Its clinical significance is that it may be misinterpreted on rectal examination for prostatic carcinoma. The calcific masses are irregular and are surrounded by fibrous tissue. The epithelial lining is intact in early stages but may be destroyed in later stages.

Tumors of seminal vesicles are very rare—fewer than 100 have been described. They may be benign or malignant, epithelial or mesenchymal. The most common tumors are papillary adenomas, fibromas, and leiomyomas. Most malignant tumors of seminal vesicles are secondary, coming usually from the prostate.

Malignant tumors. Primary carcinomas are rare. They usually occur in patients over 50 years of age, but we have seen one in a young patient. Urinary retention, dysuria, and hematuria are the usual symptoms. A high level of serum fructose has been reported in some cases.

For diagnosis of carcinoma of the seminal vesicles it is

mandatory that involvement of seminal vesicles be anatomically proven. Histologically the tumors are usually
papillary adenocarcinomas, but undifferentiated areas
may be seen in some. The tumor consists of clear columnar cells, often with brown lipofuscin pigment forming
acinar and papillary structures.

Because many reported carcinomas of the seminal vesicles are extensions from the prostate or are papillary
carcinomas of the prostate that are misdiagnosed as carcinomas of the seminal vesicles, it is essential to rule out
a primary carcinoma of the prostate; this can be done by
stains for PAP and PSA.

Sarcomas are usually of prostatic and vesical origin but
may originate in the seminal vesicles.

REFERENCES
Testes

1. Atkin, N.B.: Y bodies and similar fluorescent chromocentres in human tumours including teratomata, Br. J. Cancer **28**:275, 1973.
2. Berg, J.W.: Acid-fast lipid from spermatozoa, Arch. Pathol. (Chicago) **57**:115, 1954.
3. Brown, R.C., and Smith, B.H.: Malakoplakia of the testis, Am. J. Clin. Pathol. **47**:135, 1967.
4. Campbell, C.M., et al.: Malignant gonadal stromal tumor: case report and review of literature, J. Urol. **125**:257, 1981.
5. Capers, T.H.: Granulomatous orchitis, Am. J. Clin. Pathol. **34**:139, 1960.
6. Carr, B.I.: The variable transformation of metastases from testicular germ cell tumors: the need for selective biopsy, J. Urol. **126**:52, 1981.
7. Cohn, B.D.: Histology of the cryptorchid testes, Surgery **62**:536, 1967.
8. Dickinson, S.J.: Structural abnormalities in the undescended testis, J. Pediatr. Surg. **8**:523, 1973.
9. Dixon, F.J., and Moore, R.A.: In Atlas of tumor pathology, Section VIII, Fascicle 32, Washingston, D.C., 1952, Armed Forces Institute of Pathology.
10. Dow, J.A., and Mostofi, F.K.: Testicular tumors following orchiopexy, South. Med. J. **60**:193, 1967.
11. Friedman, N.B., and Garske, G.L.: Inflammatory reactions involving sperm and the seminiferous tubules, Urology **62**:363, 1949.
12. Friedman, N.B., and Moore, R.A.: Tumors of the testis: a report on 922 cases, Milit. Surg. **99**:573, 1943.
13. Givler, R.L.: Testicular involvement in leukemia lymphoma, Cancer **23**:1290, 1969.
14. Levin, H.S., and Mostofi, F.K.: Symptomatic plasmacytoma of the testes, Cancer **25**:1193, 1970.
15. Li, F.P., et al.: Improved survival rates among testis cancer patients in the U.S.A., J.A.M.A. **247**:825, 1982.
16. Maier, J., et al.: An evolution of lymphadenectomy in the treatment of malignant testicular germ cell neoplasms, Trans. Am. Assoc. Genitourinary Surgeons **60**:71, 1962.
17. Merrin, C., et al.: Alpha fetoprotein in testicular tumors, J. Surg. Res. **15**:309, 1973.
17a. Mostofi, F.K.: Testicular tumors: epidemiologic, etiologic and pathologic features. Cancer **32**:1186, 1973.
18. Mostofi, F.K.: Classification of tumors of testis, Ann. Clin. Lab. Sci. **9**:455, 1979.
19. Mostofi, F.K.: Pathology of germ cell tumors of testis: progress report, Cancer **45**:1735, 1980.
20. Mostofi, F.K., and Price, E.B., Jr.: Tumors of male genital system. In Atlas of tumor pathology, Series 2, Fascicle 7, Washington, D.C., 1973, Armed Forces Institute of Pathology.
20a. Mostofi, F.K., and Sesterhenn, I.A.: Testicular germ cell tumors: pathology and tumor markers. In Schroeder, F., editor: Progress and controversies in oncological urology, New York, 1984, Alan R. Liss, Inc.
21. Mostofi, F.K., and Sobin, L.H.: International histological classification of tumors of testes, Geneva, 1977, World Health Organization.
22. Mostofi, F.K., Theiss, E.A., and Ashley, D.J.B.: Tumors of specialized gonadal stroma in human male patients (androblastoma, Sertoli cell tumor, granulosa-theca cell tumor of the testis, and gonadal stromal tumor), Cancer **12**:944, 1959.
22a. Muller, K.: Cancer testis, Copenhagen, 1962, Munksgaard.
23. Pierce, G.B., Jr., and Beals, T.F.: The ultrastructure of primordial germinal cells of the fetal testes and of embryonal carcinoma cells of mice, Cancer Res. **24**:1533,1964.
24. Price, E.B., Jr.: Epidermoid cysts of the testis, J. Urol. **102**:708, 1969.
25. Price, E.B., Jr., and Mostofi, F.K.: Secondary carcinomas of the testis, Cancer **10**:592, 1957.
26. Reyes, F.I., and Faiman, C.: Development of testicular tumor during *cis*-clomiphene therapy, Can. Med. Assoc. J. **109**:502, 1973.
27. Rosai, J., Khodadoust, K., and Silber, I.: Spermatocytic seminoma. II. Ultrastructural study, Cancer **24**:103, 1969.
28. Rosai, J., Silber, I., and Khodadoust, K.: Spermatocytic seminoma. I. Clinicopathologic study of six cases and review of the literature, Cancer **24**:92, 1969.
29. Scorer, C.G.: The anatomy of testicular descent—normal and incomplete, Br. J. Surg. **49**:357, 1962.
29a. Sesterhenn, I.A., et al.: Tumor markers in 1,000 germ cell tumors of testis. (To be published.)
30. Shiffman, M.A.: Androblastoma (Sertoli cell tumor): case report, J. Urol. **98**:493, 1967.
31. Stevens, L.C.: Embryonic potency of embryoid bodies derived from a transplantable testicular teratoma of the mouse, Dev. Biol. **2**:285, 1960.
32. Teilum, G.: Oestrogen production by Sertoli cells in etiology of benign senile hypertrophy of human prostate, Acta Endocrinol. (Kbn.) **4**:43, 1950.
33. Walker, K.M.: Hunterian lecture on the paths of infection in genitourinary tuberculosis, Lancet **1**:435, 1913.
34. Westcott, J.W.: Reticulum sarcoma with primary manifestation in the testis, J. Urol. **96**:243, 1966.
35. Willis, R.A.: Pathology of tumors, ed. 4, London, 1967, Butterworth & Co. (Publishers) Ltd.
36. Young, H.H.: Radical cure of tuberculosis of seminal tract, Arch. Surg. (Chicago) **4**:334, 1922.

Epididymis; spermatic cord

37. Brosman, S.A., et al.: Rhabdomyosarcoma of testis and spermatic cord in children, Urology **3**:568, 1974.
38. Broth, G., Bullock, W.K., and Morrow, J.: Epididymal tumors, J. Urol. **100**:530, 1968.
39. Glassy, F.J., and Mostofi, F.K.: Spermatic granulomas of the epididymis, Am. J. Clin. Pathol. **26**:1303, 1956.
40. Jackson, J.R.: The histogenesis of the adenomatoid tumor of the genital tract, Cancer **11**:337, 1958.
41. Klingerman, J.J., and Nourse, M.H.: Torsion of the spermatic cord, J.A.M.A. **200**:673, 1967.
42. Kyle, V.N.: Leiomyosarcoma of the spermatic cord: a review of the literature and report of an additional case, J. Urol. **96**:795, 1966.
43. Longo, V.J., McDonald, J.R., and Thompson, G.J.: Primary neoplasms of epididymis: special reference to adenomatoid tumors, J.A.M.A. **147**:937, 1951.
44. Lundblad, R.R., Mellinger, G.T., and Gleason, D.F.: Spermatic cord malignancies, J. Urol. **98**:393, 1967.
45. Mostofi, F.K., and Davis, C.J.: Pathology of urologic cancer. In Javadpour, N., editor: Principles and management of urologic cancer, Baltimore, 1979, The Williams & Wilkins Co.
46. Mostofi, F.K., and Price, E.B.: Tumors of the male genital system. In Atlas of tumor pathology, Series 2, Fascicle 8, Washington, D.C., 1973, Armed Forces Institute of Pathology.
47. Olson, A.L.: Vasitis nodosa, Am. J. Clin. Pathol. **55**:364, 1971.
48. Rosai, J., and Dehner, L.P.: Nodular mesothelial hyperplasia in hernia sacs, Cancer **35**:165, 1975.

49. Price, E.B.: Papillary cystadenomas of the epididymis, Arch. Pathol. **91**:456, 1971.

50. Remzi, D.: Tumors of the tunica vaginalis, South. Med. J. **66**:1295, 1973.

51. Silverblatt, J.M., and Gellman, S.Z.: Mesotheliomas of spermatic cord, epididymis, and tunica vaginalis, Urology **3**:235, 1974.

52. Smith, B.A., Jr., Webb, E.A., and Price, W.E.: Carcinoma of the seminal vesicle, J. Urol. **98**:743, 1967.

53. Williams, G., and Banerjee, R.: Paratesticular tumours, Br. J. Urol. **41**:332, 1969.

Intersexuality; infertility; agonadism

54. Amelar, R.D.: Infertility in men, Philadelphia, 1966, F.A. Davis Co.

55. Ashley, D.J.B.: Human intersex, Edinburgh, 1962, Churchill Livingstone.

56. Charny, C.W.: The treatment of male infertility. In Behrman, S.J., and Kistner, R.W., editors: Progress in infertility, Boston, 1968, Little, Brown & Co.

57. Federman, D.D.: Abnormal sexual development: a generic and endocrine approach to differential diagnosis, Philadelphia, 1967, W.B. Saunders Co.

58. Goldbert, L.M., et al.: Congenital absence of testis: anorchism and monorchism, J. Urol. **11**:84, 1974.

59. Inhorn, S.L., and Opitz, J.M.: Abnormalities of sex development. In Bloodworth, J.M.B., editor: Endocrine pathology, Baltimore, 1968, Williams & Wilkins Co.

60. Jirasek, J.E.: Development of the genital system and male pseudohermaphroditism, Baltimore, 1971, The Johns Hopkins Press.

61. Jones, H.W., Jr., and Scott, W.W.: Hermaphroditism, genital anomalies, and related endocrine disorders, ed. 2, Baltimore, 1971, The Williams & Wilkins Co.

62. Jost, A.: Problems of fetal endocrinology: the gonadal and hypophyseal hormones. Rec. Progr. Horm. Res. **8**:379, 1953.

63. Paulsen, C.A. In Williams, R.H., editor: Textbook of endocrinology, ed. 4, Philadelphia, 1968, W.B. Saunders Co.

64. Wong, T.W., Straus, F.H., and Warner, N.E.: Testicular biopsy in the study of male infertility. I. Testicular causes of infertility, Arch. Pathol. **95**:151, 1973.

65. Wong, T.W., Straus, F.H., and Warner, N.E.: Testicular biopsy in the study of male infertility. II. Posttesticular causes of infertility, Arch. Pathol. **95**:160, 1973.

66. Wong, T.W., Straus, F.H., and Warner, N.E.: Testicular biopsy in the study of male infertility. III. Pretesticular causes of infertility, Arch. Pathol. **98**:1, 1974.

Scrotum

67. Borden, T.A., Rosen, R.T., and Schwartz, G.R.: Massive scrotal hematoma developing after transfemoral cardiac catheterization, Am. Surg. **40**:193, 1974.

68. Burpee, J.F., and Edwards, P.: Fournier's gangrene, J.Urol. **107**:812, 1972.

69. Dean, A.L.: Epitheliomas of scrotum, J. Urol. **60**:508, 1948.

70. Fardon, D.W., et al.: The treatment of brown spider bite, Plast. Reconstr. Surg. **40**:482, 1967.

71. Exelby, P.R.: Malignant scrotal masses in children, Cancer **24**:163, 1974.

72. Himal, H.S., McLean, A.P., and Duff, J.H.: Gas gangrene of scrotum and perineum, Surg. Gynecol. Obstet. **139**:176-178, 1974.

73. Keeler, L.L., and Harrer, W.V.: Chronic lymphedema of the scrotum and penis, J. Med. Soc. N.J. **71**:575, 1974.

74. Kickham, C.J., and DuFresne, M.: An assessment of carcinoma of the scrotum, J. Urol. **98**:108, 1967.

75. Lee, W.R., and McCann, J.K.: Mule spinners' cancer and the wool industry, Br. J. Industr. Med. **24**:149, 1967.

76. Smulewicz, J.J., and Donner, D.: Gas gangrene of the scrotum, J. Urol. **111**:621, 1974.

77. Vermillion, C.D., and Page, D.L.: Puget's disease of the scrotum: a case report with local lymph node invasion, J. Urol. **107**:281, 1972.

Penis

78. Bivens, C.H., Marecek, R.L., and Feldman, J.M.: Peyronie's disease—a presenting complaint of the carcinoid syndrome, N. Engl. J. Med. **289**:844, 1973.

79. Campbell, M.: Epispadias: report of 15 cases, J. Urol. **67**:988, 1952.

80. Dehner, L.P., and Smith, B.H.: Soft tissue tumors of the penis, Cancer **25**:1431, 1970.

81. Editorial: Med. J. Aust. **2**:1035, 1973.

82. Frew, I.D.O., Jefferies, J.D., and Swinney, T.: Carcinoma of penis, Br. J. Urol. **39**:398, 1967.

83. Graham, J.H., and Helwig, E.B.: Bowen's disease and its relationship to systemic cancer, Arch. Dermatol. **80**:133, 1959.

84. Graham, J.H., and Helwig, E.B.: Erythroplasia of Queyrat, Cancer **32**:1396, 1973.

85. Grossberg, P., and Hardy, K.J.: Carcinoma of the penis, Med. J. Aust. **2**:1050, 1973.

86. Gursel, E.O., et al.: Penile cancer, Urology **1**:569, 1973.

87. Hagerty, R.F., and Taber, E.: Hypospadias, Am. Surg. **24**:244, 1958.

88. Horton, G.E., and Devine, C.J., Jr.: Plast. Reconstr. Surg. **52**:503, 1973.

89. Johnson, D.E., Fuerst, D.E., and Ayala, A.G.: Carcinoma of the penis: experience with 153 cases, Urology **1**:404, 1973.

90. Kao, G.F., and Graham, J.H.: Bowenoid papulosis, Int. J. Dermatol. **21**:445, 1982.

91. Kaplan, C., and Katoh, A.: Erythroplasia of Queyrat (Bowen's disease of the glans penis), J. Surg. Oncol. **5**:281, 1973.

92. Masih, B.K., and Brosman, S.A.: Webbed penis, J. Urol. **111**:690, 1974.

93. Melicow, M.M., and Ganem, E.J.: Cancerous and precancerous lesions of penis, J. Urol. **55**:486, 1946.

94. Moulder, J.W.: The psittacosis group as bacteria (Ciba lectures in microbial biochemistry, 1963), New York, 1964, John Wiley & Sons, Inc.

95. Najjar, S.S.: Webbing of the penis, Clin. Pediatr. **13**:377, 1974.

96. Ngai, S.K.: Etiological and pathological aspects of squamous cell carcinoma of penis among Chinese, Am. J. Cancer **19**:259, 1933.

97. Oertel, Y.C., and Johnson, F.B.: Sclerosing lipogranuloma of male genitalia, Arch. Pathol. Lab. Med. **101**:321, 1977.

98. Poutasse, E.F.: Peyronie's disease, J. Urol. **107**:419, 1972.

99. Powley, J.M.: Buschke-Loewenstein tumor of the penis, Br. J. Surg. **51**:76, 1964.

100. Rege, P.R., and Evans, A.T.: Erythroplasia of Queyrat, J. Urol. **111**:784, 1974.

101. Smith, B.H.: Peyronie's disease, Am. J. Clin. Pathol. **45**:670, 1966.

102. Tan, R.E.: Fournier's gangrene of the scrotum and the penis, J. Urol. **92**:508, 1964.

Urethra

103. Agusta, V.E., and Howards, S.S.: Posterior urethral valves, J. Urol. **112**:280, 1974.

104. Bissada, N.K., Cole, A.T., and Fried, F.A.: Condylomata acuminata of male urethra and bladder, J. Urol. **112**:201, 1974.

105. Chambers, R.M.: Proceedings: the anatomy of the urethral structure, Br. J. Urol. **46**:123, 1974.

106. Cobb, B.G., Wolf, J.A., Jr., and Ansell, J.S.: Congenital stricture of the proximal urethral bulb, J. Urol. **99**:629, 1968.

107. Grewal, R.S., and Francis, J.: Foreign body in the urethra, Int. Surg. **48**:591, 1967.

108. Hill, B.H.: Gonorrhea and nonspecific urethritis, N.Z. Med. J. **69**:198, 1969.

109. Huvos, A.G., and Grabstald, H.: Urethreal meatal and parameatal tumors in young men, J. Urol. **110**:688, 1973.

110. Kaplan, G.W., Buckley, G.J., and Grayhack, J.T.: Carcinoma of the male urethra, J. Urol. **98**:365, 1967.

111. Klaus, H., and Stein, R.T.: Urethral prolapse in young girls, Pediatrics **52**:645, 1973.

112. Knoblich, R.: Primary adenocarcinoma of female urethra, Am. J. Obstet. Gynecol. **80**:353, 1960.

113. Malhoski, W.E., and Frank, I.N.: Anterior urethral valves, Urology **2**:382, 1973.
114. Marshall, F.C., Uson, A.C., and Melicow, M.M.: Neoplasma and caruncles of the female urethra, Surg. Gynecol. Obstet. **110**:723, 1960.
115. McEwen, C.: Reiter's disease: its nature and relationship to other diseases, Trans. Coll. Physicians Phila. **34**:39, 1966.
116. Meadows, J.A., Jr., and Quattlebaum, R.B.: Polyps of the posterior urethra in children, J. Urol. **100**:317, 1968.
117. Mitchell, J.P.: Injuries to the urethra, Br. J. Urol. **40**:649, 1968.
118. Mogg, R.A.: Congenital anomalies of the urethra, Br. J. Urol. **40**:638, 1968.
119. Morrison, A.I.: Treatment of relapses and re-infections in non-specific urethritis, Br. J. Vener. Dis. **43**:170, 1967.
120. Smith, T.F., et al.: A comparison of genital infections caused by *Chlamydia trachomatis* and by *Neisseria gonorrhea*, Am. J. Clin. Pathol. **70**:333, 1978.
121. Williams, D.I., and Retik, A.B.: Congenital valves and diverticula of the anterior urethra, Br. J. Urol. **41**:228, 1969.

Prostate

122. Baker, W.J., and Graf, E.C.: Tuberculosis in obstructive prostate gland, J. Urol. **66**:254, 1951.
123. Batson, O.V.: Vertebral veins, Ann. Surg. **112**:138, 1940.
124. Breslow, N.: Latent carcinoma of prostate at autopsy in seven areas, Int. J. Cancer **20**:680, 1977.
125. Byar, D.P., et al.: Carcinoma of the prostate: prognostic evaluation of certain pathological features in 208 radical prostatectomies, Cancer **30**:5, 1972.
126. Delaney, W.E., Burros, H.M., and Bhisitikul, I.: Eosinophilic granulomatous prostatitis simulating carcinoma, J. Urol. **87**:169, 1962.
127. Fisher, E.R., and Sieracki, J.C.: Ultrastructure of human normal and neoplastic prostate. In Sommers, S.C., editor: Pathology annual, vol. 5, New York, 1970, Appleton-Century-Crofts.
127a. Franks, L.M.: Benign nodular hyperplasia of prostate: a review, Ann. R. Coll. Surg. Engl. **14**:92, 1954.
128. Franks, L.M.: Latent carcinoma of prostate, J. Pathol. Bacteriol. **68**:617, 1954.
129. Franks, L.M.: The spread of prostatic cancer, J. Pathol. Bacteriol. **72**:603, 1956.
130. Franks, L.M.: The incidence of carcinoma of prostate: an epidemiological survey, Rec. Results Cancer Res. **39**:149, 1972.
131. Franks, L.M.: Etiology, epidemiology and pathology of prostatic cancer, Cancer **32**:1092, 1973.
132. Franks, L.M.: Recent research on prostatic pathology. In Sommers, S.C., editor: Pathology annual, vol. 5, New York, 1975, Appleton-Century-Crofts.
133. Grayhack, J.T., Wilson, J.D., and Scherbenske, M.J., editors: Benign prostatic hyperplasia, NIAMDD Workshop Proceedings, p. 63, 1975.
134. Hill, P., et al.: Environmental factors, prostatic cancer, Prev. Med. **9**:657, 1980.
135. Hoffmann, E., and Garrido, M.: Malakoplakia of the prostate: report of a case, J. Urol. **92**:311, 1964.
135a. Huggins, C., and Hodges, C.V.: Studies on prostatic cancer: the effect of castration, of estrogen and of androgen injection on serum phosphatases in metastatic carcinoma of prostate, Cancer Res. **1**:293, 1941.
136. Kadman, D., et al.: Cancer surgery and chemotherapy, J. Urol. **127**:1238, 1982.
136a. Kaufman, J.J., and Berneike, R.R.: Leiomyoma of the prostate, J. Urol. **65**:297, 1951.
137. Kovi, J., et al.: Cancer of the prostate and aging: an autopsy study in black men from Washington, D.C., and selected African cities, Prostate **3**:73, 1982.
138. Lupovitch, A.: The prostate and amyloidosis, J. Urol. **108**:301, 1972.
139. Mostofi, F.K.: Prostatic carcinoma. In Twenty-Third Clinical Conference on Cancer, Houston, M.D. Anderson Hospital and Tumor Institute, 1978.
140. Mostofi, F.K., and Morse, W.H.: Epithelial metaplasia in "prostatic infarction," Arch. Pathol. (Chicago) **51**:340, 1951.
141. Mostofi, F.K., Sesterhenn, I., and Sobin, L.H.: International histological classification of tumors of prostate, Geneva, 1981, World Health Organization.
142. Mostofi, F.K., et al.: WHO histological classification of prostate tumours, Geneva, 1975, World Health Organization.
143. Murphy, G.P., et al.: The National Survey of Prostatic Cancer in the United States, J. Urol. **127**:928, 1982.
144. Paulson, D.F., Rabson, A.S., and Fraley, E.E.: Viral neoplastic transformation of hamster prostate tissue in vitro, Science **159**:200, 1968.
145. Willis, R.A.: Carcinoma of prostate. In Pathology of tumours, London, 1948, Butterworth & Co., Ltd.

CHAPTER 22 **Lung and Mediastinum**

CHARLES KUHN III
FREDERIC B. ASKIN

PEDIATRIC LUNG DISEASE
Lung development

The lung is a foregut derivative and appears at about the twenty-sixth postovulatory day as a bud from the caudal end of the laryngotracheal sulcus.[1,2] Lung development in humans can be roughly separated into four phases: embryonic, pseudoglandular, canalicular, and terminal sac.[15,16,18] In the embryonic period (first 5 weeks) the lung buds form the lobar bronchi and the major segmental branches. The entire epithelial lining of lung airways and airspaces is of endodermal origin, but branching is apparently controlled by the mesenchymal tissues into which the lung buds grow.[24] In the pseudoglandular period (fifth to sixteenth weeks), bronchial branching continues and cartilage is formed. The distal lung-lining epithelium is composed of large cuboidal cells closely apposed around a potential space. During the canalicular period (sixteenth to twenty-fourth weeks) the pulmonary mesenchyme becomes richly vascular; septa appear in the lung and the epithelium of the distal airspaces begins to flatten. Capillaries protrude into the areas of epithelium, and the glycogen-filled cuboidal cells lining the distal airspaces begin to differentiate into recognizable type I (squamous) and type II (surfactant-producing) cells.[8] Progressive flattening of epithelium and intrusion of capillaries lead to a thin air-blood barrier, and by the end of the twenty-fifth week it should theoretically be possible to maintain respiration. Lamellar intracytoplasmic inclusions representing pulmonary surface-active material begin to appear in type II cells after the twentieth week but are present in an amount sufficient to provide lung stability only after the twenty-fourth to twenty-sixth weeks of gestaton.[12,13,17] The lung in utero is not collapsed but is distended by a distinctive fluid produced by lymphatic leakage and contributed to by the alveolar type II lung cells.[19,22] The final phase of intrauterine lung development, the terminal sac period (twenty-sixth week to term), is characterized by the development of shallow distal airspaces that have been variably termed saccules or true but immature alveoli.[10,16] Alveoli continue to form and multiply after birth.[23] With a wide range of individual variability alveoli increase approximately 10-fold in number, from 30×10^6 at birth to 300×10^6 at 8 years of age.[16] Most of the increase in numbers occurs in the first 4 years of life. After age 8, alveoli increase primarily in size until the growth of the chest wall is complete. There is some evidence that total alveolar number is related to body height.[23]

Airway branching is complete by birth, and the major cartilaginous airways have formed by the sixteenth week of intrauterine life.[15,18,20] Pulmonary artery development in the preacinar (airway) region parallels that of the bronchial tree and is complete by birth.[15,18] A pulmonary artery gives off more branches along its length than does its neighboring airway. "Conventional" branches accompany airways. "Spurious" or "supernumerary" branches pass into the adjacent alveolar region and supply the capillary bed. In the acinar (respiratory) region conventional and spurious pulmonary arteries proliferate after birth to accompany alveolar multiplication. The structure of the pulmonary arteries in infants differs markedly from that of adults in the amount and distribution of muscle in the media.[15,18] This difference is most apparent if one takes into account the location of the artery in the lung parenchyma. In children a complete muscle layer is present in the small arteries of the alveolar region by the end of the second decade of life. In terms of thickness, fetal arteries of all sizes contain more muscle than those of adults. By 4 months after birth this difference disappears. In the smaller arteries (less than 250 μm) the fall in thickness is much more rapid. The wall size of veins and the pattern of muscle distribution appear to be the same in adults and infants.[14,15] Lymphatic channels can be seen in the lungs of fetuses of 20 weeks' gestational age, and lymph nodes are seen in the peribronchial regions at birth and increase in prominence with advancing age.[15] Loose lymphoreticular aggregates appear after birth and are seen among alveoli, in peribronchiolar sites, and underneath the epithelium of bronchi, presumably representing a response to environmental antigenic stimuli.[11]

Congenital anomalies

Pulmonary agenesis may be unilateral or bilateral.[37,24,40,44,46] The former is compatible with long survival in the absence of severe infection or coexistent malformations. Tracheal agenesis has been described as well.[29,49] Abnormal pulmonary fissures and lobations and bronchial anomalies are probably the most common pulmonary malformations.[30,37,38,41,48] The azygous lobe, for example, is produced by pressure of the azygous vein on the apex of the right lung and is of little clinical significance. The relationship, however, of mirror image lobation (pulmonary isomerism) to a variety of cardiovascular anomalies has been well documented.[36,38] The horseshoe lung is fused behind the heart but anterior to the esophagus and may have abnormal venous drainage.[43] Abnormal bronchi may be either supernumerary or displaced. The most common is the tracheal bronchus, which supplies an upper lobe, usually the right, directly from the trachea.[39,47] The rare bridging bronchus joins right lower lobe airways to those of the left lung.[32] Congenital or acquired bronchial stenosis may cause either atelectasis or overinflation depending on whether the obstruction is complete or partial.[27,42]

Heterotopic tissues including adrenal cortex, striated muscle, and glial tissues have been reported in the lung.[25,26,28,35,45] Glial heterotopia in the lung parenchyma is usually found in anencephalic newborns and must be distinguished from cases in which traumatic central nervous system tissue emboli are found in pulmonary arteries.

Congenital alveolar capillary dysplasia is a developmental anomaly in which blood vessels fail to become established in the distal airspaces.[33] Extrauterine oxygen diffusion in the lung is inadequate to support life.

Hypoplasia and diaphragmatic hernia

Hypoplasia of the lung can be defined as a decrease in relative volume or weight of lung tissue appropriately mature for the patient's age. A representative group of standards is available from the work of Langston and Thurlbeck.[16] Page and Stocker[59] have found the lung weight/body weight ratio to be a reliable indicator of hypoplasia. The diminution in lung tissue may be unilateral or bilateral and may be related to a deficit of airways, acini, or alveoli, to diminished alveolar size, or to any combination of these factors. Primary pulmonary hypoplasia is a rare entity, occasionally familial, and of unknown etiology. Etiologic factors causing secondary hypoplasia can be identified and classified (Table 22-1) as related to direct intrathoracic or extrathoracic compres-

Table 22-1. Etiology of pulmonary hypoplasia

Category	Example
Unexplained	Idiopathic (isolated or familial), Down's syndrome
Compression of the lungs	
Inadequate or abnormal thoracic space	Diaphragmatic hernia, scoliosis, thoracic mass lesions, asphyxiating thoracic dystrophy, various types of dwarfism
Large extrathoracic mass	Polycystic kidneys, large bladder, abdominal masses
Decreased fetal respiratory movement	Amniotic fluid deficit (renal agenesis/dysplasia, bladder out-obstruction), amniotic fluid leak, neuromuscular disorders affecting diaphragm and other respiratory muscles, anencephaly
Metabolic defect	Renal agenesis, anencephaly, RH incompatibility, (?) other immune disorders

sion of the lung(s), deformities of the chest wall, a variety of renal, urinary tract, and placental abnormalities that lead to oligohydramnios, or one of a seemingly unrelated mixture of disorders.[50-64] More than one mechanism may be responsible in some instances. Direct compression of pulmonary parenchyma seems a straightforward cause of lung hypoplasia. It is more difficult to explain hypoplasia related to either oligohydramnios or the other factors mentioned above. Formerly it was suggested that oligohydramnios caused pulmonary hypoplasia by allowing the uterus to compress the underlying lung through the malleable chest wall. It now seems clear that other factors, especially loss of lung fluid and interference with fetal respiratory movements, can better explain the hypoplasia of the lungs associated with oligohydramnios or polyhydramnios, neuromuscular disorders, and anencephaly. It is also possible that renal agenesis may contribute to lung hypoplasia via interference with collagen metabolism.[16] The mechanism of pulmonary hypoplasia in infants with Down's syndrome is unknown.[52]

Pulmonary hypoplasia is frequently found in association with herniation of abdominal contents through a congenital, usually left-sided, diaphragmatic defect called Bochdalek hernia (Fig. 22-1). The ipsilateral lung is distorted and hypoplastic with a reduction in airways and in alveolar number and size.[57] The contralateral lung is hypoplastic as well but is not as dramatically distorted. Infants with diaphragmatic hernia appear to be particularly susceptible to the development of persistent pulmonary hypertension (see p. 866), which may be fatal. Infants who survive after surgical repair of the hernia have pulmonary function that may be close to normal. Morphologic studies in a few cases have shown a persistent deficit in alveolar multiplications and the development of compensatory emphysema.[63]

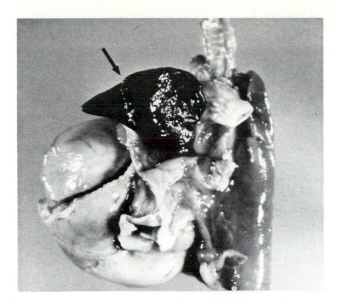

Fig. 22-1. Posterior view of hypoplastic left lung (arrow) from patient who had antenatal herniation of bowel loops into left side of chest through posterior diaphragmatic hernia. Compressed lung is hypoplastic because of diminished numbers of airways and alveoli.

Pulmonary vascular anomalies

A number of general reviews covering pulmonary vascular anomalies are available.[4,37,68,70] Arterial malformations include origin of one or both main pulmonary vessels from the aorta.[65,69,76] Absence (actually interruption) of a main artery with vascular supply to the lung via bronchial artery collaterals has been noted as well.[77] A pulmonary arterial system is present within the lung proper in these patients. In aberrant origin of the left pulmonary artery from the right pulmonary artery ("pulmonary artery sling"),[74,78,86] the anomalous vessel courses behind the trachea and may partially obstruct the airways (see discussion of congenital lobar overinflation, p. 836). Isolated or multiple discrete areas of stenosis may be found in the pulmonary artery. Some of these patients have other cardiovascular malformations.[75,80] Children with the Alagille syndrome of cholestasis and a peculiar facies often have peripheral stenoses of the pulmonary arteries.[72] Diffuse hypoplasia of pulmonary arteries has been described in patients with congenital rubella.[85]

Venous anomalies include anomalous pulmonary venous return to the heart, stenosis or atresia, and the "scimitar" syndrome. A complete review is available elsewhere.[4,37,66,81] In total anomalous venous return all four main pulmonary veins converge and then drain into the innominate vein, coronary sinus, or right atrium or they run below the diaphragm and enter the inferior vena cava or portal vein. Pulmonary lymphangioectasis (see p. 836) may be a prominent feature. Partial anoma-lous venous return has been reported as well.[81]

Isolated or multiple stenosis or even atresias may be found in the pulmonary veins and are also associated with diffuse or localized lymphangiectasis or hemorrhage and hemosiderin deposition in the lung.[71,83,84]

The "scimitar" syndrome is a multifaceted malformation characterized by a large anomalous pulmonary vein that drains from one lung, usually the right, into the inferior vena cava.[73,79] The broad roentgenographic shadow of this vein forms the scimitar. The ipsilateral lung is hypoplastic and has at least partial anomalous systemic arterial blood supply. There may be overlap in this syndrome with pulmonary sequestration (see below) or horseshoe lung (see p. 834).

Pulmonary arteriovenous fistulas may be congenital or acquired. Congenital lesions may be solitary or multiple, and between one third and one half of the patients have the Osler-Weber-Rendu syndrome with similar lesions in other organs. The blood supply of the fistula usually comes from the pulmonary artery but is occasionally derived from systemic vessels.[67,82]

Bronchopulmonary sequestration

Sequestered pulmonary lobes or segments are not connected to the airway system of the associated normal pulmonary parenchyma.[1,3,5,37] The blood supply of the sequestered area is usually via systemic vessels arising from the aorta or its branches. Two major types of sequestration occur: intralobar and extralobar.

Introlobar sequestrations occur almost equally in adults and children. The usual but not invariable location is in the posterior segment of the left lower lobe, and the sequestered area is incorporated within the pleural investment of that lobe. The disorder may be discovered when a mass lesion is seen on a routine chest roentgenogram or because of recurrent infection in the same area of the lung. Pathologically the features are frequently those of obstructive pneumonitis. Grossly the lesion may be solid or cystic, depending on the degree of inflammatory change. One or more elastic arteries supply blood to the affected area; venous drainage is usually through the pulmonary system.[87,88,91,94]

Extralobar sequestrations have also been termed accessory lobes. They are completely separate from the pleural covering of the normal lung. The usual location of extralobar sequestrations is in the left lower hemithorax, but they may occur near the esophagus or within or even below the diaphragm. Both the arterial supply and venous drainage are usually of systemic origin. In contrast to intralobar sequestration, the extralobar lesion occurs predominantly in infants and children and is frequently associated with coexisting malformations, especially diaphragmatic hernia and pectus excavatum.[37,87,88,94-96] Secondary infection and obstruction are not common features, but the basic architecture resembles that of immature lung or dysplastic bronchiolar structures.

It is likely that both types of lesion arise from an accessory lung bud from the foregut, although a small number of intralobar "sequestrations" may actually represent lesions acquired as a result of recurrent infection or as a response to the presence of abnormal systemic arterial supply to the lung.[1,37,89-91] The accessory lung bud may persist in some instances and may connect the sequestration with the esophagus, stomach, or biliary tract—the so-called bronchopulmonary foregut malformation.[34,37,90,95]

Certain vascular anomalies may mimic or actually belong in the spectrum of intralobar sequestration: isolated supply of a portion of otherwise normal pulmonary parenchyma by a systemic artery may occur and produce a large vascular shunt.[1,3,5,37,97] The scimitar syndrome (see p. 835) may also overlap with pulmonary sequestration.

Bronchogenic cyst

Bronchogenic cysts also arise from accessory lung buds from the foregut. Although they usually lack any formation of pulmonary parenchyma, transitional forms between this lesion and sequestration have been found. Bronchogenic cysts usually appear in the anterior mediastinum but can occur within the lung substance as well.[90,92,93] They are characterized by a lining of a bronchial epithelium and the presence of cartilage in their wall. These cysts are unilocular and may contain watery fluid, mucus, or, rarely, purulent material. They must be differentiated from enteric cysts lined with gastric or intestinal epithelium and, when they occur within the lung parenchyma, from a lung abscess.[92,93] The abscess has multiple airways connecting with its lumen, whereas a bronchogenic cyst does not. Bronchiectasis in young children is often misinterpreted as representing a congenital cystic disease of the lung.

Congenital adenomatoid malformation

The congenital adenomatoid malformation (Fig. 22-2, A) is an unusual lesion combining features of a hamartoma, dysplasia, and a true neoplasm in the lung.[98,104] The adenomatoid malformation usually affects a single lobe and is an expanding mass that compresses the adjacent lung and may cause severe respiratory distress and even death. Grossly a spectrum of solid to multilocular cystic lesions has been described. Multiple or bilateral lesions are rare. The malformation lacks bronchi but does appear to communicate with the airway system of the normal lung. Microscopically the cysts are lined by bronchial or cuboidal epithelium; prominent clusters of mucinous cells may be interspersed among the septa (Fig. 22-2, B and C). More solid lesions are composed of multiple curving, branched structures that resemble dysplastic or immature bronchioles. Clinically and roentgenographi-

cally, but not histologically, the differential diagnosis of adenomatoid malformation includes congenital lobar overinflation and sequestration.

Congenital pulmonary lymphangiectasis

Congenital pulmonary lymphangiectasis is a rare lesion characterized by marked distension of subpleural and septal lymphatic spaces.[105,111] Usually the disorder results from pulmonary venous obstruction, predominantly total anomalous pulmonary venous return (p. 835) and other cardiac anomalies. Rarely it may be primary in the lung or may be part of a generalized syndrome of lymphangiectasis including chylous effusions and bone destruction. Pulmonary lymphangiectasis, as a specific disorder, must be distinguished from pulmonary interstitial emphysema (see the following discussion) and from the dilated lymphatic vessels often seen in hyaline membrane disease (see p. 838).

Congenital pulmonary overinflation (lobar or segmental "emphysema")

Congenital lobar overinflation occurs in infants as a lobar disorder and in older children or adults as a segmental area of pulmonary hyperinflation without tissue destruction.[112,122] The popular term "emphysema" is not strictly correct for this entity, since the lung parenchyma is not destroyed. In infants the lesion is a rapidly enlarging mass, usually in an upper or middle lobe, causing mediastinal shift and respiratory distress. Multiple causes have been identified, the most common being partial intrinsic or extrinsic bronchial obstruction. Deficiency of bronchial cartilage in the large bronchi of the affected lobe has been identified in many cases, and in others extrinsic pressure from engorged or aberrant pulmonary vessels is presumed to be the cause.[118,120] Endobronchial trauma resulting from therapeutic suctioning has been implicated in some patients.[116] In a few cases the primary lesion appears to be an increased number of alveoli in the affected lobe.[114] Although emergency surgery may be necessary in some cases of lobar overinflation, conservative management has been possible in others.[119]

Segmental overinflation usually is diagnosed in an older child or adult and is related to segmental bronchial atresia.[113,121] The involved segment appears to enlarge because of air trapping.

In either lobar or segmental overinflation the microscopic pattern is usually simply that of normal-appearing but overinflated alveoli. Bronchial cartilage deficiency can ordinarily be demonstrated only by special dissection and staining techniques.

Adaptation to extrauterine life

The successful transition from intrauterine to extrauterine life requires a number of major changes in lung physiology.[2,12,17,32,129] The liquid that expanded alveoli

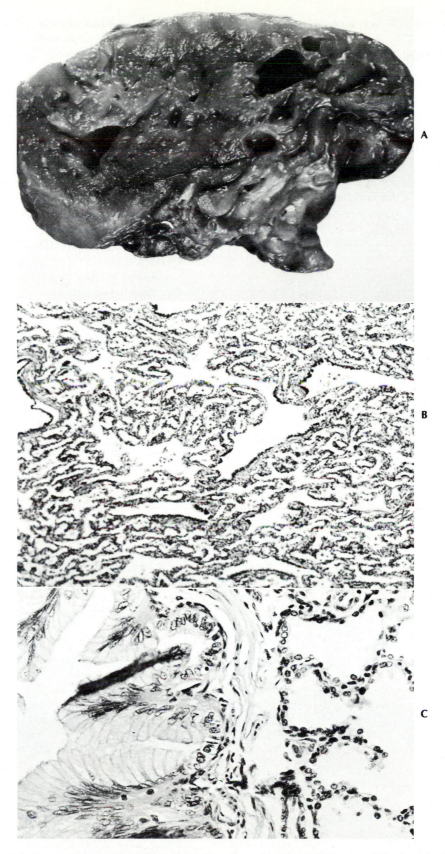

Fig. 22-2. A, Congenital adenomatoid malformation. Central portion of this upper lobe is replaced by multiple cysts. Rim of normal lung tissue is present. **B,** Low-power photomicrograph showing irregularly branching spaces lined with cuboidal epithelium. **C,** Mucigenic cells *(left)* are characteristic but are not always present in adenomatoid malformations.

in utero must be replaced by air, and surfactant must be discharged into alveoli from type II pneumocytes so that a stable residual volume can develop in the lung. The presence of surfactant ensures that alveoli do not collapse completely with each expiration.[9] In addition, the pulmonary vasculature in the newborn must change rapidly from a low-flow, high-resistance system to a low-resistance, high-flow circulation with closure of the ductus arteriosus.

Failure of one or more of these physiologic changes to occur may be associated with a variety of diseases seen only in neonates. These disorders include hyaline membrane disease and its complications (bronchopulmonary dysplasia and interstitial emphysema), meconium aspiration, massive pulmonary hemorrhage, and persistent unexplained pulmonary hypertension in the newborn (persistent fetal circulation).

Perinatal lung disease

Transient tachypnea of the newborn ("neonatal wet lung"). During the first several breaths of life, lung fluid is removed by pulmonary lymphatics and through the airways. On occasion the removal of this fluid is delayed and transient tachypnea may be seen. The chest roentgenogram shows increased interstitial vascular markings, but the condition of the infant stabilizes rapidly as parenchymal and alveolar edema fluid is resorbed. No fatalities from this condition have been reported.[123-126]

Hyaline membrane disease. Hyaline membrane disease (HMD, idiopathic respiratory disease syndrome of the newborn) is a clinical, biochemical, and pathologic entity characteristically seen in a semispecific population.* Infants at greater risk for HMD include the following:

1. Appropriate for gestational age premature infants
2. Males
3. Whites
4. Infants of mothers with a history of previously affected premature infants
5. Infants born by cesarean section before 38 weeks' gestation, mother not in labor
6. Infants of diabetic mothers
7. Infants with asphyxia or whose delivery was precipitous
8. Second born of twins

The basic cause appears to be a deficiency of pulmonary surface-active material and consequent lung instability. Whether this deficit is related to type II cell immaturity, to inhibition of production, to release or function of surfactant, or to all three or additional factors in varying proportion is not resolved. There is probably variation in the cause of individual cases.[133]

Microscopically the most important feature is the abnormal expansion pattern. The distal airspaces are col-

---

*References 2, 11, 128, 134, 144, 147.

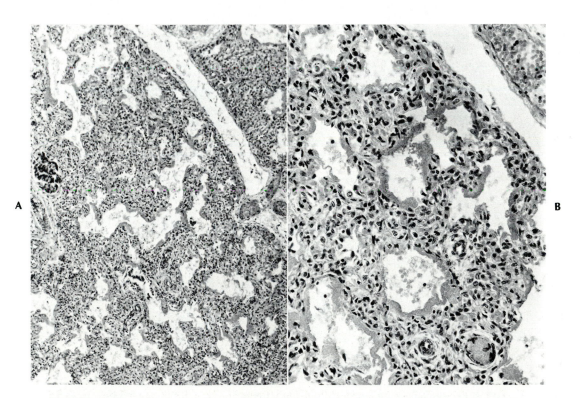

Fig. 22-3. Hyaline membrane disease. **A,** Lower-power photomicrograph shows dilated airways lined with eosinophilic ("hyaline") membranes. Distal airspaces are collapsed. Dilated lymphatics *(top)* are commonly seen. **B,** High-power view shows membranes and collapsed distal airspaces.

lapsed and the distal airways are dilated and lined by the characteristic eosinophilic ("hyaline") membranes (Fig. 22-3). Septal lymphatics are often dilated, and focal hemorrhage and edema fluid may be seen.[140] These features correlate with the roentgenographic "ground-glass" appearance and air-bronchogram effect seen on the chest film in HMD. The histologic features may be altered by the fixative employed, the time between death and autopsy, and the method of fixation.[1,140,142,146]

For the practical examination of the infant's lung at autopsy, it is generally wise to perfuse one lung with intrabronchial fixative and sample the other lung in the uninflated state. In this way both the interstitium and the expansion pattern can be examined. Fixative inflation of the lung removes the air-liquid barrier and obscures the effects of abnormally high surface tension on the lung.

Morphologic variations include the peculiar large, round airspaces described by Gruenwald[137] as "exaggerated atelectasis"; yellow staining of the membranes,[131] apparently by bilirubin; and sloughing of bronchial or alveolar epithelium to form a pseudoglandular or even giant cell pattern. The morphologic diagnosis of HMD in very small infants may be difficult because they may die before the hyaline membranes form or because the very immature lung may not be able to collapse in the recognizable HMD pattern.[135] In a tiny infant the distinction between a lung too immature to sustain respiration and HMD may be impossible to make.

It seems logical that the hyaline membranes in HMD simply represent a characteristic manifestation of diffuse alveolar damage[139] and that the abnormal expansion pattern is due to lung instability.

Methods for prenatal detection of lung maturity and pharmacologic methods for possible prevention of HMD are discussed elsewhere.[12,13,15,17,147]

Physiologic derangements in HMD include hypoxia, acidosis, pulmonary hypertension, and large right-to-left shunts through the lung and through failure of closure of the ductus arteriosus.[2] Complications include bronchopulmonary dysplasia and interstitial emphysema (see the following discussion). Problems related to therapy for HMD include subglottic stenosis and hypopharyngeal or tracheal perforation.[138,141,145]

Bronchopulmonary dysplasia. Bronchopulmonary dysplasia (BPD) is a clinical and pathologic syndrome usually found in infants treated for HMD with oxygen and artificial ventilation.[127,143,144,150] The relative importance of these two factors has been vigorously debated, but the immaturity of the lung exposed to these injurious agents may be more important than either. The alveolar septa in the immature lung are wide and cellular and seem to contain a greater potential space in which vessels and fibroblasts can proliferate. In patients who die within the first month of life the histologic features are those of diffuse alveolar damage and its repair, with the added insult of bronchiolar necrosis and florid bronchiolitis

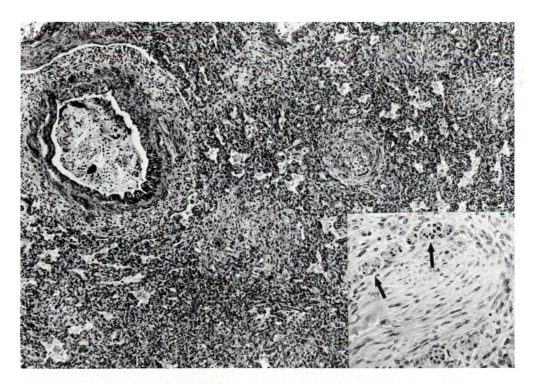

Fig. 22-4. Bronchopulmonary dysplasia in acute phase. Some bronchioles *(upper left)* show epithelial necrosis and squamous metaplasia. Lighter nodules in lung represent bronchioles whose lumen is obliterated by fibrous tissue. Inset shows such a lesion. Residual smooth muscle wall of bronchiole is outlined by arrows.

obliterans (Fig. 22-4). The question of how BPD differs from resolving untreated HMD is difficult to approach because before the use of oxygen or mechanical ventilation patients usually died within 72 hours or survived without further difficulty. Several older studies have suggested that in resolving HMD the membranes are fragmented and are phagocytosed by macrophages.[142] Why such florid bronchiolitis obliterans and interstitial fibrosis occur in treated infants is unclear.

Complications of BPD include the development of pulmonary interstitial emphysema, pneumothorax, and pneumomediastinum. Patent ductus arteriosus and intrapulmonary shunting may lead to impressive right ventricular hypertrophy. Autopsy study of long-term survivors of BPD who required continuous ventilation usually shows a pattern of chronic bronchitis and patchy interstitial fibrosis (Fig. 22-5). Areas of collapsed lung alternate with enlarged simplified airspaces that represent coalescence of groups of alveoli whose walls have been destroyed and remodeled. Interstitial vascularity is increased as well.

Complete follow-up studies of patients who survive HMD and BPD are not available. Such studies are complicated by the inability to separate deleterious effects of premature birth and therapy in general from the specific effects of lung disease at an early age. Several investigators have reported an increased incidence of subsequent pulmonary infection and of persistently abnormal chest roentgenograms with patchy fibrosis.[128,130,132,136] The presence of small airway disease has recently been documented.[136,148] Developmental and other central nervous system abnormalities are found with variable incidence in recent studies.[136,149]

Pulmonary interstitial emphysema and its complications. Although small pneumothoraces are not uncommon in newborn full-term infants, the development of significant pulmonary interstitial air with subsequent pneumomediastinum, pneumopericardium, and even pneumoperitoneum is most often seen in the premature newborn infant treated with artificial ventilation.[152-160] Most such infants also have bronchopulmonary dysplasia, and systemic air embolism has been reported as well.[156] Other clinical situations in which pulmonary instial emphysema (PIE) and its sequelae occur are the meconium aspiration syndrome; the pulmonary hypoplasias, especially those associated with severe renal abnormalities and oligohydramnios; and as a complication of amniocentesis. The pathogenesis of PIE involves dissection of air into the pulmonary interstitial space and probably into lymphatics as well.[159] Subpleural blebs rupture causing pneumothorax, or air dissects into the hilum of the lung with subsequent extension to the mediastinum, pericardium, or subcutaneous tissues. Grossly and microscopically, cystic spaces are seen around bronchovascular bundles and in the septa of the lung (Fig. 22-6), and the morphologic features may be misinterpreted as representing a cystic malformation. Extensive dissection of air around the pulmonary vessels at the hilum may

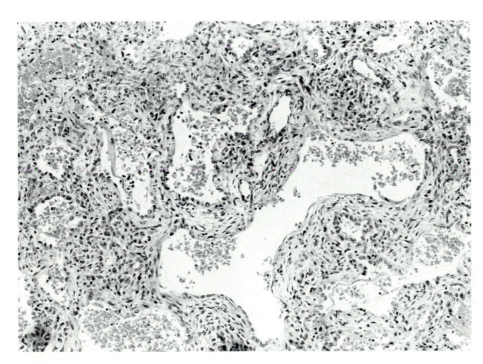

Fig. 22-5. Bronchopulmonary dysplasia, late phase. There has been extensive rearrangement of lung architecture. Interalveolar septa are fibrotic, and residual airspaces are relatively avascular. This interface does not provide efficient ventilation and perfusion matching in lung.

cause air block and circulatory compromise.[153] The large potential space available in the interalveolar (intersaccular) septa in the premature infant's lung probably contributes greatly to the more extensive PIE found in premature infants. Giant cells may be seen in the air-filled spaces and represent a response to air as an irritant.

PIE is usually a diffuse process but may occur as a predominantly localized but expanding lesion in a single lobe or lung.[154,160] Localized PIE often presents a surgical emergency. While pneumoperitoneum may be a complication of PIE, a more likely cause of pneumoperitoneum is a gastric or bowel perforation and that consideration should not be overlooked. Lung perforation can occur as a complication of treatment of pneumothorax with chest tubes.[151]

Meconium aspiration syndrome. Massive meconium aspiration is generally associated with hypoxia and fetal distress in the full-term or postmature infant.[162,163,170,173,174] Pulmonary interstitial emphysema and pneumothorax are frequent complications. On gross examination the lungs may have silvery green discoloration, and tenacious mucoid material may be expressed from the tracheobronchial tree. Microscopically, distended distal airways filled with mucus, bile pigments, and squames are the characteristic features. Since squames alone are routinely found in the distal airspaces of stillborn infants and infants dying in the neonatal peri-od, the presence of mucin obstructing the bronchioles provides a more definitive diagnosis of meconium aspiration. Polymorphonuclear cells may be present in the alveoli. Whether meconium can cause "chemical pneumonitis" is controversial.[176] Meconium does seem to enhance the development of bacterial pneumonia.[168,172]

While the amniotic fluid and placenta are usually deeply stained in cases of meconium aspiration, some reports suggest that a clinically similar syndrome can occur without external evidence of meconium staining. Although most investigators believe that meconium aspiration occurs at or after delivery, an intrauterine aspiration syndrome has been reported.[175]

Massive pulmonary hemorrhage in the newborn. Focal pulmonary hemorrhages can be seen in the lungs of neonates dying of a variety of causes.[161,165,166] Larger interstitial hemorrhages are not uncommon in the pulmonary parenchyma of stillborn infants. The term *massive pulmonary hemorrhage* (MPH) is usually employed in reference to a clinical syndrome of respiratory distress with acute collapse. Often hemorrhagic fluid pours from the nose and mouth. These infants at autopsy have pulmonary hemorrhage, predominantly intra-alveolar, involving more than one third of the total lung parenchyma. The syndrome characteristically appears in premature, small for gestational age, male infants. Infants with congenital cardiovascular disease should probably be considered as a separate population.

The etiology of MPH is unknown. Major theories advanced to date include infection (unlikely), cold injury, hemorrhagic pulmonary edema, a terminal manifestation of intracerebral damage or increased intracerebral pressure, pulmonary capillary fragility, and oxygen damage.[165,171] Most cases in the British Perinatal Study occurred between the third and seventeenth days of life.[167] MPH is not simply a severe manifestation of HMD; MPH occurs in growth-retarded infants, whereas HMD occurs in premature infants with appropriate development for their gestational age.

Wilson-Mikity syndrome. Wilson-Mikity syndrome (neonatal focal hyperaeration, pulmonary dysmaturity) is a peculiar pulmonary disorder seen almost exclusively in very small male premature infants.[164,169] Clinical features include late neonatal onset (sixth to thirty-fifth day after birth), increasing respiratory distress, and slow resolution in survivors.

Clinical and even pathologic reports of this syndrome have not clearly separated Wilson-Mikity syndrome from bronchopulmonary dysplasia. In the cases originally described, alternating areas of lobular hyperinflation and collapse were present without intervening fibrosis or bronchiolar destruction.[169]

Persistent fetal circulation. Persistent fetal circulation (PFC, unexplained persistent pulmonary hypertension

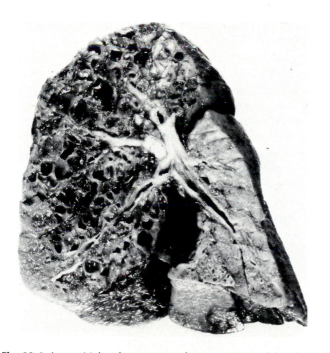

Fig. 22-6. Interstitial pulmonary emphysema. Upper lobe shows multiple coalescent cysts representing interstitial air dissecting along interlobar septa and around small and large airways. The lower lobe *(right)* shows the solid appearance associated with the collapsed airspaces of hyaline membrane disease.

of the newborn) is a clinical syndrome in which the pulmonary circulation fails to be transformed into a high-flow, low-resistance system after birth.[177-189] Infants with PFC are cyanotic and hypoxic after birth, and there is evidence of significant pulmonary hypertension with a large right-to-left shunt in the absence of a cardiovascular malformation. Some of these infants have associated hyaline membrane disease or meconium aspiration, but others have no evidence of other underlying pulmonary disorders. If the ductus arteriosus closes, right ventricular hypertrophy and heart failure may supervene.

At autopsy, morphologic evidence of pulmonary hypertension as seen in adults (see p. 866) is usually not demonstrable. Reid and associates[184] and others have demonstrated, however, that striking abnormalities may be present in the small pulmonary arteries. In patients with PFC there is an abnormal smooth muscle coat in the media of the pulmonary arteries (arterioles) in that part of the lung acinus distal to respiratory bronchioles. Ordinarily muscle is present in these vessels only after adolescence or during adult life. Less commonly, small thrombi may be seen in the pulmonary arteries of affected infants.[183,185] Other findings may reflect associated pulmonary disease and the effects of therapy. A number of infants with bilateral pulmonary hypoplasia and especially infants with hypoplastic lungs related to diaphragmatic hernia also have a clinical syndrome resembling PFC.[177,179,188,189] Infants whose mothers have taken large doses of prostaglandin inhibitors have had a similar disorder.[181]

All of these findings suggest that intrauterine and perinatal events may initiate and perpetuate PFC. Rudolph[187] has proposed a valuable clinical etiologic classification distinguishing three groups of patients with PFC. In patients with normal pulmonary vascular development, acute vasoconstriction or abnormally high blood viscosity may impede flow. In another group of patients, increased pulmonary vascular smooth muscle is present, presumably reflecting a variety of intrauterine insults. In the final group a decreased cross-sectional area of pulmonary vessels is found. These infants have pulmonary hypoplasia of varying degree. Other intrauterine events such as infection or drug exposure may also adversely affect pulmonary vascular development.

The presence of pulmonary hypertension early in the clinical course and of severity out of proportion to any associated pulmonary parenchymal changes seen on chest roentgenogram is a feature that can help to differentiate PFC from other respiratory disorders of the newborn.

Infectious disorders in the infant lung

Neonatal pulmonary infection (congenital and perinatal pneumonia) is a common finding in neonatal necropsies.[192-196,198,199,204] Pneumonia, as a primary or compli-

cating phenomenon, was found in 36% of the cases in the British Perinatal Mortality Survey in 1958 and, including the amniotic fluid infection syndrome, accounted for approximately 20% of neonatal deaths in the U.S. Collaborative Perinatal Projects.[197,200] The organisms implicated vary with the clinical features. Pneumonias in the perinatal period may be classified as the following:

1. Transplacental—part of a systemic congenital disease
2. Congenital (intrauterine)—amniotic fluid infection syndrome; usually found in stillborns, abortuses, or early postnatal deaths in full-term infants
3. Acquired during birth—signs appear in the first week; usually caused by organisms in maternal birth canal; affects premature infants especially
4. Acquired after birth—appears during the first months; caused by organisms acquired from environment

Congenital pneumonia usually accompanies the amniotic fluid infection syndrome (AFIS). The placental membranes and amniotic fluid are infected by organisms ascending from the vagina, and concomitantly clusters of polymorphonuclear cells appear in bronchi and alveoli. The isolation of bacteria or other infective agents depends on the care with which routine and special cultures are performed. The placental membranes may have ruptured before birth but may have been intact. Maternal urinary tract infection appears to be important in the pathogenesis of infection when membranes are intact.[201] Racial and socioeconomic factors appear associated with AFIS; perhaps the usual bacteriostatic activity of amniotic fluid is adversely affected in certain populations.[200-204] The presence of pulmonary vessels filled with polymorphonuclear cells has been used to differentiate true congenital pneumonia from the infant who "drowned in pus" from aspiration of infected amniotic fluid, but basically the findings seem to represent different portions of a spectrum. Whether the pulmonary disease is the cause or an accompanying phenomenon of events causing abortion, stillbirth, or neonatal death is not clear. Lung tissue or aspirated heart blood should be submitted for culture when pneumonia is suspected.

Pneumonia acquired during birth is usually caused by organisms acquired from the birth canal. Group B streptococcal infection has attracted major attention because of its rapidly fatal course if untreated and the histologic feature of hyaline membranes, which may obscure the true diagnosis.[191,198] The membranes are not present in all cases, and the lung in very early cases may show only polymorphonuclear leukocytes, gram-positive cocci, and edema. When membranes are present, the expansion pattern differs from that in HMD, and more polymorphonuclear leukocytes are seen. Pleural effusion may be seen in group B streptococcal infection and would be unusual in HMD or even other neonatal pulmonary infections.

Late-onset pneumonia is usually caused by organisms, such as staphylococci, *Pseudomonas*, or *Serratia*, acquired from human or environmental contacts.[192,194] Chlamydial pneumonitis is a distinctive pneumonitis of infants, usually appearing at 3 weeks of age with tachypnea and a staccato cough.[190,205,206] Associated conjunctivitis is seen in 50% of the infants. An absolute blood eosinophilia may be present. The course may be protracted, but recovery is the rule. Interstitial pneumonitis and florid bronchiolitis have been described as histologic features.[190] In most neonatal cases, maternal genital infection is suspected as the source.

Transplacental pneumonia appears as a part of the generalized disease associated with cytomegalovirus, herpesvirus, or other "TORCH" agents or with syphilis or certain bacterial infections such as listeriosis.[202,206,207] Evaluation of the placenta, special culture or fluorescent antibody techniques, or serum studies in mother and infant are helpful.

Bronchiolitis and bronchiolitis obliterans

In the older pediatric age groups, viral infection (adenovirus and respiratory syncytial virus) is a frequent cause of bronchiolitis.[214,215] Toxic inhalants can produce a similar picture, and both types of injury may be followed by progressive obliteration of the small airways. This bronchiolitis obliterans is essentially a syndrome caused by many reactive processes in the lung and is a descriptive term for a pattern of injury, not a specific diagnosis. Cases with apparent antenatal origin are reported.[212] Gastroesophageal reflux with aspiration of gastric acid can also produce severe bronchiolar damage in infants.[210,211]

Microscopically the acute phase consists of bronchiolar necrosis and peribronchial cuffing by inflammatory cells. Severe damage may be followed by obliteration of bronchiolar lumina by fibrous plugs.[209] In rare instances extensive obliteration of the small airways has produced the unilateral hyperlucent lung, a small lung with evidence of air trapping and generally with a small pulmonary artery (Swyer-James syndrome).[213,214] The small pulmonary artery is generally considered to be an acquired phenomenon. The bronchioles in the affected lobe are often reduced to small scars, and the lesion may be overlooked unless one makes a specific attempt to identify a bronchiole accompanying most of the small pulmonary arteries. Focal hyperlucency of the lung related to bronchial atresia is discussed on p. 834.

INFECTIONS OF THE LUNGS AND BRONCHI
Incidence

According to the U.S. vital statistics, pneumonia and influenza together account for 3% of all deaths and are the fifth leading cause of death, exceeded only by heart disease, cancer, cerebrovascular disease, and accidents. Respiratory infections are responsible for 8.5% of hospitalizations in the United States. Nosocomial pneumonias develop in 0.7% of all hospitalized patients but in as much as 13% of the critically ill patients admitted to intensive care units. With the use of potent therapies that deliberately or incidentally produce immunosuppression, there is every prospect that respiratory infections will remain a serious clinical problem. For example, pneumonia develops in one third of patients receiving chemotherapy for leukemia.[223]

Routes of infection

Pathogenic organisms gain access to the lung through the airways, through the bloodstream, by traumatic implantation, or by direct spread across the diaphragm from a subphrenic source, probably via lymphatics. The most common route is the airways. Airway spread can result from inhalation of the organism as an aerosol on droplet nuclei. This is the major mechanism of spread of many viral infections and of tuberculosis. Often, however, the development of overt infection takes place in stages with initial colonization of the upper respiratory tract by potential pathogens and subsequent aspiration into the lower respiratory tract.[219,220] This is a major mechanism for many of the gram-negative organisms. Two important determinants of the ability of a bacterium to colonize are bacterial interference by the existing flora and the binding of the bacterium to the epithelial surface, thought to be mediated by specific molecules on the epithelial cell membrane. Antibiotic therapy, by eliminating interference by the normal flora, promotes colonization by resistant organisms. Serious illness increases the ability of nasopharyngeal epithelium to bind gram-negative bacteria in vitro, and this binding activity is highly correlated with colonization of the host by these organisms.[221] The mechanism of the change is not known with certainty, but a plausible hypothesis is that proteases in saliva and airway secretions degrade certain cell surface proteins, exposing others.[226]

Pulmonary defenses

The respiratory tract has a number of protective mechanisms that dispatch most organisms deposited in the respiratory tract before they can set up an infection.[216,218,222] The trachea and bronchi are coated with a layer of mucus produced by the goblet cells of the bronchial mucosa and the glands in the lamina propria. This layer provides a physical barrier to organisms deposited in the airways and is swept upward to the oropharynx by ciliary action, removing deposited microbes. The mucus contains specific antibody, mainly IgA, produced by plasma cells in the lamina propria of the bronchus, as well as other antibacterial substances such as lysozyme and lactoferrin produced in the serous cells of the glands. At the alveolar level the main defense under ordinary circumstances is the alveolar macrophage. Most organisms that reach the alveoli are engulfed by macrophages and killed long before they are physically cleared from the lung.[217] The rate of killing varies among species of bacteria and indeed among strains of the same species. Clinically important factors that have been shown to depress macrophage function include starvation, ethanol ingestion, hypoxia, uremia, air pollutants, cigarette smoke, and antecedent viral infection.[222] The alveolar lining layer contains some antibody (mainly IgG) as well as complement components. The alveolar macrophages when stimulated can also produce a variety of chemotactic substances that recruit neutrophils and more mononuclear phagocytes.[225] With lymphoid nodules located at the branch points of small airways and in the pleura and with complete lymph nodes in the hila, the lungs are also one of the major lymphoid organs of the body.[224]

Viral infections

Viral infections are discussed in Chapter 10. The most important in terms of both morbidity and mortality is influenza, which is discussed in detail on p. 347. Viral infections early in life may also be important as a predisposing factor for the development of chronic lung disease in adulthood.

In children lethal viral infections take one of two pathologic forms, bronchiolitis or pneumonia.[227] The majority of cases of bronchiolitis are caused by respiratory syncytial virus (RSV), but parainfluenza virus, adenovirus, and *Mycoplasma pneumoniae* can also cause this syndrome.[239] Bronchiolitis is exceedingly common, comprising more than one fifth of lower respiratory infections seen in pediatric practice. Epidemics of the disease occur usually in winter, with the highest incidence in children under 2 years of age.[232] Most cases are mild, and only 1% to 2% of children require hospitalization. Among those hospitalized the mortality is only 1% to 2%. The onset of symptoms is acute with tachypnea, dyspnea, cough, and wheezing. Sternal retractions may be present. Most patients are afebrile. When patients with the rare severe cases are seen at autopsy, the lungs are well expanded and may be considered normal on gross examination. Close inspection reveals thickening of the small airways, which appear on the cut surface of the lung as 2 to 4 mm gray nodules with a pinpoint lumen barely visible. Microscopically the walls of the bronchioles are densely infiltrated with mononuclear inflammatory cells (Fig. 22-7). Early, there is necrosis of the ciliated epithelium with the formation of plugs of necrotic material and leukocytes in the bronchiolar lumen. Regeneration of the epithelium begins after 3 to 4 days and is complete by 15 days with the regeneration of cilia. The alveoli are expanded and have a round contour indic-

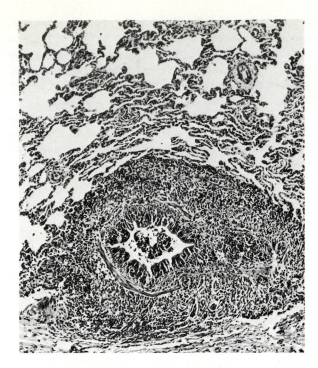

Fig. 22-7. Viral bronchiolitis. Wall of bronchiole is markedly infiltrated with mononuclear inflammatory cells, and lumen also contains exudate. Focally, alveoli are collapsed but noninflamed.

ative of air trapping. There may be limited extension of the inflammatory infiltrate into the walls of alveoli abutting the bronchioles. Bronchiolitis caused by adenovirus tends to be more severe. Necrosis of the bronchiolar epithelium is extensive and may extend into the bronchiolar wall. This probably accounts for the higher mortality of adenoviral bronchiolitis (5% to 7%) and for the high frequency of sequelae.

Viral pneumonias may occur at any age. The specific infecting virus determines the cytologic features of the infected cells, including the presence and morphology of inclusions and the tendency to form syncytia and giant cells.[228,229,236,237] However, one can make generalizations concerning the morphologic response of the lung to viruses. Most viruses that produce pneumonia infect the epithelial cells, either exclusively or in addition to infecting other cell types. The predominant tissue response is an acute interstitial pneumonia. The walls of the airspaces are thickened owing to congestion, edema, and an interstitial infiltrate predominantly of mononuclear cells. Hyaline membranes form in respiratory bronchioles and alveolar ducts, and many of the alveoli are collapsed (microatelectasis). The airspaces contain edema, fibrin, and a scanty cellular exudate of monocytes, macrophages, occasional neutrophils, and sloughed epithelial cells. There are usually focal hemorrhages. Foci of necrosis may be present, particularly with herpesviruses and adenovirus, but often are absent even in lethal infections.

The alveolar epithelial cells are enlarged and hyperplastic. In some areas they may be seen overlying or beneath hyaline membranes. Patients who have been ill for more than a few days usually have foci of epithelial regeneration and metaplastic epithelium of squamous or bronchiolar type, even in alveoli.

Bronchioles are often inflamed and may show viral inclusions in the epithelium. Occlusive plugs of necrotic material, which are common in bronchiolitis, are seen only infrequently in viral pneumonia.

Mycoplasmal pneumonia

Mycoplasmas are simple organisms, 150 nm in diameter, that occupy a taxonomic place between the large viruses and bacteria. Unlike viruses, they can be cultured on simple media in vitro. They are enclosed by a membrane but lack cell walls and therefore are difficult to demonstrate in tissue sections except by immunohistochemical methods. *Mycoplasma pneumoniae* is a common cause of upper respiratory infections. It appears that pneumonia develops in less than 10% of infected subjects.[231,235]

In large ambulatory civilian populations, 15% to 20% of pneumonias are caused by mycoplasmas. In certain closed military populations the proportion may be higher. *M. pneumoniae* is a cause of both endemic and epidemic pneumonia. The infection rate varies little with season, unlike other pneumonias. The peak age is between 5 and 15 years, and infection is relatively infrequent in those over 45 years.[233] Clinically, mycoplasmal pneumonia is a benign, self-limited disease with few complications. Usually only one lung is involved, and the process is patchy or segmental in distribution.[231]

A characteristic feature is the presence of cold agglutinins, IgM antibodies that do not react at 37° C but cause agglutination of the patient's erythrocytes at 4° C. They develop in almost all cases of mycoplasmal pneumonia but are not specific and can be seen in pneumonias caused by a variety of other organisms.[231] Occasionally they may be the cause of Raynaud's phenomenon by producing agglutination of erythrocytes in chilled extremities, and they are occasionally responsible for hemolytic anemia.[235,238]

Extrapulmonary spread of mycoplasmas has only recently been recognized. Almost any tissue can be involved; gastrointestinal disease, myocarditis, and a variety of neurologic manifestations have been described.[235]

Because of the benign course of mycoplasmal pneumonia, pathologic features of only a few cases have been described.[230,234] Grossly the lungs show a fibrinous pleurisy and patchy consolidation. Microscopically there are bronchiolitis and interstitial pneumonia. The walls of bronchioles are congested, edematous, and infiltrated with mononuclear cells. Epithelial cells degenerate and are sloughed. The parenchyma shows edema and interstitial pneumonia with hyaline membranes and mononuclear cell infiltration of the alveolar walls. The gross and histologic changes are indistinguishable from those of viral pneumonia. Culture or immunohistochemical demonstration of the organism is necessary to differentiate the diseases.

Bacterial infections
Acute tracheobronchitis

Diphtheria is discussed elsewhere. Acute bacterial infections of the large airways are a frequent complication of viral infection. In small children, owing to the small caliber of the airways, bacterial infection can cause severe obstruction. The syndrome acute tracheitis is an acute bacterial infection of the airways seen in children usually below 6 years of age. The clinical picture resembles croup but also includes stridor, high fever, and toxicity. Epiglottitis is not present. Most cases are caused by *Staphylococcus aureus*, but *Haemophilus influenzae* and other bacteria may also be responsible. Subglottic edema and thick mucopurulent exudate can cause tracheal obstruction.[247]

Bacterial pneumonia

Pneumococcal pneumonia. *Streptococcus pneumoniae* is a gram-positive facultative anaerobe that produces alpha hemolysis when cultured on blood agar. It is recognized in smears and histologic sections as a lancet-shaped diplococcus, but it can also appear in chains and clumps. The more than 80 strains that have been identified differ in the antigenic structure of their capsular polysaccharide.

The pneumococcus continues to be responsible for 30% to 80% or more of community-acquired pneumonias.[253,254] Groups at particular risk include the very young and the very old, alcoholics, diabetics, splenectomized subjects, and patients with multiple myeloma or sickle cell disease.[254] Pneumococci also cause nosocomial infections, in which case the clinical picture is often atypical. The mortality of pneumococcal pneumonia before modern therapy was 30%, but a considerable improvement was obtained with the introduction of type-specific antisera and antibiotics.[244] Even with modern antibiotic therapy, however, the mortality is 20% in those with bacteremic infection.[241,244,250]

Pathology. Pneumococcal pneumonia typically presents the picture of lobar pneumonia. One or occasionally several lobes of the lung are involved.[242] The individual involved lobes are relatively uniform in appearance, the process being rapidly spread through the lobe and limited by the lobar fissures. Occasionally a few lobules are uninvolved or at a different stage, indicating some restraint of the spread by the lobular septa. Traditionally the progress of the disease is divided into four stages: edema, red hepatization, gray hepatization, and resolution or organization.

The organisms colonize the upper respiratory tract and gain access to the lung by aspiration. Not uncommonly this follows a viral respiratory infection by several days, the way being paved by viral damage to the ciliated epithelium.[254] The initial response to the organism is an outpouring of edema fluid, which provides a rich broth in which the organisms proliferate and which spreads them throughout the lobe through pores of Kohn and bronchioles (Fig. 22-8). At this stage an involved lobe appears distended, moist, and deep red or purple. The pleura is shiny, and fluid exudes from the cut surface. With the passage of time progressively more fibrin and neutrophils enter the alveoli. Phagocytosis of bacteria begins, and within 24 hours most organisms are found within neutrophils. At first the alveolar capillaries are distended with erythrocytes and there is diapedesis of erythrocytes into the alveoli, giving the lobe a red color, while the filling of the airspaces with fibrin and leukocytes gives it a firm, liverlike consistency. Classically the lobe at this phase is described as red hepatization. With the further evolution of the process, increasing amounts of fibrin and leukocytes enter the airspaces, the alveolar capillaries appear compressed, and the lobe becomes progressively grayer in appearance, evolving into the stage of gray hepatization (Figs. 22-9 and 22-10). In untreated persons, organisms decrease in number progressively after approximately 5 days.

In the usual course of events the final stage is resolution. As a rule necrosis of alveolar walls is not a feature of

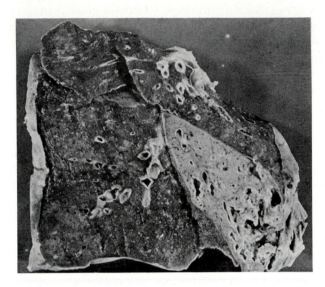

Fig. 22-9. Gray hepatization in pneumococcal pneumonia. Lobe shows beginning abscess formation.

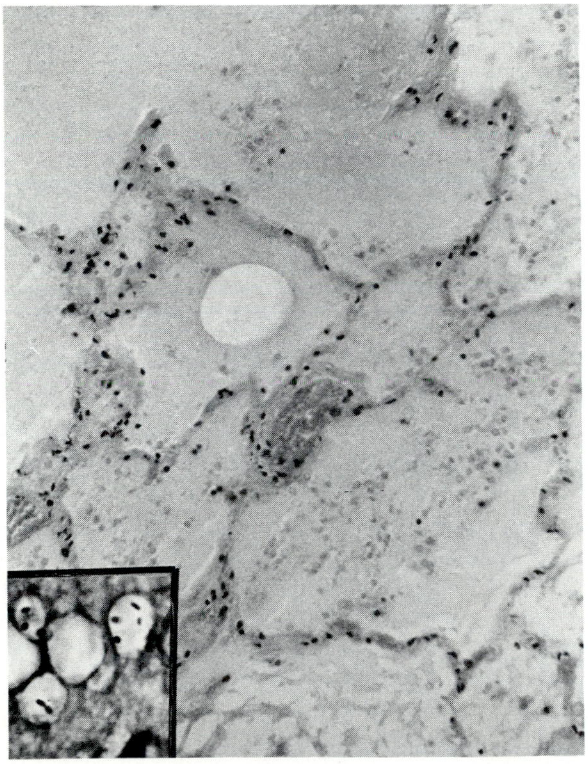

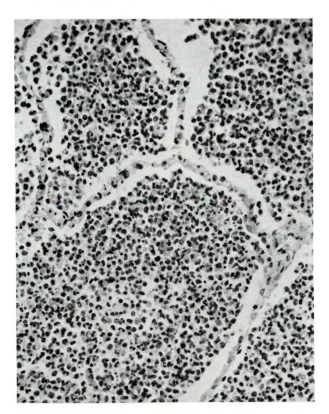

Fig. 22-8. Pneumococcal pneumonia in stage of edema. Airspaces are filled with fluid and a few erythrocytes. *Inset,* With Gram's stain, edema fluid teems with gram-positive diplococci. Halo surrounding organisms represents unstained capsular material.

Fig. 22-10. Histologic features of gray hepatization. Alveolar spaces are filled with neutrophils and fibrin. Alveolar walls are comparatively normal.

pneumococcal pneumonia except with serotype III. Since the exudation is intra-alveolar, it can be cleared through the bronchial tree, restoring the lung to normal. Macrophages are the predominant cells during this process.[252]

Beginning as early as 48 hours after onset, a few monocytes can be found in the alveolar exudate. With time they increase in number and differentiate into macrophages at a time that varies from case to case. Usually between 5 and 12 days after onset monocytes and macrophages become the predominant types of inflammatory cell. The neutrophils degenerate, and the fibrin network breaks down under the influence of proteases released from the neutrophils and newly arriving macrophages. Macrophages containing both degenerating neutrophils and organisms can be observed. Over the ensuing several days organisms disappear and empty space begins to appear progressively in the exudate, which gradually is removed by the phagocytes or is expectorated. Alveolar architecture ultimately returns to normal.

In a small proportion of cases, resolution fails to take place or is incomplete and the unresolved areas undergo organization (Fig. 22-11). The remaining exudate is invaded by fibroblasts and converted to fibrous tissue. Masses of fibroblasts invading the airspaces lay down a matrix of myxoid connective tissue rich in proteoglycan,

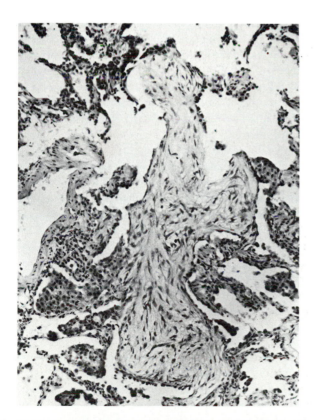

Fig. 22-11. Organizing pneumonia. Alveolar duct is filled by plug of young connective tissue containing fibroblasts and proteoglycan-rich matrix, which has replaced inflammatory exudate.

which is gradually coverted to collagenous tissue. In some areas alveolar epithelium migrates over organizing exudate within the airspaces, incorporating it into the alveolar walls and giving rise to an appearance indistinguishable from interstitial fibrosis. In other areas the airspaces remain filled, and the lung is converted to fleshy, gray, glistening, solid tissue whose meaty consistency accounts for the old term for this process, carnification.

The factors that determine whether resolution or carnification occurs are incompletely understood. The frequency with which pneumonia fails to resolve appeared to increase following the introduction of antibiotics.[240] This suggests that if the organisms are sterilized early, before the influx of phagocytic cells reaches a maximum, lysis of the fibrin by phagocyte-derived proteases will be incomplete and the residual fibrin will become organized.

Although the typical pathologic pattern of pneumococcal pneumonia is lobar consolidation, a pattern of bronchopneumonia is by no means rare. Even in preantibiotic series, atypical (that is, nonlobar) pneumonia accounted for more than 40% of fatal pneumococcal pneumonias.[245] Type III is the most common serotype causing atypical patterns, but a variety of serotypes can do so. Patients tend to be either very young or over 50 years of age and usually have underlying disease, either chronic obstructive lung disease or serious extrathoracic disease. The pneumonia is commonly bilateral and has an appearance similar to other bronchopneumonias, notably multiple foci of consolidation centered on terminal airways.

Complications. Pleural involvement occurs commonly in lobar pneumonia. In two thirds of patients there is a fibrinous pleuritis without infection of the pleural space. Pleural fluid if present has a relatively low white cell content and glucose concentration. In 15% to 25% of patients, infection of the pleural space (empyema) develops and the pleural surface becomes covered with shaggy white layers of fibrin and neutrophils. Pleural fluid becomes turbid and then frankly purulent with loculated pockets of pus. Unlike purulent exudate in the alveoli, that in the pleural cavity is not in communication with the exterior and cannot be readily cleared; instead of resolving, empyema heals by organization. This can lead to encasement of the lung by a thick fibrous peel that is several millimeters thick and ultimately may restrict lung expansion.

Bacteremia occurs in 20% to 35% of patients with lobar pneumonia and a much smaller proportion of those with bronchopneumonia. It is a serious complication that continues to have a mortality of 20% to 30% despite antibiotics. Bacteremic spread leads to metastatic infection, including meningitis, bacterial endocarditis, arthritis, or pericarditis in a small proportion of patients.

Lung abscess results from the breakdown of alveolar

walls. The frequency of this complication is twice as great with type III pneumococcus as with other types,[245,256] probably because the type III organism is protected from phagocytosis by its abundant production of capsular material.

Clinical correlations. The onset of pneumococcal pneumonia is usually abrupt with a shaking chill followed by high fever and systemic symptoms such as malaise, nausea, myalgias, and weakness. Pleuritic chest pain is common. Most patients cough up rusty or purulent sputum. Leukocytosis (up to 20,000/cu mm) is common; leukopenia is a grave prognostic sign. Before antibiotic therapy patients remained acutely ill for 5 to 6 days and then often went through a dramatic clinical change known as a crisis with profuse sweating and fall in the fever, after which they greatly improved. This change corresponded to the appearance of circulating antibodies. It did not correlate with any abrupt alteration in the morphology of the lung, which might be in the stage of red or gray hepatization. Less often clinical recovery was gradual (by lysis). The response to antibiotics is rapid, with improvement usually within 24 hours.

Beta-hemolytic streptococcal pneumonia. Beta-hemolytic streptococci are an uncommon cause of pneumonia at the present time. Lancefield group A streptococci were formerly the most prominent strains, but recently group B organisms have been assuming greater importance.[255] Infections caused by beta-hemolytic streptococci in the newborn are discussed elsewhere. Formerly many streptococcal pneumonias in older children followed the childhood viral exanthema; they are now decreasing in incidence owing to the use of vaccines against the viruses.[248] In adults, streptococcal pneumonia like other pneumonias usually occurs in elderly, severely debilitated patients.[255] Diabetes is also a risk factor.

The lower lobes are usually the site of major involvement. The airways appear thickened and are filled with a bloody or purulent exudate. The pneumonia is lobular with consolidated patches clearly centered on terminal bronchioles. The distinctive microscopic feature of streptococcal pneumonia is greater interstitial involvement than in other bacterial pneumonias. There is necrosis of the epithelium of distal airways with infiltration of the bronchial walls by neutrophils and mononuclear cells. The interstitial infiltrate also extends into the adjacent alveolar walls. The lung surrounding the pneumonic foci is edematous. The interlobular septa are swollen with edema, and the lymphatics are distended and sometimes plugged with fibrin strands. Effusions and empyema can develop with great rapidity.[248]

Staphylococcal pneumonia. *Staphylococcus aureus* commonly colonizes the nose and skin. Staphylococcal pneumonia usually occurs either in the presence of a source of bacteremia or after a viral infection. Hematog-enous pneumonia is seen in those with soft tissue infections,[251] in patients undergoing long-term dialysis, because of infected shunts, and in parenteral narcotic users, especially those with right-sided bacterial endocarditis. Hematogenous staphylococcal pneumonia most often produces multiple rounded lesions that are more numerous in the lower lung zones where blood flow is greatest. The lesions may appear as septic infarcts that are yellow and purulent but preserve to some degree the wedge-shaped configuration of infarcts and are associated with thrombosed vessels, or they may be rounded patches of necrotizing pneumonia that break down, giving rise to abscesses.

Staphylococcal pneumonia also results from spread of organisms from the colonized nasopharynx. This often follows damage to the mucociliary apparatus by viral infection, notably in influenza epidemics.[246,249] The lesions are those of a bronchopneumonia accompanied by a hemorrhagic and necrotizing bronchitis. Purulent exudate fills the bronchioles and spreads into the adjacent acini. Colonies of bacteria can usually be found without difficulty. Necrosis and breakdown of alveolar walls are early features and may result in hemorrhage in the surrounding lung.

Staphylococcal bronchopneumonia is not rare in children less than 6 months of age. A notable feature of staphylococcal pneumonia in small children is development of pneumatoceles, air-containing lesions that are seen roentgenographically within areas of confluent pneumonia and that enlarge very rapidly, often over hours. It is unlikely that they are simple abscesses because they are thin walled and can disappear over several weeks without residua. Although their morphology has rarely been described, since patients commonly recover, most radiologists assume that they arise from the trapping of air distal to partial obstruction to a bronchus, which acts as a check valve.[243]

Local complications of staphylococcal pneumonia include empyema and bronchopleural fistula.

Pneumonia caused by gram-negative aerobic bacteria. In the preantibiotic era, gram-negative pneumonias accounted for only 0.5% to 5% of pneumonias and were usually due to *Klebsiella-Enterobacter* species. Currently the incidence of gram-negative organisms as the cause of pneumonia has increased, although reliable figures are difficult to obtain and a distinction between primary pneumonia and superinfection is not always made. Between 5% and 30% of community-acquired bacterial pneumonias and up to 50% of nosocomial bacterial pneumonias are due to gram-negative organisms. Even when community acquired, gram-negative pneumonias are virtually limited to persons with underlying chronic illness.[266,268]

The routes of infection vary with the species.[270] *Escherichia coli*, *Enterobacter*, and *Pseudomonas* often reach the lung via the bloodstream. The other gram-negative bacilli usually colonize the upper airways. The spread of infection in the hospital by the use of contaminated inhalation therapy equipment has been well documented,[266] but with improvements in sterilization techniques and increased awareness of the problem it is diminishing in frequency.

Pneumonia caused by *Klebsiella pneumoniae* occurs in men far more often than in women. The predilection for alcoholics is well known; other patients are admitted to the hospital from nursing homes.[268] The organism colonizes the upper respiratory tract or oral cavity and gains access to the lung by aspiration. This undoubtedly accounts for its predilection for the right upper lobe.[257]

The onset of the disease is sudden with rigors, fever, and severe prostration and toxicity. Cough and hemoptysis are common, and the sputum is typically (although not invariably) gelatinous and brick red.[268]

The anatomic distribution of pneumonia is typically lobar and in the right lung in the majority of cases. The involved lung is bulging and gray-red and exudes slimy material. In cases of more than a few days' duration, abscesses are found. Microscopically the exudate consists of both neutrophils and macrophages, and organisms may be abundant (Fig. 22-12). Necrosis of alveolar walls appears early, and by 4 to 5 days after onset granulation tissue is forming at the margins of abscesses. The infection is more destructive than pneumococcal pneumonia, and the frequency of fibrosis in the involved tissue in survivors is much higher. The organism can be cultured from the blood in 20% to 60% of patients in the acute phase of the illness, but extrathoracic spread is unusual.

Pneumonias produced by the various species of *Proteus* are less common than *Klebsiella-Enterobacter* pneumonias but have many similar features.[273] Most patients are alcoholics with underlying chronic pulmonary disease. Pneumonia follows aspiration during a period of stupor or delirium tremens. The pneumonia most often produces consolidations of the involved lobe with multiple abscesses. Cases of bacteremic spread to the lung have also been reported.

Infections of a variety of tissues by *Haemophilus influenzae* are common in children below 3 years of age. Pneumonia caused by *H. influenzae*, however, seems to occur mainly in adults with chronic lung disease. *H. influenzae* is part of the normal flora of the upper respiratory tract and commonly colonizes the lower respiratory tract of those with chronic bronchitis. Some data have suggested that the frequency of *H. influenzae* pneumonia is increasing, but the increased rates of recovery of the organism from patients with pneumonia may also be explained by recent improvements in culture technique.[260,275]

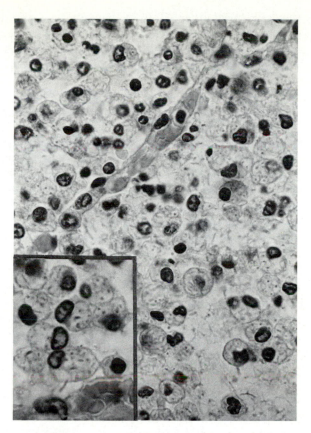

Fig. 22-12. *Klebsiella* pneumonia. Inflammatory infiltrate in airspaces consists almost entirely of macrophages containing organisms. *Inset*, Higher power showing encapsulated bacilli within macrophages.

Pneumonia caused by *H. influenzae* follows viral respiratory infection in approximately half of the patients.[262] The symptoms are similar to those of other pneumonias. Two roentgenographic patterns are recognized: a lobar consolidation, which is often associated with bacteremia, and a diffuse bronchopneumonia, often miliary in appearance, which usually is not bacteremic.[262,274] Parapneumonic (sterile) pleural effusions are common. Empyema and abscess occur in the lobar form. The prognosis of treated *Haemophilus* pneumonia is good with a mortality of less than 10%, although a mortality of 33% has been reported in septicemic cases.[262,275]

In contrast to the preceding organisms, *Pseudomonas aeruginosa* is infrequently a cause of community-acquired pneumonia but is a major agent of nosocomial infections, both primary and secondary (that is, after the institution of therapy for pneumonia caused by a different organism). The frequency with which *Pseudomonas* is isolated from patients with nosocomial bacterial pneumonia varies from 20% to 50% depending on the hospital. There are a variety of well-recognized clinical settings in which *Pseudomonas* pneumonia occurs. In the series of Lerner and Tillotson,[272] which was exceptional in the large proportion (50%) of community-acquired cases, patients had underlying chronic pulmonary disease, heart disease, and diabetes in varying combinations. Patients with hematologic malignancy or granulocytopenia, burn patients, and patients in intensive care units are important high-risk groups.[259,264] There are two types of *Pseudomonas* pneumonia with differing pathogenesis, morbid anatomy, and prognosis. Airway infection occurs as a result of colonization of the upper airways with *Pseudomonas*. This may be aided by spread from contaminated respiratory therapy equipment in some cases.[266] The frequency of colonization by *Pseudomonas* appears to increase with duration of hospitalization and severity of the underlying illness.[220] In patients with burns or hematologic disease, septicemic spread of the infection is common.

The pathologic features of airborne infection by *Pseudomonas* are not distinctive.[267,272] It is a bronchopneumonia, frequently confluent and accompanied by abscess formation. Small pleural effusions may be present, but empyema is rare. Microscopically there is intra-alveolar exudate of fibrin, neutrophils, and macrophages with focal hemorrhages and necrosis of alveolar walls. The bacteremic form of pneumonia is characterized by severe hemorrhage and necrosis.[258,263,267] Early lesions consist mainly of subpleural hemorrhages with a small, firm, necrotic center. Microscopically the hemorrhage is accompanied by necrosis of alveolar walls and contains numerous organisms. Established lesions are discrete yellow nodules a few millimeters to centimeters in size and surrounded by hemorrhage. Microscopically these lesions consist of eosinophilic coagulative necrosis in which the outlines of the underlying tissue structure remain and inflammatory cells are few (Fig. 22-13). The walls of arteries and veins are faintly basophilic and hazy, and Gram's stain shows that they are teeming with bacilli.[258,259,263,267] Teplitz[269] studied the pathogenesis of this pseudomonal vasculitis in an experimental model of *Pseudomonas* septicemia and found that the bacteria lodged in alveolar capillaries initially and then spread to involve larger vessels.[269] It might be thought that the infarctlike necrosis results from arterial occlusion, but in neither human cases nor the experimental model is thrombosis of the infected vessels conspicuous, and it is more likely that the necrosis is the result of the local effects of exotoxins and proteases produced by the *Pseudomonas*.

The prognosis for pseudomonal pneumonia is dire. Lerner and Tillotson[272] found an 80% mortality in their cases of airborne pneumonia in 1968. With the introduction of aminoglycoside antibiotics the current mortality is closer to 50%. The septicemic form remains almost invariably fatal.

Escherichia coli usually reaches the lung via the bloodstream from a site of infection in the urinary or gastrointestinal tract.[261,271] Often pneumonia follows surgery.

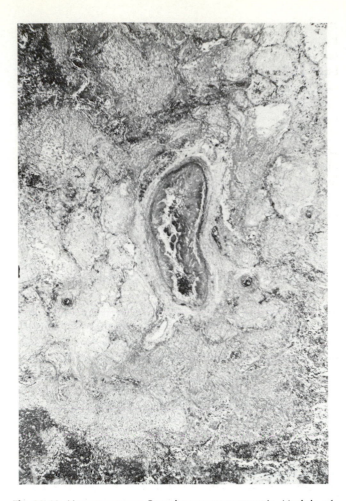

Fig. 22-13. Hematogenous *Pseudomonas* pneumonia. Nodule of infarctlike necrosis surrounded by hemorrhage. Dark haze in wall of necrotic artery *(center)* is bacteria.

The lungs are involved by a patchy, bilateral, lower lobe pneumonia. Initially the pneumonia is hemorrhagic with pronounced edema and a scanty mononuclear exudate in alveoli. In patients surviving more than a few days, the intra-alveolar cellular exudate is more pronounced but still predominantly mononuclear. Epithelial regeneration is present focally. Typical abscess with necrosis of alveolar walls and purulent exudate develops in some cases. Empyema is common in patients surviving more than 48 hours.[271]

Legionella and related pneumonias. In the 1970s a previously unknown genus of bacteria that not uncommonly causes pneumonia was discovered. The first member of the genus, *Legionella pneumophila*, was recognized as the result of investigation into a highly publicized epidemic that struck those attending an American Legion convention in Philadelphia in July 1976 and produced 29 fatalities among the 182 persons affected.[280] The causative bacterium had previously escaped detection because of its fastidious growth requirements and failure to stain by Gram's method.[277] The legionellaceae are slowly growing, motile bacteria, 2 to 4 μm in length, that resemble other gram-negative bacteria ultrastructurally. All have a single flagellum and a high content of branched-chain fatty acids.[278] There are currently six known species, which differ in antigenicity and have a DNA sequence homology of less than 30%. Each species may have several serotypes. *L. pneumophila* causes two epidemic clinical syndromes, a pneumonia with a fairly low attack rate and significant mortality and Pontiac fever, a self-limited, influenza-like, febrile illness with a high attack rate and no mortality. *L. pneumophila* also causes sporadic community-acquired and nosocomial pneumonias.[279,283,288] Other *Legionella* species also can cause nosocomial infections but are much less frequent. Data from the Centers for Disease Control indicate that *L. pneumophila* accounts for 90% of *Legionella* infections.

Epidemics usually occur in the summer months. The organism is commonly spread by aerosols of contaminated water from showerheads, air-conditioning cooling towers, and evaporative condensers.[281] As with other infections, impaired host defenses have an important role. In the original epidemic most of those affected were cigarette smokers over 50 years of age. In hospital epidemics patients with chronic disease and especially those receiving corticosteroid therapy have been affected, whereas the members of the hospital staff who were also exposed to the source rarely became ill.[283]

Although pathologic changes are limited to the lungs, the onset of the disease often is that of systemic illness with high fever and constitutional symptoms accompanied by diarrhea, leukopenia, and hyponatremia. Cough, sputum production, and signs of pneumonia may not appear until the fifth to seventh days. Whether systemic manifestations are due to a toxin or to bacteremia is unknown, but the occurrence of bacteremia has been documented.[278,287]

The gross findings in the lung are those of a confluent bronchopneumonia, usually with involvement of multiple lobes.[276-278,287] Entire lobes may be consolidated, but areas of early involvement usually show a lobular distribution. Small pleural effusions and a fibrinous pleuritis are commonly present. Abscesses are unusual but may occur.[284] The histologic findings are not distinctive. The alveoli are filled with an exudate of fibrin, neutrophils, and mononuclear phagocytes in varying proportions. Most alveolar septa show only minor changes, consisting mainly of foci of hyperplasia in the alveolar lining epithelium. Thrombosis of vessels and necrosis of alveolar walls are present in some cases. In cases of long duration, organization of the intra-alveolar exudate occurs.

The organisms are weakly gram-negative bacilli or coccobacilli that are usually invisible in sections stained by the commonly used variants of Gram's stain. With Dieterle's silver stain, however, organisms are usually numerous, appearing mainly but not exclusively in the cytoplasm of phagocytes. Dieterle's stain is nonspecific, and the diagnosis should be confirmed by immunohistochemical staining with type-specific antisera. Formalin-fixed tissue is usually satisfactory.

The relentless progression and resistance to therapy of *Legionella* pneumonia is probably a consequence of the organism's ability to survive and proliferate within phagocytes. In vitro studies indicate that the organisms can reproduce within the cytoplasm of macrophages. Specific antibodies and complement promote phagocytosis but do not promote intracellular killing. The fusion of lysosomes with phagosomes containing the bacilli is inhibited. Antibiotics such as erythromycin and rifampicin, which are effective in vivo, suppress intracellular proliferation but do not kill the organisms, which are only slowly eliminated by cellular mechanisms that are not understood.[282]

Tatlockia mcdadei, also known as the Pittsburgh pneumonia agent, is a bacterium related to *Legionella*, although serologically distinct and sharing less than 10% DNA sequence homology. The organism was originally recovered from renal transplant patients who were severely immunosuppressed and had acquired nosocomial pneumonia,[285] but it appears to be able to produce pneumonia in patients with a variety of chronic illnesses not specifically involving the immune system.[286] The pathologic features are similar to those of *Legionella* pneumonia, although there may be a greater tendency to abscess formation.[287] The organism is weakly acid fast and can be stained with modifications of the acid-fast stain in which 1% sulfuric acid is used to decolorize the carbol fuchsin.

Lung lesions caused by anaerobic bacteria. Anaerobic bacteria are plentiful in the oral cavity where they colonize the tissues beneath the gum margins and the tonsillar crypts.[282,290] They gain access to the lung by aspiration. Consequently the usual clinical context for anaerobic pulmonary infections is a combination of severe gingival disease (pyorrhea) and an altered state of consciousness such as occurs with alcohol intoxication, anesthesia, or a seizure disorder or other neurologic disease. In the past, anaerobic infections were seen after tonsillectomy in children, but with modern anesthetic techniques this complication is rare.

Aspiration introduces a mixed flora into the lung. In a large series of pulmonary infections by anaerobes, an average of 3.2 different species of bacteria was recovered per case.[290] Although many infections involved only anaerobes, in a nearly equal number of cases both aerobic and anaerobic bacteria were found. The most frequent organisms were anaerobic and microaerophilic streptococci, *Fusobacterium nucleatum*, and various species of *Bacteroides*.

Anaerobes cause four types of lesion: abscess, necrotizing pneumonia, pneumonitis, and empyema.[290] Aspirational lung abscesses are often called primary or simple lung abscesses to distinguish them from abscesses developing as a complication of another disease such as an obstructing lesion in a bronchus or pneumonia caused by one of the usual pathogens.[293,294] They occur most often in the posterior segments of the upper lobes, which are dependent when one is supine, and next most often in the basal segments of the lower lobes, which are dependent when one is erect. The right lung is involved more often than the left owing to the straighter course of the right mainstem bronchus. The lesions are usually solitary with a cavity 2 cm to several centimeters in diameter and a shaggy, irregular lining. Often they have a dirty brown appearance and fetid odor. Occasionally the cavity may contain sloughed necrotic tissue. Microscopically the cavity is lined by a pyogenic membrane and enclosed by granulation tissue. In chronic cases there may be a well-developed fibrous capsule. Partial reepithelization of the cavity, usually by metaplastic squamous epithelium, may occur. Large arteries and veins in the wall usually show fibrous intimal thickening and even complete obliteration of the lumen. Occasionally they may be thrombosed or necrotic.

Sequential roentgenographic observations suggest that abscesses begin as areas of pneumonia that undergo necrosis and cavitate over a period of 1 to 3 weeks or even longer. Patients often show signs of chronicity such as weight loss or anemia. The prognosis for primary lung abscess is good, and more than 95% of patients are cured, although one or more relapses may occur before healing is finally effected. Deaths occur rarely and result either from massive hemoptysis or occasionally from extrathoracic spread of infection. The course of secondary lung abscesses is strongly influenced by the underlying disease, and the mortality is much greater than that of primary abscesses.[293]

Like primary lung abscess, necrotizing pneumonia (pulmonary gangrene, chronic destructive pneumonia) occurs in those with severe gingivodental disease and a predisposition to aspiration and probably represents a severe form of aspiration disease.[290] Typically more than one lobe is involved, and the process includes areas of differing age or activity. The pleura is thickened and fibrotic but highly vascularized. The lung parenchyma is consolidated with multiple cavities containing pus or sloughed necrotic tissue. Histologically there is a combination of exudative and organizing pneumonia with alveolar necrosis. The bronchi show changes ranging from acute bronchitis with ulceration to bronchiectasis.[291] The organisms responsible are the same as those causing lung abscess. The clinical picture is highly variable, ranging from asymptomatic to chronic disease with fever, anemia, and weight loss to acute fulminant pneumonia. In a large series from Africa the mortality was 7.8%, a figure comparable to contemporary North American experience.[291]

Acute pneumonitis caused by anaerobes can be difficult to distinguish from other forms of bacterial pneumonia, since the characteristic fetid sputum is absent.[289] The disease is usually of short duration and responds well to antibiotic therapy. If untreated, it would probably evolve into abscesses.

Empyema is usually associated with underlying lung abscess or pneumonia and may be associated with bronchopleural fistula. Occasionally an empyema can result from spread of anaerobes from a subphrenic abscess in the absence of lung disease.

Mycobacterial infections

The mycobacteria include *Mycobacterium tuberculosis*, the causative organism of tuberculosis; *M. leprae*, which causes leprosy; and a variety of organisms found in the environment that are normally saprophytic, although many of them are potential pathogens.[297] Of these, *M. tuberculosis* and certain of the saprophytic mycobacteria cause pulmonary disease. The term *tuberculosis* should be reserved for infections with the species *M. tuberculosis*, since infections by other mycobacteria differ from tuberculosis in their epidemiology, clinical setting, and response to therapy.

Tuberculosis. Tuberculosis is a disease of great antiquity, having been identified in mummies from the fourth millenium BC. Since it is preeminently a disease of crowded conditions, it was probably unimportant in hunter-gatherer cultures but began to appear with the development of agriculture.[318] With the Industrial Revolution it assumed epidemic importance as a cause of death and disability.[307] In 1900 at least 90% of adults in Western populations had been infected with the organism as indicated by skin test reactivity to tuberculin, although many had no clinical illness. It has been estimated that 20% of all deaths in Victorian England were due to tuberculosis. With improvement in hygiene, nutrition, and social conditions the incidence of tuberculosis has been falling steadily, and the rate of decline has accelerated since the development of modern chemotherapy in the late 1940s. The incidence of tuberculosis in 1977 was 13.9 per 100,000 population in the United States, less than one third that of 25 years earlier, and the current mortality of 1.4 per 100,000 is only one tenth that of the early 1940s.[326]

Although tuberculosis is completely controllable by modern technology, it remains a major public health problem worldwide.[304] Its incidence in the developing nations of Asia, Africa, and South America is high. In parts of Southeast Asia and Oceania case rates of 300 to 500 per 100,000 are reported, 20 to 40 times the U.S. rate. In the Philippines 10% of deaths are due to tuberculosis.

Even in technically advanced countries tuberculosis remains a public health problem in certain populations.

In the United States the incidence in nonwhites is five times that in whites,[326] and in Britain the incidence in immigrants from India and Pakistan is 38 times that in native Britons.[316] In the United States tuberculosis remains the most common reportable disease, with an incidence greater than that of all other reportable diseases combined.

Causative organism. The mycobacteria occupy a taxonomic niche between the eubacteria and the actinomycetes.[297,328] The two principal species responsible for tuberculosis in humans are *M. tuberculosis* and *M. bovis.* They differ from each other in pathogenicity in different species of mammals, cultural requirements for optimum growth, and response to certain biochemical tests. A species isolated from patients in East Africa, *M. africanus,* has properties intermediate between the human and bovine strains.

The tubercle bacillus is a straight or curved rod, 0.2 to 0.5 by 2 to 5 μm, that is acid fast in Ziehl-Neelsen stains. It may stain uniformly but often takes on a beaded appearance. There are no free-living or saprophytic forms of *M. tuberculosis* in nature. In the laboratory the organism can be cultured on simple media. Usually lipid-rich media are used, although care must be taken because growth is suppressed by high concentrations of fatty acids. Growth is slow; the doubling time in culture is more than 12 hours, compared with 20 minutes for a typical pyogenic organism such as *E. coli.* Tubercle bacilli are strictly aerobic. Their dependence on molecular oxygen probably accounts in part for their propensity for growth in the lung and for the tendency for reactivation of infection in the apical regions where the alveolar Po_2 is highest. Biochemically *M. tuberculosis* is remarkable for the high lipid content of its cell wall, which accounts for its resistance to staining and, once stained, its resistance to decolorization with dilute acids or alkali. The complex chemistry of the cell wall lipids has been extensively investigated because several lipids have been implicated in important biological activities of the organism. The lipids include the mycolic acids, alpha-alkyl-beta-hydroxy fatty acids found only in the mycobacteria, corynebacteria, and nocardiae. One of the mycosides, trehalose 6,6' dimycolate or "cord factor," is responsible for the tendency of certain strains to grow in serpiginous cords and for the antitumor activity of the organism. Other mycosides are implicated in the resistance of the organism to destruction by lysosomal enzymes. A mixture of chloroform-soluble lipids, wax D, contains the materials responsible for the immunologic adjuvant activity of *M. tuberculosis.* The immunologic activity is particularly associated with the peptidoglycan components of wax D, however, and the simplest material with adjuvant activity is the peptide *N*-acyl muramyl-L-alanyl-D-isoglutamine.

A granulomatous type of histologic response similar to that seen in the disease can be produced by injection of lipid extracts, but only in doses many times larger than would be present in granulomas produced by natural infection.

Preparations of antigens from *M. tuberculosis* are known as tuberculins.[299] Following the discovery of the tubercle bacillus in 1882, Koch observed that guinea pigs exposed to killed organisms were protected against the lethal effects of a subsequent infection by living organisms. In an effort to treat tuberculous patients, he injected them with concentrates of boiled liquid cultures of tubercle bacilli, which he called "old tuberculin" (OT). Although OT was never proved to be of therapeutic benefit, Koch's observation that patients responded to injections of OT with a greater inflammatory reaction than did uninfected subjects has been of great diagnostic usefulness and is the basis for the tuberculin skin test.

A positive response to the tuberculin skin test demonstrates the presence of delayed hypersensitivity to one or more antigens in an extract of proteins from a culture of tubercle bacilli and reflects past or present infection with an organism bearing those antigens. It does not necessarily indicate the presence of disease, since the hypersensitivity persists after the healing of all active lesions. Although the tuberculins most often used currently are more refined than OT, they are still mixtures of many antigens, some of which are shared by saprophytic mycobacteria.[299] Consequently exposure to these mycobacteria can lead to false-positive reactions.

Eleven major antigens and several minor antigens are present in tuberculins. One aim of current research is to purify these antigens from tuberculins prepared from various species of mycobacteria in hopes that some will prove species specific.[299]

Transmission. The organism can be transmitted by inhalation, by ingestion, or rarely by direct implantation. A fetus can be infected in utero transplacentally. Patients with active pulmonary disease are the major source of human infection, and inhalation is overwhelmingly the most frequent route.[306,319] Droplets containing one or a few organisms become airborne during coughing, speaking, or even singing; the fluid phase evaporates, leaving particles called droplet nuclei that range from 1 to 5 μm in diameter, small enough to remain suspended in room air for hours. This is also the size that produces maximum retention in the acini of the lung. Indeed, single organisms have been demonstrated experimentally to produce infection in rabbits if inhaled on 1 to 5 μm particles, whereas aggregates of several hundred organisms may be noninfectious because they form particles larger than 10 μm, which impact on the mucus coating the walls of the large bronchi and are cleared by ciliary activity.[309]

Both the human and the bovine varieties of *Mycobacterium* can be spread by ingestion, and in the past the ingestion of raw milk from cows with tuberculous mastitis was the usual mode of transmission of the bovine type. Although bovine tuberculosis was responsible for approximately 20% of tuberculosis in 1917, it has ceased to be a public health problem owing to tuberculin testing of cattle and pasteurization of milk. Entry was either through the tonsils or more commonly through the small intestine, with spread to the cervical or mesenteric lymph nodes, respectively. The gastrointestinal tract is more resistant to infection than the lung as evidenced both by animal studies and by the rarity with which tuberculous enteritis develops in patients who swallow large numbers of organisms in their sputum.

Transplacental infection of a fetus is rare, occurring when the mother has the miliary type of tuberculosis. The fetus is surprisingly resistant to infection and may remain free of lesions even in the presence of severe placental disease.

Susceptibility. Tuberculosis is a disease of the economically disadvantaged. Crowded living conditions and poor nutrition are predisposing factors.[306,307] In addition, breeding experiments with rabbits have shown that there is a genetic influence on susceptibility to the disease.[309] Racial differences in the incidence of tuberculosis are no doubt due largely to socioeconomic factors, although inherent, presumably genetic, influences are involved. Jews appear to have a high natural resistance, probably because of natural selection over the centuries in the crowded urban ghettos of Europe. Conversely, blacks, Native Americans, and Eskimos are particularly susceptible because crowded living conditions are relatively recent in their histories and they were spared the selective influence of extensive exposure to the organism. Resistance is also lowered by certain diseases, notably silicosis and diabetes mellitus, and by gastrectomy and corticosteroid therapy.[306]

Immunity and hypersensitivity. Tubercle bacilli produce no known toxins.[298] The tissue changes caused by infection result from the host response to the organisms. It has been known since the time of Koch that the tissue response varies in its severity and tempo of development between an animal with no prior contact with tubercle bacilli and an animal that was previously infected. When Koch injected bacilli into naive guinea pigs, a localized nodule appeared at the injection site 10 days to 2 weeks later, ulcerated, and healed poorly. Tubercles appeared in the draining lymph nodes. When tubercle bacilli were injected into the skin of an animal that had been infected with tuberculosis 4 to 6 weeks earlier, an area of induration appeared at the inoculation site and grew to a diameter of 1 cm or more within 2 to 4 days. The skin over the site underwent necrosis and ulcerated but then went on to heal. Spread to the regional nodes failed to occur. In short, the previously infected animal has altered responsiveness or hypersensitivity: the altered response is more rapid and vigorous and is accompanied by necrosis. On the other hand, growth of organisms is restrained and the spread of infection is prevented. The animals have acquired relative resistance. Koch also showed that tuberculin (OT) could be used instead of living organisms to elicit the hypersensitivity response. The relationship between hypersensitivity and resistance has long been a matter of contention.[308] They are closely related. Antibodies play little role in either process. Lymphoid cells from a tuberculin-sensitive animal will transfer both hypersensitivity and resistance to a normal animal. It is now well established that both properties are transferred with specifically sensitized T lymphocytes. These T cells respond to the specific antigens in tuberculin with the elaboration of lymphokines that bring about an enhanced ability of the macrophages to kill intracellular parasites, including tubercle bacilli. The macrophages enlarge and develop increased levels of lysosomal enzymes, enhanced spreading activity on surfaces, and increased production of H_2O_2 and other oxidants that possess antimicrobial activity. The T lymphocyte responds only to the specific sensitizing antigen. The induced change in the macrophage is nonspecific. Tubercle bacilli are only one of a number of microbes whose killing by the macrophages is enhanced.[311]

Some authors regard hypersensitivity as inseparable from resistance. According to this view, the presence of sensitized T cells is beneficial when the dose of organisms is modest as with a new airborne infection or when small numbers of organisms are released from a tuberculous focus in the body. Under these conditions the macrophages are activated to engulf and dispatch the organisms with an enhanced release of oxidants and lysosomal enzymes. With massive stimulation when a very large dose of organisms is encountered, there is an overproduction of these same oxidants and hydrolases with resultant tissue damage, exudation, and necrosis. Other authors have shown that animals can be desensitized locally to the tuberculin skin test without destroying systemic resistance to infection. They argue that this militates against the view that hypersensitivity and resistance are inseparable phenomena. The answer will become clearer when it is known whether the same T cell subsets and mediators are responsible for both hypersensitivity and resistance.[308]

As a rule hypersensitivity and enhanced resistance to infection persist for many years after a clinical infection and not uncommonly they last lifelong. This may be due to the persistence of small numbers of organisms in apparently healed lesions. Hypersensitivity to tuberculin may disappear after many years, perhaps because of slow attrition among specifically sensitized T cells if organisms have disappeared. In the presence of overwhelming infection or in the terminal stages of a chronic tuberculous infection, there may also be loss of tuberculin skin reactivity, or anergy. Several mechanisms have been invoked to explain this relatively infrequent phenomenon: that very large doses of tuberculoprotein activitate suppressor cell populations; that sensitized T cells may be recruited from the skin to sites of active lesions in the viscera; or that high endogenous antigen burdens may saturate or down-regulate the available receptors.[299]

Tissue response to tubercle bacilli. The characteristic tissue response to tuberculosis is the granuloma, a compact organized collection of macrophages.[298] In a previously uninfected animal or human the earliest response to the presence of bacilli in the tissue is an influx of inflammatory cells, both polymorphonuclear leukocytes and mononuclear phagocytes that engulf the organisms. The organisms are resistant to killing by the phagocytes, owing in part to their ability to inhibit lysosome-phagosome fusion. They proliferate intracellularly, eventually killing the phagocytes. In time, mononuclear cells come to predominate in the inflammatory infiltrate and begin to form aggregates. The organisms continue to proliferate, and as macrophages containing organisms degenerate and die, new mononuclear phagocytes enter the tissue and take up the liberated organisms. Thus there is a continuous and high turnover of mononuclear phagocytes. Some of the replacement of phagocytes takes place by proliferation of local tissue macrophages, but the majority are monocytes that enter the tissue from the circulation and divide once or twice locally as they differentiate into mature macrophages. The monocytes enlarge, their nucleus becomes eccentric, their cytoplasm more abundant, and they tend to aggregate first into loose sheets of cells and then more tightly into spherical aggregates. The cells comprising these aggregates or granulomas develop eccentric vesicular nuclei and abundant pale cytoplasm. Although the cells initially remain distinct, later their cytoplasm borders become indistinct when viewed with the light microscope; with the electron microscope this is seen to be due to the close interlocking of the pseudopodia of neighboring cells. These characteristic mononuclear cells are called epithelioid cells because they are closely packed like epithelium without interposed connective tissue. They are not joined by junctional complexes, do not closely resemble epithelium morphologically, and of course are the progeny of monocytes, not epithelium. Epithelioid cells are characterized by their well-developed granular endoplasmic reticulum, as well as numerous lysosomes and high levels of lysosomal enzyme activity. They are less actively phagocytic than typical macrophages, and it has been suggested that they are macrophages specialized for secretory functions as well as for the degradation and destruction of microbes. A striking feature of the granulomas of tuberculosis and many other granulomas is the presence of multinucleated cells. Some multinucleated cells have their nuclei evenly dispersed in the cytoplasm.

These cells are called foreign body giant cells, since they are similar in appearance to the giant cells that frequently enclose foreign material in tissues. Other giant cells called Langhans' giant cells have their nuclei disposed in a ring surrounding an eosinophilic cytocenter. Both types of giant cells, formed by the fusion of several epithelioid cells, are commonly found in epithelioid granulomas irrespective of their etiology.

As the granuloma matures, it becomes surrounded by lymphocytes, plasma cells, capillaries, and fibroblasts (Fig. 22-14). Between 4 and 6 weeks after infection, necrosis begins to appear in the granulomas, the surrounding tissue may become edematous, and the number of organisms begins to diminish. The necrosis is termed caseation because its dry crumbly appearance resembles cheese. Microscopically the necrosis is granular and eosinophilic and contains nuclear debris. The outlines of the cells are usually not evident, in contrast to the coagulation necrosis of infarcts. The reticulin and elastic fibers in the tissue initially remain intact, howev-

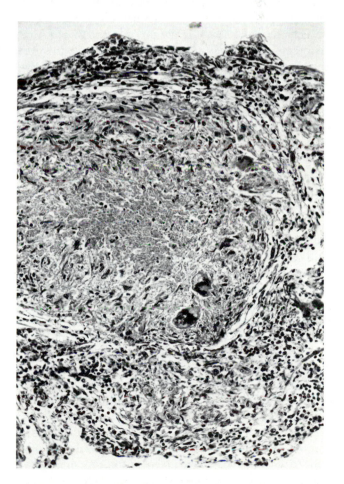

Fig. 22-14. Well-developed tubercle with caseous center surrounded by epithelioid histiocytes and giant cells. Mantle of lymphocytes, plasma cells, and monocytes surrounds epithelioid cell zone.

er, and can be demonstrated with appropriate stains. The appearance of necrosis and edema and the decrease in organisms correspond temporally with the development of a positive reaction to the tuberculin skin test and reflect the host's acquisition of delayed hypersensitivity.

The granuloma can follow several possible courses. Conditions in the necrotic caseous center are not favorable for rapid proliferation of organisms, owing to the low pH and oxygen tension and possibly other factors. Usually the number of organisms continues to decrease and a fibrous capsule forms in the surrounding zone of nonspecific inflammation. The encapsulated granuloma becomes quiescent, the inflammatory cells decrease in number, and calcium salts are usually deposited in the caseous material. Sometimes the calcium is deposited in concentric laminations known as Liesegang rings. After several years, organisms completely disappear and the contents of the granuloma are no longer infective if injected into a guinea pig.

If the organisms are particularly virulent or resistance is low, the granuloma may continue to enlarge by centrifugal growth. Satellite granulomas may form, grow, and coalesce with the original granuloma. At any time this process may cease and the lesions become arrested. Occasionally in one or more granulomas the caseous center liquefies, acquiring a more fluid, puslike consistency, mainly through the agency of proteases and other hydrolases produced by the epithelioid cells and macrophages of the granuloma.[300] When the contents of the granuloma liquefy, rapid extracellular growth of organisms ensues and the stage is set for the dissemination of disease.

The events following the introduction of a large dose of tubercle bacilli into the tissue of a highly sensitized person differ from the proliferative granuloma just described. The reaction is greatly accelerated, with a rapid outpouring of fibrin and edema, an increased influx of neutrophils and monocytes, and the more rapid and extensive development of necrosis. This is termed the exudative response (Fig. 22-15).

Natural history[296,301,314,328]

PRIMARY COMPLEX. The initial tissue response in the nonimmune host is similar regardless of the site of infection and involves the development of granulomas at the portal of entry and the formation of a secondary focus in the draining lymph nodes, the combination being known as the primary complex. In the majority of instances the primary complex involves foci in the lung and hilar lymph nodes, but it may involve tonsil and cervical nodes or intestine and mesenteric nodes in the case of ingested bacilli.

The initial infection in the lung is due to the deposition of organisms in the acini at one or more sites. The primary or Ghon's focus may develop anywhere in the lung, although usually it is within 1 cm of the pleura and not infrequently in a lower lobe where the ventilation is greater and deposition is more likely. The process probably begins as a focus of tuberculous pneumonia with some edema, fibrin, and an influx of neutrophils and mononuclear phagocytes. Some organisms or perhaps phagocytes containing engulfed bacilli reach the lymphatics and are transported to the hilar lymph nodes where they set up a secondary focus. Additional lesions may be present along the pathway of the lymphatic drainage in the lung. The primary focus in the lung usually remains less than a centimeter in size and evolves into a typical granuloma with caseation. Over several weeks or months the lesion becomes encapsulated with fibrous tissue and the necrotic contents calcify. After many years ossification may occur. The lymph node focus generally follows a parallel course. The lymph node focus is almost invariably larger than the primary parenchymal focus and heals more slowly, but it too usually undergoes eventual encapsulation and calcification.

During the early evolution of the primary complex, spread may occur to adjacent nodes, even reaching the superior mediastinal nodes or the nodes of the upper abdomen. A few bacilli commonly escape through the

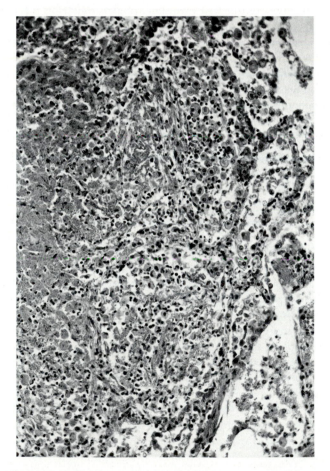

Fig. 22-15. Exudative reaction in tuberculosis. Necrosis and exudation of monocytes and macrophages without development of encapsulated granuloma.

lymphatics to the venous system whence they are taken up in the reticuloendothelial organs, liver, spleen, or bone marrow where small granulomas are established and subsequently heal. Hematogenous seeding of the lungs can result in the establishment of a new caseous focus (Simon's focus), which is distinct from the primary complex and is usually near the apex where the oxygen tension is high.

Despite the acquisition of resistance in the form of improved bacterial killing by macrophages, bacilli may remain in the acellular caseous centers of pulmonary or systemic granulomas. Such bacilli may remain dormant for months, years, or decades, becoming activated at any time by a breakdown in local immunity.

PROGRESSIVE PRIMARY TUBERCULOSIS. The pattern of transient growth, spread to lymph nodes, and subsequent encapsulation and healing of lesions is the natural history of primary tuberculous infection followed by more than 90% of patients. Symptoms are mild and nonspecific, and most primary infections pass unrecognized. In a few patients, owing to some combination of increased virulence of the organism, increased hypersensitivity, and low resistance, the primary infection is progressive. In some cases the primary focus in the lung continues to grow and caseation outstrips the rate of epithelioid cell formation and encapsulation. The caseous material may liquefy, and the liquefied material containing bacilli may become disseminated through the bronchi to other regions of the same lung and opposite lung. The dissemination of large numbers of bacteria produces a reaction of exudation of fibrin, neutrophils, and monocytes followed by the appearance of necrosis. More commonly dissemination occurs when the enlarged hilar

lymph nodes undergoing necrosis and liquefaction erode a bronchus resulting in the discharge of caseous material containing organisms. If the number of organisms is large and hypersensitivity is marked, the ensuing exudative reaction may further spread the organisms, resulting in caseous pneumonia (Fig. 22-16). Finally, if erosion of a blood vessel occurs, the dissemination of large numbers of bacteria hematogenously can result in the establishment of numerous tiny foci of tuberculosis in many organs, a form of the disease known as miliary tuberculosis (after millet seeds, which like the granulomas of severe hematogenously spread tuberculosis are 1 to 2 mm in diameter). Miliary granulomas can occur in any site but are most numerous in the liver, spleen, kidneys, bone marrow, brain, and lungs (Fig. 22-17). Although the various forms of progressive primary tuberculosis are

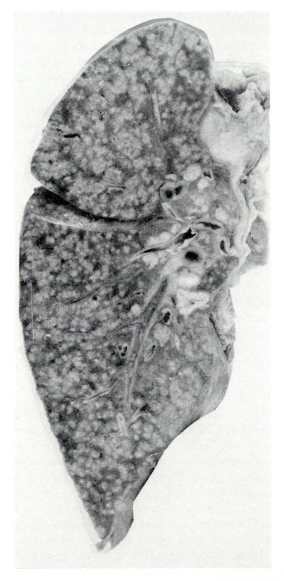

Fig. 22-17. Miliary tuberculosis. (From pathological museum of University of Manchester, U.K.)

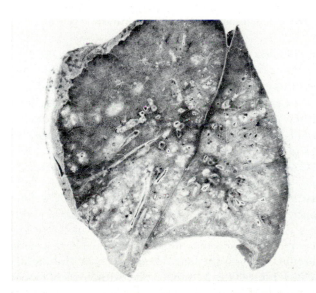

Fig. 22-16. Lung of child with a few tubercles in upper lobe and confluent areas of tuberculous pneumonia in middle and lower lobes. (From pathological museum of University of Manchester, U.K.)

serious and indeed life threatening, they may become arrested, undergo encapsulation, and heal as a result of therapy or the spontaneous development of resistance.

POSTPRIMARY TUBERCULOSIS. It is not unusual for tuberculosis to develop in adults who have been tuberculin positive for many years without evidence of clinical disease. Phthisiologists have long argued whether the new active disease is the result of a new exogenous infection or recrudescence of dormant foci. There is no reason to doubt that both occur. Stead[324] has argued persuasively on the basis of epidemiologic evidence that endogenous reactivation is the more important mechanism. In a retrospective review of published data on more than 14,000 subjects, he found only a slightly higher incidence of disease in tuberculin-positive persons (medical and nursing students) who had frequent contact with patients with active lesions than in tuberculin-positive controls with only sporadic exposure. Among tuberculin-negative persons, the highly exposed group had five times the incidence of their controls. However, when phage typing has been used to determine whether postprimary disease is due to a new strain, a new strain has been detected in 10% to 20% of cases, depending on the population studied.[312,320]

In most cases, postprimary tuberculosis is first detected in the subapical region of one or both lungs, perhaps caused by spread of viable bacteria from a Simon's focus.

The disease starts as a small area of lobular tuberculous pneumonia characterized by intra-alveolar exudate of fibrin, neutrophils, and monocytes. This area can undergo one of several courses. At this stage while the lesion is still intra-alveolar, it may resolve completely. It may progress slowly to the development of epithelioid granulomas, which gradually caseate in the center but remain encapsulated by epithelioid cells and capillaries and proliferating fibrous tissue. The granulomas may follow an irregular course, some healing and calcifying while others grow for a while, stimulating continuing fibrosis. If the original area of pneumonia undergoes necrosis, the entire area may become encapsulated or it may undergo liquefaction and slough through a patent bronchus, giving rise to a cavity (Fig. 22-18).

The formation of a cavity is an important development. The bacteria in the lining of the cavity proliferate, probably owing to the higher Po_2 than in necrotic tissue. The cavity's communication with the bronchial tree makes it an important source for spread of organisms elsewhere in the lung. When small amounts of caseous material are released from a cavity, they may be cleared harmlessly by the mucociliary mechanism and swallowed or may be aspirated into alveoli in the more dependent areas of the lung. If the dose of organisms is small, organisms reaching the alveoli set up minute new foci of tuberculous pneumonia, filling airspaces clustered about terminal

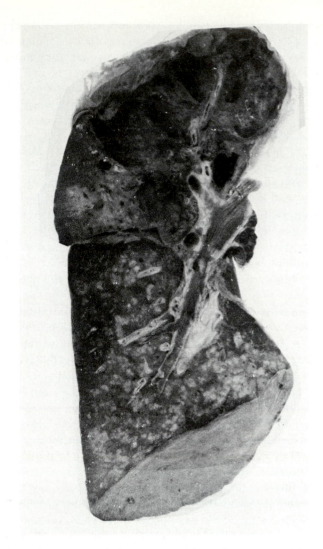

Fig. 22-18. Advanced cavitary tuberculosis. Entire upper lobe is destroyed. There are foci of acinous spread in lower lobe. (From pathological museum of University of Manchester, U.K.)

bronchioles and called acinous lesions (Fig. 22-18). If the number of organisms is large and the degree of hypersensitivity great, aspiration of infected debris produces a marked exudative reaction with an outpouring of edema, fibrin, polymorphonuclear cells, and monocytes. This rapidly progresses to necrosis, a condition known as caseous pneumonia.

Cavities in tuberculosis are generally spherical and may have a thick wall or very little encapsulation depending on their age and rate of growth. The lining appears trabeculated owing to the persistence of obliterated cordlike blood vessels. If only part of the original necrotic focus becomes liquefied, remnants of necrotic lung may also be present. Microscopically the lining of cavities typically is heterogeneous with areas of caseous necrosis with nuclear debris and organisms, pyogenic membrane of fibrin and inflammatory exudate, and granulation tissue where epithelioid cells in variable numbers are accompanied by capillaries and fibroblasts. A capsule of nonspecific fibrous tissue of variable thickness encloses the cavity. The cavity can grow by continuing necrosis or the incorporation of surrounding granulomas. Should the bronchial opening become plugged or obliterated, the necrotic contents of the cavity become inspissated, the air is absorbed, and the necrotic material remains encapsulated or eventually becomes organized into a stellate scar. Cavities that remained open rarely healed before the availability of specific antibacterial therapy. Because of this, interventions such as artificial pneumothorax or thoracoplasty were used in the past to bring about closure of the cavity. With adequate chemotherapy, open healing can occur. The cavity remains open, but the necrotic tissue, pyogenic membrane, and granulation tissue organize, leaving a fibrous wall that becomes partly or completely reepithelialized.[325]

The complications of cavities are aneurysms of the arteries that cross the cavity and extension to the pleura. Although most of the vessels in the cavity wall are obliterated, the lumen of a few may persist. Destruction of the vessel wall leads to aneurysm formation, which can cause hemoptysis and even lethal hemorrhage. Extension to the pleura can lead to bronchopleural fistula. The seeding of caseous material onto the pleural surface in a hypersensitive person leads to an acute exudative reaction with effusion or tuberculous empyema.

Just as late reactivation of primary tuberculosis occurs in the lung, activation can occur in any site in which seeding of organisms has occurred during the initial infection.[322] The pathologic features of tuberculosis in other organs are discussed in chapters dealing with those organs. Nonetheless, the lung remains the most common site of reactivation, a fact usually attributed to its higher oxygen tension. Generalized or miliary tuberculosis resulting from hematogenous spread of the organism can occur from a pulmonary or extrapulmonary source. Whereas formerly miliary tuberculosis occurred mainly in children, it is now being seen increasingly in the elderly as a manifestation of postprimary disease.

Clinical considerations. Given the potential variation in organ distribution, pathologic forms, and rate of evolution of tuberculosis, it is not surprising that the clinical manifestations are protean. In one recent series involving only 41 cases, patients were admitted to seven different clinical services and in nearly half the disease was initially misdiagnosed.[310]

Tuberculosis is now seen in an older population than formerly, most patients being over 40 years of age.[305,310] Symptoms are usually referable to the lungs (cough) or are systemic (fatigue, sweats, weight loss, fever). The initial chest roentgenogram shows classical apical changes in only two thirds of cases of pulmonary tuberculosis; in the remaining cases the roentgenographic manifestations are atypical, including such nonspecific changes as pleu-

ral effusion, solitary nodule, infiltrates in unusual locations, and miliary infiltrates.[305] As the disease becomes less common, the proportion of patients with primary tuberculosis can be expected to increase and the proportion of atypical presentations will also increase.

The course of active tuberculosis is extremely variable and in fatal cases ranges from weeks to years. Auerbach,[296] writing of the preantibiotic and early antibiotic era, gives the average duration as 1 to 2 years with wide variations. Death is usually due to pulmonary insufficiency, or general sepsis in the case of miliary tuberculosis.

Disease caused by nontuberculous mycobacteria. Mycobacteria other than *M. tuberculosis* are widely distributed in nature and infrequently cause disease, although several species are potentially pathogenic. The widely used classification of Runyon based on pigment production and growth rate has been superseded by classifications in which the organisms are grouped according to biochemical and antigenic similarities.[327] The major pathogenic groups include the following:

1. Slow-growing potential pathogens
   a. *M. avium-intracellulare*
   b. *M. scrofulaceum*
   c. *M. kansasii*
   d. *M. marinum*
2. Rapidly growing potential pathogens
   a. *M. fortuitum*
   b. *M. chelonei*

The nontuberculous or "atypical" mycobacteria are less fastidious than *M. tuberculosis* in their requirements for growth, which accounts for their ability to survive in such environments as soil, swimming pools, milk, and water taps, as well as in animals. Humans appear to acquire the organisms from the environment, and person-to-person transmission rarely if ever occurs. Familial cases can usually be explained by exposure to a common source. The organisms often colonize humans as saprophytes, and unlike the situation with *M. tuberculosis*, isolation of an atypical mycobacterium from a clinical specimen is not presumptive evidence of a pathogenic process. Disease should be attributed to nontuberculous mycobacteria when there are moderate or large numbers of organisms, multiple isolations of the same strain of mycobacterium over an extended period, a compatible clinical and roentgenographic picture, and the absence of another pathogen that would account for the condition. Isolation of atypical mycobacteria from cultures of tissue obtained under sterile conditions is also significant if the tissue contains lesions consistent with infection.

Infection with the atypical mycobacteria usually involves the lung in adults or the cervical lymph nodes in young children.[324] *M. ulcerans* and *M. marinum* produce skin infections. Osseous, renal, and meningeal disease also occur, and in the immunosuppressed patient a picture similar to miliary tuberculosis may develop.

Pulmonary infection commonly occurs in subjects with underlying chronic lung disease such as pneumoconiosis, chronic airflow limitation, bronchiectasis, or healed tuberculosis.[321] In one third of cases there is no predisposing lung disease. Men are affected three times as often as women. The majority of cases are associated with *M. kansasii*, *M. avium-intracellulare*, and *M. scrofulaceum*. Other organisms are much less common.

The pathogenesis of atypical mycobacterial infections is not well understood. Whether there is a phase analogous to the primary complex in tuberculosis has not been established. Common clinical presentations are with a solitary nodule or with upper lobe infiltrates that are frequently cavitary. It has been suggested that thin-walled cavities are more characteristic of atypical infection than of tuberculosis, but this difference is not a reliable way to distinguish the diseases.

The histologic response to the atypical mycobacteria in the lung is indistinguishable from that of tuberculosis.[313,315,323] The granulomas are similar, and caseation occurs commonly in infection with atypical mycobacteria despite their low virulence. In sections stained with the acid-fast stain the presence of large (20 μm), beaded, curved bacilli suggests *M. kansasii*,[323] but etiologic diagnosis ultimately rests on the results of culture. The histologic features of the cavities are similar to those of tuberculosis. Endobronchial granulomas are observed more commonly in infection by atypical mycobacteria than in tuberculosis, but the difference is not absolute. Atypical mycobacteria have been isolated from lungs that histologically showed only organizing pneumonia, without granulomas, but their etiologic role is unproven.

Although *M. kansasii* is sensitive to rifampin, the other mycobacteria are relatively resistant to antibiotics. Because of this, organisms may persist for years even when therapy is continued. Nevertheless, the lesions often remain of constant size or progress only very slowly. Death can result from pulmonary insufficiency but often is a consequence of underlying chronic disease.

Fungal infections

See Chapter 11.

Pneumocystis carinii pneumonia

Pneumocystis carinii is an organism, usually classified as a sporozoan, that causes pneumonia in children and adults who are debilitated or immunosuppressed.[339,341] The biologic features of the organism are not well understood. It is probably widespread in the environment, since more than two thirds of normal children develop antibodies to the organism by 4 years of age.[337] *Pneumocystis* may be able to colonize the lung without causing disease. In rabbits and rats treated with corticosteroids, interstitial pneumonia containing *Pneumocystis* organ-

isms occurs, indicating widespread latent infection in these species.

Infection with *Pneumocystis* was first recognized during World War II in Europe, where it caused a characteristic pneumonia in infants who had been born prematurely.[340] The pneumonia was characterized by a heavy infiltration of the interstitium of the lung with plasma cells and a frothy intra-alveolar exudate.[340] This form of infection, known as interstitial plasma cell pneumonia, is now rarely seen in developed countries, and the wartime cases can probably be explained by malnutrition rampant at the time.

Currently *Pneumocystis* pneumonia is seen mainly in the immunosuppressed patients, either as an isolated infection or in combination with disease caused by other agents such as cytomegalovirus. A variety of immune defects predispose to *Pneumocystis* pneumonia, including agammaglobulinemia, malnutrition, and the complex immunosuppression produced by steroids, antineoplastic drugs, or regimens used in transplantation.[339,341] *Pneumocystis* pneumonia has been recognized as one of the characteristic infections of the acquired immune deficiency syndrome (AIDS), a disorder occurring in previously healthy homosexuals, intravenous drug abusers, and hemophiliacs and characterized immunologically by a severe diminution in the T-helper subset and inversion of the T-helper/T-suppressor ratio.[330,331] Infection is limited to the lungs in most cases, but rare instances of systemic dissemination have been documented.[334]

The development of *Pneumocystis* pneumonia is manifested clinically by the rapid onset of dyspnea, tachypnea, and cyanosis, sometimes accompanied by mild nonproductive cough. There are few physical signs, but the chest roentgenogram usually shows diffuse alveolar and interstitial infiltrates. Less often, localized densities are seen. The lungs in typical cases are firm and heavy. The pleura is blue-gray and without exudate. Interlobular septa are edematous. The cut surface of the lung is dusky and uniform. The typical histologic picture is an interstitial pneumonitis with thickening and mononuclear infiltration of the alveolar walls and hyperplasia of the epithelium.[338,342] The alveolar spaces are filled with a characteristic frothy exudate, which is eosinophilic or amphophilic with round holes up to 6 or 8 μm in diameter. Some of the holes contain one or a few weakly basophilic dots no more than 1 μm in diameter. The histologic findings may be atypical in up to half the cases, showing diffuse alveolar damage with hyaline membranes, nonspecific interstitial pneumonia, or even granulomas.[342] Organisms can most easily be seen in sections stained with Gomori's methenamine-silver or sulfonated toluidine blue, which stain the cysts. Giemsa or Gram's stain demonstrates the intracystic bodies in imprints but is difficult to interpret on sections. In sections the cysts are 4 to 6 μm in diameter and often appear collapsed or cup shaped. The absence of budding helps distinguish the organisms from fungi.

A tentative life cycle for the organism, suggested by Vanek, Jirovic, and Lukes[340] based on the study of sections and imprints, has been confirmed by electron microscopy[329,332,333] and observations of cells cultured on chick embryo epithelium in vitro.[336] Organisms occur as free trophozoites and as cysts containing up to eight intracystic bodies. The vegetative trophozoites are ameboid organisms 1.5 to 2 μm in diameter. In culture they attach to the epithelial cells by short filopodia through which they apparently obtain nutrients. They grow to form large 2 to 5 μm trophozoites that contain abundant glycogen. Large trophozoites begin to encyst by laying down a cyst wall. After fission of the nucleus the cytoplasm divides, giving rise to the eight sporozoites or intracystic bodies. These are then liberated from the cyst through one or more pores as small trophozoites. In culture the entire life cycle requires 4 to 6 hours. The characteristic frothy exudate seen with light microscopy consists of organisms enmeshed in pellicular material, fibrin, and alveolar secretions, including a form of surfactant.

BRONCHIECTASIS

Bronchiectasis is irreversible dilatation of the bronchi. It is accompanied by infection of the bronchial wall and frequently by obliteration of distal airways. It occurs in a number of clinical settings: (1) after damage to the bronchi by acute infection, especially early in life, (2) distal to a lesion that produces occlusion of a major bronchus, such as a tumor, foreign body, or lymph node involved by granulomas, (3) in a heterogeneous group of conditions in which bronchial antibacterial defense mechanisms are defective, such as agammaglobulinemia, immotile cilia syndrome, and cystic fibrosis, (4) as a manifestation of allergy to certain molds (see p. 877), and (5) after inhalation of certain toxic gases.

Commonly postinfectious bronchiectasis has its onset in childhood or early adult life.[348] In over half the patients the onset follows an overt episode of infection, but in some 30% of cases the onset is insidious. In the past, pertussis, measles, and scarlet fever were prominent as antecedent infections, but as these have become rare, adenovirus infection has assumed importance. Although bronchiectasis may be asymptomatic, most patients seek medical attention because of cough, expectoration of fetid sputum, recurrent bouts of chest infection, or hemoptysis. The majority of patients have sinusitis, and many have clubbing of the fingers.

The distribution of bronchiectasis following infection has never been satisfactorily explained. Characteristically one or a few segments are involved while the rest are normal. The left lung is involved in three fourths of cases. The posterior basal segment is almost invariably involved, and the remaining two basal segments and the two lingular segments all have a high frequency of disease. Right lung involvement is relatively uncommon.[4,348]

The disease characteristically affects the first three generations of bronchi beyond the segmental bronchi; it is usually impossible to trace the bronchi past the fourth to sixth generations.[345,348] The more distal airways are obliterated. The affected bronchi are dilated nearly to the pleura, irregular in contour, and filled with mucus or more commonly mucopus (Fig. 22-19). The walls may be thickened or are sometimes in dilated saccules, abnormally thinned. The normal longitudinal ridges are replaced by transverse mucosal folds. Some authors have subclassified bronchiectasis as saccular or cylindrical according to its gross or bronchographic configuration, and others by a combination of histologic and gross features,[348] but the value of such subclasses is still not established.

Microscopically the bronchial epithelium may be normal or ulcerated or show mucous hyperplasia or squamous metaplasia. In the wall are varying degrees of chronic inflammation, fibrosis, and destruction of normal elements. The muscle and elastic tissue are destroyed

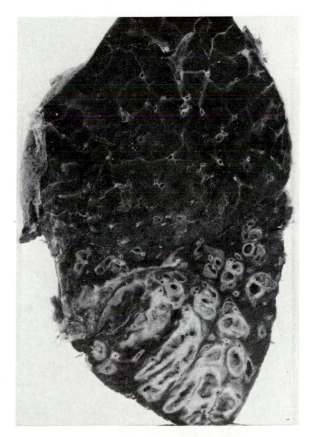

Fig. 22-19. Bronchiectasis. Marked thickening and dilatation of lower lobe bronchi. (From pathological museum of University of Manchester, U.K.)

and replaced by fibrosis, and often the cartilage is also replaced. Sometimes lymphocytic infiltrate is conspicuous and germinal centers are present. Whitwell[348] has termed this variant follicular bronchiectasis. The lung adjacent to the ectatic bronchus usually shows fibrosis.

The distribution of bronchiectasis distal to an obstruction varies depending on the cause of the obstruction. Bronchiectasis caused by compression of the bronchus by granulomatous lymph nodes is most common in the right middle lobe because the right middle lobe bronchus is relatively long and its origin is surrounded by nodes that are wedged against it by the lower lobe bronchi. The nodes at this location receive drainage from both the lower and the middle lobes, contributing to the frequency with which they are involved as part of a primary tuberculous complex. In addition to extrinsic compression, the bronchus may be obstructed by erosion of a calcified granuloma into the bronchus to form a broncholith.

Pathogenesis

Bronchiectasis results from damage to the bronchial wall, which permits the establishment of smoldering infection with destruction of the muscle and elastic tissue, and from increased traction on the bronchial wall caused by changes in the surrounding parenchyma. Varying combinations of collapse, organizing pneumonia, and obliteration of small airways result in poorly compliant lung parenchyma that efficiently transmits the negative pleural pressure to the peribronchial tissue while at the same time the inflammation and resultant destruction of muscle and elastic tissue render the bronchial wall vulnerable to the increased mechanical forces. Once dilated and distorted, the bronchi tend to retain secretions that serve as a nidus of continuing infection. A variety of organisms can be recovered from bronchiectatic secretions, including various species of streptococci, *Haemophilus influenzae*, *Staphylococcus aureus*, and anaerobic mycoplasmas.[347]

Natural history

The introduction of antibiotics has not only lowered the incidence of bronchiectasis but also dramatically changed its natural history. In the preantibiotic era almost all patients with bronchiectasis died of suppurative infections or rarely complications thereof such as amyloidosis, the majority of deaths occurring before 40 years of age. Currently, bronchiectatic patients die at an average age of 55 years, as often from a condition unrelated to bronchiectasis as one related to it. Respiratory failure caused by chronic airflow obstruction and cor pulmonale, rather than suppurative infection, are currently the important related causes of death.[346] However, 80% of patients with bronchiectasis have no greater annual loss of pulmonary function than do normal controls.[344] Accelerated decline in pulmonary function appears to be related to long bouts of lower respiratory infection.[343]

Immotile cilia syndrome

In the immotile cilia syndrome, airway clearance mechanisms are defective owing to any of a variety of structural defects in the axoneme, the internal machinery of the cilium. The axoneme is formed by nine peripheral doublet microtubules surrounding two central single microtubules together with a number of accessory structures. Arranged in rows along each doublet are paired side arms that contain dynein, an ATPase. The beating of the cilia is powered by ATP and produced by sliding shear between doublet microtubules induced by changes in the configuration of the dynein side arms that accompany the binding and hydrolysis of the ATP. The sliding shear generated by the dynein arms is converted into bending waves by rows of radial spokes that project from each doublet toward projections attached to the central microtubule pair.[352]

In the immotile cilia syndrome the cilia are usually completely inactive, but in some cases they beat slowly and ineffectively. Clearance of radiolabeled aerosols from airways is absent except during coughing. The fol-

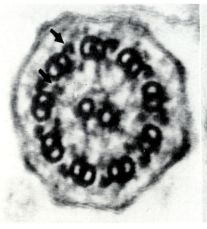
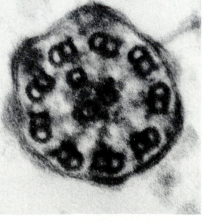

A B

Fig. 22-20. A, Cross section of normal cilium. Arrows indicate dynein arms. **B,** Immotile cilia syndrome. Dynein arms are missing. In addition, there is an extra single microtubule. Extra microtubules were present in approximately one third of the cilia. (150,000×.)

lowing abnormalities of axonemes have been reported to cause the syndrome:

1. Absent dynein arms
2. Selective absence of inner or outer arms
3. Absent radial spokes
4. Microtubule transposition
5. Combined absence of inner dynein arm and spoke head
6. Complete axonemal agenesis

The most common abnormality is absence of one or both dynein arms (Fig. 22-20). The disease appears to be hereditary, and within any one family the structural abnormality of the axoneme breeds true.[349,350]

The onset of symptoms in immotile cilia syndrome occurs soon after birth. Patients have repeated bouts of otitis, sinusitis, and chest infection. In 50% of patients there is situs inversus. Kartagener's triad of sinusitis, bronchiectasis, and situs inversus thus is a subset of immotile cilia syndrome. Bronchiectasis is present in one third of affected children but may be more common in adults.[351] Often it is of the follicular type. Since sperm flagella are powered by the same mechanism as cilia, male infertility is the rule.[349] Curiously, affected women are able to conceive despite the fact that the fallopian tube is lined with ciliated epithelium.

The diagnosis of immotile cilia syndrome can conveniently be based on phase microscopy of living ciliated cells obtained from the nasal cavity by curetting or brushing, followed by electron microscopy.[353]

Cystic fibrosis

Cystic fibrosis (CF) is a systemic disease with widespread organ involvement and an intriguing array of metabolic derangements.[354,360,376] The pulmonary involvement dominates the clinical picture in those who survive the neonatal period. Improved therapy has led to survival of many patients into late childhood and adulthood. Lung involvement occurs in virtually all patients and is the cause of death in over 95%.[361,372] The pathologic features of the pulmonary disease are well documented.* Although the lungs appear normal at birth, hypertrophy of the mucous glands can be demonstrated by an increase in the gland/wall ratio (Reid index).[356] In patients dying after the first month of life, progressively severe changes develop with metaplasia of bronchiolar epithelium to a mucus-secreting type followed by mucous plugging, bronchitis, and bronchopneumonia. After 4 months of age mucopurulent plugging of the large and small airways is universal at autopsy, and bronchiectasis is the rule. The bronchiectasis is widespread, occurring in all lobes without any particular predilection. As much as 30% to 40% of the total volume of the lung is occupied by dilated bronchi, compared with a normal value of 5%.[376]

Mild emphysema is found in the lungs of older children and adults when adequate morphologic methods are used,[356,377] but it is rarely if ever of clinical significance. Physiologically the lungs show severe airflow obstruction and abnormal distribution of ventilation but do not show the changes in lung mechanics characteristic of emphysema.[368]

The underlying basis for the lung disease is unclear, but mucus hypersecretion is evidently an early event. The observed lesions are the result of chronic relentless infection of the airways with episodes of bronchopneumonia. The increased incidence of infections in patients with CF can reasonably be attributed to their impaired mucociliary clearance.[378] The old idea that increased viscosity of the mucus was responsible for the poor clearance has been disproved. Early in the disease the viscosity of the sputum is normal and less than that of bronchitic and asthmatic adults who do not have such severe infections. Only after the sputum becomes purulent is its viscosity increased.[364,366]

The serum of patients with CF contains a factor that produces ciliary dyskinesia[373] or paralysis[357] in vitro. Its effect may be the result of mucus hypersecretion.[356,359] The factor has not been shown to affect ciliary function in vivo, but if it does, it probably does so only after the establishment of inflammation permits serum exudation onto the airway surface.[358,371] Squamous metaplasia is common in airways of CF patients and impairs mucociliary clearance, but it too is a secondary phenomenon that is probably a consequence of the infections. Malabsorption of vitamin A resulting from pancreatic steatorrhea may also be a factor in the production of metaplasia.

A curious feature of infections in patients with CF is the propensity for specific infectious agents to be involved, notably staphylococci and *Pseudomonas aeruginosa*.[367,370] As much as 50% to 90% of CF patients are colonized by mucoid variants of *Pseudomonas*. The reason for the selection of these organisms is unexplained. The immune response to *Pseudomonas* is grossly normal, although there is evidence that the IgG produced is ineffective in promoting the phagocytosis and killing of the *Pseudomonas* by macrophages.[365]

Cor pulmonale is a late complication of the lung disease in CF and affects approximately one third of all patients and half of those over 15 years of age.[374] Hypoxia is a major factor producing cor pulmonale. All the patients with clinical right-sided heart failure studied by Stern and associates[374] were severely hypoxemic, and most were hypercarbic. Morphologic muscular hypertrophy of small pulmonary arteries and arterioles occurs in the lungs of CF patients and is similar to that found in other conditions producing hypoxia.[375] Shunts between the bronchial and pulmonary arteries in the walls of ectatic bronchi[376] may also be a factor promoting pulmonary hypertension.

---

*References 356, 362, 363, 369, 377, 379.

PULMONARY VASCULAR DISEASE
Histologic features of normal pulmonary vasculature

The main pulmonary artery and its branches down to a diameter of 1 to 0.5 mm are classified as elastic pulmonary arteries.[380] Their media consists of concentric elastic lamellae separated by smooth muscle and other connective tissue matrix components. At birth the main pulmonary artery is similar to the aorta in thickness and elastic pattern, but by 2 years of age it is only half as thick as the aorta, and the elastic lamellae are fewer and appear fragmented. In the intrapulmonary branches the elastic lamellae remain intact and concentrically arranged. The number of lamellae decreases with decreasing size from 16 or 20 lamellae in lobar arteries to 3 or 4 lamellae in arteries less than 1 mm in diameter. Arteries that accompany the membranous and respiratory bronchioles and extend along proximal alveolar ducts in adults are classified as muscular arteries. They are less than 500 μm in diameter with a media defined by well-developed internal and external elastic laminae and composed mainly of smooth muscle. The arterioles less than 100 μm arise as either side branches or extensions of the muscular arteries. During their course they undergo a change in structure. Close to their origin they have a thin but complete muscular media two or three cells thick. In their terminal section, muscle is absent and the endothelium is supported only by a single elastic lamina. In the transition zone the initially complete muscle coat becomes a spiral that appears in cross section as a discontinuous muscle layer. Thus, cross sections of normal arterioles can appear muscular, partially muscular, or nonmuscular depending on the level of section. The level of the respiratory tract at which transitions occur varies with both age and disease.[383]

The arterioles give rise to a network of capillaries in the alveolar walls, which are gathered into venules similar in appearance to the nonmuscular arterioles. One can distinguish an arteriole from a venule only by serial sectioning to determine its connections to larger vessels. The venules drain into veins that lie between acini at some distance from the bronchi and bronchioles and occupy perilobular septa. Their walls consist of muscle and connective tissue with several elastic fibers that are not organized into distinct lamellae and are concentrated in the media adjacent to the adventitial connective tissue. In children there is little intima, but with aging a distinct zone of hyalinized collagen appears.

The bronchial arteries that supply the cartilage-containing airways and portions of the pleura are easily distinguished from pulmonary arteries by their smaller diameter, their thick wall characteristic of systemic vessels, and their elastic pattern. Their internal elastic lamina is well formed, but the external elastic lamina is absent or poorly developed. In addition they often have a prominent longitudinal muscle coat in the intima.

Pulmonary thromboembolism

The embolism of thrombi to the lung is considered to be both underdiagnosed[395] and overdiagnosed[393] by clinicians. Thrombi can be found in pulmonary arteries in 20% to 60% of adult autopsies, although many of these are small and probably not of clinical consequence. The general mechanisms of thrombosis and embolism are discussed on p. 717.

In principle, thrombi forming anywhere in the venous circulation can embolize to the lung. In practice more than 90% of clinically significant emboli arise in the deep veins of the legs and thighs and are associated with venous stasis.[388,390,394] In some cases of major embolism no clots can be identified in leg veins at autopsy, but if the emboli are large and the source is not evident, it is reasonable to suppose that an entire thrombus broke loose from a leg vein, leaving no residuum.

The clinical effects of thromboembolism vary depending on the volume of emboli and on the condition of both the pulmonary and systemic circulations.[384,390,394] Emboli may cause no symptoms, acute transient dyspnea, pulmonary infarcts, pulmonary hypertension, cardiac failure, or even sudden death. Some but not all of the physiologic consequences of thromboembolism can be explained by mechanical obstruction of the vascular bed. The effects of embolism on gas exchange are (1) an increment in dead space ventilation, (2) pneumoconstriction, and (3) impaired synthesis of pulmonary surfactant.[390] The ventilation of unperfused lung adds to the work of breathing and produces the tachypnea and sense of dyspnea that are such frequent symptoms of embolism. Constriction of smooth muscle in the airways and probably in the alveolar ducts may be an effect of humoral factors such as serotonin and thromboxanes released from platelets or may be mediated by reflexes. It is transient, usually lasting 20 to 30 minutes, and causes wheezing as well as contributing to acute dyspnea. Hypoxemia is common after an embolism. Since increased dead space ventilation does not cause hypoxemia, it seems likely that the explanation lies in pneumoconstriction occurring in well-perfused tissue surrounding the occluded area and leading to areas of low ventilation/ perfusion ratio. Impaired surfactant production is a delayed effect that produces edema and atelectasis, which may account for reversible roentgenographic changes in areas of embolism.[385] The hemodynamic effects of embolism are slight unless more than 50% of the vascular bed is occluded. They include a rise in pulmonary artery pressure and in severe cases congestive heart failure and shock.

Massive pulmonary embolism is a well-recognized cause of sudden death, which may be virtually instantaneous or extend over a period of a few minutes. The major pulmonary arteries are distended with clots that are often coiled or twisted and bear the imprint of venous

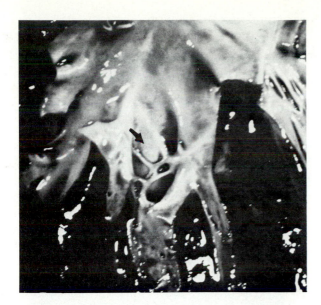

Fig. 22-21. Web in pulmonary artery *(arrow).* Such webs result from organization of pulmonary thromboemboli.

valves. The lung parenchyma shows little change except congestion, which presumably comes by way of the bronchial circulation. Sublethal thromboemboli are often recurrent. Consequently it is common to find emboli of varied age at autopsy. Fresh emboli are poorly adherent to the vessel wall but can be distinguished from postmortem clots because they distend the artery, have a drier, more granular surface, and seem less elastic. Lines of Zahn and imprints of valves are diagnostic. Older thrombi are adherent and retracted to varying degrees.

The fate of nonfatal emboli is variable. Fibrinolytic mechanisms produce dissolution of the embolus within a few days, as demonstrated by serial angiograms and lung scans.[386,396] Organization of emboli and recanalization restore the vascular lumen more slowly, within weeks. The embolus becomes invaded by myofibroblasts from the vascular intima, while endothelial cells migrate out over the surface of the clot and invade the thrombotic material to form new vascular channels within it. Gradually the clot is transformed into a ridge or into a web with multiple points of attachment to the intima (Fig. 22-21).[387,389,391] The core of the web is fibrous tissue, perhaps containing a few siderophages, and the surface is endothelialized. Occasionally such webs can be detected angiographically.[392]

Pulmonary emboli as a cause of hypertension are discussed later in the chapter.

Pulmonary infarcts

Ordinarily, emboli to the pulmonary arteries do not produce infarcts. Since the lung can obtain its oxygen from the alveolar gas and has an additional blood supply through the bronchial arteries, occlusion of a pulmonary artery does not usually produce tissue necrosis. Tissue distal to the obstructed artery may be normal or merely show congestion, hemorrhage, and intra-alveolar fibrin with intact alveolar walls. These changes may be visible roentgenographically but are reversible. In the presence of congestive heart failure or chronic pulmonary disease, however, emboli often produce tissue infarcts. This happens most often with occlusion of segmental or subsegmental arteries. Very large and microscopic occlusions are rarely associated with infarcts. Pulmonary infarcts are typically wedge-shaped, pleural-based, hemorrhagic foci, usually in the lower lung zones. Fibrinous exudate is present on the overlying pleura after several hours. With time the center of the infarct becomes brown and eventually pale as the hemorrhage breaks down and is removed. Alveolar walls undergo necrosis, and small numbers of neutrophils may be present. Over the next few weeks granulation tissue appears surrounding the necrotic tissue, which becomes encapsulated, gradually organizes, and is converted to a linear fibrous scar. During the first few weeks when granulation is taking place, there are often nests of metaplastic squamous epithelium associated with the granulation tissue, which should not be mistaken for squamous carcinoma.

Other forms of embolism

Fat emboli are discussed under the adult respiratory distress syndrome (p. 872).

Bone marrow emboli commonly follow vigorous cardiopulmonary resuscitation. Like thrombotic emboli they become adherent, endothelialized, and eventually organized.[403]

Amniotic fluid emboli are a rare complication of pregnancy. Infusion of amniotic fluid occurs during tumultuous uterine contractions when the head is in the birth canal. The amniotic fluid is forced through a rupture in the chorion into the maternal veins, precipitating severe dyspnea, tachypnea, and hypotension. Disseminated intravascular coagulation is a common consequence. At autopsy the lungs are hemorrhagic. Squamous cells are lodged in the arterioles. Amniotic debris also contains lipid and mucin, which can be identified with appropriate stains.[397] Reportedly the clinical diagnosis can be confirmed by demonstrating squamous cells in blood withdrawn by a pulmonary artery catheter.

Air embolism can be produced during inspiration if negative intrathoracic pressure draws air into an open vein, an event most likely to happen during a neurosurgical or ear, nose, and throat procedure in which the patient sits upright and the operative wound is above the level of the heart. Air bubbles become trapped in pulmonary arteries and right ventricle where they mechanically impede blood flow. Reactions at the gas-fluid interface also trigger blood clotting, and small fibrin and platelet thrombi are found in pulmonary arteries. The

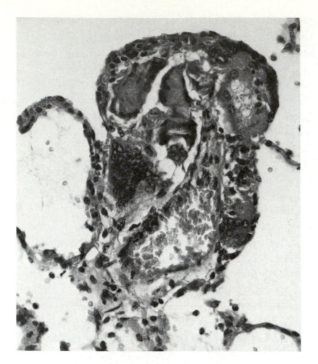

Fig. 22-22. Foreign body giant cells containing talc particles in adventitial space around small pulmonary artery. Patient had history of intravenous drug abuse.

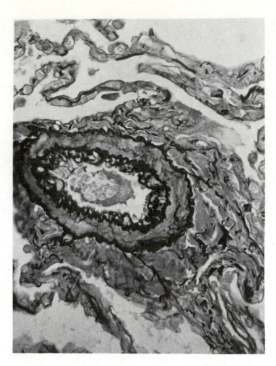

Fig. 22-23. Grade II pulmonary hypertensive change in muscular artery. Reduplication of internal elastic lamina and intimal thickening of minimal degree.

physiologic consequences include transient airway constriction and vasoconstriction with marked increases in pulmonary vascular resistance and pulmonary artery pressure. With large emboli pulmonary edema, hypoxemia, systemic hypotension, and myocardial ischemia are seen. Fatalities have been reported with embolism of 100 ml of air.[401]

Foreign body embolism can result from introduction of foreign material into the veins during medical procedures[402,404] but is also common among intravenous narcotic users. Particles of insoluble material added as "fillers" to drugs intended for oral use embolize to the lung and impact in arterioles and small muscular arteries where they cause thrombosis and proliferation of intimal cells.[399,400,405] Often they migrate into the perivascular space or interstitium where they give rise to foreign body granulomas composed of macrophages, multinucleated giant cells, and a few lymphocytes (Fig. 22-22). The process of migration appears to involve the production of a granulomatous response in the vascular wall with disintegration of muscle and elastic tissue. In cases where lesions are not numerous, their detection is aided by the use of polarizing filters, since cornstarch and talc, two of the materials commonly used as fillers, are strongly birefringent. When vascular thrombosis is widespread, pulmonary hypertension results. Lesions may resemble those of primary pulmonary hypertension, particularly in view of the cellular proliferation induced by the foreign material, but Tomashefski and Hirsch[405] could find scant morphologic evidence for an important vasoconstrictive

element to the pulmonary hypertension. Extensive interstitial granulomas can produce roentgenographic nodularity and a restrictive ventilatory defect.[348]

Pulmonary hypertension

The pressure drop across the pulmonary vascular bed equals the product of the pulmonary vascular resistance and the pulmonary blood flow.[410] This relationship can be expressed as:

$$P_{pa} = QR + P_{LA}$$

where P_{pa} is the mean pressure in the pulmonary artery, Q and R are the pulmonary blood flow and resistance, respectively, and P_{LA} is left atrial mean pressure, measurable in practice as pulmonary wedge pressure. From this relationship it is evident that pulmonary hypertension can be associated with increased flow as occurs with left-to-right shunt, with a process elevating pulmonary vascular resistance, or with increased wedge pressure as occurs with mitral stenosis, left-sided heart failure, left atrial myxoma, or diseases obstructing the pulmonary veins. Many disease processes change more than one of these variables.

In congenital heart disease with left-to-right shunt, the extent of vascular disease depends on interaction of several factors. With ventricular septal defect or patent ductus arteriosus there is increased flow because of the shunt accompanied by increased pulmonary arterial pressure because of the direct transmission of systemic pressure to the lesser circulation through the anatomic defect. The

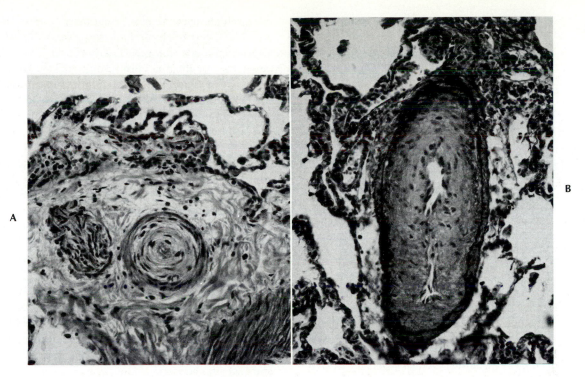

Fig. 22-24. Grade III pulmonary hypertensive change. **A,** Onion-skin hyperplasia of intima of small pulmonary artery. **B,** Severe intimal thickening with mild atrophy of media.

combination of elevated pressure and flow produces vascular damage by the time the child is several years of age and the pulmonary vascular resistance becomes elevated and eventually fixed. In atrial septal defect a large increase in pulmonary blood flow may occur with little increase in pulmonary artery pressure. Pulmonary vascular damage with the attendant rise in pulmonary vascular resistance develops only over several decades. With either type of shunt the eventual vascular damage may be severe enough to cause reversal of the shunt. Changes caused by abnormal hemodynamics have become a source of dysfunction in their own right.

The vascular changes in congenital heart disease have been of particular interest since the development of cardiac surgery, because the nature and extent of the lesions in the muscular arteries determines whether correction of the cardiac defect will relieve pulmonary hypertension. In 1958 Heath and Edwards[413] divided the vascular changes into the six grades listed below. The first three grades are reversible, but grades IV to VI generally are not.

Grade I	Muscular extension into arterioles, medial hypertrophy of muscular arteries
Grade II	Medial hypertrophy with intimal proliferation
Grade III	Progressive intimal fibrosis and occlusion
Grade IV	Plexiform lesions
Grade V	Chronic dilatation lesions with veinlike arteries
Grade VI	Arterial necrosis

The earliest changes in this scheme are muscle hypertrophy evident as distal extension of muscle in the arterioles and an increased thickness of the media of muscular arteries. Grade II changes include the preceding, but in addition some arteries show reduplication of the internal elastic lamina and proliferation of smooth muscle or myofibroblasts in the intima (Fig. 22-23). The intimal thickening of grade III changes is much more severe with marked narrowing or complete obliteration of the lumen (Fig. 22-24). The intimal proliferation often takes the form of concentrically arrayed intimal cells in a proteoglycan-rich stroma, a pattern described as onion-skin thickening. In some vessels with severe intimal thickening the media is relatively thin, indicating beginning evolution into the next stage. Grade IV changes include plexiform arterial lesions (Fig. 22-25). These are complex structures that often occur just distal to the point of branching of a muscular artery. The proximal segment of the lesion consists of an artery with a distinct muscular media and severe intimal thickening and fibrosis. The segment of artery downstream is thin walled and tortuous and has little media. At the junction between these segments there is marked cellular proliferation with complex anastomosing channels between groups of proliferated cells and often deposits of fibrin in the intercellular spaces or within the channels. The elastic laminae are often destroyed in the proliferative zone. In grade V there are numerous dilated, thin-walled, tortuous vessels that resemble veins at first glance, although serial sections show their position to be on the arterial side of

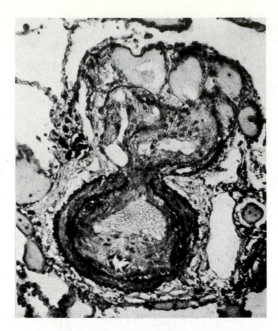

Fig. 22-25. Plexiform lesion. Muscular pulmonary artery with marked intimal fibrosis. Side branch *(top)* is filled with proliferating cells separated by anastamosing vascular channels that communicate with dilated veinlike branches.

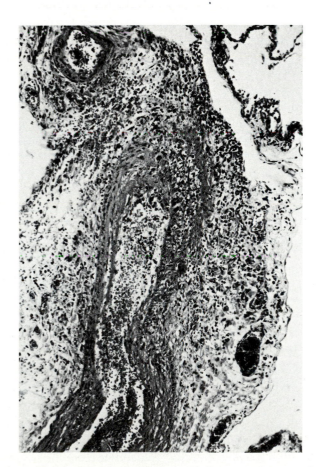

Fig. 22-26. Necrosis of muscular artery in patient with ventricular septal defect.

the circulation and in close relation to severely thickened arteries. Overt fibrinoid necrosis is the hallmark of grade VI hypertensive changes. The fiery red "fibrinoid" staining is the result of severe endothelial damage with the entry of fibrin into the media and its deposition between medial muscle cells.[415] There may or may not be an associated inflammatory reaction (Fig. 22-26). The Heath-Edwards grading scheme has been criticized by Wagenvoort[424] on three grounds. First, grades IV to VI imply a progression that may be the reverse of the actual pathogenic sequence. Plexiform lesions probably do not precede necrosis; on the contrary, there is experimental evidence that they arise after the necrosis. Arterial necrosis gives rise to medial degeneration, leading to the dilated, thin-walled vessels that are in part poststenotic dilatation of the damaged pulmonary artery and in part bronchial vessels involved in organizing the necrosis. The very cellular zone of transition with its many endothelium-lined channels may arise as an attempt at organization of the damaged vessel wall.[421] Thus grades IV to VI in Wagenvoort's view should be combined. Second, the grading is based on identification of the most severe type of lesions and takes no account of the proportion of arteries affected. Third, Reid[383] has identified loss of arteries or failure of their development that can be detected only by careful quantitative studies. The ratio of arterioles less than 10 μm in diameter to alveoli counted in sections can be used to estimate the extent of arteriolar development. Subnormal arteriolar development is an additional determinant of reversibility of the elevated vascular resistance in congenital heart disease. Thus Heath-Edwards grading must be regarded as an incomplete but rapid and convenient first estimate of prognosis.

Hypoxic vasoconstriction is one of the most common causes of pulmonary hypertension accompanied by increased vascular resistance. In contrast to the systemic circulation, in which hypoxia causes vasodilatation, alveolar hypoxia from any cause produces constriction of the small pulmonary arteries.[410,411] Physiologically this is an important mechanism for directing blood flow to well-ventilated parts of the lung, but if widespread and sustained, hypoxic vasoconstriction can lead to pulmonary hypertension and cor pulmonale. Conditions in which hypoxia is the major mechanism of pulmonary hypertension include residence at high altitude,[406] chronic hypoventilation either as a primary disease or resulting from neuromuscular disease, pathologic obesity (Pickwickian syndrome), or rarely upper airway disease such as tonsillar hypertrophy. In severe kyphoscoliosis, hypoventilation is aggravated by distortion of the arteries and areas of collapse of alveoli in which capillary resistance is elevated. In many forms of chronic lung disease hypoxic vasoconstriction is combined with destruction of the vascular bed. The histologic changes of chronic hypoxia are distal extension of smooth muscle along the arterioles and the development of a longitudinal muscle layer in the intima. Electron microscopic study of experimental hypoxia indicates that the muscle in the distal regions of arterioles arises by the differentiation of pericytes, which ordinarily are inconspicuous when viewed with the light microscope.[383] Hypertrophy of the tunica media of muscular arteries is characteristically mild.

Pulmonary hypertension of unknown cause is a clinical syndrome that can be produced by three distinct pathologic processes: multiple occult pulmonary emboli, primary pulmonary hypertension (primary-plexogenic pulmonary arteriopathy), and pulmonary veno-occlusive disease.[380,381,425]

Despite the high frequency of pulmonary emboli, they rarely present the clinical picture of slowly progressive pulmonary hypertension. Owen and associates[420] found only 12 cases in 8000 autopsies over a 20-year span. Although the chest roentgenograms had shown no abnormalities, five of the patients had small infarcts at autopsy. The histologic features of the vessels in thromboembolic pulmonary hypertension include a variable degree of muscular hypertrophy, intimal thickening that is characteristically eccentric (Fig. 22-27), and recanalized arteries.[391,425] The recanalized arteries may have multiple lumina ("collander" type) or a single fibrous septum giving it two lumina. Plexiform lesions and onion-skin intimal proliferation are not found. At autopsy most patients have some macroscopic thromboemboli in central arteries that are rarely included in biopsies.[391,420]

Primary pulmonary hypertension affects persons of all ages including young children, but a large majority of patients are young women.[427] The manifestations are usually the insidious onset of dyspnea or symptoms attributable to low cardiac output such as heart failure, syncope, or angina. One third of patients experience Raynaud's phenomenon. The chest roentgenogram shows right ventricular hypertrophy and enlarged central pulmonary arteries. Pulmonary arterial pressure can reach systemic values, but the wedge pressure is normal. The pathologic findings in the lungs cannot be distinguished from those in patients with congenital cardiac shunts. The characteristic features include onion-skin intimal proliferation in small muscular arteries, plexiform lesions, and dilatation lesions. Arterial necrosis is present in some cases. Morphometric studies of a small number of cases, conducted by Reid,[383] showed no abnormal muscular extension along arterioles but did demonstrate loss of arterioles less than 40 μm in diameter.

The cause of primary pulmonary hypertension is unknown. Familial cases have been reported. Its association with Raynaud's phenomenon suggests a hyperreactivity of the vascular system that is not limited to the lungs. Since identical histopathologic changes occur rarely in systemic lupus erythematosus, primary pulmo-

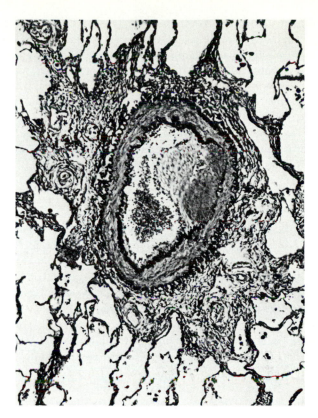

Fig. 22-27. Eccentric intimal thickening resulting from organization of thromboembolus. (Verhoef-Van Giesen stain for elastic tissue.)

nary hypertension may be related to the collagen-vascular diseases. This idea is supported by the occurrence of arthritis and autoantibodies in some patients.[418,427] Aminorex, an anorexigenic drug, caused a European epidemic of pulmonary hypertension in which the course and histopathologic changes were similar to those of primary pulmonary hypertension.[428] Some cases are associated with cirrhosis or portal hypertension, although the mechanism is unknown.[417,418,422]

The natural history of primary pulmonary hypertension is one of relentless progression despite the use of a number of vasodilatory drugs. Death is often sudden, attributable to low cardiac output. The rate of disease progression is variable. More than half of the patients die within 3 years of the onset of symptoms, but some live more than a decade.

In pulmonary veno-occlusive disease, fibrous obliteration of small veins is believed to be the cause of pulmonary hypertension, and changes in the arteries and parenchyma are secondary. There is widespread obliteration of veins and venules by eccentric or concentric fibrosis.[414,423,426] Often fibrous septa divide the lumen into one or several channels. In some cases recent and organizing thrombi were present in the veins, and it is likely that organization of thrombi is responsible for the fibrosis in many, perhaps most, cases. On the other hand, cases have been recorded in which granulomatous or other types of inflammation are responsible for the obliteration of veins.[409] The arteries show muscular hypertrophy and mild intimal fibrosis. Arterial thrombi have been reported in several cases, but whether they are in situ thrombi or emboli is uncertain. The lung parenchyma shows nodular areas of hemosiderosis and fibrosis or occasionally venous infarcts that are typically based on perilobular septa. Basophilic elastic fibers encrusted with iron and calcium are a striking feature in some cases, since affected elastic fibers act as foreign bodies, stimulating giant cell formation.

The clinical features are difficult to distinguish from those of primary pulmonary hypertension. Patients tend to be younger (most are children), and the sex incidence is equal. The chest roentgenogram may suggest the diagnosis. There are signs of interstitial edema with Kerley-B lines, but the pulmonary veins are not visible and there is no left atrial enlargement. Vascular marking is no more prominent in the upper than in the lower lobes.[423]

The etiology of veno-occlusive disease is unknown. A few features suggest that it may be triggered by infection. In many patients clinical onset has followed an influenza-like episode, and some patients have shown pathologic or serologic evidence of a preceding infection. In one case evidence of immune complex deposition in the alveolar capillaries was found by electron microscopy and immunofluorescence.[408]

In addition to the aforementioned histologic changes, which vary from disease to disease, certain morphologic features accompany chronic pulmonary hypertension irrespective of its cause. Right ventricular hypertrophy is present in almost all cases and can be evaluated at autopsy by dissecting away the atria and epicardial fat and separating the free wall of the right ventricle from the left ventricle and septum.[407,412] In adult men a weight of the free wall of the right ventricle greater than 75 g indicates hypertrophy. In children or those in whom a cause of independent left ventricular hypertrophy can reasonably be excluded, the ratio of the weight of the left ventricle and septum to the right ventricle can be used. A value less than 2 is abnormal. Measurement of the thickness of the ventricular wall is not reliable. If significant hypertension is present from birth, the elastic tissue of the pulmonary trunk does not undergo the normal fragmentation and regression, and the aorta-like elastic pattern seen in the neonate is retained.[416] If pulmonary hypertension develops after regression, the pulmonary trunk hypertrophies and may even approach the aorta in thickness if the hypertension is sufficiently severe, but the elastic lamellae continue to appear fragmented as in the normal adult. The elastic arteries also hypertrophy and develop accelerated atherosclerosis of the usual type.

PULMONARY EDEMA
General mechanisms of edema

There are few organs in which the development of edema causes greater functional impairment than in the lung. The late stages of edema with alveolar flooding are accompanied by severe disorders of gas exchange. Fortunately, involvement of the alveolar space usually develops late, following a series of sequential changes in fluid filtration in which interstitial involvement precedes airspace involvement.

The alveolar epithelium is relatively impermeable both to proteins and to small solutes.[440] The alveolar epithelial cells, which are the barrier between the air and the interstitium, are joined by tight junctions (zonulae occludentes). In freeze-fracture replicas the junctions are composed of three to five complete junctional strands. Although the endothelium of the pulmonary capillaries is nonfenestrated, the type seen in vascular beds of low permeability, the zonulae occludentes between endothelial cells are less tight than those of the epithelium. Usually they consist of two to three junctional strands, but sometimes only a single discontinuous strand is seen.[435] In consequence the capillary endothelium is more permeable than the epithelium.

The forces governing fluid filtration in the lungs, as in other tissues, are expressed in the Starling equation[434,439]:

$$Q_f = K_f (P_{mv} - P_i) - \sigma (\pi_{mv} - \pi_i)$$

where Q_f = fluid filtration rate, K_f = filtration coefficient of the microvessels, P_{mv} = the hydrostatic pressure in the microvessels, P_i = the hydrostatic pressure of the interstitial tissue, σ is a coefficient measuring the resistance of the microvasculature to the flow of protein, π_{mv} = colloid osmotic pressure of the plasma, and π_i = colloid osmotic pressure of the interstitial fluid surrounding the microvessels. Thus the main force favoring filtration of fluid and protein out of the pulmonary vascular bed is the hydrostatic pressure across the vessel wall, and that restraining it is the colloid osmotic gradient between the vessel lumen and the perivascular space.

Filtered interstitial fluid is cleared by the lymphatics. The alveolar walls themselves have no lymphatics, but there are lymphatics in the loose connective tissue spaces surrounding the bronchioles, small muscular arteries, and veins. Consequently no alveolar wall is more than 1 to 2 mm from a lymphatic. The interstitial pressures in the lung are lower in the junctions between alveoli, which helps to drain the interstitial fluid from the alveolar walls first to the junctions and thence to the perivascular and peribronchial connective tissue spaces.

The development of edema thus is a dynamic process.[438] As the filtration of fluid across the pulmonary vascular bed increases, initially the fluid is efficiently conducted to the lymphatics and removed. As the capacity of the lymphatics is exceeded, excess fluid accumulates first in the loose connective tissue spaces surrounding the bronchioles and arteries and in the lobular connective tissue septa. At this stage clinical manifestations are usually mild, but early closure of small airways owing to the peribronchiolar edema can be detected by sensitive physiologic tests of small airway function. Only occasionally is overt expiratory airflow obstruction present.

Thickening of the alveolar walls owing to interstitial edema is a late manifestation of increased fluid filtration but is accompanied by little impairment of gas exchange, since the excess fluid in the interstitial connective tissue of the alveolar wall does not materially widen the barrier for gaseous diffusion. In a section through normal alveolar wall the capillaries lie eccentrically with a space containing collagen and elastic fibers and cells on one side of the capillary but only a basement membrane shared with the alveolar epithelium on the opposite side (Fig. 22-28). When excess fluid builds up in the alveolar walls, it accumulates in the connective tissue space while the capillary remains attached to the alveolar epithelium through their shared basement membrane.

When flooding of the alveolar airspaces occurs, it tends to involve alveoli in an all-or-none manner. As fluid builds up in the corners of alveoli, the radius of the air-containing volume is reduced. In accordance with the Laplace equation the air pressure required to maintain its expansion rises, and at a critical point the air is driven out of the alveolus. Consequently, the airspaces in a lung developing edema are either at normal volume with only a minimal amount of intra-alveolar fluid or are filled with edema fluid and are at a reduced volume.

Lung in left-sided heart failure

Elevation of the pulmonary venous pressure from any cause can provoke pulmonary edema. Among its causes are left ventricular failure, disease of the mitral valve, or even mediastinal fibrosis. The lungs are heavy and moist, and frothy fluid may exude from the cut surface. Microscopically the alveolar capillaries are congested, and the perivascular spaces and interlobular septa are dilated with distended lymphatics. The alveolar spaces contain an eosinophilic coagulum of protein often with erythrocytes and macrophages in variable numbers.

Chronically elevated venous pressure produces the condition known as chronic passive congestion of the lung or brown induration. The lungs are heavy and firm, and the sectioned surface has a brown hue. Microscopically the alveolar septa are thickened and often lined with cuboidal epithelial cells, identifiable as hyperplastic type II pneumocytes by electron microscopy. The alveolar spaces contain clusters of hemosiderin-laden macrophages. The interlobular septa are thickened and the lymphatics dilated.[431]

Particularly severe cases of chronic passive congestion are commonly seen in association with rheumatic mitral stenosis. Because the stenosis develops gradually over many years, the pressure in the left atrium and pulmonary veins rises slowly. There is time for the lymphatics to hypertrophy, providing a measure of compensation for accelerated fluid filtration and permitting high venous pressures to develop without severe intra-alveolar edema. The chronic interstitial edema leads to fibrosis of the alveolar and interlobular septa and thickening of the basement membranes, which have been observed with electron microscopy.[436] Changes occurring in the pul-

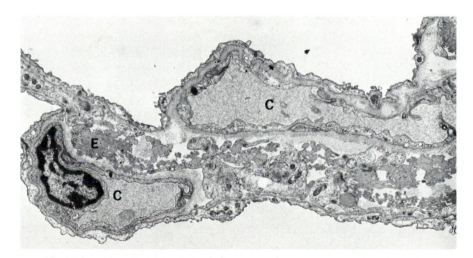

Fig. 22-28. Electron micrograph of alveolar septum of human lung. Capillaries (c) lie to side of septum, sharing basal lamina with alveolar epithelium. Connective tissue core contains elastic (E) and collagenous fibers. Interstitial edema accumulating within connective tissue space will not produce significant widening of diffusion barrier, since capillaries remain associated with shared basal lamina.

monary veins include fibrous thickening of the intima and hypertrophy of the medial smooth muscle. Sometimes the smooth muscle becomes organized into a distinct circumferential band separating elastic lamellae and resembling the tunica media of the muscular arteries.[431]

Among the consequences of venous distension is reflex constriction of the pulmonary arteries. This increase in precapillary resistance may give a small measure of protection to the pulmonary capillary bed but produces pulmonary hypertension with concomitant changes in the pulmonary arteries. The muscular pulmonary arteries develop medial hypertrophy and intimal fibrosis, while the precapillary arterioles develop a muscular media. Higher-grade hypertensive vascular changes such as those seen in congenital heart disease with left-to-right shunt, notably dilated arteries and plexiform lesions, do not occur with mitral stenosis.

Secondary changes are sometimes found in the lungs of patients with mitral stenosis or other causes of severe chronic pulmonary congestion. The elastic tissue in and around small arteries may become encrusted with calcium and ferric iron salts as a consequence of perivascular hemorrhages. The encrusted elastin fibers act as foreign bodies leading to the formation of giant cells. Small trabeculae of bone may be formed in alveolar spaces, although the mechanism for this change is not clear.[431]

Certain of the histologic changes in the chronically congested lung can be detected on the chest roentgenogram. The accumulated iron-laden macrophages give a fine nodularity to the lung fields. The thickened interlobular septa with their dilated lymphatics can be seen as fine linear shadows perpendicular to the pleura, known as septal or Kerley lines. Those lines in the depths of the lung near the hilum are the A lines. Subpleural lines are called B lines and are most clearly seen in the costophrenic angles.

Other causes of edema with a hemodynamic component

High-altitude pulmonary edema is an acute form of edema that develops in the first 48 hours after reaching high altitude in some persons with neither heart nor lung disease. The disease affects both those who live at sea level and travel for the first time at altitudes higher than 10,000 feet and dwellers at high altitude who descend to sea level for a period of time and then return to high altitude. Even in normal individuals the hypoxia of high altitude produces arteriolar constriction and pulmonary arterial hypertension, but in those with high-altitude pulmonary edema this response is greatly exaggerated.[437] Although the arterial pressure is high, pulmonary wedge and left atrial pressures are normal. These hemodynamic measurements suggest that overall capillary pressure is not elevated, and some authorities have sug-

gested that leakage of fluid takes place only in the arteries. The few autopsy cases reported had not only edema of the perivascular connective tissue septa and alveolar spaces but also hyaline membranes, indicating that the alveolar walls themselves were damaged.[429] Electron microscopic studies of animals exposed to simulated high altitude have also shown damage to alveolar capillaries.[432] To reconcile the evidence of alveolar damage with the hemodynamic findings, it has been proposed that the intense vasoconstriction responsible for the raised arterial pressure is not uniform. Those unconstricted arterioles permit transmission of the raised pressure to the capillary bed focally, producing fluid leak and capillary damage at the alveolar level.

Massive pulmonary edema develops after head injury of a wide variety of types. This neurogenic pulmonary edema can develop within seconds. In the early phase of the edema there is intense systemic and pulmonary vasoconstriction with a shift in blood volume to the pulmonary circulation. The intravascular pressures soon return to normal, but the edema may persist. The high protein content of the edema fluid indicates that microvascular permeability is increased. Evidence suggests that after head injury there is massive sympathetic discharge, resulting in the intense vasoconstriction. The consequent elevated pulmonary microvascular pressures initiate hemodynamic edema and produce capillary damage that increases microvascular permeability and maintains the leak after the pressures return to normal.

Pulmonary edema of extremely rapid onset and fatal outcome occasionally develops in users of heroin and other narcotics. The mechanism is not understood, but the high protein content of the edema fluid indicates altered permeability.

In patients with renal failure, edema may develop with a characteristic perihilar distribution seen roentgenographically. Histologic features are hemorrhage and fibrin-rich edema in the airspaces and hyaline membranes focally lining alveolar ducts. In chronic cases the fibrinous exudate may organize. Although this disorder is commonly known as uremic pneumonia, the pneumonia is not closely related to the degree of azotemia, and a variety of hemodynamic factors must contribute in individual cases. These include hypertension with left ventricular failure, fluid overload, cerebral edema in some patients, and decreased plasma colloid osmotic pressure in those with the nephrotic syndrome and hypoproteinemia.[430,433]

Altered capillary permeability

Acute injury to the alveolar capillary endothelium and epithelium leads to edema rich in proteins. The edema tends to be more prolonged than simple hemodynamic edema, in part because of the decrease in the osmotic forces favoring reabsorption and the precipitation of insoluble fibrin in the airspaces. Whether the lesions resolve, progress, or organize depends on the intensity and duration of the injury. Since the morphologic changes and pathophysiology are similar regardless of the etiology, the anatomic pattern has been called diffuse alveolar damage to emphasize its nonspecificity.[425] The early effects of injury are congestion and edema with widening of the peribronchial and perivascular spaces and filling of airspaces with proteinaceous edema and focal hemorrhages.[444,460] The alveolar walls become thickened by interstitial edema, and after 1 to 2 days hyaline membranes begin to appear, initially as deeply eosinophilic smudgy bands at the tips of alveolar septa where they protrude into the alveolar ducts.[444,451,455,461] With the passage of time the membranes grow thicker and completely line alveolar ducts and respiratory bronchioles (Fig. 22-29). Electron microscopic study of hyaline membranes shows that they occur at sites where the alveolar basement membranes are denuded by necrosis of the type I epithelial cells.[443,451] As in infants, they consist of cellular debris, membranelike fragments, and serum proteins but only rarely contain fibrin. Beneath the hyaline membranes in alveolar ducts, the alveoli are often collapsed. Inflammatory cells including small numbers of mononuclear cells and neutrophils infiltrate the alveolar septa and appear in the airspaces. In the sec-

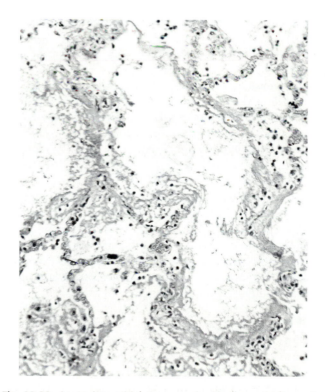

Fig. 22-29. Acute interstitial pneumonia. Hyaline membrane in alveolar duct, accompanied by a few inflammatory cells. The principal cause in this instance was hyperoxia, but similar morphologic changes could be produced by a variety of agents.

ond week reparative changes become prominent.[443,455,457,461] The alveolar epithelial cells enlarge and proliferate. Airspaces become lined with prominent cuboidal or elongated epithelial cells with atypical nuclei and abundant basophilic cytoplasm, sometimes vacuolated in appearance. Where there are hyaline membranes, these cells either cover their surface or extend along the basement membrane beneath the hyaline membranes. These epithelial changes are the general response to necrosis of type I epithelial cells. Type II cells first undergo hyperplasia to form a cuboidal lining over the denuded basement membrane, and then some of the proliferated cells spread out and differentiate into type I cells. During the transition they appear as elongated atypical epithelium.[443,451]

Fibroblastic organization occurs in two forms.[443,464] Fibroblasts proliferate and collagen is laid down within the interstitium of the lung, and fibroblasts invade the fibrinous exudate and hyaline membranes in the airspaces. In the early stages the organizing exudate is clearly within the airspaces where it appears as polypoid collections of parallel fibroblasts in a myxoid stroma. As the organizing intra-alveolar masses become collagenized and covered with regenerating epithelium, they are incorporated into the airspace walls, giving the appearance of interstitial fibrosis.

Clinically, patients with diffuse alveolar damage are tachypneic, short of breath, and cyanotic.[448,462,465] Severe hypoxemia is present, and high pressures are required to ventilate the poorly compliant lungs. The chest roentgenogram shows patchy or diffuse infiltrates. Together this group of clinical features has been called the adult respiratory distress syndrome (ARDS).[442] Although nonspecific, it is highly characteristic of patients with diffuse alveolar damage. The pathologic basis for the physiologic changes is complex and probably varies with the stage of the disease.[457] Hypoxemia is a consequence of physiologic shunting, ventilation-perfusion imbalance, and thickening of the diffusion barrier. Shunting occurs through perfusion of unventilated, edema-filled, or atelectatic airspaces. Premature closure of bronchioles cuffed by edema or directly damaged by the primary process and unequal compliance of diseased tissue lead to ventilation-perfusion inequality. Direct morphometric measurements of the thickness of the tissues to be traversed by oxygen have shown that the diffusion barrier is thickened. Early in the process, compliance is lost because of edema, abnormal surfactant synthesis, and interference with surfactant function by the serum components leaking from the damaged capillaries.[452,463] In the late phase of the process, diminished compliance is due to fibrosis.

Approximately half the patients whose disorder is clinically diagnosed as ARDS survive with modern therapy. Many survivors have residual pulmonary dysfunction.

Some of these have a restrictive ventilatory pattern as one would expect with pulmonary fibrosis. Others have expiratory airflow obstruction with hyperreactive airways for which the explanation is not obvious.[466]

The pathogenesis of the lung damage varies with the etiology. Several of the major causes of diffuse alveolar damage follow:

1. Shock
2. Infection
   a. Viral pneumonia
   b. Extrathoracic sepsis
3. Trauma
   a. Fat embolism
   b. Lung contusion
4. Aspiration
   a. Gastric acid
   b. Near drowning
   c. Hydrocarbon fluids
5. Toxic inhalants
   a. Oxygen
   b. Smoke
   c. War gases
   d. Oxides of nitrogen
   e. Metal fumes (cadmium, mercury)
   f. Other
6. Pancreatitis
7. Radiation
8. Narcotics
   a. Heroin
   b. Methadone
   c. Propoxyphene
9. Drugs
   a. Salicylates
   b. Ethchlorvynol
   c. Colchicine

Hyperoxia

The toxic effects of high concentrations of oxygen have been demonstrated repeatedly in a variety of species. When oxygen is used therapeutically, the exact level at which lung damage will occur depends on the underlying condition of the patient, but no concentrations above 50% can be regarded as entirely safe. The toxic effects of oxygen are mediated by its reduction products.[447,458] Even during normal metabolism the reduction of oxygen leads to the production of some highly reactive, short-lived intermediates such as superoxide (O_2^-), hydrogen peroxide, and hydroxyl radicals ($\cdot OH$). During exposure to oxygen the production of these radicals is increased and they can overwhelm the endogenous antioxidant defenses. The effects of oxidants that cause tissue damage include oxidation of sulfhydryl groups, DNA damage, and peroxidation of membrane lipids. Circulating neutrophils are powerful producers of oxygen radicals, which may explain why the earliest effect of hyperoxia

detectable by electron microscopy is damage to endothelium rather than to epithelium.[456]

Lung damage associated with extrathoracic injuries

ARDS is often associated with severe extrathoracic trauma, shock, intra-abdominal sepsis, burns, and pancreatitis.[448,465] Often the histopathologic changes correspond to diffuse alveolar damage. The mechanisms in such a complex clinical setting are not entirely clear. In the early phase of the process the lungs may contain thrombi in small arterioles or alveolar capillaries in addition to edema, hemorrhage, and hyaline membranes.[444] Activation of complement, agglutination of platelets, and adhesion of leukocytes in the lung with the release of oxygen radicals, vasoactive mediators, and enzymes are probably involved.[445,446,453,459,465] With major trauma, particularly if there are fractures of the long bones, fat emboli are a further factor producing lung injury. Fat embolism is the result of abrupt pressure changes in the long bones, which rupture thin-walled venous sinuses and force marrow fat into them, whence it embolizes to the lung. In addition, levels of plasma triglycerides, free fatty acids, and lipase rise as part of the stress response. Endothelial damage is caused by fatty acids released from embolized fat and by mediators released during associated blood coagulation. Fat emboli can be recognized in ordinary histologic sections as sharply delimited, empty-appearing capillary loops or arterioles, but frozen sections stained for fat are required for confirmation.[449]

Inhalation of toxic gases is another cause of diffuse alveolar damage. A variety of gases can produce the syndrome, including war gases, smoke, oxides of nitrogen as in silo-filler's disease, and others. Inhalation injury also involves conducting airways, and organizing exudates are often found in the respiratory bronchioles, a change known as bronchiolitis obliterans.

IMMUNOLOGIC LUNG DISEASE

Immunologic mechanisms play a role in a wide variety of lung diseases.[481] The diseases discussed in this section are thought in most instances to be induced by immune reactions to identifiable antigens that are not themselves directly pathogenic. Asthma has been included, although evidence suggests that immunologic reactions are only one of a number of inciting agents.

Asthma

Asthma is a disorder characterized by increased responsiveness of the airways to various stimuli, as manifested by episodes of wheezing and increased resistance to expiratory airflow. The stimuli vary widely and include antigens, infection, air pollutants, respiratory tract irritants, exercise, and emotional factors. Stimuli that cause slowing of expiration in nonasthmatic persons are effective in asthmatics at far lower concentrations. Methacholine and histamine, drugs commonly used in inhalation studies, caused bronchoconstriction in asthmatics at 1% of the normal dose.

Asthma is a common condition with an incidence in the U.S. population of approximately 4%. Clinically it has been divided into two types, extrinsic and intrinsic,[474] although the distinction is not sharp and cases with mixed features occur commonly. In extrinsic (allergic) asthma the attacks are triggered by specific identifiable allergens. The patients are usually children or young adults with an atopic history; that is, they or members of their families have histories of multiple allergies such as allergic rhinitis or urticaria. Many of these patients have elevated serum concentrations of IgE and peripheral blood eosinophilia. Asthmatic attacks typically become less frequent with time, often disappearing in adulthood.[476,478]

Most asthmatics whose symptoms develop in middle age or later do not give a history of atopy and have no identifiable allergens. The serum IgE level and white blood cell count are normal. The patient may have a history of chronic bronchitis, in which case the term "asthmatic bronchitis" is appropriate. This nonallergic or intrinsic asthma may become worse with time.[476]

Fatalities in asthma are fortunately rare. Most are caused by status asthmaticus, a severe, unremitting asthmatic episode that fails to give the usual prompt response to therapy.[474] At autopsy the lungs of patients dying of status asthmaticus appear grossly distended with air and fail to collapse as the thorax is opened. On the sectioned surface the parenchyma appears normal and the lesions of destructive emphysema are generally absent. The bronchi of segmental size and smaller are filled with ropy mucus, which may be clear and gelatinous or may have a laminated yellow appearance. On microscopic examination the bronchi and bronchioles are filled with laminated mucus that may appear eosinophilic or faintly basophilic (Fig. 22-30). The mucus is continuous with that in the cytoplasm of goblet cells and ducts of the mucous glands. The intraluminal mucus may contain sloughed epithelium, eosinophils, and crystals derived from eosinophil granules (Charcot-Leyden crystals), especially in allergic asthma. The epithelium lining the bronchi usually shows an increase in goblet cells at the expense of ciliated cells. Often there is extensive sloughing of columnar epithelium, leaving the bronchi lined only by basal cells (Fig. 22-31). This sloughing is unlikely to be an artifact, since it has been seen in biopsy specimens[470,480] and expectorated sputum,[475] as well as at autopsy.[474] The epithelium rests on an eosinophilic basement membrane that is usually 5 to 20 μm thick, compared with 1 to 2 μm normally. Electron microscopy shows that this structure consists of a basal lamina of normal thickness just beneath the epithelium and a deeper zone of cross-banded colla-

gen fibers, which accounts for the abnormal thickening.[472] The mucous glands show hypertrophy, dilated ducts, and an increased proportion of mucous cells. The bronchial muscle is hypertrophied, and all layers of the bronchial wall are infiltrated with inflammatory cells.[468] The inflammatory infiltrate may contain many eosinophils, but often eosinophils are few and plasma cells predominate. Where mast cell counts have been performed, the number of recognizable mast cells was reduced and many of those present appeared to be degranulating.[467,480]

The pathologic changes in nonfatal asthma are less well known. The rapidity with which airflow obstruction can be reversed in an acute asthmatic episode suggests that bronchospasm is the main cause of the obstruction. Biopsy specimens taken during or soon after attacks, however, show changes similar to those described in fatal status asthmaticus. Not only is there mucus hypersecretion, but a considerable degree of inflammatory infiltrate is seen.[480] It appears therefore that inflammation and mucus hypersecretion, as well as bronchospasm, contribute to the airflow obstruction in many ordinary asthmatic episodes.

The mechanisms that account for the altered airway

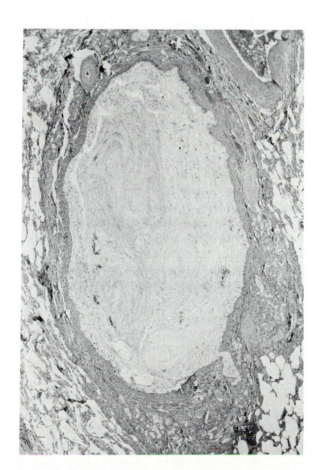

Fig. 22-30. Asthma. Laminated mucus filling small bronchus.

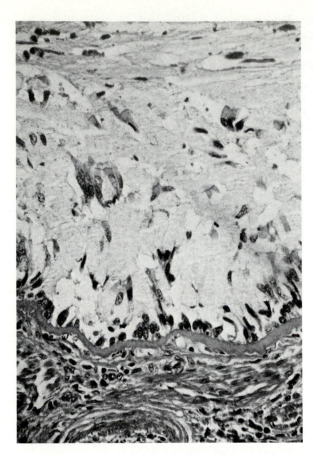

Fig. 22-31. Asthma. Higher magnification of bronchus shown in Fig. 22-30. There is sloughing of mucus-secreting and ciliated cells, leaving mainly basal cells attached to thickened basement membrane.

responsiveness probably vary.[469,479,481] Many asthmatic patients, especially those with extrinsic asthma, have antibodies capable of binding to and sensitizing lung tissue, mast cells, and blood basophils so that they promptly release mediators in response to the specific antigens.[481] These antibodies are usually of the IgE class but may be of an IgG$_4$ subclass. The sensitized tissue releases histamine, leukotriene C and D (slow-reacting substance of anaphylaxis), and platelet-activating factor (PAF; 1-O-alkyl 2-acetyl-sn-glyceryl phosphoryl choline), all potent bronchoconstrictors and stimulators of mucus secretion, as well as tetrapeptides with chemotactic activity for eosinophils (eosinophil chemotactic factor of anaphylaxis). Thus, an attractive idea is that the reaction of specific allergens with cytophilic antibody on the surface of mast cells leads to the release of mediators and the generation of the asthmatic attack. Most mast cells are in the lamina propria of the bronchus below the basal lamina, however, and this theory leaves unexplained the route by which the allergens reach the mast cells rapidly enough to produce the prompt effects observed when patients are given inhalation challenges with antigen.

Evidence suggests that the modulation of the neural regulation of bronchial muscle tone and mucus secretion is abnormal in asthma.[471] The sensory innervation of the bronchus includes small, nonmyelinated afferent nerves that terminate within the bronchial epithelium between the columnar epithelial cells. These fibers serve as irritant receptors, triggering cough and bronchospasm. The sloughing of the bronchial columnar cells commonly seen in asthmatics could contribute to airway irritability by exposing the irritant receptors.[469] The main motor innervation of the bronchi is via the vagus nerve. Presynaptic vagal fibers synapse on ganglion cells in the connective tissue sheaths around the bronchi. The ganglion cells give rise to cholinergic fibers that end on the mucous glands and bronchial smooth muscle. Acetylcholine is both a bronchoconstrictor and a stimulant of mucus secretion through its effect on muscarinic receptors. Its stimulatory activity is modulated by adrenergic influences, with alpha-adrenergic agonists such as norepinephrine enhancing bronchoconstriction and mucus secretion and beta-adrenergic agonists such as epinephrine inhibiting them. Asthmatics show increased responsiveness to cholinergic and alpha-adrenergic agonists and diminished response to beta-adrenergic agonists, but it is uncertain that any of these abnormalities is the primary defect of asthma.[471,479] Antibodies that react with beta-adrenergic receptors have been identified only in a minority of asthmatics, but in those patients they could account for diminished beta-adrenergic responsiveness.[479,482] Since cholinergic and alpha-adrenergic agonists stimulate mediator release from mast cells, whereas beta-adrenergic agonists inhibit it, similar defects in autonomic regulation could enhance both mediator release and responsiveness to vagal reflexes.

Other pathophysiologic mechanisms may be important in particular asthmatics. Some asthmatics have symptoms when exercising or exposed to cold. In these patients cooling of the airway mucosa triggers the attack.[473] Some patients have asthmatic attacks after ingesting aspirin. Commonly this type of asthma is associated with nasal polyps. An attractive explanation for the influence of aspirin came with knowledge of the metabolism of arachidonic acid. Aspirin inhibits the cyclo-oxygenase pathway to prostaglandins, increasing the metabolism of arachidonic acid via the competing lipoxygenase pathway that leads to the leukotrienes, including leukotriene C$_4$ and D$_4$ (slow-reacting substance), potent bronchoconstrictors and stimulants of mucus secretion.

Asthmatic symptoms can develop in sensitized persons in a number of industries or occupations. Fumes released during the cutting of polyvinylchloride films with a hot electric wire while wrapping produce, fumes emanating during the curing of urea-formaldehyde-based particle board, proteolytic enzymes added to detergents, and toluene diisocyanate fumes are examples of materials that can induce asthma in exposed workers.

Allergic bronchopulmonary mycosis (aspergillosis)

Colonization of the airways by certain fungi can lead to sensitization and the development of asthma complicated by disease of the parenchyma.[488,496,497,500] In most cases the colonizing fungus is *Aspergillus fumigatus* or one of the other *Aspergillus* species, although in some cases other fungi such as *Candida* or *Helminthosporium* have been isolated. Allergic aspergillosis is to be distinguished from *Aspergillus* fungus ball or mycetoma and from invasive aspergillosis. Mycetomas are aggregates of matted fungal hyphae in the lumen of a cavity such as that caused by chronic tuberculosis, histoplasmosis, or even a cavitary carcinoma. The fungi do not invade tissue and usually do not themselves cause symptoms. Invasive aspergillosis occurs in the chronically ill and especially in immunosuppressed patients and is a true infection in which organisms invade tissue and can disseminate.

Allergic bronchopulmonary aspergillosis develops in atopic persons. Signs are asthmatic episodes accompanied by eosinophilia, an elevated serum IgE level, and the appearance of parenchymal infiltrates on the chest roentgenogram. Bronchial casts containing organisms, mucus, and fibrin may be expectorated. Early in the course of the disease, roentgenograms show plugging of the bronchi and bronchiectasis involving segmental and subsegmental bronchi but sparing those more peripheral. In the late stages with severe involvement the bronchiectasis may be indistinguishable from ordinary bronchiectasis in which peripheral airways are obliterated.

Resected tissue shows severe bronchiectasis with plugging of bronchi by brown to yellow casts. The plugs consist of mucus and fibrin, and usually organisms can be stained in the intraluminal mucus but do not invade the bronchial wall. Mucus plugs usually contain large numbers of eosinophils, sloughed epithelium, and Charcot-Leyden crystals. The bronchi show mucus hypersecretion and infiltration with inflammatory cells. The lung may show obstructive pneumonia with fibrosis and lipid-laden macrophages, or infiltration with eosinophils and macrophages. Small granulomas are not unusual and consist of nodular collections of foreign body giant cells surrounding degenerated material that includes products of cell breakdown and perhaps degenerated eosinophils.

Immunologic mechanisms involve an immediate hypersensitivity, an immune complex–mediated Arthus type of reaction, or both. Patients typically have specific IgE antibodies to *Aspergillus* extracts, as well as IgG-precipitating antibody. They respond to skin tests with an immediate wheal and flare followed in many cases by a second reaction 4 to 6 hours later. When exposed to *Aspergillus* antigen by inhalation, patients show an immediate fall in vital capacity from which they recover, often followed by a second fall 4 to 6 hours later.

Bronchocentric granulomatosis

Bronchocentric granulomatosis is a response of the lung in which small airways are the site of necrotizing granulomatous inflammation.[489,491] Roughly one third to one half the patients with this histologic picture have asthmatic episodes, eosinophilia, and evidence of sensitization to *Aspergillus*. In the remainder the cause is unknown and eosinophilia absent. The tissue reaction consists of the development of necrotizing granulomas in small bronchi and bronchioles. Initially the lining of the bronchi is replaced by palisading epithelioid cells. Later the bronchi themselves are destroyed and the localization of the granulomas can be recognized only by their proximity to a pulmonary artery that is either normal or involved only by contiguity with the bronchial granuloma. The center of the granuloma may contain necrotic neutrophils, eosinophils, or simply amorphous debris surrounded by palisaded histiocytes. Rarely fungal hyphae can be found in the center of the necrotic material. Central airways are relatively spared. In addition to a nonspecific chronic inflammatory infiltrate in large bronchi, there may be small granulomas in the mucous glands and invasion and destruction of cartilage by a mononuclear inflammatory infiltrate.

Hypersensitivity pneumonitis (extrinsic allergic alveolitis)

The clinical picture of hypersensitivity pneumonitis varies depending on the nature of the exposure to antigen. An isolated exposure to a high dose of antigen produces an acute onset, whereas repetitive low-dose exposure may result in the insidious development of illness that is much more difficult for the clinician to associate with exposure. Farmer's lung is the archetype of hypersensitivity pneumonitis. The disease typically develops in a farmer who has been working in moldy hay. Four to 8 hours after exposure there is an acute onset of malaise, fever, myalgia, dyspnea, and cough. The chest roentgenogram shows patchy or miliary parenchymal shadows bilaterally. Manifestations gradually subside if further exposure is avoided. In some patients, however, the onset of disease is more insidious and a physician may not be consulted until the patient has had several attacks or chronic dyspnea has already developed.[487]

The lesions seen in biopsy specimens taken relatively early in the disease tend to be localized around terminal and respiratory bronchioles (Fig. 22-32). Alveolar walls are diffusely infiltrated with lymphocytes, plasma cells, and macrophages. In at least two thirds of cases there are granulomas consisting of aggregates of histiocytes and giant cells, which may be of foreign body or Langhans' type (Fig. 22-33). Necrosis is not a feature of the granu-

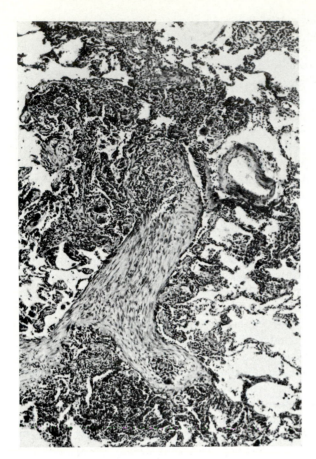

Fig. 22-32. Hypersensitivity pneumonitis. Lesion is centered on terminal airway. Respiratory bronchiole is filled in part with inflammatory cells and in part with proliferating fibrous tissue.

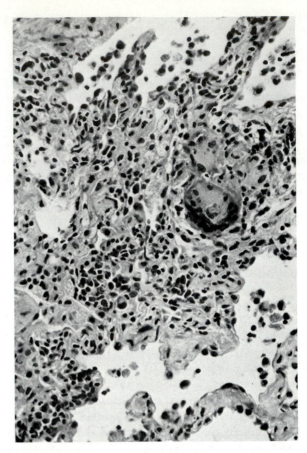

Fig. 22-33. Hypersensitivity pneumonitis. Loosely formed granuloma with giant cells.

lomas of hypersensitivity pneumonitis, and as a rule the granulomas are less compact than those of sarcoidosis. Loose organizing fibrous tissue often fills respiratory bronchioles or alveolar ducts. Alveoli may contain macrophages filled with lipid, a nonspecific change seen in association with obstruction of air passages. Eosinophils and polymorphonuclear cells are relatively few. Fragments of foreign material are present in some cases, but organisms are rarely identified.[494,499] Vasculitis is rarely seen, although it was described in one patient dying less than 2 weeks after the onset of symptoms.[483]

In chronic cases the lungs show fibrosis with or without honeycombing. Involvement is most severe in the upper lobes. The histologic changes may be entirely nonspecific with interstitial fibrosis and some inflammatory infiltrate, although frequently a few granulomas are still found.[499]

The physiologic abnormalities are those common to interstitial lung disease, including reductions in total lung capacity and its subdivisions, a low diffusing capacity, hypoxemia, and reduced compliance. A minority of

patients also have evidence of airflow obstruction[487] owing to inflammation, organizing fibrous exudate in small airways, or more rarely granulomas in their walls.

A variety of antigens can give rise to hypersensitivity pneumonitis (Table 22-2). In farmer's lung the antigens are the spores of thermophilic actinomycetes, *Thymoactinomyces vulgaris* and *Micropolyspora faeni*, which thrive in wet hay. Thermophilic actinomycetes can also grow in the fibrous residues from the processing of sugar cane (bagasse) and in mushroom compost, giving rise to the clinical syndromes of bagassosis and mushroom-worker's lung, respectively. Hypersensitivity pneumonitis caused by thermophilic actinomycetes contaminating furnace filters or domestic humidifiers causes hypersensitivity pneumonitis of insidious onset, which is often chronic by the time of clinical examinations.[486] Antigens from avian serum or droppings are responsible for bird-fancier's disease, and molds, wood dust, or animal antigens produce other clinical syndromes (Table 22-2). Despite the variety of antigens and types of environmen-

Table 22-2. Some causes of hypersensitivity pneumonitis

Syndrome	Source of antigen	Antigen
Farmer's lung	Moldy hay	*Thermoactinomyces vulgaris, Micropolyspora faeni*
Bagassosis	Moldy sugar cane	*T. vulgaris, M. faeni*
Mushroom worker's disease	Mushroom compost	*T. vulgaris, M. faeni*
Maple bark stripper's disease	Maple bark	*Cryptostroma corticale*
Sequoiosis	Redwood dust	*Graphium* sp.
Malt worker's lung	Malt dust	*Aspergillus clavatus*
Bird fancier's lung	Avian serum droppings	Avian proteins
Pituitary snuff user's lung	Pituitary powder	Bovine or porcine proteins

tal exposure involved, the clinical syndromes and histopathologic findings vary more with the intensity and duration of exposure than with the inciting antigen.[484,494,499]

The immunologic mechanisms responsible for hypersensitivity pneumonitis are incompletely understood.[481] The lag of 4 to 6 hours between exposure to antigen and the onset of symptoms is appropriate for an Arthus reaction, and patients have precipitating antibodies to the causative antigens. Since biopsies are not performed in patients ill for only hours, the earliest histologic changes are unknown. The histologic hallmarks of an Arthus reaction, vasculitis and infiltration with polymorphonuclear leukocytes, are usually absent at the time tissues are obtained, however, and immunofluorescence has usually failed to demonstrate deposition of immunoglobulin or complement. However, vasculitis was described in the lungs of a single patient dying less than 12 days after the onset of farmer's lung disease.

The microscopic characteristics of hypersensitivity pneumonitis, granulomas and mononuclear inflammatory cells, are more in keeping with delayed-type hypersensitivity than an Arthus reaction. The cells retrieved from the alveoli by bronchoalveolar lavage through a fiberoptic bronchoscope characteristically include an increased proportion of T lymphocytes.[495] Studies of persons who raise pigeons as a hobby show that most have precipitating antibodies to pigeon antigens although few have respiratory symptoms. A better correlation with respiratory symptoms was obtained when peripheral blood lymphocytes were studied to determine their ability to produce migration-inhibitory factor in response to pigeon antigen.[493] In sum, these observa-

tions suggest that the pathogenesis may involve both an Arthus reaction and delayed hypersensitivity. A defect in T-suppressor cell function in symptomatic persons offers a plausible explanation for their abnormal immune response.[490]

Pulmonary infiltration and eosinophilia

The combination of elevated eosinophil counts in the peripheral blood and infiltration of the lungs seen on the chest roentgenogram comprises the clinical syndrome of pulmonary infiltration and eosinophilia (PIE syndrome).[498] The syndrome has numerous causes, as follow:

A. Illnesses in which PIE is a major component
 1. Allergic bronchopulmonary aspergillosis
 2. Chronic eosinophilic pneumonia
 3. Drug reaction
 4. Helminth infestation
  a. Tropical eosinophilia
  b. Others
 5. Vasculitis (Churg-Strauss syndrome)
B. Illness infrequently associated with PIE
 1. Infections (bacterial and fungal)
 2. Tumors
 3. Sarcoidosis
 4. Other

When PIE syndrome is due to infestation with worms such as *Ascaris, Toxicara canis,* or *Strongyloides,* the infiltrates seen roentgenographically occur during the phase of larval migration through the lung en route to the intestine. At that time stool examination may not show ova. To make a diagnosis, it is necessary to reexamine the stool several weeks later, after the larvae have matured to adults that shed ova. Among the lesions of the lung that can be responsible for the infiltrates in PIE syndrome is eosinophilic pneumonia.[492] In eosinophilic pneumonia the predominant morphologic feature is exudate of edema fluid, monocytes, macrophages, and eosinophils into the airspaces. Infiltration of the alveolar walls takes place to a variable extent, but the predominant exudation is intra-alveolar. Collections of degenerating eosinophils known as eosinophilic abscesses are a characteristic feature. Organizing fibrous exudate infiltrated with eosinophils may be present in respiratory bronchioles.

Not all patients with eosinophilic pneumonia have the full PIE syndrome. Carrington and associates[485] described a group of nine women, predominantly middle aged, who had cough, fever, sweats, dyspnea, and roentgenographic infiltrates notable for their peripheral localization. All had eosinophilic pneumonia at biopsy, even though several had normal eosinophil counts in their peripheral blood. All responded promptly to treatment with corticosteroids.[485]

INTERSTITIAL PNEUMONIA (DIFFUSE INTERSTITIAL FIBROSIS)

Fibrosis of the lung can result from many types of lung injury. The general pathologic processes that lead to fibrosis include the organization of intra-alveolar exudates and hyaline membranes, the healing of granulomatous inflammation, and the response to chronic interstitial edema or inflammation.[506] The specific causes are too diverse and numerous to list. Despite the huge number of known causes of fibrosis, no cause is evident in half the patients who consult a physician because of diffuse interstitial pulmonary fibrosis. The diagnostic labels applied in such cases include idiopathic interstitial pneumonia or chronic idiopathic interstitial fibrosis in the United States and cryptogenic fibrosing alveolitis in Britain.

Clinical features

Persons of any age can be affected, although most cases develop in middle age or later.[509] The onset of symptoms is usually gradual with dry cough and increasing dyspnea, which initially is noticeable only on vigorous exercise but later appears on mild exertion or at rest. In some cases, however, the process begins with a febrile illness, suggesting a viral pneumonia from which the patient never fully recovers. Clubbing of the fingers is observed in over half of the patients, and a few basilar crackles can be heard on chest ausculation. The chest roentgenogram usually shows bilateral infiltrates but may be normal early in the course. The rate of progression of the process is variable. The average survival is 5 years, but the course may be more acute or much longer, even without therapy.[513] Hamman and Rich[505] were the first to record an acute course leading to death in 6 weeks to 6 months, and the term *Hamman-Rich syndrome* is sometimes used to describe the rapidly progressive form of the disease.

Pathology

The lungs are heavier than normal but reduced in volume, and the pleural surface often has a hobnail appearance. The tissue is firmer than normal and tends to retain its shape during slicing. The process is variable in character, even within a given lung. Normal areas are interspersed with foci of scarring in which the airspaces are obliterated, while in other areas the airspaces are abnormally large and thick walled (Fig. 22-34). Honeycombing, the term used to describe areas in which enlarged thick-walled airspaces predominate, can be recognized roentgenographically.

The microscopic changes vary considerably from case to case, at different stages during the course of the disease, and even from area to area in the same lung. In the early phase of the process the alveolar septa are widened by edema and a cellular infiltrate that is predominantly mononuclear but often also contains neutrophils and

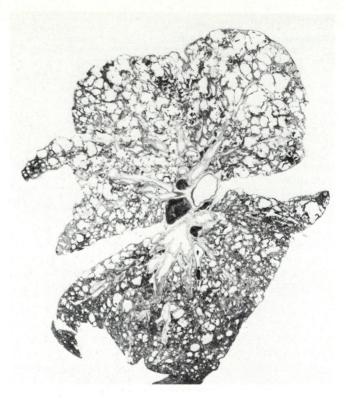

Fig. 22-34. Paper-mounted lung showing honeycombing. Airspaces are markedly enlarged and abnormal with thick fibrous walls. (Courtesy Dr. A.A. Liebow.)

sometimes eosinophils. The epithelium covering the alveolar walls is easily seen, some areas being covered by cuboidal epithelium identifiable as type II cells by electron microscopy (Fig. 22-35). Other epithelial cells are hypertrophied but partly spread over the alveolar wall and are probably transitional between type I and type II cells. They can be atypical with large nucleoli and basophilic cytoplasm.

The alveolar spaces contain an exudate that may be purely cellular—macrophages, lymphocytes, and neutrophils—or may also contain fibrin and hyaline membranes in varying stages of organization.[509] During organization, fibrin and hyaline membranes are invaded by fibroblasts, usually arrayed parallel or concentrically, and are converted to an edematous matrix initially consisting mainly of proteoglycan but gradually becoming more collagenous. Epithelial cells from the alveolar walls migrate over the surface of the organizing buds of fibrous tissue and become incorporated into the alveolar wall, contributing to the septal thickening.

In the later stages of interstitial pneumonitis, airspace walls become increasingly fibrous and alveolar capillaries disappear and are replaced by scar.[506] The number of inflammatory cells is variable but tends to decrease. The epithelium lining the fibrotic airspaces may become bronchiolar in type either by extension from bronchioles

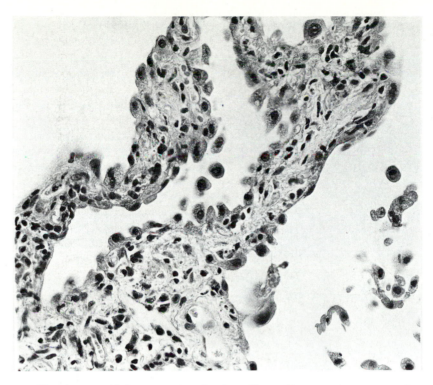

Fig. 22-35. Chronic interstitial pneumonia. Alveolar walls are fibrotic and contain predominantly mononuclear inflammatory cells. Alveolar epithelium is hyperplastic. Loss of capillaries in fibrotic septa is one factor contributing to abnormal gas exchange in this process.

or by metaplasia of the alveolar epithelium. Foci of squamous metaplasia can also be found. Arteries are thickened by a combination of medial hypertrophy and the development of an intimal layer of longitudinal muscle. Smooth muscle hyperplasia can also be striking in the interstitium, where it probably arises mainly from hyperplasia of the smooth muscle of alveolar ducts and respiratory bronchioles but possibly also from vessels or by differentiation of septa connective tissue cells.

Histologic classification

In 1965 Liebow, Steer, and Billingsley[508] classified the interstitial pneumonias into several morphologic types. They used the term *desquamative interstitial pneumonia* (DIP) to describe cases in which biopsy examination showed an apparently uniform pattern, with only modest interstitial fibrosis accompanied by hyperplasia of the alveolar lining epithelium and filling of the alveolar spaces with large mononuclear cells (Fig. 22-36). They believed the mononuclear cells to be sloughed type II epithelial cells (hence "desquamative"), but subsequent studies by electron microscopy have proved that these cells are mostly macrophages. Some interstitial lymphoid nodules and vascular thickening were present in most cases, but diffuse interstitial inflammation was not striking. They contrasted this appearance with the more heterogeneous appearance in the majority of cases of interstitial pneumonia, with greater inflammation, intra-alveolar organization, and fibrosis (usual interstitial pneumonia, UIP). Subsequent observations indicate that the DIP pattern is probably one end of a spectrum of morphologic changes.[510] There is no evidence that cases with the histologic features of DIP are separable on the basis of etiology or pathogenesis from other cases of interstitial pneumonia. The clinical course of patients with biopsy-proven DIP is more benign, however, and they respond more favorably to therapy with corticosteroids than do patients with UIP.[501]

Physiologic abnormalities

The major physiologic abnormalities of lungs with interstitial pneumonia are decreased lung volumes, decreased compliance, and impaired gas exchange.[502,504] In advanced disease, reduced lung volumes and compliance are readily explained by obliteration of airspaces by fibrous tissue and by the decreased distensibility of the tissue owing to its excess collagen content. Early in the course, edema and exudation of fibrin may also alter the surface tension properties of the lung. The irregular disposition of connective tissue produces uneven tissue compliance that, combined with inflammation around small airways, produces abnormal distribution of the

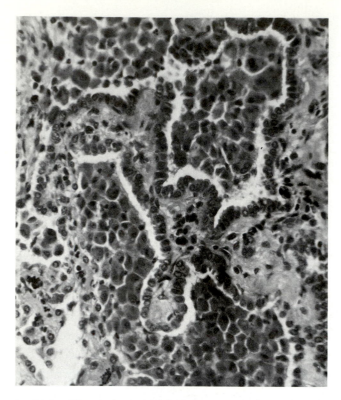

Fig. 22-36. Chronic interstitial pneumonia. This is morphologic pattern called desquamative interstitial pneumonia, in which appearance of biopsy specimen is uniform and alveoli are filled with macrophages.

inhaled air. Destruction of capillary bed in scarred alveolar septa decreases perfusion of diseased areas and probably increases flow in less-affected regions. The result of these functional changes is poor matching of ventilation to perfusion, which is measurable in the pulmonary function laboratory as widening of the gradient of oxygen tension between alveolus and arterial blood and a decreased diffusion capacity; these ultimately result in a low arterial oxygen pressure.

Pathogenesis

The pathogenesis of idiopathic interstitial pneumonia is unknown, but several lines of evidence point to an immunologic mechanism. These include the high incidence of circulating autoantibodies such as rheumatoid factor and antinuclear antibodies[514]; the occurrence of a similar interstitial pneumonia in diseases such as rheumatic fever, rheumatoid arthritis, scleroderma, polymyositis, and mixed connective tissue disease in which an immune pathogenesis is strongly suspected; the presence of elevated titers of circulating immune complexes in some patients, especially those with active disease[503]; and the immunofluorescent demonstration of the deposition of immunoglobulin and complement in some biopsy specimens.[507,511,515] The deposition of immune com-

plexes in the lungs of experimental animals leads to tissue damage and inflammation.[516] The frequency with which elevated levels of circulating immune complexes or immunofluorescent deposits can be detected is much greater early in the disease than in its late fibrotic stage. Even in studies of patients with active disease, however, medical centers vary greatly in the frequency with which these evidences of immune activity are found,[503,507,511,512,515] and no inciting antigen has been identified. It seems likely that immune complexes are responsible for some cases of idiopathic interstitial pneumonia, but this is by no means proved in all cases.

PULMONARY INVOLVEMENT IN COLLAGEN-VASCULAR DISEASE
Acute rheumatic fever

Pulmonary involvement in acute rheumatic fever is not uncommon, although reported figures vary greatly. Clinically it may be difficult to distinguish heart failure, bacterial infection, and involvement by the primary disease. In the pathologic series reviewed by Brown, Goldring, and Behrer[520] the incidence of rheumatic pneumonia varied from 12% to 50% of patients with acute rheumatic fever. Patients show tachypnea, hypoxemia, and a patchy migratory infiltrate on the chest roentgenogram. Pathologic changes are nonspecific but resemble those in other acute interstitial pneumonias with evidence of fibrous repair. The alveolar walls are thickened by edema and a mixed mononuclear infiltrate. Many alveoli and alveolar ducts are lined with hyaline membranes. Fibrin in various stages of organization is present in alveoli. Thrombosis of arterioles, alveolar septal necrosis, vasculitis, and patchy areas of infarctlike necrosis are found in a minority of cases.[536,553]

Rheumatoid disease

Pulmonary involvement in rheumatoid disease takes a number of forms including pleural effusion, interstitial pneumonitis, bronchiolitis, necrobiotic nodules, vasculitis, and rheumatoid pneumoconiosis. Pleural effusions commonly occur in male patients with high titers of rheumatoid factor. Pleural fluid glucose is reduced to below 30 mg/dl in most cases, and the pH is low.[544,550] The very low glucose concentration has been attributed to a selective block to transport of glucose from plasma into the pleural fluid. Rheumatoid arthritis (RA) cells (leukocytes containing ingested rheumatoid factor–IgG complex) have been seen in the pleural fluid in several cases.[530,545] The histologic changes in the pleura are often those of a nonspecific pleuritis, but in some cases rheumatoid granulomas similar to the subcutaneous nodules have been observed in the pleura.[530]

The frequency of interstitial fibrosis in rheumatoid arthritis is difficult to gauge. Only 1.6% have been reported to have roentgenographic changes,[536] while

30% to 40% of patients have been reported to have abnormalities of diffusion, often without symptoms.[531]

The pathologic features of pulmonary fibrosis associated with rheumatoid disease are not distinctive. At necropsy there is often honeycomb change, most marked subpleurally. The range of histologic changes is not distinguishable from those seen in patients with idiopathic interstitial pneumonia. The alveolar septa are thickened and there are a mixed, predominantly mononuclear infiltrate and epithelial hyperplasia progressing late to bronchiolar and squamous metaplasia. Nodules of lymphoid tissue are prominent in many cases and may have germinal centers. Late in the course there are often prominent smooth muscle hyperplasia and severe loss of capillaries in honeycomb areas.

The pathogenesis of the interstitial pneumonia is not clear. IgM rheumatoid factor deposits have been demonstrated in the alveolar walls by immunofluorescence,[525] and experimental studies suggest a role for such complexes in accentuating inflammation.[524]

In some cases of rheumatoid disease during treatment, the drugs rather than the primary disease may be the cause of pulmonary infiltrates.[532,535] Severe progressive obstructive lung disease caused by bronchiolitis obliterans has only recently been recognized as a complication of rheumatoid arthritis.[533] Although a relationship to penicillamine therapy has been suggested,[528] not all patients with bronchiolitis obliterans have received this drug. Minor degrees of bronchiolitis probably are not a rare complication of RA, since many patients with RA have small airway dysfunction detectable by sensitive physiologic tests.[534]

Necrobiotic nodules are pathologically the most specific manifestation of rheumatoid disease.[556] They closely resemble the more common subcutaneous nodules. They occur in patients with active disease and high titers of rheumatoid factor, may be single or multiple, and may occur as an isolated form of lung disease or against a background of pulmonary fibrosis. The center of the nodules may consist of fibrinoid necrosis or degenerating neutrophils. A band of palisading histiocytes surrounds the necrotic center. External to the palisaded cells is a zone of fibrous tissue infiltrated with lymphocytes and plasma cells (Fig. 22-37). Necrobiotic nodules developing in patients with pneumoconiosis are discussed later in the chapter (p. 908).

Necrotizing vasculitis is rare in rheumatoid disease. Pulmonary involvement usually occurs with systemic vasculitis, but it has also been described as a localized process.[518]

Systemic lupus erythematosus

Patients with systemic lupus erythematosus (SLE) commonly have lung disease during the course. Often this is due to bacterial infection, which was a well-recog-

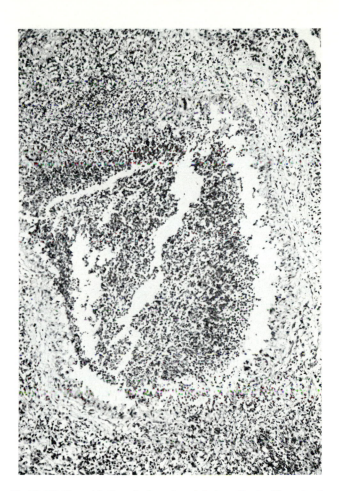

Fig. 22-37. Necrobiotic subpleural nodule in patient with systemic rheumatoid disease. Center is filled with debris of necrotic inflammatory cells and is surrounded by palisading histiocytes.

nized problem even before modern intensive immunosuppressive therapy.[537,541] Presumably hypocomplementemia and general debility were predisposing factors. The most common manifestation of SLE in the thorax is pleurisy that may be painful and is accompanied by small effusions.[537,539] The fluid has properties of an exudate and may contain L.E. cells. The histopathologic findings in the pleura are those of a nonspecific fibrous or fibrinous pleurisy. The major parenchymal manifestations of SLE are pulmonary hemorrhage, interstitial pneumonitis, and vasculitis. Pulmonary hemorrhage of varying degrees is common in the lungs of patients with SLE at autopsy. As a clinical problem it is a rare, potentially lethal manifestation that occasionally is the earliest sign of SLE.[526] Histologically the lungs show extensive intra-alveolar hemorrhage accompanied by minimal light microscopic changes in the alveolar walls, small arteries, or veins. The alveolar walls may be subtly hypercellular owing to increase of neutrophils and mononuclear cells (Fig. 22-38). Kapanci and Chamay[542] have described wire loop lesions in alveolar capillaries.[542] The alveolar

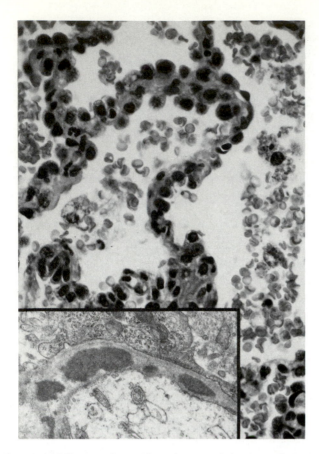

Fig. 22-38. Pulmonary hemorrhage in systemic lupus erythematosus. Alveolar walls show minimal inflammation and epithelial hyperplasia. *Inset,* Electron micrograph shows dense deposits, presumably immune complexes, in basal lamina.

epithelium is focally hyperplastic. Inflammatory cells can be found in or around small arterioles and venules.

Immunohistochemical examination reveals granular deposits of IgG in the alveolar walls, and electron microscopy shows dense deposits (Fig. 22-38) compatible with immune complexes in a subendothelial location and in the interstitium.[521,526]

Interstitial pneumonia occurs in less than 10% of patients with SLE and can be acute[546] or chronic.[527] Biopsies have been performed in relatively few cases of acute lupus pneumonitis. In retrospective autopsy studies of SLE the changes of diffuse alveolar damage are common and include inflammatory cell infiltration and edema of alveolar septa, hyaline membranes, and an intra-alveolar exudate of fibrin in various stages of organization.[537] These changes are nonspecific, and the importance of associated uremia or changes resulting from therapy has not always been critically assessed. Biopsy examination in a few cases of acute lupus pneumonitis has shown mononuclear infiltration of alveolar walls and intra-alveolar organization.[546] Immunohistochemical examination has shown the presence of DNA

and immune complexes in the alveolar walls.[540] Eluted antibody had anti-DNA activity. Chronic interstitial fibrosis in SLE may have more than one pathogenesis. Usually it is caused by low-grade interstitial pneumonia, but some cases may result from the healing of infarcts.[527]

Vasculitis involves the lung in some cases of acute SLE and may be responsible for pulmonary hypertension.[529,547] Necrobiotic nodules have been described but are very rare.[555]

Sjögren's syndrome

Sjögren's syndrome combines lymphoid infiltration of lacrimal and salivary glands with other manifestations of collagen-vascular disease, most commonly arthritis and hyperglobulinemia. Involvement of the bronchial mucous glands by a process similar to that in the salivary glands can lead to inadequate bronchial clearance and repeated infections.[554] Chronic airflow obstruction associated with bronchiolitis is common and can be disabling.[548] Whether the explanation is damage from infection or is a manifestation of a rheumatoid process is unknown. In the lung periphery, nonspecific interstitial pneumonia is present in approximately 3% to 4% of patients.[539,554] A variety of lymphoproliferative lesions also occur in the lungs in Sjögren's syndrome.[517,543] These range from lymphoid interstitial pneumonia in which the lung interstitium is heavily infiltrated by lymphocytes and plasma cells, to pseudolymphoma with nodules and masses of benign lymphoid tissue with germinal centers and a well-differentiated lymphoplasmacytic infiltrate, to frankly malignant lymphoma usually of the large cell ("histiocytic") type.[517,543] In one patient with Sjögren's syndrome, lymphomatoid granulomatosis developed, and amyloidosis has developed in several.[519]

Progressive systemic sclerosis

Progressive systemic sclerosis (PSS) is a systemic disease that frequently involves the skin, kidney, gastrointestinal tract, and skeletal muscle, as well as the lung.[538] The lung is abnormal in 80% of cases both clinically and at autopsy.[523] The most characteristic pathologic change is a myxoid thickening with concentric cellular hyperplasia of the intima of muscular arteries, which is found in 30% to 50% of patients with classical scleroderma.[523,557] In the relatively benign variant of PSS known as the CREST syndrome (calcinosis, Raynaud's phenomenon, esophageal dysfunction, sclerodactyly, telangiectasia) it occurs much less commonly.[551] In either clinical setting it can be associated with severe and progressive pulmonary hypertension. Pulmonary fibrosis, the most common form of pulmonary involvement in PSS, evolves slowly compared with the idiopathic form.[522] It usually involves the lower lobes and subpleural regions of the

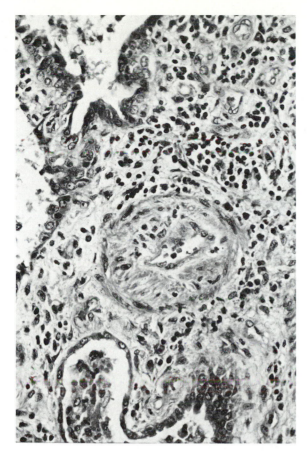

Fig. 22-39. Progressive systemic sclerosis. There is marked intimal thickening of small muscular artery. Lung shows severe interstitial fibrosis.

lung, and honeycombing is common. The vascular change and parenchymal fibrosis can occur together (Fig. 22-39) or separately. The prevalence of pneumonia is also increased in PSS, which is not surprising, since esophageal dysfunction is common and predisposes to aspiration.

Polymyositis and dermatomyositis

Interstitial pneumonitis and fibrosis may accompany polymyositis and dermatomyositis.[539,552] When the interstitial pneumonitis precedes the myopathic symptoms, the diagnosis of polymyositis may be missed and the muscular manifestations may be attributed to restricted activity and chronic illness. Involvement of the muscles of deglutition promotes aspiration.

Wegener's granulomatosis

The four components of Wegener's granulomatosis are granulomas of the upper respiratory tract, granulomas of the lung, systemic vasculitis, and a focal, usually necrotizing, glomerulonephritis.[570,571,576] Granulomas occasionally are present in other organs as well. Not all com-

ponents may be present in a given patient. The term *limited Wegener's granulomatosis* has been used to describe those who do not have glomerulitis.[564] Lesions in some cases of so-called lethal midline granuloma of the upper respiratory tract are histologically identical to Wegener's lesions and probably represent Wegener's granulomatosis without involvement of other sites.[563]

The clinical manifestations vary according to the site of involvement. Persons of any age may be affected, but most patients are middle aged. Men outnumber women by a small margin. Upper respiratory tract symptoms may be referable to the sinuses, nose, nasopharynx, or middle ear, whereas pulmonary symptoms are quite nonspecific and include cough, dyspnea, or pleurisy. Systemic manifestations such as fever, weight loss, anemia, and leukocytosis are common when multiple sites are involved but infrequent when disease is limited to one or a few sites.[567] The chest roentgenogram shows single or multiple, large, rounded densities that may cavitate and that occur predominantly in the lower lobes.

Grossly the pulmonary lesions may have the appearance of pale infarcts or vary from small to bulky necrotic nodules (Fig. 22-40).[564,574] The histologic features of upper and lower respiratory tract lesions are similar, consisting of necrotizing granulomas with an associated vasculitis. Granulomatous inflammation including macrophages, lymphocytes, plasma cells, and fibroblasts encloses geographic zones of necrosis that are often infarctlike, bland, and with preservation of the outlines of the underlying tissue, but that may be softer and contain an abundance of debris. Giant cells vary from scanty to numerous and are usually of the foreign body type. Discrete compact epithelioid granulomas like those of sarcoidosis or tuberculosis are distinctly unusual.[564,571,572,574]

Vasculitis involves both veins and arteries and vessels from millimeters to tens of micrometers in size. In some cases fibrinoid necrosis may predominate and the involved vessels closely resemble those in polyarteritis nodosa, but more often there is cellular invasion of the vessel wall by mononuclear cells that thicken the intima, replace the media, and focally destroy the elastic tissue. In larger vessels the granulomatous quality of the inflammation may be obvious with palisading histiocytes and giant cells (Fig. 22-41).[564,571,572,574]

The association of vasculitis with necrotizing granulomatous inflammation is required for the diagnosis of Wegener's granulomatosis, but it is by no means specific. Special stains and cultures are needed to rule out infection, since vasculitis is not rare in contiguity with infectious granulomas. Vasculitis in vessels remote from the actual granulomas is helpful in making the diagnosis but is not always found, especially when biopsy specimens are of limited size.

Extrapulmonary lesions, usually consisting of vasculi-

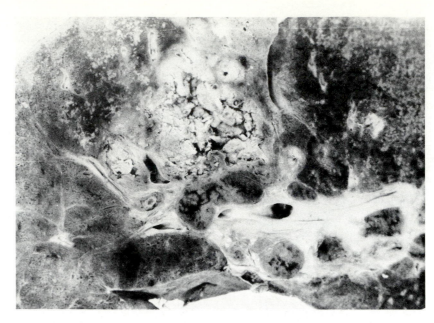

Fig. 22-40. Necrotic pulmonary lesion in Wegener's granulomatosis.

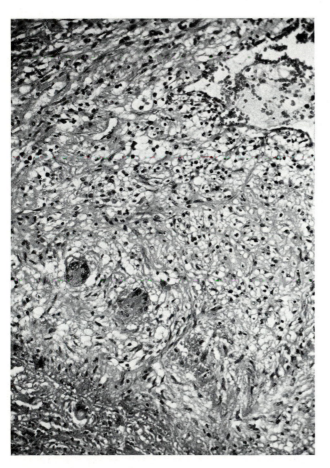

Fig. 22-41. Granulomatous vasculitis in Wegener's granulomatosis. Lumen of vessel is at upper right.

tis and sometimes of granulomas, can be found in a variety of organs. Necrosis of the spleen was mentioned in Wegener's original report, and granulomatous trabeculitis can be striking. The usual renal lesions are a segmental necrotizing glomerulitis, but cases have been described in which necrotizing granulomas were present in the kidney without glomerulitis.[564]

The pathogenesis of Wegener's granulomatosis is unknown, but as with many other forms of vasculitis, an immunologically mediated injury is likely. Elevated levels of circulating immune complexes have been detected in some cases. Immunofluorescence of the glomerular lesions gives variable results, but granular staining of immunoglobulin and complement have often been reported.[539] Therapy based on a presumption of immunologic injury has been remarkably successful. Persons with untreated, full-blown Wegener's granulomatosis with glomerulitis had a median survival of only 5 months, and 80% of patients died in the first year.[576] With vigorous immunosuppressive therapy remissions occur in as much as 80% to 90% and long-term survival is common.[570]

Allergic granulomatosis and angiitis

Like Wegener's disease, allergic granulomatosis and angiitis (Churg-Strauss syndrome) involve a combination of vasculitis and respiratory tract granulomas.[566] Asthma is usually present for several years before a systemic illness develops that resembles polyarteritis nodosa and is accompanied by eosinophilia of the peripheral blood and in most cases infiltrates or nodules on the chest roentgenogram. Clinical renal involvement is uncommon, but skin eruptions or subcutaneous nodules have been reported in two thirds of patients.[565] The pulmonary lesions include infiltrates of eosinophils and necrotizing granulomas with central fibrinoid necrosis surrounded by palisading histiocytes and giant cells.[566] Vasculitis involving small arteries and veins may be present in any organ. As a rule the vasculitis is manifest by fibrinoid necrosis and an eosinophil-rich inflammatory infiltrate, but when larger muscular arteries are involved, inflammation can be frankly granulomatous. Chumbley, Harrison, and DeRemee[565] reported a mortality of 50%. The average survival was 4½ years after the onset of symptoms.

Hypersensitivity angiitis

In 1953 Zeek[577] reviewed the vasculitides and differentiated polyarteritis nodosa, a disease affecting muscular arteries near their branch points, from hypersensitivity angiitis, which involved smaller vessels, arterioles, and venules. Polyarteritis nodosa was characterized by lesions of varying ages and had no identifiable etiology, whereas hypersensitivity pneumonitis often began after exposure to a definite allergen, usually a drug or serum, and lesions were of the same histologic age. The two conditions differed in their patterns of organ involvement: the lung and spleen were rarely involved in classic polyarteritis nodosa but were frequent targets of hypersensitivity pneumonitis. Subsequent series put the frequency of lung involvement in hypersensitivity angiitis at about 40%. Although recent writers have divided this small vessel vasculitis into subtypes,[539] the pathologic features are similar in all, consisting of fibrinoid necrosis and leukocytic infiltration of the walls of arterioles, venules, and capillaries. In the lung these usually result in hemorrhage, which may be difficult to distinguish from Goodpasture's syndrome, although antibodies to basal lamina are not found.

Goodpasture's syndrome

The development of antibodies to antigens in the basal lamina can produce either glomerulonephritis alone or pulmonary hemorrhage and glomerulonephritis, a combination known as Goodpasture's syndrome. Goodpasture's syndrome usually occurs in men between the ages of 16 and 30 years.[560] The majority of cases have been reported to be of the HLA-DRW2 haplotype. The pulmonary manifestations usually precede the renal disease.[560] Hemoptysis is the initial symptom in 95% of patients and is often accompanied by exertional dyspnea, fatigue, and weakness. Iron-deficiency anemia, hematuria, and proteinuria follow. Without therapy the disease is usually lethal within a year, but spontaneous remissions can occur.

In acute cases light microscopy shows little alteration of the lung parenchyma, whereas in more chronic cases there is interstitial fibrosis accompanied by filling of airspaces with hemosiderin-laden macrophages. Elastic fibers in the walls of small arteries and veins may be encrusted with iron salts accompanied by foreign body giant cells. Immunofluorescence shows linear deposition of immunoglobulin and complement in the basal lamina regions.[559,573] Deposition is uniform in the kidney, but focal in the lung, and can be missed if only a small lung biopsy is available for staining. Electron microscopy shows swelling, irregular lucency, and overt breaks in the basal lamina.[562,568] Gaps are present between endothelial cells, and occasional neutrophils or monocytes have been described passing through discontinuities in the alveolar-capillary membrane.

The antigens to which the antibodies form have not been fully characterized but appear to be one or more noncollagenous glycoproteins localized to the subendothelial lamina rara.[575] The antibodies are IgG in most cases, but IgA antibodies have been described.[561] The stimulus to antibody formation is unknown. The increased incidence of Goodpasture's syndrome during the year of an influenza pandemic suggests that viral injury to the alveolar basal lamina could be one stimulus.[560] Investigators have encountered a history of exposure to volatile solvents or smoke inhalation,[558] suggesting chemical injury as a stimulus.

OTHER NONINFECTIOUS GRANULOMAS
Pulmonary histiocytosis X

Histiocytosis X (well-differentiated histiocytosis) is a proliferative disease involving a subset of mononuclear phagocytes similar to the Langerhans' cells of the skin.[585] The lung can be involved either as part of disseminated histiocytosis or in a localized process limited to the lung. Disseminated histiocytosis has been described in detail by Silberberg-Sinakin, Baer, and Thorbecke.[585] The lung involvement is typically widespread and diffuse in acute disseminated histiocytosis (Letterer-Siwe type), whereas in chronic disseminated histiocytosis the lesions are focal and nodular. On healing they can result in striking honeycomb change (Fig. 22-42). The prognosis of disseminated histiocytosis depends largely on the extent and activity of the systemic process.[580,585]

Histiocytosis limited to the lung (pulmonary eosinophilic granuloma) is a disease mainly of young adults, with an average age of 30 years. Men have predominated in most series. Symptoms are variable. Some patients are asymptomatic, and the process is discovered accidentally by chest roentgenography. Some patients are first seen for pneumothorax while others have cough and gradually worsening dyspnea as a result of interstitial involvement.[508] Early chest roentgenograms show bilateral nod-

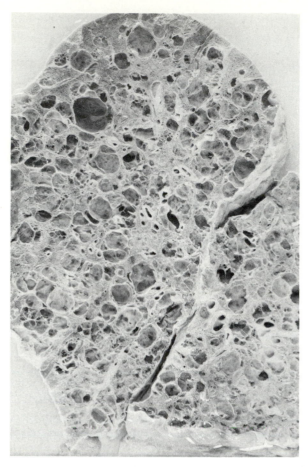

Fig. 22-42. Honeycomb lung from child with disseminated histiocytosis X.

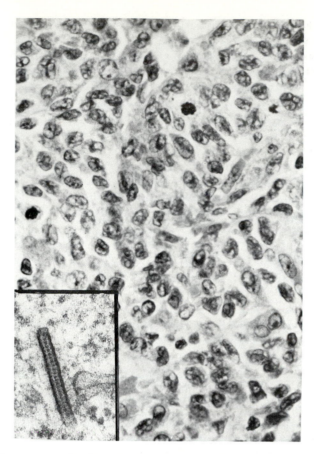

Fig. 22-43. Localized pulmonary histiocytosis X. Many nuclei have characteristic notched or folded appearance. Note mitotic figures. *Inset,* Electron micrograph of characteristic cytoplasmic organelle of Langerhans type of histiocyte.

ular infiltrates that may resolve or may become reticular with the subsequent appearance of bullae or honeycombing. Sparing of the costophrenic angles is characteristic but nonspecific.[583]

The pathologic features were well described by Auld,[578] as well as subsequent observers.[580,582] At low power a striking feature is the nodular pattern with intervening normal or near normal lung. Many lesions are centered on bronchioles or small vessels. Within the nodules the interstitium is infiltrated by a mixed cell population including lymphocytes, plasma cells, eosinophils, and some typical macrophages, as well as the characteristic histiocytosis X (Hx) cells. These cells have an indistinct pale pink or amphophilic cytoplasm and an elongated or reniform nucleus that is folded or notched (Fig. 22-43). Under the electron microscope they resemble monocytes, having few lysosomes or phagosomes. They contain characteristic cytoplasmic organelles, the Birbeck granules, which appear as pentalaminar rod-shaped structures, 35 to 40 nm wide, located both deep within the cytoplasm and at the cell periphery where they fuse with the plasma membrane. Cells with these

organelles are rarely found in other diseases of the lung.[581] Although they are not pathognomonic, their presence is strong evidence for a diagnosis of histiocytosis X. The granules can be identified by electron microscopy in bronchoalveolar lavage cells from patients with histiocytosis.[579]

The early nodular lesions are highly cellular with a predominance of Hx cells. Mitotic figures are present in some cells. Rarely invasion and obliteration of vessels by the Hx cells lead to necrosis or cavitation of the nodules, but necrosis is usually absent. With healing the center of the lesion becomes more fibrous, but at the periphery an infiltrate of Hx cells extends into the interstitium of neighboring alveolar walls, giving the lesion a stellate configuration. Ultimately the lesions heal, leaving a stellate scar. The pathologic differential diagnosis is discussed elsewhere.[5] The principal consideration is usually eosinophilic pneumonia. In eosinophilic pneumonia the low-power pattern is not nodular and the cellular infiltrate is predominantly intra-alveolar, whereas in histiocytosis it is interstitial. The eosinophilic abscesses characteristic of eosinophilic pneumonia are not found in histiocytosis. The nuclear characteristics of the mononuclear phagocytes in the two conditions differ, and in difficult cases electron microscopy can be used to confirm the nature of the mononuclear phagocytes.

The course of localized pulmonary histiocytosis is extremely variable. The majority of patients undergo spontaneous or induced arrest or remission. In some cases cysts or bullae develop leading to recurrent pneumothorax. A few, probably less than 10%, progress to disabling interstitial fibrosis and death from respiratory failure or cor pulmonale.[583]

Sarcoidosis

Sarcoidosis is a systemic disease that involves the thoracic organs in 90% of cases.[603] Scadding has defined it as a disease "characterized by the presence in all of several affected organs and tissues of non-caseating epithelioid-cell granulomas proceeding either to resolution or to conversion into featureless hyaline connective tissue."[600] This definition does not mention causation, about which nothing is known, nor an underlying alteration in immunologic reactivity, about which much remains to be learned. It is not clear whether sarcoidosis is a syndrome of many causes or a single entity.

Sarcoidosis most commonly affects adults between 20 and 40 years of age and is rare below 10 years of age. Its distribution is worldwide. In the United States the prevalence is more than 10 times higher in blacks than in whites and greater in women than in men.[596] In South Africa the prevalence is also higher in blacks.[597] In Europe the prevalence is highest in Scandinavians and there is no distinct sex predilection.

Pathology

The diagnostic feature of sarcoidosis is the noncaseating granuloma, a compact nodule of epithelioid cells with a few lymphocytes, monocytes, and macrophages (Fig. 22-44).[586,600,602] As a rule necrosis is absent, but even in cases that are clinically typical and from which infection is excluded, a few granulomas may have a small amount of granular eosinophilic necrosis in the center.[602] The epithelioid cells are generally similar to those in tuberculosis when viewed by light and electron microscopy.[578,605] By electron microscopy two types of epithelioid cells have been described,[598] one with extensively developed endoplasmic reticulum and few granules or vacuoles and the other with many vacuoles containing finely granular material. They may represent different phases in the life cycle of a single cell line, since cells with transitional ultrastructural features were seen. The epithelioid cells appear to be derived from the mononuclear phagocyte series, but owing to their paucity of phagosomes and well-developed endoplasmic reticulum they have been interpreted as a poorly phagocytic secretory form.

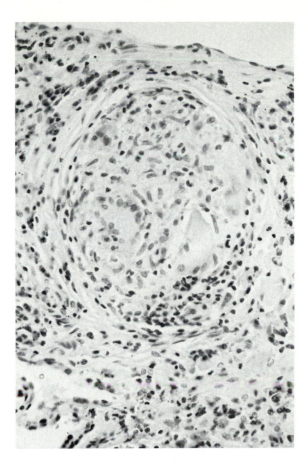

Fig. 22-44. Noncaseating granuloma in sarcoidosis. Compact epithelioid granuloma with giant cells. Early fibrous capsule has formed.

Giant cells of either foreign body or Langhans' type are common. Their ultrastructure and the results of thymidine labeling studies suggest that they form by fusion of epithelioid cells.[587] They may contain a variety of inclusions, none of which can be considered specific for sarcoidosis.[602] Asteroid bodies are stellate, strongly eosinophilic bodies that are seen in giant cells in a variety of diseases. The few ultrastructural studies indicate that they are derived from the cytosphere.[588] Schaumann or conchoidal bodies are concentric lamellae of iron- and calcium-containing material associated often with birefringent crystals that lie between the lamellae. They vary in size from 10 to 30 μm and may be either in the cytoplasm of an individual giant cell or apparently extracellular in close association with several giant cells. Some giant cells contain colorless birefringent crystals 1 to 25 μm in size. Electron probe microanalysis has shown only elements that are compatible with an endogenous origin for the crystals. Some, at least, are calcium oxalate.

The earliest stages of the sarcoid granuloma are not well known. Rosen and associates[601] observed a nongranulomatous interstitial infiltrate of mononuclear cells

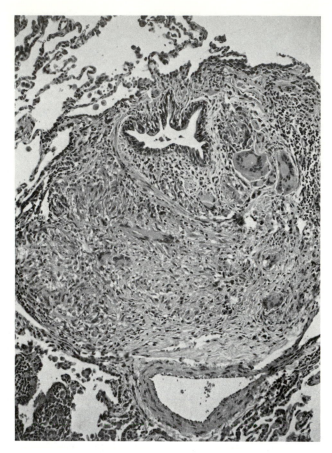

Fig. 22-45. Sarcoidosis. Involvement of bronchiole by granulomas.

Table 22-3. Frequency of major organ involvement in sarcoidosis

Organ system	United States (%)	Worldwide (%)
Thoracic	92	87
Reticuloendothelial	50	28
Ocular	15	15
Skin	23	9
Erythema nodosum	10	17
Salivary gland	7	4
Nervous system	3	4
Osseous	6	3

From James, G.D., and Neville, E.: Pathobiol. Annu. 7:31, 1977.

accompanying nonfibrotic granulomas in early sarcoidosis. They propose that the granulomas evolve from a nonspecific alveolitis.

The healing of a granuloma begins with the appearance of a thin fibrous capsule enclosing the granuloma. In cases of longer duration the capsule is thicker and formed of coarser lamellae of hyalinized connective tissue. In old and quiescent lesions the periphery of the granuloma is replaced by hyalinized connective tissue, often leaving only a few macrophages or a giant cell or two in the center. Eventually these too are replaced by fibrous tissue.

Sarcoid granulomas can involve any of the structures of the lung.[589,590,602] They can be found in airways of any size (Fig. 22-45), in walls of blood vessels, and in the pleura. Parenchymal granulomas are commonly interstitial, but some appear to develop within alveolar spaces. Conglomeration of granulomas matted together by fibrosis can give rise to large nodules. The healing and scarring late in the process can produce honeycombing, bullae, or upper lobe cavities that lack the caseous or liquefied contents of tuberculous cavities. Other organs are also involved (Table 22-3), and involvement of some,

notably the heart and nervous system, may determine the outcome of the disease.

Natural history

The natural history of sarcoidosis can be followed sequentially from study of the chest roentgenogram.[593,594] The stages are as follows:

Stage 1 Bilateral hilar lymphadenopathy
Stage 2 Hilar adenopathy with pulmonary infiltrates
Stage 3 Pulmonary infiltrates

The earliest manifestation of sarcoidosis is bilateral hilar lymph node enlargement without roentgenographic changes in the parenchyma. Some patients at this stage have the cutaneous lesions of erythema nodosum. This combination is particularly common in Scandinavia, where it is known as Löfgren's syndrome. Although the parenchyma appears normal roentgenographically, transbronchial biopsies show the presence of either nonspecific alveolitis or granulomas in a high proportion of patients. Pulmonary function is abnormal in only 20% to 30% of patients, however, and the degree of abnormality is mild.

The disease in 50% of patients at this stage will regress spontaneously within a year. In others it will take longer. In only 10% does pulmonary parenchymal disease of sufficient severity to be roentgenographically detectable develop. Patients with parenchymal infiltrates and hilar adenopathy seen on the roentgenogram usually have pulmonary dysfunction. In only half will the chest roentgenogram return to normal. Patients with parenchymal disease without hilar adenopathy (stage 3) rarely improve and usually have dysfunction. Reduced diffusion capacity and restriction of ventilation are the rule, but concomitant airflow obstruction is also common. The airflow obstruction probably results from direct involvement of bronchi and bronchioles by granulomas.

Diagnosis

The diagnosis of sarcoidosis can be based on the clinical findings plus the demonstration of noncaseating granulomas in any involved tissue.[600] Transbronchial biopsy has proved to be a valuable tool, disclosing granulomas in more than 90% of patients with roentgenographic lung involvement and roughly half of those with stage 1 disease.[602] It should be emphasized that the histologic findings are not distinguishable from those in the infectious granulomas. Staining for tubercle bacilli and fungi should always be done, and even when no organisms are seen, the pathologist would be foolish to make a stronger statement than that the lesions are "compatible with sarcoidosis."

The Kveim-Siltzbach reaction is a potentially useful diagnostic test.[586,597,600] An antigen prepared from involved lymph node or spleen is injected intradermally. Three to 6 weeks later if a nodule has appeared, biopsy is performed and the specimen is observed microscopically. The presence of noncaseating granulomas constitutes a positive result. With carefully prepared and standardized antigen there are very few false-positive reactions. False-negative results usually occur in those with chronic inactive disease. The antigen is not approved by the U.S. Food and Drug Administration and is not generally available. Laudon[598a] has said of sarcoidosis, "The only specific test is hard to spell and illegal to transport from state to state."

There are abnormalities in the serum of sarcoid patients, but none are specific. Hyperglobulinemia is common, hypercalcemia less so. Response of the hypercalcemia to corticosteroids is a helpful diagnostic feature. Elevation in angiotensin-converting enzyme (ACE) occurs in 40% to 80% of patients with sarcoidosis, more often in those with active disease. However, it also occurs in a small proportion of patients with diseases such as miliary tuberculosis, histoplasmosis, hypersensitivity pneumonitis, or idiopathic interstitial fibrosis, which can easily be confused with sarcoidosis. Consequently ACE elevation should be interpreted in the light of other clinical data. The ACE level decreases with corticosteroid therapy and is a valuable tool for following disease activity and effect of therapy.

Etiology and pathogenesis

The etiology of sarcoidosis remains unknown. The possibility of involvement by the tubercle bacillus has been raised but remains doubtful. Granules of acid-fast material are occasionally stainable in epithelioid cells, but these may be lipid sequestered in lysosomes and need not be derived from bacilli. The ingenious proposal that sarcoid patients fail to produce antibodies to common mycobacteriophages, resulting in lysis of the bacteria and hence failure to detect them, has not been confirmed. Reports of transmission of an infectious agent to animals have been difficult to repeat.[599] Although the reactivity to Kveim antigen shared by patients with active disease worldwide suggests that a single exogenous antigen

accounts for the disease, the nature of the hypothetical agent is obscure.

Immunologic abnormalities have long been recognized in patients with sarcoidosis.[604] Hyperglobulinemia, partial anergy to common skin test antigens, decreased blood lymphocyte transformation in response to phytohemagglutinin, subnormal numbers of circulating T lymphocytes, and increased numbers of circulating null cells have been relatively consistent abnormalities. Circulating immune complexes have been found in a few patients.[597] These findings pointed to a defect in cell-mediated immunity with overreactivity of B cells, a result difficult to reconcile with the histologic finding of granulomas, a hallmark of delayed-type hypersensitivity. Subsequent evidence, however, showed that some peripheral blood T cells were activated. Lymphocytes retrieved from the lungs of patients with sarcoidosis by bronchoalveolar lavage showed properties quite different from those of the circulating lymphocytes. Both total and activated T lymphocytes were increased in number, the ratio of T-helper to T-suppresser cells was increased, and cultured lymphocytes produced lymphokines and chemotactic factors for monocytes, which might be involved in the generation of granulomas.[590,591,595] Adherence of lymphocytes to macrophages has been seen in lavage cell sediments, indicating direct lymphocyte-macrophage interaction. All these observations point to an active cell-mediated immune response in the lung along with increased stimulation of the B cells modulated by helper T cells. One factor in the relatively depressed cell-mediated immune function in the circulation and skin tests may be sequestration of effector cells in sites of active inflammation. Thus much of the immunologic evidence now points to a cell-mediated immune reaction to an unknown antigen as a plausible pathogenesis for sarcoidosis.

Necrotizing sarcoid granulomatosis

The relationship between the condition that Liebow designated necrotizing sarcoid granulomatosis and ordinary sarcoidosis is unclear.[574] Kveim testing has not been reported in the former condition. Some clinical differences have been noted. Roughly half of the patients with necrotizing sarcoid granulomatosis have systemic symptoms such as fever, sweating, malaise, and weight loss. Chest pain is common, usually described as a dull ache and rarely pleuritic. A few patients are asymptomatic. The chest roentgenogram shows bilateral nodular densities or less often a miliary pattern or ill-defined infiltrates. In a few cases lesions appear to be solitary. Pathologically the lesions consist of a collection of epithelioid granulomas united in a background of fibrous tissue and nonspecific inflammatory cells. The granulomas are less discrete or encapsulated than those of typical sarcoidosis. Irregular, sometimes extensive patches of fibrinoid or coagulative necrosis are present. Central necrosis of individual granulomas, as occurs in tuberculosis, is not a feature. Vasculitis, which can take several morphologic forms, involves both veins and arteries. Vessels can be invaded or obliterated by granulomas or can be involved by an inflammatory process resembling giant cell arteritis with a preponderance of the giant cell reaction associated with the external elastic lamina, or the vasculitis can be a nonspecific mononuclear inflammatory infiltration of vessel walls. Extrapulmonary manifestations are rare. The hilar lymph nodes have been enlarged in roentgenograms of the chest in only a few patients although small granulomas in hilar lymph nodes are sometimes seen microscopically. A few patients have had hepatic granulomas or uveitis.[592] Cultures and stains have not demonstrated organisms. Although only a few patients have had adequate follow-up monitoring, the course of the disease generally has been favorable. Patients have either remained stable or have had regression of lesions with steroid or cytotoxic therapy. Recrudescences have been reported in a few instances.

The generally benign course, occurrence of epithelioid granulomas, and failure to recover an infectious agent are all properties shared with sarcoidosis. Granulomatous vasculitis is not uncommon in sarcoidosis, and nodules of confluent granulomas also occur. Necrosis is infrequent and mild in sarcoidosis but appears to be explicable in necrotizing sarcoid granulomatosis as infarction resulting from the vasculitis rather than as a characteristic of the granulomas. On the other hand, the absence of roentgenographic hilar adenopathy and the rarity with which extrapulmonary lesions have been described in necrotizing sarcoid granulomatosis are arguments against the identity of the two diseases.

MISCELLANEOUS LUNG DISEASES
Alveolar proteinosis

In 1958 Rosen, Castleman, and Liebow[617] described 27 patients with a new disease in which the distal airspaces of the lung become filled with a curious exudate consisting of granular eosinophilic material containing cholesterol clefts, occasional naked nuclei, and eosinophilic globules that are 5 to 20 μm in size and appear to be the ghosts of cells, an impression verified by electron microscopy.[611] In some areas there are numerous lipid-filled macrophages, whereas in other regions the exudate is nearly acellular (Fig. 22-46). The exudate stains strongly with the periodic acid–Schiff reaction, which led Rosen and associates to conclude that the intra-alveolar material is glycoprotein. They also had biochemical analyses that indicated a high lipid content.[617] The alveolar septa are only minimally abnormal with focal regions of type II cell hyperplasia and a few collections of lipid-filled interstitial macrophages but little inflammation. The nature of the intra-alveolar material has been stud-

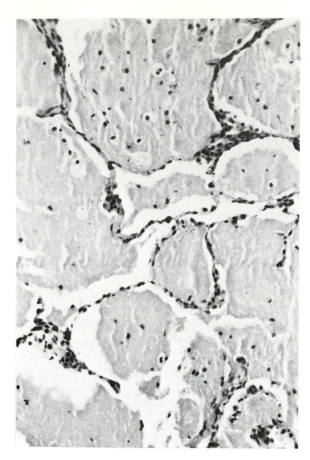

Fig. 22-46. Alveolar proteinosis. Alveoli are filled with flocculent exudate with a few nuclei, remnants of degenerated cells. Alveolar walls are normal.

ied extensively by electron microscopy and histochemical and biochemical analyses of specimens obtained by bronchoalveolar lavage.[607,610-612,614,618] The exudate contains serum proteins, some cell debris, and large amounts of alveolar surfactant including both the characteristic saturated phospholipids and specific surfactant proteins. The serum proteins present are of low molecular weight. The absence of high–molecular weight components militates against a major alteration in the permeability of the alveolar capillary membrane.

The reason for the accumulation of this material is unknown. Because other materials are present, it is probably not a simple primary overproduction of surfactant.[608] The material comprising the exudate is not itself surface active, probably because of the presence of other components that are inhibitory.[611,612] There is evidence that the intra-alveolar material turns over very slowly, suggesting a primary defect in alveolar clearance.[615] The cause of the disease is unknown. Persons of any age can be affected including young children. Increased numbers of birefringent crystals are found in the lungs of many patients, which might indicate an occupational etiology or impaired alveolar clearance.[613] The occurrence of proteinosis in patients heavily exposed to silica (p. 908) is evidence in favor of the former interpretation. An association of proteinosis with hematologic malignancy has also been observed.[606]

The clinical manifestations of alveolar proteinosis are variable, ranging from nearly asymptomatic to life-threatening hypoxemia. The chest roentgenogram in uncomplicated cases shows an alveolar filling pattern with a variable distribution but often resembling the butterfly distribution of the pulmonary edema of heart failure without cardiomegaly or effusions. As a rule disability is surprisingly mild considering the degree of roentgenographic change. Infections with fungi, nocardiae, or mycobacteria are a common and serious complication, explainable in part by the presence of a nutritious broth within the airspaces[616] and in part by an acquired defect in the function of the alveolar macrophages, which are already burdened with a heavy load of lipid and debris.[609] The course of the disease is unpredictable, with some patients having spontaneous clearing while others deteriorate.

Alveolar microlithiasis

Alveolar microlithiasis is a rare disease occurring in sporadic form and in familial groupings.[622,625,626] Persons of all ages can be affected, the youngest recorded being a premature infant of 29 weeks' gestational age and the oldest an octogenarian at the time of death. The largest number of patients become symptomatic between 30 and 60 years of age, but roughly 25% of all patients are children. The disease is characterized by the deposition of concentrically laminated calcified bodies (calcospheritis) within the alveoli. Grossly the lungs are heavy, firm, and difficult to slice. They are said to feel like sandpaper. The calcospherites, which consist mainly of calcium phosphate, range up to several hundred microns in size and by light microscopy are found predominantly within alveolar spaces. The alveolar walls are usually little affected. In some cases interstitial fibrosis is present and some of the calcospherites are in an interstitial location. Electron microscopy shows that the calcospherites seem to form in relation to collagen by a process initiated by the shedding of matrix vesicles from connective tissue cells much like other forms of ectopic mineralization. Rarely calcospherites have also been found in the submucosa of the bronchi or extrathoracic sites.

Clinically the mild dyspnea contrasts with the dramatic miliary roentgenographic shadowing, which spares only the apices. Many patients are asymptomatic when the disease is discovered. After a number of years restrictive lung disease and cor pulmonale may develop.

The calcospherites should be distinguished from other forms of pulmonary concretions. Corpora amylacea are strongly periodic acid–Schiff–positive bodies with a dense central nidus surrounded by a cortex with fine radial striations.[621] They are indistinguishable morphologically from the corpora amylacea that are common in the brain and prostate. Their cause is unknown, and they are found in both normal and diseased lungs, usually in small numbers. So-called blue bodies are laminated basophilic concretions, 12 to 25 μm in diameter, that contain calcium carbonate and small amounts of iron deposited in a mucopolysaccharide matrix. They are found in association with macrophages, usually in lungs with interstitial pneumonias of the DIP type.[620] They never attain the size of the calcospherites of microlithiasis and are not detectable as calcific density on chest roentgenograms.

Metastatic calcification and ossification

Metastatic calcification is the result of elevation of the product of ionized calcium and phosphate. It is a common finding at autopsy in patients with chronic renal disease,[619] destructive bone metastases, or multiple myeloma and has also been reported in milk-alkali syndrome and primary hyperparathyroidism. The calcific deposits are interstitial, initially localizing in basement membranes and on the elastic fibers of alveolar walls. Eventually the whole interstitial compartment and the walls of blood vessels become encrusted. The deposits are basophilic, initially appearing as fine stippling of the connective tissue fibers and eventually growing into broad bands of homogeneous brittle basophilic material. Frequently the involved alveolar septa are thickened by the presence of loose fibrillar connective tissue, and at times there is intra-alveolar fibrosis as well. It is not clear whether the fibrosis is a reaction to the calcium or conditions in tissue undergoing fibrosis favor deposition of calcium salts, but the former seems more likely.

Most cases of metastatic calcifications are clinically inapparent and are not detected roentgenographically. When severe, metastatic calcification can lead to restrictive lung disease with impaired gas exchange. The roentgenograms show nonspecific infiltrates that are usually not recognizable as calcium. The clinical diagnosis can be made by demonstrating the uptake of bone-seeking radionuclides.

Bone forms in the lung under a number of circumstances. Ossification of the bronchial cartilages is common in the aged. In tracheobronchopathia osteoplastica, nodules of cartilage and bone form in the submucosal connective tissue of the trachea and major bronchi. The affected airways are stiff, and the mucosal surface is rough and knobby. The nodules of bone and cartilage may be entirely within the submucosa or fixed to the perichondrium of the bronchial cartilages. The bone may have fatty or hemopoietic marrow. Diffuse pulmonary ossification has two forms: granular and branched.[623,624] The granular form usually occurs in the context of chronic congestion, especially that caused by mitral stenosis. Spicules of lamellar bone are found in the alveolar spaces attached to alveolar septa. The spicules are irregularly shaped and do not contain marrow. Ossification occurs in the interstitium of chronically fibrotic lung in a racemose or branched pattern. Marrow may be present but frequently is not.

Amyloidosis of the lung

Amyloidosis affecting the lung usually takes one of three forms.[632] Tracheobronchial amyloidosis is usually limited to the respiratory tract and causes bronchial obstruction manifest by wheezing, stridor, or recurrent infection distal to the obstruction.[629] A single bronchus or multiple bronchi may be affected. The gross amyloid deposits may be plaquelike, circumferential, or polypoid. The amyloid is deposited in the submucosa and may surround and compress mucous glands, which then atrophy. Nodules of amyloid occurring in the lung periphery usually appear clinically as single or multiple masses with few symptoms.[631] Multiple nodules usually appear synchronously, although in one patient two amyloid nodules developed 9 years apart.[628] Microscopically amyloid

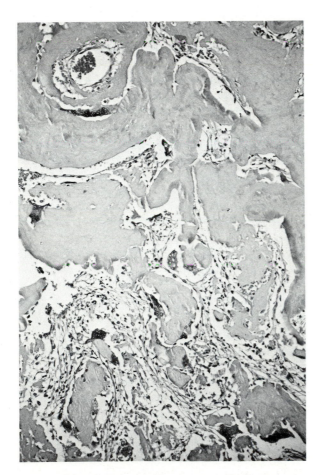

Fig. 22-47. Nodular pulmonary amyloidosis. Giant cells associated with amorphous deposits of amyloid.

nodules are composed of deposits of brittle-appearing, homogeneous eosinophilic material, usually embedded in fibrous tissue containing an infiltrate of plasma cells. Multinucleated giant cells applied to the surface of the amyloid deposits are often conspicuous (Fig. 22-47). Areas of cartilage and ossification are not unusual.

Diffuse septal amyloidosis is usually a manifestation of generalized primary amyloidosis, although in a few case reports it was limited to the lungs or part of generalized secondary amyloidosis.[627] The amyloid is deposited as homogeneous eosinophilic material in alveolar septa and vessels. The clinical manifestations in the lung are usually overshadowed by associated heart disease when septal amyloidosis is part of generalized primary amyloidosis. Because the amyloid is deposited in the interstitium displacing the capillaries, diffusion of oxygen is little affected until late when there is obliteration of capillaries.[630] The tinctorial and ultrastructural properties of amyloid are discussed elsewhere.

Lymphangiomyomatosis

Lymphangiomyomatosis is a diffuse proliferative disease of smooth muscle involving the lung and in some cases neighboring lymphatic structures including the thoracic duct.[633-635] Grossly the lungs are large but show widespread, severe honeycombing. Microscopic sections show widespread smooth muscle proliferation along the course of lymphatics in the perivenous and bronchoarterial connective tissue spaces and pleura, as well as within alveolar septa.[635] The absence of inflammation distinguishes lymphangiomyomatosis from other interstitial lung diseases, and the distribution of the smooth muscle proliferation, conforming after a fashion to anatomic structures, distinguishes it from benign metastasizing leiomyoma in which the muscle forms distinct nodules.

The clinical features of lymphangiomyomatosis are as distinctive as its morbid anatomy. The disease almost exclusively affects women of childbearing age.[635] Compression of veins by the perivenous smooth muscle proliferation leads to hemoptysis; compression of small airways results in severe expiratory airflow obstruction, air trapping, and in some cases repeated pneumothoraces. When there is involvement of neighboring lymphatics, chylous pleural effusion may develop. The chest roentgenogram shows the unique combination of severe linear reticulation, indicative of advanced interstitial lung disease, with greatly enlarged lungs and low diaphragms, indicative of severe air trapping.[634] Similar features are seen in the lungs of some patients with tuberous sclerosis.

Drug- and radiation-induced pulmonary disease

Pulmonary disease is estimated to account for only 1% to 5% of drug-induced disease. With the development of multiple drug and radiation regimens for the treatment of malignancy, it appears to be increasing in importance. Too many drugs have been implicated as pulmonary toxins to discuss individually. Recent reviews have discussed drug-induced pulmonary reactions according to drug implicated[643] and type of tissue response.[636] Some drug-induced effects on the respiratory system, such as bronchospasm or depressed ventilation, are not visible to the pathologist. The reactions that the pathologist can detect include pulmonary edema, diffuse alveolar damage, chronic interstitial pneumonia, eosinophilic pneumonia, hypersensitivity pneumonitis (allergic alveolitis), lupuslike reactions, vasculitis, and primary pulmonary hypertension.[636] As with drug reactions in other organs, some pulmonary drug reactions are toxic effects that are dose related and reproduceable in experimental animals, whereas others are idiosyncratic, occurring in only a few of the patients who receive the drug and at highly variable doses. Idiosyncratic reactions may result from either metabolic differences between individuals or immunologic (allergic) reactions. The situation is complicated by the observation that a given drug may cause disease on either a toxic or an allergic basis. For example, bleomycin, a valuable antitumor drug, causes direct dose-related toxicity that can be reproduced in a variety of animals. Ordinarily toxicity is not seen until doses of 300 to 400 mg have been given, and the histopathologic picture is that of an organizing interstitial pneumonia.[642] In an occasional patient, respiratory disease develops at much lower doses[639] or may have an atypical histologic picture suggesting hypersensitivity, such as eosinophilic pneumonia.[638] Methotrexate is implicated in both hypersensitivity pneumonitis and toxic interstitial fibrosis. Interactions between drugs or between radiation and drugs may occur.[646] Prior irradiation may predispose patients to drug reactions at doses lower than expected. Oxygen therapy also modifies the response to drugs. In experimental animals, doses of oxygen that are nontoxic in themselves can convert self-limited bleomycin-induced fibrosis to progressive fibrosis. It is now common to encounter patients with diffuse lung disease who have received multiple cytotoxic drugs and often thoracic radiation as well. Biopsy examination shows either diffuse alveolar damage or nonspecific interstitial pneumonia, and no infectious organism can be found. Although no single therapeutic agent has been given to toxic levels, lung injury probably reflects the cumulative damage produced by several agents.[644,646]

The most common morphologic response to cytotoxic drugs is diffuse alveolar damage evolving into chronic interstitial pneumonia. The pathologic sequence has been described in detail with electron microscopy in the case of busulfan[641] and bleomycin.[636] Other alkylating agents produce similar changes. Early the alveolar spaces contain cellular debris and fibrin. Hyaline membranes line many airspaces. Organization of the intra-alveolar fibrin and hyaline membranes with migration of alveolar epithelium over the surface of the hyaline membranes leads to a picture of mixed interstitial and intra-alveolar fibrosis. Marked atypism of the regenerating alveolar epithelium is characteristic of the pulmonary fibrosis seen with alkylating agents. The epithelial cells are large with irregular outlines. The cytoplasm is abundant, and the nuclei are large with prominent nucleoli. Squamous metaplasia and atypism may be found in the airways as well and can be recognized in exfoliated cells in the sputum.

The acute phase of radiation pneumonitis is difficult to distinguish histologically from other forms of acute lung injury.[640,645] The hyaline membranes, enlarged hyperplastic epithelial cells, alveolar septal edema, and sparse inflammation are nonspecific. The chronic phase is characterized by a poorly cellular fibrillar eosinophilic fibrosis affecting alveolar walls and blood vessels.[640,645] The vascular lumina are shrunken and irregular. The subendothelial space of many larger vessels is edematous with an occasional inflammatory cell. Absence of inflammatory cells other than an occasional plasma cell, fibrillar quality of the fibrosis, and atypical nuclei of the interstitial fibroblasts are all features that help distinguish radiation fibrosis from fibrosis of other causes.

The relation between dose, time, and histologic reaction is complex.[637] Jennings and Arden[640] found chronic radiation fibrosis as early as 6 months after high-dose irradiation, while in other cases acute radiation pneumonitis was still present 2 years after irradiation.

Pulmonary hemorrhage

Bleeding from pulmonary capillaries occurs in a number of settings. As noted previously, immunologic injury from either antibasal lamina antibodies or immune complex deposition can produce capillary bleeding.[654] Pulmonary hemorrhage can also occur in association with glomerulonephritis in the absence of detectable immunologic reactions in the lung. Hemorrhage is common at autopsy in severe heart failure where it probably results from a combination of hemodynamic factors and alveolar injury.[647] In thrombocytopenic patients minor alveolar injury can result in hemorrhage. This explains the occasional life-threatening hemorrhages in leukemic patients.[649,655] There remains a small group of patients in whom repeated episodes of pulmonary hemorrhage occur in the absence of any discernible predisposing illness. To this group the diagnosis of idiopathic pulmonary hemosiderosis applies. Eighty percent of patients with idiopathic pulmonary hemosiderosis are children, and most of the remainder are young adults.[656] The illness usually begins with mild episodes of intrapulmonary bleeding associated with cough and dyspnea. Occasionally the first episode is one of brisk hemoptysis. The respiratory bleeding is usually accompanied by the development of iron-deficiency anemia. Whether the anemia is entirely explicable on the basis of blood loss and sequestration of iron in the lung is controversial, but there is no evidence of hemolysis. When blood is injected into the lungs of experimental animals, they can mobilize the iron,[652] leading some to question whether there is some additional defect that prevents patients with pulmonary hemosiderosis from mobilizing their iron.

Repeated hemorrhages lead to the development of pulmonary fibrosis, the accumulation of large numbers of hemosiderin-filled macrophages (siderophages) in the alveoli, and iron deposition on the vascular elastic fibers. The basis for the bleeding is not clear, and neither auto-antibodies nor immune complexes have been demonstrable in the circulation. In a few cases abnormalities of capillary basement membranes have been seen with electron microscopy, but they have been of different types in each report.[650,651] Many investigators have failed to detect any abnormalities by electron microscopy or immunofluorescence.[648,653] The course of idiopathic pulmonary hemosiderosis is variable. Patients can die during an initial episode or survive for many years with recurring episodes leading to fibrosis and pulmonary insufficiency. Remissions of many years' duration may occur. In the cases reviewed by Soergel and Sommers[656] the average survival was 3 years.

Aspiration pneumonia

The term *aspiration pneumonia* is used to cover a number of quite different clinicopathologic processes caused by different agents that have a common means of entry to the lung.[664] The aspiration of infected material from the oral cavity can lead to bacterial pneumonia often caused by anaerobic organisms as discussed previously. The aspiration of gastric contents with a pH below 2.5 produces hemorrhagic edema in the involved region of lung and, if extensive, is rapidly fatal. The bronchi are hemorrhagic, and the lung exudes frothy fluid.[664] In patients dying rapidly there is massive pulmonary edema. Survivors for 2 to 3 days show infiltration of neutrophils, hyaline membranes, and sloughing of the bronchial epithelium. The clinical picture is that of the adult respiratory distress syndrome.

Quite different is the response of food particle aspiration that occurs in those who have difficulty swallowing because of neurologic or esophageal disease or who have undergone certain types of radical head and neck surgery.[664] Small food particles that are aspirated lodge in respiratory bronchioles. In the first few hours there is hemorrhage into the airspaces accompanied by infiltration of neutrophils and monocytes. Between 24 and 48 hours after aspiration a monocyte-macrophage response becomes predominate, and by 48 to 72 hours distinct granulomas with conspicuous foreign body giant cells

have formed about the food particles. Food particles (vegetable cells or skeletal muscle) and squamous cells can be recognized within the granulomas. The granulomas heal by fibrosis, and in the late phase the appearance of fibrous nodules with giant cells closely simulates an infectious granuloma. The clinical setting and localization strictly at the termination of the bronchial tree are helpful clues to the pathologic diagnosis. Repeated small aspirations can lead to fibrosis of the lower lung zones.

Aspiration of large particles is common in young children but also occurs in adults. Particles blocking the trachea can cause suffocation, and those lodging in major bronchi can cause air trapping or obstructive pneumonia and bronchiectasis.

Lipid pneumonia

Aspiration of lipid is the principal cause of exogenous lipid pneumonia. The lipid is usually mineral oil taken as a laxative, as a vehicle for medication, or as nose drops.[658,663] Lipid can also be inhaled while burning[661] or when added to smoking tobacco as a humectant.[660] Although relatively inert, mineral oil stimulates a chronic inflammatory response with scarring. Clinically exogenous lipid pneumonia can occur as a diffuse infiltrative

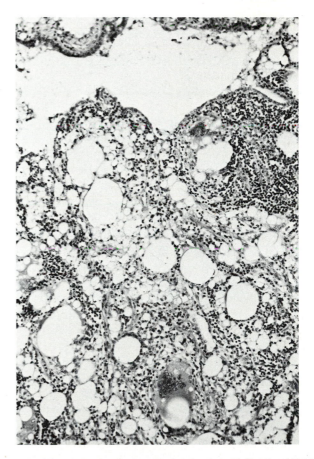

Fig. 22-48. Lipid pneumonia. Vacuoles are sites of dissolved lipid. Nodules of lymphocytes are common.

process involving the lower lobes or can form a localized mass (paraffinoma) that closely simulates a neoplasm.[658] Grossly the lesions appear as a yellow, doughy area of consolidation or as a discrete, yellow, hard mass. Retraction of the pleura over the mass enhances the resemblance to carcinoma. Microscopically much lipid is within macrophages in both the airspaces and interstitium, but in cases of long duration with severe fibrosis large extracellular lipid globules are trapped within fibrous tissue. Lipid vacuoles vary from micrometers to tens of micrometers in diameter, the largest being extracellular where they may be partly enclosed by multinucleated giant cells. Nodular aggregates of lymphocytes are almost invariably present (Fig. 22-48). The diagnosis can be made without biopsy by identifying lipid-laden macrophages in the sputum.

Lipid pneumonia arising from the retention of lipids released during the breakdown of tissue is known as endogenous lipid pneumonia. It occurs in the parenchyma distal to an obstructed bronchus or on a microscopic scale distal to blocked bronchioles and alveolar ducts. The affected tissue is consolidated and speckled bright yellow. The lipid is found in the form of uniform droplets 1 μm or less in diameter in the cytoplasm of macrophages, which are aggregated within the airspaces. Extracellular cholesteral clefts with giant cells are not unusual.

The histologic features of the two types of lipid pneumonia are distinctive, and it is rarely necessary to resort to histochemical examination to distinguish them. In frozen sections both types of lipid stain with Sudan-type stains, but only the endogenous type blackens with OsO_4.

Lung collapse and pneumothorax

The expansion of the lung is maintained by the pressure difference between the alveoli, which are normally in free communication with the atmosphere, and the subatmospheric pressure of the pleural space. The causes of collapse (atelectasis) of the lung are pleural filling, bronchial obstruction with absorption of the intraalveolar gas, and changes in surfactant function. The lung collapses when compressed by pleural effusions, tumors, other space-occupying intrathoracic lesions, or elevation of the diaphragm. Lung collapsed because of entrapment by thick pleural fibrosis can have a tumorlike roentgenographic image called rounded atelectasis. In pneumothorax the lung collapses because air gains access to the pleural space, permitting the negative pleural pressure to rise. This can occur as the result of thoracic trauma, perforation of the esophagus, extension of lung abscess or other infections through the pleura with formation of a bronchopleural fistula, or rupture of air-containing cysts or bullae associated with emphysema or other forms of diffuse or localized lung disease. In young adults without generalized underlying pulmonary disease, pneumothorax develops most often in tall slender persons who have a few localized bullae, usually in the upper lung fields.[659] The histologic changes in the walls of the bullae are nonspecific, consisting of fibrosis, chronic inflammation, focal alveolar epithelial hyperplasia, and a few hemosiderin-laden macrophages.[659] Neither the underlying cause of the bullae nor the reason for their rupture is known, but it seems doubtful that they can be explained by the greater vertical gradient in transpulmonary pressure that exists in taller persons because of gravity. A few such persons have abnormalities of connective tissue such as Marfan's syndrome or Ehlers-Danlos syndrome.

Both the parietal and the visceral pleura respond to pneumothorax by the exudation of fibrin associated with a proliferation of macrophages, giant cells, mesothelial cells, and eosinophils known as reactive eosinophilic pleuritis.[657] It is important not to confuse this nonspecific reaction to pneumothorax with the lesions of eosinophilic granuloma, which is one underlying cause of pneumothorax.

Behind a totally occluded bronchus, the absorption of alveolar gas can produce collapse of the lung. This happens rapidly in patients breathing 100% oxygen when, for example, mucus plugs an airway. In persons breathing room air, however, relatively minor volume loss follows bronchial obstruction because the nitrogen in the airspaces is absorbed only slowly and is replaced by edema fluid. Gradual occlusion of a bronchus leads to lipid pneumonia, chronic organizing pneumonia, and bronchiectasis, rather than simple collapse.

Shallow respiration also leads to alveolar collapse as a result of rising surface tension in the alveolar lining. The process is incompletely understood, but deep ventilation acts as a stimulus to surfactant secretion by type II epithelial cells and is required for the formation of a stable surface film. Collapse owing to shallow ventilation is particularly likely to occur in postoperative patients whose respiration is depressed because of anesthetics and who have a shallow pattern of ventilation because of incisional pain.[662] The administration of oxygen only compounds the problem.

If a small volume of lung is collapsed, the pleura is dark and sunken below the level of the pink, well-expanded lung. When an entire lobe or lung is affected, the pleura is wrinkled. The involved parenchyma is dark, firm, and without crepitance. Microscopically the alveolar walls are compressed, giving the tissue a solid appearance. The vascularity of the alveolar walls helps distinguish normal airless lung from fibrosis.

After collapse there is a progressive rise in pulmonary vascular resistance in the involved better-ventilated tissue. Several mechanisms are probably involved, including hypoxia, tortuosity and distortion of the vascular bed, and reflex vasoconstriction.

CHRONIC AIRFLOW LIMITATION
Definitions

The term "chronic obstructive pulmonary disease" (COPD) is an unfortunate one, since it logically should describe lesions, such as tumors, foreign bodies, and impacted secretion, that obstruct the airways to portions of the lung. However, it is too firmly embedded in clinical jargon to dislodge. The syndrome that is described as COPD or better, as chronic airflow limitation, is a functional condition in which the rate of expiratory airflow is reduced to a degree that produces disability. The entities usually associated with COPD are chronic bronchitis, emphysema, and inflammation of small bronchi and bronchioles variously called bronchiolitis or small airways disease. These three conditons commonly occur together, since they are the responses of different anatomic levels of the respiratory tract to similar irritants, and they are not always separable clinically. Asthmatic patients and many patients with bronchiectasis also manifest chronic airflow limitation, as described elsewhere. By international agreement chronic bronchitis has been defined as chronic cough and sputum production not attributable to some specific disease (such as tuberculosis or carcinoma).[686] In epidemiologic studies sputum production on most days during at least 3 months of the year in 2 consecutive years is sufficient basis for a diagnosis of chronic bronchitis. Practitioners generally make the diagnosis in patients who not only have chronic cough with sputum but also have repeated chest infections or COPD, or both. Emphysema is defined in anatomic rather than clinical terms, being an anatomic change in the acini of the lung characterized by abnormal enlargement of airspaces accompanied by destruction of airspace walls.[686] Small airways disease has only recently been documented physiologically and pathologically but is not generally used as a diagnosis in clinical practice. The term is used here to describe a group of nonspecific inflammatory changes in bronchioles and small bronchi that correlate with physiologic airflow obstruction.

Chronic bronchitis and emphysema are extremely common. They often occur together, but each can occur without the other. Small airways disease has been described accompanying each, but its prevalence has not been studied directly.

Incidence

COPD is the fifth leading cause of death in the United States and is responsible for about 2.5% of all deaths annually. Combining all deaths certified as resulting from chronic bronchitis, emphysema, and COPD, the mortality has nearly trebled since 1950. Although COPD is more common in Britain than in the United States, the mortality in Britain appears to be falling. COPD is a chronic process that progresses slowly over a period of years. It causes or contributes to 100,000 deaths each year, and more than 1.5 million new cases are diagnosed annually. The amount of disability it causes is enormous, with estimates running as high as 250 million hours lost from work annually.

Chronic bronchitis

Chronic bronchitis is a common condition that increases in prevalence at least until 40 years of age and affects men more often than women. Roughly 20% of men have cough and sputum production, but only a fraction of these have recurrent chest infections and fewer still have disabling COPD.

The microscopic finding that most consistently correlates with hypersecretion of mucus is enlargement of the mucous glands. This can be conveniently appraised using the gland/wall ratio or Reid index,[708] the ratio of the thickness of the lobules of mucous glands to the distance between the perichondrium and the basal lamina of the bronchial lining epithelium (Fig. 22-49). For normal individuals Reid obtained values of 0.14 to 0.36, whereas a group of bronchitic subjects averaged 0.59. A value of 0.4 was taken as the upper limit of normal. Subsequent work has shown that the gland/wall ratio is unimodally distributed; that is, there is a continuous distribution of gland/wall ratios rather than two distinct populations, one normal and one diseased. More accurate but laborious methods for measuring mucous gland volumes lead to the same conclusion: there is a bell-shaped distribution of mucous gland volumes, with asymptomatic subjects tending to have smaller glands and those with overt clinical bronchitis tending toward the higher end of the

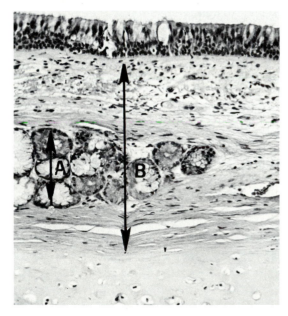

Fig. 22-49. Normal bronchus. Gland/wall ratio (A/B) is quick measure of mucous gland volume, which is increased in chronic bronchitis.

curve, but without a sharp separation between normal persons and those with disease.[710,715]

Another common abnormality in chronic bronchitis is an increase in the ratio of mucous cells to serous cells in the mucous glands. Normally, relatively equal numbers of mucous and serous cells make up the secretory tubules, but in many bronchitic patients serous cells are rare and mucous cells make up the great majority of glandular epithelium. The ducts of the glands become dilated and plugged with mucus. These dilated ducts can often be demonstrated clinically in bronchograms and have been called diverticula.

Inflammatory edema or cellular infiltration may be present in chronic bronchitis but are not constant or diagnostic features. Changes in the bronchial lining epithelium are variable. Hyperplasia of the basal cells, increased numbers of goblet cells, and foci of squamous metaplasia can all be found. The basement membrane can be thickened, and focal atrophy of the connective tissue leads to irregularity of the bronchial caliber visible on the opened bronchi as shallow depressions with transverse ridges. Increased smooth muscle has been observed in bronchitic patients who have wheezing.[714]

Patients with clinical bronchitis are often subject to repeated chest infections, probably because excessive amounts of mucus result in inefficient bronchial clearance and colonization of airways with nasopharyngeal flora. Normally the airways are sterile, but in a large proportion of bronchitic patients bacteria can be cultured from the airways. The most frequent organism to be recovered is *Haemophilus influenzae*, followed by *Streptococcus pneumoniae*. Acute infections are often associated with these organisms but also may be caused by viruses or *Mycoplasma pneumoniae*.[685,699,713] During acute infections there is often deterioration of lung function, but it is reversible, and surprisingly the long-term development of chronic airflow limitation is unaffected by intercurrent infections.[668,682,683]

Chronic airflow limitation can develop in patients with little or no emphysema and can even be lethal. Such patients usually have mucus hypersecretion of some degree, and their disability is commonly attributed to chronic bronchitis, but the relationship between the process causing chronic airflow limitation and simple chronic bronchitis is not clear. Mucous gland hyperplasia produces thickening of the bronchial wall, which narrows the bronchus and could in principal increase airway resistance, but in practice there is not a strong relationship between morphologic mucous gland hypertrophy or indices of mucus expectoration, on the one hand, and clinical outcome or results of pulmonary function tests, on the other.[715] Reid[709] observed that in patients with chronic bronchitis dying of COPD there was mucus plugging, acute obliteration of bronchioles by purulent exudate, and organizing pneumonia.[709] These observa-

tions served to focus attention on the small airways, although some of the changes she described were the result of terminal infection. Subsequent studies have shown narrowing of airways in chronic bronchitis without emphysema,[698] as well as a number of morphologic features of small airways that correlate with physiologic chronic airflow limitation, notably goblet cell metaplasia, inflammatory cell infiltration, and narrowing of the airway.[670,671,676] It should be stressed that these changes are often subtle and may be missed during inspection of histologic slides. Their importance emerges when quantitative analysis is applied to series of cases. Nevertheless, it is likely that the changes in the airways less than 2 mm in diameter are the important ones in determining airflow limitation.

The factors implicated in causing chronic bronchitis are cigarette smoking, air pollution, infection early in childhood, and a poorly defined familial tendency.[704] The most important of these is cigarette smoke. In epidemiologic studies cigarette smoking is associated with cough and phlegm, increased frequency of respiratory infections, and decreased pulmonary function. In pathologic studies it is correlated with mucous gland hyperplasia and small airways inflammation.[676] Exposure of experimental animals to cigarette smoke produces hyperplasia of the mucus-secreting apparatus. A number of effects of cigarette smoke help to account for the increased tendency to infections, including impaired mucociliary clearance owing to squamous metaplasia of the bronchial epithelium and hypersecretion of mucus and decreased antibacterial function of alveolar macrophages.[739]

The importance of community air pollution is difficult to evaluate because the powerful influence of cigarette smoking tends to overwhelm other influences. Holland and Reid[689] showed that residents of several small communities in Britain had less cough and sputum production and slightly better ventilatory function than comparable occupational groups in London. Their study was controlled for smoking. Effects of air pollution are more easily demonstrable in schoolchildren, since smoking is not a factor, but the significance of changes in respiratory symptoms in children in relation to the development of COPD in middle age is not established. Studies in both Britain and the United States have shown an increased incidence of lower respiratory infections in schoolchildren living in areas of higher pollution.[678] Experimental exposure of animals to pollutants supports a possible role for common air pollutants in chronic bronchitis. Sulfur dioxide, a major product of burning coal, causes mucus hypersecretion in animals, and nitrogen dioxide and ozone, products of the photochemical oxidation of automobile exhaust, produce inflammation in small airways. In most instances the concentrations used in animal experiments are considerably higher than those observed in even heavily polluted atmospheres, but it may be unreasonable to expect low concentrations of any single pollutant used in the laboratory to reproduce the effect of the complicated mixtures found in urban atmospheres.

Although chest infections in adults have little lasting influence on pulmonary function, some studies have found that patients with bronchitis or impaired pulmonary function more commonly have a history of lung infections early in life than do normal persons. Follow-up monitoring of young children with infections has shown poorer performance on pulmonary function testing persisting even into adolescence. Perhaps damage to the growing lung predisposes to COPD later in life.

Emphysema

With the passage of years the lung gradually loses elastic recoil, alveolar ducts dilate, and the fraction of the lung parenchyma that is composed of alveolar ducts (rather than alveoli) increases.[711,715] These changes are part of the normal process of aging and are not emphysema, which is by definition an abnormal enlargement of airspaces.

Since emphysema is defined morphologically, it is most reliably diagnosed pathologically. Mild degrees are difficult to recognize in the fresh lung. Fixation by distending the lung with fixative through the bronchi greatly improves its recognition and is adequate for routine purposes, but for optimum study and photography barium sulfate impregnation improves the recognition of emphysema and requires only a few extra minutes. In the inflation-fixed lung the alveolar ducts are at the limit of resolution for the unaided eye, although in the aged they can often be recognized as holes of up to 0.5 mm in diameter. Spaces in the parenchyma over 1 mm in size are abnormal.

Emphysema is common at autopsy, but its reported prevalence varies from 20% to 100% depending on the population studied and the technique and criteria used.[715] The prevalence and severity increase with age and are greater in men than in women. Minor degrees of emphysema are clinically inapparent, however, and as a rule subjects with less than 20% of the lung involved have no symptoms.

Classification

On the sectioned surface of an inflated lung, connective tissue septa extend inward from the pleura and outline units of parenchyma, termed secondary lobules, that are 1 to 2 cm in diameter and contain two to five acini. The acini are the functional gas-exchanging units of the lung and consist of three to five generations of respiratory bronchioles and a variable number of alveolar ducts and alveolar sacs, each with their alveoli. Emphysema is classified according to the portion of the acinus it involves.[687,715]

Centriacinar emphysema. Emphysema that initially involves the respiratory bronchioles is termed centriacinar or centrilobular emphysema (CLE). The lesions of CLE appear grossly as roughly spherical holes 1 to 5 mm in diameter near the center of the lobules and separated from the perilobular septa by a rim of normal tissue (Fig. 22-50). Usually dark pigment is associated with the lesions and in advanced lesions strands of tissue, containing vessels remaining after destruction of the alveolar walls, cross the emphysematous space (Fig. 22-51). Usually the upper lobes are involved more severely than the lower and the superior segments more than the basilar ones. The bronchioles supplying centrilobular emphysema often are inflamed, distorted, and stenotic. CLE is usually the type of emphysema found when chronic bronchitis and emphysema coexist, and patients with CLE are almost invariably smokers.

Panacinar emphysema. In panacinar emphysema all portions of the acinus are affected, but usually the alveolar ducts are involved more severely than the respiratory bronchioles. Individual lobules are variably involved, but even in minimally involved lobules abnormally enlarged airspaces reach the perilobular septa (Fig. 22-52). Both upper and lower lobes are usually involved to a

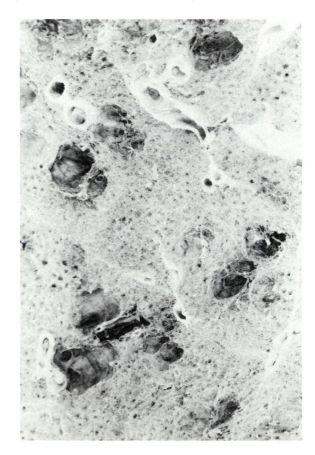

Fig. 22-50. Centriacinar emphysema. Barium sulfate–impregnated lung. Enlarged, abnormal airspaces in center of lobules are surrounded by normal tissue.

comparable degree (Fig. 22-53) but the lower zones may have the more severe lesions. Panacinar emphysema occurs most often in middle-aged cigarette smokers,[715] but it is also the characteristic form of emphysema in rare familial cases occurring in young adults, whose serum antitrypsin levels may be normal[696] or reduced.[680]

Distal acinar (paraseptal) emphysema. Distal acinar emphysema is a form that is localized along the pleura and perilobular septa. As an isolated finding it is not associated with COPD but does predispose to pneumothorax. It can also be associated with CLE.

Irregular (paracicatricial) emphysema. Enlarged and distorted abnormal airspaces are often seen surrounding scars from any cause. Since the process giving rise to the scarring may not respect acinar architecture, the lesions may be irregular in distribution within the acinus as well as within the lung as a whole.

Mixed and unclassified emphysema. It is not unusual to find emphysema of more than one type in a given lung, for example, centriacinar emphysema in the upper lobes and panacinar in the lower lobes. Many cases of emphysema do not fit unambiguously into one of the above types, either because the lesions are atypical or because they are so severe that it is impossible to recognize the portion of the acinus that was initially involved (Fig. 22-54). In one study only 27 of 122 emphysematous lungs examined by three expert pathologists unequivocally showed panacinar or centriacinar emphysema, the remainder being either mixed or unclassifiable.[700] There is general agreement that centriacinar emphysema is most severe in the upper lobes whereas panacinar emphysema is more uniformly distributed,[665,700] but there are no other clinical features that consistently distinguish them and whether they have a similar pathogenesis has not been established.

Bullae

Bullae are subpleural, air-filled, cystlike structures, greater than 1 cm in diameter, that are found most frequently along the sharp margins of the lung anteriorly and near the apices. In pathologic specimens they bulge outward from the surface of the lung, but during life they are confined by the chest wall and indent and compress the lung. They are found in association with each of the

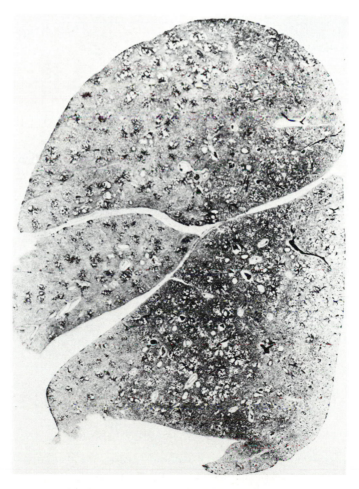

Fig. 22-51. Centriacinar emphysema. Paper-mounted lung section. (Courtesy Dr. A.A. Liebow.)

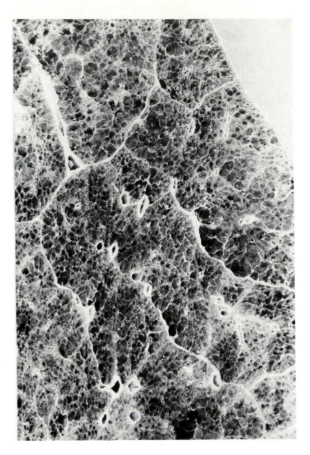

Fig. 22-52. Panacinar emphysema. Enlarged airspaces involve lobule uniformly. Barium sulfate–impregnated lung.

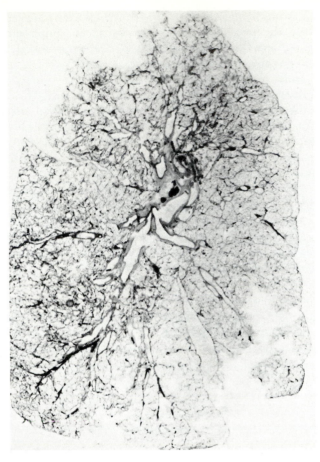

Fig. 22-53. Panacinar emphysema. Paper-mounted lung section. (Courtesy Dr. A.A. Liebow.)

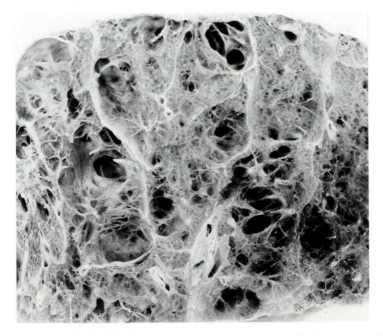

Fig. 22-54. Severe emphysema. It is difficult to discern what portion of acinus was involved initially.

other forms of emphysema and sometimes, especially in young people, in otherwise normal lungs. Some bullae appear essentially empty, but often they contain strands or remnants of tissue, indicating that they represent severely damaged lung tissue that has lost its elastic recoil. Microscopically the walls show fibrosis and chronic inflammation. The most common cause of spontaneous pneumothorax in young people is apical bullae,[659] but rupture is fortunately rare in generalized emphysema. Large bullae can also cause pulmonary dysfunction by compression of the remaining lung.

Morphogenesis of emphysematous lesions

There seem to be at least two mechanisms by which destruction of alveolar walls takes place. One mechanism, first described by Waters in 1862, is through departition of airspaces, which takes place by the enlargement and coalescence of the interalveolar pores.[693,706,707] It now is well established from observations in both humans and animals that there are small holes (pores of Kohn) in normal alveolar septa. These generally lie in the spaces between capillaries. Some enlargement of pores takes place with aging, even in nonemphysematous lungs,[707] but the process is exaggerated in emphysema. The pores encroach on and obliterate alveolar capillaries and coalesce, and gradually alveolar walls disappear leaving behind strands of tissue that often contain more resistant arteries. The abnormally large pores, called fenestrae, can be observed directly in slices of barium sulfate–impregnated lung with a stereomicroscope or in histologic sections 50 μm or more thick; their presence can be recognized in routine sections because the airspace walls between fenestrae appear to be detached from the rest of the lung parenchyma where the plane of the section passes through the fenestrae. Thus the appearance of "floating" segments of alveolar wall in ordinary sections is one reliable indicator of destruction of airspace walls.

The second mechanism, which is more difficult to understand, is a simplification of lung structure. For example, in early panacinar emphysema, Heppleston and Leopold[687] observed dilatation of alveolar ducts with shortening and effacement of the interalveolar septa, and similar morphologic changes occur in an animal model of emphysema.[693] The surface area of the lung is diminished, indicating tissue loss, but fenestration is not prominent. The mechanisms by which this rearrangement of lung structure takes place are still unclear.

Pathophysiology

Emphysema differs from other causes of chronic airflow limitation by the presence of destruction in the acinar region. The loss of gas-exchanging surface and associated vascular bed results in a decreased diffusion capacity. There are many other causes of decreased diffusion

capacity, but in a patient with COPD, magnitude of the decrease correlates well with extent of emphysema.[705] The most specific physiologic abnormality of the emphysematous lung is its loss of elastic recoil.[672,705] Two factors determine the retractive force (elastic recoil) of the lung: forces derived from surface tension in the fluid lining of small airspaces and forces derived from the stretching of connective tissue elements. In emphysema the enlarged airspaces and decreased surface area, which are a consequence of destruction of alveolar walls, tend to decrease the surface tension component of elastic recoil. Abnormalities of connective tissue are also important. Elastin is responsible for lung compliance at low and intermediate lung volumes. Collagen has little influence on lung compliance in the physiologic range but does determine the tensile strength of the tissue and provides the "mechanical stop" that limits lung expansion at total lung capacity. In the emphysematous lung the increased compliance is due in part to disruption of the elastic network, which can be seen in histologic sections.[718] Total lung capacity is increased, indicating that the collagen also is remodeled.

The basis for the airflow obstruction in emphysema has been studied intensively. Hogg and co-workers[688] showed that the major site of obstruction is in small airways. They compared the distribution of airway resistance between central airways (larger than 2 mm) and peripheral airways (smaller than 2 mm) in normal lungs and in seven emphysematous lungs. In the emphysematous lungs the resistance of the central airways was no more than twice normal but the resistance of the peripheral airways increased 10 to 40 fold. Anatomic studies point to two factors that correlate with airflow obstruction, the severity of the emphysema itself and the associated small airways disease.[701] Emphysema is associated with airway obstruction because of decreased elastic recoil. The bronchioles have thin muscular walls, and their caliber varies with lung volume. The force that holds them open during expiration is the retractive force of the surrounding lung, which of course is greater the more the lung is expanded. In emphysema the retractive force is much reduced. Physiologic studies of carefully selected emphysematous patients have shown that the conductance of their airways (the reciprocal of the resistance) is normal for the elastic recoil of their lungs, but to generate a given elastic recoil their lungs must be at higher volume than normal. In contrast, asthmatic patients with intrinsic bronchial disease had reduced conductance for a given elastic recoil. Morphologic studies showing that there are fewer alveolar walls attached to the bronchioles of emphysematous lungs provide an anatomic basis for the diminished support of small airways in emphysema.

Emphysematous patients also are likely to have associated small airways disease as a major contributor to air-

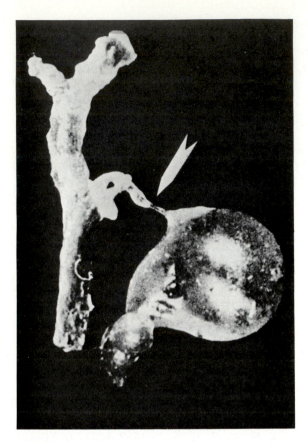

Fig. 22-55. Cast of centriacinar emphysematous space. Arrow indicates area of stenosis in bronchiole leading into space. (From Depierre, A., et al.: Chest **62:**699, 1972.)

flow limitation. This has been especially well documented in centriacinar emphysema and has been elegantly illustrated by French investigators using casts (Fig. 22-55).[698] A variety of lesions can be found, including loss of small airways, stenosis and distortion of airways, inflammation, goblet cell metaplasia, and mucus plugging.* These factors cause obstruction in various ways. Narrowing of airways increases resistance in accordance with Poiseuille's law even when flow is laminar, but distortion and abrupt stenosis convert laminar to turbulent flow. Mucus plugs may totally obstruct the airways, but goblet cell metaplasia may also impair airway function by replacing the normal bronchiolar lining of surfactant and Clara cell secretions with sticky mucus. Physiologists believe that airways close in dependent regions of the lung at the end of expiration, and the abnormal secretions in goblet cell metaplasia would be expected to impair their reopening. The diminished support of small airways resulting from the loss of elastic recoil in emphysema and the intrinsic changes in small airways reinforce each other in producing airway dysfunction when both are present in the same lung.

*References 678, 688, 694, 697, 701, 715.

Etiology

The evidence that cigarette smoking is the major cause of emphysema is overwhelming. A variety of autopsy populations from hospitals and coroners' offices have been studied, and the relationship held true.[666,667,712,715] Severity of emphysema is roughly dose related. In nonsmokers emphysema is infrequent and almost always of low grade. In smokers over 40 years of age normal lungs are unusual, and heavy smokers have more severe and extensive emphysema than do light smokers. Between 20% and 40% of those who smoke more than a pack a day have disease of relatively high grade. The activities of tobacco smoke that promote emphysema are discussed later in the chapter. In all studies, however, there are some heavy smokers who escape emphysema. This indicates that there are other factors that also determine individual susceptibility to emphysema or that cigarette smoke acts additively with other agents in the environment.

Air pollution is often mentioned as a cause of emphysema. Ishikawa and associates[690] compared paper-mounted whole lung sections from autopsies in St. Louis, Missouri, a relatively industrialized city, with a similar series from Winnipeg, Manitoba, where the pollution is less. When matched according to age, sex, and smoking history, the St. Louis patients had more severe emphysema.

There are genetic influences in emphysema. A poorly understood familial factor in COPD acts independent of any known specific disease. In addition, emphysema is a complication in a number of rare heritable diseases of connective tissue such as cutis laxa, Marfan's syndrome, and Menkes' syndrome.[692] Emphysema is also closely linked to deficiency of the serum protein alpha-1-antitrypsin or alpha-1-protease inhibitor (alpha-1-PI).[703] Although deficiency of alpha-1-PI is responsible for only about 1% of cases of emphysema, the recognition of alpha-1-PI deficiency has had such a pivotal role in shaping the modern theory of the pathogenesis of emphysema that it will be described in some detail.

Alpha-1-protease inhibitor deficiency. Alpha-1-PI is the major protein responsible for the alpha-1 band in the conventional serum electrophoretogram. A glycoprotein of mol. wt. 51,000, alpha-1-PI is synthesized in the liver and distributed in the circulating blood and a variety of body fluids including that of the lower respiratory tract. Its function is to inhibit proteases with serine at the active proteolytic site, including leukocyte elastase, chymotrypsin, cathepsin G, plasmin, and thrombin, as well as trypsin. Alpha-1-PI deficiency was first discovered in 1963 by Swedish investigators who observed a series of patients whose serum apparently lacked the alpha-1-globulin band on electrophoresis. Of the original 36 patients, 27 had chronic airflow limitation, mainly as a result of emphysema.[680] The emphysema of alpha-1-PI deficiency is of the panacinar type and predominately involves the basilar portion of the lung.[680,684] Emphysema in alpha-1-PI deficiency develops early in adult life, with an equal sex incidence, and in nonsmokers as well as smokers, although on the average smokers become symptomatic 15 years earlier than nonsmokers. COPD develops in as much as 85% of deficient subjects.

The other organ affected clinically is the liver. One half of newborn infants with the deficiency have minor abnormalities of liver function, and in one in 10 obstructive jaundice develops in the first few months of life but usually clears before the end of the first year.[703] In a small fraction of children cirrhosis develops during childhood or adolescence. The distinctive pathologic feature of the livers of these children is the presence in the cytoplasm of hepatocytes of periodic acid–Schiff–positive globules, which react with antibodies to alpha-1-PI. Electron microscopy shows the globules to be accumulations of alpha-1-PI within dilated sacs of endoplasmic reticulum in the hepatocytes. Similar globules are present in the livers of adult carriers of the gene for the deficiency even without cirrhosis. In addition, the incidence of both cirrhosis and hepatoma is increased in deficient adults, although both these complications are rare in comparison with emphysema.

The basis for the defect is now well understood.[675] Alpha-1-PI is the product of two alleles, one from each parent, located on chromosome 14. Both alleles are expressed, resulting in a codominant pattern of inheritance. The more common molecular form of alpha-1-PI found in 90% of the population has been designated M, so the protease inhibitor (Pi) phenotype of a normal individual with two M alleles is written PiMM. Over 20 abnormal variants of the alpha-1-PI molecule are known, but the one associated with most cases of clinical deficiency is designated Z. In the classic deficiency, the phenotype is PiZZ; that is, both genes code for the Z variant. The concentration of alpha-1-PI in the plasma is reduced to only 10% to 15% of normal and its electrophoretic mobility is greatly reduced. The heterozygotes, PiMZ, have a level of alpha-I-PI that is 60% of normal, a reduction in alpha-1-PI that is not of sufficient degree to be of major clinical importance, although there may be a small increase in the risk of emphysema in PiMZ heterozygotes who smoke heavily.[703]

The basic abnormality in the Z protein is a point mutation that results in the substitution of a lysine in the Z protein for a glutamic acid residue in the M protein. This reduces the negative charge on the Z molecule by two charge units, accounting for its slow electrophoretic mobility. The Z protein is as effective a protease inhibitor mole for mole as the normal M protein, and its turnover in the circulation is also normal. The deficient inhibitory activity of the serum is attributable entirely to the low concentration of inhibitor protein in the circulation of the PiZZ individual.

The periodic acid–Schiff–positive globules present in the livers of those with the Z gene have been isolated from PiZZ homozygous deficient individuals and consist of Z protein that is less glycosylated than normal, whereas the Z protein in the plasma is normally glycosylated. It appears that the primary amino acid substitution results in defective intracellular processing of the Z protein, which accumulates in the endoplasmic reticulum of the hepatocyte without being released. The small amount of protein that is fully processed is secreted and accounts for the circulating inhibitor.

The pathogenesis of the liver disease is not well understood. One theory is that the accumulation of alpha-1-PI in the endoplasmic reticulum of hepatocytes in some way predisposes the liver to injury by exogenous agents, since the presence of globules themselves does not cause hepatic dysfunction. The lung disease is the result of the low level of protease inhibitory activity in the plasma and lung, which permits proteases released from phagocytes by the inflammatory stimuli to which the lung is inevitably exposed to act unopposed on lung connective tissue. The degradation of connective tissue triggers the remodeling of lung architecture, ultimately producing emphysema.

Pathogenesis

At the same time that the association of emphysema with deficiency of alpha-1-protease inhibitor was recognized, Gross[691] reported the production of emphysema in rats by the intratracheal injection of the protease papain. These two observations indicate that the maintenance of normal lung structure requires a balance between proteases and their inhibitors and that excessive proteolytic activity in the lung because of increased protease release or decreased inhibition results in emphysema. Only proteases that degrade elastin can produce emphysema in experimental animals; attempts to use nonelastolytic proteases including bacterial collagenase have been uniformly unsuccessful.[691] Alpha-1-PI is only one of at least seven known serum protease inhibitors, but it is the major inhibitor of granulocyte elastase. Disruption of the elastic fiber network is a morphologic feature of emphysema.[718] Thus the evidence is strong that degradation of elastic fibers is a critical event in the development of emphysema.

There is evidence that cigarette smoke promotes emphysema both by increasing the amount of elastolytic protease brought to the lung and by decreasing the amount of functioning inhibitor. Cigarette smokers have four to 10 times more phagocytes in their lungs than nonsmokers. The majority of these phagocytes are macrophages, but 1% to 3% are neutrophils. There is controversy regarding which cell is the main source of the elastase that is hypothesized to initiate emphysema. Neutrophils are few in the lung but have high levels of elastase activity and turn over rapidly. Macrophages have only low levels of elastase but are associated pathologically with early emphysema. Furthermore, the earliest and most consistent lesion in the lungs of young cigarette smokers dying suddenly of nonrespiratory causes is respiratory bronchiolitis, a subtle inflammation of the wall of respiratory bronchioles accompanied by accumulation in the lumen of macrophages laden with tobacco residues. The macrophages obtained by bronchoalveolar lavage from the lungs of smokers are highly activated and have a number of properties that are germane to protease balance in the lung. They secrete a factor chemotactic for neutrophils that might indirectly increase the elastase burden in the lung, but they also can take up and sequester neutrophil proteases, both free and complexed to inhibitors, and they synthesize at least small amounts of protease inhibitors.[692] Consequently their presence in early emphysematous lesions may be either a cause of injury or a protective response.

The active inhibitory site on the alpha-1-PI molecule is a methionyl-seryl bond near the carboxy terminal end of the molecule. In vitro oxidation of the methionine destroys the inhibitory activity of alpha-1-PI for elastase.[675,692] Cigarette smoke inactivates alpha-1-PI in vitro, and a large portion of the alpha-1-PI in the lungs of smokers, as well as some of their circulating alpha-1-PI, is oxidized and nonfunctional.[669] These observations explain how cigarette smoke, which is a relatively mild inflammatory stimulus, might promote emphysema while many more formidable inflammatory stimuli do not.

Natural history of chronic airflow limitation

In normal individuals there is a decline in pulmonary function that begins around 20 years of age and continues lifelong. For the majority of cigarette smokers with cough and phlegm and even for many with recurrent chest infections, the annual rate of decline is no greater than normal. In a small number of more sensitive smokers, however, the rate of decline is accelerated. The accelerated loss of function may be detectable by spirometry by 30 or 40 years of age, long before overt COPD develops. If the smoker stops smoking, the cough may disappear and the rate of decline in pulmonary function returns to normal but the lost function is not regained and the subject functions at a lower level than normal for his or her age. With a normal rate of decline the decrease in ventilatory function does not reach clinical significance, even in advanced age. Chronic airflow limitation develops only in that minority who are unusually susceptible to cigarette smoke and whose loss of function is accelerated.[668,681,682]

By the time symptoms develop, the abnormal decline in lung function and by implication the pathologic process have been going on for many years. Survival after the development of symptoms is variable but often is for many years. Respiratory failure heralds the terminal phase of the disease, and although many patients survive their first episode of respiratory failure, two thirds will be dead within 2 years.

The pathophysiologic features of patients with COPD and bronchitis differ in some respects from those of patients with severe emphysema. Patients with COPD but little emphysema tend to produce more sputum, to have more severe hypoxemia and carbon dioxide retention for a given degree of ventilatory impairment, and to have repeated episodes of heart failure.[673] This is because bronchitic patients whose COPD is due to intrinsic disease of the conducting airways with intact lung parenchyma have many areas of lung with a low ventilation/perfusion ratio, that is, blood flow going through areas of underventilated lung, which results in hypoxemia.[717] Patients with severe emphysema have compliant lungs with loss of parenchyma and capillary bed; their ventilation/perfusion ratios are actually higher than normal, which produces wasted ventilation.[717] With increased effort they can maintain their oxygenation for many years until progression of the disease, increasing rigidity of the chest wall, and weakening of the respiratory muscles finally result in respiratory failure.

Hypertrophy and eventual failure of the right ventricle are terminal events in some COPD patients. Factors that raise pulmonary vascular resistance in COPD and contribute to cor pulmonale include hypoxic vasoconstriction, loss of capillary bed owing to emphysema, increased viscosity of the blood as a result of secondary polycythemia, and elevated alveolar pressures that may compress the alveolar capillaries during expiration against high airway resistance. Of these factors, the most important is hypoxic vasoconstriction. A large number of studies have failed to show a high degree of correlation between right ventricular weight and extent of emphysema,[677,679,702] a measure of capillary destruction, and in clinical practice the administration of oxygen usually has a rapid effect in lowering pulmonary artery pressure and improving right ventricular function.

Small airways obstruction in the absence of typical chronic bronchitis and emphysema

Although the majority of patients with COPD are middle-aged or older cigarette smokers with slowly evolving disease, a few patients differ considerably from this epidemiologic pattern. They are younger, their disease evolves more rapidly, and in some cases it seems to be traceable to episodes of chest infection in childhood. In other cases the onset seems to follow a pneumonic episode in adult life, although sometimes no history of infective onset is obtained. The chest roentgenogram often has a miliary pattern, and bronchiectasis may also be present. The bronchioles show a spectrum of changes including fibrosis, obliteration, inflammation, and mucus plugging.[695]

Byssinosis

Byssinosis is an occupational disorder of workers exposed to cotton, flax, or hemp dust. In workers returning to work on Monday after the weekend, dyspnea and a feeling of chest tightness develop during the course of the workday. Physiologic studies have documented the development of airflow obstruction during the work shift. The severity of disease in a given individual can be gauged by the number of days into the week on which symptoms recur. In more severely affected individuals airflow obstruction recurs on successive working days and after many years may become permanent.

The mechanisms underlying the bronchial reaction have not been determined and may not be uniform in all patients. There is evidence for allergy to cotton dust antigens, for the presence of pharmacologically active substances in cotton dust that directly cause histamine release, and for bacterial endotoxin contaminating the cotton dust. There are no specific pathologic changes in byssinosis. At autopsy, lungs of former workers with disability resulting from obstructive lung disease show nonspecific chronic bronchitis and emphysema. Both the smooth muscle and the mucous glands of central airways are hypertrophied.[728] However, when studies are controlled for the influence of cigarette smoking, incidence of emphysema in textile workers is not excessive, although there is an excess of mucous hyperplasia.[728] Thus it appears that the mill dust exerts its main and perhaps sole effect on airways.

PNEUMOCONIOSIS

The term *pneumoconiosis* refers to the nonneoplastic tissue responses of the lung to the presence of deposits of inorganic dusts. The dusts of concern are of limited solubility in body fluids and remain largely in the lung and draining lymph nodes. The tissue responses are of three general types: fibrous nodules exemplified by silicosis or coal worker's pneumoconiosis, interstitial fibrosis exemplified by asbestosis or aluminosis, and hypersensitivity reactions such as chronic berylliosis.

Dust deposition and clearance

The tissue response to inhaled dust depends on the chemical composition, crystalline form, and quantity of the dust and on host factors including the efficiency of the clearance mechanism, immune status of the host, and associated diseases. Some mineral dusts, such as iron oxide, produce little fibrosis, whereas others such as silica are potentially highly fibrogenic, depending on their crystalline structure. Amorphous silica and silica with an octagonal crystal lattice are usually not fibrogenic, whereas tetrahedral crystalline silicas such as quartz dust do produce fibrosis. The amount of dust deposited in the lung depends not only on the quantity of dust in the atmosphere but also on the ventilatory pattern of the subject and on the physical properties of the particles, including shape, density, electrostatic charge, hygroscopic properties, and, most important, size.[722] Particles greater than 10 μm in diameter impact on airway bifurcations and fail to reach the acini. Particles smaller than this but larger than 0.1 μm remain suspended in rapidly flowing air but settle quickly under the influence of gravity when flow is slow. Consequently they are deposited in respiratory bronchioles and proximal alveolar ducts as airflow slows at the end of inspiration. Particles less than 0.1 μm behave essentially as gases, reaching the most distal alveoli by diffusion even though these alveoli are not ventilated in normal tidal breathing. Most particles of interest to the pathologist are in the range of 0.5 to 5 μm; deposition in the acini is most efficient at about 1 μm. Particles deposited in large airways are removed within hours by the mucociliary clearance to the oropharynx to be swallowed. The clearance from the acini takes place mainly within alveolar macrophages. The uptake by alveolar macrophages also takes place within hours, but the macrophages are removed from the lung so slowly that the net half time for particles deposited in the acini is measurable in weeks. A tiny fraction of the deposited dust, typically about 1%, escapes phagocytosis by the macrophages and is transported across the alveolar epithelium to the interstitium, mainly through the cytoplasm of type I epithelial cells. Much of the dust that escapes clearance ends up either in macrophages aggregated in the connective tissue around muscular arteries, respiratory bronchioles and pleura where the lymphatic system begins or in the regional lymph nodes. Whether it is transported to these sites within the interstitial fluid or within macrophages is still uncertain.

Dusts in normal lungs

Small amounts of pigment are found in virtually all lungs after infancy. The amount increases with age and tends to be greater in persons from urban areas than in those from less polluted rural areas. The dust is found within macrophages in the adventitia of muscular arteries and bronchioles and in the pleura at the junctions with the interlobular septa. It is amorphous and contains carbon, silicon, iron, aluminum, phosphorus, and titanium, associated with a poorly characterized organic pigment.[749,755] The material incites little inflammation or fibrosis. In cigarette smokers the alveolar macrophages contain tobacco residues, including kaolinite.

Silicosis

Silicon comprises approximately 28% of the earth's crust. It occurs combined with oxygen as free silica (SiO_2) and with additional elements as silicates. Because of its ubiquitous occurrence in the earth's crust and usefulness as an abrasive, miners, quarry workers, tunnelers, sandblasters, grinders, and workers in many other trades are exposed to airborne silica. The ability of mineral dusts of cause lung disease has been recognized since the time of Hippocrates. Agricola (1556) in his treatise on mining called attention to the ability of mine dust to "corrode the lungs," and Ramazzini (1700) in his treatise on the diseases of various occupations described small "stones" in the lungs of quarrymen and stonecutters. The importance of silica in the production of disease was realized in the late nineteenth century, and the term *silicosis* was introduced by Visconte in 1870. The introduction of high-speed drills and efficient energy sources in the early twentieth century greatly compounded the problem.

Unfortunately, the effects of silica are insidious and the process often continues to progress after exposure has ended.[750,765] Usually 20 years or more of exposure is required for the development of classic chronic silicosis, but with high levels of exposure disease can be produced more rapidly. The most acute form of silicosis, acute silicoproteinosis, is seen in persons exposed to very high concentrations of free silica of small particle size. Silicoproteinosis is rare and was recognized as an entity only in 1969,[723] although disease described in the 1930s among those engaged in the production of scouring powders probably represented earlier cases. The patients in the 1969 report were sandblasters who had been employed for 3 to 6 years. The onset of symptoms was acute, with dyspnea, cough, and fever, and the course was progressive deterioration with weight loss of 20 to 30 pounds, respiratory failure, and death in an average 7½ months. The lungs at autopsy showed interstitial pneumonitis with focal alveolar septal fibrosis and interstitial collections of dust-containing macrophages but only few small fibrous nodules. The alveolar spaces were filled with a flocculent or granular periodic acid–Schiff–positive exudate indistinguishable from that of alveolar proteinosis.[723] The exudate can readily be distinguished from edema fluid by the presence of cholesterol clefts and homogeneous eosinophilic blobs, 5 to 20 μm in diameter, which are remnants of necrotic cells. The lymph nodes show little fibrosis, but pleural adhesions may be present. Since the lesions of acute silicoproteinosis have been reproduced in experimental animals, the human cases do not represent the chance occurrence of alveolar proteinosis in a patient with silicosis.

Chronic silicosis usually becomes evident roentgenographically 20 to 40 years after first exposure. Many of those with fine nodularity on chest roentgenograms have no symptoms; as in other fibrosing lung diseases, exertional dyspnea develops in symptomatic patients. In accelerated silicosis the disease becomes manifest within 5 to 10 years, but the pathologic features are similar to those of chronic silicosis.[750,765]

The chronic silicotic lung is studded with well-circumscribed, dark, hard nodules, 1 to 5 mm in size, scattered through the parenchyma and in the pleura. The nodules are round to oval with a pale center and a more heavily pigmented periphery and sometimes a laminated appearance. They are more numerous in the upper lung zones than at the bases. The hilar lymph nodes are enlarged and fibrotic and may reach sufficient size to distort the bronchi. They may contain peripheral calcium deposits, giving rise to a characteristic appearance known as "eggshell" calcifications on the chest roentgenogram.

Microscopically the nodules consist of a central zone of hyalinized fibrous tissue containing only few cells and a variable amount of dust (Fig. 22-56). Concentric bundles of collagen surround and merge with the hyaline center. A mantle of more cellular connective tissue encloses the central acellular zone and contains fibroblasts, dust-filled macrophages, and lesser numbers of lymphocytes and plasma cells. Stellate projections of fibrous tissue extend a short distance into the adjacent alveolar walls. Calcium is deposited in some hyaline nodules.

Initially the hyaline nodules form in the regions of the

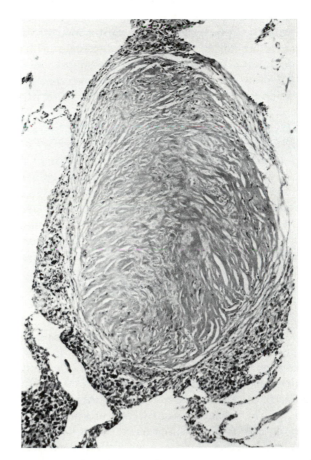

Fig. 22-56. Hyaline nodule in silicosis. Center of hyalinized collagen is enclosed by mantle of dust.

respiratory bronchioles and muscular arteries and in the pleura where the dust is concentrated. As the nodules grow and increase in number, their distribution within the acinus becomes widespread.

In some patients with severe disease individual nodules grow rapidly and coalesce to form large conglomerate masses of fibrous tissue. This process is termed complicated pneumoconiosis with the implication that some additional stimulus "complicates" the simple pneumoconiosis. In some instances the stimulus is tuberculosis and in others some other disease may produce altered immunologic responsiveness, but most often the stimulus is unknown. Conglomerate masses form predominately in the upper lobes and can grow to considerable size, cross lobar fissures, and occupy a large portion of the lung volume. Blood vessels and even bronchi can be obliterated by the process, and slitlike cavities form by ischemic degeneration. Large, ragged cavities usually indicate tuberculosis.

The functional effects of silicosis are as varied as its pathologic features. Many patients with simple pneumoconiosis detected by chest roentgenography have normal function. Symptomatic patients may have either an obstructive or a restrictive ventilatory pattern.[765] The airflow obstruction may result from involvement of bronchioles by the pneumoconiosis, an associated industrial or cigarette-induced bronchitis, or distortion of airways by larger conglomerate masses. Complicated pneumoconiosis presents a restrictive ventilatory pattern and reduced diffusing capacity owing to the replacement of lung tissue by the fibrous mass, but obstruction may also be present.

Pathogenesis

Silicosis is seen in humans in the form of established lesions. The early tissue response is inferred from animal studies, which usually involve a large single dose given by either inhalation or injection. The majority of the silica is taken up by macrophages that undergo necrosis, and new macrophages engulf the debris and released silica in a repetitive cycle of phagocytosis and necrosis. Gradually macrophages migrate or are carried to the region of respiratory bronchioles where they aggregate in alveoli and in the interstitial tissues around blood vessels. Mast cells, plasma cells, and fibroblasts become associated with the cellular aggregates, and gradually reticulin fibers and eventually mature collagen fibers are laid down. The resultant lesions resemble human hyaline nodules to a degree depending on species, technique of administration, size of particles, and dose of silica.

The mechanisms involved in the formation of these lesions are incompletely understood. There is a high correlation between the cytotoxicity of different types of silica for macrophages and their ability to produce fibrosis. This suggests that the repetitive necrosis of macrophages, release of silica, reuptake, and new cycle of necrosis are an important part of the self-perpetuating nature of the lesions. The available evidence indicates that the mechanism of cytotoxicity is related to the ability of silica to interact with cellular membranes and damage them. Hydroxyl groups on the surface of the silica particles can form hydrogen bonds with components of membranes, such as phosphoric acid residues of membrane phospholipids. Several compounds, including aluminum oxide and polyvinyl pyridine N-oxide, interact with silica to protect against its cytotoxic and fibrogenic effects.[738] These compounds share the property of being hydrogen acceptors. Regardless of the molecular details, the uptake of silica into phagosomes and phagolysosomes is followed by membrane damage, which results in the leakage of acid hydrolases from the lysosomes into the cytosol[720] and the loss of the ability of the plasma membrane to exclude extracellular calcium from the intracellular compartment. These events in turn lead to cell death.

A substantial body of experimental data suggests that stimulated or necrotic macrophages provide a stimulus for fibroblast proliferation and collagen synthesis. In 1967 Heppleston and Styles[737] reported that extracts of rat alveolar macrophages that had ingested silica stimulated collagen synthesis by chick fibroblasts. Neither extracts of normal fibroblasts nor those of fibroblasts that had been killed by freezing and thawing and then treated with silica had any effect. A number of investigators have carried out subsequent similar experiments,[751] and although their results differ in detail, they do point to a role for macrophages in the stimulation of fibroblasts in silicosis. This does not preclude an influence of other cell types such as lymphocytes, which also have been shown to produce modulators of fibroblast function.

Silicosis produces changes in the immune response, but the role of immunologic factors in the pathogenesis of silicosis is unknown.[758] Abnormalities in both humoral and cellular immunity have been observed. For example, silica acts as an adjuvant when animals are immunized. Whether it does this by adsorbing and denaturing protein on the surface of particles, by attracting macrophages and thereby increasing antigen processing, or by another mechanism is not known. In humans stimulation and abnormal regulation of the bone marrow–derived lymphocyte population are indicated by the frequent occurrence of hyperglobulinemia and autoantibodies in silicotic subjects. The prevalence of rheumatoid factor and antinuclear antibodies is approximately 30% in silicotic patients and is higher still in those with complicated pneumoconiosis. Immunoglobin has been identified in silicotic hyalin, and lung-reactive antibodies have been detected in the serum of silicotic patients, but whether the antibodies are the cause or the result of the tissue damage is unknown. Limited studies of cell-mediated immunity have been carried out in silicosis. No decrease in circulating T cells has been found, and patients do not have anergy to most common skin test antigens. Diminished reponsiveness of the peripheral blood lymphocytes to the T cell mitogen concanavalin A has been observed, however, and in silica-treated animals defective cellular immunity is shown by prolongation of skin graft survival.[758] The increased susceptibility of silicotic persons to tuberculosis suggests that a significant defect in cell-mediated immunity exists.

Tuberculosis and silicosis

Clinical and epidemiologic studies have repeatedly shown an increased risk of tuberculosis and other mycobacterial infections in silicotic persons.[756] The prevalence of tuberculosis varies depending on the prevalence of tuberculosis in the surrounding population but is always several fold higher in those with silicosis. The relative risk is greater in those with classic silicosis than in those with mixed-dust pneumoconiosis.

Typical lesions of silicosis and ordinary caseous granulomas can coexist in the lungs of silicotic persons, but the combination of silicosis and tuberculosis may also produce atypical morphologic lesions. In one form of silicotuberculosis, lesions closely resemble silicotic hyaline nodules with an outer mantle of dust-filled macrophages and fibrobasts enclosing a hyaline core that centrally appears softer and more granular than usual, reminiscent of caseous necrosis. The most dramatic form of silicotuberculosis has already been mentioned: the large conglomerate fibrous masses that form in the upper lobe of some patients. Extensive cavitation developing within massive fibrosis is presumptive evidence of tuberculosis (Fig. 22-57). Organisms are difficult to culture from sputum and even from tissue, presumably because they are trapped within the fibrous scar. Characteristically cavities are round, shaggy, and filled with black fluid that is noticeably purulent. Unlike the usual tubercular cavity, those in complicated silicosis are not trabeculated. Microscopic examination shows a thin zone of necrosis, with a few inflammatory cells and capillaries, that makes up at least a portion of the lining of the cavity.[759]

The effect of silica in modifying the response to *Mycobacterium tuberculosis* is readily demonstrable in animal experiments. Exposure of guinea pigs to silica causes enhanced growth of tubercle bacilli, reactivates healing lesions, and leads to progressive infection by ordinarily avirulent strains, including bacillus Calmette-Guérin (BCG), a strain widely used for vaccination. Interestingly the overproduction of connective tissue characteristic of progressive massive fibrosis is also reproduceable in animals. Gross, Westrick, and McNerney[734] administered nonfibrogenic quartz dust, accompanied by living or dead tubercle bacilli or tuberculin purified protein derivative (PPD), to tuberculin-sensitive guinea pigs. Fibrotic

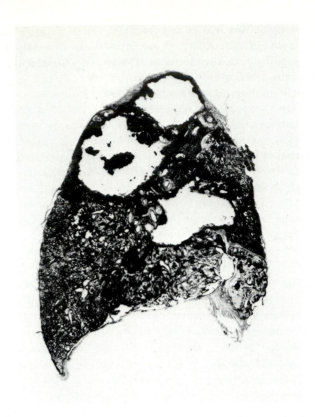

Fig. 22-57. Paper-mounted whole lung section from coal miner with tuberculosis shows massive fibrosis with extensive cavitation. (Preparation by Prof. J. Gough.)

lesions were most extensive with living organisms, less so with dead ones. Even the addition of soluble PPD increased the amount of fibrosis compared with quartz alone. Necrosis and calcification were seen only with organisms.

One reason for the increased susceptibility to tubercle bacilli is the direct action of silica on macrophages. Allison and D'Arcy Hart[719] found that cultured macrophages that had ingested sublethal amounts of silica permitted more rapid growth of tubercle bacilli and released more organisms into the culture medium than normal macrophages.

Other diseases

There is no evidence that silica increases the risk of lung cancer, nor does it enhance tobacco-induced carcinogenesis. The incidence of progressive systemic sclerosis (scleroderma) has been reported to be increased in miners. Perhaps silicosis predisposes to the development of scleroderma.

Mixed-dust pneumoconiosis

The tissue response to silica is modified by the presence of other components of a dust. When the dust contains more than approximately 18% free silica, a typical hyaline nodule is produced, but with lesser amounts of silica the tissue response is modified. Modified reactions are seen in foundry workers, hematite miners, and those engaged in removing boiler scale. The lesions are firm nodules, 2 to 5 mm in diameter, that are uniformly pigmented. Large conglomerate masses develop in some cases. As with other pneumoconioses the lesions are concentrated in respiratory bronchioles and muscular arteries and consist of a mixture of dust-laden macrophages and collagen fibers. In contrast to hyaline nodules, the dust is uniformly distributed through the nodule rather than being concentrated at the periphery, and the collagen fibers are arranged in a stellate pattern radiating into the walls of neighboring alveoli, rather than in a concentric pattern.

Pulmonary disease in coal workers

Coal worker's pneumoconiosis (CWP) is the focus of current medical and political controversy. Although few medical authorities would deny that inhalation of coal dust produces characteristic morphologic lesions, the relationship of these lesions to the development of disability is in dispute. This issue is of great economic importance. Although the coal mining population currently numbers only 120,000 miners who are at risk for CWP, the annual outlay for black lung benefits is over 1 billion dollars.[744]

For many years coal dust was considered innocuous; such disease as was acknowledged to occur in coal miners was attributed to silicosis. Coal trimmers load coal and distribute it in the holds of ships; the identification of lesions in their lungs that were similar to those of miners established that coal itself without silica could cause lesions.[731] The subsequent description of pneumoconiosis in groups working with pure carbon, electrotypers, carbon electrode workers, and graphite workers confirms the pathologic potential of carbonaceous dusts.[761] Currently three conditions are associated directly with coal mine dust: silicosis, coal worker's pneumoconiosis, and industrial bronchitis.[745,750]

Silicosis most commonly develops in anthracite miners and in certain occupational specialities among bituminous miners. Anthracite in eastern Pennsylvania occurs in narrow undulating seams, so that miners frequently are obliged to tunnel horizontally from one seam to another through hard rock, which exposes them to silica. Roof bolters and transportation workers have a high rate of silicosis, the former because they drill into hard rock and the latter because sand dusted on the tracks to provide traction for the shuttle cars is subsequently aerosolized.[745]

Coal worker's pneumociosis

CWP was first described in Britain by Gough[731] and Heppleston[736] in the 1940s. The spectrum of morphologic changes found in the lungs of coal workers has been reviewed recently.[733,741,746] The process known as simple CWP begins with the accumulation of dust-laden macrophages in the alveoli evaginating from the respiratory bronchioles, but with time the alveoli become filled and dust and macrophages also accumulate in the adventitia of the respiratory bronchioles and arteries. Small amounts of reticulin fibers are laid down, and the respiratory bronchioles become thickened and encased by solid dust-filled tissue. The alveolar ducts gradually dilate. According to Heppleston and Leopold,[687] the dust and tissue response cause atrophy of smooth muscle that leads to alveolar duct distension. Initially there is little overt destruction of airspace walls, but in more advanced cases emphysema develops in association with dust foci, the so-called focal emphysema. Heppleston and Leopold consider it a distinctive type of emphysema separable from other centriacinar emphysema by the absence of inflammation, but this opinion is not uniformly accepted in the United States.[764]

The typical dust accumulations in the respiratory bronchiolar region of miners appear grossly as dust macules, nonpalpable pigmented spots, 1 to 3 mm in diameter, in the centers of lobules (Figs. 22-58 and 22-59). Miners' lungs also may have palpable black nodules 1 to 7 mm in diameter. These are more heavily collagenized than the typical macules and may have a higher silica content.[741]

In complicated CWP or progressive massive fibrosis (PMF), masses 2 cm to several centimeters in diameter form usually in the upper zones of the lung (Fig. 22-60). Rubbery and black, they may have foci of degeneration and cavitation filled with inky fluid. The principal morphologic difference between the progressive massive fibrosis lesions of CWP and silicosis is that in CWP the lesions appear to form a single mass whereas in silicosis they arise by the fusion of several nodules bound together in a fibrous mass. The collagen in complicated CWP is laid down haphazardly, whereas in silicosis the concentric organization of the hyaline nodules is discernible.

The cause of complicated CWP is unknown in most cases. The incidence of roentgenographically diagnosed PMF varies considerably from area to area, from a high of 14% in some anthracite mines to none in Colorado bituminous mines. Tuberculosis was once held to be the major cause, but despite the dramatic fall in the prevalence of tuberculosis, no comparable fall in the frequency of PMF has occurred. Silica may play a role; PMF tends to be more frequent in lungs having a high silica content, but the correlation in individual cases is not good. PMF has been reported in carbon electrode workers exposed to little silica. The prevalence of autoantibodies such as rheumatoid and antinuclear antibodies is higher in patients with complicated CWP than in those with simple CWP, which suggests that immunologic factors may be involved. However, PMF has not been associated

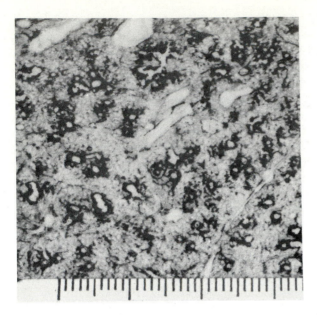

Fig. 22-58. Simple coal worker's pneumoconiosis. Paper-mounted lung section shows black dust deposits outlining respiratory bronchioles. (Preparation by Prof. J. Gough.)

with any specific HLA histocompatibility antigen, as might be expected if there were a genetic basis for abnormal immunologic response.

The diagnosis of CWP is based on a compatible occupational history and the presence of rounded opacities on the chest roentgenogram. The International Labor Organization (ILO) has devised a system of grading pneumoconiosis roentgenographically based on the size of the opacities (p, q, r in increasing size) and their profusion (increasing from 1 to 3). Complicated pneumoconiosis is diagnosed if opacities exceed 1 cm in size and is graded A, B, or C depending on size of lesions. Grading is reproducible with experienced observers and good roentgenologic technique. When Naeye and Dellinger[747] correlated the roentgenographic grading of simple CWP with the pathologic features in the tissue, the best correlations were with dust and collagen content of the tissue.

Disability in coal workers

Disability in coal workers has been discussed in detail by Morgan.[745] The mortality in coal miners is greater than in other occupational groups, but this is related largely to trauma and accidents. Mortality from respiratory disease is not demonstrably higher, a higher than

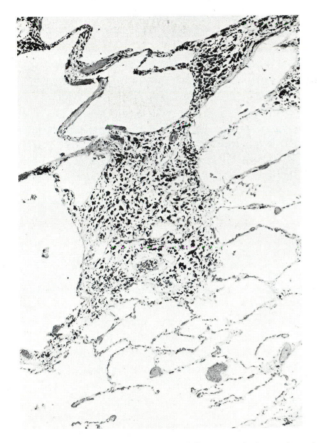

Fig. 22-59. Microscopic appearance of dust macule in coal worker.

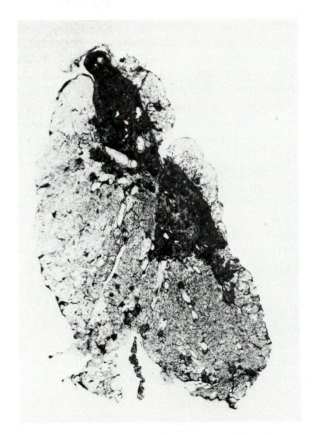

Fig. 22-60. Progressive massive fibrosis in coal worker. Paper-mounted whole lung section. (Preparation by Prof. J. Gough.)

expected number of deaths from COPD being balanced by a lower frequency of lung cancer than in comparable occupational groups. The lower frequency of lung cancer, if real, is attributable to lower levels of cigarette consumption by miners, who are prohibited from smoking underground.

Breathlessness and cough are more prevalent among miners than in controls. These symptoms show little correlation with roentgenographic category, the usual clinical index of CWP. Similarly, in pathologic studies of symptomatic and asymptomatic miners, Naeye and Dellinger[747] found no difference in the dust or collagen content or the volume of macules between the two groups. Most patients with grade 1 or 2 CWP on the chest roentgenogram have no impairment of ventilation. It is unlikely that simple CWP by itself causes disability.

Coal workers who complain of dyspnea and have impaired ventilation usually have an obstructive pattern.[745] Whether they can have hypoxemia without a reduction in expiratory flow is controversial, but currently either an $FEV_{1.0}$ below 80% of that predicted for normals or a decrease in the arterial oxygen tension can qualify a worker for compensation. Impaired ventilation is a consequence of emphysema and bronchitis as it is in the nonmining population. Right ventricular thickening, an indirect measure of hypoxemia, is also related to emphysema and unrelated to pathologic measures of CWP.[747] Although there is no doubt that cigarette smoking plays a role (some would say a predominant role) in the production of emphysema and bronchitis in most disabled miners, data indicate that coal workers have more emphysema than others who smoke a comparable amount and that some nonsmoking miners have emphysema of a degree sufficient to impair lung function. Naeye, Mahon, and Dellinger[748] found 24% of the area of lung sections of nonsmoking miners occupied by abnormal airspaces, compared with 4.8% for nonminers. Their study was retrospective and used uninflated lungs. Ryder and associates[752] in 1970 used whole lung sections of inflation-fixed lungs to determine the degree of emphysema in miners and found it to be considerably greater than in a control population, but their miner group was drawn from those receiving benefits from the Pneumoconiosis Medical Panel.[734] Cockcroft and associates[725] recently reported results of a prospective study avoiding these pitfalls that confirms the greater degree of emphysema in miners when controlled for cigarette smoking. Whether the causative agent is coal dust or some other element of the mine environment such as fumes from lamps or gases from diesel exhaust or shotfiring is uncertain.

Cough and sputum production (bronchitis) are more prevalent in miners than in nonminers and correlate with level of dust exposure, being highest in workers at the coal face where dust levels are highest and lowest in surface workers where dust is least. Slight impairment of ventilation is seen after many years of exposure.[745] Since airflows are reduced at high lung volumes but not at low lung volumes, the abnormalities appear to be in the large airways, but the mechanisms are unknown.

Whereas simple CWP does not affect life span or directly cause disability, complicated pneumoconiosis is clearly associated with airflow obstruction, reduced diffusion capacity, and restriction of ventilation. With higher grades of PMF cor pulmonale often develops. The process can progress after exposure has ceased (indeed it can first manifest itself long after exposure has ended) and life span is shortened.

Association with other diseases

Bronchogenic carcinoma does not appear to be more common in coal workers than in other groups. Some studies from both Britain and the United States point to a lesser incidence in coal workers. Tuberculosis is more common in coal workers than in the general population but less common than in patients with silicosis.

The combination of rheumatoid arthritis with CWP produces a characteristic lesion known as rheumatoid pneumoconiosis or Caplan's syndrome after the British radiologist who first recognized it.[724] Over a few months round opacities from 0.3 cm to several centimeters in diameter develop, mainly in the peripheral lung fields. The lesions evolve more rapidly than those of PMF and may finally cavitate or develop calcifications. The pathologic changes were described by Gough, Rivers, and Seal.[732] The lesions may be solitary, or several may fuse to form a large conglomerate mass. They are pale gray-yellow with concentric darker layers of pigment. The pale areas tend to liquefy, leaving clefts. Histologically the center is necrotic and often contains foci of calcium. Concentric bands of dust are found in the necrotic material. A zone of palisading fibroblasts or histiocytes surrounds the necrotic center. The outer layer consists of a capsule of circumferential collagen fibers with lymphocytes and plasma cells. Thus the lesion's characteristics are those of a rheumatoid necrobiotic nodule modified by the setting of pneumoconiosis.

Rheumatoid pneumoconiosis can appear without articular disease in miners, but circulating rheumatoid factor is invariably present. Arthritis subsequently develops in at least some such patients.

Diseases related to asbestos

Asbestos is a general term denoting any naturally occurring silicate mineral whose crystals are in the form of fibers. The major commercial types, chrysotile, crocidolite, amosite, and anthophyllite, differ in their elemental composition, fiber morphology, physical properties, and certain of their effects on cells. They probably differ also in their capacity to produce each of the various lesions associated with asbestos exposure, but since based on current knowledge none can be exonerated as a cause of any of the lesions to be discussed, no effort will be made to distinguish among them in the following discussion.

Asbestos is a ubiquitous contaminant of the urban environment and has been identified in urban air.[754] Asbestos bodies, fibers coated with iron and protein, can be found in virtually 100% of adult lungs if gram amounts of tissue are digested and the residue collected on a filter and examined with a microscope. The number of uncoated fibers is approximately 10^5 fibers per gram. The significance of this relatively low-level asbestos exposure is uncertain, but there is no evidence at present linking it to disease.

The lesions associated with exposure to elevated levels of asbestos include pulmonary fibrosis, tumors, pleural plaques, and pleural effusions.[721] Pulmonary fibrosis requires the highest levels of exposure and is practically limited to those with direct industrial exposure. Tumors and pleural plaques are induced by lower levels of exposure and can be found in those whose exposure is indirect, such as family members who handle a worker's dusty clothes or those who dwell near asbestos mines, mills, or dump sites.

Asbestosis

The term *asbestosis* should be reserved for pulmonary fibrosis caused by asbestos. Asbestosis is seen in shipyard and construction workers, insulation workers, and those engaged in the manufacture of asbestos cement, tiles, or brake linings. Disease first appears at least 10 and usually 20 or more years after first exposure.[721]

The symptoms of asbestosis are insidious and are similar to those of interstitial fibrosis of any cause: breathlessness, initially associated only with exertion, accompanied by a nonproductive cough. Physical examination usually shows basilar crackles and may show clubbing. Early in the disease the chest roentgenogram may be normal, although physiologic measurements such as vital capacity or diffusing capacity may show abnormalities. Later dyspnea becomes more severe, hyperventilation is apparent, and cor pulmonale may develop. The chest roentgenogram, which initially shows small irregular opacities at the bases, later shows honeycombing.

The lungs are small and firm with a thickened pleura.[726,727] On the sectioned surface gray zones of fibrosis enclose abnormally enlarged airspaces a few millimeters to a centimeter in size. Lesions are most prominent in the bases and the subpleural areas (Fig. 22-61).

The microscopic changes are those of a nonspecific interstitial fibrosis accompanied by the presence of characteristic structures known as asbestos or ferruginous bodies.[726,727]

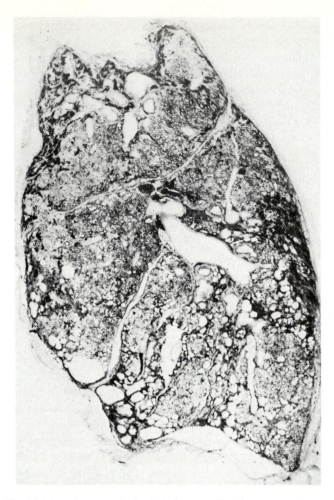

Fig. 22-61. Paper-mounted whole lung section from patient with asbestosis shows areas of honeycombing, especially in subpleural zones. (From pathological museum of University of Manchester, U.K.)

Ferruginous bodies vary in length from 10 to 50 μm or more and consist of a straight or curved translucent core of asbestos coated with globules of brown refractile material, which give the body a beaded, dumbbell, or drumstick shape (Fig. 22-62).[763] The coating stains strongly with the Prussian blue reaction for ferric iron and by electron microscopy is shown to consist of ferritin. The formation of these bodies has been observed with electron microscopy in experimental animals. Only the largest fibers give rise to ferruginous bodies; small fibers remain uncoated. The fibers are phagocytosed or, if too large to be completely phagocytosed, are enclosed by macrophage cytoplasm, forming an incomplete phagosome (Fig. 22-63). Vacuoles, probably lysosomes, containing ferritin discharge onto the surface of the fiber, leading to the buildup of coating material.[757]

The disease begins in the respiratory bronchioles, and early cases show only interstitial fibrosis in some respiratory bronchioles, accompanied by prominent hyperplastic alveolar epithelium and the accumulation of macrophages in the airspace lumina.[726] Asbestos bodies may be

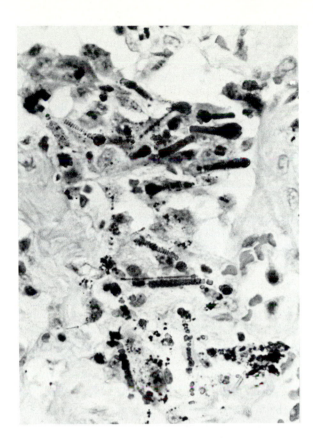

Fig. 22-62. Asbestosis. Interstitial fibrous tissue contains dust and asbestos bodies.

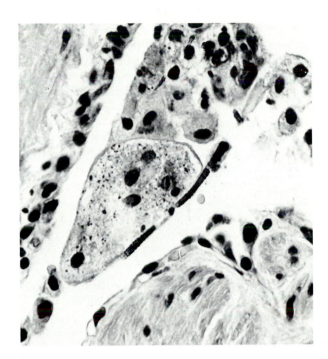

Fig. 22-63. Asbestosis. Asbestos body in alveolar space adheres to giant cell. One end appears to be within cytoplasm of a macrophage.

present either in the airspace or in the interstitium, usually in association with macrophages. With time the process extends to involve alveolar ducts, and fibrosis in neighboring lobules links up, resulting in the picture of diffuse interstitial fibrosis. The thickened alveolar walls are often infiltrated with lymphocytes and rarely with neutrophils. The alveolar epithelium is hyperplastic with areas of metaplasia to squamous or mucin-secreting epithelium. Commonly a few of the hyperplastic alveolar epithelial cells contain hyaline inclusions reminiscent of hepatic Mallory bodies, and occasionally this phenomenon is prominent (Fig. 22-64).[742] It is not specific for asbestosis, being seen occasionally in other forms of lung injury. Large numbers of macrophages, sometimes with multinucleated giant cells, are commonly present in the airspaces. Asbestos bodies are often plentiful but may be rare. One case has been reported in which no asbestos bodies were present but electron microscopy showed large numbers of uncoated fibers. In contrast to silicosis, the hilar lymph nodes show little involvement in asbestosis, although a few asbestos bodies may be present.

Pleural disease

Pleural effusions develop in as much as 5% of asbestos workers, but most are small and asymptomatic.[729] Occasionally they cause pain or fever. Pleural plaques are the

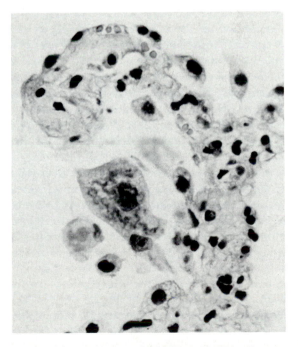

Fig. 22-64. Asbestosis. Enlarged alveolar epithelial cell apparently sloughing into alveolar space. Cytoplasm contains network of hyaline material.

most common lesion associated with asbestos.[721] They are circumscribed, usually bilateral lesions that develop on the pleural surface of the diaphragm and the parietal pleura of the chest wall. Grossly they appear as flat, ivory-colored deposits 1 mm to several millimeters thick with a smooth or knobby surface. They often calcify, which aids their roentgenographic recognition. Microscopically they consist of hyalinized collagenous tissue with few cells. Asbestos bodies are not generally found within the plaques, even when digestion techniques are used.

Plaques take many years to develop. They are infrequent in the first 20 years after exposure, but by 30 to 40 years as much as 50% of workers have calcified plaques that are seen roentgenographically. Plaques rarely cause symptoms and apparently do not restrict ventilation unless very extensive. There is no evidence that they predispose to mesotheliomas. Their importance is as a marker for exposure to asbestos.

Tumors

The association of mesothelioma with asbestos exposure was reported by Wagner, Sleggs, and Marchand[760] in 1960, and many additional cases have since been reported.[721,726,727] The asbestos exposure need not be intense, and indirect (nonoccupational) exposure is responsible for some cases. The latent period is generally more than 20 years. Either the pleura or the peritoneum may be the primary site. The pathologic features and natural history of mesothelioma are discussed elsewhere (p. 929), but it is appropriate here to reiterate that approximately 50% of mesotheliomas in men in the United States are associated with exposure to asbestos.

Bronchogenic carcinoma is the greatest single cause of excess mortality in asbestos workers.[753] The risk of bronchogenic carcinoma is slightly increased by asbestos in nonsmokers, but in smokers tobacco smoke and asbestos are synergistic. Hammond, Selikoff, and Seidman[735] found the relative risks of bronchogenic carcinoma to be 10 times greater in smokers that in nonsmokers and five times greater in asbestos-exposed nonsmokers that in other nonsmokers. The risk for asbestos workers who smoke was an appalling 50 times greater than that for nonsmoking, unexposed subjects. The bronchogenic carcinomas in asbestos-exposed patients occur more commonly in the lower lobes, whereas in the general population bronchogenic carcinoma occurs predominantly in the upper lobes. Some observers have reported adenocarcinomas to be the predominant histologic type,[762] but others have not found a preponderance of any particular histologic type.[740]

Carcinomas in other sites may also be more common in asbestos workers. The risk of carcinoma of the larynx and large intestine is greater in asbestos workers, and there are unconfirmed reports of an increase in renal cell carcinoma and hematologic malignancies.

Beryllium disease

Beryllium disease was first recognized in Europe in the 1930s. Epidemics occurred in the United States in the 1940s, particularly in the fluorescent light industry. These disappeared once the hazard was recognized and the use of beryllium in fluorescent lights was abandoned. Although the use of beryllium is increasing again because its properties of imparting lightness, hardness, and heat resistance to materials make it attractive for aerospace industries, the disease remains rare and is of interest principally for contrast with conventional pneumoconioses.

In the past, acute berylliosis was seen in the extraction industry, typically in workers who had been exposed to high concentrations for 2 to 4 weeks. The onset is acute with dyspnea, hyperpnea, and in some cases substernal pain. Most patients recover, although this may take as long as 12 weeks. The few patients examined at autopsy showed an acute chemical pneumonitis. The alveolar walls were thickened by interstitial edema and mononuclear cell infiltration. The airspaces contained edema and hyaline membranes in various stages of organization. Bronchiolitis obliterans was present in a few patients. Tissue beryllium levels were usually high.[730]

Chronic beryllium disease is a systemic disorder, although the lung, being the portal of entry, is usually the major site of clinical involvement. The symptoms may begin at any time during exposure or up to 20 years after exposure, but the majority of patients become ill in the first 5 years. Typically patients have a gradual onset of dyspnea and nonproductive cough that progress to cyanosis. Weight loss is common and may be dramatic. Other systemic manifestations include hyperglobulinemia, hypercalcemia, and occasionally renal stones.

The disease is probably not a direct manifestation of toxicity but a hypersensitivity reaction of cell-mediated type, and the histologic changes are similar to those in other types of hypersensitivity pneumonitis. The spectrum of changes ranges from diffuse interstitial pneumonitis with nonspecific infiltration of airspace walls by histiocytes, lymphocytes, and plasma cells, to mononuclear infiltration accompanied by loose or well-formed granulomas, to tightly organized noncaseating epithelioid granulomas like those of sarcoid with little interstitial infiltrate.[730] Giant cells are present with each type and frequently contain inclusions, either asteroid bodies or the concentric laminated hematoxyphilic bodies known as conchoid or Schaumann bodies. First described in sarcoid, in which they are rare, Schaumann bodies are present in 50% to 70% of patients with berylliosis, especially those with interstitial pneumonitis. Although they are by no means specific, their presence in abundance suggests a diagnosis of beryllium disease. Discrete hyalinized nodules surrounded by a fibrous capsule are present in 40% of cases and may occasionally be the predominant lesion. The center of the nodules may show infarctlike necrosis, calcification, or cholesterol clefts.

The experience of the U.S. Beryllium Disease Case Registry indicates that the course and prognosis of the disease are strongly correlated with histologic findings.[730] Among patients with diffuse interstitial pneumonia with or without granulomas, the mortality was 75% with an average survival of 8 years. Those with a sarcoid-like reaction with little interstitial infiltrate had a much better prognosis, with only a 4% mortality during an average follow-up period of 11 years.

LUNG TUMORS
Carcinomas of the lung
Incidence

The incidence of carcinoma of the lung in industrialized countries has been increasing at a phenomenal rate during the twentieth century (Fig. 22-65). Infrequent early in the century, lung cancer is now the second most common carcinoma (after skin cancer) in American men, accounting for 22% of all cancers and one third of all deaths resulting from malignancy. The incidence in women is rising 5% annually, and lung cancer is expected shortly to become the leading cause of cancer mortality in women, surpassing carcinoma of the breast before the end of the 1980s. In Britain lung cancer accounts for nearly 40% of cancer deaths in men and 13% in women. Currently the incidence is rising more rapidly in women than in men. If the present trend continues, the incidence rates for men and women will be equal by the year 2000.[812]

Cancer of the lung is a disease of middle and late life. The incidence is low in those below 35 years of age, rises to a peak at age 60, and declines slowly thereafter.

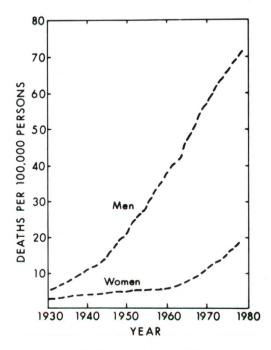

Fig. 22-65. Mortality from carcinoma of lung, 1930 to 1980.

Classification

Lung tumors are classified on the basis of histologic findings. The various histologic types of lung cancer differ in clinical presentation, natural history, and response to treatment. Evidence of more than one type of differentiation can be found in a number of lung carcinomas if special techniques such as electron microscopy are used,[769] but the practical value of standard histologic classifications based on the predominant cell type is amply justified on clinical grounds. The following is the classification recommended by an expert panel convened by the World Health Organization[859]:

1. Squamous cell carcinoma (epidermoid carcinoma)
   a. Spindle cell squamous carcinoma (variant)
2. Small cell carcinoma
   a. Oat cell carcinoma
   b. Intermediate cell type
   c. Combined oat cell carcinoma
3. Adenocarcinoma
   a. Acinar adenocarcinoma
   b. Papillary adenocarcinoma
   c. Bronchioloalveolar carcinoma
   d. Solid carcinoma with mucus formation
4. Large cell carcinoma
   a. Giant cell carcinoma (variant)
   b. Clear cell carcinoma (variant)
5. Adenosquamous carcinoma
6. Carcinoid tumor
7. Bronchial gland carcinomas
   a. Adenoid cystic carcinomas
   b. Mucoepidermoid carcinoma
   c. Others
8. Others

In common clinical usage the first four categories, squamous cell carcinoma, small cell carcinoma, adenocarcinoma, and large cell carcinoma, are grouped as "bronchogenic carcinoma." A strict histogenetic classification would group small cell carcinoma and carcinoid together as tumors of the neuroendocrine cells, but in clinical presentation small cell carcinomas resemble the other "bronchogenic" carcinomas more closely than they do carcinoid.

The diagnostic differentiation of the histologic classes of bronchogenic carcinoma can be made using either exfoliated cells or tissue sections. Both are reliable when the tumors are well differentiated. When a tumor is poorly differentiated, even expert pathologists using multiple sections may disagree.[844] In one study three experienced pathologists could agree on the classification of only 50% of poorly differentiated tumors.[862]

Bronchogenic carcinomas

Squamous cell carcinoma. Squamous cell carcinoma is probably the most common type of bronchogenic carcinoma, comprising 30% to 35% of autopsy series and 35% to 60% of surgical series,[766,832,851] although some recent studies suggest that adenocarcinoma may have overtaken it in incidence.[848] Squamous carcinomas are more common in men than in women, usually develop in middle or later life, and are strongly associated with cigarette smoking.[766] The relative risk of contracting squamous cell carcinoma was 25 times greater for smokers than nonsmokers in Kreyberg's study.[817] Roughly two thirds of squamous carcinomas are central tumors, involving the main or lobar bronchi, while one third arise in the lung periphery, either in small bronchi or in association with scars (Fig. 22-66).[782,852] However, in some patients with large bronchi involved at the time of diagnosis, serial roentgenographic observations suggest that the tumor actually arose in a more peripheral location and grew to involve the central bronchi late in its course.[834] Bronchial involvement may take the form of a warty endobronchial protrusion, or the tumor may ulcerate the bronchus and grow outward.[823] If the tumor obstructs a large bronchus, the lung distal to the tumor will often be the site of obstructive pneumonia and bronchiectasis. The gross appearance of most squamous carcinomas is not distinctive, but large, well-differentiated tumors may have

shiny caseous yellow foci where heavily keratinized. The expectoration of keratinous or necrotic material may product cavities within the tumor. Indeed, the majority of cavitary lung carcinomas are of the squamous cell type.

The microscopic diagnosis of squamous carcinoma depends on the identification of either intercellular bridges or keratinization (Fig. 22-67). Keratinized cells can be recognized in sections by their brightly eosinophilic refractile cytoplasm and pyknotic nuclei. Squamous carcinomas of the lung tend to be poorly differentiated and often vary from area to area. Typically they are composed of nests of cells that palisade at the periphery of the lobules and become enlarged and flattened centrally. Whorls or eddies of cells may be keratinized (epidermoid pearls); the whole center of the lobule may be filled with keratin, or at the other extreme only a few single cells may be keratinized.

Although most squamous cell carcinomas have at least some areas of large cells with plentiful cytoplasm, some tumors consist only of relatively small basophilic cells resembling those of basal cell carcinoma in the skin. The

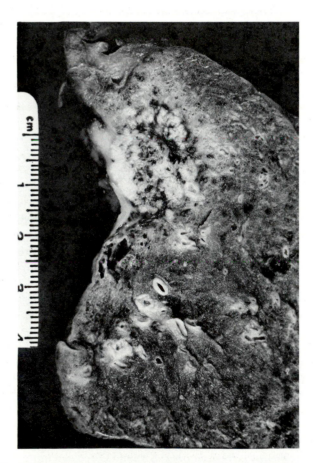

Fig. 22-66. Epidermoid carcinoma of lung. This is peripheral tumor not associated with major bronchus. Overlying pleura is thickened and retracted.

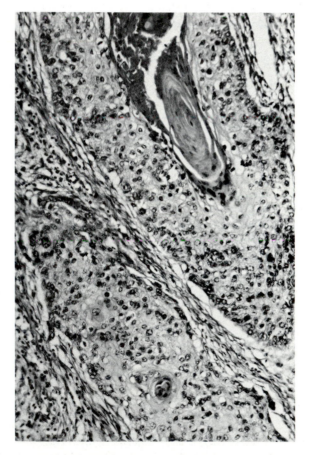

Fig. 22-67. Epidermoid carcinoma of bronchus. Note keratin nests.

distinction from small cell carcinoma is difficult in such cases. Electron microscopy and immunohistochemical studies may be helpful. The electron microscope shows that the cells of squamous carcinoma are joined by desmosomes on short projections of cytoplasm, which correspond to the intercellular bridges seen with light microscopy.[825] Secretory granules are absent, and the endoplasmic reticulum is poorly developed. Immunohistochemistry shows that keratin is invariably present and carcinoembryonic antigen is usual.[838]

Squamous cell carcinomas tend to grow more rapidly than other histologic types, with doubling times of 2 to 4 months and relatively high mitotic indices.[853,855] Despite this, they have a more favorable prognosis than other types of bronchogenic carcinoma, with a 5-year survival of 20% to 35%.[816,836,846,857]

Squamous carcinoma is believed to arise through a series of changes in the epithelium of the bronchi that includes hyperplasia of the basal cells, loss of cilia, metaplasia of the epithelium, development of a squamous type of epithelium, increasing atypism, squamous carcinoma in situ, and eventually invasion (Fig. 22-68).[768] The

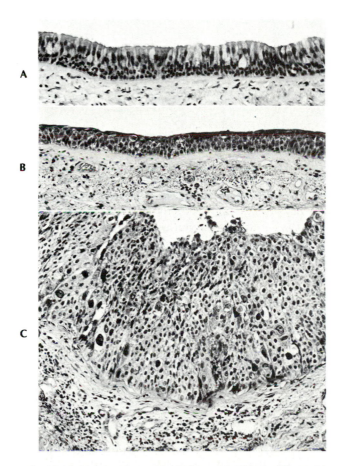

Fig. 22-68. Presumptive stages in histogenesis of epidermoid carcinoma. **A,** Normal bronchus. **B,** Squamous metaplasia. **C,** In situ carcinoma. Malignant-appearing epithelium without invasion. (130×.)

squamous cells derive either from abnormal differentiation of the basal cells or from metaplasia of mucous cells.[847] The time required for the various stages in the proposed sequence is unknown, but many patients have been observed to have cytologically malignant cells in their sputum for several years before any tumor could be detected roentgenologically.

Adenocarcinoma. Between 20% and 30% of carcinomas of the lung are adenocarcinomas, and the proportion has risen in the last 15 years.[766,832,848,851] Adenocarcinoma is the most common histologic type of bronchogenic carcinoma in women,[850] and the increasing proportion of women in the lung carcinoma population is undoubtedly a factor in the relative increase in adenocarcinomas. Although adenocarcinoma is the most common type of bronchogenic carcinoma in nonsmokers,[846,855,859] the great majority of patients with adenocarcinoma are smokers.[846] Even in Kreyberg's study,[817] which established the strong association of small cell and squamous cell carcinomas with cigarette smoking, the relative risk of adenocarcinoma was three times greater in smokers than in nonsmokers.

The majority of adenocarcinomas arise in the periphery of the lung.[766,776,852] As much as 50% may arise in scars,[832] although recent investigations suggest that the fibrosis associated with some adenocarcinomas is stroma laid down in the tumor rather than preexisting scar.[824] The association of adenocarcinoma with diffuse interstitial fibrosis[797,827] and the many instances in which a sudden change in a previously roentgenographically stable lesion turned out to be cancer leave little doubt that scarring with associated epithelial hyperplasia predisposed to carcinoma.

Adenocarcinomas appear as discrete masses, usually at the lung periphery where they often cause retraction of the overlying pleura (Fig. 22-69).[823] The borders of the tumor may be smooth, or stellate protrusions may extend into the surrounding lung. Irregular pigmentation of the tumor is not unusual, since inhaled dust and soot are not easily cleared from areas of tumor and the lymphatics are often obstructed. Microscopically adenocarcinomas are highly variable in appearance. As evidence of secretory differentiation the tumor cells may form distinct acini or have intracellular mucin (Fig. 22-70). When fibrosis is marked because of the presence of preexisting scar or excessive production of stroma, the glands and columns of tumor cells may be distorted and difficult to recognize. Papillary patterns do occur, but more often the spread of tumor through the alveolar spaces merely gives the appearance of a papillary pattern as tumor cells cover the alveolar septa where they protrude into alveolar ducts. Solid sheets of tumor cells may fill alveolar spaces.

When studied with electron microscopy, lung adenocarcinomas show moderately well-developed endoplasmic reticulum, secretory granules or vacuoles, and some-

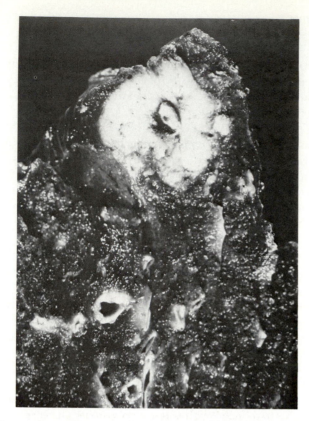

Fig. 22-69. Adenocarcinoma of lung. This tumor presumably arose in a scar. Ring of pigment in center outlines edge of calcified granuloma that occupied center of tumor.

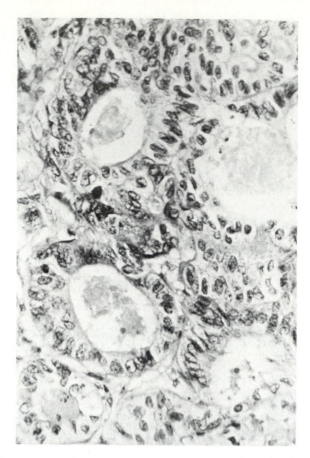

Fig. 22-70. Adenocarcinoma of lung showing well-formed glands.

times intracytoplasmic lumen formation.[779,825] Cells are often polarized with a microvillous apex where neighboring cells are joined by tight junctions, defining a lumen that may be invisible under the light microscope. Immunohistochemistry typically shows the presence of carcinoembryonic antigen, but keratin is inconspicuous.[786,838]

Adenocarcinomas are relatively slow growing, with doubling times of 4 to 10 months and low mitotic indices.[853,855] Because of their peripheral location they have a high resectability rate. Despite these seemingly favorable properties, the prognosis for primary adenocarcinoma of the lung is poor, with a 5-year survival of only 5% overall.[776,816,846,857] Treatment failure is due to the presence of metastases. Evidently because of their peripheral location, adenocarcinomas do not cause symptoms by obstructing bronchi, and the diagnosis is not made until late in the course.

Bronchioloalveolar carcinoma is a morphologic variant of adenocarcinoma in which the sole or predominant pattern of growth is spread along the existing airspace walls, which serve as the stroma for the tumor.[819] The walls of alveoli, alveolar ducts, and to a variable extent bronchioles are lined by malignant epithelial cells that vary in shape from cuboidal to columnar. The alveolar walls over

which the tumor cells spread may be normal or may be thickened by fibrosis. When they are thickened, an abrupt transition to normal thickness usually occurs precisely where the neoplastic epithelium ends, suggesting that the thickening is reaction to the tumor rather than preexisting fibrosis. The malignant epithelium may be highly atypical or closely resemble normal bronchiolar or alveolar lining cells. Some bronchioloalveolar carcinomas are composed of tall mucin-producing cells that fill the involved airspaces with mucus (Fig. 22-71). In rare instances this can lead to the clinical syndrome of bronchorrhea with electrolyte depletion.[822]

Electron microscopic studies of bronchioloalveolar carcinomas have shown differentiation along several lines. Tumors with ultrastructural features of type II alveolar epithelial cells have been described and the cells of some tumors have been shown to contain the antigens of the protein portion (apoprotein) of alveolar surfactant.[839] Other tumors are composed mainly of cells with granules like those of Clara cells. Yet a third group produces mainly mucin.[804,818]

Grossly and roentgenographically bronchioloalveolar carcinoma can appear as a discrete solitary peripheral

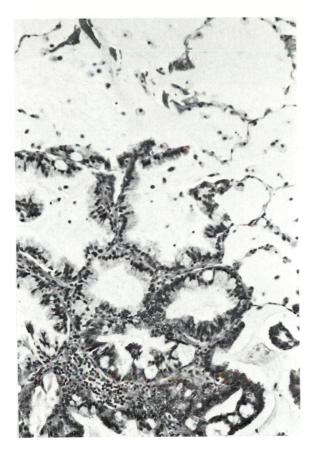

Fig. 22-71. Bronchioloalveolar carcinoma. Tall mucin-secreting epithelium spreading along alveolar septa. Airspaces are filled with mucus.

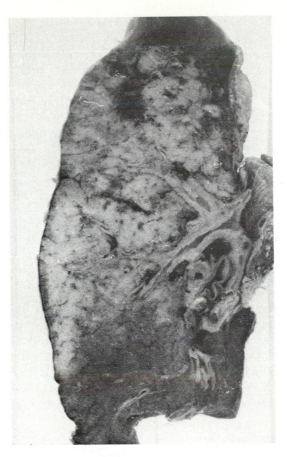

Fig. 22-72. Bronchiolalveolar carcinoma. Tumor is spreading through lung like pneumonia rather than remaining as discrete mass. (From pathological museum of University of Manchester, U.K.)

mass, as multiple small nodules in one or both lungs, or as an ill-defined area of infiltrate resembling pneumonia (Fig. 22-72).[819,822] Whether the multiple nodular form develops from multiple independent foci of origin or by metastasis of tumor cells through the airspaces is not established. The infrequent, highly secretory mucinous tumors appear shiny and gelatinous.

Whether bronchioloalveolar carcinoma is a distinct entity has engendered much controversy. Metastatic carcinoma can spread in the lung with a histologic pattern identical to that of bronchoalveolar carcinoma. However, even before markers for lung-specific differentiation such as surfactant-apoprotein were available, autopsies had established the absence of an extrapulmonary primary lesion in many cases. The differentiation of bronchioloalveolar carcinoma from other pulmonary adenocarcinomas is often difficult. Tumors occur with various proportions of solid growth and growth along alveolar walls, and the decision of where to make the separation is subjective.[775] This is one of the areas in which disagreement among pathologists is common.[862] Electron microscopy indicates that both solid or acinar adenocarcinoma and bronchioloalveolar carcinoma differentiate along similar

lines toward mucinous, Clara, or type II cells.[779] Two features supporting the idea that bronchioloalveolar carcinoma is distinct are its lack of association with cigarette smoking in some studies and that according to some reports it has a better prognosis than other adenocarcinomas when it appears as a solitary nodule.[822] The diffuse pneumonic and multinodular forms, on the other hand, are rapidly fatal.[822] In several recent reports survival has been the same for bronchioloalveolar carcinoma and other adenocarcinomas.[836]

Large cell undifferentiated carcinoma. Large cell undifferentiated carcinoma is a diagnosis by default. When viewed with the light microscope between 7% and 15% of carcinomas of the lung are composed of relatively large cells (greater than 12 μm in diameter) that lack specific features by which they could be assigned to either the squamous or the adenocarcinoma group. The tumors vary in microscopic appearance from lobules of well-formed epithelium lacking evidence of gland formation, secretion, or keratin, to anaplastic tumors formed of poorly cohesive cells scarcely recognizable as epithelium. These tumors are considered undifferentiated, but if electron microscopy or other special techniques are used, the majority of such tumors show some evidence of differentiation, indicating that they are really poorly differentiated variants of adenocarcinoma, squamous cell carcinoma, or combined adenosquamous carcinoma.[785,811]

Large cell undifferentiated carcinomas are more common in men than in women, have a peak age of onset near 60 years, and are associated with tobacco smoking in 95% of cases. They arise at the lung periphery or apex in two thirds of cases.[781,829] They grow rapidly and are usually large tumors by the time of diagnosis. The prognosis is poor, with a median survival time of only 6 months and a 5-year survival overall of 6%.[829] Tumors with ultrastructural evidence of squamous differentiation seem to have a somewhat better prognosis than those with glandular differentiation.[811]

Giant cell carcinoma is a highly malignant form of undifferentiated carcinoma composed of huge, poorly cohesive cells with eosinophilic cytoplasm and one or several large convoluted nuclei (Fig. 22-73). The tumors are often infiltrated with polymorphonuclear leukocytes, and collections of neutrophils appear within the cytoplasm of the tumor cells as if phagocytosed. Typically they are bulky, rapidly growing tumors that often involve a major bronchus. Metastases are usually evident by the time of diagnosis, and the course is rapid, with survival for more than 1 year the exception.[796,830,833]

In the preceding discussion the category of clear cell carcinoma was omitted. Although clear cell carcinoma was included as a subtype of large cell undifferentiated carcinoma in the WHO classification, adenocarcinomas, squamous carcinomas, and undifferentiated carcinomas can all be composed predominantly of cells with clear cytoplasm. The appearance of a clear cytoplasm reflects, for the most part, a high glycogen content but is also influenced by the lipid content, intracellular edema, and the type and efficiency of fixation. It does not form a useful basis for classifying bronchogenic carcinomas, since it is not known to influence the biology of the tumor.

Adenosquamous carcinoma. By light microscopy 1% to 3% of lung carcinomas have clear evidence of both keratinization and glandular or secretory differentiation.[832] Most are peripheral tumors associated with scars. Adenosquamous carcinomas should be distinguished from mucoepidermoid carcinoma of the mucous glands.

Small cell carcinoma. In the normal lung, cells con-

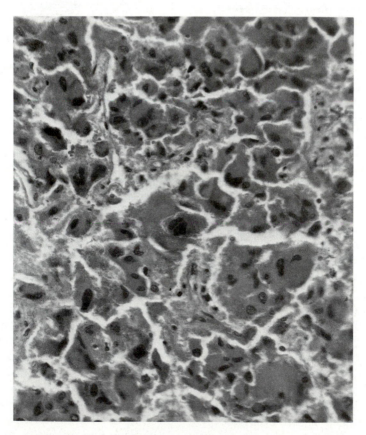

Fig. 22-73. Giant cell carcinoma. Large multinucleated cells with abundant cytoplasm. Cells are so poorly cohesive that their epithelial nature is difficult to appreciate.

taining small, electron-dense, membrane-bound granules are found at all levels of the tracheobronchial tree including the bronchi, mucous glands, and bronchioles. These cells contain serotonin and several biologically active peptides including bombesin, calcitonin, and met-enkephalin.[788] They appear to give rise to several tumors, including the highly malignant small cell carcinoma, the less malignant carcinoid, and small tumorlike proliferations known as tumorlets.

Small cell carcinomas comprise 20% to 25% of bronchogenic carcinomas.[802,815,851] They occur predominantly in middle-aged men and are strongly associated with tobacco smoking.[817] They rarely if ever occur among nonsmokers in the general population[560] but are found in some occupational groups, including uranium miners[837] and workers exposed to chloromethyl methyl ether.[795]

Small cell carcinomas appear as fleshy encephaloid tumors infiltrating and destroying the wall of a major bronchus (Fig. 22-74). Hilar and mediastinal lymph node involvement is usually extensive in untreated patients and is often more conspicuous than the primary tumor. Microscopically several patterns are recognized.[823,859] The oat cell type consists of round or elongated poorly cohesive cells 10 to 12 μm in length or slightly larger than lymphocytes (Fig. 22-75). The tumor cells have dark clumped chromatin and little recognizable cytoplasm. Necrosis is usually present and is widespread in larger tumors. Blood vessels in necrotic areas become encrusted with DNA, staining blue with hematoxylin in routine sections. The pattern of tumor growth is diffuse but with some division into lobules by vessels and stroma, which helps to distinguish oat cell carcinoma from lymphoma. The intermediate cell type of small cell carcinoma is composed of cells slightly larger than those of the oat cell type and with somewhat better intercellular cohesion and organization into lobules. Some tumors are composed of spindle-shaped cells, and some are organized into ribbons of cells or pseudorosettes closely associated with vessels, making their endocrine origin easy to recognize.[770]

By electron microscopy, 70% to 80% of small cell carcinomas contain small secretory granules of neuroendocrine type.[777,808] The characteristic granules are membrane bound, with an electron-lucent gap between the membrane and the dense granule matrix. The granules are not present in every cell, and sometimes extensive search is required for granules on which to base the diagnosis. Immunohistochemistry may prove useful for diag-

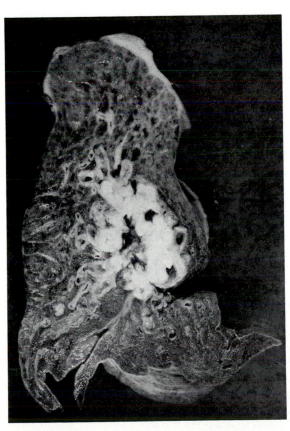

Fig. 22-74. Small cell carcinoma. This is central tumor growing within large bronchus and extending through its wall.

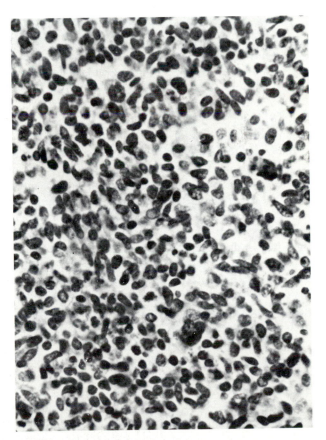

Fig. 22-75. Small cell carcinoma, oat cell type. Slightly elongated, poorly cohesive cells with scarcely any cytoplasm.

nosis, since many small cell carcinomas contain the peptide bombesin,[793] neuron-specific enolase, and a membrane antigen known as small cell carcinoma–associated antigen.[790] Keratin and carcinoembryonic antigen are infrequent.[838]

Small cell carcinoma is highly malignant and almost invariably has metastasized by the time of diagnosis. Median survival is only 4 months, and the 5-year survival with surgery is a dismal 1%, with at most only a marginal influence of histologic subtype.[783,789,831] Since these tumors are sensitive to chemotherapy and radiation, they are generally not treated surgically.[802] Therefore accurate diagnosis is mandatory to avoid unnecessary surgery, and electron microscopy or immunologic markers should be used in doubtful cases.

Spread of bronchogenic carcinoma. Carcinoma of the lung can invade contiguous structures directly and metastasize by the lymphatics and bloodstream. Lymphatic metastasis usually takes place to the hilar lymph nodes initially with spread to contiguous groups leading to mediastinal, cervical, and para-aortic involvement. When pleural adhesions are present, spread to the lymphatic plexus of the parietal pleura can lead to the appearance of tumor in axillary or supraclavicular nodes. The brain, liver, bone, and adrenal glands are the most common sites of vascular dissemination. Adrenal involvement may also develop via lymphatic connections across the diaphragm. With small cell carcinoma bone marrow involvement is common even in the absence of overt bone destruction; therefore bone scanning and marrow aspiration are useful as staging procedures.[810]

Clinical manifestations

Symptoms of lung cancer are widely variable and result from local effects of the tumor, occlusion of a bronchus, or local and distant metastases.[813] Since most patients are smokers, cough and sputum production have often been present for years. Local irritation by the tumor results in a change in the cough or sputum. Other local effects of the tumor include wheezing, hemoptysis, dyspnea, and chest pain. Infections distal to bronchial obstructions tend to resolve slowly or recur in the same location, leading to bronchiectasis and chronic pneumonia with their attendant symptoms. Pleural effusions can develop as a result of metastasis to the pleura, infection, or lymphatic obstruction. All too often the first symptoms of lung cancer are caused by distant spread: superior vena caval obstruction, recurrent nerve paralysis, painful bone lesions, neurologic symptoms resulting from brain metastases, and so forth. Indeed, in 75% of patients spread beyond the lung has occurred by the time of diagnosis.

A number of rare, so-called paraneoplastic syndromes are associated with lung cancer:

1. Endocrine
   a. Cushing's syndrome
   b. Inappropriate antidiuretic hormone (ADH) secretion
   c. Hypercalcemia
   d. Carcinoid syndrome
   e. Gynecomastia
2. Neuromuscular
   a. Polymyositis
   b. Carcinomatous myopathy
   c. Eaton-Lambert (myasthenic) syndrome
   d. Peripheral neuropathy
   e. Subacute cerebellar degeneration
3. Skeletal
   a. Clubbing
   b. Hypertrophic osteoarthropathy
4. Cutaneous
   a. Acanthosis nigricans
   b. Dermatomyositis
5. Cardiovascular
   a. Migratory thrombophlebitis
   b. Nonbacterial thrombotic endocarditis

Although some are associated with malignant tumors in many sites, others such as the Eaton-Lambert (myasthenic) syndrome and hypertrophic osteoarthropathy are particularly associated with lung cancer. Ectopic hormone production is a rare clinical problem but one that affects lung cancer patients more often than patients with cancer of other sites. Different hormonal syndromes are characteristic of different histologic types of lung cancer. Ectopic adrenocorticotropic hormone (ACTH) production, inappropriate ADH secretion, and the carcinoid syndrome are most often associated with small cell carcinoma.[771,780,807,820] Between 3% and 19% of patients with small cell carcinoma have the clinical syndrome of ectopic ACTH production,[820] which is dominated by hypokalemic alkalosis, hypertension, and signs of mineralocorticoid excess and frequently lacks the classic features of Cushing's syndrome. Up to 50% of patients with small cell carcinoma have abnormalities of adrenal function such as loss of diurnal fluctuation in plasma cortisol concentration and loss of dexamethasone suppression, but only a fraction of these have the full clinical syndrome.[780] The second most frequent endocrine abnormality with small cell carcinoma is the syndrome of inappropriate ADH secretion, characterized by low plasma sodium concentration and osmolality with a high urine osmolality.[780] Plasma ADH activity is inappropriately high for the low plasma osmolality, and if a water load is given, it is not excreted as rapidly as would be expected. Although calcitonin levels in tumor and plasma are elevated in many patients with small cell carcinoma, this does not cause symptoms.[806,807] Evidently parathyroid or other compensatory mechanisms are adequate to prevent hypocalcemia. Nevertheless, some observers have found calcitonin the most reliable of several hormones studied in following the clinical progress of small cell carcinoma. Although there is strong evidence that tumor is the source of the calcitonin in many cases,[806,807] in some instances of lung cancer the thyroid has been the apparent source of increased calcitonin production.

Parathormone production by lung tumors explains the rare occurrence of hypercalcemia in the absence of bone metastasis.[774] It is usually associated with squamous cell or large cell carcinomas. Chorionic gonadotropin production occurs with all histologic types of bronchial cancer.[787,858] Although it can be associated with gynecomastia, it is often asymptomatic. The presence of growth hormone has also been reported.[772]

Staging and prognosis

Although the overall prognosis of bronchogenic carcinoma is grim, with a cure rate of only 5% to 8%, there are a number of factors that influence prognosis in individual cases. The initial choice of therapy depends on histologic type of tumor and clinical stage, a grouping of patients according to tumor size, extent of apparent dissemination, and proximity of tumor to potential surgical margins.[784] The clinical staging of lung cancer is:

Occult carcinoma	Malignant cells in bronchopulmonary secretions without evidence of primary tumor or metastases
Stage 1	Tumor less than or larger than 3 cm without metastasis; tumor less than 3 cm with metastasis to ipsilateral hilar lymph nodes only
Stage 2	Tumor larger than 3 cm with ipsilateral hilar lymph node metastases only
Stage 3	Tumor within 2 cm of the carina or invading adjacent structures outside the lung; tumor of any size with metastasis to mediastinal lymph nodes or distant metastases

Except for patients with small cell carcinoma, those with stage 1 or 2 disease are potentially curable. For small cell carcinoma irrespective of stage, the probability of surgical cure is less than the operative mortality.

The study of the resected tissue gives additional prognostic information. Hilar lymph node metastasis has little effect on the prognosis of squamous carcinoma but has a marked deleterious effect when it occurs with the other histologic types.[816] Tumor size greater than 5 cm has a deleterious effect on prognosis that is independent of the status of the lymph nodes.[841] Mitotic rates, however, have little correlation with prognosis.[828,855]

In general, for any stage of disease, symptomatic patients fare worse than those without symptoms,[794,814] and systemic symptoms such as fever or weight loss are

particularly bad omens.[794] Performance status refers to the ability of patients to carry out their customary activities. Scales for evaluating performance, ranging from those able to carry out normal work, to disability permitting restricted activity at home, to severe disability leaving the patient bedridden, are strong predictors of survival time.[784,843] Age, sex, and smoking status also influence prognosis.[803,843]

Etiology

It has been clear at least since the mid-1950s[866] that the major cause of the epidemic increase in the incidence of lung cancer is cigarette smoking. The evidence has been summarized in the Surgeon General's reports[848] and in a report by the Royal College of Physicians.[840] Epidemiologic studies of both case-control and retrospective and prospective cohort types have documented a strong relationship between the amount of smoking and the incidence of lung cancer. Pipe and cigar smokers have a greater risk than nonsmokers but a lesser risk than cigarette smokers. The relative risk of developing lung cancer for regular cigarette smokers is 10 times greater than for nonsmokers, and the risk for smokers of more than 25 cigarettes a day is 20 times greater. The relationship with smoking is strongest for squamous and small cell carcinoma, but large cell carcinoma and adenocarcinoma are also associated with smoking. Cigarette smoke contains the following classes of known carcinogens:

1. Nitrosamines
   a. Dimethyl nitrosamine
   b. Diethyl nitrosamine
   c. Nitrosopyrolidine
   d. N-Nitrosonornicotine
   e. N'-Nitrosoanatabine
2. Polycyclic aromatic hydrocarbons
   a. Benzo(a)pyrene
   b. Benzanthracene
   c. Methylfluoranthenes
   d. Chrysenes
   e. Benzophenanthrene
3. Heterocyclic hydrocarbons
   a. Dibenzacridines
   b. Dibenzocarbazole
4. Aromatic amines
   a. Beta-naphthylamine
5. Alpha-emitting radionuclides
   a. ^{210}Pb
   b. ^{210}Po

Each of these is present in low concentration but has the potential for interactions. Smoke also contains a number of irritants, some of which have been shown to act as tumor promoters. Smoke condensate is carcinogenic for animals in standard skin-painting assays. It has been difficult to reproduce patterns of human respiratory tract cancer in animals, however, probably because of the difficulty of reproducing human smoking methods. In addition to the increased incidence of overt tumors, the bronchi of smokers have an increased prevalence of ciliary loss, epithelial hyperplasia, squamous metaplasia, and nuclear atypism, lesions thought to be precursors of carcinoma.[768] Perhaps the most compelling epidemiologic evidence comes from the effect of stopping smoking. In Doll and Peto's 20-year study of 34,000 British physicians, which began in 1951, the use of tobacco declined during the study period as physicians became convinced of the risks of smoking.[791] During this time the lung cancer mortality in the physician population fell from roughly 60% of the rate for all British men to only 40% of that for all British men. Among those who gave up smoking, the relative risk of contracting lung cancer fell with time after quitting from an initial lung cancer risk 16 times that of a nonsmoker to only twice that of a nonsmoker after 15 years. Similarly, in the United States, among those who gave up smoking the relative risk gradually declined over 13 years to the level in those who never smoked.[801] The use of filters and smoking cigarettes with a lower tar content also decrease the relative risk.[861]

Whether there is any increased risk to nonsmokers from inhaling the smoke of other people's cigarettes (passive smoking) is not clear. In one Japanese study the lung cancer mortality in nonsmoking wives of smokers was higher than that of nonsmoking wives of nonsmokers,[809] but experience in the United States has not confirmed the increased risk.[798] The carcinogenic effect of passive smoking, if any, is small.

Although tobacco has been in widespread use for centuries, cigarette smoking by men came into use starting in 1890 to 1900. Women took up the habit beginning about 1920. The average number of cigarettes consumed by the average smoker increased until the 1940s for men and until roughly 1970 for women. Thus the much earlier rise in lung cancer incidence in men is readily explained on the basis of the difference in smoking trends. Since about 1950 the tar content of cigarettes has been declining. Doll and Peto noted that for continuing smokers the amount smoked between the ages of 15 and 25 has a powerful influence on the risk of lung cancer developing past age 50. Since those currently in the age group of greatest lung cancer incidence were between 15 and 25 years of age before the decline in tar content, the effect of decreasing tar has not shown up in the general trend of lung cancer incidence or mortality. However, there are a few hopeful signs. A beginning decline in the rates of lung cancer is detectable in male smokers below age 50, that is, those who took up the habit after the start of the decline in tar content.[792] Furthermore, a recent autopsy study has shown a decline in the extent of the epithelial abnormalities suspected of being precursors of lung can-

cer compared with those in smokers of comparable numbers of cigarettes 20 years ago.[767]

Epidemiologic studies have shown a small urban-rural gradient in lung cancer rates that cannot be entirely explained on the basis of smoking habits. This suggests that air pollution may play a role in the causation of lung cancer. High local rates for lung cancer in neighborhoods near petrochemical industries indicate that specific industrial pollutants may be at fault.[800] Lung cancer rates are also inversely related to income level. Although this too may be related to a tendency for the more wealthy to live in areas of lesser pollution, other explanations such as dietary patterns could also explain the trend.

If 10% of smokers will die of lung cancer, 90% will not. One factor that seems to influence susceptibility to respiratory carcinogenesis in experimental systems is vitamin A intake. Smokers with low vitamin A intake have a greater risk of lung cancer than those with a vitamin A–rich diet.[778,826] Whether vitamin A acts through its function in maintaining epithelial differentiation, by its role in promoting cell-mediated immunity, or by some other mechanism requires further study.[842] There is also a familial influence in lung cancer; the risk to relatives of lung cancer patients is 2½ times greater than that of the general population. Some studies have suggested that the ability to metabolize carcinogenic polycyclic aromatic hydrocarbons is under genetic control, but the observations have been difficult to reproduce, and currently the nature of the familial influence is uncertain.

There are a number of well-established occupational causes of lung cancer, as follows[798]:

1. Radioisotopes (radon gas)
2. Mustard gas
3. Asbestos
4. Coal tar distillates
5. Bis(chloromethyl)ether
6. Nickel
7. Chromium
8. Arsenic

Some industrial carcinogens act synergistically with tobacco smoke.[753] Occupational lung cancers do not always follow the usual distribution of histologic types. Exposure to bis(chloromethyl)ether,[795] radon gas,[837] and perhaps chromates is associated with the development of small cell carcinoma, whereas exposure to asbestos may produce relatively more adenocarcinomas.[762]

Carcinoids

Bronchial carcinoids are tumors of low-grade malignancy that share with small cell carcinoma origin from the bronchial neuroendocrine cell.[871,889] They tend to occur at a younger age than bronchogenic carcinomas, often appearing below 40 years of age and sometimes in childhood. Bronchial carcinoids are not related to cigarette smoking and have an equal sex incidence.[923] The majority of carcinoids arise in central bronchi where they form a smooth-surfaced endobronchial polypoid growth. However, the major portion of the tumor lies outside the bronchial wall, the so-called iceberg pattern of growth (Fig. 22-76). The tumor tissue often has a yellow-tan color, especially after fixation with formaldehyde. Microscopically carcinoids are formed of uniform cells with a fairly abundant, finely granular cytoplasm and oval, centrally located nuclei with clumped chromatin. The outstanding feature is that the tumor cells are grouped in relation to regularly disposed capillaries. The grouping may be in spherical aggregates (zellballen), trabeculae, or ribbons (Fig. 22-77). The stroma is usually scant but may be plentiful and may contain hyalinized connective tissue or more rarely amyloid or bone. Mitoses are rare, and necrosis is usually absent.

Twenty percent of carcinoids arise in small bronchi or bronchioles and occur as peripheral lung nodules.[875] Often the peripheral carcinoids are composed of spindle-shaped cells with little cytoplasm. Such tumors can be mistaken for small cell carcinoma but are distinguishable by the uniformity of the cells and the absence of necrosis or mitosis.

The secretory granules of bronchial carcinoids resemble those of other foregut carcinoids.[929] They do not reduce silver in the argentaffin reaction and stain only erratically with argyrophilic stains in which the reducing agent is added. Electron microscopy, however, usually shows abundant, electron-dense, spherical granules with an average diameter of 200 nm (Fig. 22-78). The granules are readily distinguished from the larger and more irregular granules of appendiceal and ileal carcinoids.

As a rule, bronchial carcinoids produce symptoms as a result of bronchial obstruction. Only exceptionally are symptoms the result of endocrine function of the tumor, usually in the presence of distant metastases. The most characteristic endocrine syndrome resulting from bronchial carcinoids is one of severe and prolonged flushing accompanied by diarrhea, edema, lacrimation, and hypotension. Urinary excretion of the serotonin metabolite 5-hydroxyindoleacetic acid is elevated, but whether peptide hormones or serotonin is responsible for these symptoms is unknown.[805] Carcinoids can also cause ectopic ACTH syndrome.[920]

The prognosis for bronchial carcinoids is in marked contrast to that of small cell carcinoma. Of 108 patients treated at military hospitals for carcinoid tumors, more than 90% survived 10 years.[836]

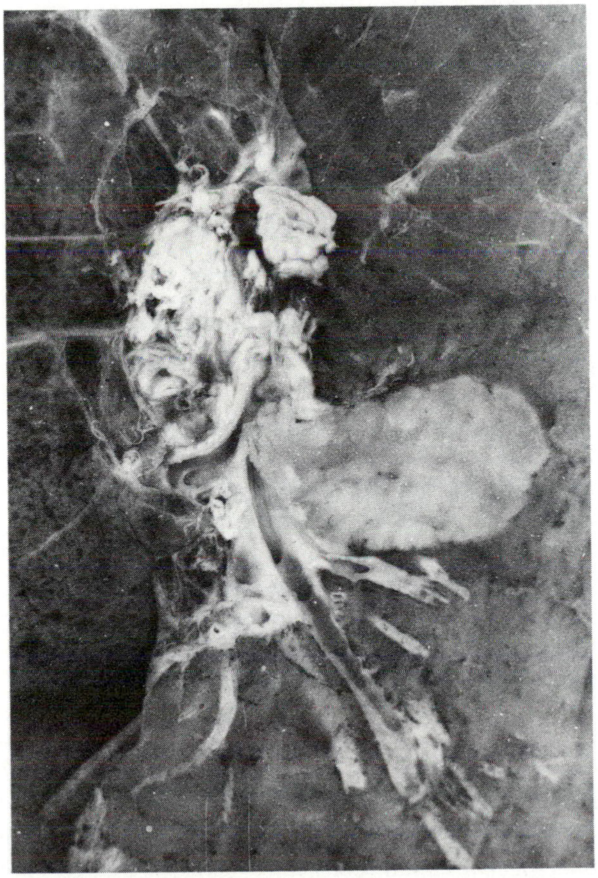

Fig. 22-76. Bronchial carcinoid. Tumor protrudes into bronchus, but its bulk lies outside bronchus.

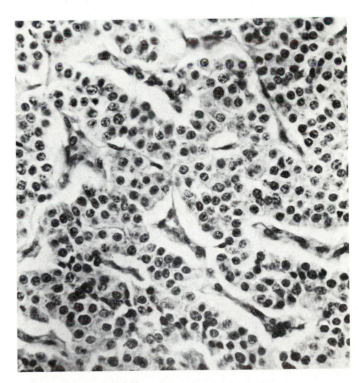

Fig. 22-77. Bronchial carcinoid. Regular ribbons of benign-appearing epithelial cells closely associated with capillaries.

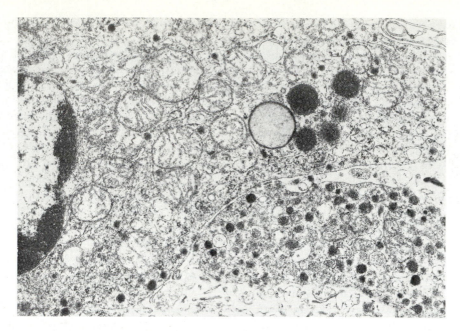

Fig. 22-78. Bronchial carcinoid. Electron micrograph illustrates granules of endocrine type.

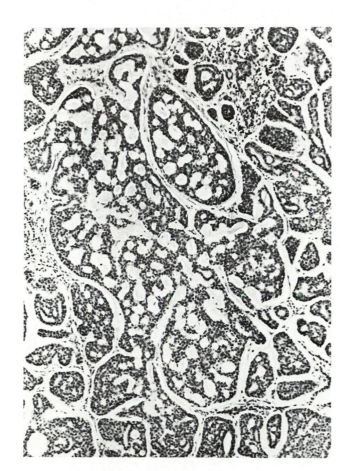

Fig. 22-79. Adenoid cystic adenocarcinoma of trachea. Lobules of epithelium are perforated by deposits of hyaline matrix in cribriform pattern.

A small number of patients have tumors with an organized pattern like that of the usual carcinoid but with greater cytologic atypism and more mitotic activity. Such tumors have been called atypical carcinoids and occupy a middle position in the morphologic spectrum from carcinoid to small cell carcinoma. Their prognosis also is intermediate.

Tumors of the mucous glands

The mucous glands give rise to a variety of tumors that mimic the morphology and biologic behavior of tumors of the salivary glands. The most common is the adenoid cystic carcinoma,[923] followed by mucoepidermoid carcinoma,[924] pleomorphic adenoma,[879,910] and rare tumors such as oncocytoma[881] and acinic cell carcinoma.[882] Adenoid cystic carcinomas arise at any level of the respiratory tract where there are mucous glands, from paranasal sinus to bronchi. They are the most common tumors in the upper third of the trachea. They grow as a smooth-surfaced submucosal endobronchial polypoid mass that invades the airway wall. In the trachea this produces stridor and airflow obstructions; in the bronchi it leads to obstructive pneumonia. Microscopically the characteristic appearance of the uniform small, slightly elongated cells arranged in a cribriform pattern is indistinguishable from that of the salivary gland tumors (Fig. 22-79). The "holes" in the cribriform sheets of cells are occupied by an eosinophilic hyaline or basophilic mucoid material, which electron microscopy has shown to be extracellular matrix separated from the tumor cells by basal lamina rather than a glandular secretion. Small ductular lumina

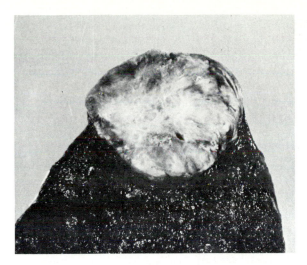

Fig. 22-80. Solitary mesothelioma. Well-circumscribed mass is adherent to visceral pleura. Sectioned surface has streaky pattern of fibrous lesion.

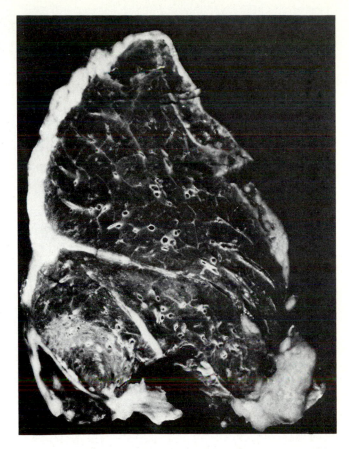

Fig. 22-81. Diffuse mesothelioma. Visceral pleura is encased by tumor, which extends into lobar fissures and to a limited extent invades interlobular septa.

with microvilli can be identified between tumor cells by electron microscopy but are too small to see with the light microscope. The evolution of adenoid cystic carcinomas is usually slow. Although they are malignant, survival for many years is not unusual, even with metastases.

Mucoepidermoid tumors of the bronchi also form smooth submucosal endobronchial masses.[866,913,924] Microscopically they are composed of three types of cells: well-differentiated squamous cells, mucous cells, and intermediate cells with a clear cytoplasm and distinct plasma membrane. Controversy surrounds their natural history. Some authors consider them slow growing and rarely metastasizing[866,913]; others have found them aggressive and rapidly fatal.[924]

Mesothelial tumors

The biologic behavior of primary pleural mesotheliomas can usually be predicted by their gross appearance.[900] Those that form a solitary discrete mass are usually benign, can be removed surgically, and rarely recur, whereas those that grow diffusely are malignant. Histologically mesotheliomas of either type may be predominantly epithelial, fibroblastic, or mixed.

Solitary mesotheliomas form circumscribed, rounded masses that are usually attached to either the parietal or the visceral pleura (Fig. 22-80).[884,909] Those arising from the pleura of the interlobar fissures may appear roentgenographically to be within the lung parenchyma, and rarely solitary mesotheliomas seem to arise entirely within the lung with at most a tenuous pedicle reaching the pleura. Solitary mesotheliomas are tough and rubbery with whorls and streaks of fibrous tissue evident on the cut surface. Microscopically they tend to be predomi-

nantly fibroblastic, with interlacing bundles of fibroblastic cells and varying amounts of extracellular matrix. Clefts lined by mesothelial cells may extend into the tumor, but only rarely are mesothelial cells predominant.

Solitary mesotheliomas cause few symptoms and usually are incidental findings on chest roentgenograms. Some patients complain of a shifting weight in the chest. Solitary mesotheliomas may be associated with systemic syndromes. The syndrome of osteoarthropathy is common,[872] but hypoglycemia is rare. Removal of the tumor is curative in both syndromes. Asbestos exposure plays no role in the etiology of solitary mesotheliomas.

Diffuse mesotheliomas are highly malignant tumors producing death in the majority of cases within a year of the onset of symptoms.[900] They appear as a nodular or homogeneous coating of white fleshy tissue over parietal and visceral pleura and diaphragm usually extending into the interlobular fissures (Fig. 22-81). Involvement of regional lymph nodes and pericardium is common at autopsy, and distant metastases sometimes occur. Clinical manifestations include chest pain, pleural effusion, and infection owing to entrapment of the lung.

Considerable variation is found histologically in the proportion of fibroblastic and mesothelial elements.[904] Mesothelial cells may form solid sheets but more often line slitlike spaces, tubules, or papillary projections (Fig. 22-82). Fibroblastic tissue varies from poorly cellular fibrous scar to frankly fibrosarcomatous.

Metastatic adenocarcinomas may closely resemble mesothelioma, grossly and microscopically, but a variety of techniques can help the pathologist make the distinction. Mesotheliomas produce hyaluronic acid that can be identified histochemically or biochemically[925]; adenocarcinomas often produce mucin. By immunohistochemistry mesotheliomas contain keratin but little carcinoembryonic antigen; adenocarcinomas typically have carcinoembryonic antigen but little keratin.[786] When viewed with the electron microscope, mesothelial cells can be recognized by their unusually long microvilli, absence of secretory vacuoles, and extensive endoplasmic reticulum and tonofilament bundles.[921]

The association of pleural and peritoneal mesothelioma with exposure to asbestos is now well recognized.[721,726,727] The period between exposure and the development of tumor varies greatly but is usually 20 to 40 years. Exposure need not be heavy; the occurrence of mesothelioma is documented in family members exposed only indirectly via the dusty clothing of workers. The evidence from both epidemiology and asbestos body counts made on lungs obtained at autopsy indicates that nearly half of the diffuse mesotheliomas in North American men are attributable to occupational exposure to asbestos.[905] There is no evidence that cigarette smoke is a factor.

Carcinosarcoma and pulmonary blastoma

There are two types of rare tumor in which both the epithelial and mesenchymal components are malignant. Carcinosarcomas are, as the name implies, tumors composed of a mixture of carcinomatous and sarcomatous elements.[872,879,880,912] The most common epithelial component is squamous carcinoma and usually the stroma fibrosarcoma, but the stroma may have osteoid or cartilaginous tissue as well. Carcinosarcomas are usually polypoid endobronchial tumors that occur in the middle aged and elderly. The prognosis is somewhat better than for bronchogenic carcinomas.

Pulmonary blastomas are peripheral lung tumors that derive their name from a resemblance to fetal lung.[886,895,911,918] The sarcomatous component resem-

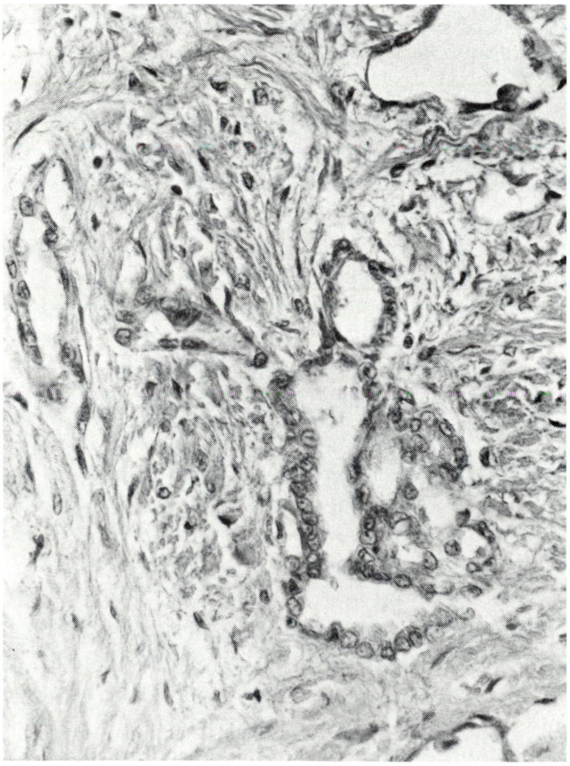

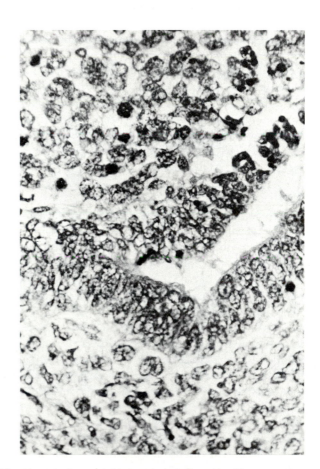

Fig. 22-82. One histologic pattern in diffuse mesothelioma. Tubules lined by flattened type of epithelium in abundant fibrous stroma. Microscopic appearance of mesotheliomas varies greatly.

Fig. 22-83. Pulmonary blastoma. Tubule is lined by primitive epithelium in highly cellular malignant stroma.

bles embryonic mesenchyme, and the epithelial component consists of primitive columnar epithelium lining branching slits and tubules (Fig. 22-83). Because of its high glycogen content, this epithelium often appears vacuolated like embryonic respiratory epithelium.[886] Although the analogy to Wilms' tumor of the kidney is sometimes made, pulmonary blastoma is not primarily a childhood tumor. It occurs at any age from childhood to old age, with the peak incidence in the fifth decade. The tumors evolve rapidly, and many patients die within a year of diagnosis. On the other hand, the 30% to 40% cure rate is much better than for bronchogenic carcinoma.

Sarcomas

The connective tissues of the lung give rise to a variety of tumors that are similar pathologically to their counterparts in the soft tissues.[907] There is one curious sarcoma of vascular origin that originates in the lung and for which no extrapulmonary counterpart is known. This is the lesion originally named intravascular bronchoalveolar tumor but better called sclerosing angiogenic tumor. Sclerosing angiogenic tumor is a multifocal lesion mani-

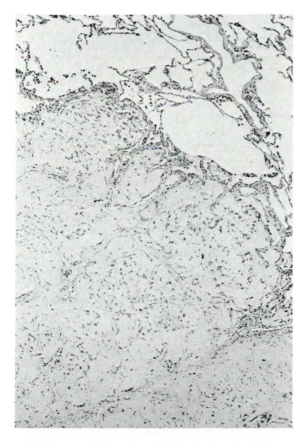

Fig. 22-84. Sclerosing angiogenic tumor. Alveoli are filled with myxoid stroma containing short rows of tumor cells.

fested clinically as slowly progressive dyspnea and multiple nodules on the chest roentgenogram. Histologically the nodules result from a process involving the filling of the alveolar spaces with accumulations of myxoid matrix containing aggregates and small chains of irregularly shaped mesenchymal cells (Fig. 22-84). In the center of the nodules the matrix becomes sclerotic and eosinophilic and the cells appear to fade out and disappear, leaving ghosts of alveoli filled with dense hyalinized matrix. At the expanding margins of the lesions where the alveoli are only partially filled with matrix, the tumor cells grow over the surface of the matrix, looking like epithelium. However, despite this appearance and a predominantly intra-alveolar pattern of growth, electron microscopy and immunohistochemical staining for the endothelial marker, clotting factor VIII antigen, have shown that the tumor cells have properties of endothelium.[873,928] The myxoid matrix contains abundant proteoglycan and a few disorganized collagenous and elastic fibers. The lesions are slowly progressive, but the tumor has the capacity to invade vessels and metastasize. Survival for many years is not unusual.

Small cell tumors involving the chest wall pleura and adjacent lung have been described in children and young adults. They are aggressive tumors composed of round or oval cells, 10 to 14 μm in diameter, arranged in compact sheets or nests. They may represent extraosseous Ewing's sarcoma or neuroblastoma, but they usually lack the glycogen characteristic of the former and only rarely have organelles compatible with the neurosecretory granules of the latter.[865] Their nature remains to be established.

Metastatic tumors

The variety of tumors that metastasize to the lungs is too great to list. Metastases usually are easily diagnosed clinically if solitary or multiple nodules appear in a patient known to have a malignancy, but lymphangitic spread of carcinoma can mimic interstitial lung disease clinically and roentgenographically. The tumor is seen pathologically as a delicate vermiform tracery on the surface of the pleura and a thickening around airways and bronchi. Microscopically tumor distends lymphatics and usually infiltrates the loose connective tissue around vessels and airways where the lymphatics are located. Patients with multiple small tumor emboli may have severe dyspnea but a normal chest roentgenogram.

Multiple nodules of well-differentiated smooth muscle sometimes appear in the lungs of women who have had a hysterectomy recently or up to several years earlier for fibromyomas. The term *benign metastasizing leiomyomas* has been applied to such lesions. Mitoses, the usual criterion for malignancy in smooth muscle tumors, are few in the lung lesions, and even on restudy the uterine lesions may not fulfill the criteria for malignancy. Nevertheless, the lung lesions probably represent metastases of a very low-grade uterine leiomyosarcoma whose malignancy is unrecognizable microscopically.[894] In some cases the pulmonary nodules have decreased in size during pregnancy and reappeared after delivery.[891] This retention of hormonal sensitivity is evidence of the müllerian origin of such smooth muscle nodules in the lung.

Benign tumors

Laryngeal papillomas seen in children and young adults sometimes spread to involve the trachea. If after multiple excisions spread extends to involve the small bronchi, usually the prognosis is grim and obstruction and pneumonia develop.[916]

In older adults solitary squamous papillomas of the bronchi occur. They consist of a branching fibrovascular stroma covered by a thick squamous epithelium that varies markedly in its degree of differentiation in different cases. Although most appear benign, atypism of some degree is present in others and some show frankly carcinomatous cytologic features.[917,919] Less commonly glandular or transitional epithelium may be found.[919]

Inflammatory polyps are rare in bronchi. Like those occurring commonly in the nose, they consist of an edematous stroma infiltrated with inflammatory cells and covered by ciliated epithelium. Symptoms result from bronchial obstruction.[864,922]

The most common benign tumors of the lung are the lesions known as hamartomas.[876] Despite their name, they appear to be acquired lesions, since they are not found in infancy and their maximum incidence is not until 60 years of age.[868] They produce no symptoms but are often discovered incidentally on chest roentgenograms and removed. They form well-circumscribed nodules, 1 to 4 cm in diameter, that shell out readily and are easily recognized grossly by their translucent cartilage-like appearance, cauliflower-like clefts, and rubbery consistency. They consist of lobules of connective tissue, usually containing cartilage, often with fat or fibrous tissue. The lobules are separated by clefts or tubules lined with columnar or cuboidal epithelium growing in from the surface of the tumor. The epithelium is probably entrapped respiratory epithelium and the connective tissue the neoplastic component.[868]

The so-called sclerosing hemangioma also causes few symptoms and is usually discovered accidentally as a rounded nodule on the chest roentgenogram.[903] Rarely it is a cause of hemoptysis. These lesions are of controversial histogenesis. They consist of a circumscribed unencapsulated nodule formed by the proliferation in the interstitium of epithelial-like cells with an oval central nucleus and a clear or pale eosinophilic cytoplasm with distinct cytoplasmic margins. Individual cells may be surrounded by fibrous tissue that in some areas compresses and replaces the tumor cells, resulting in foci of

sclerosis. Where cellular or sclerotic tumor abuts airspaces, it is covered with hyperplastic alveolar epithelium composed mainly of type II cells. In some areas involved alveolar walls protruding into alveolar ducts give the tumor a papillary appearance; hemorrhage into alveolar spaces remaining in the tumor may mimic vascular spaces, hence the original name "hemangioma."[903]

Electron microscopy shows that the characteristic tumor cells are partly enclosed by basal lamina and are partly separated by spaces into which peculiar branching microvilli extend. Thus they have some epithelial characteristics, but their exact nature remains controversial.[888,908] Some observers favor type II alveolar epithelial cells and others mesothelial cells as the cell of origin.[897]

A third tumor that occurs as an asymptomatic solitary nodule in middle-aged persons is the benign clear cell tumor, known informally as the "sugar" tumor because of its high glycogen content.[902] These lesions are circumscribed masses in the lung parenchyma formed of cords or nests of large cells with a cytoplasm sometimes entirely clear and sometimes empty but with wispy eosinophilic strands radiating from the nucleus (spider cells). The cords and nests are separated by delicate capillaries that

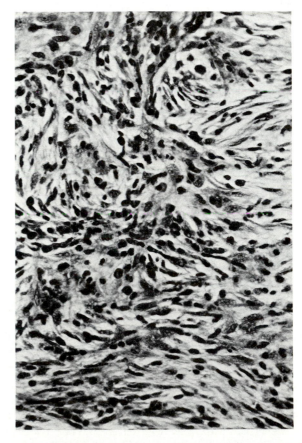

Fig. 22-85. Plasma cell granuloma. There is mixture of spindle-shaped fibroblasts and inflammatory cells, mainly plasma cells.

lead into characteristic dilated sinusoids. At first glance the lesions resemble metastatic renal cell carcinoma, but extended follow-up observation has proved their benign nature. The cytoplasm of renal cell carcinoma is clear, mainly because of fat, whereas that of benign clear cell tumor is filled with glycogen.[902] Electron microscopy characteristically shows glycogen-filled lysosomes as well as free cytoplasmic glycogen but has shown no specific feature that unambiguously establishes the histogenesis of the tumors.[869,890]

Inflammatory pseudotumors (plasma cell granulomas, fibrous xanthomas) are tumorlike lesions that are usually entirely intraparenchymal but may be attached to the pleura or even endobronchial.[867] They occur at any age but are most common in adolescents and children. They are morphologically heterogeneous, usually consisting of a background of edematous or hyalinized fibrous tissue infiltrated with varying numbers of plasma cells, Russell bodies, and lymphocytes (Fig. 22-85). Although the plasma cells are mature and well differentiated, they are often markedly distorted by fibrous tissue. Histiocytes with or without fat may be part of the solid lesions or fill adjacent obstructed airspaces. There is uncertainty whether these lesions are neoplasms or tumorlike inflammatory reactions. The recent isolation of the organism of Q fever from one such lesion favors the inflammatory origin.[893]

Lymphoproliferative diseases

Since the lung is a major lymphoid organ and nodules of lymphoid tissue are present normally at bronchiolar bifurcations and in the pleura and perilobular septa, it is not surprising that the lung is commonly involved at some time during the course of leukemia, lymphoma, and other lymphoproliferative diseases such as angioimmunoblastic lymphadenopathy. Generally infiltrates are concentrated in the perivascular and peribronchial sheaths, and the clinical presentation resembles that of interstitial disease. In multiple myeloma, pulmonary interstitial disease may be due to malignant plasma cell infiltrates, amyloidosis, or metastatic calcification. At times lymphomatous involvement takes the form of large masses or areas of consolidation. Cavitation is not unusual in Hodgkin's disease.

Sometimes malignant lymphomas arise initially in the lung. Care must be taken to distinguish malignant lymphomas from localized inflammatory masses composed mainly of lymphocytes, so-called pseudolymphomas.[887,914,915] The pseudolymphomas are characterized by a mixed population of mature lymphocytes, plasma cells, and some histiocytes. Germinal centers are often present but may be absent. The hilar lymph nodes are not involved. A mixture of B and T cell subsets was found in one case.[883] In contrast, non-Hodgkin's lymphoma shows a uniform population of lymphocytes, generally with immature forms. Germinal centers are absent. If regional lymph nodes are available for study, they may be found to be involved. Invasion of the pleura is usually more extensive with malignant lymphoma than with psuedolymphoma.

The prognosis for primary lymphomas limited to the lung is surprisingly good. Saltzstein[914,915] has suggested that this may be due to the mistaken diagnosis of cases of pseudolymphoma as malignant lymphoma. Although erroneous diagnosis may be a contributing cause, there is little doubt that local therapy can cure lymphoma limited to the lung as it can other primary visceral lymphomas.[885]

In lymphoid interstitial pneumonia the lung is more or less diffusely infiltrated by mature lymphocytes and plasma cells with or without germinal centers (Fig. 22-86).[543] The cellular populations are similar to those of pseudolymphoma, but instead of forming discrete nodules the infiltrate is exclusively interstitial and widespread. Abnormalities of serum immunoglobulins are common, taking the form of either monoclonal or polyclonal hyperglobulinemia or hypoglobulinemia.[543] Lung involvement in some patients with Sjögren's syndrome, Walden-

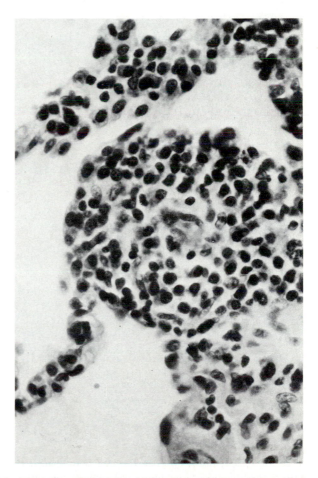

Fig. 22-86. Lymphoid interstitial pneumonia. Interstitium of alveolar walls and connective tissue surrounding a small vessel are heavily infiltrated by lymphocytes and plasma cells.

ström's macroglobulinemia, and angioimmunoblastic lymphadenopathy[892,927] fits the morphologic picture of lymphoid interstitial pneumonia.

Lymphomatoid granulomatosis is a lymphoproliferative process with a marked propensity for invading blood vessels.[896,901] Invariably the lung and frequently the skin and brain are involved. Nodular infiltrative lesions occur in the kidney and occasionally other viscera. Lethal midline reticulosis is a similar process involving the nose.

Grossly the pulmonary lesions appear as discrete unencapsulated nodules of pinkish tan tissue. Necrosis may be visible grossly. Microscopically the nodules consist of a variegated infiltrate with lymphocytes, plasma cells, histiocytes, and large atypical lymphoid cells with prominent nucleoli and a heavy rim of chromatin at the nuclear membrane. Some of the atypical cells show peripheral clumping of the chromatin reminiscent of plasma cell differentiation, suggesting that these cells are lymphoblasts. The diagnostic feature is the tendency of the atypical cells to invade small arteries and veins and expand the intima with severe reduction or obliteration of the lumen (Fig. 22-87). Although this vascular infiltra-

tion is described as a vasculitis, fibrinoid necrosis of vessels is not a feature. Large geographic areas of coagulative necrosis are common in large lesions, probably as a result of ischemia.

Patients may be of any age but are usually adults in their fourth to seventh decades. Initial symptoms are either referable to the lung, such as cough, dyspnea, hemoptysis, or chest pain, or systemic, such as fever or weight loss. Occasionally symptoms of involvement of other organs may precede pulmonary manifestations. The overall prognosis is poor; the majority of patients die of the disease with a median survival of only slightly more than 1 year. Most patients die of respiratory insufficiency. Malignant lymphoma, most commonly immunoblastic sarcoma, develops in 12% of patients.

The nature and pathogenesis of the disease are unknown. Some have suggested that it is a form of malignant lymphoma from the start, but the limited studies of lymphocyte subsets do not support this suggestion. The cellular proliferation is polyclonal in typical cases. The emergence of areas of uniform cells with monoclonal immunoglobulin heralds the development of lymphoma.[870]

Tumorlike proliferations

Whitwell introduced the whimsical term *tumorlet* to describe microscopic proliferations of epithelium either associated with inflammatory lung disease or occurring in nearly normal lung. Tumorlets are nests of small, slightly elongated epithelial cells in the walls of bronchiectatic bronchi or proliferating in the lumen of bronchioles, invading the wall or extending into adjacent alveoli. The epithelial cell nuclei have the slightly clumped regular chromatin seen in carcinoids, and electron microscopy has shown the presence of neurosecretory granules. Thus these lesions arise from the neuroendocrine cells.[874,877] Although it might be thought that these lesions are an early stage of small cell carcinoma, there is no direct evidence that this is the case, and their peripheral location and frequent multicentricity militate against such a relationship. In rare cases lymph node metastases from tumorlets have been noted but were not of clinical consequence.

Strands and whorls of epithelial-like cells are sometimes found in the connective tissue around small veins or extending into the walls of perivenous airspaces. Generally they are separated from airspaces by the alveolar capillaries. These clusters of cells have abundant cytoplasm with indistinct cell margins. They were originally designated minute pulmonary chemodectomas,[898] but with the application of electron microscopy their relation to chemoreceptor tissue became doubtful. The epithelial cells form whorls like those of meningiomas in the brain, and by electron microscopy the cells are indistinguishable from meningiomas and lack the secretory granules

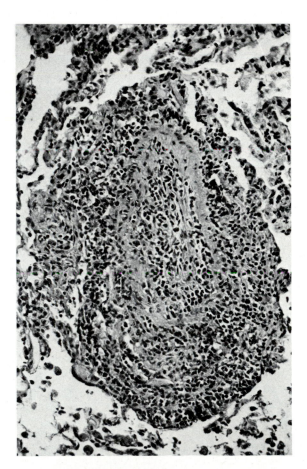

Fig. 22-87. Lymphomatoid granulomatosis. Muscular artery has been invaded by atypical lymphoid cells, which have infiltrated intima, reducing lumen.

characteristic of chemodectomas.[877,899] No plausible explanation has been offered for the appearance of meningothelial cell nests around pulmonary veins.[877,899]

The differential diagnosis between tumorlet and "minute chemodectoma" can be based on location of the abnormal cells. Tumorlets are related to airways and contact the lumen of airspaces; "minute chemodectomas" are perivenous, interstitial, and separated from airspace lumina.

MEDIASTINUM
Anatomic divisions

The central thoracic space lying between the two pleural cavities is called the mediastinum. It contains the heart, great vessels, esophagus, and trachea. The mediastinum is divided into three compartments by the pericardium. The space bounded posteriorly by the pericardium and first four thoracic vertebral bodies extending from the diaphragm to the thoracic inlet is known as the anterior mediastinum and includes the thymus, the aortic arch and its branches, the innominate veins, the vagus and phrenic nerves, and the cardiac plexus, as well as the trachea, paratracheal lymph nodes, and upper esophagus. The middle mediastinum is bounded by the fibrous pericardium and includes the heart, the ascending aorta, the pulmonary trunk, and the roots of the lungs including the tracheobronchial lymph nodes. The posterior mediastinum, between the pericardium and lower thoracic vertebrae, contains the descending aorta, the esophagus, the para-aortic lymph nodes, the paravertebral sympathetic ganglia, the azygous veins, and the thoracic duct.

Mediastinitis

Acute mediastinitis is caused by spread of infection from the neck or by perforations of the esophagus. The pretracheal fascia in the neck extends into the mediastinum to blend with the adventitia of the aortic arch. Cervical infections in front of the pretracheal fascia spread into the anterior mediastinum, whereas those behind the pretracheal fascia localize to the posterior mediastinum. Infections are usually suppurative and result in abscess formation.

Granulomatous mediastinitis is the result of spread of granulomatous infections to the mediastinal lymph nodes, usually from a primary tuberculous or histoplasmal focus in the lung.[931] This results in a mass of matted enlarged lymph nodes with caseous necrosis and fibrous encapsulation varying from a thin capsule separating the necrotic focus from the neighboring structures to an exuberant fibrous reaction up to 1 cm thick that encroaches on and compresses or invades neighboring structures. At its extreme the fibrous reaction predominates and a fibroma-like mass is produced in which the original granuloma may be overlooked.[931] This is the origin of many if not all cases of sclerosing mediastinitis.

In sclerosing mediastinitis a poorly circumscribed mass of woody white tissue surrounds and binds together mediastinal structures. Histologically, few cells are present in the tissue, which is composed of wavy thick bands and hyaline collagen separated by narrow spaces containing scattered lymphocytes and plasma cells. Foci of calcification or even ossification may be present in long-standing cases. The collagen bundles are arranged concentrically surrounding granulomas, but elsewhere the arrangement is more haphazard. The fibrous tissue entraps nerves and arteries, invades veins and bronchi, and obliterates lymphatics.[930] The clinical manifestations are highly variable depending on the structures involved but tend to fall into two groups depending on whether the paratracheal or hilar and subcarinal lymph nodes are the origin of the process.[930] Paratracheal lesions usually produce caval or innominate vein obstruction. Some patients complain of cough, hoarseness, or ill-defined discomfort. The prognosis is relatively favorable; although involvement of vital structures precludes resection, patients usually survive for years despite persistent disease. When the involvement occurs around the subcarinal lymph nodes or in the hila of lung, pulmonary veins, bronchi, or arteries may be compromised. Patients may have hemoptysis, pulmonary hypertension, and venous infarcts owing to pulmonary vein obstruction.[930,932] The arterioles and muscular arteries show marked intimal thickening and recanalization, and dilatation of perivascular lymphatics can be striking. When one pulmonary artery is compressed, volume loss occurs in the affected side.[934] With bilateral arterial compression, cor pulmonale may result.

Although many patients with sclerosing mediastinitis also have granulomatous lymphadenitis, in some cases granulomas are never found. This plausibly could be attributed to oversight, but the occasional association of sclerosing mediastinitis with retroperitoneal fibrosis or Riedel's struma suggests some sort of systemic sclerosing process.[933] Retroperitoneal and mediastinal fibrosis has also been reported as a complication of therapy with methysergide.

Pneumomediastinum

The soft tissues of the mediastinum are in communication with those of the neck through the thoracic inlet, with the peritoneum and retroperitoneum through the diaphragmatic hiatuses, and with the interstitium of the lung through the pulmonary ligaments. Interstitial emphysema of the mediastinium, or so-called pneumomediastinum, can develop as the result of perforation of a mediastinal structure or extension of air from one of these communicating compartments. Its causes include not only esophageal perforations or traumatic tears of the trachea or bronchi but also perforation of abdominal viscera, extension of subcutaneous emphysema around tracheostomy sites, and dissection of pulmonary interstitial emphysema.

Developmental cysts

A variety of developmental cystic lesions occur in the mediastinum, including cystic hygromas (lymphangiomas), meningomyeloceles, and cysts of bronchial, enteric, and pericardial origin. Pericardial cysts are usually solitary cysts adjacent to the pericardium, but 20% communicate with the pericardium.[945] Most are seen roentgenographically as smooth densities in the right cardiophrenic angle. Although they are considered to be developmental, most are detected in adult life. They consist of a fibrous wall with a thin mesothelial lining.

Bronchogenic cysts occur in the middle mediastinum behind the heart, usually below the carina. Their origin and structure are discussed on p. 836.

Enteric cysts (reduplications) occur in the posterior mediastinum along the course of the esophagus or less commonly embedded in its wall. Their wall is composed of smooth muscle, and their mucosa may recapitulate the esophageal gastric or intestinal lining. Cysts with a gastric type of lining can ulcerate and bleed or perforate.

Occasional thoracic cysts have a wall only of fibrous tissue or inflammatory tissue with no lining. Such cysts are called nonspecific, and their origin is uncertain.[945]

Tumors

Tumors and cysts arise from many of the structures of the mediastinum and have characteristic locations among the different anatomic compartments. The tumors found in each of the mediastinal compartments are listed in the following:

A. Anterior
1. Thymoma
2. Malignant lymphoma
3. Intrathoracic goiter
4. Parathyroid adenoma
5. Germ cell tumors
6. Paraganglioma
7. Lymphangioma
B. Middle
1. Malignant lymphoma
2. Developmental cysts
   a. Pericardial
   b. Bronchogenic
C. Posterior
1. Neurogenic
   a. Schwann cell
   b. Sympathetic
   c. Paraganglioma
2. Gastroenteric cyst

Table 22-4 contrasts the frequency of tumors and cysts in adults and children. In general the histopathologic fea-

Table 22-4. Relative frequency of mediastinal cysts and tumors

Type of lesion	Frequency (%)	
	Children	Adults
Neurogenic tumor	40	21
Lymphoma	18	13
Thymoma	—	19
Germ cell tumor	11	11
Mesenchymal tumor	9	7
Endocrine tumor	—	6
Cysts (pericardial, bronchogenic, enteric, and others)	18	20
Other malignancies	4	3

Data from Silverman, N.A., and Sabiston, D.C.: Surg. Clin. North Am. **60**:757, 1980.

tures and age distribution of mediastinal tumors mirror those of similarly named tumors in other parts of the body. Their natural history, however, can be influenced by their location.[935,939,945,947] Lesions of thymic origin are discussed in Chapter 31.

Lymphoproliferative disorders

Since they contain numerous lymph node groups, all three compartments of the mediastinum may be involved by malignant lymphomas and other lymphoproliferative diseases. Primary appearance of malignant lymphomas in the mediastinum is not uncommon and can run the gamut of histologic types. Non-Hodgkin's lymphomas are usually diffuse in pattern with convoluted nuclei in both adults and children.[943] Early dissemination is common. Mediastinal Hodgkin's disease is often of the nodular sclerosing type, particularly in young people, and is responsive to therapy.

A lymphoproliferative lesion that should not be mistaken for malignant lymphoma or thymoma is angiofollicular lymph node hyperplasia or Castleman's disease. Castleman originally encountered this lesion during a review of thymic tumors in 1954. He and his colleagues subsequently recognized two types, which differ in their clinical implications.[942] The more common, 80% to 90% of the total, is the hyaline-vascular type. In order of frequency, the locations for this lesion are the anterior mediastinum, the hila of the lungs, and the posterior mediastinum. Extrathoracic locations are rare. The lesion is a mass with a mean diameter of 7 cm and is composed of abnormal germinal centers in a background of vascularized and fibrous lymphoid tissue. Sinusoids are rarely retained. The germinal centers are small, composed of slightly flattened and concentrically arranged lymphoreticular cells that give a superficial resemblance to Hassal's corpuscles. They are invaded by fine capillaries or arterioles cuffed with hyaline connective tissue.

The interfollicular zones are well vascularized and contain lymphocytes, plasma cells, and activated lymphoid cells that are probably precursors of plasma cells. The hyaline-vascular type of angiofollicular lymph node hyperplasia is usually discovered accidentally on routine chest roentgenography and is asymptomatic. Patients with symptomatic disease complain of cough or a sensation of pressure. Surgery is curative.

In the less common plasma cell type of angiofollicular lymph node hyperplasia, germinal centers are larger but more typical.[942] They may be of irregular shape or confluent. The interfollicular zones contain sheets of plasma cells. Extrathoracic sites are involved more frequently than with the hyaline-vascular type, and a variety of systemic manifestations can be seen, including anemia, hyperglobulinemia, fever, growth failure, nephrotic syndrome, and peripheral neuropathy.[937,938,940]

The nature of angiofollicular lymph node hyperplasia is controversial. Some have considered it to be a hamartoma, a view disputed by Castleman and his colleagues because they detected lymph node remnants in a number of cases. In some of their patients the lesions were apparently acquired rather than developmental because chest roentgenograms made a few years earlier had been normal.[942]

Neurogenic tumors

Neurogenic tumors arise from the peripheral nerves, the sympathetic ganglia, or the aortic and pulmonary chemoreceptive glomera. Peripheral nerve tumors are unilateral paravertebral masses that usually occur in adults. Most are neurilemomas or neurofibromas. Malignant schwannomas are rare, and most occur in patients with von Recklinghausen's neurofibromatosis.[945,947] In children the majority of neural tumors are of sympathetic origin: neuroblastoma, ganglioneuroblastoma, or ganglioneuroma.[939,941] The degree of differentiation tends to vary with age: almost all tumors in patients less than 1 year of age are neuroblastomas, whereas in teenagers most are ganglioneuromas. The prognosis for malignant sympathetic nerve tumors in the mediastinum is better than for those in other locations. The cure rate is 50% for patients over 1 year of age, and the majority of those below 1 year of age can be cured with modern therapy even when metastases are present.

Paragangliomas are most common in the anterior mediastinum but can also be found in the paravertebral area. Few metastasize, but local invasion can make extirpation difficult. Most are hormonally inactive, but catecholamine-secreting thoracic paragangliomas can be a cause of hypertension.[941]

Germ cell tumors

Extragonadal germ cell tumors arise in a variety of midline structures from the retroperitoneum to the pineal gland. Those in the thorax are found in the anterior mediastinum and are similar in distribution to thymomas. Germ cell tumors are more likely than thymomas to contain calcification, however. Ninety percent are benign cystic teratomas, which are similar morphologically to the common ovarian teratomas. The sex incidence of cystic teratomas is equal, whereas malignant germ cell tumors occur almost exclusively in young men. Seminomas are locally invasive and often metastasize to the regional lymph nodes, but with well-planned management the prognosis is excellent.[946] Unfortunately, the same cannot be said for the other malignant germ cell tumors. Cures are sometimes obtained with embryonal carcinomas but are extremely rare with choriocarcinomas and solid or immature teratomas.[936,944]

Since the histologic features of mediastinal germ cell tumors are indistinguishable from those of testicular germ cell tumors, it is important to exclude the possibility of a testicular primary tumor when a mediastinal germ cell tumor is found. A mediastinal germ cell tumor may be accepted as primary if no mass has been found during careful palpation of the testis and a lymphangiogram of the retroperitoneum shows no abnormalities.

Thoracic thyroid and parathyroids

Parathyroid tissue can migrate into the chest with the thymus, with which it shares a common origin in the third and fourth branchial pouches. Consequently parathyroid adenomas occasionally occur within the anterior mediastinum or within the thymus proper. An enlarged thyroid can extend inferiorly through the thoracic inlet. Less commonly, thyroid tissue is present as a discrete mass in the anterior mediastinum.

REFERENCES
Pediatric lung disease
1. Askin, F.B.: Nose, nasopharynx, larynx and trachea; Lungs; and Thoracic parietes (three chapters). In Kissane, J.M., editor: Pathology of infancy and childhood, ed. 2, St. Louis, 1975, The C.V. Mosby Co.
2. Avery, M.E., Fletcher, B.A., and Williams, R.G.: The lung and its disorders in the newborn infant, ed. 4, Philadelphia, 1981, W.B. Saunders Co.
3. Dehner, L.P.: Pediatric surgical pathology, ed. 2, Baltimore, 1984, Williams & Wilkins Co.
4. Glenn, W.W.L., Liebow, A.A., and Linkskog, G.E.: Thoracic and cardiovascular surgery with related pathology, ed. 3, New York, 1975, Appleton-Century-Crofts.
5. Katzenstein, A.-L., and Askin, F.B.: The surgical pathology of non-neoplastic lung disease, Philadelphia, 1982, W.B. Saunders Co.
6. Kuhn, C.: The lung. In Johanessen, J.V.: Electron microscopy in human medicine, vol. 6, New York, 1979, McGraw-Hill Book Co.
7. Spencer, H.: Pathology of the lung (excluding pulmonary tuberculosis), ed. 3, Oxford, 1977, Pergamon Press.

Lung development
8. Campiche, M.A., et al.: An electron microscope of the fetal development of human lung, Pediatrics **32**:976, 1963.
9. Comroe, J.H., Jr.: Premature science and immature lungs (in three parts), Am. Rev. Respir. Dis. **116**:127,311,497, 1977.

10. Cooney, T.P., and Thurlbeck, W.M.: The radial alveolar count method of Emery and Mithal: a reappraisal. II. Intrauterine and early postnatal lung growth, Thorax 37:580, 1982.

11. Emery, J.L., and Dinsdale, F.: The postnatal development of lymphoreticular aggregates and lymph nodes in infants' lungs, J. Clin. Pathol. 26:539, 1973.

12. Farrell, P.M., editor: Lung development: biological and clinical perspectives, New York, 1982, Academic Press, Inc.

13. Hallman, M.: Fetal development of surfactant: considerations of phosphatidylcholine phosphatidylinositol, and phosphatidylglycerol formation, Prog. Respir. Res. 15:27, 1981.

14. Hislop, A., and Reid, L.: Fetal and childhood development of the intrapulmonary veins in man: branching pattern and structure, Thorax 28:313, 1973.

15. Hodson, W.A., editor: Development of the lung, New York, 1977, Marcel Dekker, Inc.

16. Langston, C., and Thurlbeck, W.M.: Lung growth and development in late gestation and early postnatal life, Perspect. Pediatr. Pathol. 7:203, 1982.

17. Perelman, R.H., Engle, M.J., and Farrell, P.M.: Perspectives on fetal lung development, Lung 159:53, 1981.

18. Reid, L.: The lung: its growth and remodeling in health and disease, Am. J. Roentgenol. 129:777, 1977.

19. Saunders, B.S., Kulovich, M.U., and Gluck, L.: Antenatal assessment of pulmonary maturation, Clin. Perinatol. 5:231, 1978.

20. Sinclair-Smith, C.C., et al.: Cartilage in children's lungs: a quantitative assessment using the right middle lobe, Thorax 31:40, 1976.

21. Spooner, B.S., and Wessels, N.K.: Mammalian lung development: interactions in formation and bronchial morphogenesis, J. Exp. Zool. 175:445, 1970.

22. Strang, L.B.: Neonatal respiration: physiological and clinical studies, Oxford, Eng., 1977, Blackwell Scientific Publications.

23. Thurlbeck, W.M.: Postnatal human lung growth, Thorax 37:564, 1982.

Congenital anomalies

24. Booth, J.B., and Berry, C.L.: Unilateral pulmonary agenesis, Arch. Dis. Child. 42:361, 1967.

25. Bozic, C.: Ectopic fetal adrenal cortex in the lung of a newborn, Virchows Arch. (Pathol. Anat.) 363:371, 1974.

26. Campo, E., and Bombi, J.A.: Central nervous system heterotopia in the lung of a fetus with cranial malformation, Virchows Arch. (Pathol. Anat.) 391:117, 1981.

27. Chang, N., et al.: Congenital stenosis of the right mainstem bronchus: a case report, Pediatrics 41:739, 1968.

28. Cox, J.N.: Respiratory system. In Berry, C.L. editor: Paediatric pathology, Berlin, 1981, Springer-Verlag.

29. Faro, R.S., et al.: Tracheal agenesis, Ann. Thorac. Surg. 28:295, 1979.

30. Foster-Carter, A.F.: Broncho-pulmonary anomalies, Br. J. Dis. Chest 40:111, 1946.

31. Gariepy, G., and Fugere, P.: Pulmonary embolization of cerebellar tissue in a newborn child, Obstet. Gynecol. 42:118, 1973.

32. Gonzalez-Crussi, F., et al.: "Bridging bronchus": a previously undescribed airway anomaly, Am. J. Dis. Child. 130:1015, 1976.

33. Janney, C.G., Askin, F.B. and Kuhn, C., III: Congenital alveolar capillary dysplasia—an unusual cause of respiratory distress in the newborn, Am. J. Clin. Pathol. 76:722, 1981.

34. Kalayoglu, M., and Olcay, I.: Congenital bronchobiliary fistula associated with esophageal atresia and tracheo-esophageal fistula, J. Pediatr. Surg. 11:463, 1976.

35. Kanbour, A.I., et al.: Anencephaly and heterotopic central nervous tissue in lungs, Arch. Pathol. Lab. Med. 103:116, 1979.

36. Landing, B.H.: Syndromes of congenital heart disease with tracheobronchial anomalies, A.J.R. 123:679, 1975.

37. Landing, B.H., and Dixon, L.G.: Congenital malformations and genetic disorders of the respiratory tract (larynx, trachea, bronchi and lungs), Am. Rev. Respir. Dis. 120:151, 1979.

38. Landing, B.H., and Wells, T.R.: Tracheobronchial anomalies in children, Perspect. Pediatr. Pathol. 1:1, 1973.

39. Maisel, R.H., et al.: Anomalous tracheal bronchus with tracheal hypoplasia, Arch. Otolaryngol. 100:69, 1974.

40. Maltz, D.L., and Nadas, D.S.: Agenesis of the lung: presentation of eight new cases and review of the literature, Pediatrics 42:175, 1968.

41. Mangiulea, V.G., and Stinghe, R.V.: The accessory cardiac bronchus: bronchologic aspects and review of the literature, Chest 54:433, 1968.

42. Nagaraj, H.S., et al.: Recurrent lobar atelectasis due to acquired bronchial stenosis in neonates, J. Pediatr. Surg. 15:411, 1980.

43. Orzan, F., et al.: Horseshoe lung: report of two cases, Am. Heart J. 93:501, 1977.

44. Ostor, A.-G., Stillwell, R., and Fortune, D.W.: Bilateral pulmonary agenesis, Pathology 10:243, 1978.

45. Remberger, K., and Hubner, G.: Rhabdomyomatous dysplasia of the lung, Virchows Arch. (Pathol. Anat.) 363:363, 1974.

46. Ryland, D., and Reid, L.: Pulmonary aplasia—a quantitative analysis of the development of the single lung, Thorax 26:602, 1971.

47. Siegal, M.J., et al.: Tracheal bronchus, Radiology 130:353, 1979.

48. Taybi, H.: Congenital malformations of larynx, trachea, bronchi and lungs, Prog. Pediatr. Radiol. 1:231, 1967.

49. Warfel, K.A., and Schulz, D.M.: Agenesis of the trachea: report of a case and review of the literature, Arch. Pathol. Lab. Med. 100:357, 1976.

Hypoplasia and diaphragmatic hernia

50. Alcorn, D., et al.: Effects of chronic tracheal ligation and drainage in the fetal comb lung, J. Anat. 123:649, 1977.

51. Chamberlain, D., et al.: Pulmonary hypoplasia in babies with severe rhesus isoimmunisation: a quantitative study, J. Pathol. 122:43, 1977.

52. Cooney, T.P., and Thurlbeck, W.M.: Pulmonary hypoplasia in Down's syndrome, N. Engl. J. Med. 307:1170, 1982.

53. Davies, G., and Reid, L.: Effect of scoliosis on growth of alveoli and pulmonary arteries and on right ventricle, Arch. Dis. Child. 46:623, 1971.

54. Goldstein, J.D., and Reid, L.: Pulmonary hypoplasia resulting from phrenic nerve agenesis and diaphragmatic amyoplasia, J. Pediatr. 97:282, 1980.

55. Hislop, A., Hey, E. and Reid, L.: The lungs in congenital bilateral renal agenesis and dysplasia, Arch. Dis. Child. 54:32, 1979.

56. Hull, D., and Barnes, N.D.: Children with small chests, Arch. Dis. Child. 47:12, 1972.

57. Kitagawa, M., et al.: Lung hypoplasia in congenital diaphragmatic hernia: a quantitative study of airway, artery, and alveolar development, Br. J. Surg. 58:342, 1971.

58. Mendelsohn, G., and Hutchins, G.M.: Primary pulmonary hypoplasia: report of a case with polyhydramnios, Am. J. Dis. Child. 131:1220, 1977.

59. Page, D.V., and Stocker, J.T.: Anomalies associated with pulmonary hypoplasia, Am. Rev. Respir. Dis. 125:216, 1982.

60. Perlman, M., Williams, J. and Hirsch, M.: Neonatal pulmonary hypoplasia after prolonged leakage of amniotic fluid, Arch. Dis. Child. 51:349, 1976.

61. Stahl, G.E., et al.: Congenital right diaphragmatic hernia: a case report and review of the literature, Clin. Pediatr. 20:422, 1981.

62. Swischuk, L.E., et al.: Bilateral pulmonary hypoplasia in the neonate, A.J.R. 133:1057, 1979.

63. Thurlbeck, W.M., et al.: Postnatal lung growth after repair of diaphragmatic hernia, Thorax 34:338, 1979.

64. Wigglesworth, J.S., Desai, R. and Guerrini, P.: Fetal lung hypoplasia: biochemical and structural variations and their possible significance, Arch. Dis. Child. 56:606, 1981.

Pulmonary vascular anomalies

65. Bahler, R.C., et al.: Absent right pulmonary artery: problems in diagnosis and management, Am. J. Med. 46:64, 1969.

66. Ben-Menachem, Y., et al.: The various forms of pulmonary varices: report of three new cases and review of the literature, Am. J. Roentgenol. Rad. Ther. Nucl. Med. 125:881, 1975.

67. Denes, D.E., Seward, J.B. and Bernatz, P.E.: Pulmonary arteriovenous fistulas, Mayo Clin. Proc. **58**:176, 1983.
68. Edwards, J.E.: Congenital pulmonary vascular disorders. In Moser, K.M., editor: Pulmonary vascular disease, New York, 1979, Marcel Dekker.
69. Edwards, J.E., and McGoon, D.C.: Absence of anatomic origin from heart of pulmonary arterial supply, Circulation **47**:393, 1973.
70. Ferencz, C.: Congenital abnormalities of pulmonary vessels and their relation to malformations of the lung, Pediatrics **28**:993, 1961.
71. Hawker, R.E., et al.: Common pulmonary vein atresia: premorten diagnosis in two infants, Circulation **46**:368, 1972.
72. Henriksen, N.T., et al.: Hereditary cholestasis combined with peripheral pulmonary stenosis and other anomalies, Acta Paediatr. Scand. **62**:7, 1977.
73. Honey, M.: Anomalous pulmonary venous drainage of right lung to inferior vena cava ("scimitar syndrome"): clinical spectrum in older patients and role of surgery, Q. J. Med. **46**:463, 1977.
74. Jue, K., et al.: Anomalous origin of the left pulmonary artery from the right pulmonary artery: report of 2 cases and review of the literature, Am. J. Roentgenol. Rad. Ther. Nucl. Med. **95**:598, 1965.
75. Kamio, A., et al.: Isolated stenosis of the pulmonary artery branches: an autopsy case with review of the literature, Jpn. Heart J. **42**:1289, 1978.
76. Keane, J.F., et al.: Anomalous origin of one pulmonary artery from the ascending aorta: diagnostic, physiological and surgical considerations, Circulation **50**:588, 1974.
77. Kieffer, S.A., et al.: Proximal interruption of a pulmonary artery: roentgen features and surgical correction, Am. J. Roentgenol. Rad. Ther. Nucl. Med. **95**:592, 1965.
78. Koopot, R., Nikaidoh, H., and Idriss, F.S.: Surgical management of anomalous left pulmonary artery causing tracheobronchial obstruction—pulmonary artery sling, J. Thorac. Cardiovasc. Surg. **69**:239, 1975.
79. Mardini, M.K., et al.: Scimitar syndrome, Clin. Pediatr. **21**:350, 1982.
80. McCue, C.M., et al.: Pulmonary artery coarctation: a report of 20 cases with review of 319 cases from the literature, J. Pediatr. **67**:222, 1965.
81. Nakib, A., et al.: Anomalies of the pulmonary veins, Am. J. Cardiol. **20**:77, 1967.
82. Przybojewski, J.E., and Maritz, F.: Pulmonary arteriovenous fistulas: a case presentation and review of the literature, South Afr. Med. J. **57**:366, 1980.
83. Sade, R.M., et al.: Stenosis of individual pulmonary veins: review of the literature and report of a surgical case, J. Thorac. Cardiovasc. Surg. **67**:953, 1974.
84. Swischuk, L.E., and L'Heureux, P.: Unilateral pulmonary vein atresia, A.J.R. **135**:667, 1980.
85. Tang, J.S., Kauffman, S.L., and Lynfield, J.: Hypoplasia of the pulmonary arteries in infants with congenital rubella, Am. J. Cardiol. **27**:491, 1977.
86. Tesler, U.F., Balsara, R.H. and Niguidula, F.N.: Aberrant left pulmonary artery (vascular sling): report of five cases, Chest **66**:402, 1974.

Bronchopulmonary sequestration and bronchogenic cyst

87. Buntain, W.L., et al.: Pulmonary sequestration in children: a twenty-five year experience, Surgery **81**:413, 1977.
88. Carter, R.: Pulmonary sequestration, Ann. Thorac. Surg. **7**:68, 1969.
89. Case reports of the Massachusetts General Hospital (Case 48-1983), N. Engl. J. Med. **309**:1347, 1983.
90. Heithoff, K.B., et al.: Bronchopulmonary foregut malformations, Am. J. Roentgenol. Rad. Ther. Nucl. Med. **126**:46, 1976.
91. O'Mara, C.S., Baker, R.R., and Jeyasingham, K.: Pulmonary sequestration, Surg. Gynecol. Obstet. **147**:609, 1978.
92. Reed, J.C., and Sobonya, R.E.: Morphologic analysis of foregut cysts in the thorax, Am. J. Roentgenol. Rad. Ther. Nucl. Med. **120**:851, 1974.

93. Salyer, D.C., Salyer, W.R., and Eggleston, J.C.: Benign developmental cysts of the mediastinum, Arch. Pathol. Lab. Med. **101**:136, 1977.
94. Savic, B., et al.: Lung sequestration: report of seven cases and review of 540 published cases, Thorax **34**:96, 1979.
95. Stocker, J.T., Drake, R.M., and Madewell, J.E.: Cystic and congenital lung disease in the newborn, Perspect. Pediatr. Pathol. **4**:93, 1978.
96. Stocker, J.T., and Kagan-Hallet, K.: Extralobar pulmonary sequestration: analysis of 15 cases, Am. J. Clin. Pathol. **72**:917, 1979.
97. Yabek, S., et al.: Aberrant systemic arterial supply to the left lung with congestive heart failure, Chest **80**:636, 1981.

Congenital adenomatoid malformation

98. Alt, B., et al.: Ultrastructure of congenital cystic adenomatoid malformation of the lung, Ultrastruct. Pathol. **3**:217, 1982.
99. Bale, P.M.: Congenital cystic malformation of the lung: a form of congenital bronchiolar ("adenomatoid") malformation, Am. J. Clin. Pathol. **71**:422, 1979.
100. Miller, R.K., Sieber, W.K., and Yunis, E.J.: Congenital adenomatoid malformation of the lung: a report of 17 cases and review of the literature, Pathol. Annu. **15**:387, 1980.
101. Moncrief, M.W., et al.: Congenital cystic adenomatoid malformation of the lung, Thorax **24**:476, 1969.
102. Nishibayashi, S.W., Andrassey, R.J., and Wolley, M.M.: Congenital cystic adenomatoid malformation: a 30-year experience, J. Pediatr. Surg. **16**:704, 1981.
103. Stocker, J.T., Madewell, J.E., and Drake, R.M.: Congenital cystic adenomatoid malformation of the lung, Hum. Pathol. **8**:155, 1977.
104. Van Poppel, H., et al.: Congenital cystic adenomatoid malformation or adenomatoid hamartoma of the lung, Acta Paediatr. Belg. **34**:83, 1981.

Congenital pulmonary lymphangiectasis

105. Brown, M.D., and Reidbord, H.E. Congenital pulmonary lymphangiectasis. Am. J. Dis. Child. **114**:654, 1967.
106. Case records of the Massachusetts General Hospital (Case 30-1980), N. Engl. J. Med. **303**:270, 1980.
107. Esterly, J.R., and Oppenheimer, E.H.: Lymphangiectasis and other pulmonary lesions in the asplenia syndrome, Arch. Pathol. **90**:553, 1970.
108. Gardner, T.W., et al.: Congenital pulmonary lymphangiectasis: a case complicated by chylothorax, Clin. Pediatr. **22**:75, 1983.
109. Hernandez, R.J.: Pulmonary lymphangiectasis in Noonan syndrome, A.J.R. **134**:75, 1980.
110. Morphis, L.G., Arcinue, E.L., and Krause, J.R.: Generalized lymphangiectasis in infancy with chylothorax, Pediatrics **46**:566, 1970.
111. Shannon, M.P., et al.: Congenital pulmonary lymphangiectasis: report of two cases, Pediatr. Radiol. **2**:235, 1974.

Congenital pulmonary overinflation

112. Buckner, D.M.: Congenital lobar emphysema, Clin. Perinatol. **5**:105, 1978.
113. Case records of the Massachusetts General Hospital (Case 41-1979), N. Engl. J. Med. **301**:829, 1979.
114. Hislop, A., and Reid, L.: New findings in emphysema of childhood. I. Polyalveolar lobe with emphysema, Thorax **25**:682, 1970.
115. Lincoln, J.C.R., et al.: Congenital lobar emphysema, Ann. Surg. **173**:55, 1971.
116. Miller, K.E., et al.: Acquired lobar emphysema in premature infants with bronchopulmonary dysplasia: an iatrogenic disease? Radiology **138**:589, 1981.
117. Murray, G.F.: Congenital lobar emphysema, Surg. Gynecol. Obstet. **124**:611, 1967.
118. Pierce, W.S., et al.: Concomitant congenital heart disease and lobar emphysema in infants: incidence, diagnosis, and other operative management, Ann. Surg. **172**:951, 1970.
119. Shannon, D.C., Todres, I.D., and Moylan, F.M.B.: Infantile lobar hyperinflation: expectant treatment, Pediatrics **59**:1012, 1977.

120. Stanger, P., Lucas, R.V., Jr., and Edwards, J.E.: Anatomic factors causing respiratory distress in acyanotic congenital cardiac disease: special reference to bronchial obstruction, Pediatrics **43**:760, 1969.
121. Talner, L.B., et al.: The syndrome of bronchial mucocele and regional hyperinflation of the lung, Am. J. Roentgenol. Rad. Ther. Nucl. Med. **110**:675, 1970.
122. Wall, M.A., Eisenberg, J.D., and Campbell, J.R.: Congenital lobar emphysema in a mother and daughter, Pediatrics **70**:131, 1982.

Adaptation to extrauterine life
Transient tachypnea of the newborn
123. Chernick, V.: Mechanics of the first inspiration, Semin. Perinatol. **1**:347, 1977.
124. Halliday, H.L., McCleve, G., and Reid, M. McC.: Transient tachypnea of the newborn: two distinct clinical entities, Arch. Dis. Child. **56**:322, 1981.
125. Swischuck, L.E., Hayden, C.K., Jr., and Richardson, C.J.: Neonatal opaque right lung: delayed fluid resorption, Radiology **41**:671, 1981.
126. Yeh, T.F., Tilien, L.D., and Pildes, R.S.: Diffuse radiographic infiltrates in a neonate, Chest **74**:291, 1978.

Hyaline membrane disease and bronchopulmonary dysplasia
127. Bonikos, D.S., et al.: Bronchopulmonary dysplasia: the pulmonary pathologic sequel of necrotizing bronchiolitis and pulmonary fibrosis, Hum. Pathol. **7**:643, 1976.
128. Boyle, R.J., and Oh, W.: Respiratory distress syndrome, Clin. Perinatol. **5**:283, 1978.
129. Chernick, V.: Fetal breathing movements and the onset of breathing at birth, Clin. Perinatol. **5**:257, 1978.
130. Coates, A.L., et al.: Long-term pulmonary sequelae of premature birth with and without idiopathic respiratory distress syndrome, J. Pediatr. **90**:611, 1979.
131. Doshi, N., et al.: Pulmonary yellow hyaline membranes in neonates, Hum. Pathol. **11**:520, 1980.
132. Driscoll, J.M., Jr., et al.: Mortality and morbidity in infants less than 1001 grams birth weight, Pediatrics **69**:21, 1982.
133. Esterly, J.R., Langegger, F., and Gruenwald, P.: Hyaline membranes in full-size infants, Virchows Arch. (Pathol. Anat.) **341**:259, 1966.
134. Farrell, P.M., and Avery, M.E.: Hyaline membrane disease, Am. Rev. Respir. Dis. **111**:657, 1975.
135. Fawcett, W.A., and Gluck, L.: Respiratory distress in the tiny baby, Clin. Perinatol. **4**:411, 1977.
136. Fitzhardinge, P.M.: Follow-up studies in infants treated by mechanical ventilation, Clin. Perinatol. **5**:451, 1978.
137. Gruenwald, P.: Exaggerated atelectasis of prematurity: a complication of recovery from the respiratory distress syndrome, Arch. Pathol. **68**:81, 1968.
138. Jones, R., et al.: Subglottic stenosis in newborn intensive care unit graduates, Am. J. Dis. Child. **135**:367, 1981.
139. Katzenstein, A., Bloor, C., and Liebow, A.: Diffuse alveolar damage: the role of oxygen, shock, and related factors, Am. J. Pathol. **85**:210, 1976.
140. Lauweryns, J.: "Hyaline membrane disease" in newborn infants: macroscopic, radiographic and light and electron microscope studies, Hum. Pathol. **1**:175, 1970.
141. Myers, A.D., Lillydahl, P., and Brown, G.: Hypopharyngeal perforations in neonates, Arch. Otolaryngol. **104**:51, 1978.
142. Robertson, B.: Pulmonary hyaline membranes of the newborn: the structure of the membranes at varying postnatal age, Acta Pathol. Microbiol. Scand. **62**:581, 1964.
143. Rosan, R.C.: Hyaline membrane disease and a related spectrum of neonatal pneumopathies, Perspect. Pediatr. Pathol. **2**:15, 1975.
144. Rosan, R.C., Lauweryns, J.M., and Brand, M.M.: Recent advances in pathologic aspects of neonatal respiratory distress, Pathol. Annu. **8**:407, 1973.
145. Schild, J.P., et al.: Tracheal perforation as a complication of nasotracheal intubation in a neonate, J. Pediatr. **88**:631, 1976.
146. Shanklin, D.R.: The influence of fixation on the histologic features of hyaline membrane disease, Am. J. Pathol. **44**:823, 1964.

147. Smith, B.T.: Prevention of hyaline membrane disease: an attempt to mimic a physiologic process. In Moss, A.J., editor: Pediatric update 1979, New York, 1979, American Elsevier, New York.
148. Smyth, J.A., et al.: Pulmonary function and bronchial hyperactivity in long-term survivors of bronchopulmonary dysplasia, Pediatrics **68**:336, 1981.
149. Vohr, B.R., Bell, E.F., and Oh, W.: Infants with bronchopulmonary dysplasia: growth pattern and neurologic and developmental outcome, Am. J. Dis. Child. **136**:443, 1982.
150. Workshop on bronchopulmonary dysplasia, J. Pediatr. **84**:1, 1979.

Pulmonary interstitial emphysema
151. Banagle, R.C., et al.: Lung perforation: a complication of chest tube insertion in neonatal pneumothorax, J. Pediatr. **94**:973, 1979.
152. Campbell, R.E., Boggs, T.R., Jr., and Kirkpatrick, J.A., Jr.: Early neonatal pneumoperitoneum from progressive massive tension pneumomediastinum, Radiology **114**:212, 1975.
153. Emery, J.L.: Interstitial emphysema, pneumothorax, and "airblock" in the newborn, Lancet **1**:405, 1956.
154. Levine, D.H., Trump, D.S., and Waterkotte, G.: Unilateral pulmonary interstitial emphysema: a surgical approach to treatment, Pediatrics **68**:510, 1981.
155. Madansky, D.L., et al.: Pneumothorax and other forms of pulmonary air leak in newborns, Am. Rev. Respir. Dis. **120**:729, 1979.
156. Opperman, H.C., et al.: Systemic air embolism in the respiratory distress syndrome of the newborn, Pediatr. Radiol. **8**:139, 1979.
157. Plenat, F., et al.: Pulmonary interstitial emphysema, Clin. Perinatol. **5**:351, 1978.
158. Stocker, J.T., and Madewell, J.E.: Persistent interstitial pulmonary emphysema: another complication of the respiratory distress syndrome, Pediatrics **59**:847, 1977.
159. Wood, B.P., et al.: Pulmonary lymphatic air: locating "pulmonary interstitial emphysema" of the premature infant, A.J.R. **138**:809, 1982.
160. Zimmerman, H.: Progressive interstitial pulmonary lobar emphysema, Eur. J. Pediatr. **138**:258, 1982.

Meconium aspiration syndrome, massive pulmonary hemorrhage,
and Wilson-Mikity syndrome
161. Ahvenainen, E.K., and Call, J.D.: Pulmonary hemorrhage in infants: a descriptive study, Am. J. Pathol. **28**:1, 1952.
162. Bacski, R.D.: Meconium aspiration syndrome, Pediatr. Clin. North Am. **24**:463, 1977.
163. Bancalari, E., and Berlin, J.A.: Meconium aspiration and other asphyxial disorders, Clin. Perinatol. **5**:317, 1978.
164. Burnard, E.D.: The pulmonary syndrome of Wilson and Mikity, and respiratory function in very small premature infants, Pediatr. Clin. North Am. **13**:999, 1966.
165. Cole, V.A., et al.: Pathogenesis of hemorrhagic pulmonary edema and massive pulmonary hemorrhage in the newborn, Pediatrics **51**:175, 1973.
166. Esterly, J.R., and Oppenheimer, E.H.: Massive pulmonary hemorrhage in the newborn. I. Pathologic considerations, J. Pediatr. **69**:3, 1966.
167. Fedrick, J., and Butler, N.R.: Certain causes of neonatal death. IV. Massive pulmonary hemorrhage, Biol. Neonate **18**:243, 1971.
168. Gregory, G.A., et al.: Meconium aspiration in infants—a prospective study, J. Pediatr. **85**:858, 1974.
169. Hodgman, J.E., et al.: Chronic respiratory distress in the premature infant: Wilson-Mikity syndrome, Pediatrics **44**:179, 1969.
170. Hoffman, R.R., Jr., Campbell, R.E., and Decker, J.P.: Fetal aspiration syndrome: clinical, roentgenologic and pathologic features, Am. J. Roentgenol. **122**:90, 1974.
171. Kotas, R.V., et al.: A new model for neonatal pulmonary hemorrhage research, Pediatr. Res. **9**:616, 1975.
172. Lauweryns, J., et al.: Intrauterine pneumonia: an experimental study, Biol. Neonate **22**:301, 1973.

173. Leake, R.D., Gunther, R., and Sunshine, P.: Perinatal aspiration syndrome: its association with intrapartum events and anesthesia, Am. J. Obstet. Gynecol. 118:271, 1975.
174. Marshall, R., et al.: Meconium aspiration syndrome: neonatal and follow-up study, Am. J. Obstet. Gynecol. 131:672, 1978.
175. Turbeville, D.F., et al.: In utero distal pulmonary meconium aspiration, South. Med. J. 72:535, 1979.
176. Tyler, D.C., Murphy, J., and Cheney, F.W.: Mechanical and chemical damage to lung tissue caused by meconium aspiration, Pediatrics 62:454, 1978.

Persistent fetal circulation

177. Bloss, R.S., Aranda, J.V., and Beardmore, H.E.: Congenital diaphragmatic hernia: pathophysiology and pharmacologic support, Surgery 89:518, 1981.
178. Fox, W.W., et al.: Pulmonary hypertension in the perinatal aspiration syndromes, Pediatrics 59:205, 1977.
179. Levin, D.L.: Morphologic analysis of the pulmonary vascular bed in congenital left-sided, diaphragmatic hernia, J. Pediatr. 92:805, 1978.
180. Levin, D.L., Weinberg, A.G., and Perkins, R.M.: Pulmonary microthrombi syndrome in newborn infants with unresponsive persistent pulmonary hypertension, J. Pediatr. 102:299, 1983.
181. Levin, D.L., et al.: Morphologic analysis of the pulmonary vascular bed in infants exposed in utero to prostaglandin synthetase inhibitors, J. Pediatr. 92:478, 1978.
182. Merten, D.F., Goetzman, B.W., and Wennberg, R.P.: Persistent fetal circulation: an evolving clinical and radiographic concept of pulmonary hypertension of the newborn, Pediatr. Radiol. 6:74, 1977.
183. Morrow, W.R., Haas, J.E., and Benjamin, D.E.: Nonbacterial endocardial thrombosis in neonates: relationship to persistent fetal circulation, J. Pediatr. 100:117, 1982.
184. Murphy, J.D., et al.: The structural basis of persistent pulmonary hypertension of the newborn infant, J. Pediatr. 98:962, 1981.
185. Oelberg, D.G., et al.: Endocarditis in high-risk neonates, Pediatrics 71:392, 1983.
186. Peckham, G.J., and Fox, W.W.: Physiologic factors affecting pulmonary artery pressure in infants with persistent pulmonary hypertension, J. Pediatr. 93:1005, 1978.
187. Rudolph, A.M.: High pulmonary vascular resistance after birth. I. Pathophysiologic considerations and etiologic classification, Clin. Pediatr. 19:585, 1980.
188. Shochat, S.J., et al.: Congenital diaphragmatic hernia: new concept in management, Ann. Surg. 190:332, 1979.
189. Weiner, E.S.: Congenital posterolateral diaphragmatic hernia: new dimensions in management, Surgery 92:670, 1982.

Infectious disorders in the infant lung

190. Arth, C., et al.: Chlamydial pneumonitis, J. Pediatr. 93:447, 1978.
191. Baker, C.J.: Group B streptococcal infections, Adv. Intern. Med. 25:475, 1980.
192. Barter, R.A., and Hudson, J.A.: Bacteriological findings in perinatal pneumonia, Pathology 6:223, 1974.
193. Bernstein, J., and Wang, J.: The pathology of perinatal pneumonia, Am. J. Dis. Child. 101:350, 1961.
194. Boyer, K.M., and Cherry, J.D.: Pneumonias in children. In Moss, A.J., editor: Pediatrics update 1979, New York, 1979, American-Elsevier New York.
195. Dudgeon, J.A.: Intrauterine infection, Proc. R. Soc. Med. 68:365, 1975.
196. Fedrick, J.: Neonatal deaths: time of death, maturity and lesion, Biol. Neonate 18:369, 1971.
197. Fedrick, J., and Butler, N.R.: Certain causes of neonatal death. III. Pulmonary infection. (A.) Clinical factors. (B.) Pregnancy and delivery, Biol. Neonate 17:458; 18:45, 1971.
198. Hammersen, G., et al.: Group B streptococci: a new threat to the newborn, Eur. J. Pediatr. 126:189, 1977.
199. Langley, F.A., and Smith, J.A.M.: Perinatal pneumonia: a retrospective study, J. Obstet. Gynecol. Br. Cmw. 66:12, 1959.
200. Naeye, R.L.: Causes of perinatal mortality in the U.S.: Collaborative Perinatal Project, J.A.M.A. 238:228, 1977.

201. Naeye, R.L.: Causes of excessive rates of perinatal mortality and prematurity in pregnancies complicated by maternal urinary-tract infections, N. Engl. J. Med. 200:819, 1979.
202. Naeye, R.L., Kissane, J.M., and Kaufman, N. editors: Perinatal diseases, Baltimore, 1981, Williams & Wilkins Co.
203. Naeye, R.L., and Peters, E.C.: Amniotic fluid infections with intact membranes leading to perinatal death: a prospective study, Pediatrics 61:171, 1978.
204. Naeye, R.L., and Tafari, N.: Risk factors in pregnancy and diseases of the fetus and newborn, Baltimore, 1983, Williams & Wilkins Co.
205. Radkowski, M.A., et al.: Chlamydia pneumonia in infants: radiography in 125 cases, A.J.R. 137:703, 1981.
206. Remington, J.S., and Klein, J.O., editors: Infectious disease of the fetus and newborn infant, ed. 2, Philadelphia, 1983, W.B. Saunders Co.
207. Rosenberg, H.S., and Bernstein, J.: Perspectives in pediatric pathology. Vol. 6. Infectious diseases, New York, 1981, Masson Publishing Co., U.S.A.
208. Schaad, U.B., and Rossi, E.: Infantile chlamydial pneumonia—a review based on 115 cases, Eur. J. Pediatr. 138:105, 1982.

Bronchiolitis and bronchiolitis obliterans

209. Azizirad, H., et al.: Bronchiolitis obliterans, Clin. Pediatr. 14:572, 1975.
210. Berquist, W.E., et al.: Gastroesophageal reflux–associated recurrent pneumonia and chronic asthma in children, Pediatrics 68:29, 1981.
211. Herbst, J.J.: Gastroesophageal reflux, J. Pediatr. 98:859, 1981.
212. Rosen, N., and Gaton, E.: Congenital bronchiolitis obliterans, Beitr. Pathol. 155:309, 1975.
213. Spigelblatt, L., and Rosenfeld, R.: Hyperlucent lung: long-term complication of adenovirus type 7 pneumonia, Can. Med. Assoc. J. 128:47, 1983.
214. Wohl, M.E.B., and Chernick, V.: Bronchiolitis, Am. Rev. Respir. Dis. 118:759, 1978.
215. Workshop on bronchiolitis, Pediatr. Res. 11(suppl.):209, 1977.

Infections of the lungs and bronchi
Routes of infection and pulmonary defenses

216. Dunnill, M.S.: Some aspects of pulmonary defense, J. Pathol. 128:221, 1979.
217. Green, G.M., and Kass, E.H.: The role of the alveolar macrophage in the clearance of bacteria from the lung, J. Exp. Med. 119:167, 1964.
218. Green, G.M., et al.: Defense mechanisms of the respiratory membrane, Am. Rev. Respir. Dis. 115:479, 1977.
219. Higuchi, J.H., and Johanson, W.G.: Colonization and bronchopulmonary infection, Clin. Chest Med. 3:133, 1982.
220. Johanson, W.G., Jr., et al.: Nosocomial respiratory infections with gram-negative bacilli: the significance of colonization of the respiratory tract, Ann. Intern. Med. 77:701, 1972.
221. Johanson, W.G., Jr., et al.: Bacterial adherence to epithelial cells in bacillary colonization of the respiratory tract, Am. Rev. Respir. Dis. 121:55, 1980.
222. Kass, E.H., Green, G.M., and Goldstein, E.: Mechanisms of antibacterial action in the respiratory system, Bacteriol. Rev. 30:488, 1966.
223. Ketchel, S.J., and Rodriguez, V.: Acute infections in cancer patients, Semin. Oncol. 5:167, 1978.
224. McDermott, M.R., Befus, A.D., and Bienenstock, J.: The structural basis for immunity in the respiratory tract, Int. Rev. Exp. Pathol. 23:48, 1982.
225. Unanue, E.R.: Secretory function of mononuclear phagocytes: a review, Am. J. Pathol. 83:396, 1976.
226. Woods, D.E., et al.: Role of salivary protease activity in adherence of gram negative bacilli to mammalian buccal epithelial cells in vivo, J. Clin. Invest. 68:1435, 1981.

Viral infections and mycoplasmal pneumonia

227. Aherne, W., et al.: Pathological changes in virus infections of the lower respiratory tract in children, J. Clin. Pathol. 23:7, 1970.

228. Archibald, R.W.R., Weller, R.O., and Meadow, S.R.: Measles pneumonia and the nature of the inclusion-bearing giant cells: a light and electron microscope study, J. Pathol. **103**:27, 1971.

229. Becroft, D.M.O.: Histopathology of fatal adenovirus infection of the respiratory tract in young children, J. Clin. Pathol. **20**:561, 1967.

230. Benisch, B.M., et al.: Mycoplasmal pneumonia in a patient with rheumatic heart disease, Am. J. Clin. Pathol. **58**:343, 1972.

231. Clinical conferences at the Johns Hopkins Hospital: mycoplasma pneumonia, Johns Hopkins Med. J. **139**:181, 1976.

232. Denny, F.W., et al.: The epidemiology of bronchiolitis, Pediatr. Res. **11**:234, 1977.

233. Foy, H.M., et al.: *Mycoplasma pneuemoniae* pneumonia in an urban area: five years of surveillance, J.A.M.A. **214**:1666, 1970.

234. Maisel, J.C., Babbett, L.H., and John, T.J.: Fatal *Mycoplasma pneumoniae* infection with isolation of organisms from lung, J.A.M.A. **202**:139, 1967.

235. Murray, H.C., et al.: The protean manifestations of myoplasma pneumoniae infection in adults, Am. J. Med. **58**:229, 1975.

236. Nash, G., and Foley, F.D.: Herpetic infection of the middle and lower respiratory tract, Am. J. Clin. Pathol. **54**:857, 1970.

237. Triebwasser, J.H., et al.: Varicella pneumonia in adults, Medicine **46**:409, 1967.

238. Turtzo, D.F., and Ghatak, P.K.: Acute hemolytic anemia with *Mycoplasma pneumoniae* pneumonia, J.A.M.A. **236**:1140, 1976.

239. Wohl, M.E., and Chernick, V.: Bronchiolitis, Am. Rev. Respir. Dis. **118**:759, 1978.

Bacterial infections

240. Auerbach, S.H., Mims, O.M., and Goodpasture, E.W.: Pulmonary fibrosis secondary to pneumonia, Am. J. Pathol. **28**:69, 1952.

241. Austrian, R., and Gold, J.: Pneumococcal bacteremia with special reference to bacteremic pneumococcal pneumonia, Ann. Intern. Med. **60**:759, 1964.

242. Berry, F.B.: Lobar pneumonia: analysis of 400 autopsies, Med. Clin. North Am. **4**:571, 1920.

243. Dines, D.E.: Diagnostic significance of pneumatocele of the lung, J.A.M.A. **204**:79, 1968.

244. Finland, M.: Pneumonia and pneumococcal infections with special reference to pneumococcal pneumonia, Am. Rev. Respir. Dis. **120**:481, 1979.

245. Finland, M., Brown, J.W., and Ruegsegger, J.M.: Anatomic and bacteriologic findings in infections with specific types of pneumocci including types I to XXXII, Arch. Pathol. **23**:801, 1937.

246. Hers, J.F., Masarel, N., and Mulder, J.: Bacteriology and histopathology of the respiratory tract and lungs in fatal Asian influenza, Lancet **2**:1141, 1958.

247. Jones, R., Santos, J.I., and Overall, J.C.: Bacterial tracheitis, J.A.M.A. **242**:721, 1979.

248. Kevy, S., and Lowe, B.A.: Streptococcal pneumonia and empyema in childhood, N. Engl. J. Med. **264**:738, 1961.

249. Miller, W.R., and Jay, A.R.: Staphylococcal pneumonia in influenza: 5 cases, Arch. Intern. Med. **109**:76, 1962.

250. Mufson, M.A., et al.: Capsular types and outcome of bacteremic pneumococcal disease in the antibiotic era, Arch. Intern. Med. **134**:505, 1974.

251. Naraqui, S., and McDonnell, G.: Hematogenous staphylococcal pneumonia secondary to soft tissue infection, Chest **79**:173, 1981.

252. Robertson, O.H., and Uhley, C.G.: Changes occurring in the macrophage system of the lungs in pneumococcus lobar pneumonia, J. Clin. Invest. **15**:115, 1936.

253. Sullivan, R.J., et al.: Adult pneumonia in a general hospital, Arch. Intern. Med. **129**:935, 1972.

254. Tuazon, C.U.: Gram-positive pneumonias, Med. Clin. North Am. **64**:343, 1980.

255. Verghese, A., et al.: Group B streptococcal pneumonia in the elderly, Arch. Intern. Med. **142**:1642, 1982.

256. Yangco, B.G., and Deresinski, S.C.: Necrotizing or cavitating pneumonia due to *Streptococcus pneumoniae*, Medicine **59**:449, 1980.

Bacterial pneumonia
Pneumonia caused by gram-negative aerobic bacteria

257. Erasmus, L.D.: Friedlander bacillus infection of the lung: with special reference to classification and pathogenesis, Q. J. Med. **25**:507, 1956.

258. Fetzer, A.E., Werner, A.S., and Hagstrom, J.W.C.: Pathology features of pseudomonal pneumonia, Am. Rev. Respir. Dis. **96**:1121, 1967.

259. Forkner, C.E., et al.: *Pseudomonas* septicemia: observations on twenty-three cases, Am. J. Med. **25**:877, 1958.

260. Hirschman, J.V., and Everett, E.D.: *Hemophilus influenzae* infections in adults: report of nine cases and a review of the literature, Medicine **58**:80, 1979.

261. Jonas, M., and Cunha, B.A.: Bacteremic *Escherichia coli* pneumonia, Arch. Intern. Med. **142**:2157, 1982.

262. Levin, D.C., et al.: Bacteremic *Hemophilus infleunzae* pneumonia in adults, Am. J. Med. **62**:219, 1977.

263. McHenry, M.C., Baggenstoss, A.R., and Martin, W.J.: Bacteremia due to gram-negative bacilli: clinical and autopsy findings in 33 cases, Am. J. Pathol. **59**:160, 1968.

264. Pennington, J.E., et al.: *Pseudomonas* pneumonia, Am. J. Med. **55**:155, 1973.

265. Pierce, A.K., and Sanford, J.P.: Aerobic gram-negative bacillary pneumonias, Am. Rev. Respir. Dis. **110**:647, 1974.

266. Pierce, A.K., et al.: An analysis of factors predisposing to gram-negative bacillary necrotizing pneumonia, Am. Rev. Respir. Dis. **94**:309, 1966.

267. Renner, R.R., et al.: *Pseudomonas* pneumonia: a prototype of hospital-based infection, Radiology **105**:555, 1972.

268. Reyes, M.P.: The aerobic gram-negative bacillary pneumonias, Med. Clin. North Am. **64**:363, 1980.

269. Teplitz, C.: Pathogenesis of *Pseudomonas* vasculitis and septic lesions, Arch. Pathol. **80**:297, 1965.

270. Tillotson, J.R., and Lerner, A.M.: Pneumonias caused by gram-negative bacilli, Medicine **45**:65, 1966.

271. Tillotson, J.R., and Lerner, A.M.: Characteristics of pneumonias caused by *Escherichia coli*, N. Engl. J. Med. **277**:115, 1967.

272. Tillotson, J.R., and Lerner, A.M.: Characteristics of nonbacteremic *Pseudomonas* pneumonia, Ann. Intern. Med. **68**:295, 1968.

273. Tillotson, J.R., and Lerner, A.M.: Characteristics of pneumonias caused by *Bacillus proteus*, Ann. Intern. Med. **68**:287, 1968.

274. Tillotson, J.R., and Lerner, A.M.: *Hemophilus influenzae* bronchopneumonia in adults, Arch. Intern. Med. **121**:428, 1968.

275. Wallace, R.J., Musher, D.M., and Martin, R.R.: *Hemophilus influenzae* pneumonia in adults, Am. J. Med. **64**:87, 1978.

Legionella and related pneumonias

276. Blackmon, J.A., Chandler, F.W., and Hicklin, M.D.: Legionnaires' disease—a review for pathologists, Pathol. Annu. **2**:383, 1979.

277. Blackmon, J.A., Hicklin, M.D., and Chandler, F.W.: Legionnaires' disease: pathologic and historical aspects of a "new" disease, Arch. Pathol. Lab. Med. **102**:337, 1978.

278. Blackmon, J.A., et al.: Review article: legionellosis, Am. J. Pathol. **103**:428, 1981.

279. England, A.C., et al.: Sporadic legionellosis in the United States: the first thousand cases, Ann. Intern. Med. **94**:164, 1981.

280. Fraser, D.W., et al.: Legionnaires' disease: description of an epidemic of pneumonia, N. Engl. J. Med. **297**:1189, 1977.

281. Helms, C.M., et al.: Legionnaires' disease associated with a hospital water system: a cluster of 24 nosocomial cases, Ann. Intern. Med. **99**:172, 1983.

282. Horowitz, M.A., and Silverstein, S.C.: Intracellular multiplication of Legionnaires' disease bacteria (*Legionella pneumophila*) in human monocytes is reversibly inhibited by erythromycin and rifampicin, J. Clin. Invest. **71**:15, 1983.

283. Kirby, B.D., et al.: Legionnaires' disease: report of sixty-five nosocomially acquired cases and review of the literature, Medicine **59**:188, 1980.

284. Lewin, S., et al.: Legionnaires' disease: a cause of severe abscess-forming pneumonia, Am. J. Med. **67**:339, 1979.

285. Meyerowitz, R.L., et al.: Opportunistic lung infection due to "Pittsburgh pneumonia agent," N. Engl. J. Med. **301**:953, 1979.
286. Muder, R.R., Yu, V.L., and Zuravleff, J.J.: Pneumonia due to the Pittsburgh pneumonia agent: new clinical perspective with a review of the literature, Medicine **62**:120, 1983.
287. Winn, W.C., and Myerowitz, R.L.: The pathology of *Legionella* pneumonias, Hum. Pathol. **12**:401, 1981.
288. Yu, V.L., et al.: Legionnaires' disease: new clinical perspective from a prospective pneumonia study, Am. J. Med. **73**:357, 1982.

Lung lesions caused by anaerobic bacteria

289. Bartlett, J.G.: Anaerobic bacterial pneumonitis, Am. Rev. Respir. Dis. **119**:19, 1979.
290. Bartlett, J.G., and Finegold, S.M.: Anaerobic infections of the lung and pleural space, Am. Rev. Respir. Dis. **110**:56, 1974.
291. Cameron, E.W.J., et al.: Characteristics and management of chronic destructive pneumonia, Thorax **35**:340, 1980.
292. Johanson, W.G., and Harris, G.D.: Aspiration pneumonia, anaerobic infections and lung abscess, Med. Clin. North Am. **64**:385, 1980.
293. Perlman, L.V., Lerner, E., and D'Esopo, N.: Clinical classification and analysis of 97 cases of lung abscess, Am. Rev. Respir. Dis. **99**:390, 1969.
294. Safron, R.D., and Tate, C.F.: Lung abscesses: a five year evaluation, Dis. Chest **53**:12, 1968.
295. Tillotson, J.R., and Lerner, A.M.: Bacterioides pneumonias: characteristics of cases with empyema, Ann. Intern. Med. **68**:308, 1968.

Mycobacterial infections

296. Auerbach, O.: The natural history of the tuberculous pulmonary lesion, Med. Clin. North Am. **43**:239, 1959.
297. Barkisdal, L., and Kim, K.S.: Mycobacterium, Bacteriol. Rev. **41**:217, 1977.
298. Boros, D.: Granulomatous inflammations, Prog. Allergy **24**:183, 1978.
299. Daniel, T.M.: The immunology of tuberculosis, Clin. Chest Med. **1**:189, 1980.
300. Dannenberg, A.M.: Liquefaction of caseous foci in tuberculosis, Am. Rev. Respir. Dis. **113**:257, 1976.
301. Dannenberg, A.M.: Pathogenesis of pulmonary tuberculosis, Am. Rev. Respir. Dis. **125**:25, 1982.
302. Dubos, R., and Dubos, J.: The white plague: tuberculosis, man and society, Boston, 1952, Little Brown & Co.
303. Green, G.M., Daniel, T.M., and Ball, W.C., editors: Koch Centennial supplement, Am. Rev. Respir. Dis. **125**:1, 1982.
304. Hershfield, E.S.: Tuberculosis in the world, Chest **176** (suppl.):805, 1979.
305. Khan, M.A., et al.: Clinical and roentgenographic spectrum of pulmonary tuberculosis in the adult, Am. J. Med. **62**:31, 1977.
306. Leff, A., and Geppert, E.F.: Public health and preventive aspects of pulmonary tuberculosis, Arch. Intern. Med. **139**:1405, 1979.
307. Leff, A., Lester, T.W., and Addington, W.W.: Tuberculosis: a chemotherapeutic triumph but a persistent socioeconomic problem, Arch. Intern. Med. **139**:1375, 1979.
308. Lefford, M.J.: Delayed hypersensitivity and immunity in tuberculosis, Am. Rev. Respir. Dis. **111**:243, 1975.
309. Lurie, M.B.: Resistance to tuberculosis: experimental studies in native and acquired defensive mechanisms, Cambridge, Mass., 1964, Harvard University Press.
310. MacGregor, R.R.: A year's experience with tuberculosis in a private urban teaching hospital in the postsanatorium era, Am. J. Med. **58**:221, 1975.
311. Mackaness, G.B.: The induction and expression of cell mediated hypersensitivity in the lung, Am. Rev. Respir. Dis. **104**:813, 1971.
312. Mankiewicz, E., and Liivak, M.: Phage types of mycobacterium tuberculosis in cultures isolated from Eskimo patients, Am. Rev. Respir. Dis. **111**:307, 1975.
313. Marchevsky, A., et al.: The spectrum of pathology of non-tuberculous mycobacterial infections in open-lung biopsy specimens, Am. J. Clin. Pathol. **78**:695, 1982.
314. Medlar, E.M.: The behavior of pulmonary tuberculous lesions: a pathological study, Am. Rev. Tuberc. **71**:1, 1955.
315. Merckx, J.J., Soule, E.H., and Karlson, A.G.: The histopathology of lesions caused by infection with unclassified acid-fast bacteria in man, Am. J. Clin. Pathol. **41**:244, 1964.
316. National survey of tuberculosis notifications in England and Wales, 1978-9: Report from the Medical Research Council Tuberculosis and Chest Diseases Unit, Br. Med. J. **281**:895, 1980.
317. Pagel, W., et al.: Pulmonary tuberculosis, ed. 4, London, 1964, Oxford University Press.
318. Perzigian, A.J., and Widmer, L.: Evidence for tuberculosis in a prehistoric population, J.A.M.A. **241**:2643, 1979.
319. Riley, R.L.: Disease transmission and contagion control, Am. Rev. Respir. Dis. **125**:8, 1982.
320. Romeyn, J.A.: Exogenous reinfection in tuberculosis, Am. Rev. Respir. Dis. **101**:923, 1970.
321. Rosenzweig, D.Y.: Pulmonary mycobacterial infections due to *Mycobacterium intracellulare-avium* complex: clinical features and course in 100 consecutive cases, Chest **75**:115, 1979.
322. Slavin, R.E.: Late generalized tuberculosis: a clinical and pathologic analysis of a diagnostic puzzle and a changing pattern, Pathol. Annu. **16**:81, 1981.
323. Snijder, J.: Histopathology of pulmonary lesions caused by atypical mycobacteria, J. Pathol. Bacteriol. **90**:65, 1965.
324. Stead, W.W.: Pathogenesis of a first episode of chronic pulmonary tuberculosis in man: recrudescence of residuals of the primary infection or exogenous reinfection? Am. Rev. Respir. Dis. **95**:729, 1967.
325. Sutinen, S.: Evaluation of activity in tuberculous cavities of the lung, Scand. J. Respir. Dis. **67** (suppl.):1, 1968.
326. U.S. Department of Health, Education and Welfare: 1977 Tuberculosis statistics: states and cities, DHEW publication no. (CDC) 79-8244, Atlanta, 1977, The Department.
327. Wolinsky, E.: Non-tuberculous mycobacteria and associated diseases, Am. Rev. Respir. Dis. **119**:107, 1979.
328. Youmans, G.P.: Tuberculosis, Philadelphia, 1979, W.B. Saunders Co.

Pneumocystis carinii pneumonia

329. Campbell, W.G., Jr.: Ultrastructure of pneumocystis in human lung: life cycle in human pneumocystis, Arch. Pathol. **93**:312, 1972.
330. Follansbee, S.E., et al.: An outbreak of *Pneumocystis carinii* pneumonia in homosexual men, Ann. Intern. Med. **96**:705, 1982.
331. Gottlieb, M.S., et al.: *Pneumocystis carinii* pneumonia and mucosal candidiasis in previously healthy homosexual men: evidence of a new acquired cellular immunodeficiency, N. Engl. J. Med. **305**:1425, 1981.
332. Ham, E.K., et al.: Ultrastructure of *Pneumocystis carinii*, Exp. Mol. Pathol. **14**:362, 1971.
333. Huang, S.-N., and Marshall, K.G.: *Pneumocystis carinii* infection: a cytologic, histologic, and electron microscopic study of the organism, Am. Rev. Respir. Dis. **102**:623, 1970.
334. LeGolvan, D.P., and Heidelberger, K.P.: Disseminated, granulomatous *Pneumocystis carinii* pneumonia, Arch. Pathol. **95**:344, 1973.
335. Masur, H., et al.: An outbreak of community acquired *Pneumocystis carinii* pneumonia: initial manifestations of cellular immune dysfunction, N. Engl. J. Med. **305**:1931, 1981.
336. Pifer, L.L., Hughes, W.T., and Murphy, M.J.: Propagation of *Pneumocystis carinii* in vitro, Pediatr. Res. **11**:305, 1977.
337. Pifer, L.L., et al.: *Pneumocystis carinii* infection: evidence for high prevalence in normal and immunosuppressed children, Pediatrics **61**:35, 1978.
338. Price, R.A., and Hughes, W.T.: Histopathology of *Pneumocystis carinii* infestation and infection in malignant disease in childhood, Hum. Pathol. **5**:737, 1974.
339. Robbins, J.B.: *Pneumocystis carinii* pneumonitis: a review, Pediatr. Res. **1**:131, 1967.

340. Vanek, J., Jirovec, O., and Lukes, J.: Interstitial plasma cell pneumonia in infants, Ann. Pediatr. **180:**1, 1953.

341. Walzer, P.D., et al.: *Pneumocystis carinii* pneumonia in United States, Ann. Intern. Med. **80:**83, 1974.

342. Weber, W.R., Askin, F.B., and Dehner, L.P.: Lung biopsy in *Pneumocystis carinii* pneumonia: a histopathologic study of typical and atypical features, Am. J. Clin. Pathol. **67:**11, 1967.

Bronchiectasis

343. Cherniack, N.S., et al.: The role of acute lower respiratory infection in causing pulmonary insufficiency in bronchiectasis, Ann. Intern. Med. **66:**489, 1967.

344. Ellis, D.A., et al.: Present outlook in bronchiectasis: clinical and social study and review of factors influencing prognosis, Thorax **36:**659, 1981.

345. Hayward, J., and Reid, L.M.: The cartilage of the intrapulmonary bronchi in normal lungs, in bronchiectasis, and in massive collapse, Thorax **7:**98, 1952.

346. Konietzko, N.F.J., Carton, R.W., and Leroy, E.P.: Causes of death in patients with bronchiectasis, Am. Rev. Respir. Dis. **100:**852, 1969.

347. Rytel, M.W., et al.: Infectious agents associated with cylindrical bronchiectasis, Dis. Chest 46:23,

348. Whitwell, F.: A study of the pathology and pathogenesis of bronchiectasis, Thorax **7:**213, 1952.

Immotile cilia syndrome

349. Afzelius, B.A.: Immotile cilia syndrome and ciliary abnormalities induced by infection and injury, Am. Rev. Respir. Dis. **124:**107, 1981.

350. Chao, J., Turner, J.A.P., and Sturgess, J.M.: Genetic heterogeneity of dynein-deficiency in cilia from patients with respiratory disease, Am. Rev. Respir. Dis. **126:**302, 1982.

351. Corkey, C.W.B., Levison, H., and Turner, J.A.P.: The immotile cilia syndrome: a longitudinal study, Am. Rev. Respir. Dis. **124:**544, 1981.

352. Gibbons, I.R.: Cilia and flagella of eukaryotes, J. Cell Biol. **91:**1075, 1981.

353. Rutland, J., and Cole, P.J.: Non-invasive sampling of nasal cilia for measurement of beat frequency and study of ultrastructure, Lancet **2:**564, 1980.

Cystic fibrosis

354. Anderson, D.H.: Cystic fibrosis of the pancreas and its relations to celiac disease, Am. J. Dis. Child. **56:**344, 1938.

355. Baur, P.S., Brinkley, B.R., and Bowman, B.H.: Effects of cystic fibrosis serum ciliary inhibitor on oyster gill ultrastructure: analysis by scanning and transmission electron microscopy, Tex. Rep. Biol. Med. **34:**155, 1976.

356. Bedrossian, C.W.M., et al.: The lung in cystic fibrosis: a quantitative study including the prevalence of pathologic findings among different age groups, Hum. Pathol. **7:**195, 1976.

357. Bowman, B., Lockhart, L., and McCombs, N.: Oyster ciliary inhibition by cystic fibrosis factor, Science **164:**325, 1969.

358. Czegledy-Nagy, E., Khan, S., and Sturgess, J.M.: Serum factor in cystic fibrosis: correlation with clinical parameters, Pediatr. Res. **13:**729, 1979.

359. Czegledy-Nagy, E., and Sturgess, J.M.: Cystic fibrosis: effect of serum factor on mucus secretion, Lab. Invest. **35:**588, 1976.

360. diSant'Agnese, P.A., and Davis, P.B.: Research in cystic fibrosis, N. Engl. J. Med. **295:**481, 534, 597, 1976.

361. diSant'Agnese, P.A., and Davis, P.B.: Cystic fibrosis in adults: 75 cases and a review of 232 cases in the literature, Am. J. Med. **66:**121, 1979.

362. Esterly, J.R., and Oppenheimer, E.H.: Cystic fibrosis of the pancreas: structural changes in peripheral airways, Thorax **23:**670, 1968.

363. Esterly, J.R., and Oppenheimer, E.H.: Observations in cystic fibrosis of the pancreas. III. Pulmonary lesions, Johns Hopkins Med. J. **122:**94, 1968.

364. Feather, E.A., and Russell, G.: Sputum viscosity in cystic fibrosis of the pancreas and other pulmonary diseases, Br. J. Dis. Chest **64:**192, 1970.

365. Fick, R.B., et al.: Cystic fibrosis *Pseudomonas* opsonins: inhibitory nature in an in vitro phagocytic assay, J. Clin. Invest. **68:**899, 1981.

366. King, M.: Is cystic fibrosis mucus abnormal? Pediatr. Res. **15:**120, 1981.

367. Kulczycki, L.L., Murphy, T.M., and Bellanti, J.A.: *Pseudomonas* colonization in cystic fibrosis, J.A.M.A. **240:**30, 1978.

368. Landan, L.I., and Phelan, P.D.: The spectrum of cystic fibrosis: a study of pulmonary mechanics in 46 patients, Am. Rev. Respir. Dis. **108:**593, 1973.

369. Oppenheimer, E.H., and Esterly, J.R.: Pathology of cystic fibrosis: review of the literature and comparison with 146 autopsied cases, Perspect. Pediatr. Pathol. **2:**241, 1975.

370. Reynolds, H.Y., diSant'Agnese, P.D., and Zierdt, C.H.: Mucoid *Pseudomonas aeruginosa:* a sign of cystic fibrosis in young adults with chronic pulmonary disease, J.A.M.A. **236:**2190, 1976.

371. Rossman, C., et al.: Cystic fibrosis–related inhibition of mucociliary clearance in vivo in man, J. Pediatr. **90:**579, 1977.

372. Shwachman, H., Kowalski, M., and Khaw, K.T.: Cystic fibrosis: a new outlook: 70 patients above 25 years of age, Medicine **56:**129, 1977.

373. Spock, A., et al.: Abnormal serum factor in patients with cystic fibrosis of the pancreas, Pediatr. Res. **1:**173, 1967.

374. Stern, R.C., et al.: Heart failure in cystic fibrosis, Am. J. Dis. Child. **134:**267, 1980.

375. Symchych, P.S.: Pulmonary hypertension in cystic fibrosis, Arch. Pathol. **92:**409, 1971.

376. Vawter, G.F., and Schwachman, H.: Cystic fibrosis in adults: an autopsy study, Pathol. Annu. **14:**357, 1979.

377. Wentworth, P., Gough, J., and Wentworth, J.E.: Pulmonary changes and cor pulmonale in mucoviscidosis, Thorax **23:**582, 1968.

378. Wood, R.E., Boat, T.F., and Doershuk, C.F.: State of the art: cystic fibrosis, Am. Rev. Respir. Dis. **113:**833, 1976.

379. Zuelger, W.W., and Newton, W.A.: The pathogenesis of fibrocystic disease of the pancreas: a study of 36 cases with special references to the pulmonary lesions, Pediatrics **4:**53, 1949.

Pulmonary vascular disease

380. Harris, P., and Heath, D.: The human pulmonary circulation: its form and function in health and disease, ed. 2, Edinburgh, 1977, Churchill Livingstone.

381. Wagenvoort, C.A., and Wagenvoort, N.: Pathology of pulmonary hypertension, New York, 1977, John Wiley & Sons, Inc., 1977.

Histologic features of normal pulmonary vasculature

382. Brenner, O.: Pathology of the vessels of the pulmonary circulation, Arch. Intern. Med. **56:**211, 1935.

383. Reid, L.M.: The pulmonary circulation: remodeling in growth and disease, Am. Rev. Respir. Dis. **119:**531, 1979.

Pulmonary thromboembolism and pulmonary infarcts

384. Bell, W.R., Simon, T.L., and DeMels, D.L.: The clinical features of submassive and massive pulmonary emboli, Am. J. Med. **62:**355, 1977.

385. Dalen, J.E., et al.: Pulmonary embolism, pulmonary hemorrhage and pulmonary infarction, N. Engl. J. Med. **296:**1431, 1977.

386. Fred, H.L., et al.: Rapid resolution of pulmonary thromboemboli in man, J.A.M.A. **196:**121, 1966.

387. Korn, D., et al.: Pulmonary arterial bands and webs: a previously unrecognized manifestation of organized pulmonary emboli, Am. J. Pathol. **40:**129, 1962.

388. LeQuesne, L.P.: Relation between deep vein thrombosis and pulmonary embolism in surgical patients, N. Engl. J. Med. **291:**1292, 1974.

389. Morell, T.M., and Dunnill, M.S.: Fibrous bands in conducting pulmonary arteries, J. Clin. Pathol. **20:**39, 1967.

390. Moser, V.–M.: Pulmonary embolism, Am. Rev. Respir. Dis. **115:**829, 1977.

391. Orell, S.R.: The fate and late effects of non-fatal pulmonary emboli, Acta Med. Scand. **172:**473, 1962.

392. Peterson, K.L., Fred, H.L., and Alexander, J.K.: Pulmonary arterial webs: a new angiographic sign of previous pulmonary thromboembolism, N. Engl. J. Med. **277:**33, 1967.

393. Robin, E.D.: Overdiagnosis and overtreatment of pulmonary embolism: the emperor may have no clothes, Ann. Intern. Med. **87**:775, 1977.

394. Rosenow, E.C., Osmundson, P.J., and Brown, M.L.: Pulmonary embolism, Mayo Clin. Proc. **56**:161, 1981.

395. Rossman, I.: True incidence of pulmonary embolization and vital statistics, J.A.M.A. **230**:1677, 1974.

396. Walker, R.H.S., Jackson, J.A., and Goodwin, J.: Resolution of pulmonary embolism, Br. Med. J. **4**:135, 1970.

Other forms of embolism

397. Attwood, H.D.: The histological diagnosis of amniotic-fluid embolism, J. Pathol. Bacteriol. **76**:211, 1958.

398. Douglas, F.G., Kafilmout, K.J., and Patt, N.L.: Foreign particle embolism in drug addicts: respiratory pathophysiology, Ann. Intern. Med. **75**:865, 1971.

399. Hopkins, G.B.: Pulmonary angiothrombotic granulomatosis in drug offenders, J.A.M.A. **221**:909, 1972.

400. Johnston, W.H., and Waisman, J.: Pulmonary cornstarch granulomas in a drug user, Arch. Pathol. **92**:196, 1971.

401. O'Quin, R.J., and Lakshminarayun, S.: Venous air embolism, Arch. Intern. Med. **142**:2173, 1982.

402. Robinson, M.J., et al.: Pulmonary granulomas secondary to embolic prosthetic valve material, Hum. Pathol. **12**:759, 1981.

403. Schinella, R.A.: Bone marrow emboli, Arch. Pathol. **95**:386, 1973.

404. Tang, T.T., et al.: Pulmonary fiber embolism and granuloma, J.A.M.A. **239**:948, 1978.

405. Tomashefski, J.F., and Hirsch, C.S.: The pulmonary vascular lesions of intravenous drug abuse, Hum. Pathol. **11**:133, 1980.

Pulmonary hypertension

406. Arias-Stella, J., Kruger, H., and Recavarren, S.: Pathology of chronic mountain sickness, Thorax **28**:701, 1973.

407. Bove, K.E., and Scott, R.C.: The anatomy of chronic cor pulmonale secondary to intrinsic lung disease, Prog. Cardiovasc. Dis. **9**:227, 1966.

408. Corrin, B., et al.: Pulmonary veno-occlusion—an immune complex disease, Virchows Arch. (Pathol. Anat.) **364**:81, 1974.

409. Crissman, J.D., Koss, M., and Carson, R.P.: Pulmonary veno-occlusive disease secondary to granulomatous venulitis, Am. J. Surg. Pathol. **4**:93, 1980.

410. Edwards, J.E.: Pathology of chronic pulmonary hypertension, Pathol. Annu. 1, 1974.

411. Fishman, A.P.: Hypoxia on the pulmonary circulation: how and where it acts, Circ. Res. **38**:331, 1976.

412. Fulton, R.M., Hutchinson, E.C., and Jones, A.M.: Ventricular weight in cardiac hypertrophy, Br. Heart J. **14**:413, 1952.

413. Heath, D., and Edwards, J.E.: The pathology of hypertensive pulmonary vascular disease, Circulation **18**:533, 1958.

414. Heath, D., Scott, O. and Lynch, J.: Pulmonary veno-occlusive disease, Thorax **26**:663, 1971.

415. Heath, D., and Smith, P.: Electron microscopy of hypertensive pulmonary vascular disease, Br. J. Dis. Chest **77**:1, 1983.

416. Heath, D., et al.: The structure of the pulmonary trunk at different ages and in cases of pulmonary hypertension and pulmonary stenosis, J. Pathol. Bacteriol. **77**:443, 1959.

417. Molden, D., and Abraham, J.L.: Pulmonary hypertension: its association with hepatic cirrhosis and iron accumulation, Arch. Pathol. Lab. Med. **106**:382, 1982.

418. Morrison, E.B., et al.: Severe pulmonary hypertension associated with macronodular (post necrotic) cirrhosis and autoimmune phenomena, Am. J. Med. **69**:513, 1980.

419. Naeye, R.I.: Hypoxemia and pulmonary hypertension: a study of the pulmonary vasculature, Arch. Pathol. **71**:447, 1961.

420. Owen, W.R., et al.: Unrecognized emboli to the lungs with subsequent cor pulmonale, N. Engl. J. Med. **249**:919, 1953.

421. Rochester, D.F., and Enson, Y.: Current concepts in the pathogenesis of the obesity-hypoventilation syndrome: mechanical and cirulatory factors, Am. J. Med. **57**:402, 1974.

422. Saldana, M.E., et al.: Experimental extreme pulmonary hypertension and vascular disease in relation to polycythemia, Am. J. Pathol. **52**:935, 1968.

423. Thadani, U., et al.: Pulmonary veno-occlusive disease, J. Med. **44**:133, 1975.

424. Wagenvoort, C.A.: Grading of pulmonary vascular lesions in a reappraisal, Histopathology **5**:595, 1981.

425. Wagenvoort, C.A., and Wagenvoort, N.: Primary pulmonary hypertension: a pathologic study of the lung vessels in 156 clinically diagnosed cases, Circulation **42**:1163, 1970.

426. Wagenvoort, C.A., and Wagenvoort, N.: The pathology of pulmonary veno-occlusive disease, Virchows Arch. (Pathol. Anat.) **364**:69, 1974.

427. Walcott, G., Burchell, H.B., and Brown, A.L.: Primary pulmonary hypertension, Am. J. Med. **49**:70, 1970.

428. Widgren, S.: Pulmonary hypertension related to aminorex intake: histologic ultrastructural and morphometric studies of 37 cases in Switzerland, Curr. Top. Pathol. **64**:2, 1977.

Pulmonary edema

429. Arias-Stella, J., and Kruger, H.: Pathology of high altitude pulmonary edema, Arch. Pathol. **76**:147, 1963.

430. Bleyl, U., Sandler, E., and Schindler, T.: The pathology and biology of uremic pneumonitis, Intensive Care Med. **7**:193, 1981.

431. Heath, D., and Edwards, J.E.: Histological changes in the lung in diseases associated with pulmonary venous hypertension, Br. J. Dis. Chest **53**:8, 1959.

432. Heath, D., Moosavi, H., and Smith, P.: Ultrastructure of high altitude pulmonary edema, Thorax **28**:694, 1973.

433. Hughes, R.T.: The pathology of butterfly densities in uremia, Thorax **22**:97, 1967.

434. Hurley, J.V.: Current views on the mechanisms of pulmonary edema, J. Pathol. **125**:59, 1978.

435. Inone, S., Michel, R.P., and Hogg, J.C.: Zonulae occludente in alveolar epithelium and capillary endothelium of dog lungs studied with the freeze fracture technique, J. Ultrastruct. Res. **56**:215, 1976.

436. Kay, J.M., and Edwards, R.: Ultrastructure of the alveolar-capillary wall in mitral stenosis, J. Pathol. **111**:239, 1975.

437. Kleiner, J.P., and Nelson, W.P.: High altitude pulmonary edema: a rare disease? J.A.M.A. **234**:491, 1975.

438. Staub, N.C.: The pathophysiology of pulmonary edema, Hum. Pathol. **1**:419, 1970.

439. Staub, N.C.: Pulmonary edema, Physiol. Rev. **54**:678, 1974.

440. Taylor, A.E., and Gaar, K.A.: Estimation of equivalent pore radii of pulmonary capillary and alveolar membranes, Am. J. Physiol. **218**:1133, 1970.

441. Theodore, J., and Robin, E.D.: Speculations on neurogenic pulmonary edema, Am. Rev. Respir. Dis. **113**:405, 1976.

Altered capillary permeability

442. Ashbaugh, D.G., et al.: Acute respiratory distress in adults, Lancet **2**:319, 1967.

443. Bachofen, M., and Weibel, E.R.: Structural alterations of lung parenchyma in the adult respiratory distress syndrome, Clin. Chest Med. **3**:35, 1982.

444. Blaisdell, F.W.: Respiratory distress syndrome, Surgery **74**:251, 1973.

445. Bone, R.C., Francis, P.B., and Pierce, A.K.: Intravascular coagulation associated with the adult respiratory distress syndrome, Am. J. Med. **61**:585, 1976.

446. Cochrane, C.C., Spragg, R., and Revak, S.D.: Pathogenesis of the adult respiratory distress syndrome: evidence of oxidant activity in bronchoalveolar lavage fluid, J. Clin. Invest. **71**:754, 1983.

447. Deneke, S.M., and Fanburg, B.L.: Normobaric oxygen toxicity of the lung, N. Engl. J. Med. **303**:76, 1980.

448. Divertie, M.D.: The adult respiratory distress syndrome, Mayo Clin. Proc. **57**:371, 1982.

449. Emson, H.E.: Fat embolism studied in one hundred patients dying after injury, J. Clin. Pathol. **11**:28, 1958.

450. Gossling, H.R., and Donohue, T.A.: The fat embolism syndrome, J.A.M.A. **241**:740, 1979.

451. Gould, V.E., et al.: Oxygen pneumonitis in man: ultrastructural observations on the development of alveolar lesions, Lab. Invest. **26**:499, 1972.

452. Hallman, M.: Evidence of lung surfactant abnormality in respiratory failure, J. Clin. Invest. **70**:673, 1982.
453. Jacob, H.S., et al.: Complement-induced granulocyte aggregation: an unsuspected mechanism of disease, N. Engl. J. Med. **302**:789, 1980.
454. Kapanci, Y., et al.: Oxygen pneumonitis in man: light and electron microscopic morphometric studies, Chest **62**:162, 1972.
455. Katzenstein, A.A., Bloor, C.M., and Liebow, A.A.: Diffuse alveolar damage: the role of oxygen, shock and related factors, Am. J. Pathol. **85**:210, 1976.
456. Kistler, G.S., et al.: Development of fine structural damage to alveolar and capillary lining cells in oxygen-poisoned rat lungs, J. Cell Biol. **32**:605, 1967.
457. Lamy, M., et al.: Pathologic features and mechanisms of hypoxemia in adult respiratory distress syndrome, Am. Rev. Respir. Dis. **114**:267, 1976.
458. McCord, J.M., and Fridovich, I.: The biology and pathology of oxygen radicals, Ann. Intern. Med. **89**:122, 1978.
459. McGuire, W.M., et al.: Studies on the pathogenesis of the adult respiratory distress syndrome, J. Clin. Invest. **69**:543, 1982.
460. Moon, V.H.: The pathology of secondary shock, Am. J. Pathol. **24**:235, 1948.
461. Nash, G., Blennerhassett, J.B., and Pontoppidan, H.: Pulmonary lesions associated with oxygen therapy and artificial ventilation, N. Engl. J. Med. **276**:368, 1967.
462. Petty, T.L., and Asbaugh, D.G.: The adult respiratory distress syndrome: clinical features, factors influencing prognosis and principles of management, Chest **60**:233, 1971.
463. Petty, T.L., et al.: Characteristics of pulmonary surfactant in adult respiratory distress syndrome associated with trauma and shock, Am. Rev. Respir. Dis. **115**:531, 1971.
464. Pratt, P.C., et al.: Pulmonary morphology in a multihospital collaborative extracorporeal membrane oxygenation project, Am. J. Pathol. **95**:191, 1979.
465. Rinaldo, J.E., and Rogers, R.M.: Adult respiratory distress syndrome, N. Engl. J. Med. **306**:900, 1982.
466. Simpson, D.L., et al.: Long term follow up of adult respiratory distress syndrome survivors, Am. Rev. Respir. Dis. **117**:449, 1978.

Immunologic lung disease
Asthma

467. Connell, J.T.: Asthmatic deaths: role of the mast cell, J.A.M.A. **215**:769, 1971.
468. Dunnill, M.S., Massarella, G.R., and Anderson, J.A.: A comparison of the quantitative anatomy of the bronchi in status asthmaticus in chronic bronchitis and in emphysema, Thorax **24**:176, 1969.
469. Empey, D.: Mechanisms of bronchial hyperreactivity, Eur. J. Respir. Dis. 63(suppl. 117):33, 1982.
470. Glynn, A.A., and Michaels, L.: Bronchial biopsy in chronic bronchitis and asthma, Thorax **15**:142, 1960.
471. Kaliner, M., et al.: Autonomic nervous system abnormalities and allergy, Ann. Intern. Med. **96**:349, 1982.
472. McCarter, J.H., and Vazquez, J.J.: The bronchial basement membrane in asthma: immunohistochemical and ultrastructural observations, Arch. Pathol. **82**:328, 1966.
473. McFodden, E.R., and Ingram, R.H.: Exercise-induced asthma: observations on initiating stimulus, N. Engl. J. Med. **301**:763, 1979.
474. Messer, J.W., Peters, G.A., and Bennett, W.A.: Causes of death and pathologic findings in 304 cases of bronchial asthma, Dis. Chest **38**:616, 1960.
475. Naylor, B.: The shedding of the mucosa of the bronchial tree in asthma, Thorax **17**:69, 1962.
476. Ogilvie, A.G.: Asthma: a study in prognosis of 1,000 patients, Thorax **17**:183, 1962.
477. Racheman, F.M.: Other factors besides allergy in asthma, J.A.M.A. **142**:534, 1950.
478. Racheman, F.M., and Edwards, M.C.: Asthma in children: a follow-up study of 688 patients after an interval of twenty years, N. Engl. J. Med. **246**:815, 858, 1952.
479. Reed, C.E.: Mechanisms of hyperreactivity of airways in asthma, Eur. J. Respir. Dis. 63(suppl. 117):88, 1982.

480. Salvato, G.: Some histological changes in chronic bronchitis and asthma, Thorax **23**:168, 1968.
481. Schatz, M., Patterson, R., and Fink, J.: Immunologic lung disease, N. Engl. J. Med. **300**:1310, 1979.
482. Venter, J.C., Fraser, C.M., and Harrison, L.C.: Autoantibodies to β2-adrenergic receptors: a possible cause of adrenergic hyporesponsiveness in allergic rhinitis and asthma, Science **207**:1361, 1980.

Other allergic lung diseases

483. Barrowcliff, D.F., and Arblaster, P.G.: Farmer's lung: a study of an early acute fatal case, Thorax **23**:490, 1968.
484. Boonpucknavig, V., et al.: Bagassosis: histopathologic study of pulmonary biopsies from six cases, Am. J. Clin. Pathol. **59**:461, 1973.
485. Carrington, C.B., et al.: Chronic eosinophilic pneumonia, N. Engl. J. Med. **280**:786, 1969.
486. Fink, J.N.: Interstitial lung disease due to contamination of forced air systems, Ann. Intern. Med. **84**:406, 1976.
487. Hapke, E.J., et al.: Farmer's lung, Thorax **23**:451, 1968.
488. Hinson, K.F.W., Moon, A.J., and Plummer, N.S.: Bronchopulmonary aspergillosis: a review and a report of eight new cases, Thorax **7**:317, 1952.
489. Katzenstein, A.-L., Liebow, A.A., and Friedman, P.J.: Bronchocentric granulomatosis, mucoid impaction and hypersensitivity reactions to fungi, Am. Rev. Respir. Dis. **111**:497, 1975.
490. Keller, R.H., et al.: Immunoregulation in hypersensitivity pneumonitis. I. Differences in T-cell and macrophage suppressor activity in symptomatic and asymptomatic pigeon breeders, J. Clin. Immunol. **2**:46, 1982.
491. Koss, M.N., Robinson, R.G., and Hochholzer, L.: Bronchocentric granulomatosis, Hum. Pathol. **12**:632, 1981.
492. Liebow, A.A., and Carrington, C.B.: The eosinophilic pneumonias, Medicine **48**:251, 1969.
493. Moore, V.L., et al.: Immunologic events in pigeon breeder's disease, J. Allergy Clin. Immunol. **53**:319, 1974.
494. Reyez, C.N., et al.: The pulmonary pathology of farmer's lung disease, Chest **81**:142, 1982.
495. Reynolds, H.Y., et al.: Analysis of cellular and protein-content of bronchoalveolar lavage fluid from patients with idiopathic pulmonary fibrosis and chronic hypersensitivity pneumonitis, J. Clin. Invest. **59**:165, 1977.
496. Richetti, A.J., et al.: Allergic bronchopulmonary aspergillosis, Arch. Intern. Med. **143**:1553, 1983.
497. Rosenberg, M., et al.: Clinical and immunologic criteria for the diagnosis of allergic bronchopulmonary aspergillosis, Ann. Intern. Med. **86**:405, 1977.
498. Schatz, M., Wasserman, S., and Patterson, R.: The eosinophil and the lung, Arch. Intern. Med. **142**:1515, 1982.
499. Seal, R.M.E., et al.: The pathology of the acute and chronic stages of farmer's lung, Thorax **23**:469, 1968.
500. Turner-Warwick, M., et al.: Immunologic lung disease due to *Aspergillus*, Chest **68**:346, 1975.

Interstitial pneumonia

501. Carrington, C.B., et al.: Natural history and treated course of usual and desquamative interstitial pneumonia, N. Engl. J. Med. **298**:801, 1978.
502. Crystal, R.G.: Idiopathic pulmonary fibrosis: clinical, histologic, radiographic, physiologic, scintigraphic, cytologic and biochemical aspects, Ann. Intern. Med. **85**:769, 1976.
503. Dreisin, R.B., et al.: Circulating immune complexes in the idiopathic interstitial pneumonias, N. Engl. J. Med. **298**:353, 1978.
504. Fulmer, J.D., et al.: Morphologic-physiologic correlates of the severity of fibrosis and degree of cellularity in idiopathic pulmonary fibrosis, J. Clin. Invest. **63**:665, 1979.
505. Hamman, L., and Rich, A.R.: Acute diffuse interstitial fibrosis of the lungs, Bull. Johns Hopkins Hosp. **74**:177, 1944.
506. Heppleston, A.G.: The pathology of honeycomb lung, Thorax **11**:77, 1956.
507. Hogan, P.G., Donald, K.J., and McEvoy, J.D.S.: Immunofluorescence studies of lung biopsy tissue, Am. Rev. Respir. Dis. **118**:537, 1978.

508. Liebow, A.A., Steer, A. and Billingsley, J.G.: Desquamative interstitial pneumonia, Am. J. Med. **39**:369, 1965.
509. Scadding, J.G.: Chronic diffuse interstitial fibrosis of the lungs, Br. Med. J. **1**:443, 1960.
510. Scadding, J.G., and Hinson, K.F.W.: Diffuse fibrosing alveolitis (diffuse interstitial fibrosis of the lungs): correlation of histology at biopsy with prognosis, Thorax **22**:291, 1967.
511. Schwartz, M.I., et al.: Immunofluorescent patterns in the idiopathic interstitial pneumonias, J. Lab. Clin. Med. **91**:929, 1978.
512. Stachura, I., Singh, G., and Whiteside, T.L.: Mechanisms of tissue injury in desquamative interstitial pneumonia, Am. J. Med. **68**:733, 1980.
513. Stock, B.H.R., Choo-Kang, Y.F.J., and Heard, B.E.: The prognosis of cryptogenic fibrosing alveolitis, Thorax **27**:535, 1972.
514. Turner-Warwick, M., and Haslam, P.: Antibodies in some chronic fibrosing lung diseases. I. Non-organ specific autoantibodies, Clin. Allergy **1**:83, 1971.
515. Turner-Warwick, M., Haslam, P., and Weeks, J.: Antibodies in some chronic fibrosing lung diseases. II. Immunofluorescent studies, Clin. Allergy **1**:209, 1971.
516. Ward, P.A.: Immune complex injury of the lung, Am. J. Pathol. **97**:85, 1979.

Pulmonary involvement in collagen-vascular disease

517. Anderson, L.G., and Talal, N.: The spectrum of benign to malignant lymphoproliferation in Sjögren's syndrome, Clin. Exp. Immunol. **9**:199, 1971.
518. Armstrong, J.G., and Steele, R.H.: Localized pulmonary arteritis in rheumatoid disease, Thorax **37**:313, 1982.
519. Bonner, H., Jr., et al.: Lymphoid infiltration and amyloidosis of lung in Sjögren's syndrome, Arch. Pathol. **95**:42, 1973.
520. Brown, G., Goldring, D., and Behrer, R.: Rheumatic pneumonia, J. Pediatr. **52**:598, 1958.
521. Churg, A., et al.: Pulmonary hemorrhage and immune-complex deposition in the lung, Arch. Pathol. Lab. Med. **104**:388, 1980.
522. Colp, C.R., et al.: Serial changes in scleroderma and idiopathic interstitial lung disease, Arch. Intern. Med. **132**:506, 1973.
523. D'Angelo, W.A., et al.: Pathologic observations in systemic sclerosis (scleroderma), Am. J. Med. **46**:488, 1969.
524. DeHoratius, R.J., and Williams, R.C.: Rheumatoid factor accentuation of pulmonary lesions associated with experimental diffuse proliferative lung disease, Arthritis Rheum. **15**:293, 1972.
525. DeHoratius, R.J., et al.: Immunofluorescent and immunologic studies of rheumatoid lung, Arch. Intern. Med. **129**:441, 1972.
526. Eagan, J., et al.: Pulmonary hemorrhage and systemic lupus erythematosus, Medicine **57**:545, 1978.
527. Eisenberg, H., et al.: Diffuse interstitial lung disease in lupus erythematosus, Ann. Intern. Med. **79**:37, 1973.
528. Elper, G.R., et al.: Bronchiolitis and bronchitis in connective tissue disease: a possible relationship to the use of penicillamine, J.A.M.A. **242**:528, 1979.
529. Fayemi, A.O.: Pulmonary vascular disease in systemic lupus erythematosus, Am. J. Clin. Pathol. **65**:284, 1976.
530. Feagler, J.R., et al.: Rheumatoid pleural effusion, Arch. Pathol. **92**:257, 1971.
531. Frank, S.T., et al.: Pulmonary dysfunction in rheumatoid disease, Chest **63**:27, 1973.
532. Geddes, D.M., and Brostoff, J.: Pulmonary fibrosis associated with hypersensitivity to gold salts, Br. Med. J. **1**:1444, 1976.
533. Geddes, D.M., et al.: Progressive airway obliteration in adults and its association with rheumatoid disease, Q. J. Med. **46**:427, 1977.
534. Geddes, D.M., et al.: Airways obstruction in rheumatoid arthritis, Ann. Rheum. Dis. **38**:222, 1979.
535. Gould, P.W., et al.: Pulmonary damage associated with sodium aurothiomalate therapy, J. Rheumatol. **4**:252, 1977.
536. Grunow, W.A., and Esterby, J.R.: Rheumatic pneumonitis, Chest **61**:298, 1972.
537. Harvey, A.M.G., et al.: Systemic lupus erythematosus: review of the literature and clinical analysis of 138 cases, Medicine **33**:291, 1954.
538. Hochberg, M.C.: The spectrum of systemic sclerosis—current concepts, Hosp. Pract. :61, 1981.

539. Hunninghake, G.W., and Fauci, A.S.: Pulmonary involvement in the collagen vascular diseases, Am. Rev. Respir. Dis. **119**:471, 1979.
540. Inoue, T., et al.: Immunopathologic studies of pneumonitis in systemic lupus erythematosus, Ann. Intern. Med. **91**:30, 1979.
541. Israel, H.L.: The pulmonary manifestations of disseminated lupus erythematosus, Am. J. Med. Sci. **266**:387, 1953.
542. Kapanci, Y., and Chamay, A.: Lesions en anse de fil de fer des capillaires pulmonaires dans le lupus erythemateux dissemine (LED), Virchows Arch. (Pathol. Anat.) **342**:236, 1967.
543. Liebow, A.A., and Carrington, C.B.: Diffuse pulmonary lymphoreticular infiltrations associated with dysproteinemia, Med. Clin. North Am. **57**:809, 1973.
544. Lillington, G.A., et al.: Rheumatoid pleurisy with effusion, Arch. Intern. Med. **128**:764, 1971.
545. Mandl, M.A.J., et al.: Pleural fluid in rheumatoid pleuritis, Arch. Intern. Med. **124**:373, 1969.
546. Matthay, R.A., et al.: Pulmonary manifestations of systemic lupus erythematosus: review of twelve cases of acute lupus pneumonitis, Medicine **54**:397, 1974.
547. Nair, S.S., et al.: Pulmonary hypertension and systemic lupus erythermatosus, Arch. Intern. Med. **140**:109, 1980.
548. Newball, H.H., and Brahim, S.A.: Chronic obstructive airway disease in patients with Sjögren's syndrome, Am. Rev. Respir. Dis. **115**:295, 1977.
549. Popper, M.S., et al.: Interstitial rheumatoid lung disease, Chest **62**:243, 1972.
550. Sahn, S.A., et al.: Rheumatoid pleurisy: observations on the development of low pleural fluid pH and glucose level, J.A.M.A. **140**:1237, 1980.
551. Salerni, R., et al.: Pulmonary hypertension in the CREST syndrome variant of progressive systemic sclerosis (scleroderma), Ann. Intern. Med. **86**:394, 1977.
552. Salmeron, G., Greenberg, D., and Lidsky, M.D.: Polymyositis and diffuse interstitial lung disease: a review of the pulmonary histopathologic findings, Arch. Intern. Med. **141**:1005, 1981.
553. Scott, R.F., Thomas, W.A., and Kissane, J.M.: Rheumatic pneumonitis: pathologic features, J. Pediatr. **54**:60, 1959.
554. Strimlan, C.V., et al.: Pulmonary manifestations of Sjögren's syndrome, Chest **70**:354. 1976.
555. Teilum, G., and Paulsen, H.E.: Disseminated lupus erythematosus: histopathology, morphogenesis and relation to allergy, Arch. Pathol. **64**:414, 1957.
556. Walker, W.C., and Wright, V.: Pulmonary lesions and rheumatoid arthritis, Medicine **47**:501, 1968.
557. Young, R.H., and Mark, G.J.: Pulmonary vascular changes in scleroderma, Am. J. Med. **64**:998, 1978.

Goodpasture's syndrome

558. Abboud, R.T., et al.: Goodpasture's syndrome: diagnosis by transbronchial lung biopsy, Ann. Intern. Med. **89**:635, 1978.
559. Beirne, A.J., et al.: Immunohistology of the lung in Goodpasture's syndrome, Ann. Intern. Med. **69**:1207, 1968.
560. Benoil, F.L., et al.: Goodpasture's syndrome: a clinicopathologic entity, Am. J. Med. **37**:424, 1964.
561. Border, W.A., et al.: IgA antibasement membrane nephritis with pulmonary hemorrhage, Ann. Intern. Med. **91**:21, 1979.
562. Botting, A.J., Brown, A.L., and Divertie, M.D.: The pulmonary lesion in a patient with Goodpasture's syndrome as studied with the electron microscope, Am. J. Clin. Pathol. **42**:387, 1964.
563. Byrd, L.J., et al.: Relationship of lethal midline granuloma to Wegener's granulomatosis, Arthritis Rheum. **12**:247, 1969.
564. Carrington, C.B., and Liebow, A.A.: Limited forms of angiitis and granulomatosus of the Wegener's type, Am. J. Med. **41**:497, 1966.
565. Chumbley, L.C., Harrison, E.G., and DeRemee, R.A.: Allergic granulomatosis and angiitis (Churg-Strauss syndrome): report and analysis of 30 cases, Mayo Clin. Proc. **52**:477, 1977.
566. Churg, J., and Strauss, L.: Allergic granulomatosis, allergic angiitis and periarteritis nodosa, Am. J. Pathol. **24**:277, 1976.
567. DeRemee, R.A., et al.: Respiratory vasculitis, Mayo Clin. Proc. **55**:492, 1980.

568. Donald, K.J., Edwards, R.L., and McEvoy, J.D.S.: Alveolar capillary basement membrane lesions in Goodpasture's syndrome and idiopathic pulmonary hemosiderosis, Am. J. Med. **59**:642, 1975.

569. Fauci, A.S., Haynes, B.F., and Katz, P.: The spectrum of vasculitis: clinical pathologic, immunologic and therapeutic considerations, Ann. Intern. Med. **89**:660, 1978.

570. Fauci, A.S., and Wolff, S.M.: Wegener's granulomatosis: studies in eighteen patients and a review of the literature, Medicine **52**:535, 1973.

571. Godman, G., and Churg, J.: Wegener's granulomatosis: pathology and review of the literature, Arch. Pathol. **58**:533, 1954.

572. Katzenstein, A.L.: The histologic spectrum and differential diagnosis of necrotizing granulomatous inflammation in the lung, Prog. Surg. Pathol. **1**:41, 1980.

573. Koffler, D., et al.: Immunologic studies concerning the pulmonary lesions in Goodpasture's syndrome, Am. J. Pathol. **54**:293, 1969.

574. Liebow, A.A.: Pulmonary angiitis and granulomatosis, Am. Rev. Respir. Dis. **108**:1, 1973.

575. Sisson, S., et al.: Localization of the Goodpasture antigen by immunoelectron microscopy, Clin. Immunol. Immunopathol. **23**:414, 1982.

576. Walton, E.W.: Giant cell granuloma of the respiratory tract (Wegener's granulomatosis), Br. Med. J. **2**:265, 1958.

577. Zeek, P.: Polyarteritis nodosa and other forms of necrotizing angiitis, N. Engl. J. Med. **248**:764, 1953.

Other noninfectious granulomas
Pulmonary histiocytosis X

578. Auld, D.: Pathology of eosinophilic granuloma of the lung, Arch. Pathol. **63**:113, 1957.

579. Basset, F., et al.: Ultrastructural examination of bronchoalveolar lavage for diagnosis of pulmonary histiocytosis X, Thorax **32**:303, 1977.

580. Basset, F., et al.: Pulmonary histiocytosis X, Am. Rev. Respir. Dis. **118**:811, 1978.

581. Basset, F., et al.: Langerhans cells and lung interstitium, Ann. N.Y. Acad. Sci. **278**:599, 1976.

582. Corrin, B., and Basset, F.: A review of histiocytosis X with particular reference to eosinophilic granuloma of the lung, Invest. Cell Pathol. **2**:137, 1979.

583. Friedman, P.J., Liebow, A.A., and Sokoloff, J.: Eosinophilic granuloma of the lung, Medicine **60**:385, 1981.

584. Newton, W.A., and Hamoudi, A.B.: Histiocytosis: a histologic classification with clinical correlation, Perspect. Pediatr. Pathol. **1**:251, 1973.

585. Silberberg-Sinakin, I., Baer, R.L. and Thorbecke, G.J.: Langerhans cells: a review of their nature with emphasis on their immunologic functions, Prog. Allergy **24**:268, 1978.

Sarcoidosis

586. Azar, H.A., et al.: Some aspects of sarcoidosis, Curr. Top. Pathol. **57**:49, 1973.

587. Black, M.M., and Epstein, W.L.: Formation of multinucleate giant cells in organized epithelioid cell granulomas, Am. J. Pathol. **74**:263, 1974.

588. Cain, H., and Kraus, B.: Asteroid bodies: derivatives of the cytosphere, Virchows Arch. (Cell Pathol.) **26**:119, 1977.

589. Carrington, C.B., et al.: Structure and function in sarcoidosis, Ann. N.Y. Acad. Sci. **278**:365, 1976.

590. Crystal, R.G.: Pulmonary sarcoidosis: a disease characterized and perpetuated by activated T-lymphocytes, Ann. Intern. Med. **94**:73, 1981.

591. Dauber, J.H., Rossman, M.D., and Daniele, R.P.: Bronchoalveolar cell populations in acute sarcoidosis, J. Lab. Clin. Med. **94**:862, 1979.

592. Churg, A., Carrington, C.B., and Gupta, R.: Necrotizing sarcoid granulomatosis, Chest **76**:406, 1979.

593. DeRemee, R.A.: The roentgen staging of sarcoidosis: historic and contemporary perspectives, Chest **83**:128, 1981.

594. Huang, C.T., et al.: Pulmonary sarcoidosis: roentgenographic, functional and pathologic correlations, Respiration **37**:337, 1979.

595. Hunninghake, G.W., and Crystal, R.G.: Pulmonary sarcoidosis: a disorder mediated by excess helper T-lymphocyte activity at sites of disease activity, N. Engl. J. Med. **305**:429, 1981.

596. Israel, H.L.: Influence of race and geographical origin on sarcoidosis. Arch. Environ. Health **20**:608, 1970.

597. James, G.D., and Neville, E.: Pathology of sarcoidosis, Pathobiol. Annu., **7**:31, 1977.

598. Jones-Williams, W., et al.: The fine structure of sarcoid and tuberculous granulomas, Postgrad. Med. J. **46**:496, 1970.

598a. Jaudon, R.G.: Editorial, Clin. Notes Respir. Dis. **20**:2, 1982.

599. Mitchell, D.N., and Rees, R.J.W.: The nature and physical characteristics of a transmissable agent from human sarcoid tissue, Ann. N.Y. Acad. Sci. **278**:233, 1976.

600. Mitchell, D.N., and Scadding, J.G.: State of the art, Sarcoidosis **110**:774, 1974.

601. Rosen, Y., et al.: Nongranulomatous interstitial pneumonitis in sarcoidosis, Chest **74**:122, 1978.

602. Rosen, Y., et al.: Sarcoidosis from the pathologist's vantage point, Pathol. Annu. **14**:405, 1979.

603. Scadding, J.G.: Sarcoidosis, London, 1967, Eyre & Spotiswoode.

604. Sones, M., and Israel, H.L.: Altered immunologic reactions in sarcoidosis, Ann. Intern. Med. **40**:260, 1954.

605. Wanstrup, J., and Christensen, H.E.: Sarcoidosis. I. Ultrastructural investigations on epithelioid cell granulomas, Acta Pathol. Microbiol. Scand. **66**:169, 1966.

Miscellaneous lung diseases
Alveolar proteinosis

606. Bedrossian, C.M.W., et al.: Alveolar proteinosis as a consequence of immunosuppression: a hypothesis based on clinical and pathologic observations, Hum. Pathol. **11**:527, 1980.

607. Bell, D.Y., and Hook, G.E.R.: Pulmonary alveolar proteinosis: analysis of airway and alveolar proteins, Am. Rev. Respir. Dis. **119**:979, 1979.

608. Carson, R.K., and Gordinier, R.: Pulmonary alveolar proteinosis: report of six cases, review of the literature and formulation of a new theory, Ann. Intern. Med. **62**:292, 1965.

609. Golde, D.W., et al.: Defective lung macrophages in pulmonary alveolar proteinosis, Ann. Intern. Med. **85**:304, 1976.

610. Hook, G.E.R., et al.: Composition of bronchoalveolar lavage effluents from patients with pulmonary alveolar proteinosis, Lab. Invest. **39**:342, 1978.

611. Kuhn, C., et al.: Pulmonary alveolar proteinosis, Lab. Invest. **15**:492, 1966.

612. McClenahan, J.B., and Mussenden, R.: Pulmonary alveolar proteinosis, Arch. Intern. Med. **133**:284, 1974.

613. McEuen, D.D., and Abraham, J.L.: Particulate concentrations in pulmonary alveolar proteinosis, Environ. Res. **17**:334, 1978.

614. Ramirez-R., J., and Harlan, W.R.: Pulmonary alveolar proteinosis: nature and origin of alveolar lipid, Am. J. Med. **45**:502, 1968.

615. Ramirez-R., J., Nuka, W., and McLaughlin, J.: Pulmonary alveolar proteinosis: diagnostic techniques and observations, N. Engl. J. Med. **268**:165, 1963.

616. Ramirez-R., J., Savard, E.V., and Hawkins, J.E.: Biological effect of pulmonary washings from cases of alveolar proteinosis, Am. Rev. Respir. Dis. **94**:244, 1966.

617. Rosen, S.H., Castleman, B., and Liebow, A.A.: Pulmonary alveolar proteinosis, N. Engl. J. Med. **258**:1123, 1958.

618. Singh, G., et al.: Pulmonary alveolar proteinosis: staining for surfactant apoprotein in alveolar proteinosis and in conditions simulating it, Chest **83**:82, 1983.

Alveolar microlithiasis and metastatic calcification and ossification

619. Conger, J.D., et al.: Pulmonary calcifications in chronic dialysis patients: clinical and pathologic studies, Ann. Intern. Med. **83**:330, 1975.

620. Koss, M.N., Johnson, F.B., and Hochholzer, L.: Pulmonary blue bodies, Hum. Pathol. **12**:258, 1981.

621. Michaels L., and Levene, C.: Corpora amylacea of lung, J. Pathol. Bacteriol. **74**:49, 1957.

622. O'Neill, R.P., Cohn, J.E., and Pellegrino, E.D.: Pulmonary alveolar microlithiasis—a family study, Ann. Intern. Med. **67**:957, 1967.

623. Pear, B.L.: Idiopathic disseminated pulmonary ossification, Radiology **91**:746, 1968.

624. Popelka, C.G., and Kleinerman, J.: Diffuse pulmonary ossification, Arch. Intern. Med. 523, 1977.

625. Prakash, L.B., et al.: Pulmonary alveolar microlithiasis: a review including ultrastructural and pulmonary function studies, Mayo Clin. Proc. **58**:290, 1983.

626. Sears, M.R., Chang, A.R., and Taylor, A.J.: Pulmonary alveolar microlithiasis, Thorax **26**:704, 1971.

Amyloidosis of the lung

627. Cellik, B.R., et al.: Patterns of pulmonary involvement in systemic amyloidosis, Chest **74**:543, 1978.

628. Dyke, P.C., et al.: Pulmonary amyloidoma, Am. J. Clin. Pathol. **61**:301, 1974.

629. Prowse, C.B.: Amyloidosis of the lower respiratory tract, Thorax **13**:308, 1958.

630. Rajan, V.T., and Kikkawa, Y.: Alveolar septal amyloidosis in primary amyloidosis, Arch. Pathol. **89**:521, 1970.

631. Rubinow, A., et al.: Localized amyloidosis of the lower respiratory tract, Am. Rev. Respir. Dis. **118**:603, 1978.

632. Thompson, P.J., and Citron, K.M.: Amyloid and the lower respiratory tract, Thorax **38**:84, 1983.

Lymphangiomyomatosis

633. Basset, F., et al.: Pulmonary lymphangiomyomatosis: three new cases studied with electron microscopy, Cancer **38**:2357, 1976.

634. Carrington, C.B., et al.: Lymphangiomyomatosis: physiologic pathologic-radiologic correlations, Am. Rev. Respir. Dis. **116**:977, 1977.

635. Corrin, B., Liebow, A.A., and Friedman, P.J.: Pulmonary lymphangiomyomatosis: a review, Am. J. Pathol. **79**:347, 1975.

Drug- and radiation-induced pulmonary disease

636. Bedrossian, C.M.W.: Pathology of drug-induced lung diseases, Semin. Respir. Med. **4**:98, 1982.

637. Gross, N.J.: Pulmonary effects of radiation therapy, Ann. Intern. Med. **86**:81, 1977.

638. Holoye, P.Y., et al.: Bleomycin hypersensitivity pneumonitis, Ann. Intern. Med. **88**:47, 1978.

639. Iacovino, J.R., et al.: Fatal pulmonary reaction from low doses of bleomycin: an idiosyncratic tissue response, J.A.M.A. **235**:1253, 1976.

640. Jennings, F.L., and Arden, A.: Development of radiation pneumonitis: time and dose factors, Arch. Pathol. **74**:351, 1962.

641. Littler, W.A., et al.: Busulphan lung, Thorax **24**:639, 1969.

642. Luna, M.A., et al.: Interstitial pneumonitis associated with bleomycin therapy, Am. J. Clin. Pathol. **58**:501, 1972.

643. Rosenow, E.C.: The spectrum of drug-induced pulmonary disease, Ann. Intern. Med. **77**:977, 1972.

644. Sostman, H.D., Matthay, R.A., and Putman, C.E.: Cytotoxic drug-induced lung disease, Am. J. Med. **62**:608, 1977.

645. Warren, S., and Spencer, J.: Radiation reaction in the lung, A.J.R. **43**:682, 1940.

646. Weiss, R.B., and Muggia, F.M.: Cytotoxic drug-induced pulmonary disease: update 1980, Am. J. Med. **68**:259, 1980.

Pulmonary hemorrhage

647. Buja, L.M., et al.: Pulmonary alveolar hemorrhage: common finding in patients with severe cardiac disease, Am. J. Cardiol. **27**:168, 1971.

648. Dordan, C.J., Srodes, C.H., and Duffy, F.D.: Idiopathic pulmonary hemosiderosis: electron microscopic, immunofluorescent and iron kinetic studies, Chest **68**:577, 1975.

649. Golde, D.W., et al.: Occult pulmonary hemorrhage in leukemia, Br. Med. J. **2**:166, 1975.

650. Gonzalez-Crussi, F., Hull, M.T., and Grossfeld, J.L.: Idiopathic pulmonary hemosiderosis: evidence of capillary basement membrane abnormality, Am. Rev. Respir. Dis. **114**:689, 1976.

651. Hukill, P.B.: Experimental pulmonary hemosiderosis: the liability of pulmonary iron deposits, Lab. Invest. **12**:577, 1963.

652. Hyatt, R.W., et al.: Ultrastructure of the lung in idiopathic pulmonary hemosiderosis, Am. J. Med. **52**:822, 1972.

653. Irwin, R.S., et al.: Idiopathic pulmonary hemosiderosis: an electron microscopic and immunofluorescent study, Chest **65**:41, 1974.

654. Morgan, P.G.M., and Turner-Warwick, M.: Pulmonary haemosiderosis and pulmonary haemorrhage, Br. J. Dis. Chest **75**:225, 1981.

655. Smith, L.J., and Katzenstein, A.L.A.: Pathogenesis of massive pulmonary hemorrhage in acute leukemia, Arch. Intern. Med. **142**:2149, 1982.

656. Soergel, K.H., and Sommers, S.C.: Idiopathic pulmonary hemosiderosis and related syndromes, Am. J. Med. **32**:499, 1962.

Aspiration pneumonia, lipid pneumonia, and lung collapse and pneumothorax

657. Askin, F.B., McCann, B.G., and Kuhn, C.: Reactive eosinophilic pleuritis: a lesion to be distinguished from pulmonary eosinophilic granuloma, Arch. Pathol. Lab. Med. **101**:187, 1977.

658. Borrie, J., and Gwynne, J.F.: Paraffinoma of lung: lipid pneumonia, Thorax **28**:214, 1973.

659. Licter, I., and Gwynne, J.F.: Spontaneous pneumothorax in young subjects: a clinical and pathological study, Thorax **26**:409, 1971.

660. Miller, G.J., et al.: The lipoid pneumonia of Blackfat tobacco smokers in Guyana, Q. J. Med. **40**:457, 1971.

661. Oldenburger, D., et al.: Inhalation lipoid pneumonia from burning fats, J.A.M.A. **222**:1288, 1972.

662. Rigg, J.R.A.: Pulmonary atelectasis after anesthesia: pathophysiology and management, Can. Anaesth. Soc. J. **28**:305, 1981.

663. Timmerman, R.J., and Schroer, J.A.: Lipoid pneumonia caused by methenamine mandelate suspension, J.A.M.A. **225**:1524, 1973.

664. Wynne, J.W., and Modell, J.H.: Respiratory aspiration of stomach contents, Ann. Intern. Med. **87**:466, 1977.

Chronic airflow limitation

665. Anderson, A.E., and Foraker, A.G.: Centrilobular emphysema and panlobular emphysema: two different diseases, Thorax **28**:547, 1973.

666. Anderson, J.A., Dunnill, M.S., and Ryder, R.C.: Dependence of the incidence of emphysema on smoking history, age and sex, Thorax **27**:547, 1972.

667. Auerbach, O., et al.: Relation of smoking and age to emphysema: whole lung section study, N. Engl. J. Med. **286**:853, 1972.

668. Bates, D.V.: The fate of the chronic bronchitic: a report of the ten-year follow-up in the Canadian Department of Veteran's Affairs coordinated study of chronic bronchitis, Am. Rev. Respir. Dis. **108**:1043, 1973.

669. Beatty, K., et al.: Determination of oxidized alpha-1-proteinase inhibitor in serum, J. Lab. Clin. Med. **100**:186, 1982.

670. Berend, N., Woolcock, A.J., and Marlin, G.E.: Correlation between the function and structure of the lung in smokers, Am. Rev. Respir. Dis. **119**:695, 1979.

671. Berend, N., et al.: Small airways disease: reproduceability of measurements and correlation with lung function, Chest **79**:263, 1981.

672. Boushy, S.F., et al.: Lung recoil pressure, airway resistance and forced flows related to morphologic emphysema, Am. Rev. Respir. Dis. **104**:551, 1971.

673. Burrows, B., et al.: The emphysematous and bronchial types of chronic airways obstruction: a clinicopathologic study of patients in London and Chicago, Lancet **1**:830, 1966.

674. Burrows, B., et al.: Quantitative relationship between cigarette smoking and ventilatory function, Am. Rev. Respir. Dis. **115**:195, 1977.

675. Carrell, R.W., et al.: Structure and variation of human α1-antitrypsin, Nature **298**:329, 1982.

676. Cosio, M.G., Hale, K.A., and Niewoehner, D.E.: Morphologic and morphometric effects of prolonged cigarette smoking on the small airways, Am. Rev. Respir. Dis. **122**:265, 1980.

677. Cromie, J.B.: Correlation of anatomic pulmonary emphysema and right ventricular hypertrophy, Am. Rev. Respir. Dis. **84**:657, 1961.

678. Depierre, A., et al.: Quantitative study of parenchyma and small conductive airways in chronic non-specific lung disease, Chest **62**:699, 1972.

679. Dunnill, M.S.: An assessment of the anatomical factor in cor pulmonale in emphysema, J. Clin. Pathol. **14**:246, 1961.

680. Eriksson, S.: Studies in alpha-1-antitrypsin deficiency, Acta Med. Scand. **177**(suppl. 432):1, 1965.

681. Ferris, B.G.: Air pollution. In Macklen, P.T., and Permutt, S., editors: The lung in transition between health and disease, New York, 1979, Marcel Dekker.

682. Fletcher, C., and Peto, R.: The natural history of chronic airflow obstruction, Br. Med. J. **1**:1645, 1977.

683. Fletcher, C., et al.: The natural history of chronic bronchitis and emphysema, Oxford, Eng., 1976, Oxford University Press.

684. Greenberg, S.D., et al.: The lungs in homozygous alpha-1-antitrypsin deficiency, Am. J. Clin. Pathol. **60**:581, 1973.

685. Haas, H., et al.: Bacterial flora of the respiratory tract in chronic bronchitis: comparison of transtracheal, fiberbronchoscopic, and oropharyngeal sampling methods, Am. Rev. Respir. Dis. **116**:41, 1977.

686. Heard, B.E., et al.: The morphology of emphysema, chronic bronchitis and bronchiectasis: definition, nomenclature and classification, J. Clin. Pathol. **32**:882, 1979.

687. Heppleston, A.G., and Leopold, J.G.: Chronic pulmonary emphysema: anatomy and pathogenesis, Am. J. Med. **31**:279, 1961.

688. Hogg, J.C., et al.: Site and nature of airway obstruction in chronic obstructive lung disease, N. Engl. J. Med. **278**:1355, 1968.

689. Holland, W.W., and Reid, D.D.: The urban factor in chronic bronchitis, Lancet **1**:445, 1965.

690. Ishikawa, S., et al.: The emphysema profile in two midwestern cities in North America, Arch. Environ. Health **18**:660, 1969.

691. Karlinksy, J.B., and Snider, G.L.: Animal models of emphysema, Am. Rev. Respir. Dis. **117**:1109, 1978.

692. Kuhn, C., Senior, R.M., and Pierce, J.A.: The pathogenesis of emphysema. In Witschi, H.P., and Nettesheim, P., editors: Mechanisms in respiratory toxicology, Boca Raton, Fla., 1982, CRC Press.

693. Kuhn, C., and Tavassoli, F.: Scanning electron microscopy of elastase-induced emphysema: a comparison with emphysema in man, Lab. Invest. **34**:2, 1976.

694. Linhartova, A., Anderson, A.E., and Foraker, A.G.: Further observations on luminal deformity and stenosis of non-respiratory bronchioles in pulmonary emphysema, Thorax **32**:53, 1977.

695. Macklem, P.T., Thurlbeck, W.M., and Fraser, R.G.: Chronic obstructive disease of small airways, Ann. Intern. Med. **74**:167, 1971.

696. Martelli, N.A.: Lower-zone emphysema in young patients without α1-antitrypsin deficiency, Thorax **29**:237, 1974.

697. Matsuba, K., and Thurlbeck, W.M.: The number and dimensions of small airways in emphysematous lungs, Am. J. Pathol. **67**:265, 1972.

698. Matsuba, K., and Thurlbeck, W.M.: Disease of small airways in chronic bronchitis, Am. Rev. Respir. Dis. **107**:552, 1973.

699. McNamara, M.J., Philips, I.A., and Williams, O.B.: Viral and *Mycoplasma pneumoniae* infections in exacerbations of chronic lung disease, Am. Rev. Respir. Dis. **100**:19, 1969.

700. Mitchell, R.S., et al.: Are centrilobular emphysema and panlobular emphysema two different diseases? Hum. Pathol. **1**:433, 1970.

701. Mitchell, R.S., et al.: The morphologic features of the bronchi, bronchioles and alveoli in chronic airway obstruction: a clinicopathologic study, Am. Rev. Respir. Dis. **114**:137, 1976.

702. Mitchell, R.S., et al.: The right ventricle in chronic airway obstruction: a clinicopathologic study, Am. Rev. Respir. Dis. **114**:147, 1976.

703. Morse, J.O.: Alpha-1-antitrypsin deficiency, N. Engl. J. Med. **299**:1045, 1099, 1978.

704. Oswald, N.C.: Chronic bronchitis: factors in pathogenesis and their clinical application, Lancet **1**:271, 1954.

705. Park, S.S., et al.: Relationship of bronchitis and emphysema to altered pulmonary function, Am. Rev. Respir. Dis. **102**:927, 1970.

706. Pump, K.K.: Fenestrae in the alveolar membrane of the human lung, Chest **65**:431, 1974.

707. Pump, K.K.: Emphysema and its relation to age, Am. Rev. Respir. Dis. **114**:5, 1976.

708. Reid, L.: Measurement of the bronchial mucous gland layer: a diagnostic yardstick in chronic bronchitis, Thorax **15**:132, 1960.

709. Reid, L.A.: Pathology of chronic bronchitis, Lancet **1**:275, 1954.

710. Restrepo, G., and Heard, B.E.: The size of the bronchial glands in chronic bronchitis, J. Pathol. Bacteriol. **85**:305, 1963.

711. Ryan, S.F., et al.: Ductectasia: an asymptomatic pulmonary change related to age, Med. Thorac. **22**:181, 1965.

712. Spain, D.M., Siegel, H., and Bradess, V.A.: Emphysema in apparently healthy adults: smoking, age and sex, J.A.M.A. **224**:322, 1973.

713. Tager, I., and Speizer, F.E.: Role of infection in chronic bronchitis, N. Engl. J. Med. **292**:563, 1975.

714. Takizawa, T., and Thurlbeck, W.M.: Muscle and mucous gland size in the major bronchi of patients with chronic bronchitis, asthma, and asthmatic bronchitis, Am. Rev. Respir. Dis. **104**:331, 1971.

715. Thurlbeck, W.M.: Chronic airflow obstruction in lung disease, Philadelphia, 1976, W.B. Saunders Co.

716. Thurlbeck, W.M., Ryder, R.C., and Sternby, N.: A comparative study of the severity of emphysema in necropsy populations in three different countries, Am. Rev. Respir. Dis. **109**:239, 1974.

717. Wagner, P.D., et al.: Ventilation-perfusion inequality in chronic obstructive pulmonary disease, J. Clin. Invest. **59**:203, 1977.

718. Wright, R.R.: Elastic tissue of normal and emphysematous lungs: a tridimensional histologic study, Am. J. Pathol. **39**:355, 1961.

Pneumoconiosis

719. Allison, A.C., and D'Arcy Hart, P.: Potentiation by silica of the growth of *Myocobacterium tuberculosis* in macrophage cultures, Br. J. Exp. Pathol. **49**:465, 1968.

720. Allison, A.C., Harington, J.S., and Birbeck, M.: An examination of the cytotoxic effects of silica on macrophages, J. Exp. Med. **124**:141, 1966.

721. Becklake, M.R.: Asbestos-related diseases of the lung and other organs: their epidemiology and implications for clinical practice, Am. Rev. Respir. Dis. **114**:187, 1976.

722. Brain, J.D., and Valberg, P.A.: Deposition of aerosol in the respiratory tract, Am. Rev. Respir. Dis. **120**:1325, 1979.

723. Buechner, H.A., and Ansari, A.: Acute silico-proteinosis: a new pathologic variant of acute silicosis in sandblasters characterized by histologic features resembling alveolar proteinosis, Dis. Chest **55**:247, 1969.

724. Caplan, A.: Certain radiological appearances in the chest of coal-miners suffering from rheumatoid arthritis, Thorax **8**:29, 1953.

725. Cockcroft, A., et al.: Postmortem study of emphysema in coal-workers and non-coal workers, Lancet **2**:600, 1982.

726. Churg, A., and Golden, J.: Current problems in the pathology of asbestos-related disease, Pathol. Annu. **17**:33, 1982.

727. Craighead, J.E., et al.: The pathology of asbestos-associated diseases of the lungs and pleural cavities: diagnostic criteria and proposed grading schema, Arch. Pathol. Lab. Med. **108**:544, 1982.

728. Edwards, C., et al.: The pathology of the lung in byssinotics, Thorax **30**:612, 1975.

729. Epler, G.R., McLoud, T.C., and Gaensler, E.A.: Prevalence and incidence of benign asbestos pleural effusion in a working population, J.A.M.A. **247**:617, 1982.

730. Freiman, D.G., and Hardy, H.L.: Beryllium disease, Hum. Pathol. **1**:25, 1970.

731. Gough, J.: Pneumoconiosis in coal trimmers, J. Pathol. Bacteriol. **51**:277, 1940.

732. Gough, J., Rivers, D., and Seal, R.M.E.: Pathological studies of modified pneumoconiosis in coal miners with rheumatoid arthritis (Caplan's syndrome), Thorax **10**:9, 1955.

733. Green, F.H.Y., and Laqueur, W.A.: Coal workers pneumoconiosis, Pathol. Annu. **15**:333, 1980.

734. Gross, P., Westrick, M.L., and McNerney, J.M.: Experimental tuberculosilicosis: a comparison of the effects produced by some of its various pathogenic components, Am. Rev. Respir. Dis. **83**:510, 1961.

735. Hammond, E.C., Selikoff, I.J., and Seidman, H.: Asbestos exposure, cigarette smoking and death rates, Ann. N.Y. Acad. Sci. **330**:473, 1979.

736. Heppleston, A.G.: The pathogenesis of simple pneumokoniosis in coal workers, J. Pathol. Bacteriol. **67**:51, 1954.

737. Heppleston, A.G., and Styles, J.A.: Activity of a macrophage factor in collagen formation by silica, Nature **214**:521, 1967.

738. Holt, P.F.: Poly(vinylpyridine oxides) in pneumoconiosis research, Br. J. Ind. Med. **28**:72, 1971.

739. Holt, P.G., and Keast, D.: Environmentally induced changes in immunological function: acute and chronic effects of inhalation of tobacco smoke and other atmospheric contaminants in man and experimental animals, Bacteriol. Rev. **41**:205, 1977.

740. Kannerstein, M., and Churg, J.: Pathology of carcinoma of the lung associated with asbestos exposure, Cancer **30**:14, 1972.

741. Kleinerman, J., et al.: Pathology standards for coal workers pneumoconiosis, Arch. Pathol. Lab. Med. **103**:375, 1979.

742. Kuhn, C., and Kuo, T.: Cytoplasmic hyalin in asbestosis, Arch. Pathol. **95**:189, 1973.

743. Lyons, J.P., et al.: Pulmonary disability in coalworkers' pneumoconiosis, Br. Med. J. **1**:713, 1972.

744. Morgan, W.K.C.: Respiratory disease in coal miners, J.A.M.A. **231**:1347, 1975.

745. Morgan, W.K.C., and Lapp, N.L.: Respiratory disease in coal miners, Am. Rev. Respir. Dis. **113**:531, 1976.

746. Naeye, R.L.: Black lung disease, the anthracotic pneumoconioses, Pathol. Annu. **8**:349, 1973.

747. Naeye, R.L., and Dellinger, W.S.: Coal workers pneumoconiosis: correlation of roentgenographic and postmortem findings, J.A.M.A. **220**:223, 1972.

748. Naeye, R.L., Mahon, J.K., and Dellinger, W.: Effects of smoking on lung structure of Appalachian coal workers, Arch. Environ. Health **22**:190, 1971.

749. Newman, J.K., Vatter, A.E., and Reiss, O.K.: Chemical and electron microscopic studies of the black pigment of the human lung, Arch. Environ. Health **5**:420, 1967.

750. Parkes, W.R.: Occupational lung disorders, London, 1974, Butterworth.

751. Reiser, K.M., and Last, J.A.: Sillicosis and fibrogenesis: fact and artifact, Toxicology **17**:51, 1979.

752. Ryder, R., et al.: Emphysema in coal workers' pneumoconiosis, Br. Med. J. **3**:481, 1970.

753. Selikoff, I.J., Hammond, E.C., and Seidman, H.: Mortality experience of insulation workers in the United States and Canada, Ann. N.Y. Acad. Sci. **330**:91, 1979.

754. Selikoff, I.J., Micholson, W.J., and Langer, A.M.: Asbestos air pollution, Arch. Environ. Health **25**:1, 1972.

755. Slatkin, D.N., et al.: The C^{13}/C^{12} ratio in black pulmonary pigment: a mass spectrometric study, Hum. Pathol. **9**:259, 1978.

756. Snider, D.E.: The relationship between tuberculosis and silicosis, Am. Rev. Respir. Dis. **118**:455, 1978.

757. Suzuki, Y., and Churg, J.: Formation of the asbestos body: a comparative study with three types of asbestos, Environ. Res. **3**:107, 1969.

758. Uber, C.L., and McReynolds, R.A.: Immunotoxicology of silica, CRC Crit. Rev. Toxicol. 303, 1982.

759. Vorwald, A.F.: Cavities in the silicotic lung: a pathological study with clinical correlation, Am. J. Pathol. **17**:709, 1941.

760. Wagner, J.C., Sleggs, C.A., and Marchand, P.: Diffuse pleural mesothelioma and asbestos exposure in the North Western Cape Province, Br. J. Ind. Med. **17**:260, 1960.

761. Watson, A.J., et al.: Pneumoconiosis in carbon electrode makers, Br. J. Ind. Med. **16**:274, 1959.

762. Whitwell, F., Newhouse, M.L., and Bennett, D.R. A study of the histological cell types of lung cancer in workers suffering from asbestosis in the United Kingdom, Br. J. Ind. Med. **31**:298, 1974.

763. Wood, W.B., and Gloyne, S.R.: Pulmonary asbestosis, Lancet **1**:445, 1930.

764. Wyatt, J.P.: Morphogenesis of pneumoconiosis occurring in southern Illinois bituminous workers, Arch. Indust. Health **21**:445, 1961.

765. Ziskind, M., Jones, R.N., and Weill, H.: State of the art: silicosis, Am. Rev. Respir. Dis. **113**:643, 1976.

Lung tumors
Carcinomas of the lung

766. Ashley, D.J.B., and Davies, H.D.: Cancer of the lung: histology and biological behaviour, Cancer **20**:165, 1967.

767. Auerbach, O., Hammond, E.C., and Garfinkel, L.: Changes in bronchial epithelium in relation to cigarette smoking, 1955-1960 as 1970-1977, N. Engl. J. Med. **300**:381, 1979.

768. Auerbach, O., et al.: Changes in bronchial epithelium in relation to cigarette smoking and in relation to lung cancer, N. Engl. J. Med. **265**:253, 1961.

769. Auerbach, O., et al.: Comparison of World Health Organization (WHO) classification of lung tumors by light and electron microscopy, Cancer **50**:2079, 1982.

770. Azzopardi, J.G.: Oat cell carcinoma of the bronchus, J. Pathol. Bacteriol. **78**:513, 1959.

771. Azzopardi, J.G., and Bellau, A.R.: Carcinoid syndrome and oat cell carcinoma of the bronchus, Thorax **20**:393, 1965.

772. Beck, C., and Burger, H.G.: Evidence for presence of immunoreactive growth hormone in cancers of lung and stomach, Cancer **30**:75, 1972.

773. Bedrossian, C.M.W., et al.: Ultrastructure of human bronchioloalveolar cell carcinoma, Cancer **36**:1399, 1975.

774. Bender, R.A., and Hansen, H.: Hypercalcemia in bronchogenic carcinoma: a prospective study of 200 patients, Ann. Intern. Med. **80**:205, 1974.

775. Bennett, D.E., and Sasser, W.F.: Bronchiolar carcinoma: a valid clinicopathologic entity? A study of 30 cases, Cancer **24**:876, 1969.

776. Bennett, D.E., Sasser, W.F., and Ferguson, T.B.: Adenocarcinoma of the lung in men: a clinicopathologic study of 100 cases, Cancer **23**:431, 1969.

777. Bensch, K.G., et al.: Oat cell carcinoma of the lung—its origin and relationship to the bronchial carcinoid, Cancer **22**:1163, 1968.

778. Bjelke, E.: Dietary vitamin A and human lung cancer, Int. J. Cancer **15**:561, 1975.

779. Bolen, J.W., and Thorning, D.: Histogenetic classification of pulmonary carcinomas: peripheral adenocarcinomas studied by light microscopy, histochemistry and electron microscopy, Pathol. Annu. **17**:77, 1982.

780. Bondy, P.K., and Gilby, E.D.: Endocrine function in small cell undifferentiated carcinoma of the lung, Cancer **50**:2147, 1982.

781. Byrd, R.B., et al.: The roentgenographic appearance of large cell carcinoma of the bronchus, Mayo Clin. Proc. **43**:333, 1968.

782. Byrd, R.B., et al.: The roentgenographic appearance of squamous cell carcinoma of the bronchus, Mayo Clin. Proc. **43**:327, 1968.

783. Carney, D.N., et al.: Influence of histologic subtype of small cell carcinoma of the lung on clinical presentation, response to therapy and survival, J. Natl. Cancer Inst. **65**:1225, 1980.

784. Carr, D.T.: The staging of lung cancer, Am. Rev. Respir. Dis. **117**:819, 1978.

785. Churg. A.: The fine structure of large cell undifferentiated carcinoma of the lung: evidence for its relation to squamous cell carcinomas and adenocarcinomas, Hum. Pathol. **9**:143, 1978.

786. Corson, J.M., and Pinhus, G.S.: Mesothelioma, profile of keratin proteins and carcinoembryonic antigen: an immunoperoxidase study of 20 cases and comparison with pulmonary adenocarcinomas, Am. J. Pathol. **108**:80, 1982.

787. Cottrell, J.C., Becker, K.L., and Moore, C.: Immunofluorescent studies in gonadotropin-secreting bronchogenic carcinoma, Am. J. Clin. Pathol. **59**:422, 1968.

788. Cutz, E., Chan, W., and Track, N.S.: Bombesin, calcitonin and leuenkephalin immunoreactivity in endocrine cells of human lung, Experientia **37**:765, 1981.

789. Davis, S., et al.: Small-cell carcinoma of the lung: survival according to histologic subtype, Cancer **47**:1863, 1981.

790. DeSchryver-Kecskemeti, K., et al.: Pulmonary oat cell carcinomas: expression of plasma membrane antigen correlated with presence of cytoplasmic neurosecretory granules, Lab. Invest. **41**:432, 1979.

791. Doll, R., and Peto, R.: Mortality in relation to smoking: 20 years' observations on male British doctors, Br. Med. J. **2**:1525, 1976.

792. Doll, R., and Peto, R.: The cause of cancer: quantitative estimates of avoidable risks of cancer in the United States today, J. Natl. Cancer Inst. **66**:1191, 1981.

793. Erisman, M.D., et al.: Human lung small cell carcinoma contains bombesin, Proc. Natl. Acad. Sci. U.S.A. **79**:2379, 1982.

794. Feinstein, A.R.: Symptoms as an index of biological behavior and prognosis in human cancer, Nature **209**:241, 1966.

795. Figueroa, W.G., et al.: Lung cancer in chloromethyl methyl ether workers, N. Engl. J. Med. **288**:1096, 1973.

796. Flanagan, P., and Roeckel, I.E.: Giant cell carcinoma of the lung: anatomic and clinical correlation, Am. J. Med. **36**:214, 1964.

797. Fraire, A.E., and Greenberg, S.D.: Carcinoma and diffuse interstitial fibrosis of lung, Cancer **31**:1078, 1973.

798. Fraumeni, J.F.: Respiratory carcinogenesis: an epidemiologic appraisal, J. Natl. Cancer Inst. **55**:1039, 1975.

799. Garfinkel, L.: Time trends in lung cancer mortality among nonsmokers and a note on passive smoking, J. Natl. Cancer Inst. **66**:1061, 1981.

800. Gottlieb, M.S., et al.: Lung cancer mortality and residential proximity to industry, Environ. Health Perspect. **45**:157, 1982.

801. Graham, S., and Levin, M.L.: Smoking withdrawal and the reduction of risk of lung cancer, Cancer **27**:865, 1971.

802. Greco, F.A., and Oldham, R.K.: Current concepts in cancer: small cell lung cancer, N. Engl. J. Med. **301**:355, 1979.

803. Green, N., Kurohara, S.S., and George, F.W.: Cancer of the lung: in-depth analysis of prognostic factors, Cancer **25**:1229, 1971.

804. Greenberg, S.D., Smith, M.N., and Spjut, H.J.: Bronchioloalveolar carcinoma—cell of origin, Am. J. Clin. Pathol. **63**:153, 1975.

805. Hammond, E.C., and Horn, D.: The relationship between human smoking habits and death rates, J.A.M.A. **155**:1316, 1954.

806. Hansen, M., Hammer, M., and Hammer, L.: ACTH, ADH and calcitonin concentrations as markers of response and relapse in small cell carcinoma of the lung, Cancer **46**:2062, 1980.

807. Hansen, M., et al.: Hormonal polypeptides and amine metabolites in small cell carcinoma of the lung with special reference to stage and subtypes, Cancer **45**:1432, 1980.

808. Hattori, S., et al.: Oat cell carcinoma of the lung: clinical and morphological studies in relation to its histogenesis, Cancer **30**:1014, 1972.

809. Hirayama, T.: Non-smoking wives of heavy smokers have a higher risk of lung cancer: a study from Japan, Br. Med. J. **282**:183, 1981.

810. Hirsch, F., et al.: Bone marrow examination in the staging of small-cell anaplastic carcinoma of the lung with special reference to subtyping: an evaluation of 203 consecutive patients, Cancer **39**:2563, 1977.

811. Hone, A., and Ohta, M.: Ultrastructural features of large cell carcinoma of the lung with reference to the prognosis of patients, Hum. Pathol. **12**:423, 1981.

812. Horne, J.W., and Asire, A.J.: Changes in lung cancer incidence and mortality rates among Americans: 1969-78, J. Natl. Cancer Inst. **69**:833, 1982.

813. Hyde, L., and Hyde, C.I.: Clinical manifestations of lung cancer, Chest **65**:299, 1974.

814. Johnston, R.N., and Smith, D.H.: Symptoms and survival in lung cancer, Lancet **2**:588, 1968.

815. Kato, Y., et al.: Oat cell carcinoma of the lung: a review of 138 cases, Cancer **23**:517, 1969.

816. Kirsch, M.M., et al.: Effect of histological cell type on prognosis of patients with bronchogenic carcinoma, Ann. Thorac. Surg. **13**:303, 1972.

817. Kreyberg, L.: Histological lung cancer types: a morphological and histological correlation, Oslor, 1962, Norwegian Universities Press.

818. Kuhn, C.: Fine structure of bronchioloalveolar cell carcinoma, Cancer **30**:1107, 1972.

819. Liebow, A.A.: Bronchiolo-alveolar carcinoma, Adv. Intern. Med. **10**:329, 1960.

820. Lokich, J.J.: The frequency and clinical biology of the ectopic hormone syndromes of small cell carcinoma, Cancer **50**:2111, 1982.

821. Lukeman, J.M.: Reliability of cytologic diagnosis in cancer of the lung, Cancer Chemother. Rep. **4**:79, 1973.

822. Marcq, M., and Galy, P.: Bronchioloalveolar carcinoma: clinical relationships, natural history, and prognosis in 29 cases, Am. Rev. Respir. Dis. **107**:621, 1973.

823. Matthews, M.J.: Morphology of lung cancer, Semin. Oncol. **1**:175, 1974.

824. McDonnell, L., and Long, J.P.: Lung scar cancer—a reappraisal, J. Clin. Pathol. **34**:996, 1981.

825. McDowell, E.M., et al.: The respiratory epithelium. V. Histogenesis of lung carcinomas in the human, J. Natl. Cancer Inst. **61**:587, 1978.

826. Mettlin, C., Graham, S., and Swanson, M.: Vitamin A and lung cancer, J. Natl. Cancer Inst. **62**:1435, 1979.

827. Meyer, E.C., and Liebow, A.A.: Relationship of interstitial pneumonia, honey combing and atypical epithelial proliferation to cancer of the lung, Cancer **18**:322, 1965.

828. Meyer, J.A.: The concept and significance of growth rates in human pulmonary tumors, Ann. Thorac. Surg. **14**:309, 1972.

829. Mitchell, D.M., Morgan, P.G.M., and Ball, J.B.: Prognostic features of large cell anaplastic carcinoma of the bronchus, Thorax **35**:118, 1980.

830. Nash, A.D., and Stout, A.P.: Giant cell carcinoma of the lung: report of 5 cases, Cancer **11**:369, 1958.

831. Nixon, D.W., et al.: Relationship between survival and histologic type in small cell anaplastic carcinoma of the lung, Cancer **44**:1045, 1979.

832. Percy, C., and Sobin, L.: Surveillance, epidemiology and end results: lung cancer data applied to the World Health Organization's classification of lung tumors, J. Natl. Cancer Inst. **70**:633, 1983.

833. Razzuk, M.A., et al.: Giant cell carcinoma of lung, J. Thorac. Cardiovasc. Surg. **59**:574, 1970.

834. Rigler, L.G.: The Heath Memorial Lecture: Peripheral carcinoma of the lung: incidence, possibilities for survival, methods of detection, identification, radiologic and other biophysical methods in tumor diagnosis, Chicago, 1975, Year Book Medical Publishers.

835. Ripstein, C.B., Spain, D.M., and Bluth, I.: Scar cancer of the lung, J. Thorac. Cardiovasc. Surg. **56**:362, 1968.

836. Rossing, T.H., and Rossing, R.G.: Survival in lung cancer: an analysis of the effects of age, sex, resectability and histopathologic type, Am. Rev. Respir. Dis. **126**:771, 1982.

837. Saccomanno, G., et al.: Histologic types of lung cancer among uranium miners, Cancer **27**:515, 1971.

838. Said, J.W., et al.: Keratin proteins and carcinoembryonic antigen in lung carcinoma: an immunoperoxidase study of 54 cases with ultrastructural correlations, Hum. Pathol. **14**:70, 1983.

839. Singh, G., Katyal, S.L., and Torikata, C.: Carcinoma of type II pneumocytes: immunodiagnosis of a subtype of "bronchioloalveolar carcinomas," Am. J. Pathol. **102**:195, 1981.

840. Smoking and health: a report of the Royal College of Physicians of London on smoking in relation to cancer of the lung and other diseases, New York, 1962, Pitman Publishing Corp.

841. Soorae, A.S., and Abbey, Smith, R.: Tumour size as a prognostic factor after resection of lung carcinoma, Thorax **32**:19, 1977.

842. Sporn, M.D., and Newton, D.L.: Chemoprevention of cancer with retinoids, Fed. Proc. **38**:2528, 1979.

843. Stanley, K.E.: Prognostic factors for survival in patients with inoperable lung cancer, J. Natl. Cancer Inst. **65**:25, 1980.

844. Stanley, K.E., and Matthews, M.J.: Analysis of a pathology review of patients with lung tumors, J. Natl. Cancer Inst. **66**:989, 1981.

845. Straus, M.J., editor: Lung cancer: clinical diagnosis and treatment, New York, 1983, Grune & Stratton, Inc.

846. Taylor, A.B., Shinton, N.H., and Waterhouse, J.A.H.: Histology of bronchial carcinoma in relation to prognosis, Thorax **18**:178, 1963.

847. Trump, B.F., et al.: The respiratory epithelium. III. The histogenesis of epidermoid metaplasia and carcinoma in situ in the human, J. Natl. Cancer Inst. **61**:563, 1978.

848. U.S. Department of Health, Education and Welfare: Smoking and health: report of the advisory committee to the Surgeon General of the Public Health Service, Washington, D.C., 1964, The Department.

849. Valaitis, J., Warren, S., and Gamble, D.: Increasing incidence of adenocarcinoma of the lung, Cancer 47:1042, 1981.

850. Vincent, T.N., Satterfield, J.V., and Ackerman, L.V.: Carcinoma of the lung in women, Cancer 18:559, 1965.

851. Walter, J.B., and Pryce, D.M.: The histology of lung cancer, Thorax 10:107, 1955.

852. Walter, J.B., and Pryce, D.M.: The site of origin of lung cancer and its relation to histological type, Thorax 10:117, 1955.

853. Weiss, W.: The mitotic index in bronchogenic carcinoma, Am. Rev. Respir. Dis. 104:536, 1971.

854. Weiss, W.: Cigarette smoke as a carcinogen, Am. Rev. Respir. Dis. 108:364, 1973.

855. Weiss, W., Boucot, K.R., and Cooper, D.A.: The histopathology of bronchogenic carcinoma and its relation to growth rate, metastasis, and prognosis, Cancer 26:965, 1970.

856. Weiss, W., et al.: Lung cancer type in relation to cigarette dosage, Cancer 39:2568, 1977.

857. Wellons, H.A., et al.: Prognostic factors in malignant tumors of the lung: analysis of 582 cases, Ann. Thorac. Surg. 5:228, 1968.

858. Wilson, T.S., et al.: Elaboration of human chorionic gonadotropin by lung tumors, Arch. Pathol. Lab. Med. 105:169, 1981.

859. World Health Organization: Histological typing of lung tumors. In International histological classification of tumors, no. 1, ed. 2, Geneva, 1981, World Health Organization.

860. Wynder, E.L., and Berg, J.W.: Cancer of the lung among nonsmokers: special reference to histologic patterns, Cancer 20:1161, 1967.

861. Wynder, E.L., Mabuchi, K., and Beattie, E.J.: The epidemiology of lung cancer: recent trends, J.A.M.A. 213:2221, 1970.

862. Yesner, R.: Observer variability and reliability in lung cancer diagnosis, Cancer Chemother. Rep. 4:55, 1973.

863. Yesner, R., et al.: Reappraisal of histopathology in lung cancer and correlation of cell types with antecedent cigarette smoking, Am. Rev. Respir. Dis. 107:790, 1973.

Other lung tumors

864. Ashley, D.J.B., Dinino, E.A., and Davies, H.D.: Bronchial polyps, Thorax 18:45, 1963.

865. Askin, F.B., et al.: Malignant small cell tumor of the thoracopulmonary region in childhood: a distinctive clinicopathologic entity of uncertain histogenesis, Cancer 43:2438, 1979.

866. Axelsson, C., Burcharth, F., and Jahansen, A.: Mucoepidermoid lung tumors, J. Thorac. Cardiovasc. Surg. 65:902, 1973.

867. Bahadori, M., and Liebow, A.A.: Plasma cell granulomas of the lung, Cancer 31:191, 1973.

868. Bateson, E.M.: So called hamartoma of the lung—a true neoplasm of fibrous connective tissue of the bronchi, Cancer 31:1458, 1973.

869. Becker, N.H., and Soifer, I.: Benign clear cell tumor ("sugar tumor") of the lung, Cancer 27:712, 1971.

870. Bender, B.L., and Jaffe, R.: Immunoglobulin production in lymphomatoid granulomatous and relation to other "benign" lymphoproliferative disorders, Am. J. Clin. Pathol. 73:41, 1980.

871. Bensch, K.G., Gordon, G., and Miller, L.: Electron microscopic and biochemical studies on the bronchial carcinoid tumor, Cancer 18:592, 1965.

872. Bergmann, M., Ackerman. L.V., and Kemler, R.L.: Carcinosarcoma of the lung: review of the literature and report of two cases treated by pneumonectomy, Cancer 4:919, 1951.

873. Bhagavan, B.S., et al.: Intravascular bronchiolo-alveolar tumor (IVBAT): a low grade sclerosing epithelioid angiosarcoma of lung, Am. J. Surg. Pathol. 6:41, 1982.

874. Bonikos, D.S., Archibald, R., and Bensch, K.G.: On the origin of the so-called tumorlets of the lung, Hum. Pathol. 7:461, 1976.

875. Bonikos, D.S., Bensch, K.G., and Jamplis, R.W.: Peripheral pulmonary carcinoid tumors, Cancer 37:1977, 1976.

876. Butler, C., and Kleinerman, J.: Pulmonary hamartoma, Arch. Pathol. 88:584, 1969.

877. Churg, A., and Warnock, M.L.: Pulmonary tumorlet: a form of peripheral carcinoid, Cancer 37:1469, 1976.

878. Churg, A.M., and Warnock, M.L.: So-called "minute pulmonary chemodectoma"—a tumor not related to paraganglioma, Cancer 37:1759, 1976.

879. Davis, P.W., et al.: Benign and malignant mixed tumours of the lung, Thorax 27:657, 1972.

880. Drury, R.A.B., and Stirland, R.M.: Carcinosarcomatous tumours of the respiratory tract, J. Pathol. Bacteriol. 77:543, 1959.

881. Fechner, R.E., and Bentinck, B.R.: Ultrastructure of bronchial oncocytoma, Cancer 3:1451, 1973.

882. Fechner, R.E., Bentinck, B.R., and Askew, J.B.: Acinic cell tumor of the lung: a histologic and ultrastructural study, Cancer 29:501, 1972.

883. Feoli, F., et al.: Pseudolymphoma of the lung: lymphoid subsets in the lung mass and in peripheral blood, Cancer 48:2218, 1981.

884. Foster, E.A., and Ackerman, L.V.: Localized mesotheliomas of the pleura: the pathologic evaluation of 18 cases, Am. J. Clin. Pathol. 34:349, 1960.

885. Freeman, C., Berg, J.W., and Cutler, S.J.: Occurrence and prognosis of extranodal lymphomas, Cancer 29:252, 1972.

886. Fung, C.H., et al.: Pulmonary blastoma: an ultrastructural study with a brief review of literature and a discussion of pathogenesis, Cancer 39:153, 1977.

887. Gibbs, A.R., and Seal, R.M.E.: Primary lymphoproliferative conditions of lung, Thorax 33:140, 1978.

888. Haas, J.E., Yunis, E.J., and Totten, R.S.: Ultrastructure of a sclerosing hemangioma of the lung, Cancer 30:512, 1972.

889. Hage, E.: Histochemistry and fine structure of bronchial carcinoid tumors, Virchows Arch. (Pathol. Anat.) 361:121, 1973.

890. Hoch, W.S., et al.: Benign clear cell tumor of the lung: an ultrastructural study, Cancer 33:1328, 1974.

891. Horstmann, J.P., et al.: Spontaneous regression of pulmonary leiomyomas during pregnancy, Cancer 39:314, 1977.

892. Iseman, M.D., Schwarz, M.I., and Stanford, R.E.: Interstitial pneumonia in angio-immunoblastic lymphadenopathy with dysproteinemia: a case report with special histopathologic studies, Ann. Intern. Med. 85:752, 1976.

893. Janigan, D.T., and Marrie, T.J.: An inflammatory pseudotumor of the lung and Q fever, N. Engl. J. Med. 308:86, 1983.

894. Kaplan, C., et al.: Multiple leiomyomas of the lung: benign or malignant? Am. Rev. Respir. Dis. 108:656, 1973.

895. Karcioglu, Z.A., and Someren, A.O.: Pulmonary blastoma: a case report and review of the literature, Am. J. Clin. Pathol. 61:287, 1974.

896. Katzenstein, A.-L.A., Carrington, C.B., and Liebow, A.A.: Lymphomatoid granulomatosis: a clinicopathologic study of 152 cases, Cancer 43:360, 1979.

897. Katzenstein, A.-L.A., et al.: So-called sclerosing hemangioma of the lung: evidence for mesothelial origin, Am. J. Surg. Pathol. 7:3, 1983.

898. Korn, D., et al.: Multiple minute pulmonary tumors resembling chemodectomas, Am. J. Pathol. 37:641, 1960.

899. Kuhn, C., and Askin, F.B.: The fine structure of so-called minute pulmonary chemodectomas, Hum. Pathol. 6:681, 1975.

900. Legha, S.S., and Muggia, F.M.: Pleural mesothelioma: clinical features and therapeutic implications, Ann. Intern. Med. 87:613, 1977.

901. Liebow, A.A., Carrington, C.R.B., and Friedman, P.J.: Lymphomatoid granulomatosis, Hum. Pathol. 3:457, 1972.

902. Liebow, A.A., and Castleman, B.: Benign clear cell ("sugar") tumors of the lung, Yale J. Biol. Med. 43:213, 1971.

903. Liebow, A.A., and Hubbell, D.S.: Sclerosing hemangioma (histiocytoma, xanthoma) of the lung, Cancer 9:35, 1956.

904. McCaughey, W.T.E.: Criteria for the diagnosis of diffuse mesothelial tumors, Ann. N.Y. Acad. Sci. 132:603, 1965.

905. McDonald, A.D., and McDonald, J.C.: Malignant mesothelioma in North America, Cancer 46:1650, 1980.

906. Melmon, K.L., Sjoerdoma, A., and Mason, D.T.: Distinctive clinical and therapeutic aspects of the syndrome associated with bronchial carcinoid tumors, Am. J. Med. 39:568, 1965.

907. Nascimento, A.G., Unni, K.K., and Bernatz, P.E.: Sarcomas of the lung, Mayo Clin. Proc. 57:355, 1982.

908. Navas Palacios, J.J., et al.: Sclerosing hemangioma of the lung: an ultrastructural study, Cancer 44:949, 1979.

909. Okike, N., Bernatz, P.E., and Woolner, L.B.: Localized mesothelioma of the pleura: benign and malignant variants, J. Thorac.
Cardiovasc. Surg. **75**:363, 1978.

910. Payne, W.S., Schier, J., and Woolner, L.B.: Mixed tumors of the
bronchus/salivary gland type 1, J. Thorac. Cardiovasc. Surg.
49:663, 1965.

911. Peacock, M.J., and Whitwell, F.: Pulmonary blastoma, Thorax
31:197, 1976.

912. Prive, L., et al.: Carcinosarcoma of the lung, Arch. Pathol.
72:351, 1961.

913. Reichle, F.A., and Rosemond, G.P.: Mucoepidermoid tumors of
the bronchus, J. Thorac. Cardiovasc. Surg. **51**:443, 1966.

914. Saltzstein, S.L.: Pulmonary lymphomas and pseudolymphomas:
classification, therapy, and prognosis, Cancer **16**:928, 1963.

915. Saltzstein, S.L.: Extranodal malignant lymphomas and pseudolymphomas. In Sommers, S.C., editor: Pathology annual, 1969,
New York, 1969, Appleton-Century-Crofts.

916. Singer, D.B., Greenberg, S.D., and Harrison, G.M.: Papillomatosis of the lung, Am. Rev. Respir. Dis. **94**:677, 1966.

917. Smith, J.F., and Dexter, D.: Papillary neoplasms of the bronchus
of low grade malignancy, Thorax **18**:340, 1963.

918. Spencer, H.: Pulmonary blastomas, J. Pathol. Bacteriol. **82**:161,
1961.

919. Spencer, H., Dail, D.H., and Arneaud, J.: Non-invasive bronchial epithelial papillary tumors, Cancer **45**:1486, 1980.

920. Strott, C.A., Nugent, C.A., and Tyler, F.H.: Cushing's syndrome caused by bronchial adenomas, Am. J. Med. **44**:97,
1968.

921. Suzuki, Y., Churg, J., and Kannerstein, M.: Ultrastructure of
human malignant diffuse mesothelioma, Am. J. Pathol. **85**:241,
1976.

922. Tedeschi, L.G., Libertini, R., and Conte, B.: Endobronchial polyp, Chest **63**:110, 1973.

923. Toole, A.L., and Stern, H.: Carcinoid and adenoid cystic carcinoma of the bronchus, Ann. Thorac. Surg. **13**:63, 1972.

924. Turnbull, A.D., et al.: Mucoepidermoid tumors of the bronchial
glands, Cancer **28**:539, 1971.

925. Wagner, J.C., Munday, D.E., and Harington, J.S.: Histochemical demonstration of hyaluronic acid in pleural mesotheliomas, J.
Pathol. Bacteriol. **84**:73, 1962.

926. Wang, N.-S.: Electron microscopy in the diagnosis of pleural
mesotheliomas, Cancer **31**:1046, 1973.

927. Weisenburger, D., Armitage, J., and Dick, F.: Immunoblastic
lymphadenopathy with pulmonary infiltrates, hypocomplementemia and vasculitis: a hyperimmune syndrome, Am. J. Med.
63:849, 1977.

928. Weldon-Linne, C.M., et al.: Angiogenic nature of the "intravascular bronchoalveolar tumor" of the lung, Arch. Pathol. Lab.
Med. **105**:174, 1981.

929. Williams, E.D., and Sandler, M.: The classification of carcinoid
tumours, Lancet **1**:238, 1963.

Mediastinum
Mediastinitis

930. Eggleston, J.G.: Sclerosing mediastinitis, Prog. Surg. Pathol. **2**:1,
1980.

931. Goodwin, R.A., Nickell, J.A., and DesPrez, R.M.: Mediastinal
fibrosis complicating healed primary histoplasmosis and tuberculosis, Medicine **51**:227, 1972.

932. Katzenstein, A.L.A., and Mazur, M.T.: Pulmonary infarct: an
unusual manifestation of fibrosing mediastinitis, Chest **77**:521,
1980.

933. Light, A.M.: Idiopathic fibrosis of mediastinum: a discussion of
three cases and review of the literature, J. Clin. Pathol. **31**:78,
1978.

934. Yacoub, M.H., and Thompson, V.C.: Chronic idiopathic pulmonary hilar fibrosis, Thorax **26**:365, 1971.

Tumors and cysts of the mediastinum

935. Benjamin, S.P. et al.: Primary tumors of the mediastinum, Chest
62:297, 1972.

936. Cox, J.D.: Primary malignant germinal tumors of the mediastinum: a study of 24 cases, Cancer **36**:1162, 1975.

937. DePaepe, M., Van der Straeten, M., and Roels, H.: Mediastinal
angiofollicular lymph node hyperplasia with systemic manifestations, Eur. J. Respir. Dis. **64**:134, 1983.

938. Fizzera, G., et al.: A systemic lymphoproliferative disorder with
morphologic features of Castleman's disease, Am. J. Surg. Pathol.
7:211, 1983.

939. Grosfeld, J.L., et al.: Primary mediastinal neoplasms in infants
and children, Ann. Thorac. Surg. **12**:179, 1971.

940. Hineman, V.L., Phyliky, R.L., and Banks, P.M. Angiofollicular
lymph node hyperplasia and peripheral neuropathy, Mayo Clin.
Proc. **57**:379, 1982.

941. Hodgkinson, D.L., et al.: Extra-adrenal intrathoracic functioning
paraganglioma (pheochromocytoma) in childhood, Mayo Clin.
Proc. **55**:271, 1980.

942. Keller, A.R., Hochholzer, L., and Castleman, B.: Hyaline-vascular and plasma cell types of giant lymph node hyperplasia of the
mediastinum and other locations, Cancer **29**:670, 1972.

943. Lichtenstein, A.K., et al.: Primary mediastinal lymphoma in
adults, Am. J. Med. **68**:509, 1980.

944. Oberman, H.A., and Libcke, J.H.: Malignant germinal neoplasms of the mediastinum, Cancer **17**:498, 1964.

945. Oldham, H.N., and Sabiston, D.C.: Primary tumors and cysts of
the mediastinum, Monogr. Surg. Sci. **4**:243, 1967.

946. Schantz, A., Sewall, W., and Castleman, B. Mediastinal germi-
noma: a study of 21 cases with an excellent prognosis, Cancer
30:1189, 1972.

947. Silverman, N.A., and Sabiston, D.C.: Mediastinal masses, Surg.
Clin. North Am. **60**:757, 1980.

CHAPTER 23 Ophthalmic Pathology

MORTON E. SMITH

ADNEXAL STRUCTURES
Lids

Most of the pathologic processes involving the eyelids are those that involve the skin in general; these are discussed in detail in Chapter 38. Some consideration, however, is given here to lesions that present particular problems.

Chalazia (lipogranulomas) (Figs. 23-1 to 23-3) and sebaceous gland carcinomas of the lid are often discussed together, although chalazia are common and carcinomas are rare. The important clinical point is that a sebaceous gland carcinoma of the lid may masquerade as a "recurrent" chalazion (Fig. 23-4).

Sebaceous gland carcinomas arise from either the meibomian glands within the tarsus (Figs. 23-5 and 23-6) or from Zeis glands closer to the skin surface. Small sebaceous gland carcinomas are usually cured with local excision. Larger ones may eventually metastasize to the preauricular, anterior cervical, or submandibular chain of lymph nodes. Distant metastasis is not common but may include the lungs.

Many localized lesions are found on the lids; these include seborrheic keratosis, papillomas, nevi, amyloid deposits, and xanthelasma. Basal cell carcinoma is more common than squamous cell carcinoma.

Orbit

The usual clinical hallmark of orbital disease is exophthalmos, although there may not be a neoplasm involved. For example, the most common cause of exophthalmos is dysthyroid ophthalmopathy (Graves' disease); rarely is a histopathologic specimen obtained in these cases.

In dysthyroid ophthalmopathy there is a dysfunction between the pituitary-thyroid axis. When examined for the ocular problem, the patient may be hyperthyroid, hypothyroid, or euthyroid by clinical and chemical manifestations. There are edema, accumulation of acid mucopolysaccharide, and chronic inflammatory cell infiltration of the extraocular muscles (Fig. 23-7). In fact, the marked thickening of the extraocular muscles is easily recognized on computed tomographic (CT) scan and ultrasound examination and is an important diagnostic sign. Eventually muscle fibers degenerate and become hyalinized.

Other systemic diseases that may involve the orbit include leukemia and malignant lymphoma, the histiocytoses, juvenile xanthogranuloma, sinus histiocytosis, metastatic carcinoma, connective tissue disorders, and Wegener's granulomatosis (Fig. 23-8).

The orbit may be secondarily invaded by lesions originating in adjacent structures such as mucoceles (Fig. 23-9) and carcinomas from the paranasal sinuses or intraocular melanomas that have broken through the sclera. The phycomycoses may spread from the sinuses to the orbit, especially in debilitated patients and in diabetics in acidosis. Localized lesions of the orbit include hemangiomas, lymphangiomas, dermoid cysts, peripheral nerve tumors, perioptic meningiomas, optic nerve gliomas, fibrous histiocytomas, inflammatory pseudotumors, and the rhabdomyosarcomas seen in children. The lacrimal gland may give rise to benign mixed cell tumors (pleomorphic adenomas), adenoid cystic carcinomas, and undifferentiated carcinomas. The benign lymphoepithelial lesion of Sjögren's syndrome may be seen in the lacrimal gland.

Conjunctiva

Most of the pathologic processes involving the conjunctiva are localized and not associated with any systemic process. The surgical pathologist would see common lesions such as cysts, pterygia, papillomas, and nevi. Localized amyloid lesions are rare.

Carcinoma in situ of the bulbar conjunctiva usually is manifested as a leukoplakic lesion at the limbus (Fig. 23-10). The histopathologic characteristics of the lesion are similar to those observed elsewhere in mucous membranes. *Text continued on p. 960.*

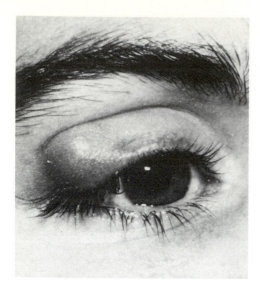

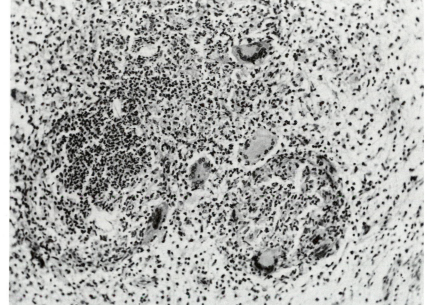

Fig. 23-1. Chalazion of right upper eyelid. (WU 79-1631; from Rosai, J.: Ackerman's surgical pathology, ed. 6, St. Louis, 1981, The C.V. Mosby Co.)

Fig. 23-2. Multiple foci of granulomatous inflammation with microabscesses and Langhans' giant cells in chalazion. (137×; AFIP 91218; from Rosai, J.: Ackerman's surgical pathology, ed. 6, St. Louis, 1981, The C.V. Mosby Co.)

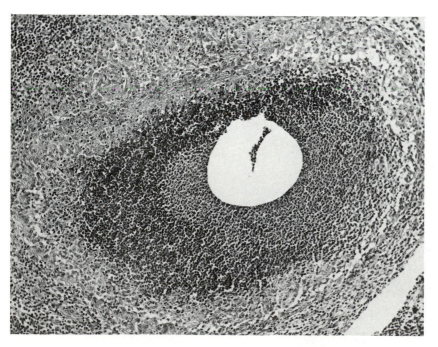

Fig. 23-3. Presence of pools of fat in center of many of granulomas is characteristic of chalazia. (115×; AFIP 732397; from Rosai, J.: Ackerman's surgical pathology, ed. 6, St. Louis, 1981, The C.V. Mosby Co.)

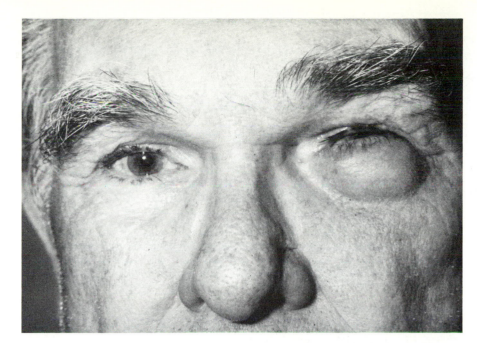

Fig. 23-4. Sebaceous gland carcinoma of left lower lid.

Fig. 23-5. Full-thickness section of eyelid showing sebaceous gland carcinoma arising from meibomian glands (*arrows*). (5×; WU 72-6065; from Rosai, J.: Ackerman's surgical pathology, ed. 6, St. Louis, 1981, The C.V. Mosby Co.)

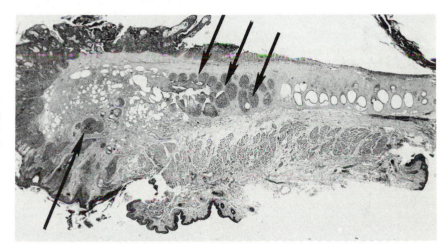

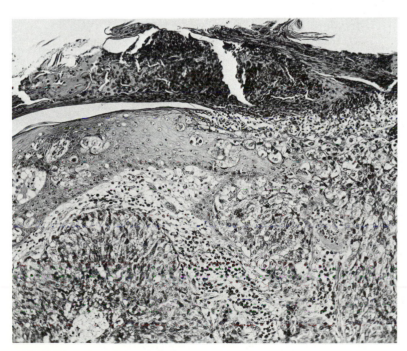

Fig. 23-6. Pagetoid invasion of epidermal surface of eyelid by sebaceous carcinoma of meibomian gland derivation. (115×; AFIP 58-13414; from Hogan, M.J., and Zimmerman, L.E.: Ophthalmic pathology, ed. 2, Philadelphia, 1962, W.B. Saunders Co.)

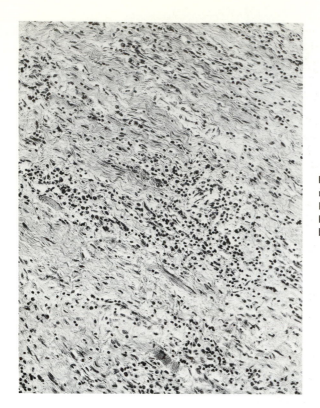

Fig. 23-7. Greatly degenerated extraocular muscles scarred and infiltrated by mononuclear inflammatory cells. (145×; AFIP 58-13128; from Zimmerman, L.E.: The eyes and ocular adnexa. In Ackerman, L.V. [in collaboration with Butcher, H.R., Jr.]: Surgical pathology, ed. 3, St. Louis, 1964, The C.V. Mosby Co.)

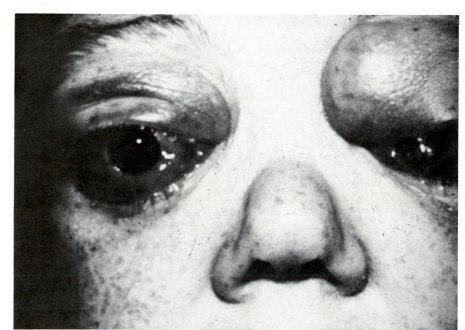

Fig. 23-8. Marked bilateral exophthalmos in Wegener's granulomatosis.

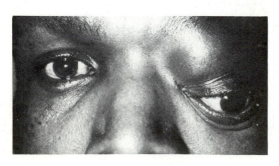

Fig. 23-9. Mucocele producing downward and lateral displacement of left eye. (WU 69-7637; from del Regato, J.A., and Spjut, H.J.: Ackerman and del Regato's cancer, ed. 5, St. Louis, 1977, The C.V. Mosby Co.)

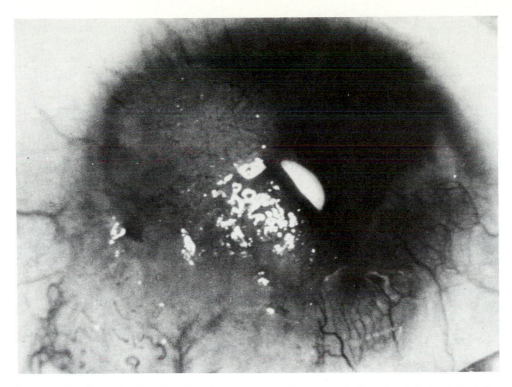

Fig. 23-10. Carcinoma in situ of conjunctiva and cornea. (WU 79-1633; from Rosai, J.: Ackerman's surgical pathology, ed. 6, St. Louis, 1981, The C.V. Mosby Co.)

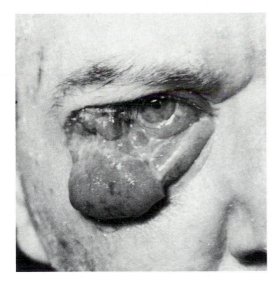

Fig. 23-11. Epidermoid carcinoma of conjunctiva. Tumor grew rapidly over 4-month period. (WU 64-3837; from Rosai, J.: Ackerman's surgical pathology, ed. 6, St. Louis, 1981, The C.V. Mosby Co.)

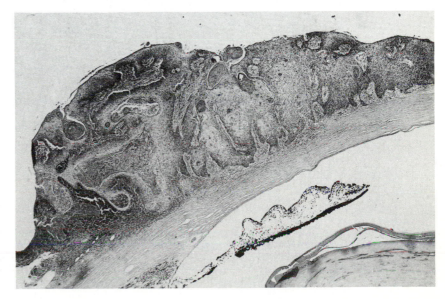

Fig. 23-12. Carcinoma of limbus. Exophytic growth pattern with formation of papillomatous mass is typical of more advanced limbal carcinomas. Even in such large tumors, corneoscleral stroma tends to prevent neoplasm from invading intraocular tissues. (18×; AFIP 785865; from Rosai, J.: Ackerman's surgical pathology, ed. 6, St. Louis, 1981, The C.V. Mosby Co.)

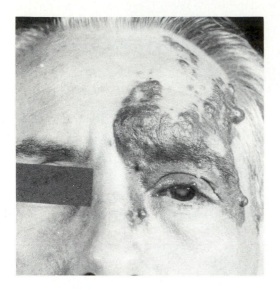

Fig. 23-13. Sturge-Weber syndrome. Patient, 42-year-old white man, had had facial hemangioma all his life and was blind in ipsilateral eye because of retinal degeneration, glaucoma, and cataract. Choroidal hemangioma was found in enucleated eye, but clinical study failed to disclose evidence of intracranial lesion. (AFIP 761707; courtesy Veterans Administration Hospital, Hines, Ill.; from Rosai, J.: Ackerman's surgical pathology, ed. 6, St. Louis, 1981, The C.V. Mosby Co.)

Invasive squamous cell carcinoma (Figs. 23-11 and 23-12) of the conjunctiva is rare. It is usually cured with simple excision, although an exenteration of all orbital contents may be necessary for extensive lesions. Metastases are rare but may include regional lymph nodes (preauricular, anterior cervical, and submandibular).

Malignant melanoma of the conjunctiva is also rare. The lesion may arise de novo, from a preexisting nevus, or from acquired melanosis. Local excision is usually curative, although extensive lesions behave similarly to squamous cell carcinoma (see previous discussion).

INTRAOCULAR LESIONS
Congenital and developmental lesions
Phacomatoses

The phacomatoses are a heredofamilial group of congenital syndromes having in common the presence of disseminated, usually benign hamartomas. The eyes are almost always involved.

In angiomatosis retinae (von Hippel's disease) hemangioblastomas may occur in any part of the retina. These are often multiple and bilateral. Severe or untreated cases may lead to retinal detachment. The combination of retinal plus central nervous system hemangioblastomas is referred to as von Hippel-Lindau disease.

Along with meningeal calcification and facial nevus flammeus (port-wine stain) (Fig. 23-13), patients with encephalotrigeminal angiomatosis (Sturge-Weber syndrome) also have congenital glaucoma and a diffuse cavernous hemangioma of the choroid (Fig. 23-14). The cho-

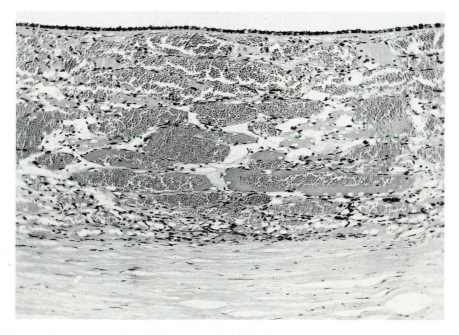

Fig. 23-14. Hemangioma of choroid in eye enucleated from 42-year-old white woman who had had a port-wine facial hemangioma since birth and ipsilateral glaucoma since early childhood. (115×; AFIP 759801; from Rosai, J.: Ackerman's surgical pathology, ed. 6, St. Louis, 1981, The C.V. Mosby Co.)

roidal hemangioma often leads to microcystoid degeneration of the overlying retina and leakage of serous fluid into the subretinal space.

Neurofibromatosis (von Recklinghausen's disease) is characterized by plexiform neurofibromas in the lid and orbit (Fig. 23-15), congenital glaucoma, multiple nevi of the iris, diffuse neurofibroma of the uveal tract, optic nerve gliomas, or absence of orbital bones leading to a pulsating exophthalmos.

In tuberous sclerosis (Bourneville's disease) there are glial hamartomas of the retina (Fig. 23-16), which are usually multiple and bilateral.

The two least frequently encountered phacomatoses are ataxia telangiectasia (Louis-Bar syndrome) and Wyburn-Mason syndrome. Telangiectasis of the conjunctiva occurs in the former and retinal arteriovenous communications in the latter.

Chromosomal aberrations

In trisomy 13 the eyes are microphthalmic. There is usually a colobomatous defect, as well as persistence and hyperplasia of the primary vitreous. Cartilage is often seen within the coloboma, and the retina is usually dysplastic. A multitude of major and minor ocular defects can occur in trisomy 18, trisomy 21, chromosome 5 deletion defect, chromosome 18 deletion defect, and mosaicism.

Retrolental fibroplasia

Retrolental fibroplasia, also referred to as retinopathy of prematurity, is an acquired developmental disorder resulting from the unique sensitivity of blood vessels of the premature retina to oxygen. There is incomplete vas-

cularization of the peripheral retina, and the exposure to oxygen inhibits the normal vascularization process. On withdrawal of oxygen, pathologic neovascularization occurs, often with leakage of blood and serum, organization, and eventual retinal detachment.

Retinitis pigmentosa

Retinitis pigmentosa is a group of diseases in which there is a generalized degeneration of the retinal pigment epithelium; they are of unknown etiology and exhibit a variety of inheritance patterns. These patients have night blindness and a decreased or absent electroretinographic response. Retinitis pigmentosa may be an associated finding in the following systemic diseases: Usher's syndrome, Laurence-Moon-Berdet-Biedl syndrome, syringomyelia, Bassen-Kornzweig syndrome, Friedreich's ataxia, Refsum's disease, and myotonic dystrophy.

Other congenital anomalies

In both Marfan's syndrome and homocystinurea, the lens of the eye is prone to dislocation.

Complete albinism involves skin, hair, and eyes, whereas incomplete albinism occurs in the ocular tissues with a deficiency but rarely a complete lack of melanin in pigment epithelium and uveal melanocytes. Poor vision, nystagmus, and photophobia are the clinical manifestations.

Other congenital anomalies include Lowe's syndrome, in which there are cataracts and glaucoma, and aniridia, in which nonfamilial cases may be associated with Wilms' tumor.

Infections and inflammations
Infections

Acute suppurative intraocular inflammation, referred to as endophthalmitis, is usually infectious in origin; it

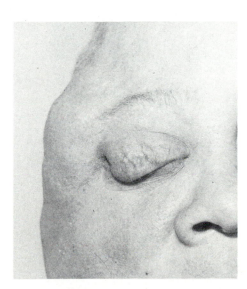

Fig. 23-15. Severe unilateral deformity of face in patient with von Recklinghausen's neurofibromatosis. (AFIP 55-17512; courtesy Dr. L.L. Calkins, Kansas City, Kan.; from Rosai, J.: Ackerman's surgical pathology, ed. 6, St. Louis, 1981, The C.V. Mosby Co.)

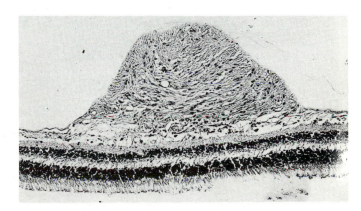

Fig. 23-16. Tuberous sclerosis showing glial nodule or hamartoma projecting against vitreous body from nerve fiber layer of retina. (90×; AFIP 511046; from Rosai, J.: Ackerman's surgical pathology, ed. 6, St. Louis, 1981, The C.V. Mosby Co.)

results from a bacterium or fungus introduced through an accidental or a surgical perforating wound (Fig. 23-17). This disease is confined to the eye and rarely includes systemic manifestations.

Occasionally endophthalmitis is endogenous, that is, via hematogenous spread. The most important lesions in this category are the "opportunistic" infections. A typical example is the patient who has received hyperalimentation following bowel surgery and in whom candidemia develops. The fungus may reach the eye and produce endophthalmitis. Other organisms that can cause opportunistic infections and produce a similar picture include *Toxoplasma*, *Nocardia*, *Aspergillus*, and *Cryptococcus* organisms.

Toxoplasmosis may be congenital or may appear in adults, in whom the retinitis is a reactivation of the organisms that have been lying dormant in the retina since birth. These patients are systemically well. Histologically the protozoan is found free in pseudocysts or in true cysts in an area of coagulative necrosis of the retina (Fig. 23-18), which usually is sharply demarcated from contiguous normal retina.

Toxocara canis infection is found principally in children between the ages of 3 and 14 years, who presumably contract the disease from puppies. These children do not have clinical evidence of systemic visceral larva migrans. Typically a single migrating larva reaches the eye hematogenously and comes to rest in the vitreous or inner surface of the retina. Severe endophthalmitis may result, and the retina may detach. Such eyes are often enucleated. A less severe reaction produces only a white fibrotic mass in the retina, often with fibrous strands in the overlying vitreous. Histologically there is a granulomatous inflammatory reaction with an intense eosinophilia (Fig. 23-19). The worm is often not seen because it has totally disintegrated.

Presumed ocular histoplasmosis syndrome occurs in healthy young adults who have decreased vision as a result of a small hemorrhagic or serous detachment of the macula. These patients often have positive histoplasmin skin test results but no evidence of systemic histoplasmosis. In fact, there has never been unequivocal demonstration of *Histoplasma capsulatum* organisms in the eyes of such patients.

Cytomegalic inclusion disease may be a congenital infection, or it may occur in adults as an opportunistic

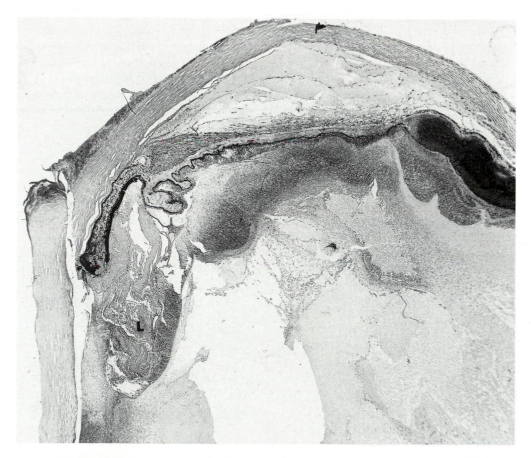

Fig. 23-17. Endophthalmitis showing infiltration of all intraocular structures by acute inflammatory cells. Lens, *L*, is necrotic. Organism presumably gained entrance through corneal wound. (15×; WU 67-4233; from Rosai, J.: Ackerman's surgical pathology, ed. 6, St. Louis, 1981, The C.V. Mosby Co.)

infection. A typical example of the latter is the leukemic patient who is receiving antibiotics and cytologic agents. The disease characteristically produces massive hemorrhage and necrosis of the retina. Histologically the typical "owl's eye" cells with large intranuclear inclusion bodies surrounded by a clear halo are found within the necrotic retina.

Subacute sclerosing panencephalitis often produces a hemorrhagic macular lesion along with progressive central nervous system findings. Histologically the retina is necrotic, is infiltrated by lymphocytes, and often shows intranuclear inclusion bodies. A similar picture can be seen in herpes simplex retinitis and encephalitis.

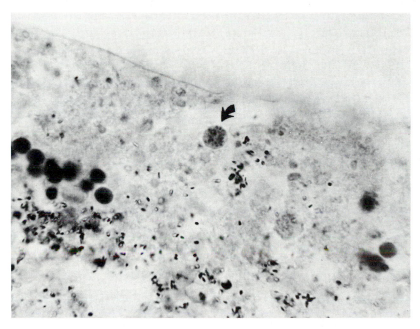

Fig. 23-18. Encysting proliferative forms (*arrow*) of *Toxoplasma gondii* found in necrotic retina. Small particles are pigment granules from necrotic retinal pigment epithelium, whereas larger round structures represent pyknotic retinal nuclei. (1000×; AFIP 754058; from Rosai, J.: Ackerman's surgical pathology, ed. 6, St. Louis, 1981, The C.V. Mosby Co.)

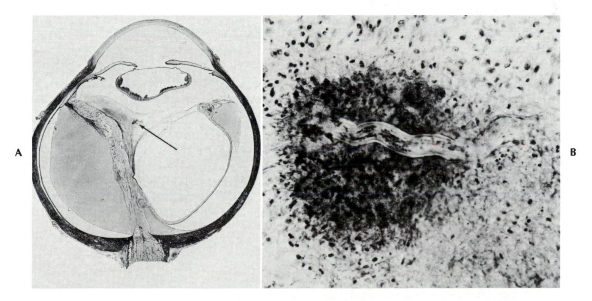

Fig. 23-19. Granulomatous endophthalmitis from *Toxocara canis*. **A,** Arrow indicates site of granuloma containing larva shown in **B.** Preretinal inflammatory membrane has led to total detachment of retina. **B,** Nematode larva in granuloma in vitreous. (**A,** 3×; **B,** 400×; **A** and **B,** from Wilder, H.C.: Trans. Am. Acad. Ophthalmol. Otolaryngol. **55:**99, 1950; AFIP 198761.)

Common ocular findings in congenital rubella syndrome include cataract, glaucoma, iritis, and a pigmentary retinopathy manifested ophthalmologically as a pigmentary stippling of the retina referred to as a salt and pepper fundus. This is caused by alternating areas of retinal pigment epithelial atrophy and hypertrophy. The cataract characteristically shows retention of lens cell nuclei in the embryonic lens nucleus.

Ocular complications occur in about 50% of cases of herpes zoster ophthalmicus. The most common problems are keratitis and iritis. The keratitis often leads to ulceration and eventual fibrosis and vascularization of the cornea. The iritis produces a patchy necrosis. There may also be involvement of the remaining uveal tract (ciliary body and choroid) as well as scleritis, retinitis, or papillitis. The characteristic histologic findings are perineural infiltration by lymphocytes, especially involving the long posterior ciliary nerves, and diffuse or patchy necrosis of the iris and pars plicata of the ciliary body.

Tuberculosis of the eye is now rare. It produces a chronic granulomatous inflammation of the uveal tract. Leprosy may involve the ocular adnexa and cornea, but intraocular involvement is rare. Syphilis may produce a nongranulomatous choroiditis, but the usual ocular manifestation is optic nerve atrophy. Congenital syphilis is the usual cause for interstitial keratitis.

Inflammations

Most cases of nongranulomatous inflammation of the uveal tract (iritis, iridocyclitis, choroiditis) are not infectious in origin and are not associated with systemic disease. An important exception is the frequent association of chronic nongranulomatous iritis in girls with juvenile rheumatoid arthritis or in young men with ankylosing spondylitis. It is rare to obtain histologic specimens of such entities, but the few that have been reported show nonspecific changes, including a diffuse nongranulomatous chronic inflammation throughout the uveal tract (Fig. 23-20). Secondary sequelae include adhesions of the iris to lens (posterior synechia) (Fig. 23-21) or to the cornea (anterior synechia). Often a cataract is present, and there is usually some degree of chorioretinal scarring.

Sympathetic uveitis (also referred to as sympathetic ophthalmia) is a diffuse granulomatous uveitis in which a penetrating injury to one eye gives rise to a granulomatous inflammation in both eyes. Fortunately, it is rare, considering the number of injuries to which eyes are subjected (50% of all enucleations are the sequelae of accidental or surgical trauma). It is believed to be caused by an autoimmunity, with uveal pigment or retinal antigen or both acting as the inciting factor.

The histology of sympathetic uveitis is characterized by a diffuse infiltration of the uvea by lymphocytes, patchy aggregations of epithelioid cells, and eosinophils (Fig. 23-22). Plasma cells are usually sparse.

Although no systemic manifestations exist in sympathetic ophthalmia, there is a closely related disease in which there are systemic manifestations. Vogt-Koyanagi-Harada disease (uveomeningoencephalitis syndrome) has similar ocular findings, but there is no history of penetrating ocular injury; these patients also have fluctuating meningeal symptoms, vitiligo, poliosis, alopecia, and dysacusis.

Phacoanaphylaxis is another granulomatous inflammation that is concentrated around a ruptured lens and therefore usually follows penetrating ocular trauma. Clinically there is an intense inflammatory reaction in the anterior chamber that resembles an acute bacterial endophthalmitis. Histologically, in the area in which the

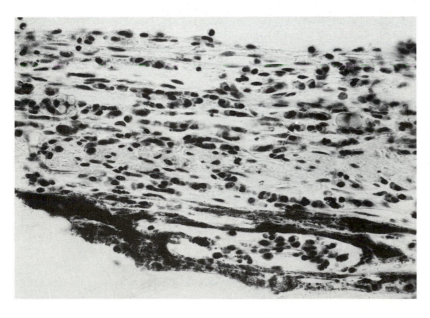

Fig. 23-20. Nongranulomatous iritis in which atrophic iris is diffusely infiltrated by plasma cells and several Russell bodies are present. Irregular degenerative and proliferative changes may be observed in pigment epithelium. (360×; AFIP 698722; from Rosai, J.: Ackerman's surgical pathology, ed. 6, St. Louis, 1981, The C.V. Mosby Co.)

lens capsule is broken, there is a massive invasion of the lens by inflammatory cells. Centrally and immediately surrounding individual lens fibers are polymorphonuclear leukocytes. Peripheral to this is a wall of epithelioid and giant cells about which is a broader zone of granulation tissue and round cell infiltration (Fig. 23-23). This disease is also thought to be autoimmune, with antilens antibodies being formed as a response to the sudden release of lens protein. No systemic manifestations are present.

About one third of patients with sarcoidosis have ocular manifestations, the most common of which is anterior uveitis. Other findings include eyelid nodules, nodular infiltrates in the palpebral conjunctiva, interstitial kera-titis, retinochoroidal granulomas, optic neuritis, papilledema, retinal periphlebitis, and tumors in the orbit or lacrimal gland. Histologically the typical noncaseating granulomatous tubercle is seen (Fig. 23-24). A biopsy of the nodular infiltrates in the conjunctiva can easily be done to establish the diagnosis (Fig. 23-25).

Granulomatous scleritis is manifested clinically by intense inflammation and pain. It is associated with rheumatoid arthritis or collagen-vascular disease in less than 25% of cases. Histologically a zonal type of granulomatous inflammatory infiltrate surrounds a nidus of necrotic scleral collagen. The lesions, which may be focal or diffuse, resemble subcutaneous rheumatoid nodules.

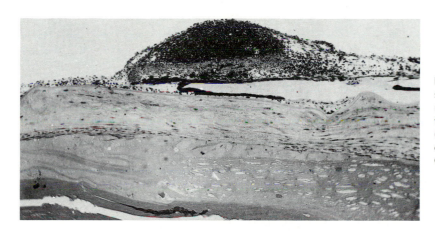

Fig. 23-21. Nongranulomatous iritis with posterior synechiae. Iris is firmly attached to lens, which reveals widespread degeneration of its cortex and fibrous metaplasia of its subcapsular epithelium. (25×; AFIP 184111; from Rosai, J.: Ackerman's surgical pathology, ed. 6, St. Louis, 1981, The C.V. Mosby Co.)

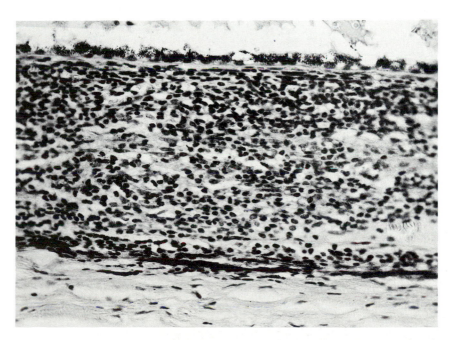

Fig. 23-22. Sympathetic uveitis. Uveal tissues are diffusely infiltrated by lymphocytes, and there are small, irregular collections of pale-staining epithelioid cells. (300×; AFIP 731769; from Rosai, J.: Ackerman's surgical pathology, ed. 6, St. Louis, 1981, The C.V. Mosby Co.)

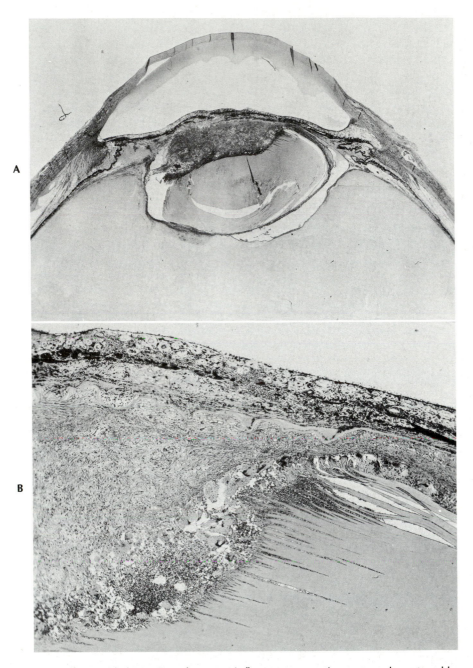

Fig. 23-23. Phacoanaphylaxis. Granulomatous inflammatory reaction surrounds ruptured lens. (**A,** 10×; AFIP 55-22260; **B,** 53×; AFIP 55-22261; from Zimmerman, L.E.: In Ackerman, L.V. [in collaboration with Butcher, H.R., Jr.]: Surgical pathology, ed. 2, St. Louis, 1959, The C.V. Mosby Co.)

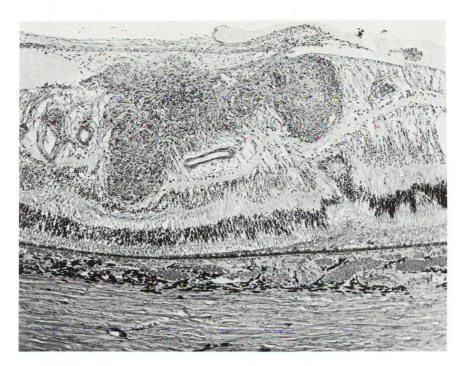

Fig. 23-24. Perivascular distribution of tubercles in patient with sarcoidosis who died as consequence of involvement of central nervous system. (50×; AFIP 63-1450.)

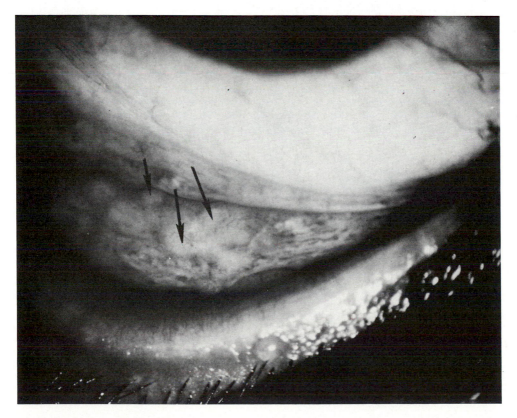

Fig. 23-25. Conjunctival granulomas in sarcoidosis. (WU 79-1632; from Rosai, J.: Ackerman's surgical pathology, ed. 6, St. Louis, 1981, The C.V. Mosby Co.)

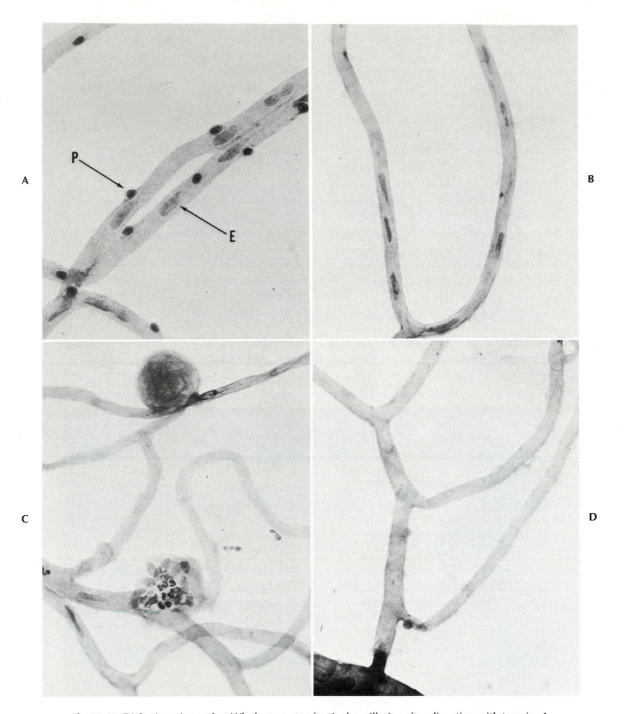

Fig. 23-26. Diabetic retinopathy. Whole mounts of retinal capillaries after digestion with trypsin. **A,** Nuclei of endothelial cells, *E,* and of pericytes or mural cells, *P,* are normally observed in about 1:1 ratio. **B,** Selective loss of mural pericytes, one of earliest changes in diabetes. **C,** Saccular microaneurysms characteristic of diabetic retinopathy. One in upper part of field is hyalinized, whereas one in lower part shows endothelial proliferation and adherent leukocytes. **D,** Many of ischemic vessels showing loss of all nuclei in advanced diabetic retinopathy. (**A,** AFIP 64-7004; **B,** AFIP 64-7010; **C,** AFIP 64-7009; **D,** AFIP 64-7008.)

Retinal vascular disease
Diabetes

Ocular diabetes is one of the leading causes of blindness in industrialized societies and is the leading cause of blindness in persons between the ages of 25 to 65 years. At present the most important factor influencing the occurrence of clinical retinopathy is the duration of the disease. Adequacy of control is probably just as important, but supportive data are only now accumulating. Retinopathy develops in many diabetics (65% or more) 15 years after the onset of the disease. There is a positive correlation between the presence of diabetic retinopathy and Kimmelstiel-Wilson nephropathy. Diabetes can cause a variety of pathologic conditions in the eye, often leading to blindness with pain, thus necessitating enucleation.

The selective retinal capillary microangiopathy appears to begin with a degeneration of the intramural pericytes and some loss of endothelial cells. Adjacent to these ischemic foci are saclike aneurysmal dilatations of the capillaries (Fig. 23-26). Diapedesis of erythrocytes occurs, producing the so-called dot hemorrhages in the deeper layers of the retina. Also developing in the deeper layers of the retina as a result of this loss of permeability of the capillaries are pockets of lipoproteinaceous material, referred to clinically as hard, waxy exudates. Soft "cotton-wool" spots may also appear, which are microinfarcts in the nerve fiber layer and are similar to those seen in hypertensive retinopathy.

All of the aforementioned changes are referred to clinically as background retinopathy. In some cases the retinopathy eventually becomes proliferative. New capillaries proliferate, often at the optic disc or along one of the retinal veins, and eventually erupt through the internal limiting membrane of the retina. Bleeding into the vitreous may then occur; this blood organizes and contracts, producing traction on the retina with consequent retinal detachment (Fig. 23-27).

In many cases the diffuse ischemia of the retina is responsible for the development of a neovascular membrane on the anterior surface of the iris. Exactly how ischemia in the posterior part of the eye causes neovascularization of the anterior part of the eye is unknown; it may be caused by some type of angiogenesis factor that is liberated from the hypoxic retina and travels forward through the vitreous. This neovascular membrane on the anterior surface of the iris (clinically referred to as rubeosis iridis) contracts, pulling the root of the iris up against the trabecular meshwork (peripheral anterior synechia), thus occluding the outflow channels of the eye and producing an intractable glaucoma (Fig. 23-28). The contraction of the neovascular membrane also pulls the pigment epithelium of the iris forward around the pupil and onto the anterior surface of the iris (ectropion uvea).

Another characteristic histologic finding in ocular diabetes is the glycogen vacuolization of the pigment epithelium layer of the iris (Fig. 23-28). This finding is analogous to Armanni-Ebstein nephropathy and is a reflection of a high serum glucose level in the 72-hour period before the specimen is obtained (either by enucleation in the living patient or at autopsy).

Hypertensive retinopathy

In hypertensive retinopathy there is generalized attenuation of retinal arterioles, often leading to retinal ischemia. Flame-shaped hemorrhages and soft cotton-wool spots are the characteristic ophthalmoscopic findings. Histologically both the hemorrhages and the cotton-wool spots are located in the inner layers of the retina, that is, in nerve fiber and ganglion cell layers. The cotton-wool spots are focal areas of ischemic infarction, producing the characteristic cytoid bodies that represent swollen axons or focal areas of axoplasmic stagnation (Fig. 23-29).

Vascular occlusive disease

Patients with generalized vascular disease, such as hypertension, arteriosclerotic cardiovascular disease, carotid artery disease, and diabetes, are prone to occlusions of the central retinal artery or vein. These patients typically complain of sudden, painless loss of vision in one eye. Sudden total occlusion of the central retinal artery is caused either by arthrosclerotic thrombosis of the artery within the lamina cribrosa portion of the optic nerve or by an embolism, usually from the carotid artery or heart valves. This vascular accident produces complete ischemic infarction of the inner layers of the retina, which are dependent for blood supply on the central retinal artery.

Histologically the retinal infarct is characterized by an early edematous thickening of the inner half of the retina with dissolution of nuclei in the ganglion cell and inner nuclear layers (Fig. 23-30). As the edema subsides, there is thinning of the inner retinal layers from which the nerve fibers, ganglion cells, and almost all of the cells of the inner nuclear layer have disappeared.

Occlusion of the central retinal vein produces a hemorrhagic infarction of the entire retina. In most of these cases the vein is narrowed and eventually closed off by a thickened arteriosclerotic artery lying adjacent to the vein within the lamina cribrosa of the optic nerve. Histologically the inner layers of the retina are involved, as in the case of central artery occlusion. However, massive hemorrhage within these layers, rather than ischemia, is present. Later, as all the blood is resorbed, the histologic picture is similar to central artery occlusion in that thinning and loss of nuclei in the ganglion cell and inner nuclear layers occur. However, a stain for iron usually reveals the presence of the hemosiderin deposition.

Eyes in which central vein occlusion has developed

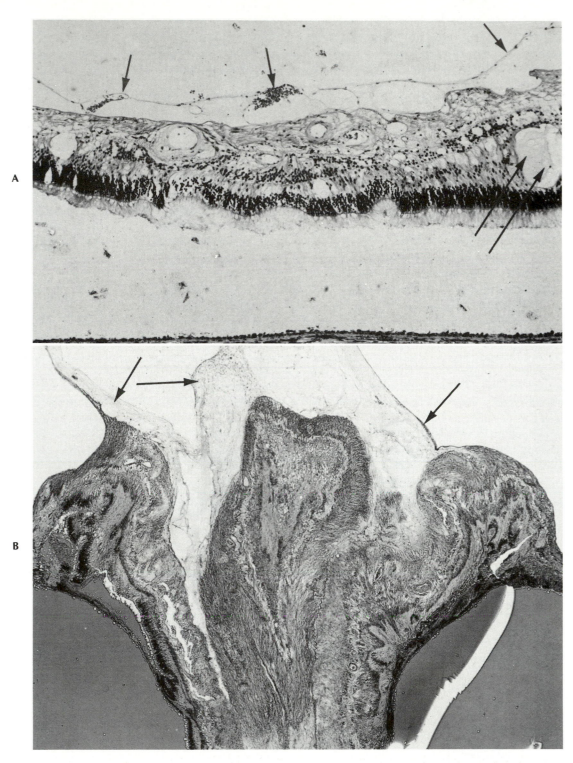

Fig. 23-27. A, Diabetic retinopathy with scattered exudates in deep retinal layers (*double arrows*) and early neovascularization extending from inner surface of retina into vitreous (*single arrows*). **B,** Diabetic proliferative retinopathy (*arrows*) has caused complete retinal detachment. (**A,** 90×; WU 72-3170; **B,** 34×; WU 72-3171; **A** and **B,** from Rosai, J.: Ackerman's surgical pathology, ed. 6, St. Louis, 1981, The C.V. Mosby Co.)

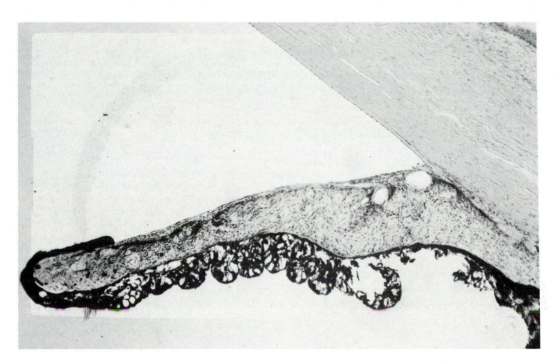

Fig. 23-28. Rubeosis iridis in diabetes. Angle of anterior chamber is occluded by peripheral anterior synechia, and fibrovascular membrane (rubeosis iridis) covers anterior surface of iris. Contraction of this membrane has pulled pigment epithelium anteriorly to produce "ectropion uvea." There is marked diabetic vacuolization of pigment epithelial cells. (90×; WU 67-4225; from Rosai, J.: Ackerman's surgical pathology, ed. 6, St. Louis, 1981, The C.V. Mosby Co.)

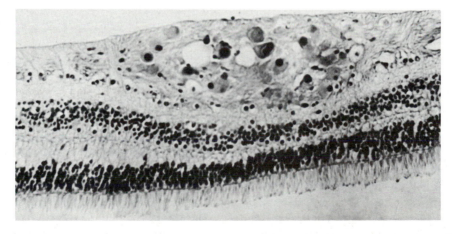

Fig. 23-29. Microinfarct of retina. "Cytoid bodies" are axonal enlargements in infarcted nerve fiber layer. (210×; AFIP 69808; from Friedenwald, J.S., et al.: Ophthalmic pathology, Philadelphia, 1952, W.B. Saunders Co.)

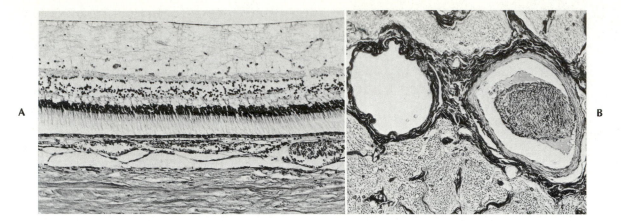

Fig. 23-30. Acute ischemic infarction of retina, **A,** produced by embolus in central retinal artery, **B,** from mural thrombus in left ventricle of patient who had sustained myocardial infarction. (AFIP 951983; **B,** from Zimmerman, L.E.: Arch. Ophthalmol. **73:**822, 1965.)

may go on to develop rubeosis iridis, the neovascularization of the anterior surface of the iris similar to that described earlier in the discussion of diabetes.

Branch retinal artery and vein occlusion, of course, cause only segmental infarctions to the retina.

Sickle cell retinopathy

Sickle cell retinopathy is most severe with sickle cell hemoglobin C disease but may also occur in other sickle hemoglobinopathies including sickle thalassemia and sickle cell disease and even in occasional cases of sickle cell trait. First, there is arteriolar occlusion in the periphery of the retina, followed by the formation of arteriolovenular anastomoses. Neovascularization then occurs, which may lead to vitreous hemorrhage, fibrous proliferations, and eventual retinal detachment.

Primary intraocular neoplasms

The two important primary intraocular malignancies considered here are melanoma and retinoblastoma.

Malignant melanoma of the uvea typically occurs in white adults. It is slow growing and metastasizes very late. Clinically it is a painless mass recognized as an incidental finding or because it has caused some visual problem.

This neoplasm arises from the pigmented or potentially pigment-producing cells of the uvea, with the choroid and ciliary body being more frequently involved than the iris.

The cytologic characteristics of uveal melanomas have been classified and are used as one criterion to determine prognostic significance. Spindle cell melanomas are a mixture of spindle A cells and spindle B cells or often only B cells. Spindle A cells are slender, spindle-shaped cells with fusiform nuclei and no nucleoli. Frequently the chromatin is arranged in a linear fashion along the central axis of the nucleus (Fig. 23-31). Spindle B cells

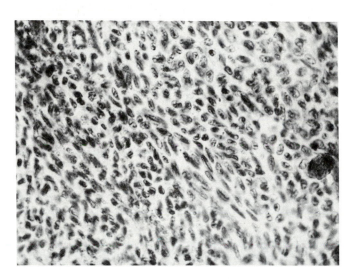

Fig. 23-31. Spindle A type of melanoma cells. (510×; AFIP 49801; from Rosai, J.: Ackerman's surgical pathology, ed. 6, St. Louis, 1981, The C.V. Mosby Co.)

are larger with ovoid nuclei containing a prominent nucleolus (Fig. 23-32). These spindle cell melanomas are cohesive and often have a fascicular pattern when viewed microscopically at low magnification (Fig. 23-33).

Epithelioid cell melanomas have cells that are larger, are irregular, and possess abundant cytoplasm. The nuclei are large, with strikingly prominent nucleoli. These cells are not cohesive (Fig. 23-34).

Most melanomas have a mixture of all of these cell types and actually represent a continuum rather than distinct groups. However, general predictions concerning prognosis can be made. Roughly two thirds to three fourths of patients with spindle cell melanomas will still be alive in 5 years, whereas roughly two thirds to three fourths of patients with epithelioid melanomas will die of their tumors within 5 years. A patient with a mixed cell

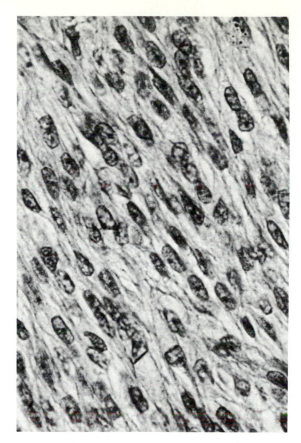

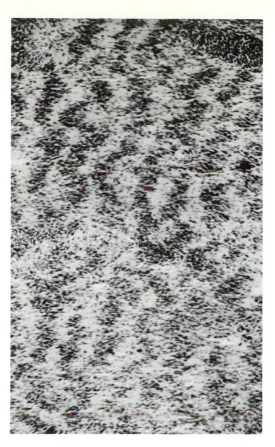

Fig. 23-32. Spindle B cells demonstrating some pleomorphism and large ovoid nuclei with prominent nucleoli. (720×; from del Regato, J.A., and Spjut, H.J.: Ackerman and del Ragato's cancer, ed. 5, St. Louis, 1977, The C.V. Mosby Co.)

Fig. 23-33. Spindle B cells with fascicular pattern. (From del Regato, J.A., and Spjut, H.J.: Ackerman and del Regato's cancer, ed. 5, St. Louis, 1977, The C.V. Mosby Co.)

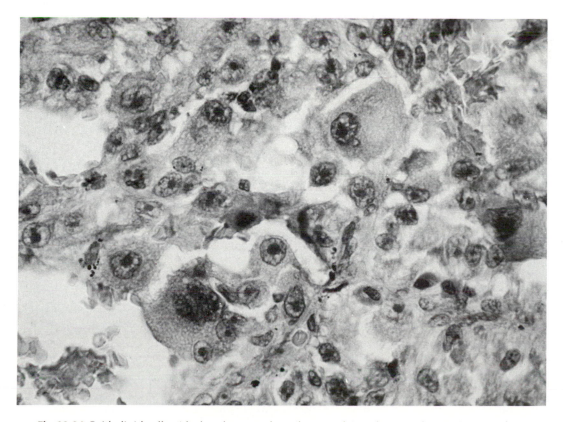

Fig. 23-34. Epithelioid cells with abundant cytoplasm, large nuclei, and extremely prominent nucleoli. (600×; WU 69-7517; from del Regato, J.A., and Spjut, H.J.: Ackerman and del Regato's cancer, ed. 5, St. Louis, 1977, The C.V. Mosby Co.)

melanoma, such as spindle plus epithelioid, has roughly a 50% chance of surviving for 5 years.

Besides cell type, the other important criteria for predicting prognosis are extraocular extension and size of the tumor; larger tumors naturally have a worse prognosis than smaller ones (Figs. 23-35 and 23-36).

Another important fact concerning the prognosis of uveal tumors is the very benign behavior of almost all melanomas of the iris. Most of these are recognized early when they are quite small, and most are spindle cell. Distant metastasis from an iris melanoma is rare.

Choroidal melanoma tends to grow inward from the

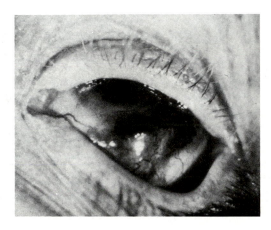

Fig. 23-35. Malignant melanoma of choroid breaking through sclera and appearing under conjunctiva. (WU 69-2213; from del Regato, J.A., and Spjut, H.J.: Ackerman and del Regato's cancer, ed. 5, St. Louis, 1977, The C.V. Mosby Co.; courtesy Registry of Ophthalmic Pathology, Armed Forces Institute of Pathology.)

choroid toward the vitreous as a discoid, globular, or mushroom-shaped mass, first elevating and then detaching the retina (Fig. 23-37). Less commonly, choroidal melanomas spread diffusely and flatly along the choroid and may extend out along scleral canals into the orbit. Rarely a patient may not seek medical attention until the tumor has grown sufficiently to become necrotic and produce such complications as endophthalmitis, massive intraocular hemorrhage, and glaucoma. Metastasis is blood borne and can occur anywhere in the body, with a particular affinity for the liver.

All of the preceding data are based on eyes that have been enucleated. A recent reappraisal of survival data on patients with uveal melanomas has led to the impression that the mortality is low before enucleation but rises abruptly following enucleation. Many ophthalmologists now do not resort to immediate enucleation of eyes with small melanomas that remain relatively stationary in growth.

Retinoblastoma, in contrast to melanoma, occurs almost exclusively in young children; no racial group is spared. Believed to be congenital and derived from incompletely differentiated retinal cells, tumors are nevertheless seldom recognized until these children are between the ages of 16 months and 2 years.

Although most cases arise sporadically, the influence of heredity is well established. Bilaterality is present in over 90% of the familial cases; survivors of bilateral retinoblastoma have a 50% chance of transmitting the disease to each of their progeny. In 80% of cases in which

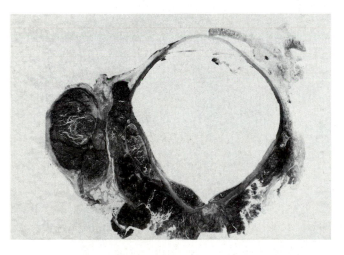

Fig. 23-36. Massive orbital extension from small choroidal melanoma that has occurred as result of diffuse spread along natural passages through sclera and optic nerve. (2×; AFIP 159090; from Friedenwald, J.S., et al.: Ophthalmic pathology: an atlas and textbook, Philadelphia, 1952, W.B. Saunders Co.)

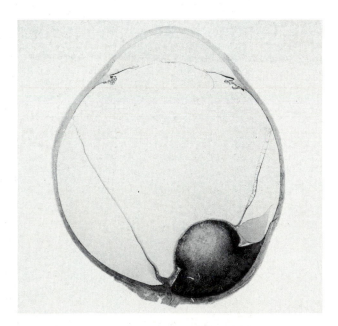

Fig. 23-37. Malignant melanoma of choroid that, by erupting through Bruch's membrane, has formed mushroom-shaped subretinal mass. (3×; AFIP 289600; from Rosai, J.: Ackerman's surgical pathology, ed. 6, St. Louis, 1981, The C.V. Mosby Co.)

the retinoblastoma is sporadic and unilateral, the mutation is considered to be somatic.

These tumors characteristically appear as a leukokoria (white pupillary reflex) (Fig. 23-38), or less often as a strabismus when the tumor is in the macula. They may protrude into the vitreous (endophytic type), often with vitreous seeding, or they may grow between the retina and the pigment epithelium (exophytic type) (Fig. 23-39).

Histologically these tumors are composed of densely packed masses of round and angulated cells with hyperchromatic nuclei and scanty cytoplasm. In the more differentiated tumors the cells are often arranged in rosettes (Fig. 23-40). There are areas of necrosis and scat-

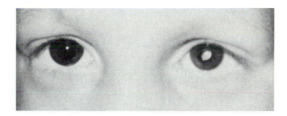

Fig. 23-38. Prominent white reflex present in dilated pupil of left eye owing to retinoblastoma. (From Rosai, J.: Ackerman's surgical pathology, ed. 6, St. Louis, 1981, The C.V. Mosby Co.)

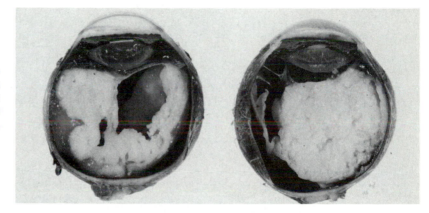

Fig. 23-39. Bilateral retinoblastoma showing presence of white mass consisting of detached retina and neoplastic tissue immediately behind lens in each eye. (AFIP 635460; from Rosai, J.: Ackerman's surgical pathology, ed. 6, St. Louis, 1981, The C.V. Mosby Co.)

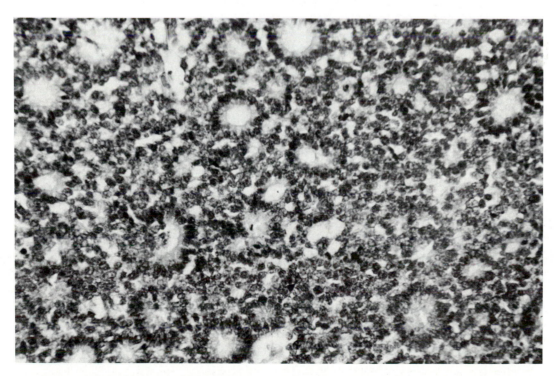

Fig. 23-40. Retinoblastoma with typical rosettes. (600×; WU 69-7513; from del Regato, J.A., and Spjut, H.J.: Ackerman and del Regato's cancer, ed. 5, St. Louis, 1977, The C.V. Mosby Co.)

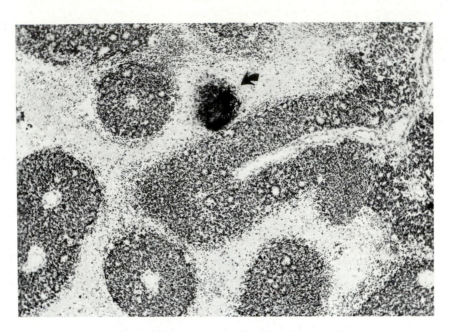

Fig. 23-41. Retinoblastoma showing typical pattern of collar of viable cells about nutrient vessels. Foci of calcification (*arrow*) occur within areas of coagulation necrosis. (80×; AFIP 147292; from Rosai, J.: Ackerman's surgical pathology, ed. 6, St. Louis, 1981, The C.V. Mosby Co.)

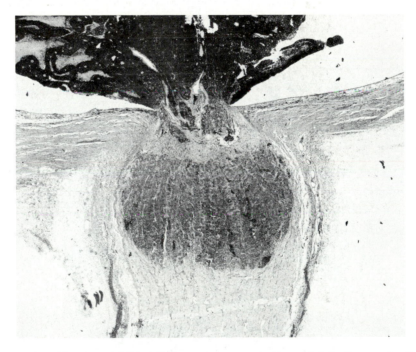

Fig. 23-42. Retinoblastomas exhibit definite tendency to spread out of globe by way of optic nerve. It is therefore of utmost importance for surgical pathologist to determine whether such optic nerve extension has occurred and, if it has, to what extent. (14×; AFIP 57-344; from Rosai, J.: Ackerman's surgical pathology, ed. 6, St. Louis, 1981, The C.V. Mosby Co.)

tered foci of calcification (Fig. 23-41). Prognosis is most influenced by the extent of the tumor and is poorest in tumors that have invaded the optic nerve, especially if the tumor is present at the surgical plane of transection (Fig. 23-42). These tumors are likely to extend along the nerve to the brain or to be carried there by the subarachnoid fluid. Another histologic finding that carries a grave prognosis is massive invasion of the uvea, in which there is a tendency for hematogenous dissemination. Survival is better than 90% in patients with unilateral retinoblastoma treated with immediate enucleation and in cases in which histologic study shows no optic nerve or uveal invasion.

Metastatic cancer

Metastatic neoplasms are the second most common intraocular neoplasms; they are second only to primary uveal melanomas. (If one were to review serial sections of autopsied eyes, the incidence of metastatic cancer would actually exceed that of melanoma.) Most metastatic neoplasms lodge in the choroid. The lids, orbit, and iris are less frequently involved. The breast is the most common primary site in women, and the lung is the most common in men. All other primary sites are relatively uncommon. Histologically these neoplasms tend to grow in a flat, diffuse manner within the choroid (Fig. 23-43).

Leukemic infiltration of the choroid or retinal hemorrhages or both are present in over 50% of patients who die of leukemia or allied disorders. Malignant lymphomas rarely involve the intraocular structures but often involve the orbit. An important exception is histiocytic lymphoma, which may involve the retina and choroid and often demonstrates characteristic vitreous. The diagnosis of histiocytic lymphoma in the vitreous can be established by withdrawing a small amount of vitreous, processing it through a membrane filter (such as millipore), and examining it after Papanicolaou staining.

Cysts of the pars plana filled with immunoglobulin are present in multiple myeloma and other paraprotein disorders.

Cataracts

The term *cataract* merely refers to opacification of the lens. This process has a variety of causes: congenital (rubella, galactosemia, familial, chromosomal defects), toxic (long-term use of systemic steroids or dinitrophenol), traumatic (contusion, penetrating wounds, or electrical injury), metabolic (diabetics are prone to senile cataracts at an earlier age), or secondary (complication of chronic intraocular inflammation). The most common cause of cataracts is aging, whereby lens fibers formed constantly throughout life become compressed into the center of the lens.

The histologic characteristics of cataracts are similar regardless of the cause. The lens fibers degenerate and become fragmented and liquefied (Fig. 23-44). The nucleus often remains intact, since it is very sclerotic. Lens epithelial nuclei have migrated posteriorly beyond the equator to lie adjacent to the posterior lens capsule. A fibrous plaque on the anterior surface of the lens is sometimes seen, especially in cases of trauma or inflammation. This plaque, referred to as anterior polar cata-

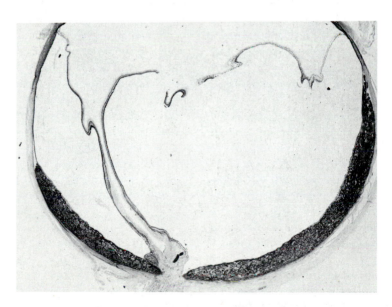

Fig. 23-43. Metastatic carcinoma from breast producing diffuse thickening of choroid posteriorly. (6×; AFIP 638509; from Rosai, J.: Ackerman's surgical pathology, ed. 6, St. Louis, 1981, The C.V. Mosby Co.)

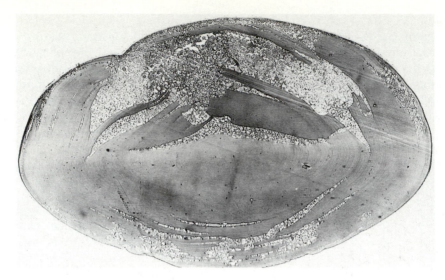

Fig. 23-44. Mature cortical and nuclear cataract. There is advanced degeneration of lens fibers, which are considerably fragmented. (27×; AFIP 66872; from DeCoursey, E., and Ash, J.E.: Atlas of ophthalmic pathology, Rochester, Minn., 1942, American Academy of Ophthalmology and Otolaryngology.)

ract, represents fibrous metaplasia of the anterior epithelial cells. Cataract extraction is one of the most successful surgical procedures performed today.

Glaucoma

The essential feature of the glaucomas is an nonphysiologic state of increased intraocular pressure, which in almost all cases is caused by an impaired outflow of aqueous humor. Aqueous humor is produced by the ciliary processes and is discharged into the posterior chamber. It flows forward between the lens and the iris, through the pupil, and into the anterior chamber. It then leaves the anterior chamber through the trabecular meshwork that is present in the deep layers of the peripheral cornea, passes into Schlemm's canal, and leaves the eye via the plexus of the intrascleral and episcleral veins (Fig. 23-45).

The glaucomas are categorized according to the reason for the impairment of the aqueous humor: congenital, primary open-angle (synonomous with chronic simple glaucoma), primary angle-closure, and secondary. In congenital glaucoma there is a malformation of the tissues in the region of the anterior chamber angle. The precise nature of this malformation is not clear, but there seems to be an incomplete separation of the iris root from the trabecular meshwork or the retention of an embryonic membrane or both.

Primary open-angle glaucoma, the most common type, appears to be a genetically determined disease that becomes evident with aging. It is characterized by an insidious onset and a slowly progressive rise in intraocular pressure resulting from an increased resistance to aqueous outflow of undetermined cause at an undetermined site. Untreated cases eventually go on to painless, progressive loss of vision.

Primary angle-closure glaucoma occurs most often in individuals who have shallow anterior chambers and narrow anterior chamber angles (the angle formed by the peripheral cornea and the iris root). These peculiar anatomic features predispose to blockage of the outflow channels by this root. During an attack of angle-closure glaucoma, the iris root actually apposes the trabecular meshwork. Chronic attacks may lead to adhesions of the iris root to the trabecular meshwork (peripheral anterior synechia), and the condition becomes permanent.

Secondary glaucoma is a complication of numerous primary processes, including trauma, inflammation, and neoplasia. The glaucoma in these secondary cases results from one or more of four main types of obstruction of the outflow of aqueous humor:

1. Adhesions of iris to lens (posterior synechiae)
2. Adhesions of iris to cornea (anterior synechiae) (Fig. 23-46)
3. Accumulation of cells or cellular debris in the anterior chamber angle (Fig. 23-47)
4. Direct damage to the outflow channels in the trabecular meshwork, canal of Schlemm, and so on

Regardless of the type and cause of glaucoma, certain degenerative changes are typically produced after periods of variable duration. When glaucoma begins in childhood, the tissues tend to stretch and the globe may become enlarged (buphthalmos). When the glaucoma occurs in adult life, the effects are mostly in the retina and optic nerve and are easily recognized microscopically. There is virtually a total loss of retinal ganglion cells and a reduction in the thickness of the nerve fiber layer,

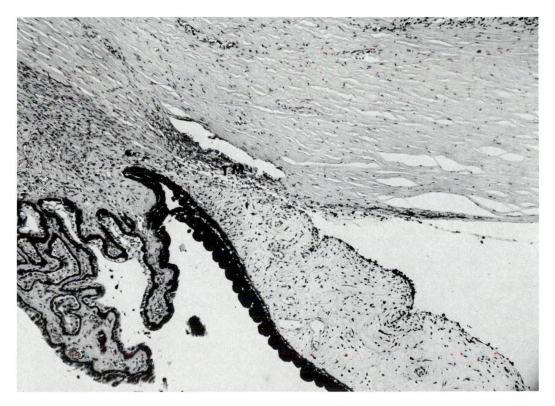

A = Angle of Anterior Chamber
C = Ciliary Processes
S = Schlemm's Canal
T = Corneoscleral Trabeculae
V = Intrascleral Veins

Cornea
Anterior Chamber
Pupil
Limbus
Iris
Conjunctiva
S
V
A
Lens
Sclera
C
Posterior
Chamber

A

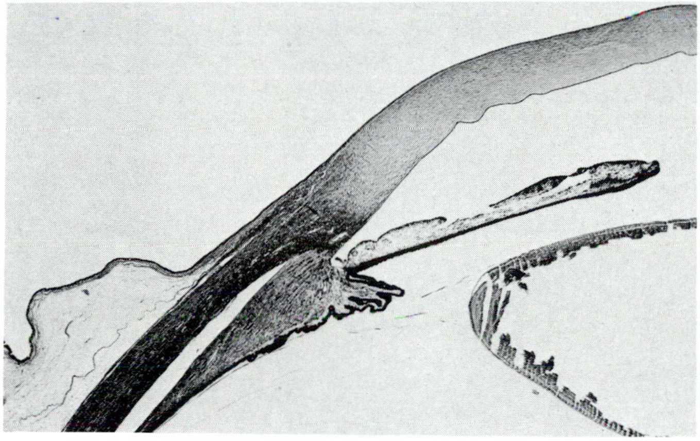

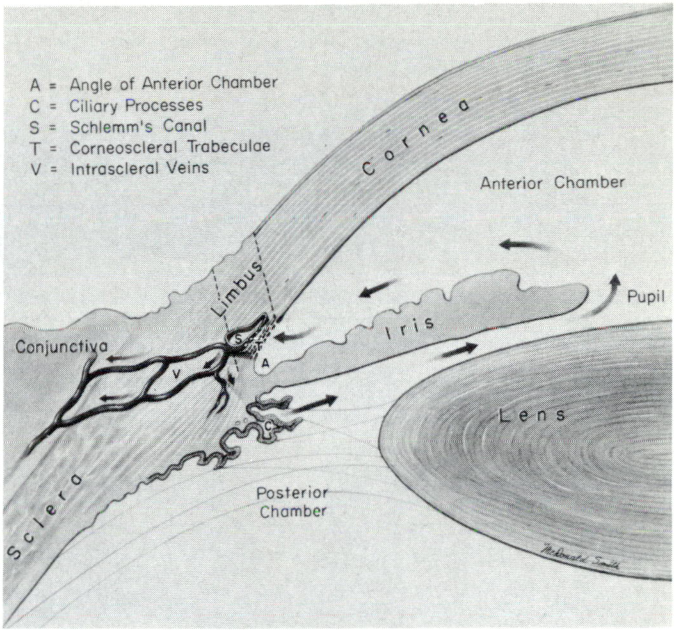

B

Fig. 23-45. Normal eye. **A,** Actual section. **B,** Artist's drawing. (**A,** 11×; AFIP 56-11490; **B,** AFIP 57-18073; from Zimmerman, L.E.: In Saphir, O., editor: A text on systemic pathology, New York, 1958-1959, Grune & Stratton, Inc.; by permission.)

TM

Fig. 23-46. Peripheral aspect of iris lying against trabecular meshwork, *TM,* producing peripheral anterior synechia and blocking outflow of aqueous humor. (90×; WU 67-4224; from Rosai, J.: Ackerman's surgical pathology, ed. 6, St. Louis, 1981, The C.V. Mosby Co.)

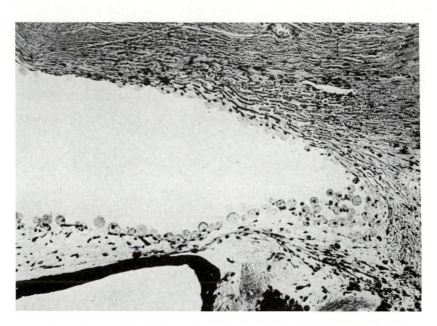

Fig. 23-47. Outflow channels blocked by macrophages in anterior chamber in phacolytic glaucoma (glaucoma resulting from lysis and escape of lens protein into aqueous humor). (75×; AFIP 609920; from Flocks, M., Littwin, C.S., and Zimmerman, L.E.: Phacolytic glaucoma: clinicopathologic study of 138 cases of glaucoma associated with hypermature cataract, Arch. Ophthalmol. **54**:37, 1955. Copyright 1955, American Medical Association.)

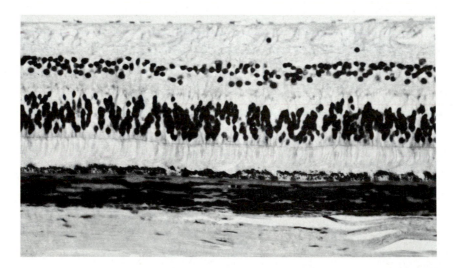

Fig. 23-48. Retina in chronic glaucoma revealing loss of ganglion cells and nerve fibers but relatively well-preserved inner nuclear and outer nuclear layers. (230×; AFIP 49729; from Friedenwald, J.S., et al.: Ophthalmic pathology: an atlas and textbook, Philadelphia, 1952, W.B. Saunders Co.)

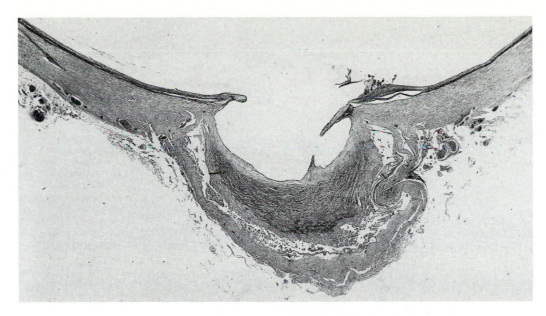

Fig. 23-49. Deep excavation (cupping) of optic disc and severe atrophy of optic nerve, which are important complications of chronic glaucoma. (12×; WU 67-4235; from Rosai, J.: Ackerman's surgical pathology, ed. 6, St. Louis, 1981, The C.V. Mosby Co.)

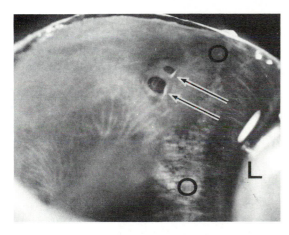

Fig. 23-50. Two holes are present in peripheral retina. Dense white retinal tissue at anterior border of each hole (*arrows*) is retracted operculum torn away in formation of holes. *O—O,* Ora serrata; *L,* posterior surface of lens. (AFIP 65-3203-1.)

while the outer nuclear layer and rods and cones remain intact (Fig. 23-48). The optic nerve shows marked excavation, posterior bowing of the lamina cribrosa, and generalized atrophy of the nerve tissue (Fig. 23-49).

Retinal degenerative diseases
Retinal detachment

Retinal detachment is a separation of the sensory retina from its normally tenuous juxtaposition to the retinal pigment epithelium. The tips of the rods and cones are normally interdigitated with villous projections from the retinal pigment epithelium, but they are not attached by any specialized structures such as desmosomes. Thus these two structures separate readily as a result of many pathologic processes.

Retinal detachment can be expected to occur as a consequence of one of three main pathogenic mechanisms: (1) traction on the retina, resulting from pathologic processes developing in the vitreous or anterior segment of the eye, (2) exudation of fluid from the choroid, opening up the potential subretinal space, for example, from inflammation or tumor in the choroid, or (3) passage of liquefied vitreous through a hole or tear in the retina (Fig. 23-50).

Because the outer layers of the retina are dependent on the choroidal circulation for nutrition and oxygenation, retinal detachment leads to a spatial separation of the retina from the choroid and a consequent ischemic loss of function. The aim of surgical reattachment of the retina is to get it back in place before irreparable damage has occurred and to prevent the detachment from spreading to the macula.

Senile macular choroidal degeneration

Senile macular choroidal degeneration accounts for most cases of central visual loss in the elderly population. It is a bilateral, painless, progressive affliction of the macula. In the earliest stages of the disease degenerative changes are seen in Bruch's membrane, the basement membrane that separates the retinal pigment epithelial layer from the choroid. These changes consist of irregular thickening and calcium deposition.

The thickened Bruch's membrane may extend into the

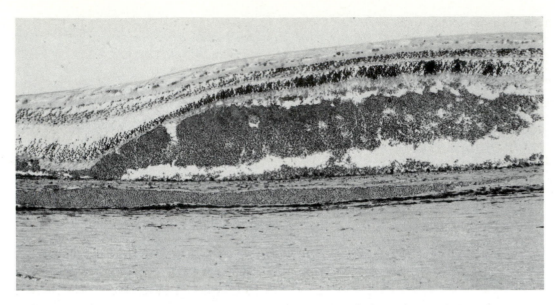

Fig. 23-51. Focal hemorrhage under retina was mistaken clinically for melanoma. (90×; WU 72-3167; from Rosai, J.: Ackerman's surgical pathology, ed. 6, St. Louis, 1981, The C.V. Mosby Co.)

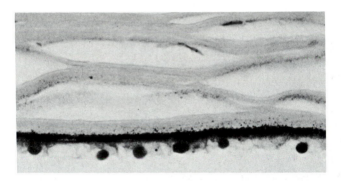

Fig. 23-52. Kayser-Fleischer ring. Dark band is copper compound that has been deposited in Descemet's membrane close to endothelium. (600×; AFIP 264768; from Hogan, M.J., and Zimmerman, L.E.: Ophthalmic pathology, ed. 2, Philadelphia, 1962, W.B. Saunders Co.)

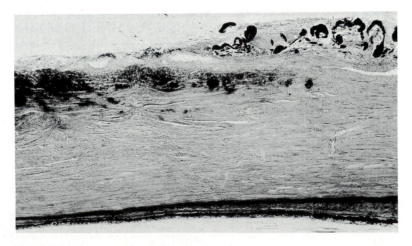

Fig. 23-53. Ochronosis. Pigmentation in degenerated elastic and collagenous tissues of sclera and episclera. (70×; AFIP 59-699; from Rones, B.: Am. J. Ophthalmol. **49:**440, 1960.)

choriocapillaris, the innermost level of blood vessels of the choroid. Portions of the choriocapillaris may be obliterated. Secondary changes in the retinal pigment epithelium then may occur, including atrophy with depigmentation or hyperplasia. Consequently there is altered function of the rods and cones, as well as development of microcystoid changes in the sensory retina.

At times the early degenerative changes of Bruch's membrane may lead to actual cracks through which small capillaries grow from the choriocapillaris. This may progress to a subretinal pigment epithelial network of neovascularization, which then may leak serous fluid or even bleed, producing a subretinal hematoma that later organizes into a fibrous mass (Fig. 23-51). Naturally there is extensive damage to the overlying sensory retina and consequent loss of central vision.

Phthisis bulbi and atrophia bulbi

The clinical term *phthisis bulbi* represents the final stages of ocular degeneration and disorganization, in which the production of aqueous humor is so reduced that the intraocular pressure is decreased (hypotony) and the globe shrinks. Histologically there is marked atrophy of all ocular structures, and often there is intraocular ossification (atrophia bulbi).

OCULAR MANIFESTATIONS OF OTHER SYSTEMIC DISEASES

In Wilson's hepatolenticular degeneration, copper is deposited in Descemet's membrane of the peripheral cornea. This is recognized clinically as a greenish brown ring in the peripheral cornea and is referred to as a Kayser-Fleischer ring (Fig. 23-52).

In cystinosis, fine scintillating polychromatic cystine crystals are deposited in the subepithelial conjunctiva and in the corneal stroma.

A brownish discoloration in the sclera occurs in ochronosis (Fig. 23-53).

In hypercalcemia calcium salts may be deposited in Bowman's membrane of the cornea. This produces the clinical picture referred to as band keratopathy.

In familial hypercholesterolemia and in certain other forms of disturbed lipid metabolism, arcus senilis becomes prominent at an early age. Clinically it is a mil-

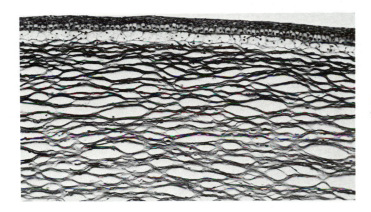

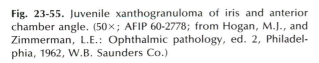

Fig. 23-54. Cells in superficial layers of corneal stroma are swollen with acid mucopolysaccharide. (90×; AFIP 68-4418.)

Fig. 23-55. Juvenile xanthogranuloma of iris and anterior chamber angle. (50×; AFIP 60-2778; from Hogan, M.J., and Zimmerman, L.E.: Ophthalmic pathology, ed. 2, Philadelphia, 1962, W.B. Saunders Co.)

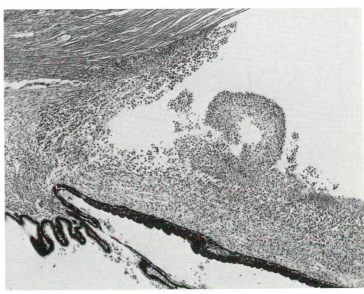

ky opacification of the peripheral cornea resulting from the accumulation of lipid in the corneal stroma.

In the mucopolysaccharidosis group of diseases, clouding of the cornea results from the accumulation of abnormal mucopolysaccharides throughout the corneal stroma and endothelium (Fig. 23-54). Haziness of the cornea also occurs in Fabry's disease.

In juvenile xanthogranuloma, along with characteristic skin lesions, there may be tumors of the conjunctiva, orbit, or uveal tract (Fig. 23-55).

Although localized amyloid tumors may occur on the lids or conjunctiva, systemic amyloidosis usually has no ocular manifestations, with the important exception of primary familial amyloidosis, in which there are dense opacities in the vitreous.

REFERENCES

1. Apple, D.J., and Rabb, M.F.: Clinicopathologic correlations of ocular disease, ed. 2, St. Louis, 1978, The C.V. Mosby Co.
2. Hogan, M., and Zimmerman, L.: Ophthalmic pathology, ed. 2, Philadelphia, 1962, W.B. Saunders Co.
3. Rosai, J., editor: Ackerman's surgical pathology, ed. 6, St. Louis, 1981, The C.V. Mosby Co.
4. Yanoff, M., and Fine, B.S.: Ocular pathology, ed. 2, New York, 1982, Harper & Row, Publishers, Inc.

Index

Page numbers in *italics* indicate illustrations.
Page numbers followed by *t* indicate tables.

A

A cells of islets of Langerhans, tumors of, 1253
Abdominal disease, suppurative, in pyogenic liver abscess, 1154
Abortion, spontaneous, 1524-1525
Abrasion, mechanical violence causing, 114, *115*
Abscess(es)
  of brain, 1903
  formation of, 41
  of liver, 1154-1156; *see also* Liver, abscesses of
  of lung
    from anaerobic bacteria, 851-852
    in pneumococcal pneumonia, 847-848
  of urethra, 815
  of vulva, 1459
Acanthamoeba, amebic meningoencephalitis from, 404
Acantholysis, definition of, 1576
Acanthosis, definition of, 1575
Acanthosis nigricans, 1578
Accelerated conduction syndrome, 651
Access in infectious disease pathogenesis, 279
Accidental vaccination of oral soft tissues, 1010
Acetabulum, dysplasia of, 1819
Acetaminophen
  hazards of, 158-159
  liver cell necrosis from, 1133
Acetophenetidin, hazards of, 159-160
Achalasia of esophagus, 1056
Achondroplasia, 1757-1758
Achromia, cutaneous pigmentation abnormalities in, 1602
Acid, bile, in liver function testing, 1099
Acidophil adenoma of pituitary gland, 1387, 1389
Acidophilic body in viral hepatitis, 1119
Acidophilic necrosis of liver cells, 1106-1107
Acidophils in adenohypophysis, 1376, 1378
Acinic cell carcinoma of salivary glands, 1042-1043
Acinus of liver, 1097
Acquired immune deficiency syndrome (AIDS), 418
  cutaneous lesions of, 1628, *1629*
Acquired tolerance, 455

Acrodermatitis chronica atrophicans, 1594
Acromegaly
  heart in, 572-573
  osteoarthrosis with, 1825
  skeleton in, 1739
Acrosclerosis, 1595
Acrospiroma, 1637
Actin in muscle contraction, 16
Actinobacillus (Malleomyces) mallei, glanders from, 312
Actinomycosis, 382-384
  of abdomen, 383
  of central nervous system, 1905
  cervicofacial, 383
  of gastrointestinal tract, 1068
  oral lesions of, 1012
  of pelvis, 383
  of thorax, 383
Acyanotic tetralogy of Fallot, 676
"Adamantinoma" of long bones, 1807-1808
Addison's disease
  adrenal glands in, 1436-1437
  cutaneous pigmentation abnormalities in, 1601
  heart in, 574
  pituitary in, 1380
Adenitis, submandibular, 1032
Adenocarcinoma
  of cervix
    metastatic, 1478
    microscopic appearance of, 1478, *1479*
  definition of, 558
  of endometrium, 1486-1488
  of fallopian tube, 1496, *1497*
  of gallbladder, 1227
  in situ of cervix, 1477
  of kidney, 768, *769*
  of lung, 919-920
  mucinous, of prostate gland, 829
  of nasal cavity, 990
  of pancreas, 1242, *1243*
  of paranasal sinuses, 990
  of salivary glands, 1043-1044
  of urethra, 816
  of vagina, 1470
    in infant, distinctive, *1471*
  of vulva, 1466
Adenofibroma of breast, architecture of, 524, *525*
Adenohypophysis; *see also* Pituitary gland
  agenesis of, 1382
  blood supply of, 1374

Adenohypophysis—cont'd
  deficiency of, 1381
  embryology of, 1372
  function of, 1376
  histology of, 1374-1378
  and hypothalamus, neural and vascular pathways between, 1374
  ischemia of, 1383-1384
  tumors of, classification of, 1387*t*
Adenoid cystic carcinoma
  of breast, 1565
  of respiratory tract, 928-929
  of salivary glands, 1041-1042
Adenoid squamous cell carcinoma of oral soft tissues, 1018
Adenolymphoma of salivary glands, 1038, *1039*
Adenoma(s)
  of adrenal glands, 1441-1443, *1444*
  adrenocortical, Cushing's syndrome and, 1439
  basal cell, of salivary glands, 1037
  bile duct, 1186-1187
  cortical tubular, 768
  definition of, 558
  hepatocellular, 1188, *1189*
  of middle ear, 996
  oxyphilic, of salivary glands, 1038-1040
  papillary, of alimentary tract, 1077, *1079*
  of parathyroid glands, 1424
  of pituitary gland, 1386-1391
    acidophil, 1387, 1389
    basophil, 1389-1390
    chromophobe, 1390-1391
    corticotroph cell, 1389-1390
    gonadotroph cell, 1390
    lactotroph cell, 1389
    oncocytic, 1391
    somatotroph cell, 1389
    thyrotroph cell, 1390
  pleomorphic
    carcinoma in, of salivary glands, 1043
    of salivary glands, 1035-1037
  of salivary glands, 1040
  of thyroid gland
    atypical, 1410
    clear cell, 1410
    follicular, 1408-1410
    Hürthle cell, 1410
Adenomatoid malformation of lung, congenital, 836, *837*

1

Bacterial diseases—cont'd
from shigellae, 289-290
from spirochetes, 313, 316-319
from vibrios, 287-289
Bacterial endocarditis, 613-619
age and, 614
bacteria-free cultures in, 618
cardiac changes in, 618
causative organisms in, 614
complications of, 618-619
death from, causes of, 619
endocardial lesions in, 615-618
extracardiac complications of, 618-619
pathogenesis of, 615
predisposing conditions for, 615, *616*
prognosis of, 619
sequelae of, 618-619
sex and, 614
subacute, focal embolic glomerulonephritis
in, 741-742
Bacterial infections
extracellular, 290-303
from *Escherichia coli*, 300
from gonococci, 298-299
from *Haemophilus*, 299-300
from *Legionella*, 301
from *Listeria*, 302-303
from meningococci, 296-298
from pneumococci, 295-296
from *Proteus*, 300
from *Pseudomonas aeruginosa*, 300-301
from staphylococci, 290-291
from streptococci, 291-295
intracellular, 303-319
from *Pasteurella*, 311-312
from salmonellae, 304-307
from *Yersinia*, 310-311
jaundice in, 1129
of lungs, 845-860
of placenta, 1527-1528
systemic, focal glomerulonephritis with, 741-
742
Bacterial pericarditis, 631-632, 635
Bacterial pseudomycosis, 387
Balanitis xerotica obliterans, 1593-1594
Balantidiasis, 404-405
Balkan nephritis, 760
Balloon cell nevus, 1616
Ballooning degeneration, definition of, 1576
Bancroftian filariasis, 435-436, *437*
Banti's syndrome, 1276
Bantu siderosis, 1168
Barbiturates in forensic pathology, toxicologic
aspects of, 212-213
Barotrauma, sinus, 136
Barr body, 5
Bartholin's gland
carcinoma of, 1466
cyst of, 1459
Basal bodies, 11
Basal cell adenoma of salivary glands, 1037
Basal cell layer of epidermis, 1572-1573
Basal cell nevus syndrome, 1613
Basal laminae, 19, *20*
Basedow's disease, 1401-1402
Basement membrane
of epidermis, 1573-1574
thickening of, in diabetes mellitus, 1249-
1250
Basophil adenoma of pituitary gland, 1389-
1390
Basophilic degeneration of heart, 562-563
Basophils
in adenohypophysis, 1378

Basophils—cont'd
in chemotaxis, 35
in inflammation, 36
Bathing trunk nevi, malignant melanoma and,
1624
Becker muscular dystrophy, 1859
Becquerel, definition of, 241-242
Beef tapeworm, 424-425
Beer-drinkers' myocardosis, 569
Behavior of tumors, 532-538
Behavioral classification of neoplasia, 519-
520
Behçet's syndrome, joint disorders in, 1837
Benign, definition of, 558
Berger's IgA focal glomerulonephritis, 742
Beriberi
alcoholic cardiomyopathy and, 569
heart in, 568-569
Berry aneurysms of central nervous system,
1884-1885
Berylliosis, 230-231, 916-917
granulomas of skin in, 1600
Beta emission decay, 240-241
Beta rays, 240
3-Beta-hydroxysteroid dehydrogenase defi-
ciency in congenital adrenal hyper-
plasia, 1431
Beta-lipoprotein deficiency, congenital, gastrointestinal manifestations of, 1077
Bilateral polycystic kidney, 766-767
Bile, peritonitis and, 1071
Bile acids in liver function testing, 1099
Bile duct adenomas, 1186-1187
Bile duct cystadenomas of liver, 1186
Bilharziasis, 420-424
Biliary atresia in infants, 1158
Biliary cirrhosis
liver in, 1150-1151
primary, 1151-1153
Biliary ducts
acquired disorders of, 1214-1218
anatomy of, 1213
congenital or developmental abnormalities
of, 1214
inflammation of
acute, 1218
chronic, 1218-1223
morphology of, 1213
noninflammatory conditions of, 1223
physiology of, 1213-1218
pseudotumors of, 1223, *1224*
tumors of, 1223-1230
benign, 1223, *1224-1225*
malignant, 1223-1224, 1226-1230; *see also*
Carcinoma(s) of biliary ducts
Biliary obstruction, liver in, 1148-1150
Biliary tract
amputation neuromas of, 1223
obstruction of, differential diagnosis of,
1184
perforation of, spontaneous, 1223
Biliary tract disease
and liver abscess, 1148
primary, 1151
Bilirubin
intracellular accumulation of, 85-86
in liver function testing, 1099
Billroth, cords of, in spleen, 1269
Biologic agents in tumor development, 549-
553
Biologic factors in radiation response, 246
Biology, radiation, cellular and molecular, 242-
247; *see also* Radiation biology, cellular and molecular

Biopsy(ies)
of myocardium, 652
needle, of liver, 1181-1183
of pericardium, 652
of skeletal muscle, 1856
Biotin, 508
Biphenyls, polychlorinated, hazards of, 222
Birth injury, cerebral, 1890
BK virus, 365
Black death, 310-311
Black piedra, 375
Blackwater fever, 415
Bladder, 775-789
calculous disease of, 776
congenital anomalies of, 775
dilatation of, 775-776
displacement of, 776
diverticula of, 776
embryonal sarcoma of, 788-789
epithelial tumors of, 781-789
carcinoma in situ as, 786
cytologic diagnosis of, 788
differential diagnosis of, 786-788
etiology of, 781-782
frequency of, 782-783
gross appearance of, 783
immunologic aspects of, 788
incidence of, 782-783
microscopic appearance of, 783-786
spread of, 788
exstrophy of, 775
fistulas of, 776
herniation of, 776
inflammation of, 776-779; *see also* Cystitis
proliferative and metaplastic mucosal lesions
of, 779-781
trauma to, 775
Von Brunn's nests in, 779, *780*
Blast cells in immune response, 450
Blast injury, 136-137
Blastoma, pulmonary, 930-931
Blastomyces dermatitidis, 386-387
Blastomycosis, 386-387
of central nervous system, 1905
South American, 395
Blastospore, definition of, 375
Bleb, definition of, 1575
Bleeding tendency in renal failure, 733-734
Bleomycin
hazards of, 180
pulmonary toxicity of, 895
Blindness, night, in vitamin A deficiency, 501
Blocking antibody in immune tolerance, 456
Blood, 1325-1346
cells of, formation of, in bone marrow, 1326
circulation of; *see* Circulation
diseases of, splenomegaly in, 1282
flagellates of, diseases caused by, 406-412
flow of
changes in, in inflammation, 25
in liver, 1108-1109
formed elements of, changes in, in inflammation, 24
peripheral, relation of bone marrow to, 1327-
1328
Blood cysts of cardiac valves, 647
Blood vessels, 684-720; *see also* Artery(ies);
Capillary(ies); Vein(s)
of bone, tumors of, 1805-1806
of bone marrow, lesions of, 1345-1346
of central nervous system, 1873-1874
diseases of, 1878-1886
malformations of, 1926-1928
neoplasms of, 1928